USI's

Clinical UROLOGY

A Practical Approach

USI's Clinical UROLOGY

A Practical Approach

Editors

Arvind Prakash Ganpule
MS (Gen Surgery), DNB (Genitourinary Surgery), MNAMS
Vice-Chairman
Department of Urology
Muljibhai Patel Urological Hospital
Nadiad, Gujarat, India

Pankaj Nandkishore Maheshwari
MS DNB MCh (Urology) FRCS (Glasgow)
Senior Consultant and Chief Urologist
Fortis Hospital
Mulund, Mumbai, India

Foreword

Sanjay Balwant Kulkarni

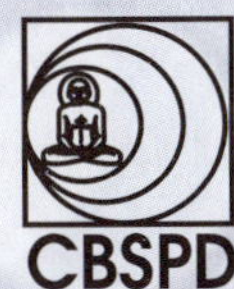

CBS Publishers & Distributors Pvt Ltd

New Delhi • Bengaluru • Chennai • Kochi • Kolkata • Lucknow • Mumbai
Hyderabad • Jharkhand • Nagpur • Patna • Pune • Uttarakhand

Disclaimer
Science and technology are constantly changing fields. New research and experience broaden the scope of information and knowledge. The editors have tried their best in giving information available to them while preparing the material for this book. Although all efforts have been made to ensure optimum accuracy of the material, yet it is quite possible some errors might have been left uncorrected. The publisher, the printer and the editors will not be held responsible for any inadvertent errors, omissions or inaccuracies.

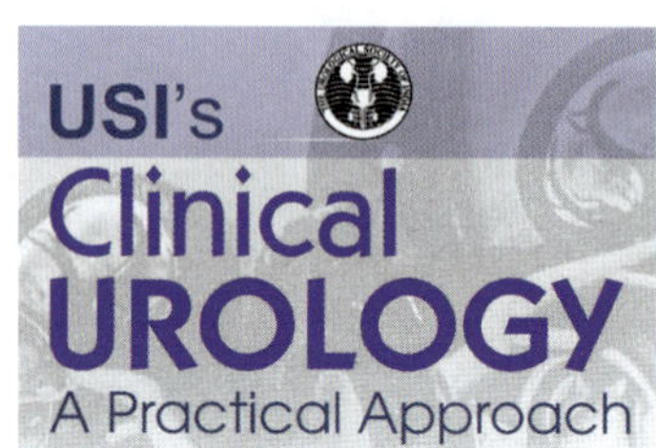

ISBN: 978-81-979822-9-3

First Edition: 2025

Published by Satish Kumar Jain and produced by Varun Jain for

CBS Publishers & Distributors Pvt Ltd
4819/XI Prahlad Street, 24 Ansari Road, Daryaganj, New Delhi 110 002, India
Ph: 011-23289259, 23266838 Website: www.cbspd.com
e-mail: delhi@cbspd.com

Corporate Office: 204 FIE, Industrial Area, Patparganj, Delhi 110 092, India
Ph: 011-4934 4934 Fax: 011-4934 4935 e-mail: publishing@cbspd.com; publicity@cbspd.com

Branches

- **Bengaluru:** Seema House 2975, 17th Cross, KR Road, Banasankari 2nd Stage, Bengaluru 560 070, Karnataka, India
  Ph: +91-80-26771678/79 Fax: +91-80-26771680 e-mail: bangalore@cbspd.com
- **Chennai:** 18/8B, Subbarayan Street, Shenoy Nagar, Chennai 600 030, Tamil Nadu, India
  Ph: +91-44-42032115, 26681266 e-mail: chennai@cbspd.com
- **Kochi:** 42/1325, 1326, Power House Road, Opposite KSEB, Power House, Ernakulum 682 018, Kochi, Kerala, India
  Ph: +91-484-4059061–65, 67 Fax: +91-484-4059065 e-mail: kochi@cbspd.com
- **Kolkata:** 147, Hind Ceramics Compound, 1st Floor, Nilgunj Road, Belghoria, Kolkata 700 056, West Bengal, India
  Ph: +91-33-25633055/56 e-mail: kolkata@cbspd.com
- **Lucknow:** Basement, Khushnuma Complex, 7 Meerabai Marg (behind Jawahar Bhawan), Lucknow 226 001, UP, India
  Ph: +91-522-4000032 e-mail: tiwari.lucknow@cbspd.com
- **Mumbai:** PWD Shed, Gala No. 25/26, Ramchandra Bhatt Marg, Next JJ Hospital Gate No. 2, Opp. Union Bank of India, Noorbaug, Mumbai 400 009, Maharashtra, India
  Ph: +91-22-66661880/89 e-mail: mumbai@cbspd.com

Representatives

- **Hyderabad** 0-9885175004
- **Jharkhand** 0-9811541605
- **Nagpur** 0-8692091830
- **Patna** 0-9334159340
- **Pune** 0-9664372571
- **Uttarakhand** 0-9716462459

Printed at: Goyal Offset Works Pvt. Ltd, Kundli, Sonipat, Haryana

to

the loving memory of

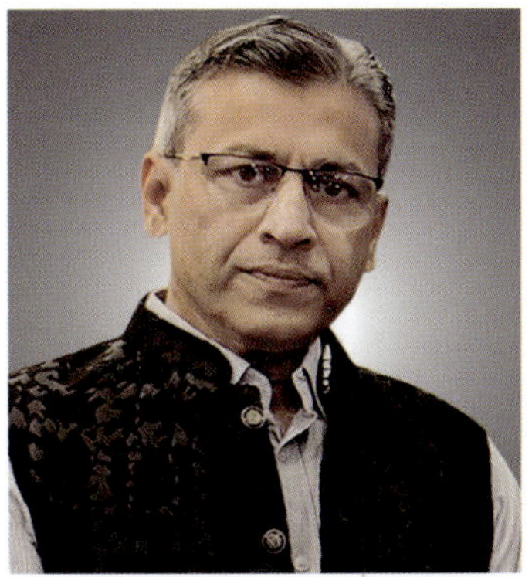

Dr GG Laxman Prabhu

He has been a constant source of inspiration to us

Editors List

Editors

Arvind Prakash Ganpule MS (Gen Surgery), DNB (Genitourinary Surgery), MNAMS
Vice-Chairman
Department of Urology
Muljibhai Patel Urological Hospital
Nadiad, Gujarat, India

Pankaj Nandkishore Maheshwari
MS DNB MCh (Urology) FRCS (Glasgow)
Senior Consultant and Chief Urologist
Fortis Hospital
Mulund, Mumbai, India

Section Editors

Uro-oncology

Abhishek Singh MS MCh (Urology)
Consultant Uro-oncologist
Muljibhai Patel Urological Hospital
Nadiad, Gujarat, India

Amandeep Arora MS MCh (Urology)
Assistant Professor, Uro-oncologist
Tata Memorial Centre, Mumbai

Pediatric Urology

Gyanendra Sharma MS MCh DNB
Consultant Urologist
Chitale Clinic Pvt Ltd, Solapur, Maharashtra

N Mallikarjuna Reddy MS MCh DNB, FEBU
Senior Consultant Urologist
Head, Department of Renal Sciences
Citizens Specialty Hospital, Hyderabad

Reconstructive Urology

Pankaj M Joshi MS DNB (Urology)
Consultant Urologist, UROKUL
Pune, Maharashtra

Venkat Arjunrao Gite MS MCh DNB
Professor and Head
Department of Urology
Government Medical College and Superspeciality Hospital
Aurangabad, Maharashtra
Dean, Government Medical College and MPGIMER
Nashik, Maharashtra

Female Urology

Sanjay Sinha MBBS MS DNB MCh
Apollo Hospitals
Hyderabad

Nikhil Khattar MS (Surgery) MCh (Urology)
The Perineourology Clinic, New Delhi
Visiting Consultant
Reconstructive Urology and Female Urology
Holy Family Hospital, New Delhi
Artemis Hospital, Gurugram (Haryana)
Ex-Professor of Urology, ABVIMS and Dr RML Hospital
New Delhi

Andrology

Vilvapathy Senguttuvan Karthikeyan
MBBS MS MCh MRCS FAIS FECSM
Microsurgical Andrologist and Urologist
Apollo Hospitals, Greams Road,Chennai

Priyank Kothari MBBS MS MCh
Assistant Professor and Microsurgical Uro-andrologist
BYL Nair Ch Hospital, Mumbai

Renal Transplant

Vikas Jain MS DNB (Urology)
Director and Unit Head, Urology, Robotics and Renal Transplantation, Fortis Hospital, Shalimar Bagh and Vasant Kunj, New Delhi

Abhijit Patil MS MCh (Urology) DNB (Urology) FACS
Consultant Urologist
Muljibhai Patel Urological Hospital
Nadiad, Gujarat, India

Prasun Ghosh
DNB (Genitourinary Surgery Urology) MS (General Surgery) MBBS MNAMS
Senior Director
Urology, Kidney Transplant and Renal Care
Medanta-The Medicity, Gurugram, Haryana

Endourology

Prashant Motiram Mulawkar
MBBS DGO MS (Gen Surgery) DNB MCh DNB (Urology) ChM (Urology) Edinburgh
Consultant Urologist
Tirthankar Superspeciality Hospital, Akola
Professor, Department of Urology
Government Medical College and
Superspeciality, Hospital, Akola
Tutor (Urology), University of Edinburgh, UK

Dilip Kumar Mishra MS MRCS MCh
Consultant and Head
Department of Urology
Pushpanjali Hospital and Research Centre
Agra, UP

General Urology

GG Laxman Prabhu MS MCh Urology
Professor, Department of Urology
Kasturba Medical College
Mangaluru, Karnataka

Rahul Gupta MS DNB (Urology)
Associate Professor
Department of Urology and Renal Transplant
GMC Jammu, Jammu and Kashmir

Contributors

Gopal Sharma MS MCh
Consultant, Urologic Oncology and Robotic Surgery
Medanta—The Medicity, Gurugram, Haryana, India

Puneet Ahluwalia MS MCh
Director and Head
Urologic Oncology and Robotic Surgery
Medanta—The Medicity, Gurugram, Haryana, India

Santosh Kumar MS MCh
Senior Professor and Head
Department of Urology Unit II
Christian Medical College, Vellore

Santhosh Nagasubramanian MS MCh
Associate Professor
Department of Urology Unit-II
Christian Medical College, Vellore

TB Yuvaraja MS MCh (Urology)
Consultant Uro-oncologist
Kokilaben Dhirubhai Ambani Hospital and Medical Research Institute
Mumbai

Santosh Subhash Waigankar
MBBS MRCS DNB [Gen Surgery] DNB [Urology]
Consultant in Urology and Uro-oncology
Derriford Hospital and UHPNT
Plymouth PL68DH UK

Sanjai Kumar Addla MBBS MRCS MD FRCS (Urol)
Consultant Uro-oncologist
Apollo Cancer Centre, Hyderabad, India

Amaresh Mohan MBBS MS (Gen Surgery) MCh (Urology)
Consultant Uro-oncologist
Basavatarakam Indo-American Cancer Hospital and Research Institute
Hyderabad, Telangana, India

Ganesh Bakshi MS MCh DNB (Urology)
Professor and Consultant Uro-oncology
PD Hinduja Hospital and Medical Research Centre
Mahim, Mumbai

Ashwin Tamankar MS MCh RCS (England)
Robotic Urology Fellowship, UK
Consultant Uro-oncologist, Apollo Hospitals
Navi Mumbai and Deenanath Mangeshkar Hospital and Research Center, Pune

Anup Kumar MS MCh DNB MNAMS
Professor and Head
Department of Robotic, Laparoscopic, Renal Transplant Surgeon, Department of Urology Robotics and Renal Transplant
Vardhman Mahavir Medical College and Safdarjung Hospital, New Delhi
Nodal Officer for Oncology Robotics and Renal Transplant

Gautam Ram Choudhary MS MCh
Additional Professor
Department of Urology, AIIMS Jodhpur

Vivek Venkatramani MS MCh (Urology)
Consultant Uro-oncologist, Mumbai, India

Gagan Prakash MS DNB (Urology)
Chief, Uro-oncology Division
Professor, Department of Surgical Oncology
Tata Memorial Centre and Homi Bhabha National Institute, Mumbai

Ginil Kumar Pooleri MS MCh (Urology) DNB (Urology)
Professor, Department of Urology
Head, Uro-oncology Division
Amrita Institute of Medical Sciences, Kochi

Shashank Agrawal MS DNB (Urology) MNAMS
Fellow in Uro-oncology and Robotic Surgery
Amrita Hospital, Kochi

Saurabh Patil MS MCh
Consultant Urologist and Robotic Surgeon
Fortis Hospital, Mulund, Mumbai

Gagan Gautam MS DNB MCh
Vice-Chairman of Uro-oncology and Robotic Surgery
Medanta Kidney and Urology Institute
Gurugram, Haryana, India

Ashish Khanna MBBS MS (Gen Surgery) MCh (Urology)
Consultant, Uro-oncology and Robotic Surgery Division
Department of Surgical Oncology
Rajiv Gandhi Cancer Institute and Research Centre
Rohini, New Delhi, India

Sudhir Kumar Rawal
MBBS MS (Gen Surgery) MCh (Urology) DNB (Urology)
Medical Director and Head, Genito-urinary Oncology
Department of Surgical Oncology
Rajiv Gandhi Cancer Institute and Research Centre
Rohini, New Delhi, India

Amandeep Arora MS MCh (Urology)
Associate Professor in Uro-oncology
Advanced Centre for Treatment, Research and Education in Cancer (ACTREC)
Tata Memorial Centre and Homi Bhabha National Institute, Navi Mumbai

Abhishek Singh MS MCh (Urology)
Consultant Uro-oncologist
Muljibhai Patel Urological Hospital, Nadiad, India

Uday Pratap Singh MS MCh
Additional Professor
Sanjay Gandhi Postgraduate Institute of Medical Sciences (SGPGIMS)
Lucknow, Uttar Pradesh, India

Sanjoy Kr Sureka DNB MCh
Additional Professor
Sanjay Gandhi Postgraduate Institute of Medical Sciences (SGPGIMS)
Lucknow, Uttar Pradesh, India

Ravimohan Mavuduru
MBBS MS (General Surgery) MCh (Urology)
Professor, Department of Urology
Advanced Urology Centre
Postgraduate Institute of Medical Education and Research, Sector 12, Chandigarh, India

Girdhar Bora MBBS MS (General Surgery) MCh (Urology)
Additional Professor
Department of Urology
Advanced Urology Centre
Postgraduate Institute of Medical Education and Research, Sector 12, Chandigarh, India

Hemang Bakshi MS MCh
Consultant Uro-oncologist
HCG Aastha Cancer Centre, Ahmedabad, India

Keval Patel MS DNB
Consultant Uro-oncologist
GCRI, Aayushyam Speciality Hospital, Ahmedabad, India

Brusabhanu Nayak MS MCh
Additional Professor, Department of Urology
All India Institute of Medical Sciences, New Delhi, India

Amlesh Seth MS MCh
Professor and Head
Department of Urology
All India Institute of Medical Sciences, New Delhi

Rajeev Kumar MS MCh
Professor
Department of Urology
All India Institute of Medical Sciences, New Delhi

Sridhar P MS MCh DrNB
Assistant Professor, Department of Urology
National Cancer Institute, Jhajjar
All India Institute of Medical Sciences, New Delhi

Bhalchandra Kashyapi MS DNB MCh DNB
Consultant Uro-oncologist
Deenanath Mangeshkar Hospital and Research Centre
Pune, Maharashtra

Mahendra Pal MS DNB (Urology)
Professor, Uro-oncology Unit
Department of Surgical Oncology
Tata Memorial Hospital, Mumbai, Maharashtra, India

Kinshuki Jain MBBS DNB DM FIPM
Head, Department of Pain and Palliative Medicine
Rajiv Gandhi Cancer Institute and Research Centre
Rohini, New Delhi

Amitabh Singh MBBS MS MCh
Senior Consultant In Department of Uro-oncology
Rajiv Gandhi Cancer Institute and Research Centre
Rohini, New Delhi, India

Vedang Murthy MBBS MD (Radiation Oncology)
Professor, Department of Radiation Oncology
Tata Memorial Centre, Mumbai

Gargee Mulye MBBS MD (Radiation Oncology)
Assistant Professor
Department of Radiation Oncology
Tata Memorial Centre, Mumbai

Sudhindra Jayasimha MS MRCS Ed MCh DNB (Urol) IntFRCS Ed (Urol)
Associate Professor, Department of Urology
Christian Medical College, Vellore

Chandra Singh J MBBS MS DNB (Surg) MCh (Urol) DNB (Urol)
Fellowship in Pediatric Urology
Professor and Head
Department of Urology
Christian Medical College, Vellore

Hemant Pathak
MBBS MS (General Surgery) MCh (Urology) DNB (Genitourinary Surgery)
Professor, Department of Urology
TNMC and BYL Nair Hospital, Mumbai
Head
Lilavati Hospital and Research Centre, Mumbai

Prasanna Matippa MS DNB (Gen Surgery) DNB (Urology)
Fellow-Paediatric Urology
Senior Consultant, Paediatric Urologist
Department of Urology, NU Hospitals, Bengaluru, India

Gyanendra Sharma MS MCh DNB
Consultant Urologist
Chitale Clinic Pvt Ltd, Solapur, Maharashtra

N Mallikarjuna Reddy MS MCh DNB FEBU
Clinical Director, Department of Urology
Yashodha Hospital, Hyderabad

Rahul Rajendra Kapoor MS MCh
Consultant Urologist
Kapoor Urology Clinic, Raipur

Amilal Bhat MS MCh
Chairman, Bhat's Hypospadias and Reconstructive Urology Hospital and Research Center
5–1, Friends Colony, Lalkothi Jaipur

Uday Sankar Chatterjee MS MCh (Ped Surg) MCh (Urology)
Nil Ratan Sircar Medical College and Hospital, Kolkata
Visiting Surgeon, Park Medical Research and Welfare Society, Kolkata

MS Ansari MS MNAMS MCh DNB
Professor, Department of Urology
Sanjay Gandhi Postgraduate Institute of Medical Sciences (SGPIMS)
Raebareili Road, Lucknow, Uttar Pradesh

Priyank Yadav MS MCh (Urology)
Associate Professor
Department of Urology and Renal Transplantation
Sanjay Gandhi Postgraduate Institute of Medical Sciences, Lucknow, Uttar Pradesh

Anil Takvani MS DNB (Urology)
Consultant Pediatric Urologist
Takvani Pediatric Urology Hospital
Ahmedabad, Gujarat

Sandesh Parab MBBS MS (General Surgery) MCh (Urology)
Assistant Professor
Department of Urology, TNMC and AMP
BYL Nair Hospital, Mumbai

Sushil Shivlal Rathi MS MCh DNB
Director and Incharge of Fellowship Program
MUHS Vishwa Institute of Urology and Kidney Centre Pvt Ltd, Nanded

Ashish Ramswarup Pardeshi DNB (Surgery) DNB (Urology)
Director
Kidney and Urology Super Speciality Institute, Pune

Hemant Goel MS MCh
Professor and Head
Department of Urology
ABVIMS and Dr Ram Manohar Lohia Hospital, New Delhi

Ajit Sawant MS MCh DNB
Professor and Head
Department of Urology
LTMMC and GH, Sion, Mumbai

Rishi Grover MS DNB (Urology)
Consultant Urologist
Icon Hospital, Surat

Sanjay B Kulkarni MS FRCS Dip in Urology
Founder and Head, UROKUL, Pune

Dhananjay Vinayak Selukar MS MCh
Professor and Head
Department of Urology
Government Medical College and Super Speciality Hospital, Nagpur

Shailesh A Shah MS MCh
Ex-Professor and Head
Institute of Kidney Diseases and Research Centre (IKDRC) and Civil Hospital, Ahmedabad
Consultant Urologist, Bodyline Hospitals, Ahmedabad

Gaurang Shah MS MCh LLB
Consultant Urologist and Head, Department of Urology
Saifee Hospital, Mumbai

Rajiv Kore MS MCh DNB FRCS (Urol, London) Dip. UROL Fellow American College of Surgeons
Consultant Reconstructive Urologist, Head-MUHS Fellowship Program in Reconstructive Urology
Director, Warana Institute of Uro-Surgery, Kolhapur

Sudheer K Devana MS MCh
Additional Professor
Department of Urology
PGIMER, Chandigarh

Martand G Patil MS MCh DNB MD (USA)
Ex-Professor and Head, Department of Urology
MGM Medical College, Aurangabad
Chief Urologist, Varun Hospital, Aurangabad

Ganesh Gopalakrishnan MS MCh FAMS FRCP
Vedanayagam Hospital, Coimbatore

Venkat Arjunrao Gite MS MCh DNB (Urology)
Professor and Head
Department of Urology, Government Medical College and Superspeciality Hospital, Aurangabad
Course Director, Fellowship in Reconstructive Urology of MUHS and Fellowship in Endourology by USI
Dean, Government Medical College and MPGIMER Nashik

Shivam Priyadarshi MS DNB MCh
Senior Professor and Head
Department of Urology
Sawai Mansingh Medical College, Jaipur

M Gopichand MS MCh DNB
Consultant Urologist and Head
Department of Urology
KIMS Hospital, Secunderabad

Vilas Sabale MS MCh DNB
Professor and Head
Department of Urology
DY Patil Medical College, Hospital and Research Centre, Pune

Umesh Sharma MS MCh DNB MNAMS
Professor and Unit Head, Department of Urology
ABVIMS and Dr Ram Manohar Lohia Hospital
New Delhi

Prakash Pawar MS MCh (Urology)
Professor, Department of Urology
LTMMC and GH, Sion, Mumbai

Bhavatej Enganti MS MCh
Consultant Urologist
Asian Institute of Nephrology and Urology
Hyderabad

Sadashiv Bhole MS MCh DNB
Consultant Urologist
Ketki Nursing Home and Urology Hospital, Nagpur

Utsav Shah MS MCh
Consultant Urologist and Uro-oncologist
Bodyline Hospitals. Ahmedabad

PVLN Murthy MS MCh MNAMS
Professor and Head
Department of Urology and Renal Transplantation
Kamineni Institute of Medical Sciences, Narketpally
Telangana

Rishikesh Kore MS DNB
Consultant Urologist
Warana Institute of Uro-Surgery, Kolhapur

Shrawan K Singh MS MCh FAMS
Ex-Professor and Head, Department of Urology
PGIMER, Chandigarh
Director, Urology
Fortis Hospital, Mohali

Tarun Jain MS MCh
Professor, Department of Urology
TN Medical College and BYL Nair Hospital, Mumbai

Suresh K Bhagat MS MCh (CMC Vellore)
Senior Consultant Urologist and Transplant Surgeon
Fortis Hospital, Mulund, Mumbai
Leelavati Hospital, Bandra (West) Mumbai

Somendra Bansal MS MCh DNB
Assistant Professor
Department of Urology
Sawai Mansingh Medical College, Jaipur

Shirish Dattatreya Yande MS FRCS
Chief Urologist and Director Academics
Ruby Hall Clinic, Pune
Director, Crystal Centre for Urodynamics and Neurourology (MMF)
Pune

Sameer Trivedi MBBS MS DNB (Urology) MCh (Urology)
Professor and Head, Department of Urology
Institute of Medical Sciences
Banaras Hindu University, Varanasi

Nikhil Khattar MS (Surgery) MCh (Urology)
The Perineo-Urology Clinic, New Delhi
Visiting Consultant Reconstructive Urology and Female Urology, Holy Family Hospital, New Delhi and Artemis Hospital Gurugram (Haryana)
Ex-Professor of Urology, ABVIMS and Dr RML Hospital
New Delhi

T Srikala Prasad MD DGO MCh (Urology)
Professor and Head, Department of Urology
Government Chengalpattu Medical College and Hospital
Tamil Nadu

N Rajamaheswari MD DGO MCh
Head, Department of Urogynaecology/Female Urology
Chennai Urology and Robotic Institute (CURI)
Chennai, Tamil Nadu

Arabind Panda MS MCh (Urology)
Senior Consultant Urologist and Renal Transplant Surgeon, AIG Hospitals
Gachibowli, Hyderabad

Ashwin Shekar P MS MCh Post-Doc Fellowship (Ped Urology)
Senior Consultant, Urologist
Program Coordinator, Dr HS Bhatt Reconstructive and Transitional Urology Fellowship
Department of Urology
Sri Sathya Sai Institute of Higher Medical Sciences
Prasanthigram, Puttaparthi, Andhra Pradesh

Pawan Vasudeva MBBS MS MRCS (Ed) UK MCh (Urology)
Professor and Head
Department of Urology and Renal Transplant
Vardhman Mahavir Medical College and Safdarjung Hospital, New Delhi

Vineet Narang MS MRCS DNB (Urology)
Senior Consultant Urologist and Transplant Surgeon
Holy Family Hospital
New Delhi

Joy Narayan Chakraborty MS FRCS Edin FRCS Eng FRCS Urol ChM Urol DNB Urol FHEA
Postgraduate Tutor Surgical and Urological Sciences
Edinburgh University, UK
Senior Consultant Urologist
Apollo Hospitals, Guwahati

Rohit Sethi MBBS MS MCh FRCS
Consultant Urologist
Department of Urology
Naruvi Hospitals, Vellore

Sanjay Sinha MCh
Honorary Professor and Consultant
Apollo Hospital, Hyderabad

Mayank Mohan Agarwal MS MRCS(Ed) MCh DNB
Senior Consultant and Head of Unit
Urology, Uro-oncology and Kidney Transplant Surgery
Apollomedics Superspeciality Hospital
Lucknow

Ankur Mittal MS MCh (Urology)
Additional Professor and Head
All India Institute of Medical Sciences
Rishikesh, Uttarakhand

Anita Patel MS MCh DNBE FRCS (Urol)
Consultant Urologist
Gleneagles Hospital, Mumbai
Endoskopik Klinik and Hospital, Mumbai
Visiting Consultant
Muljibhai Patel Urology Hospital
Nadiad, Gujarat

Rajesh Taneja MBBS MS MCh (AIIMS)
Senior Consultant and Advisor
Urology and Robotic Surgery
Indraprastha Apollo Hospitals
New Delhi

Divakar Dalela MS MCh FICS FAMS
Former Professor and Head
Department of Urology
KG Medical University, Lucknow, India

Rishi Nayyar MS MCh FMAS MAMS FIMSA
Professor
All India Institute of Medical Sciences
Ansari Nagar, New Delhi

Vijay Madduri MBBS (AIIMS, New Delhi) MS (AIIMS, New Delhi) MCh (IPGMER Kolkata)
Consultant Urologist
Robotic and Transplant Surgeon
Asian Institute of Nephrology and Urology
Banjara Hills, Hyderabad

Harini Sivamani DNB (OB&GY) MRCOG

Ahsan Ahmad
Professor, Department of Urology
Indira Gandhi Institute of Medical Sciences, Patna

Nitin Kekre MS DNB
Former Professor and Head
Department of Urology, Christian Medical College
Vellore
Senior Consultant Urologist
Naruvi Hospitals, Vellore

Deepak Kumar MS
Senior, Resident-Academics
All India Institute of Medical Sciences
Rishikesh, Uttarakhand

Lovekesh Kumar MS MCh
Department of Urology
All India Institute of Medical Sciences
New Delhi

Sanjay Pandey MS MCh DNB
Director of Urology
Head, Andrology and Reconstructive Urology
Robotic Urology and Gender
Reassignment Surgery
Kokilaben Dhirubhai Ambani Hospital and Research
Institute, Mumbai

Ajay Kanbur MS DNB MCh DNB
Consultant Urologist
Jupiter Hospital, Thane, Maharashtra

Arun Karthik P MS MCh FIAMH FECSM
Consultant Uro-Andrologist, Reproductive Microsurgeon
and Medical Director
Alpha Life UroSpeciality Clinic
Andro-One Men's Clinic, Salem and Namakkal
Tamil Nadu, India

Ashish Sabharwal MS DNB
Senior Consultant Urologist, Andrologist and Robotic
Surgeon
Indraprastha Apollo Hospital, New Delhi

Rohan Batra MS DNB (Urology)
Consultant Urologist
Muljibhai Patel Urological Hospital
Nadiad, Gujarat, India

Ashwin Mallya MS MRCS MCh (Urology)
Consultant Urologist
Sir Ganga Ram Hospital
New Delhi

Amit K Devra MS DNB (Urology)
Director, Department of Urology, Robotics and Renal
Transplantation, Jaypee Hospital
Noida, Uttar Pradesh, India

Renuka Soni
Clincial Research Associate
Kidney Transplant and Urology, Meliora Kidney and
Urology Institute, Chandigarh and Shalby Hospital
Mohali, Punjab

Sanjay P Kolte MS MCh
Director and Head
Urology and Renal Transplantation
Max Superspeciality Hospital, Nagpur
Formerly Professor, Urology
Govt Medical College and Superspeciality Hospital
Nagpur, India

Ravindra B Sabnis MS MCh
Chairman, Department of Urology
Muljibhai Patel Urological Hospital
Nadiad, Gujarat

Umesh Oza MS MCh
Professor and Head
Department of Urology
Bombay Hospital Institute of Medical Sciences
Marine Lines, Mumbai, India

Ruchir Maheshwari MS MCh
Director and Head
Urology and Kidney Transplant
Fortis Hospital, Manesar, Gurugram
Haryana, India

Ajay Oswal MS MCh DNB MNAMS
Consultant Urologist
Kamalnayan Bajaj Hospital, Aurangabad
Consultant Urologist, Seth Nandlal Dhoot Hospital
Aurangabad, (Sambhajinagar), Maharashtra

Arun Chawla MS MNAMS MCh DNB FIMS
Professor and Head
Department of Urology and Renal Transplant
Kasturba Medical College
Manipal

Abhinav Jain MS DNB
Consultant, Department of Urology
Robotic Surgery and Kidney Transplantation
Manipal Hospital, Dwarka, Delhi

Nitesh Jain MS MCh
Consultant Urologist
Apollo Hospitals, Greams Road, Chennai, Tamil Nadu
India

Muthu Veeramani MS MCh
Director and Head, Department of Urology and Renal Transplantation, SRM Institute of Renal Sciences, SIMS Hospital, Chennai, India

Kishore TA MS MCh
Consultant Urologist
Aster Medcity
Kochi, Kerala, India

Deepak Rathi MS DNB
Consultant Urologist
Medanta-The Medicity
Gurugram, Haryana

M Ramalingam MS DNB (Uro) MCh FRCS DSc
Urologist, Andrologist, Transplant and Robotic Surgery
Lead Consultant
Urology and Nephrology Unit, Hindusthan Hospitals
Nava India, Coimbatore
Tamil Nadu, India

Jamal Rizvi MS MCh
Professor of Urology
Institute of Kidney Diseases and Research Centre (IKDRC)
Ahmedabad, Gujarat

Sunil Shroff MS FRCS Dip Urol (Lond.)
Managing Trustee, MOHAN Foundation
Senior Consultant, Urology and Transplantation
Madras Medical Mission Hospital
and MGM Healthcare
Chennai, India

LP Choudhary MS MCh
Senior Consultant Urologist
Department of Urology Robotics and Renal Transplantation, Jaypee Hospital
Noida, Uttar Pradesh, India

Priyadarshani Ranjan MS MCh
Institute Director, Meliora Kidney and Urology Institute, Chandigarh
Regional Director and Chief of Urology and Kidney Transplant, Paras Hospital, Panchkula
Director, Kidney Transplant and Urology, Shalby Hospital
Mohali, Punjab
Ex-Director Kidney Transplant, Robotic Surgery and Urology, Fortis Hospital, Mohali
Former Assistant Professor, Department of Urology and Kidney Transplant, SGPGI Lucknow

Kapil Sejpal MD DM
Assistant Professor, Department of Nephrology, JNMC
Sawangi, Wardha (Maharashtra), India

Akshay Deshpande MS Senior Resident in Urology
Department of Urology
Bombay Hospital Institute of Medical Sciences
Mumbai

Anant Kumar MS MCh DNB FMGEMS
Chairman, Department of Urology, Kidney Transplantation, Robotic and Uro-oncology
Max Super-speciality Hospital, Delhi, India

Akshay Mahesh Kriplani MS MCh
Consultant Urologist
Asian Kidney Hospital and Medical Centre
Nagpur Maharashtra

Sumit Bansal MS MCh
Consultant, Department of Urology, Robotic Surgery and Kidney Transplantation, Manipal Hospital, Dwarka, Delhi

Jigish Vyas MS DNB (Urology)
Fellow, Abdominal Organ Transplant, Wake Forest Baptist Hospital, Winston-Salem, NC, USA

Varun Mittal MS MCh (Urology-SGPGIMS)
Head, Kidney Transplant and Associate Chief
Uro-oncology and Robotic Surgery, Artemis Hospital
Gurugram

V Surya Prakash MS FRCS MCh (Urology) DNB
Consultant Urologist and Transplant Surgeon
Yashoda Hospitals
Somajiguda, Hyderabad

Mudit Maheshwari MS MCh
Consultant Urologist
Manipal Hospitals, Pune

Pranjal Modi MS DNB
Professor and Head
Department of Urology
Director, Institute of Kidney Diseases and Research Centre (IKDRC)
Vice-Chancellor, Gujarat University of Transplantation Sciences (GUTS), Ahmedabad, Gujarat

Mahesh Desai MS FRCS (Eng) FRCS (Edin) FACS
Managing Trustee and Senior Consultant Urologist
Muljibhai Patel Urological Hospital
Dr Virendra Desai Road
Nadiad, Gujarat, India

Rahul Yadav MBBS MS MCh
Director
Urology, Kidney Transplant, and Robotic Uro-oncology
Tender Palm Super Specialty Hospital, Lucknow
Chief Kidney Transplant Surgeon
Charak Hospital and Research Centre, Lucknow

Janak Desai MS MCh (Urology)
Consultant Urologist
Samved Hospital, Ahmedabad

Kandarp Parikh MS MCh DNB
Chairman, Shyam Urosurgical Hospital
Ahmedabad
Director, Department of Urology
Marengo CIMS Hospital, Ahmedabad

Kaushikkumar Shah MBBS MS MCh
Consultant Urologist
Varun Hospital, Surat

Dilip Kumar Mishra MS MRCS MCh
Consultant and Head
Department of Urology
Pushpanjali Hospital and Research Centre
Agra, UP

V Chandra Mohan Vaddi
MS (AIIMS) MCh (PGI Chandigarh) MRCS DNB
Managing Director
Preeti Urology and Kidney Hospital, Hyderabad

SK Pal MS MCh
Consultant Urologist
Indraprastha Apollo Hospital, New Delhi

Ramesh Vaman Mahajan MS MCh (Urology)
Consultant Urologist, Mahajan Urology Clinic
Fortis Hospital, Zen Hospital, Mumbai

Nanjappa K Madappa MS DNB MCh DNB MNAMS
Consultant Endourologist
Cauvery Uroderm Centre
Kalyan, Maharashtra

Mukund G Andankar
MBBS, MS (General Surgery) MCh (Urology) DNB (Genitourinary Surgery)
Professor and Head
Department of Urology
TNMC and BYL Nair Hospital, Mumbai

Manoj Biswas MS (Surg) DNB (Urol)
Professor and Head
Department of Urology
Government Doon Medical College, Dehradun
Uttarakhand

Apul Goel MS (Surg) MCh (Urol) DNB (Urol)
Professor, Department of Urology
King George's Medical University, Lucknow, India

Vasudeo Ridhorkar MBBS MS DNB MCh DNB
Chief, Department of Urology, KIMS-Kingsway Hospitals
Nagpur

Rajeev TP MBBS MS MCh (AIIMS)
Director and Chief Consultant Urologist Medicity
Guwahati

Rajesh Kukreja MS DNB (Urologist)
Consultant Urologist
Urocare, Indore

Prashant Motiram Mulawkar MBBS DGO MS Gen (Surgery) DNB MCh DNB (Urology) ChM Urology Edinburgh
Consultant Urologist
Tirthankar Superspeciality Hospital, Akola
Professor, Department of Urology, GMC SSH Akola
Tutor Urology, University of Edinburgh, UK

Ajay Bhandarkar MS MCh DNB
Chief Urologist, Sujay Urological Hospital
Vadodara, Gujarat

Abhay Dinkar Mahajan MBBS MS MCh DNB MNAMS
Sai Urology Hospital and MGM Medical College and Hospital, Aurangabad

Mallikarjuna Chiruvella MS MCh
Consultant, Urologist
AINU, Hyderabad

Niramya Pathak MS DNB
Consultant Urologist
Muljibhai Patel Urological Hospital
Dr Virendra Desai Road, Nadiad, Gujarat, India

Madhu Sudan Agrawal
MS MCh (Urology) MNAMS FRCS (Glasgow)
Chairman, Urosciences, Pushpanjali Hospital, Agra

Akshay Nathani DNB DrNB
Consultant Urologist
Muljibhai Patel Urological Hospital, Nadiad, Gujarat

Aditya Parikh MS DNB
Consultant Urologist
Shyam Urosurgical Hospital

Parimalsinh Gharia MS DNB
Consultant Urologist
Icon Hospital, Surat

Karthickeyan Naganathan MS MRCS (Edin) DNB MCh
Consultant Urologist
Frontline Hospital, Trichy, Tamil Nadu

Soundarya Ganesan MS MCh Consultant Urologist
Preeti Urology and Kidney Hospital
Hyderabad

Harshawardhan Tanwar MS MCh FACS
Director, Satalkar Lotus Superspeciality Hospital
Ahmednagar

Sheshang Uday Kamat MBBS MS MCh
Consultant Urologist
Royal Darwin Hospital
Australia

Abheesh Varma Hegde MS DNB MCh DrNB FMAS
Assistant Professor, Father Muller Medical College
Mangalore, Karnataka

Prasad M Brahme MBBS MS (General Surgery) MCh (Urology)
Assistant Professor
Department of Urology
TNMC & BYL Nair Hospital, Mumbai

Siddalingeshwar Neeli MS MCh DNB
Professor and Head
Department of Urology
JN Medical College and KLE Hospital
Belgavi, Karnataka

Mohammed Taif Bendigeri MS MCh
Consultant Urologist
Asian Institute of Nephrology and Urology
Hyderabad

Sumeet Gopal Agrawal MS DNB (Urology)
Consultant Urologist
Lotus Superspeciality Hospital, Akola

Nisarg Mehta MS DNB
Consultant Urologist, Radiance Urology Hospital
Vadodara, Gujarat

Poleboyina Vamsi Krishna MS MCh (Urology)
Consultant Urologist
Care Hospitals, Hyderabad

Gopal Ramdas Tak MS DNB
Consultant Urologist, AINU
Hyderabad

Laxman Prabhu MS MCh (Urology)
Professor, Kasturba Medical College
Mangaluru

Rahul Gupta MS DrNB (Urology)
Associate Professor
Department of Urology and Renal Transplant
GMC, Jammu

Himanshu Pandey MS MCh (Urology)
Senior Professor and Head
Department of Urology and Uro-oncology
Tata Memorial Cancer Hospital, Varanasi

Ranjan Kumar Dey MCh (Urology)
Professor and Head, RG Kar Medical College and Hospital
Government of West Bengal, Kolkata

Sumantra Dey MS MCh
Junior Consultant Urologist
NH Hospital, Andul, Howrah, West Bengal

Harprit Singh MS DNB (Urology)
Clinical Director and Consultant Urologist
Urovita Hospital, Jamshedpur

Suresh Bhat MS (PGI Chandigarh) MCh
Senior Consultant, Urology
Caritas Hospital, Kottayam, Kerala

John Peter MS MCh
Senior Consultant Urologist
Dr KM Cherian Institute of Medical Sciences
Chengannur, Kerala

BM Zeeshan Hameed MS MCh
Professor and Head, Department of Urology
Kasturba Medical College, Mangalore, Karnataka

Parag Sonawane MS DNB FRCS
Consultant Urologist and Robotic Surgeon
Freeman Hospital, Newcastle, Middlesbrough
England, United Kingdom

Shruti R Sabnis MD(Pathology)
Consultant Pathologist
Muljibhai Patel Urological Hospital
Nadiad, Gujarat, India

Anwesa Chakraborty MBBS MS MCh (Pediatric Surgery)
Consultant (Pediatric Surgey and Pediatric Urology)
Medanta, Lucknow

Amit Ghose MS FRCS Dip. Urology
Consultant Uro-Oncologist
Apollo Gleneagles Hospital Limited, Kolkata, West Bengal

Venkatesh Krishnamoorthy MCh Urology FRCS Glasgow
Chairman NU Hospitals
Bengaluru

Uday Sankar Chatterjee MCh (Ped Surg) MCh (Urology)
Expert Faculty, Nilratan Sircar Medical College and Hospital, Kolkata
Visiting Surgeon, Park Medical Research and Welfare Society, Kolkata

Abhijit Patil MS MCh (Urology) DNB (Urology) FACS
Consultant Urologist
Muljibhai Patel Urological Hospital, Nadiad, Gujarat, India

Gautam Banga MBBS MS MCh (Urology)
SCI International Hospital, Greater Kailash Part 1
New Delhi

Mohsin Quadri MBBS MS DNB MNAMS
Consultant Urologist, Andrologist, Endourologist and Laparoscopic Urologist
Assistant Professor, Department of Urology
Government General Hospital, Guntur Medical College
Guntur, Andhra Pradesh, India

Prabhakar Srinivasan MBBS MS DNB MCh
Consultant Uro-Andrologist, Conceive Couple Care Clinic, Salem

Puvai Murugan P MBBS MS MCh
Professor and Head, Department of Urology, PSG Institute of Medical Sciences and Research
Coimbatore

Deepak Gupte MBBS MS MCh LLB
Bombay Hospital and Medical Research Center
Mumbai
PD Hinduja Hospital and Medical Research Center
Mumbai
LH Hiranandani Hospital

Vijayant Govinda Gupta MBBS MS MCh (Urology)
Director and Urologist
Govinda Medicenter
New Delhi

Krishna Mohan Boopathy Vijayaraghavan
MS MCh (Urology)
Assistant Professor of Urology
PSG Institute of Medical Sciences and Research
Coimbatore

Debabrat Kumar Sabat MS MCh
Professor of Urology, IMS and SUM Hospital
Bhubaneswar, Odisha

Shivakumar V MBBS MS MCh (Urology)
Associate Professor, Department of Urology
Institute of Nephro Urology, Bengaluru
Karnataka

Vineet Malhotra MBBS MS DNB
Senior Consultant Microsurgical and Prosthestic Uro-Andrologist
Director, VNA Hospitals, New Delhi
Visiting Consultant, Muljibhai Patel Urological Hospital
Nadiad, Gujarat

Vinay Chougule MCh DNB
Consultant, Jaya Urology Hospital, Kolhapur
Maharashtra

Priyank Kothari MBBS MS MCh
Assistant Professor and Microsurgical Uro-Andrologist
Dr BYL Nair Ch Hospital, Mumbai

Arun Kumar K MBBS MS DNB Surgery MCh (Urology)
Senior Consultant and Medical Director
RG Stone Urology And Laparoscopy Hospital, Chennai
Tamil Nadu

Guru Balaji Shanmugham
DNB (Gen surg) MRCS MNAMS DNB (Urology)
Gericare Hospital, Chennai, Tamil Nadu

Sanjay Prakash J MBBS MS DNB FAMH FMAS FIAGES
Microsurgical Andrologist and Urologist
Asian Institute of Nephro Urology, Chennai, Tamil Nadu

Vinod KV MS MCh (Urology)
Microsurgical Uro-Andrologist CURE, Trivandrum
Kerala

Praveen Joshi MS DNB (Urology)
Consultant Microsurgical Andrologist and Urologist
Joshi Andrology and Urology Centre, Bengaluru
Karnataka

Sitaram Mummalaneni MBBS MS MCh FIAMH
Consultant Uro-Andrologist, Androcare
Hyderabad, Telangana

Sathish Babu Pigilam MBBS MS MCh (Urology)
Consultant Urologist and Andrologist, Queen's NRI Hospital, Gurudwara
Visakhapatnam

Vilvapathy Senguttuvan Karthikeyan
MBBS MS MCh MRCS FAIS FECSM
Microsurgical Andrologist and Urologist
Apollo Hospitals, Greams Road, Chennai
Tamil Nadu

Raghavender Kosgi MCh DNB FECSM
Consultant Urologist and Andrologist
Department of Andrology and Men's Health
Apollo Hospitals, Jubilee Hills,
Hyderabad, Telangana

Ashit Shah
Chief Consultant Urologist
Aashray Urology Institute
Vadodara, Gujarat
India

Shiv Charan Navriya MBBS MS MCh
Associate Professor, AIIMS Jodhpur
Rajasthan

Datteswar Hota MBBS MS MCh
Professor and Head, Department of Urology
SCB Medical College, Cuttack
Vice-chancellor, Odisha University of Health Sciences
Odisha

Pramod Krishnappa DNB (Urol) ChM (Edinburgh)
Consultant Uro-Andrologist, Department of Urology
AndroNeo @NU Hospitals, Bengaluru
Karnataka

Chirag Gupta DNB (Urology)
Consultant Andrologist, Matratva Fertility and Andrology Clinic
Assistant Professor, Department of General Surgery
JNUIMSRC
Jaipur Rajasthan

Ashish Rawandale Patil MS MCh (Urology) DNB
Director and Head, Institute of Urology
Sakri Road, Dhule
Maharashtra

Lokesh Patni MS DNB (Urology)
Consultant Urologist
Institute of Urology, Sakri Road, Dhule, Maharashtra

Aditya Pradhan MS DNB (Urology)
Director and Head, Uro-oncology and Renal Transplantation
Venkateshwar Hospital, New Delhi

Aneesh Srivastava MS MCh (Urology)
Director, Department of Urology and Renal Transplantation, Medanta Hospital, Lucknow
Uttar Pradesh

Bipin Chandra Pal MS MCh DNB
Director and Head
Department of Urology
AIG Hospital, Hyderabad, Telangana

Jyoti Bansal MS DNB
Consultant Urologist
Fortis Hospital, Jaipur, Rajasthan

Milap Shah MS MCh
Consultant Urologist
Aarogyam Speciality Hospital, Ahmedabad
Gujarat

Ulhas V Sathaye MS MCh
Consultant Urologist
Sahyog Speciality Hospital
Jamnagar, Gujarat

Foreword

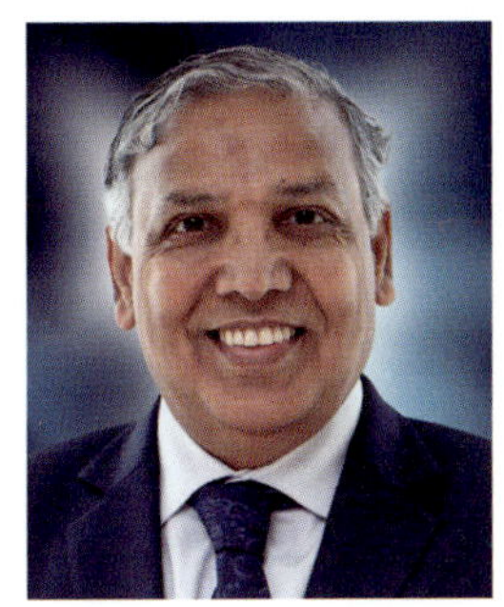

Asia is the largest populated area in the world. India is the most populous nation. This translates into high volumes in surgery and hence we are ahead in the surgical numbers game, we have presented ourselves a number of times at academic forums. The lacunae remain in presenting our experience in the form of publications.

I am happy to present this book under the auspices of the Urological Society of India. This book is meant to update yourself with the latest knowledge and practical approach to urology. It is made in India, by Indians and I am sure this will find an appeal across the world. True to the spirit of "Make in India" and makes me feel proud as an Indian.

When I became the President of the Urological Society of India, I thought of this book as my academic contribution to the society which has given me so much. We embarked on this journey by diligently picking authors who are experts in their own area.

The book has various sections and I am sure each one of you will find them interesting. I urge all residents to refer to the book for their examinations and future practice. The contributions are from the youngest resident in urology to the senior most practising urologist in the country. The textbook will be a fine example of our commitment to urology.

For me, personally, this is my biggest contribution to the Urological Society of India.

I hope this makes a great read to all of you and you enjoy the " joy " of learning.

Sanjay Balwant Kulkarni
President. Urological Society of India 2023-2024
Past President, Society International de Urologie
Past President, Genitourinary Reconstructive Surgeons

Secretary's Message

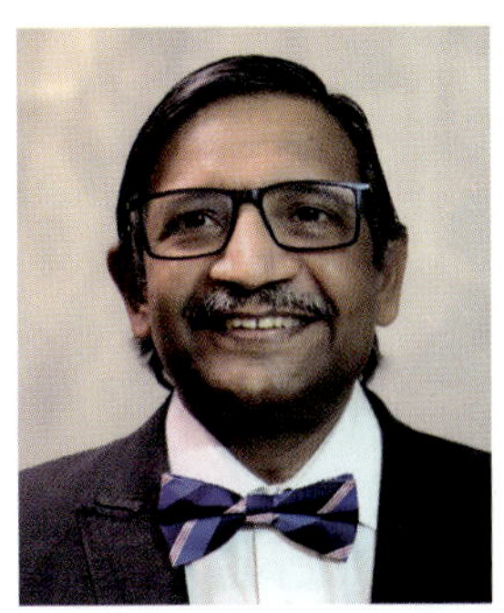

Last January our President Dr Sanjay Kulkarni gave us a task to come out with a book which would highlight practical aspects in evaluating and managing a urological case. The idea was further expanded by the able leadership of Dr Laxman. The task of putting the things together was entrusted on the editor duo. The editors and section editors have worked tirelessly in coming out with the product which you are holding in your hands. You are witnessing a first of its kind book. First in the sense that it is equally as useful to the exam going student as it is to a practising urologist. First in the sense that it is a cent percent Indian book covering most of the clinical scenarios encountered by us. First in the sense that the task of creating such a big book is accomplished in a record time of ten months. It is a not a didactic book, rather the text in the book flows like a thought process of a clinician who is evaluating a case and making a plan of management giving reasoning at each step.

The process of creating this book started with an outline of clinical scenarios which a practising urologist comes across in day to day patient care. The scenarios were made more representative and the common questions that come in mind of the treating urologist or the questions which are commonly asked by the examiners were then thought of by the contributors. The editors and contributing authors have outlined each and every aspect of the management in a great detail. Each chapter has been peer reviewed and undergone revisions so as to be more authentic and representative. More weightage has been given on reasoning the management plan as per available scientific evidence. This has created a deeper insight in the creative process of the contributors.

Unfortunately, Dr Laxman is not with us to see this dream project of the Urological Society of India being published today. We lost him midway. Aptly, this book is dedicated to his memory.

I am sure this book will help the target audience to whom it is intended and will also act as a quick reference in day to day life of a busy urologist. And it will find utility the world across.

Prashant Motiram Mulawkar
Acting Secretary, USI (2023-2024)
Consulting Urologist
Tirthankar Superspeciality Hospital, Akola
Professor, Department of Urology, GMC SSH, Akola
Tutor in Urology, University of Edinburgh, UK

Preface

"Readers and writers would be the leaders of tomorrow", these are the words which keep on echoing relentlessly in our minds as we place this book with moist eyes in the hands of our readers as a tribute to our late Secretary Prof GG Laxman Prabhu. Prof (Dr) Laxman Prabhu, would have been so happy to see his efforts see the light of the day. Nonetheless, that's destiny!!

The question that comes is why another book?

Even though there are huge and exhaustive works on urology developed from world over, there is not a single textbook available to the trainees and practitioners which deals with practical aspects of the speciality in the Indian context.

The purpose of this book was as follows: One, the Urological Society of India has a vast pool of talented writers who have done original work in their chosen domains. Secondly, a work approved, supported, scrutinized and reviewed by the nation's apex urology organisation which has international standing now, will not only have the stature of authority but also the stamp of authenticity. The book aims to provide a practical approach to both common and difficult urological disease entities along with the best treatment policies which are practical, workable and capable of producing good treatment outcomes in the Indian context. It shall hopefully be an endeavour to make assimilation of the subject easy by providing crystallized versions of difficult to cover material available in the literature of repute. The content has been carefully curated to address the needs of readers with varied interest. The volume contains 8 sections addressed to all the subspecialities in urology. Each chapter has been formatted in a question-and-answer format. In addition, there are learning points, each of which is discussed in details. The USP of this book is the QR coded videos which emphasize on different techniques in urology.

An effort of this magnitude could not have fructified, had it not been the unstinted support of President USI, Dr Sanjay Kulkarni, Late Prof (Dr) GG Laxman Prabhu and the entire USI council. We owe our gratitude to all the members of USI for entrusting us with this task.

We would like to put on record, if it was not for the enthusiasm of Mr Verma and Mr Gala, this volume would not have seen the light of the day. We would like to thank Dr Ashu Singh for being so vigilant to ensure the book maintains the required standards. A big thanks to the staff of CBS Publishers & Distributors, Mr SK Jain (CMD), Mr YN Arjuna (Senior Vice President—Publishing, Editorial and Publicity) and his entire team comprising Ms Ritu Chawla (GM—Production), Mr Neeraj Prasad (Graphic Artists), Mr Prasenjit Paul (Copy Editor) and Mr Sunil Dutt (DTP Operator) have made an excellent contribution to bring out this edition. We are really obliged to them and pray for their prosperity.

We acknowledge the help by Dr Nishanth S, consultant urologist at MPUH, Nadiad, for his inputs during copyediting of this book. We also acknowledge the fact that medical science has different views on a given subject. We urge the readers to refer to urology textbooks in case of differing views. We will try to address such issues, if any, in subsequent editions. Please feel free to send comments on Clinical.Urology.USI@gmail.com.

Last but not the least, we would be unfair if we do not acknowledge the support from all my authors and associate/assistant editors and contributors. All the bouquets and accolades should be reserved for our esteemed colleagues who have burnt the midnight oil to see the efforts fructify and brickbats if any for both of us.

Hope this makes an excellent reading for all.

Arvind Prakash Ganpule
Pankaj Nandkishore Maheshwari

The Urological Society of India

The Urological Society of India (USI) came into existence in December, 1961. At inception, a provisional Executive Committee with the late Dr GM Phadke as the Chairman and Dr BN Colabawalla as the Hon. Secretary-cum-Treasurer, were entrusted with the task of framing the rules, enrolling members. Since then, the Society has created 4 zonal chapters with the idea of spreading urology to each and every corner of India. Each zonal chapter conducts CME programmes and workshops and zonal annual conference which are attended by 300–400 delegates.

The Society holds its annual conference usually in the month of January by rotation in the four zones. The annual conference is usually attended by close to 2000 delegates. Apart from scientific deliberations, there is technical exhibition for latest equipment in urology.

The Society also publishes its own journal, Indian Journal of Urology, and a newsletter, four times a year. Indian Journal of Urology is an indexed Journal by the Excerpt Medica and PubMed (Medline).

The USI has now come of age and the membership has now crossed 5000. USI has entered the new millennium with plenty of hope and promise from younger colleagues, who will take USI to even greater heights.

Contents

SECTION 3: RECONSTRUCTIVE UROLOGY

Pankaj M Joshi and Venkat Arjunrao Gite

SECTION 4: FEMALE UROLOGY

Sanjay Sinha and Nikhil Kahttar

SECTION 5: ANDROLOGY

Vilvapathy Senguttuvan Karthikeyan VS and Priyank Kothari

ANDROLOGY

SECTION 8: GENERAL UROLOGY

Rahul Gupta and GG Laxman Prabhu

List of Videos

SECTION 1: URO-ONCOLOGY

SECTION 2: PEDIATRIC UROLOGY

SECTION 3: RECONSTRUCTIVE UROLOGY

SECTION 4: FEMALE UROLOGY

SECTION 6: RENAL TRANSPLANT

RECIPIENT

SECTION 7: ENDOUROLOGY

SECTION 8: GENERAL UROLOGY

Section

1

Uro-oncology

Chapter

1

Understanding Oncology Terminology and Statistics

• *Gopal Sharma* • *Puneet Ahluwalia*

LEARNING OBJECTIVES

- To understand the basic tenets of survival or time-to-event analysis: Basic understanding of survival and event analysis gives clinician a perspective into the disease biology.
- To define important terminologies related to survival data such as overall survival (OS) and cancer or disease-specific survival: This will help counsel the patients regarding outcome of a particular disease.
- To understand the concept of censoring which contributes to the skewing of the survival data: Different types of censoring such as left, right or interval censoring.
- How to interpret survival or Kaplan-Meier curves? They are important for understanding the survival function between the treatment groups.
- What is the hazard ratio, and how to estimate and interpret them?
- How to present survival data in a randomized control trial with a time-to-event analysis, i.e. hazard ratio, median survival and time point estimates?
- What is the Cox proportional hazard model? How is it different from logistic regression analysis? What are adjusted and unadjusted hazard ratios?

Case Scenario

Consider a hypothetical study in which patients with prostate cancer were randomized to radiation (Group 1) versus radical prostatectomy (Group 2). In each group, 50 patients were randomized from 2010–2020 and after a follow-up of 12 years results are available. The primary outcome of the study is biochemical recurrence-free survival.

1. **Which type of statistical method will you use to compare radiation versus radical prostatectomy?**
   Ans: Survival analysis.
2. **What is survival analysis?**
   Ans: Survival or time-event analysis is the study of the duration between the entry of a subject into a study to a particular event. Classically, such a type of analysis was used to study the time from receiving a particular treatment until death, hence popularized as survival analysis.[1]
3. **What can be different types of events in a study?**
   Ans: Classically, time to death was the concerned event. The time between receiving treatment till death due to any cause is called overall survival. The time between receiving treatment till disease progression or metastasis is called progression-free or metastasis-free survival. An event could be modified to include patients who died of a particular disease (disease-specific) or for cancers (cancer-specific) to give their survival rates. For prostate cancer, biochemical recurrence (BCR)-free survival is another time-related event used. It is defined as the time period between receiving treatment to documented biochemical recurrence.
4. **What is censoring?**
   Ans: Censoring is the group of patients for whom survival times are not known. In the hypothetical example provided in Fig. 1.1, patient C did not experience BCR during the study period but after it, this type of censoring is called right censoring. Some patients may be lost to follow-up, thus accounting for another reason for censoring (patient D). Some patients have to be censored as they cannot experience the said event, such as patient E who dies in the perioperative period cannot have BCR. Patients may have experienced

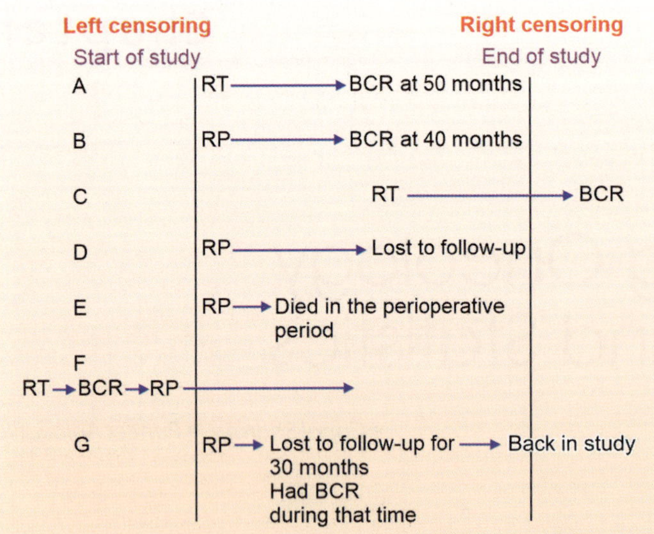

Fig. 1.1: Censoring

the event before entering the study such as patient F (called left side censoring). Patient G is an example of interval censoring, it is the interval during which the patient was lost to follow-up and had the event. Hence, we do not know exactly when he had the said event as he was lost to follow-up.[2,3]

5. **How do you calculate survival probability?**

   Ans: Kaplan-Meier (KM) survival estimate is used to estimate survival probability from observed survival times for both censored and uncensored events.[3] Plotting of survival probability or cumulative survival with time is called the KM survival curve. For the above-mentioned example, the KM curve is provided in Fig. 1.2. From the curve, if we want to know BCR-free survival after 40 months, it will correspond to 0.8 or 80% for the overall study cohort. Sometimes, the number of patients at risk is illustrated below the X-axis in some studies. It includes patients who have received treatment and have not experienced the event or have not lost to follow-up.[4,5]

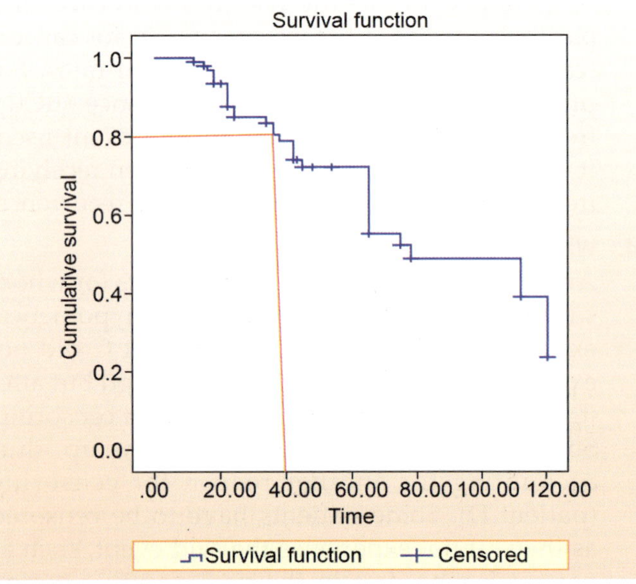

Fig. 1.2: Survival probability

6. **How do you statistically compare the two survival curves?**

   Ans: For the present example of comparing RT versus RP, the KM curve is provided in Fig. 1.3. From the visual interpretation of Fig. 1.3, not much separation between the survival curves of the two treatments could be interpreted. However, such an interpretation needs to be validated statistically using the log-rank test. For the given comparison, the p-value for the log-rank test is 0.79, thus accepting the null hypothesis, i.e. there is no difference in BCR after RT or RP.[1,3] Therefore, the log-rank test is the test used to compare the two survival curves to determine the statistical difference between them.

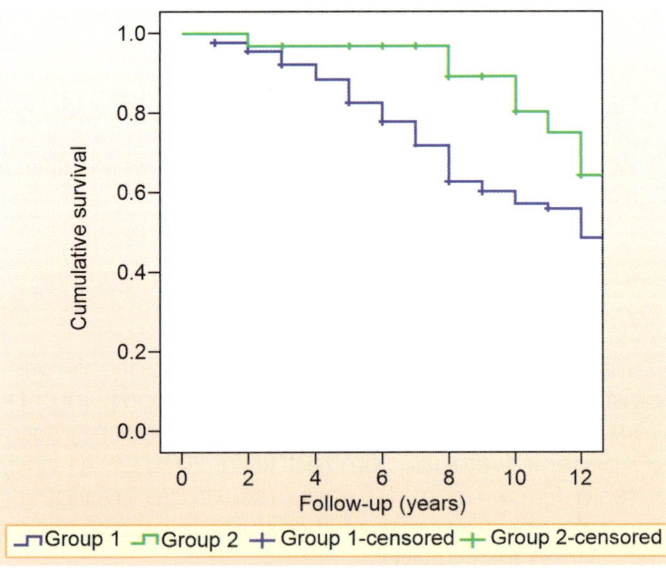

Fig. 1.3: Kaplan-Meier survival curve

7. **What is the hazard ratio (HR)?**

   Ans: The HR provides an estimate of the ratio of the hazard rates between the experimental group and a control group over the duration of the study. The hazard rate is the rate of patients experiencing the event over a time period within each of the treatment arms in the study. HRs can be interpreted as an HR = 1 means no difference in efficacy of the two treatment groups. Usually, the HR is presented so that if the experimental treatment is (i) better than the control, then the HR <1 or (ii) worse than the control, then the HR >1 (Fig. 1.4).

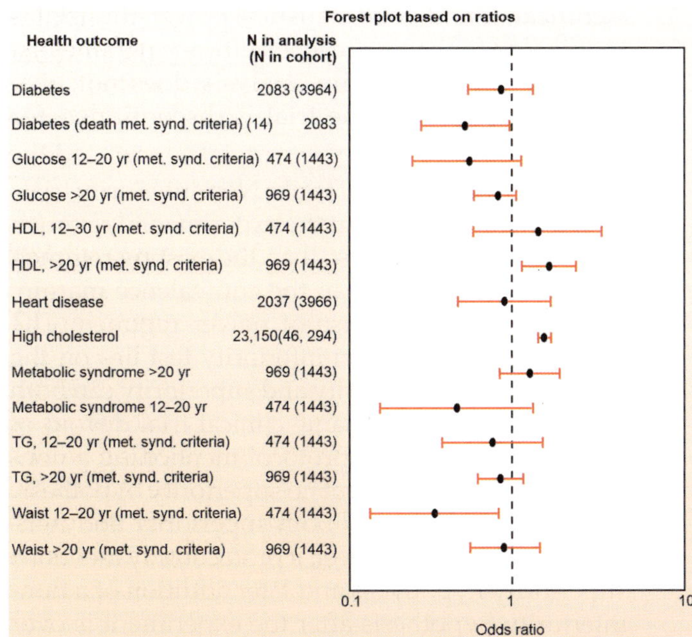

Fig. 1.4: Forest plot

(Referred from: https://www.sciencedirect.com/topics/medicine-and-dentistry/forest-plot)

8. What would you make of HR of 0.6 at the end of 4 months between abiraterone and placebo?

Ans: The HR provides an estimate of the relative efficacy between the treatment arms.[6] In this scenario, HR = 0.6 for biochemical recurrence-free survival indicates 40% lower risk of recurrence on the abiraterone treatment than the placebo.

9. What are the three main ways of estimating the magnitude and direction of survival outcomes from randomized studies?

Ans: Three important ways of estimating survival outcomes are[4] (Table 1.1):

1. HR
2. Median survival
3. Time point estimates (e.g. 1 year, 5-year or 10-year survival).

The data of present hypothetical dataset can be presented as: Hazard ratio for BCR for RT vs RP is 1.01 95% CI (0.5–2.1), p= 0.80 with median survival of 79 and 74 months respectively for RP and RT respectively. There was no difference between the two groups for RT vs. RP for 5-year (68% vs. 58%) and 10-year survival (50% vs. 33%).

10. How do we study the impact of other prognostic factors on the survival analysis?

Ans: The Cox model is preferred over the logistic model in survival analysis because logistic regression ignores survival time and censoring.[4] The Cox proportional hazards model is a regression method used in survival analysis for predicting differences in survival due to treatment and other confounding variables such as age or functional status. The Cox model is popular as it is robust, the estimated hazards are always non-negative and the hazard ratio along with confidence intervals can be calculated.

11. What are adjusted and unadjusted HRs?

Ans: Unadjusted HR is calculated from univariate, whereas adjusted HR is calculated from multivariate analysis. Unadjusted HR obtained from univariate Cox model contains treatment arm (e.g. RT vs. RP) as the covariates, whereas adjusted HRs calculated from multivariate Cox proportional hazards model also contain other covariates such as age, stage or performance status.

12. Explain Kaplan-Meier curve.

The Kaplan-Meier curve is used to estimate the survival function.[7] It shows the probability that a subject will survive up to time *t* while considering time in many small intervals. The log-rank test compares the survival curves of two or more groups (like a group that got treatment radiation, say Group 1 versus a group that got treatment radical prostatectomy, say Group 2). The curve is constructed by plotting the survival function against time. The tick marks on the curve indicate censoring and the curve moves down when the event of interest occurs (step functions). Refer to Fig. 1.3 which shows Kaplan-Meier survival curve.

13. Explain primary outcome, secondary outcome and exploratory outcomes.

Primary outcome: Primary outcome is the most highlighted parameter of interest for the study

Table 1.1: Three main ways of estimating the magnitude and direction of survival outcomes

HR	*Median survival*	*Time point estimate*
It is a relative efficacy measure that summarizes treatment effect over the duration of the study	It is an absolute efficacy measure that measures survival at one point in the KM curve, i.e. when the probability of survival is 50%	It is also an absolute efficacy measure that measures survival at one point such as 1-year, 5-year or 1-year follow-up
Trial designs such as superiority or inferiority are based on it	Median survival does not interpret data across the whole KM curve, thus trial designs are not based on it	The time point estimate method does not interpret data across the KM curve, thus trial designs are not based on it
Can be adjusted or unadjusted	Unadjusted	Unadjusted

indicated in the study protocol and power calculation is based on it. This is generally patient-centered outcome, for example, survival and recurrence of the disease.

Secondary outcome: Secondary outcomes are additional parameters of interest collected to understand and interpret at the findings of the study. The study is not specifically powered to assess the secondary endpoint.

Exploratory outcome: An outcome parameter that is of lesser importance than a primary and secondary outcome parameters but is part of a pre-specified statistical analysis plan in the protocol for evaluating the effects of the experimental treatment is specified as an exploratory or other outcome. Exploratory outcomes are useful for future studies and new hypotheses.

14. Explain subgroup analysis, interim analysis, and non-inferiority clinical trials.

Ans: Subgroup analysis: It involves subgrouping of participant data and comparing the study variables between them. The subgrouping may be demography-based (males and females), health status, type of intervention, etc. This analysis also assesses if the association between two study variables depends on the third variable. For example, comparing the biochemical recurrence-free survival between prostate cancer patients treated with radiation (Group I) and patients that underwent radical prostatectomy (Group II).

Subgroup analysis can be either pre-specified or post-hoc. Pre-specified sub-group analysis is based on a planned hypothesis that justifies an overall and subgroup effect using appropriate statistical testing. Post-hoc subgroup analyses are exploratory and help in generating a hypothesis. Differences detected in small sample size subgroups may be due to matter of chance and would not have the statistical power leading to false-negative error.

Interim analysis: The analysis of data performed before completion of data collection is termed interim analysis. The purpose of this analysis is to assess for indications for likely fulfilment of objectives, progress of the project and requirement for modification. Interim analysis is done after careful planning and not on ad hoc basis to determine the mode of action for the study. Interim analysis can be performed after 1 year of enrolment, two-thirds of sample collection, 6 months of follow-up, etc. In clinical trials, interim analysis provides sufficient evidence of efficacy or futility, thereby deciding the completion of the study. In cases where sufficient evidence is attained for a desired efficacy considering the level of significance and good statistical power, the trial is terminated for having reached efficacy parameters. However, if the interim analysis does not give sufficient evidence, the trial is discontinued for futility.

Non-inferiority clinical trials: Non-inferiority trials seek to demonstrate that the experimental regimen is not significantly worse than the existing regimen by a margin greater than the equivalence margin, thus advocating the use of newer regimen. The critical region for a non-inferiority test lies on the right side. Non-inferiority and superiority can both be determined in the same clinical trial devoid of a statistical penalty. A protocol mentioning a non-inferiority hypothesis but no superiority hypothesis is valid for performing both superiority and non-inferiority test.[8,9] However, if protocol only mentions superiority hypothesis and later addition of a non-inferiority hypothesis after the experiment is over would be challenging because the non-inferiority margin is defined subjectively. Non-inferiority margin is independent of trial sample size and statistical power of the study. The method of non-inferiority testing is similar to that for equivalence trials, however, the lower limit of the 95% CI should be more than non-inferiority margin (Snapinn, 2000 and Dunn, 2018).

15. Are all the ratios same: Risk ratios, odds ratios, and hazard ratios?

Risk ratio: This is another form of probability. Risk is defined as incidence of any unfavorable outcome like death in a defined population at any time point.[10] RR is the ratio of the risk of unfavorable outcome in a group with some specific character compared to the other group without having specific character. This is also called relative risk. For RR, we required prospective study.

In terms of probability,

$$RR = \frac{\text{Incidence of unfavourable outcome in group with specific character}}{\text{Incidence of unfavourable outcome in group without specific character}}$$

If RR = 1, indicate that there is no difference in risk between the groups, i.e. same amount of risk

RR > 1, indicate that risk is higher in subjects who had specific character

RR < 1, indicate that risk is lower in subjects who had specific character

For example, if incidence of biochemical recurrence among radiation (Group 1) for 12 years is 4% and among radical prostatectomy (Group 2) is 0.5%, then RR = 8, i.e. radiation (Group 1) have 8 times more risk of recurrence as compared to radical prostatectomy (Group 2).

Odds ratios: Odds ratio (OR) is also sometimes called the cross product ratio. Odds indicated the ratio of the number of events to nonevents. An OR is the ratio of odds of an event in a group with some specific character compared to the other group without having specific character. It means OR is the ratio of ratio. This is commonly used in a case control study. The interpretation of the OR is same as RR.[10]

$$OR = \frac{\text{Odds of an event in group with specific character}}{\text{Odds of an event in group with specific character}}$$

Hazard ratios: Hazard is the same as risk and it is the probability of occurrence of an event like death, recurrence of the disease over a time period. The hazard rate at time t is calculated by dividing the conditional probability of failure (death, recurrence) in the next instant of time by the length of that instant provided the hazard remains constant over that period. It is a rate per unit of time. The hazard ratio (HR) is the ratio of two hazard rates in the presence of a risk factor. The numerical value of the hazard ratio indicates the relative hazard reduction gained by the experimental treatment as compared to the standard of care/control treatment. An HR = 1 indicates the likelihood of the event is equally likely at any given time. An HR is not equal to 1 indicates the risk of a person in one group is different from the risk of an individual in another at any given time interval.

For example, a hazard ratio of 0.60 indicates that the experimental treatment shown the benefit and 40% risk reduction compared to the standard of care/control treatment. A hazard ratio = 1.0 indicates that the experimental treatment provides zero risk reduction, compared to the standard of care/control treatment.

16. Explain risk reduction.

Ans: The effectiveness and safety of any health related interventions is measured by relative risk reduction (RRR) and absolute risk reduction (ARR) (also called attributable risk). The RRR indicates the percentage reduction in event for those received experimental treatment as compared to those not received the experimental treatment. The ARR is a measure of risk difference and indicates the additional risk of event associated with not receiving the experimental treatment.

For example, risk of event in experimental treatment group is 15% and 30% in non-experimental treatment group. RRR is calculated as (1–Risk Ratio) × 100. The RRR in this situation is therefore (1 – 0.5) × 100 = 50%. This indicates that the experimental treatment has reduced the risk for event by 50%.

The ARR is defined as the absolute difference between the risk of event in the non-experimental treatment group and the risk of event in the experimental treatment group: ARR = Risk in non-experimental treatment group – Risk in experimental treatment group. ARR in this situation is 30% – 15% = 15%, indicating that the experimental treatment has reduced the event in 15% of the patients.

17. What is intention to treat analysis?

Ans: Intention-to-treat (ITT) analysis is a strategy used in a randomized controlled trial where all participants who were randomized in the trial are analyzed as per their initial assigned group in spite of what treatment they received subsequently. This minimizes the bias that may occur due to change in treatment group of the participants during the trial period. The findings of the study may be overestimated if ITT is not done.

18. What is number needed to treat (NNT)?

Ans: NNT provides the minimum number of patients that would need to be treated to prevent one additional bad outcome or for one additional successful outcome compared with the standard or any other treatment. For example, the NNT to prevent from biochemical recurrence one patient of prostate cancer using a radiation (Group 1) may be 8 and the NNT using radical prostatectomy (Group 2) may be 12. Then radical prostatectomy therapy would be considered more effective.

19. Explain positive predictive value and negative predictive value.

Ans: Sensitivity (Sn)/true positive rate (TPR)

Sensitivity is defined as the ability of a test to identify correctly true positives out of those who have the disease. Therefore, sensitivity is the ratio of subjects tested as positive to the total diseased subjects.

Sensitivity (Sn) = TP / (TP + FN)

This is also known as true positive rate (TPR). False negative rate or miss rate is the complement of true positive rate.

Specificity (Sp)/true negative rate (TNR)

Specificity is defined as the ability of test to identify correctly the true negatives out of those who do not have disease. Therefore, Specificity is the ratio of subjects tested as negative out of total non-diseased subjects.

Specificity (Sp) = TN / (TN + FP)

Sensitivity and specificity of a test do not change with the prevalence of disease.

Positive predictive values (PPV)/precision

Positive predictive value (PPV) of a diagnostic test is defined as the probability of a test to detect the true positive cases. Therefore, PPV represents a proportion of subjects with disease out of those tested as positive. This is calculated as

PPV = TP/(TP + FP)

When the prevalence is known, an adjusted formula for PPV is

Adj PPV = (Sn × Prevalence)/[Sn × Prevalence + (1–Sp) × (1–Prevalence)]

Negative predictive value

Negative predictive value (NPV) of a diagnostic test is defined as the probability of a test to detect the true negative cases. Therefore, NPV is defined as a proportion of subjects without the disease out of those tested as negative. This is calculated as

NPV = TN/(TN + FN)

When the prevalence is known, an adjusted formula for NPV is

Adj NPV = [(Sp × (1–Prevalence)]/[(1–Sn) × Prevalence + Sp × (1–Prevalence)]

The complement of the NPV is the false omission rate (FOR).

Diagnostic Effectiveness (Overall Accuracy)

The diagnostic accuracy of a test is expressed as the proportion of those individuals correctly diagnosed by the test. It is calculated as:

Overall Accuracy = (TP + TN)/(TP + FP + FN + TN).

This measure is affected by the prevalence of disease. An accuracy can also be determined in terms of sensitivity and specificity, when prevalence is known.

Overall Accuracy = (Sensitivity × Prevalence) + (Specificity) × (1–Prevalence)

Thus the overall accuracy of a test increases as the prevalence of disease decreases, for fixed sensitivity and specificity.

20. Explain forest plot, waterfall plot, spider plot, swimmer plot and funnel plot.

Ans: Forest plot: A forest plot is a graphical presentation of findings from a meta-analysis. First we need to identify the type of outcome either it is binary or continuous. In forest plot, a box represents the point estimate and corresponding horizontal line passing through the box represents the 95% confidence interval of the estimates (whiskers). The size of the box indicates the study weight; the bigger the box, the study provides larger information of the parameter of the interest and having greater the weight from other studies. The symbol diamond below the studies indicating the overall pooled effect from the all included studies. A vertical line in the forest plot indicating the no effect. If outcome variable is binary, then vertical line passes from 1 and if outcome parameter is continuous, then passes from 0. The I2 statistic provides the magnitude of heterogeneity among the studies. An example of a forest plot is shown in Fig. 1.4.

Waterfall plot: A waterfall plot, also known as a cascade plot or spectrogram, is a graphical representation of a three-dimensional dataset.[11,12] It is commonly used in signal processing and frequency analysis to visualize the time-varying frequency content of a signal. It is used to show or indicate how two-dimensional phenomena changes over time. It is a spectral waterfall plot where multiple curves of data are shown simultaneously. In a waterfall plot, the X-axis represents time, the Y-axis represents frequency, and the Z-axis represents the magnitude or intensity of the signal at a particular time and frequency. The plot consists of a series of stacked 2D plots, where each plot represents a snapshot of the frequency content of the signal at a specific time. Waterfall charts are visual representations of data, which can range from audio frequencies to patient data and trial findings. A waterfall plot, for instance, might be used in oncology to show how each patient responds to a specific treatment based on a criterion like tumor burden.

The magnitude or intensity of the signal is represented using different color scale, different colors indicate different magnitude or intensities. Darker colors usually represent higher magnitudes or intensities, while lighter colors represent lower magnitudes or intensities. It is an ordered histogram showing the best percentage change in tumor size, with positive values denoting tumor growth and negative ones denoting tumor shrinking. One patient is represented by each vertical column (Fig. 1.5).

Spider plot: Spider plots, also known as radar plots or spider charts, are graphical representations used to display multivariate data in a two-dimensional format.[13] They can highlight strengths and weaknesses across multiple variables and provide a quick overview of the overall profile of each outcome. Spider charts are excellent for displaying performance since they can be used to determine which variables in a dataset are scoring highly or poorly.[13]

They are particularly useful for comparing multiple variables across different dimensions or categories. In a spider plot, each variable is represented by a spoke or a line extending from a central point, like the legs of a spider. The length of each line or spoke represents the magnitude or

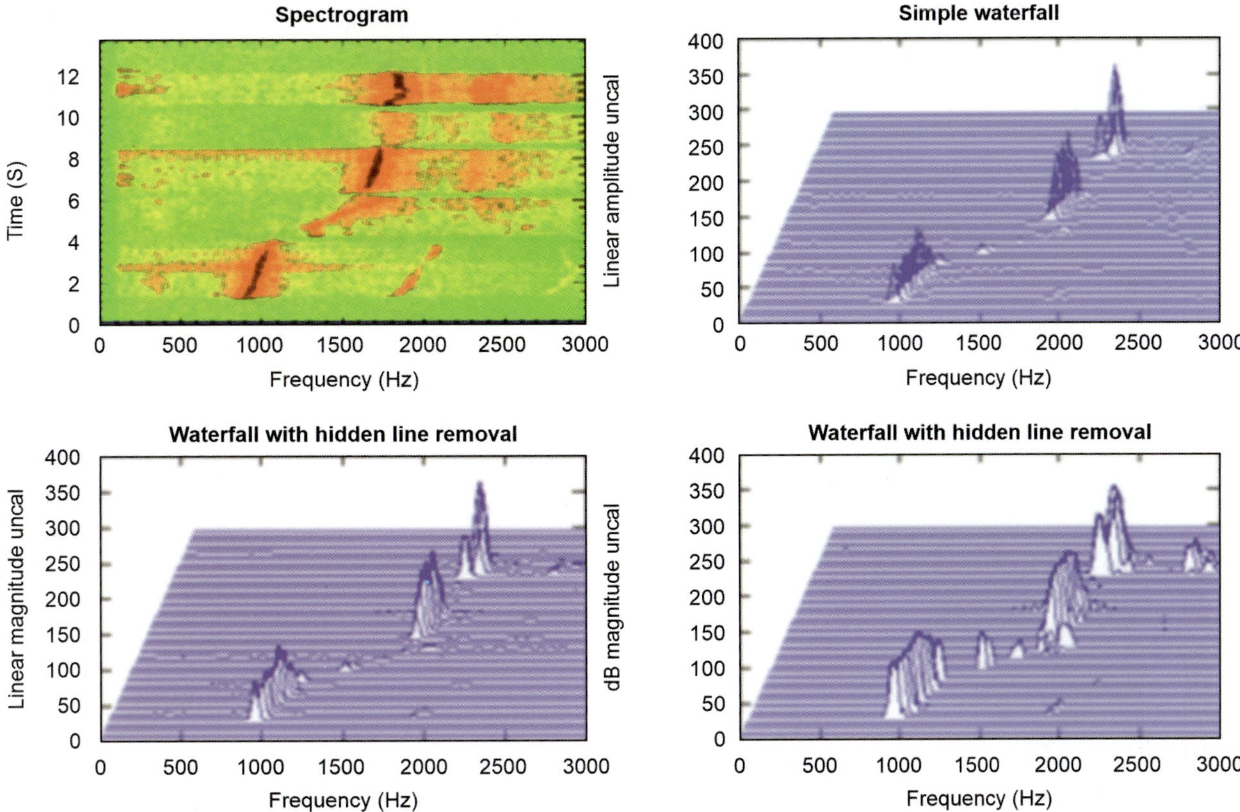

Fig. 1.5: Waterfall plot

(Referred from: https://en.wikipedia.org/wiki/File:Waterfall_plot_of_a_whistle.png#/media/File:Waterfall_plot_of_a_whistle.png)

value of the corresponding variable, and the angle of each line represents the category or dimension being measured (Fig. 1.6).

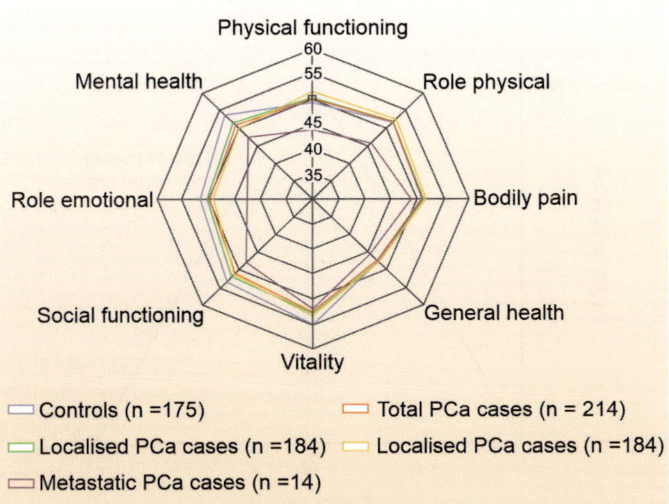

Fig. 1.6: Star plot

(Referred from: https://think.design/services/data-visualization-data-design/spider-graph/)

Swimmers plot: Swimmer plots, also known as swim lane plots or timelines, are graphical representations used to display the timelines and trajectories of individual entities or events over a certain period.[14] They are commonly used in project management, healthcare, and other fields where tracking the progress or movement of entities over time is essential.

In a swimmer plot, each entity or event is represented by a horizontal lane or swim lane, and the vertical axis represents time. Each entity's lane consists of a line or bar that indicates the duration or time period during which the entity is active or the event occurs, as well as any overlaps or interactions between them. The swim lanes are arranged vertically, and they can be grouped or categorized based on different criteria.

For example in oncology, a "swimmer plot" is the graphical representation of the overall time to tumor reaction, the degree of "complete" or "partial" response, and the length of response for a subject (Fig. 1.7).

Funnel plot: A funnel plot is a graphical representation commonly used in meta-analysis to assess publication bias or small study effects in a systematic review.[15] The funnel plot is named after its characteristic funnel shape. Funnel plots are useful tools for visualizing the potential presence of publication bias and assessing the robustness of the results in a meta-analysis. In a funnel plot,

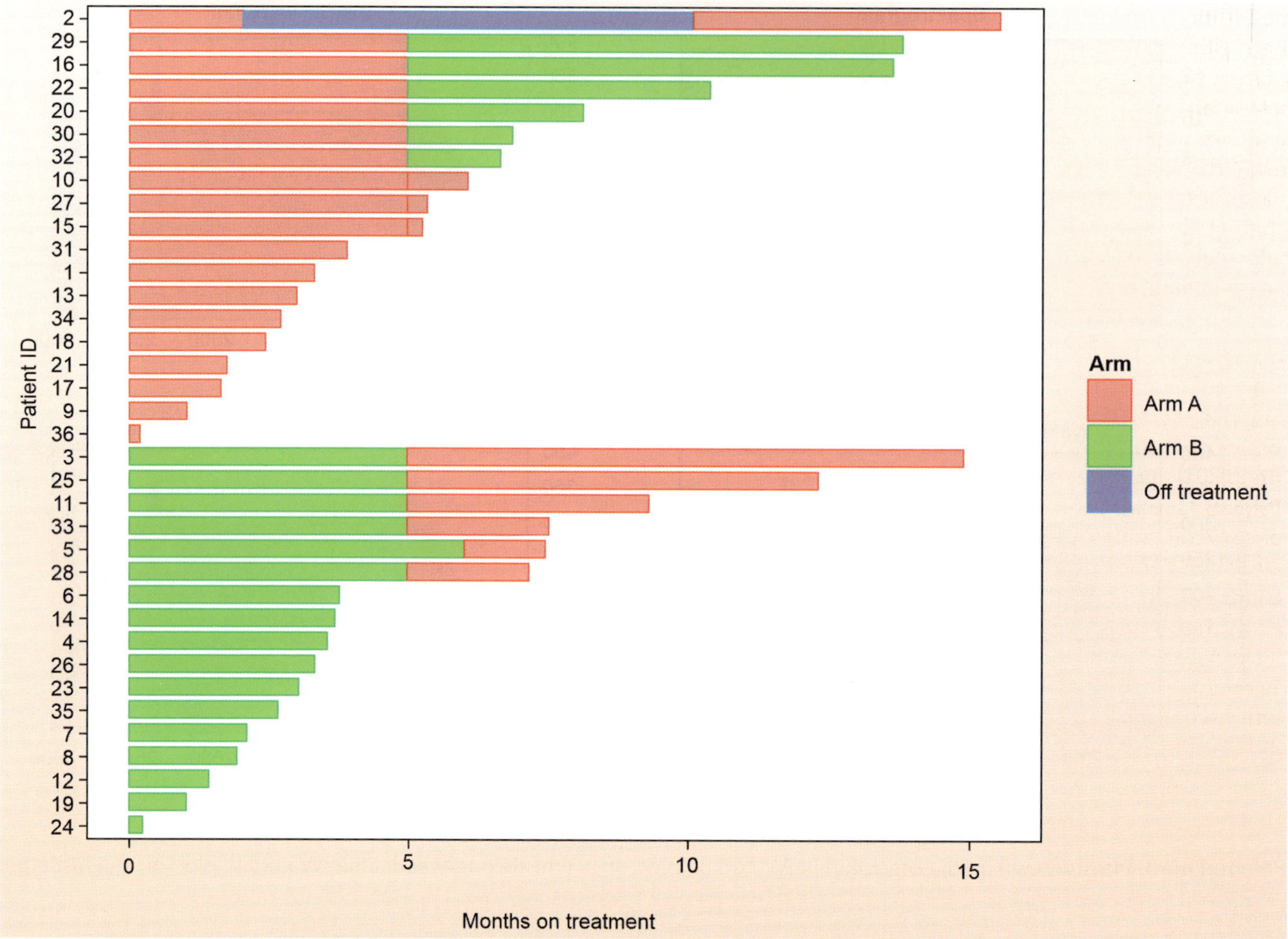

Fig. 1.7: Swimmer plot

(Referred from: https://cran.r-project.org/web/packages/swimplot/vignettes/Introduction.to.swimplot.html)

the horizontal axis represents the effect size or estimate of interest (such as the treatment effect or odds ratio), while the vertical axis represents a measure of study precision (such as the standard error or inverse of the sample size). Each study in the analysis is represented by a point or marker on the plot. In the absence of publication bias or other small study effects, it is expected that smaller studies will scatter more widely at the bottom of the funnel, while larger studies with greater precision will cluster near the top. The plot resembles a funnel because smaller studies are expected to have larger variability due to factors like sampling error, while larger studies tend to have more precise estimates (Fig. 1.8) (Lee 2012).

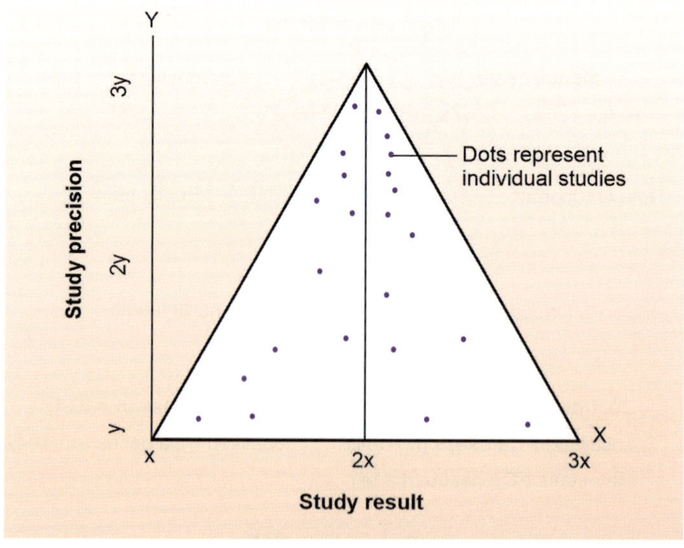

Fig. 1.8: Funnel plot

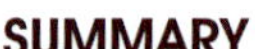
SUMMARY

- Survival analysis helps a clinician compare outcomes of various treatment modalities for a particular malignancy.
- Kaplan-Meier (KM) survival estimate is used to estimate survival probability from observed survival time.
- HR provides an estimate of the ratio of the hazard rates between the experimental group and a control group over the duration of the study.
- NNT provides the minimum number of patients that would need to be treated to prevent one additional bad outcome or for

one additional successful outcome compared with the standard or any other treatment.
- A forest plot is a graphical presentation of findings from a meta-analysis.
- Swimmer plots, also known as swim lane plots or timelines, are graphical representations used to display the timelines and trajectories of individual entities or events over a certain period.
- A funnel plot is a graphical representation commonly used in meta-analysis to assess publication bias or small study effects in a systematic review.

REFERENCES

1. Singh R, Mukhopadhyay K. Survival analysis in clinical trials: Basics and must know areas. Perspect Clin Res. 2011;2:145–8. Epub 2011/12/07.
2. Prinja S, Gupta N, Verma R. Censoring in clinical trials: review of survival analysis techniques. Indian J Community Med. 2010;35:217–21. Epub 2010/10/06.
3. Clark TG, Bradburn MJ, Love SB, Altman DG. Survival analysis part I: basic concepts and first analyses. Br J Cancer. 2003;89:232–8. Epub 2003/07/17.
4. Barraclough H, Simms L, Govindan R. Biostatistics primer: what a clinician ought to know: hazard ratios. J Thorac Oncol. 2011;6:978–82. Epub 2011/05/31.
5. Spruance SL, Reid JE, Grace M, Samore M. Hazard ratio in clinical trials. Antimicrob Agents Chemother. 2004;48:2787–92. Epub 2004/07/27.
6. Higgins JPT, Thomas J, Chandler J, Cumpston M, Li T, Page MJ, Welch VA (editors). *Cochrane Handbook for Systematic Reviews of Interventions* version 6.3 (updated February 2022). Cochrane, 2022. Available from www.training.cochrane.org/handbook.
7. Holt, Martin. (2016). A Concise Encyclopedia of Biostatistics for Medical Professionals. 10.1201/9781315372891.
8. Snapinn SM. Noninferiority trials. Curr Control Trials Cardiovasc Med. 2000;1(1):19–21. doi: 10.1186/cvm-1-1-019.
9. Dunn DT, Copas AJ, Brocklehurst P. Superiority and non-inferiority: two sides of the same coin? Trials. 2018 Sep 17;19(1):499. doi: 10.1186/s13063–018–2885-z.
10. Wexler P (ed). Encyclopedia of Toxicology, Third Edition. Waltham, MA: Academic Press, Imprint of Elsevier; 2014: pp 5,220.
11. Gillespie TW. Understanding waterfall plots. J Adv Pract Oncol. 2012 Mar;3(2):106–11. PMID: 25031936.
12. https://www.statisticshowto.com/waterfall-plot/.
13. https://think.design/services/data-visualization-data-design/spider-graph/.
14. https://www.themillerlab.io/posts/swimmer_plots/.
15. Lee, William & Hotopf, Matthew. (2012). Critical appraisal. 10.1016/B978–0–7020–3397–1.00010–0.

Chapter

2

Localized Prostate Cancer

• *Santosh Kumar* • *Santhosh Nagasubramanian*

LEARNING OBJECTIVES

- To understand the basics of PSA screening.
- To differentiate the types of PSA screening and to understand the current status of PSA screening in prostate cancer. Key findings from landmark RCTs on screening should be well understood.
- To understand the risk stratification in localised prostate cancer
- Management of localized prostate cancer varies with risk stratification hence, it should be well understood.
- To understand the role of biomarkers in the diagnostic algorithm.
- PSA in grey zone causes diagnostic dilemmas, biomarkers help clinician decide on further course of action based on the biomarkers.
- To outline the role of MRI in the diagnosis of prostate cancer—elaborate on its diagnostic performance and role in biopsy.
- To understand the role of MpMRI in appropriate decision making.
- To understand and allude to the different approaches as regards to prostate biopsy
- To be able to list the indications for PSMA PET/CT scan, and use the same appropriately in the work-up of a localized prostate cancer.
- PSMA PET scan to detect systemic spread and bony metastasis is an effective modality, indication for the same needs to be clearly understood.
- To understand the criteria and follow-up protocol of active surveillance; to differentiate between active surveillance and watchful waiting.
- To compare and contrast the outcomes of the various treatment modalities in localized prostate cancer—radical treatment (radical prostatectomy and radiotherapy) and active surveillance. In particular, to understand and synthesize the key findings from the protect trial at 15-year follow-up.
- To understand the approaches to radical prostatectomy and list the key steps of key steps of the procedure.
- To be able to follow-up a patient after a radical prostatectomy.

Case Scenario

A 61-year-old fit retired executive with well-controlled diabetes and hypertension had bothersome LUTS—poor flow, increased nighttime frequency (D-7, N3). He is sexually active with a SHIM score of 23. He does not have any family history of cancer. The digital rectal examination (DRE) did not show any obvious abnormality. The urologist evaluating him performed a serum PSA which was 4.78 ng/ml. He underwent an MRI scan which showed a 33.5 cc prostate with a PI-RADS 4/5 lesion in the right mid-peripheral zone. A systematic transrectal biopsy was performed which showed an adenocarcinoma prostate with Gleason score 3+4 (ISUP grade group 2 with <10% pattern 4), 2/12 cores positive (<50% involvement of each core) with core lenght of 3 mm, with no perineural invasion and no cribriform pattern.

1. **What is the type of PSA screening the above gentleman has had?**

   Ans: Opportunistic screening—he presented with LUTS and a PSA test was done on him.

   This is in contrast to systematic screening (population or mass screening) which is the "systematic examination of asymptomatic men to identify individuals at risk for prostate cancer" and is generally initiated by health authorities with the objective of reduction in mortality with maintained quality of life (QoL).[1]

2. What is the current status of PSA screening in prostate cancer?

Ans: Screening for prostate cancer is one of the most controversial topics in literature with contradictory results from two large randomized trials—the ERSPC (European Randomized Study of Screening for Prostate Cancer)[2] trial and the PLCO (Prostate Lung Colorectal and Ovarian) trial.[3] The salient features of these two trials have been summarized in Table 2.1.

A systematic review and meta-analysis[4] of five RCTs in 2018 showed:

Screening was associated with increased prostate cancer diagnosis (incidence ratio 1.23; 95% CI 1.03–1.48) and detection of more localized disease (RR 1.39; 95% CI 1.09–1.79) and less advanced disease (RR 0.85; 95% CI 0.72–0.99). However, there was no difference in prostate cancer specific mortality (IR 0.96 95%CI 0.85–1.08) which was the primary end point in all trials. There was no overall survival benefit as well—IR 0.99 (95% CI 0.98–1.01) even though none of the trials were designed or powered for overall survival.

TABLE 2.1: Comparison between ERSPC and PLCO trials

Variable	*ERSPC*	*PLCO*
Population	N=182,000 men 1993–2003 Age: 50–74 years 7 European countries	N=76693 1993–2001 Age: 55–74 years 10 US centres
Protocol	2–4 years repeat PSA ± DRE PSA ≥3 ng/ml (variable recruitment and PSA cut-offs)	Annual PSA, DRE PSA cut-off: 4 ng/ml
Primary outcome	Prostate cancer specific mortality (PCSM)	Prostate cancer specific mortality
Secondary outcomes	All-cause mortality, PCa incidence, clinical stage, QoL, harms	All-cause mortality, PCa incidence, clinical stage, Gleason grade, harms
Weakness	Heterogeneity of protocols and treatment bias	Highly prescreened population (nearly 50%) and high contamination in the control arm (86% at 15-year follow-up)
Result	RR: 0.80 (95% CI 0.72–0.90) About 20% reduction in PCSM NNS : 570, NNT: 18 (at 16-year follow-up)	RR: 0.97 (95% CI 0.95–1.004) No effect on PCSM

The study concluded that clinicians and patients considering PSA screening need to weigh benefits against potential short- and long-term harms of screening such as complications from biopsies and treatment (as well as risk of overdiagnosis and overtreatment).

The US Preventive Task Force (USPTF) updated the recommendation in 2018[5] to Grade C recommendation in men aged 55–69 years—offer screening based on individual circumstances (do not screen men who do not express a preference for screening) and grade D recommendation (recommends against screening) in men 70 and older (Table 2.2).

The EAU guidelines recommend a risk-adapted approach to PSA screening in well-informed men with a life expectancy of at least 10 to 15 years after adequate counseling of potential risks and benefits.[1] Further, early PSA testing is recommended in well-informed men with increased risk of prostate cancer such as—men from 45 years with a family history of prostate cancer, men of African descent from 45 years, and men carrying BRCA2 mutations from 40 years of age.[1] The EAU

TABLE 2.2: PSA screening recommendations from various groups

Group	*Recommendation*
American Academy of Family Physicians	• Age criteria in normal population: >50 Years , with life expectancy of 10 years • Age criteria in high-risk population: 45 years • PSA and DRE done • If PSA < 2.5 ng/dl, then evaluation in two years; if > 2.5 ng/dl, then annual examination.
American Cancer Society	• Age criteria in normal population: 50–69 years • PSA and DRE done • Life expectancy should be 10–15 years at least
American Urology Association	• Age criteria in normal population: 50–69 years • PSA and DRE done • Life expectancy should be 10–15 years at least • High risk patients with family history: Individualized decision
European Urology Association	• Well-informed patient with life expectancy of 10–15 years at least • PSA and DRE done • Age criteria in high-risk population: 45 years • PSA > 1 ng/dl at 40 years or >2 ng/dl at 60 years, requires 2 yearly follow-up

guidelines recommend follow-up intervals of 2 years for those initially at risk–men with PSA >1 ng/ml at 40 years of age and PSA >2 ng/ml at 60 years of age; for those not at risk the follow-up may be postponed to 8 years[1] (Table 2.2).

Shared-decision making for PSA screening is encouraged in the western world. In the shared-decision making process, the patient's own values, preferences, anticipated changes in quality of life, functional ability, expectations are considered along with the life-expectancy and general condition of the patient. The patient makes the decision after understanding the existing evidence and the balance between a small benefit of reducing prostate cancer mortality versus over diagnosis and treatment complications.

The individualized approach for offering PSA screening should consider the life-expectancy of the individual. This is not just based on the age, but also on the health status, associated comorbidities, physical and cognitive function of the individual. Tools such as the Geriatric-8 (G8) screening tools, clinical frailty score, cumulative illness score rating–geriatrics (CISR-G) and Charlson comorbidity index (CCI) may be used.

There is no good quality evidence on PSA screening from India, and the decision on PSA testing must be made on an individual basis.

3. **How would you risk stratify this case?**

Ans: Intermediate risk localized prostate cancer as per EAU risk groups (Table 2.3)[1].

Favorable intermediate risk group based on NCCN classification (Table 2.4)[6].

4. **What is PSA density (PSAD) and how do you interpret the same? Enlist the other available biomarkers in the diagnostic pathway of prostate cancer?**

Ans: PSAD is the level of serum PSA divided by the prostate volume. PSAD of >0.15 ng/ml/cc was predictive of clinically significant prostate cancer[7] while patients with PSAD <0.09 ng/ml/cc were unlikely to be detected with clinically significant prostate cancer.[8] Further, studies have shown PSAD added to mpMRI improved the diagnostic confidence of prostate cancer.[9]

Some of the biomarkers available for use in prostate cancer have been summarized in Table 2.5. Also, the algorithm for the use of biomarkers in the diagnostic and prognostic pathway is shown in Fig. 2.1.

5. **What is the role of MRI in the diagnosis of prostate cancer?**

Ans: Diagnostic performance: The sensitivity of MRI for the detection and localization of ISUP

TABLE 2.3: EAU risk stratification of localized and locally advanced prostate cancer

Definition			
Low risk	Intermediate risk	High risk	
PSA < 10 ng/mL	PSA 10–20 ng/mL	PSA >20 ng/mL	Any PSA
and GS < 7 (ISUP grade 1)	or GS 7 (ISUP grade 2/3)	or GS >7 (ISUP grade 4/5)	Any GS (Any ISUP grade)*
and cT1-2a*	or cT2b*	or cT2c*	cT3-4 or cN+**
Localised			Locally advanced

GS = Gleason score; ISUP = International Society for Urological Pathology; PSA = Prostate-specific antigen.
*Based on digital rectal examination.
**Based on CT/bone scan.

TABLE 2.4: NCCN risk stratification of localized prostate cancer

Risk group	*Clinical/pathologic features*		
Very low	Has all of the following: • cT1c • Grade group 1 • PSA <10 ng/mL • Fewer than 3 prostate biopsy fragments/cores positive, ≤50% cancer in each fragment/core[g] • PSA density <0.15 ng/mL/g		
Low	Has all of the following but does not qualify for very low risk: • cT1–cT2a • Grade group 1 • PSA <10 ng/mL		
Intermediate	Has all of the following: • No high-risk group features • No very-high-risk group features • Has one or more intermediate risk factors (IRFs): – cT2b–cT2c – Grade group 2 or 3 – PSA 10–20 ng/mL	Favorable intermediate	Has all of the following: • 1 IRF • Grade group 1 or 2 • <50% biopsy cores positive (e.g. <6 or 12 cores)[g]
		Unfavorable intermediate	Has one or more of the following: • 2 or 3 IRFs • Grade group 3 • ≥ 50% biopsy cores positive (e.g. ≥ 6 of 12 cores)[g]
High	Has no very-high-risk features and has exactly one high-risk feature: • cT3a OR • Grade group 4 OR Grade group 5 OR • PSA >20 ng/mL		
Very high	Has at least one of the following: • cT3b–cT4 • Primary Gleason pattern 5 • 2 or 3 high-risk features • >4 cores with Grade group 4 or 5		

TABLE 2.5: Summary of available tests and indications (adapted from Alford A *et al.* Rev Urol. 2017; 19(4):221–223)[10]

Test	*Specimen*	*Biomarkers*	*Clinical endpoints*	*Target patient population*	*Management guidelines*
Initial biopsy					
PHI (prostate health index)	Blood	Levels of tPSA, fPSA,p2PSA (p2PSA/fPSA) x $(tPSA)^{1/2}$	Risk of high grade cancer on biopsy (score 1–100)	Men >50 years with PSA 4–10 ng/ml and negative DRE result	Score 0–26.9: 9.8% risk of HG disease Score 27–35.9: 16.8% risk of HG disease Score 36–54.9: 33.3% risk
SelectMDx	Urine	Expression of DLX1 and HOXC6	Percent risk of Gleason >6 disease on biopsy	Men with elevated PSA value who are considering repeat biopsy	Low risk: Routine follow-up and screening High risk: Perform biopsy
Repeat biopsy					
PCA3	Urine	Ratio of PCA3 and PSA expression	Risk of Gleason >6 disease on biopsy (score 1–100)	Men age >50 y who are considering repeat biopsy after initial negative biopsy	Score 1–25: Low risk of cancer, safe to defer biopsy Score >26: High risk of cancer, perform biopsy
ConfirmMDx	Biopsy	Hypermethylation intensity of tumor suppressor genes GSTP1, RASSF1, and APC	Risk of PCa on repeat biopsy	Men who are considering a repeat biopsy after initial negative biopsy	Negative: Safe to defer biopsy Positive: Repeat biopsy
Initial or repeat biopsy					
4K score	Blood	Levels of tPSA, fPSA, intact PSA, and human kallikrein-related peptidase 2	Percent risk of HG cancer on biopsy	Men with an elevated PSA or abnormal DRE result who are considering initial or repeat biopsy	Low risk (1–7.5%): Safe to defer biopsy with follow-up of PSA High risk (>20%): Perform biopsy
MiPS	Urine	Expression of PCA3 and TMPRSS2:ERG Combined with serum PSA	Percent risk of Gleason ≥6 disease on biopsy Percent risk of HG cancer on biopsy	Men with elevated PSA value who are considering initial biopsy or repeat biopsy after initial negative result	Does not provide low and high-risk cutoffs

grade 2 cancers was good particularly when the diameter is greater than 10 mm.[11,12] In a Cochrane meta-analysis, MRI had a pooled sensitivity of 0.91 (95% CI 0.83–0.95) and pooled specificity of 0.37 (95% CI 0.29–0.46) for ISUP grade 2 cancers.[13] In ISUP grade 3 cancers, the pooled sensitivity and specificity were 0.95 (95% CI 0.87–0.99) and 0.35 (95% CI 0.26–0.46) respectively. MRI identifies less than 30% of ISUP grade 1 cancers smaller than 0.5 cc on radical prostatectomy (RP) specimens.[11] In another meta-analysis the average positive predictive value (PPV) for ISUP grade 2 cancers with PI-RADS v2.1 scores of 3, 4 and 5 were 16% (7–27%), 59% (39–78%), and 85% (73–94%) respectively.[14]

In terms of staging, MRI has a pooled sensitivity of around 0.60 and pooled specificity of around 0.90 for EPE (extraprostatic extension), SVI (seminal vesicle invasion) and T3 detection.[15] Just like CT scan, MRI has a poor sensitivity of <40% for lymph node detection.[16]

MRI in Biopsy

MRI can aid in performing targeted biopsies—this can be achieved by MRI-cognition, MRI-fusion or in-bore techniques. The current evidence shows all three techniques to be equivalent.[17]

Timing of MRI: The guidelines are variable with respect to timing of MRI and biopsy. The NICE

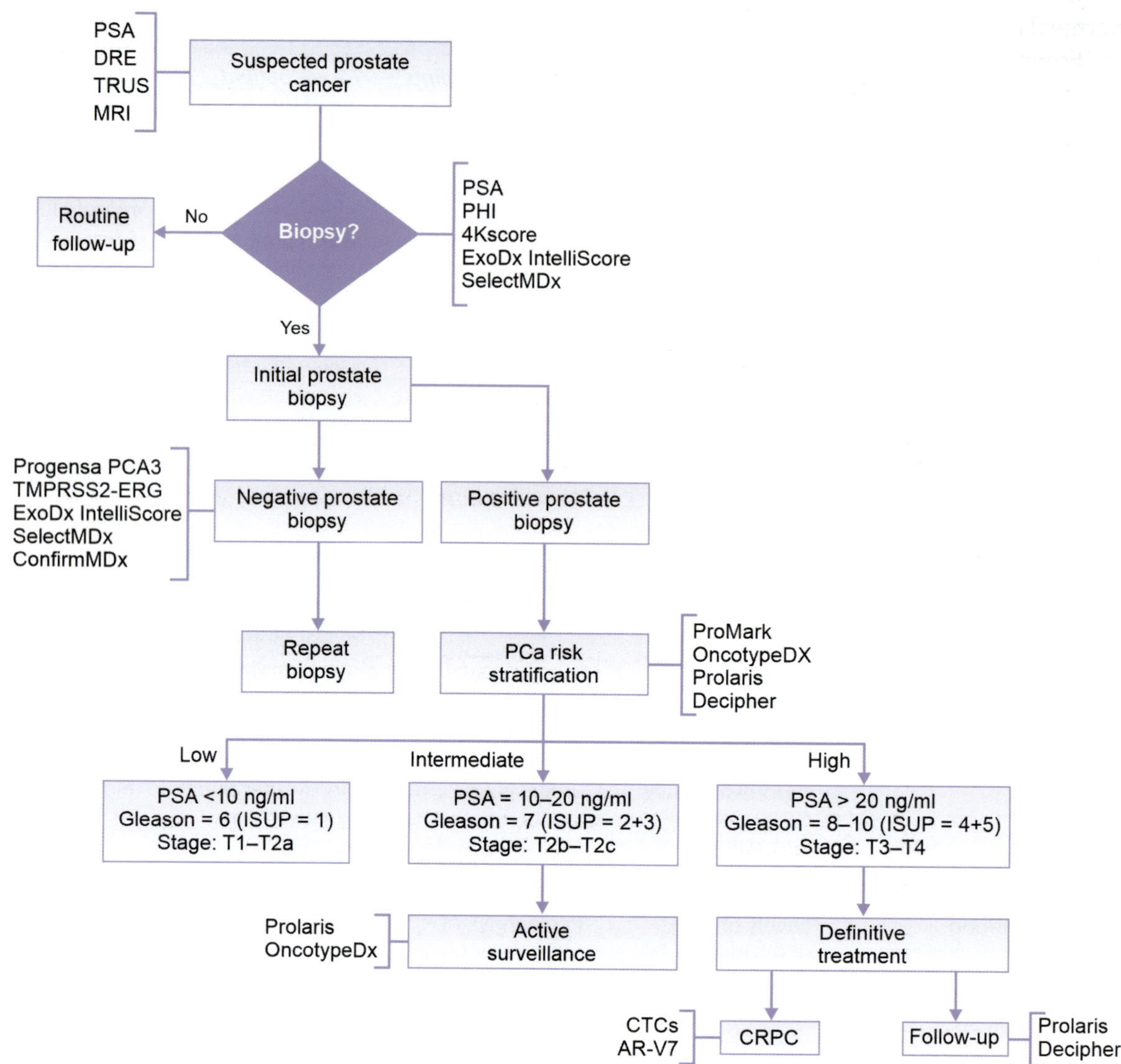

Fig. 2.1: Algorithm for the use of biomarkers in prostate cancer *(from Porzycki P et al. Cent European J Urol. 2020;73(3):300–306. doi: 10.5173/ceju.2020.0067R. Epub 2020)*

guidelines from UK suggests offering multiparametric MRI as the first-line investigation for all those with suspected clinically localized prostate cancer.[18] The EAU guidelines recommend MRI prior to biopsy (strong recommendation).[1] The NCCN guidelines recommend considering MRI but do not provide any guidelines for selection of candidates[6] while the AUA guidelines state there is insufficient evidence to consider MRI in every biopsy-naïve patient.[19]

The Urological Society of India (USI) guidelines recommend mpMRI in patients with elevated PSA and negative digital rectal examination (DRE)—strong recommendation.[20]

MRI inter-reader reproducibility is variable and hence there is a need for standardization of MRI interpretation and periodic quality checks with pathology feedback to optimize utilization of MRI.[21]

Based on the existing evidence, pre-biopsy MRI looks like the way forward in the diagnostic evaluation of pro-state cancer. Also, while performing targeted biopsy targeting the penumbra of 10 mm around the lesion may improve the diagnostic performance,[22] but current evidence indicates that systematic biopsy cannot be done away with.[1]

6. **What are the routes of prostate biopsy, and what are the differences between them?**

Ans: The two routes for prostate biopsy are—transrectal and transperineal biopsy.

The transrectal route has higher infectious complications compared to the transperineal, RR 2.48 (95% CI 1.47–4.2).[23]

One systematic review showed a higher sensitivity (86% vs. 73%) for the detection of clinically significant prostate cancer (csPCa) when the transperineal approach was used for MRI-targeted biopsy.[24] Some of the MRI fusion biopsy technologies in the horizon are summarized in Table 2.6.[25]

7. **In the above patient, is a 68Ga-PSMA PET/CT scan recommended?**

Ans: No. The patient falls in the favourable-intermediate risk prostate cancer category.

In ISUP grade 3 disease (unfavourable-intermediate), and high-risk localized/locally advanced prostate cancer, metastatic screening is recommended.[1] The USI guidelines recommend that metastatic work up is best obtained with a PSMA PET/CT scan, and suggest a bone scan and CT thorax, abdomen and pelvis as a means of cross-sectional imaging where PSMA PET/CT facility is unavailable.[20]

PSMA PET/CT has a better sensitivity compared to MRI or CT scan for lymph node staging. The sensitivity and specificity were 77% and 97% in a systematic review and meta-analysis.[26] Small lymph node metastases (<5 mm) may still be missed on PSMA PET/CT.

A multi-center study from Australia (the proPSMA study)[27] on patients with high risk prostate cancer showed 68Ga-PSMA PET/CT to have a 27% (95% CI 23–31) better accuracy than conventional CT scan and bone scan, with lesser equivocal findings, prompting management change more frequently, and having a lower radiation exposure.

Even though PSMA PET/CT scan has higher sensitivity in metastatic screening there is lack of outcome data of subsequent treatment changes.[1]

***Case Scenario** (Contd.)*

After counseling the patient regarding radical treatment options and active surveillance, he chose active surveillance.

The intent of treatment in active surveillance (AS) is curative, the follow-up schedule is predefined, and the aim is to minimize treatment-related toxicity without compromising survival in a man with good life-expectancy. The difference between active surveillance and watchful waiting is summarized in Table 2.7.

8. **What are the criteria for active surveillance, and what is the follow-up, and outcomes of active surveillance in comparison to radical treatment?**

Criteria for choosing patients for active surveillance

The criteria commonly used for selecting patients for active surveillance (AS) include: ISUP grade 1, clinical stage T1c or T2a, PSA<10 ng/dl and PSA-density (PSAD) <0.15 ng/ml/cc (all part of low-risk prostate cancer).[28]

Also, AS can be considered in low-volume ISUP grade 2 ($\geq$3 positive systematic cores and $\leq$50% core involvement) favorable-intermediate risk prostate cancers.[1,29]

ISUP grade 3, patients with intraductal or cribriform pattern on histology are exclusions to AS.

Follow-up

The follow-up schedule in AS is variable in literature. The follow-up schedule should be strictly adhered to on the basis of a predefined protocol. Follow-up commonly

TABLE 2.6: MRI fusion technologies summary

MRI fusion system	*Manufacturer*	*Hardware system*	*Fixation for biopsies*	*Elastic or rigid estimation*
Artemis	InnoMedicus Artemis	Artemis	**Stabilised, freehand unknown, semi-robotic arm**	**Both**
BioJet	Healthcare Supply Solutions Ltd.	Third party ultrasound	Stabilised, freehand (without tracking movement)	Both
BiopSee	Medcom	MedSta or third party ultrasounds	Stabilised, freehand	Both
bkFusion	BK Medical UK Ltd and MIM Software Inc.	BK 3000 or BK 5000	Stabilised, freehand	**Rigid**
Fusion Bx 2.0	Focal Healthcare	Third party ultrasounds	Stabilised, freehand, robotic arm	Both
Fusion Vu	ExactImaging	ExactVu	Stabilised, freehand	Rigid
iSR'obot™ Mona Lisa	Biobot iSR'obot	iSR'obot™ Mona Lisa	Stabilised, freehand unknown, robotic arm	**Elastic**
KOELIS Trinity	KOELIS and Kebomed	TRINITY ultrasound system	Stabilised, freehand	**Both**
UroNav Fusion Biopsy System	Phillips	Third party ultrasounds	Stabilised, freehand	**Unknown**

TABLE 2.7: Comparison of active surveillance vs. watchful waiting

	Active surveillance	*Watchful waiting*
Treatment intent	Curative	Palliative
Follow-up	Pre-defined schedule	Patient-specific
Assessment/tests used	DRE, PSA, MRI, rebiopsy	Not predefined, depends on symptoms of progression
Life expectancy	>10 years	<10 years
Aim	Minimize treatment-related morbidity without compromising survival	Minimize treatment-related toxicity
Eligible patients	Low-risk, low-intermediate risk prostate cancer	Can apply to patients with all stages

includes PSA testing (6 monthly), DRE (yearly) and repeat biopsy at 2 to 3 years.[1] MRI and repeat biopsy are recommended if PSA is rising on follow-up (PSA doubling time < 3 years).[1]

Comparison of outcomes between AS vs. radical prostatectomy (RP) vs. radiotherapy (RT)

Recently the 15-year follow-up data from the PROstate TEsting for Cancer and Treatment (ProtecT) was published.[30] The study enrolled 1643 men with PSA detected localised prostate cancer between 1999 and 2009, and randomly assigned them to receive active monitoring (less intensive follow-up to the current day active surveillance with predefined follow-up schedules), radical prostatectomy or radiotherapy. The follow-up rate was 98%. Nearly a third of the men belonged to intermediate or high-risk groups based on contemporary risk stratification. The key results have been summarized in Table 2.8.

As shown in Table 2.8, there was no difference in prostate-cancer specific mortality among different treatment modalities. Radical treatments reduced incidence of metastases, local progression and long-term androgen deprivation by half compared to active monitoring, but these reductions did not translate to differences in mortality at 15 years, a finding that reiterates the long natural history of prostate cancer.

Some of the changes to factor in the current day (compared to the ProtecT recruitment period) include advances in imaging technique like mpMRI and PSMA PET/CT, and MRI guided targeted biopsies. Also, effective salvage therapy may have masked mortality difference. Further longer follow-up may show differences in survival.

The findings of the ProtecT trial are consistent with the Prostate Cancer Intervention versus Observation Trial (PIVOT)[31] which showed no benefit of radical treatment in men with higher co-existing illnesses (the study population was less healthier). In contrast, the Scandinavian Prostate Cancer Group 4 (SPCG4) study found benefits of radical treatment as compared to watchful waiting.[32] However, about 50% of the patients

***Case Scenario** (Contd.)*

On follow-up, the PSA at 6 months was 4.82 ng/ml (from 4.78 ng/ml). On further follow-up at one year, the DRE was normal, however, the PSA had risen to 7.35 ng/ml. In view of the rising PSA (PSA density 0.219 ng/ml/cc) an mpMRI was performed which showed a new PI-RADS 5/5 lesion in the left apex. He underwent a systematic reclassification biopsy which showed a Gleason 4+3 (ISUP grade group 3) adenocarcinoma, 7/12 cores positive with maximum cancer length of 10 mm.

He was counselled regarding the radical treatment options. What are the pros and cons of various treatment options in localised prostate cancer?

The pros and cons of various treatment options of localized prostate cancer are summarized in Table 2.9.

TABLE 2.8: Summary of results from the ProtecT trial at 15-year follow-up

		Active monitoring (N = 545)	*Radical prostatectomy (N = 553)*	*Radiation therapy (N = 545)*	
Primary outcome	Prostate cancer specific mortality	17 (3.1%)	12 (2.2%)	16 (2.9%)	p = 0.53
Secondary outcomes	All cause mortality	124 (22.8%)	117 (21.15%)	115 (21.10%)	
	Metastases	51 (9.4%)	26 (4.7%)	27 (5.0%)	
	Long-term ADT	69 (12.7%)	40 (7.2%)	42 (7.7%)	
	Clinical progression	141 (25.9%)	58 (10.5%)	60 (11%)	

TABLE 2.9: Advantages and disadvantages of various treatment modalities of localized prostate cancer (*from Filson CP CA Cancer J Clin. 2015 Jul-Aug;65(4):265–82*)[33]

Treatment modality	*Advantages*	*Disadvantages*
Active surveillance	Delays/avoids treatment-associated morbidity QoL maintained Avoids overtreatment	Risk of progression Frequent monitoring and tests Increased anxiety
Radical prostatectomy	Definitive curative therapy for prostate confined disease Easy to detect PSA failure	High risk of erectile dysfunction Risk of urinary incontinence Risk of operative morbidity
External beam radiotherapy	Lower risk of urinary incontinence Option for non-surgical candidates—elderly, those with co-morbidities	High risk of erectile dysfunction Long treatment course (8–9 weeks) Bladder or bowel symptoms during treatment are common
Brachytherapy	Control rates are comparable to surgery for low-risk tumor Can be used alone or as a boost Single treatment	High risk of erectile dysfunction Bladder or bowel symptoms during treatment are common General anaesthesia

in the SPCG4 study had disease outside the prostate, and those in the watchful waiting group did not have an active surveillance.

To conclude, the choice of treatment in localised prostate cancer is a trade-off between risk of overtreatment and attendant side effects of radical treatment such as erectile dysfunction, urinary incontinence and bowel symptoms versus the risk of progression in active surveillance. The decision has to be made on an individual case basis with the knowledge about the long natural history of prostate cancer, and no differences in prostate cancer specific or overall survival among radical treatments and surveillance.

9. What are the approaches to radical prostatectomy? Mention the key steps of the procedure.

Ans: Radical prostatectomy may be performed by open, laparoscopic or robotic-assisted (RARP) approaches. Due to better surgical ergonomics and technical ease, the RARP has now become the preferred minimally-invasive approach.

RARP may be performed by standard anterior approach or Retzius-sparing (RS-RARP) approach. In RS-RARP the anterior support structures are preserved potentially improving the early post-operative continence.[1] Evidence suggests RS-RARP to show better early continence which equalizes at 12 months.[34] There was a concern of increased positive margin in RS-RARP but the evidence was of low-certainty.[34] Hence, based on current evidence one approach of RARP cannot be recommended over the other. In addition, RS-RARP may be more challenging in scenarios such as anterior tumors, post-TURP, grossly enlarged prostate and large median lobe.[1] The key steps of a standard RARP have been summarized in Box 2.1.

BOX 2.1: Key steps of a standard robotic-assisted radical prostatectomy (RARP)

Preparation of the operative field
- Patient positioning: Lithotomy position, compatible for Trendelenburg position
- Pneumoperitoneum and port placement
- Docking of the robotic arms
- Instrument insertion

Dissection of the bladder and the prostate
- Initial pre-operative preparation–adhesionolysis
- Dropping of the bladder from the anterior abdomen wall
- Defatting of the bladder and opening of the endopelvic fascia
- Bladder neck dissection
- Vas and seminal vesicles dissection
- Posterior dissection
- Neurovascular bundle (NVB) dissection/nerve sparing
- DVC and apical dissection

Anastomosis and closure
- Rocco stitch
- Vesicourethral anastomosis
- Inspection
- Instrument removal and closure

10. The patient chose to have a robotic radical prostatectomy. The final histopathology of the radical prostatectomy was pT3a adenocarcinoma prostate Gleason 4+3 (ISUP grade 3) with extraprostatic extension at the right lateral side and 3 mm left apical margin positivity. At three months post-operatively, the PSA level was undetectable, what is the follow-up of this patient after radical prostatectomy?

Ans: Following RP, the PSA is expected to be undetectable in two months after RP.

Disease-related follow-up: Serum PSA and disease-related history and examination once in 6 months for three years, and then annually.[1]

Functional outcomes follow-up: Treatment can have short-term and long-term side effects. These should be captured by validated patient-reported outcome measures (PROM) and health-related quality of life (HRQoL) questionnaires, which will lead to quality improvement, and better patient care.

SUMMARY

- The two types of PSA screening are systematic and opportunistic. PSA screening is a controversial topic. Systematic review and meta-analyses concluded that PSA screening increases the detection of prostate cancer, with more localized and less advanced diseases diagnosis. However, there was no benefit in terms of prostate cancer specific survival, cancer specific, mortality or overall survival. PSA screening has to be undertaken with a shared-decision making with the patient.
- Risk stratification based on PSA, clinical stage and ISUP grade helps to classify patient into groups to plan further diagnostic evaluation and treatment.
- PSA-density may help predicting clinically significant prostate cancer. Biomarkers in blood, urine and tissue may play a role in the diagnostic and treatment pathways.
- MRI has a good sensitivity and localization of ISUP grade 2 prostate cancer particularly >10 mm. For local staging the pooled sensitivity and specificity of MRI is around 0.60 and 0.90 respectively but the sensitivity to detect lymph nodes is poor at <40%. MRI-targeted biopsies can be performed by cognitive, MRI-fusion or in-bore techniques.
- Prostate biopsy can be performed by transperineal or transrectal routes. The transperineal route has lesser rate of infection.
- In unfavorable intermediate risk, high risk localized prostate cancer and locally advanced disease, a metastatic screening is recommended. When available, a PSMA PET/CT scan may be used, it has a better performance for detection of lymph node metastases. However, there is lack of data on the outcome of treatment changes.
- The intent of active surveillance is curative (in contrast to watchful waiting). The common inclusion criteria include low-risk prostate cancer and low-volume (≤3 positive systematic cores and 50% core involvement) favorable-intermediate risk prostate cancers. The follow-up protocol for active surveillance is variable in literature. It commonly includes PSA testing (6 monthly), DRE (yearly) and repeat biopsy in 2–3 years. MRI and repeat biopsy are recommended if PSA is rising on follow-up.
- The ProtecT trial at 15-yr follow-up showed no difference in prostate-cancer specific mortality among different treatment modalities. Radical treatments reduced incidence of metastases, local progression and long-term androgen deprivation by half compared to active monitoring, but these reductions did not translate to differences in mortality at 15 years, a finding that reiterates the long natural history of prostate cancer.
- Robotic-assisted radical prostatectomy (RARP) is now the most commonly used minimally invasive modality of prostatectomy owing to better ergonomics and technical was ease. Standard approach and Retzius sparing RARP (RS-RARP) are the two approaches to RARP.
- Follow-up after RP includes serum PSA six monthly for 3 years and then annually together with disease-related history. Functional outcomes should also be recorded at follow-up.

REFERENCES

1. Professionals SO. EAU Guidelines: Prostate Cancer [Internet]. Uroweb. [cited 2021 May 31]. Available from: https://uroweb.org/guideline/prostate-cancer/#6.
2. Hugosson J, Roobol MJ, Månsson M, Tammela TLJ, Zappa M, Nelen V, *et al.*. A 16-yr Follow-up of the European Randomized study of Screening for Prostate Cancer. Eur Urol. 2019 Jul;76(1):43–51.
3. Andriole GL, Crawford ED, Grubb RL, Buys SS, Chia D, Church TR, *et al.* Mortality results from a randomized prostate-cancer screening trial. N Engl J Med. 2009 Mar 26;360(13):1310–9.
4. Ilic D, Djulbegovic M, Jung JH, Hwang EC, Zhou Q, Cleves A, *et al.* Prostate cancer screening with prostate-specific antigen (PSA) test: a systematic review and meta-analysis. BMJ. 2018 Sep 5;362:k3519.
5. US Preventive Services Task Force, Grossman DC, Curry SJ, Owens DK, Bibbins-Domingo K, Caughey AB, *et al.* Screening for Prostate Cancer: US Preventive Services Task Force Recommendation Statement. JAMA. 2018 May 8;319(18):1901–13.
6. Search Result [Internet]. NCCN. [cited 2023 Apr 2]. Available from: https://www.nccn.org/search-result.
7. Omri N, Kamil M, Alexander K, Alexander K, Edmond S, Ariel Z, *et al.* Association between PSA density and pathologically significant prostate cancer: The impact of prostate volume. The Prostate. 2020 Dec;80(16):1444–9.
8. Yusim I, Krenawi M, Mazor E, Novack V, Mabjeesh NJ. The use of prostate specific antigen density to predict clinically significant prostate cancer. Sci Rep. 2020 Nov 17;10 (1):20015.
9. Cuocolo R, Stanzione A, Rusconi G, Petretta M, Ponsiglione A, Fusco F, *et al.* PSA-density does not improve bi-parametric prostate MR detection of prostate cancer in a biopsy naïve patient population. Eur J Radiol. 2018 Jul;104:64–70.
10. Alford AV, Brito JM, Yadav KK, Yadav SS, Tewari AK, Renzulli J. The Use of Biomarkers in Prostate Cancer Screening and Treatment. Rev Urol. 2017;19(4):221–34.
11. Bratan F, Niaf E, Melodelima C, Chesnais AL, Souchon R, Mège-Lechevallier F, *et al.* Influence of imaging and histological factors on prostate cancer detection and localisation on multiparametric MRI: a prospective study. Eur Radiol. 2013 Jul;23(7):2019–29.
12. Johnson DC, Raman SS, Mirak SA, Kwan L, Bajgiran AM, Hsu W, *et al.* Detection of Individual Prostate Cancer Foci via Multiparametric Magnetic Resonance Imaging. Eur Urol. 2019 May;75(5):712–20.
13. Drost FJH, Osses DF, Nieboer D, Steyerberg EW, Bangma CH, Roobol MJ, *et al.* Prostate MRI, with or without MRI-targeted biopsy, and systematic biopsy for detecting prostate cancer. Cochrane Database Syst Rev. 2019 Apr 25;4(4):CD012663.
14. Oerther B, Engel H, Bamberg F, Sigle A, Gratzke C, Benndorf M. Cancer detection rates of the PI-RADSv2.1 assessment categories: systematic review and meta-analysis on lesion level and patient level. Prostate Cancer Prostatic Dis. 2022 Feb;25(2):256–63.
15. de Rooij M, Hamoen EHJ, Witjes JA, Barentsz JO, Rovers MM. Accuracy of Magnetic Resonance Imaging for Local Staging of Prostate Cancer: A Diagnostic Meta-analysis. Eur Urol. 2016 Aug;70(2):233–45.
16. Hövels AM, Heesakkers R a. M, Adang EM, Jager GJ, Strum S, Hoogeveen YL, *et al.* The diagnostic accuracy of CT and MRI in the staging of pelvic lymph nodes in patients with prostate cancer: a meta-analysis. Clin Radiol. 2008 Apr;63(4):387–95.
17. Watts KL, Frechette L, Muller B, Ilinksy D, Kovac E, Sankin A, *et al.* Systematic review and meta-analysis comparing cognitive vs. image-guided fusion prostate biopsy for the detection of prostate cancer. Urol Oncol. 2020 Sep;38(9):734.e19–734.e25.

18. Overview | Prostate cancer: diagnosis and management | Guidance | NICE [Internet]. NICE; 2019 [cited 2023 Apr 8]. Available from : https://www.nice.org.uk/guidance/NG131
19. Prostate Cancer: Early Detection Guideline - American Urological Association [Internet]. [cited 2023 Apr 8]. Available from: https://www.auanet.org/guidelines-and-quality/guidelines/prostate-cancer-early-detection-guideline.
20. Kumar A, Yadav S, Krishnappa RS, Gautam G, Raghavan N, Bakshi G, *et al.* The Urological Society of India guidelines for the evaluation and management of prostate cancer (executive summary). Indian J Urol. 2022 Oct 1;38(4):252.
21. de Rooij M, Israël B, Tummers M, Ahmed HU, Barrett T, Giganti F, *et al.* ESUR/ESUI consensus statements on multi-parametric MRI for the detection of clinically significant prostate cancer: quality requirements for image acquisition, interpretation and radiologists' training. Eur Radiol. 2020 Oct;30(10):5404–16.
22. Brisbane WG, Priester AM, Ballon J, Kwan L, Delfin MK, Felker ER, *et al.* Targeted Prostate Biopsy: Umbra, Penumbra, and Value of Perilesional Sampling. Eur Urol. 2022 Sep;82(3):303–10.
23. Pradere B, Veeratterapillay R, Dimitropoulos K, Yuan Y, Omar MI, MacLennan S, *et al.* Nonantibiotic Strategies for the Prevention of Infectious Complications following Prostate Biopsy: A Systematic Review and Meta-Analysis. J Urol. 2021 Mar;205(3):653–63.
24. Tu X, Liu Z, Chang T, Qiu S, Xu H, Bao Y, *et al.* Transperineal Magnetic Resonance Imaging-Targeted Biopsy May Perform Better Than Transrectal Route in the Detection of Clinically Significant Prostate Cancer: Systematic Review and Meta-analysis. Clin Genitourin Cancer. 2019 Oct;17(5): e860–70.
25. final-protocol.pdf [Internet]. [cited 2023 May 14]. Available from: https://www.nice.org.uk/guidance/dg53/chapter/2-The-diagnostic-tests.
26. Perera M, Papa N, Roberts M, Williams M, Udovicich C, Vela I, *et al.* Gallium-68 Prostate-specific Membrane Antigen Positron Emission Tomography in Advanced Prostate Cancer-Updated Diagnostic Utility, Sensitivity, Specificity, and Distribution of Prostate-specific Membrane Antigen-avid Lesions: A Systematic Review and Meta-analysis. Eur Urol. 2020 Apr;77(4):403–17.
27. Hofman MS, Lawrentschuk N, Francis RJ, Tang C, Vela I, Thomas P, *et al.* Prostate-specific membrane antigen PET-CT in patients with high-risk prostate cancer before curative-intent surgery or radiotherapy (proPSMA): a prospective, randomised, multicentre study. Lancet Lond Engl. 2020 Apr 11;395(10231):1208–16.
28. Loeb S, Bruinsma SM, Nicholson J, Briganti A, Pickles T, Kakehi Y, *et al.* Active surveillance for prostate cancer: a systematic review of clinicopathologic variables and biomarkers for risk stratification. Eur Urol. 2015 Apr;67(4):619–26.
29. Lam TBL, MacLennan S, Willemse PPM, Mason MD, Plass K, Shepherd R, *et al.* EAU-EANM-ESTRO-ESUR-SIOG Prostate Cancer Guideline Panel Consensus Statements for Deferred Treatment with Curative Intent for Localised Prostate Cancer from an International Collaborative Study (DETECTIVE Study). Eur Urol. 2019 Dec;76(6):790–813.
30. Hamdy FC, Donovan JL, Lane JA, Metcalfe C, Davis M, Turner EL, *et al.* Fifteen-Year Outcomes after Monitoring, Surgery, or Radiotherapy for Prostate Cancer. N Engl J Med. 2023 Mar 11.
31. Wilt TJ, Brawer MK, Jones KM, Barry MJ, Aronson WJ, Fox S, *et al.* Radical prostatectomy versus observation for localized prostate cancer. N Engl J Med. 2012 Jul 19;367(3):203–13.
32. Bill-Axelson A, Holmberg L, Garmo H, Rider JR, Taari K, Busch C, *et al.* Radical prostatectomy or watchful waiting in early prostate cancer. N Engl J Med. 2014 Mar 6;370(10):932–42.
33. Filson CP, Marks LS, Litwin MS. Expectant management for men with early stage prostate cancer. CA Cancer J Clin. 2015;65(4):265–82.
34. Rosenberg JE, Jung JH, Edgerton Z, Lee H, Lee S, Bakker CJ, *et al.* Retzius-sparing versus standard robotic-assisted laparoscopic prostatectomy for the treatment of clinically localized prostate cancer. Cochrane Database Syst Rev. 2020 Aug 18;8(8):CD013641.

Chapter

3

Locally Advanced Prostate Cancer

• TB Yuvaraja • Santosh Subhash Waigankar

LEARNING OBJECTIVES

- To understand risk stratification in locally advanced prostate cancer [LACaP]:
  Treatment of LACaP is directed by risk stratification, so it is of utmost importance to do it.
- To understand the options available for treating LACaP:
  Radiotherapy traditionally has been an option for LACaP, the indications of radical prostatectomy have been increasing with the improvement in technology and surgical abilities.
- To understand the role of radical prostatectomy:
  Role of surgery has been advancing with improvement in understanding of the local anatomy and technological advancement.
- To understand the role of neo-adjuvant treatment in LACaP:
  Neoadjuvant therapy has been tried in various forms, androgen deprivation alone or in combination with androgen pathway inhibitors or with chemotherapeutic agents.
- To understand management of LNs during RP:
  Level of lymph node dissection, role of extended lymph node dissection is setting of LACaP is important to understand.
- To understand nomograms used in LACaP:
  Nomograms help prognosticate LACaP.
- To understand the role of PSMA PET/CT in understanding LN disease in LACaP:
  PSMA is a single investigation which may help stage LACaP.
- To understand the role of radiotherapy:
  External beam radiotherapy along with ADT is a standard option of treatment, but the duration of ADT, dose of EBRT and the role of brachytherapy are critical to understand.
- To understand the risk of developing biochemical recurrence (BCR):
  Timeline of BCR and the management option thereafter should be clearly known to the treating physician.
- To understand the management of cN1 disease:
  Role of prostatectomy and the evidence for RT in cN1is critical to understand.
- To understand various important trials associated with LACaP *[POP-RT trial/ RADICALS-HD trial/ ARTISTIC meta-analysis/ STAMPEDE trial/ AFU-GETUG 12 trial/ SPCG-15 trial/RAVES trial, etc.]*

Case Scenario 1

A fit and well 68-year-old man is referred to your clinic with an elevated PSA of 11.3 ng/ml. A digital rectal examination reveals a nodule in the left lobe of the prostate.

A pre-biopsy MRI prostate with contrast: PSA density 0.20. Index lesion 19 mm low signal focus (measured coronally) in the left posterolateral PZ extending apex to base, with restricted diffusion and early enhancement. There is an extended margin of contact with a likely capsular breach. PI-RADS 5 and LIKERT 3.

A targeted trans-perineal biopsy with systematic cores is performed under sedation and local anaesthetic. It confirms Gleason 4+3 [GG2], 15 mm maximum cancer core length involvement on the left. 5/5 targeted cores were positive; one systematic core from the right showed 2 mm of Gleason 7. Figure 3.1 shows MPMRI findings.

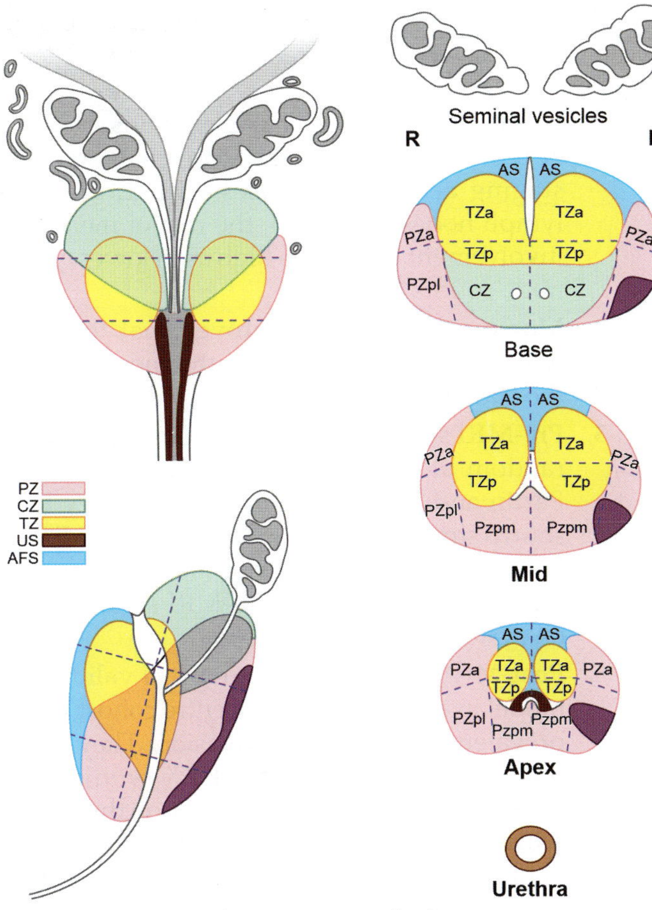

Fig. 3.1: MPMRI findings

1. **What is locally advanced prostate cancer? How would you clinically risk stratify this patient?**

   Ans: EAU risk groups for biochemical recurrence of localised and locally-advanced prostate cancer[1] are given as follows:

Definition			
Low-risk	***Intermediate-risk***	***High-risk***	
PSA <10 ng/ml and GS <7 (ISUP grade 1) and cT1-2a	PSA 10–20 ng/ml or GS 7 (ISUP grade 2/3) or cT2b	PSA >20 ng/ml or GS >7 (ISUP grade 4/5) or cT2c	Any PSA any GS (any ISUP grade) cT3-4 or cN
			Locally advanced

GS = Gleason score; ISUP = International Society for Urological Pathology; PSA = Prostate-specific antigen.

This patient can be risk stratified as a high-risk patient with possible high-risk disease, given the potential capsular extension on mpMRI [EAU risk groups]

Another risk stratification is the high-risk group as per NCCN guidelines [NCCN Clinical Practice Guidelines in Oncology (NCCN Guidelines®): Prostate Cancer. Version 1.2023].

Risk stratification schema for localized prostate cancer, according to the National Comprehensive Cancer Network (NCCN)

Risk group	***Clinical/pathological features***
Very low	T1c and Grade group 1 and PSA <10 ng/ml and Fewer than 3 prostate biopsy fragments/cores positive, ≤50% cancer in each fragment/core and PSA density <0.15 ng/ml/g
Low	T1 to T2a and Grade group 1 and PSA <10 ng/ml and Does not qualify for very low risk
Favourable intermediate	No high or very high-risk features No more than one intermediate risk factor: T2b to T2c or Grade group 2 or 3 PSA 10 to 20 ng/ml and Grade group 1 or 2 and percentage of positive biopsy cores <50%
Unfavourable intermediate	No high or very high-risk features Two or three of the intermediate risk factors: T2b to T2c Grade group 2 or 3 PSA 10 to 20 ng/ml and/or Grade group 3 and/or ≥50% of positive biopsy cores
High	No very high-risk features and T3a or Grade group 4 or 5 or PSA >20 ng/ml
Very high	T3b to T4 or Primary Gleason pattern 5 or Two or three high-risk features or >4 cores with Grade group 4 or 5

PSA: Prostate-specific antigen. *[Adapted from: NCCN Clinical Practice Guidelines in Oncology (NCCN Guidelines®): Prostate Cancer. Version 4.2018.]*

2. **What are the treatment options available for this patient?**

   Ans: Depending on life expectancy and comorbidities, the preferred treatment options are EBRT (external beam radiotherapy) with long-term ADT (androgen deprivation therapy) and RP (radical prostatectomy). However, the present literature needs more high-level evidence to support one option. A recent systematic review failed to define the most optimal treatment option.[2] Randomised controlled trials are only available for EBRT. A local treatment combined with a systemic treatment [multimodality approach] provides the best outcome, provided the patient is fit enough to receive both. A few researchers looked at a focused cohort of patients with advanced disease, like in the SCPG-15 trial. This study, which has recruited >600 men, compares radiotherapy with surgery for prostate cancer, and analysis at the time of randomisation indicates that the study will be informative and generalisable to most men with locally advanced. The initial results of the SCPG-15 trials suggested that randomisation between surgery and EBRT is feasible, but oncologic outcomes are awaited.[3]

3. What is the evidence favouring RP?

Ans:

- Radical prostatectomy surgery for locally advanced disease as part of a multi-modal therapy has been reported.[4,5]
- However, suppose one was to compare the oncological effectiveness of RP as part of a multi-modal treatment strategy as compared to upfront EBRT with ADT for locally advanced prostate cancer, the data remains to be discovered.

4. What are the oncological outcomes of RP in LACaP?

Ans:

1. Retrospective case series: The data from the retrospective case series demonstrated over 60% CSS [cancer-specific survival] at 15 years and over 75% OS [overall survival] at 10 years.[4–10]
2. Cohort studies: For cT3b disease, prostate cancer cohort studies showed 10-year CSS of over 87% and OS of 65%.[11,12]

5. If you decide to do surgery, will you do a lymph node dissection? Will you do a standard or extended lymph node dissection? How do you predict the risk of lymph node involvement?

Ans:

1. Yes. An ePLND should be considered standard if an RP is planned. The individual risk of patients harbouring positive LNs can be estimated based on validated nomograms. The nomograms available can be classified as pre-MRI and post-MRI nomograms.
2. According to the latest EAU guidelines, the ePLND template is recommended whenever PLND is required.[13–15]
3. During ePLND, at least 13 lymph nodes should be removed and investigated to achieve optimal staging accuracy. In cases with 13 or more lymph nodes examined, the rate of metastatic involvement is twice as high as in lower lymph node counts.[16]
4. Moreover, it has been proven that the more lymph nodes are removed, the more accurate the staging will be.[13,17]
5. **Pre-MRI setting:** These are based on systematic random biopsy and include The Briganti.[18,19] Partin and MSKCC nomograms.[20] They have shown similar diagnostic accuracy in predicting LN invasion.[21–23] However, these nomograms were developed in the pre-MRI setting based on systematic random biopsy.
6. **Post-MRI setting:** Gandaglia *et al* validated a model in an external multicentre cohort with a prevalence of 8% of LN invasion. They found that using a risk cut-off of 7% would have avoided LN dissection in 56% of the cohort while missing LN invasion in 2.6% of the patients below the 7% threshold.[24] Therefore, this nomogram and a 7% threshold should be used after an MRI-targeted biopsy to identify candidates for extended LN dissection (ePLND).
7. Stabile *et al* in a 2021 systematic review and meta-analysis,[25] suggest performing PLND in high-risk patients with negative PSMA PET. However, this should also be balanced against the risk of morbidity of PLND. Unfortunately, for patients with positive pelvic LNs on PSMA PET only, evidence is currently unavailable on the best treatment strategy.
8. Franklin *et al*[26] in their study on the utility of PSMA in predicting LN involvement conclude that the high-risk group would appear suitable for an extended PLND at the time of a radical prostatectomy.
9. Kordan *et al*[27] in a recent manuscript clearly mentions that using Ga-68 PSMA PET as a LNI prediction tool instead of nomograms could avoid unnecessary lymphadenectomies during RP.

6. What are the various nomograms?

Ans:

Nomograms v/s mpMRI v/s PSMA PET/CT in predicting LN metastasis

Franklin *et al* in his study found that 1. Preoperative 68 Ga-PSMA/PET/CT was more sensitive to histological pelvic LN metastasis than 3-T mpMRI. 2. Men with a negative 68 Ga-PSMA PET/CT have a lower risk of LN metastasis than predicted with CAPRA scores or MSKCC and Briganti nomograms. 3. Combination of a negative preoperative 68 Ga-PSMA PET/CT, ISUP biopsy Grade <5 and PI-RADS <5 prostate mpMRI, or an ISUP Grade 5 with PI-RADS <4 on mpMRI was associated with a <5% risk of LN metastasis. 4. The addition of CAPRA scores, MSKCC and Briganti nomograms did not improve the predictive probability within this model. 5. Conversely, men with ISUP Grade 4–5 malignancy associated with a PI-RADS 5 prostate mpMRI had a >30% risk of microscopic LNM despite a negative preoperative 68 Ga-PSMA PET/CT.[26] Table 3.1 showing various nomograms predicting lymph node metastasis.

TABLE 3.1: Variables included in nomograms predicting lymph node invasion at radical prostatectomy in patients with prostate cancer.[28]

Nomogram	*Covariates*
Briganti 2019[29]	PSA at diagnosis Clinical stage on multiparametric MRI Grade group on MRI-targeted biopsy Maximum diameter of the index lesion on multiparametric MRI Percentage of positive cores with clinically significant cancer on systematic biopsy
Briganti 2017[19]	Biopsy Gleason grade group Clinical stage Preoperative PSA Percentage of positive cores with the highest-grade disease Percentage of positive cores with the lower-grade disease
Briganti 2012[18]	PSA at diagnosis Clinical stage Primary Gleason grade Secondary Gleason grade Percentage of positive cores
MSKCC[30]	Preoperative PSA Primary biopsy Gleason grade Secondary biopsy Gleason grade Clinical stage Number of negative cores Number of positive cores
Partin 2017[31]	Preoperative PSA (0–4, 4.1–6, 6.1–10 and greater than 10 ng/ml) Gleason score (5–6, 3+4, 4+3/8, and 9–10) Clinical stage (T1c, T2a and T2b/T2c)

7. Would you rely on PSMA to omit surgical lymph node staging?

Ans:

1. Meta-analyses had shown that PSMA PET/CT before primary treatment in advanced PCa detected disease outside the prostate in 32% of cases despite prior negative conventional imaging using bone scan and pelvic CT/MRI.[32]
2. An RCT assessing PSMA-PET/CT as a staging tool in high-risk PCa confirmed these findings and showed a 32% increase in accuracy compared with conventional imaging for detecting pelvic nodal metastases.[33] Notably, more sensitive imaging also causes a stage shift with more cases classified as cN1, but with, on average, lower nodal disease burden.
3. Stabile *et al* in a 2021 systematic review and meta-analysis, showed that PSMA PET had a significantly higher sensitivity and NPV of 39% and 13%, respectively, for LN positivity in intermediate-risk vs high-risk groups.[34]

8. What is the role of neo-adjuvant treatment in LACaP?

Ans:

1. For males with LACaP who choose RP as their primary therapy, a role for any form of neoadjuvant therapy remains uncertain but is under active investigation. We concur with current guidelines from the American Society of Clinical Oncology (ASCO) and the National Comprehensive Cancer Network (NCCN) that do not recommend this as a standard approach[35] outside of the context of a clinical trial.
2. *Androgen deprivation therapy (ADT):*
   a. Neoadjuvant androgen deprivation therapy (ADT) may decrease tumor volume and improve the complete resection rate in males with clinical T3 prostate cancer[36,37] Still, there are no randomised trials compared with prostatectomy alone, and there is no high-quality evidence that long-term outcomes are improved.
   b. In a review of the available literature, neoadjuvant ADT decreased the serum PSA in almost all males and reduced the incidence of positive resection margins in six randomised prospective studies.[36] However, there were no significant differences in operative time, blood loss, transfusion rates, or length of hospital stay. Moreover, there was no improvement in the rate of lymph node metastasis, biochemical RFS, or overall survival.
3. *ADT plus newer antiandrogens:*
   a. In a single-centre randomised trial, 65 males with high-risk prostate cancer were randomly assigned to three months of abiraterone acetate plus prednisone and

an LHRH agonist or LHRH agonist alone, followed by RP.[38] Although there was no significant difference in organ confinement between the two groups, serum PSA depletion to 0.1 ng/ml was observed in >80% of males treated with abiraterone plus the LHRH agonist, and these patients had significantly lower tumour volumes.

b. At a median follow-up of four years, males receiving abiraterone had a substantially lower rate of PSA recurrence (44 versus 59%), and a lower tumour epithelial volume correlated with better outcomes.

4. *Using chemo hormonal therapy:*
   a. In a multicentre phase II trial [2021] evaluating six months of abiraterone acetate plus apalutamide and leuprolide (APAL) or abiraterone acetate plus prednisone and leuprolide (APL),[46] the median pre-prostatectomy PSA nadir was <0.01 versus 0.02 with APAL and APL, respectively, and the time to nadir was 4.2 versus 4.6 months.
   b. The combined pathological complete response and residual cancer rate was 22% with APAL and 20% with APL.[39]

9. How to manage cN0 on imaging which turn out to be positive during RP in LACaP?

Ans: In case of suspected positive LNs during RP (initially considered cN0 on conventional imaging), the procedure should not be abandoned since RP may have a survival benefit in these patients.

10. What is the role of intraoperative frozen section analysis in LACaP for suspected positive LNs during RP?

Ans: Intra-operative frozen section analysis is not justified in this case.[40]

11. Would you resort to doing LN dissection during RP for a LACaP?

Ans: Yes. An ePLND should be considered standard if an RP is planned.

12. What is the evidence favouring RT?

Ans: In locally advanced disease, RCTs have established that the additional use of long-term ADT combined with RT produces better OS than ADT or RT alone.[2]

13. What are your views about the role of ADT in combination with EBRT?

Ans:

- The combination of RT with LHRH (Luteinizing hormone—releasing hormone) ADT has proven its superiority compared with RT alone, followed by deferred ADT on relapse, as shown by phase III RCTs [41–45] (Table 3.2).
- The main message is that a longer duration of ADT, around 2–3 years, is needed for high-risk patients. Omitting ADT may result in inferior OS.[1]
- The question of the added value of EBRT combined with ADT in locally advanced patients has been clarified by 3 RCTs. All showed a clear benefit of adding EBRT to long-term ADT (Table 3.3).

14. What is the POP-RT trial?

Ans:

- The **POP-RT study**[54] was a phase 3 single-centre randomised trial that randomised patients with high-risk localised prostate cancer with estimated nodal involvement risk > = 20% (Roach formula to either prostate-only radiotherapy (68 Gy in 25 fractions) or whole pelvic

TABLE 3.2: Selected studies of the use and duration of ADT in combination with RT for PCa

Study	*Trial*	*Effect on OS*
RTOG 85-31 2005[41]	EBRT ± ADT	A significant benefit for combined treatment seems to be caused mainly by patients with ISUP grade 2–5
RTOG 94-13 2007[46]	ADT timing comparison	No significant difference between neoadjuvant plus concomitant vs adjuvant androgen suppression therapy groups
RTOG 86-10 2008[42]	EBRT ± ADT	No significant difference at 10 years.
D'Amico AV, et al 2008[43]	EBRT ± ADT	Significant benefit: Only men with no or minimal co-morbidity
RTOG 92-02 2008[47]	Short vs prolonged ADT	An overall significant benefit in the subset with ISUP grades 4–5
EORTC 22961 2009[48]	Short vs prolonged ADT	The better result with 3 years, treatment than with six months (3.8% improvement in survival at 5 years)
EORTC 22863 2010[45]	EBRT ± ADT	Significant benefit at 10 years for combined treatment
TROG 96-01 2011[44]	Neoadjuvant ADT duration	Significant benefit in OS and CSS on adding 6 months of ADT to RT
RTOG 99-10 2015[49]	Short vs prolonged ADT	Confirms LHRH as a standard
PCSIII 2020[50]	76 Gy alone vs. 76 Gy + ADT vs. 70 Gy + ADT	It significantly improved BRFS and CSS for ADT arms, with no difference in OS.

TABLE 3.3: Selected studies of ADT in combination with or without RT for PCa

Study	*Trial design*	*Effect on OS*
SPCG-7/ SFUO-3 2016[51]	ADT ± EBRT	34% (95% CI: 29–39%) vs. 17% (95% CI: 13–22% CSM at 15 years, favouring combined treatment
PRO7/NCIC 2015 [52]	ADT ± EBRT	10-yr. OS = 49% vs 55% favouring combined treatment
Sargos, et al 2020 [53]	ADT ± EBRT	Significant reduction of clinical progression; 5-yr. OS 71.4% vs. 71.5%

radiotherapy (68 Gy in 25 fractions to the prostate and 50 Gy in 25 fractions to the pelvic nodes including the common iliac). Over 80% of patients enrolled had baseline PSMA-PET scans for staging.

- The primary endpoint was biochemical recurrence-free survival at five years. At a median follow-up of 68 months, there were seven biochemical recurrences in the pelvic radiotherapy group and 29 in the prostate-only group, resulting in a 5-year biochemical recurrence-free survival of 95% vs 81.2% for pelvic radiotherapy. This corresponds to a 0.23 hazard ratio for recurrence. In an exploratory analysis, pelvic radiotherapy conferred a 0.35 hazard ratio for metastasis relative to prostate-only radiation ($p = 0.01$). Cumulative grade 2 GU toxicity was higher with whole pelvis radiotherapy, but no difference in GI toxicity was detected between the two treatment arms.
- The authors concluded that prophylactic pelvic irradiation for high-risk, locally advanced prostate cancer improved BFFS and DFS compared to PORT, but OS did not appear to differ.

15. What is unique about the POP-RT trial compared to previous trials done in this cohort of patients?

Ans: The POP-RT is unique relative to prior studies in this space because it enrolled high-risk patients, most patients had sensitive staging with PSMA-PET, it included higher radiotherapy doses to the prostate and a higher superior border for pelvic radiation, and now all patients received the standard of care two years of androgen suppression.

16. What is the role of brachytherapy?

Ans: Brachytherapy (BT) can be given as a boost along with EBRT. It can be given as a high-dose rate (HDR) or low-dose rate (LDR) brachytherapy.

17. What are the technical differences between LDR-BT and HDR-BT?[1]

Ans:

Differences in prostate brachytherapy techniques	
Low dose rate (LDR)	• Permanent seeds implanted • Uses Iodine-125 (I-125) (most common), Palladium-103 (^{103}Pd-) or Cesium-131 isotopes • Radiation dose delivered over weeks and months • Acute side effects resolve over months • Radiation protection issues for patient and carers
High dose rate (HDR)	• Temporary implantation • Iridium-192 (IR-192) isotope introduced through impanted needles or catheters • Radiation dose delivered in minutes • Acute side effects resolve over weeks • No radiation protection issues for patient or cares

18. What is low-dose rate brachytherapy?

Ans: Low-dose rate (LDR) brachytherapy uses radioactive seeds permanently implanted into the prostate.

19. What is the evidence supporting LDR-BT?

Ans: Low-dose rate brachytherapy can be combined with EBRT in high-risk patients. External beam RT (total dose of 78 Gy) has been compared with EBRT (total amount 46 Gy) followed by LDR brachytherapy boost (prescribed dose 115 Gy) in intermediate-risk and high-risk patients in the ASCENDE-RT randomised trial with 12 months of ADT in both arms.[55]

20. What are the oncological outcomes of LDR-BT?

Ans: The **LDR boost** resulted in a 5 and 7-year PSA PFS increase (89% and 86%, respectively, compared to 84% and 75%).

21. Did LDR-BT result in any side effects?

Ans: This improvement was achieved at the cost of increased late-grade 3+ GU toxicity (18% compared to 8%).[56] Toxicity resulted in the development of urethral strictures and incontinence; great care should be taken during treatment planning.

22. What is high-dose-rate brachytherapy?

Ans: High-dose-rate (HDR) brachytherapy uses a radioactive source temporarily introduced into the prostate to deliver radiation. It can be delivered in single or multiple fractions and is often combined with EBRT of at least 45 Gy.[57]

23. What is the evidence favouring HDR-BT?

Ans:

- A systematic review of non-RCTs suggests outcomes with EBRT plus HDR brachytherapy are superior to EBRT alone.[58,59]
- A 2021 single-centre RCT of EBRT followed by HDR brachytherapy has been reported.[60] The combination significantly improved the biochemical disease-free rate at 5 and 10 years (75% and 46% compared to 61% and 39%).
- TROG 03.04 RADAR trial: This trial provides supporting, but not definitive, evidence of the benefit of HDR boost. In this multicentre study, after a minimum follow-up of 10 years, HDR boost significantly reduced distant progression compared to EBRT alone and independent of the duration of ADT. HDR boost was associated with increased IPSS of 3 points at 18 months post-treatment resolving by three years but decreased rectal symptoms compared to EBRT.[61]

24. What are your views about the role of ADT in combination with HDR-BT?

Ans:

- RCT and systematic reviews show that ADT use independently predicts better outcomes regardless of radiation dose intensification.[61,62]
- Omitting ADT may result in inferior OS, and based on current evidence, ADT use and duration should be in line with that used when delivering EBRT alone.[1]

25. Are any trials looking into different treatment modalities [RP and RT] for LACaP?

Ans:

- A prospective phase III RCT (SPCG-15), which compares RP (with or without adjuvant or salvage EBRT) against primary EBRT and ADT among patients with locally advanced (T3) disease, is currently recruiting.[63] This trial, with an estimated 1200 participants, is scheduled to complete data collection by 2025.

26. What is the rationale behind the SPCG-15 trial?

Ans:

- **RP:** By adding prostatectomy to the treatment of LAPC, one removes the prostate, enabling a full pathological assessment of the tumour characteristics, and thus a better estimation of the risk of recurrence. Surgical treatment could thus reduce the numbers needed to treat with chemotherapy and radiation and thus improve quality of life after treatment. In addition, evidence also indicates that residual cancer in the prostate occurs 25% after radiation treatment,[64] and surgical removal of the prostate may improve survival beyond what can be achieved by radiation and ADT.
- **RT:** Conversely, patients treated with surgery, radiation and hormones will experience side effects of all three treatment modalities. One can provide oncological control without prior surgery by offering radiotherapy plus hormones; patients might fare much better.

Case Scenario *(Contd.)*

After counselling, the patient decides to undergo an RP despite being explained the potential risk of residual disease. Histology confirms a capsular breach on the left with a positive circumferential resection margin but negative lymph nodes. You see the patient in the OPD at four weeks and explain the histology result.

27. What is his risk of developing recurrence?

Ans: The EAU guidelines classify locally advanced prostate cancer as a high-risk group for biochemical recurrence[1] (Table 3.2). Studies have shown that 30% to 60% of patients with T3 disease will develop biochemical progression at five years.

The patient is concerned about the possible risk of residual cancer and asks if there is any further treatment that can be given.

28. What is the CAPRA-S score?

Ans:

- The risk assessment systems are not intended to replace individualised clinician-patient decision-making but to provide an instrument for facilitating disease risk classification in clinical decision-making and future research. D'Amico classification does not account for multiple risk factors and care must be taken in interpreting the predictions from the calculators/nomograms.
- To address the existing limitations of these approaches, UCSF developed the Cancer of the Prostate Risk Assessment (UCSF-CAPRA) score.[65] CAPRA is a relatively straightforward 0 to 10 score. It is nearly as easy as the D'Amico classification but with accuracy comparable to the best nomograms.
- The CAPRA score is valid across multiple treatment approaches. It helps to predict an individual's likelihood of metastasis, cancer-specific mortality, and overall mortality.
- The score is calculated using points assigned to age, PSA at diagnosis, Gleason score of the biopsy, clinical stage and percent of biopsy cores involved with cancer.
- A CAPRA score of 0 to 2 indicates *low risk*. A CAPRA score of 3 to 5 indicates *intermediate*

risk. A CAPRA score of 6 to 10 indicates *high risk [UCSF CAPRA]*

- The CAPRA-S offers good discriminatory accuracy, calibration, and ease of calculation for clinical and research settings.[65]

29. What advice would you give him?

Ans:

- The EAU guidelines advise that those patients with stage T2/T3 disease with positive margins or capsular breach can be offered immediate EBRT or clinical monitoring and salvage EBRT when the PSA is >0.2 ng/ml but <1 ng/ml.[1]

30. What is an ARTISTIC meta-analysis?[66]

Ans:

- The ARTISTIC collaborative aims to compare outcomes for adjuvant radiotherapy compared to a strategy of planned early salvage radiotherapy following radical prostatectomy. Furthermore, they relied on three randomised control trials: the RADICALS-RT, RAVES, and GETUG-AFU 17.
- The overall study question was similar, comparing adjuvant versus early salvage radiotherapy. Thus, the ARTISTIC collaborative undertook a prospective systematic review and meta-analysis utilising the FAME approach, the framework for adaptive meta-analysis.
- The outcomes of interest differed for the three included trials in RADICALS-RT, which was a time free from metastasis, and in GETAG-AFU 17, which was event-free survival, which is predominantly driven by PSA-related events, and the RAVES is the biochemical progression entirely dictated by PSA-driven events. However, to allow for pooling across these trials, the authors created an aggregate primary outcome that they deemed "event-free survival," which was the time to the first of biochemical progression defined as PSAs equal or greater than 0.4 following radiotherapy, clinical/radiological progression, initiation of non-trial treatments that was typically androgen deprivation off the trial, death from prostate cancer or any PSA greater than two at any time.
- Most patients were T3a or T3b at about three-quarters in RADICALS, almost all in GETUG and three-quarters in the RAVES study. The primary outcome measured was freedom from distant metastasis for RADICALS-RT, event-free survival for GETUG, and freedom for biochemical progression in RAVES. Interestingly, the RAVES study was a non-inferiority design, whereas the other two were superior.
- RADICALS and GETUG-AFU 17 provided event-free survival results for the meta-analysis (interim for GETUG-AFU 17). RAVES currently could only supply freedom from biochemical failure results. However, as most first events across all trials are biochemical failures, these results were pooled in a preliminary meta-analysis of event-free survival.
- So, in conclusion, adjuvant radiotherapy following prostatectomy does not improve PSA-driven event-free survival compared to early salvage radiotherapy. Early salvage radiotherapy provides the opportunity to avoid or postpone radiotherapy and associated adverse events for many men with no effect on event-free survival, and this is avoiding the overtreatment of men that would never benefit from early adjuvant radiotherapy. And finally, 88% of men remain event-free five years after radical prostatectomy.

31. What is the RAVES [Radiotherapy Adjuvant Versus Early Salvage] trial?[67–69]

Ans:

- The RAVES trial set out to assess the hypothesis that for patients with pT3 disease or positive margins following radical prostatectomy, observation with early salvage radiotherapy is non-inferior to standard treatment of adjuvant radiotherapy with respect to biochemical recurrence.
- Men were enrolled if they had positive margins, EPE, or seminal vesicle invasion. Key, unlike prior studies, men had to have undetectable PSA. This is a genuinely adjuvant use. This was phase 3 randomised controlled non-inferiority trial.
- This is unique compared to other recent publications of the GETUG-17 trial and the RADICALS-RT trial, which were both superior in design. Critical patient-level inclusion criteria included all men with prior radical prostatectomy and evidence of positive surgical margins, extraprostatic extension, or seminal vesicle invasion.
- The primary outcome of this trial was freedom from biochemical progression. That was defined as the first PSA greater than 0.4 and rising following radiotherapy. Secondary outcomes included time to the initiation of ADT, time to clinical progression, overall survival, quality of life, mental health, adverse events, and quality-adjusted life years.
- The salvage radiotherapy group was 87% biochemically disease-free at five years, and the adjuvant was 86%, so the curves overline each other. We had 75% biochemically disease-free at eight years in the salvage group and 79% in the adjuvant group. So, at eight years,

suppose you only had a 4% difference in biochemical control. In that case, the likelihood of any clinically meaningful difference between the two arms, such as metastasis or survival endpoints, will be minimal. Hence, it would not justify the additional toxicity of going through radiotherapy.

- The trial says if you wait until the PSA gets to 0.2, your patient will do just as well, plus you will better his side effect profile, plus half of the patients do not need radiotherapy. Please note that the rate of giving salvage over time in the trial was relatively uniform, but the mean was three to four years.

32. What is GETUG-AFU 17 trial?[53]

Ans:

- GETUG-AFU 17 was a randomised, open-label, multicentre, phase 3 trial. Men aged at least 18 years who had an Eastern Cooperative Oncology Group performance status of 1 or less, localised adenocarcinoma of the prostate treated with radical prostatectomy, who had pathologically staged pT3a, pT3b, or pT4a (with bladder neck invasion), pNx (without pelvic lymph nodes dissection), or pN0 (with negative lymph nodes dissection) disease, and who had positive surgical margins were eligible for inclusion in the study. Eligible patients were randomly assigned (1:1) to either immediate adjuvant radiotherapy or delayed salvage radiotherapy at the time of biochemical relapse.
- The overall median follow-up time from the random assignment was 75 months, 74 months in the adjuvant radiotherapy group and 78 months in the salvage radiotherapy group.
- Late grade 2 or worse genitourinary toxicities were 59% in the adjuvant radiotherapy group and 22% in the salvage radiotherapy group. Late genitourinary adverse events of grade 2 or worse were reported as 27% in the adjuvant radiotherapy group versus 7% in the salvage radiotherapy group. Late erectile dysfunction was grade 2 or worse in 28% of the adjuvant radiotherapy group and 8% of the salvage radiotherapy group.
- The authors concluded that there was no benefit for event-free survival in patients assigned to adjuvant radiotherapy compared with patients assigned to salvage radiotherapy. Adjuvant radiotherapy increases the risk of genitourinary toxicity and erectile dysfunction. A policy of early salvage radiotherapy could spare men from overtreatment with radiotherapy and the associated adverse events.

33. What are RADICALS-HD Trial?

Ans:

- RADICALS-HD examines the effect of different durations of androgen deprivation therapy (ADT) among men receiving postoperative radiotherapy following radical prostatectomy for prostate cancer. It is a complex trial design with multiple questions and many comparisons across two settings (adjuvant and salvage).
- The authors concluded that in patients having post-operative RT after RP, 24 months ADT vs 6 months ADT improved both times to salvage ADT and MFS. In contrast, 6 months ADT vs no ADT improved time to salvage ADT but did not improve MFS.
- In other words, adding short-term ADT to salvage RT in better-risk populations results in minor incremental improvements in MFS. However, many patients appear to do well with radiotherapy alone. Thus, longer-term follow-up is needed to understand these outcomes better and help guide patient selection.
- In patients with higher-risk disease, prolonging ADT treatment from 6 months to 2 years improved MFS. However, many patients in the short-term arm did very well. Thus, quality-of-life data may be necessary when considering the toxicity of ADT.[70]
- The trial data also indicates that the optimal duration of ADT, when given with postoperative RT, remains unclear for a specific patient.[71] There is essentially no substantial evidence in the adjuvant setting, while there is some data from RTOG 9601, GETUF-AFU-16, and RTOG 0534 regarding the use in the salvage setting for biochemical failure. However, this fails to address the question of duration.
- Thus, given this evidence void, the most recent version of the ESMO guidelines note that "concomitant ADT with LHRH agonist for six months or bicalutamide for two years may be offered" to these patients.[70]

34. What is GETUG-AFU 16 trial?[72]

Ans:

- It is an open-label, multicentre, phase 3, randomised, controlled trial that enrolled men (aged 18 years) with Eastern Cooperative Oncology Group performance status of 0 or 1, with histologically confirmed adenocarcinoma of the prostate (but no previous androgen suppression or pelvic radiotherapy), stage pT2, T3, or T4a (bladder neck involvement only) and pN0 or pNx according to the tumour, node, metastasis (TNM) staging system, whose prostate-specific antigen (PSA) concentration increased from 0 1 ng/ml to between 0 2 ng/

Section 1

ml and 2 0 ng/ml after radical prostatectomy, without evidence of clinical disease.

- The 120-month progression-free survival was 64% for patients treated with radiotherapy plus goserelin and 49% for patients treated with radiotherapy alone.
- Salvage radiotherapy combined with short-term androgen suppression significantly reduced the risk of biochemical or clinical progression and death compared to salvage radiotherapy alone. The results of the GETUG-AFU 16 trial confirm the efficacy of androgen suppression plus salvage radiotherapy in patients with increasing PSA concentration after RP for prostate cancer.

35. What is DADSPORT meta-analysis?

Ans: DADSPORT is a collaborative meta-analysis of aggregate data to assess the duration of androgen suppression with postoperative radiotherapy. The DADSPORT meta-analysis collaboration conducted a systematic review and meta-analysis of results from NRG/RTOG 9601, GETUG-AFU 16, NRG/RTOG 0534, and the RADICALS-HD trials to assess the effect of hormone therapy in men receiving radiotherapy following radical prostatectomy for localised prostate cancer.[73]

The primary analysis was a fixed-effect, inverse-variance meta-analysis stratified by hormone duration (no hormone therapy, six months, and 24 months of hormone therapy) following radiotherapy. Necessary eligibility included trials comparing radiotherapy + hormone therapy versus radiotherapy following prostatectomy in men with intermediate/high-risk localised disease, no regional or distant metastasis evidence, and published or unpublished trials.

The inferences were: 1. There was no clear evidence of a difference in survival with either 6 or 24 months of hormone therapy versus none, and there was no clear evidence of a difference between 6 versus 24 months. 2. There was evidence that six months of hormone therapy improved MFS compared to no hormone therapy (HR 0.82, 95% CI 0.70–0.96, p = 0.01), with a 5-year absolute improvement of 2%.

36. What are the EAU risk categories for biochemical recurrence?

Ans: EAU risk categories for biochemical recurrence.

These risk categories have been externally validated.[74,75]

	EAU low risk	*EAU high risk*
After RP	PSA-DT >1 year and pathological ISUP grade <4	PSA-DT <1 year or Pathological ISUP grade 4–5
After RT	Interval to biochemical failure >18 months and biopsy ISUP grade <4	Interval to biochemical failure <18 months or biopsy ISUP grade 4–5

Case Scenario *(Contd.)*

The patient was reviewed in the OPD at three months, and his PSA was <0.1 ng/ml. He was kept under regular surveillance for the next three years. His PSA remained <0.1 ng/ml. After three years, when he attends your clinic, you find that his latest PSA has increased to 0.3 ng/ml.

37. What would you tell the patient, and how would you manage this?

Ans: I counsel the patient that this likely indicates a biochemical recurrence due to residual local disease. A PSMA PET/CT would help to differentiate between local and distant recurrence.

38. What are the treatment options offered?

Ans:

- Salvage radiotherapy is an option assuming no contraindications and the recurrence is local.
- If the patient wishes to avoid the complications of radical treatment, then ADT can be given.
- ADT is best given early in systemic relapse as it has been shown to decrease the frequency of clinical metastases.[76]
- With localised recurrence, delaying ADT until the clinically evident metastatic disease is more appropriate as the median time for metastasis development is eight years, and the median time from metastasis to death is another five years.[77]

39. Is there a role for cryotherapy or HIFU?

Ans: There is no role for ablative cryotherapy or HIFU in this setting.

Case Scenario 2

A fit and well 71-year-old man is referred to your clinic with an elevated PSA of 19.1 ng/ml and an abnormal DRE. An MRI reveals a capsular breach on the left. There are synchronous suspected pelvic nodal metastases on conventional imaging (CT/bone scan) without bone or visceral metastases (cN1 M0 stage). TRUS is systematic and targeted biopsies confirm maximum Gleason 4 + 4 and overall Gleason 4 + 3 diseases.

1. **What treatment options are available?**

Approximately 5% to 10% of newly diagnosed PCa patients have synchronous suspected pelvic nodal metastases on conventional imaging (CT/bone scan) without bone or visceral metastases (cN1 M0 stage).[1]

The management of cN1M0 PCa is historically based on long-term ADT combined with a local treatment. The benefit of adding local treatment has been summarised in one systematic review.[78] The findings suggested an advantage in both OS and CSS after local treatment (RT or RP) combined with ADT compared to ADT alone.

A few retrospective studies have investigated cN1 patients and recommended local therapy in addition to long-term ADT (Table 3.4).

TABLE 3.4: Selected studies assessing local treatment in (any cT) cN1 M0 prostate cancer patients[1]

Study	*Design*	*Effect on survival*
Sarkar, *et al* 2019 [897]	Retrospective (National Veterans Affairs)	A significant benefit for RP No statistical difference for RP vs RT
Seisen, *et al* 2018 [887]	Retrospective (NCDB)	A significant benefit for combined treatment 5 years OS: 78.8% vs 49.2%. No difference between RP and RT

Based on the consistent benefit seen in retrospective studies including cN1 patients, local therapy is recommended in patients with cN1 disease at diagnosis in addition to long-term ADT.[79–84] Adding a brachytherapy boost to ADT plus EBRT was not associated with improved OS.[85]

2. **What is the role of prostatectomy in cN1?**

Ans: Only limited evidence exists supporting RP for cN1 patients. Moschino *et al* compared the outcomes of 50 patients with cN+ with 252 patients with pN1 but cN0 at preoperative staging. cN+ was not a significant predictor of CSS.[86]

3. **What is the evidence for the addition of abiraterone/docetaxel to RT in N1 disease?**

Ans:

- The intensification of systemic treatment (abiraterone acetate, docetaxel, zoledronic acid) has been assessed in unplanned sub-group analyses from the STAMPEDE multi-arm RCT by stratifying for cN1 and M1 status.[87,88] Abiraterone acetate was associated with a non-significant OS improvement (HR: 0.75) in nonmetastatic patients (N0/N + M0), but OS data were still immature.
- Adding docetaxel, zoledronic acid, or their combination did not benefit OS when stratifying by M0 and N+ status. This docetaxel arm in the STAMPEDE trial was also an underpowered subgroup analysis.
- In the AFU-GETUG 12 trial comparing the impact of docetaxel plus estramustine in addition to ADT, 29% of included high-risk nonmetastatic PCa patients had a nodal involvement (pN1). It showed a trend towards better relapse-free survival rates without OS benefits.
- A meta-analysis of docetaxel trials in N0/N1-M0 patients concluded an 8% 4-year survival advantage for docetaxel compared with ADT alone regarding failure-free survival without OS benefit.[89]
- A meta-analysis of two RCTs from the STAMPEDE platform protocol reported on men with *de novo* high-risk/locally advanced M0 disease, 39% of whom were N1 on conventional imaging.[90] The authors concluded that given the MFS and OS benefits observed in the overall population, combined ADT (for three years) and additional abiraterone (for two years) should be a SOC in cN1 patients in addition to the prostate- and whole pelvic RT.

4. **What are the techniques to reduce the rectal toxicity of RT?**

Ans:

- Rectal side effects are common after prostate cancer (PC) radiotherapy (RT). Higher radiation dose to the prostate can improve biochemical outcomes, but dose escalation significantly increases the risk of treatment toxicity.[91]
- A majority of these studies are based on a polyethylene-glycol (PEG) hydrogel (SpaceOAR®) and suggest beneficial effects of spacers in reducing the rectal dose and, subsequently, late toxicity and QoL decline.[92] Other devices used for prostate-rectal separation are rectal balloon implants[93] and collagen implants,[94] leading to decreased radiation doses to the rectum.

SUMMARY

- Patients can be risk stratified as high-risk patients with possible high-risk disease given the potential capsular extension on mpMRI [EAU risk groups]. Another risk stratification is the high-risk group as per NCCN guidelines.
- Depending on life expectancy and co-morbidities, the preferred treatment options are EBRT and RP. However, the present literature lacks high-level evidence to support one option. A recent systematic review failed to define the most optimal treatment option.
- Surgery for locally advanced disease as part of multi-modal therapy has been reported. However, if one were to compare the oncological effectiveness of RP as part of a multi-modal

treatment strategy as compared to upfront EBRT with ADT for locally advanced PCa, then the data remains unknown.

- For males with LACaP who choose RP as their primary therapy, a role for any form of neoadjuvant therapy remains uncertain but is under active investigation.
- ePLND is done as a standard template. Nomograms [pre- or post-MRI] can be used to ascertain individual patient risk.
- Pre- and post-MRI nomograms are used.
- PSMA PET had a significantly higher sensitivity for LN positivity.
- ADT using Abiraterone, Enzalutamide, etc. is being investigated
- Brachytherapy (BT) can be given as a boost along with EBRT
- The recurrence risk depends on the PSA-DT, ISUP grade and interval to biochemical failure. These factors are considered depending on the primary therapy, viz. RT or RP.
- EAU risk stratification is used to assign risk status to the patients.
- 30–60% of patients with T3 disease will develop biochemical progression at five years.
- Only limited evidence exists supporting RP for cN1 patients
- Based on the consistent benefit seen in retrospective studies, local therapy in the form of EBRT is recommended in patients with cN1 disease at diagnosis in addition to long-term ADT.
- Various ADT options have variable OS outcomes, but the overall literature does look promising.

REFERENCES

1. EAU Guidelines. Edn. presented at the EAU Annual Congress Milan 2023. ISBN 978-94-92671-19-6.
2. Moris L, Cumberbatch MG, Van den Broeck T, Gandaglia G, Fossati N, Kelly B, *et al.* Benefits and Risks of Primary Treatments for High-risk Localized and Locally Advanced Prostate Cancer: An International Multidisciplinary Systematic Review. Eur Urol. 2020 May;77(5):614–27.
3. Gongora M, Stranne J, Johansson E, Bottai M, Thellenberg Karlsson C, Brasso K, *et al.* Characteristics of Patients in SPCG-15-A Randomized Trial Comparing Radical Prostatectomy with Primary Radiotherapy plus Androgen Deprivation Therapy in Men with Locally Advanced Prostate Cancer. Eur Urol Open Sci. 2022 Jul;41:63–73.
4. Donohue JF, Bianco FJ, Kuroiwa K, Vickers AJ, Wheeler TM, Scardino PT, *et al.* Poorly differentiated prostate cancer treated with radical prostatectomy: long-term outcome and incidence of pathological downgrading. J Urol. 2006 Sep;176(3):991–5.
5. Yossepowitch O, Eggener SE, Bianco FJ, Carver BS, Serio A, Scardino PT, *et al.* Radical prostatectomy for clinically localized, high risk prostate cancer: critical analysis of risk assessment methods. J Urol. 2007 Aug;178(2):493–9; discussion 499.
6. Bastian PJ, Gonzalgo ML, Aronson WJ, Terris MK, Kane CJ, Amling CL, *et al.* Clinical and pathologic outcome after radical prostatectomy for prostate cancer patients with a preoperative Gleason sum of 8 to 10. Cancer. 2006 Sep 15;107(6):1265–72.
7. Chang K, Qin XJ, Zhang HL, Dai B, Zhu Y, Shi GH, *et al.* Comparison of two adjuvant hormone therapy regimens in patients with high-risk localized prostate cancer after radical prostatectomy: primary results of study CU1005. Asian J Androl. 2016;18(3):452–5.
8. Walz J, Joniau S, Chun FK, Isbarn H, Jeldres C, Yossepowitch O, *et al.* Pathological results and rates of treatment failure in high-risk prostate cancer patients after radical prostatectomy. BJU Int. 2011 Mar;107(5):765–70.
9. Spahn M, Joniau S, Gontero P, Fieuws S, Marchioro G, Tombal B, *et al.* Outcome predictors of radical prostatectomy in patients with prostate-specific antigen greater than 20 ng/ml: a European multi-institutional study of 712 patients. Eur Urol. 2010 Jul;58(1):1–7; discussion 10–11.
10. Zwergel U, Suttmann H, Schroeder T, Siemer S, Wullich B, Kamradt J, *et al.* Outcome of prostate cancer patients with initial PSA> or =20 ng/ml undergoing radical prostatectomy. Eur Urol. 2007 Oct;52(4):1058–65.
11. Magheli A, Rais-Bahrami S, Peck HJ, Walsh PC, Epstein JI, Trock BJ, *et al.* Importance of tumor location in patients with high preoperative prostate specific antigen levels (greater than 20 ng/ml) treated with radical prostatectomy. J Urol. 2007 Oct;178(4 Pt 1):1311–5.
12. Ward JF, Slezak JM, Blute ML, Bergstralh EJ, Zincke H. Radical prostatectomy for clinically advanced (cT3) prostate cancer since the advent of prostate-specific antigen testing: 15-year outcome. BJU Int. 2005 Apr;95(6):751–6.
13. Masterson TA, Bianco FJ, Vickers AJ, DiBlasio CJ, Fearn PA, Rabbani F, *et al.* The Association Between Total and Positive Lymph Node Counts, and Disease Progression in Clinically Localized Prostate Cancer. J Urol. 2006 Apr;175(4):1320–5.
14. Briganti A, Blute ML, Eastham JH, Graefen M, Heidenreich A, Karnes JR, *et al.* Pelvic Lymph Node Dissection in Prostate Cancer. Eur Urol. 2009 Jun 1;55(6):1251–65.
15. Touijer K, Rabbani F, Otero JR, Secin FP, Eastham JA, Scardino PT, *et al.* Standard Versus Limited Pelvic Lymph Node Dissection for Prostate Cancer in Patients With a Predicted Probability of Nodal Metastasis Greater Than 1%. J Urol. 2007 Jul;178(1):120–4.
16. Barth PJ, Gerharz EW, Ramaswamy A, Riedmiller H. The Influence of Lymph Node Counts on the Detection of Pelvic Lymph Node Metastasis in Prostate Cancer. Pathol -Res Pract. 1999 Jan 1;195(9):633–6.
17. Zheng Y, Gao Y, Cheng Y, Qi F, Zou Q. Whether extended pelvic lymph node dissection should be performed in prostate cancer: The present evidence from a systematic review and meta-analysis. Precis Med Sci. 2020;9(1):23–30.
18. Briganti A, Larcher A, Abdollah F, Capitanio U, Gallina A, Suardi N, *et al.* Updated Nomogram Predicting Lymph Node Invasion in Patients with Prostate Cancer Undergoing Extended Pelvic Lymph Node Dissection: The Essential Importance of percentage of Positive Cores. Eur Urol. 2012 Mar;61(3):480–7.
19. Gandaglia G, Fossati N, Zaffuto E, Bandini M, Dell'Oglio P, Bravi CA, *et al.* Development and Internal Validation of a Novel Model to Identify the Candidates for Extended Pelvic Lymph Node Dissection in Prostate Cancer. Eur Urol. 2017 Oct;72(4):632–40.
20. Cimino S, Reale G, Castelli T, Favilla V, Giardina R, Russo GI, *et al.* Comparison between Briganti, Partin and MSKCC tools in predicting positive lymph nodes in prostate cancer: a systematic review and meta-analysis. Scand J Urol. 2017 Oct;51(5):345–50.
21. Abdollah F, Cozzarini C, Suardi N, Gallina A, Capitanio U, Bianchi M, *et al.* Indications for pelvic nodal treatment in prostate cancer should change. Validation of the Roach formula in a large extended nodal dissection series. Int J Radiat Oncol Biol Phys. 2012 Jun 1;83(2):624–9.

22. Dell'Oglio P, Abdollah F, Suardi N, Gallina A, Cucchiara V, Vizziello D, *et al.* External validation of the European association of urology recommendations for pelvic lymph node dissection in patients treated with robot-assisted radical prostatectomy. J Endourol. 2014 Apr;28(4):416–23.
23. Hinev AI, Anakievski D, Kolev NH, Hadjiev VI. Validation of nomograms predicting lymph node involvement in patients with prostate cancer undergoing extended pelvic lymph node dissection. Urol Int. 2014;92(3):300–5.
24. Gandaglia G, Martini A, Ploussard G, Fossati N, Stabile A, De Visschere P, *et al.* External Validation of the 2019 Briganti Nomogram for the Identification of Prostate Cancer Patients Who Should Be Considered for an Extended Pelvic Lymph Node Dissection. Eur Urol. 2020 Aug;78(2):138–42.
25. Stabile A, Pellegrino A, Mazzone E, Cannoletta D, de Angelis M, Barletta F, *et al.* Can negative Prostate-specific Membrane Antigen Positron Emission Tomography/Computed Tomography Avoid the Need for Pelvic Lymph Node Dissection in Newly Diagnosed Prostate Cancer Patients? A Systematic Review and Meta-analysis with Backup Histology as Reference Standard. Eur Urol Oncol. 2022 Feb;5(1):1–17.
26. Franklin A, Yaxley WJ, Raveenthiran S, Coughlin G, Gianduzzo T, Kua B, *et al.* Histological comparison between predictive value of preoperative 3-T multiparametric MRI and 68 Ga-PSMA PET/CT scan for pathological outcomes at radical prostatectomy and pelvic lymph node dissection for prostate cancer. BJU Int. 2021 Jan;127(1):71–9.
27. Kordan Y, Köseo lu E, Sarıkaya AF, Tarım K, Kılıç M, Özkan A, *et al.* P0840 -Preoperative prediction of lymph node invasion in prostate cancer: Ga-68 PSMA PET or nomograms? Eur Urol. 2021 Jun 1;79:S1172–3.
28. Fukagawa E, Yamamoto S, Ohde S, Yoshitomi KK, Hamada K, Yoneoka Y, *et al.* External validation of the Briganti 2019 nomogram to identify candidates for extended pelvic lymph node dissection among patients with high-risk clinically localized prostate cancer. Int J Clin Oncol. 2021 Sep 1;26(9):1736–44.
29. Gandaglia G, Ploussard G, Valerio M, Mattei A, Fiori C, Fossati N, *et al.* A Novel Nomogram to Identify Candidates for Extended Pelvic Lymph Node Dissection Among Patients with Clinically Localized Prostate Cancer Diagnosed with Magnetic Resonance Imaging-targeted and Systematic Biopsies. Eur Urol. 2019 Mar 1;75(3):506–14.
30. Prostate Cancer Nomograms: Dynamic Prostate Cancer Nomogram: Coefficients | Memorial Sloan Kettering Cancer Center [Internet]. [cited 2023 Jul 1]. Available from: https://www.mskcc.org/nomograms/prostate/pre_op/coefficients
31. Tosoian JJ, Chappidi M, Feng Z, Humphreys EB, Han M, Pavlovich CP, *et al.* Prediction of pathological stage based on clinical stage, serum prostate-specific antigen, and biopsy Gleason score: Partin Tables in the contemporary era. BJU Int. 2017;119(5):676–83.
32. Perera M, Papa N, Roberts M, Williams M, Udovicich C, Vela I, *et al.* Gallium-68 Prostate-specific Membrane Antigen Positron Emission Tomography in Advanced Prostate Cancer-Updated Diagnostic Utility, Sensitivity, Specificity, and Distribution of Prostate-specific Membrane Antigen-avid Lesions: A Systematic Review and Meta-analysis. Eur Urol. 2020 Apr;77(4):403–17.
33. Hofman MS, Lawrentschuk N, Francis RJ, Tang C, Vela I, Thomas P, *et al.* Prostate-specific membrane antigen PET-CT in patients with high-risk prostate cancer before curative-intent surgery or radiotherapy (proPSMA): a prospective, randomised, multicentre study. Lancet Lond Engl. 2020 Apr 11;395(10231):1208–16.
34. Stabile A, Pellegrino A, Mazzone E, Cannoletta D, de Angelis M, Barletta F, *et al.* Can Negative Prostate-specific Membrane Antigen Positron Emission Tomography/Computed Tomography Avoid the Need for Pelvic Lymph Node Dissection in Newly Diagnosed Prostate Cancer Patients? A Systematic Review and Meta-analysis with Backup Histology as Reference Standard. Eur Urol Oncol. 2022 Feb;5(1):1–17.
35. Bekelman JE, Rumble RB, Chen RC, Pisansky TM, Finelli A, Feifer A, *et al.* Clinically Localized Prostate Cancer: ASCO Clinical Practice Guideline Endorsement of an American Urological Association/American Society for Radiation Oncology/Society of Urologic Oncology Guideline. J Clin Oncol Off J Am Soc Clin Oncol. 2018 Nov 10;36(32):3251–8.
36. Scolieri MJ, Altman A, Resnick MI. Neoadjuvant hormonal ablative therapy before radical prostatectomy: a review. Is it indicated? J Urol. 2000 Nov;164(5):1465–72.
37. Powell IJ, Tangen CM, Miller GJ, Lowe BA, Haas G, Carroll PR, *et al.* Neoadjuvant therapy before radical prostatectomy for clinical T3/T4 carcinoma of the prostate: 5-year followup, Phase II Southwest Oncology Group Study 9109. J Urol. 2002 Nov;168(5):2016–9.
38. Pietzak EJ, Eastham JA. Neoadjuvant Treatment of High-Risk, Clinically Localized Prostate Cancer Prior to Radical Prostatectomy. Curr Urol Rep. 2016 May;17(5):37.
39. McKay RR, Xie W, Ye H, Fennessy FM, Zhang Z, Lis R, *et al.* Results of a Randomized Phase II Trial of Intense Androgen Deprivation Therapy prior to Radical Prostatectomy in Men with High-Risk Localized Prostate Cancer. J Urol. 2021 Jul;206(1):80–7.
40. Engel J, Bastian PJ, Baur H, Beer V, Chaussy C, Gschwend JE, *et al.* Survival benefit of radical prostatectomy in lymph node-positive patients with prostate cancer. Eur Urol. 2010 May;57(5):754–61.
41. Pilepich MV, Winter K, Lawton CA, Krisch RE, Wolkov HB, Movsas B, *et al.* Androgen suppression adjuvant to definitive radiotherapy in prostate carcinoma-long-term results of phase III RTOG 85-31. Int J Radiat Oncol Biol Phys. 2005 Apr 1;61(5):1285–90.
42. Roach M, Bae K, Speight J, Wolkov HB, Rubin P, Lee RJ, *et al.* Short-Term Neoadjuvant Androgen Deprivation Therapy and External-Beam Radiotherapy for Locally Advanced Prostate Cancer: Long-Term Results of RTOG 8610. J Clin Oncol. 2008 Feb 1;26(4):585–91.
43. D'Amico AV, Chen MH, Renshaw AA, Loffredo M, Kantoff PW. Androgen suppression and radiation vs radiation alone for prostate cancer: a randomized trial. JAMA. 2008 Jan 23;299(3):289–95.
44. Denham JW, Steigler A, Lamb DS, Joseph D, Turner S, Matthews J, *et al.* Short-term neoadjuvant androgen deprivation and radiotherapy for locally advanced prostate cancer: 10-year data from the TROG 96.01 randomised trial. Lancet Oncol. 2011 May;12(5):451–9.
45. Bolla M, Van Tienhoven G, Warde P, Dubois JB, Mirimanoff RO, Storme G, *et al.* External irradiation with or without long-term androgen suppression for prostate cancer with high metastatic risk: 10-year results of an EORTC randomised study. Lancet Oncol. 2010 Nov;11(11):1066–73.

46. Lawton CA, DeSilvio M, Roach M, Uhl V, Kirsch R, Seider M, *et al.* An update of the phase III trial comparing whole pelvic to prostate only radiotherapy and neoadjuvant to adjuvant total androgen suppression: updated analysis of RTOG 94-13, with emphasis on unexpected hormone/radiation interactions. Int J Radiat Oncol Biol Phys. 2007 Nov 1;69(3):646–55.
47. Horwitz EM, Bae K, Hanks GE, Porter A, Grignon DJ, Brereton HD, *et al.* Ten-year follow-up of radiation therapy oncology group protocol 92-02: a phase III trial of the duration of elective androgen deprivation in locally advanced prostate cancer. J Clin Oncol Off J Am Soc Clin Oncol. 2008 May 20;26(15):2497–504.
48. Bolla M, de Reijke TM, Van Tienhoven G, Van den Bergh ACM, Oddens J, Poortmans PMP, *et al.* Duration of androgen suppression in the treatment of prostate cancer. N Engl J Med. 2009 Jun 11;360(24):2516–27.
49. Pisansky TM, Hunt D, Gomella LG, Amin MB, Balogh AG, Chinn DM, *et al.* Duration of androgen suppression before radiotherapy for localized prostate cancer: radiation therapy oncology group randomized clinical trial 9910. J Clin Oncol Off J Am Soc Clin Oncol. 2015 Feb 1;33(4):332–9.
50. Nabid A, Carrier N, Vigneault E, Van Nguyen T, Vavassis P, Brassard MA, *et al.* Androgen deprivation therapy and radiotherapy in intermediate-risk prostate cancer: A randomised phase III trial. Eur J Cancer Oxf Engl 1990. 2021 Jan;143:64–74.
51. Fosså SD, Wiklund F, Klepp O, Angelsen A, Solberg A, Damber JE, *et al.* Ten-and 15-yr Prostate Cancer-specific Mortality in Patients with Nonmetastatic Locally Advanced or Aggressive Intermediate Prostate Cancer, Randomized to Lifelong Endocrine Treatment Alone or Combined with Radiotherapy: Final Results of The Scandinavian Prostate Cancer Group-7. Eur Urol. 2016 Oct;70(4):684–91.
52. Mason MD, Parulekar WR, Sydes MR, Brundage M, Kirkbride P, Gospodarowicz M, *et al.* Final Report of the Intergroup Randomized Study of Combined Androgen-Deprivation Therapy Plus Radiotherapy Versus Androgen-Deprivation Therapy Alone in Locally Advanced Prostate Cancer. J Clin Oncol Off J Am Soc Clin Oncol. 2015 Jul 1;33(19):2143–50.
53. Sargos P, Mottet N, Bellera C, Richaud P. Long-term androgen deprivation, with or without radiotherapy, in locally advanced prostate cancer: updated results from a phase III randomised trial. BJU Int. 2020 Jun;125(6):810–6.
54. Murthy V, Maitre P, Kannan S, Panigrahi G, Krishnatry R, Bakshi G, *et al.* Prostate-Only Versus Whole-Pelvic Radiation Therapy in High-Risk and Very High-Risk Prostate Cancer (POP-RT): Outcomes From Phase III Randomized Controlled Trial. J Clin Oncol Off J Am Soc Clin Oncol. 2021 Apr 10;39(11):1234–42.
55. Morris WJ, Tyldesley S, Rodda S, Halperin R, Pai H, McKenzie M, *et al.* Androgen Suppression Combined with Elective Nodal and Dose Escalated Radiation Therapy (the ASCENDE-RT Trial): An Analysis of Survival Endpoints for a Randomized Trial Comparing a Low-Dose-Rate Brachytherapy Boost to a Dose-Escalated External Beam Boost for High- and Intermediate-risk Prostate Cancer. Int J Radiat Oncol Biol Phys. 2017 Jun 1;98(2):275–85.
56. Rodda S, Tyldesley S, Morris WJ, Keyes M, Halperin R, Pai H, *et al.* ASCENDE-RT: An Analysis of Treatment-Related Morbidity for a Randomized Trial Comparing a Low-Dose-Rate Brachytherapy Boost with a Dose-Escalated External Beam Boost for High- and Intermediate-Risk Prostate Cancer. Int J Radiat Oncol Biol Phys. 2017 Jun 1;98(2):286–95.
57. Galalae RM, Kovács G, Schultze J, Loch T, Rzehak P, Wilhelm R, *et al.* Long-term outcome after elective irradiation of the pelvic lymphatics and local dose escalation using high-dose-rate brachytherapy for locally advanced prostate cancer. Int J Radiat Oncol Biol Phys. 2002 Jan 1;52(1):81–90.
58. Pieters BR, de Back DZ, Koning CCE, Zwinderman AH. Comparison of three radiotherapy modalities on biochemical control and overall survival for the treatment of prostate cancer: a systematic review. Radiother Oncol J Eur Soc Ther Radiol Oncol. 2009 Nov;93(2):168–73.
59. Parry MG, Nossiter J, Sujenthiran A, Cowling TE, Patel RN, Morris M, *et al.* Impact of High-Dose-Rate and Low-Dose-Rate Brachytherapy Boost on Toxicity, Functional and Cancer Outcomes in Patients Receiving External Beam Radiation Therapy for Prostate Cancer: A National Population-Based Study. Int J Radiat Oncol Biol Phys. 2021 Apr 1;109(5):1219–29.
60. Hoskin PJ, Rojas AM, Ostler PJ, Bryant L, Lowe GJ. Randomised trial of external-beam radiotherapy alone or with high-dose-rate brachytherapy for prostate cancer: Mature 12-year results. Radiother Oncol J Eur Soc Ther Radiol Oncol. 2021 Jan;154:214–9.
61. Joseph D, Denham JW, Steigler A, Lamb DS, Spry NA, Stanley J, *et al.* Radiation Dose Escalation or Longer Androgen Suppression to Prevent Distant Progression in Men With Locally Advanced Prostate Cancer: 10-Year Data From the TROG 03.04 RADAR Trial. Int J Radiat Oncol Biol Phys. 2020 Mar 15;106(4):693–702.
62. Jackson WC, Hartman HE, Dess RT, Birer SR, Soni PD, Hearn JWD, *et al.* Addition of Androgen-Deprivation Therapy or Brachytherapy Boost to External Beam Radiotherapy for Localized Prostate Cancer: A Network Meta-Analysis of Randomized Trials. J Clin Oncol Off J Am Soc Clin Oncol. 2020 Sep 10;38(26):3024–31.
63. Akre O. Primary Radical Prostatectomy Versus Primary Radiotherapy for Locally Advanced Prostate Cancer: an Open Randomized Clinical Trial [Internet]. clinicaltrials.gov; 2022 Mar [cited 2023 Apr 6]. Report No.: NCT02102477. Available from: https://clinicaltrials.gov/ct2/show/NCT02102477
64. Zietman AL, Shipley WU, Willett CG. Residual disease after radical surgery or radiation therapy for prostate cancer. Clinical significance and therapeutic implications. Cancer. 1993 Feb 1;71(3 Suppl):959–69.
65. Cooperberg MR, Pasta DJ, Elkin EP, Litwin MS, Latini DM, DuChane J, *et al.* The UCSF Cancer of the Prostate Risk Assessment (CAPRA) Score: a straightforward and reliable preoperative predictor of disease recurrence after radical prostatectomy. J Urol. 2005 Jun;173(6):1938–42.
66. Vale CL, Fisher D, Kneebone A, Parker C, Pearse M, Richaud P, *et al.* Adjuvant or early salvage radiotherapy for the treatment of localised and locally advanced prostate cancer: a prospectively planned systematic review and meta-analysis of aggregate data. The Lancet. 2020 Oct;396(10260):1422–31.
67. Pearse M, Fraser-Browne C, Davis ID, Duchesne GM, Fisher R, Frydenberg M, *et al.* A Phase III trial to investigate the timing of radiotherapy for prostate cancer with high-risk features: background and rationale of the Radiotherapy-Adjuvant Versus Early Salvage (RAVES) trial. BJU Int. 2014 Mar;113 Suppl 2:7–12.
68. Kneebone A, Fraser-Browne C, Delprado W, Duchesne G, Fisher R, Frydenberg M, *et al.* A Phase III Multi-Centre Randomised Trial comparing adjuvant versus early salvage Radiotherapy following a Radical Prostatectomy: Results

of the TROG 08.03 and ANZUP "RAVES" Trial. Int J Radiat Oncol Biol Phys. 2019 Sep 1;105(1):S37–8.

69. Kneebone A, Fraser-Browne C, Duchesne GM, Fisher R, Frydenberg M, Herschtal A, *et al.* Adjuvant radiotherapy versus early salvage radiotherapy following radical prostatectomy (TROG 08.03/ANZUP RAVES): a randomised, controlled, phase 3, non-inferiority trial. Lancet Oncol. 2020 Oct;21(10):1331–40.
70. ESMO 2022: Invited Discussant: Results of RADICALS-HD [Internet]. [cited 2023 Jun 27]. Available from: https://www.urotoday.com/conference-highlights/esmo-2022/esmo-2022-prostate-cancer/139519-esmo-2022-invited-discussant-lba9.html
71. Parker CC, Clarke NW, Cook AD, Kynaston HG, Petersen PM, Catton C, *et al.* Timing of radiotherapy after radical prostatectomy (RADICALS-RT): a randomised, controlled phase 3 trial. Lancet Lond Engl. 2020 Oct 31;396(10260):1413–21.
72. Carrie C, Magné N, Burban-Provost P, Sargos P, Latorzeff I, Lagrange JL, *et al.* Short-term androgen deprivation therapy combined with radiotherapy as salvage treatment after radical prostatectomy for prostate cancer (GETUG-AFU 16): a 112-month follow-up of a phase 3, randomised trial. Lancet Oncol. 2019 Dec;20(12):1740–9.
73. Burdett S, Fisher D, Parker CC, Sydes MR, Pommier P, Sargos P, *et al.* LBA64 Duration of androgen suppression with post-operative radiotherapy (DADSPORT): A collaborative meta-analysis of aggregate data. Ann Oncol. 2022 Sep;33:S1428–9.
74. Pak S, Lee DE, You D, Jeong IG, Joung JY, Lee KH, *et al.* Validation of the European association of urology biochemical recurrence risk groups after radical prostatectomy in an Asian cohort and suggestions for refinement. Urol Oncol. 2021 May;39(5):298.e1-298.e6.
75. Tilki D, Preisser F, Graefen M, Huland H, Pompe RS. External Validation of the European Association of Urology Biochemical Recurrence Risk Groups to Predict Metastasis and Mortality After Radical Prostatectomy in a European Cohort. Eur Urol. 2019 Jun;75(6):896–900.
76. Immediate versus deferred treatment for advanced prostatic cancer: initial results of the Medical Research Council Trial. The Medical Research Council Prostate Cancer Working Party Investigators Group. Br J Urol. 1997 Feb;79(2):235–46.
77. Pound CR, Partin AW, Eisenberger MA, Chan DW, Pearson JD, Walsh PC. Natural history of progression after PSA elevation following radical prostatectomy. JAMA. 1999 May 5;281(17):1591–7.
78. Ventimiglia E, Seisen T, Abdollah F, Briganti A, Fonteyne V, James N, *et al.* A Systematic Review of the Role of Definitive Local Treatment in Patients with Clinically Lymph Node-positive Prostate Cancer. Eur Urol Oncol. 2019 May;2(3):294–301.
79. Bryant AK, Kader AK, McKay RR, Einck JP, Mell LK, Mundt AJ, *et al.* Definitive Radiation Therapy and Survival in Clinically Node-Positive Prostate Cancer. Int J Radiat Oncol Biol Phys. 2018 Aug 1;101(5):1188–93.
80. Sarkar RR, Bryant AK, Parsons JK, Ryan ST, Karim Kader A, Kane CJ, *et al.* Association between Radical Prostatectomy and Survival in Men with Clinically Node-positive Prostate Cancer. Eur Urol Oncol. 2019 Sep;2(5):584–8.
81. Tward JD, Kokeny KE, Shrieve DC. Radiation therapy for clinically node-positive prostate adenocarcinoma is correlated with improved overall and prostate cancer-specific survival. Pract Radiat Oncol. 2013;3(3):234–40.
82. Lin CC, Gray PJ, Jemal A, Efstathiou JA. Androgen deprivation with or without radiation therapy for clinically node-positive prostate cancer. J Natl Cancer Inst. 2015 Jul;107(7):djv119.
83. Seisen T, Vetterlein MW, Karabon P, Jindal T, Sood A, Nocera L, *et al.* Efficacy of Local Treatment in Prostate Cancer Patients with Clinically Pelvic Lymph Node-positive Disease at Initial Diagnosis. Eur Urol. 2018 Mar;73(3):452–61.
84. James ND, Spears MR, Clarke NW, Dearnaley DP, Mason MD, Parker CC, *et al.* Failure-Free Survival and Radiotherapy in Patients With Newly Diagnosed Nonmetastatic Prostate Cancer: Data From Patients in the Control Arm of the STAMPEDE Trial. JAMA Oncol. 2016 Mar;2(3):348–57.
85. Fischer-Valuck BW, Rao YJ, Brenneman RJ, Patel PR, Filson CP, Jani AB, *et al.* Overall survival comparison between androgen deprivation therapy (ADT) plus external beam radiation therapy (EBRT) vs ADT plus EBRT with brachytherapy boost in clinically node-positive prostate cancer. Brachytherapy. 2020;19(5):557–66.
86. Moschini M, Briganti A, Murphy CR, Bianchi M, Gandaglia G, Montorsi F, *et al.* Outcomes for Patients with Clinical Lymphadenopathy Treated with Radical Prostatectomy. Eur Urol. 2016 Feb;69(2):193–6.
87. James ND, Spears MR, Clarke NW, Dearnaley DP, Mason MD, Parker CC, *et al.* Failure-Free Survival and Radiotherapy in Patients With Newly Diagnosed Nonmetastatic Prostate Cancer: Data From Patients in the Control Arm of the STAMPEDE Trial. JAMA Oncol. 2016 Mar;2(3):348–57.
88. James ND, de Bono JS, Spears MR, Clarke NW, Mason MD, Dearnaley DP, *et al.* Abiraterone for Prostate Cancer Not Previously Treated with Hormone Therapy. N Engl J Med. 2017 Jul 27;377(4):338–51.
89. Vale CL, Burdett S, Rydzewska LHM, Albiges L, Clarke NW, Fisher D, *et al.* Addition of docetaxel or bisphosphonates to standard of care in men with localised or metastatic, hormone-sensitive prostate cancer: a systematic review and meta-analyses of aggregate data. Lancet Oncol. 2016 Feb;17(2):243–56.
90. Attard G, Murphy L, Clarke NW, Cross W, Jones RJ, Parker CC, *et al.* Abiraterone acetate and prednisolone with or without enzalutamide for high-risk non-metastatic prostate cancer: a meta-analysis of primary results from two randomised controlled phase 3 trials of the STAMPEDE platform protocol. Lancet Lond Engl. 2022 Jan 29;399(10323):447–60.
91. Hou Z, Li G, Bai S. High dose versus conventional dose in external beam radiotherapy of prostate cancer: a meta-analysis of long-term follow-up. J Cancer Res Clin Oncol. 2015 Jun 1;141(6):1063–71.
92. Miller LE, Efstathiou JA, Bhattacharyya SK, Payne HA, Woodward E, Pinkawa M. Association of the Placement of a Perirectal Hydrogel Spacer With the Clinical Outcomes of Men Receiving Radiotherapy for Prostate Cancer: A Systematic Review and Meta-analysis. JAMA Netw Open. 2020 Jun 17;3(6):e208221.
93. Melchert C, Gez E, Bohlen G, Scarzello G, Koziol I, Anscher M, *et al.* Interstitial biodegradable balloon for reduced rectal dose during prostate radiotherapy: Results of a virtual planning investigation based on the pre-and post-implant imaging data of an international multicenter study. Radiother Oncol. 2013 Feb;106(2):210–4.
94. Noyes WR, Hosford CC, Schultz SE. Human Collagen Injections to Reduce Rectal Dose During Radiotherapy. Int J Radiat Oncol. 2012 Apr;82(5):1918–22.

Chapter

4

Metastatic Hormone-sensitive Prostate Cancer

• Sanjai Kumar Addla • Amaresh Mohan

Abbreviations

- ADT: Androgen deprivation therapy
- API: Androgen receptor pathway inhibitors
- mHSPC: Metastatic hormone-sensitive prostate cancer
- PCa: Prostate cancer
- PSMA: Prostate-specific membrane antigen
- SABR: Stereotactic ablative radiotherapy

LEARNING OBJECTIVES

- To understand the principles of workup and imaging of mHSPC and current role of the PSMA PET scan: PSMA PET scan is single investigation that can aid a comprehensive diagnosis of metastatic ca prostate. PSMA PET is more sensitive in diagnosis of metastatic disease though the traditional imaging of bone scan and CT scan are better at prognostication of disease.
- To understand the prognostic factors and algorithms related to mHSPC: After initiation of initial treatment, clinicians need to understand how well the patient is going to respond to the therapy and when is he likely to need the next line of treatment.
- To understand the risk stratification based on the volume/risk of the disease: Volume of metastatic disease helps the clinician determine the intensity of initial treatment, course of future management and probability of use of local therapy.
- To understand the acute presentation of metastatic prostate cancer and the standard of care at presentation: Metastatic cancer prostate can present with spinal cord compression, bladder outlet obstruction and obstructive uropathy. Managing these emergencies are critical to the long-term outcomes of these patients.
- To understand the role of ADT: Are they all same? There are different types of medical and surgical castration modalities available, how do they compare with each other in terms of the efficacy and outcomes is important to understand for the urologist.
- To understand the novel combination treatment regimens: Doublet and Triplet therapy. Using more than one drug or modality at the outset is the current standard of care in the treatment of metastatic prostate cancer. Choice of the combination and whether three prong approach is better than doublet needs to be reviewed.
- To understand the current role of chemotherapy in the era of novel androgen pathway inhibitors: Chemotherapeutic agents have been used in metastatic cancer prostate for a long time now, with the increasing use of androgen pathway inhibitors its role and positioning needs to be redefined.
- To understand the importance of bone protective agents to prevent skeletal-related events: Metastatic cancer prostate is a high risk situations for skeletal related events and this is further increased by addition of ADT, therefore, understanding the role of bone protective agents is critical for a urologist.

Case Scenario 1

A 63 years old male, ECOG PS 1, with well-controlled hypertension and diabetes was evaluated for LUTS and was found to have an elevated sPSA of 28 ng/ml. Multi-parametric MRI was suggestive of a left PZ lesion from apex to base. TRUS-guided prostate biopsy showed adenocarcinoma of prostatic origin, Gleason grade group 3. Bone scan was suggestive of 3 spinal lesions (T10, L2, L3) and 1 near the left iliac crest.

1. **What is the next preferred imaging?**

   Ans: The next preferred investigation would be a PSMA PET/CT, this will help risk stratify the patient. PSMA PET/CT scan has better sensitivity and specificity compared to conventional cross-section imaging with CT/MRI and bone scan combined.[1]

2. **What are the various radiopharmaceuticals available to detect PCa metastases? Kindly brief about PSMA PET.**

   Ans: Table 4.1 shows the various radiopharmaceuticals available to a urologist.

TABLE: 4.1: Various radiopharmaceuticals used in Ca prostate[2]

Radiopharmaceuticals	*Target*	*Half life (min)*	*Strength*	*Weakness*	*Availability in India*
^{18}F-FDG	Glucose metabolism	100	Tracer activity may identify highly aggressive tumors	Poor performance in PCa, Prostate cancer cells are not glucose avid	Yes
^{11}C and ^{18}F-choliine	Cell membrane turnover	20	Can be utilised in both soft tissue and bone disease	Limited sensitivity for liver metastases detection because of high tracer uptake in the normal liver	Yes
^{68}Ga-PSMA	Cell membrane protein expressed in PCa	68	High sensitivity in the detection of nodal disease, promising detection rates in prostate cancer with low PSA or PSA doubling time	Limited evidence from literature on real impact on patient survival. PSMA expression is increased in anti-androgen therapy	Yes
^{18}F-PSMA	Cell membrane protein expressed in PCa	110	^{18}F-PSMA helps detect local recurrence or spread to pelvic nodes more readily as lesions are not masked by physiological urinary excretion	PSMA expression is not specific to the prostate	Yes
^{18}F-NaF	Bone turnover	109.7	High sensitivity for bone metastases detection	Bone disease specific, cannot be used to assess soft tissue disease	Yes
^{18}F-Fluciclovine	Sodium dependent amino acid transporter	109	High target to background ratio with no marked adjacent bladder accumulation. Superior to the performance of FDG	Potential false negative interpretations include low PSA levels (<1ng/ml), dense sclerotic bone metastases and early bladder activity.	No

PSMA is a transmembrane glycoprotein that is naturally present in prostate epithelial cells, renal tubular cells, celiac ganglia, and salivary glands. Because PSMA is selectively over-expressed in prostate cancer, it is a trustworthy tissue marker for staging and restaging prostate cancer. A rise in PSMA expression (measured as SUV max) is associated with higher PSA, higher tumour grade, cancer progression, and cancer relapse.

In a recent meta-analysis, Gallium-68-PSMA PET/CT demonstrated better diagnostic performance in PCa patients. The authors concluded that the majority of lymph node metastases, lung metastases, and liver metastases overexpressed PSMA, which could be directly detected.[3] Recently published results of the ProPSMA study showed the superiority of PSMA-PET/CT over conventional imaging (area under the curve of the receiver operating characteristic curve 91% vs. 59% [32% absolute difference; 28–35] for patients with pelvic nodal metastases, and 95% vs. 74% [22% absolute difference; 18–26] for patients with distant metastases.[4]

Whilst not being mentioned in the guidelines, PSMA-PET/CT is the current standard of staging investigation in India. It has been designated as the "**one-stop test**" for advanced prostate cancer because of its superior sensitivity and specificity for identifying locoregional lymph node metastases (typically 10 mm), distant visceral, and bony metastasis.

3. What is the sensitivity of a bone scan in detecting PCa bone metastases?

Ans: Bone scan (BS) has a sensitivity of 70% for detecting bony metastasis. Positive lesion on a bone scan indicates osteoblastic reaction to the presence of tumour cells. The sensitivity can be increased by using single photon emission computerised tomography (SPECT) to 87–92%.[5] 85% of prostate cancer (PCa) metastases involve the axial skeleton. A substantial correlation exists between the level of alkaline phosphatase (ALP), which is elevated in 70% of cases, and the extent of bone involvement.

The most commonly used technique for assessing bone metastases is the ^{99}Tc-MDP bone scan. The clinical stage, Gleason score, and PSA level all have a big impact on the diagnostic yield. In low-risk individuals (D'Amico low risk group), the rate of BS positive is extremely low (less than 1%), and it rises with more advanced stages of prostate cancer (stage >T3, PSA> 20, and Gleason score >7).[6] Independent of PSA level, Gleason score, or clinical stage, BS as an investigation should be considered in any symptomatic individuals.

PET/CT with ^{18}F-sodium fluoride offers higher sensitivity than BS for bony metastasis. Compared to a combined bone scan, targeted radiography, and abdominopelvic CT, diffusion-weighted whole-body and axial MRI are more sensitive and specific. In a prospective multi-centric study for high risk prostate cancers (ProPSMA) accuracy of ^{68}Ga-PSMA-PET/CT was 27% higher than that of CT and bone scintigraphy.[5]

Case Scenario *(Contd.)*

A PSMA-PET/CT scan was done in this patient confirming PSMA avid lesions in the 3 vertebrae (T10, L2, and L3) and 1 near the left iliac crest. No evidence of visceral disease.

4. How should we categorize the patient and counsel regarding further treatment?

Ans: The patient should be risk stratified based on CHAARTED criteria for low/high volume disease (Table 4.5). The description and the classification is based on conventional imaging with a CT/MRI and bone scan. PSMA-PET/CT findings are used in India for risk stratification, though this has not been validated in any study. Based on PSMA-PET scan this case can be categorised as of *de-novo* low-volume metastatic disease. As per NCCN and EAU guidelines, the patient should be counselled for systemic treatment with ADT. The add-on treatment in addition to ADT includes:

1. Local treatment of the primary with EBRT
2. Androgen pathway inhibitors like Abiraterone (+ Prednisolone)
3. Androgen receptor blockers in the form of Enzalutamide or Apalutamide
4. Chemotherapy in the form of 6 cycles of intravenous Docetaxel.

The use of EBRT as local therapy along with systemic therapy in mHSPC is based out of the results of the STAMPEDE trial where the use of EBRT for low volume disease was found to show significant improvement in overall survival and progression free survival compared to ADT alone.[7]

5. What should the patient be advised regarding ADT?

Ans: The standard of care for metastatic prostate cancer is lifelong androgen deprivation therapy (ADT). Prostate cancer cell proliferation is mostly induced by testosterone. The objective of ADT in various forms is to achieve castration levels of serum testosterone (<50 ng/ml). Patient should be counselled regarding both surgical and medical castration.

Bilateral orchiectomy: Bilateral orchiectomy (surgical castration) rapidly reduces (in 12–24 hours) serum testosterone to castrate levels. This is a simple and cost-effective procedure. Surgical castration is indicated when an urgent castration level of testosterone needs to be achieved or when the ADT is required on a life-long basis. The orchiectomy is usually done through a scrotal incision and can be a complete orchiectomy, sub-capsular or sub-epididymal. Though the cosmetic outcomes slightly different, the overall efficacy of all the three types of orchiectomy seems to be same.

Medical castration: Medical castration reduces the production of testosterone through its effects on the hypothalamic-pituitary axis. Gonadotropin-releasing hormone (GnRH) agonist or antagonist can be considered for medical castration. Antiandrogens (bicalutamide) are usually combined for 2–3 weeks with GnRH agonist to prevent the flare phenomenon, which can lead to the initial worsening of disease, especially in cases of spinal cord compression or urinary tract obstruction.

Leuprolide, goserelin and triptorelin are various types of GnRH agonists available for use (Table 4.2). GnRH antagonist (degarelix) directly suppresses testosterone production and avoids the flare phenomenon seen with use of GnRH agonists. GnRH antagonist can be considered in place of GnRH agonist when a rapid fall in testosterone levels is desired as is the case of spinal cord compression secondary to PC metastasis to vertebra and also in patients with cardiovascular and cerebrovascular comorbidity. In a randomised trial comparing GnRH agonist

TABLE 4.2 : Various LHRH agonist

Drug	*Route*	*Dosage*
Leuprolide depot	Intramuscular/ subcutaneous	22.5 mg three monthly, 45 mg six monthly
Triptorelin	Intramuscular	12.25 mg three monthly, 22.5 mg six monthly
Goserelin	Subcutaneous	10.8 mg three monthly
Degarelix	Subcutaneous	240 mg (stat dose) followed by 80 mg monthly

and antagonist for advanced prostate cancer the absolute risk reduction in major cardiovascular and cerebrovascular events at 12 months using GnRH antagonist was 18.1% (95% CI 4.6–31.2, p=0.032).[8]

6. **Does medical and surgical castration achieve equal effect?**

   Ans: Seidenfeld et al performed a meta-analysis of 24 RCTs of hormone therapy involving >6600 patients with advanced prostate cancer. Of these, 12 trials of LHRH agonists were included in the estimation of overall survival hazard ratios (HRs) relative to orchiectomy, using a comparative analysis method that allowed inclusion of trials that did not incorporate an orchiectomy arm (3 trials). The overall HR for survival with LHRH agonists relative to orchiectomy was 1.262 (95% confidence intervals [CI] 0.915–1.386) suggesting that LHRH agonists are essentially equivalent to orchiectomy in terms of overall survival.[9]

7. **Are all agonist equal in terms of survival and functional outcomes?**

   Ans: Head to head comparison of the LHRH agonist tell us that they are equally effective. In a comparative analysis of leuprolide and triptorelin at the end of 9 months, the ability to maintain castration levels of testosterone was similar.[10]

8. **Is there any role of maximal androgen blockage (MAB) in today's day and age?**

   Ans: There is currently, no role of MAB in the era of doublet and triplet therapy, even when these treatments were not available, MAB offered a modest advantage.
   - In 2000, the Prostate Cancer Trialists' Collaborative Group (PCTCG) published a meta-analysis of all the available trials of MAB versus monotherapy. The analysis included 27 trials, which incorporated 8275 men. This represented 98% of all patients ever randomised in trials of combination therapy versus monotherapy.
   - The overall survival at 5 years, for all patients receiving combination therapy, was 25.4% compared with 23.6% for patients receiving monotherapy. This equates to a 1.8% improvement but was not statistically significant.[11]

9. **What are the common side effects of ADT?**

   Ans: Common side effects of ADT are shown in Table 4.3.

TABLE 4.3 : Side effects of ADT

Symptom	*Incidence*	*Management*
Hot flushes	Very common	Can be mitigated by use of medications such as venlafaxine or gabapentin.
Osteoporosis	Very common	Long-term calcium/vitamin D supplementation is necessary along with bisphosphonates/ denosumab in selected patients
Fatigue	Very common	Anaemia correction and regular exercise is beneficial
Depression	Common	SSRI
Gynecomastia	Common	Tamoxifen/radiotherapy
Erectile dysfunction/loss of libido	Common	Referral to sexual health counselling
Metabolic syndrome	Common	Endocrinology consult, diet and exercise
Dementia	Less frequent	Encourage mentally engaging activities
Thromboembolic disease	Less frequent	Close monitoring
Cardiovasular disease	Less frequent	Primary and secondary prevention

10. **What is the role of local treatment in an oligo-metastatic setting?**

    Ans: ADT can be combined with non-curative prostate radiotherapy (using doses up to the equivalent of 72 Gy at 2 Gy per fraction) in patients with *de novo* low-volume metastatic disease. The STAMPEDE (H-Arm) study showed in a subgroup analysis that prostate radiotherapy (36 Gy/6#/6 days and 55 Gy/20#/4 weeks were the schedules used) showed improved failure-free survival in patients with low metastatic burden at baseline. However, similar evidence is not available for surgery in a metastatic setting. One cannot extrapolate these results to radical prostatectomy.

11. **How can we compare the three drugs as a first line in mHSPC?**

    Ans: Docetaxel
    - Works well with liver metastasis and other visceral metastasis
    - Only 6 cycles
    - No need for steroids
    - Cost-effective,

    Abiraterone
    - Good OS benefit in both low and high volume disease
    - Oral daily dosing therapy
    - Diabetes and hypertension may be difficult to control

    Enzalutamide
    - Good toxicity profile
    - Can be safely administered in frail patients.

There are neurological side effects. It may potentiates seizures in a patient at risk of seizure disorder. Intolerance may be a major reason for discontinuation of the drug.

12. **What is the current role of metastases-directed therapy (MDT)?**

Ans: The usage of MDT in current clinical practice is experimental. Currently, there are four recruiting or ongoing trials evaluating the role of MDT in patients with *de novo* oligo-metastatic HSPC.

1. **Phase II single-arm study (NCT03298087)** will assess the impact of stereotactic body radiotherapy directed to the metastasis in patients with 1 to 5 metastases on imaging (PSMA-PET/CT included). It will assess the effect of PSA levels at 6 months after treatment.
2. **The PLATON trial (NCT03784755),** a randomized phase III trial, will test if stereotactic body radiotherapy directed to the metastasis, in addition to systemic and/or local therapy, in patients with less than 5 metastases improves failure-free survival.
3. **The multi-arm phase II METACURE trial (NCT03436654)** includes patients from very high-risk localized to low-volume metastatic PCa, defined by less than 3 bone lesions based on conventional imaging that can be treated with radiation.

   The arms include combinations of ADT + apalutamide ± abiraterone acetate and prednisone, and the primary endpoint is pathologic complete response and minimal residual disease at radical prostatectomy. However, the secondary endpoint is undetectable PSA with non-castrate levels of testosterone, and patients with low-volume disease will further be treated with stereotactic radiotherapy.
4. Arm **M of STAMPEDE** will further clarify the role of MDT in mHSPC (oligometastatic hormone sensitive cancer prostate). Arm M will not only test if surgery as local treatment is similar to radiotherapy as a local treatment option in om HSPC but also test if the addition of stereotactic ablative body radiotherapy (SABR) to metastatic sites further improves overall survival. Arm M will exclusively consist of oligometastatic (less than 5 extra pelvic metastases) patients, relying on bone and CT scan.[12]

Trial	*Number of metastasis included*	*Imaging used*	*Modality used for treatment of metastasis*
NCT03298087	1–5	PSMA PET/CT/ bone scan	Stereotactic radiotherapy
PLATON trial	1–5	CT/MRI/bone scan	Stereotactic radiotherapy
METACURE trial	1–3	CT/bone scan	Stereotactic radiotherapy
STAMPEDE (M Arm)	1–5	CT/bone scan	Stereotactic radiotherapy

Case Scenario *(Contd.)*

The patient was started on ADT with LHRH agonist + Abiraterone 1g/day. His nadir PSA was 0.03. After 2 years of (ADT+ Abi), his PSA started rising to 3.2 ng/ml. Bone scan showed no new bone lesions, at this point,he was started on enzalutamide 160 mg/day. After 3 months his PSA was 6.9 ng/ml. Ga 68 PSMA-PET/CT-scan was suggestive of multiple small lesions in the liver.

13. **If the PSA would not have progressed, could we have stopped Abiraterone after 2 years?**

Ans: There is no consensus about when to stop abiraterone in the absence of PSA progression. One should tailor the treatment duration based on multiple factors including efficacy, any impact on blood pressure, electrolytes, liver function test, adverse reactions and lastly financial aspects into consideration.

14. **What is the absolute advantage of using 2 drugs over only ADT?**

Ans: Results of the latitude trial after a median follow-up of 30.4 months at a planned interim analysis the median overall survival was significantly longer in the abiraterone group than in the placebo group (not reached vs. 34.7 months) (hazard ratio for death, 0.62; 95% confidence interval [CI], 0.51 to 0.76; P<0.001). The median length of radiographic progression-free survival was 33.0 months in the abiraterone group and 14.8 months in the placebo group (hazard ratio for disease progression or death, 0.47; 95% CI, 0.39 to 0.55; P<0.001).

15. **How to monitor and follow-up this patient?**

Ans: Patient should be subjected to history, physical examination and PSA every 3 months.

16. **After initiation of ADT, PSA at which months has prognostic value in this patient?**

Ans: PSA at 7 months after starting ADT has prognostic value.

PSA after 7 months after start of ADT	Median survival on ADT monotherapy
< 0.2 ng/ml	75 months
0.2 < 4 ng/ml	44 months
> 4 ng/ml	13 months

17. What is the overall response rate when we shift from one API to other?

Ans: Results of the famous Kyoto Baltimore Study favours abiraterone-to-enzalutamide sequence over enzalutamide-to-abiraterone in terms of both efficacy and combined prostate-specific antigen progression-free survival, although no differences in overall survival were observed. Similar results were observed in study by Kim Chi *et al.*[13,14]

18. What are the treatment options for this patient?

Ans: The patient should be counselled about his progressing disease and further treatment intensification with docetaxel chemotherapy.

19. What are the side effects of chemotherapy?

Ans: Chemotherapy-related side effects are: Allergic reactions, fatigue, diarrhoea, stomatitis, motor neuropathy, sensory neuropathy, thromboembolism, and febrile neutropenia.[15]

Case Scenario 2

A 72 years old male patient, hypertensive on medications underwent a robotic radical prostatectomy in July 2019. Histopathology was adenocarcinoma Gleason grade group 3, non-focal EPE (pT3aNo) with negative surgical margins. On follow-up, the patient developed biochemical recurrence in May 2020 and received salvage RT + short-term ADT. Later the patient was lost to follow-up for 2 years during the Covid pandemic.

Serum PSA was 3.3 ng/ml. Bone scan and CECT abdomen was normal. After 3 months serum PSA was 7.1 ng/ml. PSMA-PET/CT scan was suggestive of PSMA avid lesions in the D5, and D7 vertebral bodies and left iliac bone.

1. How to categorize this patient?

Ans: This is a case of metachronous low-volume hormone-sensitive metastatic prostate cancer.

2. What is the current role of conventional imaging (bone scan + CT/MRI) versus PSMA-PET/CT scan?

Ans: All the trials to date have used conventional imaging (BS + CT). However, in the recent systematic review the diagnostic accuracy on a per-patient basis, measured as the area under the curve (AUC), was significantly higher for PSMA-targeted PET/CT (0.99; 95%CI: 0.96–1.00) compared to bone scintigraphy (0.85; 95%CI: 0.81–0.87). Interestingly, PSMA-targeted PET/CT correctly identified bone metastases in 22.3% of patients with negative bone scintigraphy, whereas bone scintigraphy correctly identified bone metastases in a limited percentage (1.9%) of patients with negative PSMA-targeted PET/CT findings. Bone scintigraphy is clearly inferior to PSMA-targeted PET in terms of diagnostic accuracy for detecting PC bone metastases.[16]

3. What is the role of ADT intensification in this patient?

Ans: The data on treatment recurrent mHSPC is not as strong as *de novo* mHSPC. This patient has a rapidly doubling serum PSA (<10 months). I would counsel regarding ADT + API doublet (Abiraterone 1g or enzalutamide 160 mg).

4. How to follow these patients?

Ans: Follow-up includes clinical examination, serum PSA, radiological imaging. Patients on abiraterone acetate, regular monitoring of blood pressure, liver function tests, electrolytes and lipid profile is required in view of the usage of steroid (5 mg of prednisolone).

5. What is the role of metastases-directed therapy in this setting?

Ans: STOMP is the only phase II study that enrolled 62 patients with a median follow-up of 3 years and showed a median ADT-free survival of 21 months for the MDT group vs. 13 months for the surveillance group which was statistically insignificant but with no improvement in OS.[17] The idea of MDT is to delay palliative morbid ADT and chemotherapy in this subset of patients. The recent results of ORIOLE confirmed significant improvement in PFS in favour of MDT.[18] The use of stereotactic radiotherapy in bone in oligometastases is safe with minimal toxicity and has excellent results in local control and PFS, delaying the start of the next systemic therapy.[19]

Case Scenario 3

A 63 years male with DM, HTN, CAD post-PTCA 5 years back on dual antiplatelet drugs, good ECOG performance status presented with recent onset diffuse bone pains. The patient was evaluated and found to have serum PSA of 653 ng/ml. PSMA-PET/CT scan was suggestive of PSMA/avid lesions involving both the axial and appendicular skeleton, multiple lesions in the liver.

1. How would you work up this patient? What is the role of a prostate biopsy?

Ans: This is a case of *de novo* high volume metastatic prostatic cancer. The patient needs to undergo a TRUS-guided prostate biopsy which is mandatory for confirmation of malignancy and to rule out a neuroendocrine dedifferentiation and also for medico-legal purposes. However, minimal number of cores can be taken to confirm the diagnosis.

2. **TRUS biopsy is reported as adenocarcinoma-Gleason group 5 (5+5). How would you manage this patient?**

   Ans: Firstly, IHC has to be performed to rule out de-differentiation. If the patient has good performance status (PS), I would counsel regarding ADT intensification with triplet therapy.

3. **Would you offer watchful waiting as an option of treatment modality?**

   Ans: No. Watchful waiting is not an option in metastatic prostate carcinoma especially in a symptomatic patient with poorly differentiated type of prostate cancer. The patient has good performance status, hence watchful waiting is not an option for this patient. The option of watchful waiting in the metastatic setting is offered to elderly, unfit and asymptomatic patients.

4. **What would be the ideal line of treatment? Sequential or combined? What would be the survival benefit in terms of OS and PFS with each line of treatment?**

   Ans: Based on the results from PEACE-1 and ARASENS, patient should be counselled regarding the triplet therapy.

   In view of previous cardiac intervention, LHRH antagonist should be preferred over agonist for ADT in this setting.

   Overall treatment would include ADT + Abiraterone 1 g + Prednisolone 5 mg + Docetaxel (6 cycles).

5. **What is the role of doing liver function test in this patient?**

   Ans: Patient has multiple liver lesions. LFT is important prior to starting medication as both docetaxel and abiraterone get excreted through liver.

6. **What are the trials advocating the intensification of ADT in high volume/risk mHSPC?**

   Ans: Table 4.4 showing trials using doublet, triplet and RT for metastatic hormone sensitive cancer prostate. Figure 4.1 showing median OS with various regimens for metastatic hormone sensitive prostate cancer.

7. **What are the landmark trials advocating the benefit of chemo-hormonal therapy in high volume/risk mHSPC?**

   Ans: GETUG-15, CHAARTED, STAMPEDE, PEACE 1, ARASENS

TABLE 4.4: Use of intensive ADT

ADT	*Trials*
• Chemotherapy	• **Docetaxel:** GETUG-15,CHAART-ED, and STAMPEDE arm C
• Androgen synthesis inhibitor	• **Abiraterone + Prednisolone:** Latitude and STAMPEDE Arm G
• Potent androgen receptor inhibitor	• **Enzalutamide:** ENZAMET and ARCHES • **Apalutamide :** TITAN
• Radiation to the primary prostate tumour	• **External beam radiation therapy:** HORRAD,STAMPEDE
• Potent anti-androgen chemotherapy (triple therapy)	• **Abiraterone + docetaxel + –RT:** PEACE-1 • **Darolutamide + prednisolone** • **Docetaxel:** ARASENS

8. **What are the two landmark trials advocating the benefit of androgen pathway inhibitors in mHSPC as doublet therapy?**

   Ans: LATITUDE, STAMPEDE Arm G.

9. **What are the two landmark trials published recently regarding triplet therapy?**

   Ans: PEACE-1, ARASENS

10. **What are the ideal dosage of each drug and the timing of each drug?**

    Ans:

    Docetaxel: Injectable: 75 mg/m^2—six: 3 weekly doses

    Abiraterone: 1 g OD/day (on empty stomach) + Prednisolone: 5 mg

    Apalutamide (oral tablets): 240 mg/day

    Enzalutamide (oral tablets): 160 mg OD/day

    Daroluamide (oral tablets): 600 mg BD/day

11. **Is there a role of local therapy in this patient?**

    Ans: This is a case of high volume disease. Currently, no evidence supporting any form of local therapy for survival benefit, though RT can be used for alleviation of bony pain and local symptoms. As per the results of STAMPEDE trial there was no benefit in terms of overall survival and progression free survival by addition of local EBRT in a case of high volume mHSPC.[20]

Case Scenario 4

A 64 years old male nil co-morbid was evaluated for obstructive LUTS. Serum PSA was 11 ng/ml. mpMRI suggestive of right PZ lesion in the mid-gland level. TRUS biopsy of the prostate suggestive of adenocarcinoma Gleason grade 2. PSMA PET scan suggestive of PSMA avid prostate primary with bilateral internal iliac LN and 2 cm para-aortic LN. No other metastases.

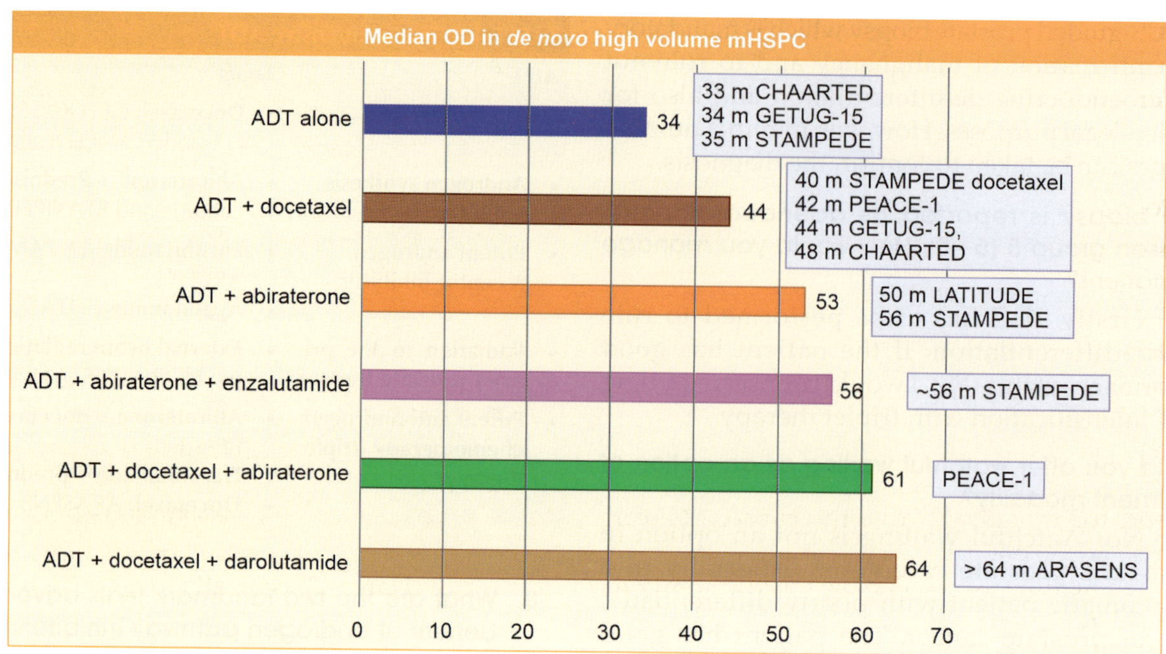

Fig. 4.1: Median OS with various regimens for metastatic hormone sensitive cancer prostate

1. **How to categorize this patient?**
   Answer: This is a case of *de novo* low-volume metastatic prostate cancer (M1a)
2. **What are the treatment options as per the current evidence?**
   Answer: Treatment of the primary with local RT + ADT + Abiraterone(1g)+ Prednisolone 5 mg the present standard of care
3. **What is the role of cytoreductive prostatectomy?**
   Ans: Moschini et al reported that cytoreductive prostatectomy (CRP) could lead to good outcomes in terms of complications and functional results. However, no survival benefit has been demonstrated for surgical patients when compared with those treated with ADT only.[21]

   One prospective randomized phase 2 trial was published after a median follow-up of 28 months where the authors reported an improved radiographic progression-free survival for the group with local therapy.[22]

   Recent studies suggest that cytoreductive surgery is safe and feasible, and may confer certain survival benefits to prostate cancer patients with oligometastatic disease. However, additional large-scale prospective randomized controlled trials will be essential to validate these results and to establish the overall benefit of such treatment to the quality of life of patients suffering from this form of cancer.[23,24] The results of the ongoing trials likely to answer the benefits of CRP would be SWOG 1802 which is a randomised phase III trial of standardised systemic therapy (SST) or SST plus definitive treatment of primary tumor in metastatic prostate cancer.
4. **What is the role of neo-adjuvant hormone therapy prior to RP?**
   Ans: At present, neoadjuvant therapy is not recommended prior to RP in men with clinically localized high-risk prostate cancer outside of a clinical trial. Robust studies including long-term oncologic outcomes will be required to establish a role for initial systemic therapy in the management of clinically localized high-risk prostate cancer. Radiotherapy with neoadjuvant/concurrent/adjuvant ADT. Thus, the current standard of care includes RP or radiotherapy with neoadjuvant/concurrent/adjuvant ADT.[25]

Case Scenario 5

A 76 years old male diabetic, old CVA on antiplatelet drugs with recent onset bilateral lower limb weakness and acute urinary retention. The patient was catheterized and evaluated elsewhere. Serum PSA was found to be 2100 ng/ml. MRI of dorsolumbar spine suggestive of cord compression at the D9 vertebral level. ECOG PS3.

1. **How to manage this patient?**
   Ans: This is a case of high volume metastatic prostate cancer with cord compression. He needs a high dose of IV steroids (dexamethasone 16 mg stat and 8 mg TID)
   a. **What is the preferred modality of ADT?**
      Ans: GnRH antagonist with Degarelix 240 mg or orchidectomy will be options in

this situation. Both these options cause rapid decline in serum testosterone to castrate levels. Considering the acute nature of the illness, it is better to go ahead with the least invasive option, i.e GNRH antagonist.

b. **Role of prostate biopsy—is it mandatory?**

Ans: Once the patient is stabilized, patient can be planned for TRUS guided prostate biopsy and imaging.

c. **How to manage if the patient cannot afford degarelix and no prostate biopsy report is available? What is the role of orchidectomy/ketoconazole in this scenario?**

Ans: We can do a two-core prostate biopsy and send for frozen to prove the cancer. We can proceed to bilateral scrotal orchidectomy at the same time. Ketoconazole has the ability to get the testosterone levels in the castrate range very quickly. However, due to its adverse effects such as hepatotoxicity it is currently not used.

d. **What is the role of immediate surgical decompression?**

Ans: Spinal cord compression is an acute surgical emergency. Urgent neurosurgeon consultation should be obtained after the administration of steroids.

2. **How to further evaluate this patient?**

Ans: Once patient is stabilized TRUS-guided prostate biopsy can be done. A bone scan or PSMA PET/CT scan should be done to risk stratify the disease.

3. **What is the role of RT to the spine in this patient?**

Ans: RT to the spine could be considered as an option if neurosurgical intervention is not appropriate.

4. **What is the role of ADT intensification?**

Ans: The performance status of the patient is poor. ADT alone would be sufficient. Once the patient is stable, one can consider adding androgen pathway inhibitors.

5. **What is the role of bone-strengthening agents?**

Ans: The skeletal system is the most predominant site of metastasis from prostate cancer. Zoledronic acid and denosumab prevent bone loss and thereby delay skeletal-related events such as osteoporosis and pathological fractures. The adverse effects of these drugs are hypocalcaemia and osteonecrosis of the mandible. One needs to monitor serum calcium and offer calcium and vitamin D supplementation when prescribing either of these medications.

6. **Which kind of regimen will you use under different circumstances of mHSPC?**

Ans: The approach should be tailored to the disease:

- Synchronous (*de novo*): High volume metastatic disease in a fit patient: Triplet therapy (ADT + Abi/Daro+ Docetaxel) (Table 4.5).

TABLE 4.5: The definition of high volume

	High	*Low*
CHAARTED (volume)	≥ 4 bone metastases including ≥ 1 outside vertebral column or pelvis **AND/OR** Visceral metastasis	Not high
LATITUDE (risk)	≥ 2 high-risk features of: • ≥ 3 Bone metastasis • Visceral metastasis • ≥ ISUP grade 4	Not high

- Synchronous (*de novo*): Low volume metastatic disease in a fit patient: Individualized (doublet therapy + local RT)
- Metachronous (Recurrent): High volume metastatic disease in a fit patient: Individualized (rare but true)
- Metachronous (Recurrent): Low volume metastatic disease in a fit patient: API doublet.
- Figure 4.2 showing median OS with various regimens for metastatic hormone sensitive cancer prostate using a doublet or triplet.

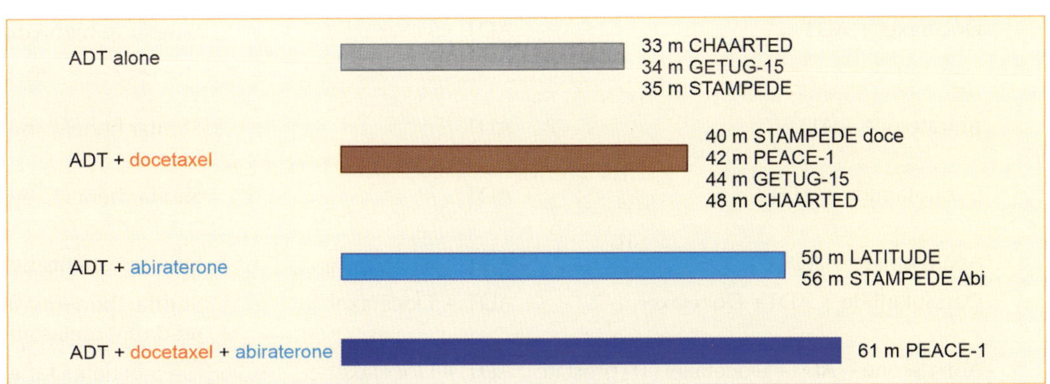

Fig. 4.2: Median overall survival (*de novo* high volume mHSPC)

- STAMPEDE showed benefit in high and low volume disease with docetaxel and abiraterone. But more benefit with abiraterone (Table 4.6).

Important points to remember:

Median overall survival with ADT alone from CHAARTED and GETUG-15 across various subgroups (Table 4.7).

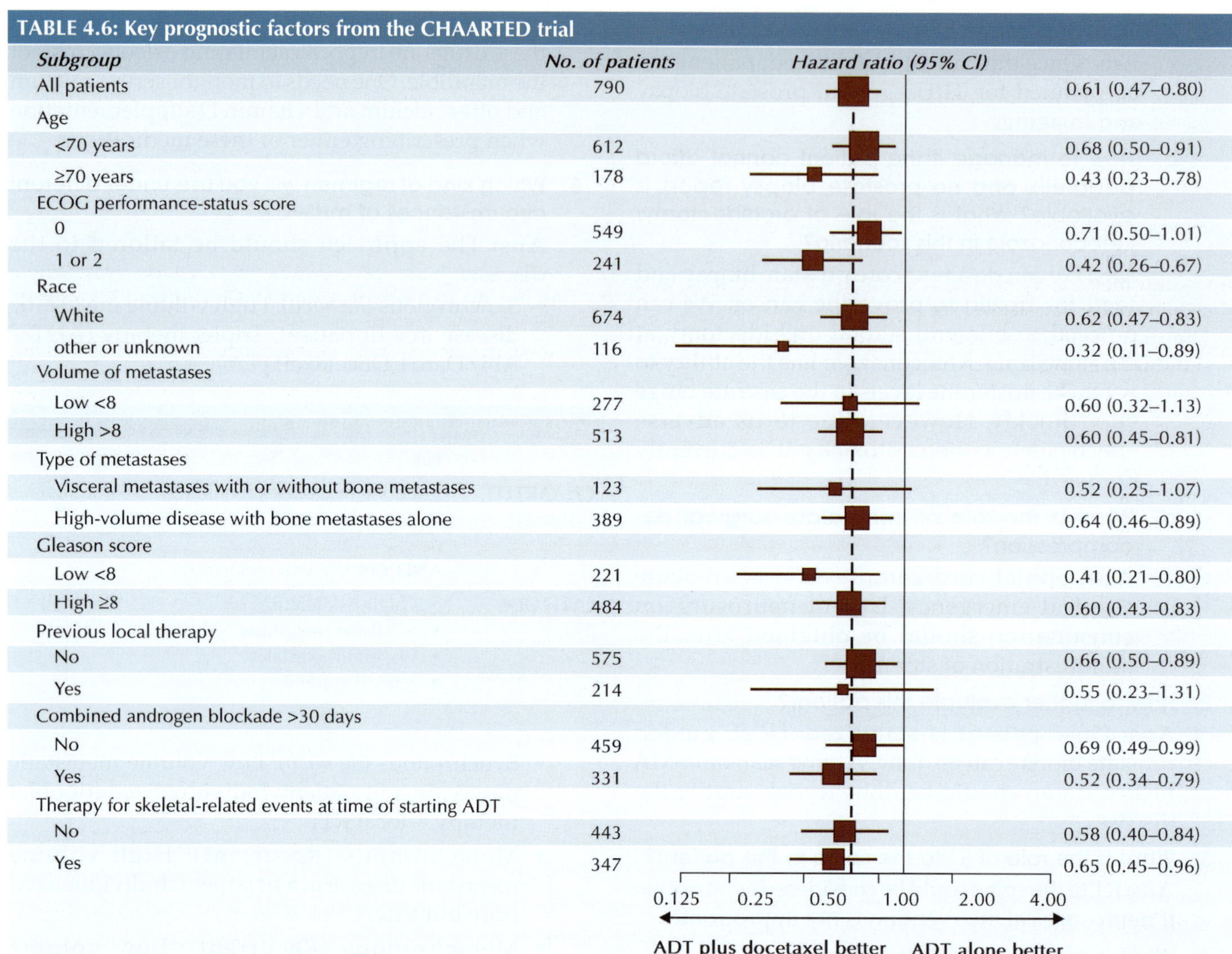

TABLE 4.6: Key prognostic factors from the CHAARTED trial

Subgroup	*No. of patients*	*Hazard ratio (95% CI)*
All patients	790	0.61 (0.47–0.80)
Age		
<70 years	612	0.68 (0.50–0.91)
≥70 years	178	0.43 (0.23–0.78)
ECOG performance-status score		
0	549	0.71 (0.50–1.01)
1 or 2	241	0.42 (0.26–0.67)
Race		
White	674	0.62 (0.47–0.83)
other or unknown	116	0.32 (0.11–0.89)
Volume of metastases		
Low <8	277	0.60 (0.32–1.13)
High >8	513	0.60 (0.45–0.81)
Type of metastases		
Visceral metastases with or without bone metastases	123	0.52 (0.25–1.07)
High-volume disease with bone metastases alone	389	0.64 (0.46–0.89)
Gleason score		
Low <8	221	0.41 (0.21–0.80)
High ≥8	484	0.60 (0.43–0.83)
Previous local therapy		
No	575	0.66 (0.50–0.89)
Yes	214	0.55 (0.23–1.31)
Combined androgen blockade >30 days		
No	459	0.69 (0.49–0.99)
Yes	331	0.52 (0.34–0.79)
Therapy for skeletal-related events at time of starting ADT		
No	443	0.58 (0.40–0.84)
Yes	347	0.65 (0.45–0.96)

TABLE 4.7: Landmark trials showing benefit of ADT intensification

Clinical trial(s)	*Intervention*	*Control*	*Comments*
STAMPEDE-H	Prostate radiation + ADT (+/- Docetaxel)		Benefit in low volume subgroup
GETUG-15 **CHAARTED** **STAMPEDE-C**	Docetaxel + ADT	ADT	Benefit in high volume subgroup
LATITUDE **STAMPEDE-G**	Abiraterone + ADT	ADT	Similar benefits by risk group
ARCHES **ENZAMET**	Enzalutamide + ADT	ADT	Similar benefits by risk group
TITAN	Apalutamide + ADT	ADT	Similar benefits by risk group
ARASENS	Darolutamide + ADT+ Docetaxel	ADT + Docetaxel	Similar benefits for *de novo* and recurrent metastatic disease
PEACE-1	Abiraterone + ADT+ Docetaxel (+/- prostate radiation) (+/- prostate radiation)	ADT + Docetaxel	r PFS benefits for all. OS benefits in high volume

a. Synchronous and high volume: 3 years
b. Synchronous and low volume: 4.5 years
c. Metachronous and high volume: 4.5 years
d. Metachronous and low volume: ~8 years

SUMMARY

- PSMA PET scan is a single investigation which can answer all the imaging related dilemmas. It has a high sensitivity and specificity in picking up metastatic lesions. In a recent meta-analysis[26] Ga-PSMA-68 PET CT was shown to be superior to that of Tc-MDP bone scan + cross-sectional imaging for the detection of PCa metastases. However, PSMA PET has not been shown to be of any prognostic significance.
- The number and location of bone metastases, presence of visceral metastases, ISUP grade, PS status, initial PSA, and alkaline phosphatase level are key prognostic factors.
- The definition of oligometastatic is variable and not standardized. The CHAARTED "volume" is the most commonly used stratification for mHSPC. The definition of high volume and risk are based on a bone scan and a cross-sectional imaging.
- Treatment of mHSPC should start with at least two modalities. Primary androgen deprivation is to be continued life long .
- No one method of androgen deprivation is better than the other. LHRH antagonists have better cardiac safety profile and quicker than the agonist. LHRH antagonists or orchiectomy are the preferred modality of ADT when urgent castration is required.
- All LHRH agonists perform equally well. They should be monitored with the castrate level of serum testosterone.
- Using a three-prong approach in mHSPC is justifiable, addition of abiraterone in addition to docetaxel and ADT in a mHSPC, especially a high volume disease has a better survival outcome.
- Local treatment with EBRT in a low volume mHSPC offers better overall survival in these patients.
- Role of surgery in the low volume metastatic disease is not yet established.
- Metastasis directed therapy in low volume disease is being studied in multiple trials, results will determine their use in future.

REFERENCES

1. Combes AD, Palma CA, Calopedos R, Wen L *et al.* PSMA PET-CT in the Diagnosis and Staging of Prostate Cancer. Diagnostics (Basel). 2022 Oct 26;12(11):2594. doi: 10.3390/diagnostics12112594. PMID: 36359439; PMCID: PMC9689635.
2. Perez-Lopez R, Tunariu N, Padhani AR, *et al.* Imaging Diagnosis and Follow-up of Advanced Prostate Cancer: Clinical Perspectives and State of the Art. *Radiology*. 2019;292(2):273–286. doi:10.1148/radiol.2019181931.
3. Zhou J, Wu R, Wang W, Zhao Y, Liu X. 68Ga-PSMA PET/CT for the evaluation of metastasis in patients with prostate cancer: A systematic review and meta-analysis. Hell J Nucl Med. 2022 Sep-Dec;25(3):297–311. doi: 10.1967/s002449912525. PMID: 36576728.
4. Yaxley JW, Raveenthiran S, Nouhaud FX, *et al* Outcomes of Primary Lymph Node Staging of Intermediate and High Risk Prostate Cancer with 68Ga-PSMA Positron Emission Tomography/Computerized Tomography Compared to Histological Correlation of Pelvic Lymph Node Pathology. *J Urol*. 2019;201(4):815–820. doi:10.1097/JU.0000000000000053.
5. Parker CC, James ND, Brawley CD, Clarke NW, Hoyle AP, Ali A, Ritchie AW, Attard G, Chowdhury S, Cross W, Dearnaley DP. Radiotherapy to the primary tumour for newly diagnosed, metastatic prostate cancer (STAMPEDE): a randomised controlled phase 3 trial. The Lancet. 2018 Dec 1;392(10162):2353–66.
6. Hofman MS, Lawrentschuk N, Francis RJ, *et al.* Prostate-specific membrane antigen PET-CT in patients with high-risk prostate cancer before curative-intent surgery or radiotherapy (proPSMA): a prospective, randomised, multicentre study. *Lancet*. 2020;395(10231):1208–1216. doi:10.1016/S0140–6736(20)30314–7.
7. Parker CC, James ND, Brawley CD, Clarke NW, Hoyle AP, Ali A, Ritchie AW, Attard G, Chowdhury S, Cross W, Dearnaley DP. Radiotherapy to the primary tumour for newly diagnosed, metastatic prostate cancer (STAMPEDE): a randomised controlled phase 3 trial. The Lancet. 2018 Dec 1;392(10162):2353–66.
8. Margel D, Peer A, Ber Y, *et al* Cardiovascular Morbidity in a Randomized Trial Comparing GnRH Agonist and GnRH Antagonist among Patients with Advanced Prostate Cancer and Preexisting Cardiovascular Disease. *J.Urol*2019;202(6):1199–1208. doi:10.1097/JU.0000000000000384.
9. Seidenfeld J, Samson DJ, Hasselblad V *et al* Single-therapy androgen suppression in men with advanced prostate cancer: a systematic review and meta-analysis. Ann Intern Med 2000; 132: 566–577.
10. Heyns CF, Simonin MP, Grosgurin P, Schall R, Porchet HC; South African Triptorelin Study Group. Comparative efficacy of triptorelin pamoate and leuprolide acetate in men with advanced prostate cancer. BJU Int. 2003 Aug;92(3):226–31. doi: 10.1046/j.1464–410x.2003.04308.x. PMID: 12887472.
11. Prostate Cancer Trialists' Collaborative Group. Maximum androgen blockade in advanced prostate cancer: an overview of the randomised trials. *Lancet* 2000; 355: 1491–1498.
12. Felix Preisser, Felix. K.H. Chun, Severine Banek, Mike Wenzel, Markus Graefen, Thomas Steuber, DeryaTilki, Philipp Mandel. Management and treatment options for patients with *de novo* and recurrent hormone-sensitive oligometastatic prostate cancer, Prostate International,Volume 9, Issue 3, 2021, Pages 113–118,ISSN2287–8882.
13. Terada N, Maughan BL, Akamatsu S, *et al.* Exploring the optimal sequence of abiraterone and enzalutamide in patients with chemotherapy-naïve castration-resistant prostate cancer: The Kyoto-Baltimore collaboration. *Int J Urol.* 2017;24(6):441–448. doi:10.1111/iju.13346.
14. Khalaf DJ, Annala M, Taavitsainen S, *et al.* Optimal sequencing of enzalutamide and abiraterone acetate plus prednisone in metastatic castration-resistant prostate cancer: a multicentre, randomised, open-label, phase 2, crossover trial. *Lancet Oncol.* 2019;20(12):1730–1739. doi:10.1016/S1470–2045(19)30688–6.
15. Kyriakopoulos CE, Chen YH, Carducci MA, Liu G *et al* Chemohormonal Therapy in Metastatic Hormone-Sensitive Prostate Cancer: Long-Term Survival Analysis of the Randomized Phase III E3805 CHAARTED Trial. J Clin Oncol. 2018 Apr 10;36(11):1080–1087. doi: 10.1200/JCO.2017.75.3657. Epub 2018 Jan 31. PMID: 29384722; PMCID.

16. Dondi F, Albano D, Bertagna F, Treglia G. Bone Scintigraphy versus PSMA-Targeted PET/CT or PET/MRI in Prostate Cancer: Lessons Learned from Recent Systematic Reviews and Meta-Analyses. Cancers (Basel). 2022 Sep 15;14(18):4470. doi: 10.3390/cancers14184470. PMID: 36139630; PMCID: PMC9496815.
17. Decaestecker K, De Meerleer G, Ameye F, Fonteyne V *et al.* Surveillance or metastasis-directed Therapy for Oligometastatic Prostate (STOMP) cancer recurrence: study protocol for a randomized phase II trial. BMC Cancer. 2014 Sep 15; 14:671. doi: 10.1186/1471–2407–14–671. PMID: 25223986; PMCID: PMC4175227.
18. Phillips R, Shi WY, Deek M, *et al* Outcomes of Observation vs Stereotactic Ablative Radiation for Oligometastatic Prostate Cancer: The ORIOLE Phase 2 Randomized Clinical Trial. *JAMA Oncol.* 2020;6(5):650–659. doi:10.1001/jamaoncol.2020.0147.
19. Sánchez-Iglesias ÁL, Morillo-Macías V, Santafé-Jiménez A, Ferrer-Albiach C. Bone-only oligometastatic prostate cancer: can SABR improve outcomes? A single-center experience. Radiat Oncol J. 2022 Sep;40(3):192–199. doi: 10.3857/roj.2022.00101. Epub 2022 Sep 27. PMID: 36200308; PMCID: PMC9535412.
20. Parker CC, James ND, Brawley CD, Clarke NW, Hoyle AP, Ali A, Ritchie AW, Attard G, Chowdhury S, Cross W, Dearnaley DP. Radiotherapy to the primary tumour for newly diagnosed, metastatic prostate cancer (STAMPEDE): a randomised controlled phase 3 trial. The Lancet. 2018 Dec 1;392(10162):2353–66.
21. Moschini M, Morlacco A, Kwon E, Rangel LJ, Karnes RJ. Treatment of M1a/M1b prostate cancer with or without radical prostatectomy at diagnosis. *Prostate Cancer Prostatic Dis.* 2017;20(1):117–121. doi:10.1038/pcan.2016.63.
22. Dai B., Zhang J., Wang H., Wang Q., Kong Y., Zhu Y. 618MO Local therapy to the primary tumour for newly diagnosed, oligo-metastatic prostate cancer: A prospective randomized, phase II, open-label trial. *Ann Oncol.2020.*
23. Mao Y, Hu M, Yang G, Gao E, Xu W. Cytoreductive prostatectomy improves survival outcomes in patients with oligometastases: a systematic meta-analysis. World J Surg Oncol. 2022 Aug 9;20(1):255. doi: 10.1186/s12957–022–02715–x. PMID: 35945562; PMCID: PMC9361652.
24. Sooriakumaran P, Wilson C, Rombach I, Hassanali N *et al* Feasibility and safety of radical prostatectomy for oligo-metastatic prostate cancer: the Testing Radical prostatectomy in men with prostate cancer and oligo-metastases to the bone (TRoMbone) trial. BJU Int. 2022 Jul;130(1):43–53. doi: 10.1111/bju.15669. Epub 2022 Jan 27. PMID: 34878715.
25. McKay RR, Xie W, Ye H, Fennessy FM *et al* Results of a Randomized Phase II Trial of Intense Androgen Deprivation Therapy prior to Radical Prostatectomy in Men with High-Risk Localized Prostate Cancer. J Urol. 2021 Jul;206(1):80–87. doi: 10.1097/JU.0000000000001702. Epub 2021 Mar 8. PMID: 33683939; PMCID: PMC9807004.
26. Zhao G, Ji B. Head-To-Head Comparison of 68Ga-PSMA-11 PET/CT and 99mTc-MDP Bone Scintigraphy for the Detection of Bone Metastases in Patients With Prostate Cancer: A Meta-Analysis. AJR Am J Roentgenol. 2022 Sep;219(3):386–395. doi: 10.2214/AJR.21.27323. Epub 2022 Apr 20. Erratum in: AJR Am J Roentgenol. 2022 Sep;219(3):529. PMID: 35441529.

Chapter

5

Castrate Resistant Prostate Cancer

• *Ganesh Bakshi* • *Ashwin Tamhankar*

LEARNING OBJECTIVES

- To define castrate resistant prostate cancer (CRPC) for decision making at appropriate time of diagnosis: The key for appropriate management of CRPC is to stage the disease at correct time and define the migration of castrate sensitive phase to resistant phase.
- To get overview on available treatment options for CRPC: With rapidly evolving landscape of options of CRPC treatment, we must ensure that clinicians and patients are well aware of the options by the clinician as well as the patient for a shared decision making.
- To know the principles of sequencing strategies of CRPC treatment and get insight on simplified algorithm for decision making: When there are multiple options, it is prudent to understand how to use them in appropriate sequence for the best interest of the patient's overall survival and other cancer related outcomes. This also includes knowledge about the various strategies and mechanisms of actions of various options and literature support for these decisions.
- To get the perspectives of quality of life parameters including bone health: In CRPC apart from survival issues, other QOL parameters are equally important and need to be addressed on priority basis.
- To understand the role of genetic testing including germline and somatic testing: Genetic testing is a recent value addition for prognostication, treatment and for understanding family repercussions of prostate cancer patient.

Case Scenario 1

Metastatic Castration Resistant Prostate Cancer [mCRPC]

A 65-year-old gentleman with ECOG 0, diagnosed oligometastatic prostate cancer in 2016 (single bone-left femur involvement on PSMA PET/CT) with sPSA levels of 48 ng/ml and biopsy GG 4 was on androgen deprivation therapy (bilateral orchiectomy). His PSA was controlled till July 2020 to the range of 0.4 ng/ml. sPSA results showed slow rise from September 2020 to 3.8 ng/ml. He was asymptomatic for the disease at time.

1. **What would you suspect at this stage?**

   Ans: Rising PSA over 2 ng/ml above nadir, flags possibility of castrate resistance and it needs to be confirmed with consecutive two more readings at a week's interval to define progression. If the criteria fits, we suspect mCRPC.

Case Scenario 2

Repeat readings: 3.9 ng/ml and 4.2 ng/ml, serum testosterone 18 ng/dl.

1. **What is the definition of castration resistant prostate cancer (CRPC)?**

   Ans: Castrate serum testosterone < 50 ng/dl or 1.7 nmol/L plus:

   a. *Biochemical progression:* Three consecutive rises in PSA at least one week apart resulting in two 50% increases over the nadir, and a PSA > 2 ng/ml.

   Or

   b. *Radiological progression:* The appearance of new lesions: Either two or more new bone lesions on bone scan or a soft tissue lesion using RECIST criteria (Response Evaluation Criteria in Solid Tumors).

Symptomatic progression alone must be questioned and subject to further investigation. It is not sufficient to diagnose CRPC.

2. **What is the acceptable level of castrate level testosterone?**

   Ans: Castrate serum testosterone < 50 ng/dl or 1.7 nmol/L

3. **What is the pathophysiology of CRPC?**

   Ans:
   - Persistent adrenal androgen biosynthesis
   - *De novo* intratumoural androgen synthesis
   - Androgen receptor (AR) associated signaling mechanisms.
   - ARs are active despite castrate levels of testosterone
   - Receptor overexpression (gene amplification and/or protein overexpression)
   - AR mutations leading to receptor promiscuity or structure-function activation
   - CYP-17 enzyme induction results in increased androgen synthesis
   - The ultimate consequence is activation of the AR signaling cascade and resulting tumor growth, survival, and proliferation despite castrate levels of androgen

4. **What would be assessment at this time?**

   Ans:
   1. Complete staging of the disease
   2. Performance status
   3. Presence of bone pain—symptomatic progression
   4. Status of bone marrow function
   5. Genetic testing—if not done before

5. **What factors are considered before deciding therapy?**

   Ans:
   - Performance status
   - Staging
   - Affordability
   - Drug side effect profile
   - Drug interactions with existing co-morbidities therapies, e.g. diabetes, thyroid
   - Prior systemic therapy

6. **Which imaging modality do you want to use at this stage?**

   Ans:
   - PSMA PET/CT for a complete staging
   - Basic blood profile (CBC, RFT, LFT, sugar, lipid profile, electrolytes)
   - Serum calcium, vitamin D levels, LDH
   - Cardiac status (ECG and 2 D Echo)

7. **Would you measure his BMD?**

   Ans: Bone mineral density should be assessed for patients starting from the day of diagnosis of metastatic prostate cancer and it should be periodically revisited, especially in CRPC stage.

   A baseline DEXA scan before the commencement of ADT should help us know the deterioration.

   T score (comparison of the density parameters to an average healthy 30-year-old adult as a standard deviation) and Z score (comparison of density parameters with a contemporary group age and gender-specific) assess the risk of fractures and extrapolates to therapeutic interventions.

Case Scenario 3

PSMA PET/CT scan showed bony progression with involvement of multiple axial and appendicular bones without any soft tissue/visceral involvement (Fig. 5.1).

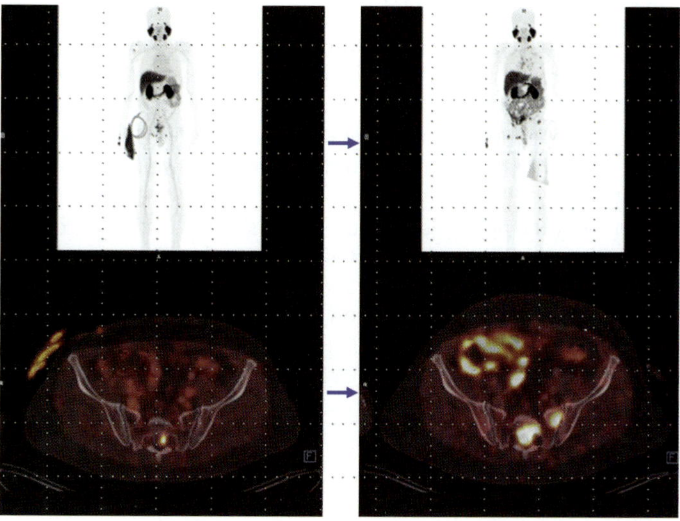

Fig. 5.1: Bony progression on CRPC

1. **What would be the goals of treatment?**

   Ans: Goals of treatment are as follows:
   1. Prolonging overall survival
   2. Relieving pain and symptoms
   3. Improving or at least maintaining QOL
   4. Evaluating the histological alterations, if suspicion in clinical parameters
   5. Understanding the sequencing strategies and defining the options which are already used and which are to be utilized
   6. Discussing about the overall prognosis and cost implications
   7. Genetic assessment and counseling.

2. **What would be your treatment strategy for this patient?**

   Ans: Summarising the present case–65-year-old, asymptomatic with ECOG 0, **mCRPC with high risk and high volume disease** as per the CHAARTED[1] and LATITUDE[2] criteria.

This individual has options of various first-line treatments as valid options and I would want to keep certain options in reserve for progression as second and third line options.

3. **Which are these first line options for mCRPC?**

Ans: The first line options for treatment of mCRPC are:

- Taxane based chemotherapy: Docetaxel
- Enzalutamide
- Abiraterone acetate with prednisolone

First Line Therapy for mCRPC

- Docetaxel chemotherapy
  - TAX 327 study Tannock *et al*[3]
  - Docetaxel + prednisone: Standard of care for men with symptomatic CRPC (Level 1: Evidence, Grade A recommendation)
  - Docetaxel 75 mg/m^2 administered intravenously every 3 weeks with 5 mg oral prednisone twice daily up to 10 cycles.
  - Docetaxel given every three weeks increased overall survival
    - Decreased risk of death by 24%
    - Absolute increase in median survival of > 2.5 months
  - Docetaxel demonstrated a higher rate of pain response, quality of life improvement and PSA.[4]
  - Docetaxel 50 mg/m^2 every two weeks can be used with much lesser AEs and is quite effective in mCRPC patients unable to tolerate the standard dose above.[4]
- Abiraterone (AA)
  - Abiraterone acetate, the prodrug of the active abiraterone, has an esterified acetate group.
  - Abiraterone is a selective, irreversible inhibitor of 17-hydroxylase/C17, 20-lyase (cytochrome P450c17 [CYP17])
  - Dose: 1000 mg daily (four 250 mg tablets)—swallowed whole with water and must not be taken with food (no food 2 hours before or 1 hour after abiraterone)
  - To be taken with 5 mg of prednisolone twice a day—prednisolone (preferably with food, prednisolone dose is 5 mg OD in mCSPC)
  - COU AA 302 trial in chemo naïve setting showed OS benefit (34.7 vs. 30.3 months, HR: 0.81, 95% CI: 0.70–0.93, $p = 0.0033$) and rPFS benefit (median 16.5 vs. 8.2 months, HR: 0.52, $p < 0.001$).[5]
  - Treatment with abiraterone acetate plus prednisone:
    - Reduces risk of disease progression by 47%
    - Decreases risk of death by 21%
    - Delays time to opiate use and chemotherapy
    - Improves quality of life measures (BPI-SF, FACT-P)
    - Remains safe and well tolerated with longer exposure
  - Clinical benefit was maintained in difficult to treat subgroups
    - Older patients
    - Patients with visceral disease
  - Precautions and contraindications

    Monitoring of LFT, serum electrolytes and blood pressure on regular basis

    Previous severe transaminitis is contraindication for abiraterone. Patients with brittle diabetes should also be kept on a close monitoring while on abiraterone.

    Low dose abiraterone 250 mg with low fat meal is been compared to standard dose 1000 mg in fasting state with a premise on financial burden of 4 pills is significantly more. It has been studied in a non-inferiority setting and found that the low dose AA with low fat meal does similar testosterone suppression in comparison to standard dose. The trial was low powered but PSA metrics did with similar pharmacodynamics in both doses.
- Enzalutamide (Enz)
  - It is a potent androgen receptor(AR) antagonist
  - Blocks DHT from binding to AR
  - Impairs nuclear translocation of AR
  - Inhibits binding to DNA
  - Dose 160 mg OD fasting (steroids are not mandatory unlike AA)
  - PREVAIL (randomized phase 3 trial) was conducted in a chemo-naïve mCRPC population of 1,717 men and showed a significant improvement in both co-primary endpoints, rPFS (HR: 0.186, CI: 0.15–0.23, $p < 0.0001$), and OS (HR: 0.706, CI: 0.6–0.84, $p < 0.001$). A $\geq$ 50% decrease in PSA was seen in 78% of patients.[6]
  - Fairly tolerated well in old population even more than 75 years.
  - Major side effects are fatigue and hypertension.
  - No significant advantage in visceral liver metastasis
  - Contraindications—previous h/o seizure disorder.

Other drugs that are available are as follows:

- Sipuleucel-T (Provenge)
  - Active cellular immunotherapy
  - "Cancer vaccine", unavailable in India
  - A phase III trial of sipuleucel-T showed a survival benefit in 512 asymptomatic or minimally symptomatic mCRPC patients. After a median follow-up of 34 months, the median survival was 25.8 months in the sipuleucel-T group compared to 21.7 months in the placebo group, with a HR of 0.78 ($p = 0.03$).[7]

Combination Therapies First Line mCRPC

- **PROpel trial:** A randomised double-blind, phase 3 trial abiraterone (1000 mg once daily) plus prednisone 5 mg/twice daily (AAP) and Olaparib (300 mg twice/daily) or placebo in patients with mCRPC in the first-line setting[8]
- **Patients were enrolled irrespective of homologous recombination repair gene mutation (HRRm) findings. Subgroup analyzed mutation positive and negative patients for outcomes.**
- Significantly positive results in favor of the combination with (imaging based) ibPFS of 24.8 vs. 16.6 mo (HR 0.66; 95% CI: 0.54 to 0.81; p = 0.001).
- The subgroup of patients with positive HRRm status showed a HR of 0.50 (CI: 0.34 to 0.73) which seems to be a major driver of the overall result.
- Survival data are still immature
- Side effects: anaemia, fatigue/asthenia, and nausea
- **MAGNITUDE trial**: Randomized, double-blind, phase 3 trial evaluating abiraterone (1,000 mg once daily) plus prednisone 5 mg twice/daily plus Niraparib (NIRA) 200 mg. This trial was again done in patients with and without HRRm mutation. Authors concluded that a combination of AA and NIRA improves rPFS and ORR in the group with HRR mutation and do not impact the outcomes in patient negative for HRRm testing.

4. **How do you decide about sequencing?**
   Ans:
   - For assessment we should look at ECOG, volume (high vs low) and risk (high vs low), visceral metastasis, prior therapies, contraindications (diabetes, seizures, prior transaminitis)
   - Overall dictum is that high volume (+/–visceral disease), younger individual or someone who has contraindication for newer androgen receptor pathway inhibitors (ARPI)—docetaxel would be considered a choice deemed fit based on the data of CHAARTED trial.
   - Medical oncology and multidisciplinary team discussion and evaluation would be necessary.
   - Someone who is not ideal candidate for taxane-based therapy [unwilling for chemotherapy and wanting tablets, hearing problems/deafness, low counts ARPI as per the eligibility would be the choice.
   - In diabetic individuals or liver dysfunction: Enzalutamide is a better choice.
   - Someone who has h/o seizures: AAP is the drug of choice

Case Scenario *(Contd.)*

- Patient was started on abiraterone acetate 1 gm plus prednisolone 5 mg BD
- PSA response: 4 months < 1 ng/ml
- Controlled PSA till May 2022 (20 months since Sept 2020)
- Regular assessment of LFT, Blood pressures, sugar, lipid profile

5. **How will you manage transaminitis caused by AA?**
   Ans: Around 13% patients on abiraterone would have some level of transaminitis and significant rise (5 times the normal value) can happen to the tune of 6%. It is related to CYP17 inhibition. It is a recommendation to monitor liver enzymes every 2 weeks for 3 months and then monthly thereafter.

   Therapy needs to be stopped for rise of levels 5 times above normal values and it should not be restarted unless the levels come back to normal. Any elevation of enzymes with jaundice should be the indication for permanent discontinuation.

6. **What would the management of other parameters apart from cancer control in this individual?**
   Ans: The following aspects need to be addressed:
   - **Bone Health**
     - Bone DEXA scan at adequate intervals, as per clinician discretion.
     - Zoledronic acid injection 4 mg zoledronic acid every 3 weeks had fewer SREs compared to the placebo group (44 vs. 33%, p = 0.021) and fewer pathological fractures (13.1 vs. 22.1%, p = 0.015).[9] Time to first SRE was longer in the zoledronic acid group than placebo.[9] It does not show any survival benefit. Jaw osteonecrosis, renal function tests and hypocalcemia need to be monitored during the therapy. Monthly zoledronic acid is recommended. The duration of therapy is not defined. A dental examination is necessary prior to starting zoledronic acid.

RANK Ligand Inhibitor

Denosumab is the humanized monoclonal antibody to RANKL which is the mediator for osteoclast function and survival. Denosumab was superior to zoledronic acid in delaying or preventing skeletal related events (SRE)—pathological fracture, radiation or surgery to bone, or spinal cord compression (HR: 0.82, p = 0.008).[10] Monthly injections of denosumab (120 mg sc) would be essential for mCRPC patients; again, after a dental examination denosumab costs 15 to 20,000 INR per 120 mg injection.

Calcium and Vitamin D Supplement

Daily calcium (>500 mg) and vitamin D (>400 IU equivalent) are recommended in all patients; especially those on above therapy.

- **Regular Cardiac Check**
  ADT and other therapies add to the toxicity and are potentially toxic for cardiac risk and hence regular assessment would be prudent.
- **Sugar, electrolytes, LFT and lipid profile monitoring for side-effect profile**
  Adequate sugar control is deemed necessary along with check on lipid profile status for these patients. LFTs and electrolytes are monitored monthly in AAP therapy.
- **High protein and calcium rich diet**
- **Regular aerobic physical activity**
- **Urinary functions and lower urinary tract symptoms**
  To continue on medical management and assess post-void residue and status of upper tracts at regular intervals to rule out any hydronephrosis.
- **Genetic testing**
  Germ line and somatic testing should be considered for all metastatic prostate cancer patients ideally at the time of initial diagnosis.
  Somatic mutations may change and it would need to be repeated again for assessment of eligibility to the PARP inhibitor therapy at the time of progression.

These Would Include Following Assessment

Tumor testing for somatic homologous recombination gene mutations (BRCA1, BRCA2, ATM, BARD1, BRIP1, CDK12, CHEK1, CHEK2, FANCL, PALB2, RAD51B, RAD51C, RAD51D, or RAD54L).

Guidelines for germline testing

Recommendations	***Strength rating***
Consider germline testing in men with metastatic PCa.	Weak
Consider germline testing in men with high-risk PCa who have a family member diagnosed with PCa at age < 60 years.	Weak
Consider germline testing in men with multiple family members diagnosed with PCa at age < 60 years or a family who dies from PCa.	Weak
Consider germline testing in men with a family history of high-risk germline mutations or a family history of multiple cancers on the same side of the family.	Weak

***Case Scenario** (Contd.)*

In May 2022, serum PSA started rising with new reading as 3.6 ng/ml with lower back pain since last 2–3 months.

7. **What would be the next step?**
   Ans: I would like to image the patient again by PSMA PET/CT scan
   PSMA PET/CT shows—progression, bony and nodal, no visceral disease (Fig. 5.2).

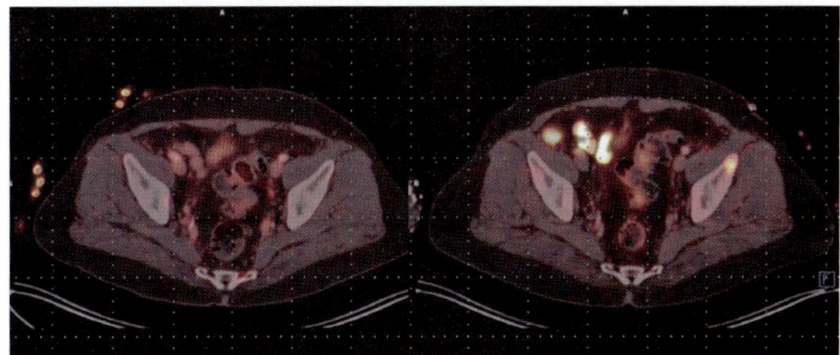

Fig. 5.2: Bony and nodal (iliac node) progression

8. **What would be the treatment option now?**
   Ans: I would like to define patient's disease at this time.
   65-year-old, ECOG 0, mCRPC with post-abiraterone progression (chemo naïve), mildly symptomatic, predominantly bony disease progression (no visceral metastasis)
   Patient's fitness and ability to tolerate docetaxel chemotherapy should be assessed. After a multi-disciplinary meeting (MDT) and discussion with medical oncologist future plan can be laid out.
   At this stage pros and cons, side effects should be discussed in details and informed decision should be taken. Cross resistance to ARPI should be considered before deciding about the sequencing and cytotoxic therapy. As it works on different mechanism, it should be considered, in case the patient is fit for the same.
   Option of chemotherapy should be strongly considered as second line in this case.
   Docetaxel can be started and continued till progression. Follow-up imaging and PSA should be done at regular intervals.
   Other second-line options for this patient are as follows:
   - Taxane-based chemotherapy.
   - PARP inhibitors (if eligible)
   - ARPI (after assessment of cross resistance): Enzalutamide
   - PSMA-based therapy—177 Lu PSMA
   - Radium 223
   - Metronomic chemotherapy

Second line therapy for mCRPC

Post First Line Docetaxel Chemotherapy Progression the Following Drugs can be Used:

- **Abiraterone acetate after docetaxel**
  Positive results—phase III trial (COU-AA-301)[10]
  Median follow-up of 20.2 months, the median survival in the AAP group was 15.8 months compared to 11.2 months in the placebo arm (HR: 0.74, $p < 0.0001$).

- **Enzalutamide after docetaxel**
  AFFIRM study[11]
  Median follow-up of 14.4 months, the median survival in the enzalutamide group was 18.4 months compared to 13.6 months in the placebo arm (HR: 0.63, $p < 0.001$)
- **Cabazitaxel**
- Tubulin binding taxane
- Active against docetaxel resistant tumors
- EAU guidelines:
  - Cabazitaxel should be considered as an effective second-line treatment following docetaxel (level of evidence A)
- **TROPIC trial:** Conclusions[12]
  - Cabazitaxel/prednisone: Significantly improved OS vs mitoxantrone/prednisone in metastatic CRPC
  - Reduced risk of death: 28% (HR: 0.72; P <.0001)
  - Significantly improved PFS, response rates, and TTP
  - Associated with acceptable safety profile
  - Febrile neutropenia and diarrhea more common
  - Cabazitaxel/prednisone first treatment to demonstrate survival benefit in patients with metastatic CRPC who failed docetaxel-based therapy.

  Docetaxel re-challenge[22] is an option if the prior chemotherapy has given good response. It gives improved overall survival especially in the high category [volume/risk] along with short duration response to ARATs.

Chemo Naïve Progression on ARPI

Considering second ARPI, post one ARPI progression should be avoided particularly if the patient had a short response to the first ARPI for mCRPC (<12 months) because of known cross resistance and the availability of chemotherapy and PARP inhibitors.[13]

Taxane based chemotherapy or PARP inhibitors would be the options in this setting.

PARP Inhibitors

PARP inhibitors can be used on the basis of PROfound trial:

A randomised phase III trial (PROfound)

Radiographic PFS by blinded independent central review in the *BRCA1/2* or *ATM* mutated population (Cohort A) was the first endpoint and significantly favoured olaparib (HR: 0.49, 95% CI: 0.38–0.63). The final results for OS demonstrated a significant improvement among men with *BRCA1/2* or *ATM* mutations (Cohort A) ($p = 0.0175$; HR: 0.69, 95% CI: 0.50–0.97). This was not significant in men with any (other) HRR alteration (Cohort B) (HR: 0.96, 95% CI: 0.63–1.49).[14]

The most common AEs were anaemia (46.1% vs. 15.4%), nausea (41.4% vs. 19.2%), decreased appetite (30.1% vs. 17.7%) and fatigue (26.2% vs. 20.8%) for olaparib vs. enzalutamide/abiraterone.

Rucaparib has been approved by the FDA for patients with deleterious *BRCA* mutations (germline and/or somatic) who have been treated with ARPI and a taxane-based chemotherapy.[15]

PSMA Based Therapy

An open-label phase III trial (VISION) [16] compared ^{177}Lu–PSMA-617 radioligand therapy with protocol-permitted SOC (i.e. excluded chemotherapy, immunotherapy, radium-223 and investigational drugs) in mCRPC patients, with PSMA expressing metastases on PET/CT, previously treated with at least one ARPI and one (around 53%) or two taxanes.

Imaging-based progression free survival and overall survival were the alternate primary endpoints. More than 800 patients were randomised. ^{177}Lu-PSMA-617 plus SOC significantly prolonged both imaging-based PFS and OS, as compared with SOC alone.

Grade 3 or above AEs were higher with ^{177}Lu-PSMA-617 than without (52.7% vs. 38.0%), but QoL was not adversely affected. ^{177}Lu–PSMA-617 has shown to be a valuable additional treatment option in this mCRPC population.

In TheraP,[17] a randomised phase II trial, patients for whom cabazitaxel was considered the next appropriate standard treatment after docetaxel and who were highly selected by 68 Ga-PSMA-11 and 18 FDG PET-CT scans, were randomised to receive 177Lu-PSMA-617 (6.0–8.5 GBq intravenously every 6 weeks for up to 6 cycles) or cabazitaxel (20 mg/m^2 for up to ten cycles) (Table 5.1).

The primary endpoint was a reduction of at least 50% in PSA. The first endpoint was met (66% vs. 37% for ^{177}Lu-PSMA-617 vs. cabazitaxel, respectively, by ITT; difference 29% (95% CI: 16–42; $p < 0.0001$; and 66% vs. 44% by treatment received; difference 23% [9–37]; $p = 0.0016$)

Case Scenario *(Contd.)*

Patient was started on Inj Docetaxel 75 mg/m^2 every 3 weeks with Prednisolone:

- After 2 cycles, PSA showed response: < 1 ng/ml
- After 6 cycles PSMA PET/CT done—showed stable disease with sclerosis (signs of healing) in bones.
- Continued for 3 more cycles—Nov 2022—PSA started rising 4 ng/ml and 13 ng/ml in 2 weeks' succession.
- PSMA PET CT—soft tissue progression including nodal disease burden in pelvic nodes and bony progression

TABLE 5.1: Summary of various treatment options and trials for mCRPC patients

Study	*Intervention*	*Comparison*	*Selection*	*Outcomes*
COU AA 302 2012	Abiraterone + Prednisolone	Placebo + Prednisolone	No prior docetaxel	OS: 34.7 vs. 30.3 months (HR: 0.81, 95% CI: 0.70–0.93, p = 0.0033) rPFS: benefit (median 16.5 vs. 8.2 months, HR: 0.52, p < 0.001)
COU-AA-301 2011	Abiraterone + Prednisolone	Placebo + Prednisolone	Prior docetaxel	OS: 14.8 vs. 10.9 months (p < 0.001 HR: 0.65; 95% CI: 0.54–0.77). FU: 12.8 months rPFS: 5.6 vs. 3.6 months
TROPIC 2013	Cabazitaxel + prednisone	Mitoxantrone + prednisone	Previous docetaxel. ECOG 0-2.	OS: 318/378 vs. 346/377 events (OR: 2.11; 95% CI: 1.33–3.33). FU: 25.5 months OS ≥ 2 yr 27% vs. 16% PFS:-
CARD 2019	Cabazitaxel (25 mg/m^2 Q3W) + prednisone + G-CSF	ARTA: Abiraterone + prednisone OR Enzalutamide	Previous docetaxel. Progression ≤ 12 months on prior alternative ARTA (either before or after docetaxel)	Med OS 13.6 vs. 11.0 month (p = 0.008, HR: 0.64, 95% CI: 0.46–0.89). rPFS 8.0 vs. 3.7 months (p < 0.001, HR: 0.54, 95% CI: 0.40–0.73). FU: 9.2 months
AFFIRM 2012	Enzalutamide	Placebo	Previous docetaxel. ECOG 0-2.	OS: 18.4 vs. 13.6 months (p < 0.001, HR: 0.63; 95% CI: 0.53–0.75). FU: 14.4 months rPFS: 8.3 vs. 2.9 months (HR: 0.40; 95% CI: 0.35–0.47, p < 0.0001).
PROfound 2020	Olaparib	Abiraterone + prednisolone or enzalutamide; cross-over allowed at progression	Previous ARPI, alterations in HRR mutated genes	rPFS: 7.39 vs. 3.55 months (p < 0.0001, HR: 0.34; 95% CI: 0.25–0.47), conf. ORR 33.3% vs. 2.3% (OR 20.86, 95% CI: 4.18–379.18). OS: 19.1 mo vs. 14.7 months (in pts with *BRCA1/2*, *ATM* alterations) (p = 0.0175; HR 0.69, 95% CI: 0.5–0.97).
VISION 2021	^{177}Lu-PSMA-617 SOC	SOC alone	Previous at least 1 ARPI and one or two taxane regimens; Mandatory: PSMA-positive gallium-68 (^{68}Ga)–labeled PSMA-PET scan	Imaging-based PFS: 8.7 vs. 3.4 months (p < 0.001; HR 0.40; 99.2% CI: 0.29–0.57) OS: 15.3 vs. 11.3 months (p < 0.001; HR 0.62; 95% CI: 0.5–0.74)
TheraP 2021	^{177}Lu-PSMA-617 (8.5 GBq i.v.q 6-weekly, decreasing 0.5 GBq/cycle; up to 6 cycles)	^{177}Lu-PSMA-617 1:1 randomisation cabazitaxel (20 mg/m^2 i.v.q 3-weekly, up to 10 cycles)	mCRPC post-docetaxel, suitable for cabaziaxel	PSA reduction of > 50%: 66 vs. 37 PSA responses; 66% vs. 37% by ITT; difference 29% (95% CI: 16–42; p < 0.0001; and 66% vs. 44% by treatment received; difference 23% [9–37]; p = 0.0016).

9. What would be the next appropriate step?

Ans: Plan third line therapy with remaining options. This would depend on the ECOG status, overall frailty assessment and prior received therapies.

Consider biopsy from the nodal disease after MDT, for somatic mutation along with germline mutations for assessment of eligibility to PARP inhibitors (if not done before). The HRR genes to be considered for use of olaparib are BRCA1, BRCA2, ATM, BARD1, BRIP1, CDK12, CHEK1, CHEK2, FANCL, PALB2, RAD51B, RAD51C, RAD51D and RAD54L

10. What are the indications of doing a biopsy?

Ans: Biopsy is usually recommended in case of rising soft tissue load without any reciprocating rise in PSA values when we suspect dedifferentiation or neuroendocrine (NEC) transformation.

Usually, NEC transformation would be disease progression with either normal or slightly elevated PSA. Biopsy proven NEC would then be treated with Carboplatin-Etoposide chemotherapy. Prognosis of NEC transformation state is poor.

For our case, having received AAP in first-line and docetaxel in second line; choice of third line is Enzalutamide, Cabazitaxel, PARP inhibitor [if HRR mutations +ve] or Lu-PSMA based therapy.

Cabazitaxel often works in third line, post-doctaxel progression but overall patient fitness is important [CARD STUDY]. Usually selected in patients with PS 0-1. If HRR +ve, PARP inhibitors is a good choice. The third option and if patient is experiencing bony site pains is Lu-PSMA therapy. In select cohort of pretreated patients, ^{117}Lu-PSMA-617 was compared with cabazitaxel in a randomised phase II trial and PSA reduction of > 50% was seen with radioligand therapy. The primary endpoint PSA reduction > 50% was in favour of the radioligand therapy.[17]

VISION study in mCRPC patients with previous ARPI and taxanes treatment showed imaging-based PFS and OS benefit. Lu-PSMA arm had higher grade 3 or above AEs but QoL was not majorly affected.[16]

11. Suppose, this case scenario was non-metastatic CRPC, how would the decisions be made?

Ans: First step: Risk stratify

Is it proven on PSMA or RADAR criteria?

Prognosticate

In nmCRPC, testosterone is in castrate range, has a rising PSA value [at least 25%] above nadir or minimum increase by 2 ng/ml and confirmed second rise and conventional imaging shows no metastatses. In India, practically this has been replaced by PSMA PET/CT which shows no metastases. SPARTAN (Apalutamide), PROSPER (Enzalutamide) and ARAMIS (Darolutamide) are the phase III RCTs and evaluated metastasis free survival (MFS) as the endpoint.[18–20] Treatment decisions are usually based on the Performance status, comorbidities, medical history and PSA doubling time [PSA-DT]. Within trials, two-thirds participants had PSA-DT <6 months [highest risk of metastases] and all showed significant MFS benefit after a median FU of 30 months. These drugs are beneficial when patients have a PSA doubling time of < 10 months. Different side-effect profile of these drugs help you choose the right drug for a given patient.

12. What is ARV 7 splice variant and what is its significance?

Ans: Androgen Receptor splice variant encodes a truncated AR protein lacking ligand-binding domain and is active in the absence of androgens.[21] Also, AR-V7 expression shows rise with ARIs. AR-V7 is one of the earliest predictive markers to predict ARI resistance, thereby giving preference to docetaxel therapy in such patients.

13. What is the role of immunotherapy?

Ans: Sipileucel-T is the only immunotherapy approved. No other immunotherapy is FDA approved (Table 5.2).

TABLE 5.2: Summary of various treatment options and trials for nmCRPC patients

Study	*Intervention*	*Control*	*Inclusion criteria*	*Outcome*
SPARTAN	ADT + apalutamide	ADT + placebo	nmCRPC; baseline PSA >2 ng/ml PSA-DT < 10 months	**72% reduction of distant progression or death Median MFS: Apalutamide 40.5 vs placebo 16.2 months; 22% reduction in risk of death** HR = 0.78 (95% CI: 0.64–0.96) p = 0.0161
PROSPER	ADT + enzalutamide	ADT + placebo	nmCRPC; baseline PSA >2 ng/ml PSA-DT < 10 months	**71% reduction of distant progression or death Median MFS: Enzalutamide 36.6 vs placebo 14.7 months; 27% reduction in risk of death** HR = 0.73 (95% CI: 0.61–0.89) p = 0.001
ARAMIS	ADT + darolutamide	ADT + placebo	nmCRPC; baseline PSA >2 ng/ml PSA-DT < 10 months	**59% reduction of distant progression or death Median MFS: Darolutamide 40.4 vs placebo 18.4 months; 31% reduction in risk of death** HR = 0.69 (95% CI: 0.53–0.88) p = 0.003

SUMMARY

- Nearly all patients with mHSPC will progress to CRPC on ADT
- Androgen deprivation needs to be continued for life in patients with metastatic cancer prostate even when they become castrate resistant.
- Sequencing of the drugs depends on multitude of factors, in general, one androgen receptor inhibitor should not follow the other. Chemotherapeutic agent should be sandwiched between the two.
- Genetic testing, both somatic and germline, should be offered to CRPC patients.
- HRR mutation positive CRPC patients can be treated with Olaparib.
- Cabazitaxel is an effective drug even in the third line, if the performance status of the patient is good.
- Radiological soft tissue progression with static PSA is a strong indication of biopsy to rule out neuroendocrine transformation.
- Bone health management to prevent skeletal related events is important. Zolendronic acid and denosumab should be used at least once a month to prevent skeletal related events.

REFERENCES

1. Sweeney, C.J., *et al.* Chemohormonal Therapy in Metastatic Hormone-Sensitive Prostate Cancer. N Engl J Med, 2015. 373: 737.
2. Fizazi, K., *et al.* Abiraterone plus Prednisone in Metastatic, Castration-Sensitive Prostate Cancer. N Engl J Med, 2017. 377: 352.
3. Tannock, I.F., *et al.* Docetaxel plus prednisone or mitoxantrone plus prednisone for advanced prostate cancer. N Engl J Med, 2004. 351: 1502.
4. Kellokumpu-Lehtinen, P.L., *et al.* 2-Weekly versus 3-weekly docetaxel to treat castration-resistant advanced prostate cancer: a randomised, phase 3 trial. Lancet Oncol, 2013.14:117.
5. Ryan, C.J., *et al.* Abiraterone acetate plus prednisone versus placebo plus prednisone in chemotherapy-naive men with metastatic castration-resistant prostate cancer (COU-AA-302): Final overall survival analysis of a randomised, double-blind, placebo-controlled phase 3 study. Lancet Oncol, 2015. 16: 152
6. Beer, T.M., *et al.* Enzalutamide in metastatic prostate cancer before chemotherapy. N Engl J Med, 2014. 371: 424.
7. Kantoff, P.W., *et al.* Sipuleucel-T immunotherapy for castration-resistant prostate cancer. N Engl J Med, 2010. 363: 411.
8. Clarke, N.W., *et al.* Abiraterone and Olaparib for Metastatic Castration-Resistant Prostate Cancer. NEJM Evidence, 2022. 1: EVIDoa2200043.
9. Saad, F., *et al.* A randomized, placebo-controlled trial of zoledronic acid in patients with hormone-refractory metastatic prostate carcinoma. J Natl Cancer Inst, 2002.94: 1458.
10. Fizazi, K., *et al.* Abiraterone acetate for treatment of metastatic castration-resistant prostate cancer: final overall survival analysis of the COU-AA-301 randomised, double-blind, placebo-controlled phase 3 study. Lancet Oncol, 2012. 13: 983.
11. Scher, H.I., *et al.* Increased survival with enzalutamide in prostate cancer after chemotherapy. N Engl J Med, 2012.367: 1187.
12. de Bono, J.S., *et al.* Prednisone plus cabazitaxel or mitoxantrone for metastatic castration-resistant prostate cancer progressing after docetaxel treatment: a randomised open-label trial. Lancet, 2010. 376: 1147.
13. Mori, K., *et al.* Sequential therapy of abiraterone and enzalutamide in castration-resistant prostate cancer: a systematic review and meta-analysis. Prostate Cancer Prostatic Dis, 2020. 23: 539.
14. Hussain, M., *et al.* Survival with Olaparib in Metastatic Castration-Resistant Prostate Cancer. N Engl J Med, 2020. 383: 2345.
15. Abida, W., *et al.* Rucaparib in Men With Metastatic Castration-Resistant Prostate Cancer Harboring a BRCA1 or BRCA2 Gene Alteration. J Clin Oncol, 2020. 38: 3763.
16. Sartor, O., *et al.* Lutetium-177-PSMA-617 for Metastatic Castration-Resistant Prostate Cancer. N Engl J Med, 2021. 385: 1091.
17. Hofman, M.S., *et al.* [(177)Lu]Lu-PSMA-617 versus cabazitaxel in patients with metastatic castration-resistant prostate cancer (TheraP): a randomised, open-label, phase 2 trial. Lancet, 2021. 397: 797.
18. Smith, M.R., *et al.* Apalutamide Treatment and Metastasis-free Survival in Prostate Cancer. N Engl J Med, 2018. 378: 1408.
19. Hussain, M., *et al.* Enzalutamide in Men with Nonmetastatic, Castration-Resistant Prostate Cancer. N Engl J Med, 2018. 378: 2465.
20. Fizazi, K., *et al.* Darolutamide in Nonmetastatic, Castration-Resistant Prostate Cancer. N Engl J Med, 2019. 380: 1235.
21. Zhang T, Karsh LI, Nissenblatt MJ, Canfield SE. Androgen Receptor Splice Variant, AR-V7, as a Biomarker of Resistance to Androgen Axis-Targeted Therapies in Advanced Prostate Cancer. Clin Genitourin Cancer. 2020 Feb;18(1):1-10. doi: 10.1016/j.clgc.2019.09.015. Epub 2019 Sep 26. PMID: 31653572.
22. Ref-Hung SC, Chang LW, Li JR, Wang SS, Yang CK, Chen CS, Lu K, Chen CC, Wang SC, Lin CY, Cheng CL, Ou YC, Chiu KY. Docetaxel Rechallenge Improves Survival in Patients With Metastatic Castration-resistant Prostate Cancer: A Retrospective Study. In Vivo. 2021 Nov-Dec;35(6):3509-3519. doi: 10.21873/invivo.12653. PMID: 34697189; PMCID: PMC8627717.

Chapter
6

Non-Muscle Invasive Bladder Cancer

• Anup Kumar • Gautam Chowdhary

LEARNING OBJECTIVES

- To know the risk factors of carcinoma urinary bladder (UB): Tobacco smoking and occupational exposure are the two most important risk factors and genetic factors play a minor role.
- To understand the workup of a patient with Ca UB: Urine cytology and cystoscopy is performed in all patients. CT urography and MRI are the cross-sectional imaging options available to the urologist to choose from.
- To understand different techniques of TURBT: TURBT can be performed in the traditional piecemeal method or in en-bloc method, both have recently been shown to have similar outcomes.
- To understand the methods to prevent obturator jerk: General anesthesia with muscle relaxation and/or obturator nerve blocks are methods to prevent jerk. Bipolar cautery has not shown to reduce obturator jerk substantially.
- To understand the indications and rationale behind restage TURBT: Restage TURBT identifies residual tumour in about 50% of the cases and leads to upstaging in around 10%, hence it has a very important role to play in high-risk disease.
- To understand the risk stratification of patients with NMIBC: Patients are stratified on the basis of the risk of recurrence and progression into low, intermediate, high and very high-risk groups. This helps to plan the further treatment.
- To understand the rationale behind post-operative intra-vesical adjuvant therapy: Intravesical adjuvant therapy is instilled with an aim of reducing the recurrence and progression.
- To understand how BCG failure is defined: BCG failure can be categorized into BCG refractory, BCG relapse, BCG unresponsive and BCG intolerant groups based on the time of recurrence of tumor and its histology.
- To understand the indications of radical cystectomy (RC) in NMIBC: "Early" RC can be performed in the very high-risk group of patients or in BCG unresponsive patients.
- To understand the upcoming and new combination chemotherapy and also immunotherapy in NMIBC: The sequential combination of gemcitabine + docetaxel instilled intravesically has shown a lot of promise for NMIBC so has systemic pembrolizumab in patients with BCG-unresponsive CIS.

Case Scenario

A 60-year-old hypertensive male, smoker for past 30 years, presented with a single episode of gross painless hematuria. The local examination was normal. An ultrasonography scan was performed which revealed a 3 × 3 cm mass in the bladder on the right posterolateral wall with internal vascularity.

1. What is the presentation of patient with bladder cancer?

Ans: Most common presentation of Ca UB is painless gross hematuria, associated with amorphous clots.

- Any patient > 50 years, even on antiplatelets or anticoagulants, with gross hematuria should be evaluated for Ca UB.

2. What are the risk factors for carcinoma bladder?

Ans: Several risk factors have been shown to increase the risk of Ca UB.

1. **Tobacco smoking** accounts for approximately 50% of the cases of Ca UB. Current smokers –3.14 times increased risk.[1] Risk is dose dependent, reaches a plateau at around 15 cigarettes/day and 50 pack years.[1] Increasing duration after cessation of smoking-reduces the risk, however, former smokers remain at 50% higher risk.[1]

2. **Occupational exposure** accounts for 10% of the cases, being second most important cause. Exposure to aromatic amines, polycyclic aromatic hydrocarbons and chlorinated hydrocarbons in industrial plants which process paint, metal, dye and petroleum products increase the risk.
3. **Genetic:** No clinically relevant genetic mutation found. Genetic predisposition increases the susceptibility to other risk factors and may explain the increased risk among first and second degree relatives.[2]
4. **Dietary factors:** Consumption of Mediterranean diet rich in fruits and vegetables, selenium and vitamin A supplementation reduces the risk.[1] Western diet rich in saturated fats and meat increases the risk.[1]
5. **Environmental exposure:** Chlorine and arsenic in drinking water increases the risk. Exposure to personal hair dyes in subjects with slow *NAT2* acetylation phenotype was believed to increase the risk of Ca UB, but a recent study could not confirm this.[3]
6. **Others**: Schistosomiasis increases the risk of squamous cell cancer of bladder. Ionising radiation to the pelvis and cyclophosphamide chemotherapy also increase the risk.

3. What other investigations would you want to perform in this patient?

Ans: Urine cytology and imaging in the form of a computed tomography urography.

4. What is the role of cytology in evaluation of patients with Ca UB?

Ans: Shedding of malignant cells in urine support the diagnosis of Ca UB.

- Overall sensitivity and specificity vary from 31–100% (median 48%) and 62–100% (median 94%), respectively.[4]
- Has high sensitivity (84%) in high grade tumors, low grade tumors the sensitivity is low (16%). For CIS the sensitivity ranges from 28 to 100%.[5]
- The specificity exceeds 90%.[5]
- Gross hematuria, active UTI, foreign body in UB, prior intravesical therapy, and prior pelvic radiation therapy can affect the cytology report.
- The Paris Reporting System for urinary cytology is being used for reporting.

Category 1	Non-diagnostic/ unsatisfactory
Category 2	Negative for high-grade urothelial carcinoma (NHGUC)
Category 3	Atypical urothelial cells (AUC)
Category 4	Suspicious for high grade urothelial carcinoma (SHGUC)
Category 5	High grade urothelial carcinoma (HGUC)
Category 6	Low grade urothelial neoplasm (LGUN)
Category 7	Other: primary and secondary malignancies of the bladder and miscellaneous lesions

5. Enumerate a few benign lesions of urinary bladder.

Ans: Epithelial metaplasia, papilloma and inverted papilloma, nephrogenic adenoma, leukoplakia, cystitis cystica and cystitis glandularis (can transform into adenocarcinoma UB, regular follow-up is required).

6. What are the indications of ordering a computed tomography scan?

Ans: All cases with a suspicion of Ca UB should undergo a CT IVU. Typically, CT is indicated in tumors >3 cm, multiple tumors or hydronephrosis or tumors located at the trigone.[6]

- These patients are at higher risk for co-existent upper tract urothelial malignancy or advanced disease.

7. What is the role of multiparametric MRI and VI-RADS score in the diagnosis of cancer bladder?

Ans: Reporting of multiparametric MRI (mpMRI) using the Vesical Imaging Reporting and Data System (VI-RADS) has high accuracy in predicting MIBC.[7]

- mpMRI in predicting MIBC: 83% sensitivity and 90% specificity.
- Excellent pooled inter-reader agreement of VI-RADS recently confirmed.[8]
- The role of mpMRI and VI-RADS is still being defined. CT is still considered the investigation of choice.
- Identification of MIBC on mpMRI cannot replace the histological confirmation of MIBC at TURBT prior to proceeding to definitive management.
- VI-RADS scoring system is a 5-point Likert scale (VI-RADS 1 to 5) based on the likelihood of muscle invasion. VI-RADS 1: Muscle invasion is highly unlikely, VI-RADS 2: Muscle invasion is unlikely to be present, VI-RADS 3: Muscle invasion is equivocal, VI-RADS 4: Muscle invasion is likely to be present and VI-RADS 5: Invasion of muscle and beyond the bladder is highly likely.

8. How does it compare with a CT scan?

Ans: As compared to a CT scan, mpMRI has higher accuracy in suggesting T2 disease and differentiating T1 from T2 disease.

- CT scan is unable to differentiate between stages from Ta to T3a.
- Either of the investigations can be used to assess locally invasive disease, that is T3b or T4.
- For pelvic nodal metastasis, the accuracy is similar with a sensitivity of 60% and 40% and

specificity of 91% and 92% for MRI and CT scans, respectively for associated upper tract disease, CECT has an advantage.[9]

Case Scenario (Contd.)

Urine cytology was positive for high-grade urothelial cancer. A contrast-enhanced computed tomography scan of the abdomen and pelvis was performed which revealed a 3.5 x 4.5 cm mass in the right posterolateral wall of the bladder with no gross extra-vesical extension, normal kidneys, no evidence of mass lesion in the pelvicalyceal system and the ureters in the excretory phase, no evidence of nodal or distant metastasis (Fig. 6.1).

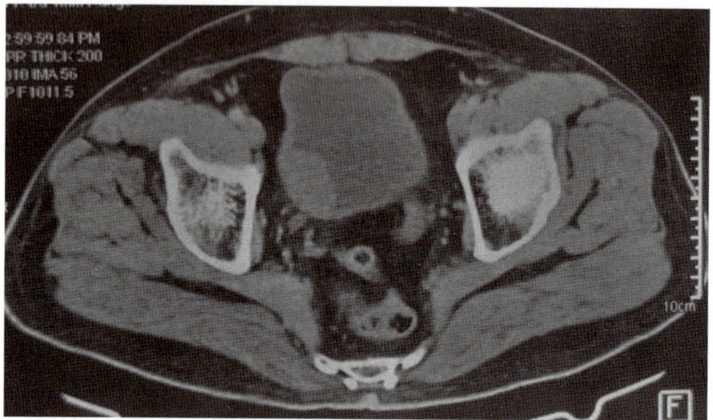

Fig. 6.1: Axial section of computed tomography through the bladder showing mass on the right posterolateral wall.

9. What is the next plan for this patient?

Ans: The patient should be planned for evaluation under anaesthesia, cystoscopy and trans-urethral resection of the bladder tumor (TURBT).

10. How is examination under anesthesia done and what is its role in the present era?

Ans: Examination under anesthesia has been traditionally recommended as the first step when a patient is taken for a TURBT. The bladder is emptied with a catheter. The left hand is placed supra-pubically on the bladder. The right index finger is inserted per rectally in males and per vaginally and the bladder mass is palpated between the left hand and the index finger of the right hand. This is done both prior to the resection and at the end of resection. The following findings have been described:

- Palpable prior to TURBT but not palpable after a complete TURBT: T2 disease
- Palpable prior to TURBT and some induration felt after TURBT: T3 disease
- Invading prostate/vagina/rectum but still mobile: T4a disease
- Invading prostate/vagina/rectum and not mobile (fixed to pelvic walls): T4b disease

These findings were described more than 5 decades ago and in the present era of high-quality imaging, examination under anesthesia does not add much to the information already available from imaging.

11. What are the goals of TURBT?

Ans: TURBT is a diagnostic, staging as well as therapeutic procedure.

- Goals of TURBT-histological diagnosis, assigning the disease risk (number of tumours, size and presence of CIS), assessment of clinical stage (bimanual examination under anaesthesia) and to completely resect all the visible tumours (if clinically safe and feasible).

12. Do the cystoscopy findings predict the stage and grade of the disease?

Ans: There is high correlation between the cystoscopic appearance of the tumor and stage and grade of disease.

- Tumors with long branches or fronds are likely to be low grade and those with short fronds with overlying calcification or necrosis are likely to be high grade.
- A solid broad-based tumor is likely to be muscle invasive, whereas one with narrow stalk is more likely to be NMIBC.
- Tumors which appear like corals (inner circle radius is smaller than outer branch length) are likely to be NMIBC, whereas those which appear like crumbs (inner circle radius larger than outer branch length) are likely to be muscle-invasive (Fig. 6.2).[10]

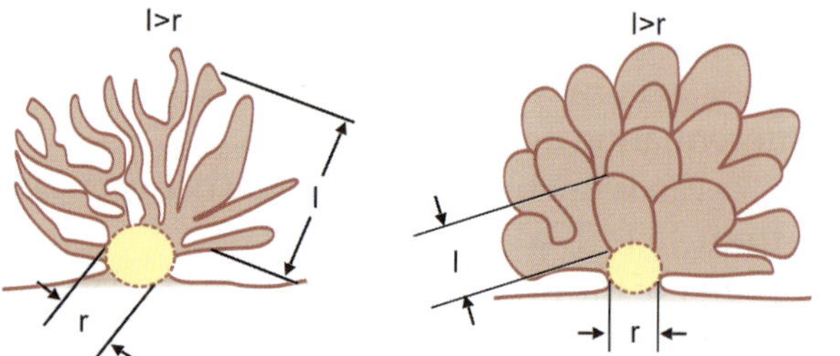

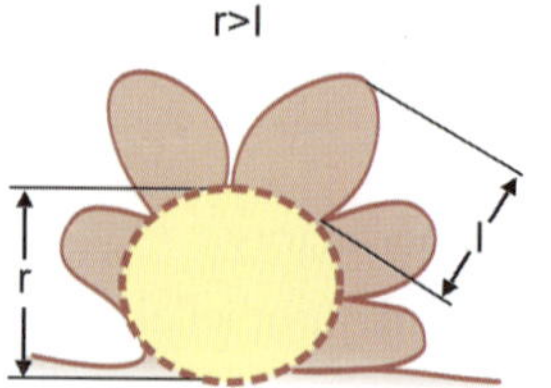

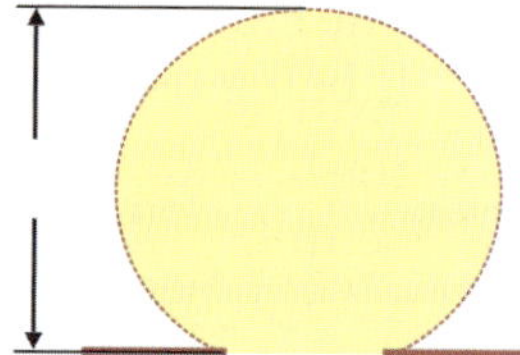

Fig. 6.2: Coral and crumb-like appearance of bladder tumor. Tumors with inner circle radius smaller than the outer branch length are corals, whereas those with inner circle radius larger than the outer branch length are crumbs (l = length and r = radius).

- Overall, the accuracy of correctly predicting the stage and grade ranges from 60 to 80%.

13. What are the different energy sources for TURBT?

Ans: Either mono-polar or bipolar electrocautery.

- Both the energy modalities have similar complication rates such as obturator jerk and bladder perforation rates as well as blood transfusion rates.[11] However, the fall in hemoglobin and the thermal artefacts are lesser with bipolar.
- Recently, both holmium and thulium lasers have also been used for en-bloc TURBT.

14. What are the different techniques of TURBT?

Ans: Traditional piece-meal fashion or as an en-bloc resection.

- En-bloc resection with monopolar or bipolar loop or with lasers such as holmium or thulium fibre laser (TFL) or KTP laser.
- En-bloc was theorized to have a superior representation of the deep muscle on the final histopathology; however, no difference was found.[12]
- En-bloc resection is suitable for small tumors at select locations and require considerable surgical expertise.[13]

15. What is obturator jerk and how can it be prevented?

Ans: While resecting a tumor on the lateral wall, the electric current can stimulate the nearby obturator nerve resulting in a spasm of the adductor muscles of the leg, called "obturator jerk".

- The best way to prevent either general anesthesia (GA) with muscle relaxation or a combination of spinal anesthesia with an obturator nerve block (ONB).
- GA: Depolarizing neuromuscular blockade with succinylcholine is superior to non-depolarizing neuromuscular blockade with vecuronium or atracurium.
- Obturator nerve can be blocked distally in the thigh or proximally in the pelvis or even transvesically.
- Distal ONB using a nerve stimulator is the most optimal method, superior to all other techniques of ONB.[14]
- Other surgical steps to reduce the jerk include reducing the inflow of irrigation fluid and keeping the bladder partially filled, reducing the cautery settings, making small superficial cuts or using LASER.
- Shifting to bipolar cautery was theorized to reduce obturator jerk, however, recent studies have shown similar rates with mono and bipolar cautery.[11]

16. What are the steps to improve the outcomes of TURBT?

Ans: The outcomes can be improved by reporting the cystoscopy findings on a bladder diagram, following a checklist and by offering an early restage TURBT.

- A 10-point checklist has been proposed that comprises assessment of prognostic factors on initial cystoscopy and visual inspection and bimanual palpation after the resection.[15] A high-quality TURBT is one which has obtained all the information necessary for accurate classification of clinical stage and cancer risk, has visually confirmed resection of all bladder tumors and has carefully assessed the integrity of bladder at the end of the procedure.[15]

17. What precautions should be taken while resecting tumors over ureteric orifice?

Ans: Pure cutting current with pin point coagulation should be used.

- The chances of developing ureteric stricture are low, 5–16%.[16]
- Typically, a stent is not placed and the patients are followed up with an ultrasonography to assess for the development of hydronephrosis.
- Placing a stent increases the risk of metachronous upper tract recurrence by 3.4 times and thus prophylactic stenting should be avoided.[17]

18. What is the current role of NBI and PDD during TURBT?

Ans: The standard TURBT is performed under white light and has the potential to miss some lesions.

- **Narrow band imaging:**
  - Filters white light into 2 different bandwidths —blue (415 nm) and green (540 nm) spectrum.
  - In NBI mode, the light is strongly absorbed by hemoglobin and only penetrates the superficial tissues. As bladder tumors are vascular, they appear brown or green over a white background.
  - NBI increases the detection of tumors during surgery—lower recurrence rates at 3 and 12 months.
  - NBI has a pooled sensitivity of 96% and a pooled specificity of 65% as compared to 71% and 71%, respectively, for white light in detection of the pri mary tumor, and improves the RFS (HR= 0.76).[18,19]
  - However, another meta-analysis, that included patients with a single post-operative instillation of chemotherapy, was unable to show the benefit in RFS with NBI.[20]

- **Photodynamic diagnosis / blue light cystoscopy**
  - 5-aminolaevulinic acid (ALA) or hexaminolaevulinic acid (HAL) is instilled in the bladder and cystoscopy is performed with blue light (380–450 nm) after 1 hour.
  - Due to abnormalities of metabolism in the malignant cells, there is accumulation of protoporphyrin IX in the mitochondria, whereas the drug is eliminated from the normal cells. The incident blue light induces the protoporphyrin to emit red fluorescence and thus the tumors appear red over a blue background of normal cells.
  - Blue light cystoscopy increases the detection of tumors with a pooled sensitivity of 93% and specificity of 63% as compared to 71% and 71%, respectively, for the white light in the detection of the primary tumor, and has also been shown to improve the RFS (HR: 0.73).[18,19]
  - Also, this improvement in RFS at 12 months appears to be maintained in patients who received single postoperative instillation of chemotherapy, unlike that with NBI.[20]
  - PDD with HAL is superior than that with 5-ALA.
  - A recent randomized control trial (PHOTO) showed that PDD guided not reduce the recurrence rates as compared to white light cystoscopy.[21] However, several shortcomings of this trial have been pointed out while the authors of the trial continue to maintain that the results are satisfactory. The most recent Cochrane review, published prior to this study, which included 16 RCTs, found a favorable impact on the recurrence and the progression of the disease.[22,23]

19. How would you collect the TURBT specimen and why?

Ans: While collecting the TURBT specimen, the bulk of the tumor is collected and sent in one container and the deep muscle is taken separately and sent in a separate container. This helps in accurate identification of deep muscle as well as identification of deep muscle invasion.

20. Would you advise post-operative intra-vesical instillation of chemotherapy in this particular patient and why?

Ans: Immediate post-operative single instillation of chemotherapy destroys the circulating cells after the TURBT and has a chemo-ablative effect on the residual tumor cells at the site of resection and any small tumor that may have been overlooked.

- Single instillation of chemotherapy reduces the 5-year recurrence rate by 14%.[24]
- Recommended in patients with primary tumors (presumably low risk) and in intermediate-risk tumors with a recurrence rate of <1/year and those with an EORTC recurrence score of <5.
- High-risk tumors or >1 recurrence/year do not derive a benefit.
- Avoided in patients with bladder perforation, extensive resection or bleeding with clots.
- MMC (40 mg) and Gemcitabine (2 grams) are most commonly used. Epirubicin and pirarubicin have also been used, with no evidence of superiority of one over the other.
- Implantation of the tumor cells starts within the first few hours after surgery and later gets covered by extracellular matrix, making the chemotherapy ineffective.
- Thus, chemotherapy should be instilled as soon as possible, preferably within the first two hours after surgery.

21. What is the dose, timing and dwell duration of a single dose chemotherapeutic instillation post-TURBT?

Ans: The single immediate post-operative intra-vesicle instillation should be administered as soon as possible, either inside the operation theatre or preferably within 2 hours of surgery. There is probably no benefit of post-operative instillation after 24 hours of surgery.[5]

- The dose of single instillation depends on the agent used and MMC is the most commonly used in dose of 40 mg in 50 ml and the dwell time is 1–2 hours. Other options are gemcitabine 2 g in 100 ml and epirubicin 50 mg in 50 ml.

22. Would you give this patient saline irrigation or a distilled water irrigation post-operatively?

Ans: Yes as it would prevent clot formation and also wash out the cancer cell and decrease the probability of cancer seeding and recurrence.[5]

23. What is the role of random bladder biopsies and prostatic urethral biopsies?

Ans: Random bladder biopsies and biopsies from normal-looking prostatic urethra are recommended in patients with positive cytology or urine molecular markers in the absence of visible tumor in the bladder. Prostatic urethral biopsies are also recommended in patients with possibly muscle-invasive disease near the bladder neck or trigone to help choose the choice of urinary diversion at the subsequent radical cystectomy.

Case Scenario (Contd.)

On cystoscopy, the tumor was around 3.5 × 3.5 cm in size on the right posterolateral wall, away from the ureteric orifice and was completely resected. The histology report showed high grade urothelial cancer invading the sub-epithelial connective tissue (T1 HG), deep muscle was submitted separately and was free of tumor.

24. What else do you want to know in histology and cystoscopy finding?

Ans: I would want to know whether there were CIS changes and whether a biopsy was taken from the same. Also, on histology, whether LVI was present or not. Presence of CIS places the patients into the very high-risk group according to the EAU and AUA risk stratification, whereas the LVI places the patient into very high risk according to the AUA risk stratification.

25. What should be the next plan of this patient?

Ans: Restage TURBT.

26. What are the indications and benefits of restage TURBT?

Ans: Indications:

1. All patients with T1 lesions, irrespective of deep muscle being present in the specimen
2. When the deep muscle was not included in the specimen with the exception of TaLG and CIS.
3. A repeat TURBT may also be required in patients who had incomplete resection on the first sitting.

Rationale:

- There is significant risk of residual disease and disease under staging in patients with T1 lesions or in those where the deep muscle was not adequately sampled.
- On restage TURBT, up to 29% of patients thought to have early-stage disease may be upstaged and the rates of residual tumor detection ranges from 55 to 76%, with being ~20% when muscle was present in the specimen and >50% when it was not.[25–27]
- Recent systematic reviews have found the residual tumor rate to be 17–67% in patients with TaHG disease and 20–71% in T1 tumors.[28]
- In patients with T1 disease, who had deep muscle in the biopsy, the rate of residual disease was found to be 47% and there was a 10% chance of upstaging at the restage TURBT.[29]
- Restage TURBT has been shown to improve the recurrence free survival and outcomes after BCG and also to provide prognostic information.

27. What is the recommended time frame in which restage TURBT should be performed?

Ans: 2–6 weeks after the initial surgery.

Case Scenario (Contd.)

The restage TURBT showed no mass in the bladder and the biopsy from the previous scar site showed no evidence of malignancy

28. What is the next step in the management of this patient?

Ans: The next step is to risk-stratify the patient. This patient falls in the high-risk group category of NMIBC and thus should be advised adjuvant intravesical treatment with full dose of BCG for three years, i.e. 6 weekly doses of induction followed by maintenance.

29. How do you risk stratify non-muscle invasive cancer bladder?

Ans: Risk stratification is based on the probability of recurrence and progression. The risk classification commonly used include the EAU 2021 or the AUA 2016 or the EORTC 2016 risk calculator (Tables 6.1–6.3).

TABLE 6.1: EAU 2021 risk stratification

Low risk	A primary, single, Ta/T1, LG/G1 tumour < 3 cm in diameter without CIS in a patient ≤ 70 years
	A primary Ta LG/G1 tumour without CIS with at most ONE of the additional clinical risk factors
Intermediate risk	Patients without CIS who are not included in either the low-, high-, or very high-risk groups
High risk	All T1 HG/G3 without CIS, EXCEPT those included in the very high-risk group All CIS patients, EXCEPT those included in the very high-risk group
	Stage and grade with additional clinical risk factors: Ta LG/G2 or T1G1, no CIS with all 3 risk factors Ta HG/G3 or T1 LG, no CIS with at least 2 risk factors T1G2 no CIS with at least 1 risk factor
Very high risk	Stage and grade with additional clinical risk factors: Ta HG/G3 and CIS with all 3 risk factors T1G2 and CIS with at least 2 risk factors T1 HG/G3 and CIS with at least 1 risk factor T1 HG/G3 no CIS with all 3 risk factors
Clinical risk factors	Age >70 years, multiple papillary tumors, tumor diameter >3 cm

The EAU risk stratification can be accessed at www.nmibc.net. This risk stratification gives an individual patient's risk of progression if he/she does not receive adjuvant intravesical BCG.

TABLE 6.2 : AUA 2016 risk stratification

Low risk	Papillary urothelial neoplasm of low malignant potential Low grade urothelial cancer: • Ta and • ≤3 cm and • solitary
Intermediate risk	Low grade Ta: • Solitary >3cm or • Multifocal or • Recurrence within 1 year • HG Ta < 3 cm or LG T1
High risk	High grade T1 HG Ta: • Recurrent • With CIS • >3 cm or • Multifocal
High risk	Very high-risk features (any): • BCG unresponsive • Variant histologies • Lymphovascular invasion • Prostatic urethral invasion

This provides the risk of recurrence and progression for individual patients.

TABLE 6.3: EORTC risk calculator

Factor		***Recurrence Score***	***Progression Score***
Number of tumors	Single	0	0
	2–7	3	3
	>7	6	3
Tumor diameter	<3	0	0
	>3	3	3
Prior recurrence rate	Primary	0	0
	≤ 1 Recurrence/year	2	2
	>1 Recurrence/year	4	2
Category	Ta	0	0
	T1	1	4
Concurrent CIS	No	0	0
	Yes	1	6
Grade	G1	0	0
	G2	1	0
	G3	2	5
Total score		0–17	0–23

After the scores have been calculated, the actual risk of recurrence and progression at 1 and 5 years can be found out on https://www.eortc.be/tools/bladdercalculator.

30. **What is the risk stratification-wise management of NMIBC?**

Ans: Figure 6.3 shows the flowchart of management.

- **Low-risk disease:** There is negligible risk of disease progression—single post-operative instillation of chemotherapy is sufficient.[5] Additional adjuvant intra-vesical chemotherapy is not recommended. Check cystoscopy is recommended at 3 months, if negative then at 9 months later, and then yearly for 5 years.
- **Intermediate risk disease:**The patients should be prescribed either full dose of intravesical BCG for one year (induction plus 3-weekly instillations at 3, 6 and 12 months) or intra-vesical chemotherapy instillation for a period of one year, the schedule of which is not yet defined. The choice between the two depends on the risk of recurrence and progression and the possible adverse events associated with each. The first follow-up check cystoscopy and cytology are performed at 3 months. If negative, an individualized follow-up schedule between high and low-risk cancer is recommended, usually 3 monthly for the first 2 years and then 6 monthly thereafter.
- **High-risk disease:** In these patients, full-dose intravesical BCG for 3 years (induction plus 3-weekly instillations at 3, 6, 12, 18, 24, 30 and 36 months), is indicated. Because of high risk of progression, the option of immediate radical cystectomy should also be discussed. Check cystoscopy and urine cytology is recommended at 3 months, if negative, 3 monthly for 2 years, 6 monthly for up to 5 years and then yearly. Upper tract imaging in the form of a USG KUB or a CECT should be performed annually.
- **Highest risk disease:** The option of radical cystectomy should be discussed. If not feasible or refused, full-dose intravesical BCG for 3 years is indicated.

31. **What is the role of BCG in NMIBC?**

Ans: BCG reduces the risk of tumor recurrence and delays and reduces the risk of progression.

- Has superior efficacy as compared to intravesical chemotherapy.
- The risk of recurrence is reduced by 32%, whereas the progression is reduced by 27% in patients receiving induction and maintenance of BCG as compared to chemotherapy.[30,31]
- BCG induction should always be followed by maintenance doses, as induction doses alone were found to be inferior to intravesical chemotherapy (Fig. 6.3).

32. **What is the mechanism of action of BCG?**

Ans: BCG activates the innate as well as adaptive immune response, both of which play a role in

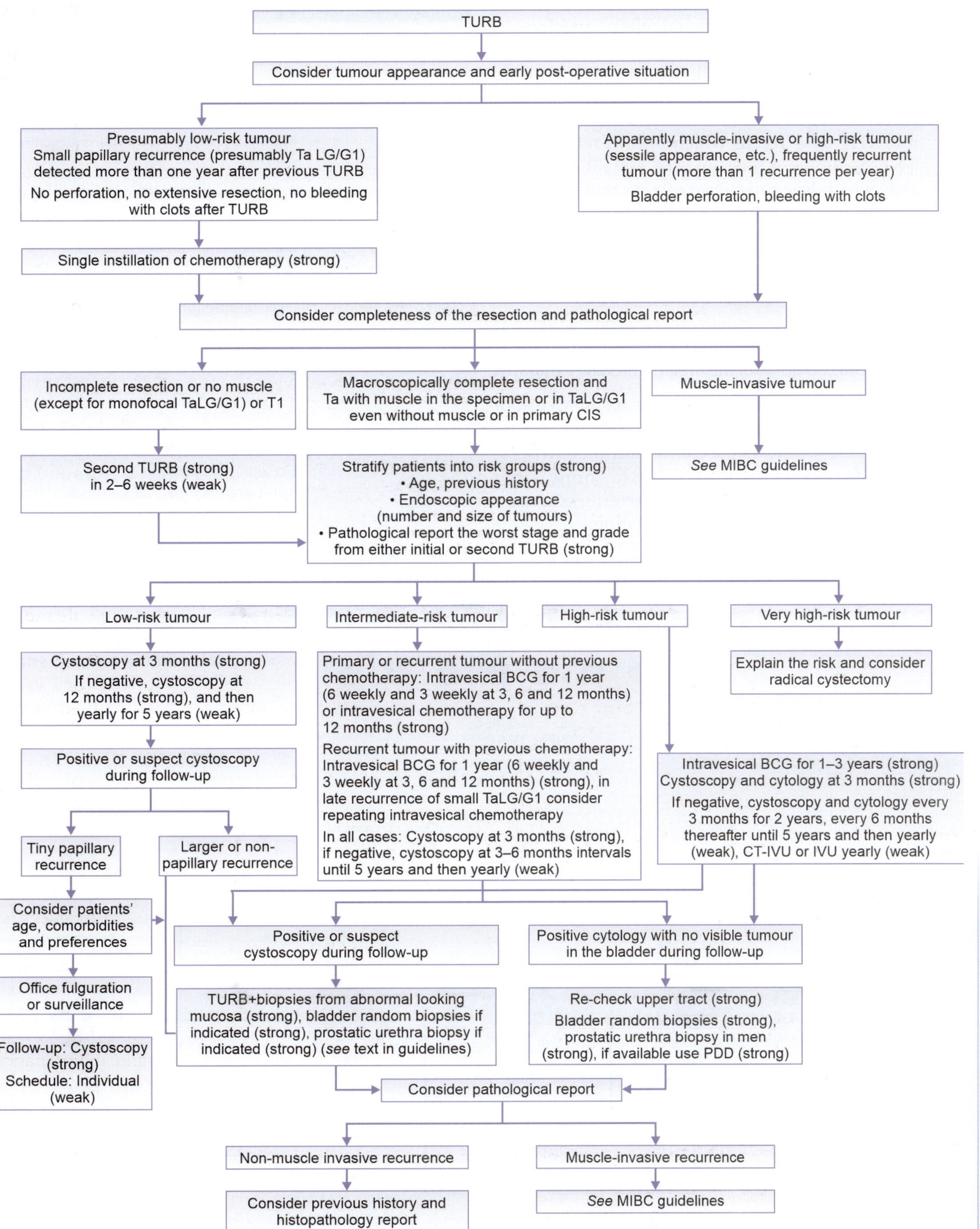

Fig. 6.3: Treatment flowchart based on risk category in patients without prior BCG

its anti-tumor effect. Once instilled, the BCG is internalized into the urothelial cells by attaching to fibronectin and results in an influx of granulocytes, macrophages, natural killer (NK) cells, dendritic cells and lymphocytes. Activated dendritic cells present antigen to CD4 T cells and stimulate them into TH1 CD4 T cells which in turn release IL-2, TNF-α, IFN-γ, which in turn activated CD8 T cells which has anti-tumor effects. Stimulation of neutrophils and activation into natural killer cells, a part of innate immunity, has been shown to have anti-tumor effect[32] (Fig. 6.4).

33. What is the definition of adequate BCG?

Ans: Adequate BCG is defined as the completion of at least 5 of 6 doses of an initial induction course plus at least 2 out of 3 doses of the first maintenance therapy.

34. What are the contraindications for intravesical BCG?

Ans: Table 6.4 shows the contraindication to BCG.

- The presence of leukocyturia, nonvisible hematuria or asymptomatic bacteriuria is not a contraindication of BCG instillation.

TABLE 6.4: Contraindications to intravesical BCG therapy

Absolute contraindications	Immediately after transurethral resection on the basis of risk of intravasation and septic death Personal history of BCG sepsis Gross hematuria (intravasation risk) Traumatic catheterization (intravasation risk) Total incontinence (patient will not retain agent) Immunosuppressed and immunocompromised patients
Relative contraindications	UTI (intravasation risk) Liver disease (precludes treatment with isoniazid if sepsis occurs) Personal history of TB (risk theorized but unknown) Poor overall performance status Advanced age
Insufficient data	Patients with prosthetic materials Ureteral reflux Anti-tumor necrosis factor medications (can predispose to BCG sepsis)

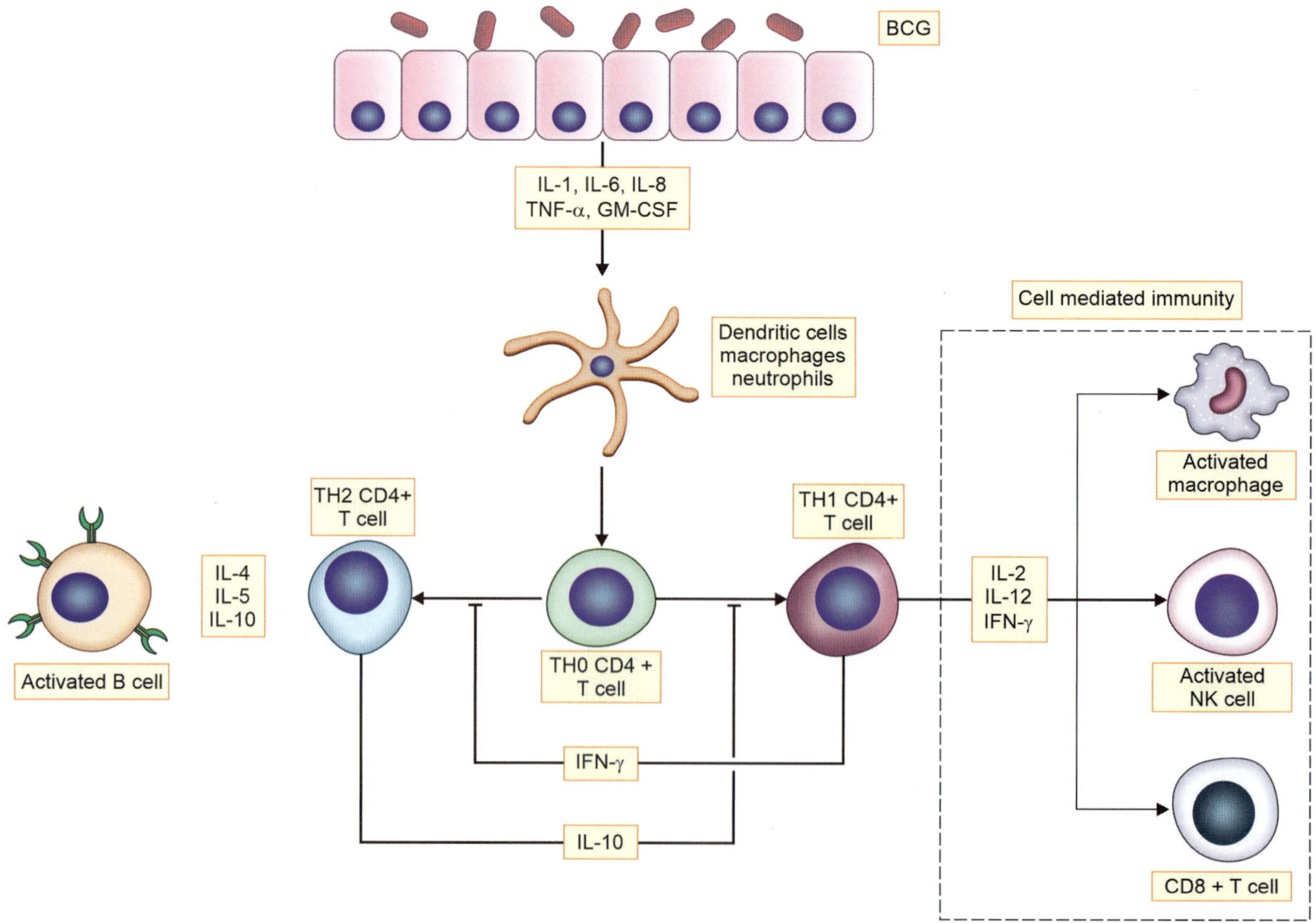

Fig. 6.4: Mechanism of action of BCG

35. What pre-instillation preparation and post-instillation advise will you give to your patient?

Ans: Pre-procedure advise—avoid caffeinated beverages and diuretics for 4 hours prior to instillation and void prior to instillation to ensure bladder is empty. Also, ensure at least 2 weeks have passed post-surgery and there is no hematuria or symptoms suggestive of active urinary tract infection.

Procedure—the parts are cleaned and prepared, an infant feeding tube or small size Foley's catheter is placed, carefully ensuring no trauma to the urethra and urine, if present, is drained to ensure empty bladder. If there is trauma to urethra while catheterization, the procedure is abandoned. Desired dose of BCG is diluted in 50 ml of normal saline and instilled in bladder ensuring no spillage onto the penis.

Post -procedure—patient is asked not to void for a total of 2 hours. Long duration courses of fluoroquinolone, doxycycline and gentamycin antibiotics are avoided.

Usually, post-instillation antibiotics are avoided, however, there is some evidence that a single dose of fluoroquinolone, administered 6 hours after instillation, can reduce symptoms while maintaining the efficacy.[33]

Post-instillation, the patient is asked to keep well hydrated, avoid public toilets, avoid splashing while voiding and after voiding, add 2 cups of undiluted bleach to the toilet, close the lid, wait 15 to 20 minutes prior to flushing.

36. What is the recommended dose and regime for intravesical BCG?

Ans: Current recommendation: Full dose of BCG (80 or 120 mg as suggested by the manufacturer), instilled as per SWOG regime. (An induction phase of six weekly instillations followed by a maintenance phase of three weekly instillations at 3, 6 and 12 months for intermediate-risk patients which is continued at 18, 24, 30 and 36 months for high-risk patients. followed by maintenance dose—3-weekly instillations at 3, 6, 12, 18, 24, 30 and 36 months.)

- The 3 years of maintenance was found to reduce the recurrence rate when compared to one year in patients with high-risk disease, but in not those with intermediate-risk disease, however, there was no difference in the progression or OS.
- Reduced number of instillations either in the induction or in the maintenance settings have been found to be inferior to standard SWOG regimen.[34–36]
- **Dose of BCG**
- BCG is a vaccine constituting of live attenuated bacteria-dosing comes in colony forming units (CFU) rather than in mg.
- The original data from Morales and Lamm with Pasture and Armand Frappier strains indicate that a dose of 10^8–10^9 is effective standard dose, traditionally counted as 120 mg.
- In India, Danish 1331 strain was available till the middle of the last decade and was available as a 40 mg vial containing 1–8 x 10^8 CFU and 3 vials were used for each instillation.
- Currently, Moscow strain manufactured at Serum Institute of India, Pune is available in 40 mg vials containing 1–19 × 10^8 CFU.[37] Since the number of CFU in each vial has a wide range, the full dose needs to be adequately defined and is commonly used as either 2 or 3 vials per instillation depending on institutional practices.
- A recent study comparing 120 mg of Moscow strain to 120 mg of Danish 1331 strain showed similar efficacy but higher adverse events.[38]
- Another recent study compared 80 mg and 120 mg of Moscow strain and found similar oncological outcomes with 80 mg dose.[39]

37. What are the different strains of BCG and is there a difference in their efficacy?

Ans: Some of the noticeable strains are Armand Frappier, Pasture, Connaught, Tice, Tokyo-172, RIVM, Danish 1331, Moreau, Moreau Rio and Moscow.

- There is inadequate evidence to suggest that one strain is superior to the other.

38. What are the side effects of BCG?

Ans: The incidence of serious side effects is 5% and the incidence of BCG infection after BCG instillation is 1% (Table 6.5).

TABLE 6.5: Side effects of intravesical BCG therapy

Local adverse effects	*Systemic adverse effects*
Symptoms of cystitis and LUTS	Generalized malaise, fever
Hematuria	Arthralgia / arthritis
Symptomatic granulomatous prostatitis	Persistent high grade fever
Epididymo-orchitis	BCG sepsis

- A recent study showed reduction in the high-grade adverse events when combining 2 doses of levofloxacin with each instillation of BCG.[40]

39. What is the follow-up protocol for high risk NMIBC?

Ans: Cystoscopy and cytology is performed at 3 months.

- If negative, cystoscopy and cytology is performed every 3 months till 2 years, then every 6 months until 5 years and then yearly.
- Upper tract imaging either in form of USG or CT IVU is recommended annually.

40. What are the options for intravesical therapy in NMIBC?

Ans: Table 6.6 describes the available options for intravesical therapy for NMIBC, however, majority of these are not in clinical use these days, except, MMC, BCG and gemcitabine.

41. What is the mechanism of action for mitomycin C?

Ans: MMC is an alkylating agent. It cross-links the complementary strands found in DNA with absolute specificity and high efficiency for CPG sequence and kills the cell independent of a particular cell cycle phase.

42. What is the efficacy of adjuvant intravesical instillation MMC in patients with NMIBC and how does it compare with BCG?

Ans: Adjuvant intravesical instillations of MMC has been shown to reduce the risk of recurrence at 1 year by 44% when compared with TURBT alone, resulting in an absolute reduction of 14%.

- However, MMC has no effect on the risk of progression.[41]
- As compared to MMC, BCG is superior in reducing the risk of recurrence and also reduces the risk of progression.
- BCG results in 32% reduction in the risk of recurrence and a 27% reduction in the risk of progression when compared to MMC.[30,31]

43. What are the methods to improve the efficacy of MMC?

Ans: The traditional dose of MMC is 40 mg mixed in 40 ml of sterile water retained in the bladder for one hour. Various methods have been described to improve the efficacy.

Optimization of drug delivery

- Fasting for 6 hours reduces the urine output and prevents the dilution of the drug.
- Administration of oral desmopressin 0.2 mg 1 hour prior to instillation also reduces the drug dilution by 38%.[42]
- Administration of oral doses of 1.3 gm of sodium bicarbonate, the night before, the morning and 30 min prior to instillation leads to urine alkalinisation and improves efficacy.
- Draining the bladder with a Foley's catheter prior to drug administration prevents dilution.
- Dissolving 40 mg of MMC in 20 ml of sterile water increases drug concentration and prevents dilution.

Device assisted intravesical chemotherapy: Conductive hyperthermia (hyperthermic intravesical chemotherapy with mitomycin C-HIVEC), electromotive drug administration (EMDA) and microwave-induced hyperthermia—used to increase drug permeability and improve the efficacy.

44. What is HIVEC and how does it compare to MMC?

Ans: HIVEC is recirculating hyperthermic intravesical chemotherapy (HIVEC), which involves a recirculation system with a conductive aluminum heat exchanger that heats MMC solution to 43°C; the solution is then recirculated through the bladder at a constant flow rate via a three-way catheter.

- Initial studies showed promising results. HIVEC II, the only phase II RCT comparing HIVEC to passive chemotherapy in patients with intermediate-risk disease failed to demonstrate an improvement in DFS at 24 months over standard adjuvant intravesical chemotherapy (61% vs. 60%) and had a higher risk of treatment discontinuation (59% vs. 89%).[43]

TABLE 6.6: Various options of intravesical therapy

Agent	*Perioperative use*	*Risk group*	*Cystitis (%)*	*Other toxicity*	*Dropout (%)*	*Concentration and dose*
Doxorubicin (Adriamycin)	Yes	Low to intermediate	20–40	Fever, allergy, contracted bladder, 5%	2–16	50 mg/50 ml
Epirubicin	Yes	Low to intermediate	10–30	Contracted bladder rare	3–6	50 mg/50 ml
Thiotepa	yes	Low to intermediate	10–30	Myelosuppression 8–19%	2–11	30 mg/30 ml
Mitomycin	Yes	Low to intermediate	30–40	Rash 8–19%, contracted bladder 5%	2–14	40 mg/20–40 ml
BCG	No	Intermediate to high	60–80	Serious infection, 5%	5–10	1 vial/50 ml
Interferon	No	Salvage	<5	Flulike symptoms 20%	Rare	50–100 MU/50 ml
Gemcitabine	Yes	Salvage	Mild	Occasional nausea	<10	1–2 g/50–100 ml
Valrubicin	No	Salvage	Mild	UTI, abdominal pain, asthenia	<10	800 mg/55 ml

- HIVEC-HR is the only phase II pilot study that compares HIVEC with BCG in high-risk patients and has shown comparable outcomes at 2 years.[44]

Case Scenario *(Contd.)*

The patient was started on intravesical BCG and regular check cystoscopy. At 6 months cystoscopy he was found to have a 1x1cm growth in the bladder on the posterior wall. He underwent TURBT for the same and the histopathology revealed it as high-grade urothelial cancer limited to epithelium.

45. What are the current possible options for this patient?

Ans: The patient has BCG refractory disease and is unlikely to respond to further BCG. Radical cystectomy (RC) is the preferred option in this patient.[5] For a patient unwilling or unfit for a radical cystectomy, the option of sequential gemcitabine and docetaxel may be offered after discussing the risk of disease recurrence and/or progression.

46. How is BCG failure defined?

Ans: Several categories of BCG failure have been defined:

BCG refractory	• If T1 HG/G3 tumour is present at 3 months • If Ta HG/G3 tumour is present after 3 months and/or at 6 months, after either re-induction or first course of maintenance • If CIS (without concomitant papillary tumour) is present at 3 months and persists at 6 months after either re-induction or first course of maintenance. If patients with CIS present at 3 months, an additional BCG course can achieve a complete response in > 50% of cases • If HG tumour appears during BCG maintenance therapy
BCG relapsing tumour	• Recurrence of HG/G3 tumour after completion of BCG maintenance, despite an initial response
BCG unresponsive	• BCG—unresponsive tumours include all BCG refractory tumours and those who develop T1/Ta HG recurrence within 6 months of completion of adequate BCG exposure or develop CIS within 12 months of completion of adequate BCG exposure
BCG intolerant	• Severe side effects that prevent further BCG instillation before completing treatment

- Patients who do not respond to BCG are categorized as BCG refractory, whereas those who relapse after initial response are BCG relapsing.
- BCG relapsing tumors have better outcomes as compared to BCG refractory.
- BCG unresponsive tumours—patients where additional BCG is unlikely to provide benefit and comprises BCG-refractory and some of the BCG-relapsing tumours (early relapses before 6 months).
- Patients with low grade recurrence during or after BCG are not considered as BCG failures.
- Adequate BCG is defined as the completion of at least 5 of 6 doses of an initial induction course plus at least 2 out of 3 doses of the first maintenance therapy within a period of 6 months (Fig. 6.5).

47. What are the Indications of cystectomy in NMIBC?

Ans: Cystectomy prior to documenting muscle invasion can be offered for:

- **Upfront RC prior to any intravesical therapy:** For patients belonging to very high-risk group.
  - Rationale-staging accuracy of TURBT is low and 25–50% of patients may be upstaged to MIBC at RC. Besides, these patients have very high risk of progression to MIBC, 50% at 10 years, and the oncological outcomes of those who progress to MIBC are worse than those who present with MIBC.
- **Timely RC:** In patients who have BCG unresponsive tumors. They are unlikely to respond to further BCG and should be offered RC.
- **Other indications:** Variant histology (micropapillary, squamous, plasmacytoid, nested), endoscopically unresectable disease

48. What are the options in this patient if he refuses for RC?

Ans: Table 6.7 depicts options of intravesical chemotherapy post-BCG failure:

- These patients can usually be offered re-induction with BCG or proceed with maintenance therapy.

TABLE 6.7: Intravesical chemotherapy post-BCG failure

Single-agent chemotherapy	• Gemcitabine • Docetaxel • Valrubicin
Combination therapy	• Gemcitabine + MMC • Gemcitabine + docetaxel • Valrubicin + docetaxel
Device assisted instillations	• HIVEC • EMDA
Intravesical immunotherapy	• Reinduction with BCG • BCG + interferon • BCG + MMC
Systemic immunotherapy	• Pembrolizumab
Gene therapy	• Intravesical nadofaragene firadenovec gene therapy

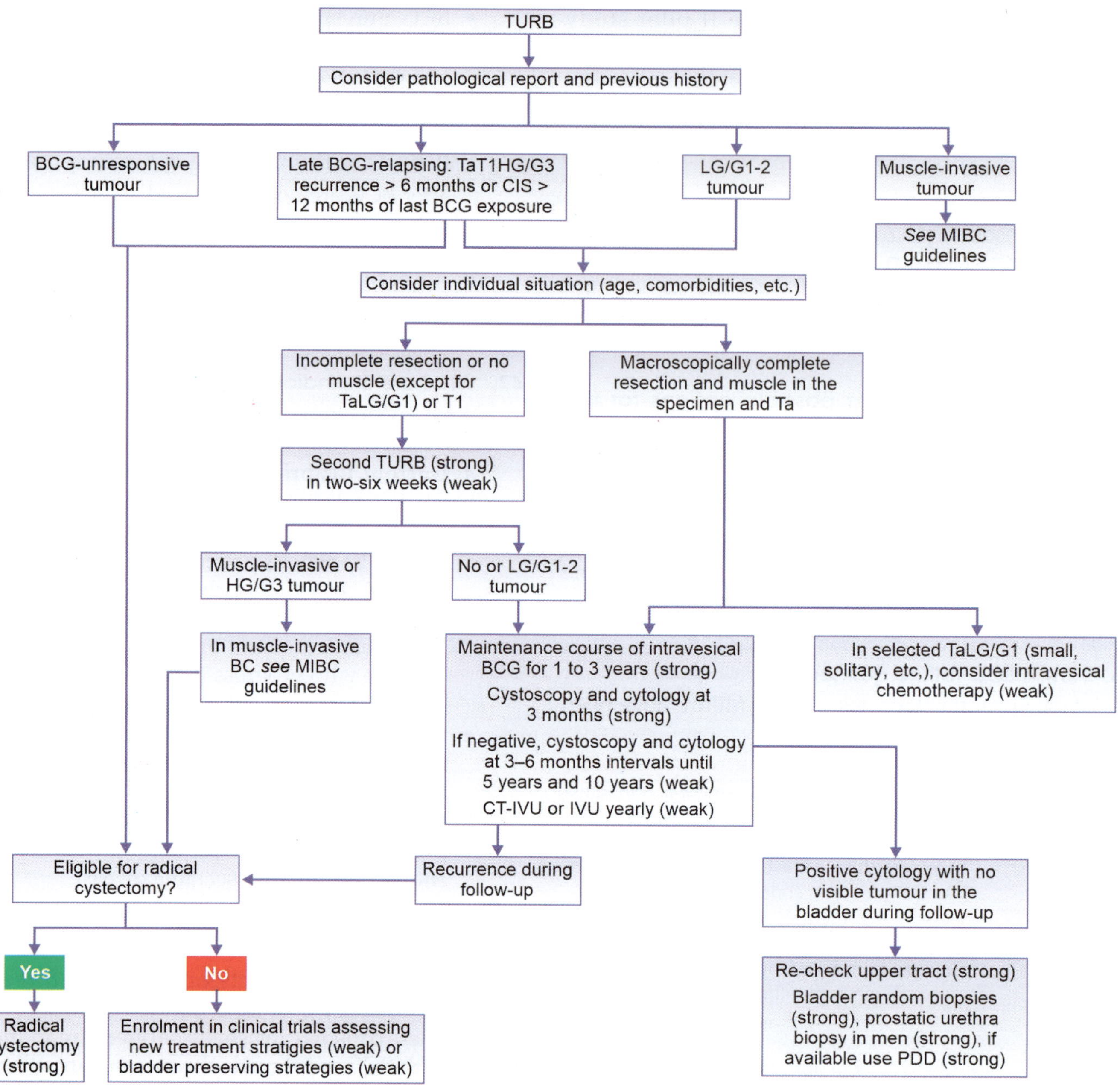

Fig. 6.5: Treatment strategy after recurrence on BCG

However, patients who recur or have persistent disease after two induction courses or induction plus maintenance in general should not receive additional BCG.

- A combination of BCG + MMC has been shown to have superior efficacy than BCG alone but with higher adverse effects. BCG + IFN was not consistently found to be superior to BCG alone, thus is seldom used.
- **Gemcitabine**: In patients with 1 failed course of BCG, as compared to re-induction BCG, gemcitabine showed improved 2-year DFS, but progression and cystectomy rates were similar. Gemcitabine has also shown a 2-year DFS of 21% in patients who failed 2 courses of BCG. However, single agent chemotherapy is seldom used in this setting.
- **Gemcitabine + Docetaxel:** 1 gm gemcitabine in 50 ml sterile water (or normal saline) for 90 minutes followed by 37.5 mg docetaxel dissolved in 50 ml normal saline for 90–120 minutes.
- Combination has shown 1 and 2-year RFS rates of 60% and 46%, and high grade RFS rates of 65% and 52%, respectively, in BCG unresponsive patients.[45] The combination was also found to be of similar efficacy as BCG+ INF in patients who failed on 1st BCG.[46] Recently, in wake of BCG shortage in the West, Gem + Doce combination has been tried in BCG naive settings also, and a RFS of 89%, 85% and 82% at 6, 12 and 24 months,

respectively, has been reported. No patient died of Ca UB and OS was 84%.[47] Thus, sequential instillations with gemcitabine and docetaxel is an emerging treatment concept awaiting further prospective scientific evaluation. Combination chemotherapy is frequently employed currently in this clinical setting.

- **Systemic Immunotherapy:** A recent phase II trial, evaluating patient's BCG unresponsive CIS with or without concomitant papillary tumors, showed complete response in 40% of the patients with intravenous Pembrolizumab leading to its FDA approval.[48]
- **Gene therapy:** With intravesical nadofaragene firadenovec showed a complete response in 53.4% of patients with BCG-unresponsive CIS.[49]

49. What is the role of Erdafitinib in non-muscle invasive bladder cancer?

Ans: Erdafitinib is an oral selective pan-FGFR tyrosine kinase inhibitor approved in metastatic urothelial cancer in adults with FGFR3/2alt who have progressed on platinum-containing chemotherapy. It is being evaluated in patients with BCG unresponsive high risk NMIBC and intermediate risk NMIBC after incomplete TURBT with FGFR3/2 alterations in the THOR-2 trial, which has recently published its interim analysis and showed good response with good safety profile.[50]

50. Elaborate on the management of variant histology in non-muscle invasive bladder cancer.

Ans: NMBIC with variant histology are regarded as high risk tumors due to the high rate of progression in up to 40%. The rate of understaging ranges from 27% to 57% and thus re-stage TURBT is recommended in all cases of T1 variant histology regardless of the presence of detrusor in the biopsy, if conservative therapy with BCG is planned.[51]

Variant histologies are usually associated with advanced disease and poor oncological outcomes. Upfront radical cystectomy is the recommended treatment option for squamous, micropapillary, sarcomatoid and plasmacytoid variants as conservative measures have been shown to have poorer survival. Highly selected patients with glandular variant and nested variant with small tumors, no LVI, no disease at restage can be managed with BCG, alternatively these can be offered upfront radical cystectomy. Those managed conservatively must understand that there is a high risk of progression with conservative therapies and will require close follow-up and may require radical surgery at a later date.[51]

SUMMARY

- Tobacco use and occupational exposure are the two most important risk factors for bladder cancer.
- Urine cytology, cystoscopy and a CECT should be performed in all patients presenting with gross painless hematuria.
- About 75% of bladder cancers are non-muscle invasive at presentation.
- A well-performed TURBT is a crucial component of staging and treating NIMBC. It should provide information about the number, location and appearance of the bladder tumors.
- The pathology report of a TURBT should provide information about the tyoe of tumor (urothelial vs variant), grade of the tumor, the depth of invasion (non-invasive vs lamina propria vs deep muscle) and the presence of CIS.
- Immediate post-operative chemotherapy instillation has been shown to be beneficial in reducing early recurrences in patients with low and intermediate risk NMIBC.
- Intravesical BCG therapy is the standard of care for high grade intermediate risk and high risk NMIBC. The instillation schedule consists of an induction phase of six weekly instillations followed by three weekly instillations at 3, 6 and 12 months for intermediate risk patients which is continued at 18, 24, 30 and 36 months for high-risk patients.
- Early cystectomy should be offered to patients with very high risk NMIBC. Intravesical BCG may be offered to these patients if they are unfit for or refuse a cystectomy.
- BCG refractory NMIBC patients should also proceed to a radical cystectomy.
- Intravesical sequential Gemcitabine-Docetaxel has shown promise in BCG refractory patients who refused a cystectomy or were unfit for a cystectomy. Recently this therapy has also been tried in BCG naive patients and has shown acceptable results.

REFERENCES

1. Al-Zalabani AH, Stewart KF, Wesselius A, Schols AM, Zeegers MP. Modifiable risk factors for the prevention of bladder cancer: a systematic review of meta-analyses. Eur J Epidemiol 2016;31:811.
2. Zhong JH, Zhao Z, Liu J, Yu HL, Zhou JY, Shi R. Association between APE1 Asp148Glu polymorphism and the risk of urinary cancers: a meta-analysis of 18 case-control studies. Onco Targets Ther 2016;9:1499.
3. Zhang Y, Birman BM, Han J, Giovanucci EL, Speizer FE, Stampfer MJ, *et al.* Personal use of permanent hair dyes and cancer risk and mortality in US women: prospective cohort study. BMJ 2020;370:m2942.
4. Wood DP. Tumors of the bladder. In Wein AJ, Kavoussi LR, Partin AW, Peters CA, editors. Campbell-Walsh Urology, Eleventh edition. Philadelphia: Elsevier; 2016. Page 2198.
5. Gontero P, Comperat E, Dominguez Escrig JL, Liedberg F, Mariappan P, Masson-Lecomte A, *et al.* EAU Guidelines on muscle invasive bladder cancer. Edn. presented at the EAU Annual Congress Milan 2023. ISBN 978-94-92671-19-6.
6. Galgano SJ, Porter KK, Burgan C, Rais-Bahrami S. The Role of Imaging in Bladder Cancer Diagnosis and Staging. Diagnostics (Basel). 2020 Sep 16;10(9):703.
7. Woo S, Panebianco V, Narumi Y, Giudice FD, Muglia VF, Takeuchi M, *et al.* Diagnostic Performance of Vesical Imaging Reporting and Data System for the Prediction of Muscle-

invasive Bladder Cancer: A Systematic Review and Meta-analysis. Eur Urol Oncol 2020;3:306–15.

8. Del Giudice F, Pecoraro M, Vargas HA, Cipollari S, Berardinis ED, Bicchetti M, *et al.* Systematic Review and Meta-Analysis of Vesical Imaging-Reporting and Data System (VI-RADS) Inter-Observer Reliability: An Added Value for Muscle Invasive Bladder Cancer Detection. Cancers (Basel), 2020. 12: 2994.
9. Crozier J, Papa N, Perera M, Ngo B, Bolton D, Sengupta S. Comparative sensitivity and specificity of imaging modalities in staging cancer prior to radical cystectomy: a systematic review and meta-analysis World J Urol 2019;37:667–90.
10. Chen H, Hong Y, Yu B, Ruiqian L, Jun L, Ziyong W, *et al.* Retrospective analysis of bladder cancer morphology and depth of invasion under cystoscopy. BMC Urol 2022;22:12.
11. Sharma G, Sharma AP, Mavuduru R, Bora GS, Devana SK, Singh SK, *et al.* Safety and efficacy of bipolar versus monopolar transurethral resection of bladder tumor: a systematic review and meta-analysis. World J Urol 2021;39:377–87.
12. Gallioli A, Diana P, Fontana M, Territo A, Rodriguez-Faba O, Gaya JM, *et al.* En Bloc Versus Conventional Transurethral Resection of Bladder Tumors: A Single-center Prospective Randomized Noninferiority Trial. Eur Urol Oncol 2022;5:440.
13. Croghan SM, Compton N, Manecksha RP, Cullen IM, Daly PJ. En bloc transurethral resection of bladder tumors: A review of current techniques. Can Urol Assoc J. 2022 May;16(5):E287–E293.
14. Wu J, Gao Y, Xiong Z, Xiao X, Yang J, yang X, *et al.* Comparison of different methods of obturator nerve block in transurethral resection of bladder tumors: A systematic review and network meta-analysis. Cancer Med 2023;12:5420–35.
15. Anderson C, Weber R, Patel D, Lowrance W, Mellis A, Cookson M, *et al.* A 10-item checklist improves reporting of critical procedural elements during transurethral resection of bladder tumor. J Urol 2016;196:1014–20.
16. Mano R, Shoshany O, Baniel J, Yossepowitch O. Resection of ureteral orifice during transurethral resection of bladder tumor: functional and oncologic implications. J Urol 2012;188:2129–33.
17. Sountoulides P, Pyrgidis N, Brookman-May S, Mykoniatis I, Karasavvidis T, Hatzichristou D. Does Ureteral Stenting Increase the Risk of Metachronous Upper Tract Urothelial Carcinoma in Patients with Bladder Tumors? A Systematic Review and Meta-analysis. J Urol 2021;205:956–66.
18. Russo GI, Sholklapper TN, Cocci A, Broggi G, Caltabiano R, Smith AB, Lotan Y, *et al.* Performance of Narrow Band Imaging (NBI) and Photodynamic Diagnosis (PDD) Fluorescence Imaging Compared to White Light Cystoscopy (WLC) in Detecting Non-Muscle Invasive Bladder Cancer: A Systematic Review and Lesion-Level Diagnostic Meta-Analysis. Cancers (Basel) 2021;17:4378.
19. Li H, Cao Y, Ma P, Ma Z, Li C, Yang W, *et al.* Novel Visualization Methods Assisted Transurethral Resection for Bladder Cancer: An Updated Survival-Based Systematic Review and Meta-Analysis. Front Oncol 2021;11:644341.
20. Sari Motlagh R, Mori K, Laukhtina E, Aydh A, Katayama S, Grossmann NC, *et al.* Impact of enhanced optical techniques at time of transurethral resection of bladder tumour, with or without single immediate intravesical chemotherapy, on recurrence rate of non-muscle-invasive bladder cancer: a systematic review and network meta-analysis of randomized trials. BJU Int 2021;128: 280–89.
21. Heer R, Lewis R, Vadiveloo T, Yu G, Mariappan P, Creswell J, *et al.* A Randomized Trial of Photodynamic Surgery in Non–Muscle-Invasive Bladder Cancer. NEJM Evidence, 2022. 1: 10.
22. Liedberg F, Bobjer J. Re: Rakesh Heer, Rebecca Lewis, Thenmalar Vadiveloo, *et al.* A Randomized Trial of PHOTOdynamic Surgery in Non-muscle-invasive Bladder Cancer. NEJM Evid. In press. https://doi.org/10.1056/EVIDoa2200092. Eur Urol Open Sci, 2022. 46: 53.
23. Maisch P, Koziarz A, Vajgrt J, Narayan V, Kim MH, Dahm P. Blue vs white light for transurethral resection of non-muscle-invasive bladder cancer: an abridged Cochrane Review. BJUI 2022;130:730–40.
24. Sylvester RJ, Oosterlink W, Holmag S, Sydes MR, Birtle A, Gudjonsson S, *et al.* Systematic Review and Individual Patient Data Meta-analysis of Randomized Trials Comparing a Single Immediate Instillation of Chemotherapy After Transurethral Resection with Transurethral Resection Alone in Patients with Stage pTa-pT1 Urothelial Carcinoma of the Bladder: Which Patients Benefit from the Instillation? Eur Urol 2016;69:231.
25. Miladi M, Peyromaure M, Zerbbib M, Saighi D, Debre B. The Value of a Second Transurethral Resection in Evaluating Patients with Bladder Tumours. Eur Urol 2003;43:241–45.
26. Huang J, Fu J, Zhan H, Xie K, Liu B, Yang F, *et al.* Analysis of the absence of the detrusor muscle in initial transurethral resected specimens and the presence of residual tumor tissue. Urol Int 2012;89:319–25.
27. Herr HW. The value of a second transurethral resection in evaluating patients with bladder tumors. J Urol 1999;162:74–6.
28. Cumberbatch MGK, Foster B, Catto JWF, Kamat AM, Kassouf W, Jubber I, *et al.* Repeat Transurethral Resection in Non-muscle-invasive Bladder Cancer: A Systematic Review. Eur Urol 2018;73:925.
29. Naselli A, Hurle R, Paparella S, Buffi NM, Lughezzani G, Lista G, *et al.* Role of Restaging Transurethral Resection for T1 Non-muscle invasive Bladder Cancer: A Systematic Review and Meta-analysis. Eur Urol Focus 2018;4:558.
30. Malmstrom PU, Sylvester RJ, Crawford DE, Friedrich M, Krege S, Rintala E, *et al.* An individual patient data meta-analysis of the long-term outcome of randomised studies comparing intravesical mitomycin C versus bacillus Calmette-Guerin for non-muscle-invasive bladder cancer. Eur Urol 2009;56:247.
31. Sylvester RJ, van der Meijden APM, Lamm DL. Intravesical bacillus Calmette-Guerin reduces the risk of progression in patients with superficial bladder cancer: a meta-analysis of the published results of randomized clinical trials. J Urol 2002;168:1964–70.
32. Maruf M, Brancato SJ, Agarwal PK. Nonmuscle invasive bladder cancer: a primer on immunotherapy. Cancer biology and medicine 2016;13:194–205.
33. Colombel M. The effect of ofloxacin on bacillus Calmette-Guerin induced toxicity in patients with superficial bladder cancer: results of randomised, prospective, double-blind, placebo controlled, multicenter study. J Urol 2006;176:935–39.
34. Ojea A, Nogueira JL, Solsona E, Flores N. Gomez JMF, Molina JR, *et al.* A multicentre, randomised prospective trial comparing three intravesical adjuvant therapies for intermediate-risk superficial bladder cancer: low-dose bacillus Calmette-Guerin (27 mg) versus very low-dose

bacillus Calmette-Guerin (13.5 mg) versus mitomycin C. Eur Urol 2007;52:1398–406.
35. Oddens J, Brausi M, Sylvester R, Bono A, van de Beek C, van Andel G, Hoeltl W, *et al.* Final results of an EORTC-GU cancers group randomized study of maintenance bacillus Calmette-Guerin in intermediate-and high-risk Ta, T1 papillary carcinoma of the urinary bladder: one-third dose versus full dose and 1 year versus 3 years of maintenance. Eur Urol 2013;63:462–72.
36. Grimm MO, van der Heijden AG, Colombel M, Muilwijk T, Martínez-Piñeiro N, Babjuk MM. *et al.* Treatment of High-grade Non-muscle-invasive Bladder Carcinoma by Standard Number and Dose of BCG Instillations Versus Reduced Number and Standard Dose of BCG Instillations: Results of the European Association of Urology Research Foundation Randomised Phase III Clinical Trial "NIMBUS". Eur Urol 2020;78:690–98.
37. Arora A, Bakshi G, Pal M, Addla S, Waigakar S, Prakash G. Tailoring the dose of Moscow strain of intravesical bacillus Calmette-Guerin for Indian patients: A plea for urgent action. Indian J Urol 2022;38:165.
38. Thyavihally YB, Dev P, Waigankar S, Pednekar A, Athikari N, Raut A, *et al.* Intravesical bacillus Calmette-Guerin (BCG) in treating non-muscle invasive bladder cancer–Analysis of adverse effects and effectiveness of two strains of BCG (Danish 1331 and Moscow). Asian J Urol 2021;8:315–23.
39. Sood R, Sharma H, Sharma B, Parekh S, Pujari P, Shewale S. A prospective comparative study to assess the efficacy and tolerability of 2 different doses of intravesical bacillus Calmette-Guerin (BCG) in patients with non-muscle-invasive bladder cancer. Urol Oncol 2020;38:433–39.
40. Numakura K, Kobayashi M, Ishida T, Okane K, Suzuki K, Shimoda N, *et al.* Effect of Levofloxacin on the Efficacy and Adverse Events in Intravesical Bacillus Calmette-Guerin Treatment for Bladder Cancer: Results of a Randomized, Prospective, Multicenter Study. Eur Urol Focus 2022; 6:1666–72.
41. Huncharek M, McGarry R, Kupelick B. Impact of intravesical chemotherapy on recurrence rate of recurrent superficial transitional cell carcinoma of the bladder: results of a meta-analysis. Anticancer Res 2001;21:765–9.
42. Cliff AM, Heatherwick B, Scoble J, Parr NJ. The effect of fasting or desmopressin before treatment on the concentration of mitomycin C during intravesical administration. JU Int 2000;86:586–47.
43. Tan WS, Prendergast A, Ackerman C, Yogeswaran Y, Cresswell J, Mariappan P, *et al.* Adjuvant Intravesical Chemohyperthermia Versus Passive Chemotherapy in Patients with Intermediate-risk Non–muscle-invasive Bladder Cancer (HIVEC-II): A Phase 2, Open-label, Randomised Controlled Trial. Eur Urol 2022;S0302–2838(22)025520.
44. Guerrero-Ramos F, González-Padilla DA, González-Díaz A, de la Rosa-Kehrmann F, Rodríguez-Antolín A, Inman BA. *et al.* Recirculating hyperthermic intravesical chemotherapy with mitomycin C (HIVEC) versus BCG in high-risk non-muscle-invasive bladder cancer: results of the HIVEC-HR randomized clinical trial. World J Urol 2022;40:999–1004.
45. Steinberg RL, Thomas LJ, Brooks, Mott SL, Vitale A, Crump T, *et al.* Multi-Institution Evaluation of Sequential Gemcitabine and Docetaxel as Rescue Therapy for Nonmuscle Invasive Bladder Cancer. J Urol 2020;203:902–09.
46. Steinberg RL, Packiam VT, Thomas LJ, Brooks N, Vitale A, Mott SL, *et al.* Intravesical sequential gemcitabine and docetaxel versus bacillus calmette-guerin (BCG) plus interferon in patients with recurrent non-muscle invasive bladder cancer following a single induction course of BCG. Urol Oncol 2022;40:9.e1-9.e7.
47. McElree IM, Steinberg RL, Martin AC, Richards J, Mott SL, Gellhaus PT, *et al.* Sequential Intravesical Gemcitabine and Docetaxel for bacillus Calmette-Guérin-Naïve High-Risk Nonmuscle-Invasive Bladder Cancer. J Urol 2022;208 :589-99.
48. Balar AV, Kamat AM, Kulkarni GS, Uchio EM, Boormanns JL, Roumiguié M, *et al.* Pembrolizumab monotherapy for the treatment of high-risk non-muscle-invasive bladder cancer unresponsive to BCG (KEYNOTE-057): an open-label, single-arm, multicentre, phase 2 study. Lancet Oncol 2021;22:919–30.
49. Boorjian SA, Alemozaffar M, Konety BR, Shore ND, Gomella LG, Kamat AM, *et al.* Intravesical nadofaragene firadenovec gene therapy for BCG-unresponsive non-muscle-invasive bladder cancer: a single-arm, open-label, repeat-dose clinical trial. Lancet Oncol 2021;22:107–17.
50. Daneshmand S, Zaucha R, Gartrell BA, Lotan Y, Hussain SA, Lee EK, *et al.* Phase 2 study of the efficacy andsafety of Erdafitinib in patients with intermediate risk non-muscle invasive bladder cancer (IR-NMIBC) with FGFR3/2alterations in THOR-2: Cohort 3 interim analysis. J Clin Oncol 2023;41
51. Sanguedolce F, Calo B, Mancini V, Zanelli M, Paliccelli A, Zizzo M, *et al.* Non-muscle invasive bladder cancer with variant histology: Biology features and clinical implications. Oncology 2021;99:345–58.

Chapter 7

Muscle Invasive Bladder Cancer

• *Vivek Venkatramani* • *Gagan Prakash*

LEARNING OBJECTIVES

- To understand the basic work-up of a patient diagnosed with muscle-invasive bladder cancer (MIBC) on a TURBT: A complete metastatic evaluation should be done for all patients detected with MIBC.
- To understand the evolving role of MRI in the evaluation of bladder cancer: The VI-RADS score as reported in MRI has shown high accuracy in differentiating T1 from T2 lesions. However, its integration into the algorithm for MIBC will require more studies.
- To understand the role of neoadjuvant therapy: Neoadjuvant chemotherapy has proven survival benefit and should be offered to all patients diagnosed with MIBC. Neoadjuvant immunotherapy is currently being evaluated in trials.
- To understand the surgical aspects of management of MIBC: Radical cystectomy is the standard of care for patients with MIBC. All surgical approaches (open, laparoscopic and robotic) have similar oncological and functional outcomes.
- To understand about the indications, contraindications and complications associated with various urinary diversions: Apart from certain contraindications, both ileal conduit and neobladder can be offered to most patients undergoing a radical cystectomy.
- To understand the indications for adjuvant therapy after radical cystectomy: Adjuvant chemotherapy is recommended for patients who did not receive neoadjuvant chemotherapy and still have ≥T3 or N+ disease after cystectomy.
- To understand about the option of bladder preservation: Bladder preservation in the form of trimodal therapy has shown equivalent results to radical cystectomy in well-selected patients. It may also be offered to patients who are unfit to undergo a radical cystectomy.
- To understand the role of immunotherapy in MIBC: Immunotherapy is being evaluated in the neoadjuvant setting either as monotherapy or in combination with chemotherapy. Adjuvant nivolumab is recommended for patients who have yp≥T2 or ypN+ disease.
- To understand the follow-up following a radical cystectomy: Patients need to remain on long-term follow-up as recurrences have been described even after an initial disease-free period of a couple of years.

Case Scenario

A 55-year-old otherwise healthy gentleman (40 pack-years smoker) was evaluated for gross hematuria and found to have a 4 cm sessile right lateral wall bladder tumor on computed tomography (CT) with urography. There was no hydroureteronephrosis. Sub-centimeter right obturator and iliac lymph nodes were noted. Blood investigations were within normal limits.

He underwent a TURBT which revealed high grade urothelial carcinoma of the urinary bladder with invasion of the detrusor muscle. There was a small component (<10%) of squamous differentiation in the specimen.

1. **How will you proceed further?**

   Ans: After counseling the patient, I would like to complete the metastatic work up by imaging the chest. A general work up of the patient as a pre-treatment evaluation will also be done. A geriatric and frailty assessment is also done when indicated. Involvement of occupational therapist, nutritionist and rehabilitation should be commenced as early as feasible. Consultation with medical oncologist for discussion on neoadjuvant chemotherapy is also considered.

2. **What is a maximal TURBT?**

   Ans: Maximal TURBT involves removal of as much tumor tissue as possible (potentially complete resection) which is considered an essential part of trimodality therapy involving chemo-therapy and radiotherapy additionally. The aim is to remove all visible tumor tissue, while also sampling the surrounding bladder tissue to ensure that no additional tumors are present.

3. **What is the role of FDG PET-CT?**

Ans:

- FDG PET-CT has low sensitivity (but higher than CT) and high specificity for detection of metastatic lymph nodes.
- FDG PET-CT can provide important staging information which may impact clinical management of MIBC patients, though it is not recommended as the initial imaging of choice in all patients with MIBC.[6]
- In patients with deranged renal function, where contrast is to be avoided, a non-contrast FDG PET/CT can be done for staging.

4. **Is MRI useful before or after TURBT?**

Ans:

- MRI is promising in the pre-TURBT setting, as tissue architecture has not been distorted by surgery.
- TURBT or intravesical therapy causes edema and inflammation in the bladder wall and the surrounding perivesical tissue, making it difficult to distinguish normal tissues from bladder cancer and resulting in an overestimation of the local stage. Therefore, MRI study is best performed before the procedure or at least 2 weeks after transurethral resection, biopsy, or intravesical treatment.[7] Inflammatory artifacts can be mistaken for T3 disease.
- Air in the bladder (from cystoscopy or indwelling catheter) can cause distortion of diffusion-weighted imaging (DWI) due to susceptibility artifact. A 2 or 3-day interval between cystoscopy or removal of Foley catheter and MRI examination is recommended.
- MRI has superior soft tissue contrast resolution than CT. The accuracy of MRI for primary staging ranges from 75 to 95%.
- Pre-operative MRI provides useful information regarding tumor response. In the neoadjuvant setting, DWI has been shown to have higher specificity than T2W and DCE MRI in assessing therapeutic response to induction chemotherapy. The high specificity of DWI indicates that it is useful for accurate prediction of a complete histopathological response, allowing better patient selection for bladder sparing protocols.

5. **Is there any other modality by which one can stage the bladder tumor locally apart from TURBT and CT scan?**

Ans:

- Yes, VI-RADS scoring system has been introduced by using mpMRI to differentiate T1 vs T2.
- T2-weighted (T2W) image, DWI, and dynamic contrast-enhanced image (DCE MRI) are key components of mpMRI examination.
  - Definitive muscular invasion is decided by DWI and DCE
  - Images must include the whole bladder, proximal urethra, pelvic nodes, and prostate if the patient is a male. In females, adjacent pelvic viscera (uterus, ovaries, fallopian tubes, and vagina) should also be included.
  - T1-weighted (T1W) image is used to identify hemorrhage and clot in the bladder, and bone metastasis.
  - It has got high diagnostic accuracy to differentiate T1 vs T2.
  - A five-point VI-RADS score is generated using the individual T2W, DWI, and DCE MRI categories and suggests the possibility of muscle invasion.[4,5]
  - VI-RADS 1: Muscle invasion is highly unlikely
  - VI-RADS 2: Muscle invasion is unlikely
  - VI-RADS 3: Muscle invasion: Equivocal
  - VI-RADS 4: Muscle invasion likely
  - VI-RADS 5: Invasion of muscle and beyond is very likely
- The potential role of mpMRI as 1st line test for local staging of bladder cancer rather than TURBT has been demonstrated by Bryan *et al.*[8]
- The **Bladder Path study** is exploring the utility of MRI in the management pathway. If the MRI reliably confirms muscle invasion, it can potentially obviate the need of a TURBT and reduce the time to definitive management. The downside of this pathway, however, is that it is based on reliability of VI-RADS reporting and that in some patients, variant histology can be missed if TURBT is skipped.
- Although cystoscopy remains the standard means of post-treatment follow-up, the need for frequent repeat examinations has driven mpMRI as a noninvasive alternative. DWI is superior to DCE MRI in identifying tumor recurrence following either TURBT or partial cystectomy. Larger studies are required to consider using mpMRI for treatment response and to standardize it for regular usage.

6. **Is neoadjuvant chemotherapy recommended in this case?**

Ans:

- Yes, neoadjuvant chemotherapy (NAC) is recommended in this case considering it to be a muscle invasive bladder cancer which has proven survival advantage.

- Cisplatin based combination NAC is recommended for patients with T2-T4a, cN0, M0.
- It can be used in patients with mixed urothelial carcinoma histology.
- Urothelial carcinoma plus squamous differentiation, adenocarcinoma differentiation, micropapillary, nested, plasmacytoid, and sarcomatoid should be identified because of the potential to have a more aggressive natural history. These are usually treated in a similar manner to pure urothelial carcinoma of the bladder.
- Micropapillary, plasmacytoid, and sarcomatoid histologies are generally at higher risk for progression to muscle invasive disease and a more aggressive approach should be considered.
- Majority of subtypes are MIBC with around 15–30% being NMIBC at presentation.
- NAC has been reported to have the following advantages:[3]
  i. Improve overall survival by 5–8% at 5 years.
  ii. 16% reduction in mortality risk
  iii. Improvement in 10-year survival from 30% to 36%
  iv. Pathological complete response rate: 30–40%

7. Is there any difference in the role of NAC in cT2 vs ≥cT3?

Ans:

- In a recent meta-analysis, it was found that for patients with cT2, NAC before RC showed no significant effect on overall survival, but showed significantly increased rates of pathological complete response (ypT0N0).
- For patients with cT3-4, NAC showed remarkable improvements in both OS and pathological complete response.[9]

8. What are the contraindications, advantages and disadvantages of NAC?

Ans:

- **Contraindications**: Those who are unfit or having contraindication for cisplatin usage (First 5 of the following constitutes the **Galsky criteria** for cisplatin ineligibility for metastatic bladder cancer):[10]
  i. ECOG PS >1,
  ii. GFR <60 ml/min,
  iii. Audiometric hearing loss grade ≥2
  iv. Peripheral neuropathy grade ≥2,
  v. NYHA class III heart failure
  vi. Allergy to agents that contain platinum/mannitol,
  vii. HIV/AIDS with CD4 count <200/microliter
- Selected patients with GFR <60 ml/min can be treated by using split doses of cisplatin and aggressive hydration.
- **Advantages**
  - Chemotherapy can be delivered early when the burden of micro metastases is low.
  - Potential reflection of *in vivo* chemosensitivity allowing assessment of individual
  - Tumor downstaging
  - Proven survival advantage
  - Better tolerability before surgery; patients can receive full dose and cycles (40% patients show decline in renal function after cystectomy)
  - Does not increase surgical morbidity.
- **Disadvantages**
  - Delayed definitive treatment for up to 3 months with potential compromise of outcome in unresponsive patients
  - Over treatment in some patients
  - No benefit seen for loco-regional control and loco-regional DFS
  - In Indian patients,[1] bilateral obstructive uropathy and consequent cisplatin ineligibility is quite common due to delayed presentation. In such situations, if a diversion procedure improves the GFR, then NAC should be reconsidered; otherwise, opting for RC followed by adjuvant chemotherapy could be an alternative approach.[11]
  - Optimal pathological response after NAC: Attainment of ypT0N0/ypTisN0 at radical cystectomy.
  - Chemotherapy alone as primary therapy for localized bladder cancer is not recommended and a local therapy (radical cystectomy or RT) has to be added even if complete radiological response is seen post-NAC.

9. Which drugs are used for neoadjuvant chemotherapy and how many cycles are recommended?

Ans:

- NAC should only be used in patients eligible for cisplatin-combination based chemotherapy.
  - **MVAC**: Methotrexate + Vinblastine + Adriamycin + Cisplatin (Adriamycin also known as Doxorubicin)
  - **ddMVAC** (3–6 cycles) (with primary G CSF-Filgrastim): Higher rates of downstaging, higher rates of pathological complete response rate (38% as against 26% with GC) and a significantly longer time to progression. Preferred regimen in healthy patients <70 years age.
  - **GC** (4 cycles; Each cycle to be repeated every 21 days for a total of two cycles prior to restaging): Better toxicity profile compared to ddMVAC.

i. Standard single dose Cisplatin regimen: Gemcitabine 1000 mg/m on day 1 and 8; Cisplatin 70 mg/m on day 1; repeat cycle every 21 days.

ii. Split dose Cisplatin regimen (For those with GFR 45–60 ml/min): Cisplatin 35 mg/m and gemcitabine 1000 mg/m on days 1 and 8 of each cycle.

iii. A 28-day cycle can also be used where Gemcitabine can be given in a dose of 1000 mg/m^2 on day 1, 8 and 15. Cisplatin is given in the dose of 70 mg/m^2 on day 2.

- *Gemcitabine:* To be given IV in 250 ml NS over 30 min.
- *Cisplatin*: Prehydrate with 1000 ml NS over 1 hour, then Cisplatin IV in 500 ml NS with 20 mEq potassium chloride, 1g magnesium sulfate, 30 g mannitol over 1 hour.
- *VESPER trial:* 500 patients were randomly assigned in 28 French centers and received either 6 cycles of ddMVAC once every 2 weeks or 4 cycles of GC once every 3 weeks before surgery (neoadjuvant group) or after surgery (adjuvant group). It was found that the 3-year progression free survival (64% vs 56%), time to progression and overall survival was better for patients in the ddMVAC arm compared to those receiving GC.[12]
- *Other less commonly used regimens:*

  i. MVEC: Methotrexate + Vinblastine + Epirubicin + Cisplatin

  ii. CMV: Cisplatin + Methotrexate + Vinblastine

  iii. CM: Cisplatin + Methotrexate

  iv. CA: Cisplatin + Adriamycin

  v. CF: Cisplatin + 5-fluorouracil

- Radical cystectomy should be performed after 2–3 weeks and definitely within 6 weeks after completion of NAC.

10. What is the role of neoadjuvant immunotherapy in MIBC?

Ans:

- Neoadjuvant immunotherapy is recommended only within a clinical trial setting.
- Pembrolizumab and atezolimumab have shown positive results in conducted trials.
- Also, neoadjuvant chemo-immunotherapy is showing promising pathological response rates in patients with MIBC. The concern with adding therapies together is the increase in the toxicity profile.

11. What is the role of radiotherapy in MIBC?

Ans:

- **Preoperative radiotherapy**: It is not recommended for localized operable MIBC, as there is no contemporary data showing survival benefit. However, a few studies have shown downstaging after 4–6 weeks of preoperative RT.
- **Role of RT as definitive therapy**: EBRT alone is not as effective as surgery or trimodality therapy, however, it can be an alternative treatment in patients unfit for RC or concurrent chemotherapy. The target total dose for curative EBRT is 64–66 Gy in 32 fractions (reasonable alternative is 55 Gy in 20 fractions which is found to be non-inferior to 64 Gy).
- Radiotherapy alone is inferior to radiotherapy combined with chemotherapy for patients with an invasive bladder tumor, and is not considered standard for patients who can tolerate combined therapy. Also, chemotherapy alone is considered to be inadequate without additional treatment to the bladder and it remains investigational. However, concurrent chemoradiotherapy should be considered as potentially curative therapy in selected patients especially in medically MIBC patients unfit for a cystectomy.[13]
- Trimodality therapy is discussed in a subsequent answer.
- **Evolving role of adjuvant RT**: It can be considered in addition to adjuvant CT in patients with pT3b/4 or N+ or positive margins (weak recommendation, EAU 2023).[3] There is evolving interest in considering adjuvant RT. Bladder cancer adjuvant radiotherapy trial (BART) is one such ongoing prospective randomized trial (TMH, Mumbai) of adjuvant radiotherapy following RC and chemotherapy in patients with MIBC; primary outcome being improvement in loco-regional relapse free survival in 2 years.
- RT can also be used to stop bleeding from the tumor when local control cannot be achieved by transurethral procedures.

12. What are the steps of radical cystectomy?

Ans:

- No recommendation for bowel preparation preoperatively.
- In males, RC involves removal of the bladder, perivesical soft tissue, terminal ureters, prostate, seminal vesicles and regional lymph nodes.
- In women, along with the bladder, perivesical tissue and terminal ureters, the ovaries, fallopian tubes, uterus with cervix and anterior vaginal wall (anterior exenteration) are also removed. In organ-confined MIBC with no cancer in

the bladder base, trigone or bladder neck, preservation of the vaginal wall and/or uterus may be considered.

- Patient position: Supine, with or without mild flexion at the anterior superior iliac spine.
- If urethrectomy is planned, lithotomy position is preferable. In females, low lithotomy may be used to provide access to the vagina.
- First, a midline incision is made from the umbilicus to the symphysis pubis. The space of Retzius is entered, and the bladder is released from pelvic sidewall attachments bilaterally using blunt dissection. This is done in a cephalad direction until the level of the vas deferens in men and the round ligament in women is reached. The urachus is then controlled and divided as high as possible, and the peritoneum between the two median umbilical ligaments is included in the dissection. Mobilization is done on both sides to expose the great vessels and the ureters. The bilateral ureters are dissected free and divided close to the bladder. The superior vesical artery can be ligated and divided for ureteral dissection.
- The utilization of frozen section analysis to evaluate the presence of urothelial carcinoma in the distal ureteral margin remains a controversial practice. While research has established a correlation between positive findings of carcinoma in the ureteral margin and a heightened likelihood of upper tract recurrence, its impact on overall survival has yet to be fully established. Notably, a study has reported that in cases where sequential resection was employed to achieve a negative margin following an initial positive ureteral margin, upper tract recurrence was not always prevented, especially in patients with CIS.[2]
- In males, after completely ligating vascular pedicles, the peritoneum is incised over the seminal vesicles. The rectum is dissected from the midline, and dissection is carried out at the level of the prostate. Sharp dissection is preferred to avoid rectal injury. Dissection is then carried out laterally, and the posterior vesical pedicles are identified. After dissection, the surgeon should be able to reach the prostate and palpate the urethra. Anterior dissection is similar to radical prostatectomy. After ligation of the dorsal venous complex, the anterior urethra is identified, and dissection is completed. Preservation of maximal urethral length is important if a neobladder is planned. A frozen section of the urethral margin is mandatory in case of a neobladder.
- In females, the procedure includes anterior pelvic exenteration, which encompasses the bladder, urethra, anterior vagina, uterus, and cervix. Most of the steps are similar to radical cystectomy in males. However, knowledge of the steps of hysterectomy and identification of the posterior fornix, gaining entry into the vaginal canal, dissection of the uterus, cervix, anterior vaginal cuff, and bladder is essential. The urethral meatus can be excised from the pelvis or the vagina. Closure of the vaginal defect is necessary. At times, vaginal sparing surgery is done in the absence of bladder neck involvement.
- Radical cystectomy should not be delayed beyond 3 months after diagnosis as it increases the risk of progression and cancer specific mortality, unless the patient receives NAC.

13. When is urethrectomy indicated?

Ans:

- Diffuse CIS of prostatic urethra or ducts.
- Prostatic stromal invasion.
- T4 tumors involving urethra and/or vagina in females.
- Positive apical margin on RC specimen.
- Urethrectomy is to be done at the time of cystectomy or subsequently as a separate procedure if the tumor involves the bladder neck in females or prostatic urethra in males, or if the urethral cut margin is positive at the end of cystectomy.

14. What is the extent of lymphadenectomy?

Ans:

- Lymphadenectomy provides optimal staging of bladder cancer and might be curative in a small proportion of patients. It remains an essential component of radical cystectomy.
- The optimal extent of lymphadenectomy has not been established to date.
- **Primary lymphatic zone** for bladder cancer includes: Hypogastric (internal iliac), obturator, presacral and external iliac (HOPE).
- **Secondary lymphatic zone**: Common iliac, paracaval, paraaortic, interaortic.
- Bilateral pelvic lymphadenectomy should be performed and include common, internal iliac, external iliac, and obturator nodes.[13]
  - **Standard LND** is recommended: Includes internal iliac, presacral, obturator fossa and external iliac nodes.[14] The template extends:
    i. *Cranially:* Common iliac bifurcation or till the level of the ureter crossing the common iliac.

ii. *Caudally:* Circumflex iliac vein, lacunar ligament and the LN of Cloquet.
iii. *Medially:* Obturator nerve caudally; internal iliac artery and ureter superiorly.
iv. Laterally: Genitofemoral nerve

- **Limited LND**: Includes the nodes from the true pelvis, but excluding the deep obturator nodes.[15]
- **Extended LND**: Same boundaries as standard LND, except for the cranial limit which is the bifurcation of the aorta.
- **Super extended LND**: Cranial extent is till the inferior mesenteric artery.[16]
- Extended and super-extended LND did not show a significant advantage over limited LND for RFS, cancer-specific survival, or OS.[13]
- In a phase III multicenter RCT, Gschwend *et al* observed that the **extended LND** (obturator, internal and external iliac nodes, deep obturator, common iliac, presacral, paracaval, interaortocaval, and para-aortal nodes up to the inferior mesenteric artery) failed to show superiority over **limited LND** (obturator, and internal and external iliac nodes) with regard to RFS, CSS and OS. Clavien grade ≥3 lymphoceles were also more frequently reported in the extended LND group within 90 days after surgery. Inclusion of T1 high grade tumors may have contributed to the negative study result.[17]
- Recently, at ASCO 2023, results of the SWOG 1011 trial were presented. This trial compared standard LND with extended LND and showed no benefit in DFS or OS with the extended dissection. The full manuscript is awaited for a more detailed review of the results.

15. What is the minimum number of nodes to be dissected? How do you optimize lymph node yield?

Ans:

- No guidelines are established for the minimum number.
- **10–12 lymph nodes** on pathology indicates an adequate dissection. Submission of lymph nodes in separate packets is associated with increased yield.[18]
- Two important studies have demonstrated the limited utility of node count as a surrogate marker of the completeness of dissection, supporting a "template-based LND".
- It is suggested that the LN density and the presence of extra nodal extension are more important for OS.[19] (Lymph Node density = No. of positive LN/Total number of LN). Various lymph node density figures (<20%, <15%) have been found to be associated with better survival.

16. What approach would you choose: Open vs robotic–benefits and trade-offs?

Ans:

- Robotic RC has been studied and compared with open cystectomy across randomized trials and has a high quality of evidence supporting its use. It is associated with:
  i. Equivalent oncologic outcomes (PFS, OS, positive margins, lymph node yields)
  ii. Reduced blood loss and transfusion rates
  iii. Around 1–1.5 hours longer OR time
  iv. Around 1–2 days shorter hospital stay
  v. Reduced opiate requirement
  vi. Reduced need of TPN
  vii. Similar grade 3–5 complication rates
  viii. No significant difference in quality of life
  ix. Higher healthcare costs
- Surgeon experience and institutional volume are considered the key factors for the outcome of both RARC and open RC, not the approach.
- Two major trials have compared: Open RC and robotic RC.
  - **RAZOR trial**: Open RC with urinary diversion was compared with robotic RC with extracorporeal urinary diversion. Primary endpoint was progression free survival (PFS) at 2 years. The PFS at 2 years was comparable in both the arms (robotic RC and open RC: 72.3% and 71.6%).[20]
  - **iROC trial**: Open RC with urinary diversion was compared with robotic RC with intracorporeal urinary diversion. The primary outcome was the median number of days "alive and outside of the hospital" within 90 days of surgery which was found to be 82 days and 80 days for patients undergoing robotic radical cystectomy and open surgery respectively. At a median follow up of 18.4 months, absence of cancer recurrence was comparable in either of the groups (Robotic RC and open RC: 82% and 84%). However, the thromboembolic (1.9% vs 8.3%) and wound (5.6% vs 16%) complications were less common in the robotic surgery group.[21]

17. Is there any proven benefit of intracorporeal approach to diversion?

Ans:

- No clear benefits have been demonstrated with intracorporeal diversion.

- Intracorporeal diversion is known to be associated with higher OR time.[21]
- **Purported advantages**:
  i. Avoidance of mini laparotomy
  ii. Reduced bowel handling with quicker return of bowel function
  iii. Less intraoperative blood loss
  iv. Reduced mobilization of ureters (thus possibly less ischemic strictures)
  v. Lower readmission rate at 30 and 90 days
  vi. Less gastrointestinal and infectious complications
- **Disadvantages/Challenges**:
  i. Increased OR time
  ii. Very steep learning curve

18. What is the role of indocyanine green (ICG) in radical cystectomy?

Ans:

- ICG fluorescence can be used to assess the vascularity of the terminal ureters during intracorporeal urinary diversion which may reduce the risk of ischemic uretero-enteric strictures significantly.[22]
- ICG can be prepared by reconstituting 25 mg powdered ICG in 5 mL distilled water.
- Following isolation and preparation of the ileal conduit or neobladder and just before spatulation and creation of the uretero-enteric anastomosis, 1–2 mL ICG is injected I.V. The distal ureteric segments are examined using the near infrared camera system which are available for open surgery, in laparoscopy carts and in robotic system as an integrated feature (Firefly technology in the Xi da Vinci Robotic system).
- The vascularity of the bowel is also examined during the same time with the same dose of ICG.
- Examination of the ureter is made during arterial and perfusion phases of ICG as initially the small periureteric arteries fluoresce, followed by fluorescence in the ureteric wall as the ICG perfuses into the ureteric tissue. It takes ~30 s after injection to assess arterial flow and ~5 min to get a good idea of perfusion.[22]

19. What are the types of urinary diversion?

Ans:

- The two most common urinary diversions are ileal conduit and orthotopic neobladder (Table 7.1).
  - **Camey II**: Transverse U
  - **Ghoneim**: 40 cm ileum in W configuration and ureters are brought into reservoir through extramural serous lined tunnels preventing reflux
  - **Hautmann pouch:** 70 cm ileum used in W configuration
  - **Studer** pouch: 60 cm ileum used; 44 cm placed in an inverted U configuration to form reservoir and proximal 15 cm segment of ileum is used as afferent limb
  - **Mainz pouch:** Ileum-cecum
  - **Le-Bag pouch:** Ileum-cecum-colon
  - **Indiana pouch:** Right colon pouch with tapered ileum as efferent limb; most reliable of all reservoirs, easy to construct, low complication rate.

TABLE 7.1: List of various urinary diversions

Continent diversions	*Continent cutaneous diversions*	*Non-continent diversions*
Orthotopic neobladder: **Ileal:** 1. Camey II 2. Ghoneim 3. Hautmann pouch 4. Studer pouch 5. T pouch **Ileocolonic:** 1. Mainz pouch (Ileum-cecum) 2. Le-Bag pouch (Ileum-cecum-colon)	**Non-orthotopic/heterotopic:** Continent catheterizable pouches on abdominal wall (Low pressure detubularised bowel reservoirs): 1. Using right colon: a. Indiana pouch b. Florida pouch c. Miami pouch d. Penn pouch 2. Using ileum: a. Kock pouch b. Double T pouch c. Mainz I pouch	**Non-continent conduits:** 1. Ileal 2. Jejunal 3. Colonic
Colonic: 1. Right colon pouch 2. Sigmoid pouch	**Rectal bladder urinary diversions:** 1. Uretero-sigmoidostomy 2. Folded rectosigmoid bladder 3. Augmented valves rectum 4. Hemi-Kock and T Kock procedure 5. Sigma rectum pouch (Mainz II)	**Cutaneous ureterostomy**

- **Penn pouch:** Ileocolonic pouch with appendix as efferent limb
- **Kock pouch:** 15 cm terminal ileum used with nipple valve intussusception.
- **Mainz I pouch:** Ileocecal pouch with intussuscepted ileal segment as efferent limb
- Non-continent **ileal conduit:** Gold standard non-continent diversion. Terminal 10–15 cm ileum is preserved to maintain adequate absorption of bile salts, vitamin B_{12} and fat-soluble vitamins.
- **Cutaneous ureterostomy:** Preferred in old and frail and those with solitary functioning kidney (least burdensome type of diversion as it avoids bowel resection—anastomosis and ureteroileal anastomosis). High rate of stenosis and UTI.[23]

20. What are the principles for creating a neobladder?

Ans:

- Adequate external sphincter mechanism
- Non-obstructed healthy urethra
- Bowel segment should be detubularised and reconstructed into a spherical shape
- Reservoir must be sufficiently compliant to maintain low pressure throughout filling phase
- Reservoir must have adequate storage volume once the pouch is mature (300–500 ml) to allow reasonable voiding intervals.[2]

21. What are the advantages of small bowel over large bowel for neobladder?

Ans:

- Small bowel has
  i. Better compliance
  ii. Ability to stretch
  iii. Reduced mucus formation

22. What are the prerequisites before considering neobladder?

Ans:

- Patient should agree for close long-term follow-up.
- **Patient related factors**:
  - Patient should be active and independent
  - Adequate external urethral sphincter function
  - Adequate renal function (creatinine <1.6–2 mg/dl; eGFR > 35–40 ml/min)
  - Adequate liver function (reabsorbed ammonia can lead to hyperammonemia and possible hepatic encephalopathy)
  - Obesity is not a contraindication
  - Manual dexterity and willingness to do self-catheterisation (CIC is needed in around 30–60% females and 10–15% males)
  - Patent urethra
- **Tumor-related factors**:
  - Intraoperative frozen cut margin of the urethra should be negative in both males and females.
  - CIS, multifocal tumor and extravesical disease should not preclude orthotopic neobladder if frozen section of urethral margin is negative.[2]

23. What are the contraindications for neobladder?

Ans:

- **Absolute contraindications**:
  - GFR <40–50 ml/min or serum creatinine >2 (urinary electrolytes gets reabsorbed and metabolic acidosis can happen)
  - Severe hepatic dysfunction
  - Inadequate intellectual capacity, dexterity and mobility preventing performance of self-catheterisation
  - Positive prostatic apical margin on frozen section
  - Positive proximal urethral margin
  - If urethrectomy is indicated
  - Inadequate bowel length
- **Relative contraindications**:
  - Inflammatory bowel disease
  - Non-compliant patient
  - >80 years
  - Complex urethral stricture
  - High dose preoperative RT
  - Severe urethral sphincter related incontinence
- In men with a prior positive transurethral prostatic biopsy, subsequent orthotopic neobladder construction should not be denied, unless an intraoperative frozen section of the distal urethral stump shows malignancy at the level of urethral dissection.[24,25]

24. What are the advantages and disadvantages of conduit and neobladder?

Ans:

- **Advantages of ileal conduit**:
  i. Simple
  ii. Easy to maintain
  iii. Low reoperation rates
- **Disadvantages of ileal conduit**:
  i. Stoma on abdominal wall may be associated with affected QOL and body-image issues
  ii. Stoma related complications
- **Advantages of neobladder**:
  i. Naturally situated reservoir with good QOL
  ii. Process of urination closely matches the natural process (continence depends on the external urethral sphincter; voiding is done

by increased intra-abdominal pressure and relaxation of pelvic floor muscles)

iii. No stoma bag (cosmesis maintained)

- **Disadvantages of neobladder**:
  i. Increased OR time
  ii. Technically demanding
  iii. Chance of urinary retention and need for CIC
  iv. Urinary incontinence especially nocturnal in the initial period
  v. Patient counseling regarding conversion to ileal conduit intraoperatively is needed.

25. What are the early and late complications of ileal conduit?

Ans:

- **Early complications** (within 30 days)[26]
  i. UTI, pyelonephritis
  ii. Uretero-ileal leak
  iii. Stoma related issues: Stomal necrosis, give way of mucocutaneous sutures.
- **Late complications**:
  i. Stoma complications (24%)
  ii. Upper tract functional damage
  iii. Uretero-ileal stricture
  iv. Metabolic disorders
  v. Parastomal hernia
  vi. Stomal stenosis

26. What are the early and late complications of orthotopic neobladder ?

Ans:

- **Early complications**:
  i. UTI
  ii. Uretero-ileal anastomosis leak
  iii. Bleeding, thromboembolic events, cardiovascular and pulmonary complications
  iv. Postoperative ileus: Nasogastric tube insertion, chewing gum, avoid fluid excess, avoid hypovolemia (provoke splanchnic hypoperfusion)
  v. Postoperative nausea and vomiting
  vi. Ileal anastomosis leakage (ileostomy as soon as possible)
- **Late complications**:
  i. Anastomotic stricture
  ii. Urinary retention (because of neobladder-urethral anastomotic stricture, tumor recurrence, ventral hernia—decrease in intra-abdominal pressure, posterior prolapse of pouch) → Needs drainage and self-catheterisation education
  iii. Need for CIC (5–25%; F>M)
  iv. Incontinence (diurnal 8–10%; nocturnal 20–30%)
    - Daytime continence develops gradually in 6–12 months
    - Nighttime incontinence is troublesome, persistent in 20–50% patients.
    - Physiotherapy with Kegel's exercises helps
  v. Electrolyte disturbances associated with ileum and colon are: Metabolic acidosis with hypokalemia, hyperchloremia, hypocalcaemia, hypomagnesemia. Treatment includes hydration, alkalizing agents, oral $NaHCO_3$, nicotinic acid (Cl transport inhibitor), vitamin B_{12} supplementation.
  vi. Malabsorption (vitamin B_{12})
  vii. Upper tract functional damage
  viii. Pouch rupture (Needs nephrostomy and indwelling catheter/surgery for drainage of neobladder)
  ix. Calculi in the neobladder
  x. Non-compressive lymphocele (managed by observation); compressive lymphocele (needs percutaneous drainage or marsupialisation)
  xi. Mucus block (catheterize and rinse the bladder)
  xii. Ureteral reflux (no treatment required if it is asymptomatic).[2,3]

27. What are the types of uretero-Ileal anastomosis?

Ans:

- **Refluxing anastomosis:**
  - Bricker (most commonly performed): Simple end to side ureter-ileal anastomosis
  - Wallace: The two ureteric opening are anastomosed to each other and the common opening is then anastomosed with the bowel wall in an end to side manner.
- **Non-refluxing anastomosis:**
  - Split-nipple technique
  - Le-Duc technique
  - Hammock anastomosis
  - Ureteral dipping technique
- "Intermittent" uretero-ileal anastomosis suturing technique is linked to a lower incidence of strictures, but a higher incidence of leaks when compared to "continuous" uretero-ileal anastomosis.[27, 28]

28. What are the complications of uretero-ileal anastomosis?

Ans:

- Urinary fistula (3–9%): Within 5–7 days of surgery. Usually urine leak will heal by fibrosis and then subsequently can form anastomotic stricture.
- Uretero-ileal anastomotic stricture: Higher incidence in non-refluxing techniques.

Those strictures which are especially formed within 1 year of the procedure, or >1.5 cm long or are left sided are best treated by re-exploration, removal of stenotic segment and re-anastomosis of the ureter.

- Another site of ureteric stricture is where the left ureter crosses the aorta and angulates beneath the inferior mesenteric artery.
- Pyelonephritis can be early or recurrent.

29. What are important preoperative and postoperative components of ERAS protocol for RC patients?

Ans:

- **Fast tract/ERAS protocol**= Early Recovery After Surgery.
  - **Preoperative recommendations**:
    i. Preoperative counseling and education about the surgery, stay and discharge
    ii. Preoperative medical optimization (correction of anemia and other comorbidities, nutritional support, smoking cessation and reduction of alcohol intake 4 weeks before surgery)
    iii. No need of bowel preparation
    iv. Same day admission
    v. Early discharge planning
    vi. Decreased fasting (solid food till 6 hours before surgery; clear liquids till 2 hours before surgery)
    vii. Carbohydrate loading to all nondiabetic patients [no specific guidelines; For example, 6 cartons of clear, non-carbonated lemon flavoured, iso-osmolar carbohydrate containing, liquid oral nutritional supplement providing 100 kcal/200 ml over the 18 hours prior to surgery.[29] Preoperative carbohydrate loading is known to decrease insulin resistance, thirst and helps in maintaining muscle strength and lean body mass.[30]
    viii. Preoperative exercise program (walking for 1 hour/day)
    ix. Pre-warming
    x. Avoidance of long-acting sedatives
  - **Preoperative recommendations**:
    i. Active warming
    ii. Opioid sparing
    iii. Epidural anesthesia
    iv. Minimally invasive surgery
    v. Avoiding prophylactic NG tube and drains
  - **Postoperative recommendations**:
    i. Early oral nutrition (oral sips on POD 0 evening; oral fluids on POD 1)
    ii. Early ambulation (6 hours out of bed on POD 1; Walk 10–20 m on POD 1; Walk 100 m on POD 2; Walk >100 m on POD 3+)
    iii. Use of Alvimopan—not available in India
    iv. Pain management
       - Reduced usage of opioids.
       - Thoracic epidural analgesia is considered superior to systemic opioids for pain and should be continued for 72 hours.
       - Increased usage of high dose acetaminophen and/or ketorolac (only as breakthrough pain medication).
    v. Venous thromboembolism prophylaxis
  - With ERAS protocol, it has been found that patients have better emotional and physical functioning scores, less wound healing issues, less fever, less thrombosis and less postoperative ileus (7.3% as against 22% without ERAS).[31]

30. Is venous thromboembolism (VTE) prophylaxis recommended in patients undergoing RC?

Ans:

- **VTE prophylaxis** may be implemented as a part of ERAS protocol.
- Patients should wear well-fitting compression stockings.
- VTE prophylaxis such as LMWH to be given to the patients undergoing RC, starting from the 1st day pre-surgery, for a period of at least 4 weeks.[3]
- If BMI >30, extended (90 days) heparin prophylaxis is to be considered.

31. When would sexual preservation techniques be offered and what are the techniques?

Ans:

- Sexual preservation techniques may be offered to eligible men who are very motivated to preserve their sexual function.
- It can be offered if the disease is organ confined and when there is absence of any kind of tumor at the level of the prostate, prostatic urethra or at the bladder neck.
- Sexual preserving techniques:[3]
  - Prostate-sparing cystectomy
  - Prostatic capsule sparing cystectomy
  - Seminal vesicle sparing: Seminal vesicles, vas and neurovascular bundles are preserved.
  - Nerve sparing cystectomy
- These techniques are associated with better preservation of continence and erection.
- If prostate preserving is considered, TUR sampling of the bladder neck and prostatic urethra is required.

32. Is there any role of partial cystectomy in MIBC?

Ans:

- MIBC patients who are unfit for radical cystectomy and who have a small solitary lesion which is amenable to wide resection with 2 cm margin and away from the ureteric orifices (ideally at the dome), without extravesical spread with negative random mucosal biopsies (to rule out CIS) and negative surgical margin on frozen can be considered for partial cystectomy.[2] It must be remembered that even for such patients, the standard treatment option would be a radical cystectomy.
- Advantage over only radical TURBT is that, in partial cystectomy, full pelvic lymphadenectomy is done and also full thickness bladder wall and perivesical fat is removed.
- Contraindication: Presence of CIS.
- Partial cystectomy has a place in management of urachal adenocarcinoma, but removal of the urachus, posterior peritoneum and lymph node dissection is critical along with partial cystectomy.

33. What is Trimodal therapy?

Ans:

- Trimodal therapy is an important type of bladder preservation treatment for bladder cancer.
- Trimodal therapy can be offered to selected well informed and compliant patients, especially for whom radical cystectomy is not an option or not acceptable.
- It should be a limited burden disease: Solitary, <4 cm, <cT3, N0, absence of CIS, no hydronephrosis and should be totally resectable with good bladder function.[2]
- Trimodal therapy combines maximal safe TURBT + chemotherapy + radiotherapy.
- Rationale for combining TURBT with RT is to achieve maximal local tumor control in the bladder and adjacent nodes.
- Micro-metastases are targeted by chemotherapy.
- 55% 5-year OS.
- Two types:
  - **Continuous course therapy**: TURBT + full course of CT and RT followed by restage TURBT after 6 months.
  - **Split course therapy**: TURBT + Induction CT + RT (40 Gy) followed by imaging + restage TURBT. If there is no persistent invasive disease, consolidative CT/RT (64 Gy) to be given. If there is persistent invasive disease, RC to be considered.
  - Salvage cystectomy rates are around 8–33%.

34. What are the recommendations for the assessment of the tumor specimen?

Ans:

- To record the depth of invasion of the entire specimen.
- To record the margins with focusing on the radial margin, prostate, ureter, urethra, peritoneal fat, uterus and vaginal vault.
- The percentage of subtype in the specimen should be reported since it has been shown to be of prognostic value.
- To record the total number of lymph nodes, number of positive lymph nodes and extranodal spread.
- To record lymphovascular invasion.
- To record the presence of CIS.[3]

35. How is the management of variant histologies different from a pure urothelial carcinoma of bladder?

Ans:

- **Muscle invasive pure squamous cell carcinoma (SCC)** of the bladder should be treated with primary radical cystectomy and lymphadenectomy. Adjuvant RT is the standard of care for pT3 + or pN + or in case of positive margins.
- **Muscle invasive pure adenocarcinoma of bladder** is also treated with primary radical cystectomy and lymphadenectomy.
- There is no proven role of neoadjuvant/adjuvant CT in both pure SCC and pure adenocarcinoma of the bladder.
- **Bladder urothelial carcinoma with small cell neuroendocrine variant** should be treated with NAC (which is the mainstay) followed by RC or RT regardless of the stage. NAC with cisplatin + etoposide has been found to improve OS. Brain imaging is recommended if there is a small cell component.

36. When is adjuvant therapy needed?

Ans:

- Adjuvant CT after RC is recommended for pT3/4 and/or pN+ disease if NAC was not given (strong recommendation, EAU 2023).
- Adjuvant CT to be given within 3 months of cystectomy; preferably 6–8 weeks (MVAC or GC for 4 cycles).
- **Benefits of adjuvant CT** are:
  - No delay in definitive surgery
  - Chemotherapy is administered after accurate pathological staging, thus avoiding chemotherapy in patients with low risk of micro-metastases.

- A fraction of patients who were ineligible for cisplatin due to obstructive uropathy at presentation can be reconsidered for chemotherapy as an adjuvant. In the adjuvant setting, even carboplatin may be given if the patient is still cisplatin ineligible.

- **Drawbacks of adjuvant CT**:
  - Delay of or intolerability to chemotherapy due to postoperative morbidity
  - Assessment of *in vivo* chemosensitivity of the tumor is not possible
- Adjuvant immunotherapy (nivolumab) can be offered in selected patients with pT3/4 and/or pN+ disease who are not eligible for adjuvant cisplatin-based chemotherapy or who declined it.

37. What is the average 5-year survival rate of T2 bladder cancer?

Ans:

- Average 5-year survival rate of T2 is around 55%.
- 5-year survival rate of T3-T4a is around 30%.[2]

38. What are the chances of local recurrence and distant recurrence after radical cystectomy?

Ans:

- **Local recurrence**:
  - Local recurrences take place in the soft tissues of the original surgical site or LNs.
  - 5–15% probability of pelvic recurrence which usually occurs within 2 years (most commonly within 6–18 months after RC).[32]
  - An Indian study of 188 patients who underwent RC with perioperative chemotherapy found that the incidence of recurrence was 29% overall with 16% of the patients having loco-regional recurrence. Loco-regional recurrence is a significant problem post-RC, with a cumulative incidence as high as 35% in the high-risk group. The median time to loco-regional recurrence was 8.2 months.[33]
- **Distant recurrence**: Seen in up to 50% patients after RC, 90% of which occur within 3 years (especially within 2 years).[34] Systemic recurrence of 30–60% in pT3/4 and 50–70% in N+ patients.[35] Non-regional lymph nodes, lungs, liver and bone are common sites of distant recurrence.

39. What is the risk of urethral recurrence and upper tract urothelial cancer after RC?

Ans:

- After RC, there is around 4.4% risk of a metachronous urethral tumor.
- Risk factors for secondary urethral tumors are: Urethral malignancy in the prostatic urethra/prostate (in males) and bladder neck (in females).
- Orthotopic neobladder is associated with a significantly lower risk of urethral tumors after RC.[36]
- Upper tract urothelial cancer is seen in 4–10% of cases and these constitute the most common site of late recurrence.[37]

40. How will you follow-up a case after radical cystectomy?

Ans:

- **Oncological follow-up of pure urothelial carcinoma**:
  - CT scan every 6 months until 3rd year, followed by annual imaging thereafter.[3]
  - Physical examination including pelvic and rectal examination, CBC and comprehensive metabolic panel: 4 monthly for 1 year, 6 monthly for 2nd and 3rd year, and annually thereafter.
  - Voided urine cytology, urethral wash cytology and vitamin B_{12} levels once a year.
- Oncological follow-up of variant histology tumors (including urothelial variants, non-urothelial variants and mixed variants): Patients younger than 60 years to have extended surveillance for >10 years as they have greater recurrence risk than pure urothelial carcinoma.[38]
- Patients with multifocal disease, NMIBC with CIS, positive ureteral margins: Higher risk of developing UTUC, which can develop late after 3 years.

41. How do stoma societies help?

Ans:

- *Stoma society*: "Ostomy India" is a not-for-profit association affiliated to Indian Cancer Society which serves ostomates across the Indian subcontinent. It offers the following services:
  - Preoperative and postoperative counseling of ostomy patients
  - Free of charge stoma care and counseling by entero-stomal therapists
  - Ostomy material distribution at subsidized rates or free for poor patients
  - Ostomate to ostomate talk/family counseling
  - Align existing ostomates to new ostomates
  - Arranging meetings/events for the ostomates

42. Are there any societies dedicated to bladder cancer research and patient advocacy?

Ans:

- There are a few dedicated societies which concentrate on the bladder cancer research and awareness.

- The International Bladder Cancer Group (**IBCG**) is a widely recognized organization that has published numerous peer-reviewed articles addressing gaps in bladder cancer knowledge and offering recommendations for managing the disease.
- The International Bladder Cancer Network (**IBCN**) is another organization dedicated to enhancing the diagnosis, prevention, and treatment of bladder cancer.
- The Global Society of Rare Genitourinary Tumors (**GSRGT**) is committed to both education and research, aiming to establish evidence-based standards for diagnosing and treating rare genitourinary tumors worldwide. They also focus on education and research related to variants of bladder cancer.
- The World Bladder Cancer Patient Coalition (**WBCPC**) serves as the global advocate for individuals affected by bladder cancer. It brings together patient organizations from around the world that strive to raise awareness and provide support to bladder cancer patients. Recently, an Indian chapter has been established, which also included bladder cancer awareness videos in Hindi language.
- The month of May is globally recognized as World Bladder Cancer Awareness Month.

SUMMARY

- Muscle invasive bladder cancer (MIBC) is an aggressive and potentially lethal disease that often requires multimodal management.
- **Painless visible hematuria** is the most common presenting complaint.
- **CECT** imaging of abdomen, pelvis and chest.
  - For local staging (useful in detecting cT3b), lymph nodes and liver metastasis
  - Hydronephrosis suggests invasive disease
  - 5% of bladder cancers are associated with upper tract urothelial carcinoma.
- **MRI** for diagnosing the T-stage non-invasively is showing promise (Accuracy: 75–95%). For local staging, MRI is superior to CT for differentiating T1 vs T2. MRI is better than CT for local tumor depth and for detecting liver metastases; however, CT outperforms MRI for detecting nodal and lung metastases.
- FDG PET/CT is showing promise in providing important staging information which may impact clinical management of MIBC patients.
- **Radical cystectomy (RC)** is the gold standard for treatment for MIBC, however, it is a morbid procedure, and requires urinary diversion with its potential long-term implications. Minimally-invasive techniques like robotic surgery have been introduced with a view to reduce surgical morbidity and the use of orthotopic urinary diversions may help in body-image and quality-of-life after cystectomy.
- **Neoadjuvant chemotherapy (NAC)** is an essential component of treatment in cisplatin fit patients and has been shown to improve overall survival (5–8% survival benefit). Neoadjuvant radiotherapy or immunotherapy is not recommended.
- **Adjuvant chemotherapy** is used in certain cases depending on the final histopathology, only if neoadjuvant chemotherapy was not given.
- **Adjuvant immunotherapy** in selected patients.
- **Trimodal therapy** with chemo-radiation and maximal TURBT can also be used as an alternative to RC in selected cases.

REFERENCES

1. Prakash G, Pal M, Odaiyappan K, Shinde R, Mishra J, Jalde D, Rajkumar B, Prabhash K, Joshi A, Noronha V, Murthy V. Bladder cancer demographics and outcome data from 2013 at a tertiary cancer hospital in India. Indian Journal of Cancer. 2019 Jan 1;56(1):54–8.
2. Partin AW, Wein AJ, Kavoussi LR, Peters CA, Dmochowski RR. Campbell Walsh Wein Urology, E-Book. Elsevier Health Sciences; 2021.
3. EAU Guidelines. Edn. presented at the EAU Annual Congress Milan 2023. ISBN 978-94-92671-19-6.
4. Huang, L., *et al.* The Diagnostic Value of MR Imaging in Differentiating T Staging of Bladder Cancer: A Meta-Analysis. Radiology, 2018. 286: 502.
5. Panebianco, V., *et al.* Multiparametric Magnetic Resonance Imaging for Bladder Cancer: Development of VI-RADS (Vesical Imaging-Reporting And Data System). Eur Urol, 2018. 74: 294.
6. Voskuilen, C.S., *et al.* Staging (18)F-fluorodeoxyglucose Positron Emission Tomography/Computed Tomography Changes Treatment Recommendation in Invasive Bladder Cancer. Eur Urol Oncol, 2022. 5: 366.
7. Sim KC, Sung DJ. Role of magnetic resonance imaging in tumor staging and follow-up for bladder cancer. Translational Andrology and Urology. 2020 Dec;9(6):2890.
8. Bryan RT, Liu W, Pirrie SJ, Amir R, Gallagher J, Hughes AI, Jefferson KP, Knight A, Nanton V, Mintz HP, Pope AM. Comparing an imaging-guided pathway with the standard pathway for staging muscle-invasive bladder cancer: preliminary data from the BladderPath study. European urology. 2021 Jul 1;80(1):12–5).
9. Liu S, Yao Y, Guan F, Sun L, Zhang G. Neoadjuvant chemotherapy for different stages of muscle-invasive bladder cancer: A systematic review and meta-analysis. Disease Markers. 2022 Mar 2;2022.
10. Jiang DM, Gupta S, Kitchlu A, Meraz-Munoz A, North SA, Alimohamed NS, Blais N, Sridhar SS. Defining cisplatin eligibility in patients with muscle-invasive bladder cancer. Nature Reviews Urology. 2021 Feb;18(2):104–14.
11. Srivishnu S., *et al.* Patterns of utilisation and outcomes of Perioperative chemotherapy in Patients with locally advanced urothelial bladder cancer (LABC)—real world data from an Indian tertiary care cancer center. Clinical genitourinary cancer, 2023 (Article in press).
12. Pfister C, Gravis G, Fléchon A, Chevreau C, Mahammedi H, Laguerre B, Guillot A, Joly F, Soulié M, Allory Y, Harter V. Dose-dense methotrexate, vinblastine, doxorubicin, and cisplatin or gemcitabine and cisplatin as perioperative chemotherapy for patients with nonmetastatic muscle-invasive bladder cancer: results of the GETUG-AFU V05

VESPER trial. Journal of Clinical Oncology. 2022 Jun 20;40(18):2013–22.

13. NCCN clinical practice guidelines in oncology version 1.2023
14. Simone G, *et al.* Stage-specific impact of extended versus standard pelvic lymph node dissection in radical cystectomy. Int J Urol, 2013. 20: 390.
15. Jensen JB, *et al.* Extended versus limited lymph node dissection in radical cystectomy: impact on recurrence pattern and survival. Int J Urol, 2012. 19: 39.
16. Zehnder P, *et al.* Super extended versus extended pelvic lymph node dissection in patients undergoing radical cystectomy for bladder cancer: a comparative study. J Urol, 2011. 186: 1261.
17. Gschwend JE, Heck MM, Lehmann J, Rübben H, Albers P, Wolff JM, Frohneberg D, de Geeter P, Heidenreich A, Kaelble T, Stöckle M. Extended versus limited lymph node dissection in bladder cancer patients undergoing radical cystectomy: survival results from a prospective, randomized trial. European urology. 2019 Apr 1;75(4):604–11.
18. Chang SS, Bochner BH, Chou R, *et al.* Treatment of Non-Metastatic Muscle-Invasive Bladder Cancer: AUA/ASCO/ASTRO/SUO Guideline. J Urol. 2017;198(3):552–559. doi:10.1016/j.juro.2017.04.086.
19. Ku, J.H., *et al.* Lymph node density as a prognostic variable in node-positive bladder cancer: a meta-analysis. BMC Cancer, 2015. 15: 447.
20. Parekh DJ, Reis IM, Castle EP, *et al.* Robot-assisted radical cystectomy versus open radical cystectomy in patients with bladder cancer (RAZOR): an open-label, randomised, phase 3, non-inferiority trial. Lancet. 2018;391(10139):2525–2536.
21. Catto JWF, Khetrapal P, Ricciardi F, *et al.* Effect of robot-assisted radical cystectomy with intracorporeal urinary diversion vs open radical cystectomy on 90-day morbidity and mortality among patients with bladder cancer: a randomized clinical trial. JAMA. 2022;327(21):2092–2103.
22. Ahmadi N, Ashrafi AN, Hartman N, Shakir A, Cacciamani GE, Freitas D, Rajarubendra N, Fay C, Berger A, Desai MM, Gill IS. Use of indocyanine green to minimise uretero-enteric strictures after robotic radical cystectomy. BJU international. 2019 Aug;124(2):302–7.
23. Deliveliotis, C., *et al.* Urinary diversion in high risk elderly patients: modified cutaneous ureterostomy or Ileal conduit? Urology, 2005. 66:299.
24. von Rundstedt FC, *et al.* Transurethral biopsy of the prostatic urethra is associated with final apical margin status at radical cystoprostatectomy. J Clin Urol, 2016. 9: 404.
25. Kates M, *et al.* Accuracy of urethral frozen section during radical cystectomy for bladder cancer. Urol Oncol, 2016. 34: 532.e1.
26. Rezaee ME, *et al.* Ileal Conduit Versus Continent Urinary Diversion in Radical Cystectomy: A Retrospective Cohort Study of 30-day Complications, Readmissions, and Mortality. Urology, 2022.
27. Prakash G, Bakshi G, Shinde R, Niyogi D, Pal M, Menon S, Murthy V, Joshi A, Sable N. Complications following continous and interrupted suturing for ureteroileal anastomosis in patients undergoing radical cystectomy for bladder cancer. European Urology Supplements. 2017 Nov 1;16(10):e2793.
28. Large MC, Cohn JA, Kiriluk KJ, Dangle P, Richards KA, Smith ND, Steinberg GD. The impact of running versus interrupted anastomosis on ureterointestinal stricture rate after radical cystectomy. The Journal of urology. 2013 Sep 1;190(3):923–7.
29. Pang KH, Groves R, Venugopal S, Noon AP, Catto JW. Prospective implementation of enhanced recovery after surgery protocols to radical cystectomy. European urology. 2018 Mar 1;73(3):363–71.
30. Mir MC, Zargar H, Bolton DM, Murphy DG, Lawrentschuk N. Enhanced recovery after surgery protocols for radical cystectomy surgery: review of current evidence and local protocols. ANZ Journal of Surgery. 2015 Jul;85(7–8):514–20.
31. Xu W, *et al.* Postoperative Pain Management after Radical cystectomy: Comparing Traditional versus Enhanced Recovery Protocol Pathway. J Urol, 2015. 194: 1209). (Pang KH, Groves R, Venugopal S, Noon AP, Catto JW. Prospective implementation of enhanced recovery after surgery protocols to radical cystectomy. European urology. 2018 Mar 1;73(3): 363–71.
32. Huguet J. Follow-up after radical cystectomy based on patterns of tumour recurrence and its risk factors. Actas Urol Esp, 2013. 37: 376.
33. Murthy V, Bakshi G, Manjali JJ, Prakash G, Pal M, Joshi A, Dholakia K, Bhattacharjee A, Talole S, Puppalwar A, Srinivasan S. Locoregional recurrence after cystectomy in muscle invasive bladder cancer: Implications for adjuvant radiotherapy. In Urologic Oncology: Seminars and Original Investigations 2021 Aug 1 (Vol. 39, No. 8, pp. 496-e9). Elsevier.
34. Ghoneim MA, *et al.* Radical cystectomy for carcinoma of the bladder: 2720 consecutive cases 5 years later. J Urol, 2008. 180:121
35. Donat SM. Staged based directed surveillance of invasive bladder cancer following radical cystectomy: valuable and effective? World J Urol, 2006. 24: 557.
36. Fahmy, O., *et al.* Urethral recurrence after radical cystectomy for urothelial carcinoma: A systematic review and meta-analysis. Urol Oncol, 2018. 36: 54.
37. Gakis G, *et al.* Systemic review on the Fate of the Remnant Urothelium after Radical Cystectomy Eur Urol, 2017.71: 545
38. Martini A, *et al.* Oncologic Surveillance for Variant Histology Bladder Cancer after Radical Cystectomy. J Urol, 2021. 206: 885.

Chapter

8

Metastatic Bladder Cancer

• Amit Ghose

LEARNING OBJECTIVES

- To understand the importance of complete staging in a patient with advanced bladder cancer: Every patient with a diagnosis of a muscle invasive bladder cancer should have a complete metastatic staging evaluation performed with either a CECT thorax + abdomen + pelvis or a FDG PET CT.
- To understand the importance of identifying the histological type of the bladder cancer: The histological type of the metastatic bladder cancer dictates the chemotherapy regimen and also the prognosis.
- To know the criteria for platinum eligibility: Platinum-based chemotherapy is the standard of care for metastatic urothelial bladder cancer. It is important to assess the patient if he is fit to receive cisplatin or carboplatin or neither of them.
- To know the standard chemotherapy regimens for first line therapy for metastatic bladder cancer: MVAC and Gem-Cis are the two regimens which have similar survival benefit. Gem-Cis is more commonly used as it is better tolerated.
- To know the options for cisplatin-ineligible patients: Gemcitabine-carboplatin is the standard of care for these patients. They may also be offered pembrolizumab/atezolizumab if they are PD-L1 positive.
- To know the options for platinum-ineligible patients: Single agent chemotherapy options offer modest survival benefit. These patients may also be offered pembrolizumab/atezolizumab irrespective of the PD-L1 status.
- To understand maintenance therapy after initial chemotherapy: Maintenance therapy with avelumab is the standard of care following initial platinum-based chemotherapy.
- To know of the newer agents available for disease progression following chemotherapy/immunotherapy: Enfortumab vedotin, sacituzumab govitecan and erdafitinib are the newer agents approved for second line therapy.
- To know the options available for managing intractable hematuria for metastatic bladder cancer: Endoscopic procedures, hemostatic radiation therapy, angioembolization and palliative cystectomy are the options that can be employed for managing intractable hematuria.

Case Scenario

A 67-year-old female came with gross hematuria, lower abdomen discomfort and weight loss for 2 months. She has smoked for the past 20 years. She does not have diabetes or hypertension and has an ECOG score of 1. A contrast enhanced CT of the abdomen and pelvis revealed a 10 x 8 cm bladder mass with metastasis to pelvic and retroperitoneal lymph nodes and the liver.

1. What is the next step in the evaluation of this patient?

Ans:

- A complete staging evaluation is required. This is best done by the addition of a CT chest to the abdomen + pelvis CT that has already been done.
- The abdominal CT will also tell about the upper tracts. Two percent of individuals with bladder urothelial carcinoma will have an upper tract tumour at the time of presentation, and six percent will acquire a metachronous lesion.[1]
- A FDG PET scan may also be performed in place of the CT chest. At present we do not have definite evidence to say that one is superior to the other. This is discussed a bit more in the chapter in muscle invasive bladder cancer.
- Once staging is done, the next step would be to establish a histological diagnosis of cancer.

2. How would you establish the histological diagnosis for the patient and why is it important?

Ans:

- A histological diagnosis is necessary to determine the pathology of the bladder cancer that we are dealing with as this will have implications on what chemotherapy drugs we use and also the prognosis.

- The histological diagnosis can be made on a transurethral biopsy. If there are concerns with tumor bleed, an image guided biopsy can be done from the most accessible metastatic site.

3. What are the prognostic factors for metastatic bladder cancer?

Ans:

- The MSKCC group has developed a prognostic model based on two risk factors—Karnofsky Performance Status <80% and presence of visceral metastasis (liver, lung and bone).
- The median OS for patients with none, one and two risk factors was 33, 13.4 and 9, 3 months respectively.[2]
- They published an updated version with two additional risk factors–serum albumin and hemoglobin level.[3]

4. What is the first line systemic therapy for metastatic urothelial cancer?

Ans:

- Cisplatin-based combination chemotherapy is the optimal first therapy for individuals with metastatic urothelial carcinoma. However, certain criteria need to be satisfied for a patient to be eligible to receive cisplatin. Patients who are unfit for cisplatin are then assessed if they are fit to receive carboplatin. Some patients may not be able to receive platinum-based therapy.[4] These criteria are outlined in Table 8.1.
- Some patients with obstructive uropathy may become platinum eligible after insertion of PCN.

5. What is the first line therapy for patients who are cisplatin eligible?

Ans:

- Two cisplatin-combination regimens are used:
  a. **GC:** Combination of cisplatin (70 mg/m^2 on day 2) and gemcitabine (1000 mg/m^2 on days 1, 8, and 15), repeated every 28 days for a maximum of six cycles.
  b. **MVAC:** Methotrexate (30 mg/m^2 on days 1, 15, and 22), vinblastine (3 mg/m^2 on days 2, 15, and 22), doxorubicin (30 mg/m^2 on day 2), and cisplatin (70 mg/m^2 on day 2) are the components. Six cycles of this treatment are administered every 28 days.
- Overall response rates are around 50% for both regimens. They both achieve a similar median survival of 14–15 months.[5] However, the GC regimen is less toxic and is thus more preferred.[6]
- Dose-dense MVAC (**ddMVAC**) is better tolerated than MVAC with similar survival benefit.[7]
- Another regimen that was tried in an RCT was **PGC** (paclitaxel, gemcitabine and cisplatin). However, the addition of paclitaxel to GC did not show a survival benefit compared to GC alone; and hence is not routinely used.[8]
- The recently reported CALGB 90601 (Alliance) trial tested if adding bevacizumab to GC could improve the survival benefit. However, this was a negative trial.[9]

6. Is carboplatin as effective as cisplatin?

Ans: Multiple studies have found that carboplatin is not as effective as cisplatin and hence they should not be used interchangeably in patients who are cisplatin eligible.[10]

7. What are the chemotherapy options for patient who are not eligible for cisplatin?

Ans:

- About half the patients with metastatic bladder cancer may be unfit for cisplatin.
- There could be various reasons for this: advanced age, comorbid status, obstructive uropathy, etc. The criteria for cisplatin ineligibility are listed in Table 8.1.
- The standard regime for these patients is Gemcitabine + carboplatin (Gem-Carbo). It has shown a response rate of around 40%.[11]
- Single agent chemotherapy leads to inferior outcomes and is not recommended as the standard option.

TABLE 8.1: Criteria for platinum eligibility

Platinum-eligible		***Platinum-ineligible***
Cisplatin-eligible	Carboplatin-eligible	
ECOG PS 0-1 and	ECOG PS 2 or GFR 30–60 ml/min	Any of the following:
GFR > 50–60 ml/min and	or not fulfilling other cisplatin-eligibility criteria	GFR < 30 ml/min
Audiometric hearing loss grade < 2 and		ECOG PS >2
Peripheral neuropathy grade < 2 and		ECOG PS 2 and GFR <60 ml/min
Cardiac insufficiency NYHA class < III		Comorbidities > Grade 2

ECOG = Eastern Cooperative Oncology Group; GFR = Glomerular filtration rate; NYHA = New York Heart Association; PS = Performance status.

8. What are the chemotherapy options for patients who are unfit to receive any platinum-based therapy?

Ans:

- When the patient does not satisfy criteria for platinum therapy, the performance status of the patient is anyway very poor and such patients do not do well.
- There is very little data about such patients as most trials have not included them.
- As noted above, single agent chemotherapy may be tried but with marginal benefit.

9. What is the role of immunotherapy in metastatic urothelial bladder cancer?

Ans: Immunotherapy for metastatic bladder cancer has been evaluated in the following settings:

A. Combination with chemotherapy for platinum-eligible patients.

- Three trials have evaluated immunotherapy agents in combination with cisplatin/carboplatin-based chemotherapy as the first line treatment.
- **IMvigor 130**[12]
  - Compared atezolizumab + chemotherapy combination vs atezolizumab alone vs chemotherapy alone.
  - Primary endpoint was PFS which was significantly longer in the combination arm was 8.2 months vs 6.3 months in the chemotherapy alone arm.
  - Overall survival for the combination was 16 months in the combination arm which was numerically greater than the 13.4 months seen in the chemotherapy alone arm. Although this p value was 0.027 with a HR of 0.83, it did not achieve the pre-specified statistical significance level of 0.007. Thus, the benefit with the combination was deemed to be statistically insignificant.
  - Since the OS benefit with the combination was not superior to chemotherapy alone, OS comparison between atezolizumab alone vs chemotherapy was not performed.
- **Keynote 361**[13]
  - Similar trial design as above.
  - No benefit for the combination of pembrolizumab + Gem-platinum chemotherapy over chemotherapy alone for PFS and OS.
- **DANUBE**[14]
  - Tested the combination of durvalumab + tremelimumab vs chemotherapy.
  - No benefit of immunotherapy combination over standard chemotherapy.
- As a result, combining immunotherapy agents with standard of care chemotherapy is not recommended.

B. First line immunotherapy in patients unfit for cisplatin-based chemotherapy

- All the three trials mentioned above had an arm with single agent immunotherapy also. In none of these trials did the single agent immunotherapy arm show any benefit over the standard of care chemotherapy arm.
- Two phase 2 trials evaluated pembrolizumab and atezolizumab respectively in cisplatin-ineligible patients.[15,16] Based on the results on these two trials which showed an overall response rate of 23–29%, the US FDA has approved these drugs for first line therapy in cisplatin-ineligible patients with positive PD-L1 status.
- However, in patients who are cisplatin-ineligible but eligible for carboplatin, gemcitabine-carboplatin chemotherapy is the recommended treatment option.

C. Maintenance with immunotherapy following response to chemotherapy

- **JAVELIN Bladder 100 study**[17]
  - Patients with stable disease or response to 4–6 cycles of platinum-based chemotherapy were randomized to either best supportive care or maintenance with avelumab.
  - OS in the avelumab maintenance arm was 21.4 months compared to 14.3 months in the best supportive care group.
  - Thus, avelumab maintenance therapy is the standard of care for stable/responsive disease following platinum-based chemotherapy for metastatic urothelial cancer.

10. Is there any role of immunotherapy for patients who are not fit for cisplatin and also carboplatin?

Ans: Pembrolizumab and atezolizumab have been approved as first line therapy for platinum ineligible patients, irrespective of the PD-L1 status.

11. What are the options for second line therapy for patients who have progression following first line therapy?

Ans: Second line options can either be chemotherapy or immunotherapy drugs.

A. Second line chemotherapy

- Most are phase 2 studies.
- Single agent treatment with paclitaxel/docetaxel/gemcitabine/oxaliplatin/ifosfamide has shown response rates of 0–28%.[18]

- The combination of gemcitabine and paclitaxel has been tried in a RCT but the results were not satisfactory with high toxicity.[19]
- A large retrospective study looked at patients who were rechallenged with platinum-based chemotherapy if they had a disease-free interval of 6–12 months between the initial platinum-based chemotherapy and the progression. These patients had a better OS compared to those who had received non-platinum based chemotherapy after progression (7.9 vs 5.5 months).[20]
- Vinflunine was tested in a phase 3 trial against best supportive care, but showed only modest results in a subset of patients.[21]

B. Second line immunotherapy for patients previously treated with platinum-based chemotherapy.

- In the Keynote 045 trial, pembrolizumab showed a significantly better OS (10.3 months vs 7.4 months) as compared to single agents chemotherapy in patients who had progressed following platinum based therapy.[22] This was independent of PD-L1 expression. Thus, pembrolizumab is the standard of care immunotherapy option in the second line setting after platinum-based chemotherapy.
- However, in the same setting, atezolizumab did not show a survival benefit.[23]

12. What are the novel agents being tried in metastatic bladder cancer?

Ans:

Antibody drug conjugates

1. Enfortumab vedotin (EV)

- EV consists of a monoclonal antibody which is directed against Nectin-4, an extracellular adhesion protein which is highly expressed in urothelial cancers. The antibody is attached to monomethyl auristatin E (MMAE), a chemotherapeutic microtubule-disrupting agent, via a protease-cleavable linker. EV binds to urothelial cells expressing Nectin-4 and the resulting complex is internalized into the urothelial cancer cell. Once internalized, proteolytic cleavage results in release of MMAE which then goes on to disrupt the microtubule network within the cell leading to cell cycle arrest and apoptosis.[24] The mechanism of action is also depicted in Fig. 8.1.
- In a phase 3 RCT of patients who had progressed on prior platinum-based chemotherapy or immunotherapy, EV showed a significant survival benefit compared to single-agent chemotherapy (12.8 months vs 8.9 months).[25]
- The US FDA has approved EV for patients progressing after first line chemotherapy or immunotherapy.[26]
- An ongoing trial (EV-302) is investigating the combination of EV and pembrolizumab as first-line therapy for metastatic urothelial cancer.

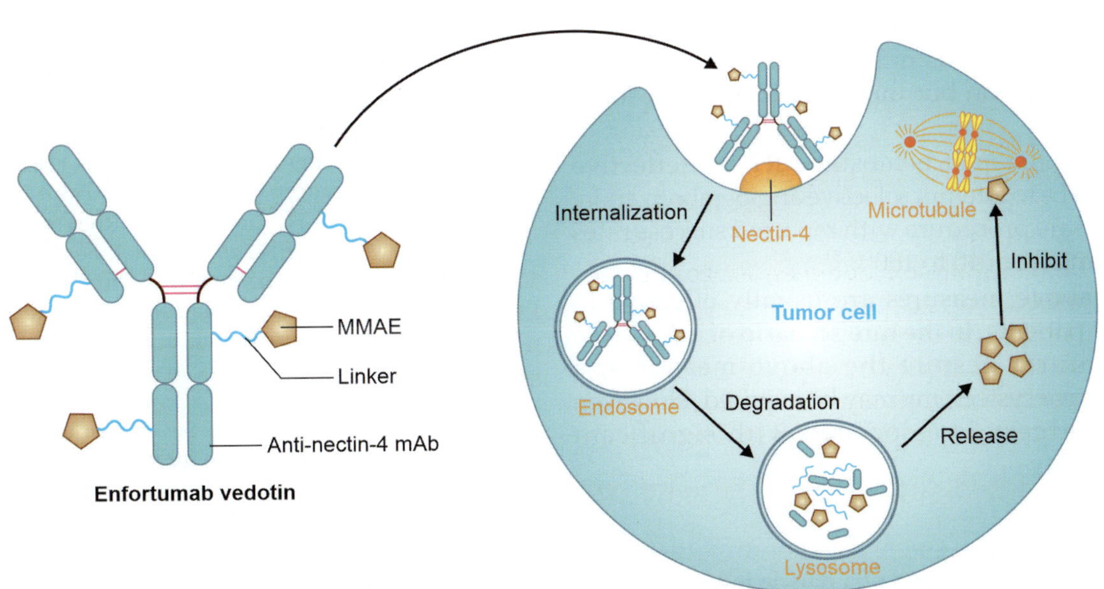

Fig. 8.1: Mechanism of action of enfortumab vedotin

Source: https//www.creativebiolads.net//enfortumabvedotinoverview.htm

2. **Sacituzumab govitecan**
   - Here the antibody is targetted against trophoblast cell surface antigen 2 (Trop-2). The antibody is conjugated to SN-38 which is the active metabolite of irinotecan.
   - It has also received accelerated FDA approval for use in metastatic urothelial bladder cancer patients who have received prior chemotherapy/immunotherapy.[27]
   - **FGFR inhibitors**
     - Alterations in FGFR gene have been identified as potential targets for treatment.
     - Erdafitinib is FDA approved in the post-chemotherapy setting for metastatic urothelial cancer patients whose tumors harbour FGFR 2/3 alterations.[28]

13. What are the options for patients with variant histology?

Ans:

- Very limited data exists for these patients.
- Patients with mixed histology with a predominant urothelial component should be managed like those with pure urothelial cancer.[29]
- Those with a predominant non-urothelial component should be managed with appropriate chemotherapy as used in the setting of muscle invasive variant bladder cancer.

14. How will you manage intractable hematuria in a patient with metastatic bladder cancer?

Ans:

- If the mass in the bladder is not too large and is amenable for a transurethral resection or fulguration, then this should be attempted.
- Hemostatic radiation therapy is an option in large masses. It is quite effective with a rapid onset of action but the effect is not very long-lasting.[30]
- The next step if hemostatic RT is ineffective would be to attempt selective angioembolization. It is a safe procedure with reported success rates ranging from 40 to 100%.[31]
- The above measures are usually effective in most patients. In the rare scenario of intractable hematuria despite the above measures, a palliative cystectomy may be required. However, this surgery is associated with significant morbidity.

SUMMARY

- Every patient with a diagnosis of a muscle invasive bladder cancer should have a complete metastatic staging evaluation performed with either a CECT thorax + abdomen + pelvis or a FDG PET CT.
- The histological type of the metastatic bladder cancer dictates the chemotherapy regimen and also the prognosis.
- Platinum-based chemotherapy is the standard of care for metastatic urothelial bladder cancer. It is important to assess the patient if he is fit to receive cisplatin or carboplatin or neither of them.
- MVAC and Gem-Cis are the two regimens which have similar survival benefit. Gem-Cis is more commonly used as it is better tolerated.
- Gemcitabine-carboplatin is the standard of care for these patients. They may also be offered pembrolizumab/atezolizumab if they are PD-L1 positive.
- Single agent chemotherapy options offer modest survival benefit. These patients may also be offered pembrolizumab/atezolizumab irrespective of the PD-L1 status.
- Maintenance therapy with avelumab is the standard of care following initial platinum-based chemotherapy
- Enfortumab vedotin, sacituzumab govitecan and erdafitinib are the newer agents approved for second line therapy.
- Endoscopic procedures, hemostatic radiation therapy, angioembolization and palliative cystectomy are the options that can be employed for managing intractable hematuria.

REFERENCES

1. Browne RFJ, Meehan CP, Colville J, Power R, Torreggiani WC. Transitional cell carcinoma of the upper urinary tract: spectrum of imaging findings. Radiographics. 2005;25(6):1609–27.
2. Bajorin DF, Dodd PM, Mazumdar M, Fazzari M, McCaffrey JA, Scher HI, *et al.* Long-term survival in metastatic transitional-cell carcinoma and prognostic factors predicting outcome of therapy. J Clin Oncol. 1999 Oct;17(10):3173–81.
3. Sonpavde G, Pond GR, Rosenberg JE, Bajorin DF, Choueiri TK, Necchi A, *et al.* Improved 5-factor prognostic classification of patients receiving salvage systemic therapy for advanced urothelial carcinoma. J Urol. 2016 Feb;195(2):277–82.
4. Galsky MD, Hahn NM, Rosenberg J, Sonpavde G, Hutson T, Oh WK, *et al.* A consensus definition of patients with metastatic urothelial carcinoma who are unfit for cisplatin-based chemotherapy. Lancet Oncol. 2011 Mar;12(3):211–4.
5. von der Maase H, Sengelov L, Roberts JT, Ricci S, Dogliotti L, Oliver T, *et al.* Long-term survival results of a randomized trial comparing gemcitabine plus cisplatin, with methotrexate, vinblastine, doxorubicin, plus cisplatin in patients with bladder cancer. J Clin Oncol. 2005 Jul 20;23(21):4602–8.
6. von der Maase H, Hansen SW, Roberts JT, Dogliotti L, Oliver T, Moore MJ, *et al.* Gemcitabine and cisplatin versus methotrexate, vinblastine, doxorubicin, and cisplatin in advanced or metastatic bladder cancer: results of a large, randomized, multinational, multicenter, phase III study. J Clin Oncol. 2000 Sep;18(17):3068–77.
7. Sternberg CN, de Mulder P, Schornagel JH, Theodore C, Fossa SD, van Oosterom AT, *et al.* Seven year update of an EORTC phase III trial of high-dose intensity M-VAC chemotherapy and G-CSF versus classic M-VAC in advanced urothelial tract tumours. Eur J Cancer. 2006 Jan;42(1):50–4.
8. Bellmunt J, von der Maase H, Mead GM, Skoneczna I, De Santis M, Daugaard G, *et al.* Randomized phase III study comparing paclitaxel/cisplatin/gemcitabine and gemcitabine/cisplatin in patients with locally advanced or metastatic urothelial cancer without prior systemic therapy:

EORTC Intergroup Study 30987. J Clin Oncol. 2012 Apr 1;30(10):1107–13.

9. Rosenberg JE, Ballman KA, Halabi S, Atherton PJ, Mortazavi A, Sweeney C, *et al.* Randomized Phase III Trial of Gemcitabine and Cisplatin With Bevacizumab or Placebo in Patients With Advanced Urothelial Carcinoma: Results of CALGB 90601 (Alliance). J Clin Oncol. 2021 Aug 1;39(22):2486–96.
10. Galsky MD, Chen GJ, Oh WK, Bellmunt J, Roth BJ, Petrioli R, *et al.* Comparative effectiveness of cisplatin-based and carboplatin-based chemotherapy for treatment of advanced urothelial carcinoma. Ann Oncol. 2012 Feb;23(2):406–10.
11. De Santis M, Bellmunt J, Mead G, Kerst JM, Leahy M, Maroto P, *et al.* Randomized phase II/III trial assessing gemcitabine/carboplatin and methotrexate/carboplatin/vinblastine in patients with advanced urothelial cancer "unfit" for cisplatin-based chemotherapy: phase II--results of EORTC study 30986. J Clin Oncol. 2009 Nov 20;27(33):5634–9.
12. Galsky MD, Arija JÁA, Bamias A, Davis ID, De Santis M, Kikuchi E, *et al.* Atezolizumab with or without chemotherapy in metastatic urothelial cancer (IMvigor130): a multicentre, randomised, placebo-controlled phase 3 trial. Lancet. 2020 May 16;395(10236):1547–57.
13. Powles T, Cs szi T, Özgüro lu M, Matsubara N, Géczi L, Cheng SYS, *et al.* Pembrolizumab alone or combined with chemotherapy versus chemotherapy as first-line therapy for advanced urothelial carcinoma (KEYNOTE-361): a randomised, open-label, phase 3 trial. Lancet Oncol. 2021 Jul;22(7):931–45.
14. Powles T, van der Heijden MS, Castellano D, Galsky MD, Loriot Y, Petrylak DP, *et al.* Durvalumab alone and durvalumab plus tremelimumab versus chemotherapy in previously untreated patients with unresectable, locally advanced or metastatic urothelial carcinoma (DANUBE): a randomised, open-label, multicentre, phase 3 trial. Lancet Oncol. 2020 Dec;21(12):1574–88.
15. Balar AV, Castellano D, O'Donnell PH, Grivas P, Vuky J, Powles T, *et al.* First-line pembrolizumab in cisplatin-ineligible patients with locally advanced and unresectable or metastatic urothelial cancer (KEYNOTE-052): a multicentre, single-arm, phase 2 study. Lancet Oncol. 2017 Nov;18(11):1483–92.
16. Balar AV, Galsky MD, Rosenberg JE, Powles T, Petrylak DP, Bellmunt J, *et al.* Atezolizumab as first-line treatment in cisplatin-ineligible patients with locally advanced and metastatic urothelial carcinoma: a single-arm, multicentre, phase 2 trial. Lancet. 2017 Jan 7;389(10064):67–76.
17. Powles T, Park SH, Voog E, Caserta C, Valderrama BP, Gurney H, *et al.* Avelumab Maintenance Therapy for Advanced or Metastatic Urothelial Carcinoma. N Engl J Med. 2020 Sep 24;383(13):1218–30.
18. Raggi D, Miceli R, Sonpavde G, Giannatempo P, Mariani L, Galsky MD, *et al.* Second-line single-agent versus doublet chemotherapy as salvage therapy for metastatic urothelial cancer: a systematic review and meta-analysis. Ann Oncol. 2016 Jan;27(1):49–61.
19. Albers P, Park SI, Niegisch G, Fechner G, Steiner U, Lehmann J, *et al.* Randomized phase III trial of 2nd line gemcitabine and paclitaxel chemotherapy in patients with advanced bladder cancer: short-term versus prolonged treatment [German Association of Urological Oncology (AUO) trial AB 20/99]. Ann Oncol. 2011 Feb;22(2):288–94.
20. Wong RL, Ferris LA, Do OA, Holt SK, Ramos JD, Crabb SJ, *et al.* Efficacy of Platinum Rechallenge in Metastatic Urothelial Carcinoma After Previous Platinum-Based Chemotherapy for Metastatic Disease. Oncologist. 2021 Dec;26(12):1026–34.
21. Bellmunt J, Théodore C, Demkov T, Komyakov B, Sengelov L, Daugaard G, *et al.* Phase III trial of vinflunine plus best supportive care compared with best supportive care alone after a platinum-containing regimen in patients with advanced transitional cell carcinoma of the urothelial tract. J Clin Oncol. 2009 Sep 20;27(27):4454–61.
22. Bellmunt J, de Wit R, Vaughn DJ, Fradet Y, Lee JL, Fong L, *et al.* Pembrolizumab as Second-Line Therapy for Advanced Urothelial Carcinoma. N Engl J Med. 2017 Mar 16;376(11):1015–26.
23. Powles T, Durán I, van der Heijden MS, Loriot Y, Vogelzang NJ, De Giorgi U, *et al.* Atezolizumab versus chemotherapy in patients with platinum-treated locally advanced or metastatic urothelial carcinoma (IMvigor211): a multicentre, open-label, phase 3 randomised controlled trial. Lancet. 2018 Feb 24;391(10122):748–57.
24. Alt M, Stecca C, Tobin S, Jiang DM, Sridhar SS. Enfortumab Vedotin in urothelial cancer. Ther Adv Urol. 2020;12:1756287220980192.
25. Powles T, Rosenberg JE, Sonpavde GP, Loriot Y, Durán I, Lee JL, *et al.* Enfortumab Vedotin in Previously Treated Advanced Urothelial Carcinoma. N Engl J Med. 2021 Mar 25;384(12):1125–35.
26. Chang E, Weinstock C, Zhang L, Charlab R, Dorff SE, Gong Y, *et al.* FDA Approval Summary: Enfortumab Vedotin for Locally Advanced or Metastatic Urothelial Carcinoma. Clin Cancer Res. 2021 Feb 15;27(4):922–7.
27. Tagawa ST, Balar AV, Petrylak DP, Kalebasty AR, Loriot Y, Fléchon A, *et al.* TROPHY-U-01: A Phase II Open-Label Study of Sacituzumab Govitecan in Patients With Metastatic Urothelial Carcinoma Progressing After Platinum-Based Chemotherapy and Checkpoint Inhibitors. J Clin Oncol. 2021 Aug 1;39(22):2474–85.
28. Loriot Y, Necchi A, Park SH, Garcia-Donas J, Huddart R, Burgess E, *et al.* Erdafitinib in Locally Advanced or Metastatic Urothelial Carcinoma. N Engl J Med. 2019 Jul 25;381(4):338–48.
29. JaW, MB, JB, Hm B, Tm DR, M DS, *et al.* EAU-ESMO Consensus Statements on the Management of Advanced and Variant Bladder Cancer-An International Collaborative Multistakeholder Effort†: Under the Auspices of the EAU-ESMO Guidelines Committees. European urology [Internet]. 2020 Feb [cited 2023 Jul 19];77(2). Available from: https://pubmed.ncbi.nlm.nih.gov/31753752/
30. Lacarrière E, Smaali C, Benyoucef A, Pfister C, Grise P. The efficacy of hemostatic radiotherapy for bladder cancer-related hematuria in patients unfit for surgery. Int Braz J Urol. 2013;39(6):808–16.
31. Taha DE, Shokeir AA, Aboumarzouk OA. Selective embolisation for intractable bladder haemorrhages: A systematic review of the literature. Arab J Urol. 2018 Mar 2;16(2):197–205.

Chapter 9

Upper Tract Urothelial Cancer

• Ginil Kumar • Shashank Agrawal

LEARNING OBJECTIVES

- To understand the aspects of imaging and staging in upper tract urothelial cancer (UTUC): A CECT provides the best assessment of the locoregional disease. A chest CT should be performed in all cases of high grade UTUC.
- To understand the indications of flexible ureteroscopy: Any kind of ureteric instrumentation is known to increase the risk of a future bladder recurrence.
- To understand risk stratification of UTUC: All patients with UTUC should be classified as either low or high risk UTUC to decide if nephron sparing options can be offered.
- To know the kidney sparing options available for low risk UTUC: Low risk UTUC patients can be offered kidney sparing treatment options if the size and location of the tumor permits.
- To understand the management of high risk UTUC: Radical nephroureterectomy with bladder cuff excision is the standard of care for high risk UTUC.
- To understand the importance of lymph node dissection during RNU: Regional lymph node dissection (depending on the location of the UTUC) is recommended for all patients undergoing a RNU.
- To understand about post-operative intravesical mitomycin instillation: A single post-operative intravesical mitomycin C instillation has been shown to reduce the risk of future bladder recurrences.
- To understand the role of chemotherapy in UTUC: We have level 1 evidence from the POUT trial for benefit of adjuvant chemotherapy for patients with ≥pT2 or pN+ disease after RNU.

Case Scenario

62 years old diabetic female presented with history of two episodes of gross painless hematuria in past three weeks. Her serum creatinine was 1.1 mg/dl while urine routine and microscopy showed 10–20 RBCs/HPF. Her performance score was ECOG: 0.

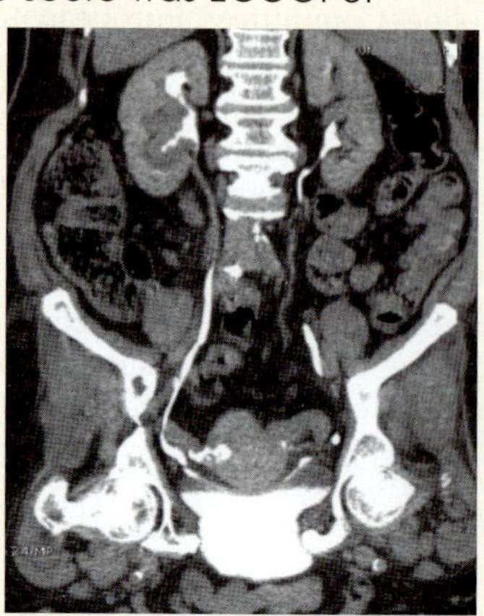

CT urography showed 4 × 3.3 cm lesion in axial plane and 3.9 cm in coronal plane which was homogeneously enhancing soft tissue density lesion involving mid and lower pole of right kidney which is extending into renal pelvis on delayed phase images. There were no enlarged retroperitoneal lymph nodes.

1. **What is the differential diagnosis of filling defect in pelvicalyceal system on IVU?**

   Ans: Blood clots, radiolucent stones like matrix stone, sloughed papillae, fungus ball, overlying bowel gas and upper tract urothelial carcinoma.[1]

2. **Which radiological imaging will you prefer in patient with suspected UTUC?**

   Ans:

   - Among imaging techniques, computed tomography urography (CTU) offers the highest accuracy in UTUC diagnosis, with a pooled sensitivity of 92% and a pooled specificity of 95%.[2,3] Urothelial cancers have an average density of 46 Hounsfield units (HU) and range between 10 and 70 HU.

- Magnetic resonance urography (MRU) has been proven to be inferior to CTU and is indicated in patients who cannot undergo CTU where use of iodinated contrast media or radiation is contraindicated. MRU can be done in compromised renal function patients as group II gadolinium-based contrast agents like gadobenate dimeglumine, gadobutrol, gadoterate meglumine are safe in chronic kidney disease patients.[4]
- Direct comparison of MRU and CTU showed a sensitivity of 82.8–86.2% and a specificity of 83.1–83.3% for MRU compared to 96.6% and 87–91.5% of CTU, respectively[5], so present guidelines indicate CTU as the imaging of choice.

3. **What are the various appearances of UTUC on CTU?**

Ans: Based upon morphology UTUC can be papillary tumor, flat lesion and invasive carcinoma.

- Papillary tumor can appear as single or multiple filling defects in collecting system varying from the millimetric to wide base tumors.
- Flat lesion can be visualized as a concentric or eccentric pyelocaliceal or ureteric wall thickening.
- Invasive UTUC can present as infiltrative pattern with increased attenuation and stranding of periureteral and renal sinus fat.

4. **What is "oncocalyx" and "phantom calyx"?**

Ans: When tumors involve the calyceal system, a calyx could be entirely missing in the excretory phase due to complete filling by solid tissue, it is known as "oncocalyx". If tumor develops in the infundibular neck resulting in calyceal amputation and its dilatation with absence of urine opacification, it is known as "phantom calyx".[6]

5. **How will you differentiate intrarenal TCC from centrally located renal cell carcinoma?**

Ans: Table 9.1 shows radiological differentiation between RCC and upper tract TCC.

6. **What are the risk factors for development of upper tract urothelial cancer?**

Ans:

- Smoking: Tobacco exposure increases the relative risk of developing UTUC from 2.5 to 7.0.
- Aristolochic acid, which is commonly used in Chinese herbal medicine.
- Industrial carcinogens, phenacetin (analgesic), cyclophosphamide, arsenic
- Prior bladder cancer (2–4% develop UTUC)
- Lynch syndrome

7. **What is Lynch syndrome?**

Ans: Lynch syndrome is characterized by an increased risk for colorectal cancer (CRC) and cancers of the endometrium, ovary, stomach, small bowel, urinary tract, biliary tract, brain (usually glioblastoma), skin (sebaceous adenomas, sebaceous carcinomas, and keratoacanthomas),

TABLE 9.1: Radiological differentiation between RCC and upper tract TCC

S.No.	Characteristics	Intrarenal TCC	Centrally located RCC
	Representative image		
1.	Tumor centre	Within collecting system	Within renal parenchyma
2.	Filling defect in PCS	Present	Absent
3.	Enhancement pattern	Homogenous and less enhancing than RCCs	Heterogenous
4.	Renal shape	Preserved	May be distorted
5.	Continuity between mass and collecting system	Present	Absent
6.	Extension towards uretero-pelvic junction	Present	Absent
7.	Necrotic or cystic changes	Less likely	More likely
8.	Calcification (seen on unenhanced phase)	Less likely	More likely
9.	Renal vein invasion	Very rare	More common
10.	Lymph node involvement	More common	Less common

pancreas. The Amsterdam criteria are a set of diagnostic criteria to help identify families which are likely to have Lynch syndrome.[7] Patients identified at high risk for Lynch syndrome should undergo germline DNA sequencing for patient and family counselling.

8. When to select patients with UTUC for Lynch syndrome screening?

Ans: Germline DNA sequencing of the patients need to be performed when the suspicion for hereditary UTUC is high. Following are the risk factors:

- Personal history of Lynch-spectrum cancer.

  Or
- First-degree relative <50 years with Lynch-spectrum cancer.

  Or
- Two first-degree relatives with Lynch-spectrum cancer.

9. At which stage patients with UTUC usually present?

Ans: At diagnosis, 60% of UTUC patients have an invasive tumor versus 20–25% of carcinoma bladder.[8] Hence, the prognosis of UTUC is poor with a 5-year overall survival (OS) of approximately 70%; for invasive disease the 5-year OS is less than 40%, which is lower than reported for UCB patients treated with radical cystectomy.[9]

10. What are the percentage of concomitant bladder cancer in patients with UTUC and vice versa?

Ans: The incidence of concomitant urothelial carcinoma bladder at the time of diagnosis of primary UTUC is 17%[10] while the risk of developing an UTUC following the diagnosis of a primary non-muscle invasive bladder cancer is approximately 2.6% although the proportion was higher in multifocal and high-risk tumors.[11]

11. What will be the next appropriate step?

Ans: Voided urine cytology and urethrocystoscopy. Urethrocystoscopy is done to rule out bladder tumour because up to 17% of UTUC present with concurrent bladder cancer.

12. What is the role of urine cytology?

Ans: Examination of freshly voided urine for examination of exfoliated cancer cell has high sensitivity in high grade UTUC. Sensitivity of cytology has been estimated at about 20% for grade 1, 45% for grade 2, and 75% for grade 3 tumours. However, cytology is less sensitive for UTUC than bladder tumours. Ureteroscopic biopsy of any identified lesion and cytologic washing from selective upper tract system is performed in patients with negative voided cytology but suspected UTUC on imaging.

The Paris System, standardised reporting system, published in 2022 redefined urinary cytology diagnostic categories as:[12]

a. No adequate diagnosis possible (no diagnosis).
b. Negative for UC (negative).
c. Atypical urothelial cells (atypia).
d. Suspicious for HG UC (suspicious).
e. High-grade/G3 UC (malignant).

Limitations of cytology: (a) User dependent (b) Hampered assessment in low cellular yield, urinary tract infection.

Although the traditional teaching has been to avoid sending urine for cytology during active haematuria, an experienced cytopathologist can still detect urothelial cancer cells amidst of the RBCs. Also, adding acetic acid to the urine sample lyses RBCs, making it easier to identify the cancer cells. The sample for urine cytology has to be a freshly voided sample. It can be given at any time of the day.

13. What is the role for retrograde pyelography (RGP) in patients with UTUC?

Ans: RGP can be done in the following scenarios:

a. Poorly functioning kidney.
b. In patients with contrast allergy.
c. Intraluminal filling defect can be seen.
d. Goblet sign (also called champagne glass sign): Appearance of ureter when it is focally dilated with intraluminal mass (Fig. 9.1).

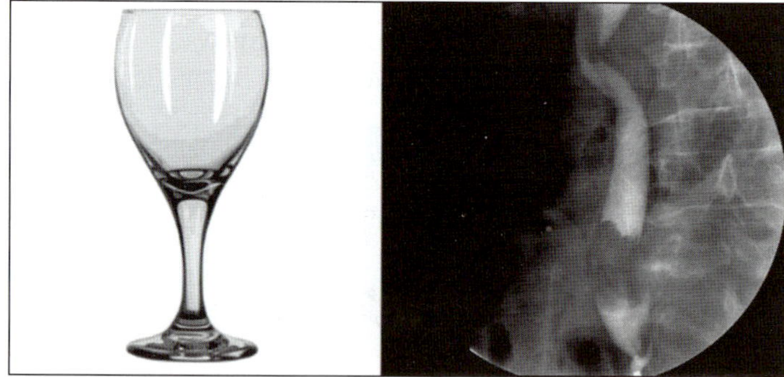

Fig. 9.1: Champagne glass sign on RGP

14. What are the indications of diagnostic ureteroscopy?

Ans: Flexible ureteroscopy(fURS) can be considered in situation where diagnosis remains unclear after imaging and/or voided urine cytology as ureteroscopy increases the diagnostic accuracy of excretory or retrograde urography alone from 75% to 85–90%. It will help map the disease, risk stratify it and plan management.

15. How will you perform ureteroscopy (if indicated)?

Ans:

- Ureteroscopic examination of the affected side commences with "no touch" technique.

- The smallest flexible ureteroscope (preferably digital scopes) available should be passed.
- Ureter is examined and complete ureterorenoscopy should be performed in a systematic manner from the upper pole to lower pole, to ensure direct examination of all the potential space of the intraluminal collecting system.[13]
- In patients with existing ureteric strictures or difficult access to the upper tract, the risk of ureteric injury can be minimized by using gentle dilatation techniques like temporary stenting. Use of ureteral access sheaths should be discouraged.

16. What will you do if you find a bladder tumor during process of ureteroscopy?

Ans: In patients who have concomitant lower tract tumors (bladder/urethra) discovered at the time of ureteroscopy, the lower tract tumors should be managed in the same setting as ureteroscopy.

17. What do you look for in ureteroscopy?

Ans: I will look for focality of tumor, its location, appearance, and size.

18. What will you do if the flexible ureteroscope does not reach the upper tract despite all the measures?

Ans: In cases where flexible ureteroscopy is not possible, an attempt for selective upper tract washing or barbotage for cytology can be made. Retrograde ureteropyelography can also be performed in cases where good quality imaging such as CT or MR urography are not available.

19. What is the role of upper tract tumour biopsy and how it can be performed?

Ans:

- Identification of grade of tumour which helps in risk stratification of patient. This is required only when voided cytology or selected cytology is negative for high grade and kidney sparing surgery can be offered in case of low grade TCC. If size or location of tumor preclude kidney sparing treatment, then tumor biopsy has no role.
- Ureteroscopic biopsy technique: When a lesion is encountered, cytology washings are taken via the irrigation channel of the ureteroscope. Then biopsy can be performed using 3-F cold cup forceps or basket. Choice of cold cup forceps versus basket depends on the nature of the lesion; with the cold cup biopsy forceps being superior for sessile lesions, while the basket is useful for large friable tumours. Once the biopsy is obtained, the tumor sample, biopsy device and ureteroscope are removed together as one unit, to avoid shearing and loss of the sample.

  However, stage assessment using ureteroscopic biopsy can be inaccurate.

20. This patient's urine cytology shows high-grade malignant cells. How will you further assess this patient?

Ans: Given the CTU and the positive urine cytology, I would like to complete the metastatic staging work-up with CT scan of the chest.

21. What are you assessing while reading the CT scan of this patient?

Ans: I will look for the following mentioned points on CTU:[14]

- Soft tissue mass on unenhanced phase which will show homogenous enhancement in arterial phase and filling defect(s) or luminal narrowing in the urinary tract in excretory phase.
- Size of the mass and its morphology which can be flat, papillary, or invasive carcinomas. Flat lesions could manifest as concentric or eccentric pyelocaliceal or ureteral wall thickening.
- Hydronephrosis may be present when tumor occlude ureteral or calyceal lumen.
- Renal sinus fat or periureteral stranding may indicate infiltrative pattern of tumor.
- Retroperitoneal lymph node: Number and size of involved lymph nodes in the largest dimension.
- Visceral metastasis.

22. How do you risk stratify UTUC?

Ans: Risk stratification of non-metastatic UTUC[15] (Table 9.2):

TABLE 9.2: Risk stratification of non-metastatic UTUC

Low-risk UTUC (All of the below factors need to be present)	*High-risk UTUC (Any of the below factors need to be present)*
• Unifocal disease • Tumor size < 2 cm • Low-grade cytology • Low grade URS biopsy • Non-invasive on CTU	• Hydronephrosis • Tumor size >2 cm • High-grade cytology • High-grade URS biopsy • Multifocal disease • Previous radical cystectomy for bladder cancer • Variant histology

23. What treatment option will you offer to this patient?

Ans: I will offer right radical nephroureterectomy (RNU) with excision of a cuff of bladder tissue at the ureteric orifice with regional lymphadenectomy with perioperative intravesical instillation of mitomycin 2–10 days after the surgery.

24. How to assess risk of post-RNU CKD or dialysis in patients with UTUC?

Ans: A median decline in renal function after NU up to 32% has been reported which can induce or exacerbate a state of CKD, affect a patient's candidacy to receive adjuvant chemotherapy.[16] Predictive factors for post-operative development of CKD or progression of pre-existing CKD include older age, diabetes mellitus, hypertension, as well as male sex, obesity, tobacco use, larger tumor size, and post-operative acute kidney injury.[17,18]

With significant nephron mass loss, hyper-filtration can occur resulting in glomerular damage, exacerbation of proteinuria and progressive sclerosis with further decline in GFR. Therefore, repeat assessment of blood pressure, eGFR, and proteinuria should be performed soon after nephrectomy then again in three to six months to assess for development or progression of CKD.

25. What are the principles of doing radical nephroureterectomy (RNU)?

Ans: Oncological principles preventing tumour seeding should be followed.

- Early clipping of the ureter.
- Kidney and ureter must be removed en bloc with the bladder cuff.
- Procedure should be performed in a closed system. Avoid morcellation of the tumour and use an endobag for tumour extraction.
- Inadvertent entry into the urinary tract should be avoided, except when performing a bladder cuff excision and only after prior clipping of the ureter and complete drainage of the bladder.

26. What are the various approaches of performing radical nephroureterectomy?

Ans:

- **Open approach:** Traditional approach for the open technique is the loin incision. A second Pfannenstiel or lower midline incision can also be used to facilitate excision of the bladder cuff. The entire renal unit and collecting system can also be removed through a midline abdominal incision which is preferred in case of bulky retroperitoneal lymph nodes. Open approach is preferred in cT3/T4 or N+ tumors.
- Laparoscopic RNU can be performed with either a transperitoneal or retroperitoneal approach.
- Robot-assisted laparoscopic approach.
- **Combined approach:** Nephrectomy part is dealt with laparoscopic approach and then lower midline, or Gibson's incision is placed for distal ureterectomy and bladder cuff removal.

27. Why complete removal of distal ureter along with bladder cuff is recommended?

Ans:

- Complete removal of ureter including intra-mural portion of ureter and bladder cuff offers superior oncological outcomes to those off incomplete resection.
- Risk for tumour recurrence in the remaining ureteral stump is 30–75%. Additionally, cystoscopy surveillance of residual ureteric stump is not possible.

28. What are various ways to manage distal ureter and bladder cuff during radical nephroureterectomy?

Ans: Only the traditional methods of either an extravesical or trans-vesical resection of the intramural ureter with bladder cuff excision are recommended (Table 9.3).

29. What is the status of lymph node dissection in patients with UTUC?

Ans: Risk of LN metastasis increases with advancing tumour stage. Lymph node dissection appears to be unnecessary in cases of TaT1 UTUC because of the low risk of LN metastasis,[19,20] however, tumour staging is inaccurate pre-operatively; therefore, a template-based LND should be offered to all patients who are scheduled for RNU for high-risk non-metastatic UTUC.

30. What is the template of lymphadenectomy?

Ans: Template-based and completeness of LND improves CSS in patients with muscle-invasive disease and reduces the risk of local recurrence.[21] Kondo and Tanabe proposed an extended lymphadenectomy template based on the location of the tumor[22] (Fig. 9.2).

31. What is the indication of kidney-sparing treatment and options available in patients of UTUC?

Ans: Indications of nephron-sparing treatment:

- Kidney-sparing surgery can be offered in low-risk UTUC as it reduces the morbidity associated with radical surgery (e.g. loss of kidney function), without compromising oncological outcomes.[23]
- High grade tumours in solitary kidney.
- High-risk patients with imperative indications such as bilateral UTUC, chronic kidney disease or any other comorbidity compromising the use of RNU.

Treatment options:

1. Ureteroscopic:[24]
   - Basket or biopsy forceps used to debulk tumor if large.
   - Laser or Bugbee used to completely ablate small tumors or base of larger tumors.
   - Risk of disease progression remains → stringent surveillance is required.
2. Percutaneous access:[25]
   - Allows for treatment of larger tumors.

TABLE 9.3: Management of lower ureter in upper tract TCC

Traditional open distal ureterectomy (Extravesical approach)	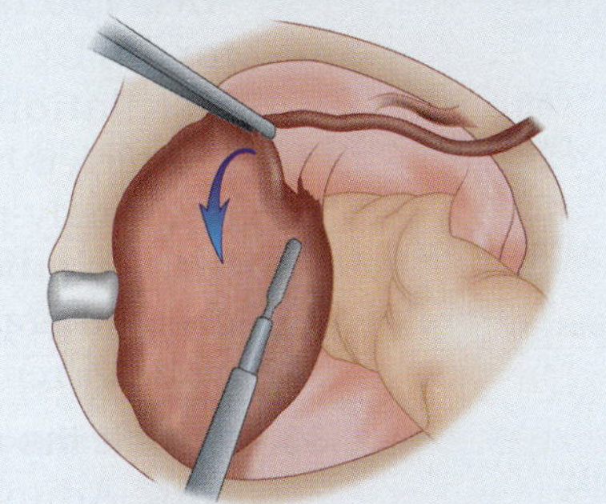	Distal ureter is freed till the intramural ureter and ipsilateral lateral pedicle of the bladder is ligated and divided. Cuff of bladder is removed en bloc with the ureter by applying a clamp to bladder wall and excising the full intramural portion of the ureter. Care is taken to stay away from the contralateral ureteral orifice.
Traditional open distal ureterectomy (Transvesical approach)	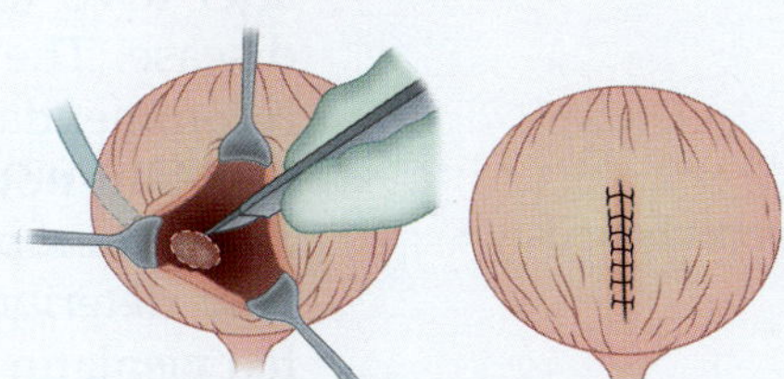	Anterior cystotomy is made, and intravesical dissection of ureter is performed, including a traditional 1 cm mucosal cuff around the orifice. Cystotomy defects are closed in two layers with interrupted or running absorbable sutures. First layer should incorporate mucosa, second layer should include detrusor muscle and adventitia.
Transvesical ligation and detachment technique	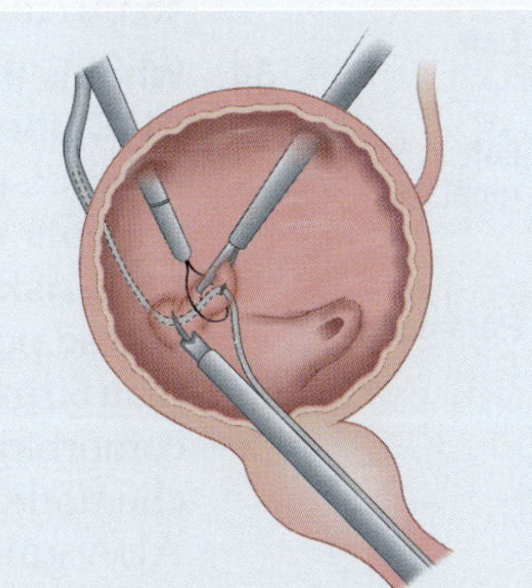	Via cystoscopy: Bladder is filled. Two 5 mm trocars placed intravesically. Endoloop is placed around ureteric orifice and ureteral catheter is advanced into ureter. With Collins knife bladder cuff is incised up to extravesical space. After freeing ureter, Endoloop is clinched around the ureter and ureteral catheter is simultaneously removed.
Intussusception (stripping) technique	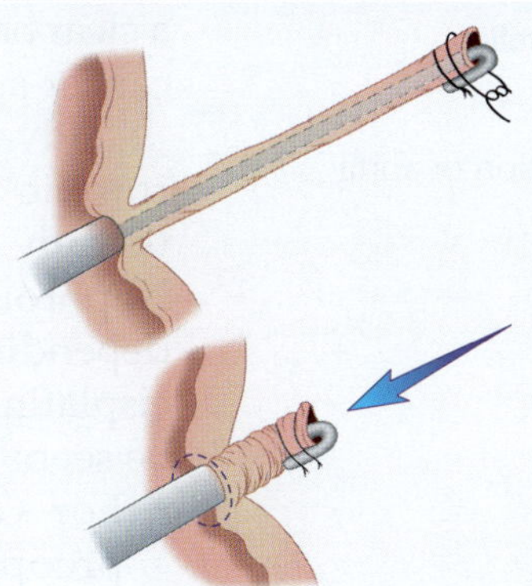	After nephrectomy ureter is divided and ureteral catheter is secured to distal end of ureter. Patient is changed to Lithotomy posture: Ureter is intussuscepted into bladder with retrograde traction. A resectoscope is used to excise the attached orifice.
Total laparoscopic approach		

- Access location is key, i.e. calyceal tumor, renal pelvis.
- Less used due to the availability of improved flexible ureteroscopes.
- Risk of tumour seeding remains with percutaneous access.

3. Ureterectomy:[26,27]
   - **Segmental ureterectomy** with primary reanastamosis for smaller low-grade and focal high-grade tumors in the mid-ureter.
   - **Distal ureterectomy** with bladder cuff removal and ureteroneocystostomy for low-risk tumors in the distal ureter that cannot be removed completely endoscopically. Distal ureterectomy +/-LND +/-peri-operative chemotherapy is also an option for high-risk tumors involving the distal ureter.
   - **Total ureterectomy** with ileal interposition for upper ureteral tumors.
4. Renal autotransplantation with pyelocystostomy.

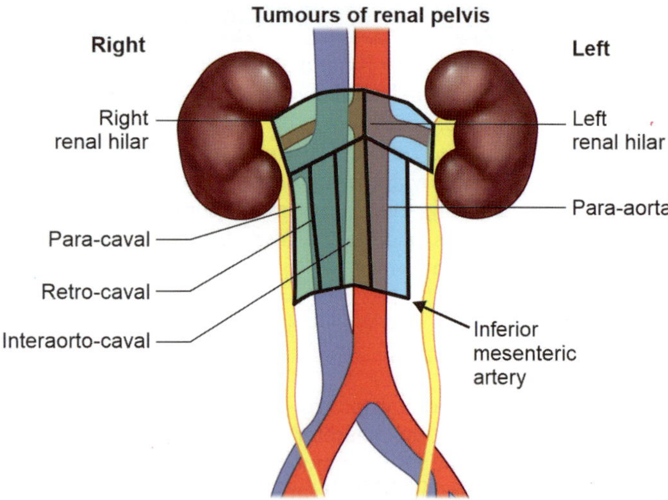

Fig. 9.2A: The inferior mesenteric artery marks the inferior boundary of the template

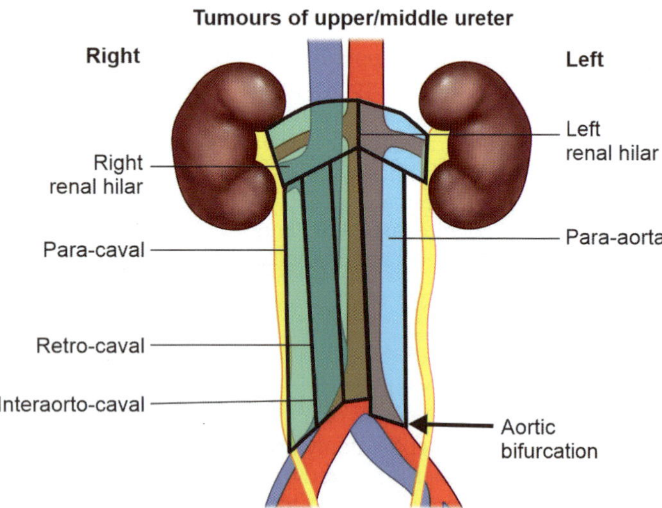

Fig. 9.2B: Template is extended to the level of bifurcation of aorta

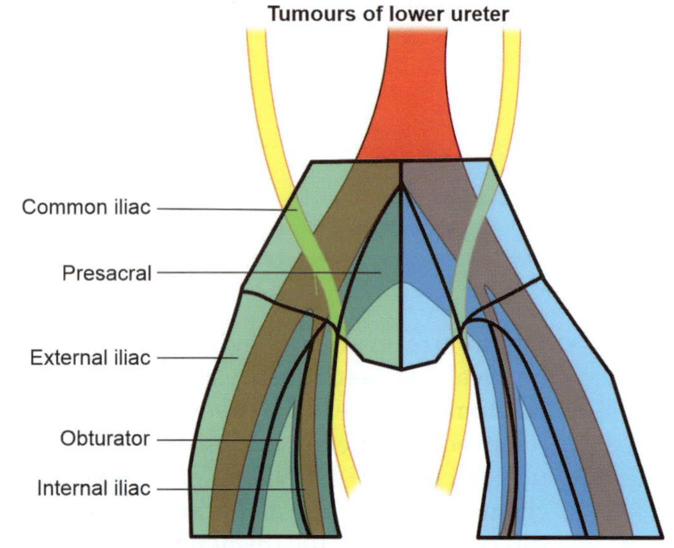

Extended lymphadenectomy template for tumors in the distal ureter includes ipsilateral common, external and internal iliac, obturator, and presacral nodes.

Fig. 9.2C: Lymph node dissection templates for UTUC

32. What is the role if adjuvant bladder instillation?

Ans: The rate of bladder recurrence after RNU for UTUC is 22–47%. Post-operative bladder instillation of chemotherapy (mitomycin C, pirarubicin) to lower the intravesical recurrence rate is strongly recommended in EAU guidelines.[28,29] Many studies support peri-operative intravesical chemotherapy 2–10 days post-RNU or at time of catheter removal.

33. What is the role of adjuvant chemotherapy?

Ans: Adjuvant platinum-based chemotherapy after RNU to patients with pT2–T4 and/or pN+ disease. The EAU2023 guidelines give a strong recommendation for the same.

Main potential limitation of using adjuvant chemotherapy is the concern that renal function may deteriorate after RNU. However, fractionated cisplatin may be considered up to a GFR of 45 ml/min.

34. What is the status of neoadjuvant chemotherapy (NAC) therapy in UTUC?

Ans: Cisplatin-based NAC should be offered to patients undergoing RNU or ureterectomy with high-risk UTUC, particularly in those patients whose post-operative eGFR is expected to be less than 60 m/min/1.73 m^2 or those with other medical comorbidities that would preclude platinum-based chemotherapy in the post-operative setting (The AUA guidelines given a strong recommendation for the same). Recent meta-analysis has also shown a clear benefit of NAC in both overall survival and cancer-specific survival.[30]

Advantage of administering potentially nephrotoxic cisplatin-based combination chemotherapy when patients still have both kidneys. Nephroureterectomy reduces GFR by 24%, and depending on the GFR cut-off used to administer cisplatin-based chemotherapy, the following can be seen:[31]

- For GFR of 60 ml/min: 49% are eligible preoperatively while only 19% are eligible postoperatively.
- For GFR of 45 ml/min: 80% are eligible preoperatively while only 55% are eligible postoperatively.

Disadvantages of NAC: (a) Needs biopsy for confirmation of disease (b) Delay in definitive RNU leading to inadvertent disease progression, particularly in chemo-resistant patients. (c) Toxicities related to chemotherapy may delay surgery even further. (d) Overtreatment can occur in patients without pathologically proven muscle-invasive disease.

Overall, NAC seems to be promising given the favourable response and tumour downstaging rates.

35. Is there any role of adjuvant immunotherapy in UTUC?

Ans: Adjuvant nivolumab in patients unfit for, or who declined, platinum-based adjuvant chemotherapy for > pT3 and/or pN+ disease after RNU alone or > ypT2 and/or ypN+ disease after neoadjuvant chemotherapy, followed by RNU can be discussed.[32] However, recent meta-analysis suggests superior oncological benefit for adjuvant platinum-based chemotherapy over immune checkpoint inhibitors in patients treated with radical surgery for UTUC.[33]

36. What is UGN-101 (Jelmyto™ or mitomycin gel)?

Ans:

- UGN-1016–9 (Jelmyto™, formerly MitoGel, UroGen Pharma, Israel) has been approved by the US Food and Drug Administration (FDA) as the first treatment for low-risk UTUC.[34]
- It is temperature sensitive, reverse thermosensitive gel composed of hydrogel polymer base and MMC. It remains in liquid state at room temperature and converts to a gel at body temperature, thereby conforming to each patient's distinct pelvicalyceal and ureteric anatomy. It is dissolution continuous urinary bathing results in slow-release, sustained drug delivery.
- Preliminary results of a phase III trial (OLYMPUS study) demonstrated its efficacy as a successful chemo-ablative agent for low-grade upper tract tumors. Further details of this trial is discussed in later part of this chapter.

37. What information do you want in histopathology report?

Ans: In histopathological report I would like to know the tumour site, size and focality on gross examination and histological type, grade, tumour configuration, tumor extension, margins, lymph node status on microscopic examination.

38. What are the chances of tumour recurrence following RNU?

Ans: Following RNU intra-vesical recurrence within the first 2 years following surgery is found in 22% to 47% of the patients, whereas 2–6% patients develop a recurrence in the contralateral upper urinary tract following RNU.[35]

39. What should be the follow-up of patients?

Ans: As per the EAU 2023 guidelines: Follow-up protocol of UTUC (Fig. 9.3):[15]

40. Six years later this woman came with complaints of weight loss, anorexia and loin pain. A repeat CT scan is performed and shows a local recurrence in the renal bed. How will you proceed further?

Ans: I will do re-staging with a CT scan of her chest. As she is symptomatic, so further treatment is needed. If on imaging the lesion seems to be resectable, then I will go for resection of lesion, otherwise I will do the biopsy of the lesion and will discuss chemotherapy option (Fig. 9.4).

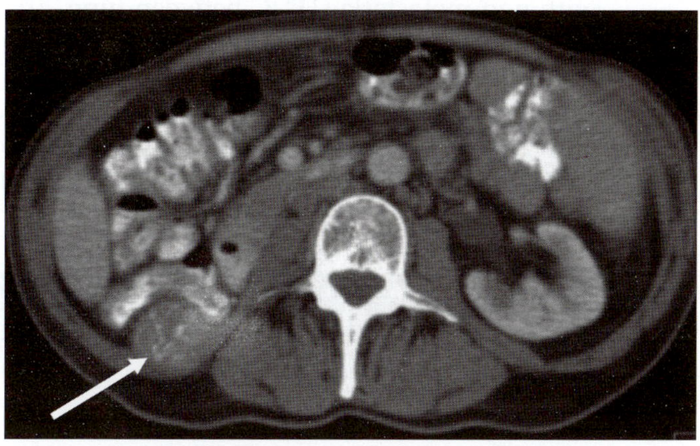

Fig. 9.4: Follow-up CT showing residual lesion

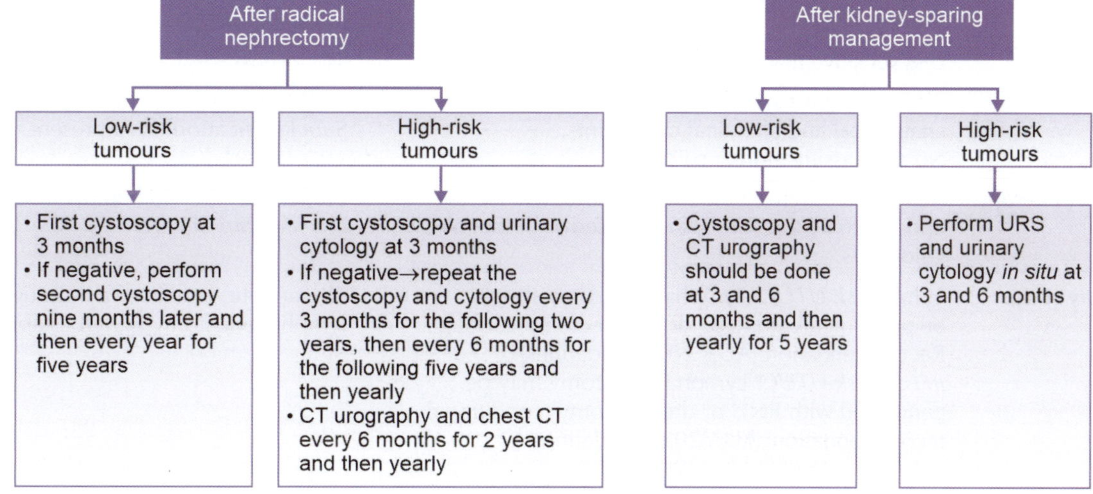

Fig. 9.3: Follow-up protocol of UTUC

Uro-oncology

41. What is the contemporary conditional cancer-specific survival (CSS) after RNU in patients with nonmetastatic UTUC?

Ans: 5-year cancer-specific survival (CSS) of UTUC patients as per stage is as follows:[36]

T_1LGN_0	93.4%
T_1HGN_0	86.2%
T_2N0	77.5%
T_3N0	63%
$T_4N_0/T_{any}\ N_{1-3}$	38.8%

42. How does UTUC differ from bladder cancer?

Ans: Urothelial carcinoma of the bladder and the upper tract: Disparate twins[37] (Table 9.4).

IMPORTANT TRIALS

Pout Trial[38]

- Multicentric phase III open label RCT of perioperative chemotherapy versus surveillance in UTUC.
- 261 patients of age ≥16 years and diagnosed with non-metastatic UTUC between June 2012 and November 2017: Underwent en-bloc RNU with lymphadenectomy.
- Patients with pT2-pT4 N0M0 or pTanyN1-3M0 randomized to adjuvant chemotherapy (ACT) (Four cycles of three weekly schedule) vs observation.
- Chemo arm with Gemcitabine (1000 mg/m^2 on Day 1 and 8) + Cisplatin (70 mg/m^2 when eGFR>50 mg/dl) or Carboplatin (eGFR 30–<50 mg/ml) on day 1 of each cycle.
- Follow-up three monthly to twelve months and six monthly to 36 months and annually thereafter with scopy and CT abdomen/pelvis.
- Primary endpoint: Disease free survival (DFS).
- 3-years DFS were 71% versus 46% in chemotherapy and surveillance arm respectively. At median follow-up of 30.3 months, ACT significantly improved DFS (HR = 0.45; p = 0.0001)
- In chemotherapy arm, 44% of the patients had grade 3 treatment related adverse effect which were managed conservatively and there was no treatment related death.

OLYMPUS TRIAL (Optimized deLiverY of Mitomycin for Primary UTUC study):[39]

- Single-arm phase III trial, patients with primary low-grade upper tract urothelial carcinoma underwent 6 once-weekly instillations of UGN-101 (JELMYTO), a reverse-thermosensitive polymer gel containing 4 mg/ml of mitomycin, into upper tract via retrograde catheter followed by once-monthly maintenance instillations for up to 12 months in complete responders which was assessed 4-6 weeks following last instillation of MMC.

TABLE 9.4: Differences between upper tract TCC and carcinoma bladder

	UTUC	*Carcinoma bladder (UCB)*
Embryological origin	Mesoderm-derived epithelium	Endoderm derived epithelium
Gender distribution	Male: Female =2:1	Male: Female =3-4:1
Risk factors	Unique association with Lynch syndrome and Aristolochic acid exposure.	No such unique association.
Presentation	60% are invasive at presentation.	15–20% are invasive at the time of presentation.
Urine cytology	Less sensitive than in UCB.	More sensitive than UTUC
Staging differences	Biopsy samples are of lower quality because of anatomical and technical constraints. No subclassification of pT3.	TURBT provides good sampling. Subclassification of T3 present.
Endocavitary chemotherapy/ Immunotherapy	Antegrade or retrograde BCG or mitomycin-C in upper urinary tract are sparsely used without any clear guidelines.	Intravesical chemotherapy/immunotherapy are standard of care.
Lymphadenectomy status	*In high-risk UTUC:* Lymphadenectomy should be performed with RNU or ureterectomy. (Strong Recommendation: AUA 2023 guidelines) *In Low-risk UTUC:* Lymphadenectomy may be performed with RNU or ureterectomy (conditional recommendation: AUA 2023 guidelines)	Therapeutic benefit of a thorough lymphadenectomy is well established.
Neo-adjuvant therapy	Limited prospective studies.	Recommended in Guidelines (T2-4N0M0)

- Inclusion and exclusion criteria:

Inclusion Criteria
- 18 years or older.
- Biopsy proven, new or recurrent LG, non-invasive UTUC superior to UPJ
- Minimum of 1 papillary tumor 0.5–1.5 cm in size
- Partial resection allowed for tumors >1.5 cm in size
- Wash urine-cytology negative for HG UTUC

Exclusion Criteria
- Receipt of BCG therapy for urothelial cancer (UC) within six months.
- Untreated UC in other location.
- History of CIS
- History of invasive UC within 5 years
- History of HG UC within 2 years

- Primary end point results:

Response	***N***	**%**
Complete response (CR)	42/71	59.2
No complete response:		
No response	12/71	16.9%
Partial response	8/71	11.3%
Emergence of high-grade disease	6/71	8.5%
Indeterminate	3/71	4.2%

ODMIT C TRIAL[40]

- 284 patients with no previous or concurrent history of bladder cancer undergoing nephro-ureterectomy for suspected UTUC were prospective, randomised, nonblinded trial to receive single postoperative intravesical dose of MMC (40 mg in 40 ml saline) immediately prior to removal of the urethral catheter **or** standard management on removal of the urinary catheter.
- By treatment as per protocol analysis, 17 of 105 patients (16%) in the MMC arm and 31 of 115 patients (27%) in the standard treatment arm developed a recurrence (p = 0.03).
- A single postoperative dose of intravesical MMC appears to reduce the risk of a bladder tumour within the first year following nephroureterectomy for UUTUC. The absolute reduction in risk is 11%, the relative reduction in risk is 40%.

SUMMARY

- Conduct a urethrocystoscopy to check for the presence of a bladder tumor.
- Consider diagnostic ureteroscopy if imaging and voided urine cytology do not provide
- sufficient information for diagnosing or risk-stratifying patients suspected of having UTUC.
- Utilize prognostic factors to classify patients by risk for guiding treatment decisions.
- Offer kidney-sparing management as the first-line treatment option for patients with low-risk tumors.
- Perform RNU in patients with high-risk non-metastatic UTUC.
- Recommend adjuvant platinum-based chemotherapy following RNU to eligible patients with pT2–T4 and/or pN+ disease, as it improves disease-free survival.
- A single post-operative intravesical chemotherapy instillation reduces the recurrence rate of bladder cancer in patients with no prior history of the disease.
- Consider discussing adjuvant nivolumab with patients who are either unsuitable for or have declined platinum-based adjuvant chemotherapy, particularly for those with >pT3 and/or pN+ disease after prior RNU alone or >ypT2 and/or ypN+ disease following neoadjuvant chemotherapy and subsequent RNU.
- Recommend Enfortumab vedotin combined with pembrolizumab as a first-line treatment for patients with advanced or metastatic disease.
- Provide platinum combination chemotherapy to patients who are eligible for platinum-based treatment but not suitable for Enfortumab + pembrolizumab

REFERENCES

1. Pollack, HM, *et al.* Computed tomography of renal pelvic filling defects. 1981. 138(3): p. 645–651.
2. Janisch, F., *et al.* Diagnostic performance of multidetector computed tomographic (MDCTU) in upper tract urothelial carcinoma (UTUC): a systematic review and meta-analysis. 2020. 38: p. 1165–1175.
3. Cowan, N.C., *et al.* Multidetector computed tomography urography for diagnosing upper urinary tract urothelial tumour. 2007. 99(6): p. 1363–1370.
4. Schieda, N., *et al.* Gadolinium-based contrast agents in kidney disease: a comprehensive review and clinical practice guideline issued by the Canadian Association of Radiologists. 2018. 5: p. 2054358118778573.
5. Martingano, P., *et al.* Magnetic resonance urography vs computed tomography urography in the evaluation of patients with haematuria. 2013. 118(7): p. 1184–1198.
6. Browne, R.F., *et al.* Transitional cell carcinoma of the upper urinary tract: spectrum of imaging findings. 2005. 25(6): p. 1609–1627.
7. Vasen, H.J.F.c., Clinical description of the Lynch syndrome [hereditary nonpolyposis colorectal cancer (HNPCC)]. 2005. 4: p. 219–225.
8. Rouprêt, M., *et al.* European Association of Urology guidelines on upper urinary tract urothelial carcinoma: 2020 update. 2021. 79(1): p. 62–79.
9. Adibi, M., *et al.* Oncological outcomes after radical nephroureterectomy for upper tract urothelial carcinoma: comparison over the three decades. 2012. 19(12): p. 1060–1066.
10. Cosentino, M., *et al.* Upper urinary tract urothelial cell carcinoma: location as a predictive factor for concomitant bladder carcinoma. 2013. 31: p. 141–145.
11. Millan-Rodriguez, F., *et al.* Upper urinary tract tumors after primary superficial bladder tumors: prognostic factors and risk groups. 2000. 164(4): p. 1183–1187.
12. Wojcik, E.M., D.F. Kurtycz, and D.L. Rosenthal, The Paris system for reporting urinary cytology. 2022: Springer.

13. Smentkowski, K.E., *et al.* Ureteroscopic biopsy of upper tract urothelial carcinoma and role of urinary biomarkers. 2020. 9(4): p. 1809.
14. Martingano, P., *et al.* CT Urography findings of upper urinary tract carcinoma and its mimickers: a pictorial review. 2020. 56(12): p. 705.
15. Rouprêt, M., *et al.* European association of urology guidelines on upper urinary tract urothelial carcinoma: 2023 update. 2023.
16. Kaag, M., *et al.* Preoperative predictors of renal function decline after radical nephroureterectomy for upper tract urothelial carcinoma. 2014. 114(5): p. 674–679.
17. Malcolm, J.B., *et al.* Comparison of rates and risk factors for developing chronic renal insufficiency, proteinuria and metabolic acidosis after radical or partial nephrectomy. 2009. 104(4): p. 476–481.
18. Li, L., *et al.* Risk of chronic kidney disease after cancer nephrectomy. 2014. 10(3): p. 135–145.
19. Zareba, P., *et al.* Association between lymph node yield and survival among patients undergoing radical nephroureterectomy for urothelial carcinoma of the upper tract. 2017. 123(10): p. 1741–1750.
20. Moschini, M., *et al.* Trends of lymphadenectomy in upper tract urothelial carcinoma (UTUC) patients treated with radical nephroureterectomy. 2017. 35: p. 1541–1547.
21. Dominguez-Escrig, J.L., *et al.* Potential benefit of lymph node dissection during radical nephroureterectomy for upper tract urothelial carcinoma: a systematic review by the European association of urology guidelines panel on non–muscle-invasive bladder cancer. 2019. 5(2): p. 224–241.
22. Kondo, T. and K.J.I.j.o.u. Tanabe, Role of lymphadenectomy in the management of urothelial carcinoma of the bladder and the upper urinary tract. 2012. 19(8): p. 710–721.
23. Seisen, T., *et al.* Oncologic outcomes of kidney-sparing surgery versus radical nephroureterectomy for upper tract urothelial carcinoma: a systematic review by the EAU non-muscle invasive bladder cancer guidelines panel. 2016. 70(6): p. 1052–1068.
24. Cutress, M.L., *et al.* Ureteroscopic and percutaneous management of upper tract urothelial carcinoma (UTUC): systematic review. 2012. 110(5): p. 614–628.
25. Rouprêt, M., *et al.* Upper urinary tract transitional cell carcinoma: recurrence rate after percutaneous endoscopic resection. 2007. 51(3): p. 709–714.
26. Jeldres, C., *et al.* Segmental ureterectomy can safely be performed in patients with transitional cell carcinoma of the ureter. 2010. 183(4): p. 1324–1329.
27. Ou, Y.-C., *et al.* Long-term outcomes of total ureterectomy with ileal-ureteral substitution treatment for ureteral cancer: a single-center experience. 2018. 18(1): p. 1–7.
28. Hwang, E.C., *et al.* Single-dose intravesical chemotherapy after nephroureterectomy for upper tract urothelial carcinoma. 2019(5).
29. Freifeld, Y., *et al.* Intraoperative prophylactic intravesical chemotherapy to reduce bladder recurrence following radical nephroureterectomy. in Urologic Oncology: Seminars and Original Investigations. 2020. Elsevier.
30. Leow, J.J., *et al.* Neoadjuvant and adjuvant chemotherapy for upper tract urothelial carcinoma: a 2020 systematic review and meta-analysis, and future perspectives on systemic therapy. 2021. 79(5): p. 635–654.
31. Kaag, M.G., *et al.* Changes in renal function following nephroureterectomy may affect the use of perioperative chemotherapy. 2010. 58(4): p. 581–587.
32. Bajorin, D.F., *et al.* Adjuvant nivolumab versus placebo in muscle-invasive urothelial carcinoma. 2021. 384(22): p. 2102–2114.
33. Laukhtina, E., *et al.* Chemotherapy is superior to checkpoint inhibitors after radical surgery for urothelial carcinoma: a systematic review and network meta-analysis of oncologic and toxicity outcomes. 2022. 169: p. 103570.
34. Kokorovic, A. and S.F.J.T.A.i.M.O. Matin, UGN-101 (mitomycin gel): a novel treatment for low-grade upper tract urothelial carcinoma. 2020. 12: p. 1758835920937950.
35. van Doeveren, T., *et al.* Synchronous and metachronous urothelial carcinoma of the upper urinary tract and the bladder: are they clonally related? A systematic review. in Urologic Oncology: Seminars and Original Investigations. 2020. Elsevier.
36. Rosiello, G., *et al.* Contemporary conditional cancer-specific survival after radical nephroureterectomy in patients with nonmetastatic urothelial carcinoma of upper urinary tract. 2020. 121(7): p. 1154–1161.
37. Green, D.A., *et al.* Urothelial carcinoma of the bladder and the upper tract: disparate twins. 2013. 189(4): p. 1214–1221.
38. Birtle, A., *et al.* Adjuvant chemotherapy in upper tract urothelial carcinoma (the POUT trial): a phase 3, open-label, randomised controlled trial. 2020. 395(10232): p. 1268–1277.
39. Kleinmann, N., *et al.* Primary chemoablation of low-grade upper tract urothelial carcinoma using UGN-101, a mitomycin-containing reverse thermal gel (OLYMPUS): an open-label, single-arm, phase 3 trial. 2020. 21(6): p. 776–785.
40. O'Brien, T., *et al.* Prevention of bladder tumours after nephroureterectomy for primary upper urinary tract urothelial carcinoma: a prospective, multicentre, randomised clinical trial of a single postoperative intravesical dose of mitomycin C (the ODMIT-C Trial). 2011. 60(4): p. 703–710.

Chapter
10

Localised Kidney Cancer

• Saurabh Patil • Gagan Gautam

LEARNING OBJECTIVES

- To understand primary work-up in localized kidney cancers: Most small renal masses are incidentally detected on USG. Further characterization of the mass is done on a CECT or MRI.
- To know the various pathological types of RCC: Clear cell, papillary and chromophobe RCC are the most common types. Various other less common types exist and it is important to be aware of their clinical presentations
- To know the role of renal biopsy in SRMs: A biopsy for a SRM is only required for masses which are indeterminate on CT or when there is a clinical suspicion of abscess, lymphoma or metastasis from another site.
- To understand the surgical principles of partial nephrectomy: Partial nephrectomy is the standard of care for T1a renal masses and also for T1b masses when feasible. It aims to preserve normal functional renal parenchyma to delay progression to CKD.
- To understand the complications of partial nephrectomy: Post-operative bleeding and urine leak are the two main complications that can occur following a partial nephrectomy.
- To understand the follow-up protocol following surgery for localized renal cancer: Based on the pathology report, patients are classified into low, intermediate or high risk and this then decides the intensity of the follow-up.
- To understand the option of active surveillance: Active surveillance may be offered to elderly patients with co-morbidities who are not candidates for surgery.
- To understand the option of thermo-ablation: Thermal ablation in the form of RFA or cryoablation may be offered to patients with masses less than 3 cm. They have a higher recurrence rate than partial nephrectomy.

Case Scenario

A 32 years old male, without any co-morbidities or a significant family history, during a routine health check-up, was incidentally detected to have a solid/cystic mass 5 × 4.5 × 4.3 in the interpolar to lower pole of left kidney on ultrasonography.

1. **What are the types of renal cysts? Can we predict the risk of malignancy on CT images?**

   Ans: Renal cysts can be simple (benign) or complex (malignant). The Bosniak classification helps in differentiating benign from malignant cysts, with recent 2019 updates clarifying previously undefined features[1] (Table 10.1). Originally developed based on CT findings, Bosniak classification can also be used with MRI and contrast-enhanced ultrasound (Fig. 10.1).

2. **What are the different pathological types of RCCs?**

   Ans: The types of RCC are shown in Table 10.2.

3. **What are the imaging modalities for such a lesion (an incidentaloma) in the kidney?**

   Ans:

   - Contrast-enhanced triple-phase computed tomography scan.

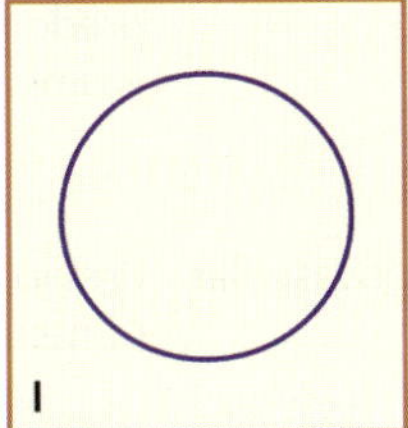

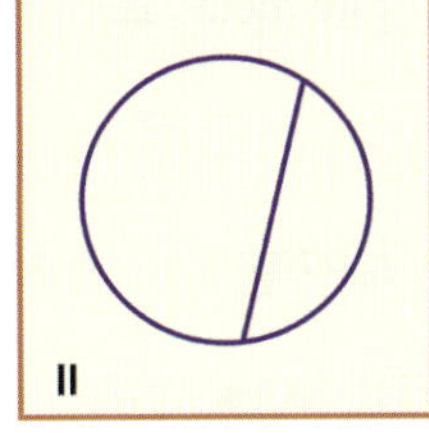

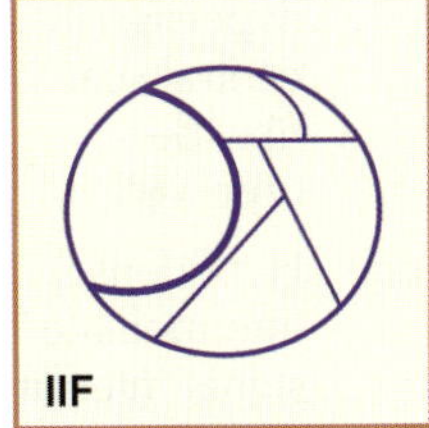

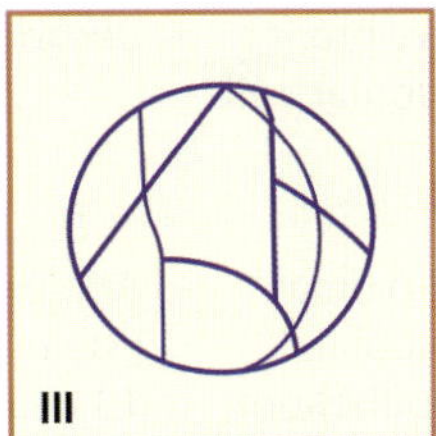

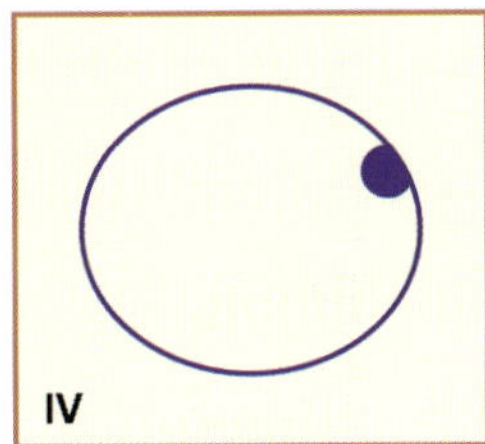

Fig. 10.1: Bosniak classification of renal cysts

TABLE 10.1: Bosniak classification of renal cystic masses (Version 2019)[1]

Bosniak stage	*Risk of malignancy*	*Features*
I	0	Thin wall without septa or solid components. No internal enhancement
II	0	Few (≤3) thin septa. It may show minimal enhancement of the septa. Hyperintense on T1 without enhancement.
IIF	5	Few (>3) thin septa. Smooth mild thickening of the wall or septa. It may contain minimal enhancement of the septa.
III	50	Thickened (>3 mm) wall or septa with enhancement. Irregular wall or septa with enhancement.
IV	90	Soft tissue enhancing mass independent from the wall

TABLE 10.2: Enumerates the different pathological types of RCC

Subtype	*Incidence (%)*	*Origin, histology*	*Age (Years)*	*Signal/density pattern*	*Biological behaviour*	*Hemodynamic pattern*	*Association and predisposition*
Clear cell	75	Proximal nephron, tubular epithelium	>50	Heterogeneous density/signal	Aggressive, according to the stage, Fuhrman's grade, sarcomatoid transformation	Hypervascular	von Hippel-Lindau (25–45%), tuberous sclerosis (2%)
Papillary	10	Distal nephron, tubular epithelium	>50	Low T2 signal/ hypodense	Aggressive, according to the stage, Fuhrman's grade, sarcomatoid transformation	Hypovascular	Hereditary papillary RCC
Chromophobe	5	Distal nephron, intercalated cells of distal tubule	>50	Hypodense/ intermediate signal density	Low mortality (10%)	Hypovascular	Birt-Hogg-Dube syndrome (in association with oncocytoma)
Cystic-solid	1–4	Similar to clear cell, without solid nodules	4th and 5th decade	High T2 signal intensity, fluid density	Indolent without metastasis	Septal and solid portions enhancement	Predominance in men
Collecting ducts (Bellini)	1	Collecting tubules	>50	Low T2 signal, heterogeneous	Very aggressive, mortality 70% in two years	Hypovascular	Subtle Predominance in men
Medullary	1	Distal nephron	2nd and 3rd decade				
3rd decade	Heterogeneous, infiltrating	Extremely aggressive	Hypovascular	Associated with sickle cell disease			
Xp11 translocation	Rare	Distal/ proximal nephron, may be similar to papillary/clear cell RCC	Early childhood	Hypodense, intermediate T2 signal intensity	Indolent	Hypovascular	TFE 3 gene involved in the tumor genesis
Mucinous tubular and spindle cell	Rare	Distal nephron/ tubular cells	4th and 5th decade	Subtle T2 hypersignal, central scar may be observed	Slow growing rare metastasis	Hypovascular	Mucinous predominance in women
Associated with neuroblastoma	Rare	Proximal tubular epithelium	Adolescence (Mean 13 years)	Hypodense, intermediate T2 signal intensity	Indolent	Hypovascular	Previous history of neuroblastoma
Non-classified	4–6	Variable	Variable	Variable	High mortality	Variable	-

Phases of CT scan

Plain, corticomedullary (20–40 seconds post IV contrast injection), nephrographic (100–150s after) and the excretory phase (180–300s after). A change of 15 HU in the solid tumour parts, before, and after contrast administration, is suggestive of malignant masses.

CT provides useful information on function of the contralateral kidney, venous involvement, and enlargement of locoregional LNs (Fig. 10.2). In SRMs, CT (especially renal angiography/CT renal protocol) helps in understanding tumor extension, its relationship with the calyceal system, vascular anatomy and thus in planning surgical steps and in anticipating complications.

Imaging findings like perinephric fat stranding, thickened perirenal fascia and visualization of ill-defined margins between tumour tissue and the perinephric fat may suggest perirenal fat invasion.[9]

4. **Can CTU/CECT abdomen and pelvis be done at all levels of creatinine clearance?**

Ans: No, one should calculate the creatinine clearance and then decide about the contrast use. If the CrCl> 60 ml/min, then you can directly go ahead. If CrCl is between 45–60 ml/min, one should consider hydration and then do the study.

Q. What is the role of MRI in the imaging of renal lesions?

Ans: MRI also helps in diagnosing complex renal cysts better (higher sensitivity and specificity 71% and 91% vs 36% and 76% respectively for MRI and CT).

MRI can also help in predicting the histology of RCC, clear cell RCC appears hyperintense, and papillary appears hypointense on the T2 sequence. Recently a scoring system has been proposed using multiparametric MRI, which helps in diagnosing clear cell RCC in cT1 masses.[2] This system, known as clear cell likelihood score (ccLS), has been validated and found to be highly accurate.[3]

CT or MRI allows diagnosis of RCC, but cannot reliably distinguish oncocytoma and fat-free AML from malignant renal neoplasms.

MRI with contrast can now be used in CKD and even ESRD with advent of generation 2 gadolinium (available in India). In a CKD situation, it scores over CT with contrast.

5. **How can imaging help to distinguish between oncocytoma and RCC?**

Ans: Oncocytoma can be differentiated from RCC by using a ^{99}Tc-sestamibi scan. ^{99}Tc-sestamibi accumulates in cells with high content of mitochondria as it is lipophilic. Oncocytomas cells have a high content of mitochondria so it lights up on this scan; similarly, RCC do not concentrate ^{99}Tc-sestamibi.[4]

6. **What is the role of contrast enhanced ultrasound (CEUS) in the evaluation of small renal masses?**

Ans: Contrast-enhanced ultrasound, which uses intravenous contrast agents consisting of microbubbles/nanobubbles of gas, is mainly used to differentiate between cystic and solid lesions with equivocal features on sonography and for a detailed characterization of complex cystic masses.[5] CEUS is more sensitive than CT in detecting tumor microvasculature, i.e. blood flow, especially in hypovascular lesions and in detecting enhancement of the cyst wall, septa, and solid components in complex cystic lesions.[5] Because of the high sensitivity (100%) and specificity (97%), the recent EAU guidelines strongly recommend its use in characterisation of SRMs especially when CT results are indeterminate.[2] But, there has been a concern that CEUS may increase the detection of septa, causing overdiagnosis of Bosniak III cysts which would have otherwise been classified as Bosniak II, leading ultimately to increase in the number of surgical procedures.[6]

Scan QR Code for Video on
Contrast enhanced ultrasound

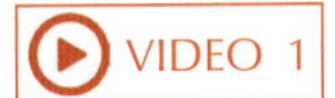

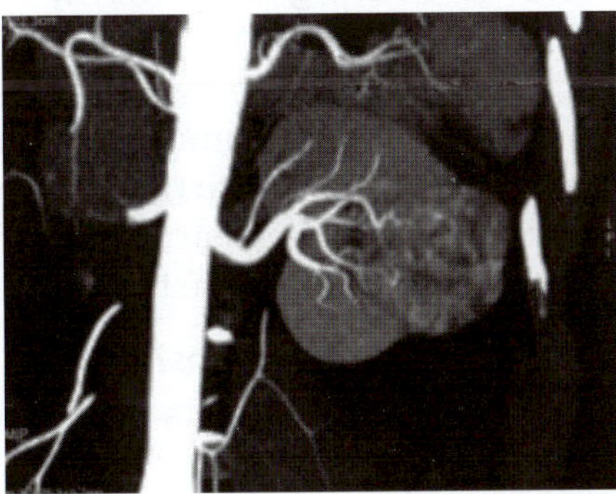

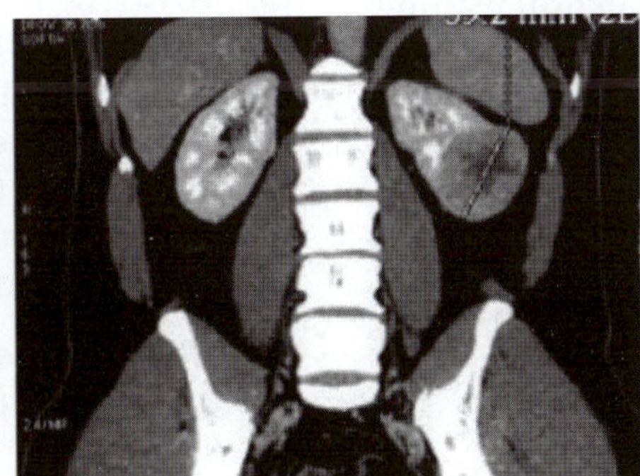

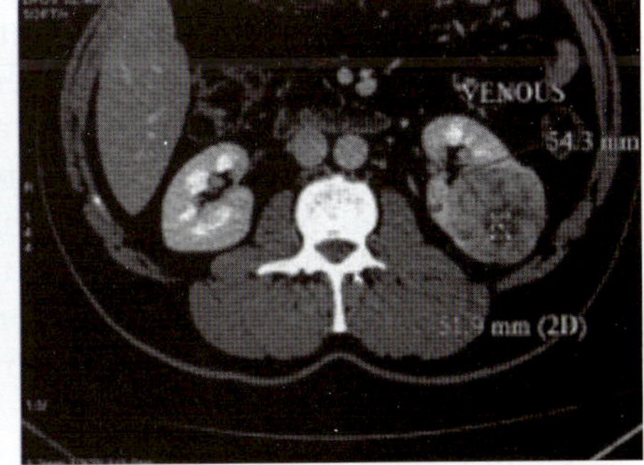

Fig. 10.2: Left interpolar renal mass 5.1 × 5.4 cm, heterogeneously enhancing, has areas of necrosis, supplied by a single artery and vein, abutting the mid pole calyx, no venous invasion and showing no lymphadenopathy

7. Which investigations would you ask to evaluate metastases?

Ans: Chest CT is accurate for ruling out pulmonary metastases. However, chest CT may be omitted in cT1aN0 patients without chest symptoms due to low malignant potential of T1a tumors.[4] Most bone metastases are symptomatic at diagnosis, and thus, routine bone imaging is not generally indicated.[1] FDG PET/CT has a low sensitivity and specificity for detection and characterisation of malignant renal masses, hence its routine use is not recommended.[1]

8. What are the newer advances in imaging for RCC? Discuss the ZIRCON trial in brief?

Ans: ZIRCON is a phase 3 open-label multicentre clinical trial of 89Zr-DFO-girentuximab for PET/CT imaging of renal masses intended to help in differentiating clear cell RCC from other pathologies.[10] Girentuximab is a monoclonal antibody against carbonic anhydrase IX (CAIX), an antigen expressed on the cell surface of 95% of clear cell RCC (ccRCC) and minimally expressed on normal kidney cells. Radiolabelled 89Zr-DFO-girentuximab is highly specific for carbonic anhydrase IX and can be used with PET/CT scan for the detection of clear cell RCC. ZIRCON was a positive study as it met its primary endpoint exceeding the sensitivity and specificity thresholds, proving a promising role of girentuximab PET/CT in management of indeterminate SRMs especially in limiting biopsies or over treatment of benign lesions.[10]

9. What are the indications of AS for renal masses in clinical practice?

Ans: With the evolving understanding of natural history of SRMs, there has been increasing interest in surveillance as an active management strategy for SRMs especially low-risk groups which are known to be indolent, slow growing and of low metastatic potential. However, it has to be understood that 'watchful waiting' is not the same as 'active surveillance'; though both are non-surgical treatment options. Watchful waiting, mainly planned for old patients who are poor surgical candidates, is a less intensive mode with no need for repeated imaging, and intervention is only intended for symptom relief (palliative). Active surveillance, on the other hand, is a deferred treatment option with a curative aim, where intervention is done based on progression of the disease as evident on frequent imagings.[6–8]

So watchful-waiting is done in

1. Elderly patients with significant co-morbidities.
2. Life expectancy <5 years
3. Patients with very high risk for anaesthesia:

AS can be considered in patients with marginal renal functions with a significant risk of ESRD and also in young healthy patients with small masses <3 cm, tumor growth rate <5 mm per year, non-infiltrative low complexity on imaging, favourable histology on biopsy.[6,12]

A biopsy is not mandatory, but preferable, prior to putting a patient under active surveillance as this can help tailor the intensity of follow-up.

10. What are the other indications for doing renal biopsy in SRMs?

Ans:

1. In a radiologically indeterminate renal mass to differentiate between hematogenous (lymphomatous), infective and malignant masses (primary vs metastasis from other organs).
2. To obtain histology before ablative treatments
3. To select the most suitable medical treatment strategy (targeted therapy) in the setting of metastatic disease.

Multiple core biopsies should be performed and are preferred over fine needle aspiration.[11]

11. What are the progression criteria/triggers for intervention?

Ans: Progression criteria for intervention are:[6]

1. Small renal mass-related symptoms
2. Size >4 cm
3. Unfavourable histology
4. Stage progression
5. Growth rate >5 mm/year

12. How frequently would you follow-up these patients put under AS?

Ans: As per the standard guidelines, initial cross-sectional imaging in form of CT/MRI (preferred) or USG at 3–6 months after diagnosis and then 6–12 monthly, with a chest X-ray annually till trigger points are observed.[6–8]

13. What is the role of scoring systems in the management of localised renal masses?

Ans: Scoring systems help surgeons in understanding the complexity of the tumor and thus anticipate the intra-operative difficulty and complications while performing a partial nephrectomy, especially by minimal invasive techniques.

14. What are the different scoring systems?

Ans: Renal nephrometry score is given in Table 10.3.[13]

Using the renal nephrometry score, renal masses can be classified as low (≤ 6), intermediate (7–9),

TABLE 10.3: Renal nephrometry score

Feature	Points		
	1	2	3
Radius (Max diameter)	≤4 cm	>4 but <7 cm	≥7 cm
Exophytic proportion	≥50%	<50%	0% (100% endophytic)
Nearness to the renal collecting system or fat sinus	≥7 mm	>4 but <7 cm	≤4 mm
Anterior or posterior	No point, mass assigned a descriptor of anterior or posterior		
Location relative to polar lines	Entirely above the upper pole line or entirely below the lower pole line	Mass crosses a polar line	>50% of the mass is above the upper pole line or below the lower pole line, the mass crosses the axial renal midline; or the mass is entirely between the polar lines

or high (≥ 10) complexity. Renal score is the most widely used score because of its easy applicability in practice.

Other reported scoring systems: PADUA (Pre-operative Aspects and Dimensions Used for Anatomical classification) score, centrality index, NePhRO, MAP (Mayo Adhesive Probability) score.

Tables 10.4 and 10.5 depict the other scoring systems such as PADUA (Table10.4) and MAP (Table 10.5a) score:

TABLE 10.4: PADUA score[14]

Parameter	*1 point*	*2 points*	*3 points*
Longitudinal (polar) location	Superior/ inferior	Middle	NA
Exophytic vs endophytic	≥50% exophytic	<50% exophytic	Entirely endophytic
Renal rim	Lateral	Medial	NA
Renal sinus	Not involved	Involved	NA
Collecting system	Not involved	Dislocated/ infiltrated	NA
Tumor size	≤4 cm	4.1–7 cm	>7 cm

TABLE 10.5a: Mayo adhesive probability (MAP) score[15]

Posterior perinephric fat thickness (cm)	*MAP score*
<1.0	0
1.0–1.9	1
≥2 cm	2
Perinephric fat satranding	
None	0
Type 1	2
Type 2	3

Risk stratification for PADUA score: Low = 6–7, Moderate = 8–9, High ≥ 10. Suffix 'a' or 'p' is used to indicate location of the tumor-anterior versus posterior.[14]

15. **What would be your treatment of choice for localised RCC?**

Ans: Surgical excision is the curative treatment for localised kidney cancers.

Partial nephrectomy (PN) or nephron sparing surgery (NSS) should be the preferred option for localised renal masses over radical whenever feasible as recommended by guidelines.[1,6] Compared to radical nephrectomy, PN is known to reduce the risk of development of chronic kidney disease in future and thus of cardiovascular mortality.

16. **Can you describe the procedure in brief?**

Ans:

Procedure: Partial nephrectomy

Position: Lateral decubitus

Approach:

Irrespective of the approach, open or minimal invasive, the principles and the basic steps remain the same.

Key steps:

- For open technique, an extraperitoneal flank incision approach is preferred. A traditional 11th rib bed incision with/without resection of 11th rib is taken. Alternatively mini-flank incision can be taken in which 8–10 cm incision is made superior to the 11th or 12th rib, giving comparable oncologic outcomes and fewer wound related complications.[10]
- Once retroperitoneum is entered, kidney is mobilized all around to gain access to hilum.
- Artery and vein are looped separately.
- Ureteric dissection should be kept to the minimal to avoid injury and devascularization.
- Perinephric fat is cleared to score the margins all around keeping peritumoral fat intact. Use

of intra-operative USG helps in understanding the extent endophytic part of the mass.

- Renal vascular clamping (arterial only in most of the cases) can be done using bulldog clamp, vascular clamp, loop tourniquet or finger compression of the adjacent parenchyma.
- Venous clamping is preferred only in centrally locating/hilar tumors as venous congestion may increase the bleeding in peripheral tumors.[18]
- Cold ischemia is then achieved by surface cooling with ice slush.
- Tumor excision is done by sharp cutting with scissors ensuring a good margin from tumor capsule.
- Intermittent suction irrigation enables clear operative field and avoids the risk of inadvertent entry into the tumor.
- Different methods and suture materials are described for renorrhaphy in literature. Most widely practised is a two-layer renorrhaphy: Inner and outer layer renorrhaphy. If the pelvicalyceal is system is breached, it can, in addition, be sutured with 3–0/4–0 polydiaoxanone suture.
- For inner renorrhaphy, a barbed suture is used as a hemostatic suture, continuous suturing is done along the cut surface of the kidney securing small blood vessels and breaches in collecting system. Bleeders on the cut surface of the kidney, especially arterial, can be identified and oversewn individually with absorbable sutures like PDS (polydioxanone suture). Clamps can be removed at this stage, known as early unclamping.
- Outer renorrhaphy is done using sliding Hem-o-lok clip technique with absorbable suture like polydiaoxanone on a CT1/CT2 needle. Once haemostasis is achieved and instrument count is confirmed, nephropexy is done to avoid flipping of the kidney especially in cases where kidney was mobilised completely all around.
- Drain placement is at surgeon's discretion. Closure is done in layers.
- In laparoscopic/robotic trans-peritoneal app-roach, positioning and port placements are same as for other kidney surgeries. Surgery starts by reflecting colon medially to develop a plane between posterior mesocolon and Gerota's fascia. Minimal handling of mesocolonic fat reduces the chances of post-operative ileus. After colon is reflected, on right side duodenum is kocherized to define the lateral margin of IVC and to identify the renal vein. Once vein is identified and dissected, attention is diverted towards the artery which is dissected and looped. On left side, identification of gonadal vein and following it cranially helps finding the renal vein and hilum. Gonadal vein dissection is not necessary on right side. After control of hilum rest of the steps are same as those in open PN.

17. What are trifecta and pentafecta outcomes after partial nephrectomy?

Ans. Trifecta outcomes consist of achievement of:

1. Negative surgical margins
2. No postoperative complications
3. Warm ischemia time 25 minutes

Pentafecta includes two other variables, namely, > 90% estimated glomerular filtration rate preservation and no chronic kidney disease stage progression 1 year after surgery[11].

18. What are the methods to maintain/improve global renal function after PN?

Ans:

1. Pre-operative optimisation (involvement of nephrology services whenever indicated)
2. Zero clamping
3. Selective arterial clamping
4. Early unclamping
5. Enucleation of tumour rather than resection

These ways have been described to minimize renal ischemia; however, they may not necessarily translate into superior functional outcomes.

The most important parameters affecting long-term renal function are preoperative renal functional status and the amount of parenchyma preserved after PN.[12]

Ischemia time, techniques of vessel clamping or surgical approach do not have significant impact as far as long-term renal function is concerned.[2]

The final histology for this case showed 5.1 × 4.6 × 4.2 cm clear cell carcinoma with ISUP grade 2. The tumor margin was negative. No LVI, necrosis.

19. How would you risk stratify this disease?

Ans: The renal tumours are risk stratified as follows (Table 10.5b):

TABLE 10.5b: Risk stratification[12]

Low risk (LR)	pT1 and Grade 1/2
Intermediate risk (IR)	pT1 and Grade 3/4, or pT2 any grade
High risk (HR)	pT3 any grade
Very high risk	pT4 or pN1, or sarcomatoid/rhabdoid dedifferentiation, or macroscopic positive margin

20. Describe Leibovich, SSIGN and UISS prognostic models.

Ans: Different prognostic models have been developed and found useful in predicting clinically relevant oncological outcomes. Following are the most relevant prognostic models, currently there is no evidence to recommend one model over the other.[2]

UISS (UCLA Integrated Staging System): For all histopathological subtypes

1. ECOG PS
2. T classification
3. N classification (N+ classified as metastatic)
4. Grade
   T1N0M0G1–2, ECOG PS 0: Low-risk disease
   T3N0M0G2–4, ECOG PS > 1 OR T4N0M0: High-risk disease

Any other N0M0: Intermediate-risk disease

Leibovich score/model 2018: Different for different pathologies:

i. **ccRCC (Clear cell)**
   Progression (9 factors): Constitutional symptoms, grade, tumour necrosis, sarcomatoid features, tumour size, perinephric or sinus fat invasion, tumour thrombus level, extension beyond kidney, nodal involvement (Table 10.6).
   Cancer-specific survival (12 factors): Age, ECOG PS, constitutional symptoms, adrenalectomy, surgical margins, grade, tumour necrosis, sarcomatoid features, tumour size, perinephric or sinus fat invasion, tumour thrombus, nodal involvement.
   For both of the above, a score is calculated based on the presence or absence of the respective enumerated factors. This score is then used to estimate the progression free survival and cancer specific survival at 5, 10 and 15 years.

ii. **pRCC**
   Low risk (group 1): Grade 1–2, no fat invasion, no tumour thrombus.
   Intermediate risk (group 2): Grade 3, no fat invasion, no tumour thrombus.
   High risk (group 3): Grade 4 or fat invasion or any level tumour thrombus.

iii. **chRCC**
   Low risk (group 1): No fat invasion, no sarcomatoid differentiation, no nodal involvement.
   Intermediate risk (group 2): Fat invasion and no sarcomatoid differentiation and no nodal involvement.
   High risk (group 3): Sarcomatoid differentiation or nodal involvement.

TABLE 10.6: SSIGN (Stage Size Grade Necrosis) score

Feature	*Score*
T stage	
pT1	0
pT2	1
pT3	2
pT4	4
N stage	
pNx	0
pN0	0
pN1	2
M stage	
M0	0
M1	4
Tumor size	
<5 cm	0
≥5 cm	2
Grade	
1–2	0
3	1
4	3
Necrosis	
Absent	0
Present	2

21. Discuss the findings of the EORTC 30904 trial.

Ans: In 2011, the European Organization for Research and Treatment of Cancer (EORTC) did a randomized trial (30904) of NSS (nephron sparing surgery) versus RN (radical nephrectomy) for SRMs (5 cm), with a prospective assessment of renal function, oncologic outcomes, and overall and cause-specific survival followed by an exploratory analyses of the same cohort in 2013.[19] Over a median follow-up of 6.7 years for eGFR, authors found out that NSS reduced the risk of moderate renal dysfunction compared with RN, however, this beneficial impact of NSS on eGFR did not result in improved survival and overall survival was better in the RN arm. The incidence of advanced kidney disease (eGFR <30) and of kidney failure (eGFR <15) were nearly identical in both the arms. This study was, however, criticised for being underpowered and its premature closure due to slow accrual. It is known that the pre-existing medical comorbidities causing pre-surgical chronic kidney disease remains more important cause of adverse overall survival than the renal function impairment following surgery. This was also not taken into account in this trial. Taken together, survival advantages for RN vs NSS remains a controversial issue. Recent guidelines encourage for partial nephrectomy as long as oncological principles are maintained.

22. In which cases would you prefer open approach over minimal invasive?

Ans: In the following conditions open surgery may be beneficial:

1. Previous renal surgery
2. Solitary kidney with a complex mass
3. CKD patient
4. Expected prolonged ischemia time
5. Multiple tumors

23. Can PN be done in cT3a masses?

Ans: Partial nephrectomy, compared to radical, has comparable cancer specific, recurrence free and overall survival, including risk of positive surgical margins and complications. Hence whenever feasible, PN should be considered for functional benefits.[16] However, when the tumor has increased oncologic potential and/or risk of high perioperative morbidity with PN due to increased tumor complexity, predicting NBGFR (New Baseline GFR) would be helpful in choosing RN. So, in these circumstances when NBGFR is >45 ml/min/1.73 m^2, RN can safely be considered over PN.[17]

Predicted NBGFR = Global GFR pre-RN × SRF contralateral × 1.24. (SRF+ split renal function).[21]

24. Would you like to perform lymph node dissection also?

Ans: Because there is no strong evidence about survival advantage of doing LND and no defined templates, routine LND is not recommended in localised RCC with clinically negative nodes (on imaging and/or intraoperative).[1] AUA recommends LND in clinically concerning masses for staging purpose.[6]

25. When would you also perform adrenalectomy along with radical nephrectomy?

Ans: As per AUA guidelines, adrenalectomy can be performed if imaging and/or intraoperative findings suggest metastasis or direct invasion of the adrenal gland.[7] Upper pole location is not predictive of adrenal involvement and thus adrenalectomy is not always indicated for upper pole tumors.[1] EAU guidelines clearly state that "ipsilateral adrenalectomy during RN or PN has no survival advantage in the absence of clinically evident adrenal involvement".[1]

26. How would you treat positive surgical margins (PSM) found on final post-operative histopathology report?

Ans: PSM can be seen in around 2–8% of cases after PN. Most studies in the literature state that PSMs do not translate into a higher risk of metastases or a decreased cancer-specific survival.[1, 13] Local bed tumor recurrence can also be seen in around 3% of cases with negative surgical margins. Radical nephrectomy or re-resection of margins may lead to over-treatment in some cases. Best way to manage these cases would be a patient counselling, consider the risk group of this patient to be a group higher and a stringent surveillance done as per the next higher group protocol.

27. Would you prefer a routine intra-operative frozen section to avoid PSMs?

Ans: Most trials have shown no significant beneficial role in avoiding the risk of PSMs, so its routine use is not recommended.[1]

28. What are the likely and significant surgical complications?

Ans:

- Intra-operative
  - Hemorrhage
  - Damage to other organs (e.g. spleen, liver, intestines)
  - Pleural injury (open PN)
- Early post-operative
  - AKI (acute kidney injury)
  - Urinary leak
  - Hemorrhage
  - Chest infection/atelectasis
  - Ileus
- Late post-operative
  - Urinary fistula
  - Arteriovenous fistula
  - Incisional hernia

29. What are the possible risk factors for development of urinary fistula after PN?

Ans: The risk factors for urinary fistula are: Size >4 cm, complex tumors (high nephrometry scores), tumor proximity to the PCS, surgeon's initial experience, moderate and severe CKD, laparoscopic approach.[15–17]

30. How will you manage a urinary fistula after PN?

Ans: Observation, keeping a watch on volume of leak, signs and symptoms of infection, would be sufficient in most of the cases.

Constant/increasing volume of discharge, pain, fever, ileus needs imaging and active intervention.

Insertion of double J ureteric stent with a per-urethral catheter in place improves the urinary outflow, decreases the pressure inside PCS which contributes to the healing of the PCS defect. In rare instances, further intervention is required in forms of simultaneous installation of two stents, percutaneous nephrostomy, retrograde or percutaneous application of fibrin glue, percutaneous cryoablation of the fistulous passage and re-exploration.[15,16]

31. How will you manage post-operative bleed following partial nephrectomy?

Ans: Bleeding complications after PN are reported in as many as 10% of patients and these bleeds may result in life-threatening hemorrhage.[23] Arterial malformations (AM), resulting from pseudoaneurysm (PA) or arteriovenous fistula (AV fistula) accounts for the most cases of post-operative hemorrhage following PN.[23]

Most of these patients are symptomatic and present with symptoms like gross hematuria, flank pain with or without anemia, presenting a mean of 15 days after surgery, more commonly after minimal invasive PN than open.[24] CT with angiography or MRI remain the preferred modes for diagnosis. The options of treatment are observation, angioembolisation and nephrectomy in the desperate situations. Percutaneous super-selective embolization of the feeding interlobar arteries with microcatheters, using micro coils or polyvinyl alcohol particles, is successful in most of the patients.

32. How will you manage a patient in early CKD?

Ans: Loss of functional renal parenchyma is associated with an increased long-term risk of progressive CKD (eGFR <60 ml/min per 1.73 m^2), end-stage renal disease with all-cause and cardiovascular mortality.[20] Contrary to the old beliefs, CKD due to surgical nephron loss is equally harmful and life-threatening as CKD from medical causes and regardless of underlying aetiology, risk of adverse outcomes increases significantly with lower eGFR (<45 ml/min per 1.72 m^2).[21]

Patients in early CKD stages should be counselled and monitored regularly after surgery by evaluating serum creatinine, eGFR, and albumin-creatinine ratio.[20] In initial stages measures like good control of blood pressure, sugar levels, dyslipidemia, avoidance of nephrotoxic drugs, good hydration and involvement of a nephrologist, help maintaining the renal function. A nomogram model is available online to predict the occurrence of early CKD after nephrectomy (https://dongy.shinyapps.io/aki_ckd).

33. What is the risk of recurrence of this disease?

Ans: The risk of recurrence is given in Table 10.7.[22]

TABLE 10. 7: Risk of recurrence in RCC

	Recurrence risk	
Low risk (LR)	~ 9.2%	pT1 and Grade 1/2
Intermediate risk (IR)	~ 32%	pT1 and Grade 3/4, or pT2 any grade
High risk (HR)	~ 49%	pT3 any grade
Very high risk (VHR)	~ 70%	pT4 or pN1, or sarcomatoid/rhabdoid dedifferentiation, or macroscopic positive margin

34. What are the standard follow-up protocols after treatment of localised renal cancer?

Ans: Aim of follow-up after treatment for RCC is to monitor or identify:

- Post-operative complications/morbidity
- Kidney function
- Residual or recurrent lesion
- Recurrence in the contralateral kidney
- Distant metastases
- Cardiovascular events (Table 10.8).

35. Can thermo-ablative technique be used for the management of SRMs?

Ans: Thermo-ablative (TA) technique, in the form of cryosurgery or radiofrequency ablation, is an alternative therapy for management in those T1 patients who are poor candidates for surgery (old, poor PS, severe coagulopathy, multiple co-morbidities). When compared, heat-based thermal ablation has a twofold higher cancer-specific mortality than after cryoablation in masses sized 3.1 to 4 cm, however, for tumors 3 cm outcomes are similar.

Renal mass biopsy is required prior to any TA procedure. For less than 3 cm masses, all types of

TABLE 10.8: EAU guidelines follow-up protocol

Risk profile	*Treatment*	*Surveillance*						
		6 months	*1 year*	*2 years*	*3 years*	*4 years*	*5 years*	*After 5 years*
Low	RN/PN	US and chest X-ray	US and chest X-ray	US and chest X-ray	US and chest X-ray	US and chest X-ray	US and chest X-ray	Stop
Intermediate	RN/PN/cryotherapy/RFA	CT	US and chest X-ray	CT	US and chest X-ray	US and chest X-ray	CT	US and chest X-ray annually
High	RN/PN/cryotherapy/RFA	CT	CT	CT	CT	CT	CT	CT/chest X-ray alternate years

thermal ablations provide acceptable oncologic outcomes. If the tumor is > 3 cm, cryoablation or MWA (microwave ablation) is better as they create a larger ablation area than RFA using a single electrode. When the mass is centrally located or protruding into the renal sinus, cryoablation is more helpful in reducing urothelial damage.[27]

Oncological outcomes after cryoablation are reported to be better for cT1a tumours, with a local recurrence rate of 7.7% in cT1a tumours vs. 34.5% in cT1b. The risk of disease progression increases by 32% with each 1 cm increase in tumour size. For T1b tumors, local clearance is poor with 5-year CSM rates of 7.6–9%.[29,30]

Oncological outcomes after RFA are better for cT1a tumors than cT1b, the 5-year OS rate being 73–79% for T1a and 5-year DFS 74.5% to 81% for T1b tumors.

The approach (percutaneous vs laparoscopic) for doing TA has comparable results, with percutaneous being less invasive and requires only local anaesthesia. Common complications associated with TA are bleeding (usually self-limiting), urothelial injury, ureteric strictures, adjacent organ injuries.

The long-term oncological effectiveness of TA compared to PN is not clear, so EAU guidelines recommend TA only to frail and/or comorbid patients with SRMs.

NCCN guidelines recommend following follow-up protocol for surveillance after ablative therapies:

- History and physical examination annually
- Laboratory tests annually, as clinically indicated
- **Abdominal imaging:** Abdominal CT or MRI with and without IV contrast (unless otherwise contraindicated) at 1–6 months following ablative therapy, then CT or MRI (preferred) annually for 5 years or longer as clinically indicated.

  If there is imaging or clinical concerns for recurrence, then more frequent imaging, renal mass biopsy, or further treatment may be indicated.
- **Chest imaging:** Chest X-ray or CT annually for 5 years for patients who have biopsy-proven low-risk pathologic features (no sarcomatoid, low-grade [grade 1/2]) renal cell carcinoma (RCC), nondiagnostic biopsies, or no prior biopsy.

  Stereotactic ablative radiotherapy (SABR) is an emerging technique for localised RCC patients who are not fit for surgery. The reported local failure rate is around 3–8% at 4 years, progression free survival 65–90% and overall survival 69–92%. The decrease in eGFR is in the range of 7–8.7% with grade 3 or 4 toxicities in 1.5% of patients.[33–35] However, viable tumour cells are often seen in post-radiation biopsies.

SUMMARY

- The incidence of small renal masses in on the rise due to the higher number of USGs being performed. Further characterization of the mass is done on a CECT or a MRI.
- A renal mass biopsy is not required unless the mass appears indeterminate on the CT or if the patient is planned for focal therapy.
- The renal nephrometry score is the most commonly used score for grading the complexity of small renal masses.
- Post-operative bleed and urine leak are two complications specific to partial nephrectomy.
- Partial nephrectomy has been shown to reduce the rate of progression to CKD. However, whether this translates to lesser mortality is not unequivocally proven.
- Open, laparoscopic and robotic approached have equivalent oncological and functional outcomes for partial nephrectomy.
- Once the final pathology report is available, patients should be classified into low/intermediate/high risk groups to tailor the intensity of follow-up.
- Following a partial or radical nephrectomy for localized renal cancer, patients are followed up as per the protocol for their respective risk categories.
- Thermo-ablative techniques may be used in patients with small renal masses who are not candidates for surgery.
- For elderly patients with SRMs with poor performance status who are not candidates for surgery or even thermoablation, active surveillance may be offered.

REFERENCES

1. Silverman SG, Pedrosa, I, Ellis JH, Hindman NM, Schieda, N, Smith AD, Remer EM, Shinagare AB, Curci NE, Raman SS, *et al.* Bosniak classification of cystic renal masses, version 2019: An update proposal and needs assessment. Radiology 2019, 292, 475–488.
2. EAU Guidelines. Edn. presented at the EAU Annual Congress Milan 2023. ISBN 978-94-92671-19-6.
3. Johnson BA, Kim S, Steinberg RL, de Leon AD, Pedrosa I, Cadeddu JA. Diagnostic performance of prospectively assigned clear cell Likelihood scores (ccLS) in small renal masses at multiparametric magnetic resonance imaging. Urol Oncol. 2019 Dec;37(12):941–946. doi: 10.1016/j.urolonc.2019.07.023. Epub 2019 Sep 17. PMID: 31540830; PMCID: PMC6934987.
4. Campbell SP, Tzortzakakis A, Javadi MS, Karlsson M, Solnes LB, Axelsson R, Allaf ME, Gorin MA, Rowe SP. 99mTc-sestamibi SPECT/CT for the characterization of renal masses: a pictorial guide. The British Journal of Radiology. 2018 Apr;91(1084):20170526.
5. Bertolotto M, Cicero C, Perrone R, Degrassi F, Cacciato F, Cova M.A. Renal masses with equivocal enhancement at CT: Characterization with contrast-enhanced ultrasound. Am. J. Roentgenol. 2015, 204, W557–W565.
6. Clevert D.A, Minaifar N, Weckbach S, Jung E.M, Stock K, Reiser M, Staehler M. Multislice computed tomography versus contrast-enhanced ultrasound in evaluation of complex cystic renal masses using the Bosniak classification system. Clin. Hemorheol. Microcirc. 2008, 39, 171–178.
7. Steinberg RL., *et al.* Prospective performance of clear cell likelihood scores (ccLS) in renal masses evaluated with multiparametric magnetic resonance imaging. Eur Radiol, 2021. 31: 314.

8. Voss, J., *et al.* Chest computed tomography for staging renal tumours: validation and simplification of a risk prediction model from a large contemporary retrospective cohort. BJU Int, 2020. 125: 561.
9. Sokhi HK, Mok WY, Patel U. Stage T3a renal cell carcinoma: staging accuracy of CT for sinus fat, perinephric fat or renal vein invasion. Br J Radiol 2015;88(1045):20140504.
10. Shuch BM, Pantuck AJ, Bernhard J-C, *et al.* Results from phase 3 study of 89Zr-DFO-girentuximab for PET/CT imaging of clear cell renal cell carcinoma (ZIRCON). J Clin Oncol. 2023;41(suppl 6; abstr LBA602).
11. Finelli A, Ismaila N, Bro B, et al.: Management of small renal masses: American Society of Clinical Oncology clinical practice guideline. J Clin Oncol 35:668–680, 2017.
12. Campell SC, Clark PE, Chang SS *et al.* Renal Mass and Localized Renal Cancer: Evaluation, Management, and Follow-Up: AUA Guideline Part I. J Urol 2021; 206: 199.
13. Motzer RJ, Jonasch E, Agarwal N, *et al.* Kidney Cancer, Version 3.2022, NCCN Clinical Practice Guidelines in Oncology. J Natl Compr Canc Netw. 2022;20(1):71–90.Kutikov A, Uzzo RG. The R.E.N.A.L. nephrometry score: a comprehensive standardized system for quantitating renal tumor size, location and depth. J Urol 2009;182:844–53.
14. Ficarra V, Novara G, Secco S, *et al.* Preoperative aspects and dimensions used for an anatomical (PADUA) classification of renal tumours in patients who are candidates for nephron-sparing surgery. Eur Urol 2009;56(5):786–793.
15. Davidiuk AJ, Parker AS, Thomas CS, *et al.* Mayo adhesive probability score: an accurate image-based scoring system to predict adherent perinephric fat in partial nephrectomy. Eur Urol 2014;66:1165–71.
16. Wang H, Zhou L, Guo J, Sun LA, Long Q, Ma Y, Zhang L, Lin Z, Zhu T, Wang G. Mini-flank supra-12th rib incision for open partial nephrectomy compared with laparoscopic partial nephrectomy and traditional open partial nephrectomy. PLoS One. 2014 Feb 21;9(2):e89155.
17. Castellucci R, Primiceri G, Castellan P, Marchioni M, D'Orta C, Berardinelli F, Neri F, Cindolo L, Schips L. Trifecta and Pentafecta Rates After Robotic Assisted Partial Nephrectomy: Comparative Study of Patients with Renal Masses <4 and 4 cm. J Laparoendosc Adv Surg Tech A. 2018 Jul;28(7):799–803. doi: 10.1089/lap.2017.0657. Epub 2018 Mar 1. PMID: 29493436.
18. Volpe A, Blute ML, Ficarra V, *et al.* Renal ischemia and function after partial nephrectomy: a collaborative review of the literature. Eur Urol 2015;68:61–74.
19. Scosyrev E, Messing EM, Sylvester R, Campbell S, Van Poppel H. Renal function after nephron-sparing surgery versus radical nephrectomy: results from EORTC randomized trial 30904. Eur Urol. 2014;65(2):372–377.
20. Liu, H., *et al.* A meta-analysis for comparison of partial nephrectomy vs. radical nephrectomy in patients with pT3a renal cell carcinoma. Transl Androl Urol, 2021. 10: 1170.
21. Rathi N, Palacios DA, Abramczyk E, *et al.* Predicting GFR after radical nephrectomy: the importance of split renal function. World J Urol. 2022;40(4):1011–1018.
22. Lopez-Costea, M.A., *et al.* Oncological outcomes and prognostic factors after nephron-sparing surgery in renal cell carcinoma. Int Urol Nephrol, 2016. 48: 681.
23. Meeks JJ, Zhao LC, Navai N, Perry KT Jr, Nadler RB, Smith ND. Risk factors and management of urine leaks after partial nephrectomy. J Urol. 2008;180(6):2375–8.
24. Kundu SD, Thompson RH, Kallingal GJ, Cambareri G, Russo P. Urinary fistulae after partial nephrectomy. BJU Int. 2010;106(7):1042–4.
25. Zargar H, Khalifeh A, Autorino R, Akca O, Brandao LF, Laydner H, Krishnan J, Samarasekera D, Haber GP, Stein RJ, Kaouk JH. Urine leak in minimally invasive partial nephrectomy: analysis of risk factors and role of intraoperative ureteral catheterization. Int Braz J Urol. 2014;40(6):763–71.
26. Selli C, De Maria M, Manica M, Turri FM, Manassero F. Minimally invasive treatment of urinary fistulas using N-butyl-2-cyanoacrylate: a valid first line option. BMC Urol. 2013;13:55.
27. Ward TJ, Ahmed O, Chung BI, Sze DY, Hwang GL. Percutaneous Cryoablation for Successful Treatment of a Persistent Urine Leak after Robotic-Assisted Partial Nephrectomy. J Vasc Interv Radiol. 2015;26(12):1867–70.
28. Gill IS, Kavoussi LR, Lane BR, *et al.* Comparison of 1,800 laparoscopic and open partial nephrectomies for single renal tumors. J Urol. 2007;178(1):41–46.
29. Jain S, Nyirenda T, Yates J, Munver R. Incidence of renal artery pseudoaneurysm following open and minimally invasive partial nephrectomy: a systematic review and comparative analysis. J Urol. 2013;189(5):1643–1648.
30. Ellis RJ. Chronic kidney disease after nephrectomy: a clinically-significant entity? Transl Androl Urol. 2019 May;8(Suppl 2):S166–S174.
31. Ellis, R.J., Cameron, A., Gobe, G.C. *et al.* Kidney failure, CKD progression and mortality after nephrectomy. Int Urol Nephrol 54, 2239–2245 (2022). https://doi.org/10.1007/s11255–022–03114–7.
32. Park BK, Shen SH, Fujimori M, Wang Y. Thermal Ablation for Renal Cell Carcinoma: Expert Consensus from the Asian Conference on Tumor Ablation. Korean J Radiol. 2021;22(9):1490–1496.
33. Pickersgill, N.A., *et al.* Ten-Year Experience with Percutaneous Cryoablation of Renal Tumors: Tumor Size Predicts Disease Progression. J Endourol, 2020. 34: 1211.
34. Pecoraro, A., *et al.* Cryoablation Predisposes to Higher Cancer Specific Mortality Relative to Partial Nephrectomy in Patients with Nonmetastatic pT1b Kidney Cancer. J Urol, 2019. 202: 1120.
35. Andrews J.R. *et al.* Oncologic Outcomes Following Partial Nephrectomy and Percutaneous Ablation for cT1 Renal Masses. Eur Urol, 2019. 76: 244.
36. Psutka, S.P., *et al.* Long-term oncologic outcomes after radiofrequency ablation for T1 renal cell carcinoma. Eur Urol, 2013. 63: 486
37. Chang, X., *et al.* Radio frequency ablation versus partial nephrectomy for clinical T1b renal cell carcinoma: long-term clinical and oncologic outcomes. J Urol, 2015. 193: 430.
38. Correa, R.J.M., *et al.* The Emerging Role of Stereotactic Ablative Radiotherapy for Primary Renal Cell Carcinoma: A Systematic Review and Meta-Analysis. Eur Urol Focus, 2019. 5: 958.
39. Siva S, Correa RJ, Warner A, Staehler M, Ellis RJ, Ponsky L, Kaplan ID, Mahadevan A, Chu W, Gandhidasan S, Swaminath A. Stereotactic ablative radiotherapy for T1b primary renal cell carcinoma: A report from the International Radiosurgery Oncology Consortium for Kidney (IROCK). International Journal of Radiation Oncology Biology Physics. 2020 Nov 15;108(4):941–9.
40. Siva S, Louie AV, Warner A, Muacevic A, Gandhidasan S, Ponsky L, Ellis R, Kaplan I, Mahadevan A, Chu W, Swaminath A. Pooled analysis of stereotactic ablative radiotherapy for primary renal cell carcinoma: A report from the International Radiosurgery Oncology Consortium for Kidney (IROCK). Cancer. 2018 Mar 1;124(5):934–42.

Chapter

11

Locally Advanced Renal Cell Carcinoma

• *Ashish Khanna* • *Sudhir Kumar Rawal*

LEARNING OBJECTIVES

- To understand the spectrum of locally advanced renal cell carcinoma (LA-RCC).
- To understand common clinical presentations of patients with LA-RCC and learn about patho-physiology behind these presentations.
- To understand the principles of imaging in a case of LA-RCC and their utility in treatment planning.
- To understand clinical implications of nodal involvement in RCC and the role of lymphadenectomy in RCC.
- To understand clinical implications of venous system involvement in RCC and role of thrombectomy.
- To understand the role of neoadjuvant and adjuvant therapy in LA-RCC.

Case Scenario

A 60-year-old gentleman presented with left flank pain and intermittent hematuria for the past 20 days. The pain was colicky in nature accompanied with gross hematuria and passage of linear serpiginous clots. The pain was often accompanied by vomiting. There was no history of loss of weight or appetite. On examination, the patient was pale, BP was normal, however, tachycardia (pulse 110/min) was present. Abdominal examination was normal; however, the patient had a left-sided varicocele which did not reduce in supine position. There was mild pitting edema in bilateral lower limbs. Ultrasound abdomen done outside revealed a left renal mass with suspicion of a thrombus in the left renal vein and IVC and 20 cc clots in the bladder. After stabilization, the patient underwent a CECT (triple phase) chest and abdomen which revealed 8 x 8 cm exophytic left upper polar renal mass with left renal vein and IVC thrombus extending up to the IVC-right atrium junction.

Check out the cystoscopy findings of this case.

1. What is the TNM staging of renal cell carcinoma (RCC)?

Ans: RCC is currently staged as per American Joint Committee on Cancer (AJCC) Cancer Staging 8th edition (2016) (Fig. 11.1) which has important prognostic survival implications in patients with RCC (Table 11.1).

2. What constitutes locally advanced RCC?

Ans: Following TNM characteristics are classified as **"locally advanced"** (Table 11.2):

Tumor:

cT3: Involving major veins [renal vein (RV) or IVC]/perinephric tissues (not beyond Gerota's fascia)/pelvicalyceal system/renal sinus fat (cT3)

or

cT4: Extending beyond Gerota's fascia (including contiguous infiltration of ipsilateral adrenal gland)

and/or

Node:

cN1: Regional lymph node involvement

and

Metastasis:

M0: No distant metastasis

Note: **"Contiguous"** infiltration of ipsilateral adrenal is T4, whereas "**non-contiguous**" ipsilateral adrenal involvement or contralateral adrenal involvement constitutes M1 (Fig. 11.2).

Clinical Staging Renal Cell Carcinoma : AJCC 8th Edition

T Category	*T Criteria*
TX	Primary tumor cannot be assessed
T0	No evidence of primary tumor
T1	Tumor ≤ 7 cm in greatest dimension, limited to the kidney
T1a	Tumor ≤ 4 cm in greatest dimension, limited to the kidney
T1b	Tumor > 4 cm but ≤ 7 cm in greatest dimension limited to the kidney
T2	Tumor > 7 cm in greatest dimmension, limited to the kidney
T2a	Tumor > 7 cm but ≤ 10 cm in greatest dimension limited to the kidney
T2b	Tumor > 10 cm, limited to the kidney
T3	Tumor extends into major veins or perinephric tissues, but not into the ipsilateral adrenal gland and not beyond Gerota's fascia
T3a	Tumor extends into the renal vein or its segmental branches, or invades the pelvicalyceal system, or invades perirenal and/or renal sinus fat but not beyond Gerota's fascia
T3b	Tumor extends into the vena cava below the diaphragm
T3c	Tumor extends into the vena cava above the diaphragm or invades the wall of the vena cava
T4	Tumor invades beyond Gerota's fascia (including contiguous extension into the ipsilateral adrenal gland)

N Category	*N Criteria*
NX	Regional lymph nodes cannot be assessed
N0	No regional lymph node metastasis
N1	Metastasis in regional lymph node(s)

M Category	*M Criteria*
M0	No distant metastasis
M1	Distant metastasis

Stage	*T*	*N*	*M*
I	T1	N0	M0
III	T1	N1	M0
II	T2	N0	M0
III	T2	N1	M0
III	T3	NX, N0	M0
III	T3	N1	M0
IV	T4	Any N	
IV	Any T	Any N	M1

Locally advanced renal cell carcinoma

Fig. 11.1: AJCC TNM (8th edition, 2016) classification for renal cell carcinoma

TABLE 11.1: Tumor, node, metastasis (TNM) stage and 5-year survival for renal cell carcinoma

Findings	*TNM (2009)*	*5-year survival (%)*
Organ-confined (overall)	T1-2N0MO	70–90
≤4.0 cm	T1aN0M0	90–100
<4.0 cm to 7.0 cm	T1bN0M0	80–90
>7.0 to 10.0 cm	T2aN0M0	65–80
>10.0 cm	T2bN0M0	50–70
Invasion of perinephric or renal sinus fat	T3aN0M0	50–70
Invasion of renal vein or branches	T3aN0M0	40–60
Invasion of IVC below diaphragm	T3bN0M0	30–50
Invasion of IVC above diaphragm or invasion of IVC wall	T3cN0M0	20–40
Direct adrenal involvement	T4N0M0	0–30
Locally advanced (invasion beyond Gerota fascia)	T4N0M0	0–20
Lymph node involvement	(Any)TN1M0	0–20
Systemic metastases	(Any)T(any)NM1	0–10

Stage	T	N	M
I	T1	N0	M0
III	T1	N1	M0
II	T2	N0	M0
III	T2	N1	M0
III	T3	NX, N0	M0
III	T3	N1	M0
IV	T4	Any N	
IV	Any T	Any N	M1

Locally advanced renal cell carcinoma

Fig. 11.2: Spectrum of locally advanced RCC as per AJCC TNM 8th edition

3. What are the common presentations of patients with locally advanced RCC?

Ans: The common clinical presentations are listed in Table 11.2.

The "classical triad: Too late triad "of flank pain, gross hematuria and palpable abdominal masses is now rarely found (6–10%).[1]

TABLE 11.2: Common clinical presentations of patients with locally advanced RCC

Clinical Presentation	*Causes/Comment*
Abdominal mass	Due to retroperitoneal location renal masses remain non-palpable until locally advanced
Flank pain	Stretching of renal capsule by mass effect
	Clot colic (with hematuria)
	Spontaneous retroperitoneal hemorrhage
	Infiltration of the posterior abdominal wall/nerve roots/paraspinous muscles
Hematuria	Infiltration of pelvicalyceal system
	Renal vein/IVC thrombus
	Arterio-venous shunts/malformations within the tumor
Bilateral lower limb edema	IVC thrombus
	Hypoalbuminemia
	Retroperitoneal/pelvic LN masses causing venous compression/thrombus
	Deep vein thrombus (usually unilateral)
Varicocele *	Renal vein/IVC thrombus
Constitutional symptoms (weight loss, fever, and night sweats)	Indicative of advanced/metastatic disease

*Note: Right sided and/or non-reducing varicocele (persisting in supine position) more suspicious.

4. **Define paraneoplastic syndromes and describe paraneoplastic manifestations associated with RCC.**

   Ans: Paraneoplastic syndromes are defined as signs and symptoms that cannot readily be explained by the anatomic distribution of the tumor or by the elaboration of hormones indigenous to the tissue from which the tumor arose.[2]

   These manifestations are seen in approximately 10–20% patients with RCC and are commonly seen with advanced and metastatic disease states.[3] Table 11.3 lists the common paraneoplastic manifestations associated with RCC.[4]

TABLE 11.3: Incidence of paraneoplastic manifestations with RCC

Syndrome	%
Elevated erythrocyte sedimentation rate	55.6
Hypertension	37.5
Anemia	36.3
Cachexia, weight loss	34.5
Pyrexia	17.2
Abnormal liver function	14.4
Hypercalcemia	4.9
Polycythemia	3.5
Neuromyopathy	3.2
Amyloidosis	2.0

5. **What is Stauffer's syndrome?**

   Ans: Stauffer syndrome (named after Herbert Stauffer who first reported it in 1961[5] refers to non-metastatic hepatic dysfunction associated with RCC. This paraneoplastic manifestation is seen in 3–20% patients with RCC.[6,7] Production of IL-6 and other cytokines from the primary tumor are believed to play a pathogenic role. Almost all patients have raised alkaline phosphatase levels, two-thirds have deranged prothrombin time values or hypoalbuminemia and a little less than one-third (20–30%) have elevated serum bilirubin/transaminase levels. Nephrectomy leads to normalization of liver functions in 60–70% patients. Residual or recurrent disease can lead to persistence or recurrence of hepatic dysfunction.

6. **Explain the pathogenesis of hypercalcemia in RCC, describe its clinical manifestations and treatment.**

   Ans: The incidence, pathophysiology and manifestations of hypercalcemia associated with RCC are listed in Table 11.4.

Management

The key components in the management of malignancy associated hypercalcemia are listed in Table 11.5.

Nodal Disease

7. **What are the regional lymph nodes for kidney?**

   Ans: There is no systematic pattern of lymphatic drainage of the kidney. However, mapping studies[9] have suggested the following regions as sites of regional lymph nodes (Table 11.6).

8. **What is the incidence of nodal involvement in RCC?**

   Ans: RCC is known for early hematogenous dissemination rather than a predictable lymphatic

TABLE 11.4: Incidence, pathophysiology, and manifestation of hypercalcemia in RCC

Incidence	*Up to 13% patients with RCC*[3]
Mechanism	a. Osteolytic metastasis b. Paraneoplastic: Tumor secretion of parathormone related peptide **(PTH-rP) {most common}**, 1,25 dihydroxy cholecalciferol, prostaglandins.
Manifestations (dependent on serum levels of calcium)	a. Gastrointestinal: Nausea, anorexia, peptic ulcer, constipation, pancreatitis b. Neurological: Lethargy, altered sensorium, coma c. Renal: Nephrogenic diabetes insipidus, acute kidney injury d. Cardiac: Short QT interval, arrhythmias

TABLE 11.5: Key strategies to correct hypercalcemia related to malignancy[8]

Agent	*Regimen*	*Onset*	*Duration*
0.9% Sodium chloride	2–4 L IV/day	Immediate	2–3 days
Calcitonin	4–8 units/kg SQ q 6–12 hours	4–6 hours	Up to 3 days
Bisphosphonates			
Pamidronate	60–90 mg IV over 2–6 hours	48 hours	3–4 weeks
Zoledronic acid	3–4 mg IV over 15–30 minutes	48 hours	3–4 weeks
Corticosteroids	200–400 mg hydrocortisone IV/day for 3–5 days	7 days	Unclear, perhaps 1 week
Gallium nitrate	200 mg/m^2 daily for 5 days	4 days	2 weeks
Denosumab	120 mg SQ weekly for 4 weeks, then monthly thereafter	7–10 days	3–4 months

Abbreviations: IV, intravenous; q, every; SQ, subcutaneous

TABLE 11.6: Regional lymph node stations for right and left kidney

Right kidney	*Left kidney*
Hilum	Hilum
Paracaval	Paraaortic
Precaval	Preaortic
Retrocaval	Retroaortic
Inter-aortocaval	Inter-aortocaval

Note: Drainage of lymph into the thoracic duct without passing through any lymph nodes is also seen

spread.[10] Overall reported incidence of nodal involvement in RCC is quite variable reported from 1% to as high as 35%. Recruitment of different patient populations and utilization of variable dissection templates may account for this observation. Contemporary literature suggests that incidence of pathological node involvement in low risk, cN0, cM0 RCC ranges from 1 to 5%.[10]

9. What are the factors that predict lymph nodal involvement in RCC?

Ans:

a. **Lymph node size:** In a series of patients at high-risk of lymph node metastases, the rates of metastatic nodes were 20%, 29%, and 90% for nodes 7, 10 and 30 mm in size, respectively.[11] Even in patients with radiographic adenopathy (defined as ≥ 1 cm), only 30% to 43% of clinically enlarged lymph nodes contain metastatic deposits.[12]

b. **Primary tumor related factors:** Several studies have reported that probability of lymph node metastasis increases with increasing T stage (T1/T2 vs T3/T4)[13–15] and grade of disease (Fuhrman grade 1/2 vs 3/4).[13,14,16]

In clinically node negative patients, Blute *et al* proposed criteria for increased risk (greater than 40%) of lymph node metastasis.[17,18]

The "Blute's Criteria" include:

1. Large primary tumor (>10 cm)
2. Clinical stage T3/T4
3. High tumor grade (grade 3/4)
4. Sarcomatoid features
5. Histologic tumor necrosis.

≥ 2 high risk features in the primary tumor required. Some may be known only if preoperative biopsy has been done

10. What is the prognostic implication of lymph nodal involvement in RCC?

Ans: Pathological nodal involvement is considered a dire prognostic sign with 5- and 10-year survival rates of 5% to 30% and 0% to 5%, respectively.[18,19]

Although better survival outcomes are expected in patients with a low number of positive LNs (< 4) and absence of extra-nodal extension.[1]

11. What is the current role of lymph node dissection for RCC at the time of radical nephrectomy?

Ans: Although lymphadenectomy for RCC provides accurate staging, the therapeutic benefits of routine lymphadenectomy are controversial. Based on the evidence at hand, there is no role of LND in clinically localized RCC with no evidence of nodal enlargement. LND may be of clinical benefit in locally advanced cases and those with clinically enlarged lymph nodes.[1]

Multiple retrospective studies have suggested a possible benefit to regional lymphadenectomy for carefully selected patients.[14,17,18,20]

The European Organization for Research and Treatment of Cancer (EORTC) 30881 is the only prospective RCT published addressing this issue till date.[21] An overall lymph node involvement of 4% was reported in the 772 patients included. However, the study failed to demonstrate any oncological benefit of LND. Critical appraisal of the trial showed that a very high percentage of patients with low risk of nodal involvement (81% were grade I/2 and 72% were organ confined) were included. In addition, only 25% of patients with pT3 tumors underwent a complete LND and the LN template used by the authors was not clearly stated.

More recently, Luo *et al* reported a systematic review and meta-analyses showing a survival benefit in patients with locally advanced disease treated with LND.[22] More specifically, thirteen studies on patients with LND and non-LND were identified and included in the analysis. In the subgroup of locally-advanced RCC (cT3–T4NxM0), LND showed a significantly better OS rate in patients who had undergone LND compared to those without LND (HR: 0.73, 95% CI: 0.60–0.90, p = 0.003).

12. What are the current indications of LND in RCC?

Ans: The indications are

1. Enlarged lymph nodes on imaging, or intraoperatively (cN+ disease)
2. Renal tumor size greater than 10 cm
3. Presence of tumor necrosis on imaging
4. Extrarenal tumor extension
5. Tumor thrombus cT3-T4 disease } cT3–T4 disease
6. Direct tumoral invasion of adjacent organs. } cT3–T4 disease
7. Nuclear grade 3 or greater } if biopsy available preoperatively
8. Sarcomatoid histology } if biopsy available preoperatively

13. What is the template for lymph node dissection for RCC?

Ans: Currently, there is no consensus on the anatomical extent and adequacy of LND in RCC management. However, templates have been suggested in Table 11.7.

Rule of thumb: Inter-aorto-caval lymph nodes + Lymph nodes around ipsilateral great vessel

At least 15 LN should be removed for LND to be considered adequate,[1] although, variable cut offs have been suggested.

TABLE 11.7: Description of template for lymph node dissection in RCC

Side	*Right*	*Left*
Great vessel	IVC	Aorta
Groups to be removed	Inter-aortocaval *	Inter-aortocaval*
	Precaval	Preaortic
	Paracaval	Paraaortic
	Retrocaval	Retroaortic
Cranial limit	Crus of diaphragm	Crus of diaphragm
Caudal limit	Right common iliac artery or bifurcation of IVC	Left common iliac artery or bifurcation of aorta

* Involvement of inter-aortocaval LNs without regional hilar involvement is reported in up to 35–45% of cases[23–25] hence included in both templates.

Venous involvement

14. Enumerate common tumors associated with IVC thrombus.

Ans: RCC is the most common cause associated with IVC tumor thrombus, accounting for 18% of all tumors that have venous thrombi.[26] Other causes are listed in Table 11.8.[3]

TABLE 11.8: Common tumors associated with IVC thrombus

Children	*Adults*
Wilms tumor	Renal cell carcinoma
Clear cell sarcoma of kidney	Angiomyolipoma
Adrenocortical carcinoma	Urothelial carcinoma renal pelvis
Neuroblastoma	Adrenocortical carcinoma
	Pheochromocytoma
	Lymphoma
	Retroperitoneal sarcoma

15. What is the incidence of venous involvement in RCC?

Ans: Overall, involvement of the venous system with RCC occurs in 4% to 10% of patients.[3]

16. What clinical symptoms and signs may help suspect IVC thrombus?

Ans: IVC tumor thrombus should be suspected in patients with a renal tumor who also have

- Lower extremity edema
- Isolated right-sided varicocele or one that does not collapse with recumbency
- Dilated superficial abdominal veins
- Pulmonary embolism
- Right atrial mass
- Nonfunction of the involved kidney.
- Proteinuria

17. What is the role of various imaging modalities in patients of RCC with venous thrombus?

Ans: In addition to characterization of the primary renal mass and other nodal/metastatic deposits, imaging modalities used should answer the following points about the venous thrombus:

- Absence or presence of venous thrombus
- Tumor thrombus vs bland thrombus
- Cranial extent of tumor thrombus
- Relation with hepatic vein ostium (when applicable)
- IVC/renal vein wall involvement
- Presence of collateral vessels

USG Color Doppler

- Commonly used modality due to non-invasive nature and easy availability
- Can comment on
  - Exact length of thrombus
  - Distance of thrombus from inferior liver edge/hepatic vein: IVC junction/cavo-atrial junction
  - Good blood flow and space between the thrombus and IVC wall: Indicate low possibility of IVC wall invasion by tumor thrombus
- Some authors suggest getting fresh color Doppler in the evening prior to surgery as progression of the tumor thrombus may mandate important changes in intraoperative management plan.

Computed tomography (CT)

- **Contrast enhanced triple phase multidetector CT** preferred
- Venous extension optimally visualized during **cortico-medullary phase** when contrast enhancement of vein is at its peak.[27]
- CT findings suggestive of venous involvement include
  - Venous enlargement
  - Abrupt change in the caliber of the vein
  - Filling defects in the vein
- The sensitivities of CT for detection of renal venous tumor thrombus and IVC involvement are 78% and 96%, respectively.[28,29]
- Contrast administration allows tumor thrombus to be differentiated from bland thrombus, because the latter does not demonstrate enhancement.

Magnetic Resonance Imaging (MRI)

- MRI with gadolinium enhancement has been preferred diagnostic study for the past few decades.
- However, recent studies suggest that multiplanar CT is equally effective as an MRI especially for presence of thrombus and cranial extent of thrombus.[29, 30]
- Currently preferred in the following cases:
  - Equivocal thrombus level/wall invasion assessment on CT scan.
  - Intravenous contrast administration for CT scan not possible (e.g. deranged renal function tests): In such cases high definition T2 images provide valuable information. Generation 2 gadolinium-based contrasts can now be used in patients with renal dysfunction.
- Conventional angiography/venography:
  - Invasive contrast-enhanced imaging, such as venacavography, is rarely used and reserved for patients in whom MRI and CT findings are equivocal or for whom MRI and CT are contraindicated.
- Trans-esophageal echocardiography (TEE):
  Due to the availability of CT/MRI and invasive nature of TEE, it is seldom needed in the preoperative setting. However, TEE is a valuable tool intraoperatively where it can serve the following purposes.[31,32]

a. Accurately identify the level of IVC thrombus and thus aid in surgical planning (may even obviate need of bypass in certain cases)
b. Characterize thrombus nature: Floating, fragility and adherence
c. Identify completeness of thrombus removal
d. Identify migration of thrombus
e. Intraoperative cardiovascular and fluid management
f. Aid in central venous access placement (avoid shear to thrombus by guidewire or line)

18. What are the imaging features suggestive of IVC wall involvement?

Ans: Findings reported in various studies that **may** suggest IVC invasion

- Preoperative IVC (AP) diameter on MRI > 18 mm (measured at the level of renal vein ostium).[33]
- Preoperative renal vein (AP) diameter on MRI > 14 mm (measured at the level of renal vein ostium).[33]
- Tumor signal on both sides (intraluminal and extraluminal) of IVC wall on MRI: **Most reliable sign with 92% accuracy.**[34]
- Complete occlusion of IVC with failure of contrast to pass around thrombus.[33, 35]
- Preoperative IVC diameter on CT scan > 40 mm.[36]

19. How do you classify the level of venous tumor thrombus and what is its clinical implications?

Ans: In the AJCC TNM classification, venous thrombi are classified as

T3a: Renal vein thrombus

T3b: IVC thrombus below the diaphragm

T3c: IVC thrombus above the diaphragm/IVC wall invasion.

These subclassifications hold key clinical implications as 5-year survival drops with increasing thrombus level (Fig. 11.1) and in planning surgical approaches (discussed later)

Neves and Zincke classified IVC thrombus originally into level I–IV.[37] Blute *et al* modified this classification by addition of a level 0: Renal vein thrombus and proposed the Mayo staging system for venous thrombi[26] (Fig. 11.3).

Ciancio *et al*[38] classified level III IVC thrombi (defined as thrombus involving the retrohepatic and suprahepatic IVC but not extending into the atrium) into the following (Fig. 11.4).

IIIa: Intrahepatic IVC not reaching up to hepatic vein ostium.

IIIb: Retrohepatic IVC reaching up to ostium of major hepatic veins and may extend into hepatic veins (causing Budd-Chiari syndrome).

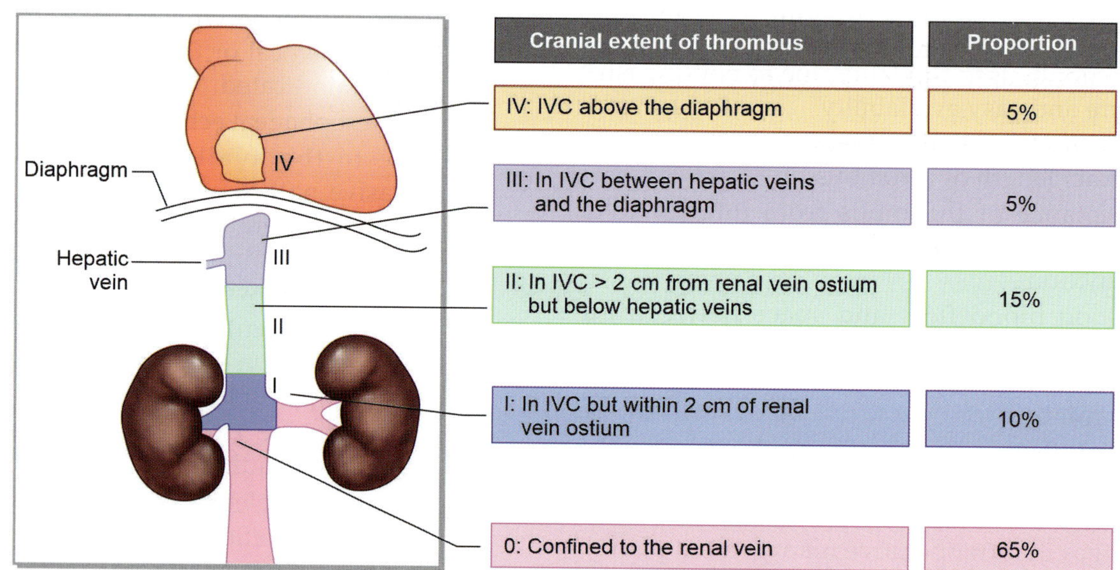

Fig. 11.3 Mayo staging system for IVC thrombus classification

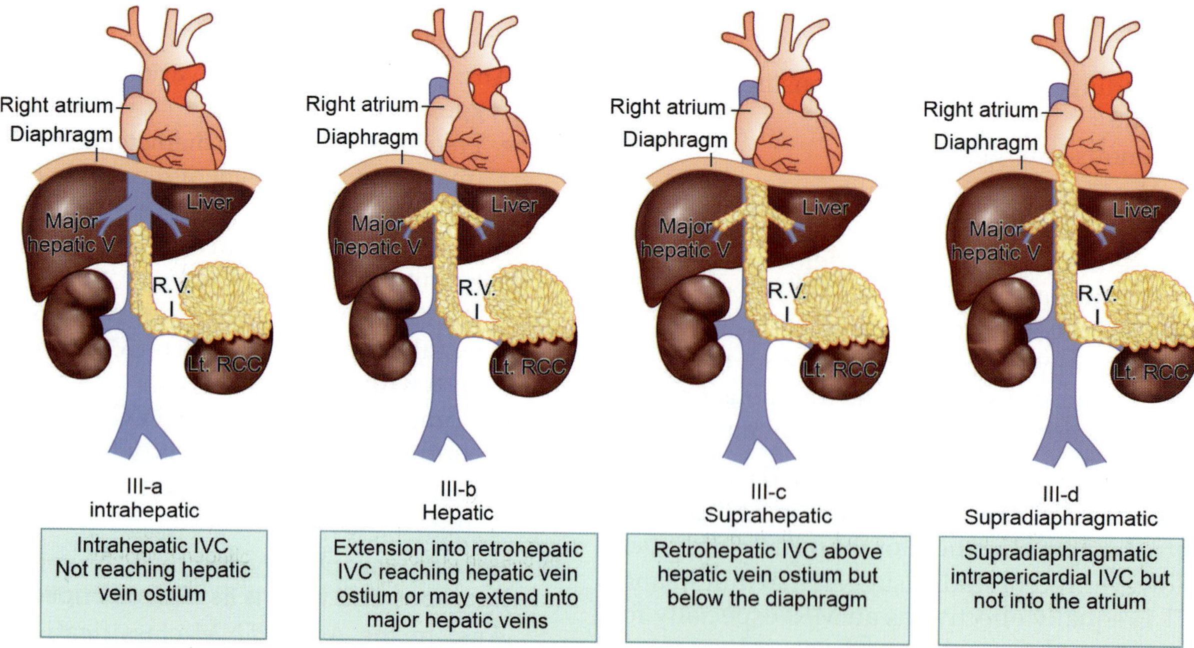

Fig. 11.4: Ciancio classification of level III IVC thrombus

IIIc: Retrohepatic IVC above hepatic vein ostium but below the diaphragm.

IIId: Supradiaphragmatic intrapericardial IVC but not into atrium.

And tumors extending into atrium were classified at level IV. This classification system has important clinical implications on surgical strategies taken to deal with them (discussed later).

20. What is the overall prognosis of patients with IVC thrombus? Should IVC thrombectomy be aggressively pursued?

Ans: Older reports reported poor prognosis of patients with venous involvement. However, contemporary literature[26,39] reports 45–69% 5-year survival of patients with venous tumor thrombus treated with aggressive surgical approaches if cancer is localized to the kidney.

Patients with venous tumor thrombi and concomitant lymph node (10% patients) or systemic metastases (25% patients) have markedly decreased survival, and those with tumor extending into the perinephric fat (50% patients) have intermediate survival.

The exact prognostic significance of the cranial extent of tumor thrombus is still debatable. IVC wall invasion appears to be a more adverse prognostic factor than thrombus level.

21. What is the current role of preoperative angioembolization of renal artery?

Preoperative angioembolization is neither essential nor recommended for routine management of IVC thrombus. It has its own advantages and disadvantages (Table 11.9):

TABLE 11.9: Advantages and disadvantages of preoperative angioembolization

Advantages/indications	*Disadvantages*
Allows early control of renal vein/ IVC without searching for the artery	Post-embolization/infarction pain syndrome
Bulky hilar/retroperitoneal lymphadenopathy IVC thrombus	Tumor lysis syndrome Tumor thrombus embolism
May help reduce level of thrombus and extent of thrombectomy (As in almost one-third cases direct arterial supply from renal artery/aorta to thrombus seen)	Vascular trauma
May reduce extent of nephrectomy by theoretically reducing size of tumor	Costly procedure
Bleeding renal tumor	
Theoretical reduction in intraoperative blood loss	

When used should be preferably undertaken within 24 hours of nephrectomy, although ideal time is yet a matter of debate.

22. What is the current role of IVC filter placement prior to radical nephrectomy?

Ans: Currently placement of preoperative suprarenal IVC filters is not recommended due to risk of contralateral renal and hepatic vein thrombosis, the risk for provoking embolization, and the impediment posed to future IVC thrombectomy.

23. What are the common incisions used for RN in locally advanced RCC?

Ans:

- Chevron incision (bilateral subcostal)
- Midline laparotomy incision (preferred in tall thin individuals)
- Modified Makuuchi incision (preferred in cases requiring hepatic mobilization)

The vertical limb extends from the tip of xiphoid process to 1 cm cranial to the umbilicus in the midline. This then curves laterally to join the horizontal limb which runs parallel to the anatomical abdominal fold and the dermatomal distribution of nerves to end midway between the lowest part of the rib cage and anterior superior iliac spine[40] (Fig. 11.5).

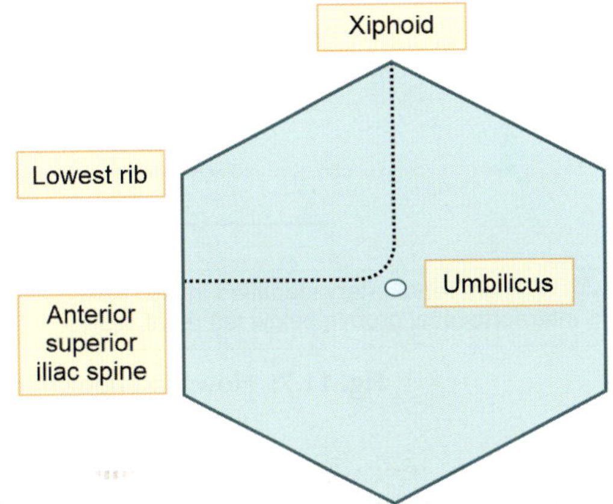

Fig. 11.5: Depiction of right sided modified Makuuchi incision

When simultaneous intra-abdominal and intra-thoracic interventions are planned (Fig. 11.6).

- Midline laparotomy with sternotomy
- Chevron laparotomy with sternotomy
- Thoracoabdominal incision

24. What is early arterial control/early arterial ligation and how is it accomplished?

Ans:

- Renal tumors are highly vascular with large thin-walled collaterals that are fragile and may

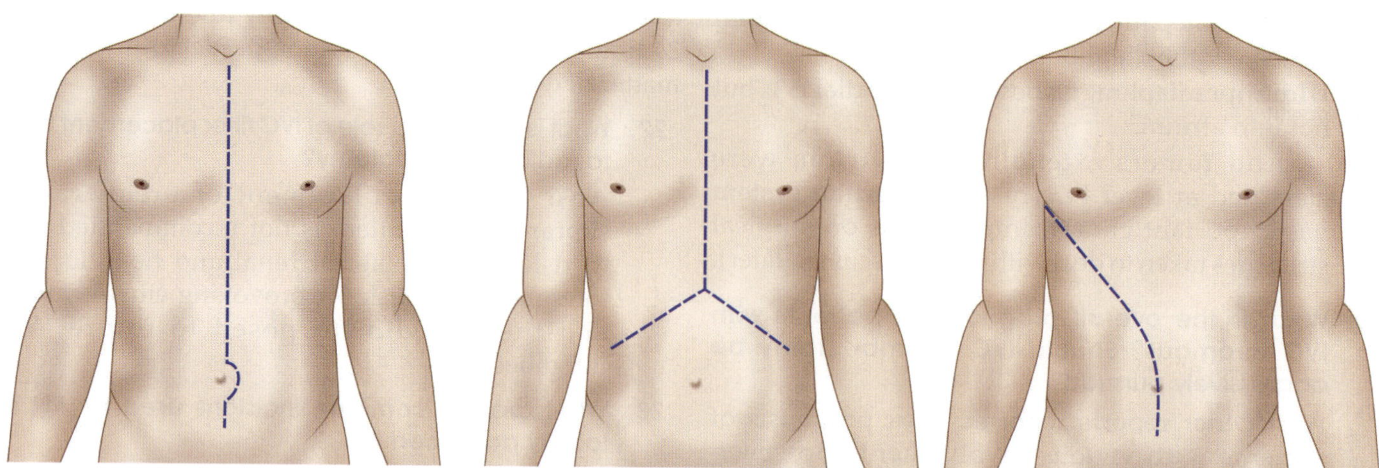

Fig. 11.6: Surgical incisions for combined intra-abdominal and intrathoracic approach to vena caval tumor thrombi

cause significant blood loss if they rupture prior to arterial control.

- Early arterial ligation refers to ligation of respective renal arteries early in the radical nephrectomy without much dissection. Figure 11.7 describes key steps.
- This may not be always possible in larger tumors and/or associated retroperitoneal lymphadenopathy around the great vessels. In such cases arterial control is taken after colonic mobilization.

25. What are the key steps in IVC thrombectomy?

Ans: The key steps are related to the level and side of renal mass and are described in Table 11.10.

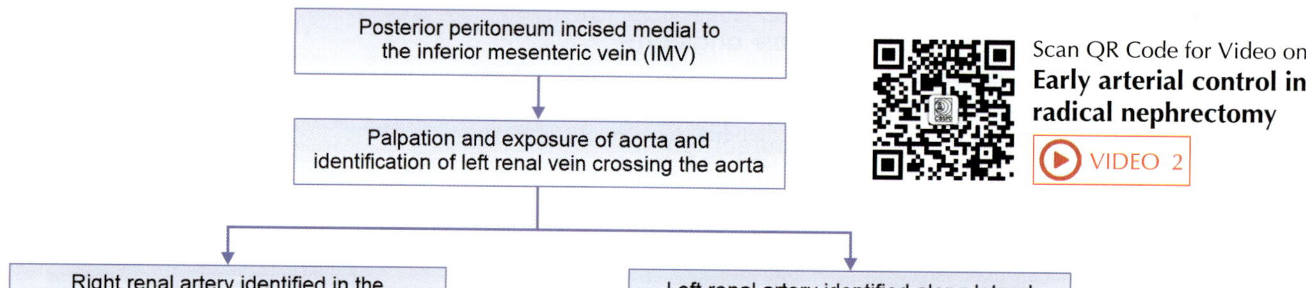

Fig. 11.7: Flowchart depicting steps for early arterial control during nephrectomy

TABLE 11.10: Key steps in IVC thrombectomy

Level	*Comment/Steps*
I	• Satinsky clamp/vascular stapler on IVC • Preserve at least 50% IVC lumen • Can be approached by flank incision for right-sided tumors
II	• Ligate lumbar veins# • Clamping sequence: Infrarenal IVC → Contralateral RV@ → Suprarenal IVC above thrombus • Un-clamping sequence: Infrarenal IVC → Contralateral RV → Suprarenal IVC above thrombus (essentially same as clamping sequence)
IIIa	Additional steps: • Ligate SHV draining the caudate lobe of liver • Mobilize right lobe of liver (divide right triangular/coronary ligaments and Makuuchi ligament) • Rest as in level II

(Contd.)

TABLE 11.10: Key steps in IVC thrombectomy *(Contd.)*

Level	*Comment/Steps*
IIIb/Some IIIc	Additional steps: • Mobilize both right and left lobes of liver • High control of suprahepatic IVC • Clamping sequence: Infrarenal IVC → Contralateral RV@ → Porta hepatis**(Pringle maneuver) → Suprahepatic IVC (also known as total hepatic vascular occlusion) • Unclamping sequence: Infrarenal IVC → Contralateral RV@ → Porta hepatis → Suprahepatic IVC
IIIc/IIId	Transabdominal approach by division of central tendon of diaphragm and taking control of the intra-pericardial IVC or transthoracic approach by sternotomy
IV	Combined transabdominal and transthoracic approach. Bypass techniques either by venovenous bypass or cardiopulmonary bypass with or without deep hypothermia are needed.

#Lumbar veins are important sources of bleed during IVC thrombectomy. It is a must to ligate (not necessarily divide) them to have a bloodless field.
@For left-sided tumors, also clamp right renal artery to avoid engorgement of the right kidney as right renal vein does not have collateral drainage via the adrenal or gonadal veins.
**Under normothermic conditions, Pringle maneuver can be safely done up to 60 minutes, however, clamping time of 20 minutes or less is preferred to reduce ischemic hepatic injury, portal vein thrombosis and splenic engorgement/rupture.
For cases where the caval wall is infiltrated by the tumor and primary closure results in luminal compromise, graft replacement can be done.

26. What are the hemodynamic changes seen during total hepatic vascular occlusion or during clamping of suprahepatic IVC?

Ans:

10% to 20% reduction in mean arterial blood
40% reduction in cardiac output
50% increase in heart rate
60% reduction in cardiac preload
80% increase in peripheral vascular resistance

The patient will not tolerate suprahepatic IVC clamping if the cardiac output drops by more than 50% or the mean arterial BP drops more than 30%.

27. In what cases are bypass techniques employed/ preferred?

Ans: Bypass (veno-venous or cardiopulmonary bypass) should be considered in patients in whom

- IVC cross-clamping trial causes significant hypotension
- Patients with preoperative cardiac or hepatic dysfunction, contralateral renal dysfunction, or portal venous hypertension (IVC clamping can precipitate decompensation)
- Major intraoperative bleeding that is difficult to control.

28. Enumerate important complications encountered in IVC thrombectomy?

Ans:

- Air embolism
- Pulmonary embolism
- Massive hemorrhage
- Hepatic dysfunction
- Complications related to cardiopulmonary bypass:
  1. Coagulopathy
  2. Stroke
  3. Perioperative mortality

29. What is bland thrombus, its pathophysiology, classification systems and management?

Ans: Bland thrombus refers to a blood coagulum devoid of tumor cells. The tumor thrombus impedes venous flow in the infrarenal IVC, and common iliac veins and this stasis promotes bland thrombus formation. The Mayo Clinic Thrombus Grouping system[26] classifies bland thrombi and suggests possible management strategies (Fig. 11.8).

Case Scenario* *(Contd.)

This patient underwent open radical nephrectomy with IVC thrombectomy utilizing median sternotomy and laparotomy incision and cardiopulmonary bypass. Post-operative recovery was uneventful. Final biopsy report was suggestive of clear cell RCC, grade 4 (sarcomatoid areas seen), pelvicalyceal system invasion seen, margins negative, IVC thrombus involved by tumor, renal vein margins negative. The patient and attendants are apprehensive about the prognosis, risk of recurrence and wish to know the further course of action.

Recurrence Risk and Adjuvant Therapy in RCC

Between 20% and 40% of all patients with non-metastatic kidney cancer experience a recurrence following surgery, with nearly 50% of the highest risk patients recurring within 6 years.[41–43]

Most commonly recurrences occur within 3 years of complete resection, however, many occur even 10 years after surgery.[44,45] Local recurrences after RN occur in 2–4%.

The most common systemic recurrences occur in lung (64%), liver (11%), bone (15%), regional lymph nodes (9%).[46]

A variety of factors have been studied that impact the prognosis and risk of recurrence and progression. Table 11.11 lists several such factors.[47,48]

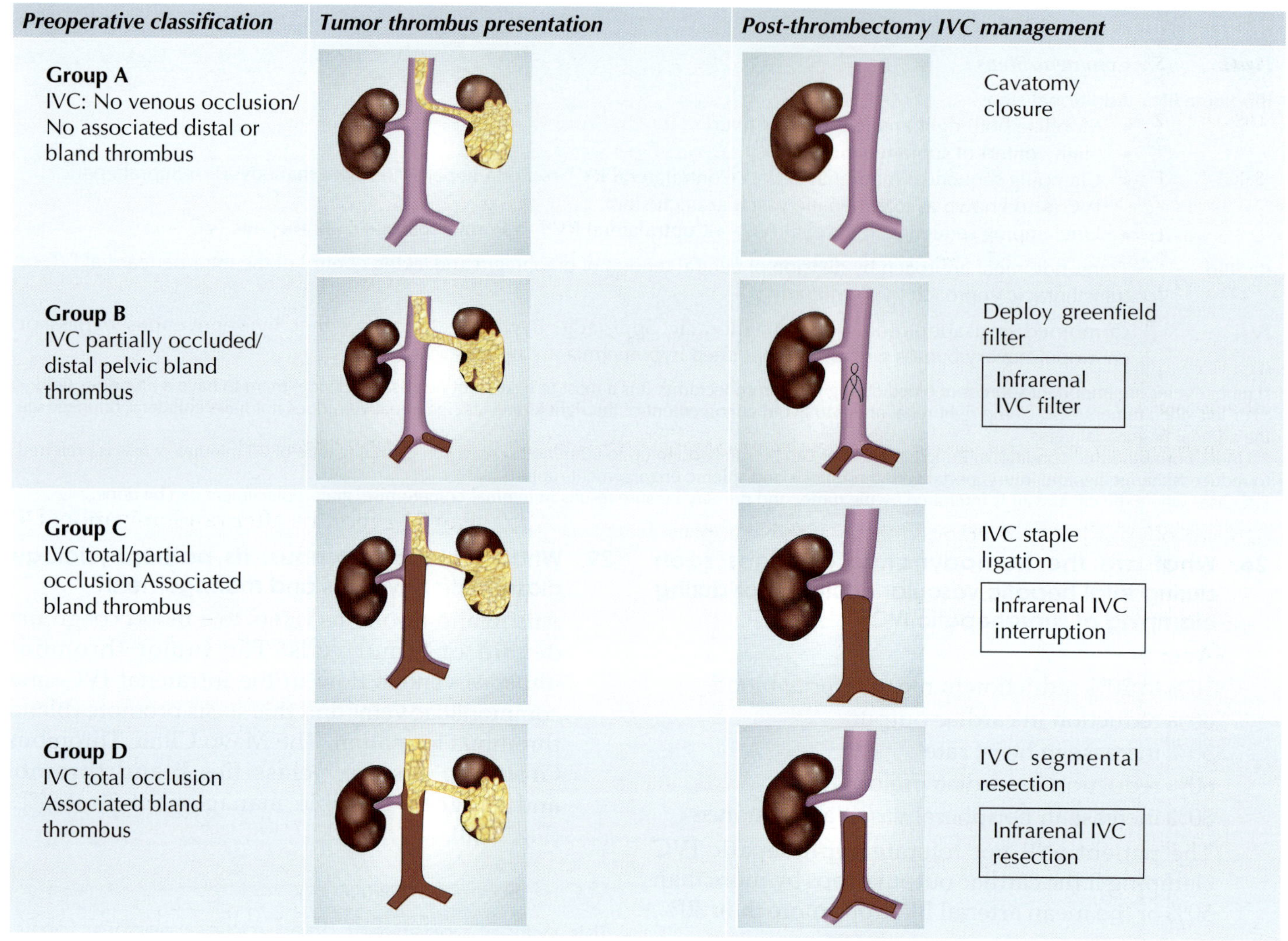

Fig. 11.8: Mayo clinic thrombus staging system and suggested management strategies for infrarenal IVC post-tumor thrombectomy

TABLE 11.11: Adverse prognostic factors for renal cell carcinoma

Clinical	*Anatomic*	*Histologic*
Poor performance status Systemic symptoms Anemia Hypercalecemia Elevated lactate dehydrogenase Elevated erythrocyte sedimentation rate Eevated C-reactive protein Thrombocytosis Elevated alkaline phosphatase	Larger tumor size Venous involvement Extension into contiguous organs, including adrenal gland Lymph node metastases Distant metastases and greater metastatic burden	High nuclear grade Certain histologic subtypes Sarcomatoid features Presence of histologic tumor necrosis Vascular invasion Invasion of perinephric or renal sinus fat Collecting system invasion Positive surgical margin

Data from Lane BR, Kattan MW: Prognostic models and algorithms in renal cell carcinoma. *Urol Clin North Am* 35(4):613–625, 2008; Sun M, Vetterlein M, Harshman LC, at a;.: Risk assessment in small renal masses: a review article. *Urol Clin North Am* 44(2):189–202, 2017.

A variety of nomograms[49–53] have also been developed that predict risk of recurrence and disease-free survival (Table 11.12). Majority of these are based on surgical pathology report of the radical nephrectomy specimen.

The goal of adjuvant drug therapy is to provide additional therapy following treatment of the primary tumor to reduce the risk of disease recurrence and death by eliminating residual micro metastatic disease that is destined to recur.

30. What is the current evidence in favour of adjuvant therapy in RCC?

Ans: Summary and recommendations as per EAU 2023.[1]

TABLE 11.12: Components of various nomograms predicting risk of recurrence post-nephrectomy

System	Study	T Stage	N Stage	M Stage	Tumor Size	Grade	Necrosis	Histology	ECOG	MVI	Clinical Symptoms	Gender
UISS	Zisman et al,[49] 2002	1997 T stage	×	×	–	–	–	–	×	–	–	–
SSIGN	Frank et al,[50] 2002	2002 T stage	×	×	(< or ≥5 cm)	×	×	–	–	–	–	–
Leibovich	Leibovich et al,[51] 2003	2002 T stage	×	–	(0 or ≥ 10 cm)	×	×	–	–	–		–
MSKCC	Kattan et al, [52] 2001	1997 T stage	–	–	Continuous	×	×	Clear cell, papillary, chromophobe	–	×	×	–
Raj[a]	Raj et al,[53] 2008	–	×	–	Continuous	–	×	–	–	–	×	×

Abbreviations: ECOG, Eastern Cooperative Group performance status; MSKCC, Memorial Sloan Kettering Cancer Center; MVI, microvascular invasion; SSIGN, stage, size, grade, and necrosis; UISS, University of California, Los Angeles, intergrated staging system.
[a]Used prenephrectomy, thus N status, tumor size, and necrosis based on imaging; all others used postnephrectomy and use pathologic data.

Recommendation	Strength
Do not offer adjuvant therapy with sorafenib, pazopanib, everolimus, girentuximab, or axitinib.	Strong
Do not offer adjuvant sunitinib following surgically resected high-risk clear-cell renal cell carcinoma (ccRCC).	Weak
Offer adjuvant pembrolizumab to ccRCC patients, preferably within 12–16 weeks post-nephrectomy, with a recurrence risk as defined in the Keynote-574 trial: • Intermediate-high risk: – pT2, grade 4 or sarcomatoid, N0, M0 – pT3, any grade, N0 M0 • High risk: – pT4, any grade, N0, M0 – any pT, any grade, N+, M0 • M1 no evidence of disease (NED): – NED after resection of oligometastatic sites ≤ 1 year from nephrectomy	Weak

Several trials with classical immunotherapy agents such as IFN-α 2b, IFN-α, high dose IL-2 and tumor vaccines failed to show any clinical benefit of the various trials using tyrosine kinase inhibitors like sorafenib, sunitinib, axitinib and pazopanib and m-TOR inhibitors like everolimus only the S-TRAC study[54] using sunitinib demonstrated a DFS (6.2 years vs 4 years) benefit HR:0.76 CI:0.59–0.98 with non-significant difference in OS. Based on this sunitinib was given FDA approval in adjuvant setting.

Keynote-564[55] evaluated pembrolizumab (17 cycles of 3-weekly therapy) vs. placebo as adjuvant therapy in 994 patients with

a. Intermediate-high risk: pT2, grade 4 or sarcomatoid, N0, M0; or pT3, any grade, N0, M0
b. High risk: pT4, any grade, N0, M0 or pT any stage, and grade, or N+, M0
c. M1 (no evidence of disease [NED] after primary tumor plus soft tissue metastases completely resected < one year from nephrectomy) disease.

At median 24.1 months after randomization, DFS was significantly better with pembrolizumab vs placebo (HR: 0.68, 95% CI: 0.53–0.87, p = 0.001). The estimated 24-month DFS rate was 77% vs. 68% for pembrolizumab and placebo, respectively. This benefit was seen across all 3 groups.

In an updated analysis[56] with median follow-up of 30 months, pembrolizumab continued to demonstrate a DFS benefit over placebo (HR: 0.63, CI 0.50-0.80). In this analysis, the authors explored the efficacy of patient subgroups as per the UISS risk group and disease states. Approximately 75% of patients in each arm were UISS intermediate risk, with 5.9% of the total cohort M1 NED. Almost 88% of patients had AJCC stage 3 disease.

Other trials like IMmotion010 (Atezolizumab vs placebo) and CheckMate 914 (Nivolumab vs Placebo), however, failed to demonstrate any clinical benefit.

31. Given resource limited settings such as the Indian subcontinent, what is your take on utilization of sunitinib as adjuvant therapy?

Ans: Unlike immunotherapy, where studies have demonstrated persistent effect despite discontinuation of therapy with durable responses, the inhibition of VEGF induced angiogenesis by sunitinib and other TKI has been seen to reverse rapidly on discontinuation.[57] Thus, in cases of RCC where relapses may be seen after many years, a temporally limited use of TKI is unlikely to have positive impact on risk of relapse. In other words, continued use of these agents over prolonged periods may be required to have demonstrable benefits. The antecedent toxicities of these agents preclude such prolonged usage, as demonstrated by high number of patients requiring dose reductions (34.3%), dose interruptions (46.4%) and discontinuation (28.1%) in the S-TRAC trial.[53]

Due to concerns regarding toxicity, lack of demonstrable OS survival benefit and conflicting results across various trials (STRAC/ASSURE/ATLAS/PROTECT), the NCCN has given a category 3 level of recommendation for use of adjuvant sunitinib for patients with stage III, clear cell disease and high risk of relapse.

32. What is the current evidence for adjuvant therapy in non-clear cell histologies of RCC?

Ans: Currently there is lack of evidence of adjuvant therapy in non-clear cell histologies of RCC.

33. What is the recommended follow-up schedule for patients with locally advanced RCC?

Ans: The NCCN recommends the following follow-up schedule for patients with locally advanced disease

a. History, physical examination, comprehensive metabolic panel every 3–6 months for 3 years, then annually for up to 5 years.
b. CT/MRI 3–6 months after surgery followed by CT/MRI/USG every 3–6 months for 3 years, then annually for up to 5 years.
c. CT chest MRI 3–6 months after surgery followed by CT/MRI/USG every 3–6 months for 3 years, then annually for up to 5 years

It is suggested that follow-up can continued beyond 5 years if clinically indicated.

34. What is the current role of neoadjuvant therapy in the management of locally advanced RCC?

Ans: The role and evidence for neoadjuvant therapy in management of RCC is evolving. The aim of neoadjuvant treatment is:

1. Improve oncological outcomes (DFS, MFS, OS)
2. Facilitate resection of surgically complex tumors
    a. Making unresectable masses resectable and reduce need for adjacent organ resection.
    b. Change surgical plan from radical nephrectomy to partial nephrectomy. This may be useful in patients with imperative indication for renal preservation such as:
        i. Tumours in patients with renal insufficiency
        ii. Bilateral renal tumours in the setting of locally advanced disease
        iii. Locally advanced disease in a solitary kidney.
        iv. Complex renal masses: High renal score (10–12)
    c. Downsize IVC tumor thrombus thus impacting surgical plan, reducing surgical morbidity and/or need for major vascular resection.

SUMMARY

- Clinical stage cT3-T4, N1, M0 RCC as per the AJCC TNM 8th edition constitutes locally advanced RCC. This holds important prognostic survival implications and in addition may also guide surgical strategies required for treatment. Clinical presentations of patients with LA-RCC are often attributable to local mass effect/infiltration of adjacent structures (renal vein, IVC, retroperitoneal nerves and musculature, etc.) or by paraneoplastic manifestations. Ultrasonography (USG), multiplanar contrast enhanced CT, MRI are crucial preoperative imaging modalities used to stage RCC and to plan surgical interventions. Intra-operative trans-esophageal echocardiography (TEE) can be of immense utility in selective cases. Pathological nodal involvement in RCC is a poor prognostic factor with survival similar to metastatic disease. Although lymphadenectomy for RCC provides accurate staging, the therapeutic benefits of routine lymphadenectomy are controversial.
- Venous system involvement is seen in 4–10% cases of RCC. There are multiple systems for classification of level of renal vein/IVC tumor thrombus such as the TNM, Neves and Zincke, Mayo, Ciancio. Level of thrombus has prognostic survival impact and holds key importance in surgical planning. Forty-five to seventy percent patients with venous tumor thrombus can be cured with nephrectomy and thrombectomy, including patients with tumor thrombus extending to the cardiac atrium. Multidisciplinary care is often required in management of such cases.
- Neoadjuvant therapy in RCC is still evolving. It aims to improve oncological outcomes and facilitate resection in surgically complex tumors. Although primarily still a surgical disease, there is an unmet need for adjuvant therapy to improve oncological outcomes post-nephrectomy with/without metastatectomy.
- In view of toxicity and controversial oncological benefit, tyrosine kinase inhibitors (TKI) such as sunitinib are not preferred for adjuvant therapy. However, they may have role in resource limited settings where immunotherapy may not be available/affordable. Pembrolizumab has shown to have benefit in adjuvant setting as seen in the Keynote 564 trial.

REFERENCES

1. EAU Guidelines. Edn. presented at the EAU Annual Congress Milan 2023. ISBN 978-94-92671-19-6.
2. Kumar V, Abbas AK, Aster JC. Robbins & Cotran Pathologic Basis Of Disease. 10th ed. S.L.: Elsevier-Health Science; 2021
3. Partin AW, Meredith Fairfax Campbell, Walsh PC, Wein Alan J. Campbell-Walsh-Wein Urology. Volume I. Amsterdam: Elsevier, Cop; 2021.
4. Gold PJ, Fefer A, Thompson JA. Paraneoplastic manifestations of renal cell carcinoma. In Seminars in urologic oncology 1996 Nov 1 (Vol. 14, No. 4, pp. 216–222).
5. Stauffer MH. Nephrogenic hepatosplenomegaly. Gastroenterology. 1961;40:694–6.
6. Kranidiotis GP, Voidonikola PT, Dimopoulos MK, *et al.* Stauffer's syndrome as a prominent manifestation of renal cancer: a case report. Cases J 2009;2:49.
7. Giannakos G, Papanicolaou X, Trafalis D, *et al.* Stauffer's syndrome variant associated with renal cell carcinoma. Int J Urol 2005;12:757–9.

8. Sternlicht H, Glezerman IG. Hypercalcemia of malignancy and new treatment options. Therapeutics and clinical risk management. 2015 Dec 4:1779–88.
9. Karmali RJ, Suami H, Wood CG, Karam JA. Lymphatic drainage in renal cell carcinoma: back to the basics. BJU Int. 2014;114(6):806–17
10. van Hattem MW, Roussel E, Van Poppel H, Albersen M. Role of Lymphadenectomy in renal cell cancer. Renal Cancer: Contemporary Management. 2020:281–94.
11. Gershman B, Takahashi N, Moreira DM, Thompson RH, Boorjian SA, Lohse CM, *et al.* Radiographic size of retroperitoneal lymph nodes predicts pathological nodal involvement for patients with renal cell carcinoma: development of a risk prediction model. BJU Int. 2016;118(5):742–9.
12. Capitanio U, Deho F, Dell'Oglio P, *et al*: Lymphadenopathies in patients with renal cell carcinoma: clinical and pathological predictors of pathologically confirmed lymph node invasion, World J Urol 34(8):1139–1145,2016.
13. Sun M, Bianchi M, Hansen J, Abdollah F, Trinh QD, Lughezzani G, *et al.* Nodal involvement at nephrectomy is associated with worse survival: a stage-for-stage and grade-for-grade analysis. Int J Urol. 2013;20(4):372–80.
14. Capitanio U, Suardi N, Matloob R, Roscigno M, Abdollah F, Di Trapani E, *et al.* Extent of lymph node dissection at nephrectomy affects cancer-specific survival and metastatic progression in specific sub-categories of patients with renal cell carcinoma (RCC). BJU Int. 2014;114(2):210–5.
15. Giuliani L, Giberti C, Martorana G, Rovida S. Radical extensive surgery for renal cell carcinoma: long-term results and prognostic factors. J Urol. 1990;143(3):468–73. discussion 73–4.
16. Pantuck AJ, Zisman A, Dorey F, Chao DH, Han KR,Said J, *et al.* Renal cell carcinoma with retroperitoneal lymph nodes: role of lymph node dissection. J Urol.2003;169(6):2076–83.
17. Blute ML, Leibovich BC, Cheville JC, Lohse CM, Zincke H. A protocol for performing extended lymph node dissection using primary tumor pathological features for patients treated with radical nephrectomy for clear cell renal cell carcinoma. J Urol. 2004;172(2):465–9.
18. Crispen PL, Breau RH, Allmer C, Lohse CM, Cheville JC, Leibovich BC, *et al.* Lymph node dissection at the time of radical nephrectomy for high risk clear cell renal cell carcinoma: indications and recommendations for surgical templates. Eur Urol. 2011;59(1):18–23.
19. Phillips CK, Taneja SS. The role of lymphadenectomy in the surgical management of renal cell carcinoma. In Urologic Oncology: Seminars and Original Investigations 2004 May 1 (Vol. 22, No. 3, pp. 214–223). Elsevier.
20. Sun M, Trinh QD, Bianchi M, Hansen J, Abdollah F, Tian Z, *et al.* Extent of lymphadenectomy does not improve the survival of patients with renal cell carcinoma and nodal metastases: biases associated with the handling of missing data. BJU Int.2014;113(1):36–42.
21. Blom JH, van Poppel H, Maréchal JM, Jacqmin D, Schröder FH, de Prijck L, Sylvester R. Radical nephrectomy with and without lymph-node dissection: final results of European Organization for Research and Treatment of Cancer (EORTC) randomized phase 3 trial 30881. European urology. 2009 Jan 1;55(1):28–34.
22. Luo, X., *et al.* Influence of lymph node dissection in patients undergoing radical nephrectomy for non-metastatic renal cell carcinoma: a systematic review and meta-analysis. Eur Rev Med Pharmacol Sci, 2019. 23: 6079.
23. Capitanio U, *et al.* Lymph node dissection in renal cell carcinoma. Eur Urol, 2011. 60: 1212.
24. Herrlinger A, *et al.* What are the benefits of extended dissection of the regional renal lymph nodes in the therapy of renal cell carcinoma. J Urol, 1991. 146: 1224.
25. Chapin BF, *et al.* The role of lymph node dissection in renal cell carcinoma. Int J Clin Oncol, 2011.16: 186.
26. Blute ML, Leibovich BC, Lohse CM, *et al.* The Mayo Clinic experience with surgical management, complications and outcome for patients with renal cell carcinoma and venous tumour thrombus, BJU Int 94:33–41, 2004b.
27. Tsili AC, Argyropoulou MI. Advances of multidetector computed tomography in the characterization and staging of renal cell carcinoma. World J Radiol. 2015 Jun 28;7(6):110–27.
28. Herts BR: Role of three-dimensional imaging in surgical planning for kidney surgery, BJU Int 95(Suppl 2):16–20, 2005.
29. Ng CS, Wood CG, Silverman PM, *et al*: Renal cell carcinoma: diagnosis, staging, and surveillance, Am J Roentgenol 191(4):1220–1232, 2008.
30. Guzzo TJ, Pierorazio PM, Schaeffer EM, Fishman EK, Allaf ME. The accuracy of multidetector computerized tomography for evaluating tumor thrombus in patients with renal cell carcinoma. The Journal of Urology. 2009 Feb 1;181(2):486–91.
31. Calderone CE, Tuck BC, Gray SH, Porter KK, Rais-Bahrami S. The role of transesophageal echocardiography in the management of renal cell carcinoma with venous tumor thrombus. Echocardiography. 2018 Dec;35(12):2047–55.
32. Souki FG, Demos M, Fermin L, Ciancio G. Transesophageal echocardiography-guided thrombectomy of intracardiac renal cell carcinoma without cardiopulmonary bypass. Annals of cardiac anaesthesia. 2016 Oct;19(4):740.
33. Zini L, Destrieux-Garnier L, Leroy X, Villers A, Haulon S, Lemaitre L, *et al.* (2008). Renal vein ostium wall invasion of renal cell carcinoma with an inferior vena cava tumor thrombus: prediction by renal and vena caval vein diameters and prognostic significance. *J Urol* 179: 450–454.
34. Aslam Sohaib S, Teh J, Nargund V, Lumley J, Hendry W, Reznek R. (2002) Assessment of tumor invasion of the vena caval wall in renal cell carcinoma cases by magnetic resonance imaging. *J Urol* 167: 1271–1275.
35. Psutka SP, Boorjian SA, Thompson RH, Schmit GD, Schmitz JJ, Bower TC, Stewart SB, Lohse CM, Cheville JC, Leibovich BC. Clinical and radiographic predictors of the need for inferior vena cava resection during nephrectomy for patients with renal cell carcinoma and caval tumour thrombus. BJU international. 2015 Sep;116(3):388–96.
36. Gohji K., Yamashita C., Ueno K., Shimogaki H., Kamidono S. (1994) Preoperative computerized tomography detection of extensive invasion of the inferior vena cava by renal cell carcinoma: possible indication for resection with partial cardiopulmonary bypass and patch grafting. *J Urol* 152: 1993–1996.
37. Neves RJ, Zincke H. Surgical treatment of renal cancer with vena cava extension. British Journal of Urology. 1987 May;59(5):390–5.
38. Ciancio G, Vaidya A, Savoie M, Soloway M. Management of renal cell carcinoma with level III thrombus in the inferior vena cava. The Journal of Urology. 2002 Oct;168 (4 Part 1): 1374–7.

39. Martinez-Salamanca JI, Huang WC, Millan I, *et al*: Prognostic impact of the 2009 UICC/AJCC TNM staging system for renal cell carcinoma with venous extension, Eur Urol 59(1):120–127, 2011.
40. Chang SB, Palavecino M, Wray CJ, Kishi Y, Pisters PW, Vauthey JN. Modified Makuuchi incision for foregut procedures. Archives of surgery. 2010 Mar 1;145(3):281–4.
41. Haas NB, Manola J, Uzzo RG, *et al.* Adjuvant sunitinib or sorafenib for high-risk, non-metastatic renal-cell carcinoma (ECOG-ACRIN E2805): a double-blind, placebo-controlled, randomised, phase 3 trial. Lancet 2016;387(10032):2008–16.
42. Ravaud A, Motzer RJ, Pandha HS, *et al.* Adjuvant sunitinib in high-risk renal-cell carcinoma after nephrectomy. N Engl J Med 2016;375(23):2246–54.
43. Haas NB, Manola J, Dutcher JP, *et al.* Adjuvant treatment for high-risk clear cell renal cancer: updated results of a high-risk subset of the ASSURE randomized trial. JAMA Oncol 2017;3(9):1249–52.
44. Wood Erika L, Adibi M, Qiao Wei, *et al.* Local tumor bed recurrence following partial nephrectomy in patients with small renal masses. J Urol 2018;199(2):393–400.
45. Abara E, Chivulescu I, Clerk N, *et al.* Recurrent renal cell cancer: 10 years or more after nephrectomy. Can Urol Assoc J 2010;4(2):E45–9.
46. Eggener SE, Yossepowitch O, Pettus JA, *et al.* Renal cell carcinoma recurrence after nephrectomy for localized disease: predicting survival from time of recurrence. J Clin Oncol 2006; 24(19):3101–6.
47. Lane BR, Kattan MW. Prognostic models and algorithms in renal cell carcinoma. Urologic Clinics of North America. 2008 Nov 1;35(4):613–25.
48. Sun M, Vetterlein M, Harshman LC, Chang SL, Choueiri TK, Trinh QD. Risk assessment in small renal masses: a review article. Urologic Clinics. 2017 May 1;44(2):189–202.
49. Zisman A, Pantuck AJ, Wieder J, *et al.* Risk group assessment and clinical outcome algorithm to predict the natural history of patients with surgically resected renal cell carcinoma. J Clin Oncol 2002;20(23):4559–66.
50. Frank I, Blute ML, Cheville JC, *et al.* An outcome prediction model for patients with clear cell renal cell carcinoma treated with radical nephrectomy based on tumor stage, size, grade and necrosis: the SSIGN score. J Urol 2002;168(6):2395–400.
51. Leibovich BC, Blute ML, Cheville JC, *et al.* Prediction of progression after radical nephrectomy for patients with clear cell renal cell carcinoma. Cancer 2003; 97(7):1663–71.
52. Kattan MW, Reuter V, Motzer RJ, *et al.* A postoperative prognostic nomogram for renal cell carcinoma. J Urol 2001;166(1):63–7.
53. Raj GV, Houston TR, Leibovich Bradley C, *et al.* Preoperative nomogram predicting 12-year probability of metastatic renal cancer. J Urol 2008;179(6): 2146–51.
54. Ravaud A, Motzer RJ, Pandha HS, George DJ, Pantuck AJ, Patel A, Chang YH, Escudier B, Donskov F, Magheli A, Carteni G. Adjuvant sunitinib in high-risk renal-cell carcinoma after nephrectomy. New England Journal of Medicine. 2016 Dec 8;375(23):2246–54.
55. Choueiri TK, Quinn DI, Zhang T, Gurney H, Doshi GK, Cobb PW, Parnis F, Lee JL, Park SH, Semenov A, Chang WY. KEYNOTE-564: A phase 3, randomized, double blind, trial of pembrolizumab in the adjuvant treatment of renal cell carcinoma.
56. Powles T, Tomczak P, Park SH, Venugopal B, Ferguson T, Symeonides SN, Hajek J, Gurney H, Chang YH, Lee JL, Sarwar N. Pembrolizumab versus placebo as post-nephrectomy adjuvant therapy for clear cell renal cell carcinoma (KEYNOTE-564): 30-month follow-up analysis of a multicentre, randomised, double-blind, placebo-controlled, phase 3 trial. The Lancet Oncology. 2022 Sep 1;23(9):1133–44.
57. Mancuso MR, Davis R, Norberg SM, O'Brien S, Sennino B, Nakahara T, Yao VJ, Inai T, Brooks P, Freimark B, Shalinsky DR. Rapid vascular regrowth in tumors after reversal of VEGF inhibition. The Journal of clinical investigation. 2006 Oct 2;116(10):2610–21.

Chapter 12

Metastatic Renal Cell Carcinoma

• *Abhishek Singh* • *Amandeep Arora*

LEARNING OBJECTIVES

- To understand the principles of workup and imaging in a case of metastatic RCC: Contrast-enhanced CT of the chest, abdomen and pelvis is the most commonly ordered investigation for advanced RCC. The role of FDG PET scan is evolving. RCC has limited FDG-avidity.
- To understand the principles of renal mass biopsy in large renal mass: Renal mass biopsy should be done percutaneously under image guidance. Ultrasound guidance is the preferred choice as it is a dynamic investigation. The risk of tract-seeding is theoretical.
- To understand the risk stratification of metastatic RCC: Risk stratification of metastatic RCC enables prognostication and helps clinicians choose the best possible therapeutic option between upfront surgery vs systemic therapy.
- To understand the role of cytoreductive nephrectomy: The role of cytoreductive nephrectomy has definitely gone down as compared to the cytokine era. Even in the era of tyrosine kinase inhibitors and immunotherapy, patients with an IMDC risk score of 0/1 may benefit with a cytoreductive nephrectomy.
- To understand the implication of various histological subtypes on management of metastatic RCC: Clear cell renal cell carcinoma is the most common histological variant and it responds well to both TKI and immunotherapy. Patients with sarcomatoid differentiation respond poorly to all types of therapies.
- To understand the choice and sequencing of drugs in metastatic RCC: A combination of immunotherapy and tyrosine kinase inhibitors has now become the first therapeutic choice for metastatic RCC. A combination of two immune checkpoint inhibitors can also be used.
- To understand the role of genetic work-up in metastatic RCC patients: A younger patient with a positive family history or with a symptom-complex suggestive of a syndrome should definitely undergo genetic analysis.
- To understand the basis and role of immune check point inhibitors (ICIs) in metastatic RCC: ICIs are now the first-line agents in metastatic RCC. They alone or in combination with TKIs significantly improve the PFS and OS across all the groups of risk stratification.
- To understand the follow-up of a metastatic RCC patient on systemic therapy: Patients on systemic therapy require a clinical and radiological follow-up between 6 and 16 weeks. If the disease is stable, 4 monthly follow-up is acceptable. A baseline imaging and imaging at suspected progression and before changing the line of therapy should be strongly considered.
- To understand the role of best supportive care in metastatic RCC: Supportive care is focused on maintaining the quality of life during and after the exhaustion of drug therapy directed at improving overall survival. Components of supportive care include pain management, use of bisphosphonates and RANK-L inhibitors to prevent skeletal-related events, and local radiation for spinal/brain metastasis.

Case Scenario

A 65-year-old hypertensive and diabetic male, post-CABG and on blood thinners, was evaluated for weight loss and headache and was found to have a left renal mass (on a screening USG abdomen). A CT scan of the chest, abdomen and pelvis was suggestive of a 9.6 cm heterogeneously enhancing left renal mass with multiple pulmonary metastases (largest measuring 2.9 cm), multiple liver metastases in the right lobe, largest measuring 6.6 × 6.2 cm and also brain metastasis measuring 3.1 × 1.7 × 2.6 cm. His ECOG score was 0 (Fig.12.1A to 12.1C).

1. **What would be the next appropriate action?**
   Ans: A biopsy to establish the diagnosis.
2. **Where would you do a biopsy from?** (Video link)
   Ans: Biopsy in any malignancy should be done from the most representative and most accessible site. In this case, it happens to be the kidney which has a mass of 9.6 cm and can be easily targetted.

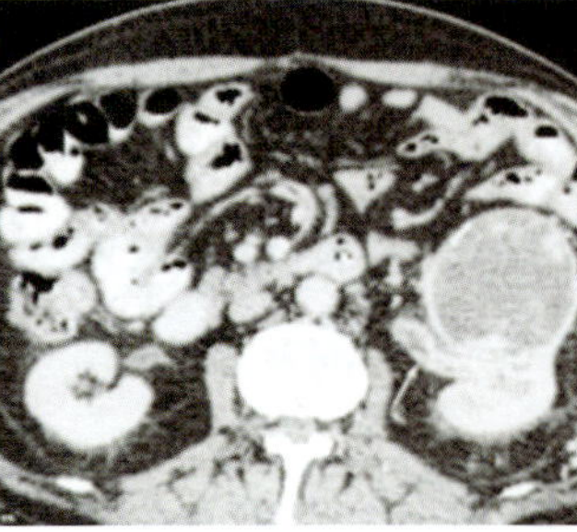

Fig. 12.1A: The left renal mass

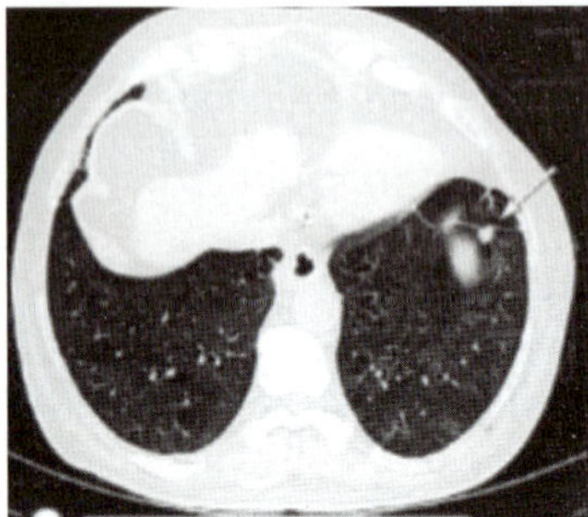

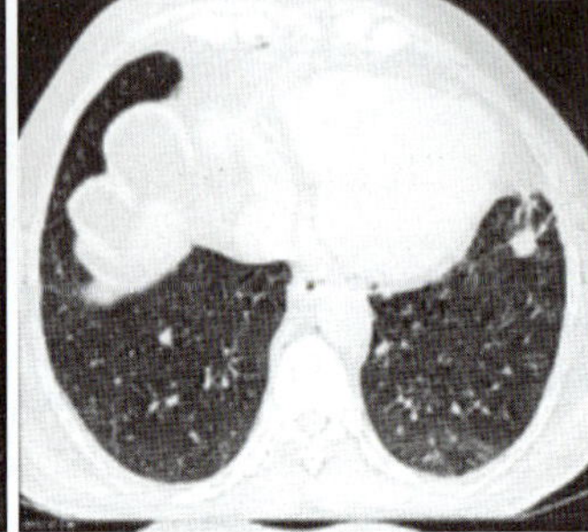

Fig. 12.1B: Pulmonary metastasis

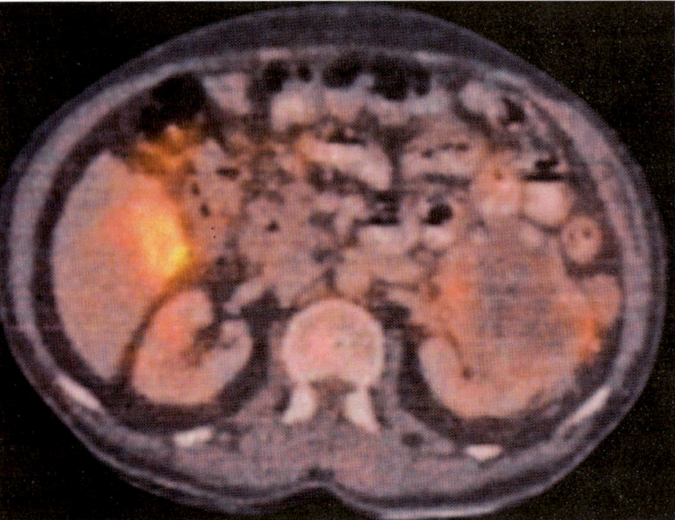

Fig. 12.1C: FDG uptake in the liver lesion

A USG-guided biopsy is easier to perform than a CT-guided biopsy. USG is dynamic and real-time visualization is possible. The Doppler mode can be used to avoid vessels.

The biopsy is done in using a dedicated puncture guide on the USG machine and a biopsy gun. A 15 mm core is good for renal biopsy. Two to three cores are adequate to achieve the diagnosis.

3. **What are the common complications of renal biopsy and is tract seeding of malignancy a possibility?**

Ans: Hemorrhage is the most common complication; however, even this is quite rare. It is usually self-limiting; occasionally, the patient may have significant hematuria and may go into clot retention or develop a peri-nephric hematoma. Rarely (<1%), the patient may require angioembolization.

The risk of tract seeding is very low and the incidence reported is < 0.01%, though a handful of case reports have been published.[1]

4. **What is the importance of performance status and how is it measured?**

Ans: Performance status is a metric to evaluate whether the patient is in a position to tolerate the therapy that is going to be offered.

Scales used include: ECOG (Eastern Co-operative Oncology Group) score and the Karnofsky performance index[2,3] (Table 12.1).

TABLE 12.1: Comparison of the ECOG and Karnofsky performance status

ECOG performance status	*Karnofsky performance status*
0: Fully active, able to carry on all pre-disease performance without restriction	100: Normal, no complaints; no evidence of disease 90: Able to carry on normal activity; minor signs or symptoms of disease
1: Restricted in physically strenuous activity but ambulatory and able to carry out work of a light or sedentary nature, e.g. light house work, office work	80: Normal activity with effort, some signs or symptoms of disease 70: Cares for self but unable to carry out normal activity or to do active work
2: Ambulatory and capable of all self-care but unable to carry out any work activities; up and about more than 50% of waking hours	60: Requires occasional assistance but is able to care for most of personal needs 50: Requires considerable assistance and frequent medical care
3: Capable of only limited selfcare; confined to bed or chair more than 50% of waking hours	40: Disabled; requires special care and assistance 30: Severely disabled; hospitalization is indicated although death not imminent
4: Completely disabled; cannot carry on any selfcare; totally confined to bed or chair	20: Very ill; hospitalization and active supportive care necessary 10: Moribund
5: Dead	0: Dead

5. **What was the histology report of the biopsy?**

Ans: It was a clear cell RCC with ISUP grade 4.

6. **What do you want to know in a biopsy report of a suspected RCC?**

Ans:

1. Histological type: Clear cell, papillary, chromophobe, etc.
2. Grade of the tumour.

The histological type determines the aggressiveness, prognosis and response to therapy.

7. What are the subtypes of RCC and what are the clinico-pathological implications of each?

Ans: The histological types of RCC have been discussed in the chapter on "localised renal cell cancer".

8. What is the role of FDG PET scan in a patient with metastatic RCC?

Ans:

- FDG PET/CT is not the standard recommendation in most of the major guidelines for the evaluation of RCC, mainly because of the physiological excretion of ^{18}F-fluoro-2-deoxy-2-d-glucose (FDG) from the kidneys, which decreases the contrast between renal lesions and normal tissue, and may obscure or mask the lesions of the kidneys.[4]
- However, with the advent of newer hybrid PET/CT scanning systems, this modality has shown increased efficacy in the evaluation of primary renal masses along with the detection of extrarenal metastases, restaging recurrent RCC, and also in monitoring response to targeted therapy.[5–7]

VARIOUS UTILITIES OF FDG PET/CT IN METASTATIC RCC

1. *Detection of extrarenal synchronous or metachronous metastases:* Sensitivity and specificity of FDG PET in detecting metastasis from RCC ranges from 63% to 75% and from 90% to 100%, respectively. It has a sensitivity and specificity of close to 100% when it comes to detecting both osteoblastic and osteolytic metastases.
2. *Monitoring therapeutic response of metastatic RCC to systemic therapy*[8]*:* The metabolic activity of metastatic RCC lesion, reflected as standardized uptake value (SUV_{max}), gets affected in patients undergoing treatment with TKIs (tyrosine kinase inhibitors) or ICIs (immune checkpoint inhibitors).

   Partial metabolic response correlates well with the PFS and/or the OS. The highest survival rates are seen in patients who show the greatest post-therapeutic reduction in SUV_{max}. This is true for both bony and soft tissue lesions.
3. *Postoperative surveillance and in diagnosing recurrent RCC:* Three meta-analyses which included 1168 patients showed that FDG PET-CT has a sensitivity of 80–100%, specificity of 70–100%, accuracy of 90% and PPV of 95–100% in detecting all metastatic and recurrent lesions, smallest of which was a 7 mm lymph node. There was a change in therapeutic plan in 43% patients based on the scan.
4. *Predictive Role in the prognosis of Primary RCC:* FDG PET helps in predicting metastases. A primary RCC with a high SUV_{max} >8.8 was shown to have a higher likelihood of having occult metastasis.[9]
5. *It also has a role in differentiating benign or bland emboli from tumor thrombosis.*

CURRENT ADVANCES IN PET-CT IN RCC

- Mutation of the VHL gene leads to CA-IX over-expression in most cases of clear cell RCC. MAb G250 is a monoclonal antibody that binds to CA-IX and 124I-cG250 immuno-PET/CT has been used with promising results in both localized and metastatic RCC.
- ^{18}F-Fluoromisonidazole PET has been used to delineate hypoxic tumors, which have a poorer response to TKI therapy.[10]
- ^{18}F-Fluorothymidine (FLT) enables PET evaluation of cell proliferation and its greatest advantage over the ^{18}F-FDG is its ability to more accurately distinguish inflammation from tumors. FLT uptake and higher initial FLT uptake are prognostic indicators in RCC and FLT PET allows to evaluate the response to TKI therapy earlier than the FDG PET scan.[11]
- The role of radiotracers such as the 68Ga-labeled 1, 4, 7, 10-tetraazacyclo-dodecane-N, N′, N″, N‴-tetraacetic acid-D-Phe1-Tyr3-octreotide, 124I geruntuximab, 89Zr geruntuximab, 18F sodium fluoride, and 89Zr bevacizumab in metastatic RCC is promising but is still experimental.
- The ZIRCON study is a phase III study that evaluated the utility of 89Zr-DFO-girentuximab (TLX250 CDx) in detection of RCC. It is a chimeric antibody and have affinity for CA IX . In this study 300 patients who were planned for nephrectomy or partial nephrectomy received the 89Zr-DFO-girentuximab in the dose of 10 mg, 5 days prior to PET scanning and the scan were evaluated by 3 independent observers. The sensitivity and specificity 86% [80%, 90%] and 87% [79%, 92%] respectively. As the expression of CA IX is significant in ccRCC it helps in differentiating ccRCC from other variants with a threshold value of SUV_{max} > 24.1. Based on this data the trace was approved by FDA in February 2023.[12]
- ^{Ga}68-PSMA PET scan has been the most widely investigated of the experimental radiotracers, in both newly diagnosed and recurrent RCC, and also to evaluate the response to therapy, due to the expression of PSMA on the neovasculature of the renal tumors. The branch of "theranostics" has seen PSMA ligands labeled with both β- and α-emitters with impressive results in prostate cancer patients refractory to multiple lines of chemotherapy. This thought and line of action can be carried forward to

other cancers expressing PSMA, including RCC and dosimetry-driven clinical studies are certainly the way to go forward.
- The REMAP study is an ongoing single-center prospective observational study that aims to compare the efficacy of FDG PET/MRI with DWI with the standard of care CECT to evaluate response in patients with advanced RCC on TKI therapy, in order to provide timely and personalized treatment decisions.[13]

9. How will you risk stratify this patient?

Ans: Patient can be risk stratified using IMDC risk stratification.

IMDC RISK STRATIFICATION

Heng *et al* presented a new risk-stratification model in 2009 that was based solely on patients treated with VEGFRi; also termed the International Metastatic Renal-Cell Carcinoma Database Consortium (IMDC) criteria-for use in patients with metastatic RCC for prognostication and treatment selection.[14–16]

Based on six risk factors, the IMDC risk group categorizes patients as having favorable risk (no factors), intermediate risk (one or two factors), or poor risk (at least three factors) with their median overall survival being 43.2 months, 22.5 months and 7.8 months respectively.

Validated in the following settings

1. Patients with clear cell and non-clear cell metastatic renal cell carcinoma.
2. Patients undergoing targeted therapies and immune checkpoint inhibitor therapy.

Memorial Sloan Kettering Cancer Center (MSKCC) Prognostic model

Prognostic Factors

1. Interval from diagnosis to treatment <1 year
2. Karnofsky performance status < 80%
3. Serum LDH > 1.5 times the upper normal limit
4. Corrected calcium greater than upper normal limit
5. Serum hemoglobin < lower limit of normal

International Metastatic Renal Cell Carcinoma Database Consortium (IMDC) Model Criteria

Prognostic factors

1. Interval from diagnosis to treatment <1 year
2. Karnofsky performance status < 80%
3. Serum hemoglobin < lower limit of normal (normal = 12 gm/dl)
4. Corrected calcium greater than upper normal limit (normal range 8.5 to 10.2 mg/dl)
5. Neutrophil > upper limit of normal (normal 2.0 to 7.0 × 109)
6. Platelets > upper limit of normal (150000 to 400000).

Prognostic risk groups for both the models

1. *Favourable risk:* No prognostic factors present
2. *Intermediate risk:* 1–2 prognostic factors present
3. *Poor risk:* > 3 prognostic factors present

10. What should be the first line of this patient?

Ans: According to the NCCN guidelines, the choice of first-line systemic therapy for metastatic RCC is based on the risk category of the patient[17–24] (Tables 12.4 and 12.5).

The first line of treatment in today's day and age should be a combination of a TKI with an ICI. The earlier standard of care which were the TKIs have been replaced by a combination of TKI and IO. The combinations which are available are as follows:

- Axitinib + Pembrolizumab
- Cabozantinib + Nivolumab
- Lenvatinib +Pembrolizumab
- Axitinib + Avelumab

The PD-1 inhibitors seem to be more effective than PD-L1 inhibitors, though conclusive evidence for the same seems to be lacking.

A combination of two immunotherapy agents can also be used as the first line therapy, i.e Ipilimumab +Nivolumab.

A. Axitinib + Pembrolizumab combination was the first to be approved on the basis of the Keynote-426 trial. In this trial, pembrolizumab + axitinib was compared to sunitinib in advanced ccRCC. The ORR was 55.8% vs 29.5% in favour of the combination in intermediate and poor risk groups. The 18-month OS favored the combination group (82.3% vs 72.1%) with an HR (hazard ratio) of 0.53 (95% CI 0.38–0.74, p>0.0001).[17]

B. The CheckMate 214 study established the role of IO + IO combination; in this case, the combination of nivolumab + ipilimumab was studied against sunitinib. In the intermediate and high-risk patients, it was found that ORR was 42% vs 27% in favour of combination treatment. A 9% complete response rate was achieved in the combination group in intermediate and poor risk as compared to 1% in the sunitinib group. In the good risk patients, the ORR for sunitinib was better starting the debate that is TKI alone a better option in good risk disease (Table 12.2).[22]

C. Another combination in the TKI + IO segment is Lenvatinib + Pembrolizumab. The data for this comes from the CLEAR trial (Table 12.3). This trial compared lenvatinib + pembrolizumab (n=355) with lenvatinib + everolimus (n=357),

TABLE 12.2: Comparison of the Keynote-426 and CheckMate 214 studies

Keynote 426	*Intermediate/poor risk*		*Checkmate 214*	*Intermediate/poor risk*	
	Pembro + Axi n=294	Sunitinib n = 298		Nivo + Ipi n=425	Sunitinib n=422
ORR (%)	55.8	29.5	ORR (%)	42	27
p value	–	–	*p* value	< 0.001	
CR (%)	4.8	0.7	CR (%)	9	1
Median PFS months	12.6	8.8	Median PFS months	11.6	8.4
Hazard ratio (95% CI)	0.67 (0.53-0.85)		Hazard ratio (95% CI)	8.2 (0.64-1.05)	
p Value	–		*p* Value	0.03	
12-month OS (%)	87	71	12-month OS (%)	80	72
Hazard ratio (95% CI)	0.52 (0.37-0.74)		Hazard ratio (95% CI)	0.63 (0.44-0.99)	
p Value	–	–	*p* Value	<0.001	

TABLE 12.3: Current landscape of the first line agents used in management of advanced clear cell renal carcinoma

	Checkmate 214 Nivolumab+ Ipilimumab n = 550	***Keynote 426 Axitinib + Pembrolizumab n = 432***	***Checkmate 9ER Cabozantinib + Nivolumab n = 323***	***CLEAR Lenvatinib + Pembrolizumab n = 357***
Favourable/Intermediate/poor risk (%)	23/61/17	32/55/13	23/58/19	31/59/9
Prior nephrectomy	80	83	69	74
Sarcomatoid features	11	18	11	8
Follow-up in months	67.7	42.8	32.9	33.7
Mean progression free survival (PFS) in months	12.4	15.7	16.6	23.3
PFS (intermediate/poor risk) HR(CI)	0.73 (0.61-0.87)	0.67 (0.55-0.81)	I: 0.58 (0.45-0.76)	
P: 0.36 (0.23–0.56)	0.36 (0.26-0.47)			
Overall response rate/complete response, %	39 (12)	60 (10)	56 (12)	71 (16)
Grade 3–5 adverse effects	46	68	65	82

and sunitinib (n = 357). The lenvatinib + pembrolizumab arm showed longer progression free survival of 23.9 months as compared to 14.7 months and 9.2 months respectively by lenvatinib + everolimus and sunitinib groups. The objective response rate was highest for the lenvatinib + pembrolizumab group 71% (66.3–75.7%) vs 53.5% (48.3–58.7) for lenvatinib + everolimus group vs 36.1% (31.2–41.1) for the sunitinib group. Complete response was seen in 16.1% vs 9.8% vs 4.2%, respectively, which was clearly in favour of the penvatinib + pembrolizumab group. The trial concluded that lenvatinib and pembrolizumab combination is better than sunitinib with respect to progression free survival and overall survival.[24]

D. In a phase III, open label randomized control trial, 651 patients were studied to compare the combination of nivolumab + cabozantinib against sunitinib. At a median follow-up of 18.1 months, the progression free survival was 16.6 months (12.5–24.9) vs 8.3 months (7.0–9.7) in favour of the combination group. The combination group also had an objective response rate of 55.7% vs 27.1% in the sunitinib group. The overall survival at 12 months favored the combination group at 85.7% (95% CI, 81.3 to 89.1) vs 75.6% (95% CI, 70.5 to 80.0)[19] (Table 12.4).

Note:

- Active surveillance can be used in certain favourable risk patients
- Temsirolimus can be used in certain poor/intermediate risk patients
- Axitinib single agent and high dose IL-2 can be used in all the risk group in certain situations

TABLE 12.4: First line therapy for metastatic clear cell RCC (Adapted from NCCN guideline 2023)

Risk	*Preferred regimen*	*Other options*
Favorable risk	Axitinib + Pembrolizumab (Category 1) Cabozantinib + Nivolumab (Category 1) Lenvatinib +Pembrolizumab (Category 1)	Axitinib + Avelumab Cabozantinib (Category 2B) Ipilimumab +Nivolumab Pazopanib Sunitinib
Intermediate and poor risk	Axitinib + Pembrolizumab (Category 1) Cabozantinib + Nivolumab (Category 1) Lenvatinib +Pembrolizumab (Category 1) Ipilimumab +Nivolumab (Category 1) Cabozantinib	Axitinib + Avelumab Pazopanib Sunitinib

11. What are the treatment choices in case on non-clear cell renal cell carcinoma?

Ans: For advanced non-clear cell disease, cabozantinib is a promising option. It was studied in a randomized study at 65 centers in North America and 147 patients were randomised to receive cabozantinib, sunitinib, crizotinib or salvotinib. The crizotinib and the salvotinib arms were halted after futility analysis. The response rate was 23% in cabozantinib group vs 4% in sunitinib group. The progression free survival favored the cabozantinib group 9 months (6–12 months) vs 5.6 months (3–7 months). Hence, it is now accepted as a drug of choice for non-clear cell advanced RCC[25] (Table 12.5).

Other drugs that can be useful in certain circumstances are:

1. Axitinib
2. Bevacizumab

TABLE 12.5: Treatment options for non-clear cell RCC

Preferred treatment	*Other regimens*
Clinical Trial	Lenvatinib + Everolimus
Cabozantinib	Nivolumab
Sunitinib	Nivolumab + Cabozantinib
	Pembrolizumab

3. Bevacizumab+ Erlotinib (For advance papillary RCC including HLRCC)
4. Bevacizumab + Everolimus
5. Erlotinib
6. Everolimus
7. Nivolumab +ipilimumab
8. Pazopanib
9. Temsirolimus (category 1 for poor risk group)

Case Scenario *(Contd.)*

Patient was started on T. Sunitinib. He took the drug for 2 months and then developed intolerance.

12. On what basis can one start use of TKI after the first line use of TKI?

Ans: Several phase III randomized controlled trials have shown superiority of TKIs over placebo for advanced ccRCC after initial use of TKI (Table 12.6).

13. What is the dose and duration of sunitinib and is it recommended as the first line for stage 4 disease?

Ans: Sunitinib is at present recommended as the first line option only for non-clear cell stage IV RCC who are not getting enrolled for clinical trial. It can be used as a second line in the clear cell RCC stage 4.

Dose: 50 mg/day

Regimen and Cycle:

1. 4 weeks continuous and 2 weeks rest: 6 weeks equals one cycle.
2. 2 weeks continuous and 1 week rest x 2: 6 weeks equals one cycle.

TABLE 12.6: Role of TKI after first line TKI in advance RCC

Parameter	*RECORD-1[26] Everolimus vs Placebo*	*AXIS[27] Axitinib vs Sorafenib*	*METEOR[28] Cabozantinib vs Everolimus*	*CheckMate 025[29] Nivolumab vs Everolimus*	*LEN EVE[30] Lenvatinib +Everolimus vs Everolimus*
Patients	410	723	658	821	153
MSKC risk (%)					
Good risk	29	28	46	36	23
Intermediate risk	56	37	42	49	36
Poor risk	15	33	13	15	40
Prior TKI	Anti-VEGF	Sunitinib	Anti-VEGF	Anti-VEGF	Anti-VEGF
ORR %	2 vs 0	19 vs 9	21 vs 5	25 vs 5	43 vs 3
Median OS (months)	14.8 vs 14.0	20.1 vs 19.2	vs 17.1	25 vs 19.6	

Dose reduction to 37.5 mg and subsequently 25 mg is possible.

14. When should you consider dose reduction of sunitinib?

Ans:

1. Intolerance
2. Absolute neutrophil count 1000/mm^3: Delay treatment
3. Platelet count: <75,000/microliter: Delay treatment.
4. CTC grade 3–4 toxicity: Delay treatment or reduce dose by 1 level.
5. Cardiac: If the decrease in left ventricular ejection fraction is more than 10%, consider holding the drug and lowering the dose. Evaluate 4 weekly if the trend is decreasing
6. Renal dysfunction: Can be given in mild renal dysfunction as its excretion is hepatic. Creatinine less than or equal to 2x the upper limit of normal is acceptable. No data is available for severe renal impairment.
7. Hepatic dysfunction: The excretion is hepatic, despite this fact, sunitinib can be given in mild liver dysfunction, meaning, if the bilirubin is less than or equal to 1.5 times the upper limit of normal, it can be safely administered.
8. Sunitinib-induced hypothyroidism: TSH levels should be checked at the start of every cycle for the 1st 4 cycles and then 3 monthly. Levothyroxine should be initiated at 25–50 μg orally if symptomatic and if TSH rises to more than 20 mU/L.
9. Hypertension: Hypertension may be caused and requires a rigorous control. Dose reduction may be required if the blood pressures are not getting controlled.

***Case Scenario** (Contd.)*

Was shifted to Tab. Axitinib for 1.5 years as he had intolerance to sunitinib. The disease remained radiologically stable on the same for 1.5 years.

15. The patient had brain metastasis at the outset. Is systemic therapy enough or are any extra measures required?

Ans: Brain metastasis occur in 17% metastatic RCC patients. The blood–brain barrier restricts the penetration of systemic therapy to these lesions. Surgical resection is often extremely challenging due to the patients' poor performance status.

Radiation therapy is an appealing treatment option. Traditionally, whole brain radiation was done (WBRT). With the advances in radiation technology, the paradigm has shifted towards stereotactic radiosurgery (SRS).[31]

SRS for RCC metastasis allows a greater dose per fraction to combat a traditionally radio-resistant tumor. With SRS, the neurocognitive toxicity is less and the outcome in terms of overall survival are comparable to whole brain radiation.[32] Local control rates have been very promising, ranging from 98 to 100%. SRS is a day-care procedure, can be delivered in very sick patients and can also be delivered at difficult locations deemed unfit for surgical resection.[33–36]

16. When would you consider genetic work-up of these patients?

Ans: The following are the indications to do a genetic work up:[37,38]

1. An individual with a close blood relative with a known pathogenic/likely pathogenic variant in a cancer susceptibility gene
2. Diagnosed at age of 46 years
3. Bilateral or multifocal tumors
4. 1 first-or second-degree relative with RCC
5. Multifocal papillary histology
6. HLRCC-associated RCC, RCC with fumarate hydratase (FH) deficiency or other histologic features associated with HLRCC
7. Birt-Hogg-Dubé syndrome (BHDS)-related histology (multiple chromophobe, oncocytoma, or oncocytic hybrid)
8. Angiomyolipomas of the kidney and one additional tuberous sclerosis complex (TSC) criterion in the same person
9. Succinate dehydrogenase (SDH)-deficient RCC histology
10. 2 first-or second-degree relatives with RCC (on the same side of the family)

Important Syndromes with their Features (Tables 12.7 and 12.8).

***Case Scenario** (Contd.)*

The patient progressed on axitinib at the end of 1.5 years

17. What should be the next line of treatment?

Ans: The patient should be started on immunotherapy.

- Patient received Inj. Nivolumab (6 cycles) + Lenvatinib and then Inj. Nivolumab (6 cycles) + Cabozantinib (Table 12.9).

18. What is the principal mechanism of action of modern-day immunotherapy?

Ans: Modern-day immunotherapy revolves around immune checkpoint inhibition. T cells are the cells responsible for destroying tumour cells. Immune checkpoints are a normal part of the immune mechanism of the human body. Immune

TABLE 12.7: Features of tuberous sclerosis complex

Major features	*Minor features*
Renal angiomyolipoma	Multiple renal cysts
Cardiac rhabdomyoma	Confetti lesion (multiple 1–3 mm hypopigmented macules scattered over regions of body such as arms and legs)
Cortical dysplasia, including tubers and cerebral white matter migration lines	Dental enamel pits (>3)
Angiofibromas (≥3) or fibrous cephalic plaque	Intraoral fibromas (≥2)
Hypermelanotic macules (3 to >5 mm in diameter)	Non-renal hamartomas
Lymphangioleiomyomatosis Multiple retinal nodular hamartomas Shagreen patch Subependymal nodules (SENs) Subependymal giant cell astrocytoma (SEGA) Ungual fibromas > 2	Retinal achromic patch

checkpoints have a role in regulating the immune response so that it does not destroy normal healthy cells. Checkpoint proteins, namely PD-1 on T cells and PD-L1 on tumour cells, modulate the immune response. The binding of PD-L1 to PD-1 sends an "off" signal to the T cell and prevents it from destroying the tumour cells. Immune checkpoint inhibitors work on the principle of blocking the

TABLE 12.8: Features of von Hippel-Lindau (vHL) disease

Major features	*Minor features*
Hemangioblastoma of the retina, spine or brain	Endolymphatic sac tumors
Clear cell RCC (ccRCC) diagnosed < 40 years of age or multiple bilateral ccRCC tumors diagnosed at any age	Papillary cystadenomas of the epididymis or broad ligament
PCCs	Pancreatic serous cystadenoma >1
Paraganglioma of abdomen, thorax or neck	Pancreatic neuroendocrine tumor (pNET) or multiple pancreatic cyst >1
Renal angiomas	

checkpoint proteins from binding to their partner proteins. When this happens, the "off" signal is not sent and hence the T cell kills the tumour cell[39] (Fig. 12.2).

Commonly used checkpoint inhibitors are:

Anti PD-1: Pembrolizumab and nivolumab

Anti PD-L1: Atezolizumab, avelumab and durvalumab

Anti CTLA-1: Ipilimumab, tremelimumab

19. What are the side effects of IO and TKI therapy?

Ans:

Common side effects of TKI therapy are:

- Diarrhoea
- Hypertension
- Stomatitis

TABLE 12.9: Subsequent lines of treatment for clear cell RCC

Past history of ICI	*Current recommendation*	*Can be considered*
No	Axitinib + pembrolizumab	Axitinib
	Cabozantinib	Everolimus
	Cabozantinib + nivolumab	Pazopanib
	Nivolumab + ipilimumab	Sunitinib
	Lenvatinib + everolimus	Tivozanib
	Lenvatinib + pembrolizumab	Belzutifan
	Nivolumab	Bevacizumab
Yes	Axitinib	Axitinib + Pembrolizumab
	Cabozantinib	Cabozantinib + nivolumab
	Lenvatinib +everolimus	Nivolumab + ipilimumab
	Tivozanib	Lenvatinib + pembrolizumab
		Everolimus
		Pazopanib
		Sunitinib

Note: Some other drugs that can be useful include
- High dose IL-2 for selected patients
- Temsirolimus
- Axitinib + avelumab
- Belzutifan and bevacizumab can be considered in patients treated with ICI in the past.

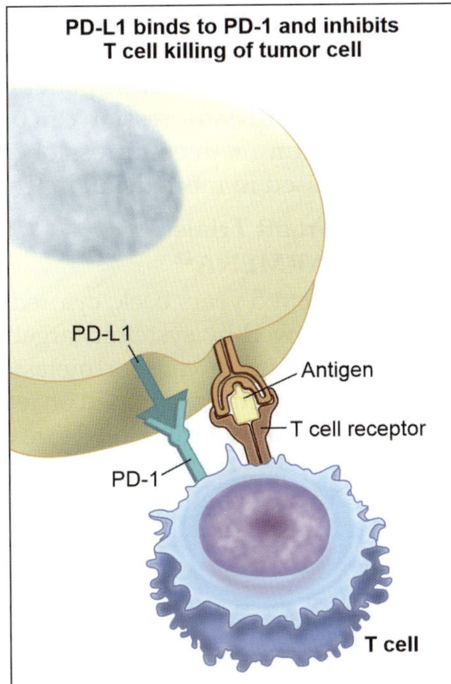

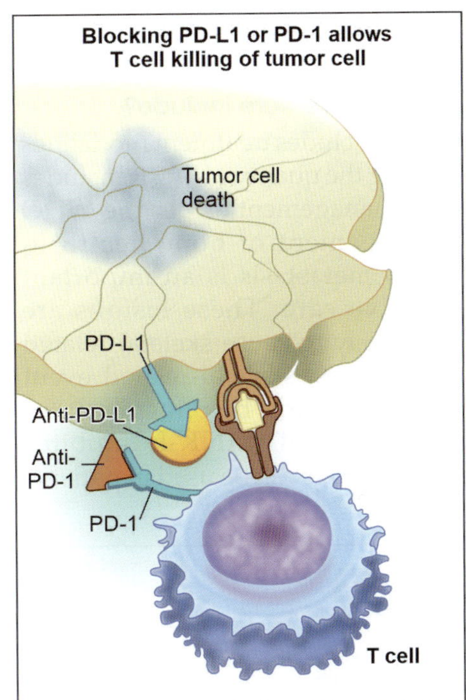

Fig. 12.2: Mechanism of action of immune checkpoint inhibitors

- Hypothyroidism
- Fatigue
- Hand-foot syndrome
- Decreased appetite
- Nausea
- Protienurea
- Dysgeusia
- Asthenia
- Rash
- Dysphonia.

Side effects of IO therapy are:

- Local: Pain, swelling, soreness, redness, rash, itchiness
- Flu-like symptoms: Chills, fever, weakness, dizziness, nausea/vomiting, muscle and joint pain, headache, breathing difficulty, hyper-hypotension
- Swelling and weight gain from water retention
- Palpitation
- Sinus congestion
- Organ inflammation: Pneumonitis, pancreatitis, gastroenteritis, hepatitis, colitis, hypophysistis, adrenalitis, thyroiditis, myocarditis.

Management of IO toxicity

- Withholding the drug
- Starting steroids for grade 3–4 toxicity
- Appropriate hormone replacement may be required.

20. How should you follow-up these patients?

Ans: These patients should be followed up every 6–16 weeks with detailed history and physical examination. Imaging should be done at the onset of any significant clinical finding or symptom. Before initiation of any new treatment regimen, a CT or MRI scan should be done. Subsequent imaging can again be done between 6 and 16 weeks at the discretion of the clinician. Bone scan at baseline and then at clinician's discretion. FDG PET is not recommended by guidelines but may have a potential role. Other laboratory evaluations may be carried out as per the requirements for the therapeutic agent being used.

21. The disease progressed on immunotherapy after 12 cycles. What is the best course of action now?

Ans: Third-line agents like a combination of Lenvatinib and everolimus can be used. Also, single agent Tivozanib and high dose IL-2 are options (Table 12.8). It is critical to evaluate the performance status and general health of the patient. Patients who have poor tolerance to systemic therapy should also be counselled for best supportive care.

22. What is Belzutifan?

Ans: Belzutifan is a HIF-2α inhibitor and has been approved in VHL patients. About 90% of the patients with sporadic ccRCC have a defective pVHL. HIF-2α is involved in activation of vascular endothelial growth factor, angiogenesis, metabolism and growth. So, it may be helpful in managing advanced RCCs. Also its combination with cabozantinib may potentially be useful in the near future.

23. **What does best supportive care include?**

Ans: Supportive care includes treatment modalities targeted at improving the quality of life. It includes symptomatic pain management as per the WHO pain ladder. Management of bone health in patients with bony metastasis is an important aspect of supportive care. These lesions are osteolytic and are likely to cause skeletal-related events.[40] Time to the first skeletal-related event can be prolonged by using bisphosphonates (e.g., zoledronic acid) and RANK-L inhibitor (Denosumab).[41] Both drugs can be used in patients with a creatinine clearance of >30 ml/min. Daily supplementation of calcium and vit D is strongly recommended in these patients. Pain arising from spinal cord compression can be mitigated by local radiation or decompression. Supportive care is discussed in more detail in Chapter 19.

Important Trials

A. CARMENA[42]

About 5 years back, cytoreductive nephrectomy followed by systemic targetted therapy was the standard of care for metastatic RCC. However, this practice was based on retrospective data. The CARMENA trial aimed to test this in a prospective RCT (Fig. 12.3 and Tables 12.10 to 12.12).

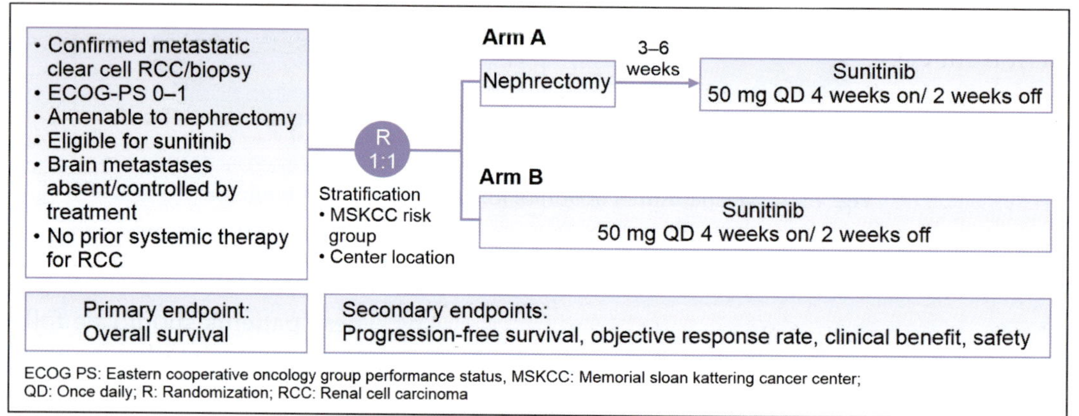

Fig. 12.3: CARMENA: Prospective, multicenter, open-label, randomized, phase-3 non-inferiority study

TABLE 12.10: Overall survival in the two arms of CARMENA

Population	*Arm A*			*Arm B*			*HR (95% CI), analysed by IMDC risk group*
	n	*Events, n (%)*	*Median (95% CI), months*	*n*	*Events, n (%)*	*Median (95% CI), months*	
Intention to treat	226	179 (79)	15.6 (12.5–18.6)	224	179 (80)	19.8 (15.6–24.8)	0.97 (0.79–1.19)

TABLE 12.11: Median overall survival in IMDC intermediate risk patients

Median OS, months (95% CI)	*Arm A: Nephrectomy + Sunitinib (n = 127)*	*Arm B: Sunitinib alone (n=139)*	*HR (95% CI)*	*p*
IMDC 1 risk factors	(*n* = 63) 31.4 (17.3–45.5)	(*n* = 63) 25.2 (19.6–35.4)	1.29 (0.85–1.98)	0.232
IMDC 2 risk factors	(*n* = 64) 17.6 (13.7–21.5)	(*n* = 76) 31.2 (20.5–40.4)	0.63 (0.44–0.97)	0.033

TABLE 12.12: Overall survival stratified by number of metastatic sites

Median OS, months (95% CI)	*Arm A: Nephrectomy + Sunitinib (n = 226)*	*Arm B: Sunitinib alone (n=224)*	*HR (95% CI)*	*p*
1 site	(*n* = 75) 23.2 (13.9–43.4)	(*n* = 68) 22.7 (17.5–33.1)	1.09 (0.75–1.59)	0.655
> 1 site	(*n* = 148) 14.4 (11.8–17.6)	(*n* = 155) 16.7 (13.8–24.8)	0.87 (0.70–1.20)	0.284

Conclusions

At a median follow-up of 50 months, sunitinib alone was found to be non-inferior to cytoreductive nephrectomy followed by sunitinib.

Upfront cytoreductive nephrectomy may be beneficial in patients with one IMDC risk factor. Presence of >3 sites of metastasis and liver metastasis were associated with poor survival.

Critical analysis of CARMENA

- Included only intermediate and poor risk patients
- Accrual was slow (<1 per year per centre) and incomplete (planned for 576), this reflects difficulty in enrolment and selection bias.
- Previous retrospective studies had already indicated that poor risk patients do not benefit from CN
- Considerable shorter OS in both arms compared to previously reported similar cohorts
- Median size of primary was 88 mm and median total tumor burden was 140 mm. So metastatic disease contributed 40% to the total tumor burden. Thus, cytoreduction in the true sense was not possible for many patients.

B. SURTIME[43]:

The SURTIME trial aimed to determine the right sequencing of cytoreductive nephrectomy and sunitinib for metastatic RCC (Figs 12.4 and 12.5).

- Median OS of 32.4 months in the deferred CN arm and 15 months in the immediate CN arm.
- In the deferred CN arm, 48 of 49 patients received sunitinib vs 40 of 50 in the immediate arm.

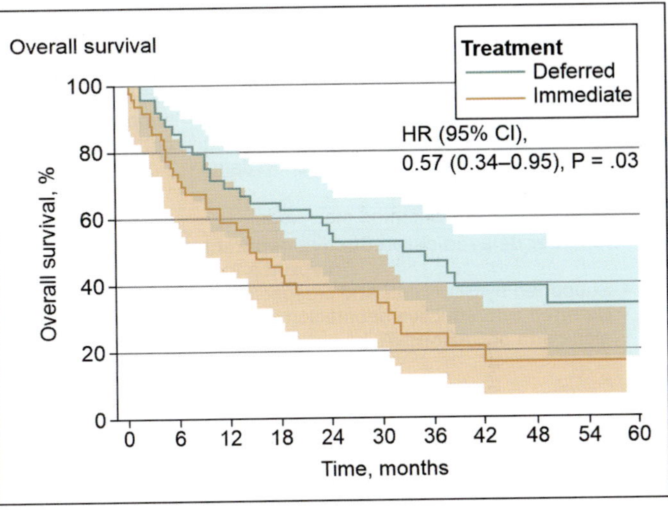

Fig. 12.5: Results of surtime trial

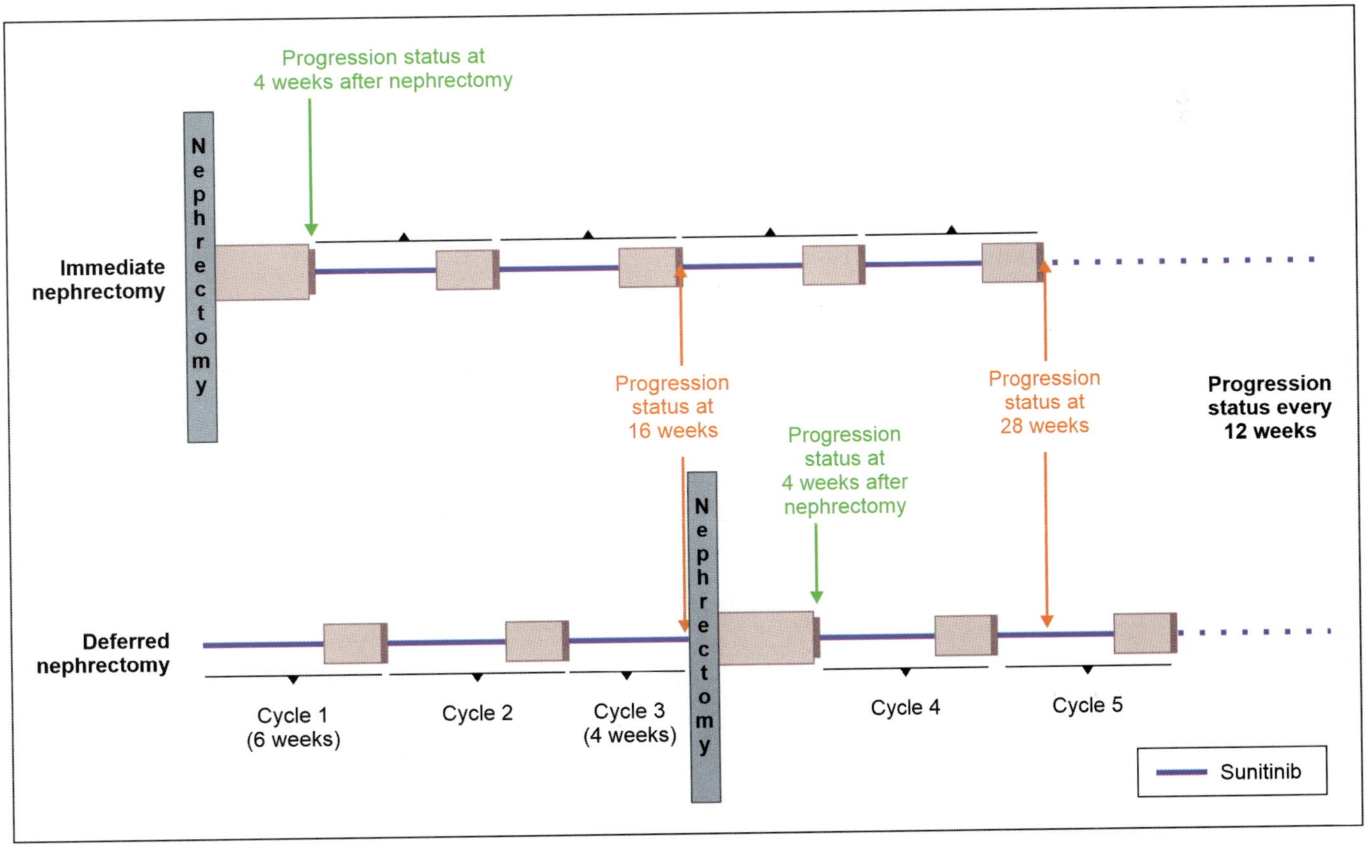

Fig. 12.4: Trial design of SURTIME trial

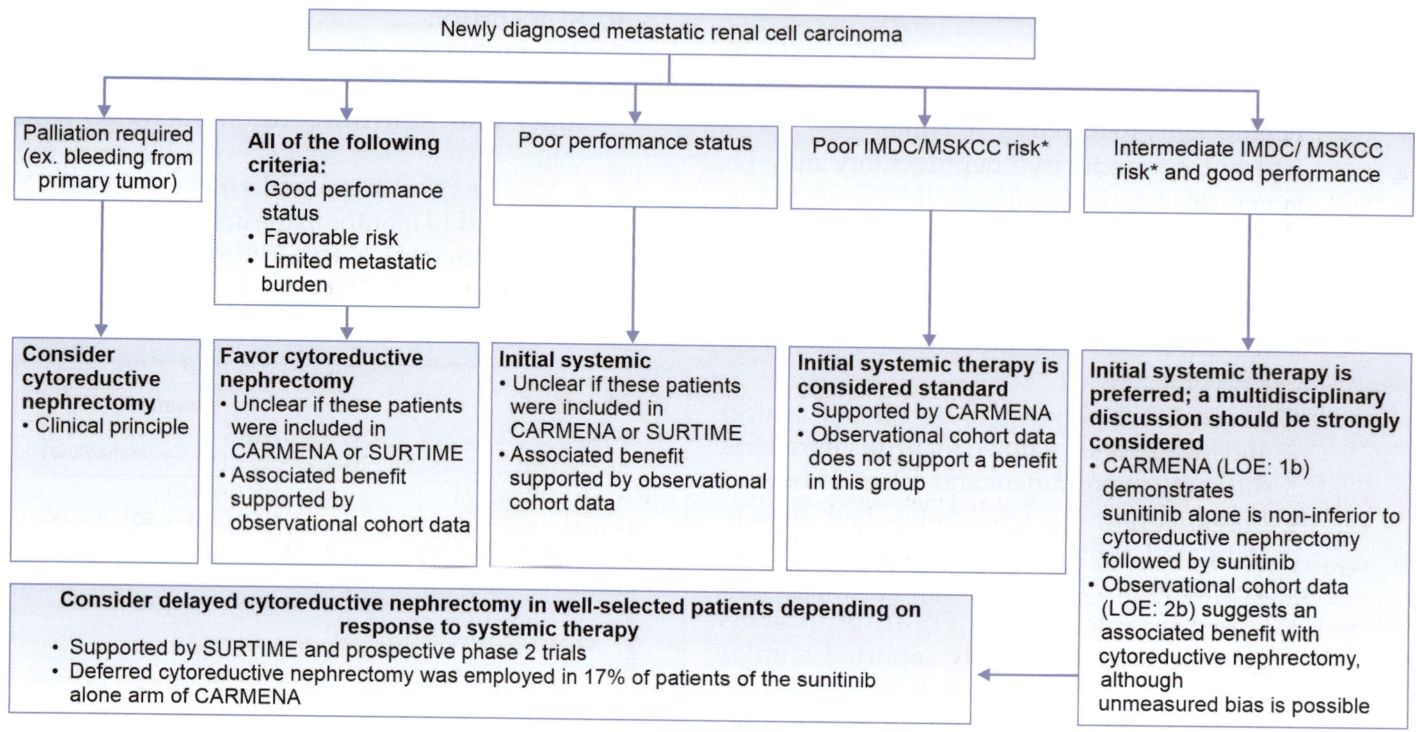

Fig. 12.6: Individualised decision making for metastatic RCC patients

- Systemic progression before planned CN in the deferred arm resulted in a recommendation against nephrectomy in 14 patients (29%).

Conclusions

- With the deferred approach, more patients received sunitinib and OS results were higher.
- Pretreatment with sunitinib may identify patients with inherent resistance to systemic therapy before planned CN.

Critical analysis of SURTIME

- Poor accrual—only 99 patients
- 19% of patients did not receive the therapy that they were assigned (Fig. 12.6).

SUMMARY

- Contrast-enhanced CT of the chest, abdomen and pelvis is the most commonly ordered investigation for advanced RCC. The role of FDG PET scan is evolving. RCC has limited FDG-avidity.
- Renal mass biopsy should be done percutaneously under image guidance. Ultrasound guidance is the preferred choice as it is a dynamic investigation. The risk of tract-seeding is theoretical.
- Risk stratification of metastatic RCC enables prognostication and helps clinicians choose the best possible therapeutic option between upfront surgery vs systemic therapy.
- The role of cytoreductive nephrectomy has definitely gone down as compared to the cytokine era. Even in the era of tyrosine kinase inhibitors and immunotherapy, patients with favorable and intermediate risk may benefit with a cytoreductive nephrectomy.
- Clear cell renal cell carcinoma is the most common histological variant and it responds well to both TKI and immunotherapy. Patients with sarcomatoid differentiation respond poorly to all types of therapies.
- A combination of immunotherapy and tyrosine kinase inhibitors has now become the first therapeutic choice for metastatic RCC. A combination of two immune checkpoint inhibitors can also be used.
- A younger patient with a positive family history or with a symptom-complex suggestive of a syndrome should definitely undergo genetic analysis.
- ICIs are now the first-line agents in metastatic RCC. They alone or in combination with TKIs significantly improve the PFS and OS across all the groups of risk stratification.
- Patients on systemic therapy require a clinical and radiological follow-up between 6 and 16 weeks. If the disease is stable, 4 monthly follow-up is acceptable. A baseline imaging and imaging at suspected progression and before changing the line of therapy should be strongly considered.
- Supportive care is focused on maintaining the quality of life during and after the exhaustion of drug therapy directed at improving overall survival. Components of supportive care include pain management, use of bisphosphonates and RANK-L inhibitors to prevent skeletal-related events, and local radiation for spinal/brain metastasis.

REFERENCES

1. Caoili EM, Davenport MS. Role of Percutaneous Needle Biopsy for Renal Masses. Semin Intervent Radiol. 2014 Mar;31(1):20–6.
2. Oken MM, Creech RH, Tormey DC, Horton J, Davis TE, McFadden ET, *et al.* Toxicity and response criteria of the Eastern Cooperative Oncology Group. Am J Clin Oncol. 1982 Dec;5(6):649–55.

3. Karnofsky D. The clinical evaluation of chemotherapeutic agents in cancer. In 1949 [cited 2023 Mar 8]. Available from: https://www.semanticscholar.org/paper/The-clinical-evaluation-of-chemotherapeutic-agents-Karnofsky/ee9f2644a4ef6a7b18f787b5d46a32b131791d66
4. Karivedu V, Jain AL, Eluvathingal TJ, Sidana A. Role of Positron Emission Tomography Imaging in Metabolically Active Renal Cell Carcinoma. Curr Urol Rep. 2019 Aug 29;20(10):56.
5. Elahmadawy MA, Elazab MSS, Ahmed S, Salama M. Diagnostic value of F-18 FDG PET/CT for local and distant disease relapse surveillance in surgically treated RCC patients: Can it aid in establishing consensus follow up strategy? Nucl Med Rev Cent East Eur. 2018;21(2):85–91.
6. Ma H, Shen G, Liu B, Yang Y, Ren P, Kuang A. Diagnostic performance of 18F-FDG PET or PET/CT in restaging renal cell carcinoma: a systematic review and meta-analysis. Nucl Med Commun. 2017 Feb;38(2):156–63.
7. Ferda J, Ferdova E, Hora M, Hes O, Finek J, Topolcan O, *et al.* 18F-FDG-PET/CT in potentially advanced renal cell carcinoma: a role in treatment decisions and prognosis estimation. Anticancer Res. 2013 Jun;33(6):2665–72.
8. Caldarella C, Muoio B, Isgrò MA, Porfiri E, Treglia G, Giovanella L. The role of fluorine-18-fluorodeoxyglucose positron emission tomography in evaluating the response to tyrosine-kinase inhibitors in patients with metastatic primary renal cell carcinoma. Radiol Oncol. 2014 Jul 10;48(3):219–27.
9. Namura K, Minamimoto R, Yao M, Makiyama K, Murakami T, Sano F, *et al.* Impact of maximum standardized uptake value (SUV_{max}) evaluated by 18-Fluoro-2-deoxy-D-glucose positron emission tomography/computed tomography (18F-FDG-PET/CT) on survival for patients with advanced renal cell carcinoma: a preliminary report. BMC Cancer. 2010 Dec 3;10:667.
10. Hugonnet F, Fournier L, Medioni J, Smadja C, Hindié E, Huchet V, *et al.* Metastatic renal cell carcinoma: relationship between initial metastasis hypoxia, change after 1 month's sunitinib, and therapeutic response: an 18F-fluoromisonidazole PET/CT study. J Nucl Med. 2011 Jul;52(7):1048–55.
11. Horn KP, Yap JT, Agarwal N, Morton KA, Kadrmas DJ, Beardmore B, *et al.* FDG and FLT-PET for Early measurement of response to 37.5 mg daily sunitinib therapy in metastatic renal cell carcinoma. Cancer Imaging. 2015 Sep 3;15(1):15.
12. Phase 3 ZIRCON Study Shows High Sensitivity/Specificity With 89Zr-DFO-girentuximab in ccRCC [Internet]. Targeted Oncology. 2023 [cited 2023 May 24]. Available from: https://www.targetedonc.com/view/phase-3-zircon-study-shows-high-sensitivity-specificity-with-89zr-dfo-girentuximab-in-ccrcc
13. Kelly-Morland C, Rudman S, Nathan P, Mallett S, Montana G, Cook G, *et al.* Evaluation of treatment response and resistance in metastatic renal cell cancer (mRCC) using integrated 18F–Fluorodeoxyglucose (18F–FDG) positron emission tomography/magnetic resonance imaging (PET/MRI); The REMAP study. BMC Cancer. 2017 Jun 2;17:392.
14. Motzer RJ, Bacik J, Murphy BA, Russo P, Mazumdar M. Interferon-alfa as a comparative treatment for clinical trials of new therapies against advanced renal cell carcinoma. J Clin Oncol. 2002 Jan 1;20(1):289–96.
15. Heng DYC, Xie W, Regan MM, Warren MA, Golshayan AR, Sahi C, *et al.* Prognostic factors for overall survival in patients with metastatic renal cell carcinoma treated with vascular endothelial growth factor-targeted agents: results from a large, multicenter study. J Clin Oncol. 2009 Dec 1;27(34):5794–9.
16. Mekhail TM, Abou-Jawde RM, Boumerhi G, Malhi S, Wood L, Elson P, *et al.* Validation and extension of the Memorial Sloan-Kettering prognostic factors model for survival in patients with previously untreated metastatic renal cell carcinoma. J Clin Oncol. 2005 Feb 1;23(4):832–41.
17. Rini BI, Plimack ER, Stus V, Gafanov R, Hawkins R, Nosov D, *et al.* Pembrolizumab plus Axitinib versus Sunitinib for Advanced Renal-Cell Carcinoma. New England Journal of Medicine. 2019 Mar 21;380(12):1116–27.
18. Powles T, Plimack ER, Soulières D, Waddell T, Stus V, Gafanov R, *et al.* Pembrolizumab plus axitinib versus sunitinib monotherapy as first-line treatment of advanced renal cell carcinoma (KEYNOTE-426): extended follow-up from a randomised, open-label, phase 3 trial. Lancet Oncol. 2020 Dec;21(12):1563–73.
19. Choueiri TK, Powles T, Burotto M, Escudier B, Bourlon MT, Zurawski B, *et al.* Nivolumab plus Cabozantinib versus Sunitinib for Advanced Renal-Cell Carcinoma. New England Journal of Medicine. 2021 Mar 4;384(9):829–41.
20. Cella D, Motzer RJ, Suarez C, Blum SI, Ejzykowicz F, Hamilton M, *et al.* Patient-reported outcomes with first-line nivolumab plus cabozantinib versus sunitinib in patients with advanced renal cell carcinoma treated in CheckMate 9ER: an open-label, randomised, phase 3 trial. Lancet Oncol. 2022 Feb;23(2):292–303.
21. Motzer RJ, Powles T, Burotto M, Escudier B, Bourlon MT, Shah AY, *et al.* Nivolumab plus cabozantinib versus sunitinib in first-line treatment for advanced renal cell carcinoma (CheckMate 9ER): long-term follow-up results from an open-label, randomised, phase 3 trial. The Lancet Oncology. 2022 Jul 1;23(7):888–98.
22. Motzer RJ, Tannir NM, McDermott DF, Arén Frontera O, Melichar B, Choueiri TK, *et al.* Nivolumab plus Ipilimumab versus Sunitinib in Advanced Renal-Cell Carcinoma. N Engl J Med. 2018 Apr 5;378(14):1277–90.
23. Motzer RJ, Penkov K, Haanen J, Rini B, Albiges L, Campbell MT, *et al.* Avelumab plus Axitinib versus Sunitinib for Advanced Renal-Cell Carcinoma. N Engl J Med. 2019 Mar 21;380(12):1103–15.
24. Motzer R, Alekseev B, Rha SY, Porta C, Eto M, Powles T, *et al.* Lenvatinib plus Pembrolizumab or Everolimus for Advanced Renal Cell Carcinoma. N Engl J Med. 2021 Apr 8;384(14):1289–300.
25. Pal SK, Tangen C, Thompson IM, Balzer-Haas N, George DJ, Heng DYC, *et al.* A comparison of sunitinib with cabozantinib, crizotinib, and savolitinib for treatment of advanced papillary renal cell carcinoma: a randomised, open-label, phase 2 trial. Lancet. 2021 Feb 20;397(10275):695–703.
26. Motzer RJ, Escudier B, Oudard S, Hutson TE, Porta C, Bracarda S, *et al.* Phase 3 trial of everolimus for metastatic renal cell carcinoma : final results and analysis of prognostic factors. Cancer. 2010 Sep 15;116(18):4256–65.
27. Rini BI, Escudier B, Tomczak P, Kaprin A, Szczylik C, Hutson TE, *et al.* Comparative effectiveness of axitinib versus sorafenib in advanced renal cell carcinoma (AXIS): a randomised phase 3 trial. Lancet. 2011 Dec 1;378(9807):1931–9.
28. Choueiri TK, Escudier B, Powles T, Mainwaring P, Rini BI, Donskov F, *et al.* Cabozantinib versus everolimus in advanced renal cell carcinoma. N Engl J Med. 2015 Nov 5;373(19):1814–23.

29. Cella D, Grünwald V, Nathan P, Doan J, Dastani H, Taylor F, *et al.* Quality of life in patients with advanced renal cell carcinoma given nivolumab versus everolimus in CheckMate 025: a randomised, open-label, phase 3 trial. Lancet Oncol. 2016 Jul;17(7):994–1003.
30. Motzer RJ, Hutson TE, Glen H, Michaelson MD, Molina A, Eisen T, *et al.* Lenvatinib, everolimus, and the combination in patients with metastatic renal cell carcinoma: a randomised, phase 2, open-label, multicentre trial. Lancet Oncol. 2015 Nov;16(15):1473–82.
31. Du Y, Pahernik S, Hadaschik B, Teber D, Duensing S, Jäger D, *et al.* Impact of resection and systemic therapy on the survival of patients with brain metastasis of metastatic renal cell carcinoma. J Neurooncol. 2016 Oct;130(1):221–8.
32. Chang EL, Wefel JS, Hess KR, Allen PK, Lang FF, Kornguth DG, *et al.* Neurocognition in patients with brain metastases treated with radiosurgery or radiosurgery plus whole-brain irradiation: a randomised controlled trial. Lancet Oncol. 2009 Nov;10(11):1037–44.
33. Wardak Z, Christie A, Bowman A, Stojadinovic S, Nedzi L, Barnett S, *et al.* Stereotactic Radiosurgery for Multiple Brain Metastases From Renal-Cell Carcinoma. Clin Genitourin Cancer. 2019 Apr;17(2):e273–80.
34. Shuto T, Matsunaga S, Suenaga J, Inomori S, Fujino H. Treatment strategy for metastatic brain tumors from renal cell carcinoma: selection of gamma knife surgery or craniotomy for control of growth and peritumoral edema. J Neurooncol. 2010 Jun;98(2):169–75.
35. Muacevic A, Kreth FW, Mack A, Tonn JC, Wowra B. Stereotactic radiosurgery without radiation therapy providing high local tumor control of multiple brain metastases from renal cell carcinoma. Minim Invasive Neurosurg. 2004 Aug;47(4): 203–8.
36. Noel G, Valery CA, Boisserie G, Cornu P, Hasboun D, Marc Simon J, *et al.* LINAC radiosurgery for brain metastasis of renal cell carcinoma. Urol Oncol. 2004;22(1):25–31.
37. Hampel H, Bennett RL, Buchanan A, Pearlman R, Wiesner GL, Guideline Development Group, American College of Medical Genetics and Genomics Professional Practice and Guidelines Committee and National Society of Genetic Counselors Practice Guidelines Committee. A practice guideline from the American College of Medical Genetics and Genomics and the National Society of Genetic Counselors: referral indications for cancer predisposition assessment. Genet Med. 2015 Jan;17(1):70–87.
38. Shuch B, Vourganti S, Ricketts CJ, Middleton L, Peterson J, Merino MJ, *et al.* Defining early-onset kidney cancer: implications for germline and somatic mutation testing and clinical management. J Clin Oncol. 2014 Feb 10;32 (5):431–7.
39. Francis DM, Thomas SN. Progress and opportunities for enhancing the delivery and efficacy of checkpoint inhibitors for cancer immunotherapy. Adv Drug Deliv Rev. 2017 May 15;114:33–42.
40. Zekri J, Ahmed N, Coleman RE, Hancock BW. The skeletal metastatic complications of renal cell carcinoma. Int J Oncol. 2001 Aug;19(2):379–82.
41. Roza T, Hakim L, van Poppel H, Joniau S. Bone-targeted therapies for elderly patients with renal cell carcinoma: current and future directions. Drugs Aging. 2013 Nov;30(11): 877–86.
42. Méjean A, Ravaud A, Thezenas S, Colas S, Beauval JB, Bensalah K, *et al.* Sunitinib Alone or after Nephrectomy in Metastatic Renal-Cell Carcinoma. New England Journal of Medicine. 2018 Aug 2;379(5):417–27.
43. Bex A, Mulders P, Jewett M, Wagstaff J, van Thienen JV, Blank CU, *et al.* Comparison of Immediate vs Deferred Cytoreductive Nephrectomy in Patients With Synchronous Metastatic Renal Cell Carcinoma Receiving Sunitinib: The SURTIME Randomized Clinical Trial. JAMA Oncology. 2019 Feb 1;5(2):164–70.

Chapter
13

Stage I Germ Cell Tumor

• Uday Pratap Singh • Sanjoy Surekha

LEARNING OBJECTIVES

- To know how to evaluate a patient with a testicular lesion/swelling: Every patient with a testicular lesion should be viewed with suspicion for testicular cancer and should be evaluated with a testicular ultrasound and tumor markers.
- To know the role of tumor markers: AFP, β-hCG and LDH are the three tumor markers used to evaluate testicular cancer. These should be performed before and after the orchidectomy.
- To understand the role of imaging: Every patient with a diagnosis of testicular cancer should be imaged with a CECT of the chest, abdomen and pelvis to complete staging evaluation.
- To know how to perform a high inguinal orchidectomy: High inguinal orchidectomy is the standard of care for a testicular mass with the clinical diagnosis of testicular malignancy.
- To understand the high risk features of stage 1 GCTs: Patients with certain high risk features on pathology have a higher chance of micrometastatic disease and should be offered active treatment.
- To understand the treatment options for stage 1 seminoma: Surveillance, radiation therapy and single agent carboplatin are the three options for stage 1 seminoma patients. The choice of treatment depends on the risk factors seen on the pathology of the orchidectomy specimen.
- To understand the treatment options for stage 1 NSGCT: Surveillance, RPLND and one cycle of BEP are the options for stage 1 NSGCT. The choice of treatment depends on the risk factors seen on the pathology of the orchidectomy specimen.
- To understand the follow-up protocol for stage 1 GCT patients: These patients need to be on a strict follow-up protocol with physical examination, tumor markers and imaging.

Case Scenario

A 29-year-old male, married with one child, with no medical risk factors, was evaluated for swelling in the left hemi-scrotum and was found to have a left testicular mass. Ultrasound scrotum reported a hetero-echoic rounded mass of 5 × 5 cm in the left scrotal sac with multiple internal cystic areas and increased internal vascularity. Serum tumor markers were elevated (β-hCG—41.82 mIU/ml, alpha-fetoprotein—357 ng/ml and LDH—350).

1. How does testicular cancer clinically present?

Ans:

- The usual presentation is that of a painless testicular mass. Sometimes it may present as an incidental finding on ultrasound. Pain in the scrotum, abdomen, or back due to other etiology may cause a delay in diagnosis. Some patients may have gynecomastia. Patients may also present with a lump in the abdomen or chest-related symptoms in the advanced stages of the disease.
- A comprehensive assessment should include an abdominal, chest, and supraclavicular examination.

2. What are the risk factors for testicular cancer?

Ans:

- The testicular dysgenesis syndrome, which includes cryptorchidism, hypospadias, reduced spermatogenesis, impaired fertility, and disorders/differences in sex development, are epidemiological risk factors for testicular cancer.
- First-degree relatives with a history of testicular cancer and the existence of a contralateral testicular tumor or GCNIS (germ cell neoplasia *in situ*) are additional risk factors.

- At diagnosis, 1–2% are bilateral. For patients with non-seminomatous germ cell tumors (NSGCT) and mixed germ cell tumors, the peak incidence occurs in the third decade of life; for those with seminoma testis (ST), it occurs in the fourth decade.

3. What is the role of various imaging modalities in assessing testicular cancer?

Ans:

- ***USG:***
  - High frequency (7.5/10 MHz, linear probe) testicular USG to determine the mass location, volume, and internal vascularity and screen the contralateral testicle.
  - Men presenting with retroperitoneal or visceral mass with or without raised serum tumor markers without palpable testicular mass should also undergo a scrotal ultrasound.[5]
  - USG testis should be done in all individuals with testicular swelling as it will help diagnose the lesion and also help screen the opposite testis.
  - On ultrasound, the typical GCT is hypoechoic, with heterogeneous echotexture more commonly associated with NSGCT. Seminomas usually have a homogenous echotexture.
  - The association between testicular microlithiasis and GCT is not clearly defined, and this alone should not prompt further evaluation.
  - In men with advanced GCT and a normal testicular examination, scrotal ultrasonography should be performed to rule out the presence of a small, impalpable scar or calcification, indicating a "burned-out" primary testis tumor.
  - In 5% of GCT patients, the primary site is at an extragonadal location, with no tumor on USG (primary retroperitoneal GCT).
- ***Contrast-enhanced computed tomography (CECT) chest, abdomen, and pelvis*** is recommended in all patients for staging before or after orchidectomy.[6]
  - The CT gives information about the N and M staging, the location of the retroperitoneal nodal lesions and status of the kidneys.
- ***Magnetic resonance imaging (MRI):***
  - Scrotal MRI can be used in patients with indeterminate findings on ultrasound. It helps differentiate between para-testicular and intratesticular tumors and characterize intratesticular masses.[7]
  - MRI of the abdomen can be used for staging purposes if there is a contraindication to radiation or iodine-based media with an accuracy similar to CECT in detecting the retroperitoneal lymph nodes.[6]
- ***Fluorodeoxyglucose-positron emission tomography (FDG-PET):*** There is currently no role of FDG-PET in the initial staging of testicular cancer.[8]

4. What staging system is used for carcinoma testis?

Ans: The 2016 Tumor, Node, Metastasis (TNM) classification of the International Union Against Cancer (UICC) is recommended to assess the anatomical extent of the disease[1] (Table 13.1).

TABLE 13.1: TNM classification for testicular cancer (adapted from UICC, 2016, 8th edn.)

pT	Primary tumor
pTx	Primary tumor cannot be assessed
pT0	No evidence of a primary tumor
pTis	Intratubular germ cell neoplasia
pT1	Tumor limited to testis and epididymis without vascular/lymphatic invasion; tumor may invade tunica albuginea but not tunica vaginalis
pT2	Tumor limited to testis and epididymis with vascular/lymphatic invasion, or tumor extending through tunica albuginea with involvement of tunica vaginalis
pT3	Tumor invades spermatic cord with or without vascular/lymphatic invasion
pT4	Tumor invades scrotum with or without vascular/lymphatic invasion
N	**Regional lymph nodes—clinical**
Nx	Regional lymph nodes cannot be assessed
N0	No regional lymph node metastasis
N1	Metastasis with a lymph node mass 2 cm or less in the greatest dimension or multiple lymph nodes, none more than 2 cm in the greatest dimension

(Contd.)

TABLE 13.1: TNM classification for testicular cancer (adapted from UICC, 2016, 8th edn.) *(Contd.)*

N2	Metastasis with a lymph node mass more than 2 cm but not more than 5 cm in greatest dimension; or more than five nodes positive, not more than 5 cm; or evidence of extranodal extension of tumor		
N3	Metastasis with a lymph node mass of more than 5 cm in the greatest dimension		
pN	**Regional lymph nodes—pathological**		
pNx	Regional lymph nodes cannot be assessed		
pN0	No regional lymph node metastasis		
pN1	Metastasis with a lymph node mass 2 cm or less in the greatest dimension and five or fewer positive nodes, not more than 2 cm in the greatest dimension		
pN2	Metastasis with a lymph node mass more than 2 cm but not more than 5 cm in greatest dimension; or more than five nodes positive, not more than 5 cm; or evidence of extranodal extension of tumor		
pN3	Metastasis with a lymph node mass of more than 5 cm in the greatest dimension		
M	**Distant Metastasis**		
Mx	Distant metastasis cannot be assessed		
M0	No distant metastasis		
M1	Distant metastasis M1a—non-regional lymph node(s) or lung metastasis M1b—distant metastasis other than non-regional lymph nodes and lung		
S	**Serum Tumor Markers (Prechemotherapy)**		
Sx	Serum marker studies not available or not performed		
S0	Serum marker study levels within normal limits		
	LDH (U/l)	**hCG (mIU/ml)**	**AFP (ng/ml)**
S1	<1.5 times the upper normal limit and	<5000 and	<1000
S2	1.5–10 times the normal upper limit or	5000–50000 or	1000–10000
S3	>10 times the normal upper limit	>50000	>10000

LDH: Lactate dehydrogenase; hCG: Human chorionic gonadotrophin; AFP: Alpha-fetoprotein

5. Which tumors are included in stage I?

Ans: Patients with primary tumors are limited to testis and epididymis or a more locally invasive primary tumor but no sign of metastatic disease[1] (Table 13.2).

Stage IA: Primary tumor limited to testis and epididymis, with no evidence of vascular or lymphatic invasion, no sign of metastases on imaging, and post-orchidectomy serum tumor markers within normal limits.

Stage IB: Patients have more locally invasive primary tumors, but no sign of metastatic disease.

Stage IS: Patients have persistently elevated serum tumor markers after orchidectomy, indicating the presence of subclinical metastatic disease.

6. What are the risk factors for relapse in clinical stage I testicular cancer?

Ans:

- In ***seminoma***, primary testicular tumor size and stromal invasion of rete testis are associated with the risk of relapse.[2] The absence of both risk factors is associated with a low rate of recurrence (6%).[3]
- LVI, tumor size, and rete testis invasion are not yet validated as prognostic factors as per the NCCN 2023 guidelines.
- In **NSGCT**, lymphovascular invasion (LVI) is strongly associated with the risk of disease relapse.[4] The risk of relapse at five years is 50% for LVI-positive tumors, while it is 15% for LVI-

TABLE 13.2: Prognostic groups for testicular cancer (UICC, 2016, 8th ed.)

Stage grouping	*T*	*N*	*M*	*S*
Stage I	pT1-T4	N0	M0	Sx
Stage IA	pT1	N0	M0	S0
Stage IB	pT2–pT4	N0	M0	S0
Stage IS	Any pT/Tx	N0	M0	S1–3

negative tumors. Also, undifferentiated cells, infiltration of the tunica albuginea, and the absence of yolk sac elements are associated risk factors for relapse.

7. What are the different serum tumor markers associated with testicular cancer, and what is their role?

Ans: Serum alpha-fetoprotein (AFP), beta subunit of human chorionic gonadotropin (β-hCG), and LDH are the serum tumor markers. Their levels should be assessed before and after orchidectomy (Table 13.3).

- ***Pre-operative serum tumor markers*** support the diagnosis of testicular cancer and may indicate GCT histology. Up to 90% of NSGCT have raised AFP or β-hCG at diagnosis, with 39% having increased serum levels of both. Sometimes, pure seminomas may have modestly elevated β-hCG levels at diagnosis in up to 30%. Significant elevation of AFP in seminomas may raise concerns for a missed NSGCT component.[9] However, serum tumor markers are known to have low sensitivity, and their normal levels do not exclude the presence of disease.[10] Serum LDH indicates the burden of disease.
- ***Post-orchidectomy serum tumor markers*** help in staging and prognostication.[11] Post-operatively normalization of tumor marker levels may take several weeks. If still elevated, metastatic disease is a possibility. The normalization of marker levels cannot always exclude metastatic disease. They also help in assessing treatment response as well as the detection of disease relapse.[12]
- Micro-RNAs (miRNAs) are potential new biomarkers emerging as tools with better accuracy than conventional tumor markers.[13] These are non-coding RNAs that regulate gene expression. miRNAs bind to complementary sequences in the 3′–untranslated region (UTR) of target mRNA and cause gene silencing. This, in turn, causes the induction of mRNA degradation and inhibition of protein translation. Increases in miRNA-371a-3p in GCT have been seen to correlate with stage, response to therapy, relapse, and residual significant malignant GCT (not teratoma).

8. What is the procedure done for histopathologically diagnosing testicular cancer?

Ans:

- Standard procedure for histopathological diagnosis is a high inguinal orchidectomy. The spermatic cord is ligated with a non-absorbable suture at the deep inguinal ring. A scrotal approach for orchidectomy is avoided when testicular cancer is suspected as it violates natural planes of progression and upstages the disease with a higher local recurrence rate.[14]
- **Steps of high inguinal orchidectomy:**
  1. **Preparation and positioning:** Supine—lower abdomen area cleaned with a scrub and sterile drape placed to expose the ipsilateral inguinal region and hemiscrotum.
  2. **Incision:** Oblique incision starting 2 cm above and lateral to the pubic tubercle along Langer's line parallel to the inguinal ligament extending laterally towards the anterior superior iliac spine (ASIS), length of incision may range from 3 to 10 cm and guided by the size of the testicular mass. The inguinal incision can be extended towards the scrotum to facilitate a large testicular tumor delivery.
  3. **Exposure:** External oblique (EO) aponeurosis is exposed and cleaned of subcutaneous fat. It is sharply incised to open the roof of the inguinal canal from the superficial inguinal ring to the deep inguinal ring.

TABLE 13.3: Serum tumor markers associated with testicular carcinoma

Tumor marker (normal range)	*Raised in GCT*	*Half-life*	*Comments*
AFP (<40 μg/L)	NSGCT (embryonal carcinoma, yolk sac tumor, teratoma) Never raised in seminoma or choriocarcinoma	5–7 days	Any patient with elevated AFP must have a non-seminomatous component
hCG (<5 IU/L)	All NSGCT; higher levels are associated with worse prognosis 15% of seminomas	24–36 hours	In both seminomas and NSGCT, cancerous cells can transform into syncytiotrophoblasts and secrete hCG. Cross-reactive with LH. Falsely elevated in hypogonadal men.
LDH (1.5–3.2 μkat/L)	No specific association	24 hours	Less specific than others; correlate to high tumor burden

The ilioinguinal nerve is identified on the anterior surface of the spermatic cord and freed from the external spermatic fascia and cremasteric muscle. Injury to this nerve can cause chronic post-operative pain and paraesthesia of the upper thigh.

4. **Dissection of the spermatic cord:** Spermatic cord mobilized at the level of the pubic tubercle using blunt dissection to develop the plane between the cord and the floor of the inguinal canal. Dissection through the inguinal canal floor can cause a risk of post-operative direct inguinal hernia. Once mobilized, the spermatic cord is encircled with a Penrose drain and secured with a clamp just distal to the internal inguinal ring. This causes early control over vasculature and helps in the traction of the cord to facilitate delivery of the testis.
5. **Delivery of the testicle:** Gentle traction is applied to the spermatic cord in the cephalad direction along with external pressure at the ipsilateral hemiscrotum, and the testis, with its tunica vaginalis, is pushed into the surgical field. Investing fascial layers over the tunica vaginalis are dissected. Gubernaculum is divided at the most inferior aspect of the testis. The testis, with its tunica vaginalis, is free and attached only by the spermatic cord.
6. **Ligation of the spermatic cord:** The spermatic cord is mobilized to the level of the deep inguinal ring. The proximal point of mobilization is taken at the point of peritoneal reflection, where the vas deferens diverge from the spermatic vessels. This is important as it facilitates complete resection of the inguinal spermatic cord. High cord ligation gives oncological control and facilitates subsequent RPLND if required, as cord structures retract in the retroperitoneal space.
   The spermatic cord is advised to be divided using a triple-clamp approach, in which two clamps are positioned at the level of the internal ring proximal to the Penrose tourniquet, and a third clamp is positioned distally to the tourniquet.
   The cord can then be transected, the specimen removed, and non-absorbable sutures applied to the proximal stump, which retracts in the retroperitoneum.
   Individually ligating the vas deferens from the remainder of the cord structures facilitates easy retrieval of the spermatic cord stump during RPLND where the vas deferens is not taken and helps to minimize the risk of scrotal or retroperitoneal hematoma.
7. **Hemostasis and closure:** After meticulous hemostasis, the testicular prosthesis can be placed in the testicular fossa if the patient desires. EO aponeurosis closed with a running absorbable suture with caution to avoid the ilioinguinal nerve. The closure of subcutaneous fascial layers and skin follows this.

9. What is Chevassu manoeuvre?

Ans:

- Traditionally, before freeing the testicle in the scrotum, the spermatic cord vessels are occluded by a bowel clamp or a tourniquet to prevent tumor cell seeding. This method was introduced in 1906 and named after its inaugurator. It was based on the theory that metastatic dissemination of testicular neoplasms could occur via the cord vessels. As the clinical prognosis of testicular tumors is predominantly influenced by systemic therapy, the oncological value of the Chevassu maneuver is difficult to clarify and has never been systematically evaluated. However, there is no detrimental effect on the orchidectomy result, and it may be performed as a precautionary measure.

10. What is the Chevassu procedure?

Ans:

- Occasionally patients present with a small palpable intra-testicular swelling with normal tumor markers.
- In such cases, it is difficult to establish a clinical diagnosis of testicular cancer as the swelling may also be a benign pathology.
- In such cases, a Chevassu procedure is performed. Here, the inguinal canal is opened and the spermatic cord is looped and clamped. The testis is then delivered. The tunica is opened at the site of the palpable lesion. An intra-op USG may also be used. The lesion is then excised and sent for frozen section analysis. If the frozen report suggests a benign disease, then the tunica is closed after achieving hemostasis. If the frozen suggests malignancy, then the cord is cut at the deep ring and the high orchidectomy is completed.

11. Can Testis-sparing surgery be offered in these patients?

Ans:

- There is no role of testis-sparing surgery (TSS) in a patient with a normal contralateral testis. It can be considered sparingly in synchronous bilateral tumors or tumors in solitary testis with proper counseling.[15]

- It is performed only if the tumor is less than 30% of the testis volume and testosterone levels are normal. At least two additional testicular biopsies should be taken to exclude germ cell neoplasia *in situ* (GCNIS).
- However, limited data exists as of now regarding the oncological safety of TSS.
- TSS can be offered together with frozen section examination (FSE), which is highly reliable and concordant with the final histopathology report.[16] Delayed orchidectomy is offered in case of discordance between FSE and final histopathology.

12. Is there any need for a biopsy from the contralateral testis?

Ans:

- Routine contralateral biopsy is not a norm. There is a low incidence of GCNIS (9%) and metachronous contralateral testicular tumors (2.5%).[17] However, testicular cancer patients at high risk for contralateral GCNIS, i.e. testicular volume 12 mL, poor spermatogenesis (Johnson score 1–3), or a history of cryptorchidism, should be informed of the risks and advantages of a biopsy of the contralateral testis.
- Patients should be aware that despite a negative biopsy, a future germ cell tumor may still occur.[18] When necessary, the technical method advised is a two-site surgical testicular biopsy.[19]

13. How would you detect and treat germ cell neoplasm *in situ* (GCNIS)?

Ans:

- GCNIS cannot currently be diagnosed using either a serological test or an imaging technique. A surgical sample is used to diagnose GCNIS; this specimen should be 3 mm in diameter and have at least 30–40 tubules on a histological cross-section to be representative of the entire testis. A testicular biopsy carries a 3% risk of edema, superficial hemorrhage, or infection; problems are more likely to arise in small testes and after orchidopexy.
- Ultrasonography is a supplemental technique to identify patients at risk for GCNIS since testes harboring the disease may have an irregular echo pattern with so-called microliths that ultrasound can pick up. Ultrasound-guided FNAC may help make a cytopathological diagnosis.
- Even though microlithiasis can be seen in testes without GCNIS, their existence, particularly in people with smaller testes, implies a higher risk of GCNIS.
- AUA Guidelines (2013). Germ cell neoplasia *in situ*
  - In patients with GCNIS, clinicians should inform patients of the risks/benefits of surveillance, radiation, and orchiectomy. (Moderate recommendation; Evidence level: Grade C)
  - Clinicians should recommend surveillance in patients who prioritize the preservation of fertility and testicular androgen production. (Moderate recommendation; Evidence level: Grade C)
  - Clinicians should recommend testicular radiation (18–20 Gy) or orchiectomy in patients who prioritize reducing cancer risk, considering that radiation reduces the risk of hypogonadism compared to orchiectomy. (Moderate recommendation, Evidence level: Grade C).

14. Is there any need for screening?

Ans:

- There is no quality evidence supporting screening protocols in this subset of patients. However, physical self-examination must be taught in young males, especially those with risk factors, including a history of cryptorchidism or a male relative with testicular cancer.[20]
- The testicular self-examination should be performed before a mirror during or immediately following a warm shower or bath. The exam is made simpler by relaxing the scrotum from the heat.
- One should observe for any obvious scrotal swelling. It is typical to have one testicle that appears somewhat larger than the other, or that hangs lower than the other.
- Both hands are put on each testicle to examine it. The testicle is rolled firmly yet softly between the fingers while holding it between the thumb and middle finger.
- One should be aware of any hard lump or nodule or any change in the testis size, shape, and consistency.
- Gentle handling should be done; there should be no pain during self-examination. Normally, the testis should be smooth and firm to the touch.
- The examination should be done once a month, and any suspicious finding should be reported to the consulting urologist.

15. What fertility-related issues should be discussed with the patient?

Ans:

- Sperm-related anomalies are quite commonly found in patients with TC. Up to 24% may be azoospermic, and almost 50% are oligozoospermic before treatment.[21]

- Orchidectomy may harm reproductive function. Both chemotherapy and radiation therapy (RT) also harm fertility. After RT, long-term infertility is uncommon and dose-dependent with chemotherapy.[22]
- The most economical method for preserving fertility should be made available to all patients, which is semen preservation. This should be provided before orchidectomy to increase the likelihood of fertilization and lower the danger of a non-functioning residual testis. If not scheduled before orchidectomy, it should be done before chemotherapy or radiation therapy.[23]
- Both chemotherapy and radiotherapy are teratogenic. Hence, it is necessary to utilize contraception throughout therapy and at least six months after it ends.[24]

16. What is the management of stage I seminoma germ cell tumor?

Ans:

- Approximately 20% of stage I Seminoma have subclinical metastatic disease, usually in the retroperitoneum, that will relapse after orchidectomy alone.[25] After extensive consultation with the patient, considering both potential risks and benefits and the specifics of each patient, decisions on adjuvant therapy should be made.
- ***Surveillance:*** For early detection of individuals experiencing recurrence who must get salvage treatment, this necessitates a stringent regimen of repeated cross-sectional imaging, monitoring of blood tumor markers, and clinical assessment.
  - **Rationale:** On "active surveillance," the cancer-specific survival (CSS) rate for CS I Seminoma is greater than 99%.[26]
  - **Surveillance protocol:** European Association of Urology (EAU) recommends minimal follow-up for seminoma clinical stage I on active surveillance, measuring tumor markers biannually for three years, followed by yearly study for years 4 and 5.
  - Imaging is done with abdominopelvic magnetic resonance imaging (MRI)/ computed tomography (CT) biannually for two years, once in year three and once in year 5. Follow-up after five years can be decided on the case to case basis.
  - Recently, to reduce the frequency and burden of surveillance, an individualized follow-up protocol was suggested based on the conditional risk of relapse as opposed to static protocols.[27]
  - **Advantages:** Avoids side effects of chemotherapy and radiation. This modality also helps in maintaining the quality of life.
  - **Disadvantages:** Due to the requirement for frequent imaging of the retroperitoneum and clinic visits, surveillance might be burdensome for the patient. Patient compliance, which is essential to an active surveillance approach, may be impacted by these.
- ***Adjuvant chemotherapy:***
  - **Rationale:** One cycle of carboplatin is recommended as the appropriate dose if adjuvant chemotherapy is planned. The time to recurrence following carboplatin may be greater than with active surveillance. There is no difference between adjuvant RT and one cycle of carboplatin in terms of relapse-free rates (95% and 96%), time to recurrence, or survival.[28]
  - **Dose of chemotherapy:** One cycle of carboplatin reaching the area under a curve of 7 mg/mL/min (AUC 7)
  - **Advantages:** Most patients relapsing after adjuvant carboplatin can be successfully treated by standard, stage-adapted cisplatin-based chemotherapy
  - **Disadvantages:** Myelosuppression due to adjuvant carboplatin is common with leukopenia and thrombocytopenia rates of 30%.
  - Normalization of sperm counts, morphology, and motility during carboplatin chemotherapy could last up to 4 years after carboplatin therapy.
- ***Adjuvant radiotherapy (RT) / post-operative radiotherapy (PORT):***
  - **Rationale:** In general, radiotherapy should only be used on a very small number of patients who would not benefit from systemic chemotherapy in the case of relapse.
  - **Dose and field of RT:** Paraaortal area; Testicular tumors located at the left side tend to relapse around the insertion of the left testicular vein into the left renal vein, so the left para-aortic region has to be included in the irradiated volume.The recommended adjuvant RT dose in CSI testicular seminoma is 20 Gy in 2 Gy fractions.
  - **Advantages:** Side effects of chemotherapy are avoided. To reduce the acute and side effects, novel techniques, such as intensity modulated radiation therapy (IMRT) and spot scanning

proton therapy, may play a role in particular clinical situations, such as one kidney and another needing tissue sparing.
- **Disadvantages:** This pertains to the long-term danger of non-germ cell malignancies in the radiation field and, more specifically, the toxicity of RT.[29] Acute toxicity of paraaortic field radiation for CS I seminoma includes significant gastrointestinal toxicity such as nausea (46%), leukopenia (14%), diarrhea (7%) as well as a peptic ulcer (7%). Depending on the pretreatment sperm counts, it takes about 13 to 24 months after RT for sperm to return to the normal posttreatment sperm count ranges.

17. What is a risk-adapted treatment for stage I seminoma testis?

Ans:

- Patients may be divided into low- and high-risk groups based on tumor size > 4 cm and stromal rete testis invasion. Those with no risk factors have a very low risk of recurrence and do not require adjuvant treatment.[30]

18. What is the management of stage I non-seminomatous germ cell tumors?

Ans:

- Adjuvant chemotherapy and surveillance are two treatment options for non-seminomatous germ cell tumors that have reached clinical stage I (CS I-NSGCTs).
- In certain circumstances, retroperitoneal lymph node dissection (RPLND) has a restricted role. Overall, orchidectomy alone can cure about 70% of CS I-NSGCTs.
- History has shown that relapse occurs 50% more frequently in those with the high-risk feature of LVI than in people without. A full conversation about the potential benefits and drawbacks of various treatment options, as well as specific co-morbidities, should be had with the patient.
- *Surveillance:*
  - **Rationale:** Repeated cross-sectional imaging, monitoring of serum tumor markers, and clinical evaluation are all required for CS I-NSGCT surveillance to identify patients experiencing relapse early enough to require salvage therapy.
  - **Surveillance protocol:** EAU guidelines recommend measurement of serum tumor markers every three months for the first two years, followed by biannually in the year 3, 4, and 5.

    Chest X-ray is to be done biannually for the first two years, then once a year for year 3, in case of positive lymphovascular invasion, and last at year 5.

    Imaging with abdominopelvic MRI/CT is done biannually in year 1, followed by the next CT at 24 months, 36 months, and 60 months.
  - **Advantages:** Avoids side effects of chemotherapy and radiation. This modality also helps in maintaining the quality of life.
  - **Disadvantages:** According to the largest surveillance reports, the cumulative risk of recurrence for CS I-NSGCT is around 30% (for high- and low-risk CS I-NSGCT, the five-year conditional risk of relapse is 42% and 17%, respectively).[31] As a result of the requirement for frequent imaging of the retroperitoneum and clinic visits, surveillance might be burdensome for the patient. Patient compliance, which is essential to an active surveillance approach, may be impacted by these.
- *Retroperitoneal lymph node dissection:*
  - **Rationale:** Men with teratomas with a malignant somatic component or patients who are unable or unwilling to receive chemotherapy in the event of a recurrence, particularly in cases where lympho-vascular invasion is present, are just a few examples of stage I disease indications.

    If the specimen is positive for the disease, the recommended treatment is adjuvant chemotherapy, consisting of two cycles of bleomycin, etoposide, and cisplatin (BEP).
  - **Surgery:** Nerve-sparing and minimally invasive techniques are methods to lower the morbidity of primary RPLND. This can only be done at high-volume RPLND facilities with the necessary minimally invasive surgery training.
  - **Advantages:** The advantages are good efficacy of treatment, less costly follow-up, and reduced need for cross-sectional imaging.
  - **Disadvantages:** Data from high-volume and specialized centers show that primary RPLND is linked to a 15% chance of relapse.[32] According to more current research, 10% of negative node patients experience relapse.[33]

    In light of the high CSS rates of surveillance, the low recurrence rates with adjuvant treatment, and the poorer reproducibility of primary RPLND on a broad scale, RPLND for CS I-NSGCT has lost some of its significance.[34]

- *Adjuvant chemotherapy:*

  In stage 1A, surveillance is preferred over chemotherapy or RPLND, while in stage 1B, chemotherapy with BEP for one or two cycles or RPLND scores over surveillance.

  - **Rationale:** Single-cycle BEP, which is now the advised course of action if adjuvant chemotherapy is necessary, prevents > 90% of relapses and improves the risk-benefit ratio of chemotherapy.
  - **Dose of chemotherapy:** Clinical stage I NSGCT patients with evidence of venous invasion by the primary tumor receive two courses of adjuvant chemotherapy, as follows: Cisplatin 20 mg/m^2 on days 1 to 5, etoposide 100 mg/m^2 on days 1 to 5, and bleomycin 30 U by push injection on days 2, 9, and 16 (PEB). This course was repeated on day 22.
  - **Advantages:** In the CS I-NSGCT, adjuvant chemotherapy has been assessed with both one and two cycles of BEP with low recurrence rates (2–3%).[35,36]
  - **Disadvantages:** Chemotherapy-related side effects are alopecia, myelosuppression, nausea/vomiting, and fever.

19. What is the risk-adapted approach for Stage I non-seminomatous germ cell tumors?

Ans:

- Although certain patients with major comorbidities or worries about salvage chemotherapy with multicycle cisplatin-based chemotherapy may choose adjuvant therapy, patients without LVI should be advised to consider surveillance.
- The high risk of relapse (up to 50%) for those with LVI should be emphasized, and they should be advised to seek adjuvant chemotherapy with BEP × 1 as the "preferred" choice.
- Some patients could be interested in primary RPLND. However, they should be aware of the 10% chance of systemic relapse even with pN0, necessitating further chemotherapy treatment, and the potential additional need for adjuvant chemotherapy if nodes have an active disease (pN1) (BEP × 3). National Comprehensive Cancer Network (NCCN) advises surveillance for pN0 disease after primary RPLND in stage I NSGCT. In pN1 disease, surveillance is preferred, while chemotherapy with Etoposide/Cisplatin (EP) for two cycles is another option that can be discussed. Similarly, in pN2 disease, surveillance and chemotherapy are options, the preferred chemotherapy with EP for two cycles. In pN3 disease, BEP for three cycles or EP for four cycles is advised.
- Retrospective datasets of CS I patients with post-pubertal teratomas with malignant somatic components (TSMC) were analyzed in a multi-institutional study. The results showed that these patients had a five-year OS of 10% lower than other CS I-GCT patients. The primary RPLND in CS I-NSGCT with TSMC is supported by this work.[37]

SUMMARY

- Stage I germ cell tumors have a fairly favorable prognosis.
- Bilateral testicular ultrasound should be performed in patients with suspicion of testicular cancer.
- Serum tumor markers should be measured both before and after orchidectomy.
- Orchidectomy provides the specimen for histopathological diagnosis.
- CECT of the chest, abdomen, and pelvis should be performed for staging in all patients of TC. MRI can be performed when CT is contraindicated.
- The pathological risk factors denoting occult metastatic disease in stage I GCT are tumor size and rete testis invasion in seminoma and lymphovascular invasion in nonseminoma.
- Patients should be informed about all available management options, including surveillance or adjuvant therapy (chemotherapy or radiation) after orchidectomy, treatment-specific recurrence rates, and acute and long-term side effects.
- Discuss sperm banking with all men prior to starting treatment for testicular cancer.
- Use a risk-adapted approach for choosing treatment options in stage I GCT.

REFERENCES

1. Bertero L, Massa F, Metovic J, Zanetti R, Castellano I, Ricardi U, Papotti M, Cassoni P. of the UICC Classification of Malignant Tumours: an overview of the changes in the pathological TNM classification criteria—What has changed and why?. Virchows Archiv. 2018 Apr;472:519–31.
2. Warde P, Specht L, Horwich A, Oliver T, Panzarella T, Gospodarowicz M, von der Maase H. Prognostic factors for relapse in stage I Seminoma managed by surveillance: a pooled analysis. Journal of clinical oncology. 2002 Nov 15;20(22):4448–52.
3. Aparicio J, Germà JR, del Muro XG, Maroto P, Arranz JA, Sáenz A, Barnadas A, Dorca J, Gumà J, Olmos D, Bastús R. Risk-adapted management for patients with clinical stage I Seminoma: the Second Spanish Germ Cell Cancer Cooperative Group study. Journal of clinical oncology. 2005 Dec 1;23(34):8717–23.
4. Blok JM, Pluim I, Daugaard G, Wagner T, Jó wiak K, Wilthagen EA, Looijenga LH, Meijer RP, Bosch JR, Horenblas S. Lymphovascular invasion and presence of embryonal carcinoma as risk factors for occult metastatic disease in clinical stage I nonseminomatous germ cell tumour: a systematic review and meta-analysis. BJU international. 2020 Mar;125(3):355–68.

5. Angulo JC, González J, Rodríguez N, Hernández E, Núñez C, Rodríguez-Barbero JM, Santana A, López JI. Clinicopathological study of regressed testicular tumors (apparent extragonadal germ cell neoplasms). The Journal of urology. 2009 Nov;182(5):2303–10.
6. Laguna MP, Albers P, Algaba F, Bokemeyer C, Boormans JL, Fischer S, Fizazi K, Gremmels H, Leão R, Nicol D, Nicolai N. Testicular cancer. InEAU Annual Congress Amsterdam 2020.
7. Tsili AC, Argyropoulou MI, Dolciami M, Ercolani G, Catalano C, Manganaro L. When to ask for an MRI of the scrotum. Andrology. 2021 Sep;9(5):1395–409.
8. Oechsle K, Hartmann M, Brenner W, Venz S, Weissbach L, Franzius C, Kliesch S, Mueller S, Krege S, Heicappell R, Bares R. [18F] Fluorodeoxyglucose positron emission tomography in nonseminomatous germ cell tumors after chemotherapy: the German multicenter positron emission tomography study group. Journal of Clinical Oncology. 2008 Dec 20;26(36):5930–5.
9. Dieckmann KP, Simonsen-Richter H, Kulejewski M, Anheuser P, Zecha H, Isbarn H, Pichlmeier U. Serum tumour markers in testicular germ cell tumours: frequencies of elevated levels and extents of marker elevation are significantly associated with clinical parameters and with response to treatment. BioMed research international. 2019 May 28;2019.
10. Barlow LJ, Badalato GM, McKiernan JM. Serum tumor markers in the evaluation of male germ cell tumors. Nature Reviews Urology. 2010 Nov;7(11):610–7.
11. Mead GM, Stenning SP. The International Germ Cell Consensus Classification: a new prognostic factor-based staging classification for metastatic germ cell tumours. Clinical oncology (Royal College of Radiologists (Great Britain)). 1997 Jan 1;9(4):207–9.
12. Gilligan TD, Seidenfeld J, Basch EM, Einhorn LH, Fancher T, Smith DC, Stephenson AJ, Vaughn DJ, Cosby R, Hayes DF. American Society of Clinical Oncology Clinical Practice Guideline on uses of serum tumor markers in adult males with germ cell tumors. J Clin Oncol. 2010 Jul 10;28(20):3388–404.
13. Almstrup K, Lobo J, Mørup N, Belge G, Rajpert-De Meyts E, Looijenga LH, Dieckmann KP. Application of miRNAs in the diagnosis and monitoring of testicular germ cell tumours. Nature Reviews Urology. 2020 Apr;17(4):201–13.
14. Patel HD, Gupta M, Cheaib JG, Sharma R, Zhang A, Bass EB, Pierorazio PM. Testis-sparing surgery and scrotal violation for testicular masses suspicious for malignancy: A systematic review and meta-analysis. In Urologic Oncology: Seminars and Original Investigations 2020 May 1 (Vol. 38, No. 5, pp. 344–353). Elsevier.
15. Nason GJ, Aditya I, Leao R, Anson-Cartwright L, Jewett MA, O'Malley M, Sweet J, Hamilton RJ. Partial orchiectomy: The Princess Margaret cancer centre experience. In Urologic Oncology: Seminars and Original Investigations 2020 Jun 1 (Vol. 38, No. 6, pp. 605–e19). Elsevier.
16. Fankhauser CD, Roth L, Kranzbühler B, Eberli D, Bode P, Moch H, Oliveira P, Ramani V, Beyer J, Hermanns T. The role of frozen section examination during inguinal exploration in men with inconclusive testicular tumors: a systematic review and meta-analysis. European urology focus. 2021 Nov 1;7(6):1400–2.
17. Andreassen KE, Grotmol T, Cvancarova MS, Johannesen TB, Fosså SD. Risk of metachronous contralateral testicular germ cell tumors: A population-based study of 7,102 Norwegian patients (1953–2007). International journal of cancer. 2011 Dec 15;129(12):2867–74.
18. Souchon R, Gertenbach U, Dieckmann KP, Hahn E, Ruwe M, Stambolis C, Loy V, Claßen J. Contralateral testicular cancer in spite of TIN-negative double biopsies and interval cisplatin chemotherapy. Strahlentherapie und Onkologie. 2006 May 1;182(5):289.
19. Dieckmann KP, Kulejewski M, Pichlmeier U, Loy V. Diagnosis of contralateral testicular intraepithelial neoplasia (TIN) in patients with testicular germ cell cancer: systematic two-site biopsies are more sensitive than a single random biopsy. European urology. 2007 Jan 1;51(1):175–85.
20. Thornton CP. Best practice in teaching male adolescents and young men to perform testicular self-examinations: a review. Journal of Pediatric Health Care. 2016 Nov 1;30(6):518–27.
21. Rives N, Perdrix A, Hennebicq S, Saïas-Magnan J, Melin MC, Berthaut I, Barthélémy C, Daudin M, Szerman E, Bresson JL, Brugnon F. The semen quality of 1158 men with testicular cancer at the time of cryopreservation: results of the French National CECOS Network. Journal of andrology. 2012 Nov 12;33(6):1394–401.
22. Brydøy M, Fosså SD, Klepp O, Bremnes RM, Wist EA, Bjøro T, Wentzel-Larsen T, Dahl O. Sperm counts and endocrinological markers of spermatogenesis in long-term survivors of testicular cancer. British journal of cancer. 2012 Nov;107(11):1833–9.
23. Gilbert K, Nangia AK, Dupree JM, Smith JF, Mehta A. Fertility preservation for men with testicular cancer: is sperm cryopreservation cost effective in the era of assisted reproductive technology?. InUrologic Oncology: Seminars and Original Investigations 2018 Mar 1 (Vol. 36, No. 3, pp. 92–e1). Elsevier.
24. Arnon J, Meirow D, Lewis-Roness H, Ornoy A. Genetic and teratogenic effects of cancer treatments on gametes and embryos. Human reproduction update. 2001 Jul 1;7(4):394–403.
25. Kollmannsberger C, Tandstad T, Bedard PL, Cohn-Cedermark G, Chung PW, Jewett MA, Powles T, Warde PR, Daneshmand S, Protheroe A, Tyldesley S. Patterns of relapse in patients with clinical stage I testicular cancer managed with active surveillance. J Clin Oncol. 2015 Jan 1;33(1):51–7.
26. Tandstad T, Smaaland R, Solberg A, Bremnes RM, Langberg CW, Laurell A, Stierner UK, Ståhl O, Cavallin-Ståhl EK, Klepp OH, Dahl O. Management of seminomatous testicular cancer: a binational prospective population-based study from the Swedish Norwegian testicular cancer study group. Journal of clinical oncology. 2011 Feb 20;29(6):719–25.
27. Gariscsak PJ, Anson-Cartwright L, Atenafu EG, Jiang DM, Chung P, Bedard P, Warde P, O'Malley M, Sweet J, Glicksman RM, Hamilton RJ. Safety of minimizing intensity of follow-up on active surveillance for clinical stage I testicular germ cell tumors. European Urology Open Science. 2022 Jun 1;40:46–53.
28. Oliver RT, Mead GM, Rustin GJ, Joffe JK, Aass N, Coleman R, Gabe R, Pollock P, Stenning SP. Randomized trial of carboplatin versus radiotherapy for stage I Seminoma: mature results on relapse and contralateral testis cancer rates in MRC TE19/EORTC 30982 study (ISRCTN27163214). Journal of Clinical Oncology. 2011 Mar 10;29(8):957–62.
29. Patel HD, Srivastava A, Alam R, Joice GA, Schwen ZR, Semerjian A, Allaf ME, Pierorazio PM. Radiotherapy for stage I and II testicular seminomas: secondary malignancies and survival. In Urologic Oncology: Seminars and Original Investigations 2017 Oct 1 (Vol. 35, No. 10, pp. 606–e1). Elsevier.

30. Tandstad T, Ståhl O, Dahl O, Haugnes HS, Håkansson U, Karlsdottir Å, Kjellman A, Langberg CW, Laurell A, Oldenburg J, Solberg A. Treatment of stage I Seminoma, with one course of adjuvant carboplatin or surveillance, risk-adapted recommendations implementing patient autonomy: a report from the Swedish and Norwegian Testicular Cancer Group (SWENOTECA). Annals of Oncology. 2016 Jul 1;27(7):1299–304.
31. Kollmannsberger C, Tandstad T, Bedard PL, Cohn-Cedermark G, Chung PW, Jewett MA, Powles T, Warde PR, Daneshmand S, Protheroe A, Tyldesley S. Patterns of relapse in patients with clinical stage I testicular cancer managed with active surveillance. J Clin Oncol. 2015 Jan 1;33(1):51–7.
32. Donohue JP, Thornhill JA, Foster RS, Rowland RG, Bihrle R. Retroperitoneal lymphadenectomy for clinical stage A testis cancer (1965 to 1989): modifications of technique and impact on ejaculation. The Journal of urology. 1993 Feb 1;149(2):237–43.
33. Nelson JB, Chen RN, Bishoff JT, Oh WK, Kantoff PW, Donehower RC, Kavoussi LR. Laparoscopic retroperitoneal lymph node dissection for clinical stage I nonseminomatous germ cell testicular tumors. Urology. 1999 Dec 1;54(6):1064–7.
34. Foster RS, Roth BJ. Clinical stage I Nonseminoma: surgery versus surveillance. InSeminars in oncology 1998 Apr 1 (Vol. 25, No. 2, pp. 145–153).
35. Chevreau C, Mazerolles C, Soulié M, Gaspard MH, Mourey L, Bujan L, Plante P, Rischmann P, Bachaud JM, Malavaud B. Long-term efficacy of two cycles of BEP regimen in high-risk stage I nonseminomatous testicular germ cell tumors with embryonal carcinoma and/or vascular invasion. European urology. 2004 Aug 1;46(2):209–15.
36. Tandstad T, Ståhl O, Håkansson U, Dahl O, Haugnes HS, Klepp OH, Langberg CW, Laurell A, Oldenburg J, Solberg A, Söderström K. One course of adjuvant BEP in clinical stage I Nonseminoma mature and expanded results from the SWENOTECA group. Annals of oncology. 2014 Nov 1;25(11):2167–72.
37. Giannatempo P, Pond GR, Sonpavde G, Albany C, Loriot Y, Sweeney CJ, Salvioni R, Colecchia M, Nicolai N, Raggi D, Rice KR. Treatment and clinical outcomes of patients with teratoma with somatic-type malignant transformation: an international collaboration. The Journal of Urology. 2016 Jul 1;196(1):95–100.

Chapter

14

Metastatic Germ Cell Tumors

• Ravimohan Mavuduru • Girdhar Bora

LEARNING OBJECTIVES

- To know the staging evaluation for a patient with germ cell tumors (GCTs): Every patient with a diagnosis of a testicular tumor should have a contrast enhanced CT scan of the chest, abdomen and pelvis.
- To understand the risk stratification of patients with advanced GCTs: The international Germ Cell Cancer Collaboration Group (IGCCCG) risk stratification system is used to classify patients into good/intermediate/poor risk GCT. This guides further management and is also prognostic.
- To know about the chemotherapy regimens for advanced GCTs: The BEP (Bleomycin, Etoposide and Cisplatin) regimen is the most commonly used for GCTs. The number of cycles depends on the IGCCCG risk category of the patient.
- To understand the peri-chemotherapy precautions: Hydration, thromboembolic prophylaxis, and monitoring for pulmonary and renal toxicity are the considerations when the patient is on chemotherapy.
- To understand the management of post-chemotherapy residual lesions in seminoma: It is still not very clear what is the best management for patients with post-chemotherapy residual masses in seminoma. Most decisions are guided by the findings of a FDG PET-CT.
- To understand the management of post-chemotherapy residual lesions in NSGCT: A post-chemotherapy retroperitoneal lymph node dissection (RPLND) is the standard of care for all residual lesions larger than 1 cm.
- To know of the settings in which RPLND is performed: The different settings in which a RPLND is performed include: Primary RPLND for stage 1 and stage 2A GCTs with normal tumor markers, post-chemotherapy RPLND, salvage RPLND, desperation RPLND and RPLND for growing teratoma syndrome.
- To know the templates for RPLND: A standard bilateral template RPLND entails removal of all nodal tissue within a template bounded by the left renal vein superiorly, the crossing of the ureters over the common iliac arteries inferiorly and both ureters laterally.
- To understand the concept of modified template RPLND: A modified template RPLND may be performed in patients with low burden of disease in an attempt to limit surgical morbidity.
- To know about the follow-up protocol: All patients following completion of treatment for advanced GCTs should be asked to follow-up as per a fixed protocol which includes regular evaluation with tumor markers, physical examination and imaging.

Case Scenario

A 23-year-old unmarried male presented with a right testicular swelling. On scrotal ultrasound, a well-defined enhancing mass of 4 x 3 cm size was seen in the right testis; the left testis was normal. The tumor markers for this patient were as follows: AFP 393, bHCG 16,355 and LDH 741. A CT scan of the chest, abdomen and pelvis showed multiple retroperitoneal nodal masses, largest being a 5.8 × 4 cm para-aortic node. There were also 3 lung nodules, largest being a 1.7 × 1.4 cm lesion in the left upper lobe (Fig. 14.1A and B).

1. **What is the next step?**

   Ans:

   - Patients with metastatic GCT require chemotherapy and RPLND which may affect their fertility potential.[1]

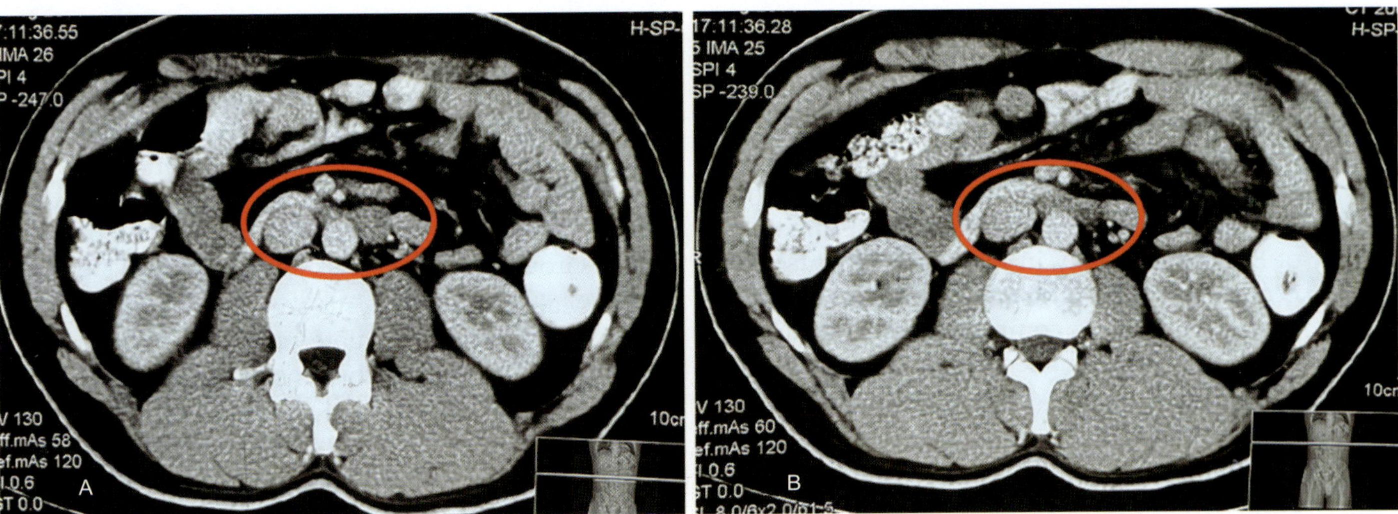

Fig. 14.1A and B: CT Image showing retroperitoneal nodes

- A baseline sperm count should be done and sperm banking should be discussed where family is not completed apart from radical orchiectomy.

2. **Is orchiectomy always the first step?**

Ans:

- For males who present with clinically advanced disease, we perform a radical orchiectomy prior to chemotherapy whenever possible.
- Despite this, there are some males who present with life-threatening advanced disease who undergo systemic chemotherapy prior to orchiectomy ("delayed orchiectomy"). This chemotherapy is started on the basis of raised tumor markers which suggest the diagnosis of NSGCT. For patients with only raised LDH, where the clinical suspicion is of a seminoma, a biopsy of the retroperitoneal mass is performed and the presence of seminoma is confirmed prior to starting the chemotherapy.
- Brain and testis are considered immune-privileged sites owing to a blood–brain barrier and a blood–testis barrier (BTB) respectively making them less penetrable to systemic chemotherapy. However, whether this BTB remains working in a disease-infiltrated testis is questioned and the need for post-chemotherapy delayed orchidectomy is being revisited.[2–4]
- Histopathological examination of tissue from retroperitoneum as well as from the testis in patient undergoing delayed orchiectomy and RPLND have shown disparity for response to chemotherapy.
- Complete resolution of tumor in the testis and residual tumor in the retroperitoneum cannot be answered by BTB only and possibly could be due to tumor heterogeneity.
- A delayed orchiectomy should be performed later in such select patients where the chemotherapy was given upfront.[3,4]

3. **What is the imaging done for systemic staging?**

Ans:

- A high-resolution computed tomography (CT) scan of the chest, abdomen and pelvis is recommended for staging.
- MRI of the brain is performed if brain metastases are suspected. (Neurologic symptoms, β-hCG >5000 IU/L, AFP >10,000 ng/ml, choriocarcinoma or extensive disease like multiple lung metastasis, non-pulmonary visceral metastasis.)
- Positron emission tomography (PET) scan is of limited utility in the initial staging of patients with testicular germ cell tumors (GCTs).

4. **What is the pattern of lymph node involvement and how to identify malignant node on a CT?**

Ans:

- CT is essential for accurately determining the extent of nodal and metastatic spread in GCTs.
- GCTs primarily spread to retroperitoneal lymph nodes through lymphatic and venous pathways originating from the gonads. The spread follows on right-side along the gonadal vein, involving aortocaval or paracaval nodes, and since left gonadal vein drains into left renal vein, left-sided GCTs typically metastasize to left paraaortic nodes below the left renal hilum. Contralateral spread is rare without ipsilateral nodal involvement.
- Nodal disease above the level of renal hila is considered metastatic and falls under M staging.[6,7]

- The accuracy of CT in identifying malignant nodes depends on the size cut-off. Using a threshold of 4 mm or larger, sensitivity is excellent (>90%), but specificity decreases to 58%. Raising the cut-off to 10 mm increases specificity to almost 100%, but sensitivity drops to 37–47%. A recommended short axis diameter of 8 mm, especially in high-risk patients with lymph-vascular invasion or an embryonal predominance, is commonly used to define suspicious lymph nodes on CT.
- Additionally, morphologic features like shape (round or spiculated) and enhancement (heterogeneous, central necrosis) provide suspicion of positive lymph nodes.
- Also, surrounding organ involvement and ureteral obstruction with hydronephrosis can be identified.

5. What is the risk stratification of advanced germ cell tumor?

Ans:

- For males with advanced GCTs, management does not differ for seminoma and NSGCTs. Instead, treatment is selected based on the International Germ Cell Cancer Collaborative Group (IGCCCG) risk stratification system.
- Males with seminoma are categorized as having good- or intermediate-risk disease. Males with NSGCTs are categorized as having good-, intermediate-, or poor-risk disease based on the sites of disease involvement and tumor marker levels.
- With the advancement in chemotherapy, the 5-year survival rates have increased for both metastatic seminoma and non-seminomatous tumors from the initial IGCCCG series [9–11] (Table 14.1).

TABLE 14.1: The International Germ Cell Cancer Collaboration Group (IGCCCG) classification of advanced germ cell tumors (GCTs)

Seminomas		*Non-seminomas*	
Good risk		**Good risk**	
All of the following:		**All of the following:**	
Any primary site	5-year PFS: 89% (CI, 87–90)	Testicular or retroperitoneal primary tumors	5-year PFS: 90% (95% CI, 89–91)
No metastases to organs other than the lungs and/or lymph nodes	OS: 95% (CI, 94–96)	No metastases to organs other than the lungs and/or lymph nodes	OS: 96% (95–96%)
Normal serum AFP		Serum AFP <1000 ng/ml, β-hCG <5000 mIU/ml, and LDH <3 times the upper limit of normal	
Intermediate risk		**Intermediate risk**	
All of the following:		**All of the following:**	
Any primary site	5-year PFS: 79% (95% CI, 70–85)	Testicular or retroperitoneal primary tumors	5-year PFS: 78% (76–80%)
Metastases to organs other than the lungs and/or lymph nodes	OS: 88% (95% CI, 80–93)	No metastases to organs other than the lungs and/or lymph nodes Serum AFP 1000 to 10,000 ng/ml or Serum β-hCG 5000 to 50,000 mIU/ml or	OS: 89% (88–91%)
		LDH 3 to 10 times the upper limit of normal	
Normal serum AFP			
		Poor risk	
No patients classified as poor risk		**Any of the following:**	
		Mediastinal primary with or without metastases	5-year PFS: 54% (95% CI, 52–56)
		Metastases to organs other than the lungs and/or lymph nodes	
		Serum AFP >10,000 ng/ml or β-hCG >50,000 mIU/ml or LDH >10 times the upper limit of normal	OS: 67% (95% CI, 65–69)

- These recent studies also identified lactate dehydrogenase (LDH) proved to be an additional adverse prognostic factor for patients with advanced seminomas. Good prognosis patients with LDH above 2.5 x upper limit of normal had a 3-year PFS of 80% (95% CI, 75 to 84) and a 3-year OS of 92% (95% CI, 88 to 95) versus 92% (95% CI, 90 to 94) and 97% (95% CI, 96 to 98) in the group with lower LDH[10] (Table 14.1).
- For NSGCTs, a prognostic model was developed and independently validated. This model identified a new cutoff of lactate dehydrogenase at a 2.5 upper limit of normal and increasing age and presence of lung metastases as additional adverse prognostic factors. An online calculator is provided (https://www.eortc.org/IGCCCG-Update).[11]

6. What is the chemotherapy regimen for advanced GCTs?

Ans:

- **Good-risk disease**: For males with good-risk GCTs, three cycles of bleomycin, etoposide, and cisplatin (BEP) are recommended. For those with compromised pulmonary function, four cycles of EP is recommended to avoid bleomycin-related toxicity.
- **Intermediate-or poor-risk disease:** For males with intermediate-risk or poor-risk disease, four cycles of BEP are recommended. An alternative regimen of etoposide, ifosfamide, and cisplatin (VIP) is preferred for patients at risk of bleomycin-induced lung injury.
- Table 14.2 depicts the BEP regimen.[12]
- Table 14.3 depicts the VIP regimen:[13] Similar efficacy as BEP but causes more myelotoxicity

7. What are criteria monitored by the medical oncologists while administration of chemotherapy for GCTs?

Ans:

- **Pre-treatment considerations:**
  - *Hydration:* Induce diuresis with at least 2000 ml of NS to minimize cisplatin nephrotoxicity. Maintain urine flow of at least 100 ml/hour for 2 hours before and after cisplatin administration.
  - Emesis risk is high (>90% frequency of emesis). Prior use of antiemetics is a must.
  - *Vesicant/irritant properties:* Bleomycin, etoposide, and cisplatin are irritants. Avoid extravasation.
  - *Myelo-stimulation prophylaxis:* Primary prophylaxis with G-CSF is not indicated.
  - *Dose adjustment for liver/renal dysfunction:* Bleomycin contraindicated if baseline creatinine >2.0 mg/dl. Consider lower initial doses of cisplatin or etoposide for hepatic or renal dysfunction.
- **Monitoring parameters:**
  - CBC with differential and platelet count weekly during treatment.
  - Basic metabolic panel prior to each treatment cycle.
  - Baseline pulmonary function tests (PFTs), including DLCO, before and during bleomycin therapy.
- **Toxicity:**
  - *Myelotoxicity:* Begin each cycle on schedule. Reduce etoposide dose by 25% if febrile neutropenia or thrombocytopenic bleeding occurs. Administer G-CSF if neutrophil count 2500 cells/µl or platelets 100,000/µl.

TABLE 14.2: The BEP regimen

Drug	*Dose and route*	*Administration*	*Days*
Bleomycin	30 units IV per dose	Dilute in 50 ml NS and administer over 10 minutes	1, 8, 15
Etoposide	100 mg/m² IV per day	Dilute in 500 ml NS (concentration < 0.4 mg/ml) and administer over one hour	1–5
Cisplatin	20 mg/m² IV per day	Dilute in 250 ml NS and administer over two hours	1–5

Repeat the cycle every 21 days

TABLE 14.3: The VIP regimen

Drug	*Dose and route*	*Administration*	*Days*
Etoposide	75 mg/m² IV per day	Dilute in 500 ml NS and administer over one hour	1–5
Ifosfamide	1200 mg/m² IV per day	With Mesna protection	1–5
Cisplatin	20 mg/m² IV per day	Dilute in 250 ml NS and administer over two hours	1–5

Repeat the cycle every 21 days

- *Pulmonary toxicity:* Maximum lifetime bleomycin dose should not exceed 400 mg. Discontinue if clinical/radiographic evidence of pulmonary injury or DLCO decline 25%.
- *Neurologic toxicity:* Discontinue cisplatin if neuropathy interferes with function. Peripheral neuropathies may occur after prolonged courses. Consider benefit–risk balance.
- *Renal toxicity:* Discuss treatment goals and risks of cisplatin nephrotoxicity in the setting of renal impairment (creatinine >2.0 mg/dl or GFR <50 ml/min).

Case Scenario *(Contd.)*

The patient received 4 cycles of BEP. Tumor markers 4 weeks after the completion of chemotherapy had normalized. A response evaluation CECT revealed that 2 of the three lung lesions had completely resolved while one lesion in the left upper lobe showed no interval decrease in size. The size of the para-aortic LN had decreased to 3 × 2 cm. There were no new lesions. Figure 14.2 showing residual retroperitoneal node.

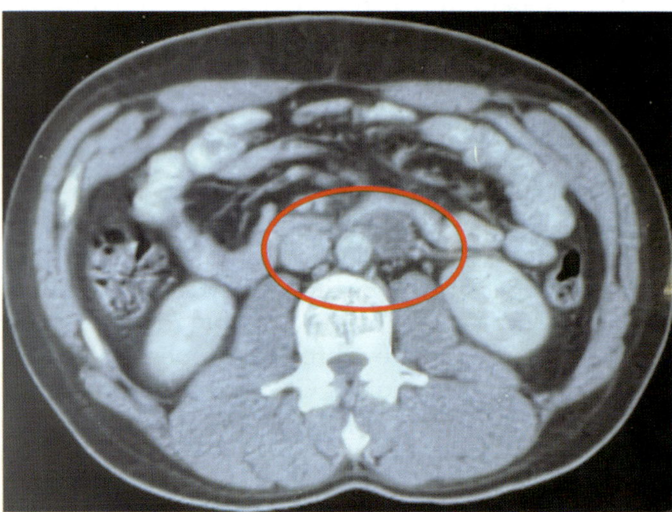

Fig. 14.2: Residual retroperitoneal node

8. What is the management of post-chemotherapy residual lesions?

Ans: The management of post-orchiectomy/post-chemotherapy depends on the histologic type of germ cell tumor (GCT):

A. Seminoma[14,15]

For seminomas, the response evaluation scan is a FDG PET/CT which is performed 8–10 weeks after the completion of the chemotherapy.

- No evidence of residual disease: Surveillance
- Residual mass < 3 cm: Masses <3 cm invariably have necrosis or fibrosis only, therefore, surveillance is a reasonable option.
- Residual mass >3 cm: FDG PET has a high NPV for these lesions, meaning that residual masses with no FDG uptake, even if larger than 3 cm, can be safely observed.[16] However, the PPV of FDG PET is only around 25–30% and thus irradiating all lesions which are >3 cm with FDG uptake would lead to considerable overtreatment. The results of the SEMPET trial have not been replicated in other multicentric cohort studies. Studies are evaluating if any cut-off value of SUV_{max} can predict if the residual mass has actual residual disease.
- If there is progressive disease accompanied with high β-hCG, then salvage chemotherapy should be initiated.
- If there is progressive disease without elevation of β-hCG, then a biopsy from the mass should be performed before starting salvage chemotherapy.
- RPLND for post-chemotherapy seminoma is rarely performed in the present day because of the high morbidity associated with the surgery as a result of severe desmoplastic reaction.

B. Nonseminomatous germ cell tumor

- In contrast to seminoma, there is no role for FDG-PET scans in the work-up of residual disease seen on CT of males with NSGCT.[17] FDG-PET is neither sufficiently sensitive in detecting nodes that contain viable tumor nor can it reliably differentiate teratoma from fibrosis.
- The role of surgery for residual retroperitoneal lesions of <1 cm is uncertain, the alternative option is close surveillance, with risk of recurrence up to 6–9%.[18]
- For males who have normalized their serum tumor markers but have imaging evidence of retroperitoneal lymph node(s) larger than 1 cm, a retroperitoneal lymph node dissection (RPLND) is recommended.[5,14] RPLND should be performed within 6–8 weeks of the last chemotherapy, within 4 weeks of a CT scan and 7–10 days of markers assessment.
- Second line chemotherapy is offered when the tumour markers show elevation after completion of the first line chemotherapy.

9. What histopathology one can except following the resection of residual masses for NSGCT?

Ans:

- The differential diagnosis of residual masses present at the completion of chemotherapy includes:[19]
  - Necrosis or fibrosis (40 to 50%)

  - Mature or immature teratoma (30 to 40%)
  - Residual non-teratomatous germ cell tumor (GCT) (10 to 15%)
- Unfortunately, it is generally not possible to distinguish these possibilities on imaging. For example, multiple factors may predict the histology of residual retroperitoneal masses in males with NSGCT, including the presence of teratomatous elements in the primary tumor, levels of serum tumor markers prior to chemotherapy, and the degree of reduction in mass size during chemotherapy.[20]

10. Why is resection of residual masses in NSGCT done when the possibility of residual tumor is only 10–20%?

Ans:

- The goal of resecting residual masses is to remove any residual teratoma or viable germ cell tumor (GCT). In addition, the resection of residual cancer is necessary in order to guide decisions about whether to administer additional chemotherapy.
- There are multiple reasons to resect residual teratoma even though most teratomas behave in an indolent manner:
  - Teratomas are relatively resistant to the chemotherapy and radiation therapy (RT) regimens for testicular GCTs because they are relatively slow growing tumors. Therefore, surgery is the only reliable way to eliminate them.
  - Viable GCT may coexist with teratoma, which can lead to clinical recurrence if not resected.
  - Malignant transformation of mature teratoma can occur. Sarcomas or carcinomas arising from a teratoma are resistant to chemotherapy and are associated with a poor prognosis.
  - Indolent growth of a teratoma may compromise vital organ function and/or cause pain and other symptoms (growing teratoma syndrome).

11. What is growing teratoma syndrome?

Ans:

- Benign teratomatous elements may enlarge during or after chemotherapy, mimicking progressive or relapsed disease first described by Logothetis.[21]
- Two primary theories have been put forth: The first suggests that chemotherapy selectively targets immature malignant cells while leaving teratoma cells unaffected, and the second proposes that chemotherapy accelerates the process of de-differentiation, leading malignant cells to transform into benign mature teratoma cells.
- In patients who meet Logothetis' criteria, suspicion should arise for the presence of growing teratoma syndrome, which includes three key elements: Progressive enlargement of masses during or following systemic chemotherapy, a return to normal levels of previously elevated serum tumor markers, and the identification of mature teratoma in prior histological analyses.
- Complete surgical resection is indicated rather than additional chemotherapy.

12. What are the different settings in which RPLND is performed in GCTs?

Ans:

1. **Primary RPLND:** This is done for stage 1 and stage 2A GCTs with normal tumor markers. It is an established option for stage 1 NSGCT when the patient has high risk featured in the pathology of the orchidectomy. Although traditionally, primary RPLND has not been utilized for stage 1 seminoma, recent studies like SEMS, COTRIMS have evaluated the role primary RPLND in stage 1 seminoma and have demonstrated its feasibility and acceptable oncological outcomes.
2. **Post-chemotherapy RPLND:** This is done for all advanced NSGCTs which have a residual lesion more than 1 cm in size after completion of first-line chemotherapy with normalized tumor markers.
3. **Salvage RPLND:** When the tumor markers fail to normalize after completion of first-line chemotherapy, second-line chemotherapy is the standard of care. If the tumor markers have normalized or reduced to very low levels after the second-line chemotherapy, then salvage RPLND is performed. This is done even if the residual lesion is less than 1 cm in size.
4. **Desperation RPLND:** Occasionally, tumor markers continue to rise during chemotherapy and the RPLND needs to be performed as a desperate measure.
5. **RPLND for growing teratoma syndrome:** Occasionally, the retroperitoneal nodal mass continues to grow even though the tumor markers have normalized. This suggests the presence of teratoma in that nodal mass.

13. What is the template for a RPLND?

Ans:

- The standard of care for a post-chemotherapy RPLND is a complete bilateral template RPLND
- The boundaries are as follows:
  - Cranial: The left renal vein

- Caudal: The point of crossing of the ureters over the common iliac arteries
- Laterally: Both ureters

- A standard bilateral template RPLND entails removal of the following nodal packets: Paracaval, precaval, inter-aortocaval, pre-aortic, para-aortic.
- Retrocaval and retro-aortic tissue is removed if there was disease prior to initiation of chemotherapy.

14. What are the indications for a modified template RPLND?

Ans:

- The concept of modified template has come into being in an attempt to reduce the morbidity associated with extensive dissection and also to allow for at least one side nerves to be preserved during a RPLND.
- The right-side template includes removal of the paracaval, precaval and inter-aortocaval lymph nodes.
- The left template includes removal of the para-aortic and inter-aortocaval lymph nodes.
- Studies have shown that in well-selected patients, a modified template RPLND is not oncologically inferior to standard template dissection.[22,23]
- These patients are those with IGCCCG good risk disease who have residual nodal burden less than 5 cm.

15. What is the role of nerve-sparing RPLND?

Ans:

- A bilateral nerve-sparing RPLND should be performed whenever feasible.
- These nerves are the post-ganglionic sympathetic nerve fibres which are responsible for bladder neck closure at the time of ejaculation. Damage to these nerves will lead to retrograde ejaculation.
- A modified template RPLND aims to preserve one-side nerves which has also been shown to result in antegrade ejaculation in 70% patients.
- However, preservation of the nerve fibres should never be given priority over removing all nodal tissue in the described template.

16. What are the surgical approaches for RPLND?

Ans:

- The most commonly used approach is the open midline transperitoneal one.
- However, this requires bowel mobilization which leads to post-operative ileus in some patients.
- The midline extraperitoneal approach avoid bowel mobilization and is associated with earlier bowel recovery.
- The laparoscopic and robotic approaches have also been described. These are usually utilized for primary RPLNDs and in post-chemotherapy RPLNDs with small residual disease.[24]

17. What is the role of resection of extra-retroperitoneal disease in GCTs?

Ans:

- **Lung lesions:** Patients with persistent intrathoracic masses following cisplatin-based chemotherapy should undergo resection of disease if technically feasible. Prognosis following resection is favourable; over 80 percent can be expected to achieve long-term survival. Lung lesions should be resected, if feasible, irrespective of the pathology of the RPLND specimen as the degree of concordance between the 2 sites is only 60–70%.
- **Mediastinal disease:** In contrast to GCTs that are metastatic to the mediastinum, GCTs that arise in the mediastinum carry a very poor prognosis despite chemotherapy or a multimodality approach.

18. How are these patients followed up?

Ans: Patients are followed up as given in Table 14.4.

TABLE 14.4: Germ cell tumours

Modality	*Year 1*	*Year 2*	*Year 3*	*Years 4 and 5*
Tumor markers + doctor visit	4 times	4 times	2 times	2 times
Chest X-ray	1–2 times	Once	Once	Once
Abdominopelvic magnetic resonance imaging (MRI)/ computed tomography (CT)	1–2 times	At 24 months	Once at 36 months	Once at 60 months
Thorax CT	1–2 times	At 24 months	Once at 60 months	Once at 60 months

Fertility and Sexual Aspects

Testicular tumors and its treatment with chemotherapy/ RPLND affect the fertility potential of the patients.

Patients should be counselled regarding future infertility and need for semen cryopreservation. Patients may recover from the chemotherapy and have an improvement in their semen parameters and regain fertility. However, semen cryopreservation should be offered to all patients of testicular cancer as it is more cost-effective than other treatments for fertility in the future. Usually, 2–3 semen samples are used for cryopreservation depending on the semen quality. With advancements in *in-vitro* fertilization techniques, any cryopreserved semen sample, even when it contains only a few sperms, could be used for subsequent infertility treatment. However, the utilization rates of preserved semen are low, possibly due to regaining normal fertility, use of cryopreserved semen after the follow-up period of the study or death due to disease or treatment.[1,25]

SUMMARY

- A contrast enhanced CT scan of the chest, abdomen and pelvis is the standard imaging evaluation for patients with GCTs.
- Patients with advanced GCTs are classified as per the IGCCCG risk stratification.
- Bleomycin + Etoposide + Cisplatin (BEP) is the most commonly used chemotherapy regimen for advanced GCTs. The number of cycles depend on the IGCCCG risk category.
- Patients with IGCCCG good risk disease receive 3 cycles of BEP while intermediate and poor risk patients receive 4 cycles.
- For seminomas, a FDG PET/CT is done 8–10 weeks after completion of the chemotherapy. FDG PET CT has a high NPV but low PPV for the presence of residual seminoma.
- For non-seminomas, a CECT of the chest, abdomen and pelvis is done 4 weeks after completion of chemotherapy. Any residual disease more than 1 cm in size warrants a RPLND.
- Persistently raised tumor markers after first line chemotherapy warrants the use of second line chemotherapy like VIP or TIP. If markers normalize after the second line chemotherapy, then a salvage RPLND is performed.
- If the retroperitoneal mass continues to grow in size even after normalization of tumors markers, then this suggests a growing teratoma syndrome, for which a RPLND is performed.
- The standard template of RPLND is bounded by the left renal vein superiorly, the crossing of the ureters over the common iliac arteries inferiorly and the two ureters laterally.
- A modified template RPLND may be performed in patients with good risk IGCCCG disease and limited nodal burden.
- A unilateral or bilateral nerve sparing RPLND helps preserve antegrade ejaculation.
- Lung lesions should always be resected when feasible.
- A strict follow-up schedule with physical examination, tumor markers and imaging should be followed.

REFERENCES

1. Sharma AP, Mavuduru RS. Oncofertility and Fertility Preservation in Males: Current Perspective. JPMER,Volume 53, Issue 4 (October-December, 2019).
2. Bart J, Hollema H, Groen HJ, De Vries EG, Hendrikse NH, Sleijfer DT, Wegman TD, Vaalburg W, Van Der Graaf WT. The distribution of drug-efflux pumps, P-gp, BCRP, MRP1 and MRP2, in the normal blood–testis barrier and in primary testicular tumours. European Journal of Cancer. 2004 Sep 1;40(14):2064–70.
3. Dave DS, Leppert JT, Rajfer J. Is the testis a chemo-privileged site? Is there a blood-testis barrier? Reviews in Urology. 2007;9(1):28.
4. Gupta A, Noronha J, Bakshi G, Menon S, Pal M, Joshi A, Prabash K, Noronha V, Murthy V, Krishnattry R, Patil A. Blood–testis barrier revisited—Analysis of post-chemotherapy germ cell tumor orchidectomy and retroperitoneal lymph node dissection specimens. Journal of Surgical Oncology. 2021 Mar;123(4):1157–63.
5. Gilligan T, Lin DW, Aggarwal R, *et al.* Testicular Cancer, Version 2.2020, NCCN Clinical Practice Guidelines in Oncology. J Natl Compr Canc Netw. 2019;17(12):1529–1554. doi:10.6004/jnccn.2019.0058
6. Ray B, Hajdu SI, Whitmore Jr WF. Distribution of retroperitoneal lymph node metastases in testicular germinal tumors. Cancer. 1974 Feb;33(2):340–8.
7. Jamieson JK, Dobson JF. The lymphatics of the testicle. The Lancet. 1910 Feb 19;175(4512):493–5.
8. Pierre T, Selhane F, Zareski E, Garcia C, Fizazi K, Loriot Y, Patrikidou A, Naoun N, Bernard-Tessier A, Baumert H, Lebacle C. The Role of CT in the Staging and Follow-Up of Testicular Tumors: Baseline, Recurrence and Pitfalls. Cancers. 2022 Aug 17;14(16):3965.
9. Mead G. Group ftIGCCC. International Germ Cell Consensus Classification: a prognostic factor-based staging system for metastatic germ cell cancers. International Germ Cell Cancer Collaborative Group. J Clin Oncol. 1997;15:594–603.
10. Beyer J, Collette L, Sauvé N, Daugaard G, Feldman DR, Tandstad T, Tryakin A, Stahl O, Gonzalez-Billalabeitia E, De Giorgi U, Culine S. Survival and new prognosticators in metastatic seminoma: results from the IGCCCG-update consortium. Journal of clinical oncology. 2021 May 10;39(14):1553–62.
11. Gillessen S, Sauvé N, Collette L, Daugaard G, de Wit R, Albany C, Tryakin A, Fizazi K, Stahl O, Gietema JA, De Giorgi U. Predicting outcomes in men with metastatic nonseminomatous germ cell tumors (NSGCT): results from the IGCCCG update consortium. Journal of Clinical Oncology. 2021 May 5;39(14):1563.
12. Saxman SB, Finch D, Gonin R, Einhorn LH. Long-term follow-up of a phase III study of three versus four cycles of bleomycin, etoposide, and cisplatin in favorable-prognosis germ-cell tumors: The Indiana University Experience. J Clin Oncol 1998;16:702–706.
13. Nichols CR, Catalano PJ, Crawford ED, *et al.* Randomized comparison of cisplatin and etoposide and either bleomycin or ifosfamide in treatment of advanced disseminated germ cell tumors: An Eastern Cooperative Oncology Group, Southwest Oncology Group, and Cancer and Leukemia Group B Study. J Clin Oncol 1998;16:1287–1293.
14. Patrikidou A, Cazzaniga W, Berney D, Boormans J, de Angst I, Di Nardo D, Fankhauser C, Fischer S, Gravina C, Gremmels H, Heidenreich A. European Association of Urology Guidelines on Testicular Cancer: 2023 Update. European Urology. 2023 May 12.
15. Puc HS, Heelan R, Mazumdar M, Herr H, Scheinfeld J, Vlamis V, Bajorin DF, Bosl GJ, Mencel P, Motzer RJ. Management of residual mass in advanced seminoma: results and

recommendations from the Memorial Sloan-Kettering Cancer Center. Journal of clinical oncology. 1996 Feb;14(2):454–60.

16. De Santis M, Becherer A, Bokemeyer C, *et al.* 2-18fluoro-deoxy-D-glucose positron emission tomography is a reliable predictor for viable tumor in postchemotherapy seminoma: an update of the prospective multicentric SEMPET trial. J Clin Oncol 2004; 22:1034.
17. Oechsle K, Hartmann M, Brenner W, *et al.* [18F]Fluoro-deoxyglucose positron emission tomography in nonseminomatous germ cell tumors after chemotherapy: the German multicenter positron emission tomography study group. J Clin Oncol 2008; 26:5930.
18. Ehrlich Y, Brames MJ, Beck SDW, Foster RS, Einhorn LH. Long-term follow-up of cisplatin combination chemotherapy in patients with disseminated nonseminomatous germ cell tumors: is a postchemotherapy retroperitoneal lymph node dissection needed after complete remission? J Clin Oncol 2009;28:531–6
19. Carver BS, Serio AM, Bajorin D, *et al.* Improved clinical outcome in recent years for men with metastatic nonseminomatous germ cell tumors. J Clin Oncol 2007; 25:5603.
20. Spiess PE, Brown GA, Pisters LL, *et al.* Viable malignant germ cell tumor in the postchemotherapy retroperitoneal lymph node dissection specimen: can it be predicted using clinical parameters? Cancer 2006; 107:1503.
21. Logothetis, C.J.; Samuels, M.L.; Trindade, A.; Johnson, D.E. The growing teratoma syndrome. Cancer 1982, 50, 1629–1635
22. Fitzgerald JP, Ercole B, Parekh DJ. Management of post-chemotherapy residual mass in patients with metastatic nonseminomatous germ cell tumors of the testis. Indian Journal of Urology. 2010 Jan 1;26(1):98–101.
23. Lavery HJ, Bahnson RR, Sharp DS, Pohar KS. Management of the residual post-chemotherapy retroperitoneal mass in germ cell tumors. Therapeutic Advances in Urology. 2009 Oct;1(4):199–207.
24. Rosenvilde JJ, Pedersen GL, Bandak M, Lauritsen J, Kreiberg M, Wagner T, Aagaard M, Daugaard G. Oncological outcome and complications of post-chemotherapy retroperitoneal surgery in non-seminomatous germ cell tumours–a systematic review. Acta Oncologica. 2021 Jun 3;60(6):695–703.
25. Gilbert K, Nangia AK, Dupree JM, Smith JF, Mehta A. Fertility preservation for men with testicular cancer: is sperm cryopreservation cost effective in the era of assisted reproductive technology?. In Urologic Oncology: Seminars and Original Investigations 2018 Mar 1 (Vol. 36, No. 3, pp. 92-e1). Elsevier.

Chapter 15

Node Negative Penile Cancer

• Hemang Bakshi • Keval Patel

LEARNING OBJECTIVES

- To understand the importance of clinical examination of the primary tumour and inguinal regions.
  - Clinical examination is one of the most sensitive modalities to detect lymph adenopathy.
- To define and characterize various premalignant conditions with their treatment.
  - Premalignant lesion can be subjected to penile preservation and surveillance, therefore, need to be well identified.
- To understand the indications and technique of penile tumor biopsy.
  - Penile biopsy is the first step in management of ca penis and needs to be well done.
- To understand the role and methods of staging ca penis.
  - All penile lesion should be appropriately staged for standardized management.
- To define the key steps of partial penectomy.
  - Partial penectomy is a ablative and reconstructive procedure, a strong consideration for functional outcomes, helps surgeon deliver the best results.
- To understand the importance of risk stratification.
  - Risk stratification is important for decision making, especially in a N0 groin situation.
- To define the role of inguinal node dissection and understand the boundaries and techniques of the procedure.
  - Inguinal node dissection is a surgery associated with high morbidity so the template needs to be well understood.
- To understand the follow-up protocols and outcomes of groin negative ca penis.

Case Scenario

A 40-year-old male patient presented with ulcer over penis since 3 months (Fig.15.1). It was painless, and bled on touch. He had a history of whitish discolouration of glandular skin since 10 years and recent circumcision. He had no comorbidities.

1. **How will you proceed?**

   Ans: Local examination of the tumour, the penis, the surrounding structures and the groins would be the first step.

   On examination, the ulcer was a 3 × 2 cm in size, involving the glans up to the corona, with a normal meatus.

2. **What will you look for in local examination?**

   Ans: On examination you should look for the following:

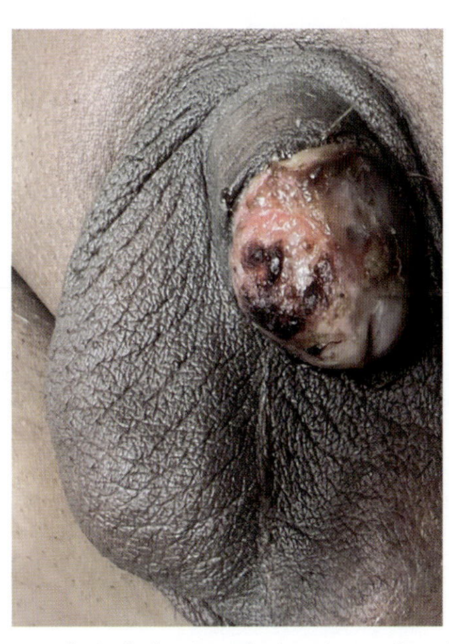

Fig.15.1: Clinical photograph showing a glans lesion

- **Ulcer:** Note the size, shape, number, location (prepuce/glans/shaft), extension and depth (groin/scrotal skin), margins (regular/irregular), induration, bleeding to touch, tenderness.
- **Mass**: Evaluate the size, shape, number and site, the characteristics (exophytic/endophytic), consistency (hard/soft/firm), extension to base of penis and scrotum are documented. Look for the remainder of normal penis, as planning for partial penectomy.
- **Groin:** The examination is done in a frog leg position, i.e. in supine position, thigh is abducted and externally rotated. Look for the following:
  - Presence of palpable lymph nodes
  - Number
  - Consistency
  - Laterality
  - Mobility/fixity and from/to underlying structures
  - Involvement of the overlying skin
  - Palpation of the underlying femoral vessels

In this patient the clinical examination showed no palpable groin nodes.

3. What is the accuracy of clinical examination in predicting nodal metastases?

Ans: In rural Indian population, due to habit of walking barefoot, 30% to 60% of patients have palpable groin nodes at presentation, of which half are metastatic and half are inflammatory.[1] Clinical examination for nodal assessment is subjective and inaccurate, especially in obese patients, with a specificity of 61%, a PPV of 67% and an NPV of 77%.[2]

4. What are the conditions that are considered premalignant for carcinoma penis?

Ans: About 10% of penile lesions at initial presentation are premalignant conditions or Penile Intraepithelial Neoplasia (PeIN),[3] which can be HPV related or HPV non-related.

The characteristics of PeIN, their common sites, clinical findings, viral association, risk of progression and treatment are described in Table 15.1 and Fig. 15.2.

TABLE 15.1: Precancerous lesion of penis

PeIN	*Site*	*Clinical features*	*Viral association and risk of progression*	*Treatment*
Erythroplasia of Queyrat (Fig. 15.2)	Glans, prepuce, urethral meatus	Single, well-demarcated, slightly raised bright red and moist plaque with bleeding[5]	5–33% Associated with HPV 16[4]	1st line: 5-fluorouracil cream.[6] Imiquimod cream. Solasodine glycosides (BEC5) purified extract from an Australian plant (*Solanum sodomaeum*) CO_2 laser vaporisation. Photodynamic therapy with topical methyl aminolevulinate (ALA–PDT) Mohs micrographic surgery[7] total glans resurfacing.
Bowen's disease	Shaft, inguinal and pubic regions	Isolated and well-defined reddish scaly plaque with surface fissures and sometimes presenting foci of pigmentation resembling melanoma	5% Associated with HPV 16[8]	Best-surgical excision. Cryotherapy—effective but painful, bleeding, infection and meatal stenosis common. CO_2 laser—both primary and recurrence ALA–PDT—for larger lesions.
Bowenoid papulosis	Mostly shaft, but can involve prepuce, glans and perianal region	Multiple, small, darkly pigmented flat papules or patches	Sporadic (<1%) but high risk in immunocompromised patients Associated with HPV 16[9]	Main therapy—local destruction using electrocautery, cryo, CO_2 laser, 5-FU cream, imquimod cream. Topical 0.05% tazarotene (retinoid prodrug).
Leukoplakia	Glans, prepuce and balano-preputial sulcus	Thick, whitish, and slightly infiltrated verrucous plaque	Associated with HPV 16, 18 and 33[10] 10–20% have dysplastic changes Especially in diabetics	CO_2 laser vaporisation Circumcision[10]

(Contd.)

TABLE 15.1: Precancerous lesion of penis *(Contd.)*				
PeIN	***Site***	***Clinical features***	***Viral association and risk of progression***	***Treatment***
Pseudoepitheliomatous keratotic, and micaceous balanitis	Glans	Hyperkeratotic, silvery-white plaques with mica-like crust on the glans penis associated with phimosis	Rare	5-FU cream and cryotherapy surgery if evidence of malignancy[11]
Penile horn	Glans	Occurs over warts or nevi or chronic abrasion and chronic balanoposthitis	Sporadic Risk increases if recurrent disease	Wide surgical excision with an area of base.[12]
Giant condyloma (Buschke–Löwenstein tumor, verrucous carcinoma)	Anorectal region, glans, prepuce and shaft	Large (>5 cm), slow growing, locally destructive highly recurrent cauliflower like growth associated with fistulas[13]	Rare Associated with HPV 6 and 11. Increased risk in immumocompromised patients.[14]	Wide surgical excision (high risk of recurrence) Combined approach (few authors) surgery plus oral acitretin and topical imiquimod Nd:YAG or CO_2 laser with interferon[15]
Extramammary Paget's disease (adenocarcinoma of skin)	Shaft Scrotum[16]	Red, moist, eroded plaque with a sharp border between normal and affected skin	Usually spreads to lymph nodes and internal malignancy.[17]	Wide local excision using the Mohs micrographic surgery and immediate reconstruction with skin grafting or a local skin flap is the current preferred treatment.
Kaposis sarcoma	Neoplastic vascular lesion of multifocal origin occurring primarily on the lower extremities. glans penis, foreskin, coronal sulcus, penile shaft, and the urethral meatus[18]	Single or multiple, red-to-purple, macular lesions or skin-colored nodules	Associated with Epstein–Barr family, human herpesvirus 8 (HHV-8)[19]	Small/solitary lesion: Surgery or local therapy Large/multiple lesions: Radiotherapy Systemic therapy for disseminated disease
Lichen sclerosus et atrophicus (balanitis xerotica obliterans)	Glans, prepuce and meatus of uncircumcised patients	Pale atrophic plaques causing phimosis and meatal stenosis	2.3–8%	Circumcision if prepuce involved. Close observation.

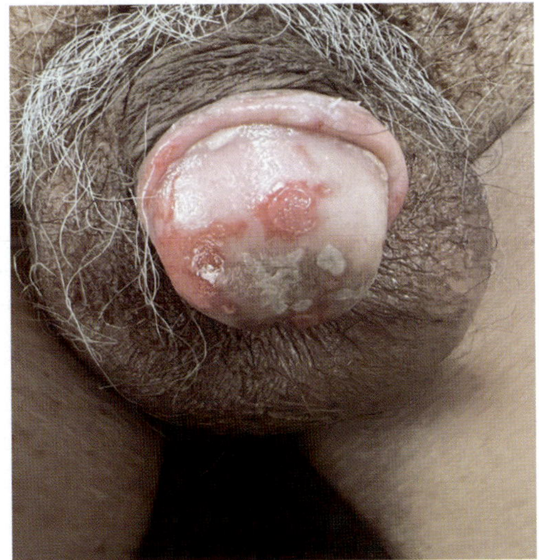

Fig 15.2: A clinical image of erythroplasia of Queyret

5. **What is the technique of penile biopsy?**

Ans: Penile biopsy can be done in one of three ways:[20]

- **Incisional biopsy**: A small piece of abnormal area including a normal portion is sampled with a knife or scissors and forceps.
- **Punch biopsy**: Linear samples of tissues are taken using a biopsy gun.
- **Excisional biopsy**: In a small lesion, the whole lesion is excised enbloc, with a circumferential margin of normal tissue.

  This is done under local or general anaesthesia, in supine position.
- When the lesion involves only the preputial skin a circumcision can be curative.
- A dorsal slit may be needed in some cases with phimosis, to expose the tumour.

- For large tumours, a wedge resection of the tumour along with normal skin may be needed.
- In the case discussed, an incisional biopsy was taken, which showed moderately differentiated squamous cell carcinoma.

6. How do you stage a case of carcinoma of penis?

Ans: The UICC/AJCC 8th edition TNM clinical and pathological classifications are given in Table 15.2.[21]

7. What radiological investigations would you like to perform?

Ans:

- **Staging investigations for the primary tumour**
  1. **Magnetic resonance imaging:** Physical examination is as good as an MRI to distinguish between T1 and T2 stages.[22] To assess cavernosal involvement (T3), especially when organ sparing approach

TABLE 15.2: TNM staging of ca penis

	Clinical classification	*Pathological classification*
T-primary tumour	Tx: Primary tumour cannot be assessed T0: No evidence of primary tumour Tis: Carcinoma *in situ* (Penile Intraepithelial Neoplasia: PeIN) Ta: Non-invasive verrucous carcinoma (verrucous) T1: Tumour invades subepithelial connective tissue T1a: Tumour invades subepithelial connective tissue without lymphovascular invasion or perineural invasion and is not poorly differentiated T1b: Tumour invades subepithelial connective tissue with lymphovascular invasion or perineural invasion or is poorly differentiated T2: Tumour invades corpus spongiosum with or without invasion of the urethra. T3: Tumour invades corpus cavernosum with or without invasion of the urethra T4: Tumour invades other adjacent structures	
N-regional lymph nodes	cNx: Regional lymph nodes cannot be assessed	pNx: Regional lymph nodes cannot be assessed
	cN0: No palpable or visibly enlarged inguinal lymph nodes	pN0: No regional lymph node metastasis
	cN1: Palpable mobile unilateral inguinal lymph node	pN1: Metastasis in one or two inguinal lymph nodes
	cN2: Palpable mobile multiple or bilateral inguinal lymph nodes	pN2: Metastasis in more than two unilateral inguinal nodes or bilateral inguinal lymph nodes
	cN3: Fixed inguinal nodal mass *or* pelvic lymphadenopathy, unilateral or bilateral	pN3: Metastasis in pelvic lymph node(s), unilateral or bilateral or extra nodal extension of regional lymph node metastasis
M-distant metastasis	M0: No distant metastasis M1: Distant metastasis	

G	Histopathological grading
Gx	Grade of differentiation cannot be assessed
G1	Well differentiated
G2	Moderately differentiated
G3	Poorly differentiated
G4	Undifferentiated

Evaluation of HPV by assessment of p16 (immunohistochemistry marker) is recommended.

The UICC/AJCC 8th edition TNM cancer staging groups

Stage	T	N	M
0	Tis	N0	M0
	Ta	N0	M0
I	T1a	N0	M0
IIA	T1b	N0	M0
	T2	N0	M0
IIB	T3	N0	M0
IIIA	T1–3	N1	M0
IIIB	T1–3	N2	M0
IV	T4	Any N	M0
	Any T	N3	M0
	Any T	Any N	M1

is planned, MRI is superior to physical examination.[23,24] MRI, with or without artificial erection, has a pooled sensitivity of 80% and specificity of 96% in predicting corpora cavernosal involvement as per a recent meta-analysis.[25]

An MRI may help in planning resection in T4 disease.

2. **Penile Doppler ultrasound**: It can be a useful alternative when MRI is not available, with a sensitivity and specificity of 96% in a prospective study of 200 patients.[26]

- **Staging Investigations for Lymph Nodes in cN0:**
  1. **Radiological investigations:** For patients having nonpalpable inguinal nodes, 1 out of 4 (25%) will have microscopic metastases in inguinal nodes.[27] The actual risk depends on the T stage and grade of the primary tumor. **No accurate imaging methods are available for nonpalpable nodes less than 1 cm.**[28] US, CT, MRI or PET can be useful in cases where physical examination is difficult, like morbid obesity, history of prior inguinal surgery or radiation. Ultrasonography with FNAC has reported a sensitivity and specificity of 39% and 100% respectively.[29]

     All patients with non-palpable or non-bulky palpable inguinal LNs should undergo a USG of both inguinal regions with a FNAC of any suspicious lymph node. Patients with reactive appearing nodes on USG or with a negative FNAC report for indeterminate/suspicious nodes on USG are staged as clinically node negative, irrespective of whether the nodes are palpable or not. There is no role of giving a trial of antibiotics in patients with suspiciously palpable inguinal nodes.
  2. **Invasive nodal surgical staging:** In form of **dynamic sentinel lymph node biopsy** and **modified or superficial lymph node dissection** are available.
- **Staging Investigations for Distant Metastasis:** For clinically negative groins, further investigations for metastasis in form of chest and abdominal CT or PET scan are **not recommended.**

Wide local excision

There is no clear consensus on the width of a safe negative margin for wide local excisions and even for glansectomy/penectomy. A negative margin of 1–5 mm for low risk tumors and 5–10 mm for high risk tumors should be aimed for.

8. What are the treatment options for the primary tumour?

Ans: Tables 15.3 and 15.4 show the treatment options for carcinoma (ca) penis.

TABLE 15.3 Treatment options for ca penis

Disease stage	Treatment options
PeIN, Tis, Ta	Topical therapy, LASER excision, circumcision (if on the prepuce), radiation therapy
T1, T2	Wide local excision, glans resurfacing, glansectomy, partial penectomy, radiation therapy
T3	Partial/total penectomy

TABLE 15.4 Topical therapy for ca penis

	5 Fluorouracil	Imiquimod
Mechanism of action	Inhibits thymidylate synthase leading to DNA damage	Activate toll-like receptor resulting in activation of immune system
Application	Leave it on for 12 hours every 48 hours for 4–6 weeks	Thrice weekly for 12 weeks
Complete response	40–60%	55–65%
Toxicity	Erythema, erosions, crusting	

Response assessment is done clinically and by a biopsy in suspicious cases. Failure of topical treatment should lead to more invasive treatment Table 15.5 depicting LASER ablation for ca penis.

TABLE 15.5 LASER ablation for ca penis

	CO_2 LASER	Nd:YAG LASER
Type	**Vaporizing** (Cutting action allows histologic analysis of resected tissue)	**Coagulative** (Coagulative action prevent histologic analysis leading to understaging)
Wavelength	10,600 nm	1060 nm
Skin depth	2–2.5 mm	3.5.mm
Healing time	5–8 weeks	8–12 weeks
Recurrence rate	10–26%	3–48%

External beam radiotherapy

- For lesions up to T1 and infrequently for T2 lesions
- With the patient supine, penis is supported vertically in a chamber
- Treated volume includes full thickness of the penis with a 1 cm margin around the lesion
- 66 to 70 Gy over 7 weeks
- 5-year local control rate: 40–70%
- S/E: Erythema, desquamation, edema → resolve in 2–4 weeks
- Most frequently used in old debilitated patients
- Local failures are treated with salvage excision

Brachytherapy

- Sterile technique under anesthesia
- Indwelling Foley catheter
- Needles avoid the urethra
- Needles placed at 12–15 mm intervals
- 3 Gy twice daily 6 hours apart
- Total dose 45–51 Gy over 7–8 days
- Penile preservation rate 80–100%

Decision regarding a glansectomy vs partial penectomy vs total penectomy is made following a clinical assessment for the size of the tumor and the length of the residual penile stump. Conventionally, it has been aimed to have at least a 2 cm stump length after resection to allow the patient to have a stump for erect voiding. In obese patients with suprapubic fat and in those with a scrotal webbing, suprapubic defatting and taking down the scrotal webbing respectively, can help 'gain' some corporal length and avoid a total penectomy in some patients.

9. What are the techniques and rationale for invasive nodal staging?

Ans: When inguinal node dissection is done after and if the nodes become palpable, the advantage would be sparing the morbidity of groin dissection in those patients who will have negative lymph nodes after surgery. This would mean node dissection could be avoided in up to 75% men with clinically negative groins.

However, delayed treatment of occult nodal metastases leads to a significantly lower cancer-specific survival: 84% vs 35%,[31] so we should not wait for nodes to become clinically positive before doing groin dissection.

Since imaging cannot reliably pick up lymph node metastasis in clinically negative groins, invasive nodal staging is done to accurately identify micrometastases in inguinal nodes in a predictable, superficial nodal area. These nodes are sent for frozen section and a full dissection is done if the frozen section is positive. Various techniques for this include dynamic sentinel node biopsy (DSNB)[31,32] modified inguinal lymph node dissection (MILD) and superficial inguinal lymph node dissection (SILD).

10. What are the steps of partial penectomy?

Ans: The surgery is performed in supine position, usually under spinal anaesthesia. A tourniquet at the base of penis may be used to reduce bleeding although it is not routinely done.[34]

1. The tumour is first isolated using a glove or a gauze to cover the lesion.
2. The skin incision is marked circumferentially, 2 cm proximal to the tumour and deepened.
3. After incising is the Buck's fascia laterally, superficial and deep dorsal venous plexuses are ligated and divided.
4. The neurovascular bundles are ligated and divided after developing a plane between tunica albuginea and neurovascular structures.
5. A plane is developed between corpus spongiosum and corpora cavernosa by sharp dissection to separate urethra from the corpora.
6. The corpora cavernosa are clamped using Kocher's clamps and divided sharply with cautery. The specimen is left hanging over the urethra and the urethra is transected 1 to 1.5 cm distal to the corpora to remove specimen. A frozen section for negative margins is not mandatory,[35] but can be done when there is clinical suspicion of a positive margin.
7. The corpora are closed transversely with interrupted or continuous horizontal mattress sutures of 2–0 polydioxanone or polyglactin.
8. The penile skin is closed vertically over the corpora cavernosa with 3–0 polyglactin interrupted sutures. After dorsal spatulation of the urethra, the cut edges are sutured to penile skin with 3-0 or 4–0 polyglactin sutures to create

a ventral neo-meatus. A Foley catheter is placed for 3–5 days.

Case Scenario (Contd.)

This patient underwent a partial penectomy. The pathology report showed pT2 moderately differentiated squamous cell carcinoma with negative surgical margins.

11. How will you risk stratify penile cancer cases?

Ans: Risk stratification is based on T stage, grade of differentiation, and the presence of lympho-vascular/peri-neural invasion in the primary tumour[36–37] (Table 15.6).

TABLE 15.6 Risk stratification of ca penis

Risk category	Primary tumor	Risk of inguinal nodal micro-metastasis
Low	Tis, Ta, T1a (without LVI) and grade 1	Almost 0%
Intermediate	T1a (without LVI) with grade 2	6–8%
High	T1b (with LVI), T2-4 of any grade and any grade 3 tumors	22–30%

Patel *et al*[38] studied 176 patients and developed a risk scoring system based on 8 factors—size of growth more than 3 cm, ulcero-infiltrative growth, involving shaft, palpable lymph nodes, ultrasound size of lymph nodes more than 1 cm with loss of fatty hilum, moderate or poor differentiation and presence of lympho-vascular/peri-neural invasion. Each risk factor is assigned a score of 0 or 1 based on the presence or absence of the factors and a total score for each patient is calculated further categorising them into three groups of low, intermediate and high-risk category. Based on the occurrence of lymph node involvement of 0%, 41.4% and 89.5% in low, intermediate and high-risk groups respectively in their study, the authors recommended avoiding lymph node dissection in low risk, and performing it in high-risk cases, whereas in intermediate risk group, they recommended FNAC for palpable lymph nodes and sentinel lymph node biopsy for non-palpable lymph nodes.

12. What are the indications for groin dissection in clinically negative groins?

Ans: Invasive inguinal staging is recommended for all patients with a high-risk primary tumor. For patients with intermediate risk tumors, both surveillance and invasive inguinal staging can be offered.[30]

13. What are the options for invasive inguinal staging?

Ans: The three options for invasive inguinal staging include (Figs 15.3–15.5):

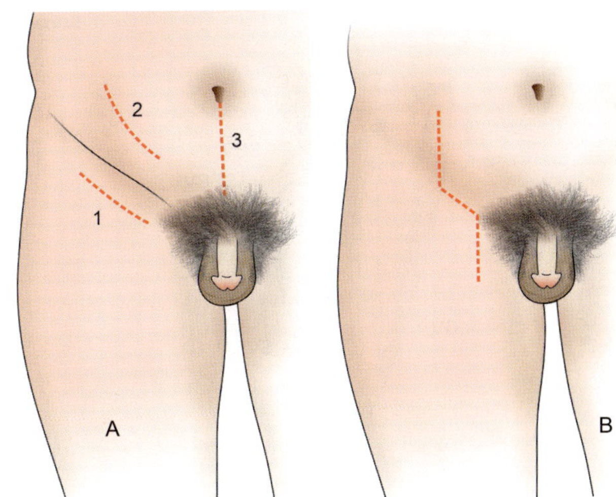

Ilioinguinal lymph node dissection. A, incisions for inguinofemoral lymph node dissection (1), unilateral pelvic lymph node dissection (2), and bilateral pelvic lymph node dissection (3). B, single-incison approach for ilioinguinal lymph node dissection. (Reprinted with permission, Cleveland Clinic Center for Medical Art and Photography © 2003–2010. All rights reserved.)

Fig. 15.3A and B: Various incisions used for groin node dissection

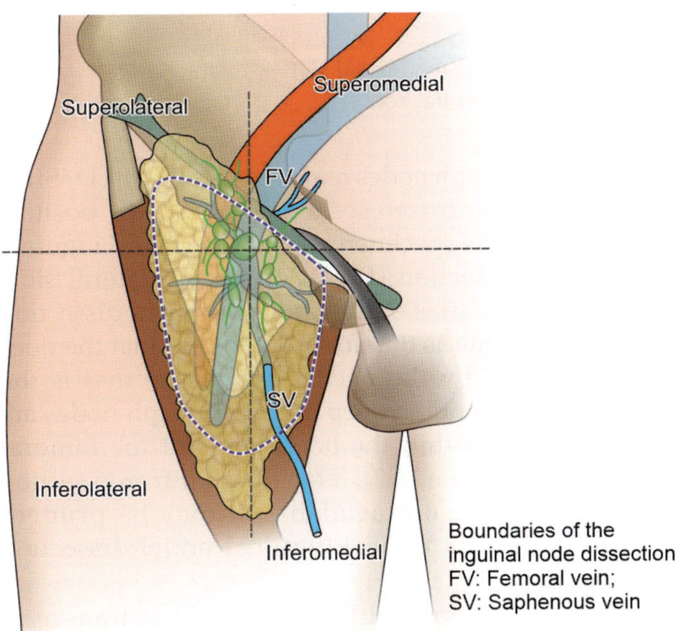

Fig. 15.4: Boundaries of groin node dissection

1. Modified inguinal lymph node dissection (MILD)[39]
2. Superficial inguinal lymph node dissection (SILD)[39]
3. Dynamic sentinel lymph node biopsy (DSNB)[31]

The boundaries of dissection for MILD and SILD are summarized in Table 15.7.

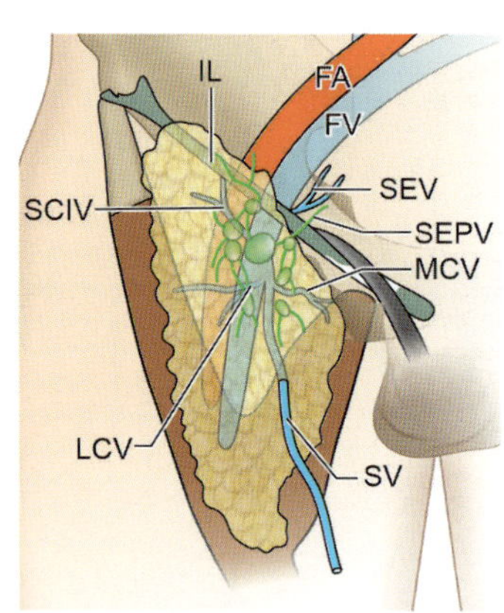

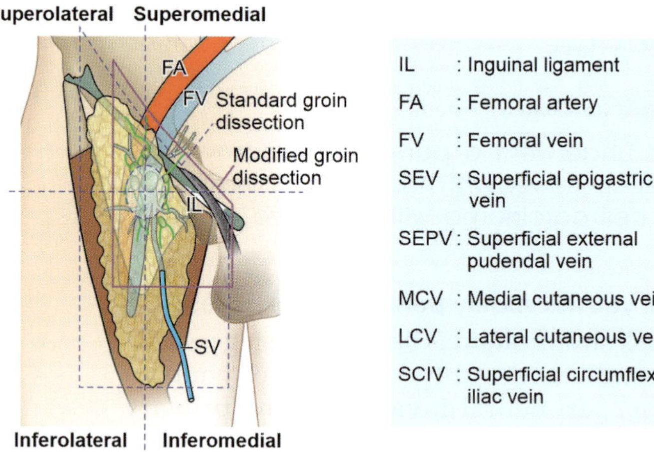

Fig. 15.5: Landmarks observed during inguinal nodal dissection

TABLE 15.7: The boundaries of dissection for MILD and SILD

	MILD	*SILD*
Superior limit	Inguinal ligament	
Medial limit	Adductor longus	
Inferior limit	Fossa ovalis	Apex of femoral triangle
Lateral limit	Femoral artery	Sartorius
Floor	Fascia lata	
Nodes removed	Supero-medial and central zones	All superficial inguinal LNs

The lymph nodes removed during MILD/SILD are sent for frozen section analysis. Any positive node in this specimen warrants a radical inguinal nodal dissection (RILD) on the ipsilateral side. The boundaries of the radical inguinal dissection are the same as that for SILD, except that the floor is formed by the pectineus muscle, that is the fascia lata and all deep inguinal lymph nodes are removed within the boundaries of the femoral triangle (Table 15.7). If facilities for frozen section analysis are not available, it may be prudent to perform a radical inguinal nodal dissection straightaway.

Incision for MILD/SILD/RILD: A transverse incision about 2 finger breadths below and parallel to the inguinal crease is the preferred incision. A vertical or the 'lazy S' incision are associated with higher rates of wound-related complications (Fig. 15.3A and 15.3B).

14. How is DSNB performed?

Ans:

- Intradermal injection of radiolabelled colloid 4 hours before surgery
- USG-guided FNAC from palpably enlarged nodes that fail to pick up colloid activity
- Intradermal injection of blue dye/ICG just before surgery
- Use a gamma probe during surgery to identify "hot" nodes and NIRF camera for green nodes[31]
- Intraoperative palpation of the inguinal region
- Excision of all "hot," blue/green and palpable nodes for frozen section examination
- Serial sectioning and immune-histochemical staining of the nodes instead of routine paraffin sections

15. What is the role of minimally invasive surgery in ILND?

Ans: Laparoscopic lymphadenectomy since 2006 and robotic lymphadenectomy (Figs 15.6A to C) since 2009 are recent techniques having advantages of lower morbidity as compared to open surgery. The lymph node yields are comparable to open surgery.

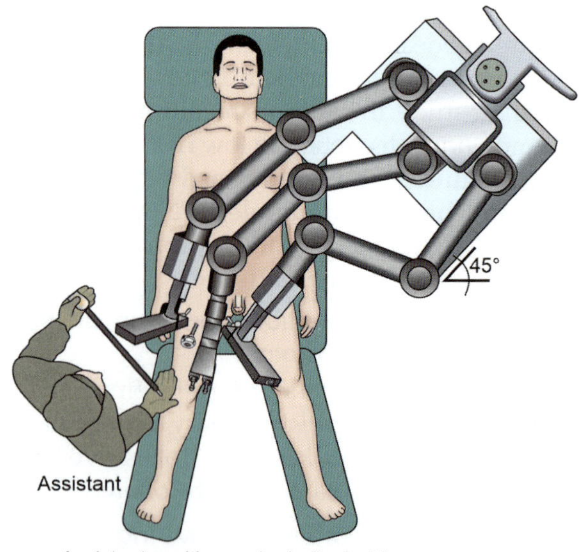

Assistant position and robotic docking for right inguinal node disection

Fig.15.6A: Robotic setup

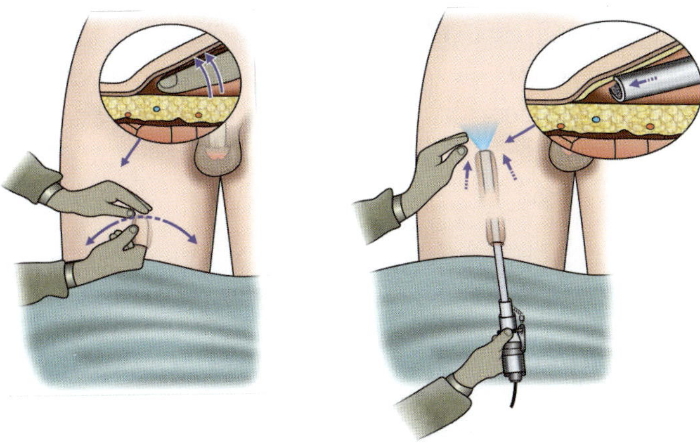

Fig. 15.6B: Creating space for robotic VEIL

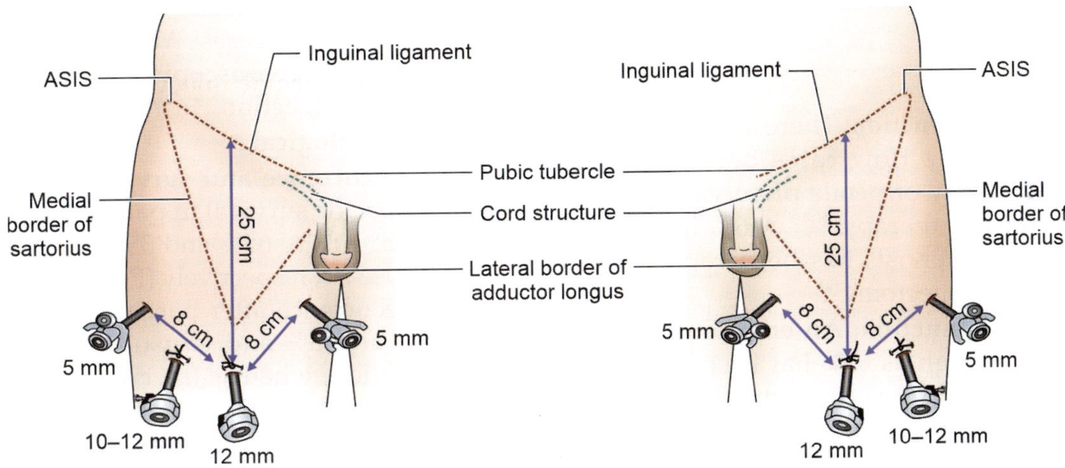

Fig. 15.6C: Port positioning for robotic VEIL

Long-term data and large volume series are yet to emerge but early data is encouraging. Complication rates have been low between 20 and 27% as shown by Sotelo *et al* in 2009 and Master *et al* in 2012.[40–42] The major limitations are the availability of instrumentation and the costs. A recent meta-analysis of 10 studies with 290 procedures showed clear advantages in reducing wound complications and lymphedema.[43]

The data in Indian scenario is similar with lower complications in robotic inguinal lymphadenectomy.[44] ICG dye can be used to identify inguinal lymphatics and nodes (Fig. 15.7).

The evidence for minimally invasive inguinal nodal dissection is higher for cN0 patients.

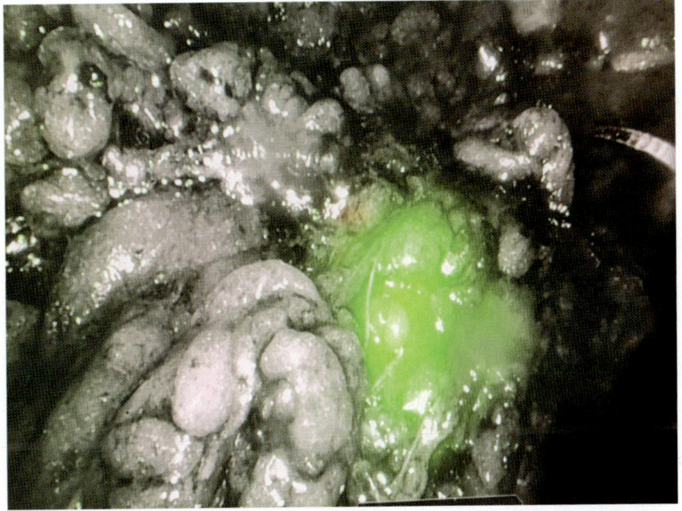

Fig.15.7: Metastatic inguinal node coloured green after ICG injection during robot assisted inguinal lymphadenectomy

16. How do the various techniques of invasive inguinal nodal dissection compare?

Ans: Comparison of the various techniques of invasive inguinal nodal dissection is given in Table 15.8.

17. How do you follow-up the cases of carcinoma penis?

Ans: Follow-up is important to detect recurrences early. Data from an Indian institute report most recurrences occur early, 52.3% within two years and 79.5% within three years.[45] Most of the

Table 15.8: Comparing various techniques of LND

	MILD	SILD	DSNB	VEIL
False negatives	15–20%	Should be 0%	4–8%	Not known
Wound related complications	++	+++	+	+
Evidence	Poor	Poor	Highest	Evolving
Needs expensive equipment	×	×	✓	✓
Possible in non-centralized care	✓	✓	×	×

recurrences after 5 years are local or new primary lesions.[46] Based on these facts a follow-up strategy has been formulated by EAU guidelines 2023[47] which is shown in Table 15.9.

18. What are the outcomes in cases of carcinoma penis?

Ans:

- **Functional**
  1. **Urinary function:** There are no differences in urinary flow rates between partial penectomy or penile preservation surgery or brachytherapy.[48,49] A 6% incidence of meatal stenosis has been reported after partial penectomy.[50]
  2. **Sexual function:** An erectile dysfunction rate as high as 67% has been reported by one RCT,[51] however, contradictory findings were reported by a study[52] where 64% could perform sexual intercourse normally after partial penectomy. Some studies have also reported negative impact on every domain of IIEF score after partial penectomy.[53]
  3. **Complications of groin dissection:** A recent meta-analysis[54] have reported complications of groin dissection. Skin necrosis was reported in between 4 and 30% and wound infection in range of 2 to 60%. Lymphedema was reported for 5.6 to 37% of the cases. **All complications were less in laparoscopic and robotic lymph node dissection.**
- **Oncological**

  Recurrence and survival: The 5-year disease-specific survival in patients was approximately 95%, 80%, 65% and 35% for N0, N1, N2 or N3 disease, respectively (P<0.001).[55] The risk of local recurrence after partial penectomy is between 4 and 5% and is usually detected on examination, whereas the risk of nodal recurrence is 9% if the patient is on surveillance and 2.3% if the patient has undergone groin dissection with pN0.[56] These can be detected by ultrasound or FNAC. A local recurrence rate of 0% has been reported for patients with T1 tumours and 18% to 21% for T2 lesions.[46]

TABLE 15.9: Follow-up schedule formulated by EAU

	Interval of surveillance		*Examinations and investigations*	*Minimum duration of follow-up*
	Years 1–2	Years 3–5		
Recommendations for follow-up of the primary tumour				
Penile-preserving treatment	3-monthly	6-monthly	Regular physician or self-examination. Repeat biopsy after topical or laser treatment for PeIN (optional).	5 years
Amputation	3-monthly	Annually	Regular physician or self- examination.	5 years
Recommendations for follow-up of the inguinal lymph nodes				
Surveillance	3-monthly	6-monthly	Regular physician or self-examination. US +/-FNAC optional.	5 years
pN0	3-monthly	Annually	Regular physician or self-examination. US +/-FNAC optional.	5 years
pN+	3-monthly	6-monthly	Regular physician or self-examination. US +/-FNAC, CT chest/abdomen/ pelvis or 18FDG-PET/CT optional.	5 years

Outcomes after external beam radiation: Local control and penile preservation is 60% to 65%

SUMMARY

- Penile malignancy may present ranging from a spectrum of pre-malignant disease to a florid metastatic disease.
- Penile preservation is an objective whenever possible.
- Local therapy, lasers, radiation therapy and surgery can all be used for penile preservation.
- Role of imaging in difficult groin, i.e operated, fatty groin is justified.
- Margin for oncological clearance in a moderate risk disease is 5 mm and should be increased to 8 mm in a high risk disease.
- Partial penectomy is an oncological and functional surgery and requires utmost due diligence.
- N0 groin should be risk stratified.
- High risk group should be subjected to modified or superficial groin node dissection.
- At present from a literature standpoint, minimal access techniques are not better than open surgery.

REFERENCES

1. Ornellas, AA, Seixas AL, Marota A, Wisnescky A, Campos F, de Morales JR . Surgical treatment of invasive squamous cell carcinoma of the penis: Retrospective analysis of 350 cases. J Urol 1994 ; 151: 1244–9.
2. Senthil Kumar MP, Ananthakrishnan N, Prema V. Predicting regional lymph node metastasis in carcinoma of the penis: A comparison between fine needle aspiration cytology, sentinel lymph node biopsy. Br J Urol 1998;81;453–7.
3. Partin AW, Wein AJ, Kavoussi LR. Urology. 14th ed. Vol. 3. Philadelphia: Elsevier; 2012.
4. Malek RS (1992) Laser treatment of premalignant and malignant squamous cell lesions of the penis. Lasers Surg Med 12:246–253.
5. Graham JH, Helwig EB (1973) Erythroplasia of Queyrat, A clinicopathologic and histochemical study. Cancer 32: 1396–1414.
6. Porter WM, Francis N, Hawkins D, Dinneen M, Bunker CB (2002) Penile intraepithelial neoplasia: Clinical spectrum and treatment of 35 cases. Br J Dermatol 147:1159–1165.
7. Mohs FE, Snow SN, Larson PO (1992) Mohs micrographic surgery for penile tumors. Urol Clin North Am 19:291–304.
8. Cox NH, Eedy DJ, Morton CA (2007) Guidelines for management of Bowen's disease: 2006 update. Br J Dermatol 156:11–21.
9. Hama N, Ohtsuka T, Yamazaki S (2006) Detection of mucosal human papillomavirus DNA in bowenoid papulosis, Bowen's disease and squamous cell carcinoma of the skin. J Dermatol 33:331–337.
10. Aynaud O, Bergeron C (2004) Penile intraepithelial neoplasia. Prog Urol 14:100–104.
11. Murthy PS, Kanak K, Raveendra L, Reddy P (2010) Pseudo-epitheliomatous, keratotic, and micaceous balanitis. Indian J Dermatol 55:190–191.
12. Solsona E, Algaba F, Horenblas S, Pizzocaro G, Windahl T (2004) EAU guidelines on penile cancer. Eur Urol 46:1–8.
13. Gholam P, Enk A, Hartschuh W (2009) Successful surgical management of giant condyloma acuminatum (Buschke-Lowenstein tumor) in the genitoanal region: a case report and evaluation of current therapies. Dermatology 218:56–59.
14. Boshart M, zur Hausen H (1986) Human papillomaviruses in Buschke-Lowenstein tumors: physical state of the DNA and identification of a tandem duplication in the noncoding region of a human papillomavirus 6 subtype. J Virol 58:963–966.
15. Erkek E, Basar H, Bozdogan O, Emeksiz MC (2009) Giant condyloma acuminata of Buschke-Lowenstein: successful treatment with a combination of surgical excision, oral acitretin and topical imiquimod. Clin Exp Dermatol 34:366–368.
16. Zhao W, Li ZH, Kong CZ (2010) Diagnosis and management of scrotal Paget's disease: report of 23 cases. Zhonghua Nan Ke Xue 16:453–455.
17. Zhu Y, Ye DW, Yao XD, Zhang SL, Dai B, Zhang HL, Shen YJ, Mao HR (2009) Clinicopathological characteristics, management and outcome of metastatic penoscrotal extramammary Paget's disease. Br J Dermatol 161:577–582.
18. Micali G, Nasca MR, De Pasquale R, Innocenzi D (2003) Primary classic Kaposi's sarcoma of the penis: report of a case and review. J Eur Acad Dermatol Venereol 17:320–323.
19. Chang Y, Cesarman E, Pessin MS, Lee F, Culpepper J, Knowles DM, Moore PS (1994) Identification of herpesvirus-like DNA sequences in AIDS-associated Kaposi's sarcoma. Science 266:1865–1869.
20. https://www.cancerresearchuk.org/about-cancer/penile-cancer/getting-diagnosed/tests/biopsy.
21. Brierley J, *et al.* TNM Classification of Malignant Tumours, 8th Edn. 2016.
22. Lont AP, *et al.* A comparison of physical examination and imaging in determining the extent of primary penile carcinoma. BJU Int, 2003. 91: 493.
23. Kayes O, *et al.* The role of magnetic resonance imaging in the local staging of penile cancer. Eur Urol, 2007. 51: 1313.
24. Hanchanale V, *et al.* The accuracy of magnetic resonance imaging (MRI) in predicting the invasion of the tunica albuginea and the urethra during the primary staging of penile cancer. BJU Int, 2016. 117: 439.
25. Krishna S, *et al.* Diagnostic Accuracy of MRI in Local Staging (T Category) of Penile Cancer and the Value of Artificial Erection: A Systematic Review and Meta-Analysis. AJR Am J Roentgenol, 2022. 219: 28.
26. Bozzini G, *et al.* Role of Penile Doppler US in the Preoperative Assessment of Penile Squamous Cell Carcinoma Patients: Results From a Large Prospective Multicenter European Study. Urology, 2016. 90: 131.
27. Srinivas V, *et al.* Penile cancer: relation of extent of nodal metastasis to survival. J Urol, 1987. 137: 880.
28. Jakobsen JK, *et al.* DaPeCa-7: comparative assessment of fluorodeoxyglucose positron emission tomography/computed tomography (CT) and conventional diagnostic CT in diagnosis of lymph node metastases, distant metastases and incidental findings in patients with invasive penile cancer. BJU Int, 2021. 127: 254.
29. Lee EWC, *et al.* High diagnostic accuracy of inguinal ultrasonography and fine-needle aspiration followed by dynamic sentinel lymph node biopsy in men with impalpable and palpable inguinal lymph nodes. BJU Int, 2022. 130: 331
30. EAU-ASCO guidelines on penile cancer 2023.
31. Kroon BK, Horenblas S, Lont AP, *et al.* Patients with penile carcinoma benefit from immediate resection of clinically occult lymph node metastasis. J Urol 2005b; 173:816–9.

32. Pettaway CA, *et al.* Sentinel lymph node biopsy for penile squamous carcinoma: The MD Anderson Cancer center experience. J Urol 1995; 154:1999–2003.
33. Paolo Dell Oglio *et al.* Hybrid indigo cyanine Green-99 mTc-nanocolloid for Single–photon emission computed tomography and combined Radio-and fluorescence-guided sentinel node biopsy in penile cancer. European urology 78(2020) 865–872.
34. David S. Sharp, Kenneth W. Angermeier. Surgery of Penile and Urethral Carcinoma. Campbell-Walsh Urology, 11th edition,vol 1, chapter 39:973.
35. Sri,D *et al.* A study into the association between local recurrence rates and surgical resection margins in organ sparing surgery for penile squamous cell cancer.BJU Int,2018.122:576.
36. Solsona E, Iborra I, Rubio J, Casanova JL, Ricós JV, Calabuig C. Prospective validation of the association of local tumor stage and grade as a predictive factor for occult lymph node micrometastasis in patients with penile carcinoma and clinically negative inguinal lymph nodes. J Urol. 2001 May;165(5):1506–9.
37. Slaton JW, Morgenstern N, Levy DA, Santos MW Jr, Tamboli P, Ro JY, Ayala AG, Pettaway CA. Tumor stage, vascular invasion and the percentage of poorly differentiated cancer: independent prognosticators for inguinal lymph node metastasis in penile squamous cancer. J Urol. 2001 Apr;165(4):1138–42.
38. Patel KN, Bhirud C, Dipin J, Nandy K, Venugopal V, Salunke A, Pandya SJ. A proposed Clino-radio-pathological Risk Scoring System (CRiSS) for prediction and management of inguinal lymph-nodes metastasis in squamous cell carcinoma of the penis. Surg Oncol. 2021 Mar;36:147–152.
39. Catalona WJ. Modified inguinal lynphadenectomy for carcinoma of the penis with preservation of saphenous veins: Technique and preliminary results.J Urol 1988;140:306–10.
40. K Angermeier,Rene Sotelo, David Sharp. Inguinal Node Dissection. Campbell-Walsh Urology, 11th edition,vol 1, chapter 39:895,902–903.
41. Master VA, Jafri SM, Moses KA, *et al.* Minimally invasive inguinal lymphadenectomy via endoscopic groin dissection: comprehensive assessment of immediate and long-term complications. *J Urol.* 2012;188:1176–1180.
42. Matin SF, Cormier JN, Ward JF, *et al.* Phase 1 prospective evaluation of the oncological adequacy of robotic assisted video-endoscopic inguinal lymphadenectomy in patients with penile carcinoma. *BJU Int.* 2013;111:1068–1074.
43. Patel KN, Salunke A, Bakshi G, Jayaprakash D, Pandya SJ. Robotic-Assisted Video-Endoscopic Inguinal Lymphadenectomy (RAVEIL) and Video-Endoscopic Inguinal Lymphadenectomy (VEIL) versus Open Inguinal Lymph-Node Dissection (OILND) in carcinoma of penis: Comparison of perioperative outcomes, complications and oncological outcomes. A systematic review and meta-analysis. Urol Oncol. 2022 Mar;40(3):112.e11–112.e22.
44. Thyavihally,Y.B. *et al.* Comparative study of perioperative and survival outcomes after video endoscopic inguinal lymphadenectomy(VEIL) and open inguinal lymph node dissection(0-ILND) in the management of inguinal lymph nodes in carcinoma of the penis.J Robot Surg 2021.15:905.
45. Arora, A., *et al.* A0694-Patterns of recurrence in penile cancer: Implications for surveillance strategies. Eur Urol, 2022. 81: S1033.
46. Leijte, J.A., *et al.* Recurrence patterns of squamous cell carcinoma of the penis: recommendations for follow-up based on a two-centre analysis of 700 patients. Eur Urol, 2008.54:161.
47. EAU-ASCO Penile Cancer Guidelines. Edn. presented at the EAU Annual Congress Milan 2023. ISBN 978–94–92671–19–6.
48. Pérez, J., *et al.* Oncological and Functional Outcomes After Organ-Sparing Plastic Reconstructive Surgery for Penile Cancer. Urology, 2020. 142: 161.
49. Martz, N., *et al.* High-dose rate brachytherapy in localized penile cancer: 5-Year clinical outcome analysis. Clin Transl Radiat Oncol, 2021. 27: 89.
50. Horenblas S, van Tinteren H, Delemarre JF, *et al.* Squamous cell carcinoma of the penis. II. Treatment of the primary tumor. J Urol 1992;147: 1533–8.
51. Monteiro, L.L., *et al.* Erectile function after partial penectomy for penile cancer. Int Braz J Urol, 2021. 47: 515.
52. D'Ancona, C.A., *et al.* Quality of life after partial penectomy for penile carcinoma. Urology, 1997. 50: 593.
53. Sedigh, O., *et al.* Sexual function after surgical treatment for penile cancer: Which organ-sparing approach gives the best results? Can Urol Assoc J, 2015. 9: E423.
54. Patel KN, Salunke A, Bakshi G, Jayaprakash D, Pandya SJ. Robotic-Assisted Video-Endoscopic Inguinal Lymphadenectomy (RAVEIL) and Video-Endoscopic Inguinal Lymphadenectomy (VEIL) versus Open Inguinal Lymph-Node Dissection (OILND) in carcinoma of penis: Comparison of perioperative outcomes, complications and oncological outcomes. A systematic review and meta-analysis. Urol Oncol. 2022 Mar;40(3):112.e11–112.e22.
55. Zhu Y, Ye DW. Lymph node metastases and prognosis in penile cancer. Chin J Cancer Res. 2012 Jun;24(2):90–6.
56. Kroon, B.K., *et al.* Patients with penile carcinoma benefit from immediate resection of clinically occult lymph node metastases. J Urol, 2005. 173: 816.

Chapter

16

Node Positive Penile Cancer

• *Brusabhanu Nayak* • *Amlesh Seth*

LEARNING OBJECTIVES

- To understand the initial workup required in a case of node positive penile cancer:: Initial assessment includes a thorough clinical examination of the primary and the groin. Biopsy of the primary tumor confirms diagnosis.
- To recognize important prognostic factors in the management of penile carcinoma: Lymph node metastasis is the single most important prognostic factor in the management of penile carcinoma.
- To appreciate the management options for clinically node positive patients with penile cancer: Patients with clinically positive nodes require aggressive management either by doing a radical lymph node dissection or by starting chemotherapy followed by consolidative surgery.
- To know the types of inguinal lymph node dissection used in the management of penile cancer: Staging lymphadenectomy, radical ILND and pelvic LND are the three types of lymph node dissections that can be used in various situations.
- To know the rationale and the extent of lymphadenectomy in node positive penile cancer: The extent of lymphadenectomy depends on the presence of metastasis in the lymphadenectomy specimen on frozen section. The natural spread is from superficial inguinal to deep inguinal and then to pelvic nodes.
- To understand the boundaries of lymphadenectomy in penile cancer: The boundaries of lymph node dissection varies with the indication, i.e staging vs a therapeutic lymphadenectomy.
- To recognize the role of chemotherapy in node positive penile cancer: Chemotherapy can be used in three scenarios: Neoadjuvant chemotherapy, adjuvant therapy and palliation.
- To understand the follow-up of patients with penile carcinoma: Clinical examination and cross sectional imaging form the cornerstone of the follow-up of a patient with cancer penis.

Case Scenario

A 66-year-old gentleman came with a 4×3 cm ulceroproliferative lesion over the distal penile shaft for the past 6 months. He also has bilateral palpable inguinal lymph nodes, largest being 2×2 cm on the right side. He is a known hypertensive and diabetic with an ECOG score of 0.

1. **How would you evaluate the patient further?**

   Ans: Clinical examination of the penis and groin

   - Carcinoma of the penis is usually clinically obvious lesions present as ulcero-proliferative growths which can be locally destructive and foul smelling. It is important to note the under surface of the foreskin in case of phimosis.
   - Examination should include inspection and palpation of the entire penis to identify potential skip lesions. The dimensions, anatomic location, and extent of local invasion should be noted along with the assessment of stretched penile length.
   - Careful palpation of both groins for enlarged inguinal lymph nodes (LN) is recommended. Enlarged LNs secondary to infection of the primary tumour (rather than metastasis) can occur.
   - For physical examination of the groin the patient can be placed in a frog leg position, thigh abducted and externally rotated.
   - The number (single/multiple), unilateral/bilateral, size, fixity (mobile/fixed) to underlying structure, and overlying skin should be noted. Relation to the groin vessels should also be assessed.

2. What are your differential diagnoses for this lesion?

Ans: 1. Carcinoma penis
2. Verrucous tumour
3. Condyloma acuminatum

3. What would you do next to confirm your diagnosis?

Ans: Biopsy

- An edge wedge biopsy along with some normal tissue is taken for histopathology examination.
- Usually done under local anaesthesia

4. What information is looked for in the biopsy of penile lesions?

Ans:

- Type of tumour: Squamous cells carcinoma constitute ~95% of penile cancers.
- Grade of tumours: Well differentiated or poorly differentiated squamous cell carcinoma
- Depth of invasion of the tumour (Table 16.1).

5. How would you ascertain the groin node status in carcinoma penis patient?

Ans:

- At the initial presentation, clinically palpable inguinal lymphadenopathy is present in approximately 50–60% of patients with squamous cell penile cancer. More than 50% of these lymphadenopathy harbor metastatic disease.[1]
- Inguinal lymph nodes that become palpable during follow-up harbor metastatic disease in nearly all cases.[2]
- Physical examination is the best method to evaluate the groin nodes except in certain situations like obese patients and patients with prior groin surgery.
- In such cases ultrasound guided fine needle aspiration cytology (FNAC) of suspicious nodes, CECT scan, MRI and PET scan can be of use for evaluating the node status.
- Lymphotrophic nanoparticle MRI (LN-MRI) has shown good results in identifying occult metastases in small series. It had a sensitivity of 100% and specificity of 97%.[3] However, it is not routinely recommended for evaluating the groin node status.

6. What investigations are required in patients with clinically node positive groins?

Ans:

- In patients with palpable inguinal nodes, nodal metastases are present in approximately 45–80% of cases.[4] It is preferable to confirm whether the nodes are involved or not by a USG-guided FNAC (Table 16.2). This may not be necessary in bulky or hard or fixed nodal disease.
- The sensitivity of fine needle aspiration cytology for clinically palpable lymph nodes is 93% and the specificity is 91% so is highly recommended.[4,5]
- It is recommended to stage the pelvis and rule out distant metastases. A CECT of chest, abdomen and pelvis for the detection of pelvic lymph nodes (sensitivity–20 –40%) and distant metastases is recommended.[6]
- MRI is an alternative to CECT with comparable sensitivity. FDG-PET has a sensitivity and specificity of 91% and specificity of 100%, respectively, for the detection of pelvic metastases in patients with confirmed positive inguinal LN.[6]
- In patients initially staged as cN0 and who are subsequently upstaged to pN+ at surgical.

7. How is the primary tumour managed?

Ans:

- The management of the primary tumour includes both surgical and non-surgical options.
- Non-surgical modalities are reserved for tumors up to T1a (G1 and G2). Options include topical therapy, laser ablation and radiotherapy (Table 16.2).
- Surgical options include glansectomy, wide local excision, partial penectomy or a total penectomy.

8. How much surgical margin is considered adequate?

Ans:

- Traditionally, a surgical margin of 2 cm was considered essential for disease control.
- However, this has been challenged by recent studies which show acceptable outcomes with lesser margins.
- Agrawal *et al* studied 64 penectomy specimens and showed that the maximum tumour spread

TABLE 16.1: Grades of penile cancer

Features	*Grade 1*	*Grade 2*	*Grade 3*	*Sarcomatoid*
Cytological atypia	Mild	Moderate	Anaplasia	Sarcomatoid
Keratinisation	Abundant	Less prominant	+/-	Absent
Intercellular bridges	Prominent	Occasional	Few	Absent
Mitotic activity	Rare	Increased	Abundant	Abundant
Tumour Margins	Pushing/Well-defined	Infiltrative/Ill-defined	Infiltrative/Ill-defined	Infiltrative/Ill-defined

TABLE 16.2: Stagewise management of ca penis	
Stage	Management options
Tis	Topical therapy; Laser ablation; Penile preservation
Ta, T1a	
(G1 and G2)	Laser ablation; Penile preservation; Radiotherapy (<4 cm)
T1b (G3) and T2	Wide local excision with reconstruction; Glansectomy with reconstruction; Radiotherapy (<4 cm)
T3	Glansectomy with distal corporectomy; Partial penectomy; Total penectomy (if urethral involvement)
T4	Total penectomy; Neo-adjuvant chemotherapy followed by surgery in unresectable; palliative chemotherapy

was 5 mm for grade I tumours and 10 mm for tumour grades II and III.[7] Philippou *et al* followed up 179 patients who underwent limited margin excision and the local recurrence rate was 8.9%.[8]

- These findings suggest that a 2 cm margin might not be always necessary, especially in small low-grade tumours.
- *Guidelines currently recommend a 3 to 5 mm margin which is tailored based on the grade of tumor (Grade I: 3 mm; Grade II: 5 mm; Grade III: 8 mm).*[9]

9. How is a partial penectomy performed and what are its outcomes (Figs. 16.1A to C)?

Ans:

- Partial penectomy provides local control, enables patient to void in a standing position and might allow satisfactory sexual performance.
- The procedure is performed under a torniquet control to reduce blood loss.
- The distal growth is wrapped with a surgical glove and isolated to avoid wound seeding.
- A per urethral catheter is placed and the skin is incised circumferentially proximal to the growth after preserving adequate skin for closure.
- The dorsal neurovascular bundles are ligated, and the corpora is transected.
- The urethra is transected 1 to 1.5 cm distal to the corporal bodies.
- A horizontal mattress closure of the corporal bodies is done with 1–0 vicryl suture.
- The urethra is spatulated and is sutured to the penile skin with 4–0 absorbable sutures.
- Spatulation prevents the late complication of neomeatal stenosis which is seen in 6% of patients.
- The local recurrence following partial penectomy ranges from 4 to 13%.[10–12]

10. What is the indication and how is a total penectomy performed?

Ans:

- A total penile amputation is indicated in penile tumours which are large and are extend proximally (Fig. 16.2).
- A perineal urethrostomy is fashioned for urinary diversion.
- Unlike radical penectomy where the corporal bodies are excised entirely, total penectomy

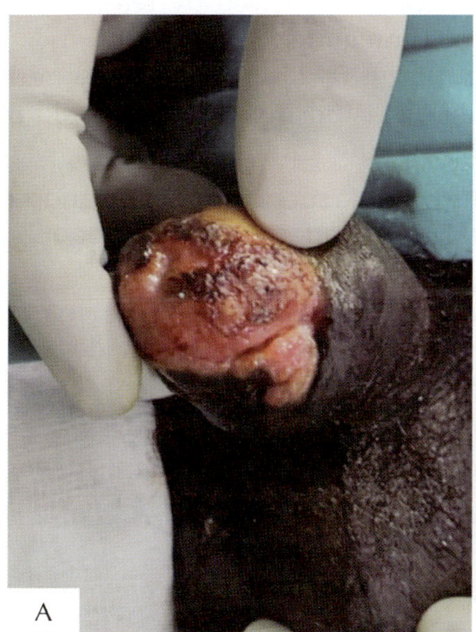

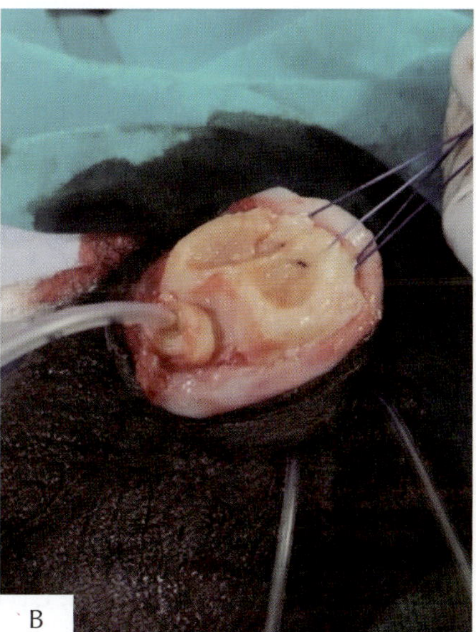

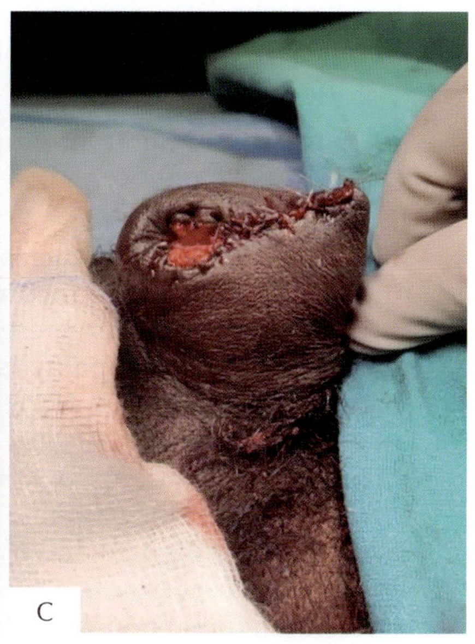

Fig. 16.1: A: Distal penile growth involving corona, B: Post-excision of growth, C: Spatulated urethra with skin closure

Uro-oncology

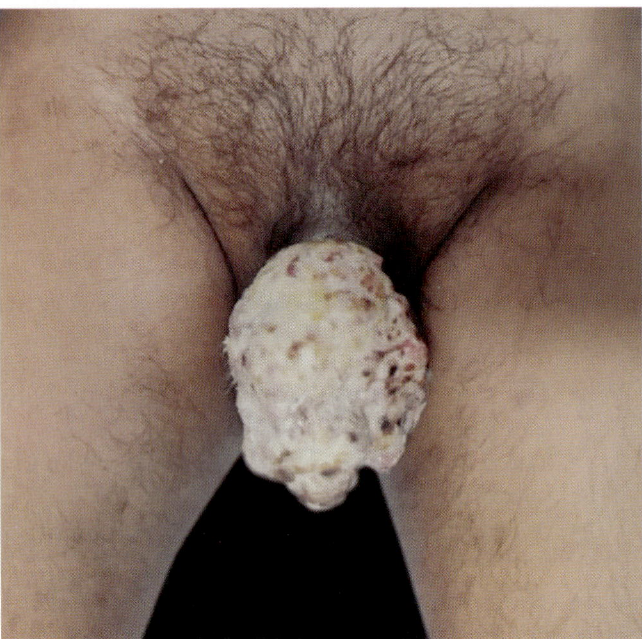

Fig. 16.2: Penile growth involving the entire shaft

involves in amputation of penis at the level of the suspensory ligament of penis.

- A diamond-shaped incision is given at the base of the penis.
- Following which the suspensory ligament is divided and proximal crural amputation is achieved.
- The urethra is mobilized ventrally until adequate length is obtained to reach the perineum.
- A perineal skin flap is raised and is sutured to the full thickness spatulated urethra with 3–0 sutures over a per urethral catheter which is removed after a week.
- The diamond-shaped skin defect is closed transversely.
- Local recurrences following total penectomy are less than 10%.[13,14]

11. What is the most important prognostic factor for survival in penile cancer?

Ans:

- Inguinal lymph nodal metastasis is the most important prognostic factor for survival in penile cancer. At index presentation, palpable inguinal lymphadenopathy is noted in 60% of patients and up to 85% of them end up having nodal metastasis.
- On the other hand, up to 30% of patients who have no clinically palpable inguinal lymph nodes are shown to have occult inguinal micrometastasis.
- Bilateral inguinal nodal involvement is seen in up to 80% of patients.

12. What is the natural history of nodal metastasis in penile cancer?

Ans:

- Squamous cell carcinoma of penis has a prolonged locoregional phase prior to distant spread.
- This window offers an opportunity and for the clinician to intervene and provide surgical cure with lymphadenectomy.
- Moreover, the lymphatic spread occurs in a predictable manner. It follows a distinct pathway—initially to the superficial inguinal nodes, then to deep inguinal and finally to the pelvic nodes.
- Unlike other urologic cancers where lymphadenectomy helps in staging and prognosticating the disease, lymphadenectomy in penile cancer, when performed appropriately, in select patients with limited nodal disease has a curative potential.
- Involvement of retroperitoneal nodes is regarded as metastatic disease.

13. What is the role of antibiotic in patients with palpable nodes in penile cancer?

Ans:

- Historically, a course of antibiotics was recommended for patients with suspicious nodes to differentiate from infective adenopathy.[15]
- However, this causes significant delay of curative treatment and is not recommended at present.[14,16]
- This is indicated only in some specific situations like Tis and Ta disease with clinically palpable lymph nodes. The chances of nodal metastasis is very low in these situations and hence a 4 weeks antibiotic course followed by reassessment of groin is recommended.
- Definite diagnosis by FNAC of whether a palpable node is positive or not, should not be delayed by giving antibiotics.

14. What are the possible scenarios in the management of regional lymph nodes in penile cancer?

Ans:

- There are three possible scenarios in the management of regional lymph nodes
  - Clinically node negative patients
  - Clinically palpable lymph nodes and
  - Enlarged fixed or ulcerated lymphadenopathy.

15. What is the management of cN1 and cN2 penile cancer?

Ans: Up to 50% of clinically negative contralateral groins in patients with N1 or N2 disease are found to have occult metastasis. Hence, a bilateral inguinal LND is offered in all patients with N1 and N2 disease.[17] However, both groins are treated on their own merit. If the USG guided FNAC had identified positive nodes on either side, then a bilateral radical inguinal lymph node dissection is performed. However, if only one side nodes are positive on the FNAC, then a superficial inguinal lymph node dissection (for staging) is performed on the contralateral side, and we proceed to a radical inguinal dissection only if the frozen section identifies positive nodes.

Management of pelvic nodes is discussed in question 19.

16. Describe the procedure of modified inguinal lymph node dissection and radical ILND.

Ans:

- The boundaries include the medial edge of sartorius laterally, lateral edge of adductor longus muscle medially, the apex of the femoral triangle inferiorly, the muscular floor of the femoral triangle posteriorly (formed by the pectineus muscle), and by the inguinal ligament superiorly.
- The skin incision in radical inguinal LND is 2 cm inferior and parallel to the inguinal ligament. Alternatively, a lazy S incision can also be used in case of concomitant PLND, however, this has been shown to result in a higher chance of flap-related complications post-operatively. Thus, a transverse incision is preferred (Fig. 16.3). A separate Gibson or lower midline incision may be taken for the pelvic nodal dissection is required. Skin flaps are raised below the Scarpa's fascia.
- Boundaries of dissection: Lateral—20 cm down from anterior superior iliac spine, Medial—15 cm below pubic tubercle.
- The areolar tissue is dissected from the external oblique aponeurosis and the spermatic cord till the inferior border of the inguinal ligament. This forms the superior nodal pocket.
- The femoral vessels are identified at the apex of the femoral triangle which is the inferior nodal pocket.
- The saphenous vein is usually preserved unless this is deemed to be oncologically unsafe.
- Within these boundaries, all lymphatic tissue, superficial and deep, including the Cloquet node are removed. A sartorius transposition is usually performed to cover the femoral vessels.[18]
- Standard lymph node dissection: Dressler's quadrangle (Fig. 16.4) is the area bounded[19] superiorly by a line connecting the anterior superior iliac spine and the pubic tubercle. Laterally a line measuring 20 cm is dropped caudally from the ASIS, medially a line from pubic tubercle is dropped to a distance of 15 cm, base of the quadrilateral is formed by the apex of femoral Triangle. Skin flaps is created in the plane just below Scarpa's fascia.
- Modified lymphadenectomy was proposed by **Catalona**. The limits of the modified inguinal lymphadenectomy are the abductor[20] longus muscle medially, the femoral artery laterally,

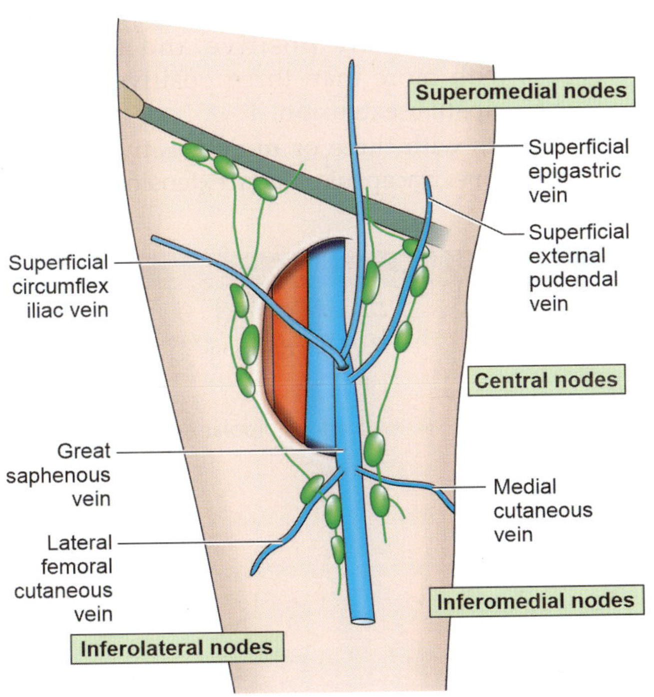

Fig. 16.3: Lymph node anatomy of the groin

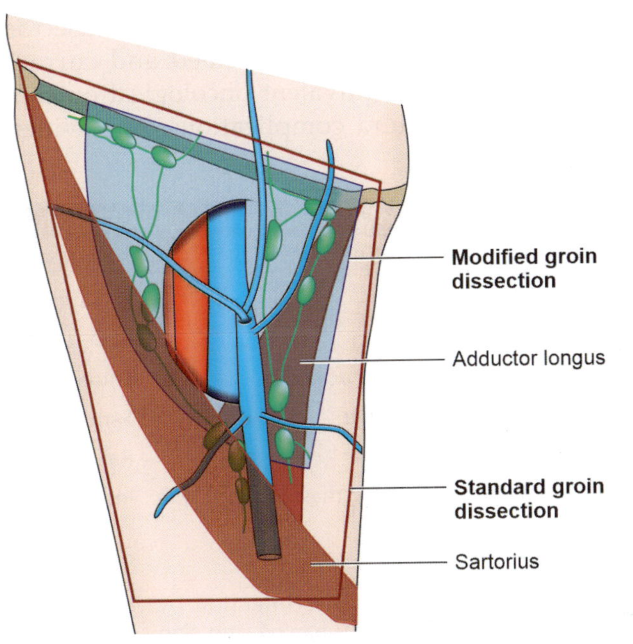

Fig. 16.4: Dressler's quadrilateral

and the inguinal ligament with the fossa ovalis as superior, and inferior limits, respectively. The four modifications include a smaller skin incision, limitation of dissection medial to the femoral artery, preservation of the saphenous vein and omitting the transposition of sartorius muscle. Superficial and deep nodes within this region including the Cloquet node are removed bilaterally and sent for histopathological examination. If metastasis is present, the procedure is converted to standard LND on the corresponding side.[21] The blue marked area represents the boundaries of modified inguinal lymph node dissection and yellow lines represent boundaries of radical lymph node dissection.

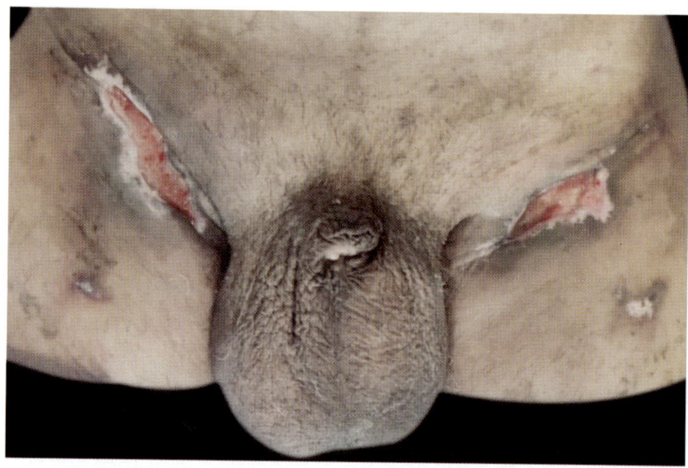

Fig. 16.5: Flap necrosis following inguinal lymph node dissection

17. What are the complications of Inguinal lymph node dissection?

Ans: ILND results in impaired lymphatic drainage from the lower limbs. The morbidity following ILND is as high as 50%. BMI is a significant risk factor for wound complications. Contemporary series show a reduced morbidity of 25%. Meticulous tissue handling and ligation of all lymphatic channels are recommended. Post operatively, compression stockings, bandages, inguinal compression dressings and suction drains can be used to mitigate morbidity. Common complications include surgical site infection (1.4%), flap necrosis (4.7%), lymphedema (13.9%) and lymphocele formation (4%).[18] (Table 16.3 and Fig. 16.5). Table 16.3 showing modalities to decrease complications.

18. What are the minimally invasive methods of inguinal lymph node dissection?

Ans: Video endoscopic inguinal lymphadenectomy (VEIL) has been well described and currently practiced with equivalent oncological outcomes and lesser wound complications. The evidence for VEIL is higher in clinically node negative patients and it is not standard practice in clinically node-positive patients. This can be done by pure laparoscopic approach or robotic approach.

Scan QR Code for Video on
Robot assisted video endoscopic inguinal lymph node dissection (RA-VEIL)

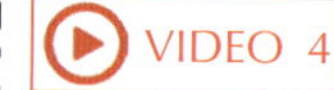

19. What is the role of pelvic lymph node dissection in penile carcinoma?

Ans: Management of pelvic nodes is discussed below:

- The probability of PLN involvement in solitary inguinal nodal involvement is up to 5%. This increases to 25% when two or more inguinal lymph nodes are positive and further to 56% with more than three positive nodes or extracapsular extension.
- Patients with three or more positive inguinal nodes or extracapsular nodal extension in a single

TABLE 16.3: Prevention of complication in inguinal lymph node dissection: ASCO 2023

Positive Impact	*Negative impact*	*Uncertain effect*
Linear transverse incision	S-shaped incision, vertical incision	Vacuum dressings
Saphenous sparing	Time-controlled drainage	Fibrin glue
Volume controlled drainage	Ultrasonic device	Advanced bipolar device
Minimally invasive technique	Sartorius transposition	
Fascial sparing	Raised BMI	
Lymphedema prevention by massage and skin care	Increased disease burden	
DVT prophylaxis	Sacropenia	
Prevention of the surgical site infection by using antibiotic prophylaxis, shaving and skin preparation		

node are recommended to undergo ipsilateral pelvic lymph node dissection (PLND).[22,23]

- Nodal metastasis more than 4 cm are associated with extranodal extension. These patients should also undergo a PLND.
- PLND can be either done along with ILND or as a secondary procedure. In case of bilateral PLND, a midline suprapubic extraperitoneal incision is preferred.
- The extent of PLND includes the distal common iliac, external iliac, obturator, internal iliac, and presacral lymph nodal groups.
- The decision for a PLND depends on the nodal status of the ipsilateral groin only.

20. What is the management of cN3 penile cancer?

- There are two 'types' of cN3 patients → those with fixed inguinal nodes and those with enlarged pelvic nodes on imaging (Fig. 16.6).

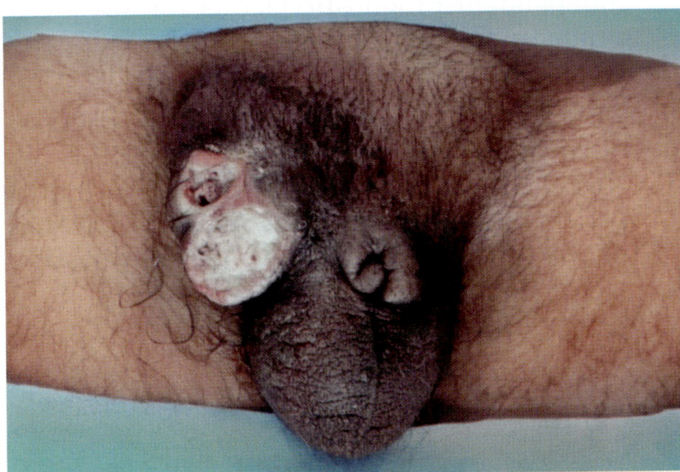

Fig. 16.6: Ulcerated lymphadenopathy

- Survival in patients with bulky fixed nodal metastasis is dependent upon complete eradication of the disease. This is seldom achieved by surgery or chemotherapy as standalone management options.
- N3 disease carries a poor prognosis and multimodal therapy is recommended in these patients. Neoadjuvant chemotherapy followed by consolidation surgery has shown benefit in advanced penile carcinoma. Studies have shown up to 60% response rates with chemotherapy and up to 20% showing complete response in patients undergoing consolidative ilioinguinal LND (Table 16.4).
- Neoadjuvant paclitaxel, ifosfamide and cisplatin (TIP) chemotherapy (4 cycles) resulted in an overall response rate of 50% with 30% pathologic complete response. TIP regimen was better tolerated and had a higher response rate compared to single agent cisplatin chemotherapy.
- Thus, a 4-cycle course of platinum and taxane based triple combination regimen is recommended.
- In patients who do not respond or progress on NACT, a multidisciplinary team should evaluate the benefit of surgical resection, as the bad biology of the disease here points towards poor prognosis.

21. What is the role of adjuvant therapy in node positive penile carcinoma?

Ans:

- Patients with pN2/pN3 disease require adjuvant chemotherapy following LND.
- The disease-free survival in patients undergoing adjuvant chemotherapy is reported to be 84%

TABLE 16.4 : Management of lymph node metastasis

Nodal status	*Management*
cN0 (No palpable inguinal nodes)	Tis, Ta, T1G1: Surveillance T1G2 and above: Invasive lymph node staging (dynamic sentinel node biopsy or bilateral modified inguinal lymphadenectomy)
cN1/cN2 (Palpable inguinal nodes)	• FNAC should be done irrespective of the stage of the primary, course of antibiotic may have some role in Tis and Ta • Bilateral FNAC positive—B/L radical inguinal lymph node dissection and proceed SOS to pelvic nodal dissection • Unilateral FNAC positive: Ipsilateral radical ILND and contralateral SILD or DSNB and frozen section analysis • Bilateral FNAC negative: B/L Superficial inguinal lymph node dissection or DSNB and frozen section and proceed further as per frozen findings.
cN3	• Neoadjuvant chemotherapy followed by radical inguinal lymphadenectomy if responsive. • Consider upfront radical ilioinguinal node dissection (if resectable on imaging) followed by chemotherapy in patients with infected or ulcerated lesions who may not be able to receive NACT
Pelvic nodes	Ipsilateral pelvic lymphadenectomy if three or more inguinal nodes are positive (pN2) or in extranodal extension (pN3)

compared to 39% in historical controls without any adjuvant therapy.[24]

- Better toxicity profile and outcomes were found with three to four cycles of a cisplatin, 5-FU and taxane (paclitaxel or docetaxel) regimen (TPF).
- At a median follow-up of 42 months, 52% of patients were disease free with TPF chemotherapy.[25]
- For patients with pN1 disease, no data exists concerning adjuvant therapy and is therefore not routinely provided.
- The International Penile Advanced Cancer Trial (InPACT) is the first randomized trial aiming to evaluate treatment options in penile cancer. It is a multi-institutional trial which is currently underway in the UK, US, Canada, and Columbia. The study sets to answer two important questions via 2 independent randomizations. First is the role of NACT prior to standard surgical therapy. Patients are being randomized into three arms (chemotherapy, chemoradiotherapy and no NACT). Second is the role of prophylactic pelvic lymphadenectomy in patients who receive inguinal lymphadenectomy with high risk pathologic factors.[26] The results of this RCT will throw light in the sequence of multimodal therapy in PSCC.
- Although level I evidence is lacking, adjuvant RT in patients with cN2/N3 disease has been shown to improve overall survival in patients who have >2 positive inguinal nodes but negative pelvic nodes.[27] The dose of radiation that benefits these patients is 54 Gy (extra nodal extension) and up to 57–60 Gy (for gross residual disease). This is higher than the conventional dose of 50 Gy. The in-field recurrences were almost doubled for patients who received lower doses of RT.[28] Adjuvant RT improves disease specific survival by 6 months and delays the time to recurrence.[29]

22. What is the management of nodal recurrence in penile carcinoma?

Ans:

- Patients who have a nodal recurrence should be managed the same way as cN1/cN2 disease. Among patients with prior DSNB or a modified ILND, the natural lymphatic drainage is absent, and the disease spread is erratic.
- The survival of patients who have a recurrence after radical ILND is 16% and multimodal therapy is recommended in these patients.
- In patients who are under observation, new onset unilateral lymphadenopathy signifies metastatic spread. New onset unilateral recurrence after 6 months is considered interval recurrence. Considering the cross over lymphatic drainage and assuming equal growth rates of metastatic disease, the absence of lymphadenopathy after a prolonged surveillance period suggests absence of disease in clinically negative groin. Hence a unilateral inguinal lymph node dissection is recommended. Contralateral nodal disease is reported in up to 30% of patients with an ipsilateral bulky recurrence. Therefore, in addition to radical ILND on the ipsilateral side, a contralateral modified ILND is recommended in patients with bulky nodal metastases even for recurrence after 6 months.[30]
- However unilateral recurrence within 6 months is considered early and rapid recurrence. Hence, should be managed like CN1/CN2 disease.

23. What is the management of advanced penile cancer?

Ans: The presence of visceral metastases and an ECOG score of greater than one are considered independent prognostic factors for advanced penile cancer. Cisplatin based regimen is preferable and has better outcomes.

24. What are the survival in patients with node negative and node positive penile cancer?

Ans: The five-year survival in node negative patients is 90 to 100%. This reduces to 60% in patients with positive inguinal nodal metastasis which are resected (Fig. 16.6).[31]

- Survival in node positive patients also depends upon the number, size, histopathologic features. There is an 80% survival after lymphadenectomy in patients with unilateral, limited (up to 2 nodes) disease with no extra nodal extension or pelvic nodes.[15]
- This figure drops to 25% in patients with more than 2 positive nodes or presence of extra nodal extension.[32]
- The survival in patients with positive pelvic nodes is less than 10%[22] (Table 16.5).

TABLE 16.5: Cancer specific outcomes at 2 years

	2-year CSM rates
Node negative	1.9%
≤2 Inguinal node metastases without extra nodal extension (ENE)	19.0%
≥3 inguinal metastases and/or ENE	43.3%
Pelvic lymph node involvement	68.6%

25. What is the recommended follow-up in penile cancer patients?

Ans:

- Recurrent penile cancer can be local or regional which usually occurs within the first two years

Section 1

of primary treatment. Early detection of local recurrences and prompt treatment before metastasis to inguinal nodes has survival advantage.

- This calls for an intensive follow-up in the first two years followed by three years of less intensive follow-up amounting to a total of 5 years.
- In patients with cN0 disease, physical examination of penis and groins is recommended. Imaging does not provide an added advantage. In patients who underwent laser ablation or topical therapy, confirmatory biopsies are taken following completion of treatment course.
- Following management of node positive disease, cross-sectional imagining is recommended every three months for the first two years. After 5 years, surveillance can be omitted provided the patient is educated about self-examination.

SUMMARY

- Positive inguinal node and pelvic nodal positivity in a case of ca penis, merits a complete metastatic workup.
- Lymphadenectomy not only helps in staging the disease, but is also curative in node positive disease.
- Patients with mobile inguinal lymph nodes (cN1/cN2) are managed with bilateral inguinal lymph node dissection (ILND). Patients with fixed inguinal lymph nodes (cN3) should be managed with neoadjuvant chemotherapy followed by consolidation surgery.
- Staging/modified ILND involves removing the superficial inguinal lymph nodes medial to the femoral artery. Radical ILND includes superficial and deep lymphadenectomy. PLND involves in removing the common, external and internal iliac along with obturator and presacral nodes.
- If staging lymphadenectomy for superficial inguinal nodes is positive for metastasis, radical ILND is performed. If more than two nodes are positive or if there is extra nodal extension in radical ILND, an ipsilateral pelvic lymph node dissection is recommended.
- Neoadjuvant chemotherapy is recommended for fixed/ulcerated inguinal nodes, whereas adjuvant therapy is recommended in all pN2 and pN3 disease following ILND. Palliative chemotherapy is used in advanced disease and in the presence of visceral metastases. Cisplatin based chemotherapeutic regimens are preferred (TPF: Cisplatin, 5-FU and paclitaxel).
- Following management of node positive disease, cross-sectional imagining is recommended every three months for the first two years. After 5 years, surveillance can be omitted in self-motivated patients.

REFERENCES

1. Hegarty PK, Kayes O, Freeman A, Christopher N, Ralph DJ, Minhas S. A prospective study of 100 cases of penile cancer managed according to European Association of Urology guidelines. BJU Int. 2006 Sep;98(3):526–31.
2. Kroon BK, Horenblas S, Lont AP, Tanis PJ, Gallee MPW, Nieweg OE. Patients with penile carcinoma benefit from immediate resection of clinically occult lymph node metastases. J Urol. 2005 Mar;173(3):816–9.
3. Tabatabaei S, Harisinghani M, McDougal WS. Regional lymph node staging using lymphotropic nanoparticle enhanced magnetic resonance imaging with ferumoxtran-10 in patients with penile cancer. J Urol. 2005 Sep;174(3):923–7; discussion 927.
4. Saisorn I, Lawrentschuk N, Leewansangtong S, Bolton DM. Fine-needle aspiration cytology predicts inguinal lymph node metastasis without antibiotic pretreatment in penile carcinoma. BJU Int. 2006 Jun;97(6):1225–8.
5. Scher B, Seitz M, Reiser M, Hungerhuber E, Hahn K, Tiling R, *et al.* 18F-FDG PET/CT for staging of penile cancer. J Nucl Med. 2005 Sep;46(9):1460–5.
6. Jakobsen JK, Frahm Nielsen T, Ipsen P, Albrecht-Beste E, Cardoso Costa J, Alslev L, *et al.* DaPeCa-7: comparative assessment of fluorodeoxyglucose positron emission tomography/computed tomography (CT) and conventional diagnostic CT in diagnosis of lymph node metastases, distant metastases and incidental findings in patients with invasive penile cancer. BJU Int. 2021 Feb;127(2):254–62.
7. Agrawal A, Pai D, Ananthakrishnan N, Smile SR, Ratnakar C. The histological extent of the local spread of carcinoma of the penis and its therapeutic implications. BJU Int. 2000 Feb;85(3):299–301.
8. Philippou P, Shabbir M, Malone P, Nigam R, Muneer A, Ralph DJ, *et al.* Conservative surgery for squamous cell carcinoma of the penis: resection margins and long-term oncological control. J Urol. 2012 Sep;188(3):803–8.
9. Solsona E, Algaba F, Horenblas S, Pizzocaro G, Windahl T. EAU Guidelines on Penile Cancer. European Urology. 2004 Jul 1;46(1):1–8.
10. Piva L, Nicolai N, Di Palo A, Milani A, Merson M, Salvioni R, *et al.* [Therapeutic alternatives in the treatment of class T1N0 squamous cell carcinoma of the penis: indications and limitations]. Arch Ital Urol Androl. 1996 Jun;68(3):157–61.
11. Lümmen G, Sperling H, Pietsch M, Otto T, Rübben H. [Treatment and follow-up of patients with squamous epithelial carcinoma of the penis]. Urologe A. 1997 Mar;36(2):157–61.
12. Korets R, Koppie TM, Snyder ME, Russo P. Partial penectomy for patients with squamous cell carcinoma of the penis: the Memorial Sloan-Kettering experience. Ann Surg Oncol. 2007 Dec;14(12):3614–9.
13. Greenberg RE. Surgical Management of Carcinoma of the Penis. Urologic Clinics. 2010 Aug 1;37(3):369–78.
14. Horenblas S, Newling DW. Local recurrent tumour after penis-conserving therapy. A plea for long-term follow-up. Br J Urol. 1993 Dec;72(6):976.
15. Srinivas V, Morse MJ, Herr HW, Sogani PC, Whitmore WF. Penile cancer: relation of extent of nodal metastasis to survival. J Urol. 1987 May;137(5):880–2.
16. Richter S, Ruether JD, Wood L, Canil C, Moretto P, Venner P, *et al.* Management of carcinoma of the penis: Consensus statement from the Canadian Association of Genitourinary Medical Oncologists (CAGMO). Can Urol Assoc J. 2013;7 (11–12):E797–811.
17. Ekstrom T, Edsmyr F. Cancer of the penis; a clinical study of 229 cases. Acta Chir Scand. 1958 May 23;115(1–2):25–45.
18. Margulis V, Sagalowsky AI. Penile Cancer: Management of Regional Lymphatic Drainage. Urologic Clinics of North America. 2010 Aug 1;37(3):411–9.
19. Daseler EH, Anson BJ, Reimann AF. Radical excision of the inguinal and iliac lymph glands; a study based upon

450 anatomical dissections and upon supportive clinical observations. Surg Gynecol Obstet. 1948 Dec;87(6):679–94.

20. Jacobellis U. Modified Radical Inguinal Lymphadenectomy for Carcinoma of the Penis: Technique and Results. The Journal of Urology. 2003 Apr 1;169(4):1349–52.
21. Catalona WJ. Modified inguinal lymphadenectomy for carcinoma of the penis with preservation of saphenous veins: technique and preliminary results. J Urol. 1988 Aug;140(2):306–10.
22. Lont AP, Kroon BK, Gallee MPW, van Tinteren H, Moonen LMF, Horenblas S. Pelvic lymph node dissection for penile carcinoma: extent of inguinal lymph node involvement as an indicator for pelvic lymph node involvement and survival. J Urol. 2007 Mar;177(3):947–52.
23. Liu JY, Li YH, Zhang ZL, Yao K, Ye YL, Xie D, *et al.* The risk factors for the presence of pelvic lymph node metastasis in penile squamous cell carcinoma patients with inguinal lymph node dissection. World J Urol. 2013 Dec;31(6):1519–24.
24. Pizzocaro G, Piva L. Adjuvant and neoadjuvant vincristine, bleomycin, and methotrexate for inguinal metastases from squamous cell carcinoma of the penis. Acta Oncol. 1988;27(6b):823–4.
25. Giannatempo P, Paganoni A, Sangalli L, Colecchia M, Piva L, Catanzaro M, *et al.* Survival analyses of adjuvant or neoadjuvant combination of a taxane plus cisplatin and 5-fluorouracil (T-PF) in patients with bulky nodal metastases from squamous cell carcinoma of the penis (PSCC): Results of a single high-volume center. JCO. 2014 Feb;32(4_suppl):377–377.
26. Canter DJ, Nicholson S, Watkin N, Hall E, Pettaway C, InPACT Executive Committee. The International Penile Advanced Cancer Trial (InPACT): Rationale and Current Status. Eur Urol Focus. 2019 Sep;5(5):706–9.
27. Jaipuria J, Kohli T, Venkatasubramaniyan M, Singh A, Gupta S, Pathak P, *et al.* Adjuvant radiation compares favorably to chemotherapy in patients with carcinoma penis and nodal positivity restricted to groin. Urol Oncol. 2020 Jul;38(7):641.e9–641.e18.
28. Ager M, Njoku K, Serra M, Robinson A, Pickering L, Afshar M, *et al.* Long-term multicentre experience of adjuvant radiotherapy for pN3 squamous cell carcinoma of the penis. BJU Int. 2021 Oct;128(4):451–9.
29. Tang DH, Djajadiningrat R, Diorio G, Chipollini J, Ma Z, Schaible BJ, *et al.* Adjuvant pelvic radiation is associated with improved survival and decreased disease recurrence in pelvic node-positive penile cancer after lymph node dissection: A multi-institutional study. Urol Oncol. 2017 Oct;35(10):605.e17–605.e23.
30. Horenblas S, van Tinteren H, Delemarre JF, Moonen LM, Lustig V, van Waardenburg EW. Squamous cell carcinoma of the penis. III. Treatment of regional lymph nodes. J Urol. 1993 Mar;149(3):492–7.
31. Margulis V, Sagalowsky AI. Penile cancer: management of regional lymphatic drainage. Urologic Clinics. 2010 Aug 1;37(3):411–9.
32. Ravi R. Prophylactic lymphadenectomy vs observation vs inguinal biopsy in node-negative patients with invasive carcinoma of the penis. Jpn J Clin Oncol. 1993 Feb;23(1):53–8.

Chapter

17

Adrenal Tumors

• *Rajeev Kumar* • *Sridhar P*

LEARNING OBJECTIVES

- To understand the basic anatomy and physiology of the adrenal glands: Each adrenal gland consists of two parts which are embryologically and functionally very distinct from each other. The cortex, which itself consists of three zones, is mesodermal in origin and responsible for the production of steroid hormones. The medulla is a part of the autonomic nervous system and consists of chromaffin cells. It secretes the catecholamines epinephrine, nor-epinephrine and dopamine. The glands are located within the Gerota's fascia on either side and have a variable and plentiful blood supply, making them extremely vascular.
- To understand the epidemiology of adrenal lesions: Adrenal tumors may occur in around 2% of people above the age of 50 years and are thus among the most common tumors. A very small proportion of these lesions is symptomatic and around 1 in 4000 of them are malignant. Thus, the majority of these lesions may not require any intervention.
- To learn the presentation of adrenal tumors: Adrenal tumors may be detected either incidentally on routine radiologic imaging of the abdomen or through symptoms produced by their mass effect or the actions of the hormones or catecholamines secreted by them.
- To define incidental adrenal tumors: Tumors of the adrenal gland that are detected during routine abdominal imaging are called incidental tumors. Incidentally detected tumours are the most common lesions of the adrenal gland. Since most of them are benign and asymptomatic, investigations are targeted to identify those that require intervention, e.g. those that are functional or malignant.
- To understand the importance of size of the lesion in determining etiology: The incidence of malignancy rises with size and while less than 2% of lesions below 4 cm are malignant, 25% of those above 6 cm have cancer.
- To recollect the imaging strategies for evaluating incidental tumors: Myelolipomas can be clearly identified on imaging as they contain macroscopic fat. Such lesions may not require any further functional evaluation. Adrenal adenomas contain intracytoplasmic fat which can be detected on tailored washout studies on CT. These lesions have a low Hounsfield value on plain CT imaging, may enhance on contrast administration, but show rapid washout of the contrast. Such changes are also seen on chemical shift imaging on an MRI. Pheochromocytomas are very bright on T2 weighted MRI images which can be diagnostic.
- To understand the functional work-up of adrenal lesions: All solid lesions other than myelolipomas should also undergo a basic hormonal evaluation for hypersecretion of cortisol and catecholamines. Patients with hypertension or hypokalemia should also be evaluated for aldosterone hypersecretion.
- To recollect the value of concomitant malignancy for adrenal tumor

  History of cancer: In patients who have a history of concomitant or recent cancer elsewhere, around 50% of the adrenal lesions harbour a metastasis.
- To enumerate the indications of biopsy.

  Biopsy: Most adenomas and functional tumors should not be biopsied. Lesions suspected to have cancer, infection, or those that remain indeterminate may undergo a fine-needle aspiration cytology once the diagnosis of pheochromocytoma has been ruled out.
- To enumerate the common hereditary syndromes for adrenal tumors: Hereditary syndromes account for a significant number of adrenal tumors. These include the VHL syndrome, tuberous sclerosis, and MEN syndromes among others. Evaluating the family history and screening of the family in case a syndrome is identified are important components of the valuation and management of these tumors.
- To outline the management strategies for adrenal tumors: Management of adrenal tumors is largely surgical. All benign lesions that are functional or have symptoms related to the size of the lesion require removal. Surgery is the primary intervention modality for adrenal carcinomas. Unfortunately, many of these cancers are large at the time of diagnosis and may have locally advanced or metastasized. Surgery remains the intervention of choice where feasible with a limited role of adjuvant therapy.

- To discuss pre-operative preparation of patients with pheochromocytomas: Patients with pheochromocytoma require pre-operative preparation to decrease operative morbidity and mortality. This involves administration of α-adrenergic blockade to decrease blood pressure and reverse the action of catecholamines on peripheral vasculature. They also require fluids, salt and additional medication to control blood pressure and diabetes which may be present.
- To describe various surgical approaches to adrenalectomy: Traditionally, open surgery was recommended for adrenal lesions greater than 4 cm in size. However, with greater expertise and improved technology, minimally invasive surgery has become the standard of care for most adrenal tumors. Both transperitoneal and retroperitoneal approaches have been used successfully. While pure laparoscopy is the most frequently used minimally invasive approach, robotic-assistance has also been used for adrenalectomies.

Case Scenario

24-year-old male undergoing pre-employment screening ultrasound is found to have 3 cm, solid lesion in his right adrenal gland.

1. **What are the differential diagnoses for such a lesion?**

   Ans: Lesions of the adrenal gland that are detected on routine abdominal imaging, or imaging for unrelated conditions without symptoms and measure ≥1 cm are called adrenal incidentalomas. These lesions may be cystic, solid or solid lesions with necrosis or cystic degeneration (Table 17.1). Among the solid lesions, most common are benign adenomas which are non-functioning. Functioning tumors may secrete steroid hormones or catecholamines. Catecholamine secreting tumors are called pheochromocytomas. Less common benign tumors include myelolipomas and ganglioneuromas. Malignant lesions could be adrenocortical carcinoma or metastasis. Rarely, tuberculosis or fungal infections may present as mass lesions but are unlikely to be incidental or asymptomatic.

2. **Which portion of adrenal gland secretes catecholamines?**

   Ans: Each adrenal gland consists of two parts which are embryologically and functionally very distinct from each other. The cortex, which itself consists of three zones, is mesodermal in origin and responsible for the production of steroid hormones. The medulla is a part of the autonomic nervous system and consists of chromaffin cells. It secretes the catecholamines epinephrine, nor-epinephrine and dopamine. The glands are located within the Gerota's fascia on either side and have a variable and plentiful blood supply, making them extremely vascular.

3. **What symptoms should be sought?**

   Ans: Adrenal tumors may manifest symptoms due to their size, production of hormones or catecholamines or infiltration of adjacent organs. Benign non-functional adenomas may have no symptoms. Cortisol producing lesions will present with Cushing's syndrome and features of hypercortisolism including weight gain, easy bruisability, facial puffiness, abdominal striae, etc (Table 17.2). Lesions that produce

TABLE 17.1: Lesions of the adrenal gland
A. Cysts: Pure cysts do not require further evaluation or management unless they are symptomatic due to size.
B. Benign tumors:
1. Non-functional adenomas
2. Functional adenomas
a. Cortisol producing (Cushing's syndrome)
b. Mineralocorticoid producing (Conn's syndrome)
c. Catecholamine producing (Pheochromocytoma)
3. Myelolipoma
4. Ganglioneuroma
5. Hematoma
6. Infectious lesions (Tuberculosis, fungal)
C. Malignant lesions:
1. Adrenocortical carcinoma
2. Metastases

TABLE 17.2: Symptoms to be assessed while working up a case of adrenal incidentaloma

Condition	History	Physical Exam
Hypercortisolism (Cushing's syndrome)	Weight gain, central obesity, Severe hypertension, diabetes, Proximal girdle weakness, depression, sleep disturbance, menstrual irregularities and virilisation (in female) and pathological fractures	Hypertension, central obesity, supraclavicular fat deposition, dorsolumbar fat pad, facial plethora, thinned skin, purple straie, acne, ecchymoses, hirsuitism and proximal girgle weakness
Aldesteronism	Hypertension, hypokelemia, muscle cramps and wasting, intermittent or periodic paralysis	Hypertension, fluid retension
Pheochromocytoma	Headaches, anxiety attacks, sweating, palpitations, family history of VHL, MEN II, neurofibromatosis type II, familial paraganglioma syndrome	Severe hypertension, tachycardia,arrhythmias, congestive heart failure, excessive sweating, anxiety and pallor
Adrenocortical carcinoma	Flank pain, vague abdominal discomfort, hypercortisolism, virilization, feminization or aldesteronism	Weight loss, hirsuitism, gynecomastia, signs of hypercortisolism
Metastasis	Personal and family history of malignant lesion, weight loss, unexplained fevers, smoking	Lymphadenopathy, lung mass, breast mass, renal mass, skin lesion s/o melanoma, any other cancer specific findings

mineralocorticoids will present with Conn's syndrome with weakness, hypertension, periodic paralysis due to hypokalemia. Pheochromocytomas may be asymptomatic or may have hypertension, fatigue, blurring of vision, stroke, myocardial ischemia or hyperglycemia. Adrenocortical carcinomas may have excess androgen production with hirsutism anorexia, weight loss or may manifest with metastasis. Women with androgen-secreting tumors would have features of virilization and conversely men with estrogen secreting tumors would have features of feminization.

Tumors which are a part of hereditary syndromes may also have symptoms related to the syndrome including brain or spinal lesions, renal, parathyroid and pancreatic pathologies.

TABLE 17.3: Features suggesting tumors which may not require intervention

A. Asymptomatic

B. Tumor characteristics on imaging:

1. Size less than 4 cm
2. Cystic
3. Presence of fat suggestive of myelolipoma
4. Low baseline HU (<10), lack on enhancement on contrast, high washout of contrast

C. Lack of functionality

1. Negative 1 mg dexamethasone suppression test
2. Normal 24-hour urinary or serum catecholamines
3. Non-hypertensive, normal serum potassium

D. No history of other cancers, tuberculosis, immunocompromised state

4. Do all of these lesions require active surgical treatment?

Ans: Adrenal tumors may occur in around 2% of people above the age of 50 years and are thus among the most common tumors. A very small proportion of these lesions is symptomatic and around 1 in 4000 of them are malignant. Thus, the majority of these lesions may not require any intervention (Table 17.3).

5. What is the role of family history in this condition?

Ans: Family history plays a very important role in patients with adrenal tumors. Many of these are a part of hereditary syndromes such as VHL, tuberous sclerosis, MEN and succinate dehydrogenase enzyme deficiencies. A detailed family history, particularly if the patient has evidence of a syndromic manifestation, helps in identifying the familial condition.

6. What specific examination is required?

Ans: In all patients, physical examination should evaluate the blood pressure in different postures and manifestation of steroid excess such as hirsutism and gynaecomastia. In the presence of symptoms, specific findings related to the pathology such as obesity, abdominal striae, palpable abdominal mass, etc. may be found. In patients with a syndromic condition, findings may include fibromas, hypopigmented macules, angiomas, etc. Cardiovascular, ophthalmological and neurological evaluation are also required in patients with complications of hormone excess or familial syndromes.

7. What are the evaluation guidelines for adrenal incidentalomas?

Ans: Evaluation of adrenal incidentalomas aims to separate benign, non-functional lesions from those that are functional or may be malignant., Cystic lesions or those which radiologically appear to be myelolipomas do not require further functional evaluation. All other lesions require a minimal functional evaluation. An outline of the evaluation strategy is given in Fig. 17.1.

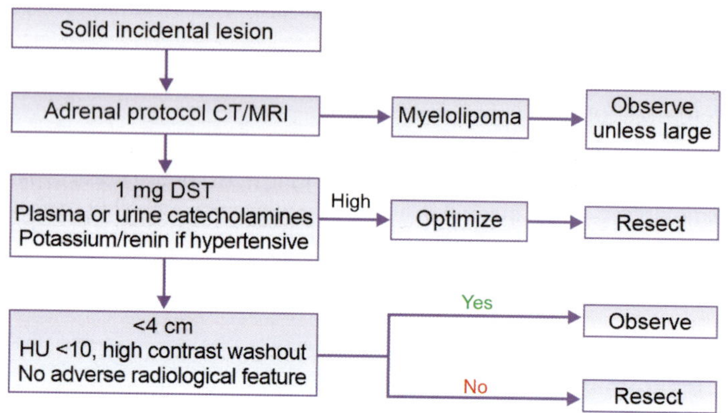

Fig. 17.1: Work-up of an adrenal incidentaloma

8. What functional investigations are required?

Ans:

- Functional evaluation aims to rule out production of excessive hormone steroids or catecholamines. All patients with adrenal incidentaloma should undergo assessment for hypercortisolism and hyperaldosteronism and excess secretion of catecholamine. Hypertensive patients should also be assessed for elevated mineralocorticoids. The investigations are given in Table 17.4.
- Both plasma and urinary metanephrines have a high sensitivity and specificity for diagnosing pheochro-mocytomas. While release of catecholamines from the tumors may be sporadic, conversion into their metabolites, the metanephrines (metanephrine and nor-metanephrine) is continuous and thus measurement of metanephrines in either plasma or urine is a much more sensitive and specific test.

9. What imaging should be obtained?

Ans: Once a lesion is identified, usually on ultrasound, an adrenal protocol CT scan may be the most appropriate next imaging study. This includes a non-contrast CT, a contrast-enhanced scan at 60–90 seconds, followed by a delayed scan at 15 minutes.

Benign adenomas have a baseline non-contrast HU <10 with high washout of contrast (absolute >60%, relative >40%) which are fairly specific findings. The combination of these two characteristics is useful for both lipid rich and lipid poor adenomas. Pheochromocytomas have a baseline HU of >10, typically around 35 and do not show washout which differentiates them from non-functional benign adenomas.

If the CT is indeterminate, MRI scans with chemical-shift or out-of-phase imaging can also detect adenomas with reasonable certainty (Table 17.5). Adenomas show loss of signal intensity on out-of-phase images compared with in-phase images. Pheochromocytomas show intense brightness on T2-weighted images, sometimes called a 'light-bulb' appearance. PET scans are generally not required for suspected

TABLE 17.4: Functional investigations for adrenal incidentalomas

Disease	*Screening test*
Cushing's syndrome	1 mg overnight dexamethasone suppression test (DST)
Conn's syndrome	Plasma aldosterone to renin ratio
Pheochromocytoma	24-hour urinary fractionated metanephrins or plasma free metanephrines
Adrenocortical cancer	Sex steroids and precursors like androstenedione, testosterone, DHEA-S, and 17 β-estradiol

TABLE 17.5 Comparing CT and MRI

Washout CT	Chemical shift MRI
+ve Adenomas have high washout AW > 60% and RW >40%. ACC have low washout and it is widely available test.	**+ve** Can detect adenomas based on SI drop with good sensitivity and specificity. No risk of radiation
-ve: False positives, 1/3rd lipid poor adenoma do washout in the adenoma range	-ve: Decreased performance on lesion with unenhanced > 30 HU
-ve: False negative. 1/3rd pheochromocytoma washout in adenoma range. Metastasis especially RCC and HCC can washout in adenoma range	-ve: High cost and lower availability

benign lesions. 18F-FDG PET/CT scans have excellent sensitivity for most pheochromocytomas and are also helpful in patients with suspected malignancy and metastasis.

The patient is not hypertensive or diabetic and has no family history of similar disease. His plasma nor-metanephrine and 24-hour urinary metanephrin level is elevated more than 3 times above normal. All other investigations are normal. The CT shows a 3 cm, enhancing lesion in the right adrenal gland (Fig. 17.2).

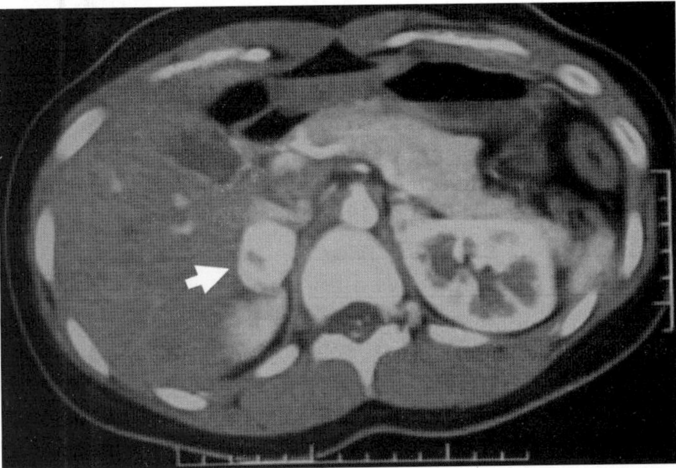

Fig. 17.2: 3 cm, right adrenal lesion on contrast enhanced CT scan

10. Between urine and blood, which tests are better for catecholamine measurement?

Ans: Both plasma free metanephrines or 24-hour urinary fractionated metanephrines level are recommended as screening tests for the diagnosis of pheochromocytoma and paraganglioma without any superiority of one over the other.[4,] Eisenhofer *et al* showed that the diagnostic performance of plasma free metanephrines was higher than the urinary measurements, despite the low false negativity rate of both plasma and urine free metanephrines measurements in pheochromocytoma and paraganglioma diagnosis. However, serum measurement is more convenient and the compliance is better compared to 24-hour urinary measurement.

11. Which functional imaging should be acquired if needed?

Ans: An I-131 MIBG scan has a very high sensitivity for detecting pheochromocytomas. However, it lacks spatial resolution and it is difficult to detect small tumors or tumors with extensive necrosis/haemorrhage, leading to false-negative results.[9]

Expression of somatostatin receptors by pheochromocytoma enables DOTANOC PET/CT imaging.[68]Ga-DOTANOC PET/CT has a high diagnostic accuracy in patients with a suspicion of pheochromocytoma, and is superior to MIBG imaging. It has better signal-to-noise ratios than 18F-FDG PET.[11]

The patient undergoes an MIBG scan that shows specific uptake in the lesion. All other regions show only physiological uptake.

12. What is the diagnosis?

Ans: This patient has a pheochromocytoma. The combination of an anatomic lesion in the adrenal gland, functionality demonstrated by elevated catecholamines, and uptake on the MIBG scan confirm the diagnosis.

Pheochromocytomas comprise around 5% of all adrenal masses but less than 0.5% of all causes of hypertension.[12,13] These are thus rare tumors. Tumors arising outside the adrenal gland are called paragangliomas and may arise from neural crest tissue along the ganglia. Pheochromocytomas arise from the adrenal medulla. Conversion of nor-epinephrine to epinephrine occurs in the adrenal gland through the enzyme phenylethanolamine-N-methyltransferase. This is one of the few organs that possess this enzyme and thus elevated metanephrine, a metabolite of epinephrine, suggests the origin from the adrenal gland. The classic teaching of pheochromocytoma being a '10%' tumor is not valid as more than 20% may occur outside the adrenal gland and the incidence of familial tumors exceeds 25%.

13. What is the preoperative preparation required?

Ans: Tumor handling is associated with catecholamine surges that can result in large blood pressure spikes, predisposing patients to cardiovascular events such as strokes and myocardial infarction. Such surges can also occur during endotracheal intubation and creation of pneumoperitoneum. Thus, preoperative stabilization is considered an essential part of preparation for pheochromocytoma surgery.[15]

Prazosin, a selective α-adrenergic blocker, is the preferred drug to initiate control of blood pressure. It is titrated as per need to a blood pressure that is normal for age with mild postural hypotension. Additional drugs such as β-blockers and calcium channel blockers may occasionally be required in some patients. The index patient does not have hypertension and though there is some evidence that such patients may not require-adrenergic blockade, most centres would continue to administer a small dose before surgery.[16] Hydration and salt intake to expand the intravascular volume is also started at the same time.

In addition, patients should be evaluated for cardiovascular fitness including an echocardiogram, particularly if they are elderly or have severe hypertension. Sugar control is required in subjects with preoperative diabetes which may also be a manifestation of catecholamine excess.[17]

14. What is the intervention planned?

Ans: The patient should undergo surgery after preoperative preparation. All pheochromocytomas require surgical removal.[18] Even though manifest symptoms such as hypertension and diabetes can be controlled by medication, the excessive catecholamines produced by these tumors result in cardiomyopathy, vascular changes, affect glucose metabolism among other changes and thus simply control of blood pressure and sugar is not a valid outcome measure.

15. Which approach is ideal?

Ans: Laparoscopic adrenalectomy is the current standard of care for pheochromocytomas. Traditionally, open surgery was considered the best approach. Recent surveys of surgical practice continue to show open surgery to be common, however, laparoscopy has been shown to have similar or better outcomes when performed by expert teams.[19] The deep-seated gland requires extensive surgical incisions which are no longer essential. Minimally invasive surgery allows quick, safe excision of these tumors with attendant benefits to the patients.[20] Both the transperitoneal and retroperitoneal approaches can be used with similar outcomes.[21]

The patient underwent a transperitoneal, laparoscopic adrenalectomy.

16. What are the precautions and complications of this surgery?

Ans: Despite the preoperative preparation, these patients are prone to significant hemodynamic changes during the surgery. While some of these can be predicted, many occur despite all precautions and the anaesthetist must be aware of these.[22] For the surgeon, it is important to be aware of the anatomy and be quick and efficient in his dissection. Since this patient's tumor is on the right side, in the transperitoneal approach, the liver should be retracted to allow exposure of the tumor. Dissection from the liver under-surface and the vena cava should be careful, without placing any traction or pressure on the tumor. The short adrenal vein at the cranio-medial border of the gland should be identified and clipped. Early vein ligation is useful but not essential as there may be additional draining veins apart from the principal vein.

Intraoperative complications include injury to adjacent organs, primarily the liver on the right side, bleeding from an avulsed vein or the gland itself, and incomplete resection of the gland. In order to avoid these, the gland should not be directly handled as far as possible as it is friable and vascular. Separation from the liver must be done after clearly identifying the cranial end of the gland which can extend significantly under the liver. On the medial side, separation from the vena cava must follow strict anatomic plains while being aware of variable venous drainage patterns.

Post-operatively, the most common complications are related to prolonged hypotension and hypoglycemia.[23] The patients may require extensive inotropic support and close monitoring of blood sugars.[24] Atelectasis, hematoma and fluid collections are rare complications for 3 cm pheochromocytomas but can be seen with larger tumors.

17. What would be the management if the lesion had been located outside the adrenal gland?

Ans: The management of paragangliomas is similar to pheochromocytomas with some differences. Paragangliomas are closely associated with large blood vessels, particularly the aorta, with significant adhesions, requiring careful sharp separation. This may make laparoscopic surgery difficult. Additionally, they are often close to the ipsilateral renal hilum and if the renal vessels cannot be carefully separated from the tumor, may result in injury to these vessels.[25] Large tumors and those located in inter-aorto-caval regions may necessitate upfront open surgery.[26]

18. What would be done if the lesions were bilateral?

Ans: Partial adrenalectomy has been recommended for patients with bilateral pheochromocytoma. These may occur synchronously or metachronously, particularly in patients with hereditary syndromes such as MEN or VHL. This can help avoid the need for hormone replacement (cortisol and mineralocorticoids) in these patients and prevent episodes of adrenal insufficiency or excess. In a large review of bilateral surgeries, it was noted that partial adrenalectomy could be achieved in 73% of whom 13% developed a recurrence in the residual gland while 23% required hormone replacement despite adrenal sparing surgery.[27]

The histology reported a 3 cm, well encapsulated pheochromocytoma.

19. How is malignancy diagnosed in such lesions?

Ans: There are no histopathological features in a resected adrenal specimen that can diagnose malignant pheochromocytoma and the diagnosis is based only on the demonstration of metastasis. A high Ki-67 proliferative index may indicate malignancy but is not diagnostic.[28] A mutation in the SDHB gene, particularly in paragangliomas may be an indicator of higher risk of metastasis.[29]

20. What would be the management if the lesion was suspected to be malignant?

Ans: The primary treatment for suspected malignant pheochromocytomas remains surgery. Metastasis is rarely present at diagnosis and usually appears metachronously, often many years after resection of the primary lesion. Many such patients will progress or recur and will require palliative care. Some patients may benefit from ^{131}I-MIBG radioactive therapy and chemotherapy using cyclophosphamide, vincristine and dacarbazine has also been used with limited results.[30]

Adrenocortical cancers are rare aggressive tumors where surgery is the mainstay of therapy. Surgery is often insufficient to cure the disease and patients will require palliative radiation or chemotherapy along with symptomatic control of accompanying hormone excess.

21. What are the expected outcomes of this surgery?

Ans: Adrenalectomy results in significant resolution of symptoms. Many patients with hypertension and diabetes will require fewer or no medication. However, the resolution may not be complete and patients must be aware of the potential need for continuing therapy after surgery.[12,31]

22. What is the follow-up of such lesions?

Ans: Patients should be followed up for hypertension and sugar control and tested for resolution of increased catecholamine levels after surgery. Repeat imaging is indicated in case of incomplete resolution of symptoms. Follow-up should be prolonged as recurrences may occur many years after surgery.[20]

23. What would you do if the lesion is > 4 cm and not secreting?

Ans: Since in this patient, the lesion is incidental and there is no suspicion of it being malignant or infective, it can be observed with a diagnosis of non-functional benign adenoma. There is no indication for a biopsy. Imaging should be repeated at 6–12 months. If the lesion grows at > 5 mm/year, surgery may be considered..

24. When do you suspect and how do you diagnose aldosterone secreting adenomas?

Ans: Aldosterone secreting adenomas can present with hypertension and hypokalaemia. To diagnose the condition a serum aldosterone to serum renin ratio needs to be calculated. 20 ng/dl per ng/ml/hr has a sensitivity of > 90% in diagnosing hyperaldosteronism. Saline suppression and salt loading with 24-hour urine aldosterone measurement will help establish a diagnosis. Adrenal vein sampling is recommended prior to adrenalectomy for lateralisation in patients with primary hyperaldosteronism.[31]

25. What is MACS?

Ans: MACS stands for mild autonomic cortisol secretion, previously known as subclinical Cushing's disease. It does not progress to overt Cushing's disease but may be associated with type 2 diabetes, hypertension, cardiovascular events, vertebral fracture and mortality. Patient who have metabolic comorbidities attributable to cortisol excess can be subjected to adrenalectomy. About 25% improvement can be expected in the control of diabetes, also improvement in hypertension and dyslipidaemia can be expected[4].

26. What are the hormonal test suggested in a case of suspected ACC?

Ans: In a suspected case of ACC serum DHEAS (dehydroepiandrosterone sulfate) and serum testosterone should be tested. Increased leaves suggest increased burden of disease.[4]

CASE SUMMARY

- 24-year-old male
- Incidental 3 cm right solid adrenal lesion
- Does not have any symptoms or signs of functionality
- CT scan is required to characterise lesion
  - CT suggests a pheochromocytoma due to intense brightness
- Functional evaluation shows elevated metanephrines, confirming a pheochromocytoma
- Preoperative preparation may be recommended even though he is normotensive
- Laparoscopic excision is standard of care for such lesions
  - Transperitoneal laparoscopic adrenalectomy is performed
- Histology shows pheochromocytoma
  - Malignancy cannot be determined in the absence of metastasis
- Follow-up catecholamine levels and imaging should be obtained

CHAPTER SUMMARY

- Adrenal tumors may occur in around 2% of people above the age of 50 years and are thus among the most common tumors. A very small proportion of these lesions is symptomatic and around 1 in 4000 of them are malignant. Thus, the majority of these lesions may not require any intervention. Adrenal tumors may be detected either incidentally on routine radiologic imaging of the abdomen or through symptoms produced by their mass effect or the actions of the hormones or catecholamines secreted by them.

- Tumors of the adrenal gland that are detected during routine abdominal imaging are called incidental tumors. Incidentally detected tumours are the most common lesions of the adrenal gland. Since most of them are benign and asymptomatic, investigations are targeted to identify those that require intervention, i.e. those that are functional or malignant. The incidence of malignancy rises with size and while less than 2% of lesions below 4 cm are malignant, 25% of those above 6 cm have cancer.
- Myelolipomas can be clearly identified on imaging as they contain macroscopic fat. Such lesions may not require any further functional evaluation. Adrenal adenomas contain intracytoplasmic fat which can be detected on tailored washout studies on CT. These lesions have a low Hounsfield value on plain CT imaging, may enhance on contrast administration, but show rapid washout of the contrast. Such changes are also seen on chemical shift imaging on an MRI. Pheochromocytomas are very bright on T2 weighted MRI images which can be diagnostic. All solid lesions other than myelolipomas should also undergo a basic hormonal evaluation for hypersecretion of cortisol and catecholamines. Patients with hypertension or hypokalemia should also be evaluated for aldosterone hypersecretion. History of cancer: In patients who have a history of concomitant or recent cancer elsewhere, around 50% of the adrenal lesions harbour a metastasis.
- Biopsy: Most adenomas and functional tumors should not be biopsied. Lesions suspected to have cancer, infection, or those that remain indeterminate may undergo a fine-needle aspiration cytology once the diagnosis of pheochromocytoma has been ruled out.
- Hereditary syndromes account for a significant number of adrenal tumors. These include the VHL syndrome, tuberous sclerosis, and MEN syndromes among others. Evaluating the family history and screening of the family in case a syndrome is identified are important components of the valuation and management of these tumors. Management of adrenal tumors is largely surgical. All benign lesions that are functional or have symptoms related to the size of the lesion require removal Surgery is the primary intervention modality for adrenal carcinomas. Unfortunately, many of these cancers are large at the time of diagnosis and may have locally advanced or metastasized. Surgery remains the intervention of choice where feasible with a limited role of adjuvant therapy.
- Patients with pheochromocytoma require pre-operative preparation to decrease operative morbidity and mortality. This involves administration of α-adrenergic blockade to decrease blood pressure and reverse the action of catecholamines on peripheral vasculature. They also require fluids, salt and additional medication to control blood pressure and diabetes which may be present.Traditionally, open surgery was recommended for adrenal lesions greater than 4cm in size. However, with greater expertise and improved technology, minimally invasive surgery has become the standard of care for most adrenal tumors. Both transperitoneal and retroperitoneal approaches have been used successfully. While pure laparoscopy is the most frequently used minimally invasive approach, robotic-assistance has also been used for adrenalectomies.

REFERENCES

1. NIH state-of-the-science statement on management of the clinically inapparent adrenal mass ("incidentaloma"). NIH Consens State Sci Statements. 2002;19:1–2.
2. Kutikov A, Crispen P, Uzzo R. Pathophysiology, Evaluation, and Medical Management of Adrenal Disorders. In Partin AW, Dmochowski RR, Kavoussi LR, Peters CA Eds. Campbell-Walsh Urology, 12 Ed, Elsevier, Philadelphia 2021 pp.
3. Zeiger MA, Thompson GB, Duh QY, Hamrahian AH, Angelos P, Elaraj D, *et al.* American Association of Clinical Endocrinologists; American Association of Endocrine Surgeons. American Association of Clinical Endocrinologists and American Association of Endocrine Surgeons Medical Guidelines for the Management of Adrenal Incidentalomas: executive summary of recommendations. Endocr Pract. 2009;15:450–3.
4. Fassnacht M, Arlt W, Bancos I, Dralle H, Newell-Price J, Sahdev A, *et al.* Management of adrenal incidentalomas: European Society of Endocrinology Clinical Practice Guideline in collaboration with the European Network for the Study of Adrenal Tumors. Eur J Endocrinol. 2016;175:G1-G34.
5. Park JJ, Park BK, Kim CK. Adrenal imaging for adenoma characterization: imaging features, diagnostic accuracies and differential diagnoses. Br J Radiol. 2016;89:20151018.
6. Lenders JW, Keiser HR, Goldstein DS, Willemsen JJ, Friberg P, Jacobs MC, *et al.* Plasma metanephrines in the diagnosis of pheochromocytoma. Ann Intern Med. 1995;123:101–9.
7. Eisenhofer G, Prejbisz A, Peitzsch M, Pamporaki C, Masjkur J, Rogowski-Lehmann N, *et al.* Biochemical Diagnosis of Chromaffin Cell Tumors in Patients at High and Low Risk of Disease: Plasma versus Urinary Free or Deconjugated O Methylated Catecholamine Metabolites. Clin Chem. 2018;64:1646–56.
8. Bombardieri E, Giammarile F, Aktolun C, Baum RP, Bischof Delaloye A, Maffioli L, *et al.* European Association for Nuclear Medicine. 131I/123I-metaiodobenzylguanidine (mIBG) scintigraphy: procedure guidelines for tumour imaging. Eur J Nucl Med Mol Imaging. 2010;37:2436–46.
9. Sharma P, Dhull VS, Arora S, Gupta P, Kumar R, Durgapal P, *et al.* Diagnostic accuracy of (68)Ga-DOTANOC PET/CT imaging in pheochromocytoma. Eur J Nucl Med Mol Imaging. 2014;41:494–504.
10. Chang CA, Pattison DA, Tothill RW, Kong G, Akhurst TJ, Hicks RJ, Hofman MS. 68Ga-DOTATATE and 18F-FDG PET/CT in paraganglioma and pheochromocytoma: utility, patterns and heterogeneity. Cancer Imaging. 2016;16:1–12.
11. Lenders JW, Eisenhofer G, Mannelli M, Pacak C. Phaeochromocytoma. Lancet. 2005;366:665–675.
12. Young WF Jr. Management approaches to adrenal incidentalomas. A view from Rochester, Minnesota. Endocrinol Metab Clin North Am. 2000;29:159–185.
13. Benn DE, Robinson BG. Genetic basis of phaeochromocytoma and paraganglioma. Best Pract Res Clin Endocrinol Metab.2006;20:435–450.
14. Waingankar N, Bratslavsky G, Jimenez C, Russo P, Kutikov A. Pheochromocytoma in Urologic Practice. Eur Urol Focus. 2016;1:231–240 .
15. Shao Y, Chen R, Shen ZJ, Teng Y, Huang P, Rui WB, *et al.* Preoperative alpha blockade for normotensive pheochromocytoma: is it necessary? J Hypertens. 2011;29:2429–32.
16. Khatiwada S, Agarwal S, Kandasamy D, Jyotsna VP, Kumar R, Bansal VK, *et al.* Diabetes mellitus in pheochromocytoma and paraganglioma: Prevalence, dynamics of insulin secretion, sensitivity and predictors of remission. Diabetes & Metabolic Syndrome: Clinical Research & Reviews. 2020;14: 2169–2175.

17. Khorram-Manesh A, Ahlman H, Nilsson O, *et al.* Long-term outcome of a large series of patients surgically treated for pheochromocytoma. J Intern Med. 2005;258:55–66.
18. Rao N, Ramachandran R, Tandon N, Singh P, Kumar R. Laparoscopic adrenalectomy for pheochromocytoma-does size matter? A single surgeon comparative study. Transl Androl Urol . 2016;5:780–783.
19. Singh P, Kumar R. Laparoscopic Adrenalectomy for Large Tumors. Recent Adv Endourology. 2013;16:13–24.
20. Hemal AK, Kumar R, Mishra MC, Gupta NP, Chumber S. Retroperitoneoscopic adrenalectomy for pheochromocytoma: a comparison with retroperitoneal open surgery. JSLS. 2003;7:341–345.
21. Ramachandran R, Rewari V, Sharma A, Kumar R, Trikha A. Laparoscopic Surgery for Pheochromocytoma and Paraganglioma Removal: A Retrospective Analysis of Anaesthetic Management. Curr Hypertens Rev. 2016;12:222–227.
22. Prakash P, Ramachandran R, Tandon N, Kumar R. Changes in blood pressure, blood sugar, and quality of life in patients undergoing pheochromocytoma surgery: a prospective cohort study. Indian J Urol. 2019;35:34–40.
23. Ramachandran R, Rewari V, Jain S, Kumar R. Refractory hypotension after paraganglioma removal- Reason to worry. Ind J Anesth. 2016;60:606–7.
24. Kumar R, Desai P, Rao N. Laparoscopic nephron-sparing excision of hilar paraganglioma: tips and technique. J Urol. 2015;193 (Supp):e909.
25. Prakash P, Ramachandran R, Tandon N, Kumar R. Open surgery for pheochromocytoma: Current indications and outcomes from a retrospective cohort. Indian J Urol. 2020;36:21–5.
26. Neumann HPH, Tsoy U, Bancos I, Amodru V, Walz MK, Tirosh A, *et al.* Comparison of Pheochromocytoma-Specific Morbidity and Mortality Among Adults With Bilateral Pheochromocytomas Undergoing Total Adrenalectomy vs Cortical-Sparing Adrenalectomy. JAMA Netw Open. 2019;2:e198898.
27. Pacak K, Eisenhofer G, Ahlman H, Bornstein SR, Gimenez-Roqueplo AP, Grossman AB, *et al.* International Symposium on Pheochromocytoma. Pheochromocytoma: recommendations for clinical practice from the First International Symposium. October 2005. Nat Clin Pract Endocrinol Metab. 2007;3:92–102.
28. Pacak K. Preoperative management of the pheochromocytoma patient. J Clin Endocrinol Metab. 2007;92:4069–79.
29. Scholz T, Eisenhofer G, Pacak K, Dralle H, Lehnert H. Clinical review: Current treatment of malignant pheochromocytoma. J Clin Endocrinol Metab. 2007;92:1217–25.
30. Amar L, Servais A, Gimenez-Roqueplo AP, Zinzindohoue F, Chatellier G, Plouin PF. Year of diagnosis, features at presentation, and risk of recurrence in patients with pheochromocytoma or secreting paraganglioma. J Clin Endocrinol Metab. 2005;90:2110–6.
31. Kempers MJ, Lenders JW, van Outheusden L, van der Wilt GJ, Schultze Kool LJ, Hermus AR, Deinum J. Systematic review: diagnostic procedures to differentiate unilateral from bilateral adrenal abnormality in primary aldosteronism. Annals of internal medicine. 2009 Sep 1;151(5):329–37.
32. Further Reading : Rowe NE, Kumar RM, Schieda N, Siddiqi F, McGregor T, McAlpine K, Violette PD, Bathini V, Eng M, Izard J, Jana K. Canadian Urological Association guideline: Diagnosis, management, and followup of the incidentally discovered adrenal mass. Canadian Urological Association Journal. 2023 Feb;17(2):12.

Chapter 18

Urethral Cancers

• *Balchandra Kashyapi* • *Mahendra Pal*

LEARNING OBJECTIVES

- To understand the clinical evaluation and imaging of urethral cancer.
- To understand the urethral malignancy which is a rare disease and requires a diligent work up.
- To understand how to differentiate urethral malignancy from other diseases with similar symptoms: Urethral bleed can occur due to stone disease, inflammatory and irritative urethral pathology and needs to be differentiated from malignancy.
- To understand staging of male and female urethral cancers: Staging of urothelial malignancy of urethra is different from the rest of the urinary tract and variant treatment application.
- To understand treatment options including surgery/chemotherapy, RT, both in neoadjuvant and adjuvant settings.
- To understand approach for diagnosis and management of urethral recurrence post-radical cystectomy.

Case Scenario 1

A 67-year-old diabetic and hypertensive male, who is a chronic smoker, with a history of angioplasty 6 months back and now on blood thinners, presented in the OPD with decreased flow of urine since 4 months. He also gave history of reddish staining of undergarments off and on along with dysuria since 2 months. No definitive history of gross total painless haematuria. History of prior endoscopic interventions (thrice) for stricture urethra in the past 10 years.

1. **What is clinical diagnosis?**

   Ans:
   1. Recurrent stricture urethra with UTI
   2. BPE with UTI with or without vesical calculus
   3. Recurrent stricture urethra with secondary urethral malignancy
   4. Urogenital cancer in view of long smoking history, origin may be urinary bladder or upper urinary tracts.
   5. Coagulation abnormality as patient is on blood thinners (very unlikely).

2. **Are there any specific findings you want to ask?**

   Ans: I would like to know if urinary stream is deviated or splayed as it suggests toward urethral or penile lesion. I would also like to ask if any mass or nodule is felt on penile under surface.

3. **What are the findings you can expect in urethral cancer?**

   Ans: In males: Urethra may be absolutely normal on palpation, there is possibility of induration in the course of the urethra or a palpable firm to solid lesion along localized or entire course of urethra and penile shaft, which can be tender with or without purulent or bloody discharge if infected.

   Bilateral inguinal palpation should be done to assess the presence of enlarged LNs, describing location, size, and mobility.[1]

   A digital rectal examination would allow assessment of perineal body and extra urethral spread of the disease.

   A bimanual examination, when necessary, under general anaesthesia, should be performed for local clinical staging and to assess whether colorectal or gynaecological malignancies are present (Fig. 18.1).

   In females: Visible or palpable friable mass at external urethral meatus

   Indurated urethra and tenderness along the anterior vaginal wall

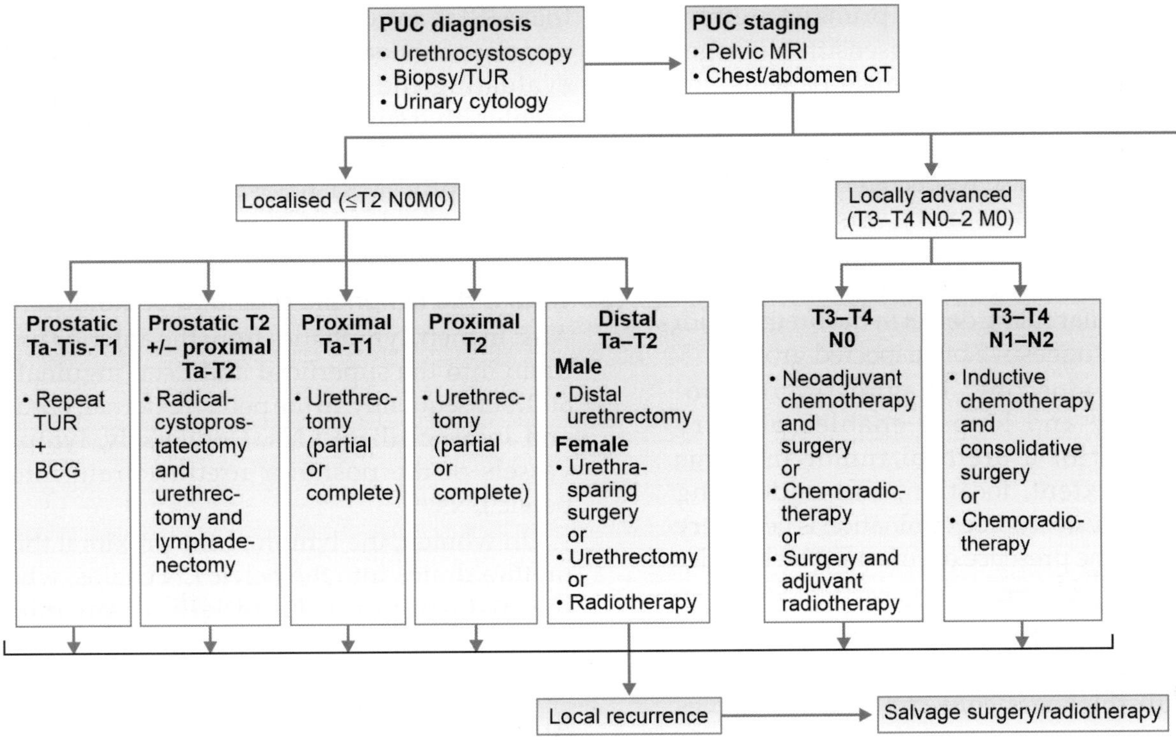

PUC diagnosis
- Urethrocystoscopy
- Biopsy/TUR
- Urinary cytology

→ **PUC staging**
- Pelvic MRI
- Chest/abdomen CT

Localised (≤T2 N0M0)

Prostatic Ta-Tis-T1
- Repeat TUR + BCG

Prostatic T2 +/– proximal Ta-T2
- Radical-cystoprostatectomy and urethrectomy and lymphadenectomy

Proximal Ta-T1
- Urethrectomy (partial or complete)

Proximal T2
- Urethrectomy (partial or complete)

Distal Ta–T2

Male
- Distal urethrectomy

Female
- Urethra-sparing surgery or
- Urethrectomy or
- Radiotherapy

Locally advanced (T3–T4 N0–2 M0)

T3–T4 N0
- Neoadjuvant chemotherapy and surgery or
- Chemoradiotherapy or
- Surgery and adjuvant radiotherapy

T3–T4 N1–N2
- Inductive chemotherapy and consolidative surgery or
- Chemoradiotherapy

Distant metastasis
- Systemic therapy according to underlying histology

Local recurrence → Salvage surgery/radiotherapy

Fig. 18.1: Management of primary urethral carcinoma

From EAU 2023
* Ensure complete circumferential assessment if penile-preserving/urethra-sparing surgery or partial urethrectomy is intended.
** Squamous cell carcinoma.
*** Regional lymphadenectomy should be considered in clinically enlarged lymph nodes. **** Consider neoadjuvant chemotherapy.
***** In extensive or BCG-unresponsive disease: Consider (primary) cystoprostatectomy +/-urethrectomy + lymphadenectomy.
BCG = bacillus Calmette-Guérin; CT = computed tomography; MRI = magnetic resonance imaging; PUC = primary urethral carcinoma; TUR = transurethral resection

4. What other way urethral cancer can present?

Ans: When becoming clinically apparent, most patients (45–57%) with primary urethral carcinoma present with symptoms associated with locally-advanced disease (T3/T4). At initial presentation visible haematuria or bloody urethral discharge is reported in up to 62% of the cases. Further symptoms of locally-advanced disease include an extra-urethral mass (52%), bladder outlet obstruction (48%), pelvic pain (33%), urethra-cutaneous fistula (10%), abscess formation (5%) or dyspareunia.[2]

5. What are the aetiology/risk factors associated with urethral cancer?

Ans: Aetiology for male primary urethral carcinoma includes:
1. Recurrent urethral strictures
2. Chronic irritation after intermittent catheterization/urethroplasty[3]
3. External beam irradiation therapy (EBRT)
4. Radioactive seed implantation
5. Chronic urethral inflammation/urethritis following sexually transmitted diseases (e.g. condylomata associated with human papillomavirus 16)
6. Lichen sclerosis[4]

Aetiology/risk factors for female primary urethral carcinoma include:
- Recurrent UTI/recurrent urethral dilatations
- Radiation therapy
- Urethral diverticula with recurrent infections
- Mid-urethral sling meshes have not been associated with an increased risk of primary urethral carcinoma.[5]

6. What are the differential diagnosis of female urethral carcinoma?

Ans:
1. Urethral diverticula
2. Recurrent urinary tract infections have been associated with primary urethral carcinoma.

7. What investigations would you do?

Ans:
1. Urinary cytology is part of the standard work-up of a patient with hematuria. However, the

role of urinary cytology in primary urethral carcinoma is limited since its sensitivity ranges between 55% and 59%. In male patients, the sensitivity for urothelial carcinoma (UC) and squamous cell carcinoma (SCC) was reported to be 80% and 50%, respectively, whereas in female patients, sensitivity was found to be 77% for SCC and 50% for UC.

2. Ascending urethrogram/retrograde urethrogram: Irregular filling defect in the urethra with stricture is suggestive of suspected growth.
3. Urethro-cystoscopy: Diagnostic urethro-cystoscopy and biopsy enables primary assessment of a urethral tumor in terms of tumor extent, location, and underlying histology. Cystoscopic examination is necessary to exclude the presence of concomitant bladder tumors.[6,7]

8. How can you maximize the tissue yield during urethral biopsy?

Ans: A full thickness cold-cup biopsy enables accurate tissue retrieval for histological analysis and avoids tissue damage. In patients with larger lesions, transurethral resection (optionally in men under penile blood arrest using a tourniquet) can be performed for histological diagnosis.[8]

9. Any special circumstance you can expect?

Ans: In patient with stricture urethra, ureteroscope can use for urethro-cystoscopy and biopsy.

10. How to take tissue from prostatic urethra?

Ans: In patients with UC of the prostatic urethra or ducts, resectoscope loop biopsy of the prostatic urethra (between the five and seven o'clock position from the bladder neck and distally around the area of the verumontanum) can contribute to an improved detection rate.[9]

11. What is the epithelial lining of urethra?

Ans: From the bladder neck to the membranous urethra the urethra is lined by urothelial cells and squamous cells line the urethra from bulbous urethra to urethral meatus.

12. What imaging you do to stage the urethral cancer?

Ans: To assess local staging and to detect lymphatic and distant metastatic spread. Imaging work-up should include computed tomography (CT) of the chest, abdomen and pelvis for staging, including CT urography for urothelial evaluation was found to be 72.9% and 70.6%, respectively.[10] Magnetic resonance imaging (MRI) can be used to evaluate tumor location and size, as well as local tumor extent and presence of regional LN metastases, focusing in particular on inguinal and pelvic LNs for local staging, there is evidence that MRI is an accurate tool for monitoring tumor response to neoadjuvant chemoradiotherapy and evaluating the extent of local disease prior to exenterative surgery.[11,12]

18F-Fluorodeoxglucose positron emission tomography/MRI has shown to improve the diagnostic evaluation in patients with metastatic disease.[13]

13. What is the lymphatic drainage of urethra?

Ans: In men, lymphatics from the anterior urethra drain into the superficial and deep inguinal LNs and, subsequently, to the pelvic (external, obturator and internal iliac) LNs. Conversely, lymphatic vessels of the posterior urethra drain into the pelvic LNs.[14]

In women, the lymph of the proximal third of urethra drains into the pelvic LN chains, whereas the distal two-thirds initially drain into the superficial and deep inguinal nodes.[15,16]

14. How does grading of urethral cancer is done?

Ans: It is done based on histopathology.

Urothelial urethral carcinoma:

a. PUNLMP: Papillary urothelial neoplasm of low malignant potential
b. Low grade: Well differentiated
c. High grade: Poorly differentiated

Non-urothelial urethral carcinoma: Squamous cell/adenocarcinoma

a. Gx: Tumor grade not assessable
b. G1: Well differentiated
c. G2: Moderately differentiated
d. G3: Poorly differentiated

15. What is the common cancer in urethra?

Ans: Urothelial carcinoma (UC) of the urethra is the predominant histological type of primary urethral cancer (54–65%), followed by squamous cell carcinoma (SCC) (16–22%) and AC (10–16%). Primary UC with unconventional histological subtypes are very rare and exhibit a dismal prognosis.[17]

16. What is the TNM staging for urethral TCC?

Ans: NCCN Guidelines Version 2.2023 Bladder Cancer (Tables 18.1 and 18.2).

17. This patient had distal urethral squamous cell carcinoma with right inguinal palpable lymph node. How will you manage?

Ans: As distal urethral tumors exhibit significantly improved survival rates compared with proximal tumors treatment of distal urethral carcinoma focuses towards improving functional outcomes and quality of life (QoL), while preserving

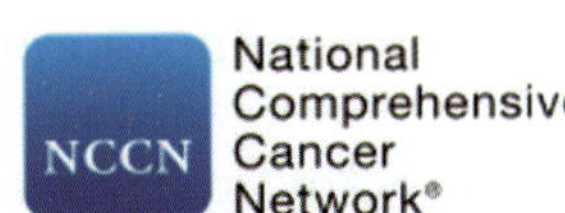

NCCN Guidelines Version 2.2023
Bladder Cancer

NCCN Guidelines Index
Table of Contents
Discussion

TABLE 18.1: American Joint Committee on Cancer (AJCC)

TNM Staging System for Urethral Carcinoma (8th ed., 2017)

Male Penile Urethra and Female Urethra

T	Primary Tumor
TX	Primary tumor cannot be assessed
T0	No evidence of primary tumor
Ta	Non-invasive papillary carcinoma
Tis	Carcinoma *in situ*
T1	Tumor invades subepithelial connective tissue
T2	Tumor invades any of the following: corpus spongiosum, periurethral muscle
T3	Tumor invades any of the following: Corpus cavernosum, anterior vagina
T4	Tumor invades other adjacent organs (e.g. invasion of the bladder wall)

Prostatic Urethra

T	Primary Tumor
TX	Primary tumor cannot be assessed
T0	No evidence of primary tumor
Ta	Non-invasive papillary carcinoma
Tis	Carcinoma *in situ* involving the prostatic urethra or periurethral or prostatic ducts without stromal invasion
T1	Tumor invades urethral subepithelial connective tissue immediately underlying the urothelium
T2	Tumor invades the prostatic stroma surrounding ducts either by direct extension from the urothelial surface or by invasion from prostatic ducts
T3	Tumor invades the periprostatic fat
T4	Tumor invades other adjacent organs (e.g., extraprostatic invasion of the bladder wall, rectal wall)

X	Regional lymph nodes
NX	Regional lymph nodes cannot be assessed
N0	No regional lymph node metastasis
N1	Single regional lymph node metastasis in the inguinal region or true pelvis [perivescial, obturator, internal (hypogastric) and external illiac, or presacral lymph node
N2	Multiple regional lymph node metastasis in the inguinal region or true pelvis [perivesical, obturator, internal (hypogastric) and external iliac], or presacral lymph node

M	Distant metastasis
M0	No distant metastasis
M1	Distant metastasis

Histologic Grade (G)

Grade is reported by the grade value. For urothelial histology, a low and high-grade designation is used to match the current WHO/ISUP recommended grading system:

LG	Low grade
HG	High grade

For squamous cell carcinoma and adenocarcinoma, the following grading schema is recommended:

GX	Grade cannot be assessed
G1	Well differentiated
G2	Moderately differentiated
G3	Poorly differentiated

TABLE 18.2: AJCC Progonostic group

	T	B	N
Stage 0is	Tis	N0	M0
Stage 0a	Ta	N0	M0
Stage I	T1	N0	M0
Stage II	T2	N0	M0
Stage III	T1	N1	M0
	T2	N1	M0
	T3	B0	M0
	T3	N1	M0
Stage IV	T4	N0	M0
	T4	N1	M0
	Any T	N2	M0
	Any T	Any N	M1

oncological safety. Penile-preserving surgery with iliac/inguinal lymphadenectomy (LND) for clinically suspected LN disease or presence of LVI and PNI.[18,19]

18. What are the margins that you keep in mind while doing a penile preservation for urethra malignancy, are they any different from ca penis? Also does it differ with the change in histology?

Ans: A minimum of 5 mm margin is required while doing a penile preservation for urethra malignancy if partial/total penectomy is planned. There is no data available about the relation of histology and safe margin for penile preservation for urethra malignancy.[20]

19. Is there any role of prophylactic LND in urethral cancer in clinically N0 inguinal node?

Ans: Currently, there is still no clear evidence supporting prophylactic bilateral inguinal and/or pelvic LND in all patients with urethral carcinoma. However, in patients with clinically enlarged inguinal/pelvic LNs or invasive tumors, regional LND should be considered as initial treatment since cure might still be achievable with limited disease with an OS benefit.[21,22]

20. What is the status of adjuvant therapy in urethral cancer?

Ans: Positive pathologic nodes or pT3 disease can be managed with adjuvant chemotherapy/RT after surgical management of primary.

21. What if tumor involves prostatic urethra?

Ans: Local conservative treatment with extensive TUR and subsequent BCG instillation is effective in patients with Ta or Tis prostatic urethral carcinoma with a higher disease-free survival (80–100% vs. 63–89%) and progression free survival (PFS) (90–100% vs. 75–94%).[23]

Radical cysto-prostatectomy should be offered as a primary treatment option in patients with ductal involvement and prostatic stromal invasion.[24]

22. What is the role of intravesical therapy in superficial tumours of prostatic urethra?

Ans: A systematic review and meta-analysis of intravesical BCG for treatment of noninvasive urothelial carcinoma of the prostate found that the complete response rate for prostatic disease was 88% (95% CI, 0.81–0.96).[25]

23. Is there a role of neo-adjuvant chemotherapy in management of invasive prostatic urethral urothelial carcinoma?

And: Yes in locally-advanced primary urethral carcinoma (> cT3 and/or cN+) neo-adjuvant chemotherapy. The 3-year OS for this locally advanced subset of patients (cT3 and/or cN+) who received NAC (N = 5), N-CRT (N = 3), surgery-only (N = 10) and surgery plus ACH (N = 8) was 100%, 100%, 50% and 20%, respectively (P = 0.016). Among these 26 patients, receipt of neoadjuvant treatment was significantly associated with improved 3-year relapse-free survival (RFS) (P = 0.022) and OS (P = 0.022).[26]

24. Is there any difference between urothelial cancer of prostatic urethra, bulbar urethra and pendulous urethra?

Ans: Proximal tumour location correlated with inferior 3-year RFS and OS (P = 0.056/0.005).[26]

25. What is the current status of adjuvant therapy in urothelial cancer of urethra?

Ans: Adjuvant chemotherapy and RT both are feasible option, NAC or chemoradiotherapy demonstrated improved survival compared to those who underwent upfront surgery with or without adjuvant chemotherapy **and** RT and surgery vs. surgery alone demonstrated that the addition of RT improved OS.[26,27]

26. Is management of female urethral cancer is same as male urethral cancer?

Ans: In female with localized urethral carcinoma, partial urethrectomy is associated with recurrence rate of 22–60%.[28]

Primary radical urethrectomy with removal of all the peri-urethral tissue from the bulbocavernosus muscle bilaterally and distally, with a cylinder of all adjacent soft tissue up to the pubic symphysis and bladder neck with bladder neck closure and appendico-vesicostomy or permanent SPC for primary distal urethral lesions has been shown to provide satisfactory functional results.[1]

27. What would be the treatment options for a small, exophytic cT2N0 female urethral carcinoma located near the urethral meatus?

Ans: Small exophytic distal female urethral cancers can be effectively treated with surgical excision or radiation with or without chemotherapy. Radical urethrectomy can usually be avoided for distal tumors. The distal 1/3 of the female urethra can be safely excised without compromising urinary continence, but excision of the distal 2/3 will likely cause incontinence and is not a good option.

As the node positivity rate in patients with T1 to T4 and N0 is 9%, much lower than reported in penile cancer with a high-risk primary tumor, there is currently no role for prophylactic inguinal lymphadenectomy for cN0 female distal urethral cancer. Most distal urethral tumors can be biopsied transurethrally.[22]

28. What is the predictor of recurrence and survival in urethral cancer?

Ans: Cancer-specific survival (CSS) rates at five and ten years were 68% and 60%, respectively. Female patients showed higher stage disease and 5-year CSM despite higher use of multimodal therapy.

Prognostic factors of worse survival in patients with primary urethral carcinoma are:

- Advanced age (> 65 years) and black race.
- Higher stage, grade, nodal involvement and metastasis.
- Increased tumor size and proximal tumor location.
- Underlying (non-urothelial or unconventional) histology.
- Presence of concomitant bladder cancer.
- Extent of surgical treatment and treatment modality.
- Location of recurrence (urethral vs. non-urethral).

29. Is there any role of radiotherapy?

Ans: With a median cumulative dose of 65 Gy (range 40–106 Gy), the 5-year local control rate was 64% and 7-year CSS was 49%.[29]

Most local failures (95%) occurred within the first two years after primary treatment.[76] The extent of urethral tumor involvement was found to be the only parameter independently associated with local tumor control but the type of RT (EBRT vs. interstitial brachytherapy) was not.

Addition of brachytherapy to EBRT reduced the risk of local recurrence by a factor of 4.2.[30]

30. Is there any role of multi-modal therapy in urethral Ca?

Ans: Chemo + RT seems to work well of SCC of the urethra as combination chemoradiation offers the potential for genital preservation and is an alternative therapeutic choice in patients not seeking surgery or considered surgical candidates. It provides 5-year overall, disease specific and disease-free survival rates were 52% (S/E 10.6%), 68.4% (S/E 10%) and 43.2% (S/E 10.2%), respectively.[31]

31. What are the side effects of RT?

Ans: Pelvic toxicity in those achieving local control was considerable (49%), including urethral stenosis, fistula, necrosis, cystitis and/or hemorrhage, with 30% of the reported complications graded as severe.[29,32]

32. Is there any role of multimodal treatment in urethral cancer?

Ans: Multimodal treatment in locally-advanced urethral carcinoma in both males and females consists of definitive surgery plus chemotherapy with additional RT. It results in improved OS in patients with locally advanced primary urethral carcinoma.[26] Neoadjuvant chemotherapy was reported to decrease the risk of all-cause mortality, while adjuvant chemotherapy was not associated with an OS benefit.[26]

33. What is the salvage treatment in recurrent primary urethral carcinoma?

Ans: Salvage treatment in recurrent primary urethral carcinoma after surgery for primary treatment with re-surgery or RT-based salvage treatment for recurrent solitary or concomitant urethral disease, demonstrated similar survival rates compared to patients who never developed recurrence after primary treatment.[33]

34. Discuss the management of metastatic urethral cancer.

Ans: Systemic therapy in metastatic disease should be selected based on the histology of the tumor.

Such as for UC chemotherapy for metastatic MIBC can be followed. No subgroup analyses are available for immunotherapy.[34]

35. How will you follow-up this case?

Ans: Follow-up: Given the low incidence of primary urethral carcinoma, follow-up has not been systematically investigated. Therefore, it seems reasonable to tailor surveillance regimens to patients' individual risk factors:

- Advanced age (> 65 years) and black race
- Higher stage, grade, nodal involvement and metastasis.
- T3/T4 and proximal tumour location.
- Non-urothelial or unconventional histology
- Presence of concomitant bladder cancer.
- Extent of surgical treatment and treatment modality
- Treatment in academic centres
- Location of recurrence (urethral vs. non-urethral)

In patients undergoing urethra-sparing surgery, it seems prudent to advocate a more extensive follow-up with urinary cytology, urethracystoscopy and cross-sectional imaging despite the lack of specific data.

Case Scenario 2

A 45 years old male underwent radical cystectomy (RC) and ileal conduit (IC) 9 months back, now he is complaining of bloody discharge through urethra.

1. What are the causes of urethral bleeding after RC?

Ans: The usual cause of urethral bleeding after RC is tumor recurrence at proximal stump of urethra. Other rare causes are trauma, urethritis or stone.

2. Discuss incidence and risk factors for tumor recurrence.

Ans: Urothelial recurrences: After RC, the incidence of new urethral tumors was 4.4% (1.3–13.7%).

Risk factors:

In men: Positive urethral margin, cutaneous diversions and urethral malignancy in the prostatic urethra/prostate. *In female:* Bladder neck involvement and a positive urethral margin.

Orthotopic neobladder was associated with a significant lower risk of urethral tumors after RC (OR: 0.44).[35]

3. Can urethral recurrence be identified early?

Ans: Routine surveillance with urethral wash and urine cytology may help in identification of urethral recurrence.

4. What are the present day indication for urethral wash cytology ?

Ans: Urethral wash cytology is reserved for patients with high-risk disease. High-risk disease includes: Positive urethral margin, multifocal CIS, and prostatic urethral invasion with sensitivity of 55%.[36]

5. **How will you proceed?**

   Ans: Would like to do urethral wash, urethroscopy for diagnosis of recurrence and MRI for staging the disease, including the extent of local invasion and presence of pelvic nodal metastasis.

6. **Are there any prognostic factors?**

   Ans: Yes, it depends upon type of recurrence. If noninvasive, single, low-grade recurrence have better prognosis compare to invasive, multiple and high-grade recurrence. Also, there is a significant survival advantage in men with urethral recurrence diagnosed asymptomatically vs. symptomatically.[37]

7. **What are the treatment strategies for urethral recurrence?**

   Ans: Treatment options based on local stage and grade of urethral occurrence.

   Patients with non-invasive urethral recurrences have a favourable prognosis and can often be managed with transurethral resection and topical BCG, thus avoiding radical urethrectomy in some cases. BCG instillations have success rates of 83%.[38]

   In invasive disease, radical urethrectomy should be performed if the urethra is the only site of disease; in case of distant disease, systemic chemotherapy is indicated.[39]

8. **Should we not do a radical urethrectomy in all cases of urethral cancer developing after a cystectomy, irrespective of whether it is invasive or not?**

   Ans: Yes we can offer radical urethrectomy in all cases of urethral cancer developing after a cystectomy based on type and time of recurrence. Early, high grade, multiple and proximal recurrence should offer radical urethrectomy. Late, low grade, single and distal recurrence can be managed by conservative management after adequate counselling.[40]

9. **What is the role of lymphadenectomy or penectomy in urethral recurrence?**

   Ans: There is no role for routine inguinal lymphadenectomy, and penectomy is not required unless the urethral tumor is invasive into the deep structures of the penis. If penile tissue is involved, radical penectomy is warranted.

10. **What are the steps of radical urethrectomy post-RARC? Enumerate measures to identify the proximal end of urethra and ensuring a complete resection.**

    Ans: Radical urethrectomy can be performed prophylactically: Simultaneously during radical cystectomy/as interval radical urethrectomy based on indications, or later if recurrence in urethra during follow-up.

    Principle remains same to excise complete length of urethra along with radical cystectomy specimen in toto or later as condition mentioned above. Urethra from external meatus to prostatic apex must be removed.

    It is easy to identify proximal end of urethra during radical cystectomy as prostatic apex is identifiable landmark, but in interval urethrectomy proximal end fibrosed so to ensure complete removal of urethra at proximal end, its fibrosed part must be removed by identifying the non-absorbable suture at the proximal end of urethra which placed during radical cystectomy or remove the proximal end of urethra as much as possible beyond the levator ani muscle with taking utmost care not to injured rectum if stitch was not placed.

11. **Discuss the management of urethral recurrence after orthotopic neobladder.**

    Ans: After urethrectomy in patients with orthotopic neobladders, bowel from the neobladder can often be reconfigured and used for a cutaneous diversion.

SUMMARY

- Urethral cancers are rare, they can be urothelial, squamous or adenocarcinoma
- The more proximal the lesion, the more aggressive it is likely to be.
- All urethral bleeds should be investigated for urethral cancer
- Post-cystectomy urethral surveillance is important in all symptomatic patient
- Urethral recurrence, merits a radical urethrectomy
- Posterior dissection in case of secondary urethrectomy is extremely challenging.

REFERENCES

1. Blaivas, J.G., *et al.* Periurethral masses: etiology and diagnosis in a large series of women. Obstet Gynecol, 2004. 103: 842. https://pubmed.ncbi.nlm.nih.gov/15121554/.
2. Gheiler, E.L., *et al.* Management of primary urethral cancer. Urology, 1998. 52: 487. https://pubmed.ncbi.nlm.nih.gov/9730466/.
3. Mohanty, N.K., *et al.* Squamous cell carcinoma of perineal urethrostomy. Urol Int, 1995. 55: 118.https://pubmed.ncbi.nlm.nih.gov/8533195/.
4. Wiener, J.S., *et al.* Oncogenic human papillomavirus type 16 is associated with squamous cell cancer of the male urethra. Cancer Res, 1992. 52: 5018. https://pubmed.ncbi.nlm.nih.gov/1325290/.
5. Thomas, A.A., *et al.* Urethral diverticula in 90 female patients: a study with emphasis on neoplastic alterations. J Urol, 2008. 180: 2463. https://pubmed.ncbi.nlm.nih.gov/18930487/.

6. Touijer, A.K., *et al.* Role of voided urine cytology in diagnosing primary urethral carcinoma. Urology, 2004. 63: 33. https://pubmed.ncbi.nlm.nih.gov/14751342/.
7. Gakis, G., *et al.* Oncological Outcomes of Patients with Concomitant Bladder and Urethral Carcinoma. Urol Int, 2016. 97: 134. https://pubmed.ncbi.nlm.nih.gov/27462702/.
8. Samm, B.J., *et al.* Penectomy: a technique to reduce blood loss. Urology, 1999. 53: 393. https://pubmed.ncbi.nlm.nih.gov/9933061/.
9. Donat, S.M., *et al.* The efficacy of transurethral biopsy for predicting the long-term clinical impact of prostatic invasive bladder cancer. J Urol, 2001. 165: 1580. https://pubmed.ncbi.nlm.nih.gov/11342921/.
10. Schubert, T., *et al.* MP11–20 The predictive accuracy between clinical staging and pathological staging in patients with primary urethral carcinoma. J Urol, 2019. 201: e135. https://www.auajournals.org/doi/abs/10.1097/01.JU.0000555184.87550.3c.
11. Itani, M., *et al.* MRI of female urethra and periurethral pathologies. Int Urogynecol J, 2016. 27: 195.https://pubmed.ncbi.nlm.nih.gov/26209954/.
12. Gourtsoyianni, S., *et al.* MRI at the completion of chemoradiotherapy can accurately evaluate the extent of disease in women with advanced urethral carcinoma undergoing anterior pelvic exenteration. Clin Radiol, 2011.66: 1072. https://pubmed.ncbi.nlm.nih.gov/21839430/.
13. Laudicella, R., *et al.* (18)F-FDG PET/MR Refines Evaluation in Newly Diagnosed Metastatic Urethral Adenocarcinoma. Nucl Med Mol Imaging, 2019.
14. Chapter11. Urethra, Victor E. Reuter, Hikmat A. Al-Ahmadie. Urologic Surgical Pathology (Fourth Edition) 2020, Pages 534–548, 548.e1–548.e5.
15. Carroll, P.R., *et al.* Surgical anatomy of the male and female urethra. Urol Clin North Am, 1992. 19: 339.https://pubmed.ncbi.nlm.nih.gov/1574824/.
16. Sharp, D., *et al.* Surgery of penile and urethral carcinoma, In: Campbell's Urology, D. McDougal, A. Wein, L. Kavoussi, A. Novick, A. Partin, C. Peters and P. Ramchandani, Editors. 212, Saunders Elsevier: Philadelphia, PA, USA.
17. Current Disease Management of Primary Urethral Carcinoma. Florian Janisch *et al.* European Urology Focus Volume 5, Issue 5, September 2019, Pages 722–734).
18. RARECARENet. Surveillance of Rare Cancers in Europe. 2019. Access date Dec 2022.http://www.rarecare.eu/default.asp.
19. Smith, Y., *et al.* Penile-preserving surgery for male distal urethral carcinoma. BJU Int, 2007. 100: 82. https://pubmed.ncbi.nlm.nih.gov/17488307/.
20. Current Perspectives on the Diagnosis and Management of Primary Urethral Cancer: A Systematic Review. M Ryan Farrell Jonathan T Xu Alex J Vanni. Research and Reports in Urology 2021:13 325–334.
21. Torbrand, C., *et al.* Diagnosing Distal Urethral Carcinomas in Men Might Be Only the Tip of the Iceberg. Clin Genitourin Cancer, 2017. 15: e1131. https://pubmed.ncbi.nlm.nih.gov/28784424/.
22. Werntz, R.P., *et al.* The role of inguinal lymph node dissection in men with urethral squamous cell carcinoma. Urol Oncol, 2018. 36: 526 e1. https://pubmed.ncbi.nlm.nih.gov/30446445/.
23. Patschan, O., *et al.* Systematic Review of the Role of BCG in the Treatment of Urothelial Carcinoma of the Prostatic Urethra. Bladder Cancer, 2021. 7: 213. https://content.iospress.com/articles/bladder-cancer/blc201516.
24. Vazina, A., *et al.* Stage specific lymph node metastasis mapping in radical cystectomy specimens. J Urol, 2004. 171: 1830. https://pubmed.ncbi.nlm.nih.gov/15076287/.
25. REF: Kokorovic A, Westerman ME, Krause K, *et al.* Revisiting an Old Conundrum: A Systematic Review and Meta-Analysis of Intravesical Therapy for Treatment of Urothelial Carcinoma of the Prostate. Bladder Cancer 2021;7:243–252.
26. G Gakis *et al.* Impact of perioperative chemotherapy on survival in patients with advanced primary urethral cancer: results of the international collaboration on primary urethral carcinoma. Ann Oncol 2015 Aug;26(8):1754–9).
27. Son, C.H., *et al.* Optimizing the Role of Surgery and Radiation Therapy in Urethral Cancer Based on Histology and Disease Extent. Int J Radiat Oncol Biol Phys, 2018. 102: 304).
28. Dimarco, D.S., *et al.* Surgical treatment for local control of female urethral carcinoma. Urol Oncol, 2004. 22: 404. https://pubmed.ncbi.nlm.nih.gov/15464921/18 PRIMARY URETHRAL CARCINOMA-LIMITED UPDATE MARCH 2023.
29. Garden, A.S., *et al.* Primary carcinoma of the female urethra. Results of radiation therapy. Cancer, 1993. 71: 3102. https://pubmed.ncbi.nlm.nih.gov/8490839/.
30. Milosevic, M.F., *et al.* Urethral carcinoma in women: results of treatment with primary radiotherapy. Radiother Oncol, 2000. 56: 29. https://pubmed.ncbi.nlm.nih.gov/10869752/.
31. Kent, M., *et al.* Combined chemoradiation as primary treatment for invasive male urethral cancer. J Urol, 2015. 193: 532).
32. Zinman, L.N., *et al.* Management of Proximal Primary Urethral Cancer: Should Multidisciplinary Therapy Be the Gold Standard? Urol Clin North Am, 2016. 43: 505. https://pubmed.ncbi.nlm.nih.gov/27717436/.
33. Gakis, G., *et al.* The prognostic effect of salvage surgery and radiotherapy in patients with recurrent primary urethral carcinoma. Urol Oncol, 2018. 36: 10 e7. https://pubmed.ncbi.nlm.nih.gov/29055518/.
34. Galsky, M.D., *et al.* Society for Immunotherapy of Cancer (SITC) clinical practice guideline on immunotherapy for the treatment of urothelial cancer. J Immunother Cancer, 2021. 9. https://pubmed.ncbi.nlm.nih.gov/34266883/
35. Fahmy, O., *et al.* Urethral recurrence after radical cystectomy for urothelial carcinoma: A systematic review and meta-analysis. Urol Oncol, 2018. 36: 54. https://pubmed.ncbi.nlm.nih.gov/29196179/.
36. Boorjian SA, Kim SP, Weight CJ, Cheville JC, Thapa P, Frank I. Risk factors and outcomes of urethral recurrence following radical cystectomy. Eur Urol 2011; 60: 1266–72.
37. Soukup, V., *et al.* Follow-up after surgical treatment of bladder cancer: a critical analysis of the literature. Eur Urol, 2012. 62: 290. https://pubmed.ncbi.nlm.nih.gov/22609313.
38. Varol, C., *et al.* Treatment of urethral recurrence following radical cystectomy and ileal bladder substitution. J Urol, 2004. 172: 937. https://pubmed.ncbi.nlm.nih.gov/15311003.
39. Gakis, G., *et al.* EAU Guidelines on Primary Urethral Carcinoma. In: EAU Guidelines published at the 38th Annual Congress Milan 2023. European Associaton of Urology Guidelines Office, Arnhem, the Netherlands.
40. G Gakis *et al.* Systematic Review on the Fate of the Remnant Urothelium after Radical Cystectomy. Eur Urol. 2017 Apr; 71(4): 545–557.

Chapter 19

Pain Management, Palliation and Best Supportive Care

• *Amitabh Singh* • *Kinshuki Jain*

LEARNING OBJECTIVES

- Identification and assessment of pain : Pain is the most distressing symptom in cancer patients.
- Impact of untreated pain: Pain can cause physiological and psychological distress
- Management of pain: Pain should be managed in a stepladder fashion.
- Assessment for palliative care: Palliative care is an important pillar of terminal cancer management.
- Provision of palliative care is to improve quality of life:

Case Scenario

A 55-year-old male patient is diagnosed case of carcinoma urinary bladder. Post-TURBT, post-chemotherapy with Gem-Cis 6 cycles. He has a c/o severe, dull aching pain in lower abdomen and pelvis persisting throughout the day, increased on micturition and defecation with strong burning and stretching and cramping sensation, radiating to thigh. He also has C/O tingling sensation in both feet, increased after 4th cycle of chemotherapy. Patient is unable to sleep due to pain. His blood investigations show normal liver and kidney functions. Complete blood count reveals anaemia with Hb of 8 gm%. Urine examination shows presence of RBCs in urine. There is a little relief in pain with paracetamol 1 gm thrice daily.

1. **What is the definition of pain?**

   Ans: Pain is defined as "an unpleasant sensory and emotional experience associated with, or resembling that associated with, actual or potential tissue damage".[1]

2. **How do you assess pain in a patient with urological malignancy?**

   Ans: Assessing pain in urological malignancy involves a thorough evaluation of the patient's pain symptoms, medical history, physical examination, and diagnostic imaging studies. Here are some steps involved in assessing pain in urological malignancy:

Patient history: Ask the patient about their pain symptoms, including the type, location, intensity, duration, and any factors that make the pain worse or better. Also ask about the patient's medical history, including any prior cancer treatments and other medical conditions.

Physical examination: To assess the patient's general health and identify any local signs of cancer, such as lumps or swelling in the affected areas cause of pain.

Diagnostic imaging: Diagnostic imaging studies such as X-rays, CT scans, and MRI scans may be ordered to visualize the tumour and assess its size, location, metastasis and invasion of surrounding tissues.

Pain assessment tools: Various pain assessment tools such as the numeric rating scale (NRS) or the brief pain inventory (BPI) may be used to quantify the patient's pain intensity and monitor changes in pain over time.

NRS: The numerical rating scale (NRS) is a subjective measure in which individuals rate their pain on an eleven-point numerical scale where 0 signifies "no pain at all" to 10, signifying "worst imaginable pain". It is a simple, easily comprehensible and reproducible tool.[2] (Fig. 19.1).

Brief Pain Inventory (BPI): A useful self-reporting pain assessment tool for cancer patients which aims not only to assess the level of pain but also its

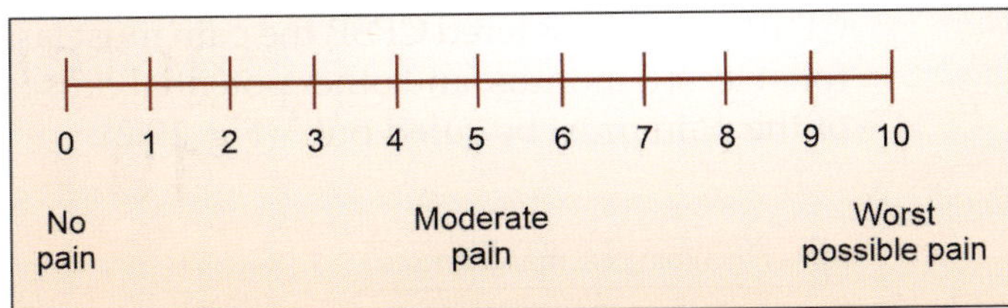

Fig. 19.1: Numeric rating scale (NRS)

impact on patient's life and response to treatment. It is albeit time consuming which limits its use in busy practice.[3]

Psychological assessment: Psychological assessment may be conducted to identify any emotional or psychological factors that may be contributing to the patient's pain, such as anxiety or depression.

Evaluation of pain-related functional impairment: The healthcare provider may evaluate the patient's ability to perform daily activities and assess any functional impairment related to their pain.

Overall, the goal of pain assessment in urological malignancy is to obtain a comprehensive understanding of the patient's pain symptoms and to develop an individualized pain management plan that addresses their specific needs and preferences.

3. What are the causes of pain in urological malignancies?

Ans: The causes of pain in urological malignancies are varied (Fig. 19.2) and may include the following:

1. **Tumour growth**: Tumours in the urinary tract can cause pain by obstructing the flow of urine, putting pressure on surrounding tissues, e.g. rectum, or invading nearby structures such as nerves and bones.
2. **Pain due to metastasis**
3. **Treatment of cancer**: Chemotherapy, radiation therapy, and surgery can all cause pain in patients with urological malignancies.

   Pain due to chemotherapy can be caused by various factors, including the direct toxicity of chemotherapy drugs to nerves, inflammation, and tissue damage. Here are some common types of pain experienced by patients undergoing chemotherapy:

   Chemotherapy-induced peripheral neuropathy (CIPN): CIPN is a common side effect of chemotherapy that affects the peripheral nerves, resulting in symptoms such as numbness, tingling, burning, and shooting pain in the hands and feet.

   Mucositis: Mucositis is a condition that causes inflammation and painful sores in the mouth, throat, and gastrointestinal tract. It can be caused by chemotherapy drugs that damage the lining of the digestive system.

   Headaches and body aches: Chemotherapy drugs can cause headaches and myalgias, which can be mild or severe depending on the individual.

   Bone pain: Chemotherapy drugs can cause bone pain, which can be felt as a deep, dull ache in the bones.

   Pain at the injection site: Chemotherapy drugs are often administered through an intravenous (IV) infusion, which can cause pain or discomfort at the injection site.

   The immune checkpoint inhibitors (CPIs) ipilimumab (targeting CTLA-4), pembrolizumab and nivolumab(PD-1), and avelumab, atezolizumab and durvalumab (PD-L1) are approved for urothelial and renal cell carcinomas, as either palliative or adjuvant therapies cause immune-related adverse events (IrAEs) which may affect any organ and can be life-threatening or compromise quality of life. These agents also cause peripheral neuropathies, mucositis, myalgias, arthralgias, tenosynovitis, and rheumatological arthritis.[4]

- **Radiation therapy** is a common treatment for cancer, but it can also cause various side effects, including pain syndromes. Some of the pain syndromes associated with radiation therapy include:
  - **Acute radiation dermatitis:** This is a common side effect of radiation therapy that causes redness, itching, and burning of the skin in the treated area. The skin may also become dry and peel.
  - **Chronic radiation dermatitis:** This is a long-term side effect of radiation therapy that can cause persistent redness, itching, and burning of the skin in the treated area. The skin may also become thickened, dry, and discoloured.
  - **Radiation-induced peripheral neuropathy:** This is a nerve disorder that can occur after radiation therapy, causing pain, numbness, tingling, or weakness in the limbs or other parts of the body.
  - **Radiation-induced fibrosis:** This is a condition that can occur months or years after radiation therapy, causing scarring and thickening of the tissues in the treated area. This can cause pain and stiffness in the affected area.
  - **Radiation-induced enteritis:** This is inflammation of the small intestine that can occur after radiation therapy to the abdomen or

pelvis, causing pain, diarrhoea, and other digestive symptoms.

Radiation-induced proctitis is a condition that can occur after radiation therapy to the pelvis, specifically to the rectum or the prostate gland. It is caused by damage to the lining of the rectum from the radiation, and can result in symptoms such as pain, bleeding, diarrhoea, and a sensation of incomplete bowel movements.

- **Radiation-induced myopathy:** This is a rare condition that can occur after radiation therapy, causing muscle weakness and pain in the affected area.
- **Radiation-induced osteoporosis:** This is a condition that can occur after radiation therapy, causing the bones to become weak and brittle, leading to pain and increased risk of fractures.
- **Radiation-induced neuropathic pain:** This is a type of chronic pain that can occur after radiation therapy, causing tingling, burning, or shooting pain in the affected area.
- **Radiation-induced arthropathy:** This is a condition that can occur after radiation therapy, causing joint pain, stiffness, and swelling in the affected area.
- **Radiation-induced fibromyalgia:** This is a chronic pain condition that can occur after radiation therapy, causing widespread pain, fatigue, and other symptoms.

Post-surgical pain

Acute post-surgical pain: It is usually experienced at the site of surgery—incisional and visceral. Referred pain may be experienced in certain situations like shoulder pain due to pneumoperitoneum in laparoscopic or robotic surgeries. Failure to appropriately manage acute pain can have negative consequences on various aspects of a patient's health, delayed recovery, and potentially lead to the development of chronic pain.

Chronic postsurgical pain (CPSP) is a significant and widespread clinical issue that can adversely affect postoperative recovery and overall quality of life. This type of pain is typically experienced in the area where the surgery was performed (localized) or in other parts of the body (referred), and it often persists beyond the normal period of healing and increases in intensity over time. The incidence of CPSP after surgery can range from 3% to 85% depending on the type of surgical procedure, with up to 25% of patients experiencing severe CPSP. To be considered CPSP, the pain must last for at least 3 months, and other potential causes of the pain must be ruled out.[5] (Fig. 19.2).

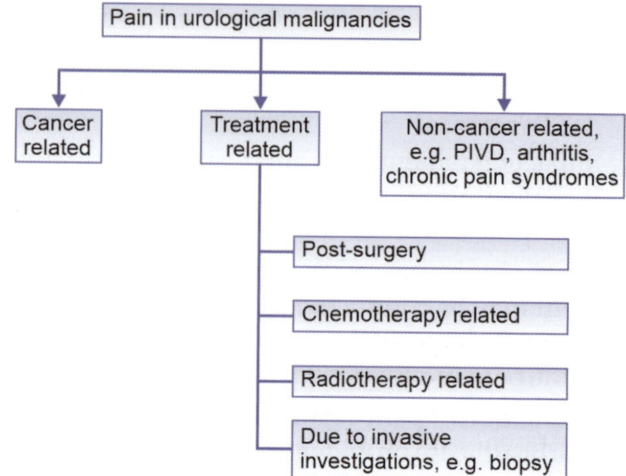

Fig. 19.2: Causes of pain in urological malignancies. (PIVD: Prolapsed intervertebral disc)

4. **Comorbidities**: Patients with urological malignancies may also suffer from other conditions such as arthritis or chronic pain syndromes, which can exacerbate their pain.

4. What are the adverse effects of poorly controlled post-surgical pain?

Ans: Poorly controlled pain can have several adverse effects on a patient's health and recovery, including:

Delayed wound healing: Pain can increase the levels of stress hormones in the body, which can delay the process of wound healing.

Respiratory complications: Pain can cause shallow breathing or respiratory depression, which can lead to respiratory complications such as pneumonia or atelectasis.

Cardiovascular complications: Pain can cause an increase in heart rate, blood pressure, and cardiac output, which can increase the risk of cardiovascular complications such as myocardial infarction or stroke.

Gastrointestinal complications: Pain can cause a decrease in intestinal motility, which can lead to nausea, vomiting, and constipation.

Immune system suppression: Pain can suppress the immune system, which can increase the risk of infections and delay recovery.

Development of chronic pain: Poorly controlled acute pain can lead to the development of chronic pain, which can have long-term negative effects on a patient's physical and mental health.

5. **What are adverse effects of poorly controlled chronic pain?**

Ans: Poorly controlled chronic pain can have several adverse effects on a patient's health, including:

Decreased quality of life: Chronic pain can significantly impact a patient's quality of life, making it difficult to perform daily activities and negatively affecting their social, occupational, and personal functioning.

Mental health issues: Chronic pain can lead to the development of mental health issues such as depression, anxiety, and irritability.

Physical deconditioning: Chronic pain can cause a patient to avoid physical activity, leading to physical deconditioning and a further decrease in functional capacity.

Sleep disturbances: Chronic pain can cause sleep disturbances such as insomnia or frequent awakenings, which can lead to fatigue and decreased daytime functioning.

Decreased immune function: Chronic pain can lead to a decrease in immune function, making patients more susceptible to infections and illnesses.

Risk of medication overuse: Patients with chronic pain may be at risk of medication overuse, leading to further adverse effects such as gastrointestinal bleeding, liver damage, or kidney damage.

6. **Elaborate on the management of pain in urological malignancies.**

Ans: The management of pain in urological malignancies should be individualized based on the underlying cause of the pain, the severity of the pain, and the patient's overall health status. A multidisciplinary approach is often necessary, involving the input of urologists, oncologists, pain specialists, and other healthcare professionals.

Acute post-operative pain can be managed using three strategies:

Pre-emptive analgesia: It works by preventing central sensitization and hyper-excitability which prevents wind-up and thus decreases post-operative pain. It should be started before incision, continue through the surgical period and the initial post-operative period.[6]

Regional analgesia: It can be attained through central neuraxial blockade (viz. epidural or intrathecal drug delivery) or peripheral nerve blocks (for example—Quadratus lumborum block, transversus abdominis plane block, intercostal nerve block, dorsal penile nerve block).

Systemic analgesia: Using multimodal analgesia approach is preferred to minimize adverse effect profile. It combines use of opioids, NSAIDs, and other adjuvants (for example—local anaesthetics, anti-depressants, anti-convulsant, magnesium, paracetamol).

Chronic cancer pain can be managed using following approaches:

I. **Pharmacological interventions:** Pharmacological interventions are often necessary in the management of pain in urological malignancies, and may include the following:
   a. **Non-steroidal anti-inflammatory drugs (NSAIDs):** NSAIDs may be useful in the management of nociceptive pain in patients with urological malignancies. However, caution should be exercised when prescribing NSAIDs to patients with renal impairment.
   b. **Opioids:** Opioids are often necessary in the management of moderate to severe pain in patients with urological malignancies. The choice of opioid and the dose should be individualized based on the patient's pain severity, comorbidities, and overall health status. The use of opioids in the management of pain in urological malignancies should be monitored closely due to the risk of addiction, tolerance, and adverse effects.
   c. **Adjuvant medications:** Adjuvant medications such as antidepressants, anticonvulsants, muscle relaxants and steroids may be useful in the management of neuropathic pain in patients with urological malignancies.

   The World Health Organization (WHO) developed a pain ladder in 1986 for the management of cancer pain. This ladder consists of three steps, with the goal of achieving pain relief using the least invasive and safest interventions.

Recent advances in pain management have led to some modifications and updates to the WHO pain ladder (Fig. 19.3), including the following:

1. **Individualized approach:** Pain management is becoming increasingly individualized based on the patient's pain characteristics, underlying cause of the pain, and overall health status. The concept of "**total pain management**" utilizes addressing all components of pain—physical, emotional, social and spiritual.
2. **Multimodal approach:** A multimodal approach to pain management involves using a combination of interventions, such as

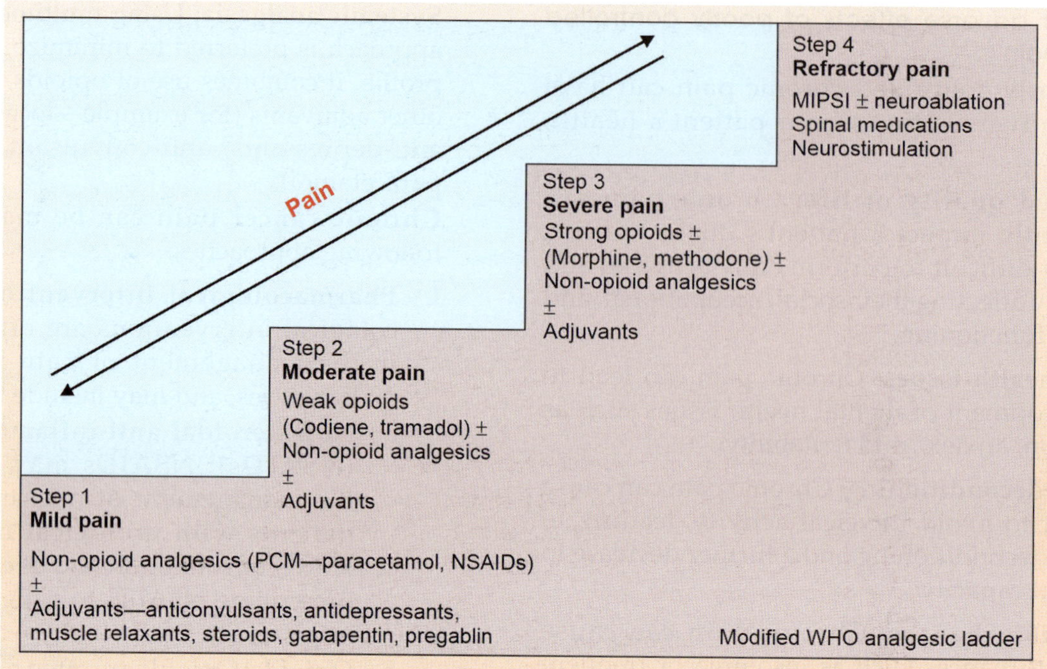

Fig. 19.3: Modified WHO analgesic ladder

(MIPSI: Minimally invasive pain and spine interventions, NSAIDs: Non-steroidal anti-inflammatory drugs)

non-opioid analgesics, opioids, adjuvant medications, and interventional procedures, to achieve pain relief. This approach can be more effective and lead to fewer side effects than using opioids alone. Opioid therapy is associated with the risk of addiction, tolerance, and adverse effects. Therefore, risk assessment and monitoring are necessary to ensure that patients receive appropriate and safe pain management.

3. **Non-pharmacological interventions:** Non-pharmacological interventions such as cognitive-behavioural therapy, relaxation techniques, and physical therapy can also be useful in the management of cancer pain.
4. **Interventional procedures:** Interventional procedures such as nerve blocks, radiofrequency ablation, and spinal cord stimulation can be effective in the management of cancer pain, and may be used earlier in the treatment algorithm.

7. How do you follow the pain ladder in practice?

Ans: Conventionally, the analgesics are *stepped up* in a graded manner according to the patient's pain. Practically, pain management requires thorough assessment of all dimensions of pain ("total pain") and the analgesics and adjuvants prescribed accordingly. If a patient presents with mild pain, paracetamol, with or without NSAIDs may be first line of treatment, which may be stepped up in case of partial relief. But, if a patient presents with severe pain, then the treatment directly goes according to third step of ladder. The interventions may be added at any step. Moreover, if a patient has resolution of the causative factor, e.g. post-surgery or after good tumour response to definitive treatment modalities, then *stepping down* the analgesic ladder is warranted.

8. Elaborate on use of morphine in cancer pain management.

Ans: When using morphine for cancer pain management, it is important to follow specific guidelines and work closely with a pain physician to ensure safe and appropriate use. Here are general considerations for using morphine in cancer pain management:

Prescription and dosage: Morphine is available only by prescription from a healthcare provider. The dosage will be determined based on the individual patient's pain intensity, pain characteristics, previous analgesic use, and overall medical condition. The pain physician will start with a conservative dose and adjust it as needed to achieve optimal pain relief with minimal side effects.

Administration: Morphine can be administered in various forms, including immediate-release (IR) formulations for immediate relief and extended-release (ER) formulations for around-the-clock pain control. The specific formulation and route of administration (oral, subcutaneous, intravenous, etc.) will depend on the patient's condition, pain level, and treatment goals.

Titration: Finding the appropriate dosage of morphine for pain control often involves a process called titration. It can be through intravenous or oral route, depending upon patient's condition.

Individualized approach: Pain management is highly individualized, and the response to morphine can vary from person to person. Factors such as age, weight, liver function, and kidney function may influence the choice of dose and frequency.

Side effects and monitoring: Morphine use may be associated with side effects, including sedation, constipation, nausea, vomiting, dizziness, and respiratory depression. Close monitoring for these side effects is crucial.

Safety considerations: It is important to store morphine securely, away from children and individuals without a prescription. Never share morphine with others or use someone else's prescription. Educating a patient regarding morphine is of prime importance for ensuring safe and effective usage.

Withdrawal and discontinuation: If morphine has been used for a prolonged period and is no longer needed, it is important to gradually reduce the dosage under supervision to avoid withdrawal symptoms. Abruptly stopping morphine can lead to withdrawal symptoms such as anxiety, restlessness, sweating, and insomnia.

9. What is the role of transdermal drug delivery system (patches) in cancer pain management?

Ans: Transdermal drug delivery system (patches) are a convenient way of administering analgesics. Common drugs available in the form of patches are fentanyl (12/25/ 50 μg), buprenorphine (5/10/20 μg/hr), diclofenac (100/200 mg), etc. While they provide advantages of being non-invasive route, along with controlled, sustained delivery and better patient compliance, there are certain points of caution while using it in oncology set up:

- Slow onset of action—not good choice for acute pain conditions
- Variability of drug absorption—very important in oncology patients undergoing active treatments which lead to recurrent fever episodes. High or low body temperatures lead to erratic drug absorption, e.g. a patient with neutropenic fever may suffer from overdose of narcotic (e.g. fentanyl) if patch is not removed in time.
- Limited dose flexibility—therefore, usually preferred after titration, whenever possible, to avoid over and under-dosing. Also, not all patches can be cut to modify dose administration.
- Skin irritation, especially in sensitive skin conditions, due to chemotherapy and radiotherapy.
- Proper adherence to skin—timely inspection needed in conditions of sweating, friction over applied area, improper technique of application, etc.

Thus, use of patches should be done after proper patient selection, proper type of patch, proper drug selection, proper patient education and monitoring, preferably by a pain physician.

10. What are other non-pharmacological interventions available to treat pain?

Ans: Non-pharmacological interventions may be useful in the management of pain in urological malignancies, and may include the following:

a. **Physical therapy:** Physical therapy may help to improve mobility and reduce pain in patients with urological malignancies. For example, pelvic floor muscle exercises may be useful in reducing pain in patients with bladder cancer.

b. **Acupuncture:** Acupuncture may help to reduce pain and improve overall well-being in patients with urological malignancies.

c. **Transcutaneous electrical nerve stimulation (TENS):** TENS is a non-invasive treatment that uses electrical stimulation to reduce pain and may be useful in the management of pain in patients with urological malignancies. It is to be noted that it should be avoided over sites of tumour or metastasis.

d. Other modalities which may be utilized include tai chi, yoga, stretching modalities, heat and cold, behavioural medicine approaches, cognitive behavioural therapy, meditation, hypnosis, relaxation techniques, guided imagery, music interventions, massage therapy and so forth.

11. Mention a few interventional procedures to treat pain.

Ans: Interventional procedures may be useful in the management of pain in urological malignancies, and may include the following:

a. **MIPSI:** Minimally invasive pain and spine interventions include nerve blocks which involve the injection of local anaesthetics or steroids into the nerves that are causing pain or minimally invasive spinal interventions such as endoscopic spinal decompression, spinal cord stimulation and central neuraxial pain procedures. For example, a ganglion impar block, hypogastric plexus block or caudal epidural steroid injection may be useful in reducing pain in patients with urological malignancies. These also include neuromodulating procedures (pulsed radiofrequency ablations), as well as neuroablative procedures (chemical, thermal, or cryoablation)

b. **Radiofrequency ablation (RFA):** RFA is a minimally invasive procedure that uses heat to destroy the nerves that are causing pain. For example, RFA may be useful in reducing pain in patients with renal cell carcinoma who have metastases to the bones.
c. **Surgical interventions:** May be utilized for painful bone metastasis (for example, kyphoplasty or vertebroplasty) or other palliative surgeries (viz. percutaneous nephrostomy for symptomatic urinary obstruction).

12. What are available radiopharmaceutical therapies to treat pain in cancer patients?

Ans: Radiopharmaceutical agents are radioactive substances which deliver targeted radiation to cancer cells, which can lead to tumour destruction and improved pain in bone metastasis in urological malignancies. Various agents used for bone pain associated with prostate cancer include radium-223 dichloride, lutetium-177-PSMA-617, Actinium-225-PSMA-617, thorium-227-PSMA-617, Iodine-131-MIP-1095, and copper-64-PSMA.

13. Describe the role of radiotherapy in management of pain and palliative care.

Ans: Palliative radiotherapy plays a pivotal role in the comprehensive management of advanced prostate cancer and other urological malignancies, offering targeted symptom relief and substantial improvements in patients' quality of life. This therapeutic approach mitigates pain associated with bone metastases. Also, it can effectively manage localized symptoms such as urinary obstruction or rectal bleeding in case of organ infiltration. Furthermore, hemostatic radiotherapy is invaluable in managing prostate cancer-related bleeding, in cases of intractable bleeding, especially in locally progressing disease. The dosage of radiation used for this is 8 Gy in a single fraction, 20 Gy in 5, or 30 Gy in 10 fractions. Additionally, the utilization of radiotherapy, including stereotactic body radiotherapy (SBRT), exhibits significant efficacy in controlling tumour burden and providing symptomatic relief in cases of bony metastases. This technique offers precise radiation at a very high dose per fraction. The radiobiological property of this fractionation essentially ablates the disease offering durable symptom relief with negligible adverse effects. However, for SBRT, the volume of disease should be small. The usual dose fractionation is 30 Gy in 5 or 24 Gy in 3 fractions on alternate days of the week. The judicious integration of palliative radiotherapy within the overall treatment strategy enables comprehensive care for advanced cancer patients, encompassing pain management, symptom control, and therapeutic interventions targeting localized and metastatic disease sites.

Palliative care: Palliative care is an important aspect of the management of pain in patients with urological malignancies. Palliative care focuses on improving the quality of life for patients with serious illnesses, and may include the management of pain, symptom management, and emotional support.

14. What is the definition of palliative care?

Ans: Palliative care is defined as approach to patient/family/healthcare provider that engages on alleviating patient's distressing symptoms while incorporating psychosocial and spiritual care according to patient/family/caregiver needs, values, beliefs, and cultures.[7]

Here, family persons are also counselled and prepared for the same goal. At the same time, psychosocial and spiritual care incorporated accordingly. The objective is to anticipate, prevent, and reduce suffering and to promote adaptive coping with the support for the best quality of life for patient, family and caregivers.

15. What is the difference between supportive care and palliative care?

Ans: Even though terms "Supportive" and "Palliative" are used interchangeably, because their intents and goals far outweigh their differences, palliative care is a subset of supportive care. Where "supportive" care can go along with any cancer treatment (curative or non-curative), "palliative" care is conventionally used where curative intent is not possible (Fig. 19.4).

16. Is palliative care, end of life care ?

Ans: End of life care is a subset of palliative care. Conventionally, "end of life care" is used for patient with life expectancy of less than 6 months. End of life care is also known as "hospice care".

17. What are the advantages of early integration of palliative care?

Ans: Early integration of palliative care has shown better quality of life, better survival, symptoms

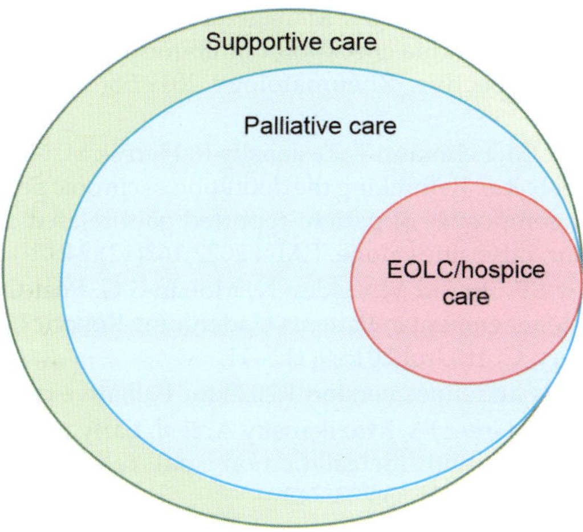

Fig: 19.4: Relationship between various aspects of supportive care

intensity.[8] it also reduces chemotherapy and futile life sustaining treatment at the end of life. Home base palliative care also reduces need of intensive care unit admission as well as duration of stay and frequency of hospitalisation.[9]

18. When should a specialist palliative/supportive care consult be sought?

Ans: (1) Unmanaged symptoms; (2) moderate to severe distress related to cancer diagnosis and therapy; (3) serious comorbid physical, psychiatric, and psychosocial conditions; (4) complex psychosocial needs; (5) poor prognostic awareness; (6) potentially life-limiting disease; (7) advanced cancers (≥ stage 3) associated with high morbidity and mortality; (8) patient/family/caregiver concerns about the course of disease and decision-making; (9) patient or family requests for palliative care; and/or (10) patient request for hastened death.

19. How do we classify our patients to decide delivery of various palliative care interventions?

Ans: The patients are divided into four groups to address the effect of life expectancy on the delivery of palliative care interventions: (1) Patients with years to months to live; (2) patients with months to weeks to live; (3) dying patients in their final weeks to days; and (4) Patients in their final hours of life are referred to as *"imminently dying"* and may require special interventions.

20. What are the indications of worsening prognosis ?

Ans: There are many uncontrolled symptoms which indicate worsening prognosis like, decreased performance status (ECOG score 3; KPS score 50), persistent hypercalcemia, central nervous system metastases, delirium, malignant bowel obstruction, superior vena cava syndrome, spinal cord compression, cachexia, malignant effusions, need for palliative stenting, potentially life-limiting disease, or other serious comorbid conditions.

21. What are the commonly observed symptoms at end of life?

Ans: Most commonly observed symptoms are pain, dyspnoea, anorexia/cachexia, nausea and vomiting, constipation, diarrhoea, malignant bowel obstruction, fatigue, delirium, and psychological distress. Detailed treatment protocol of all these distressing symptoms has been given in NCCN guideline for palliative care.[10]

22. Should palliation of major symptoms be dealt with in sequential manner?

Ans: Commonly observed clinical conditions in urogenital malignancy requiring palliative procedure (Table 19.1).

SUMMARY

- Pain management is an integral management of cancer care.
- Understanding the pathophysiology of pain in a given situation is critical to pain management .
- Pre-emptive pain management, can prevent pathological effects of pain.

TABLE 19.1: Palliative procedures in common urological malignancies

Clinical scenario	*Urogenital malignancy*	*Palliative procedure*
Gross hematuria	Kidney, ureter, urinary bladder, prostate	Continuous saline irrigation, cystofulguration, angioembolisation, hemostatic radiation, hemostatic medication administration
Obstructive uropathy	Urinary bladder, prostate, testis, penis	DJ stenting (metallic/silicon/polyurethrane)
Percutaneous nephrostomy		
Paraparesis/severe pain	All	Surgical decompression, palliative radiation, kyphoplasty
Acute urinary retention	Urinary bladder, prostate	Per urethral catheterisation, suprapubic catheterisation
Lower limb edema	All	Diuretics, massage, compression pumps or garments, LMWH in case IVC thrombosis
Deep venous thrombosis	All	LMWH, IVC filter

- A "peaceful death" has many definitions. But, it should constitute freedom from pain, being at spiritual peace, and being with family.
- Comprehensive palliative care continues for patients' family and caregiver even after death of patient because they are uniquely at risk of developing psychosocial dysfunction.
- Bereavement care is best provided by hospice team or a mental healthcare professional.

REFERENCES

1. Raja SN, Carr DB, Cohen M, Finnerup NB, Flor H, Gibson S, *et al.* The revised International Association for the Study of Pain definition of pain: concepts, challenges, and compromises. PAIN 2020;161(9):1976.
2. Serlin RC, Mendoza TR, Nakamura Y, Edwards KR, Cleeland CS. When is cancer pain mild, moderate or severe? Grading pain severity by its interference with function. Pain 1995;61(2):277–84.
3. Cleeland CS, Ryan KM. Pain assessment: global use of the Brief Pain Inventory. Ann Acad Med Singapore 1994;23(2):129–38.
4. Steven NM, Fisher BA. Management of rheumatic complications of immune checkpoint inhibitor therapy–an oncological perspective. Rheumatology 2019;58(Supplement_7): vii29–39.
5. Hofer DM, Lehmann T, Zaslansky R, Harnik M, Meissner W, Stüber F, *et al.* Rethinking the definition of chronic postsurgical pain: composites of patient-reported pain-related outcomes vs pain intensities alone. PAIN 2022;163(12):2457.
6. Batley SE, Prasad V, Vasdev N, Mohan-S G. Post-Operative Pain Management in Patients Undergoing Robotic Urological Surgery. Curr Urol 2015;9(1):5–11.
7. NCCN Guidelines version 1.2023 for Palliative care.
8. Temel JS, Greer JA, Muzikansky A, *et al.* Early palliative care for patients with metastatic non-small-cell lung cancer. N Engl J Med 2010;363:733-742
9. McNamara BA, Rosenwax LK, Murray K, Currow DC. Early admission community-based palliative care reduces use of emergency departments in the ninety days before death. J Palliat Med 2013;16:774-779
10. NCCN Guidelines version 1.2023 for Palliative care. Page no. PAL 1-5.

Chapter 20

Application of Radiation Therapy in Uro-Oncology

• *Vedang Murthy* • *Gargee Mulye*

LEARNING OBJECTIVES

- To learn about the fundamentals of radiation therapy in oncology: Radiation therapy uses ionizing radiation, mostly in the form of photons to induce DNA damage in cells, which induces cell death in cancer cells which are rapidly dividing and have lost DNA repair mechanisms.
- To learn about fractionation in radiation therapy: Convention fractionation has been the most utilized traditionally. However, hypofractionation allows for shorter treatment durations.
- To understand the use of radiation therapy in non-metastatic prostate cancer: Radiation therapy with/without hormonal therapy is an established treatment modality for nonmetastatic prostate cancer. In fact, for node-positive cancer, there is higher evidence for RT rather than radical prostatectomy.
- To learn about the role of RT in metastatic prostate cancer: RT to the primary in low-volume prostate cancer has shown survival benefit. Additionally, RT may be used for the metastatic sites in the palliative setting.
- To understand the role of RT in bladder cancer: Bladder preservation using trimodal therapy seems to be an oncologically equivalent option to radical cystectomy in well selected patients with muscle invasive bladder cancer. The role of adjuvant RT after cystectomy is being explored in RCTs; however, adjuvant RT is the standard of care for squamous bladder cancers.
- To know about the application of RT for renal cancers: SBRT to the primary renal tumor has shown encouraging results and is being evaluated in multiple studies. Local control rates appear to be very satisfactory.
- To understand the role of RT in the management of penile cancer: Brachytherapy to the primary penile tumor is a valid alternative to surgery in well selected and motivated patients. Also, adjuvant RT to the inguinal regions following surgery for node-positive disease has also shown survival benefit.
- To learn about the use of RT in adrenocortical cancer: Adjuvant RT to patients with adverse histopathological features has shown to have survival benefit.

1. What is the physics behind the use of radiation therapy for cancer treatment?

Ans:

- Radiation oncology is the use of ionizing radiation for the treatment of malignant diseases.
- Ionizing radiation is of two types—electromagnetic waves comprising of packets of energy (photons) or charged particles like electrons, protons, etc. Photons are the most used ionizing radiation in clinical practice and may be in the form of gamma rays or X-rays.
- Gamma rays are produced by radioactive sources such as Co-60 and therapeutic X-rays are produced by linear accelerators. Virtually all photon treatments in the current era are in the form of X-rays produced by medical linear accelerators. Therapeutic X-rays, however, have a much higher beam energy (megavoltage range), as opposed to CT scanner which produces X-ray energy in the kilovoltage range.
- A medical linear accelerator is in essence a sophisticated cathode ray tube that has been augmented to deliver precise treatment with the required properties. Modern linear accelerators can produce a continuous supply of X-rays with required characteristics; coupled with beam modifying devices (e.g. wedges, tissue compensators and multi-leaf collimators) that modify the shape and intensity of the beam. These advances have allowed the development of treatment techniques that accurately target the tumour and minimize radiation dose to the surrounding normal tissues.

- The dose in therapeutic radiation is measured as absorbed dose with SI unit Gray (Gy) where 1 Gy is equal to 1 joule of energy absorbed per kg of material.

2. How does radiation therapy induce damage to cancer cells?

Ans:

- The damage caused by radiation to the cells can be divided into direct and indirect damage. DNA is the major target of radiation damage.
- Direct damage results from breakage of DNA strands. Indirect damage is caused by transfer of energy to water molecules resulting in formation of reactive oxygen species which then cause DNA damage.
- DNA damage leads to cell death, both for normal and cancer tissues. However, intact DNA repair mechanism in normal tissues and lower rate of cell division allow recovery, resulting in relatively more cell-kill in cancer cells. This differential cell-kill is called the therapeutic ratio and forms the basis of radiation oncology.

3. What are the target volumes used in radiotherapy?

Ans:

- The clinical or radiological tumour is called gross tumour volume; the microscopic subclinical disease extent is labeled as clinical target volume (CTV).
- Planning target volume (PTV) is formed by applying a geometric margin to the CTV to account for daily organ motion (e.g. internal motion due to rectal or bladder filling) and set up errors due to daily minor irregularities in the patient's position on the treatment machine. The organs at risk include any adjacent normal tissue which needs to be spared from radiation and have no disease involvement.

4. How is the radiation dose administered and what are the different types of dose fractionations possible?

Ans:

- Radiation is usually given once daily in the form of equal sized fractions of the required dose. With increase in dose/fraction, effect of radiation on normal tissues increases. Types of fractionations are:
  - *Conventional fractionation*: Daily doses of 1.8–2 Gy/fraction. This is the most used fractionation regimen.
  - *Hyper-fractionation*: Multiple daily fractions (2–3) are given with a low dose/fraction of < 1.5 Gy/# (= fraction). It may reduce normal tissue toxicities, however, is rarely used due to the logistical challenge of treating a patient multiple times a day.
  - *Hypofractionation:* Treatment with a high dose/fraction (>2.4 Gy/#). Moderate hypofractionation delivers dose at >2.4–5 Gy/# and is used in cases where the normal tissue is more radiosensitive in comparison to the tumour, e.g. prostate, breast.
  - *Extreme hypofractionation*: Also known as SBRT/SABR, it uses high dose/fraction; ≥5 Gy/# up to five total fractions of treatment.

5. What are the techniques of delivering radiation therapy?

Ans:

- **EBRT/IMRT/VMAT/IGRT:** These are the techniques of delivering external beam radiotherapy (EBRT), where the radiation source is outside the body. IMRT is a technique where differential dose can be delivered across the beam profile, and this decreases toxicity. Volumetric arc therapy (VMAT) is a type of IMRT where the gantry rotates continuously while the treatment beam is on. Image guided radiotherapy (IGRT) comprises on-board imaging. IMRT-IGRT are pre-requisites for SBRT. These treatments can be delivered on most modern, advanced linear accelerators. The make/company of the machine is not of critical significance.
- **Proton therapy:** It uses charged particles in the form of protons (H^+), i.e. the hydrogen nucleus to deliver extremely targeted radiation with significantly reduced normal tissue dose compared to photons.
- **Brachytherapy:** Also known as internal radiation, it is a technique where radioactive sources are placed within or at the surface of the tumour. It is based on the principle of the 'inverse square law' wherein the radiation dose decreases as an inverse of the square of the distance between the source and the reference point. There is rapid fall of dose beyond the target. Brachytherapy sources can be temporarily (Ir-192, Cs 137) or permanently (Pd-103) implanted within the tumour. Urological tumours amenable for brachytherapy are selected cases of prostate cancer and early penile cancers.

6. What is the role of radiation therapy in non-metastatic prostate cancer?

Ans:

- Radiation can be used as the principle curative treatment in low, intermediate, high risk and node-positive prostate cancer with or without androgen deprivation therapy (short-term for intermediate risk and long-term ADT for high-risk and node positive disease).

- Treatment volumes comprise the prostate and seminal vesicles with the addition of pelvic lymph nodes in high-risk and node positive cancer.
- Moderate hypofractionation (2.5–4 Gy/#) is the standard of care. The standard dose is 60–68 Gy in 20–25 fractions delivered to the prostate/seminal vesicles along with 50 Gy to the pelvic lymph nodes.
- Ultra-hypofractionation or SBRT (>5 Gy/#) is evolving in prostate cancer. It allows for treatment to be completed in 5–7#, thus optimizing use of radiotherapy resources and increasing patient convenience. Dose given in SBRT is 36.25–40 Gy/5# to the prostate and 25 Gy/5# to the pelvic nodes.
- IMRT has been proven to significantly reduce both acute and late toxicities and hence is the current standard in prostate.[1]
- Radiotherapy is typically started 1–6 months after the start of ADT. This allows for shrinkage of bulky disease and resolution of urinary symptoms that may be aggravated with radiotherapy. ADT is also purported to act as a radiosensitizer and should be continued during RT.
- A TURP may be required in patients with severe obstructive symptoms at baseline, and this is not a contraindication for radiotherapy including SBRT. A gap of 3–6 months between TURP and radiotherapy (particularly SBRT) reduces the probability of a urethral stricture.[2]
- Clinical outcomes with radiotherapy are equivalent to surgery, however, the side effect profile is different.[3] Similarly, use of modern radiation techniques has reduced incidence of clinically significant late radiation toxicities (>/= Gr 3) to about 5%.[4]

7. Does brachytherapy have a role in the management of non-metastatic prostate cancer?

Ans:

- Brachytherapy can be used as monotherapy in low and intermediate risk or as a boost post EBRT in high-risk prostate cancer.
- Dose escalation to the discrete lesion within the prostate (also known as DIL-dominant intraprostatic lesion) significantly reduces local recurrence. Escalation can be achieved both with EBRT and brachytherapy.[5]

8. Following radical prostatectomy, how does one select patients for adjuvant/salvage RT?

Ans:

- Selection of patients for adjuvant radiotherapy depends on histopathological findings of the surgical specimen. High Gleason's grade, presence of extra capsular extension and positive surgical margins portend higher chances of biochemical failure and need for further treatment.
- These factors, with the addition of pre-op PSA, seminal vesicle involvement and lymph node invasion are components of the CAPRA-S score, that estimates the risk of recurrence post prostatectomy.[6]
- Recent evidence supports the use of salvage RT (RT at biochemical failure, PSA >0.2 ng/mL) as opposed to immediate adjuvant RT to avoid overtreatment in men who are likely to never fail post-prostatectomy.[7]
- However, adjuvant RT still has a role in patients with a very high risk of recurrence, especially those with persistent PSA (PSA > 0.1 ng/ml at 6 weeks post-surgery) or a high CAPRA-S score.
- Along with irradiation of the prostate bed, addition of radiation to the pelvic nodal areas with or without ADT has shown greater benefit in selected cases.[8] Dose to the prostate bed can either be 64 Gy/32# or 52.5 Gy/20#. Dose escalation is no longer indicated in salvage RT.[9]

9. What is the application of RT in metastatic prostate cancer?

Ans:

- Radiotherapy to the prostate improves overall survival in low volume metastatic prostate.[10] Low volume is defined as absence of visceral disease, any number of nodal metastases and up to 3 bone metastases restricted to the axial.[11] The rationale is that treatment of the primary will prevent further seeding of cancer cells to new metastatic sites.
- Alternately, irradiation of the metastases to ablative doses provides a chance of cure in patients with limited metastases, i.e. oligometastatic disease. Dose to the metastatic site will depend on the tumour size; a higher dose/fraction and higher total equivalent dose can be delivered in smaller tumours. Commonly used dose fractionations are 24 Gy/2#, 27 Gy/3# and 30 Gy/5.[12]
- RT is also an excellent option for palliation of painful bony metastases and a symptomatic prostatic primary.

10. What is the role of RT in bladder preservation for muscle invasive bladder cancer?

Ans:

- Radical cystectomy has long been the gold standard in bladder cancer with radiotherapy restricted to old unfit patients unable to undergo surgery. Results with radiotherapy have largely been suboptimal due to selection of cases with advanced disease and unfit patients.

- SPARE was the only randomized trial which aimed to compare radiotherapy and surgery in bladder cancer. However, it was closed prematurely due to unacceptably slow accrual and the cross-over of a large proportion of patients (24%) from the surgery to radiotherapy.[13]
- We do have data from well conducted sysematic reviews and meta-analyses that show that surgery and radiotherapy have equivalent outcomes. Kaushik, *et al* conducted a meta-analysis of nearly 10,000 bladder cancer patients treated in 8 studies wherein there was no difference in the 5-year or 10-year (HR 1.02, favoring cystectomy, 95% CI 0.73–1.42; P= 0.905) overall survival. Disease-free survival and progression-free survival were also comparable at 5 and 10 years.[14]
- Radiotherapy to the bladder is done in the form of trimodality therapy-TURBT followed by radiotherapy with concurrent chemotherapy.[15] Complete TURBT is associated with better outcomes. Radiotherapy volumes consist of the bladder and pelvic lymph nodes. The prostate is included in tumours in the bladder base or gross prostatic involvement.
- Definitive RT can also be considered selectively in recurrent/very high risk NMIBC in patients unwilling or unfit for.[16]
- Post-radiotherapy patients are kept on regular follow up with cystoscopies, urine cytology and routine/microscopy. In cases of non-muscle invasive recurrence, the bladder can still be preserved with TURBT and intravesical therapy.
- In cases of a muscle invasive local recurrence, salvage cystectomy is the treatment of choice. Pelvic nodal dissection, as part of salvage cystectomy, need not be done if the nodes have been irradiated.
- Dose used for bladder radiotherapy is 64 Gy/32# to the bladder and 55 Gy/32# to the pelvis. Alternatively, 55 Gy/20# to the bladder and 44 Gy/20# to the pelvis is used. Adaptive radiotherapy which takes into account daily variability in bladder filling is a necessary part of bladder RT.[17]

11. Is there any role for RT in the adjuvant setting following a radical cystectomy?

Ans:

- The use of adjuvant radiation had gone out of vogue due to unacceptably high bowel toxicities with conventional techniques. The advent of IMRT has renewed interest in this setting.
- Grade 3 and higher toxicity in recent series is seen in 5–7%.[18]
- Adjuvant RT should be offered as standard for patients with squamous cell cancer.[19]
- In urothelial cancers, evidence for adjuvant RT is evolving. Patients with high-risk features in the cystectomy specimen such as >= T3 disease, nodal involvement, positive margins, LVI or poor lymph node yield predict increased chances of locoregional failure and may be offered adjuvant RT in addition to systemic therapy (if indicated).[20] Significant relapses occur in the cystectomy bed despite negative margins and in the common iliac lymph node region which may be outside the standard surgical template.[21]
- Randomised trials are ongoing to establish the role of RT in urothelial cancers: BART trial (India) NCT02951325, GETUG AFU 30 (France)-NCT03333356, NCI Cairo.[22]

12. When is radiation therapy offered in germ cell tumors of the testis?

Ans:

- Seminomas are more radiosensitive as compared to non-seminomatous germ cell tumors (NSGCT) and thus radiotherapy has role in management across all seminoma stages.[22]
- Radiotherapy is equivalent to chemotherapy (SA Carboplatin AUC7) as a treatment option in stage IA seminoma.[23] Treatment volume is restricted to the retroperitoneal lymph nodes.[24] A dose of 20 Gy/10# with the goal of targeting occult disease is used.[25] Horseshoe kidney and history of inflammatory bowel disease are scenarios wherein radiotherapy should be avoided.[26]
- In stage IIA/IIB seminomas, radiotherapy is given to a larger volume encompassing retroperitoneal and ipsilateral pelvic lymph nodes.[26,27] Additionally, ipsilateral inguinal nodes should be included for patients with prior scrotal or pelvic surgery.[26] Radiotherapy doses used in stage IIA and IIB disease are 30 Gy and 36 Gy, respectively.[28] Cisplatin-based chemotherapy (3 cycles of BEP/4 cycles of EP) is an alternative option for stage IIA, however, the preferred one for stage IIB seminoma.[29]
- The novel SAKK 01/10 regimen of using de-escalated chemotherapy (one cycle carboplatin as opposed to 3 cycles BEP) and de-escalated radiotherapy (similar doses as standard radiotherapy to involved node only) has the potential to reduce toxicity in stage II seminoma.[30]
- Radiotherapy in advanced seminoma stage IIC–III is a salvage option in post-chemotherapy

recurrence.[28] Its use in residual disease post-chemotherapy is under investigation. No further therapy is recommended for patients with complete response on PET-CT scan at 8–10 weeks.[28] There may be benefit in irradiating patients with >3 cm residual disease with SUV_{max} >3 in the response PET-CT.

- Radiotherapy has limited role in NSGCTs at present, primarily, only in the palliative setting.[30] Second malignancies have always been a concern for RT in seminomas. However, modern series report 1% rate of second malignancies with a relative risk of 1.8.[32]

13. Can RT be considered for the management of the penile primary?

Ans:

- Men with primary tumour limited to the glans and less than 4 cm in diameter or with recurrent disease limited to distal penile shaft are well-suited for brachytherapy.[32,34]
- An ultrasound for inguinal nodal involvement, circumcision to allow for full tumor exposure and to reduce the risk of paraphimosis and necrosis are done prior to brachytherapy.
- In appropriately selected cases brachytherapy offers similar 5-year local control (84 vs 86%) and overall-survival (79 vs 78%) to penectomy.[34] Over three-fourths of the patients achieve penile preservation with effective surgical salvage available in case of a local recurrence.[34,35]
- With the modern brachytherapy treatment planning techniques, previously seen late toxicities of soft tissue necrosis (0–26%) and urethral stenosis (1–45%) can be minimized.[36]

14. Is there any role of adjuvant RT in advanced node-positive penile cancer?

Ans:

- Adjuvant radiotherapy to nodal basins in penile cancer has fast evolved from being a intuitively practiced modality to now being a guideline-recommended one.[36]
- The important questions to answer in this regard are the patients who will benefit most, the optimum dose, volume and technique of adjuvant radiotherapy.
- Patients with pN3 disease benefit most with a multimodal approach of adjuvant chemotherapy followed by chemo-radiotherapy with a 2-year DFS and OS of 93%.[38] Radiotherapy dose higher than 50 Gy reduces in-field recurrences by roughly half as compared to less than 50 Gy in pN3 penile cancers and extended-field radiotherapy (involved basin plus one pelvic echelon) significantly reduces regional failures as compared to involved-field volumes (4% versus 55%).[39,40]
- This has been aided by the use of IMRT that has reduced rates of severe skin toxicity and lymphedema previously associated with groin irradiation.[33,41]
- The EAU-ASCO penile cancer guidelines 2023 have incorporated recommendation for adjuvant radiotherapy (with or without chemo-sensitization) to patients with ENE, multiple or bilateral inguinal nodes or PLN metastases (pathological N2/N3 disease).[37]

15. Does radiation therapy have any role in the management of renal cancer?

Ans:

- Traditionally RCC was thought to be a radio-resistant tumor. There is emerging data suggesting that the apparent radio-resistance of RCC can be overcome with the use of SBRT.
- SBRT is indicated in medically inoperable or unwilling patients, those with a single functioning kidney, unfit for thermal ablation and operable but at risk for dialysis post-surgery.
- A very high dose of 10–15 Gy is given 3–5 times using precise planning and delivery. RT is associated with a local control of 95% at 5 years, negligible toxicity and a mean fall in GFR of 7 ml/min. Post-SBRT renal masses are usually stable with slow regression. Post-SBRT biopsies are not helpful and monitoring is done with imaging, usually MRI.[42]

16. Does adjuvant radiotherapy help following surgery for adrenocortical cancer?

Ans:

- Adjuvant radiotherapy improves recurrence-free survival in patients with adrenocortical carcinoma.
- The Weiss score is calculated using 9 histological features on the surgical specimen-nuclear grade, number of mitoses per 10 HPF, abnormal mitoses, % of clear cells, fraction of tumour with diffuse architecture, necrosis, presence or absence of venous, sinusoidal and capsular invasion.
- Patients with a Weiss score >3 and/or residual disease are likely to benefit with radiotherapy. Radiotherapy is given to the adrenal bed to a dose of 45–50 Gy/25# over 5 weeks.[43]

SUMMARY

- Radiation therapy uses ionizing rays to induce DNA damage in cancer cells.

- Hypofractionation allows for the desired dose to be delivered in lesser fractions, allowing for shorter treatment duration.
- External beam radiation therapy to the prostate with or without hormonal therapy is one of the first line options for non-metastatic prostate cancer.
- RT to the prostate is also recommended in low volume metastatic prostate cancer.
- Bladder preservation using trimodal therapy with TURBT and CT/RT is the first line option for well-selected patients with muscle invasive bladder cancer.
- Adjuvant RT following cystectomy is the standard line of treatment for squamous bladder cancer. This is being explored in on-going trials for urothelial cancers as well.
- Following encouraging results from smaller series, SBRT to the renal primary is being evaluated in larger studies.
- Brachytherapy to the penile tumor is a penile-preserving option for well-selected patients.
- Adjuvant RT to the inguinal regions has shown survival benefit following surgery for node-positive penile cancer.
- Adjuvant RT following surgery for adrenocortical cancer has shown benefit for patients with adverse pathological features.

REFERENCES

1. Viani GA, Viana BS, Martin JEC, Rossi BT, Zuliani G, Stefano EJ. Intensity-modulated radiotherapy reduces toxicity with similar biochemical control compared with 3-dimensional conformal radiotherapy for prostate cancer: A randomized clinical trial. Cancer. 2016 Jul 1;122(13):2004–11.
2. Murthy V, Sinha S, Kannan S, Datta D, Das R, Bakshi G, *et al.* Safety of Prostate Stereotactic Body Radiation Therapy after Transurethral Resection of Prostate (TURP): A Propensity Score Matched Pair Analysis. Pract Radiat Oncol. 2019;9(5):347–53.
3. Hamdy FC, Donovan JL, Lane JA, Metcalfe C, Davis M, Turner EL, *et al.* Fifteen-Year Outcomes after Monitoring, Surgery, or Radiotherapy for Prostate Cancer. N Engl J Med. 2023 Apr 27;388(17):1547–1558
4. Murthy V, Maitre P, Kannan S, Panigrahi G, Krishnatry R, Bakshi G, *et al.* Prostate-Only Versus Whole-Pelvic Radiation Therapy in High-Risk and Very High-Risk Prostate Cancer (POP-RT): Outcomes From Phase III Randomized Controlled Trial. J Clin Oncol Off J Am Soc Clin Oncol. 2021 Apr 10;39(11):1234–42.
5. Kerkmeijer LGW, Groen VH, Pos FJ, Haustermans K, Monninkhof EM, Smeenk RJ, *et al.* Focal Boost to the Intraprostatic Tumor in External Beam Radiotherapy for Patients With Localized Prostate Cancer: Results From the FLAME Randomized Phase III Trial. J Clin Oncol Off J Am Soc Clin Oncol. 2021 Mar 1;39(7):787–96.
6. Cooperberg MR, Pasta DJ, Elkin EP, Litwin MS, Latini DM, DuChane J, *et al.* The UCSF Cancer of the Prostate Risk Assessment (CAPRA) Score: a straightforward and reliable preoperative predictor of disease recurrence after radical prostatectomy. J Urol. 2005 Jun;173(6):1938–42.
7. Vale CL, Fisher D, Kneebone A, Parker C, Pearse M, Richaud P, *et al.* Adjuvant or early salvage radiotherapy for the treatment of localised and locally advanced prostate cancer: a prospectively planned systematic review and meta-analysis of aggregate data. Lancet Lond Engl. 2020 Oct 31;396(10260):1422–31.
8. Pollack A, Karrison TG, Balogh AG, Gomella LG, Low DA, Bruner DW, *et al.* The addition of androgen deprivation therapy and pelvic lymph node treatment to prostate bed salvage radiotherapy (NRG Oncology/RTOG 0534 SPPORT): an international, multicentre, randomised phase 3 trial. Lancet Lond Engl. 2022 May 14;399(10338):1886–901.
9. Dose-intensified Versus Conventional-dose Salvage Radiotherapy for Biochemically Recurrent Prostate Cancer After Prostatectomy: The SAKK 09/10 Randomized Phase 3 Trial-PubMed [Internet]. [cited 2023 Apr 19]. Available from: https://pubmed.ncbi.nlm.nih.gov/34140144/
10. Parker CC, James ND, Brawley CD, Clarke NW, Hoyle AP, Ali A, *et al.* Radiotherapy to the primary tumour for newly diagnosed, metastatic prostate cancer (STAMPEDE): a randomised controlled phase 3 trial. Lancet Lond Engl. 2018 Dec 1;392(10162):2353–66.
11. Chemohormonal Therapy in Metastatic Hormone-Sensitive Prostate Cancer: Long-Term Survival Analysis of the Randomized Phase III E3805 CHAARTED Trial-PubMed [Internet]. [cited 2023 Apr 19]. Available from: https://pubmed.ncbi.nlm.nih.gov/29384722/
12. Zilli T, Achard V, Dal Pra A, Schmidt-Hegemann N, Jereczek-Fossa BA, Lancia A, *et al.* Recommendations for radiation therapy in oligometastatic prostate cancer: An ESTRO-ACROP Delphi consensus. Radiother Oncol J Eur Soc Ther Radiol Oncol. 2022 Nov;176:199–207.
13. Huddart RA, Birtle A, Maynard L, Beresford M, Blazeby J, Donovan J, *et al.* Clinical and patient-reported outcomes of SPARE–a randomised feasibility study of selective bladder preservation versus radical cystectomy. Bju Int. 2017 Nov;120(5):639–50.
14. Vashistha V, Wang H, Mazzone A, Liss MA, Svatek RS, Schleicher M, *et al.* Radical Cystectomy Compared to Combined Modality Treatment for Muscle-Invasive Bladder Cancer: A Systematic Review and Meta-Analysis. Int J Radiat Oncol Biol Phys. 2017 Apr 1;97(5):1002–20.
15. Portner R, Bajaj A, Elumalai T, Huddart R, Murthy V, Nightingale H, *et al.* A practical approach to bladder preservation with hypofractionated radiotherapy for localised muscle-invasive bladder cancer. Clin Transl Radiat Oncol. 2021 Nov;31:1.
16. Rodrigues Pessoa R, Mueller AC, Boxley P, Flaig TW, Piper C, Konety B, *et al.* Systematic review and meta-analysis of radiation therapy for high-risk non-muscle invasive bladder cancer. Urol Oncol. 2021 Nov;39(11):786.e1–786.e8.
17. Murthy V, Master Z, Adurkar P, Mallick I, Mahantshetty U, Bakshi G, *et al.* "Plan of the day" adaptive radiotherapy for bladder cancer using helical tomotherapy. Radiother Oncol J Eur Soc Ther Radiol Oncol. 2011 Apr;99(1):55–60.
18. Fonteyne V, Dirix P, Van Praet C, Berghen C, Albersen M, Junius S, *et al.* Adjuvant Radiotherapy After Radical Cystectomy for Patients with High-risk Muscle-invasive Bladder Cancer: Results of a Multicentric Phase II Trial. Eur Urol Focus. 2022 Sep;8(5):1238–45.
19. Zaghloul MS, Christodouleas JP, Smith A, Abdallah A, William H, Khaled HM, *et al.* Adjuvant Sandwich Chemotherapy Plus Radiotherapy vs Adjuvant Chemotherapy Alone for Locally Advanced Bladder Cancer After Radical Cystectomy: A Randomized Phase 2 Trial. JAMA Surg. 2018 Jan 17;153(1):e174591.
20. Jp C, Bc B, J H, Wt H, Kn T, Je B, *et al.* Optimizing bladder cancer locoregional failure risk stratification after radical

cystectomy using SWOG 8710. Cancer [Internet]. 2014 Apr 15 [cited 2023 Jan 7];120(8). Available from: https://pubmed.ncbi.nlm.nih.gov/24390799/

21. Murthy V, Bakshi G, Manjali JJ, Prakash G, Pal M, Joshi A, *et al.* Locoregional recurrence after cystectomy in muscle invasive bladder cancer: Implications for adjuvant radiotherapy. Urol Oncol. 2021 Aug;39(8):496.e9–496.e15.
22. Boujelbene N, Cosinschi A, Boujelbene N, Khanfir K, Bhagwati S, Herrmann E, *et al.* Pure seminoma: A review and update. Radiat Oncol. 2011 Aug 8;6(1):90.
23. Mead GM, Fossa SD, Oliver RTD, Joffe JK, Huddart RA, Roberts JT, *et al.* Randomized trials in 2466 patients with stage I seminoma: patterns of relapse and follow-up. J Natl Cancer Inst. 2011 Feb 2;103(3):241–9.
24. Fosså SD, Horwich A, Russell JM, Roberts JT, Cullen MH, Hodson NJ, *et al.* Optimal planning target volume for stage I testicular seminoma: A Medical Research Council randomized trial. Medical Research Council Testicular Tumor Working Group. J Clin Oncol Off J Am Soc Clin Oncol. 1999 Apr;17(4):1146.
25. Jones WG, Fossa SD, Mead GM, Roberts JT, Sokal M, Horwich A, *et al.* Randomized trial of 30 versus 20 Gy in the adjuvant treatment of stage I Testicular Seminoma: a report on Medical Research Council Trial TE18, European Organisation for the Research and Treatment of Cancer Trial 30942 (ISRCTN18525328). J Clin Oncol Off J Am Soc Clin Oncol. 2005 Feb 20;23(6):1200–8.
26. Wilder RB, Buyyounouski MK, Efstathiou JA, Beard CJ. Radiotherapy Treatment Planning for Testicular Seminoma. Int J Radiat Oncol Biol Phys. 2012 Jul 15;83(4):e445–52.
27. Classen J, Schmidberger H, Meisner C, Souchon R, Sautter-Bihl ML, Sauer R, *et al.* Radiotherapy for Stages IIA/B Testicular Seminoma: Final Report of a Prospective Multicenter Clinical Trial. J Clin Oncol [Internet]. 2016 Sep 21 [cited 2023 Apr 15]; Available from: https://ascopubs.org/doi/pdf/10.1200/JCO.2003.06.065?role=tab
28. Chung P, Warde P. Contemporary management of stage I and II seminoma. Curr Urol Rep. 2013 Oct;14(5):525–33.
29. Honecker F, Aparicio J, Berney D, Beyer J, Bokemeyer C, Cathomas R, *et al.* ESMO Consensus Conference on testicular germ cell cancer: diagnosis, treatment and follow-up. Ann Oncol. 2018 Aug 1;29(8):1658–86.
30. Papachristofilou A, Bedke J, Hayoz S, Schratzenstaller U, Pless M, Hentrich M, *et al.* Single-dose carboplatin followed by involved-node radiotherapy for stage IIA and stage IIB seminoma (SAKK 01/10): a single-arm, multicentre, phase 2 trial. Lancet Oncol. 2022 Nov 1;23(11):1441–50.
31. Francolini G, Trodella LE, Marvaso G, Matrone F, Nicosia L, Timon G, *et al.* Radiotherapy role in non-seminomatous germ cell tumors, radiobiological and technical issues of an unexplored scenario. Int J Clin Oncol. 2021 Oct;26(10):1777–83.
32. Heinzelbecker J, Schmidt S, Lackner J, Busch J, Bokemeyer C, Classen J, *et al.* Therapy of clinical stage IIA and IIB seminoma: a systematic review. World J Urol. 2022 Dec;40(12):2829–41.
33. Patel A, Naghavi AO, Johnstone PA, Spiess PE, Grass GD. Updates in the use of radiotherapy in the management of primary and locally-advanced penile cancer. Asian J Urol. 2022 Oct;9(4):389–406.
34. Hasan S, Francis A, Hagenauer A, Hirsh A, Kaminsky D, Traughber B, *et al.* The role of brachytherapy in organ preservation for penile cancer: A meta-analysis and review of the literature. Brachytherapy. 2015;14(4):517–24.
35. Martz N, Bodokh Y, Gautier M, Thamphya B, Schiappa R, Lam Cham Kee D, *et al.* High-dose rate brachytherapy in localized penile cancer: 5-Year clinical outcome analysis. Clin Transl Radiat Oncol. 2021 Jan 17;27:89–95.
36. Scheltes D, Mohanty S, Smits G, van der Steen-Banasik E, Murthy V, Hoskin P. Improving Quality of Life with Brachytherapy for Urological Malignancies. Clin Oncol [Internet]. 2023 Jan 31 [cited 2023 Apr 19]; Available from: https://www.sciencedirect.com/science/article/pii/S0936655523000225
37. Brouwer OR, Albersen M, Parnham A, Protzel C, Pettaway CA, Ayres B, *et al.* European Association of Urology-American Society of Clinical Oncology Collaborative Guideline on Penile Cancer: 2023 Update. Eur Urol. 2023 Mar 7;S0302–2838(23)02638–6.
38. Khurud P, Krishnatry R, Telkhade T, Patil A, Prakash G, Joshi A, *et al.* Impact of Adjuvant Treatment in pN3 Penile Cancer. Clin Oncol R Coll Radiol G B. 2022 Mar;34(3):172–8.
39. Ager M, Njoku K, Serra M, Robinson A, Pickering L, Afshar M, *et al.* Long-term multicentre experience of adjuvant radiotherapy for pN3 squamous cell carcinoma of the penis. BJU Int. 2021 Oct;128(4):451–9.
40. Khurud P, Gupta A, Krishnatry R, Panigrahi G, Phurailatpam RD, Menon S, *et al.* Optimizing Target Volume for Adjuvant Radiation Therapy in Penile Cancer. Pract Radiat Oncol. 2022 Nov 30;S1879–8500(22)00365–4.
41. Mittal R, Krishnatry R, Maitre P, Murthy V. Recommendations and Clinical Validation of Inguinal Clinical Target Volume Delineation in Penile Cancer. Int J Radiat Oncol Biol Phys. 2021 Nov 1;111(3):741–53.
42. Siva S, Ali M, Correa RJM, Muacevic A, Ponsky L, Ellis RJ, *et al.* 5-year outcomes after stereotactic ablative body radiotherapy for primary renal cell carcinoma: an individual patient data meta-analysis from IROCK (the International Radiosurgery Consortium of the Kidney). Lancet Oncol. 2022 Dec;23(12):1508–16.
43. Ho J, Turkbey B, Edgerly M, Alimchandani M, Quezado M, Camphausen K, *et al.* Role of Radiotherapy in Adrenocortical Carcinoma. Cancer J Sudbury Mass. 2013;19(4):288–94.

Section

2

Pediatric Urology

Chapter

1

Antenatal Hydronephrosis in the Second Trimester: Evaluation and Counselling

• *Sudhindra Jayasimha*

LEARNING OBJECTIVES

- To describe the incidence, natural history and aetiology of antenatal hydronephrosis (ANH).
- To list the classification systems in ANH.
- To describe foetal urine production and the basis for pre-natal and post-natal evaluation.
- To risk-stratify, prognosticate and explain treatment algorithms used in ANH (pre and postnatal).

INTRODUCTION

This chapter discusses the implication of antenatally detected hydronephrosis, prenatal evaluation, counselling and management. The following case scenarios and the ensuing discussion highlight the salient features of ANH.

Case Scenario

Scenario 1: Second trimester scan at 24 weeks reveals bilateral hydroureteronephrosis with APD of 19 mm on both sides. Bladder appears distended. Amniotic fluid index (AFI): 6 cm. No other anomalies visualised (Fig. 1.1).

Scenario 2: Second trimester scan at 24 weeks shows unilateral hydronephrosis with APD of 42 mm. The contralateral kidney and bladder appear normal. There is no evident ureteric dilatation. AFI: 14 cm. No other anomalies seen (Fig. 1.2).

1. **How common is antenatal hydronephrosis?**
   Ans: Antenatal hydronephrosis is the second commonest condition detected in pregnancy after cardiac anomalies. It is seen in 1–5% of all antenatal

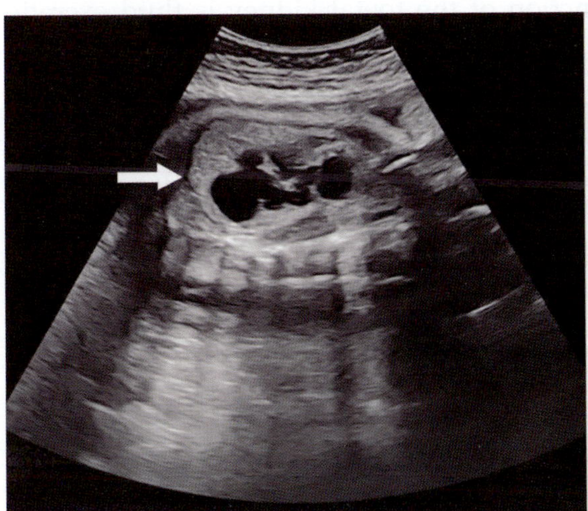
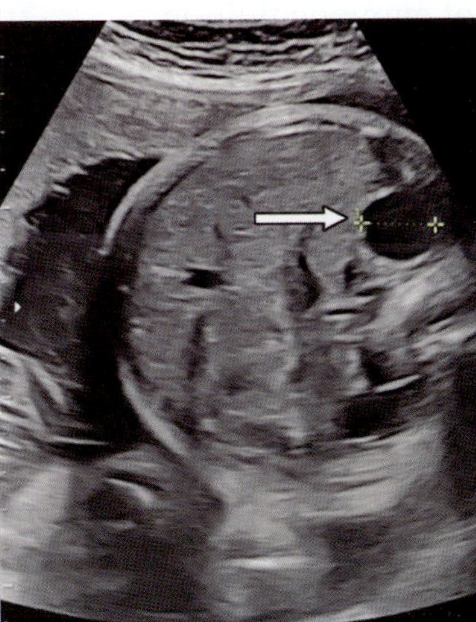
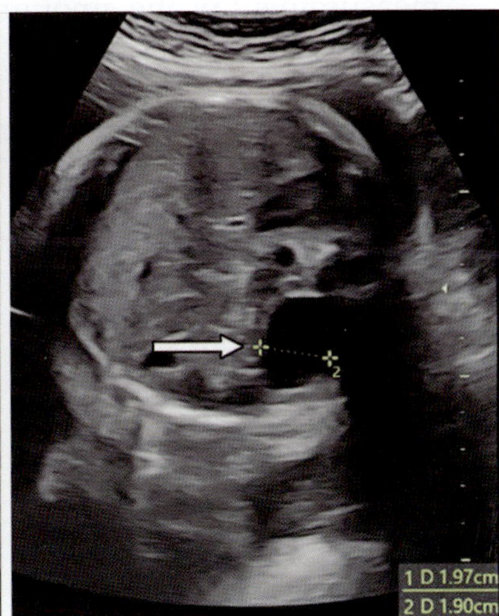

Fig. 1.1: Antenatal ultrasound images, scenario 1

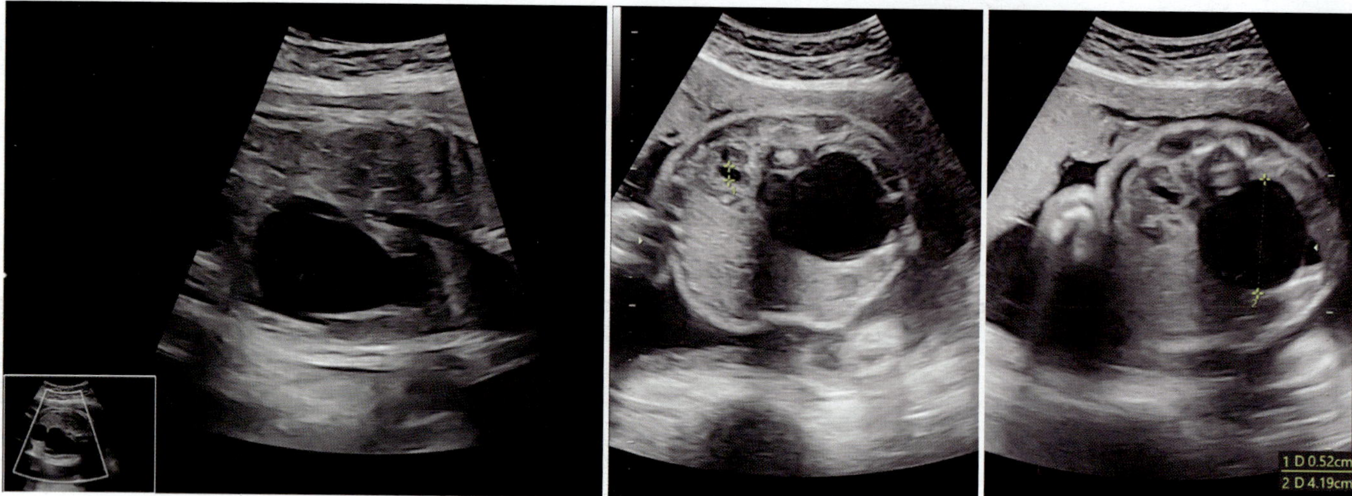

Fig. 1.2: Antenatal ultrasound images, scenario 2

ultrasound scans. Most are diagnosed in the second trimester and the majority will show spontaneous resolution[1] on follow-up.

2. **What features will you look for in an antenatal scan that reports upper tract dilatation?**

   Ans: Table 1.1.

3. **What is megacystis?**

   Ans: It is abnormally distended bladder. In the *first trimester*, megacystis is most commonly defined as a longitudinal bladder dimension of ≥7 mm. Later in pregnancy, a sagittal dimension (in mm) greater than gestational age (in weeks) + 12 is often accepted. Suspect outlet obstruction (posterior urethral valve, urethral atresia) and prune-belly/triad syndrome if the bladder does not empty even after 45 minutes of observation on ultrasound.[3]

4. **What is amniotic fluid index (AFI)? How is it calculated and interpreted?**

   Ans: Amniotic fluid index is an objective measurement of the amount of amniotic fluid in the gestational sac. It is the sum total of the depth of four pockets of fluid surrounding the foetus.[4]

   i. Normal: 8–18 cm (amniotic volume 500–1500 ml)
   ii. Oligohydramnios: <5–6 cm (amniotic volume <500 ml)
   iii. Polyhydramnios: >20–24 cm (amniotic volume >1500 ml)

5. **Describe foetal urine production.**

   Ans: The ureteric bud fuses with metanephric mesenchyme by 28 days. Lobulated kidneys ascend between six and nine weeks and are seen on scans by the 12th week. Renal architecture is evident by 20 weeks. Nephrogenesis occurs as a result of reciprocal induction and is completed by 34 weeks. Each kidney contains about 1 million nephrons by then. Urine production starts at 10 weeks and is seen on ultrasound scans by 14 weeks. Prenatally, the composition of urine is regulated by the placenta and the principal function of the foetal kidney is fluid excretion.

TABLE 1.1: Ultrasound parameters in antenatal hydronephrosis (ANH)[2]

Sl No.	*Parameter*	*Comment*
1	Antero-posterior diameter (APD) of the renal pelvis	Maximal width of intrarenal pelvis in transverse plane (mm)
2	Calyceal dilatation	Major/minor calyx dilated (Y/N)
3	Parenchymal thickness	Normal/abnormal
4	Appearance of parenchyma	Echogenicity, cortico-medullary differentiation, cysts
5	Ureter	Dilated/not dilated
6	Bladder/urethra	Normal/abnormal (thick wall, keyhole sign, ureterocoele)
7	Laterality	Unilateral/bilateral
8	Amniotic fluid index	Normal/oligohydramnios/polyhydramnios
9	Associated anomalies (e.g., cardiac, spine, limb)	Present/absent

Tubular maturation starts from the 14th week onwards.[1,4] Urine output increases from 5 ml/hour at 20th week to 50 ml/hour by week 40.

6. **What are the implications of oligohydramnios?**

Ans: The foetal urine forms amniotic fluid and is responsible for alveolar development by means of mechanical expansion and induction via renal derived growth factors.[3] Lower urinary tract obstruction and renal dysplasia both impair foetal urine production causing oligohydramnios which in turn leads to pulmonary hypoplasia. Potter's syndrome is a characteristic set of deformities in a foetus with severe oligohydramnios and includes flat nose, retrognathic chin, low-set ears, small thorax/hands and bow legs with talipes equinovarus due to external compression.[4]

7. **What are the possible differential diagnoses for ANH? How do they differ in scenarios 1 and 2?**

Ans: In Tables 1.2 and 1.3, aetiology of ANH and possible differential diagnoses for ANH are discussed in detail.

TABLE 1.2: Aetiology of ANH[2]

Cause	*Frequency*
Physiological transient hydronephrosis	50–70%
Pelvi-ureteric junction obstruction	10–30%
Vesico-ureteric reflux	10–40%
Megaureter	5–15%
Multicystic dysplastic kidney	2–5%
Posterior urethral valve	1–5%
Ureterocoele, duplex, ectopic ureter, prune-belly/triad syndrome, urethral atresia	Rare

TABLE 1.3: Differential diagnosis in unilateral and bilateral ANH[3]

Unilateral	*Bilateral*
Physiological transient hydronephrosis	Posterior urethral valve
Pelvi-ureteric junction obstruction	Prolapsed ureterocoele with outlet obstruction
Vesico-ureteric reflux	Urethral atresia
Megaureter	Prune belly syndrome
Multicystic dysplastic kidney	Bilateral presence of unilateral pathology
Ureterocoele, duplex, ectopic ureter	

8. **How is ANH classified?**

Ans: Tables 1.4 to 1.6 depict classification of ANH.

TABLE 1.4: Society for fetal urology grading of ANH[5]

Grade	*Description*	
	Kidney	*Ureter*
0	No pelvi-calyceal dilatation	Not seen
1	Splitting of the pelvis	<7 mm
2	Dilatation of pelvis and major calyces	7–10 mm
3	Dilatation of pelvis major and minor calyces with normal parenchyma	>10 mm
4	Dilatation of pelvis major and minor calyces with thin parenchyma	

TABLE 1.5: Onen grading of ANH[6]

Grade	*Description*
1	Pelvis dilated
2	Pelvis and calyces dilated
3	Pelvis and calyces dilated Medulla is thin Corticomedullary differentiation is maintained **Total parenchymal thickness:** – 2nd trimester: 2–5 mm – 3rd trimester: 2.5–6 mm – Post-natal : 3–7 mm
4	Pelvis and calyces dilated Cortex is thin Loss of corticomedullary differentiation **Total parenchymal thickness:** – 2nd trimester: <2 mm – 3rd trimester: <2.5 mm – Post–natal : <3 mm

9. **What is the natural history of ANH?**

Ans: The natural history of ANH is variable and depends on gender, laterality, severity and age at detection. The main causes of mortality in severe ANH are oligohydramnios resulting in pulmonary hypoplasia, prematurity and renal dysplasia.[8] However, the majority of ANH is mild (P1/SFU 1–2) and resolves with time.[1] The resolution rates at 3 years follow-up, are as follows:[9]

SFU grade 1: 98% SFU grade 2: 87%	UTD P1: 90%
SFU grade 3: 76%	UTD P2: 81%
SFU grade 4: 57%	UTD P3: 71%

Longitudinal follow-up studies have shown that 5% of children with SFU grade 3/4 developed features of renal impairment (hypertension, proteinuria, reduced eGFR) over a median follow-up period of 6.4 years. Creatinine, parenchymal thickness and recurrent UTI were predictive of renal impairment in those with SFU 3/4 ANH.[10] Children with APD <7 mm, no calyceal/ureteral dilatation and normal bladders/renal parenchyma showed no deterioration of renal function on follow-up.[11]

TABLE 1.6: UTD classification[7]

	Antenatal		*Postnatal*		
	UTD A1	**UTD A2/3**	**UTD P1**	**UTD P2**	**UTD P3**
Anteroposterior diameter (APD) of renal pelvis	<28 weeks: 4–7 mm ≥28 weeks: 7–10 mm	<28 weeks: ≥7 mm ≥28 weeks: ≥10 mm	10–15 mm	≥15 mm	≥10 mm
		OR	OR	OR	OR
Calyceal dilation	Central	Any	Central	Peripheral	Any
		OR		OR	OR
Ureteral dilatation (>4 mm)		Present and APD ≥4 mm		Present and APD ≥10 mm	Any
		OR			AND
Abnormal renal parenchyma/abnormal bladder/oligohydramnios (modified from Ref.7)		Present			Present

10. How do you prognosticate ANH?

Ans: ANH may be prognosticated with biochemical and ultrasound-based assessment.

Biochemical parameters

Serial assessment of foetal urine is performed using ultrasound guided vesicocentesis. Complete bladder aspiration is recommended at 24–48-hour intervals (minimum 3 times over 5–7 days) at 18–22 weeks gestational age.

First sample: Urine in the bladder from an undetermined period

Second sample: Urine drained from foetal upper tracts

Third sample: Actual urine produced by foetal kidneys

If renal function is poor, solute absorption is poor and urine continues to remain concentrated. The values used for prognostication are given in Table 1.7.

TABLE 1.7: Biochemical parameters for prognostication of ANH

Biochemical parameter	*Good prognosis*	*Poor prognosis*
Sodium	<90 mmol/L	>100 mmol/L
Chloride	<80 mmol/L	>90 mmol/L
Osmolality	<180 mOsm/L	>200 mOsm/L
Calcium	<7 mg/dl	>8 mg/dl
Total protein	<20 mg/dl	>40 mg/dl
Beta-2 microglobulin	<6 mg/dl	>10 mg/dl

Ultrasound findings predicting adverse outcome

- Presence of other life-threatening congenital anomalies (e.g. cardiac or neural tube defects)
- Small, echogenic kidneys with cysts
- Severe oligohydramnios[8]

11. What are the indications for prenatal intervention?

Ans: The eligibility for prenatal intervention is assessed based on karyotype, detailed ultrasound and serial evaluation of foetal urine biochemistry Karyotyping is performed using amniocentesis, or in case of anhydramnios, using transabdominal chorionic villus sampling or cordocentesis. In case of oligo/anhydramnios, 150–250 ml of warmed 5% Dextrose with Ringer's lactate is used to perform amnioinfusion to aid visualisation and to prevent pressure related deformities of the limbs and face. The inclusion criteria for prenatal intervention are as follows:

- Singleton pregnancy between 16 and 24 weeks
- Male karyotype*
- Absence of other major congenital anomalies
- Isolated lower urinary tract obstruction
- Oligo/anhydramnios
- Favourable foetal urinary biochemical parameters[8,12]

The Ruano staging system may be used to guide prognostication and therapy.[13] Foetal intervention is usually limited to stages I and II. Foetal intervention is difficult in stages III and IV as they have end stage renal disease before birth with an under-filled bladder. Most of these children die within the first week of birth due to pulmonary hypoplasia (Table 1.8).

12. What are the various types of prenatal intervention?

Ans:

1. **Vesico-amniotic shunting (VAS)**
   - Foetal bladder is diverted into the amniotic sac as a temporary measure to relieve outlet obstruction

*To be addressed in keeping with the prenatal sex determination laws of the country—not legally permissible in india

TABLE 1.8: Ruano staging

Stage	Ultrasound	Foetal urine biochemistry	Management
I	AFI normal, no renal cysts or dysplasia	Favourable 3 successive samples	Weekly ultrasound
II	Oligohydramnios, no renal cysts or dysplasia. Severe bilateral dilatation	Favourable 3 successive samples	VAS/cystoscopy
III	Oligo/anhydramnios, echogenic kidneys with cysts and dysplasia	Unfavourable successive samples	VAS +/- amnioinfusion
IV	Anhydramnios and anuria after monitoring for bladder filling. echogenic, dysplastic kidneys	Unfavourable samples, anuria	Amnioinfusion

- Maternal local anaesthesia with intravenous sedation (morphine, diazepam) is used
- A trocar is introduced under ultrasound guidance through the abdominal wall and the uterus
- Once the trocar enters the foetal bladder, the shunt is deployed between bladder and amniotic sac
- In anhydramnios, amnioinfusion is needed to create space to place the shunt
- Types of shunt: Harrison's, Rodeck, rocket of London

2. **Foetal cystoscopic valve ablation**
   - The foetal bladder is accessed via a suprapubic route to directly visualise posterior urethral valves
   - A neodymium yttrium aluminium garnet laser was used to ablate the valves under vision[1,8]
   - In a retrospective comparative study, valve ablation showed better 6-month survival and renal function compared to controls, whereas VAS was only associated with better 6-month survival and no improvement in renal function.[13]

13. **Are there any trials that have evaluated prenatal intervention? What were the outcomes?**

    Ans: Table 1.9 depicts randomized trials of prenatal intervention.

14. **What are the complications of prenatal intervention?**

    Ans: Complication rates up to 44% were described in early series. The possible adverse outcomes include the following:[1,12,14,16]
    - Direct injury to the foetus (rare)
    - Bleeding, infection, preterm rupture of membranes and abortion (1–2%)

TABLE 1.9: Randomized trials of prenatal intervention in ANH[14,15]

	PLUTO (Morris)	*MOMS (Adzick)*
Patient	**Foetal lower urinary tract obstruction**	**Foetal meningomyelocoele**
Intervention	**Vesico-amniotic shunt (VAS)** 16 (randomized) 13 VAS 2 intra-uterine death 1 termination	**Prenatal repair** 91 randomised 77 repaired
Comparison	**Conservative management** (n = 15)	**Postnatal repair** 92 randomized 80 repaired
Outcome	**Survival at 28 days** VAS arm: 8 Conservative arm: 4 (ITT: RR 1.88, 0.71-4.96, p = 0.27) (Per-protocol: RR 3.2, 1.06–9.62, p = 0.03) **86% better survival with VAS at 28 days** **Only 2 VAS survived to 2 years with normal renal function**	**Death/need for CSF shunt** 68% intervention arm 98% control arm (RR 0.7, 0.58–0.84, p<0.001) **Mental and motor development** Better score with intervention
Complications of intervention	Spontaneous membrane rupture 3 Dislodged stent 3 Blocked stent 1 Pregnancy loss 4 (27%)	Uterine dehiscence (13 vs. 6%) Abruption (6 vs. 0%) Pulmonary oedema (6 vs. 0%) Preterm delivery (46% vs. 5%) Perinatal death similar (3 vs. 2%)
Comments	**Poor recruitment, sample not reached** Neonatal deaths: pulmonary hypoplasia **Significant morbidity** Severe long-term effects of CKD	**Better foetal outcome at the cost of higher morbidity**

- Displacement/loss of function of shunt (up to 40%)
- Urinary ascites (7%)
- Bladder and intestinal herniation through the puncture site used for VAS
- Umbilical strangulation (rare)
- Perinatal death up to 33%
- Urethro-cutaneous and recto-urethral fistulae with foetal cystoscopy

15. How should one counsel parents about prenatal intervention? How would this differ in scenario 1 and 2?

Ans:

- Prenatal intervention carries significant risk of morbidity (>40%) and foetal loss (as detailed above).
- Relieving lower tract obstruction may restore amniotic fluid volume and facilitate lung development. This may improve the odds of survival by 2.5 times.
- Although initial studies did not show improvement in renal outcomes with prenatal intervention, a meta-analysis of multiple studies has shown that prenatal intervention may improve the odds of good renal function in the first 2 years of life by 2 times.
- It is only indicated in a singleton, foetus 16 and 24 weeks with isolated lower tract obstruction, oligohydramnios and favourable urinary biochemical parameters.
- One of two procedures may be employed (VAS/foetal cystoscopy and valve ablation) based on local expertise with no clear advantage of one over the other.
- Shared, individualised decision making in a multi-disciplinary setting is indicated. The team should include maternal-foetal obstetrics, paediatric urology, paediatric nephrology and neonatology.[1,8,17]

Based on the above, antenatal intervention may be discussed in scenario 1. However, it is not indicated in scenario 2 as the clinical picture is suggestive of unilateral obstruction with normal amniotic fluid volume.

16. What happens to serum creatinine after birth?

Ans: There is biochemical balance between the mother and the foetus in-utero leading to equilibration of creatinine levels. Once the neonate is separated from the maternal circulation, there is excretion of creatinine in the urine coupled with its backflow across the immature, permeable renal tubules of the neonate into the blood-stream. This leads to a high creatinine level which gradually decreases over a period of 1–2 weeks. The more premature the infant, the higher the creatinine.[18] Creatinine is higher in males and the fall is more rapid in term compared to preterm neonates.[19]

17. When should ultrasound be performed after birth and why?

Ans: The neonatal kidney has a low glomerular filtration rate and concentrating ability. During the first 48 hours of life, there is relative fluid deprivation compounded by insensible losses. Coupled with the inability to concentrate urine, there is fluid depletion and a decrease in intravascular volume. This in turn, leads to low urine volumes and apparently decreased dilatation of the urinary tract which may erroneously underestimate the degree of hydronephrosis.[20] Therefore, ultrasound should only be performed after 48 hours unless there is suspicion of lower urinary tract obstruction leading to renal dysfunction.[1]

18. What are the indications for MCU in ANH?

Ans:

i. Ureteric dilatation
ii. Thick, abnormal bladder
iii. SFU grade 3 or 4 (UTD P2 or P3) ANH

If outlet obstruction is suspected, this will have to be performed before discharge within the first few days of life.[1]

19. What is the role of renal scintigraphy in ANH?

Ans: The role of renal scintigraphy in the immediate post-natal management of ANH is limited as the neonatal nephrons are immature with a low GFR and do not respond well to diuretics which may result in a technically inadequate study.[21] It may be employed in severe/UTD P3 upper tract dilatation. Scintigraphy may confirm absence of renal function in a multi-cystic dysplastic kidney (Tc-99m DMSA) or obstruction at the pelvi-ureteric or vesico-ureteric junction (Tc-99m MAG3 or EC).[3,4]

20. What is the role of MRI in ANH?

Ans: In case of uncertainty in diagnosis, MRI provides accurate anatomical information and the ability to assess differential function and drainage without exposure to radiation especially in complex congenital anomalies such as cloaca, exstrophy and urogenital sinus.[1,3]

21. Describe the role of postnatal antibiotic prophylaxis in ANH.

Ans: Studies in ANH included heterogeneous groups of patients and systematic reviews have not been able to draw firm conclusions on the utility of antibiotics due to conflicting results of individual studies. However, they may be of benefit in the following:[22,23]

- High grade hydronephrosis especially with abnormal renal parenchyma (up to 76% increased risk)
- Ureteric dilatation >7 mm (up to 4.5 times higher risk)
- Uncircumcised infants (up to 88% higher risk of UTI)
- Female infants

Using the information above, describe the concerns, timeline of antenatal and postnatal management and follow-up in the two scenarios provided.

Case Scenario

Scenario 1: UTD A2-3, bilateral, ureteral dilatation. Concern for bladder outlet obstruction. Pregnancy and delivery to be planned at a tertiary centre with neonatal intensive care. Pros and cons of foetal intervention may be discussed. An additional ultrasound is recommended at 32 weeks of gestation. The neonate needs early ultrasound followed by appropriate lower tract drainage (e.g. catheterisation, puncture of prolapsed ureterocoele), initiation of prophylactic antibiotics, followed by management as outlined in Fig. 1.3.

Scenario 2: UTD A2-3, unilateral, no ureteral dilatation. No evidence of outlet obstruction. Pregnancy and delivery to be planned at a tertiary centre with neonatal intensive care. Foetal intervention not indicated. Ultrasound may be performed after 48 hours and if there is no evidence of ureteral dilatation, management is as outlined in Fig. 1.4.[3]

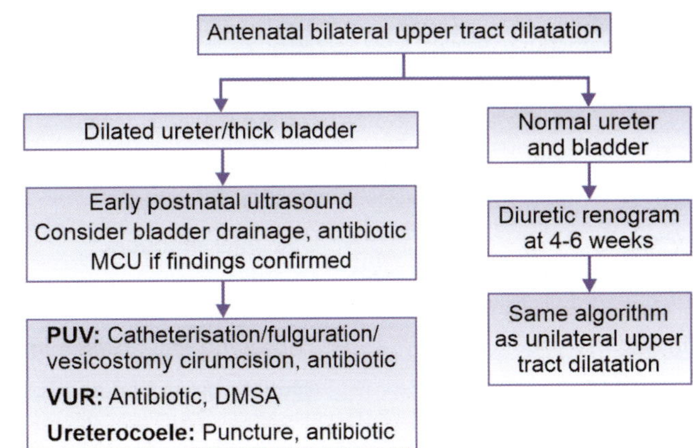

Fig. 1.3: Management of bilateral upper tract dilatation (modified from Ref.3)

The suggested follow-up (antenatal and postnatal) as per UTD classification is presented in Table 1.10.[2]

SUMMARY

- ANH is common and is usually diagnosed in the second trimester
- The majority of ANH is mild (SFU grade 1/2) and resolves by 3 years of age

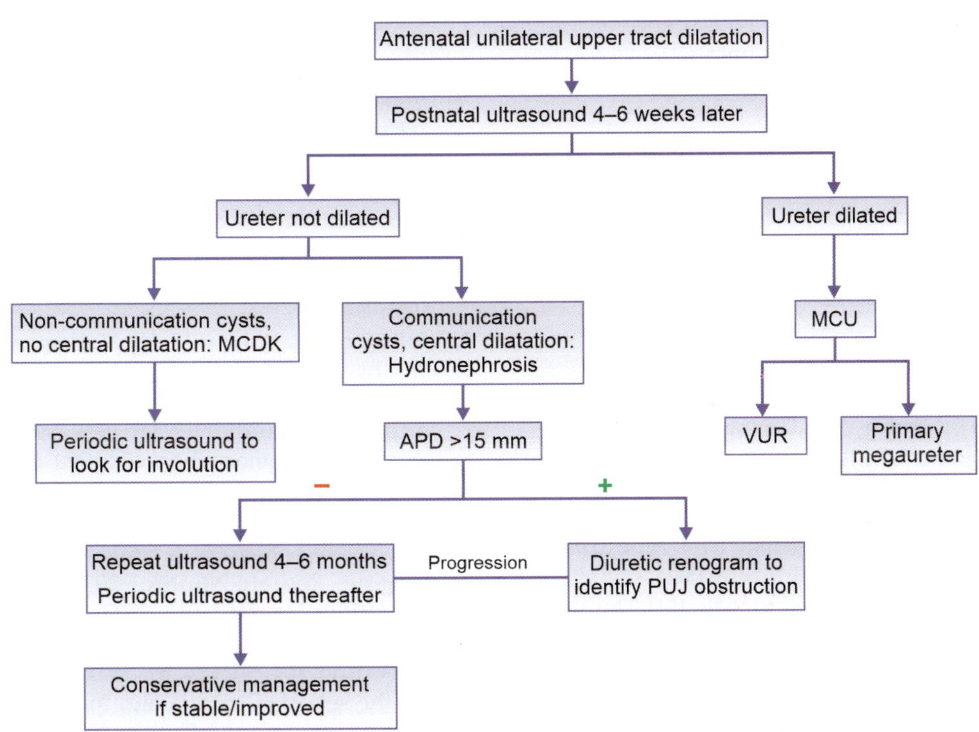

Fig. 1.4: Management of unilateral upper tract dilatation (modified from Ref.3)

TABLE 1.10: Management of ANH

	Antenatal			*Postnatal*		
	UTD A1	*UTD A2/3*		*UTD P1*	*UTD P2*	*UTD P3*
Risk	Low	Increased	Risk	Low	Intermediate	High
Prenatal	USG at 32 weeks	USG in 4–6 weeks	MCU	Optional	Optional	Yes
Postnatal	USG: – 48 hours–1 month – 1–6 months	USG after 48 hours	Antibiotic	Optional	Optional	Yes
Others		Consult urology, nephrology	Renogram	No	Optional	Optional
		(Outlet obstruction needs urgent USG)	Review	1–6 months	1–3 months	1 month

(Modified from Ref.7)

- Creatinine, parenchymal thickness, APD, ureteral dilatation and recurrent UTI predict renal dysfunction
- Foetal urine forms the majority of amniotic fluid and is responsible for lung maturation
- ANH may be classified using SFU grading, Onen grading and UTD classification
- ANH may be prognosticated using ultrasound and biochemical assessment of foetal urine. Along with karyotype, these parameters are used to decide on prenatal intervention
- Renal dysfunction results in poor absorption and concentrated urine
- A singleton foetus with isolated lower urinary tract obstruction, oligohydramnios and favourable serial urinary biochemical parameters is eligible for prenatal intervention between 16 and 24 weeks
- Vesico-amniotic shunting and foetal cystoscopic valve ablation showed better 6-month survival and post-natal renal function.
- Prenatal intervention is associated with >40% risk of maternal and foetal morbidity and 33% perinatal mortality
- Ultrasound is performed 48 hours after birth or later due to insensible losses, immature tubules and fluid depletion leading to decreased dilatation of the urinary tract
- MCU is indicated if there is ureteric dilatation, thick bladder and significant (SFU 3/4) ANH
- MRI may provide added anatomical and functional information in complex anomalies
- Renal scintigraphy is indicated in UTD P3 ANH
- High grade hydronephrosis, ureteric dilatation >7 mm, uncircumcised male and female infants may benefit from post-natal antibiotic prophylaxis.

REFERENCES

1. Wein AJ. Campbell-Walsh-Wein Urology. Elsevier; 2020.
2. Nguyen HT, Benson CB, Bromley B, Campbell JB, Chow J, Coleman B, *et al.* Multidisciplinary consensus on the classification of prenatal and postnatal urinary tract dilation (UTD classification system). J Pediatr Urol 2014;10:982–98. https://doi.org/10.1016/j.jpurol.2014.10.002.
3. Docimo SG, Canning D, Khoury A, Salle JLP. The Kelalis-King-Belman Textbook of Clinical Pediatric Urology. CRC Press; 2018.
4. Nguyen HT, Herndon CDA, Cooper C, Gatti J, Kirsch A, Kokorowski P, *et al.* The Society for Fetal Urology consensus statement on the evaluation and management of antenatal hydronephrosis. J Pediatr Urol 2010;6:212–31. https://doi.org/10.1016/j.jpurol.2010.02.205.
5. Fernbach SK, Maizels M, Conway JJ. Ultrasound grading of hydronephrosis: introduction to the system used by the society for Fetal Urology. Pediatr Radiol.1993;23(6).478–80.
6. Onen A. Grading of Hydronephrosis: An Ongoing Challenge. Front Pediatr 2020;8:458. https://doi.org/10.3389/fped.2020.00458.
7. Nguyen HT, Phelps A, Coley B, Darge K, Rhee A, Chow JS. 2021 update on the urinary tract dilation (UTD) classification system: clarifications, review of the literature, and practical suggestions. Pediatr Radiol 2022;52:740–51. https://doi.org/10.1007/s00247-021-05263-w.
8. Wu S, Johnson MP. Fetal lower urinary tract obstruction. Clin Perinatol 2009;36:377–90, x. https://doi.org/10.1016/j.clp.2009.03.010.
9. Braga LH, McGrath M, Farrokhyar F, Jegatheeswaran K, Lorenzo AJ. Society for Fetal Urology Classification vs Urinary Tract Dilation Grading System for Prognostication in Prenatal Hydronephrosis: A Time to Resolution Analysis. J Urol 2018;199:1615–21. https://doi.org/10.1016/j.juro.2017.11.077.
10. Costa FP, Simões E Silva AC, Mak RH, Ix JH, Vasconcelos MA, Dias CS, *et al.* A clinical predictive model of renal injury in children with isolated antenatal hydronephrosis. Clin Kidney J 2020;13:834–41. https://doi.org/10.1093/ckj/sfz102.
11. Herthelius M, Axelsson R, Lidefelt K-J. Antenatally detected urinary tract dilatation: a 12–15-year follow-up. Pediatr Nephrol 2020;35:2129–35. https://doi.org/10.1007/s00467-020-04659-4.
12. Johnson MP, Bukowski TP, Reitleman C, Isada NB, Pryde PG, Evans MI. In utero surgical treatment of fetal obstructive uropathy: a new comprehensive approach to identify appropriate candidates for vesicoamniotic shunt therapy. Am J Obstet Gynecol 1994;170:1770–6; discussion 1776–1779. https://doi.org/10.1016/s0002-9378(94)70353-1.
13. Ruano R, Dunn T, Braun MC, Angelo JR, Safdar A. Lower urinary tract obstruction: fetal intervention based on prenatal staging. Pediatr Nephrol 2017;32:1871–8. https://doi.org/10.1007/s00467-017-3593-8.
14. Farrugia MK, Braun MC, Peters CA, Ruano R, Herndon CD. Report on The Society for Fetal Urology panel discussion on the selection criteria and intervention for fetal bladder outlet obstruction. J Pediatr Urol 2017;13:345–51. https://doi.org/10.1016/j.jpurol.2017.02.021.

15. Morris RK, Malin GL, Quinlan-Jones E, Middleton LJ, Hemming K, Burke D, *et al.* Percutaneous vesicoamniotic shunting versus conservative management for fetal lower urinary tract obstruction (PLUTO): a randomised trial. The Lancet 2013;382:1496–506. https://doi.org/10.1016/S0140–6736(13)60992–7.
16. Adzick NS, Thom EA, Spong CY, Brock JW, Burrows PK, Johnson MP, *et al.* A Randomized Trial of Prenatal versus Postnatal Repair of Myelomeningocele. New England Journal of Medicine 2011;364:993–1004. https://doi.org/10.1056/NEJMoa1014379.
17. Elder JS, Duckett JW, Snyder HM. Intervention for fetal obstructive uropathy: has it been effective? Lancet 1987;2:1007–10. https://doi.org/10.1016/s0140–6736(87)92567–0.
18. Saccone G, D'Alessandro P, Escolino M, Esposito R, Arduino B, Vitagliano A, *et al.* Antenatal intervention for congenital fetal lower urinary tract obstruction (LUTO): a systematic review and meta-analysis. J Matern Fetal Neonatal Med 2020;33:2664–70. https://doi.org/10.1080/14767058.2018.1555704.
19. Guignard J-P, Drukker A. Why Do Newborn Infants Have a High Plasma Creatinine? Pediatrics 1999;103:e49. https://doi.org/10.1542/peds.103.4.e49.
20. Savory DJ. Reference ranges for serum creatinine in infants, children and adolescents. Ann Clin Biochem 1990;27 (Pt 2):99–101. https://doi.org/10.1177/000456329002700201.
21. Maclaurin JC. Changes in body water distribution during the first two weeks of life. Arch Dis Child 1966;41:286–91. https://doi.org/10.1136/adc.41.217.286.
22. Conway JJ, Maizels M. The "well tempered" diuretic renogram: a standard method to examine the asymptomatic neonate with hydronephrosis or hydroureteronephrosis. A report from combined meetings of The Society for Fetal Urology and members of The Pediatric Nuclear Medicine Council-The Society of Nuclear Medicine. J Nucl Med 1992;33:2047–51.
23. Silay MS, Undre S, Nambiar AK, Dogan HS, Kocvara R, Nijman RJM, *et al.* Role of antibiotic prophylaxis in antenatal hydronephrosis: A systematic review from the European Association of Urology/European Society for Paediatric Urology Guidelines Panel. J Pediatr Urol 2017;13:306–15. https://doi.org/10.1016/j.jpurol.2017.02.023.
24. Holzman SA, Braga LH, Zee RS, Herndon CDA, Davis-Dao CA, Kern NG, *et al.* Risk of urinary tract infection in patients with hydroureter: An analysis from the Society of Fetal Urology Prenatal Hydronephrosis Registry. J Pediatr Urol 2021;17:775–81. https://doi.org/10.1016/j.jpurol.2021.09.001.

Chapter

2

Posterior Urethral Valve in Neonate

• *Chandra Singh J*

LEARNING OBJECTIVES

- To describe the pathophysiology, classification and epidemiology of posterior urethral valve.
- To describe the presentation and evaluation of posterior urethral valve.
- To discuss the pros and cons of various options for definitive management.
- To present the long-term implications and follow-up.
- To explain the role of renal transplantation in boys with posterior urethral valve.

INTRODUCTION

Posterior urethral valves are one of the most common causes of urinary tract obstruction in the pediatric population, an important etiology of end-stage renal disease in children. A posterior urethral valve (PUV) is one of the most devastating anomalies that occur in the urinary tract. Though the structural anomaly of the valve is small and the operative intervention is relatively minor in a vast majority of boys, the pre-operative optimization or management following fulguration or both, need to be meticulously carried out to get optimal outcomes. This chapter focuses on these aspects, highlighting the essential aspects of evaluation, optimization, operative intervention and postoperative follow-up.

Case Scenario

A three-day-old boy was brought with poor feeding, high grade fever and drowsiness. Mother did not have any antenatal scans. He was born at home and was noted to have straining to void since birth. On examination, he was febrile, drowsy and tachypnoeic. His bladder was palpable and ultrasonogram revealed bilateral hydroureteronephrosis and grossly distended bladder. VCUG after optimisation revealed a thickened bladder, dilated posterior urethra, gross vesicoureteric reflux (Fig. 2.1).

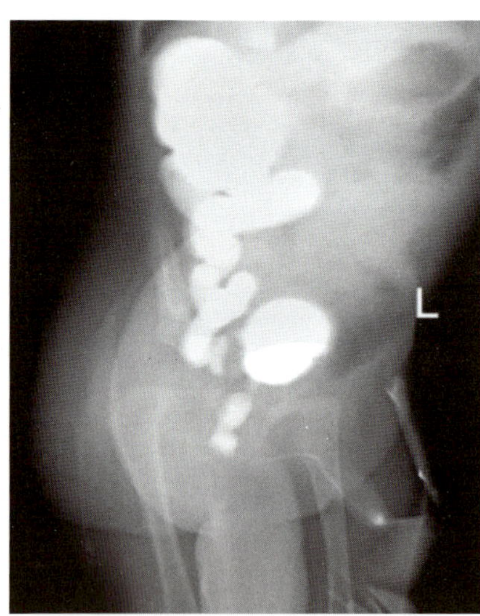

Fig. 2.1: VCUG in a 3-day old child

1. **What is the most likely cause of presentation in this child?**

   Ans: The child has presented with lower urinary tract obstruction that is most likely due to posterior urethral valve (PUV).

2. **What are the effects of PUV?**

   Ans: Due to lower urinary tract obstruction during organogenesis, several structural and functional changes affect the developing bladder, upper urinary tract and glomeruli, resulting in long-term impact in a large number of children as well as impacted lung development causing respiratory distress at birth. This can result in lifelong disabilities including progressive renal failure and urinary incontinence despite optimal treatment.[1,2]

3. What findings in prenatal ultrasonogram will point towards a diagnosis of PUV?

Ans: Unilateral or bilateral hydroureteronephrosis are often noted. Concomitant bladder wall thickening and poor bladder emptying may be noted. Key hole sign is highly indicative and oligohydramnios is suggestive of the severity.[1]

4. How is PUV classified?

Ans: The original classification by Hugh Hampton Young is the most commonly used classification even today.[2] He described three categories: Type I, type II and type III. However, today, only type I and type III are found to be obstructive. As type II seems to be more like a fold and not obstructive, it is no longer referred to as a valve. Hampton Young's descriptions of type I and III are as follows:

Type I (90–95%). 'In the most common type there is a ridge lying on the floor of the urethra, continuous with the verumontanum, which takes an anterior course and divides into two fork-like processes in the region of the bulbomembranous junction. These processes are continued as thin membranous sheets, direct upward and forward which may be attached to the urethra throughout its entire circumference. It is generally supposed that the valves have complete fusion anteriorly, leaving only an open channel at the posterior urethral wall. Yet, the fusion of the valves anteriorly may not be complete in all cases, and at this point a slight separation of the folds exists'.

Type III. There is a third type which has been found at different levels of the posterior urethra and which apparently bears no such relation to the verumontanum. This obstruction was attached to the entire circumference of the urethra, with a small opening in the center. However, this classification has been challenged. Dewan suggested that types I and III described by Young are the same structure that only appears to be distinct entities following a central defect rupturing antenatally naturally or due to iatrogenic instrumentation.[3]

5. What is the epidemiology of PUV?

Ans: 1:5000 live male births commonly quoted, with 50% progressing to ESRD within ten years.[4] In specific populations, this incidence has decreased over the years in which prenatal diagnosis and subsequent termination of affected fetuses are performed. In one report, 46% of fetuses diagnosed with valves were electively terminated.[5]

6. What are the poor prognostic factors at presentation?

Ans: These include oligohydramnios (low amniotic fluid volume defined as the maximum vertical pocket 2.0 cm), urinary ascites, perinephric urinoma (maybe pop off), increased renal echogenicity, and cortical cysts. Diagnosis of PUV up to the second trimester is associated with high perinatal mortality and risk of end-stage renal disease (ESRD), particularly if there is severe bilateral hydronephrosis with oligohydramnios, and findings suggestive of renal dysplasia.[6] When oligohydramnios is detected in the second trimester, the mortality may be as high as 90–95%.[7] Other poor prognostic factors include respiratory distress at birth, urinary sepsis, dyselectrolytemia and bilateral VUR.

7. What are the structural effects of PUV?

Ans: PUVs are membranous folds that obstruct the lumen of the posterior urethra. Depending on the extent of obstruction, the effects may be manifested in the rest of the urinary tract—the bladder neck is often hypertrophied. Bladder is grossly trabeculated and there may be many diverticula. Due to high pressure in the prostatic urethra, there may be urinary reflux into the ejaculatory duct. Most patients have gross hydroureteronephrosis which may or may not be associated with secondary vesicoureteric reflux. Other pop off mechanisms include perinephric urinomas and abdominal distension secondary to urinary ascites and a patent urachus presenting as umbilical discharge. In severe cases, oligohydramnios occurs due to decreased fetal urine, which in turn may cause pulmonary hypoplasia.[8]

8. What are the ways of post-natal presentation in PUV?

Ans: If the diagnosis of PUVs has not been made prenatally, the most severely affected patients with PUVs present in the newborn period with a urinary tract infection or urosepsis. Neonates with lesser impact may present with delayed voiding, weak stream or dribbling of urine, urosepsis, or a palpable bladder. Premature neonates with respiratory distress and renal failure should be regarded as having PUV unless proven otherwise. Those discharged after delivery may present with lethargy, poor feeding, or failure to thrive. In severe cases, they may present with respiratory distress due to pulmonary hypoplasia.[6] Most infants or older children with a new diagnosis of PUVs presented with urinary tract infections, voiding complaints, urosepsis or renal failure. Therefore, boys with these presentation should be evaluated for PUV especially recurrent urinary tract infections, poor urinary stream, obstructive uropathy or overflow incontinence.[9] Though prenatal ultrasonography is extensively performed, a study performed at Children's Hospital of Philadelphia showed that 43% of patients with PUVs presented after 6 months of age,[10] hence in boys with these presentations, even if the prenatal ultrasonography was normal they have to be evaluated appropriately.

9. What clinical findings need to be looked for?

Ans: Physical examination may be entirely normal. Abdominal palpation may reveal poor muscle tone and the abdomen may be distended because of distended bladder or urinary ascites or secondary to hydronephrosis. Sick neonates may have features suggestive of respiratory distress, sepsis or azotemia. Observed urinary stream may be poor.

10. What is the differential diagnosis for a neonate with bladder outflow obstruction?

Ans: Commonest include urethral atresia, prune-belly syndrome, anterior urethral valves, congenital megalourethra and obstructing ureterocele. Other rare causes include isolated megacystis and megacystis-megaureter association. In a large population based study,[1] PUV accounted for 63% of LUTO, with a prevalence of 2.1 per 10,000 live births. Urethral atresia was 9.9% with 0.33 per 10,000 live births. Urethral stenosis was 7% with 0.23 per 10000 live births, Prune belly was 2.5% with 0.08 per 10,000 live births and other unspecified causes were 17.6% with a prevalence of 0.59 per 10000 live births.

11. What is the initial management of boys with PUV soon after birth?

Ans: Initial management, summarized in[11] Fig. 2.2 is tailored based on the presentation—birthweight, renal dysfunction, sepsis and acidosis. Bladder drainage is initially achieved with a suitable feeding tube, the maximum size that would be admitted by the urethra. If available, a soft feeding tube may be placed to reduce the bladder spasm. It is essential to ensure that the catheter is in the bladder and not coiled in the roomy posterior urethra. Intense bladder spasm, hypertrophic bladder neck and roomy posterior urethra often hamper successful per-urethral placement of catheter into the bladder. Ultrasonogram is an excellent modality to document the correct placement of the catheter. Rarely, failure to establish adequate bladder drainage with a urethral catheter may warrant placement of a suprapubic catheter under ultrasound guidance—especially in sick neonates. Clinical monitoring including daily weight, urine output, blood pressure, and signs of infection is crucial. Twice daily monitoring of creatinine, urea and electrolytes is advisable, as the initial readings may be misleading. In the initial few days after birth, deficiency of the neonates intrinsic renal function may be obscured by placental exchange and clearance by maternal kidneys.

Following relief of obstruction, diuresis may ensue, especially in the neonates with renal failure. Often there is tubular dysfunction, resulting in an inability to concentrate the urine or normally absorb solutes (sodium and potassium). In addition, some patients with PUV due to urinary obstruction may have type IV renal tubular acidosis. Input of the pediatric intensivist is critical, to ensure fluid replacement is appropriate and electrolyte imbalance is corrected. Urine output, serum and urinary electrolytes, serum osmolality and body weight should be closely monitored until renal failure and fluid shifts stabilize. Adequate intravenous access is critical to ensure fluid replacement can keep pace with diuresis in those with marked tubular dysfunction. Undiagnosed neonates may present later with septicemia and dyselectrolytemia and acidosis. The metabolic disturbances and underlying sepsis demand vigorous treatment, which should be undertaken in cooperation with a pediatric nephrologist. If the bladder drainage is satisfactory, definitive intervention may be planned a few days later, once the neonate is optimized metabolically (Fig. 2.2).

12. Once the neonate is optimized, what are the imaging modalities to be carried out?

Ans: Renal and bladder ultrasonography is performed to assess the kidneys, ureter and the bladder. A dilated posterior urethra and valve leaflet may be documented. Voiding cystourethrography (VCUG) is the gold standard imaging modality for the diagnosis of posterior urethral valves. The detailed description of the procedure, adapted from Sharma et[12] is given in Table 2.1. Features suggestive of posterior urethral valves include a thickened trabeculated bladder, elongated and dilated posterior urethra, circumferential filling defect at the level of the pelvic floor; and a prominent bladder neck and vesicoureteric reflux in many infants.[6]

13. What is the role of renal scintigraphy?

Ans: Nuclear scintigraphy allows estimation of the differential function and to plan further

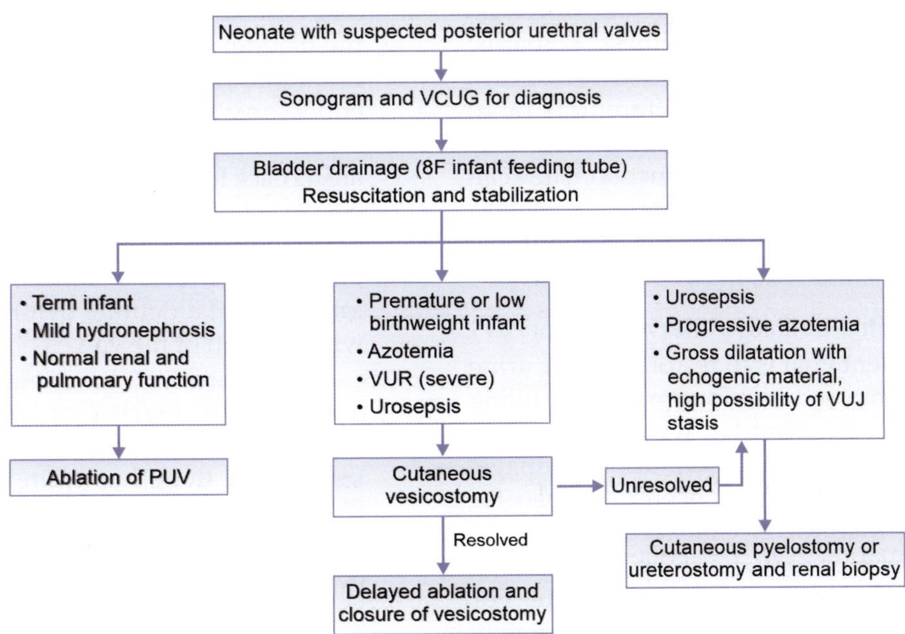

Fig. 2.2: Algorithm for evaluation and management of a neonate suspected to have posterior urethral valves

TABLE 2.1: Procedure for doing micturating cystourethrogram in a neonate	
1.	Counselling parents regarding the study, positioning of the baby during the study, etc helps to reduce the time spent in the fluoroscopy suite as well as radiation exposure recapturing images.
2.	Keep all equipment ready prior to starting the study. The major concern is hypothermia in the exposed neonate and can be avoided if delays are circumvented.
3.	Two attendants should hold the newborn in the supine position. A plain skiagram covering the kidneys, ureters and bladder region and the lumbosacral spine is taken in anterior-posterior and lateral position to assess the spine and bowel gases. Prior to the study, the child is hydrated, ensure normoglycemia and normothermia. The table should be covered with a warm sheet as most fluoroscopy suites have air conditioning which needs to be turned off during the duration of the study. Antibiotics are administered as per institutional protocols.
4.	The genitalia should be cleaned with betadine scrub and dried.
5.	2% sterile lignocaine jelly is layered over an infant feeding tube no. 6/8 French (Fr). The feeding tube should be inserted gradually till it reaches the bladder. In some neonates, with a dilated posterior urethra, the tube may get coiled. The study may still be performed successfully. Care should be taken not to force the catheter which may result in creation of a false passage in the urethra as well as traumatise the urethra. Urine is collected after successful insertion for bacterial culture and sensitivity.
6.	Bladder is filled gradually with the baby held in supine position. The contrast to sterile saline dilution is 1:1 initially. This ensures detection of ureterocoeles in the filling phase. The dilution may be increased in older children and if there is reflux with significant PVR causing dilution intrinsically.
7.	The contrast volume is calculated as 7 ml/kg body weight and filling is stopped if the bladder neck opens or the child starts voiding. After full bladder filling is achieved, right oblique and left oblique views are taken to determine minor grades of reflux and presence of diverticula, trabeculations and sacculation.
8.	The volume filled is documented. Furthermore, the side and volume at which any reflux starts is also documented as this helps guide decision making regarding construction of ureterostomy, if indicated later on.
9.	The catheter is then slowly removed (inject saline during removal) and a container is placed below the baby to collect the urine. The baby is encouraged to pass urine (dripping saline over the genitals or feet) and the voiding film is captured in the right or left oblique manner.
10.	During the procedure, intermittent still shots are captured and saved by radiographer on the machine. Relevant fluoroscopic videos may also be obtained.
11.	A post-void film is taken in supine position to look for post-void residuals and to assess whether the ureters with VUR are draining (obstructed refluxing megaureter). Bladder volume as well as PVR should be interpreted cautiously (pseudopost-void residue) in the presence of major reflux.
12.	If PUV is confirmed, to catheterize with the infant feeding tube till definitive intervention.
13.	Dry the baby and wrap in prewarmed sheets at the end of the study and shift back to NICU immediately.

management based on function, degree of reflux, status of infection and general fitness. Dynamic studies such as DTPA or MAG 3 renogram allows for the estimation of differential renal function. DMSA scan helps identifying any photopenic areas and split renal function. They can demonstrate differential renal function as well as focal parenchymal defects as it is extracted in the proximal tubules and remains in these cells.

14. How to carry out the definitive intervention for PUV?

Ans: The treatment goal is to restore flow of urine through the urethra and enable normal cyclic filling and emptying of the bladder, which is superior to urinary diversion and passive urine drainage. A variety of techniques have been described for PUV ablation including: Cold knife ablation, hook diathermy electrode, hot loop resectoscope and valve ablation using bugbee electrode. For neonates weighing less than 3 kg, the urethra may accommodate 6.5 Fr endoscope. If the urethra admits a 8/9 Fr cystoscope that has a 5 Fr working channel, fulguration may be carried out using a bugbee electrode to fulgurate the valves under vision. In babies over 3.5 kg, 9.5 Fr resectoscope may be used for fulguration/incision of the valves. The sickle-shaped cold knife is preferred by most surgeons. Others may use the cutting loop, hook with or without ball-tip electrode, sharp-angled electrode, or blunt-angled electrode. The valve may be either incised, ablated or to resected at 4–5, 7–8 or 12 o'clock position, or at all three positions, depending on the surgeon's preference (Video 5). It is important to avoid extensive electrocoagulation, as the most common complication of this procedure is stricture formation. Cold knife incision has been shown to have lesser incidence of urethral stricture compared to fulguration using diathermy electrode.[13] Holmium or thulium fiber laser to ablate valves is an alternate option with a lower risk of urethral stricture due to limited tissue penetration, short catheterization time and less irritative symptoms when compared to thermal ablation.[14] Often the urethral catheter is retained for at least 24 to 48 hours. In those with obstructive uropathy, catheter may be retained longer to monitor urine output.

Scan QR Code for Video on
Technique of PUV ablation
VIDEO 5

15. What are the indications for vesicostomy?

Ans: In preterm infants or low birth weight neonates where the urethra would not admit 8 Fr cystoscope, vesicostomy is an option to drain the bladder temporarily. With the miniaturization of endoscopes, most boys can be managed with endoscopic ablation but in case of severe sepsis in an infant presenting months after delivery, if they are too sick for anesthesia, bedside vesicostomy may be carried out under local anesthesia. Vesicostomy drainage serves as a bridging therapy to allow patients to preserve renal function and somatic growth until a definite treatment can be provided with incision of the valves.[15]

Vesicostomy closure and toilet training are typically carried out at 3–5 years of age, after maximal optimization of the upper tracts. Intuitively, there has been a concern regarding the effects of vesicostomy on bladder compliance and capacity but this assumption has not been confirmed by longitudinal studies.[16] Vesicostomy in addition to valve ablation, was not noticed to be of any added benefit in boys with stage 3 CKD.[17] These conflicting data about the value of diversion, like many other debates in the field of PUV, highlight the obvious limitations of PUV literature including insufficiently powered studies comparing heterogeneous patient populations with variable baseline characteristics, outcome definition and follow-up protocols. Additionally, the choice of primary treatment as well as subsequent management is clearly subject to selection bias. In summary, every PUV patient should be evaluated thoroughly and on individual basis in order to select patients who could potentially benefit from urinary diversion and also to optimize the timing, duration and choice of the diversion technique.

16. How do we follow-up to ensure adequacy of valve ablation?

Ans: Repeating the VCUG 1 to 3 months after valve ablation is recommended, to ensure that the valves are no longer visible. Other findings that suggest satisfactory ablation include diminished bladder pressures, improvement in renal dilation and in the volume of vesicoureteral reflux.[18]

17. When do you consider supravesical diversion?

Ans: In cases of persistent sepsis or upper tract dilatation and elevated creatinine, upper urinary tract diversion by a cutaneous ureterostomy or pyelostomy enables direct decompression of the kidney. An easy guide to follow is persistent upper tract dilatation noted on USG, in the presence of adequate bladder drainage via a percutaneous catheter. As the upper tracts are grossly dilated, options to choose include high-loop ureterostomy, ring ureterostomy, end ureterostomy or pyelostomy, with each technique having advantages and disadvantages. The most common technique followed is the low-loop ureterostomy. As the bladder is completely defunctionalized in case of bilateral supravesical diversion, it may affect bladder cycling and as a result, adversely affect bladder function. But supravesical diversion is the last resort if the baby continues to be unwell with urosepsis, dilated upper tracts and renal failure. The cumulative incidence of ESRD was not significantly different among those who had primary valve ablation alone or with supravesical diversion, with longer follow-up. Though diversion may not prevent or decrease the ultimate risk of ESRD, possibly delay the progression to ESRD and the need for renal replacement therapy in a select patient population is beneficial.[19] Delaying the onset of ESRD should not be underestimated since dialysis management in infants and small children is challenging and carries a high mortality risk. As renal transplantation is more challenging in smaller children, delay in the onset of ESRD postpones the requirement of renal replacement therapy.

18. What is the association between PUV, vesicoureteric reflux and nonfunctioning kidney?

Ans: Reflux is very common in PUV patients (up to 72%). Half of these will have unilateral reflux and the other half would be bilateral. Relief of obstruction will decrease the pressures, resolve reflux in 25% to 40% of patients, and improve bladder trabeculation in most cases.[20] During the first few months of life, antibiotic prophylaxis may be given to prevent febrile UTI, especially in those with high-grade reflux.[21] Cotrimoxazole is avoided in children less than 4 months, preferably up to a year, because of risk of kernicterus. Cefalexin (10 mg/kg every night at bedtime) is a safe alternative. In those with phimosis, circumcision can be discussed to reduce the risk of UTIs. High-grade reflux is often associated with a poorly functioning or nonfunctioning kidney. However, nephrectomy is not essential.

19. How do you follow-up boys with PUV?

Ans: All boys with posterior urethral valves require long-term follow-up. Within the first year, three monthly follow-up is advisable and subsequent follow-up may be annual, depending upon the response to initiated measures. Parameters to be monitored are summarized in Table 2.2.

TABLE 2.2: Parameters to be seen during follow-up
• Every visit – Height and weight – Blood pressure – Ultrasonogram of the kidneys – Creatinine – Electrolytes • As indicated – Uroflowmetry – Pressure flow studies – Voiding cystourethrogram – DTPA renogram

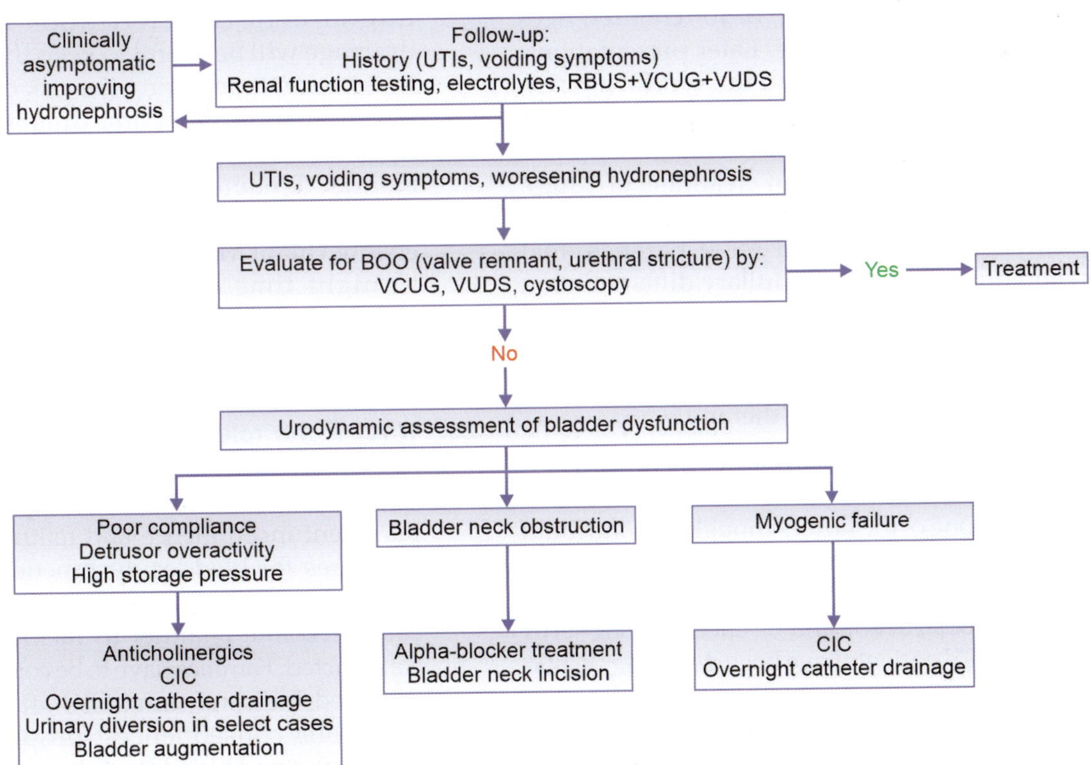

Fig. 2.3: Follow-up for posterior urethral valves[21]

The protocols may vary from center to center but the objective remains the same (Fig. 2.3). Goals of follow-up are to minimize urinary infections, address factors that may accelerate loss of function and to identify any changes in bladder behavior and make appropriate recommendations.

20. What are the indications for pressure flow studies?

Ans: During follow-up, if there are findings suggestive of bladder dysfunction, urodynamic studies are very useful to decide on further interventions. In the following situations, urodynamics often play a definite role in management.[22]

1. Persistent daytime urinary incontinence beyond the age of 5 years
2. Deterioration in renal function (rising creatinine or drop in GFR) with no obvious cause such as growth spurt
3. Increase in upper tract dilatation in the absence of ongoing outflow obstruction
4. Before renal transplantation to ensure a safe, compliant low-pressure urinary tract
5. To assess the efficacy of treatment or intervention
6. As a research tool to study the evolution or natural history of developing bladder function in boys with successfully treated PUV
7. Functional problems—detrusor-sphincter discoordination or suspected dyssynergia.

21. What are the poor prognostic factors in PUV noted after initiating follow-up?

Ans: A serum creatinine of 0.3–0.7 mg/dl for children under age 3 and 0.5–1.0 mg/dl for children ages 3–18 years is considered safe. Later presentations, especially those who have had uneventful infancy, tend to have a better outcome. Persistently elevated serum creatinine after definitive intervention is a risk factor for ESRD. A serum creatinine of 1 mg/dl or above at 1 year of age is poor prognosis. Renal parenchyma quantity (total renal parenchymal area) and quality (corticomedullary differentiation and renal echogenicity) on initial postnatal US also have prognostic value.[23] High creatinine nadir (>1 mg/dl) and severe bladder dysfunction are risk factors for renal replacement therapy.[24]

22. How should the bladder neck hypertrophy be addressed?

Ans: Though one of the factors thought to contribute to bladder dysfunction in PUV patients is bladder neck hypertrophy,[25] the true existence of secondary bladder neck obstruction and its effect on long-term outcome of PUV patients have been debated.[26] While there is prospective literature to justify bladder neck incision stating improved urodynamic parameters and higher VUR resolution rates, there is literature to refute this claim.[27,28]

23. What is the role of anticholinergics?

Ans: Oxybutynin is the anticholinergic extensively studied and approved for use in children. Commonly used dose is 0.1–0.2 mg/kg BID or TID. Higher doses were given in older children up to 5 mg three times daily. With oxybutynin, infants with reduced bladder capacity and poor compliance were noticed to have improvement from a mean of 47.7% to 216% of expected bladder capacity for age.[29] Though dry mouth and constipation are common with anticholinergics, frequently they are mild.

They should be screened for increase in post-void residues after the initiation of anticholinergics.

24. How should these boys be followed up in the long term?

Ans: Most boys have long-term consequences even after documented complete valve ablation. Intrinsic bladder dysfunction, high storage pressure, poor bladder compliance and decreased sensation may lead to worsening upper tracts.[19] In addition to this, as these boys may have high residual volumes and bladder pressures, they may have incontinence and dribbling.

25. What are the measures that may help retard progression?

Ans: Initially, for those with polyuria and incomplete voiding, timed and frequent voiding may be beneficial. If the residual volume progressively increases and there is myogenic failure, clean intermittent catheterization and night time drainage will be useful to keep the bladder empty. In addition to reducing the risk of UTI and upper tract dilatation, night time drainage could provide a period of bladder rest and subsequently improve bladder dynamics and upper tract outcomes.[30] As these boys have a sensate urethra, catheterizable channel like a Mitrofanoff may improve adherence to night time drainage or clean intermittent catheterization.[31] The lifetime prevalence of end-stage renal disease (ESRD) in boys with PUVs is between 20% and 50%.[32]

26. What is the role of augmentation cystoplasty in PUV?

Ans: If there is worsening upper tract changes, persistent incontinence and failure to conservative measures for bladder dysfunction, augmentation cystoplasty may be required. Concomitantly, catheterizable channel to facilitate CIC may be constructed. Families have to be counselled regarding the need for continuing CIC after augmentation, metabolic consequences, propensity to mucus production and bladder washes, need for additional compliance and follow-up, risk of malignancy and stone formation. Augmentation cystoplasty may not alter the natural history of CKD in PUV patients with renal dysplasia.

27. How do these children fare when renal transplantation is required?

Ans: PUV if one of the frequent indications of renal transplantation in children. Ensuring that the bladder is suitable to receive the graft is highly essential. Evaluation includes video urodynamics and cystoscopy. If the compliance is poor, bladder augmentation may be required. Those with hypocontractile bladder will need to continue clean intermittent catheterization with its attendant risk in immunosuppressed children following transplant. Many contemporary series have documented comparable graft survival in those who required transplant.[33] However, in another study, patients with PUV had significantly higher serum creatinine at 10 years relative to controls. Although not statistically significant, urological complications, especially ureteral obstruction, were more common in PUV.[34]

QR Code:

SUMMARY

- PUVs are a heterogeneous birth defect with varying degrees of severity and correspondingly, different clinical manifestations.
- To optimize the sick neonates, it is crucial to have the input of pediatric intensivist and nephrologist.
- After optimization timely intervention is possible when suitable endourological instruments are available.
- For preterm or small birth weight infants, vesicostomy for decompression enables quicker recovery.
- Life-long monitoring is mandatory in all boys, as bladder dysfunction can occur as a result of renal pathology which in turn may worsen outcome by causing progressive upper tract deterioration.
- Up to 50% of these children may develop renal failure in the long term. Renal transplantation may be safely carried out after optimizing their lower urinary tract.

REFERENCES

1. Malin G, Tonks AM, Morris RK, Gardosi J, Kilby MD. Congenital lower urinary tract obstruction: a population-based epidemiological study. BJOG Int J Obstet Gynaecol. 2012 Nov;119(12):1455–64.
2. Young HH, Frontz WA, Baldwin JC. Congenital obstruction of the posterior urethra. J Urol, 3: 289–365, 1919. J Urol. 2002 Jan;167(1):265–7; discussion 268.
3. Dewan PA, Zappala SM, Ransley PG, Duffy PG. Endoscopic reappraisal of the morphology of congenital obstruction of the posterior urethra. Br J Urol. 1992 Oct;70(4):439–44.
4. Casella DP, Tomaszewski JJ, Ost MC. Posterior urethral valves: renal failure and prenatal treatment. Int J Nephrol. 2012;2012:351067.
5. Lloyd JC, Wiener JS, Gargollo PC, Inman BA, Ross SS, Routh JC. Contemporary epidemiological trends in complex congenital genitourinary anomalies. J Urol. 2013 Oct;190(4 Suppl):1590–5.
6. Nasir AA, Ameh EA, Abdur-Rahman LO, Adeniran JO, Abraham MK. Posterior urethral valve. World J Pediatr WJP. 2011 Aug;7(3):205–16.
7. Hutton KA, Thomas DF, Arthur RJ, Irving HC, Smith SE. Prenatally detected posterior urethral valves: is gestational age at detection a predictor of outcome? J Urol. 1994 Aug;152(2 Pt 2):698–701.
8. Sarhan OM. Posterior urethral valves: Impact of low birth weight and preterm delivery on the final renal outcome. Arab J Urol. 2017 Jun;15(2):159–65.
9. Schober JM, Dulabon LM, Woodhouse CR. Outcome of valve ablation in late-presenting posterior urethral valves. BJU Int. 2004 Sep;94(4):616–9.
10. Engel Dl, Pope JC, Adams MC, Brock JW, Thomas JC, Tanaka ST. Risk factors associated with chronic kidney disease in patients with posterior urethral valves without prenatal hydronephrosis. J Urol. 2011 Jun;185(6 Suppl):2502–6.
11. Gonzales, Edmond. Common Problems in Pediatric Urology. First. Mosby; 1991.
12. Sharma S, Joshi M, Gupta DK, Abraham M, Mathur P, Mahajan JK, *et al.* Consensus on the Management of Posterior Urethral Valves from Antenatal Period to Puberty. J Indian Assoc Pediatr Surg. 2019;24(1):4–14.
13. Babu R, Kumar R. Early outcome following diathermy versus cold knife ablation of posterior urethral valves. J Pediatr Urol. 2013 Feb;9(1):7–10.
14. Stuhldreier G, Schweizer P, Hacker HW, Barthlen W. Laser resection of posterior urethral valves. Pediatr Surg Int. 2001;17(1):16–20.
15. Narasimhan KL, Kaur B, Chowdhary SK, Bhalla AK. Does mode of treatment affect the outcome of neonatal posterior urethral valves? J Urol. 2004 Jun;171(6 Pt 1):2423–6.
16. Kim YH, Horowitz M, Combs A, Nitti VW, Libretti D, Glassberg KI. Comparative urodynamic findings after primary valve ablation, vesicostomy or proximal diversion. J Urol. 1996 Aug;156(2 Pt 2):673–6.
17. Chua ME, Ming JM, Carter S, El Hout Y, Koyle MA, Noone D, *et al.* Impact of Adjuvant Urinary Diversion versus Valve Ablation Alone on Progression from Chronic to End Stage Renal Disease in Posterior Urethral Valves: A Single Institution 15-Year Time-to-Event Analysis. J Urol. 2018 Mar;199(3):824–30.
18. Fishberg SE, Landau EH, Duvdevani M, Gofrit ON, Friedman SE, Hidas G. Posterior Urethral Valves: Prenatal, Neonatal, and Long-Term Management. NeoReviews. 2018 Dec 1;19(12):e753–61.
19. Ghanem MA, Nijman RJM. Long-term follow-up of bilateral high (sober) urinary diversion in patients with posterior urethral valves and its effect on bladder function. J Urol. 2005 May;173(5):1721–4.
20. Scott JE. Management of congenital posterior urethral valves. Br J Urol. 1985 Feb;57(1):71–7.
21. Abdelhalim A, Hafez AT. Antenatal and postnatal management of posterior urethral valves: where do we stand? Afr J Urol. 2021 Dec;27(1):140.
22. Desai DY. A review of urodynamic evaluation in children and its role in the management of boys with posterior urethral valves. Indian J Urol IJU J Urol Soc India. 2007 Oct;23(4):435–42.

23. Odeh R, Noone D, Bowlin PR, Braga LHP, Lorenzo AJ. Predicting Risk of Chronic Kidney Disease in Infants and Young Children at Diagnosis of Posterior Urethral Valves: Initial Ultrasound Kidney Characteristics and Validation of Parenchymal Area as Forecasters of Renal Reserve. J Urol. 2016 Sep;196(3):862–8.
24. Ansari MS, Gulia A, Srivastava A, Kapoor R. Risk factors for progression to end-stage renal disease in children with posterior urethral valves. J Pediatr Urol. 2010 Jun;6(3):261–4.
25. Androulakakis PA, Karamanolakis DK, Tsahouridis G, Stefanidis AA, Palaeodimos I. Myogenic bladder decompensation in boys with a history of posterior urethral valves is caused by secondary bladder neck obstruction? BJU Int. 2005 Jul;96(1):140–3.
26. Glassberg KI. The valve bladder syndrome: 20 years later. J Urol. 2001 Oct;166(4):1406–14.
27. Kajbafzadeh AM, Payabvash S, Karimian G. The effects of bladder neck incision on urodynamic abnormalities of children with posterior urethral valves. J Urol. 2007 Nov;178(5):2142–7; discussion 2147–2149.
28. Singh SK, Sharma V, Singh A. Urodynamic Changes after Valve Fulguration Alone and Valve Fulguration with Bladder Neck Incision. J Indian Assoc Pediatr Surg. 2019;24(1):31–5.
29. Abdelhalim A, El-Hefnawy AS, Dawaba ME, Bazeed MA, Hafez AT. Effect of Early Oxybutynin Treatment on Posterior Urethral Valve Outcomes in Infants: A Randomized Controlled Trial. J Urol. 2020 Apr;203(4):826–31.
30. Koff SA, Mutabagani KH, Jayanthi VR. The valve bladder syndrome: pathophysiology and treatment with nocturnal bladder emptying. J Urol. 2002 Jan;167(1):291–7.
31. Sultan S, Hussain I, Ahmed B, Aba Umer S, Saulat S, Naqvi SAA, *et al.* Clean intermittent catheterization in children through a continent catheterizable channel: a developing country experience. J Urol. 2008 Oct;180(4 Suppl):1852–5; discussion 1855.
32. Sarhan OM, El-Ghoneimi AA, Helmy TE, Dawaba MS, Ghali AM, Ibrahiem EHI. Posterior urethral valves: multivariate analysis of factors affecting the final renal outcome. J Urol. 2011 Jun;185(6 Suppl):2491–5.
33. Hebenstreit D, Csaicsich D, Hebenstreit K, Müller-Sacherer T, Berlakovich G, Springer A. Long-term outcome of pediatric renal transplantation in boys with posterior urethral valves. J Pediatr Surg. 2018 Nov;53(11):2256–60.
34. Salomon L, Fontaine E, Gagnadoux MF, Broyer M, Beurton D. Posterior urethral valves: long-term renal function consequences after transplantation. J Urol. 1997 Mar; 157(3):992–5.

Chapter 3

Valve Bladder Syndrome

• *Hemant Pathak* • *Sandesh Parab*

LEARNING OBJECTIVES

- Etiopathogenesis and evolution of valve bladder syndrome.
- Presentation—history and examination.
- Diagnosis and evaluation.
- Management.
- Follow-up.

INTRODUCTION

Posterior urethral valves (PUV) are the most common cause of bladder outlet obstruction (BOO) in male infants (93%), occurring in 2.6 per 10,000 live births.[1] Presentation is often identified antenatally (35%) with evidence of a key-hole sign, bladder distension, associated bilateral hydroureteronephrosis and possible oligohydramnios on ultrasound.[1,2]

Valve bladder syndrome (VBS) was first described by Mitchell. It defines the pathophysiological bladder changes, which occur after valve ablation in boys with PUV.

It should be suspected in boys with history of PUV with a presentation of urinary incontinence with or without elevated postvoid urine residual volumes and persistent hydroureteronephrosis after adequate valve ablation.[3] Evaluation of voiding dysfunction and polyuria starts with a voiding diary and uroflowmetry to assess incontinence, bladder functional capacity, and voiding habits. For further evaluation, videourodynamics (VUDS) is the best imaging study to evaluate bladder filling pressures and voiding dynamics.[3,4]

With this background, we will discuss a case of a child who had undergone PUV fulguration and now presented with dribbling and raised creatinine.

Case Scenario

A 2½-year-old child presented with dribbling and serum creatinine of 1.2 mg%. He had undergone PUV fulguration at 1.5 years of age. The mother gave the history that he was passing urine with a good stream but had recent onset dribbling and would wet his underpants. He has been on regular follow-up.

1. What aspects of symptomatology should be covered in such cases?

Ans:

- Urine flow, urgency, daytime incontinence, bedwetting, breakthrough infections.
- At what age PUV fulguration was done, complains at that time, baseline creatinine at that time?
- Antenatally detected hydronephrosis.
- Overall development and milestones of the child.

2. What examination findings would you like to note in this child?

Ans:

- P/A examination to look for palpable bladder or tenderness.
- External genitalia to look for circumcision status.

3. How will you investigate this child?

Ans:

Baseline investigations to be done are:

- Complete blood count which were—Hb:10.5, WBC: 10,500, platelets: 2.2 lacs
- Serum creatinine: 1.2 mg/dl
- Urine R/M: Normal
- Sonography of KUB region with PVR.
- Uroflowmetry

Ultrasonography images of this patient showed these findings (Fig. 3.1)**:**

- There was bilateral hydronephrosis with calyceal dilatation
- Bladder is thick walled with irregular walls suggestive of pseudo-diverticula. The posterior urethra is dilated—'key hole' sign.
- Post-void residue is 35 cc

Visual uroflow was very good and child would not void on command in urodynamic lab.

4. Any further investigations would you like to suggest?

Ans: Micturating cystourethrogram (MCU) or voiding cystourethrogram (VCUG) should be performed in patients suspected to have PU valves (Fig. 3.2).

This patient's recent VCUG films showed trabeculated bladder with multiple diverticula and dilated posterior urethra. There is no post-void residual on VCUG. There is no VUR.

5. What is posterior urethra: anterior urethra ratio on VCUG and what is its role?

Ans:

Posterior urethra: anterior urethra ratio (PAR) is computed by dividing maximum posterior urethral diameter by anterior urethral diameter. Distances should be measured by an on-screen distance measurement tool and should be done in well-exposed oblique films where posterior and anterior urethra are well delineated.

Improvement in PAR on repeat VCUG after 3 months of PUV fulguration may be associated with successful fulguration and in these patients repeat cystoscopy can be avoided.[5] A urethral ratio less than a range of 2.2–3.5 has been shown to be a beneficial predictor of ablation success.

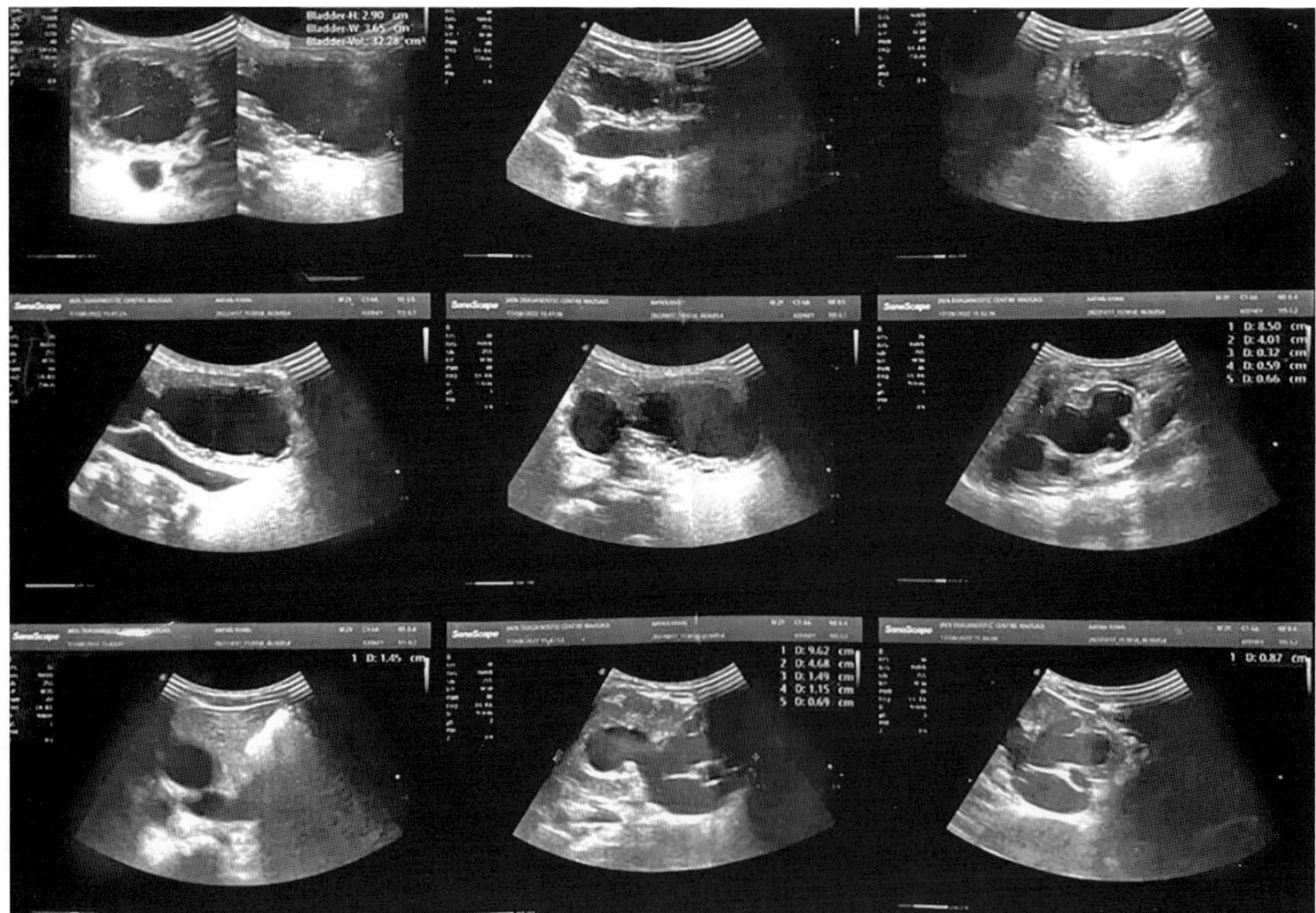

Fig. 3.1: Ultrasonography images

Section 2

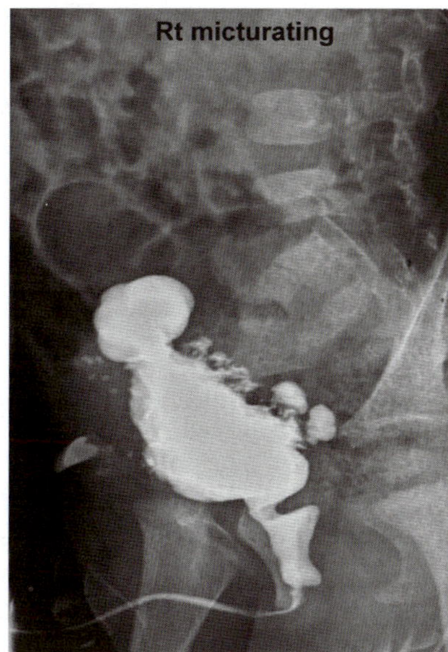

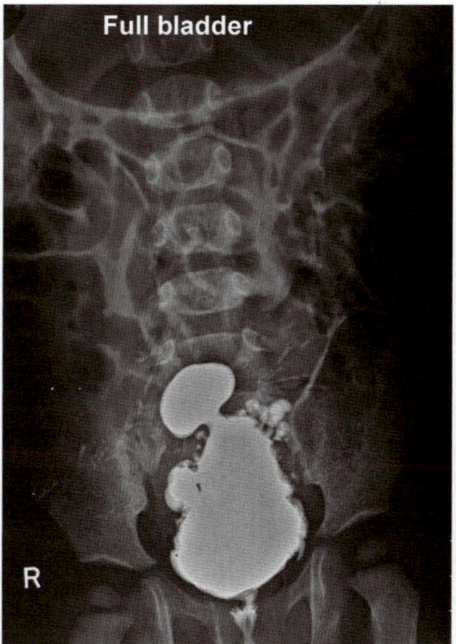

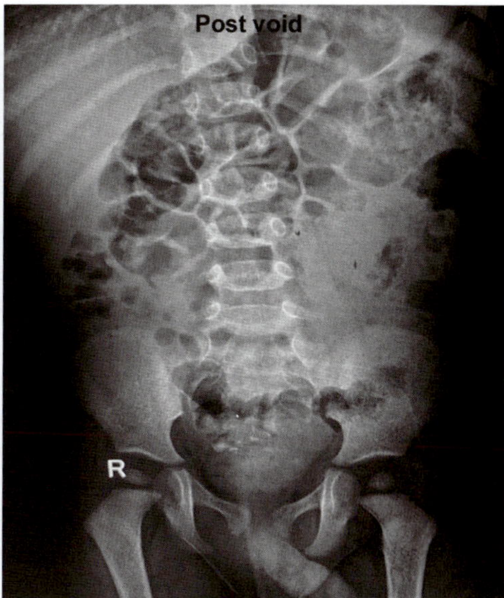

Fig. 3.2: Micturating cystourethrogram

6. **Would you like to do urodynamic study in this patient?**

   Ans: Urodynamic study is integral part of the evaluation of this patient. The fact that there is recent change in the voiding pattern of the child along with the VCUG showing irregular bladder suggests that there is a strong possibility of voiding dysfunction (Fig. 3.3).

7. **How will you describe this UDS?**

   Ans:

   - As the filling began, there was immediate rise in the detrusor pressures to 20 cm of H_2O.
   - During the filling phase, there is rise in detrusor pressure. Pdet going till 60 cm of H_2O with intermittent leak.
   - Bladder is poorly compliant. Maximum cystometric capacity could not be commented because of intermittent leak.

8. **What difficulties you may come across while performing UDS in pediatric age group and how should those be tackled?**

   Ans: It is difficult to carry urodynamics study in pediatric age group especially in a child less than 5 years. Various common technical difficulties faced are:

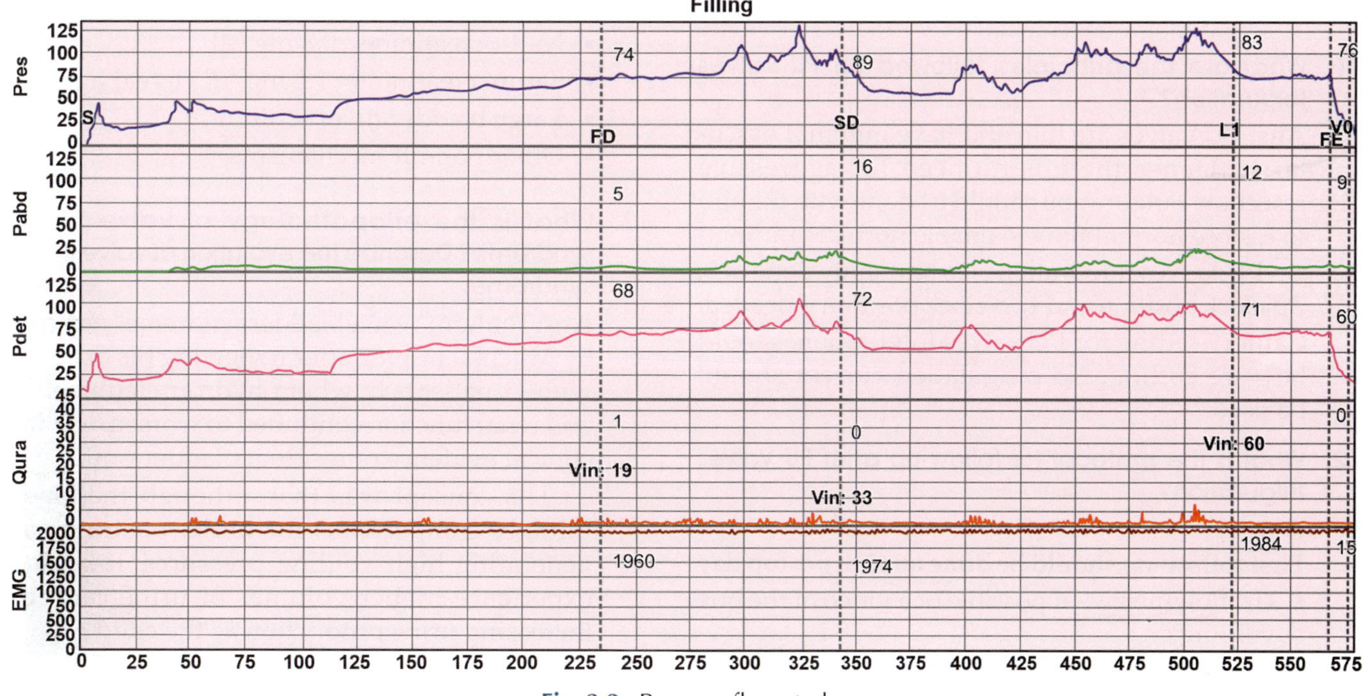

Fig. 3.3: Pressure flow study

- Difficulty in accommodating two catheters in urethra—this problem can be solved by using smaller diameter catheters or inserting 4 Fr double lumen catheter for filling and cystometry phase.
- Many times, an anxious child may not allow to conduct UDS; in such a scenario, videos and television are acceptable distraction techniques. If child is not co-operative, UDS can also be done under mild sedation.
- It is difficult to distinguish between sensations of normal urge, strong desire and pain in children while doing UDS as they are too young to describe what they are feeling. Crying during procedure can erroneously increase abdominal pressure, hence signs such as curling of the toes and tightening of the abdomen, can be helpful to know about urge and desire to void in children.

9. What further investigations to be done for evaluation of PU valves patient?

Ans: DTPA/EC scan or DMSA scan for quantification of renal function.

10. What is the clinical presentation in such cases?

Ans: Clinical presentation may vary as per severity of urinary obstruction.

If child presents at young age, then patient's parents usually complain about child's poor urinary stream and sometimes dribbling of urine. The affected patients may also present with urinary tract infections, sepsis, impaired renal function, anaemia, and failure to thrive.

In the older age group, patient may present with urinary incontinence.

11. What are the principles followed for PU valves fulguration?

Ans: PU valves are thin and have minimal vascularity. Hence there is no need for aggressive resection. Fulguration should be done with the aim to restore normal flow to enable normal voiding.

PU Valves fulguration is to be mainly done at 5, 7 o'clock position and 12 o'clock position if needed. Cautery setting for PU valves fulguration, should be pure cutting. No coagulation current should be used.[6]

12. What is the protocol for follow-up after PU Valves fulguration?

Ans:

First follow-up should be done on 15th postop day

- Uroflowmetry—if possible or a video of the boy voiding
- Check for any complaints
- Urine routine and microscopy
- Ultrasound for upper tracts and bladder

Second follow up to be planned at 3rd month

- Symptoms
- Uroflowmetry
- Urine routine and microscopy
- Ultrasound for upper tracts and bladder
- VCUG
- Some centres perform cystoscopy depending on their institutional protocol.

Lifelong follow-up to prevent valve bladder syndrome.

13. What are the long-term sequelae of PUV fulguration?

Ans: Valve bladder syndrome and end stage renal disease are the long-term sequelae of PUV fulguration.

14. What should be the aim of treatment for this patient?

Ans: Treatment should be aimed at preservation of bladder function by maintaining low bladder pressures. If bladder function is preserved, it can prevent damage to upper tracts.

15. How should be the line of treatment for this child?

Ans: Currently the child should be started on oxybutynin on 2.5 mg BD and dose titration should be done depending on the response. Dose will be escalated to 5 mg later if needed.

Option of Botox injection 100 units also can be considered.

16. What are the factors for assessment of prognosis?

Ans: Good prognostic factors are:

- Nadir creatinine< 0.8 mg/dl
- Serum creatinine< 1.2 mg/dl (1 year age)
- Large bladder diverticulum
- Other pop-off mechanisms[7,8]

17. What is the etiopathology of valve bladder syndrome? Describe the evolution of valve bladder syndrome.

Ans: The term "valve bladder syndrome" was coined by Mitchell in 1982 after reviewing his experience with 11 patients in whom hydroureteronephrosis and renal function continued to worsen despite no clinical evidence of residual bladder outlet.

His concept was that although the bladder initially compensates for outlet obstruction by generating high voiding pressures, it begins to experience higher volumes of urine caused by increasing urine production as the child grows.

The polyuria caused by nephrogenic diabetes insipidus secondary to evolving renal impairment augments the urine volumes entering a bladder that is increasingly unable to empty completely.

As the postvoid residue increases, the bladder no longer enjoys periods of complete relaxation, and the detrusor fibers are continuously in a state of partial or complete stretch, beginning a cascade of genotypic and phenotypic changes that further impair contractility of the bladder.[9]

When the bladder does empty partially, the urine already stored in the hydronephrotic kidneys quickly empties into the bladder, once again denying the detrusor muscle periods of relaxation.

The impaired contractility and increasing PVRs then transmit the increasing bladder pressures to the kidneys, potentially worsening the already impaired renal function.

There are three processes that contribute toward the devolution of a bladder into a valve bladder:

1. Polyuria;
2. Bladder insensitivity; and
3. Residual urine volume.[10]

These three factors—all secondary to the original insult of impaired bladder compliance creating high wall tension caused by increases in collagen and matrix-conspire to sustain bladder overdistension that ultimately leads to the valve bladder.

There is collagen deposition in the muscular wall of the ureter as well which hampers the peristalsis. Upper tracts and bladder pressures equalise, normal falling pressure gradient from renal pelvis to bladder is lost.

- The bladder in boys with PUV undergoes a phase of initial hypertrophy, a subsequent compensation phase, and a later decompensation phase.
- During the hypertrophy stage, mechanical stress results in smooth muscle hypertrophy and hyperplasia and deposition of extracellular matrix, causing focal areas of hypoxia.
- Angiogenesis is initially able to compensate for detrusor hypertrophy during the compensation phase, but eventually reaches a limit.
- Additional mechanisms by which persistently elevated residual bladder volumes occur are through pseudo-residual (mediated by unilateral or bilateral vesicoureteral reflux), and pseudo-pseudo-residual urine (functional ureterovesical junction obstruction during filling secondary to poor bladder compliance).[10]
- By puberty, boys with VBS can develop myogenic failure: Hypercompliant bladders without the ability to sustain an effective emptying detrusor contraction.
- The process by which myogenic failure develops has been described by Fusco *et al*—result of cyclical ischemia–reperfusion injury during the micturition phase and is associated with urothelial dysfunction, neuronal and smooth muscle degeneration, and high levels of extracellular matrix deposition.[11]
- The development of VBS is influenced by the severity of the PUV (degree of residual bladder outlet obstruction), timing of diagnosis, and initial interventions, which are dictated by the severity of the valves.
- Antenatal diagnosis is associated with greater renal dysfunction and renal dysplasia and potentially a greater likelihood of VBS.

18. How will you manage valve bladder syndrome?

Ans:

1. Behavioural therapy and catheterization
2. Medications
3. Surgical options
4. Experimental therapy

1. Behavioural therapy and catheterization

- Behavioural management options to minimize overdistension include timed and frequent voiding, as well as double voiding.
- For patients who are unable to empty their bladders secondary to poor sensation or voiding dysfunction, clean intermittent catheterization (CIC) may be recommended.
- Nocturnal bladder drainage is instituted if ureteral dilation and hydronephrosis does not respond to behavioural modification or an affected child develops worsening renal function or recurrent urinary tract infections.
- The continuous bladder drainage, achieved by leaving a urinary catheter in the bladder over a 7-to 10-hour period, allows an extended period of bladder decompression.
- This simple step interrupts the "vicious cycle" of bladder remodeling and consequent renal effects caused by chronic bladder distension.
- Patients with sensate urethra and major compliance issue, Mitrofanoff procedure may be needed.[12]

2. Medical

- The primary role of anticholinergics in VBS is to improve bladder compliance and reduce detrusor overactivity during filling. Use of anticholinergics may decrease the risk of myogenic failure by reducing smooth muscle cell hypertrophy and hyperplasia that occurs during bladder wall remodelling in the hypertrophy phase.[13,14]

- Alpha-adrenergic blockade has been used to relieve secondary bladder neck obstruction due to sphincteric hypertonicity. Tamsulosin and terazosin have been used.[15,16]
- Botox-single dose of 100 units of botulinum toxin into the hypertrophied bladder neck at 3, 6, and 9 o'clock can be tried.[17]

3. **Surgical**
   - Bladder neck incision (BNI) with valve ablation (VA)—there are mixed opinions as it may be associated with incontinence or dry ejaculation.
   - BNI did not show any improvements in renal function, urodynamic, or upper urinary tract outcomes.[18]
   - Bladder augmentation using intestinal segments or dilated ureter may be considered for patients with poorly compliant bladders to reduce bladder filling pressures in boys with PUV and significant VBS.[19]

Transplants in patients with VBS

- There is significantly higher complication rate and graft loss in boys in whom bladder dysfunction is incompletely managed or bladder reservoir is not optimized.
- Videourodynamics should be obtained for transplant candidates to determine the safe storage pressures and contractile function of the future reservoir.
- Overnight bladder drainage or CIC may be initiated before transplant to optimize the reservoir and establish proper bladder management skills that will be essential for graft success after transplant.

4. **Experimental therapy**
   - Mesenchymal stem cells may have potential therapeutic implications in the management and prevention of myogenic failure in VBS.[20]
   - Sodium tanshinone IIA sulfonate, derived from the Chinese herb *Salvia miltiorrhiza* has been used to assess whether bladder fibrosis secondary to obstruction can be reduced by inhibiting growth factor signaling pathway activation in rats.[21]
   - 17-DMAG, a hypoxia inducible factor (HIF) inhibitor, prevents the development of detrusor overactivity and improves the urodynamic parameters in mice with obstructed bladders.[22]
   - Oxybutynin and Tadalafil administration resulted in significant improvements in bladder capacity and compliance, and less detrusor hyperactivity.
   - Oral Losartan (ARB) (angiotensin II type 1 receptor antagonist) partially prevented the urodynamic and structural changes that occur with BOO in a mouse model.[23]
   - These experimental treatments represent potential therapeutic options to prevent and manage the development of VBS in boys with PUV.

SUMMARY

- In unobstructed animal models, the compliance improves with gestational age in which type I collagen increases (good collagen).
- In paediatric patients with anatomic and functional obstruction, type III collagen (bad collagen) infiltrates the detrusor muscle and hampers the compliance.
- Underlying primary renal dysplasia in utero cannot be altered by postnatal interventions, although bladder function can be preserved, thereby avoiding cascading effects of VBS.
- Bladder dysfunction, even when not detected on clinical history alone, must always be suspected in children with a history of valve ablation.
- Active, appropriate intervention to effectively drain the overdistended bladder could alter the course toward decompensation and preserve bladder functionality.
- Reliance on clinical examination or patient questionnaires alone may grossly underestimate bladder dysfunction, and obtaining a uroflow, checking PVRs, UDS,MCU and electrolyte evaluations should be a routine part of follow-up in toilet-trained children with a history of PUVs.
- Behavioural, medical, surgical options to be utilised as appropriate.

REFERENCES

1. Brownlee E, Wragg R, Robb A, Chandran H, Knight M, McCarthy L, *et al.* Current epidemiology and antenatal presentation of posterior urethral valves: outcome of BAPS CASS National Audit. J Pediatr Surg. 2019;54:318–21.
2. Robyr R, Benachi A, Daikha-Dahmane F, Martinovich J, Dumez Y, Ville Y. Correlation between ultrasound and anatomical findings in fetuses with lower urinary tract obstruction in the first half of pregnancy. Ultrasound Obstet Gynecol. 2005;25:478–82.
3. Glassberg KI, Combs A. The valve bladder syndrome: 35+ years later. J Urol. 2016;196:16–7.
4. Riah L, Belhaj K, Lmidmani F, el Fatimi A, el Kettani Y, el Ayoubi M, *et al.* Urodynamic profile of voiding disorders persisting after treatment of posterior urethral valve. Prog Urol. 2015;25:217–23.
5. Babu R, Hariharasudhan S, Ramesh C. Posterior urethra: Anterior urethra ratio in the evaluation of success following PUV ablation. Journal of Pediatric Urology. 2016 Dec 1;12(6):385-e1.
6. Sarhan O, El-Ghoneimi A, Hafez A, Dawaba M, Ghali A, Ibrahiem el-H. Surgical complications of posterior urethral valve ablation: 20 years experience. J Pediatr Surg. 2010 Nov;45(11):2222–6.

7. Drozdz D, Drozdz M, Gretz N, Möhring K, Mehls O, Schärer K. Progression to end-stage renal disease in children with posterior urethral valves. Pediatr Nephrol. 1998 Oct;12(8): 630–6
8. DeFoor W, Clark C, Jackson E, *et al.* Risk factors for end stage renal disease in children with posterior urethral valves, J Urol 180(4 Suppl):1705–1708, discussion 1708, 2008.
9. Kirsch AJ, Macarak EJ, Chaqour B, *et al.* Molecular response of the bladder to obstruction, Adv Exp Med Biol 539(Pt A):195–216, 2003.
10. Koff SA, Mutabagani KH, Jayanthi VR: The valve bladder syndrome: pathophysiology and treatment with nocturnal bladder emptying, J Urol 167(1):291–297, 2002.
11. Fusco F, Creta M, De Nunzio C, *et al.* Progressive bladder remodeling due to bladder outlet obstruction: a systematic review of morphological and molecular evidences in humans. BMC Urol. 2018;18:15.
12. McLeod DJ, Szymanski KM, Gong E, Granberg C, Reddy P, Sebastião Y, *et al.* Pediatric Urology Midwest Alliance (PUMA). Renal Replacement Therapy and Intermittent Catheterization Risk in Posterior Urethral Valves. Pediatrics. 2019 Mar;143(3):e20182656.
13. Lopez Pereira P, Martinez Urrutia MJ, Espinosa L, Lobato R, Navarro M, Jaureguizar E. Bladder dysfunction as a prognostic factor in patients with posterior urethral valves. BJU Int. 2002;90: 308–11.
14. Glassberg KI, Combs A. The valve bladder syndrome: 35+ years later. J Urol. 2016;196:16–7.
15. Abraham MK, Nasir ARA, Sudarsanan B, Puzhankara R, Kedari PM, Unnithan GR, *et al.* Role of alpha adrenergic blocker in the management of posterior urethral valves. Pediatr Surg Int. 2009;25: 1113–5.
16. Skenazy J, Horowitz M. Alpha adrenergic blockade in neonates with posterior urethral valves. J Urol. 1618;187.
17. Mokhless I, Zahran AR, Saad A, Yehia M, Youssif ME. Effect of Botox injection at the bladder neck in boys with bladder dysfunction after valve ablation. J Pediatr Urol. 2014;10:899–904.
18. Sarin YK, Sinha S. Efficacy of bladder neck incision on urodynamic abnormalities in patients with posterior urethral valves. Pediatr Surg Int. 2013;29:387–92.
19. Lopez Pereira P, Martinez Urrutia MJ, Espinosa L, Jaureguizar E. Long-term consequences of posterior urethral valves. J Pediatr Urol. 2013;9:590–6.
20. Wiafe B, Adesida AB, Churchill T, *et al.* Mesenchymal stem cell therapy inhibited inflammatory and profibrotic pathways induced Curr Bladder Dysfunct Rep by partial bladder outlet obstruction and prevented high-pressure urine storage. J Pediatr Urol. 2019;15:254.e1–254.e10.
21. Jiang X, Chen Y, Zhu H, *et al.* Sodium tanshinone IIA sulfonate ameliorates bladder fibrosis in a rat model of partial bladder outlet obstruction by inhibiting the TGF-β/Smad pathway activation. PLoS One. 2015;10:e0129655.
22. Iguchi N, Dönmez M , Malykhina AP, Carrasco A Jr, Wilcox DT. Preventative effects of a HIF inhibitor, 17-DMAG, on partial bladder outlet obstruction-induced bladder dysfunction. Am J Physiol Ren Physiol. 2017;313:F1149–60.
23. Comiter C, Phull HS. Angiotensin II type 1 (AT-1) receptor inhibition partially prevents the urodynamic and detrusor changes associated with bladder outlet obstruction: a mouse model. BJU Int. 2012;109:1841–6.

Chapter

4

Ectopic Ureter

• *Venkatesh Krishnamoorthy*

LEARNING OBJECTIVES

- Incidence of ectopic ureters, associated anatomy of the upper tract, and location of the ectopia.
- Differences in clinical presentation in male and female children.
- Differential diagnosis, and evaluation.
- Management planning based on anatomy, renal function, and clinical presentation.

INTRODUCTION

An ectopic ureter is defined as a ureteric opening anywhere, except into the trigone of the urinary bladder.

In males, the ectopic opening can be in the following locations:

- Bladder neck
- Prostatic urethra
- Vas deferens or
- Seminal vesicles and ejaculatory duct

In females, the ectopic opening may be in the following locations[1]

- Bladder neck
- Urethra
- Gartner's duct
- Vaginal vestibule and uterus
- Rectum

In males, the ectopic ureter opening is superior to the external sphincter, and therefore does not cause urinary incontinence, but may present as urinary infection and pain. In females the opening in the Gartner's duct and vaginal vestibule may present with persistent incontinence.[2]

To explain this embryologically, this ectopic location results from the ureter not being incorporated into the posterior part of the urinary bladder. It gets carried caudally with the mesonephric duct and gets incorporated into the caudal portion of the urogenital sinus. This part becomes a prostatic urethra in males, and vagina in females, and therefore explains the typical location of the ectopic openings, and their clinical presentations.

In autopsy studies, the incidence of ectopic ureters is approximately 1 in 2000. The actual incidence is difficult to determine, as many remain asymptomatic.[3] In females, the incidence is 2–3 times more common than in males.[4,5] In females, more than 80% of ectopic ureters have duplex systems while in males, about 75% have single systems.[6,7] Overall, 70–80% of ectopic ureters are associated with complete duplication. In such cases, it is the upper moiety ureter that becomes ectopic (Weigert Meyer Rule). Nearly 20% of patients with ectopic ureters, have bilateral involvement.[4]

In males, the posterior urethra is the commonest site of drainage (57%). The seminal vesicle is involved in about 33%. Ectopic opening into the ejaculatory duct, and vas are rare (10%). In females, the commonest site of drainage (69%) is the urethra and vestibule. Vaginal ectopic openings occur in about 25%. Opening into the rectum is very rare.[4]

Case Scenario

A 5-year-old girl presented with a history of urinary frequency both day and night, and continuous small amount of urinary incontinence. She also voids separately normally, and wears diapers for the leak.

There is no history of urinary tract infection.

At age 3, she had undergone corrective surgery for a patent ductus arteriosus.

Physical examination revealed wetness in the genital area. No obvious site of urine leak could be identified.

(Contd.)

(Contd.)

Her blood and urine tests were normal. Urine culture was sterile.

An ultrasound study reported left duplex kidney, with dilated upper moiety. There was a dilated tubular structure, probably the lower ureter, near the left pelvic adnexa. The bladder was reported to be normal. There was no post-void residual urine (Fig. 4.1A to 4.1C).

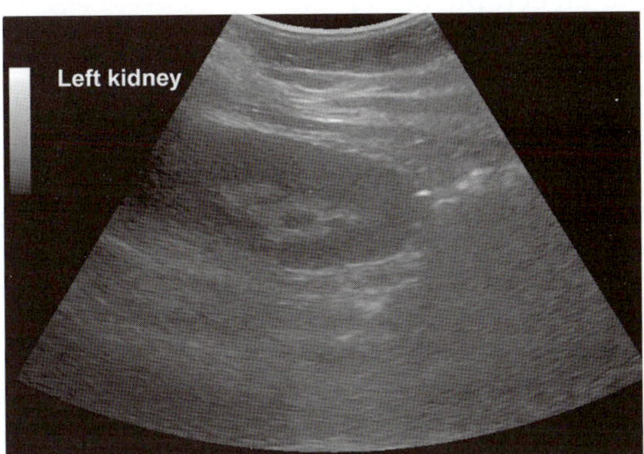

Fig. 4.1A: Left kidney

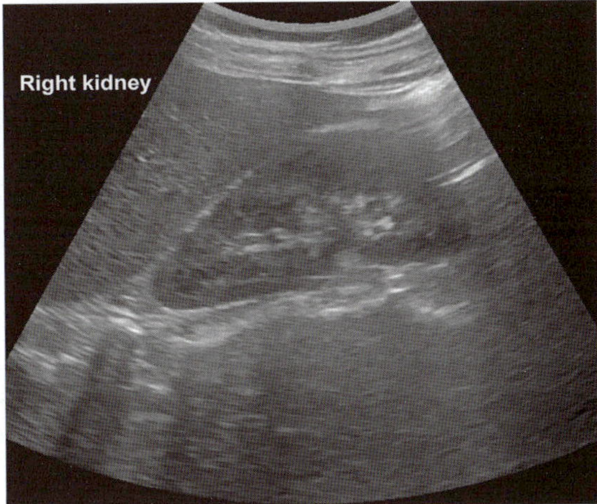

Fig. 4.1B: Right kidney

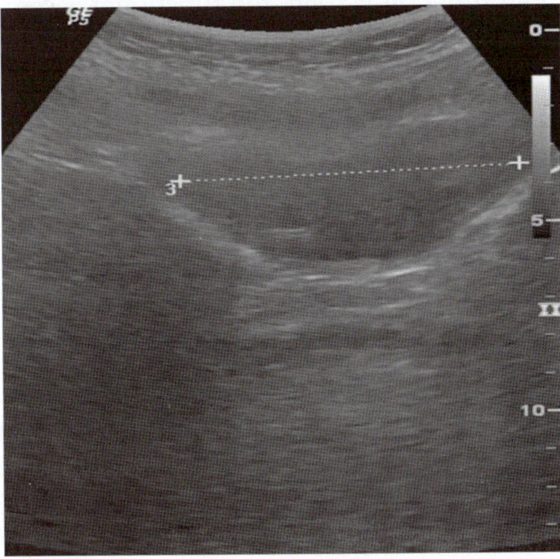

Fig. 4.1C: Bladder

A DMSA scan reported the left kidney to be contributing only 31% of the total function, of which the upper moiety was contributing 13%.

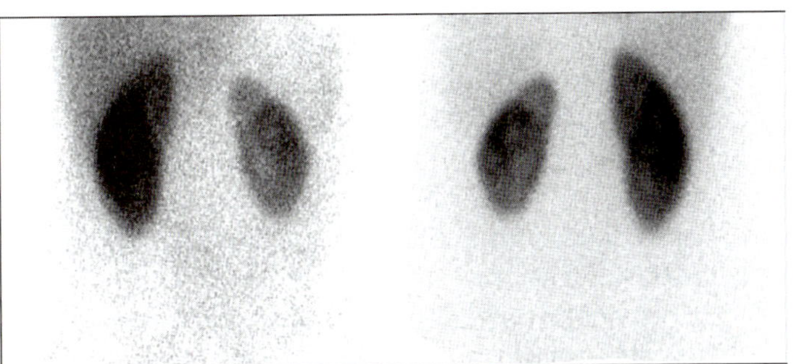

IMPRESSION

Well-perfused and normal functioning right kidney. No evidence of pyelonephritic foci/scarring in the right kidney.

Left kidney (duplex moiety): Small-sized kidney.

Small sized upper moiety. Generalized reduced tracer uptake in this moiety. No obvious focal scars on this side. (upper moiety contributes to 13% of left kidney function)

Lower moiety is perfused and shows preserved functional parenchaymal volume. No evidence of pyelonephritic foci/scarring in the lower moiety.

	Left	Right
Relative Function:	31%	69%

Examination under anesthesia revealed vaginal pooling of urine. However, no ectopic ureteric orifice could be identified. Urethroscopy revealed an ectopic ureteric opening about 1 cm distal to the bladder neck. The bladder neck was normal. The other left ureteric orifice was close to the bladder neck. A ureteric catheter was passed over a guidewire into the upper moiety. A stent was placed in the lower moiety ureter (Fig. 4.2).

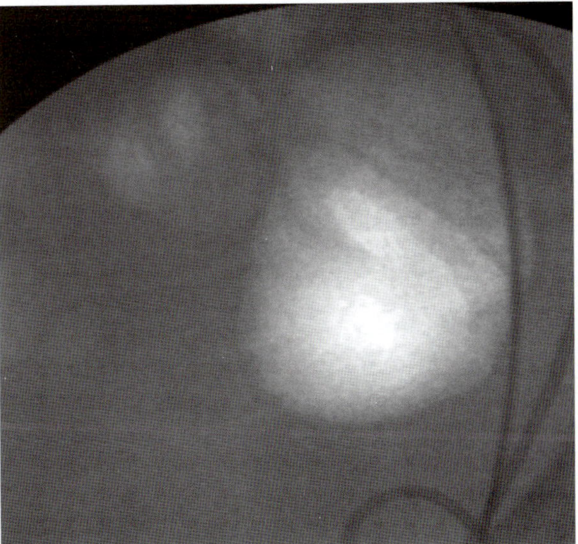

Fig. 4.2: C arm image of stent placed in lower moiety

Exploration of the left kidney revealed a thick and dilated upper moiety, pelvis, and ureter. The lower moiety ureter was normal in calibre. There was thick, healthy parenchyma in the upper moiety also. An ipsilateral end-to-side ureteroureterostomy was done about 5 cm below the PUJ. The distal part of the upper moiety ureter was left open.

She has recovered well.

1. **What is the clinical presentation of ectopic ureters?**

   Ans: Antenatal detection: Is by identification of hydronephrosis. This leads to repeat postnatal imaging, and better characterization of the condition. In the absence of dilatation, the prenatal identification of an ectopic ureter, or a duplex system is difficult.

   Postnatal detection: In the absence of symptoms, it is an incidental finding of hydronephrosis/hydroureteronephrosis, when evaluation is done for some other abdominal symptom.

   Urine infection remains a significant and important reason for clinical presentation of ectopic ureters. An ultrasound study will then help identify the abnormality.

   Urinary incontinence is the usual presentation in girls. Commonly there is a low-volume dampness in the diapers, associated with normal voiding at other times. However, this is usually identifiable and confirmatory, only after toilet training is complete.

   Pain is generally not an associated symptom of an ectopic ureter. If present, it is usually associated to acute infection or pain of the affected organs (testicles and epididymis).

2. **What do you look for in the physical examination?**

   Ans: Genital examination generally does not yield results, other than confirming dampness or urine leak. Even for openings outside of the urethra it may be difficult to detect. The examination, however, must include looking for palpable kidneys. The differential diagnosis invariably is that of an ureterocele, or urinary fistula.

3. **What imaging studies are necessary for planning management?**

   Ans:

   Ultrasonography

   Ultrasound imaging helps differentiate between single system and duplex moieties; it also helps in differentiating between an ureterocele, and a plain ectopic ureter, during bladder imaging. The study may not be able to give information on the location of the ectopic orifice. A suggestion of such an entity is possible because the ureter can be seen coursing well beyond the bladder walls. Sometimes, a grossly dilated ectopic ureter may impinge on the bladder, and appear as an intravesical structure—"pseudoureterocele".[8] It is important to distinguish between a ureterocele and a pseudoureterocele. The wall of the pseudoureterocele is bilaminar, irregular and much thicker (range from 2 to >5 mm) than the wall of a typical ureterocele.[9]

   Voiding cystourethrogram (VCUG)

   This gives a definitive evaluation of the lower urinary tract. It provides recognition of VUR as the cause of a dilated ureter, as well as provides definitive differentiation between an ureterocele and an ectopic ureter.

   Magnetic resonance imaging (MRI)

   While this provides the most detailed images of the entire urinary tract, in young children it requires sedation, and typically does not add any vital information. It is generally reserved for patients with complex anatomy, that cannot be defined by simpler imaging methods.

   Functional assessment

   Functional assessment of renal function forms the foundation in the management algorithm, for renal preservation versus excision of the affected moiety/kidney. While a good ultrasound imaging of renal parenchymal thickness can suggest poor function or adequate function of the moiety, nuclear imaging with dimercaptosuccinic acid (DMSA) remains the gold standard for renal functional assessment. While there is no definition of what normal function of an affected moiety should be, it is very helpful when the decision is between 'no function', and 'some function'.

   Intravenous urogram (IVU)

   It was the mainstay for evaluation in earlier days, with classic descriptions such as the 'drooping lily, missing calyx, lateralisation of the lower moiety ureter' and so on. However, now it is not used often, because of radiation concerns, and as it offers no details on a poorly functioning moiety. Even when function is seen, the functional assessment is only qualitative, and therefore, the IVU is a less useful baseline study.

   Endoscopic evaluation

   The final step of the evaluation will be an endoscopic study of the lower urinary tract. It can be done separately or at the same time as definitive surgical intervention. During the urethrocystoscopy, a detailed study should be made of the character of the urethra, the bladder neck, and the trigone. The location of the orthotopic ureteric orifices should be noted. The orifice of the ectopic ureter should be looked for but may not be identified. An ectopic orifice at the bladder neck level is often patulous.

   Locating the opening of an ectopic ureter can be challenging. While there are several tips and techniques described, that can assist in identifying the ectopic opening, these vary depending on the specific case and the patient's individual characteristics. Some general guidelines to consider are as follows:

- Get a detailed history, especially symptoms related to urinary incontinence. The areas to search for narrow down to the vestibules, to the vagina, and in the distal urethra. Look for urine pooling or dampness in the vaginal area or external urethral meatus, which may provide clues to the location. Oral pyridium has been described to look for urine staining in the ectopic ureter with incontinence. The utility of this test is directly proportional to the degree of function in that kidney/moiety, and the volume of the urine leak.
- Injection of methylene blue into a dilated moiety, and looking for its efflux either by visual examination or endoscopy can be of help. For endoscopy, utilise a scope which permits good visualisation of the entire circumference of the urethra. A neonatal scope is ideal, even for the older child. The urethra must distend well with irrigant fluid, to permit examination of all the walls. Locating the ectopic orifice is less important in an obstructed system, than in a refluxing system.

4. What are the options in clinical management?

Ans: Ectopic ureters are managed surgically in nearly all patients, especially if associated with symptoms. Observational treatment has been reported for asymptomatic patients.

The goals of therapy are as follows:

- Preservation of renal function
- Elimination of urinary incontinence
- Elimination of infection, obstruction, and reflux

There is no role for fetal management in the ectopic ureter.

Neonatal management

Most ectopic ureters do not need any urgent management in the neonatal period. At most, in the presence of infection, antibiotic prophylaxis can be considered. In the event of significant hydronephrosis with obstruction, a renal function study can be obtained after the age two months.

Urgent management is indicated only in the presence of sepsis due to urinary infection, and is best managed with a temporary end-ureterostomy/ endoscopic ureteral meatal incision/stenting/ nephrostomy, in addition to antibiotics.[10]

Early decompression of infected urine permits good recovery of function in the renal unit, before definitive management. Percutaneous drainage has also been reported to be effective.[11]

5. What is the basis for definitive management of an ectopic ureter?

Ans: Decision making for definitive management of ectopic ureter is very straightforward. It will depend on the answers to the following questions:

1. Is the affected ureter single or a portion of a duplex system?
2. Is the affected ureter obstructed or refluxing?
3. Is the other ipsilateral ureter affected by the primary anomaly?
4. What is the functional status of the contralateral kidney and ureter?

6. What is the functional status of the kidney or portion of the kidney associated with the ectopic ureter?

Ans: Nearly 90% of kidneys that accompany single system ectopic ureters do not have any appreciable function. Nephrectomy is the treatment of choice. The commonly cited cut off limit of 10–15% function, has very little meaning, adding value, only in the presence of an impaired contralateral renal function.

In a duplex moiety, the presence of reflux in the lower pole matters.[12] If present, and the upper moiety function is good, a common sheath re-implantation is the best option. An alternative is reimplantation of the lower pole ureter with ipsilateral ureteroureterostomy (IUU).

If there is no lower pole reflux, proximal IUU is performed. Even if the degree of function is ambiguous or low, an upper ureteroureterostomy is a good option. Size mismatch between the two ureters does not seem to impede a satisfactory anastomosis.[13] A high anastomosis is preferable to a lower anastomosis, as there is a theoretical risk of yo-yo reflux in the lower anastomosis.

Upper pole nephrectomy for poorly functioning moieties, though not necessary, is the preferred treatment, but carries the risk of damage to the lower pole function[14–16] and vascularity of the lower moiety ureter. In 20% of patients an upper pole urinoma is reported after upper pole nephrectomy, which in most cases needs no intervention.[16–18]

If there is significant reflux, the distal ureter may also be excised, taking care not to damage the bladder neck.

SUMMARY

- An ureteric opening anywhere except into the trigone of the bladder, is termed an ectopic ureter.
- The incidence of ectopic ureter is 2–3 times more common in females.
- 70–80% of ectopic ureters are associated with complete duplication. In females the clinical presentation is commonly

of incontinence. In males it is of obstruction and/or urinary tract infection.

- It is difficult to identify an ectopic ureteric opening during physical examination, though an ultrasonography is a simple imaging method to identify duplex moieties and possible location of the ectopic ureter.
- Definitive management of the ectopic ureter is based on single or duplex systems and functional status of the affected moiety.

REFERENCES

1. Ghosh B, Shridhar K, Pal DK, *et al.* Ectopic ureter draining into the uterus. *Urol Ann.* 2016;8(1):105–107.
2. Williams DI. The ectopic ureter: diagnostic problems. Br J Urol. 1954;26(3):253–260).
3. Prewitt LH Jr., Lebowitz RL (1976) The single ectopic ureter. AJR Am J Roentgenol 127: 941–8
4. Ellerker AG (1958). The Extravesical Ectopic Ureter. Br J Surg 45: 344.
5. Malek R S, Kelalis PP, Stickler GP (Reza S. Malek, Panayotis P. Kelalis, Gunnar B. Stickler, and Edmund C. Burke) *et al.* (1972b) Observations on ureteral ectopy in children. J Urol 107:308.
6. Schulmann CC (1976) The single ectopic ureter. Eur Urol 2:64
7. Ahmed S, Barker A (Saeed Ahmed, Andrew Barker) (1992) Single-system ectopic ureters: a review of 12 cases. J pediatric Surg 27:491.
8. Sumfest JM, Burns MW, Mitchell ME. Pseudoureterocele: potential for misdiagnosis of an ectopic ureter as a ureterocele. Br J Urol. 1995;75(3):401–405.,
9. Lee MD, Lin CC, Chang BP, Lin PY, Tsai JD. Pseudoureterocele. Pediatr Neonatol. 2018;59:104–5. doi: 10.1016/j.pedneo.2017.09.002.)
10. Ortiz R, Parente A, Burgos L (Ruben Ortiz, Alberto Parente, Laura Burgos, and Jose Maria Angulo), *et al.* Endoscopic urinary diversion as initial management of symptomatic obstructive ectopic ureter in infants. Front Pediatr. 2017;5:208.
11. Bilen CY, Aygun C, Ozkaya O (Cenk Y Bilen, Canan Aygün, Ozan Ozkaya, O uz Aydin, Nevzat Gürmen, Saban Sarikaya), *et al.* Percutaneous ureterostomy as an effective diversion in a newborn. Int J Urol. 2006;13(5):622–624.
12. Michael A. Keating, A Barry Belman, Lowell R. King, Stephen A. Kramer, Clinical Pediatric Urology 4th edition page 703
13. el Ghoneimi A, Lottmann H, Odet E, Bonnin F, Aigrain Y. Ureteropyelostomy for obstructed duplicated ureter an easy and reliable operation in infants. Ann Urol (Paris). 1998;32(4):241–6.
14. Mandell J, Colodny AH, Lebowitz R (James Manbell, Arnold H. Colobny, Robert Lebowitz, Stuart B. Bauer, Alan B. Retik), *et al.* Ureteroceles in infants and children. J Urol. 1980;123(6):921–926.
15. Wallis MC, Khoury AE, Lorenzo AJ (M. Chad Wallis, Antoine E. Khoury, Armando J. Lorenzo, Joao L. Pippi-Salle, Darius J. Bägli, and Walid A. Farhat), *et al.* Outcome analysis of retroperitoneal laparoscopic heminephrectomy in children. J Urol. 2006;175(6):2277–2280 [discussion 2280–2272].
16. You D, Bang JK, Shim M (Dalsan You, Jeong Kyoon Bang, Myungsun Shim, Dong Soo Ryu, Kun Suk Kim), *et al.* Analysis of the late outcome of laparoscopic heminephrectomy in children with duplex kidneys. BJU Int. 2010.
17. Valla JS, Breaud J, Carfagna L (Jean-Stéphane Valla, Jean Breaud, Luanna Carfagna, Stefano Tursini, Henri Steyaert), *et al.* Treatment of ureterocele on duplex ureter: upper pole nephrectomy by retroperitoneoscopy in children based on a series of 24 cases. Eur Urol. 2003;43(4):426–429.
18. Mason MD, Anthony Herndon CD, Smith-Harrison LI (Matthew D Mason, C D Anthony Herndon, L I Smith-Harrison, Craig A Peters, Sean T Corbett), *et al.* Robotic-assisted partial nephrectomy in duplicated collecting systems in the Pediatric population: techniques and outcomes. J Pediatr Urol. 2014;10(2):374–379.

Ureterocele

• Prasanna Matippa

LEARNING OBJECTIVES

- Embryological background of the development of ureterocele.
- Use of correct imaging techniques in evaluation of ureterocele with functional renal studies.
- Appropriate management at various stages from fetal period through the childhood.
- Appropriate management protocols when dealing with ureterocele in the setting of sepsis or when dealt with electively.

INTRODUCTION

Identification and management of ureteroceles in very young children have always flummoxed physicians treating them, as they have such a varied presentation. Better understanding of the steps of evaluation and management of ureteroceles would definitely improve outcomes.

Case Scenario

On routine pre-natal ultrasound at eight months gestation, right urinary tract dilatation along with a cystic lesion in the bladder was detected. A follow-up ultrasound prior to delivery reported antero-posterior diameter (APD) of right renal pelvis measuring 1.4 cm with a suspicion of duplicated system and a ureterocele measuring 2.6 cm x 2 cm. The findings were persistent on a post-natal ultrasound reporting a tortuous dilated right ureter measuring 9.8 mm in diameter with normal parenchymal thickness and a 4 cm x 4 cm right ureterocele along with gross hydroureteronephrosis of upper pole and a minimal hydronephrosis of the lower pole. The child was started on continuous antibiotic prophylaxis (CAP) and advised follow-up.

There were recurrent episodes of breakthrough urinary tract infections, while on CAP with a follow-up ultrasound at 3 months reporting an infected ureterocele measuring 2.9 cm with debris in the dilated right ureter, with a significantly increased renal pelvis APD of 23 mm and parenchymal thickness of 4 mm. The patient had undergone a deroofing of the ureterocele elsewhere. Post-surgery, DTPA (Diethylenetriamine pentaacetate) scan revealed 32% split function on the right side (eGFR 12 ml/min). The child continued to have breakthrough UTIs even after deroofing of ureterocele. A repeat imaging with ultrasound revealed right upper pole renal pelvis APD measuring 2 cm, dilated proximal and distal ureter, and ureterocele measuring 2.5 cm × 2.5 cm × 1.6 cm at right vesico-ureteric junction (VUJ). DMSA (Dimercapto succinic acid) scan revealed right kidney split function of 45% (upper moiety function of 20.58% and lower moiety 79.1%). The function was falsely over-estimated by the nuclear scan due to background activity. A voiding cystourethrography (VCUG) was suggestive of large right ureterocele (as shown in Fig. 5.1). Cystoscopy revealed a large caeco-ureterocele at the bladder neck with ureteric orifice opening at the summit of the ureterocele. The other right ureteric orifice and left ureteric orifice were normal. A repeat ureterocele incision was then performed. The child was continued on CAP post-operatively. At 6 months follow-up, the child is voiding normally with no breakthrough UTIs.

1. **How do we define a ureterocele?**

   Ans: Ureterocele is a cystic dilatation that develops in the intravesical part of the submucosal ureter.[1] It may be associated with a single system, i.e. a kidney with one ureter or with a duplex system where the ureterocele invariably belongs to the upper moiety.

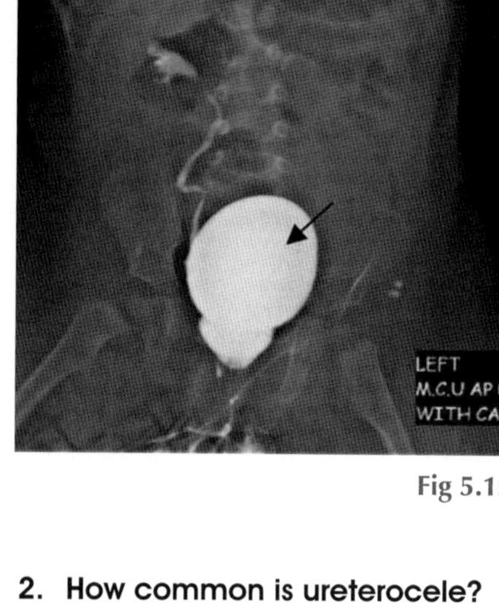

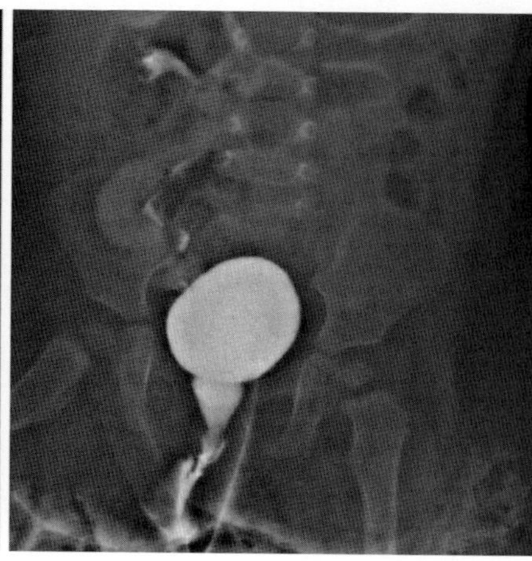
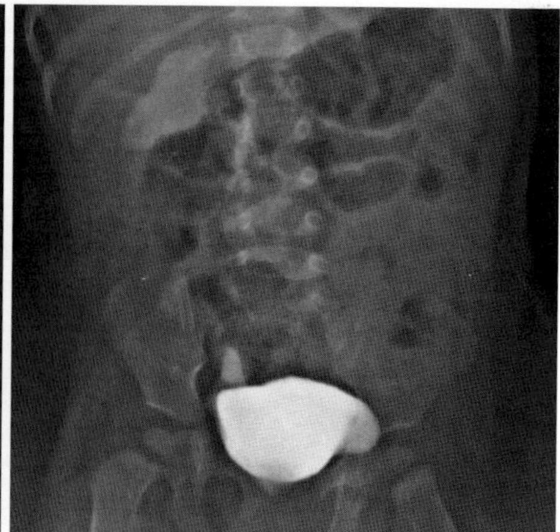

Fig 5.1: VCUG demonstrating a large right ureterocele (arrow)

2. **How common is ureterocele?**

Ans:

- Ureteroceles are known to occur in approximately 1 in 4000 children and are most common in Caucasians.[2]
- Ureteroceles are 4–6 times more common in females both in children and adult population.
- There is a slight predominance on the left side with bilateral incidence being reported in 10% of cases.
- An ectopic ureterocele has been reported to be four times more common than an intravesical ureterocele.
- 80% ureteroceles in infants are associated with the upper pole moiety of a duplex system and 60% of these have an ectopic location. The upper pole in these cases tends to be dysplastic or poorly functioning.
- Single-system ectopic ureteroceles are less common and are most often found in males.[3]
- Reflux into ureterocele is uncommon.[4]
- **Weigert-Meyer rule**. It describes the inverse relationship of the duplex ureteral orifices in which the ectopic ureter or ureterocele associated with the upper pole is caudal to the lower pole ureteral orifice.

3. **What is the embryological background in the development of the ureterocele?**

Ans: The classic explanation of ureterocele formation was described by Chwalle (1927) who described that distal ureteral expansion is produced by failure of rupture of a distal membrane at the ureteral orifice called the "Chwalle membrane".

During the ureteral bud formation, the caudal portion of the mesonephric duct becomes the common nephric duct (CND). Ureteral maturation begins with the most distal portion of CND merging with the urogenital sinus and undergoing apoptosis which occurs over several days. The ureter is initially occluded by cells that undergo apoptosis. These cells correspond to the Chwalle membrane. If the apoptosis is abnormal, this is thought to result in formation of the ureterocele.[5]

4. **What are the types of ureteroceles?**

Ans: The ureteroceles were first classified into either simple or ectopic depending on the location of the ureteric orifice by Ericsson in 1954.[6] Subsequently there were various classification systems described as:

- **American Academy of Paediatrics classification (most commonly used)**
  a. **Orthotopic (intravesical) ureterocele**
     The intravesical or orthotopic ureterocele is completely located in the bladder. Intravesical ureteroceles are mostly combined with a single kidney system and account for about 15% of cases. It is seen more in older children or adults.
  b. **Ectopic (extravesical) ureterocele**
     If any portion of the ureterocele extends into the bladder neck or urethra, it is called an ectopic ureterocele. Ectopic ureterocele is the most common form of ureterocele (> 80%). It can be voluminous, dissociating the trigone and slipping into the urethra, and may prolapse through the urethral meatus.
- **Stephens classification (1968)**:
  Classified into 4 categories depending on the size and location of the ureteric orifice:
  a. **Stenotic:** Narrow orifice within the bladder
  b. **Sphincteric:** Wide orifice within the internal sphincter
  c. **Sphinctero-stenotic:** Narrow orifice within the internal sphincter
  d. **Caeco-ureterocele:** Blind ending ureterocele extending down the urethra.

5. **What is the clinical presentation of ureterocele?**

Ans:

- **Prenatal detection**
  - Usually suspected on prenatal ultrasonography. A duplication anomaly should be suspected in the presence of ureteral dilation that is greater than associated renal pelvis dilation. Ultrasonography may detect a cystic mass within the bladder that is more easily identified on postnatal bladder ultrasonography.
- **Incidental post-natal detection**
  - Diagnosed based on the findings of hydronephrosis when imaging was performed for unrelated reasons as trauma or abdominal pain.
  - There have been reports of presumed ovarian cysts which were actually markedly dilated ureters. Hence, it is important to consider the dilated ureter as part of the differential diagnosis while evaluating dilated structures in pelvis.[7]
- **Infection/urosepsis**
  - **Pain**. Pain is uncommon. However, it may be related to the acute infection or bladder pain caused by an obstructing ureterocele.
  - **Prolapse**. Prolapse is unusual but distinct presenting sign. It is generally a smooth, congested, mucosal covered interlabial mass associated with difficulty in voiding.

6. **How do you evaluate and diagnose a child with ureterocele?**

Ans:

Clinical Examination

A prolapsed ureterocele is diagnostic, however, it is not a common presentation. Sometimes, dilated upper pole of the ectopic ureterocele may be palpable in a relaxed infant, but it is difficult to appreciate this in an older child.

Imaging Studies

Ultrasonography

There are no characteristics that permit differentiation between a dilated ectopic ureter and ureterocele above the level of the bladder.

Usually USG shows a thin walled, cystic dilation within the bladder and not extending beyond its walls (Fig. 5.2). In case of ectopic ureters the lumen will extend well outside the bladder walls. The laterality of the ureterocele can be usually apparent but it may appear as midline structure if it is large. A large ureterocele may completely fill a bladder with no urine in the bladder itself. A full bladder with an effaced ureterocele may be mistakenly considered an ectopic ureter.

Voiding cystourethrogram

The voiding cystourethrogram (VCUG) is an obligatory imaging test. An initial VCUG should always be obtained before any intervention to know the baseline situation. The presence of reflux may determine initial treatment and is an important parameter in clinical management after initial decompression of the ureterocele. After incision of an ureterocele, the presence of reflux either ipsilaterally or contralaterally will be critical in therapeutic decision making.

Magnetic resonance imaging

Generally, not required as it does not add any additional information. It may be useful in patients in whom other imaging techniques fail to define the anatomical complexities.

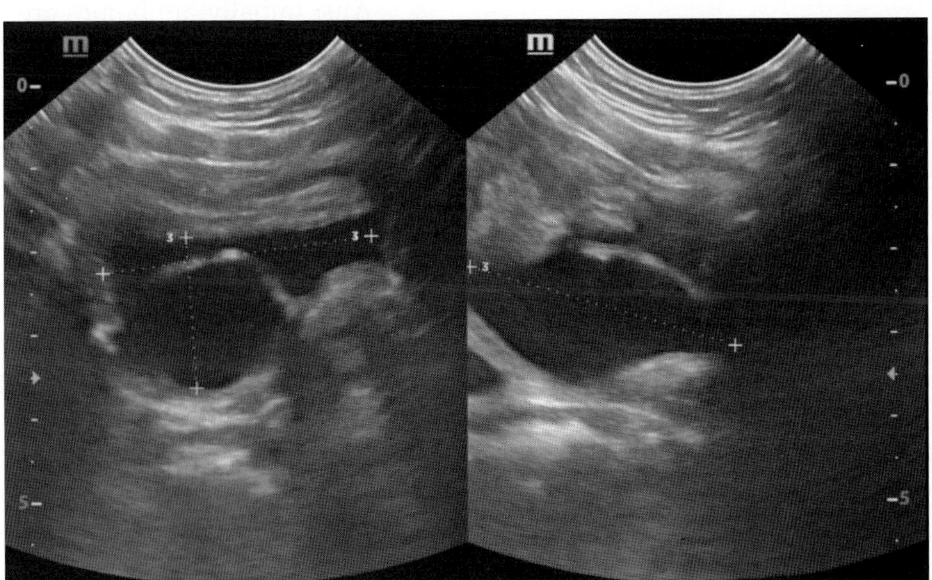

Fig. 5.2: USG image of a right ureterocele (arrow)

Functional Assessment

Nuclear scan

A diuretic renal scan will help in assessment of ureteroceles in which an observational approach may be considered. This provides both functional and drainage measurements. This has been shown to be of some clinical value in ureteroceles in which drainage is adequate, and ultimate resolution of the hydronephrosis has been reported.[8]

7. **Is endoscopic evaluation of ureterocele required before surgical intervention? What points are to be noted during an endoscopic evaluation?**

Ans: Endoscopic evaluation is important, if not essential, before deciding on the surgical intervention for ureterocele. When an endoscopic incision is to be performed, an evaluation should be performed thoroughly before incision to permit selection of the most effective site.

Following things should be noted during the endoscopic evaluation:

- Characteristics of the urethra, bladder neck, and trigone in relation to the ureterocele.
- The location of the other ureteral orifice.
- The orifice of the affected ureter should be searched for; however, it may not be identified.
- If the ureteral orifice is not seen in the bladder, then the urethra must be carefully examined to look for location of the orifice.
- The ureterocele examination should be done with slow bladder filling as its appearance will vary with bladder filling (slow flattening of the ureterocele with increasing bladder volume). With partial filling of the bladder, true limits of the borders can be appreciated better which will expose the lowest portion (which is the best site for incision).
- A cecoureterocele may be detected and this indicates the need to make sure this portion does not cause obstruction with incision. Retrograde contrast injection can confirm the presence of ureterocele disproportion.

8. **What are the goals of management of a ureterocele?**

Ans:

- Preservation of the renal function
- Elimination of infection, obstruction and reflux
- Maintenance of urinary continence

9. **What is the role of fetal intervention in management of ureterocele?**

Ans: Fetal surgical intervention for ureterocele is rarely done especially when the ureterocele is large causing obstruction of both renal units. In these cases, puncturing of the ureterocele, fetoscopy with laser ablation or laser ablation through an ultrasound guided needle have been used as treatment modalities.[9]

10. **What are the management modalities for the ureterocele in the neonatal period?**

Ans: Most of the children present in a non-emergency situation as follow-up for prenatally detected sonographic abnormality. The starting of prophylactic antibiotics is considered to minimize the risk of infection in the setting of hydroureteronephrosis with obstruction even with the absence of reflux. A VCUG is necessary. If the child is more than 2 months of age, a renal functional study should also be considered.

If the size of the ureterocele is small with minimal degree of hydronephrosis and with no or a little demonstrable obstruction, the child can be observed.

If the hydronephrosis is significant with obstruction along with compromised parenchyma in the obstructed segment, surgical intervention should be considered.

- **Low transverse incision**
- **Watering-can incision:** Use of holmium laser is used to puncture multiple holes in the ureterocele with a possibility of lower risk of *de novo* VUR when compared to a traditional incision.[10]
- **Cutaneous distal ureterostomy:** If an endoscopic approach cannot be undertaken, then a cutaneous diversion with distal ureterostomy, followed by a formal re-implantation once the child is old enough for the surgery.

11. **How will you manage a neonate with ureterocele who presents with sepsis?**

Ans: Initially antibiotics are usually sufficient to stabilize the child clinically. However, if the child fails to respond promptly, then trans-urethral incision (TUI) of an obstructing ureterocele or a nephrostomy of the obstructing moiety or a cutaneous distal ureterostomy needs to be done.

If a surgical procedure was not required in an emergency with adequate response to the conservative management with antibiotics, a drainage procedure should be undertaken in an elective setting once the child is stabilized to prevent future infections as the child is prone to infections subsequently.

12. **What are the management options for a child presenting with ureterocele?**

Ans: The general goals of treatment remain the same as described earlier with a principle concern for preserving the renal parenchyma.

The decision on preservation of renal parenchyma is largely empirical with a few objective criteria to indicate how much residual function is worth preserving. In a duplex system with ureterocele, the upper pole contributes a little to the overall renal function, but there are no fixed criteria as to what should be the normal upper pole function for preserving the moiety.

Observation: This modality can be an appropriate strategy with careful case selection. Parental education and counseling regarding potential for later acute presentations of infection and sepsis is important. A broad criteria for observation include a child in the setting of no obstruction of the ipsilateral lower pole or contralateral kidney and limited reflux to the lower pole (grade 3 or less), no functional deterioration of the upper pole and with no obstruction on nuclear scan.[8,11,12] These children can be observed for a period without intervention and there have been reports of resolution of upper pole dilatation and lower pole reflux.

Total reconstruction: Total reconstruction of both upper and lower tracts including upper pole partial nephrectomy with ureterocele excision and re-implantation has been advocated by some as the most definitive procedure for ureteroceles.

13. **What are the complications associated with upper pole nephrectomy?**

Ans: Complications related to upper pole nephrectomy include loss of function of the lower pole and development of postoperative upper pole urinoma (20%).

14. **What is the effect on lower pole reflux in duplex system with ureterocele following upper pole nephrectomy?**

Ans: Following upper pole nephrectomy, the resolution of reflux in the lower pole may be expected in around 20% of patients and a new reflux may be noticed in 15–50% of patients in whom there was no reflux preoperatively.[13]

15. **What is the unique concern with surgical management of caeco-ureterocele?**

Ans: Following caeco-ureterocele excision and re-implantation, the distal aspect of the ureterocele can act like an obstructive flap valve during voiding. This can be avoided by ensuring the distal segment is excised. This is aided by the placement of traction sutures, on the distal segment to deliver it into the operative field of vision and then an excision can be done. If the overall size is not too large, the opening can be closed in two layers. Alternatively, marsupialization of the intravesical portion of the ureterocele can be done.

SUMMARY

An algorithm for the management of the duplex system ureteroceles (DSU) as per the European Association of Urology guidelines 2023 is given in Fig. 5.3.

REFERENCES

1. EAU guidelines on Pediatric Urology. European Association of Urology 2023.
2. Shah H, Tiwari C, Shenoy NS, Dwivedi P, Gandhi S. Transurethral incision of ureteroceles in paediatric age group. Turk J Urol. 2017 Dec; 43 (4):530–535.
3. Upadhyay J, Bolduc S, Braga L, Farhat W, Bägli DJ, McLorie GA, Khoury AE, El-Ghoneimi A. Impact of prenatal diagnosis on the morbidity associated with ureterocele management. J Urol. 2002 Jun;167 (6):2560–5.

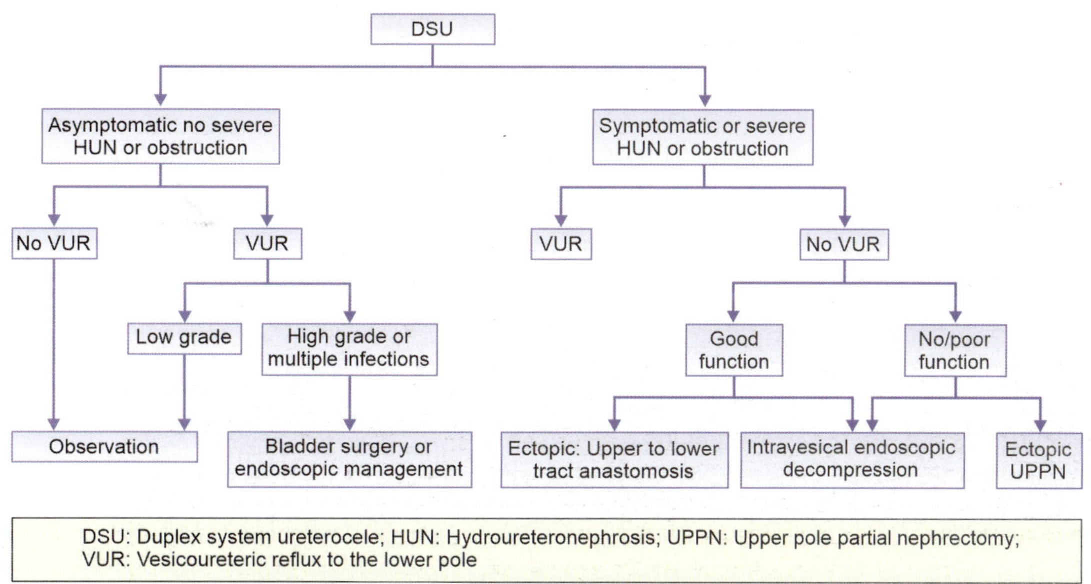

Fig. 5.3: Algorithm for the management of duplex system ureteroceles

4. Monfort G, Guys JM, Coquet M, Roth K, Louis C, Bocciardi A. Surgical management of duplex ureteroceles. J Pediatr Surg. 1992 May; 27 (5):634–8.
5. Chwalle R. The process of formation of cystic dilatations of the vesical end of the ureter and of diverticula at the ureteral ostium. UrolCutan Rev. 1927; 31:499.
6. Ericsson NO. Ectopic ureterocele in infants and children; a clinical study. Acta Chir Scand Suppl. 1954; 197:1–93.
7. Mason MD, Peters CA, Schenkman NS. Robot-assisted upper pole nephrectomy in adult patients with duplicated renal collecting systems. J Endourol. 2012 Jul;26 (7):838–42.
8. Han MY, Gibbons MD, Belman AB, Pohl HG, Majd M, Rushton HG. Indications for non operative management of ureteroceles. J Urol. 2005 Oct;174(4 Pt 2):1652–5; discussion 1655–6.
9. Persico N, Berrettini A, Fabietti I, Dallagiovanna C, Minoli D, Mosca F, Fedele L, Manzoni G. New minimally invasive technique for cystoscopic laser treatment of fetal ureterocele. Ultrasound Obstet Gynecol. 2017 Jul; 50(1):124–127.
10. Joseph Haddad, Bhalaajee Meenakshi-Sundaram, Nathan Rademaker, Hubert Greger, Christopher Aston, Blake W. Palmer, Bradley P. Kropp, Dominic Frimberge. "Watering Can" ureterocele puncture technique leads to decreased rates of *de novo* vesico ureteral reflux and subsequent surgery with durable results. Urology.2017; 108:161–165.
11. Direnna, Tania and Michael P. Leonard. "Watchful waiting for prenatally detected ureteroceles." *The Journal of urology 175 (4) (2006): 1493–5; discussion 1495.*
12. Shankar KR, Vishwanath N, Rickwood AM. Outcome of patients with prenatally detected duplex system ureterocele; natural history of those managed expectantly. J Urol. 2001 Apr; 165 (4):1226–8.
13. Husmann D, Strand B, Ewalt D, Clement M, Kramer S, Allen T. Management of ectopic ureterocele associated with renal duplication: a comparison of partial nephrectomy and endoscopic decompression. J Urol. 1999 Oct;162 (4):1406–9.

Chapter

6

PUJ Obstruction in a 3-Month-Old Male Child

• *Gyanendra Sharma*

LEARNING OBJECTIVES

- Use of correct terminology to describe prenatally detected hydronephrosis.
- Ultrasonography—technique and parameters to be assessed.
- Indications for antibiotic prophylaxis.
- Diuretic renogram—indications, timing, different types and their interpretation.

INTRODUCTION

Since the widespread use of ultrasonography in the evaluation of obstetric patients, the number of genitourinary anomalies detected during the prenatal period has significantly gone up. Nearly 1–5% of all pregnancies have a diagnosis of fetal hydronephrosis made during the prenatal scans.[1,2] Most of the time this hydronephrosis is transient in nature and disappears in the postnatal period but some may persist. Amongst the various causes of hydronephrosis which persists in the postnatal period, pelvi-ureteric junction (PUJ) obstruction is the most common cause. Management of these infants with postnatal persistence of prenatally detected hydronephrosis is a cause for concern both for the treating clinician as well as the parents. The fear of surgery hangs like a sword of Damocles on the psyche of the parents. Majority of these hydronephrosis do not need surgical intervention and subside or stabilize in due course of time. From the clinicians' point of view it is imperative to distinguish those hydronephrosis which are likely to subside, from those which would need surgical intervention. The current chapter aims to provide guidelines for the evaluation of these children using sonography and interpretation of renogram to diagnose obstruction and to differentiate it from non-obstructive dilatation.

Case Scenario

A 3-month-old male child is brought by parents with a history of left side hydronephrosis detected in the prenatal ultrasonography performed during the second trimester. They gave the history that there was some increase in the hydronephrosis in the third trimester scan but the amniotic fluid was normal. The mother had a full-term normal delivery and the baby has been asymptomatic since birth. The parents were advised by their family physician to seek a urology consultation at the age of 3 months; hence they have come for opinion regarding the further management.

1. **How common is PUJ like obstruction in prenatally detected hydronephrosis?**

   Ans: It is seen in 10–30% of all cases of prenatally detected hydronephrosis.[3]

2. **What terminology should be used to describe these patients with PUJ obstruction?**

   Ans: Hydronephrosis is aseptic dilatation of the pelvicalyceal system. It may be due to obstruction or it could be a non-obstructive dilatation. Hence it is erroneous to use terminology like PUJ obstruction for all hydronephrosis. The correct terminology as proposed by Nguyen *et al* is urinary tract dilatation.[3]

3. **What should be the sonography protocol to follow-up these patients postnatally?**

   Ans: Usually the first postnatal sonography is done at least 48 hours after birth. The neonate is relatively dehydrated immediately after birth, hence sonography done within the first 48 hours may underestimate the degree of hydronephrosis.[3] To look for the persistence of hydronephrosis, another sonography is warranted at 4 weeks. If this sonography also shows hydronephrosis then depending on the degree of hydronephrosis a renogram is indicated or further follow-up with sonography is advisable.

4. What precautions should be taken while doing sonography in these infants and what all should be reported?

Ans: The infant should be well hydrated. Degree of bladder fullness can affect the dilatation of the pelvicalyceal system, hence a good practice is to ask the sonologist to start the sonography by scanning the bladder first. The gentle pressure of the ultrasound probe provides the stimulus for a reasonably full bladder to evacuate itself; then the kidneys can be scanned.[4]

5. What are the points which a sonologist should report while doing ultrasonography in an infant with prenatally detected hydronephrosis?

Ans: The sonologist should provide information as per the urinary tract dilatation (UTD) system.[3]

- The degree of central dilatation
- The degree of peripheral dilatation
- The parenchymal thickness at upper, mid and lower pole
- The parenchymal echotexture
- The presence or absence of dilatation of ureters
- The bladder wall thickness and post-void residual urine

The most important amongst these is the providing information of the degree of pelvicalyceal dilatation. There are many ways in which this has been described: Society of Fetal Urology (SFU) classification, the antero-posterior penal pelvic diameter (APRPD), Onen's classification and modified Onen's classification, etc. Out of all these the one which is commonly followed is measurement of APRPD. The urinary tract dilatation (UTD) system described by Ngyuen *et al*[3] utilizes the APRPD along with detailed description of other parameters.

6. Is the UTD classification reproducible?

Ans: This classification system has been found to have inter- and intra-observer correlation.[5] Measurement of antero-posterior diameter is the most dynamic of the various parameters described in this system and it is also associated with good intra- and inter-observer correlation.[6]

7. How should antero-posterior renal pelvic diameter be measured?

Ans: Very often these hydronephrotic kidneys are associated with significant dilatation of the pelvis. One should keep in mind that the degree of hydration, position and degree of bladder fullness can all affect the measurement of APRPD.[4] Ideally the APRPD is measured at the level of the renal hilum in a well-hydrated child on an empty bladder. The measurement should be within the confines of the renal parenchyma so that the extra renal dilated renal pelvis does not affect the measurement and leads to a very high APRPD. The accompanying video demonstrates this. Ideally the same sonologist should do the sonography on every follow-up so that consistency is maintained and the sonologist should mention how the measurements were taken.[3,7]

8. Above what cut-off value of APRPD should follow-up be done?

Ans: APRPD > 10 mm in the postnatal sonography warrants follow-up. Even if there is no hydronephrosis in the first postnatal scan, a repeat sonography at 4 and 12 weeks is needed as at times subsequent scans may show dilatation which was not evident initially.[3]

9. In what position should sonography be done?

Ans: As there are pros and cons of imaging the kidneys in either the prone or supine position, the current recommendation is that the same position be used in the same patient during each follow-up measurement to make for more accurate comparisons.[3]

10. Does measurement of APRPD in supine and prone position have any significance?

Ans: It is a well-established fact that the pelvicalyceal system drains better in a prone position. Studies have shown that those kidneys which show a decrease in the APRPD in a prone position are less likely to need surgical intervention.[4] Based on the changes in the diameter of the renal pelvis and calyces in supine and prone position, a classification has been pro-posed which categorizes these hydronephrotic kidneys into those having good, partial or poor drainage.[8]

The renal pelvis is considered to have a poor drainage if the anteroposterior diameter increases by >10% in prone position with or without increase in calyceal dilatation The renal pelvis is supposed to have a good drainage into the ureters if the anteroposterior diameter decreases by >10% in prone position as compared to the supine position and whatever falls between the two is supposed to have partial drainage.

Scan QR Code for Video on **Measurement of APRPD in prone position**

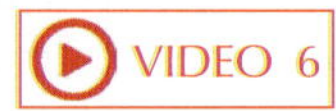

Scan QR Code for Video on **Measurement of APRPD in supine position**

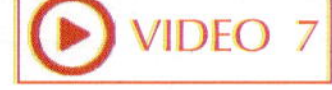

11. Can we identify the renal units at risk of damage due to suspected PUJ obstruction on sonography?

Ans: In cases having hydronephrosis suggestive of PUJ like obstruction, a renal unit will be at risk of damage, i.e. deterioration of renal function if it will have poor drainage into the ureter. The UTD classification as well as the measurement of APRPD in supine and prone position (on an empty bladder) help in categorizing these children into those with good, partial and poor drainage of the pelvicalyceal system.[3,4,8]

Figure 6.1 describes this combining both these parameters.

12. How do you identify increasing hydronephrosis on ultrasonography?

Ans: The following parameters suggest increase in hydronephrosis.

- Increase in APRPD
- Increase in APRPD by > 10% in prone position as compared to supine position
- Increase in calyceal dilatation especially the peripheral calyces
- Decrease in the parenchymal thickness

13. Should these children be kept on antibiotic prophylaxis?

Ans: This has been a controversial issue. Previously it was probably a natural reflex of the clinicians to start chemoprophylaxis in all patients with dilatation of the urinary tract, However, many studies have proved the lack of usefulness of this approach. Nowadays antibiotic prophylaxis is advised in infants at risk of developing infection. They are those with UTD P3, or in other words antibiotic prophylaxis is indicated[9,10] if the antero-posterior renal pelvic diameter (APRPD) is >15 mm with peripheral calyceal dilatation and/or if the

- Parenchymal thickness < 4 mm
- Parenchymal appearance is abnormal
- There is dilatation of ureter
- Sonography is suggestive of poor drainage of the pelvicalyceal system.

14. What should be the choice of antibiotics for chemoprophylaxis?

Ans: Most commonly amoxycillin is used in the dose of 15 mg/kg in the first couple of months after birth followed by cephalexin 10–15 mg/kg. They are given once at bedtime. Alternatively, cephalexin can be used right from the neonatal period.

15. Should a voiding cystourethrogram (VCUG) be routinely done in these patients?

Ans: Again this is a contentious issue. The opinions of clinicians have ranged from doing VCUG in all cases to selectively advising it to kids with moderate to severe hydronephrosis especially in UTD P3 category. Many investigators refrain from advising it routinely in all cases as VCUG is an invasive procedure with a small but significant risk of infection. Many pediatric urologists recommend it only when the infant presents with documented UTI or there is hydroureter or parenchymal abnormality suggestive of scarring.[3,10] The aim is to diagnose associated higher grades of vesico-ureteric reflux which can impact the management. Routine VCUG in all the patients with hydronephrosis may diagnose low grade reflux that may not necessitate any change in the treatment strategy. Whenever done, VCUG should be done under cover of antibiotics with all aseptic precautions.

16. Should intravenous urography or CT urography be done in these infants?

Ans: Sonography provides good anatomical details of the pelvicalyceal system and the functional component is best studied by doing radionuclide studies. There is no benefit of doing IVU or CT urography in these children suspected of having PUJ like obstruction. These studies give excess

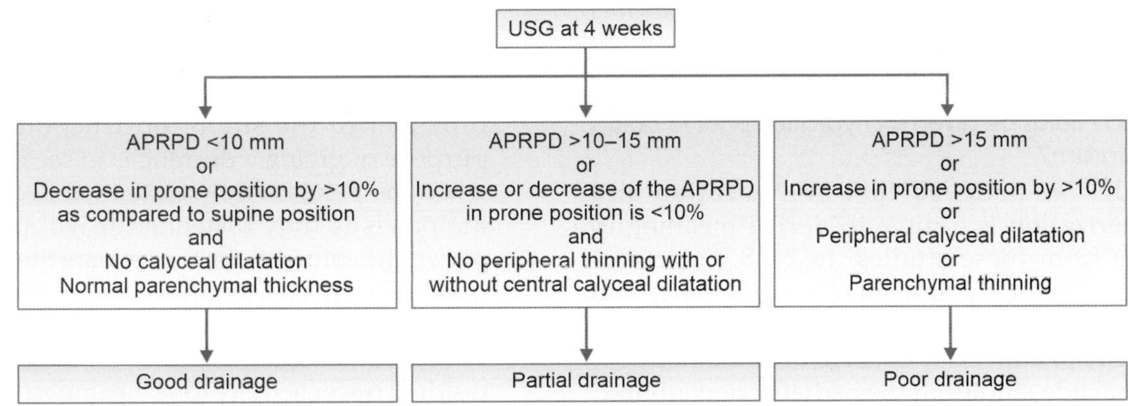

Fig. 6.1: Sonography criteria to differentiate kidneys at risk of deterioration of renal function from those where this risk is less

undesirable and unwarranted radiation to these children.

17. What is the ideal time to do renogram in these patients?

Ans: If the second USG (done at 4 weeks) shows central and peripheral calyceal dilatation without any parenchymal thinning, then another USG is warranted at 3 months, and if the sonography picture is the same, then renogram is advisable. If the serial sonography shows a decrease in the dilatation of the pelvicalyceal system, then renogram can be further deferred or avoided.[3,8] However, if the sonography at 4 weeks shows increase in the dilatation as compared to the first sonography and/or if there is parenchymal thinning then renogram should be advised at 4–6 weeks.

18. What precautions should be taken while advising renogram?

Ans: The infant should be well hydrated and should not be having a urinary tract infection. If there is pyelonephritis, then the differential renal function (DRF) can be compromised which can lead to erroneous interpretation and subsequent management.

19. Which radionuclide tracer should be used for the diuretic renogram?

Ans: Ideally Technetium-99m mercaptoacetyl triglycine (Tc-99m MAG3) should be used but it is not routinely available in most centers in India. Hence diethylene-cysteine, i.e. EC should be used. Technetium-99m diethylene triamine penta-acetic acid (Tc-99m DTPA) should be avoided in children especially during the first 2 years of life due to the high background activity which can falsely result in increased DRF. The reason for this is that both MAG3 and EC are excreted by tubules while DTPA is excreted by glomerular filtration. Agents having tubular excretion have a higher renal uptake giving rise to a higher renal to background image. Thus it is recommended that radiopharmaceuticals having tubular secretion should be used.

20. Should IV fluids be given for hydration prior to doing a renogram?

Ans: It was believed that IV hydration and catheterization is a must to derive meaningful results from these studies. In 2018, Society of Nuclear Medicine and Imaging (SNMMI) and European Association of Nuclear Medicine (EANM) produced a consensus statement for radionuclide studies in the pediatric age group.[12] They suggested that good oral hydration is mandatory prior to the procedure and IV hydration is indicated only if the procedure is being done under sedation or general anesthesia. For IV hydration, DNS in a dose of 15–20 ml/kg is to be given, Two-thirds of the dose should be given before the injection of furosemide.

21. Should bladder drainage be done to keep the bladder empty during a renogram?

Ans: Bladder drainage by an indwelling catheter is recommended in infants and children who have hydroureteronephrosis, suspected reflux, posterior urethral valves or neuropathic bladder. Though continuous bladder drainage helps in better drainage of the upper tracts and decreases radiation to the gonads, its routine use is not recommended.

22. What renogram protocol should be followed?

Ans: There are many different protocols which have been described and followed. Since Conway *et al* described the 'well-tempered' renogram, much has been discussed regarding the usefulness of various protocols. The different protocols are based on their timing of furosemide in relation to the timing of the injection of radiopharmaceutical agent. The various protocols followed are F – 15, F0, F + 10, F + 20 or F + 30. Studies have shown that the F0 protocol in which furosemide is injected along with the radiopharmaceutical is superior to F – 15 and F + 20 protocol.[13]

23. What is the dose of furosemide?

Ans: Recommended dose of furosemide is 1 mg/kg with a maximum of 40 mg. However, at most center a dose of 1 mg/kg is used in children below the age of 2 years and dose of 0.5 mg/kg is used for children > 2 years of age.

24. Why is a diuretic given?

Ans: Diuretic is administered to distinguish between good from poor drainage of the pelvi-calyceal system. A non-obstructed system would drain when the system is stressed by diuresis, while the drainage in obstructed system would get hampered, the washout would remain slow with a prolonged retention of radiopharmaceutical proximal to the site of obstruction. The basic purpose of giving a diuretic is to see the drainage when the pelvis is fully distended because unless the pelvis is fully distended it will not generate peristaltic contractions to evacuate the urine in the ureter. For this reason, furosemide should ideally be injected after the entire collecting system is filled with radioactive urine and there is adequate residual tracer activity for a meaningful evaluation of post-diuresis drainage parameters. In massively dilated systems one may need to wait even beyond 20–30 minutes before furosemide is injected.[14] Practically it is not possible at most centers to decide precise timing of furosemide and hence the F0 protocol is commonly followed.

25. Does full bladder and gravity affect drainage of urine from the ureters and thus also the interpretation of renogram?

Ans: Drainage can be affected by the supine position of the patient and, in the absence of indwelling bladder catheter, by varying degrees of bladder filling. Therefore, if drainage at the end of dynamic imaging shows high residual activity, then the child should be kept upright for 15 minutes and a static 1 minute image obtained preferably on an empty bladder. Likewise, in the absence of an indwelling catheter, a static 1 minute image is obtained in 60 minutes (or even longer) after the radiopharmaceutical has been injected. This gravity assisted postvoid drainage evaluation is of paramount importance to assess whether the drainage is good or poor.[15]

26. What are the important parameters one should look at in the renogram?

Ans: The diuretic renogram mentions the differential renal function, T half values and depicts the drainage curves. But in infants and young children, parameters evaluating gravity assisted postvoid drainage and parameters describing the transit of the radionuclide tracer through the renal parenchyma are more important.

27. Which parameter describes gravity assisted post-void drainage?

Ans: With the increasing importance of gravity assisted postvoid drainage, NORA, i.e. normalized residual activity should be calculated and mentioned. NORA is a ratio between the residual decay corrected kidney counts over one minute at a predefined time point to the kidney counts in the second minute of the parenchymal phase. Typically, the NORA is calculated on the 60th minute, post-void post-gravity assisted image. NORA >1.8 indicate poor drainage while NORA <0.5 indicates good drainage while the values between 0.5 and 1.8 indicate partial drainage.[12,16,17]

28. What parameter describes the passage of the radionuclide tracer through the renal parenchyma and what is its significance?

Ans: Another parameter which is gaining significance is the cortical transit time. It is the time taken by the radiotracer to traverse the renal parenchyma and appear in the pelvicalyceal system. CTT >3 minutes is considered to be abnormal. It can be calculated visually or by the software. It is considered by many to the only parameter which can identify the renal units at increased risk of the loss of function due to obstruction.[18]

29. What are the indications for pyeloplasty?

Ans: Pyeloplasty is indicated when there is clinically significant obstruction.

The well-accepted indications for pyeloplasty are[19]

- DRF <40%.
- Drop in DRF by >10% in serial renograms.
- Increasing hydronephrosis.
- Symptomatic patient.

One big dilemma is to identify renal units with DRF > 40% on the initial renogram which are at risk of deterioration in future. In other words, how to differentiate non-obstructive dilatation from obstructive dilatation before irreversible damage to renal function occurs.

30. How to interpret renograms to diagnose an obstructed system?

Ans: Diuretic renogram typically provides a drainage pattern. Quite erroneously the words obstructed or nonobstructed drainage patterns have become established and are commonly used. What the renogram suggests is good, partial or poor drainage of the urine from the pelvis into the ureter.[20] The system would be classified as obstructed only and only if the degree of drainage is poor enough to cause back pressure effects leading to deterioration of renal function.[21] The correct terminology would be good, partial or poor drainage. Traditionally T½ values >20 minutes have been described to be associated with obstruction while value below 10 minutes suggests nonobstructed system and the T½ values between 10–20 minutes are considered to be equivocal. However, what has got overlooked over a period of time is that these values were arrived at during studies done for adults or older symptomatic children who have much less compliant pelvis.[22] Nowadays the majority of cases of PUJ like obstruction are diagnosed prenatally. Postnatally the baby is born with a presumptive diagnosis rather than a symptom. The pelvis of these infants is much more compliant. Due to the reservoir effect very often the pelvis will not drain till it is completely full. For the same reason drainage curves are also not indicative of obstruction. Recent studies have suggested that T½ values <5 minutes suggest good drainage, value >75 minutes suggest poor drainage while the values between 5–75 minutes suggest indeterminate range. Practically, no diuretic renogram is done for >75 minutes. Also, injection of furosemide is suggested to be given if the pelvis does not drain for >30 minutes[14,15] (again something which is not done in practice). A better way to categorize good, partial or poor drainage is by calculating NORA which takes into consideration both the gravity assisted and postvoid drainage films.[12,23]

31. **How to differentiate a dilated system which is obstructed from the one which is non-obstructed?**

Ans: Gravity assisted drainage provides the answer to whether the renal pelvis is having good, partial or poor drainage. NORA is the best parameter to assess gravity assisted drainage. Once the question of drainage of the renal pelvis is addressed, the next question to be answered is whether it is a dilated but non-obstructive or a dilated and obstructed system. Poor drainage will result in backpressure effects. The pathophysiological changes that occur are a decrease in the concentrating and excreting ability of the kidneys. Decrease in the concentrating ability manifests as decrease in DRF. Hence a DRF <40% or drop in DRF between two renograms of >5–10% are absolute indications for pyeloplasty. In cases where the initial DRF is >40%, the clinician relies on increasing hydronephrosis as seen on sonography or serial renograms to see for a drop in DRF. Many investigators have attempted to objectively evaluate the decrease in the excreting ability of the renal parenchyma by calculating the cortical transit time. Many studies have found this to be the most reliable parameter to diagnose obstruction.[18]

32. **What are key points in the radiological evaluation of these children with prenatally detected hydronephrosis?**

Ans:
- T ½ values >20 minutes does not confirm obstruction.
- T ½ values <5–10 minutes definitely suggest good drainage and suggest a non-obstructed system.
- Drainage curves are not predictive of obstruction.[24]
- NORA is a more reliable parameter as it takes into account gravity assistance and postvoid drainage. NORA >1.8 suggests poor drainage while value <0.5 suggests good drainage.[16,17,23]
- Often sequential renogram are needed to decide about surgical intervention.
- CTT >3 minutes suggests impairment of the excreting ability of the kidney.[18]
- Increasing hydronephrosis on sonography is suggestive of impaired drainage of the renal pelvis.

33. **How long should follow-up be advised in patients who have not been advised surgery initially but some hydronephrosis is persisting beyond the first year of life?**

Ans: This question has not been categorically answered by the current available literature. Usually a child is followed until the age of 6 years. If the hydronephrosis has subsided by this time, then no further follow-up is needed. Also, if hydronephrosis persists but has been stable for the last 1 year then further follow-up is not needed till puberty. The increase in the body mass during puberty results in an increase in the urine output. By this time the dilated renal pelvis also becomes less compliant and a latent obstruction can become manifest. At this stage some renal units which showed an equivocal pattern of drainage on renograms may show deterioration in the renogram parameters necessitating surgical intervention. Hence a hydronephrosis which is stable in early childhood needs a close follow-up during the adolescent years.[26]

34. **What is supranormal differential renal function?**

Ans: Supranormal differential renal function is a DRF of >55% in a hydronephrotic kidney often with APRPD of >30 mm associated with altered renal geometry. These kidneys need close monitoring as DRF alone cannot determine the need of surgery in such cases.[27]

35. **Summary and Take Home Message.**

Ans:
- All neonates with prenatally detected hydronephrosis should undergo a sonography between 2 and 5 days after birth. The exceptions to this are: those with bilateral hydronephrosis, those suspected of having infravesical obstruction and those with a solitary kidney especially if the AP diameter was >15 mm on the third trimester scan.
- The grading of hydronephrosis should be done as described below:[26]
  - UTD P1–APRPD is 10–15 mm or there is central dilatation of calyces
  - UTD P2–APRPD is >15 mm or there is peripheral dilatation of calyces
  - UTD P3–APRPD is >10 mm with any calyceal dilatation and parenchymal thinning of abnormal echotexture of parenchyma
- Chemoprophylaxis is advised if there is bilateral hydronephrosis with or without hydroureter or there is unilateral hydroureteronephrosis or there is hydronephrosis with parenchymal thinning or abnormal appearance of parenchyma.

- A repeat USG is advisable at 4 weeks after birth.
- In patients with no hydronephrosis, a repeat sonography at 12 weeks is advisable.
- If sonography at 4 weeks shows UTD P2, then patient should be advised follow-up and a sonography is advisable at 3 months. If a similar picture is seen, then a diuretic renogram should be done at 3 months.
- If sonography at 4 weeks shows a picture suggestive of UTDP3 then a renogram is advisable at 4 weeks.
- There is no role of doing IVU or CT Urography in infants with suspected PUJ like obstruction.
- Diuretic renogram should be done taking care of the following things:
  - It should be EC or MAG3
  - Child should be free of infection
  - Child should be well-hydrated prior to the study
  - F0 protocol should be used
  - The nuclear medicine department should mention the DRF, T½, NORA and provide 1 minute images so that the cortical transit time can be ascertained
- T½ values > 20 minutes or upgoing drainage curve do not indicate obstruction and surgery should not be advised based only on these parameters
- T½ values < 5–10 minutes indicate good drainage and rule out any significant obstruction
- Pyeloplasty is indicated in these infants if the DRF is < 40%
- Figures 6.2 to 6.4 describe the strategy to manage infants with prenatally detected PUJ like obstruction. [8,16–18,20,23]

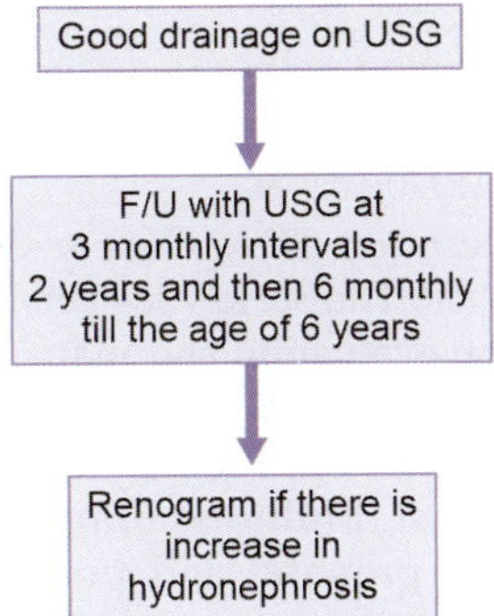

Fig. 6.2: Management algorithm of those kidneys which show good drainage on sonography and are at least risk of deterioration of renal function

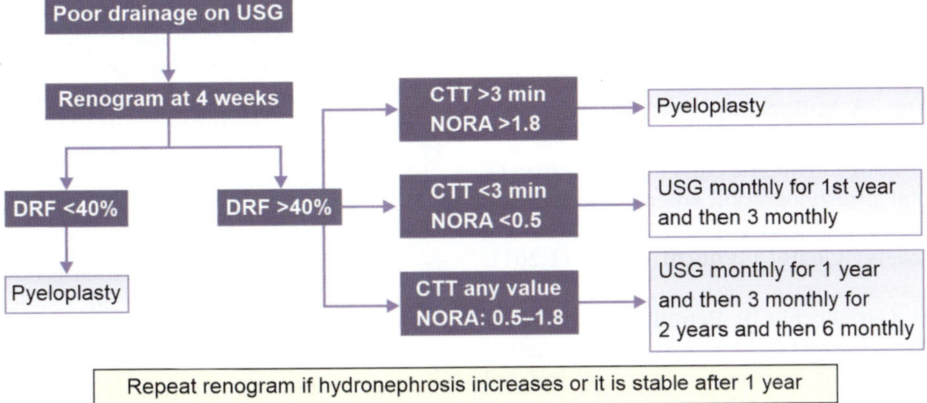

Fig. 6.3: Management algorithm for kidneys which show poor drainage pattern on sonography and are at high risk of functional deterioration

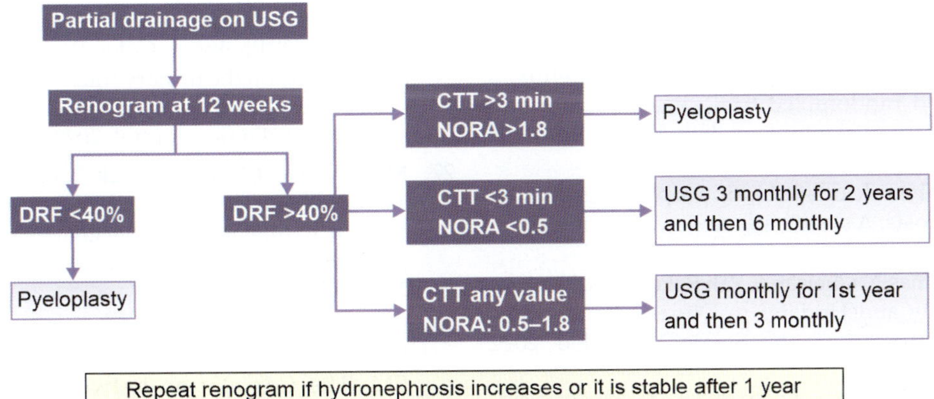

Fig. 6.4: Management of kidneys which show equivocal drainage pattern on sonography

- Renal units with UTD P2 or those having partial drainage pattern on sonography or those which show DRF > 40% at the initial renogram and are followed up using sonography should also undergo renogram if there is increasing hydronephrosis or after 1 year if the hydronephrosis remains stable. This is important as even those renal units with seemingly stable hydronephrosis can deteriorate over a period of time.[28]

REFERENCES

1. Garre WJ, Grunwald G, Robinson DE. Prenatal diagnosis of fetal polycystic kidney by Ultrasound.Aust NZ J ObstetGynaecol1970;10:7–9.
2. Nguyen HT, Herndon CDA, Cooper C, Gatti J, Kirsch A, Kokorowski P, *et al.* The Society for Fetal Urology consensus statement on the evaluation and management of antenatal hydronephrosis. J Pediatr Urol. 2010 Jun;6(3):212–31.
3. Nguyen HT, Benson CB, Bromley B, Campbell JB, Chow J, Coleman B, *et al.* Multidisciplinary consensus on the classification of prenatal and postnatal urinary tract dilation (UTD classification system). J Pediatr Urol. 2014 Dec;10(6):982–98.
4. Sharma G, Sharma A, Maheshwari P. Predictive value of decreased renal pelvis anteroposterior diameter in prone position for prenatally detected hydronephrosis. J Urol. 2012 May;187(5):1839–43.
5. Nelson CP, Lee RS, Trout AT, Servaes S, Kraft KH, Barnewolt CE, Logvinenko T, Chow JS. Interobserver and Intra-Observer Reliability of the Urinary Tract Dilation Classification System in Neonates: A Multicenter Study. J Urol. 2019 Jun;201(6):1186–1192.
6. Pereira AK, Reis ZS, Bouzada MC, de Oliveira EA, Osanan G, Cabral AC. Antenatal ultrasonographic anteroposterior renal pelvis diameter measurement: is it a reliable way of defining fetal hydronephrosis? Obstet Gynecol Int. 2011;2011: 861865.
7. Hodhod A, Eid H, Capolicchio JP, Petrella F, Sadri I, El-Sherbiny M, Jednak R, Lacroix C. How can we measure the renal pelvic anteroposterior diameter in postnatal isolated hydronephrosis? J Pediatr Urol. 2023 Feb;19(1):75–82.
8. Sharma G, Sharma A. Usefulness of Ultrasonography and Cortical Transit Time to Differentiate Nonobstructive From Obstructive Dilatation in the Management of Prenatally Detected Pelvic Ureteric Junction Like Obstruction. Urology. 2017 Dec;110:208–212.
9. Craig, J., *et al.* Long-term antibiotics to prevent urinary tract infection in children with isolated vesicoureteric reflux: a placebo-controlled randomized trial., in Australian and New Zealand Society of Nephrology 38th Annual Scientific Meeting 2002: Sydney.
10. Silay, M.S., *et al.* The role of antibiotic prophylaxis in antenatal hydronephrosis: A systematic review. J Pediatr Urol, 2017.13: 306.
11. Bar-Sever Z, Shammas A, Gheisari F, Vali R. Pediatric Nephro-Urology: Overview and Updates in Diuretic Renal Scans and Renal Cortical Scintigraphy. Semin Nucl Med. 2022 Jul;52(4):419–431.
12. Majd M, Bar-Sever Z, Santos AI, De Palma D. The SNMMI and EANM Procedural Guidelines for Diuresis Renography in Infants and Children. J Nucl Med. 2018 Oct;59(10): 1636–1640.
13. Babu R, Venkatsubramaniam D, Venkatachalapathy E. F+0 diuretic protocol is superior to F-15 and F+20 for nuclear renogram in children. Indian J Urol. 2015 Jul-Sep;31(3):245–8.
14. Sussman RD, Blum ES, Sprague BM, Majd M, Rushton HG, Pohl HG. Prediction of Clinical Outcomes in Prenatal Hydronephrosis: Importance of Gravity Assisted Drainage. J Urol. 2017 Mar;197(3 Pt 2):838–844.
15. Hodhod A, Turpin S, Petrella F, Jednak R, El-Sherbiny M, Capolicchio JP. Validation of modified diuretic drainage times criteria in congenital hydronephrosis. J Pediatr Urol. 2021 Dec;17(6):832.e1–832.e8.
16. Piepsz A, Tondeur M, Ham H. NORA: a simple and reliable parameter for estimating renal output with or without furosemide challenge. Nucl Med Commun. 2000;21:317–323.
17. Piepsz A, Kuyvenhoven JD, Tondeur M, Ham H. Normalized residual activity: usual values and robustness of the method. J Nucl Med. 2002;43:33–38.
18. Sharma GR, Panda A, Sharma AG. Renal cortical transit time in the evaluation of prenatally detected presumed pelvi ureteric junction like obstruction: A systematic review. Indian J Urol. 2021 Apr-Jun;37(2):116–124.
19. EAU Guidelines. Edn. presented at the EAU Annual Congress Milan, 2023.
20. Piepsz A. Antenatal detection of pelviureteric junction stenosis: main controversies. Semin Nucl Med. 2011 Jan;41 (1):11–9.
21. Koff SA. Problematic ureteropelvic junction obstruction. J Urol. 1987 Aug;138(2):390.
22. Bayne CE, Majd M, Rushton HG. Diuresis renography in the evaluation and management of pediatric hydronephrosis: What have we learned? J Pediatr Urol. 2019 Apr;15(2):128–137. doi: 10.1016/j.jpurol.2019.01.011.
23. Sharma GR, Sharma AG, Sharma NG. Comparison of two drainage parameters on diuretic renogram in predicting the fate of prenatally detected pelvi-ureteric junction-like obstruction. Indian J Urol. 2022 Jul-Sep;38(3):216–219.
24. Gordon I, Colarinha P, Fettich J, Fischer S, Frökier J, Hahn K, Kabasakal L, Mitjavila M, Olivier P, Piepsz A, Porn U, Sixt R, van Velzen J; Paediatric Committee of the European Association of Nuclear Medicine. Guidelines for standard and diuretic renography in children. Eur J Nucl Med. 2001 Mar;28(3):BP21–30.
25. Jacobson DL, Flink CC, Johnson EK, Maizels M, Yerkes EB, Lindgren BW, Liu DB, Rosoklija I, Cheng EY, Gong EM. The Correlation between Serial Ultrasound and Diuretic Renography in Children with Severe Unilateral Hydronephrosis. J Urol. 2018 Aug;200(2):440–447.
26. Nguyen HT, Phelps A, Coley B, Darge K, Rhee A, Chow JS. 2021 update on the urinary tract dilation (UTD) classification system: clarifications, review of the literature, and practical suggestions. Pediatr Radiol. 2022 Apr;52(4):740–751.
27. Martín-Solé O, Soria-Gondek A, Pérez-Bertólez S, Paredes P, Tarrado X, García-Aparicio L. Value of supranormal function on 99m Tc-mercaptoacetyltriglycine renal scan in paediatric patients with obstructive hydronephrosis. BJU Int. 2019 Nov;124(5):842–848.
28. Jacobson DL, Flink CC, Johnson EK, Maizels M, Yerkes EB, Lindgren BW, Liu DB, Rosoklija I, Cheng EY, Gong EM. The Correlation between Serial Ultrasound and Diuretic Renography in Children with Severe Unilateral Hydronephrosis. J Urol. 2018 Aug;200(2):440–447.

Chapter

7

Urinary Incontinence in a 5-Year-Old Male Child with Myelomeningocele

• N. Mallikarjuna Reddy

LEARNING OBJECTIVES

- Evaluation of a child with neurogenic incontinence.
- Step by step management of the child.
- Appropriate doses of medications.
- When to change the treatment parameters?
- Long-term follow-up.

INTRODUCTION

The incidence of myelodysplasia is about 9.1 per 10,000 births. About 12% of infants with myelodysplasia do not have symptoms at birth. Neurogenic bladder due to myelodysplasia in children is a debilitating illness. It has many connotations of upper tract damage, social, psychological, and sexual implications. Majority of children have normal upper tracts at birth. Untreated, 60% would develop upper tract dysfunction. Almost 50% of these children, if remain untreated, will develop ESRD (end stage renal disease). The variations of presentation are multitude. Arriving at a proper diagnosis is the cornerstone for long-term well-being.[1]

1. **What are the *goals of treatment*?**

   Ans:
   - Newborn: Preservation of renal function
   - School age: Urinary and fecal continence
   - Adolescent: Sexual function.

Case Scenario

A 5-year-old boy was brought to the clinic with a complain of incontinence of urine. He had a history of being operated for meningomyelocele at the age of 1 year.

2. **What history should be elicited in such a case?**

   Ans:

   Frequency of urination, incontinence, and type of incontinence like stress, urgency incontinence, and continuous incontinence should be elicited. Associated febrile urinary tract infection (UTI) needs to be assessed and the need for admission for the treatment of UTI should be ascertained. If the child is on CIC (clean intermittent catheterization), we need to ask the frequency of CIC and ask for history of episodes of incontinence in between the CIC. If the child is on medications, then the medications and the dosages need to be checked.

   History pertaining to the bowel habits needs to be elicited. Presence or absence of sensation of flatus and stool, constipation, and encopresis should be asked in the history.[1–5]

3. **What should be looked for while examining such a patient?**

   Ans: General appearance with physical growth, gait, and the body habitus need to be checked.

   Blood pressure needs to be checked and if hypertensive should be placed on appropriate medication. The coordination of upper limbs needs to be assessed so that we get an idea whether, as the child grows, CIC is possible. Abdominal bloating may be a sign of constipation.

   Palpation of the abdomen is essential to check for palpable stool in the colon, palpable bladder, and a renal mass. External genitalia needs to be examined thoroughly for any anatomical abnormality. The examination of spine is a must.

A focused neurological examination assessing the bulbocavernosus reflex, anal reflex and the presence of anal and urethral sensation needs to be performed. The examination of the spine is important. (Figs 7.1 and 7.2).

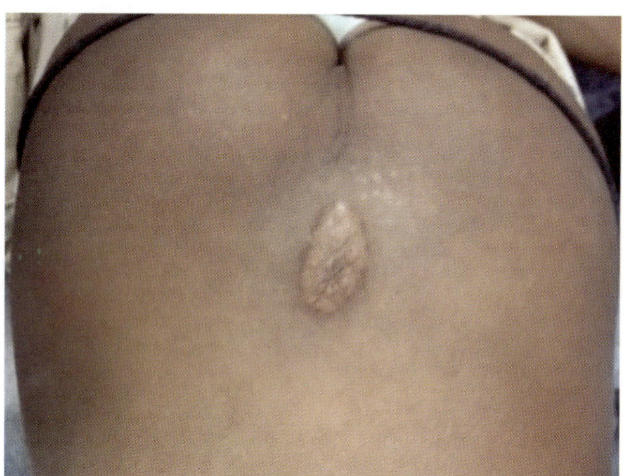

Fig. 7.1: Spina bifida occulta

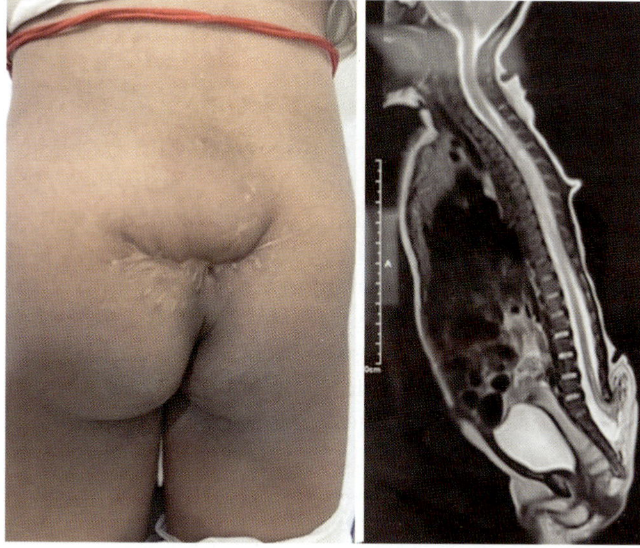

Fig. 7.2: Post-operative scar of operated MMC, MRI showing lipomeningocele

4. **What are the investigations to be done in such a case?**

   Ans:

   a. Laboratory investigations

      Renal function tests, complete blood counts, urine examination[6] and urine culture need to be performed. If there is any abnormality it needs to be further evaluated. Asymptomatic patients on CIC are bound to have pyuria and even if their urine culture is positive it does not warrant treatment with antibiotics. Presence of albuminuria is an early marker of renal disease.

   b. Frequency volume chart should be done whenever possible preferably for 3 days.

   c. Ultrasonography

      The following things should be diligently looked at and noted.

   - Presence or absence of upper tract dilatation—if present, then the grade of hydronephrosis.
   - Prevoid volume of urine on a full bladder.
   - Postvoid volume of urine if the child is voiding and is not on CIC.
   - Detrusor wall thickness is to be measured. Anything more than 4 mm is significant.

   d. Uroflowmetry

      All patients whenever possible should get a uroflowmetry done.

      Uroflowmetry with external sphincter EMG with surface electrode is a limited noninvasive urodynamics but has limited value. This modality provides assessment of the relaxation of the sphincter during voiding and provides an idea of discordance of the external sphincter.

5. **What are the indications for voiding cysto-urethrogram (VCUG)?**

   Ans: Almost all patients will need to have a VCUG done for evaluation.

   Only patients with normal upper tracts, minimal residual volume and mild symptoms can avoid a VCUG.

6. **What are the parameters to be seen in VCUG?**

   Ans:

   - Spine, bony shadows, and soft tissue shadows (Fig. 7.3).
   - Bladder capacity
   - Bladder contour
   - Presence of diverticulae
   - Presence of VUR
   - Posterior urethra (Fig. 7.4)
   - Anterior urethra and the
   - Residual urine volume (Fig. 7.5).

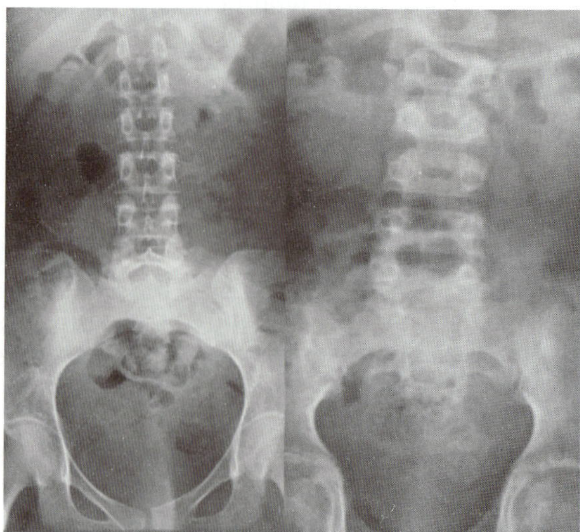

Fig. 7.3: Sacral agenesis and spina bifida

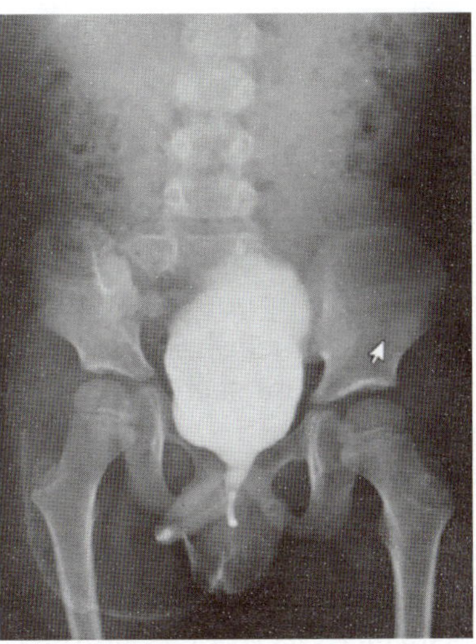

Fig. 7.4: Lax bladder neck with spina bifida

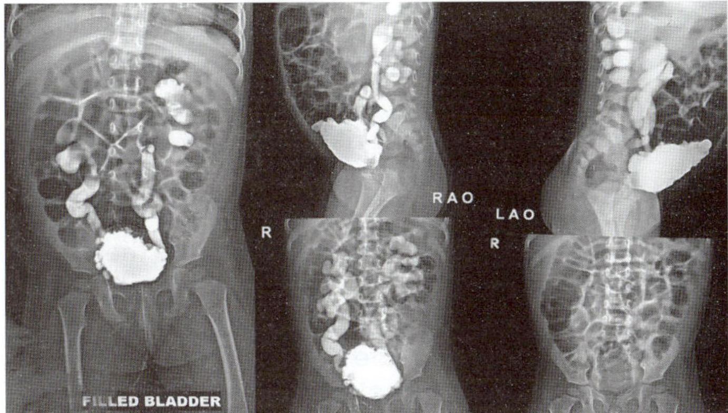

Fig. 7.5: VCUG with bilateral reflux and firtree bladder representative of neurogenic bladder

7. **What is the role of urodynamics (UDS)?**

Ans: All patients should get a baseline urodynamics preferably video urodynamics with EMG. This should be under cover of antibiotics the choice of which is based on the urine culture or the antibiotic profile of the area and the hospital.[7,8]

The general parameters evaluated in the urodynamic studies are:

- Cytometric capacity
- Filling pressure
- Bladder compliance
- Pressures during voiding
- Detrusor overactivity
- Competence of internal and external sphincters
- Sphincter dyssynergia
- Postvoid residue.

8. **What are the red flags in UDS studies?**

Ans:

1. Detrusor leak point pressure (DLPP) of > 40 cm of water in the absence of abdominal straining or detrusor contractions
2. Bladder compliance less than 20 ml/cm H_2O (such patients are 4.3 times more likely to have VUR than when it is less than 20 ml/cm H_2O)
3. Detrusor sphincter dyssynergia. (72% of children may develop complications if not properly treated)
4. Decreased bladder capacity and elevated storage pressure which are manifestations of detrusor overactivity.

9. **Do we need urodynamics in all cases?**

Ans: The emphatic answer is yes, and it is mandatory.

In cases where the facilities are not available it is safe to start on CIC. The usage of anticholinergics will be debatable as they need 2 weeks for washout before the urodynamic studies are performed and the bladder and lower urinary tract is assessed.

Baseline urodynamic parameters need to be assessed to treat and prognosticate and follow-up these children.

10. **What is the status of doing DMSA scan in these patients?**

Ans: It is indicated in children showing VUR to look for the presence or absence of scars.

DTPA/MAG3

These scans would help in the assessment of individual renal function and is also indicated where obstruction of the upper urinary tract is suspected.

The indications would be:

1. Hydronephrosis unilateral or bilateral
2. Scarred kidneys
3. To evaluate differential function of kidneys
4. Assessment of function prior to reconstructive surgery

Practical classification of neurogenic bladder (Table 7.1).

TABLE 7.1: Practical classification of neurogenic bladder

	Detrusor overactivity	*Detrusor underactivity*
Sphincter overactivity	SO/DO With sphincter dyssynergia	SO/DU Incomplete bladder emptying
Sphincter underactivity	SU/DO Incontinence not deleterious to renal function	SU/DU Incontinence incomplete emptying risk of UTI

1. Overactive bladder with overactive sphincter
2. Overactive bladder with underactive sphincter
3. Underactive bladder with overactive sphincter
4. Underactive bladder with underactive sphincter

The level of myelodysplasia does not correlate with the extent of neurological damage of the bladder and the sphincter.

11. What is the most important aspect in treating these children?

Ans:

- CIC is the cornerstone of conservative management.
- All patients except those with a lax urinary sphincter, mild symptoms and insignificant postvoid residue need to be initiated on CIC.
- It should be done 3–4 hourly. In the night, the child needs to be woken up at least once to do CIC
- The amount of fluid intake should be restricted appropriately and significantly restricted at night to decrease nocturia[9,10] (Table 7.2).

TABLE 7.2: Overview of treatment of neurogenic bladder

UDS variables or imaging findings	*CIC*	*Anticholinergics*
Poor compliance	Y	Y
DO	Y	Y
DSD	Y	Y
LPP>40	Y	Y
Incoming emptying	Y	
VUR/HDN	Y	Y

12. How do you evaluate a newborn with myelomeningocele?

Ans:

- Anal reflex/ARM
  - Absence
  - Presence intact sacral cord DSD alert
- Emptying ability and residual urine
  - 4-hour voiding observation.
- UDS: The expected bladder capacity is
  - The fill rate should be kept at 1 ml/kg/min and the bladder filling done
- Parameters to be evaluated
  - Residual volume, compliance, contractility, leak point pressure, sphincter EMG
- Care of performing UDS in newborn
  - Child needs oral sedation
  - Saline should be warm
  - Avoid anaesthesia
  - Need to do at least 3 runs to get proper information
- Other investigations
  - Ultrasonography,
  - MCUG
  - DMSA or MAG3

13. What are the management options in a neonate?

Ans:

- Bladder empty, upper tracts: Normal
  - No intervention
- Retention with normal upper tracts
  - CIC every 3 hours
- Retention with upper tract dilation
  - CIC with anticholinergics like oxybutynin, tolterodine (*see* section on CIC for detailed dosages)
- Vesicostomy

14. What are the takeaway in prenatal of myelomeningocele study (MOMS) trial?

Ans:

- Decreased need for VP shunting
- The urological improvement is not clear
- Carr found that 18.5% success for toilet training in prenatally closed compared to 8.3%
- Delaying closure beyond 72 hours increased the incidence of febrile UTI and VUR and poor UDS parameters.
- Flowchart 7.1 for evaluation of a child with neurogenic bladder according to the age of diagnosis.

15. What is the appropriate method of performing CIC with a reusable catheter?

Ans:

1. Wash hands or sanitize hands before touching the catheter.
2. Clean the genitals with saline or water. Do not use sanitizer.
3. Pick the catheter (do not wash it as water is not sterile), apply lubricant jelly.
4. Insert the catheter into the urethra and push it 1 cm beyond the distance when first drops of urine are seen.
5. Allow the bladder to empty fully.
6. Pull the catheter slowly to empty the residual urine.
7. Wash the catheter and place it in a dry cloth in a dry place so that there are no traces of water externally or internally in the catheter.
8. Measure the quantity of urine every time one catheterizes once a week for 24 hours.

16. What is the age to start CIC?

Ans:

1. CIC should be started in the newborn age. Even if the sphincter is lax this will allow the mother and child to get used to the procedure.
2. It is easy to stop CIC rather than starting it.[9]

Flowchart 7.1: Algorithm of treatment of neurogenic bladder (*Courtesy*: ESPU Guidelines 2023)

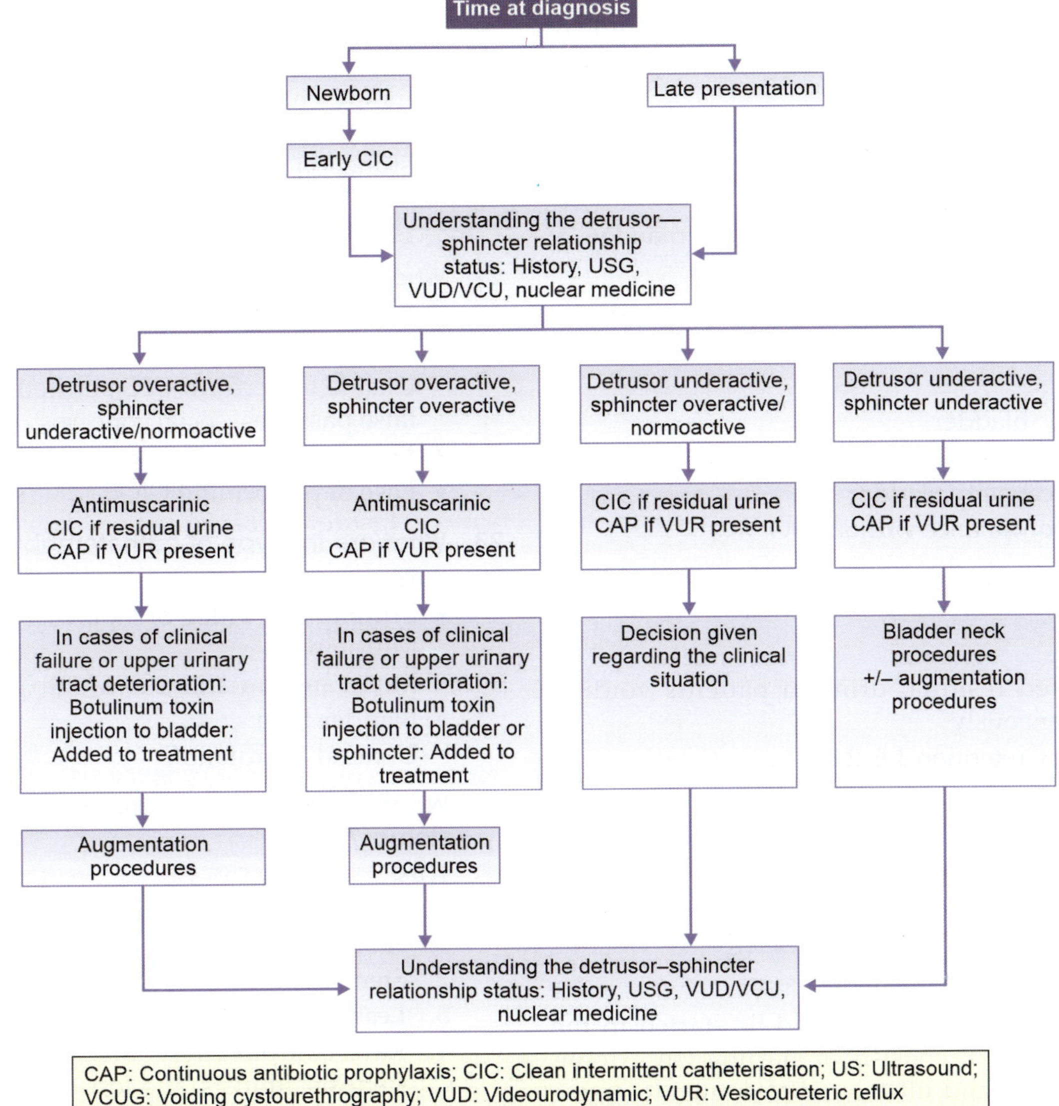

CAP: Continuous antibiotic prophylaxis; CIC: Clean intermittent catheterisation; US: Ultrasound; VCUG: Voiding cystourethrography; VUD: Videourodynamic; VUR: Vesicoureteric reflux

17. What are the medications used?

Ans:

Anticholinergics

The anticholinergics which are approved for pediatric usage are.

1. Oxybutynin 0.2/0.4/0.6 mg/kg/day in 2–4 divided doses per day
2. Tolterodine 0.5–4.0 mg/day or 0.1 mg/kg/day to a max of 8 mg/day
3. Propioverine 0.7–0.8 mg/kg/day
4. Solifenacin 1.25–10 mg/day
5. Mirabegron 12.5–50 mg/day
6. Intravesical oxybutynin 10 mg showed to be safe and equally efficacious with decreased side effects.

The drugs must be administered till the maximum dosage is reached or adequate response is obtained, or significant side effects develop where the dosage is de-escalated.[11–14]

Double anticholinergic therapy

In cases with inadequate response the addition of tolterodine, Solifenacin or mirabegron to oxybutynin is a safe alternative and is tolerated well. The adjusted dose regime is safe and is efficacious than the single drug regimen.[13]

Alpha blockers have a limited role in cases with detrusor sphincter dyssynergia. Most used drug is tamsulosin 0.2–0.4 mg/day.[15]

18. When is intra-detrusor onabotulinum toxin A indicated?

Ans:

1. Inadequate response to anticholinergics. Leak in between CIC intervals, upper tract dilatation not responding to CIC and anticholinergics.
2. Detrusor sphincter dyssynergia. 100 IU of Botox is given intradetrusor and 100 units are injected

into the sphincter via cystoscope or perineum in males and periurethral in females.[16–22]

3. Multiple sittings can be given to a maximum of 12. Minimum gap needs to be 3 months before a retreatment is done.
4. The second dose is given around 4–6 months after the first dosage and from the 3rd dose onwards 9–12 monthly.
5. Reassessment of the urinary tract is mandatory before every reinjection on Botox.[16–20]

19. What are the contraindications for intra-detrusor Botox injection?

Ans:
- Fibrotic bladder
- Acontractile bladder
- Small capacity bladder
- Poor compliance without DO

20. What are the adverse effects of Botox?

Ans:
- UTI
- Elevated residual urine in patients voiding spontaneously
- Urinary retention 1.6–2.8%

21. Is DEFLUX injection for VUR indicated?

Ans: Yes, in a very few situations where there is significant VUR associated with recurrent febrile UTI and renal damage. It is generally combined with Botox to the detrusor muscle.

Overview of management...

Proactive management should be started in the newborn age. It consists of starting CIC, doing urodynamics and ultrasound abdomen to assess the bladder and the upper tracts. If the bladder is hostile anticholinergic medication needs to be started. This is the preferred mode of treatment.

Expectant management is also recommended line of therapy where the treatment is started once there are changes in the upper tract. This has a disadvantage of having higher rate of upper tract dysfunction and incontinence episodes.

Surgical Management

22. What are the indications for catheterisable stomas?

Ans:
- Sensate urethra
- Unable to perform CIC perurethrum, stricture, false passages, social concerns.
- Independence from caregivers
- Ease of performing CIC

23. What are the type of catheterisable stomas?

Ans:
- Mitrofanoff (Video of laparoscopic and robotic Mitrofanoff)
- Monti and variations of Monti
- Bladder tube
- Ureteral Mitrofanoff

24. What are the complications of catheterisable stomas?

Ans:
1. Stenosis seen in 25–30% of Mitrofanoff stomas (Fig. 7.7).
2. Stenosis 12% in Monti stomas (Fig. 7.6).
3. Leak through the stoma (6% will needful revision)
4. Rare complications are kinks, anastomotic stenosis, fibrosis, and loss of stoma (Fig. 7.8). (Video of Mitrofanoff to be included)

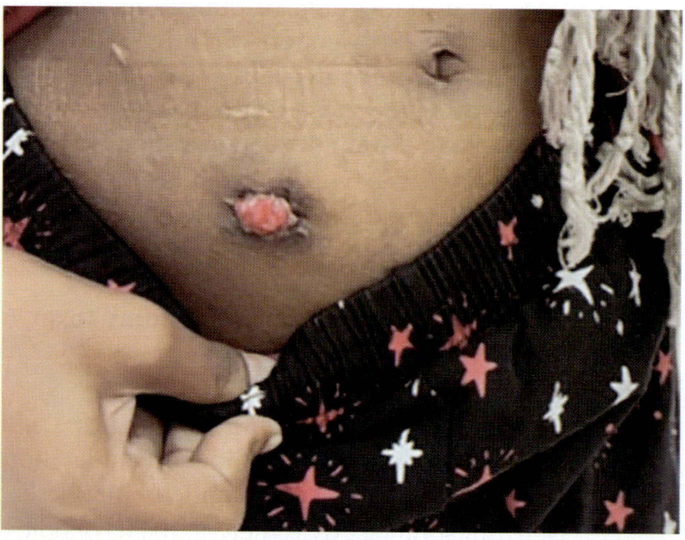

Fig. 7.6: Monti stoma

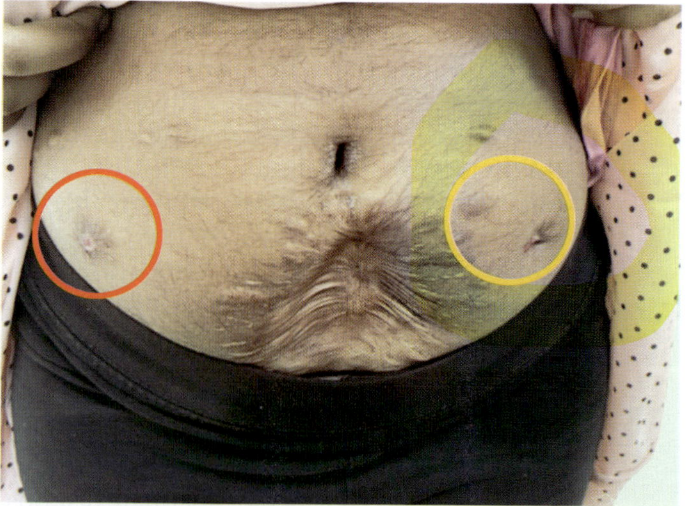

Fig. 7.7: Yellow mark Monti and red mark MACE stoma with scarred abdomen following augmentation

Fig. 7.8: Images of external appearance Mitrofanoff operative

25. What are the indications for augmentation cystoplasty?

Ans:

1. Small capacity bladder not responding to medications (Fig. 7.9).

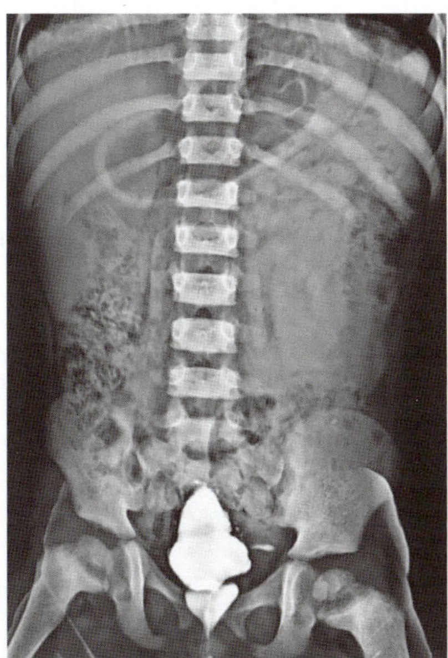

Fig. 7.9: Post-augmentation cystoplasty

2. Poorly compliant with deteriorating upper tracts
3. Intractable incontinence
4. Incompetent bladder neck where bladder neck is transected and closed, or a sling is placed to occlude the bladder neck.

26. What are the contraindications for augmentation cystoplasty?

Ans:

1. Creatinine more than 2 mg% or GFR less than 30 ml
2. Patients whose follow-up is questionable.
3. Crohn's disease and ulcerative colitis
4. Patients who cannot catheterize or lack of constant caregivers.[23–27]

27. What should be the management of constipation in these children?

Ans:

Laxatives

First line Polyethylene glycol

Second line Magnesium sulphate

Enemas

Dietary recommendation on increase in fibre diet.

MACE

Refractory fecal incontinence MACE is an appropriate operation to perform antegrade enemas to empty the colon and prevent fecal soiling (Fig. 7.10).

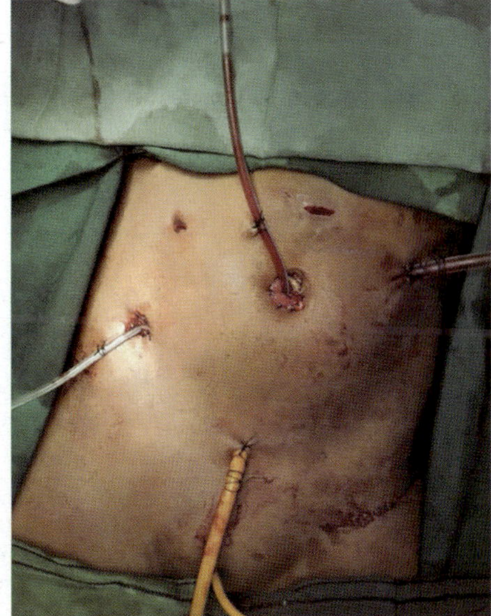

Fig. 7.10: Immediate postoperative image with MACE in the flank and Monti in the umbilicus

28. What should be follow-up strategy in these children?

Ans: These children need lifelong follow-up. Flowchart 7.2 illustrates the follow-up protocol.

SUMMARY

- Neurogenic detrusor-sphincter dysfunction (NDSD) may result in different forms of LUTD and ultimately result in incontinence, UTIs, VUR, and renal scarring.
- Bladder sphincter dysfunction correlates poorly with the type and level of the spinal cord lesion.
- Urodynamic, and functional classifications are more practical in defining the extent of the pathology and in guiding treatment planning.
- Children with neurogenic bladder can have disturbances of bowel function as well as urinary function which require monitoring and, if needed, management.
- The main goals of treatment are prevention of urinary tract deterioration and achievement of continence at an appropriate age.
- Urodynamic studies should be performed in every patient with spina bifida as well as in every child with high suspicion of a neurogenic bladder to estimate the risk for the upper urinary tract and to evaluate the function of the detrusor and the sphincter.
- In all newborns, intermittent catheterisation (IC) should be started soon after birth. In those with a clear underactive sphincter and no overactivity, starting IC may be delayed. If IC is delayed, closely monitor babies for urinary tract infections, upper tract changes (US) and the lower tract (UD).
- Start early anticholinergic medication in the newborns with suspicion of an overactive detrusor.
- The use of suburothelial or intradetrusor injection of onabotulinum toxin A is an alternative and a less invasive option in children who are refractory to anticholinergics in contrast to bladder augmentation.
- Treatment of faecal incontinence is important to gain continence and independence. Treatment should be started with mild laxatives, rectal suppositories as well as digital stimulation. If not, sufficient trans anal irrigation is recommended, if not practicable or feasible, a Malone antegrade colonic enema

Flowchart 7.2: Algorithm of treatment of neurogenic bladder (*Courtesy:* ESPU Guidelines 2023)

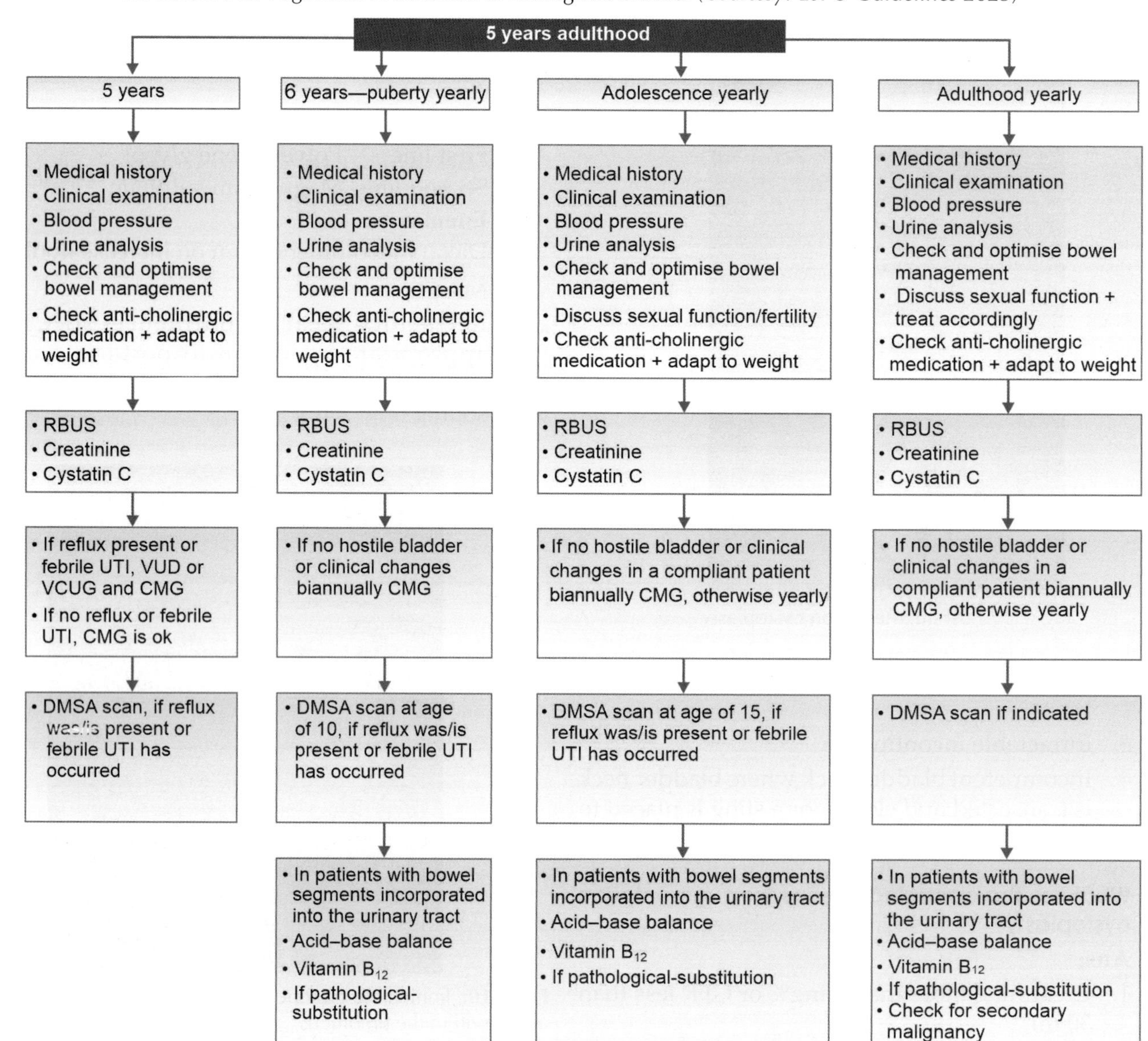

(MACE)/antegrade continence enema (ACE) stoma should be discussed.

- Ileal or colonic bladder augmentation is recommended in patients with therapy resistant overactivity of the detrusor, small capacity, and poor compliance, which may cause upper tract damage and incontinence. The risk of surgical and nonsurgical complications and consequences outweigh the risk of permanent damage of the upper urinary tract +/-incontinence due to the detrusor.
- In patients with a neurogenic bladder and a weak sphincter, a bladder outlet procedure should be offered. It should be done in most patients together with a bladder augmentation.
- Creation of a continent cutaneous catheterisable channel should be offered to patients who have difficulties in performing an IC through the urethra.
- A life-long follow-up of renal and reservoir function should be available and offered to every patient. Addressing sexuality and fertility starting before/during puberty should be offered.
- Urinary tract infections are common in children with neurogenic bladders, however, only symptomatic UTIs should be treated.

REFERENCES

1. Stuart B Bauer, Paul F Austin, Yazan F Rawashdeh, Tom P de Jong, Israel Franco, Charlotte Siggard, *et al.* International Children's Continence Society's recommendations for initial diagnostic evaluation and follow-up in congenital neuropathic bladder and bowel dysfunction in children. Neurourology and Urodynamics, 2012. 31: 610.
https://pubmed.ncbi.nlm.nih.gov/22532312/
2. Bauer, S.B. The argument for early assessment and treatment of infants with spina bifida. Pediatr Urol, 2000. 23: 2. [No abstract available].
3. Jessica C Lloyd, Unwanaobong Nseyo, Ramiro J Madden-Fuentes, Sherry S Ross, John S Wiener, Jonathan C Routh. Reviewing definitions of urinary continence in the contemporary spina bifida literature: A call for clarity. J Pediatr Urol,2013. 9: 567.
https://pubmed.ncbi.nlm.nih.gov/52491875/
4. SB Bauer, M Hallett, S Khoshbin, R L Lebowitz, KR Winston, S Gibson., *et al.* Predictive value of urodynamic evaluation in newborns with myelodysplasia. Jama, 1984. 252: 650.
https://pubmed.ncbi.nlm.nih.gov/6737668/
5. David B Joseph, Michelle A Baum, Stacy T Tanaka, Dominic C Frimberger, Rosalia Misseri, Rose Khavari., *et al.* Urologic guidelines for the care and management of people with spina bifida.
J Pediatr Rehab Med, 2020. 13: 479.
https://pubmed.ncbi.nlm.nih.gov/33252091
6. Rachel O Millner, Janae Preece, Ann Salvator, Daryl J McLeod, Christina B Ching, Brian Becknell., *et al.* Albuminuria in Pediatric Neurogenic Bladder: Identifying an Earlier Marker of Renal Disease. Urology, 2019. 133: 199.
https://pubmed.ncbi.nlm.nih.gov/31454657/
7. Richard Foon, Philip Toozs-Hobson, Pallavi Latthe., *et al.* Prophylactic antibiotics to reduce the risk of urinary tract infections after urodynamic studies. Cochrane Database Syst Rev, 2012. 10: CD008224.
https://pubmed.ncbi.nlm.nih.gov/23076941/
8. Devon C Snow-Lisy, Elizabeth B Yerkes, Earl Y Cheng, Update on Urological Management of Spina Bifida from Prenatal Diagnosis to Adulthood. J Urol, 2015. 194: 288.
https://pubmed.ncbi.nlm.nih.gov/25839383/
9. Wael Elzeneini, Ramy Waly, David Marshall, Alan Bailie. Early start of clean intermittent catheterization versus expectant management in children with spina bifida. J Pediatr Surg, 2019. 54: 322.
https://pubmed.ncbi.nlm.nih.gov/30558962/
10. KN Moore, M Fader, K Getliffe. Long-term bladder management by intermittent catheterisation in adults and children. Cochrane Database Syst Rev, 2007: CD006008.
https://pubmed.ncbi.nlm.nih.gov/17943874/
11. Karl-Erik Andersson, Christopher R Chapple, Linda Cardozo, Francisco Cruz, Hashim Hashim, Martin C Michel., *et al.* Pharmacological treatment of overactive bladder: report from the International Consultation on Incontinence. Curr Opin Urol, 2009. 19: 380.
https://pubmed.ncbi.nlm.nih.gov/19448545
12. Pramod P Reddy , Niels G Borgstein, Rien J M Nijman, Pamela I Ellsworth. Long-term efficacy and safety of tolterodine in children with neurogenic detrusor overactivity. J Pediatr Urol,2008. 4: 428.
https://pubmed.ncbi.nlm.nih.gov/50195955
13. Geneviève Nadeau, Annette Schröder, Katherine Moore, Lucie Genois, Pascale Lamontagne, Micheline Hamel., *et al.* Double anticholinergic therapy for refractory neurogenic and nonneurogenic detrusor overactivity in children: Long-term results of a prospective open-label study. Can Urol Assoc J, 2014. 8: 175.
https://pubmed.ncbi.nlm.nih.gov/25024786
14. Cristian Sager, Marianela Sanmartino, Carol Burek, Yesica Ruth Gomez, Mariana Vazquez Patiño, Santiago Weller., *et al.* Efficacy and safety of Mirabegron as adjuvant treatment in children with refractory neurogenic bladder dysfunction. J Pediatr Urol,2020.16: 655.
https://pubmed.ncbi.nlm.nih.gov/32800710
15. P F Austin, Y L Homsy, J L Masel, M P Cain, A J Casale, R C Rink. alpha-Adrenergic blockade in children with neuropathic and nonneuropathic voiding dysfunction. J Urol, 1999. 162: 1064.
https://pubmed.ncbi.nlm.nih.gov/10458432/
16. Maya Horst, Daniel M Weber, Christine Bodmer, Rita Gobet. Repeated Botulinum-A toxin injection in the treatment of neuropathic bladder dysfunction and poor bladder compliance in children with myelomeningocele. Neurourol Urodyn, 2011. 30: 1546.
https://pubmed.ncbi.nlm.nih.gov/51478950/
17. Yavuz Onur Danacioglu, Ferhat Keser, Cevper Ersoz, Salih Polat, Ali Egemen Avci, Senad Kalkan., *et al.* Factors predicting the success of intradetrusor onabotulinum toxin A treatment in children with neurogenic bladders due to myelomeningocele: The outcomes of a large cohort. J Pediatr Urol, 2021.
https://pubmed.ncbi.nlm.nih.gov/33712371/
18. Juliette Hascoet, Andrea Manunta, Charlène Brochard, Alexis Arnaud, Mireille Damphousse, Hélène Menard., *et al.* Outcomes of intra-detrusor injections of botulinum toxin in patients with spina bifida: A systematic review. Neurourology and Urodynamics., 2016.
https://pubmed.ncbi.nlm.nih.gov/27187872/
19. Cristian Sager, Carol Burek, Juan Bortagaray, Juan Pablo Corbetta, Santiago Weller, Victor Durán., *et al.* Repeated

injections of intradetrusor onabotulinumtoxinA as adjunctive treatment of children with neurogenic bladder. Pediatric Surgery International, 2014. 30: 79.
https://pubmed.ncbi.nlm.nih.gov/52736614

20. S Tiryaki, I Yagmur, Y Parlar, K Ozel, C Akyildiz, A Avanoglu., *et al.* Botulinum injection is useless on fibrotic neuropathic bladders. J Pediatr Urol,2015. 11: 27.e1.
https://pubmed.ncbi.nlm.nih.gov/25448589/

21. Israel Franco, Lori Landau-Dyer, Ginger Isom-Batz, Therese Collett, Edward F Reda. The Use of Botulinum Toxin A Injection for the Management of External Sphincter Dyssynergia in Neurologically Normal Children. J Urol, 2007. 178: 1775.
https://pubmed.ncbi.nlm.nih.gov/47368508

22. I Mokhless, S Gaafar, K Fouda, M Shafik, A Assem. Botulinum A toxin urethral sphincter injection in children with nonneurogenic neurogenic bladder. J Urol, 2006. 176: 1767.
https://pubmed.ncbi.nlm.nih.gov/16945643/

22. Raimund Stein, Annette Schröder, Joachim W Thüroff. Bladder augmentation and urinary diversion in patients with neurogenic bladder: surgical considerations. J Pediatr Urol, 2012.8:153.
https://pubmed.ncbi.nlm.nih.gov/22264521

23. S Herschorn, R J Hewitt. Patient perspective of long-term outcome of augmentation cystoplasty for neurogenic bladder. Urology, 1998. 52:672.
https://pubmed.ncbi.nlm.nih.gov/9763092/

24. Ricardo Medel, Adolfo C Ruarte, Marcela Herrera, Roberto Castera, Miguel L Podesta. Urinary continence outcome after augmentation ileocystoplasty as a single surgical procedure in patients with myelodysplasia. J Urol, 2002. 168: 1849.
https://pubmed.ncbi.nlm.nih.gov/12352374/

25. Alexander Kavanagh, Kourosh Afshar, Heidi Scott, Andrew E MacNeily. Bladder neck closure in conjunction with enterocystoplasty and Mitrofanoff diversion for complex incontinence: Closing the door for good. J Urol, 2012.188: 1561.
https://pubmed.ncbi.nlm.nih.gov/52167570

26. Alice Faure, Rebecca Cooksey, Aurore Bouty, Alan Woodward, John Hutson, Mike O'Brien., *et al.* Bladder continent Catheterisable conduit (the Mitrofanoff procedure): Long-term issues that should not be underestimated. J Pediatr Surg, 2016.11.
https://pubmed.ncbi.nlm.nih.gov/27707652/

Chapter

8

Nocturnal Enuresis

• *Rahul Rajendra Kapoor*

LEARNING OBJECTIVES

- How to differentiate primary nocturnal enuresis from other causes (non-monosymptomatic enuresis)?
- Learn the indication and choice of therapy.
- Choice of drug therapy at right dose and right time to achieve maximum benefit.

INTRODUCTION

Nocturnal enuresis (NE) (bedwetting) or monosymptomatic nocturnal enuresis is a common childhood problem, defined as presence of intermittent bed wetting usually more than 2 episodes/week. To avoid confusion the international children's continence society has updated in 2014 and defined enuresis as wetting that occurs at night and no longer refers to daytime incontinence as diurnal enuresis.[1] The term diurnal enuresis should be avoided; instead, daytime incontinence should be used.

NE is a benign condition, twice more common in boys than girls, present in around 5–10% of the children by seven years of age. The data on Indian prevalence of nocturnal enuresis is limited but is around 7.61–16.3%.[2] Prevalence is found to be higher in children from poor socio-economic class than upper middle class in rural Indian population.[3] Other contributing factors are living with a single parent, living with stepparents, parents with health problems, conflicts at home, stress due to enuresis, scolding, and poor scholastic performance.[2] Also, enuresis is found to be more common with history of birth asphyxia, cesarean section, low birth weight and lack of breastfeeding. Studies have suggested autosomal dominant type of inheritance with 90% penetrance.[4] Hereditary predisposition is suggested by three to five times increased incidence if one or both parents have had similar childhood history.

NE continues to resolve at 15% per year and persists in around 1–2/100 in adolescent age group. There can be primary or secondary nocturnal enuresis. In primary enuresis, there is no nocturnal dry period of 6 months, while in secondary nocturnal enuresis, dry spell of around 6 months exists with recurrence of symptoms. Primary nocturnal enuresis contributes to 80% of the cases.

Even though benign in nature, it demands treatment as it is associated with social stigma in the form of emotional stress, social restriction, and embarrassment both for the child and the family. These children will avoid social participation like school camp, sleep over due to fear of embarrassment. It is also responsible for depression, lack of self-esteem and poor academic results. Usually, medical treatment is offered once child is more than 5 years of age.

Case Scenario

A 7-year-old male child came to the OPD accompanied by parents for bedwetting. He wets his bed since birth, usually 2–3 times a week. His elder brother also had a similar history but became dry by 5 years. There are no daytime symptoms. He can hold urine for some time and does not have to run to pass urine. Usually, undergarments are not wet during daytime. No constipation or fecal soiling of clothes is mentioned by parents. There is no episode of febrile urinary tract infection in the past. As his symptoms were present even at 7 years of age urology consultation was taken.

1. **Is there any demographic difference seen in enuresis?**

   Ans: No prevalence difference is seen among various cultures. The prevalence and resolution rates stand to remain same. Though it is more common in boys than girls, this difference decreases after the age of 10 years.

2. **What is the pathophysiology for primary nocturnal enuresis?**

Ans: The pathophysiology of nocturnal enuresis is multi-factorial as high arousal threshold, vasopressin deficiency and nocturnal overactive bladder, all tends to play a role.[5] These factors tend to be present in various combinations in every patient, explaining why one treatment does not work in all patients. Two hypotheses are put forth as a reason for nocturnal enuresis (Flowchart 8.1).

Flowchart 8.1: Pathophysiology

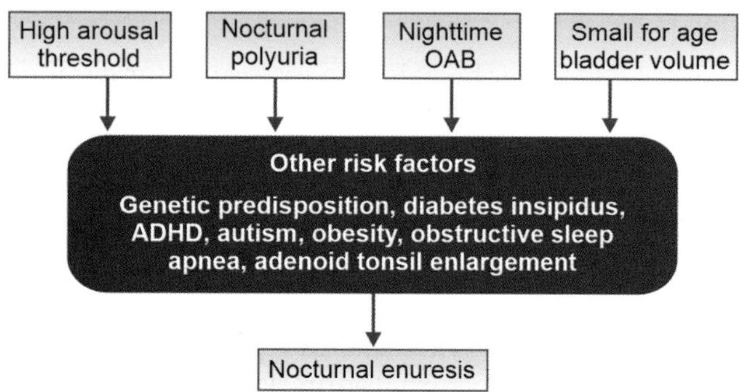

First is high arousal threshold from sleep. NE occurs early in the sleep, primarily in sleep stage 2 and deep sleep.[6] It is considered that these children are deep sleepers, and it is difficult to wake them up. Contrary to this belief, children with higher arousal threshold from sleep are paradoxically associated with disturbed sleep pattern. Sleep fragmentation and periodic limb movement which is suggestive of cortical arousal is seen more frequently in children with nocturnal enuresis.[7] Also, high arousal threshold is not only seen as a contributing factor but as an outcome of disturbed sleep due to obstructed sleep or contracting bladder (OAB).

Multiple studies have shown correlation between NE and obstructive sleep apnea (OSA). OSA is defined as repetitive partial or complete airway closure that disrupt breathing during sleep and leading to repetitive arousal. Reasons for OSA can be obesity or adeno-tonsillar hypertrophy. Children with NE were found to have higher apnea-hypopnea index, snoring, and other sleep disordered breathing (SDB) symptoms like anxiety and sweating.[8] This is proven by the fact that treatment for OSA with adenotonsillectomy leads to resolution or improvements of NE in 33–74% and 23–31% of children, respectively[9]. There is increased association of nocturnal enuresis with obesity. Increased intra-abdominal and intra-vesical pressure, hyperglycemia, sleep disordered breathing and psychological stress all due to obesity tend to play a role for nocturnal enuresis.[10]

Imbalance in nighttime urine production and bladder capacity is another etiological factor. This can be in the form of "nocturnal polyuria", "nighttime OAB" or "small for age bladder volume". Nocturnal polyuria is due to vasopressin deficiency or altered circadian rhythm[11]. Impaired or deficient growth hormone release may inhibit vasopressin release, causing excess urine production at night[3]. But nocturnal polyuria does not explain why these children do not wake up to full bladder stimulus, as not all children with nocturnal polyuria are enuretic. Many non-polyuric children with enuresis often pass urine in small volume, suggestive of nocturnal detrusor overactivity.[12]

3. **How to evaluate a child in the OPD?**

Ans: Usually the child feels embarrassed to talk and developing a rapport with the child is of paramount importance. Complete family history should be elucidated from parents.

In every case both parents and child should be interviewed. Focus during the history taking is to rule out symptoms indicating non-mono symptomatic nocturnal enuresis. Following points should be noted:

1. Frequency and pattern of nocturnal enuresis (wet night during week or months, approximate time, and number of times child wets bed during every night)
2. Family history (similar history in parents and other siblings)
3. Details of previous treatment taken
4. Daily fluid intake and urination including the time of the day when child drinks maximum water.
5. Stool frequency and habits
6. Sleeping arrangement at home
7. Psychological effect on the child. What bring the parents to urologist?

Bowel bladder dysfunction (BBD) or dysfunctional voiding syndrome can present with lower urinary tract symptoms (LUTS) in daytime, recurrent UTI or bowel dysfunction.

Symptoms suggestive of BBD (dysfunctional voiding) could be during storage or voiding phase:

1. Abnormal urinary frequency (>8 or <3 per day),
2. Urgency
3. Wetting of undergarments
4. Intermittent or continuous urine leak
5. Straining to pass urine or

6. Abnormal holding maneuver like leg crossing, standing on tip toe while passing urine.

History suggestive of bowel dysfunction are
1. Bowel movement less than 3 per week
2. Fecal soiling of clothes.

Parents should be counseled to pay attention regarding the presence of the above symptoms.

4. What other signs or symptoms should be paid attention to besides bowel bladder symptoms?

Ans: Associated findings seen in these children are:
1. Obesity, obstructive sleep apnea, snoring, mouth breathing, sweating during sleep[13] or increase limb movements. Obesity[10] and allergic diseases are frequently seen in these children.
2. Adeno-tonsillar hypertrophy can also be present.
3. Neurodevelopmental disorders like attention deficit/hyperkinetic syndrome, autism spectrum disorder and learning disabilities are associated with incontinence and daytime urinary and bowel symptoms.[14] Behavioral disorder like ADHD, depression should be looked for diligently and their presence suggests poor treatment outcome.[15] Delayed milestone and other learning abilities should be looked for. Stressful situations in the family, e.g. loss of loved one, arrival of newborn, parental disputes can also trigger secondary NE. All these behavioral and psychological signs should be looked for. In the presence of above signs or symptoms, it is important to involve a psychiatrist.

5. What physical examination is needed in children with nocturnal enuresis?

Ans: Usually, the physical examination is normal in enuretic child. But a quick and focused assessment should be done (Flowchart 8.2).
1. Abdominal examination to look for palpable bladder or loaded colon is done.
2. External genitalia are examined for any anatomical anomalies or presence of excoriation of skin.
3. The lower back is also inspected for cutaneous lesions, dimple, or tuft of hair suggestive of spina bifida or its variants.
4. Attention is paid to clothes if they are wet or fecal soiling is present.
5. Height and weight of the child should be noted. Growth abnormality can point toward renal impairment.
6. Signs suggestive of sexual abuse should be looked which can be the cause of secondary or persistent enuresis.[3]

Flowchart 8.2: Treatment algorithm

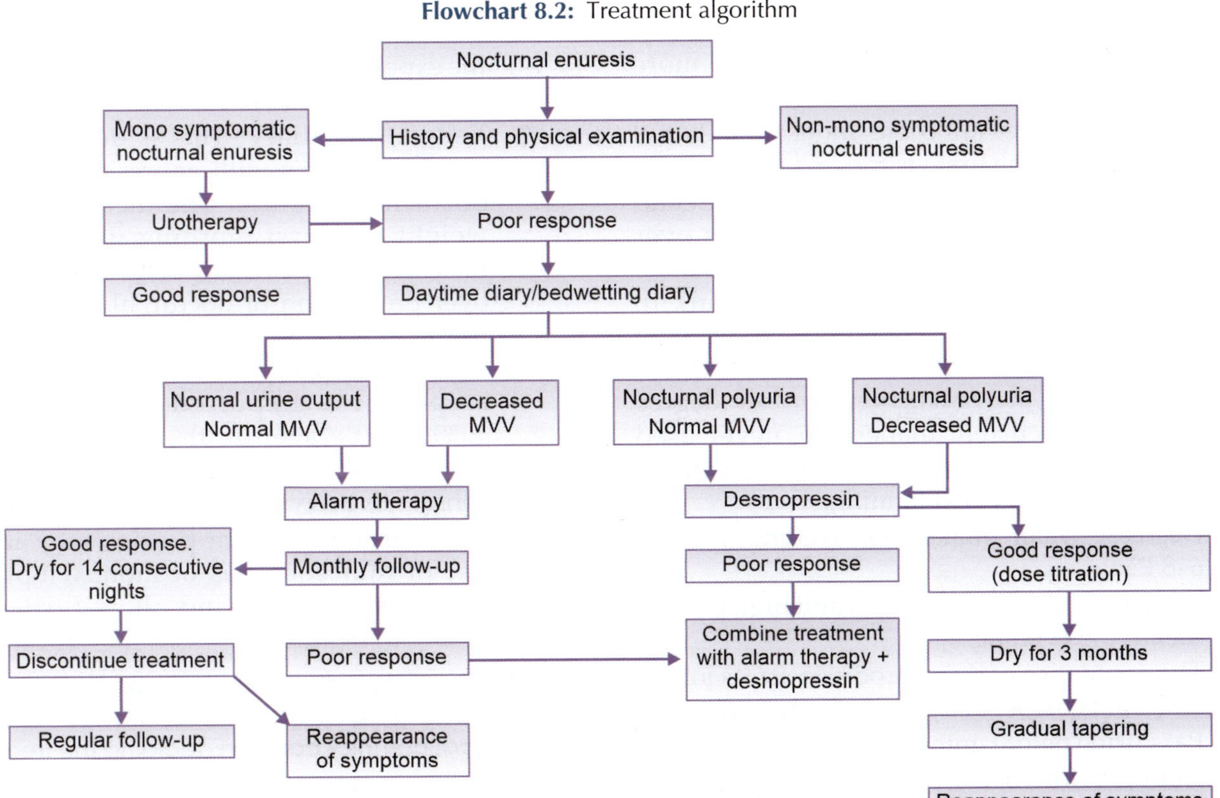

6. What investigations should be done on the first visit?

Ans: Usually no investigations are needed during the first visit. There is controversy regarding performance of urine routine and microscopy. Urine analysis can be performed to rule out ketoacidosis, diabetes insipidus, sudden onset of NE and urinary tract infection (UTI).[16] Uroflowmetry and ultrasound does not give any additional information and are usually not indicated.[17] Other investigation like voiding cystourethrogram or urodynamics are also indicated only in non-monosymptomatic nocturnal enuresis children only.

7. What should be the management plan during the first OPD visit?

Ans: Counseling of the parents and the child is most important. Usually telling that in most of the children symptoms disappear with time with annual cure rate of 15% will allay the anxiety. Treatment is recommended only when child is more than 5 years age. Parents should be told not to punish, humiliate, or compare with other children. As suggested besides urine analysis no further tests are indicated. Usually, urotherapy is offered as a primary therapy during the first visit.

8. What are the components of urotherapy?

Ans: Simple behavioral methods may be superior to no active treatment but appear to be inferior to enuresis alarm therapy and some drug therapy (such as imipramine and amitriptyline). Simple behavioral therapies could be tried as the first line treatment before considering enuresis alarm therapy or drug therapy, which may be more demanding and have adverse effects.[18]

Following measures (all come under urotherapy) can be offered at the first visit:

1. Dry–bed training: It involves waking the child on a schedule of decreasing intervals over several nights. The child is made to change clothes and bedding (if wet) and walk to the toilet if voiding is required. Predictor of successful outcome after 6 months of dry-bed training are female gender, low degree of enuresis, current diaper use, never used anticholinergics in past and degree of enuresis 6 weeks after dry-bed training.[19]
2. Decrease water intake after evening (around 6–8 PM)
3. Restrict salt intake (fast food) and high protein diet in the evening
4. The avoidance of dairy products, fruits juices, and fluids before bedtime is also beneficial.
5. Pass urine before going to bed
6. Get up before usual time of bed wetting and pass urine.
7. Restricting electronic device usage.
8. Treating constipation.

Other therapies like acupuncture and hypnotherapy were found to be better than placebo in reducing the number of bed wetting episodes, but found to be inferior to alarm therapy.[20,21]

9. How to proceed if child did not get relief and visits again?

Ans: Active intervention in the form of alarm therapy or desmopressin are indicated only when urotherapy failed to demonstrate any benefit even after 3–6 months. At this point, physical examination and history needs to be repeated. Physical examination (back and spine) to look for occult neurological disease should be done. Ask for any subtle signs of daytime lower urinary tract symptoms (LUTS). Urine routine and examination can be performed. Voiding and drinking habit (frequency–volume chart) for 2 days should be asked for. Constipation is more common than thought in the children and Bristol stool chart can be used to document presence of constipation. Uroflowmetry or ultrasound KUB is indicated in unusual cases only.

10. What are the various types of voiding diaries?

Ans:

1. **Daytime diary:** This is usually asked to assess the child's bladder capacity by measuring MVV (maximum voided volume). The first morning void is excluded. It can be small (if less than 65%) or large (if more than 150%) of the expected bladder capacity. The diary needs to be prepared over 2 weekends (Table 8.1).
2. **Bedwetting diary:** This is done to register number of days with enuresis and diagnose nocturnal polyuria. The increase in diaper weight and first morning urine sample is measured. Nocturnal polyuria is defined as over production of nocturnal urine. Usually, nighttime urine production of more than 130% of expected bladder capacity is defined as polyuria. Expected bladder capacity = 30 + [30 × age] till the age when capacity reached 400 ml. Diary is made over seven consecutive days/night (Table 8.2).

Information from diaries may identify one of four subtypes of monosymptomatic nocturnal enuresis and allow further fine-tuning of treatment.

11. How to divide patients into various categories according to the voiding diaries and what implications they carry on deciding the treatment?

Ans: After complete evaluation, we can divide children into either 4 categories as follows:

TABLE 8.1: Voiding diary (Frequency volume chart)

	Monday	Tuesday	Wednesday	Thursday	Friday	Saturday	Sunuday
Time to bed							
Wake up time							
Dry night							
Wet night							
Got up to pass urine. Measure volume							
Volume to first urine passed in morning							
Clear bowel							
Total night time urine production Night time urine volume + first morning urine volume/increase diaper weight							

TABLE 8.2: Bed wetting diary

	Water intake (ml)	Urine output (ml)	Episode of urine leak
Time			

1. Children with a normal urine output during the night and normal bladder capacity—they can be given either the alarm or desmopressin. It is good to start with alarm therapy first.
2. Children with smaller than expected bladder capacity for age—they will likely be desmopressin-resistant and more sensitive to the alarm.
3. Children with nocturnal polyuria and normal bladder volume will be more sensitive to desmopressin.
4. Children with both excessive urine output and reduced bladder capacity may find combined therapy of alarm and desmopressin to be successful. This strategy lessens the burden of alarm treatment as the alarm is triggered several times per night.

12. What is alarm therapy and how does it work?

Ans: The first step usually is alarm treatment. There is level 1, grade-A ICI recommendation. It was first introduced by Meinhard von Pfaundler, a German pediatrician in 1907. Though there are many devices, the principle remains the same. The first drops of urine moisten the fabric separating two electrodes, thereby completing the circuit, and setting off the alarm that the child is wearing. When triggered on getting wet, it produces either a sound or a vibration. It may happen that initially the child might not wake up when the alarm is triggered, and parents must wake the child up. Gradually the child starts getting up with alarm and finally the sensation of full bladder awakens the child before wetting. Due to this reason response is usually not immediate and alarm needs to be used for at least 3 months. The recommended treatment duration is around 2–3 months and, in some cases, up to 5 months. The success rate is around 50% with lowest relapse rate among active interventions, even after removing alarm. Positive reinforcement by increasing fluid intake before going to bed has positive result of alarm therapy.[22] Intermittent reinforcement where the child uses the alarm therapy every alternate day before discontinuing is recommended. It is usually indicated in older children with motivated families.[23] If the child is dry for 14 consecutive days, alarm use can be withdrawn.

Alarm therapy is not indicated:

1. When parents or the child is not motivated.
2. Nocturnal enuresis is infrequent, e.g. 1–2 days/week.
3. Fast results are needed.

During the whole session, urotherapy should be continued. Child should be rewarded with every positive change.

13. What are the various medical treatment options available?

Ans: There are two drugs available, either desmopressin (tablet/sublingual) or anticholinergic. Desmopressin, also available as nasal spray, is not indicated due to erratic absorption and high side effects.

Tricyclic antidepressant is not recommended during the initial therapy due to their cardiotoxicity. They are also less effective than other drugs with response rate around 20% with high relapse rate after discontinuation of the drug. They are known to block fast sodium channels that can result in cardiac arrhythmia. Hence some recommend use of cardiac monitoring during their use.

14. What is the first line of medical treatment?

Ans: Desmopressin is the first line of treatment for primary nocturnal enuresis.[24,25] It is the synthetic form of arginine vasopressin. It is found to be suitable in the following cases:[26]

1. Child with nocturnal polyuria, normal maximum voided volume, older children, or less severe symptoms.
2. Alarm therapy has failed or not suitable.
3. Sometime when rapid treatment or short-term improvement is needed, e.g. during night out, family vacation.

15. How the desmopressin dosage is planned and what precautions should be told to family?

Ans: Its available in two forms.

Sublingual (fast melting oral lyophilizate): (>5 years, sublingual, initially 120 μg at bedtime; if needed, after 4 weeks increase to a maximum of 240 μg at bedtime). This is the recommended formulation in children as its absorption is not affected by nasal congestion, gastrointestinal transit and does not require fluid intake as in tablet forms.

Oral (>5 years, oral, initially 200 μg at bedtime; if needed, increase to 400 μg at bedtime).

As already mentioned, intranasal spray is not indicated due to uncontrolled absorption and high chances of hyponatremia.

16. What precautions should be followed in children prescribed with desmopressin?

Ans: Some general precautions given to all children are:

1. Restrict water intake 1 hour before and 8 hours after desmopressin dosage.
2. Drug to be given 1 hour before bedtime and 2 hours after food.
3. Restrict fluid intake to usually <200 cc.

17. What are the side effects of desmopressin?

Ans: Most serious side effects of desmopressin are related to overhydration. Desmopressin is contraindicated in children who cannot restrict fluid intake. Look diligently for hyponatremia symptoms—nausea, headache, and vomiting. This can lead to convulsion or cerebral edema.[27] One should not increase the dose if child is not going for urination in the morning after getting up.

18. How to follow children on desmopressin?

Ans: Beside symptoms suggestive of side effects, children are called once a month. Around 30% of children are full responders and 40% have partial response.[28] In children with partial response, dose can be increased after 1 month. Increasing the dose from 0.2 to 0.4 mg resulted in a further 31.1% of children responding. In case the child is dry for 3 months, dose can be withdrawn gradually.[29] Relapse rates are high up to the tune of 60–70%.

19. What is the difference in treatment outcome of various therapies?

Ans: In comparison to the alarm therapy, treatment benefit is not sustained after discontinuation of the desmopressin. Relapse rate between desmopressin and alarm therapy is 60–70% versus 50%. Though tricyclic antidepressant (TCA) is as effective as desmopressin, it is less likely to achieve 14-day dry night. Relapse rate with TCA is not known but they are associated with higher toxicity.

20. How is failure to therapy defined?

Ans: Inability to achieve >50% improvement in symptoms is defined as treatment resistance.

21. What precaution to be taken in non-responders to desmopressin?

Ans: Every effort should be made to find the cause of poor response. Following could be the reason for poor desmopressin response:

1. Poor compliance
2. Not passing urine before sleep
3. Taking drug less than 1 hour before sleep
4. Not restricting nighttime fluid intake is often seen.
5. High protein or salt intake in the form of fast food.

Besides above reasons, non-monosymptomatic nocturnal enuresis, persistent constipation, overactive bladder, diabetes mellitus, diabetes insipidus, desmopressin resistant nocturnal enuresis should be thought.

In case of partial response, desmopressin dose can be increased. In child with night OAB, anticholinergic drug can be added.

In children with behavioral signs suggestive of ADHD, sleep disorder, autism tricyclic antidepressant can be added after psychiatric consultation. Atomoxetine use in ADHD has been found to be effective in decreasing bedwetting frequency.[30]

Consultation with the ENT surgeon to look for adeno-tonsillar hypertrophy should be made. Surgery should be considered in appropriate children.[9]

22. What is the role of anticholinergic drugs?

Ans: Various anticholinergic drugs act by decreasing uninhibited detrusor contractions. Combination of anti-cholinergic with desmopressin is more effective than desmopressin alone in children with NE.[31]

23. What is the role of tricyclic antidepressant in management of nocturnal enuresis?

Ans: TCA is used as a third line treatment usually as a single bedtime dose of 1–2.5 mg/kg. Various TCA used are imipramine, desipramine or amitryptiline. It has anti-cholinergic and nonadrenergic effect. It decreases the amount of time spent in REM sleep, stimulate vasopressin secretion, and relax the detrusor muscle. Major rare significant adverse effects include cardiotoxicity and hepatotoxicity. Minor side-effects are related to their anti-cholinergic actions and include postural hypotension, dry mouth, constipation, perspiration, tachycardia, nausea, lethargy, and insomnia. A pretreatment electrocardiogram may be obtained to detect any underlying rhythm disorder. Treatment can be continued for 4–6 months. In a systematic review, compared with placebo, treatment with TCA was associated with reduction of approximately one wet night per week.[32] In view of their cardiotoxicity, poor outcome and high relapse rate, ICS has given Grade 1C recommendation for the use of imipramine. Also, World Health Organization (WHO) and National Institute for Health and Care Excellence (NICE) guideline does not recommend TCA (e.g. imipramine) or its combination with anticholinergic as a first line treatment for bedwetting in children.[33,34]

24. What other drugs can be used in case of failure of response to desmopressin or TCA?

Ans: Besides various anti-cholinergic, frusemide can be used as an early morning therapy to decrease nighttime diuresis.[35] Other drugs used were diclofenac, indomethacin, atropine amphetamines, but none of the drugs were more effective than desmopressin.

KEY POINTS

- For nocturnal polyuria—start desmopressin
- For reduced maximum voided volume–alarm therapy
- Combine—both works well
- Use of anticholinergic, tricyclic antidepressant in selected condition only

SUMMARY

- Nocturnal enuresis is a common pediatric urology problem.
- Treatment is required for children >5 years old.
- History taking and physical examination is of paramount importance.
- Features suggestive of non-monosymptomatic enuresis should be looked for.
- Urotherapy should be offered as treatment on the first visit.
- If no response, voiding diary should be ordered. On this basis, children are catergorized into four types.
- Alarm therapy is usually offered first when nocturnal polyuria is not present. It results in 50% improvement with lower relapse rate when treatment is stopped.
- Desmopressin is the drug of choice in patient with nocturnal polyuria. Precautions for using desmopressin should be adhered to.
- Tricyclic anti-depressant is used for nocturnal enuresis along with psychiatric consultation only.

REFERENCES

1. Austin PF, Bauer SB, Bower W, Chase J, Franco I, Hoebeke P, Rittig S, Walle JV, von Gontard A, Wright A, Yang SS, Nevéus T. The Standardization of Terminology of Lower Urinary Tract Function in Children and Adolescents: Update Report from the Standardization Committee of the International Children's Continence Society. *J Urol.* 2014; 191:1863–5. doi: 10.1016/j.juro.2014.01.110.
2. De Sousa A, Kapoor H, Jagtap J, Sen M. Prevalence and factors affecting enuresis amongst primary schoolchildren. *Indian J Urol.* 2007; 23:354–7.
3. Reddy NM, Malve H, Nerli R, Venkatesh P, Agarwal I, Rege V. Nocturnal Enuresis in India: Are We Diagnosing and Managing Correctly? Indian J Nephrol. 2017 Nov-Dec;27(6):417–426.
4. Thurber S. Childhood Enuresis: Current Diagnostic Formulations, Salient Findings, and Effective Treatment Modalities. Arch PsychiatrNurs. 2017 Jun;31(3):319–323.
5. Nevéus T. Pathogenesis of enuresis: Towards a new understanding. Int J Urol. 2017 Mar;24(3):174–182.
6. Pedersen MJ, Rittig S, Jennum PJ, Kamperis K. The role of sleep in the pathophysiology of nocturnal enuresis. Sleep Med Rev. 2020 Feb; 49:101228.
7. Dhondt K, Van Herzeele C, Roels SP, Raes A, Groen LA, Hoebeke P, Walle JV. Sleep fragmentation and periodic limb movements in children with monosymptomatic nocturnal enuresis and polyuria. Pediatr Nephrol. 2015 Jul;30(7):1157–62.
8. Bascom A, McMaster MA, Alexander RT, MacLean JE. Nocturnal enuresis in children is associated with differences in autonomic control. Sleep. 2019 Mar 1;42(3): zsy239.
9. Firoozi F, Batniji R, Aslan AR, Longhurst PA, Kogan BA. Resolution of diurnal incontinence and nocturnal enuresis

after adenotonsillectomy in children. J Urol. 2006 May;175(5): 1885–8.

10. Ma Y, Shen Y, Liu X. Association between enuresis and obesity in children with primary monosymptomatic nocturnal enuresis. Int Braz J Urol. 2019 Jul-Aug;45(4):790–797.
11. Rittig S, Knudsen UB, Nørgaard JP, Pedersen EB, Djurhuus JC. Abnormal diurnal rhythm of plasma vasopressin and urinary output in patients with enuresis. Am J Physiol. 1989 Apr;256(4 Pt 2): F664–71.
12. Fonseca EG, Bordallo AP, Garcia PK, Munhoz C, Silva CP. Lower urinary tract symptoms in enuretic and nonenuretic children. *J Urol.* 2009;182(4 Suppl):1978–1983.
13. Martinez cayuelas, L *et al*. Evaluation of sleep hygiene and prevalence of sleep disorders in patients with monosymptomatic enuresis. Usefulness of the BEARS sleep screening tool. ActasUrolEsp (Engl Ed), 2020.44:477.
14. De Sena Oliveira AC, Athanasio BDS, Mrad FCC, Vasconcelos MMA, Albuquerque MR, Miranda DM, Simões E Silva AC. Attention deficit and hyperactivity disorder and nocturnal enuresis co-occurrence in the pediatric population: a systematic review and meta-analysis. Pediatr Nephrol. 2021 Nov;36(11):3547–3559.
15. Von Gontard A, Hussong J, Yang SS, Chase J, Franco I, Wright A. Neurodevelopmental disorders and incontinence in children and adolescents: Attention-deficit/hyperactivity disorder, autism spectrum disorder, and intellectual disability-A consensus document of the International Children's Continence Society. Neurourol Urodyn. 2022 Jan;41(1):102–114.
16. Sinha R, Raut S. Management of nocturnal enuresis–myths and facts. World J Nephrol. 2016 Jul 6;5(4):328–38.
17. Cayan S, Doruk E, Bozlu M, Akbay E, Apaydin D, Ulusoy E, Canpolat B. Is routine urinary tract investigation necessary for children with monosymptomatic primary nocturnal enuresis? *Urology.* 2001; 58:598–602.
18. Caldwell PH, Nankivell G, Sureshkumar P. Simple behavioural interventions for nocturnal enuresis in children. Cochrane Database Syst Rev. 2013 Jul 19;(7):CD003637.
19. Hofmeester I, Kollen BJ, Steffens MG, van Capelle JW, Mulder Z, Feitz WF, Blanker MH. Predictors for a positive outcome of adapted clinical dry bed training in adolescents and adults with enuresis. Neurourol Urodyn. 2016 Nov;35(8):1006–1010.
20. Lv ZT, Song W, Wu J, Yang J, Wang T, Wu CH, *et al*. Efficacy of acupuncture in children with nocturnal enuresis: A systematic review and meta-analysis of randomized controlled trials. *Evid Based Complement Alternat Med.* 2015; 2015:320701.
21. Seabrook JA, Gorodzinsky F, Freedman S. Treatment of primary nocturnal enuresis: A randomized clinical trial comparing hypnotherapy and alarm therapy. Paediatr Child Health. 2005 Dec;10(10):609–10.
22. Kosilov KV, Loparev SA, Ivanovskaya MA, Kosilova LV. Night diuresis stimulation increases efficiency of alarm intervention. *J Pediatr Urol.* 2015; 11:261.e1–5.
23. Glazener CM, Evans JH, Peto RE. Alarm interventions for nocturnal enuresis in children. *Cochrane Database Syst Rev.* 2005;18:CD002911.
24. Tekgul S, Nijman R, Hoebeke P, Canning D, Bower W, von Gontard A (2009) Diagnosis and management of urinary incontinence in childhood. Report from the 4th International Consultation on Incontinence. Health Publication Ltd.
25. Lottmann H, Froeling F, Alloussi S, El-Radhi AS, Rittig S, Riis A, Persson BE. A randomised comparison of oral desmopressin lyophilisate (MELT) and tablet formulations in children and adolescents with primary nocturnal enuresis. *Int J Clin Pract.* 2007; 61:1454–1460.
26. Predictive parameters of response to desmopressin in primary nocturnal enuresis.VanHerzeele C, Evans J, Eggert P, Lottmann H, Norgaard JP, VandeWalle J. J Pediatr Urol. 2015 Aug; 11(4):200.e1–8.
27. Donoghue MB, Latimer ME, Pillsbury HL, Hertzog JH. Hyponatremic seizure in a child using desmopressin for nocturnal enuresis. *Arch Pediatr Adolesc Med.* 1998; 152:290–292.
28. Neveus T, Eggert P, Evans J, Macedo A, Rittig S, Tekgül S, VandeWalle J, Yeung CK, Robson L; International Children's Continence Society. Evaluation of and treatment for monosymptomatic enuresis: a standardization document from the International Children's Continence Society. J Urol. 2010 Feb;183(2):441–7. doi: 10.1016/j.juro.2009.10.043. Epub 2009 Dec 14.
29. Marschall-Kehrel D, Harms TW. Structured desmopressin withdrawal improves response and treatment outcome for monosymptomatic enuretic children. *J Urol.* 2009; 182: 2022–2026.
30. Shatkin JP. Atomoxetine for the treatment of pediatric nocturnal enuresis. *J Child Adolesc Psychopharmacol.* 2004; 14:443–447.
31. Park SJ, Park JM, Pai KS, Ha TS, Lee SD, Baek M Korean. Children's Continence and Enuresis Society. Desmopressin alone versus desmopressin and an anticholinergic in the first-line treatment of primary monosymptomatic nocturnal enuresis: A multicenter study. *Pediatr Nephrol.* 2014; 29: 1195–200.
32. Glazener CM, Evans JH, Peto RE. Tricyclic and related drugs for nocturnal enuresis in children. *Cochrane Database Syst Rev.* 2003;(3):CD002117.
33. National Institute for Health and Care Excellence. Nocturnal Enuresis–The Management of Bedwetting in Children and Young People.
34. World Health Organization. Guidelines for the Management of Conditions Specifically Related to Stress. Geneva: World Health Organization; 2013.
35. A. De Guchtenaere, C. Vande Walle, P. Van Sintjan, R. Donckerwolcke, A. Raes, J. Dehoorne, E. Van Laecke, P. Hoebeke, J. Vande Walle. Desmopressin Resistant Nocturnal Polyuria May Benefit from Furosemide Therapy Administered in the Morning. J Urol.Vol. 178, Issue 6,2007, 2635–39.

Chapter

9

Hypospadias Cripple

• *Amilal Bhat*

LEARNING OBJECTIVES

- To evaluate a case of hypospadias with multiple failed surgeries and also having unilateral undescended testis.
- Surgical decision making in such cases.
- How to correct chordee and torsion in such cases?
- How to plan urethroplasty—one stage or two stage?
- Which healthy tissue to be interposed between skin and neourethra?
- How to plan skin cover in these cases?

INTRODUCTION

The results of hypospadias repair have improved significantly with advancements in hypospadialogy, still complications are inevitable regardless of technique applied for hypospadias repair and they vary with surgical experience. It is more difficult to treat patients with multiple complications. Multiple surgeries are likely to leave significant deformities worse than the primary congenital anomaly itself. Failure of multiple surgeries may lead to functional loss of the penis and lead to a stage is called 'hypospadias cripple'. Horton and Devine used the term hypospadias cripple for the patient who had undergone multiple unsuccessful hypospadias repairs. The exact prevalence of the hypospadias cripple is unknown, but the best available estimate shows it occurs in 5–7% of patients after multiple failed attempts of repair. The initial repair goals are to reconstruct an adequate size and straight penis for successful intercourse and a forward-directed projectile urinary stream. This can be achieved by chordee correction, urethroplasty, meatoplasty/glansplasty, scrotal transposition repair and skin coverage. The complications are considerably more significant in redo surgeries than for primary repairs with the same surgical technique. It becomes more complicated when it is associated with disorders of sexual differentiation (DSD) or undescended testis. These facts guide us to think about careful patient selection, modification in the techniques, adding supportive and healthy tissue cover, designing skin flaps for skin cover and choosing a procedure that may not commonly be used for primary repair.[1–3]

Case Scenario

A twelve years old boy with multiple failed repairs for proximal hypospadias—with non-palpable testis. Records of earlier surgeries are not available. At present patient complains of passing urine from ventral side like a shower with straining. He also has ventral bending of penis which is painful. One side of testis was not seen in the scrotum since birth. On examination, patient is having multiple urethral fistulae. The penis shows rotation, i.e. torsion on the left side along with and chordee and a bifid scrotum. Secondary sexual characters are normal.

1. **How will you evaluate such a patient?**

   Ans: These patients may come to the hospital with complains of fistula, chordee, torsion, penile deformity, complex psychosexual problems, and urinary or ejaculatory problems. The details of the original type of hypospadias; type of previous surgery and the reason of failure, if available will help in planning the surgery. Careful and systematic evaluation is an essential step in the workup of these patients. The size of the penis and glans, present location and size of the meatus, chordee, penile torsion, multiple openings suggestive of fistulae, presence of scars, the pliability of the tissue, preputial hood or residual preputial skin, palpable thickening of the urethra, ballooning of ventral side during micturition are evaluated and recorded. Urethrogram is done in cases of failed proximal hypospadias confirm stricture, diverticula, mullerian duct remnant and a large prostatic utricle. Patients with undescended testis and features suggestive of DSD also needs endocrine evaluation. Most of the DSD patients have dimple, bifurcation of median raphe discoloration of skin in midline and longer ano-scrotal distance (Fig. 9.1). MRI of pelvis and a genitogram are useful to evaluate the remnant of mullerian duct (Fig. 9.2). The photograph taken during erection by the patient or parents is helpful to evaluate the residual curvature or recurrence of curvature or penile torsion. Clinical examination and an artificial erection with pharmacological agents and curvature measurement may help decide the plan: either plication procedure or ventral lengthening procedures. Endoscopy is mandatory in these cases to observe for stricture, diverticula, fistula specially the mullerian duct remanent like vagina and prostatic utricle (Fig. 9.1). Diagnostic laparoscopy can be done to confirm the mullerian duct remnants. The patient should be counselled before surgery, considering their aspirations and realistic expectations about the penile size and shape, urinary and sexual functions. Other issues frequently seen in seemingly simple cases are—fistulae, scarring, recurrent chordee, and an abnormal meatus, often related to a small glans and nearly always with a deficiency of the dartos layer often with underlying associated psychosexual problems. The assessment is an important step in the planning of the surgery, and alternatives in the surgical approach as second or third line.[4,5]

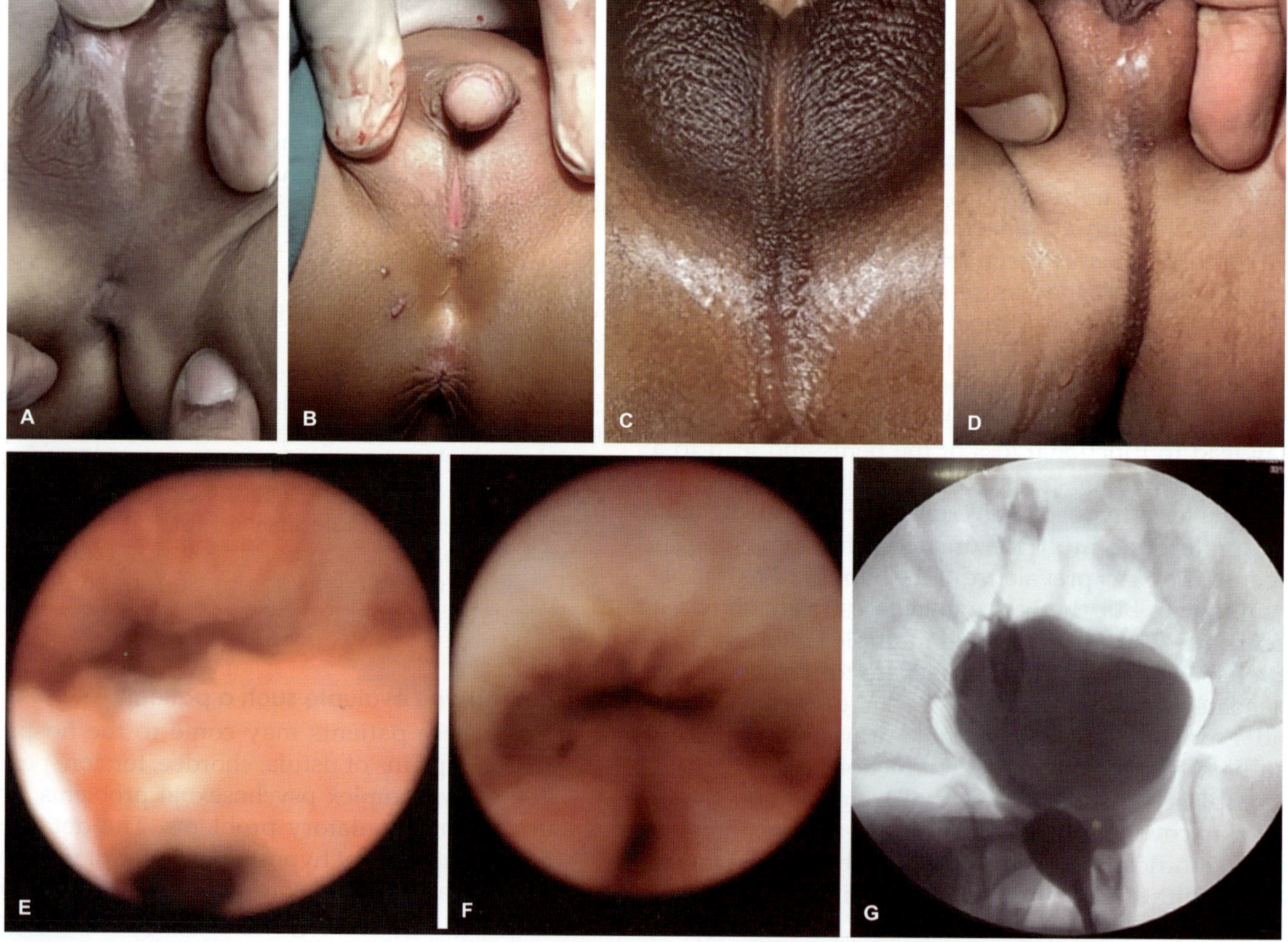

Fig. 9.1A to G: Clinical radiological and endoscopic evaluation: (A) A dimple in the perineum; (B) Dimple and discoloration in the perineum; (C) Bifurcation of median raphe; (D) and (E) Two opening in the urogenital canal: Dorsal one of urethra and ventral of vagina and (F) Genitogram showing Mullerian duct remnant; (G) Imaging cystogram

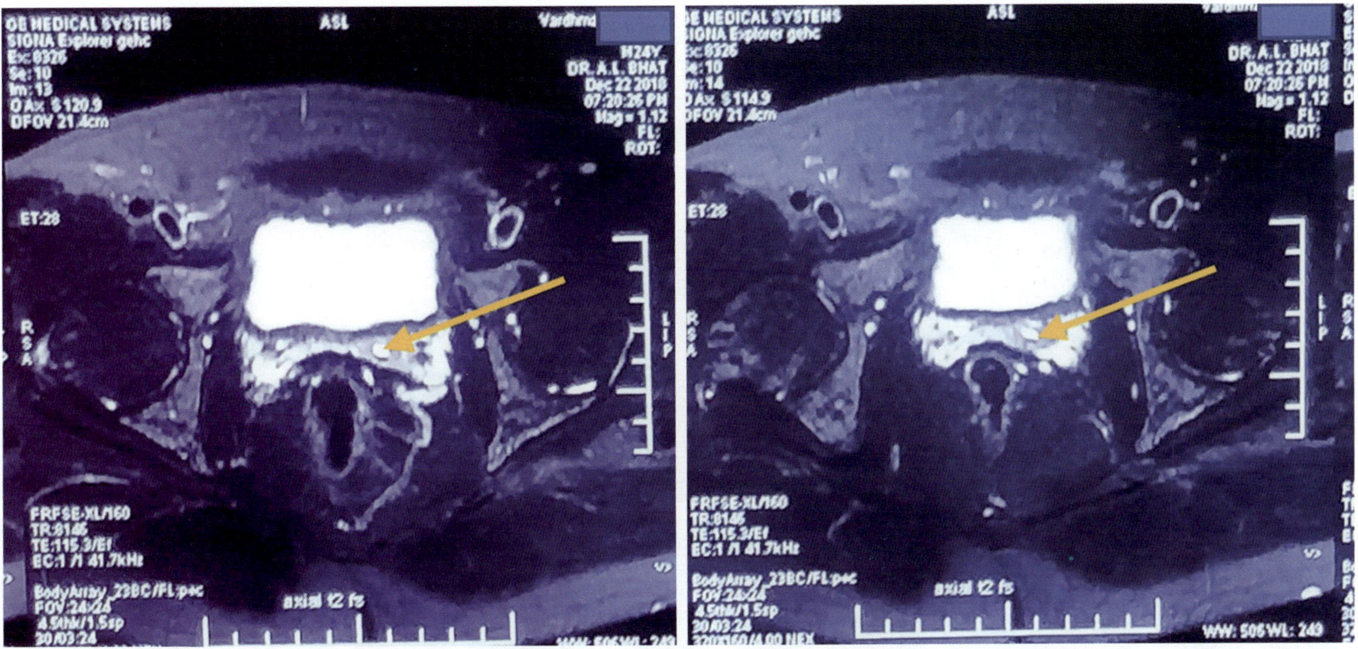

Fig. 9.2: MRI showing DSD. Arrows showing Mullerian duct remnant

2. **What are the causes of a residual chordee?**

   Ans: The causes of the recurrent curvature in hypospadias cripple are fibrosis of the periurethral tissue, short ventral skin, shortening of the reconstructed urethra and disproportionate dorso-ventral corpora.

3. **How will you manage the chordee?**

   Ans: Chordee due to skin fibrosis is likely to be corrected after penile skin degloving itself, but it is to be confirmed by Gittes test before proceeding for urethroplasty. The urethra or urethral plate is examined to see whether it is healthy or fibrotic. Shortening due to urethral plate or urethra can be corrected by mobilization of urethral plate/urethra (Figs 9.3 and 9.4). But the fibrotic urethra/tethered urethral plate causing the chordee is to be transected or resected to correct the ventral curvature. Chordee less than 30 degrees due to corporal disproportion is managed by dorsal plication (Fig. 9.4) or superficial corporotomy if the penile length is inadequate. Transection of urethral plate/urethra and corporoplasty is done in cases of chordee more than 30 degrees; buccal mucosal or skin graft is placed in order to reconstruct urethral plate and can be tubularized in the second stage. If needed, ventral shortening of the skin can be covered by Z plasty, double Z plasty or multiple Z plasties.[1,2,6]

4. **What are the causes of penile torsion?**

   Ans: Penile torsion results from traction on the vascular pedicle of the inner preputial flap, traction on the tunica flap used for interposing healthy tissue during previous surgery, intrinsic corporal shortening and unequal skin flap closure.

5. **How will you correct the penile torsion?**

   Ans: Torsion can be corrected by penile degloving, (Fig. 9.5 A–H) release of vascular pedicle traction by mobilization of the pedicle according to the cause of torque. If it still persists, then counter traction by dartos wrap, plication procedures, and final adjustment with skin closure is done.[7]

6. **What causes urethral stricture in such patients?**

   Ans: Stricture is the second most common long-term complication in hypospadias repair and the site of the strictures is anastomotic, sub-meatal, incision of the urethral and proximal healthy urethra due to urethrotomy or injury to urethra due to long catheterization. The factors responsible for stricture urethra are poor design of the neourethra, insufficient calibre, tension on suture lines, deep incision in the urethral plate, inadequate spatulation of the urethra at the site of anastomosis, trauma, infection and tissue ischemia.

7. **How will you confirm the diagnosis of urethral stricture?**

   Ans: Diagnosis of the stricture with depiction of its exact location and length is done by urethrogram and is confirmed by cystoscopic examination with a 0-degree lens under anaesthesia. Proximal dilation of the urethra (Fig. 9.6 A–F) may be delineated in the urethrogram and help to plan the treatment.

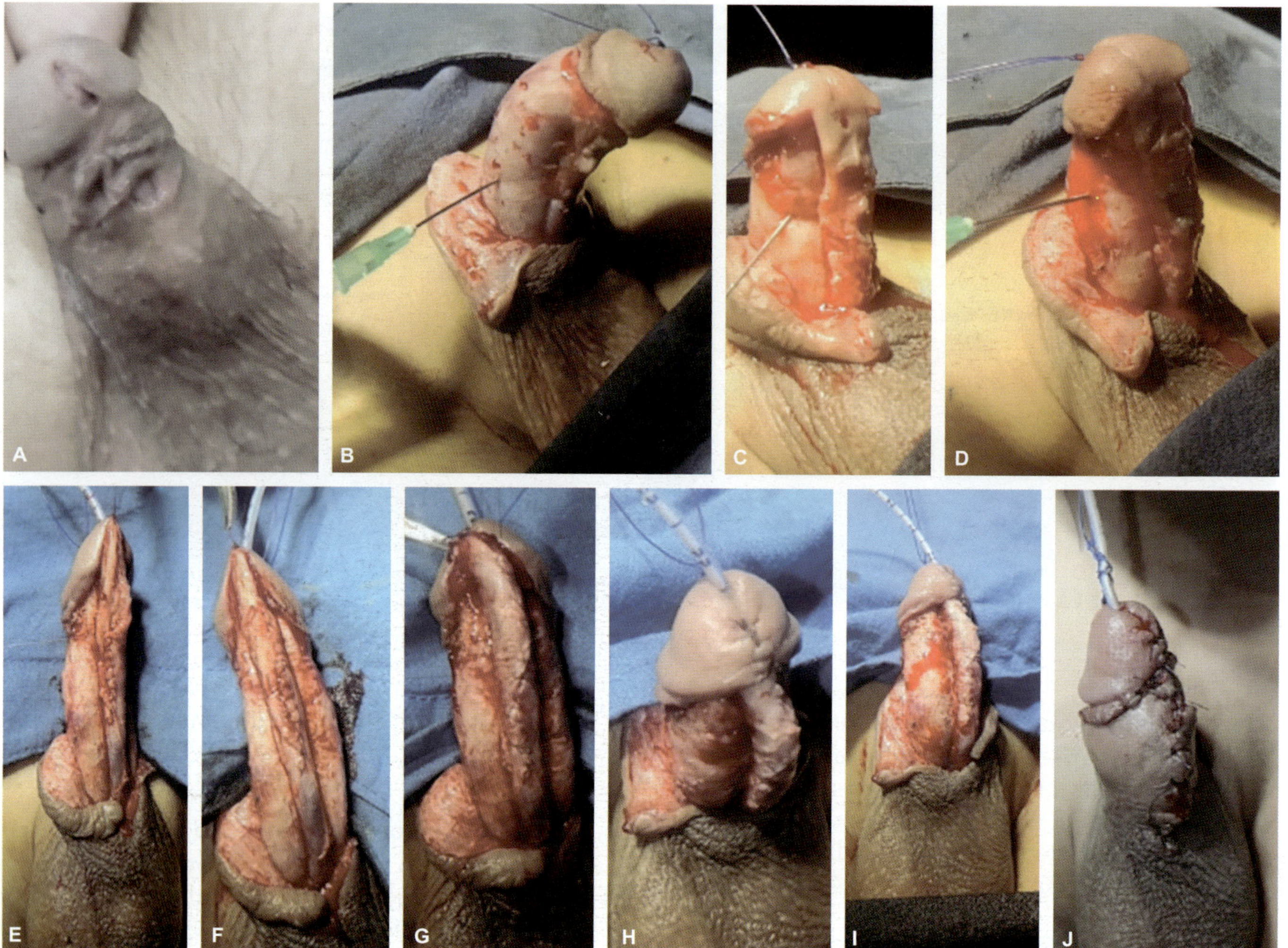

Fig. 9.3A to J: Chordee correction by mobilization of urethral plate and spongiosum: (A) Chordee, fistula and distal laid open urethra; (B) Gittes test showing moderate chordee after penile degloving; (C) and (D) Gittes test showing correction chordee after penile degloving and mobilization of urethral plate and spongiosum; (E) Tubularization of urethral plate; (F) and (G) Double breasting spongioplasty; (H) and (I) Glansplasty and (J) Skin closure

8. How will you manage post-hypospadias repair strictures?

Ans: Methods applied for the management of stricture are:

1. Urethral dilatation
2. VIU: Visual internal urethrotomy
3. Excision and primary anastomosis
4. Replacement urethroplasty using adjacent skin flaps, free pedicle or tube grafts, or buccal mucosa grafts—single/two-stage.

We proposed an algorithm for management of post-hypospadias strictures (Fig. 9.7).[1,2]

9. How common are urethral fistula?

Ans: Urethrocutaneous fistula is the commonest complication of hypospadias repair. The urethral fistula incidence varies from 4% to 28% according to the type of hypospadias and repair. With the use of microsurgical equipment and improved operative technique the incidence of fistula is steadily decreasing.

10. What are the causes of development of urethral fistula?

Ans: The factors implicated in the development of urethral fistula are technical factors like overlapping suture lines, improper approximation or eversion of the epithelium, or late or non-absorbable suture material, distal urethral obstruction/meatal stenosis. Factors affecting wound healing like edema, attenuated vascular supply, infection and hematoma are also important etiological factors.

11. What are the common sites where fistula occur?

Ans: The site of the fistula depends upon the type of hypospadias and the surgical technique used for repair (Fig. 9.8). Sub-coronal fistulae are most common in tubularized incised plate

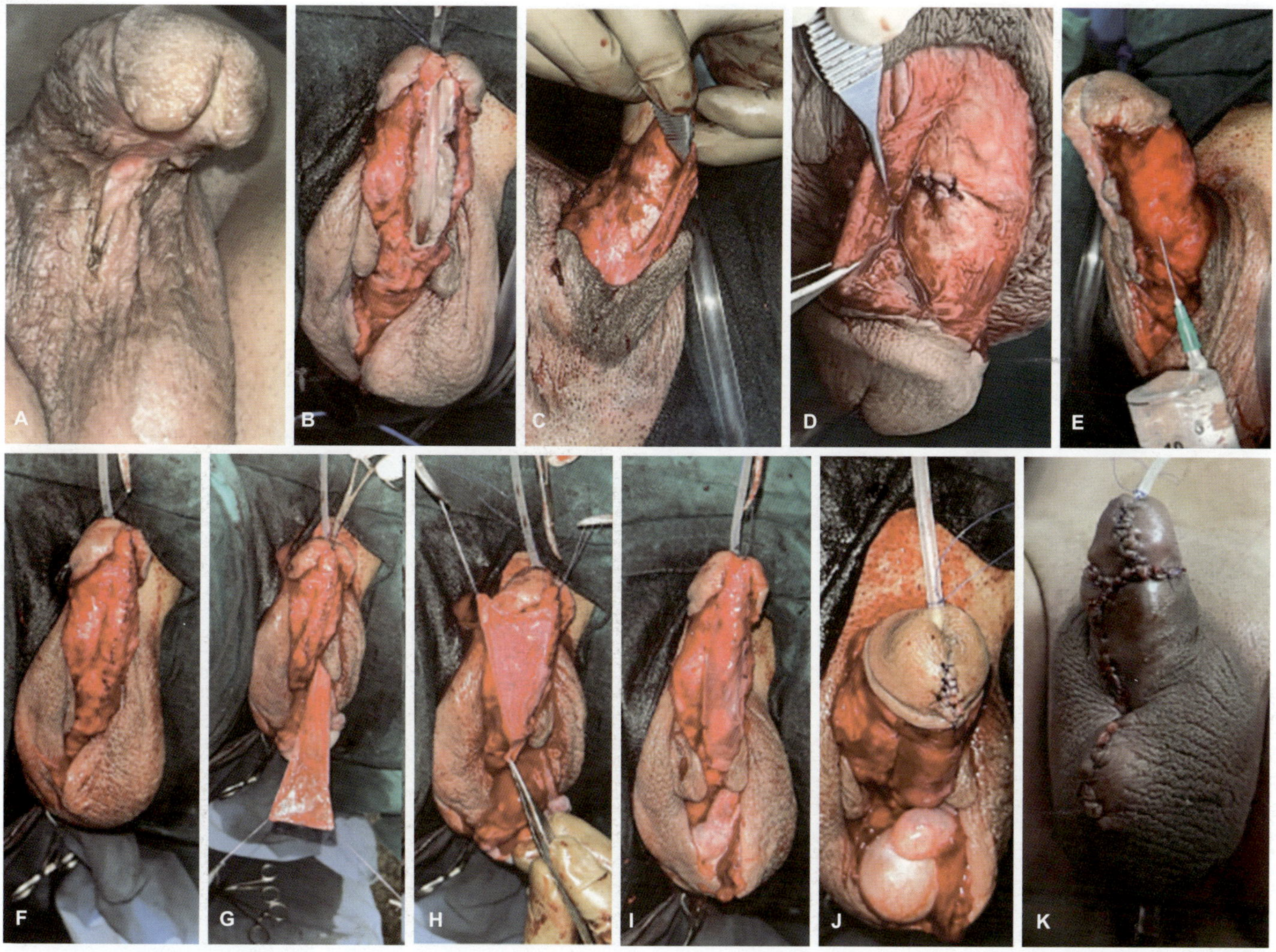

Fig. 9.4A to K: Chordee correction by mobilization of urethral plate, spongiosum; (A) And dorsal plication; (B) Chordee, and open urethra; (C) Moderate chordee after penile degloving and mobilization of spongiosum; (D) Mobilization of neurovascular bundle; (E) Gittes test showing correction of chordee; (F) Tubularization of urethral plate; (G) Mobilization of tunica vaginalis flap; (H) and (I) Suturing the tunica flap over the neo-urethra; (J) Glansplasty and (K) Skin closure

urethroplasty (TIPU)/augmented repair. They are seen at anastomotic site in flap repair, but may occur anywhere.

12. **How should these fistulas be treated?**

    Ans: Small fistulae without distal obstruction are likely to heal spontaneously but larger fistulae, persisting beyond several weeks, associated with stricture and meatal stenosis invariably require surgery. The proper time for fistula repair is 6–12 months after the surgery depending upon the suppleness of the tissue.

13. **What are the main surgical principles in the surgical repair of these urethral fistulas?**

    Ans: Excision of the fistulous tract, closure of the fistula with fine sutures, covering it with a healthy interposing tissue layer and skin closure, avoiding superimposition suture line are the critical steps in fistula repair.

14. **How will you manage these fistulae?**

    Ans: A small coronal fistula is excised, and penile shaft skin is advanced to cover the defect. If there is a retrusive meatus with fistula, the ledge between meatus and fistula is excised, and TIPU with spongioplasty (Fig. 9.9 A–F) is done. If the urethral plate is not wide, then dorsal inlay skin graft/buccal mucosal graft (Fig. 9.10 A–G) or onlay flap urethroplasty is done to avoid the stricture and tension-free closure. Larger fistulas may require coverage with a trap-door or island flap of penile shaft skin. Multiple fistulae can be combined, and closure is done with or without the dorsal inlay. If the defect is larger after connecting all fistulae, then onlay flap urethroplasty is done. In general, better results can be achieved when a second layer or flap coverage is possible, especially in cases having history of failed repairs of fistula. Skin coverage can be obtained by several methods to

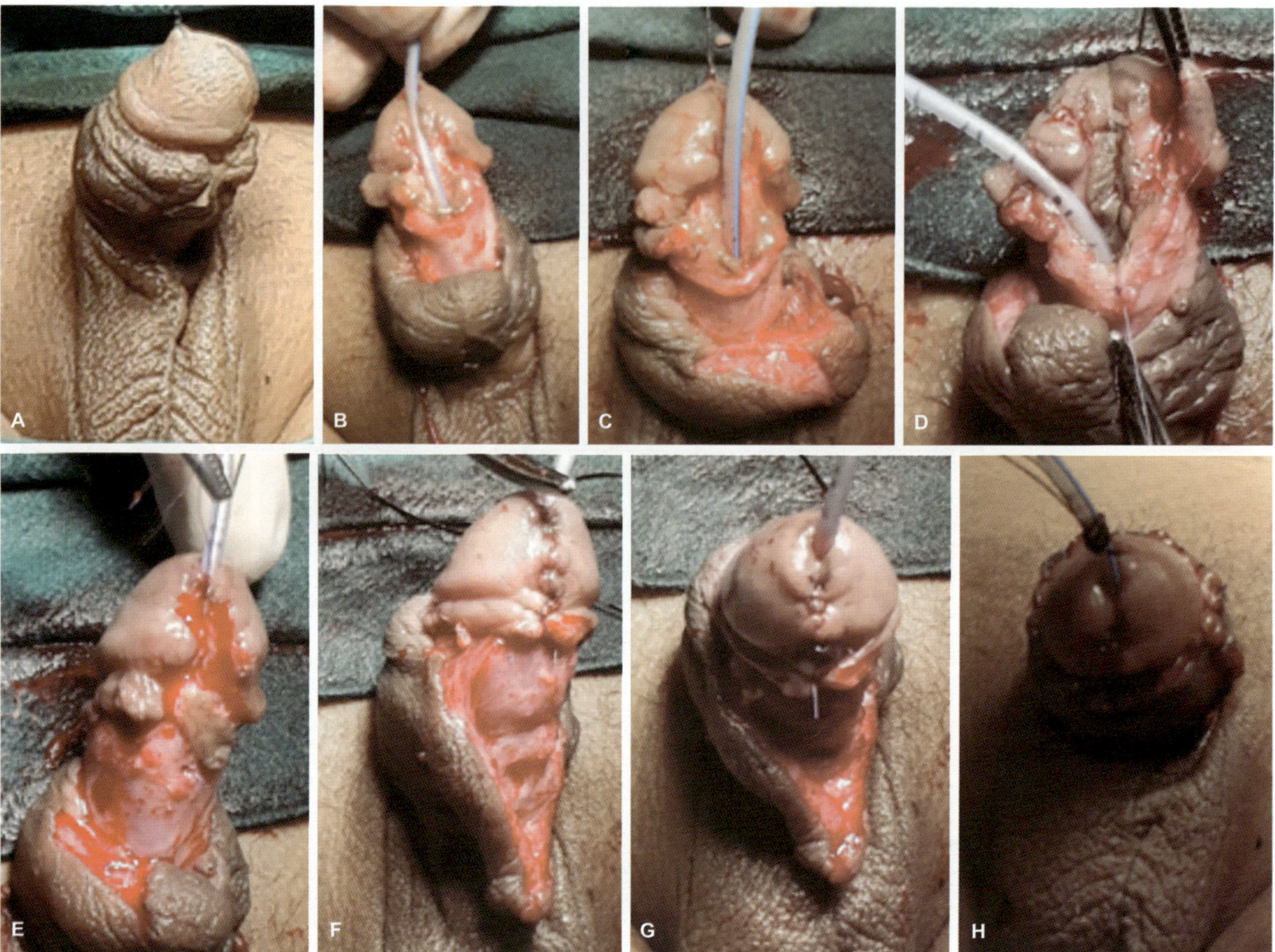

Fig. 9.5A to H: Torsion correction in a three-year-old male child with distal laid open urethra with TIPU and dartos cover (with permission Bhat AL. Reference [1] @ copyright Springer Nature Singapore); (A) Failed hypospadias repair showing torque; (B) and (C) Correction of torque after penile degloving; (D) Urethral plate tubularization started; (E) Urethral plate and spongioplasty tubularization; (F) and (G) Coverage with dartos flap and glansplasty and (H) Skin closure

avoid overlap of urethral and skin suture lines. There was no statistically significant relationship between the fistula site, size and number of the fistula with success rate.[8]

15. How do urethral diverticula develop in such cases?

Ans: Diffuse dilation of either the neourethra or the native urethra is termed diverticula. They occur due to lack of supporting tissue over neourethra, turbulence during micturition due to poor fixity of urethra, distal stricture or meatal stenosis, and wider neourethra leading to a sudden step-off at the level of the neo-urethral anastomosis. Surprisingly, sometimes distal obstruction is not seen with post-hypospadias surgery diverticula.

16. How common are urethral diverticula following hypospadias surgery?

Ans: The diverticula are more frequently observed in patients with onlay flaps and two-stage repairs because of the lack of spongiosum and a longer urethroplasty. The reported incidence of urethral diverticula in flap and flap tube urethroplasties is 7–12%. The urethral diverticula rarely occur in TIPU; Snodgrass reported in only three patients (0.33%) of 885 cases of TIPU and 1.43% in two-stage graft repairs. Snyder *et al* found stricture only in one out of thirteen cases. Snodgrass reported diverticula in 5 patients out of nine who underwent Byars flap repair in proximal hypospadias, but none had distal obstruction.[1,2, 9,10]

17. How will you manage these diverticula?

Retrograde and micturating urethrogram helps to diagnose distal obstruction and shows the site and size of the diverticula along with any associated fistula. Cystourethroscopy before a repair will make the surgeon wiser about the status of the urethra, diverticula, stones in diverticula, prostatic utricle and any secondary changes in the bladder (Fig. 9.11C). Repair is done

Fig. 9.6A to F: Stricturoplasty with skin flap from the dilated skin urethra: (A) RGU and MCU showing stricture at the anastomotic site; (B) MCU showing the dilated proximal urethra; (C) Laid open stricture and distal skin tube; (D) Skin flap taken and stricturoplasty; (E) and (F) Postoperative results well-formed glans meatus at tip and good flow

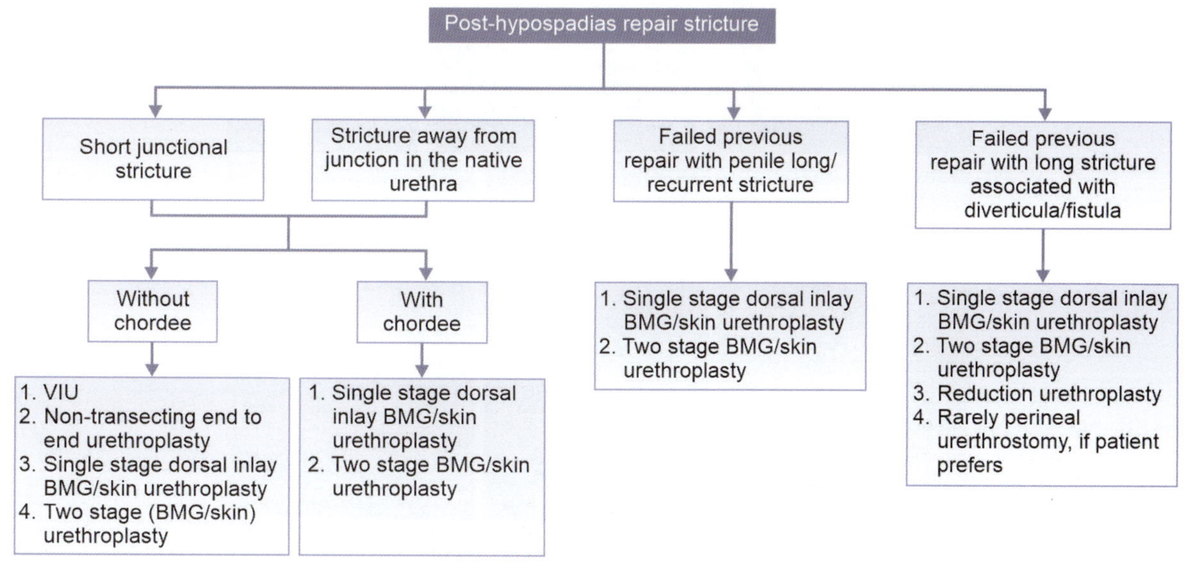

Fig. 9.7: Algorithm stricture (with permission Bhat AL. Reference [2] @ copyright Springer Nature Singapore)

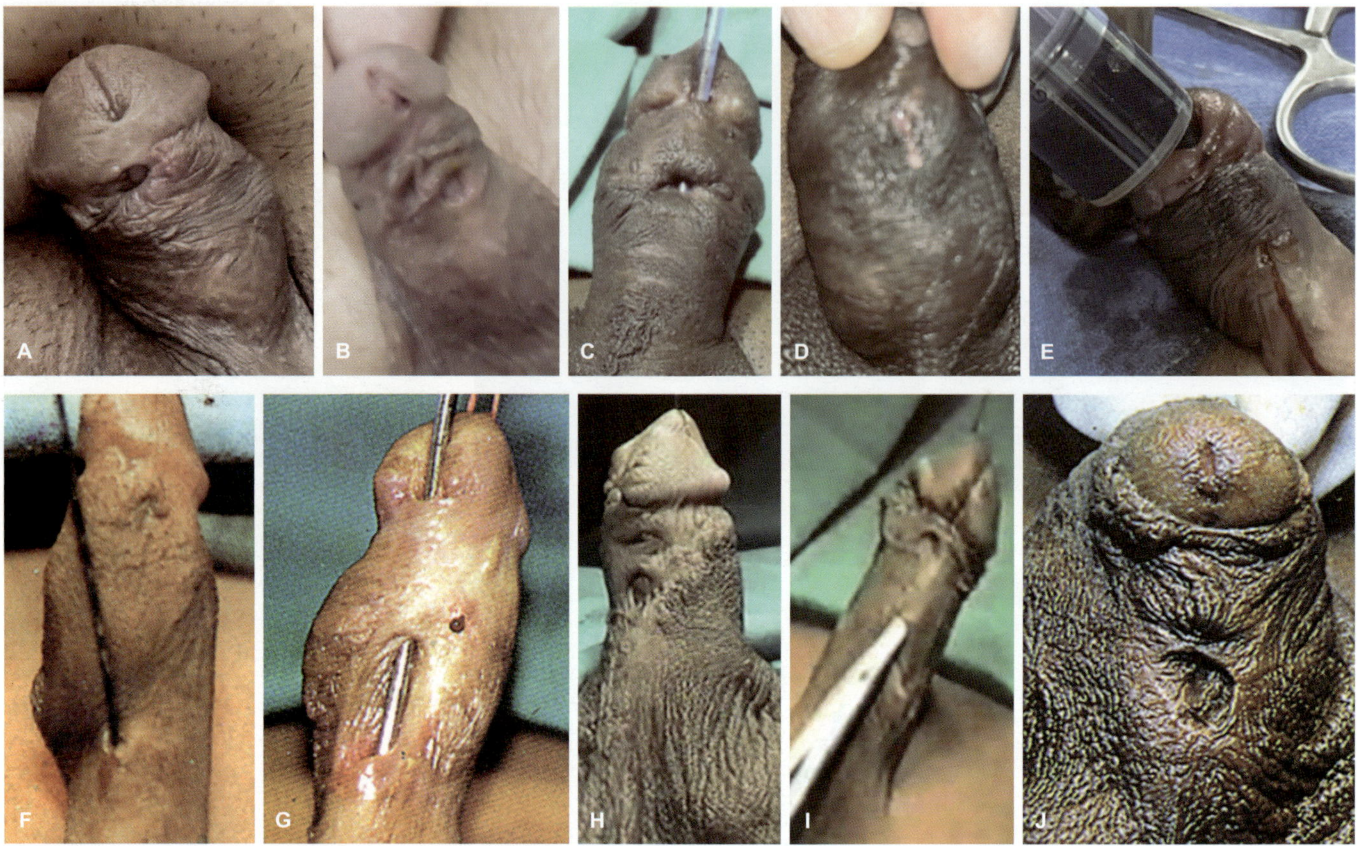

Fig. 9.8A to J: Different types of fistula; (A) Subcoronal; (B to D) Distal penile (E) Mid-penile (F) and (G) Proximal penile and (H to J) Multiple

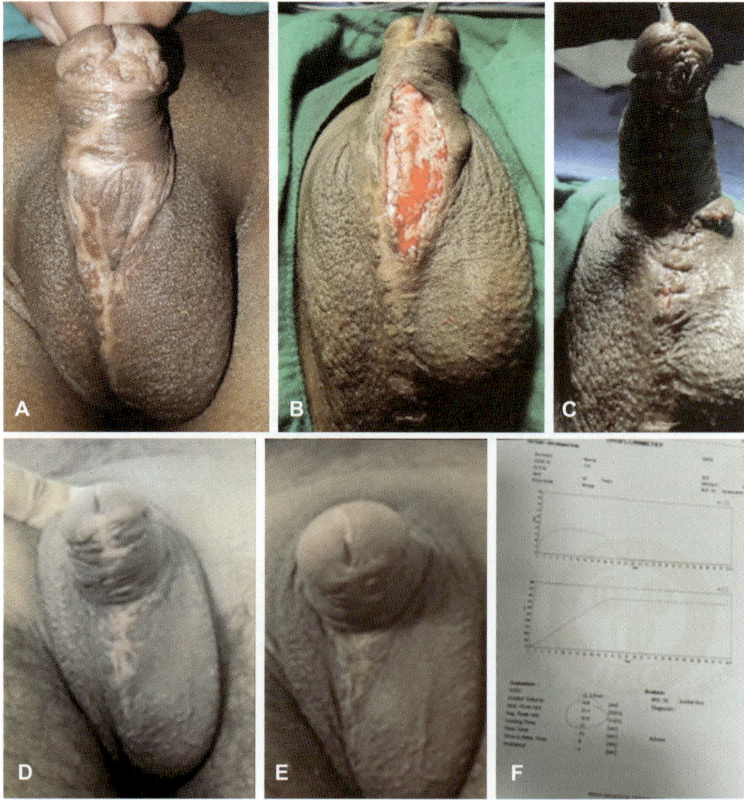

Fig. 9.9A to F: Fistula closure with repair of distal laid open urethra in failed hypospadias with undescended testis: (A) Distal laid open urethra penoscrotal fistula right undescended testis (B) Fistula closure with dartos cover; (C) TIPU for distal laid open urethra (D) and (E) Postoperative picture with normal meatus at tip of the well-formed glans and (F) Postoperative uroflowmetry at 2 years

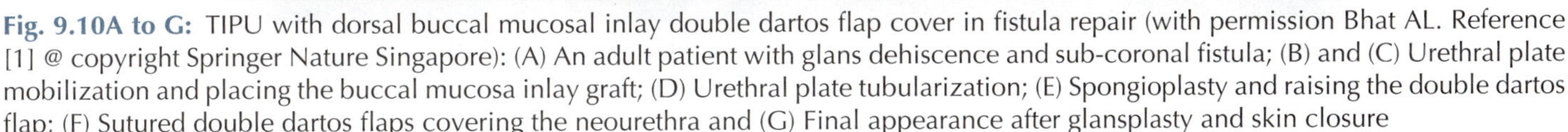

Fig. 9.10A to G: TIPU with dorsal buccal mucosal inlay double dartos flap cover in fistula repair (with permission Bhat AL. Reference [1] @ copyright Springer Nature Singapore): (A) An adult patient with glans dehiscence and sub-coronal fistula; (B) and (C) Urethral plate mobilization and placing the buccal mucosa inlay graft; (D) Urethral plate tubularization; (E) Spongioplasty and raising the double dartos flap; (F) Sutured double dartos flaps covering the neourethra and (G) Final appearance after glansplasty and skin closure

by excising the excessive part of the diverticular skin wall. A portion of it is denuded to cover the suture line and neo-urethra, creating a pseudospongiosum (Fig. 9.11 A–F). The technique is called pseudospongioplasty. A tunica vaginalis flap cover over the repair effectively decreases the urethrocutaneous fistula rate. Alternatively, a dartos flap (Fig. 9.12 A–G) or a de-epithelialized flap may be employed. Results of diverticula repair are good, but there are chances of fistula and recurrence of the diverticula. Snyder et al. repaired the diverticula in 13 cases with a success rate of 76.23%.[9]

18. What is the importance of knowing the history of the type of repair done previously?

If previous surgery notes/information are available; then knowing whether plate preservation procedure (TIPU, augmented TIPU or onlay flap) or tubularized flap urethroplasty was done will help in planning the reconstruction of urethra.

19. How will you manage cases where the urethral plate was preserved previously?

Ans: If previous urethral plate is available, then redo TIPU is feasible. If the urethral plate is not wide enough, dorsal inlay or buccal mucosal graft can be used to augment the urethral plate.

Advantage in these cases is that the spongiosum is available, so spongioplasty can be done after tubularization of the urethral plate. Healthy tissue like dartos, double dartos, scrotal dartos and need be tunica vaginalis can be used for interposition between the skin and the neourethra[1,2] (Fig. 9.13A–G).

20. How will you utilize the dorsal hood?

Ans: If dorsal hood is available then it may be utilized to reconstruct the urethra as onlay flap (Fig. 9.14 A–F) or tubularized flap urethroplasty or dorsal dartos can be used as an healthy intervening healthy tissue. Skin cover may be an issue in multiple failed surgery; dorsal hood may prove very useful to cover skin in these redo cases.[1,2]

21. What are the possible diagnosis on evaluation of hypospadias with undescended testis?

Ans: The possibilities of the different diagnosis are:

1. Hypospadias with undescended testis.
2. Hypospadias with atrophic testis due to torsion.
3. Hypospadias with undescended testis and mullerian duct remnant.
4. Hypospadias with ovotestis and mullerian duct remnant.

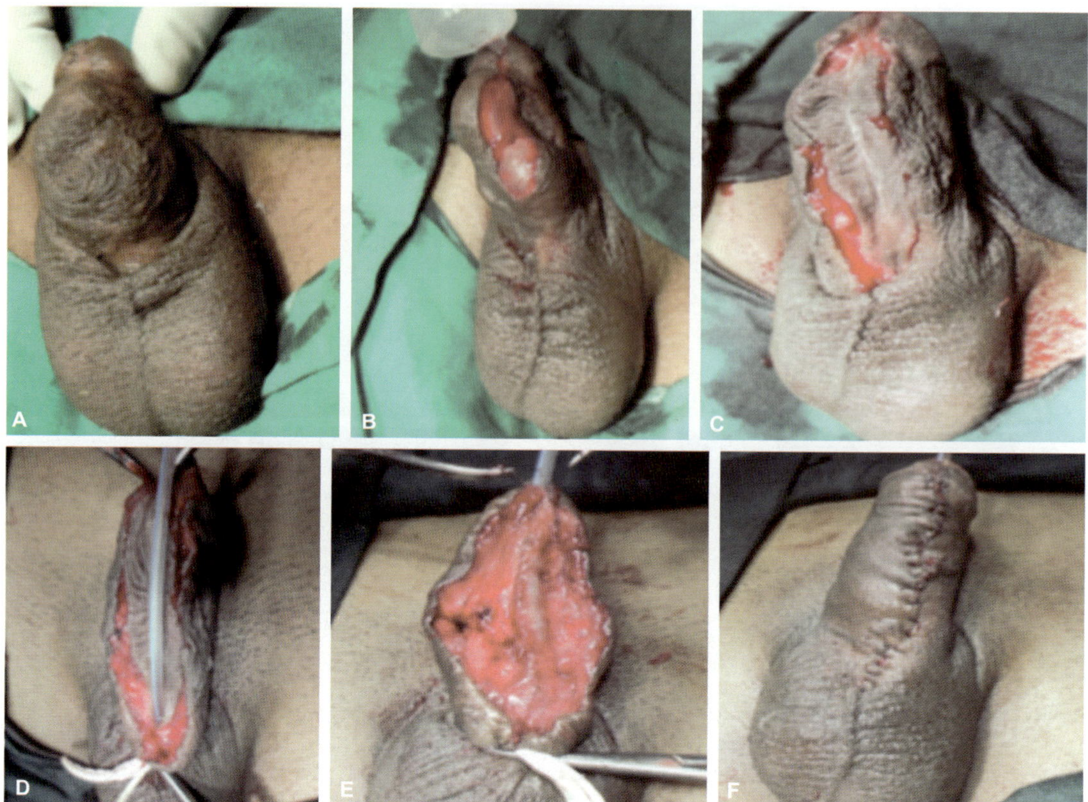

Fig. 9.11A to F: Reduction urethroplasty in urethral diverticula (with permission Bhat AL. Reference [2] @ copyright Springer Nature Singapore): (A) An adult patient with a urethral diverticulum; (B) Skin incision showing saline-filled diverticulum; (C) Laid-open diverticula; (D)Urethral skin trimmed to create the urethral plate of adequate size; (E) Urethral plate tubularization and covering it with dartos and (F) Skin closure

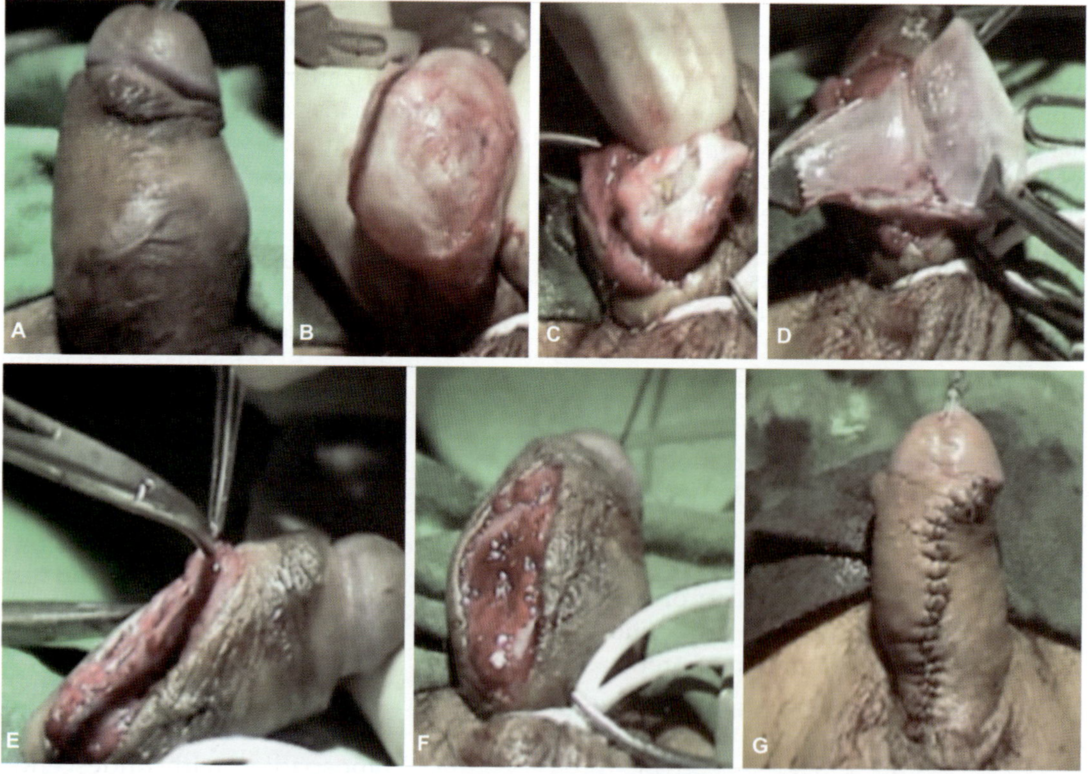

Fig. 9.12A to G: Diverticula, torsion and urethral stones (with permission Bhat AL. Reference [1] @ copyright Springer Nature Singapore): (A) Deformed shaft, torsion and ballooning of ventral surface of the shaft; (B) Mobilized urethral diverticula; (C) Urethral stones in opened diverticula; (D) Excision of urethral diverticula closure of the neck of diverticula; (E and F) Supporting the urethra with dartos and (G) Skin closure and final picture

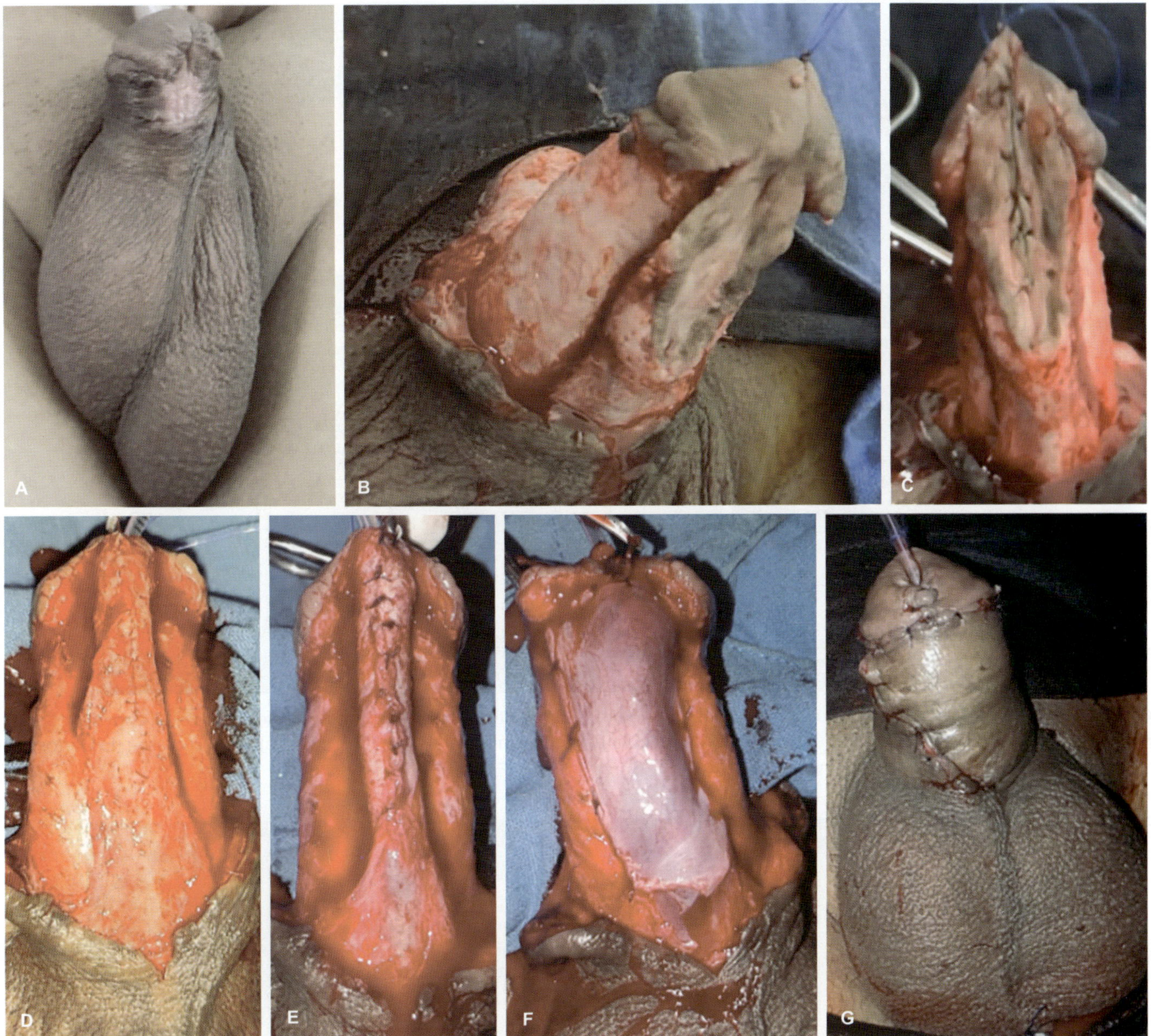

Fig. 9.13A to G: Distal laid open urethra augmented TIPU and tunica vaginalis. Flap: (A) Distal laid open urethra; (B) Penile degloving and mobilization of urethral plate and spongiosum; (C) Dorsal inlay graft; (D) Tubularization of urethral plate; (E) Spongioplasty; (F) Tunica vaginalis. Flap cover and (G) Skin closure

22. How will you manage them?

Ans: For simple undescended testis orchiopexy or orchidectomy in atrophic testis has to be done along with hypospadias repair. But cases with DSD or mullerian duct remnant; excision of vaginal pouch or hysterectomy with unilateral oophorectomy or excision of ovotestis is required (Fig. 9.15). Removal of intraperitoneal mullerian duct remnant can be done with laparoscopy or with open surgery.[1]

23. How will you plan surgery in a hypospadias cripple?

Ans: No single technique is considered standard of care for crippled hypospadias repair; they have multiple problems of variable deformities and the consequent functional abnormality. The surgeon's experience with all surgical techniques of hypospadias repair is an important factor in a successful outcome. Problems can be grouped in as follows and treated accordingly:

1. Residual chordee and/or penile torsion can be managed by Penile de-gloving, urethra/urethral plate/vascular pedicle mobilization, plication procedures of corporotomy and corporoplasty.
2. Reconstruction of the urethra: Urethroplasty can be done in single if tissue (previous urethra, residual urethral plate, peri fistula skin flap,

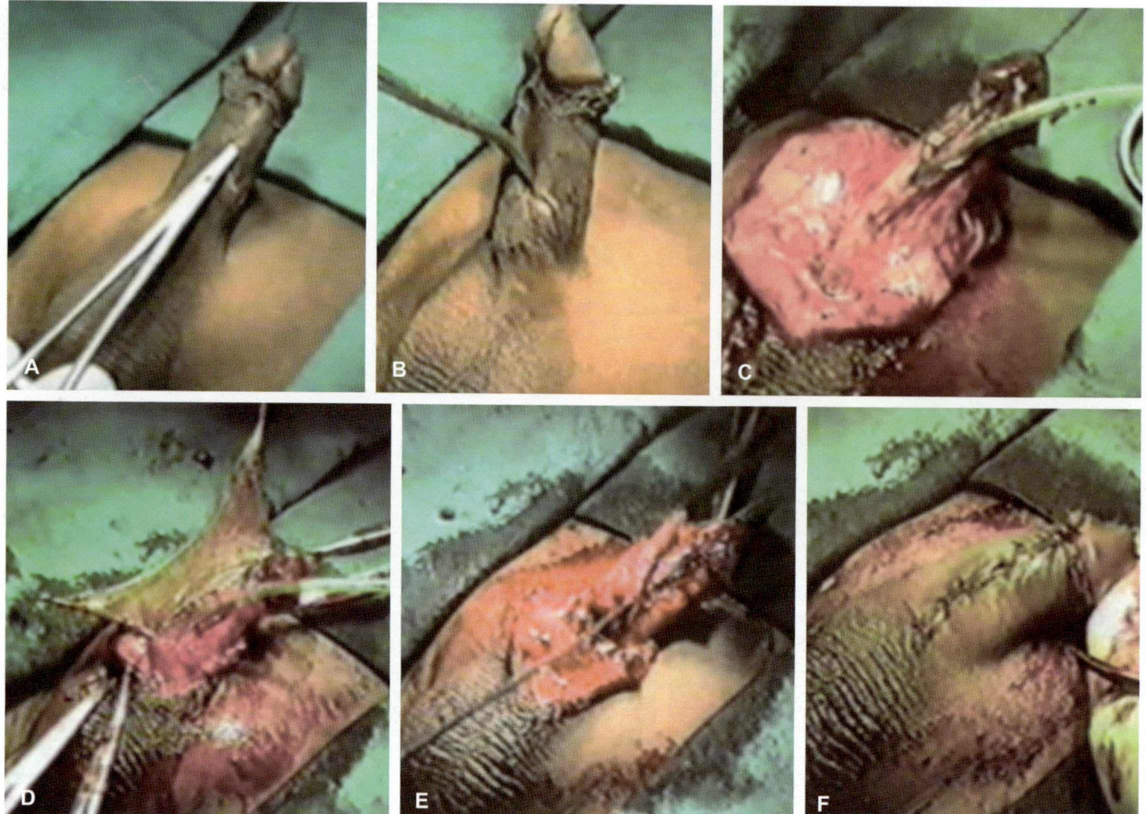

Fig. 9.14A to F: (A and B) Multiple fistulae and distal laid open urethra (with permission Bhat AL. Reference [1] @ copyright Springer Nature Singapore); (C) Penile degloving and creating urethral plate by combining all fistula; (D) Onlay flap urethroplasty; (E) Dartos cover over neo-urethra and (F) Glansplasty and skin closure

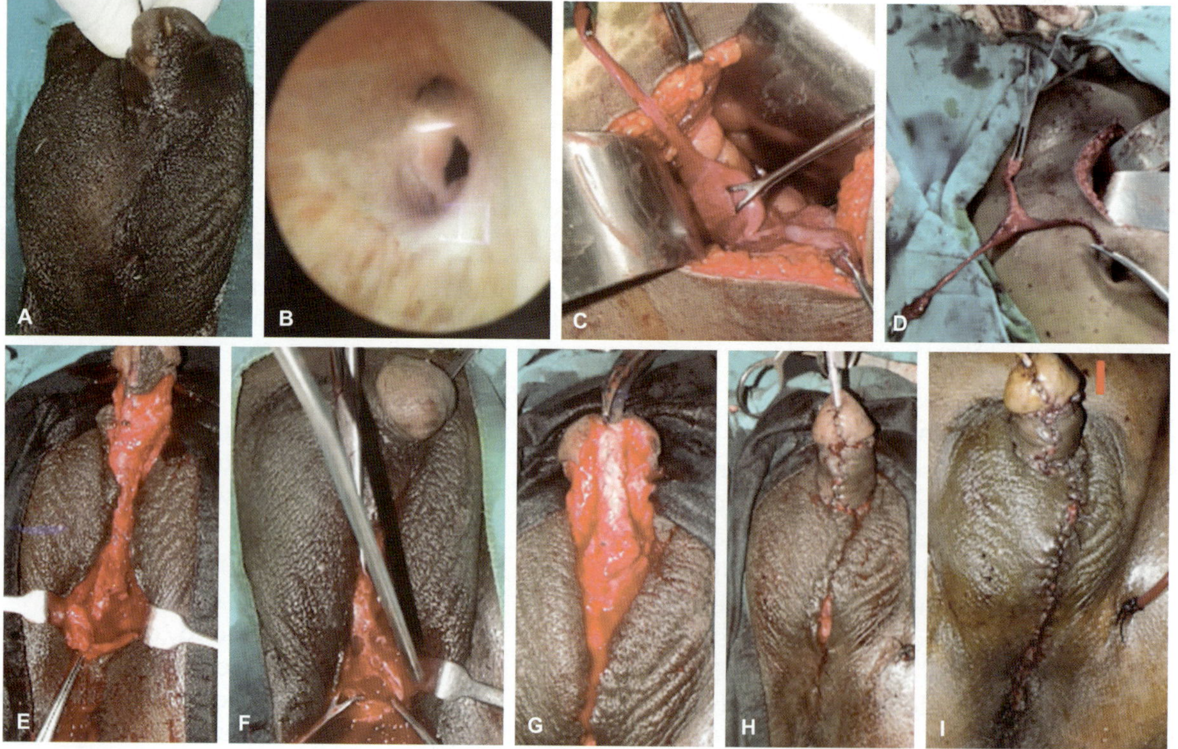

Fig. 9.15A to I: Urethroplasty with excision of Mullerian duct remnant; (A) Distal laid open urethra with bifid scrotum with perineal fistula; (B) Urethroscopy showing dorsal urethra and ventral vaginal opening; (C) Mullerian duct mobilized after laparotomy; (D) Mullerian duct remnant excised; (E) Perineal fistula mobilized; (F) Vaginal cavity opened and mobilized; (G) Urethral opening from urethra closed distal opened urethra tubularized and spongioplasty done; (H) Scrotoplasty done and (I) Skin closure done

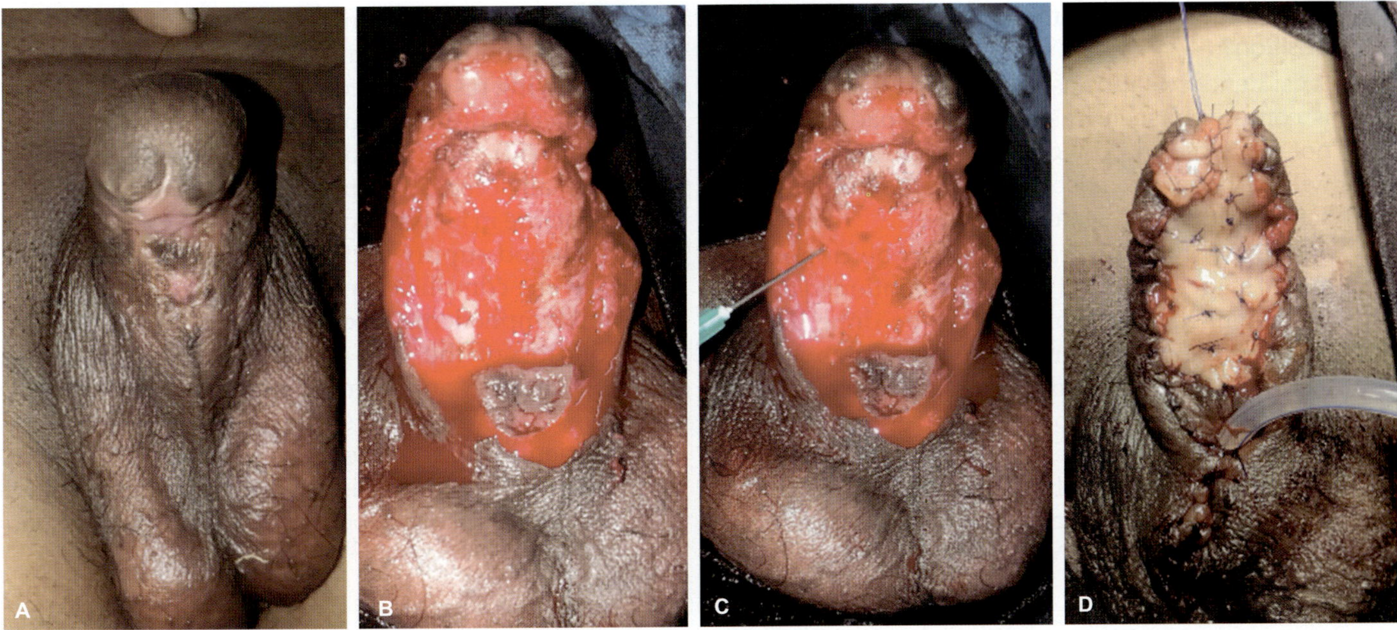

Fig. 9.16: Hypospadias cripple operated five times failed buccal mucosal graft (with permission Bhat AL. Reference [1] @ copyright Springer Nature Singapore): (A) Failed hypospadias repair with proximal meatus, chordee, contracture of buccal graft and unhealthy ventral skin; (B) Chordee correction after excising the fibrous tissue; (C) Gittes test to confirm chordee correction and (D) Buccal mucosal graft and quilting on the ventral aspect of the penis up to the glans' tip.

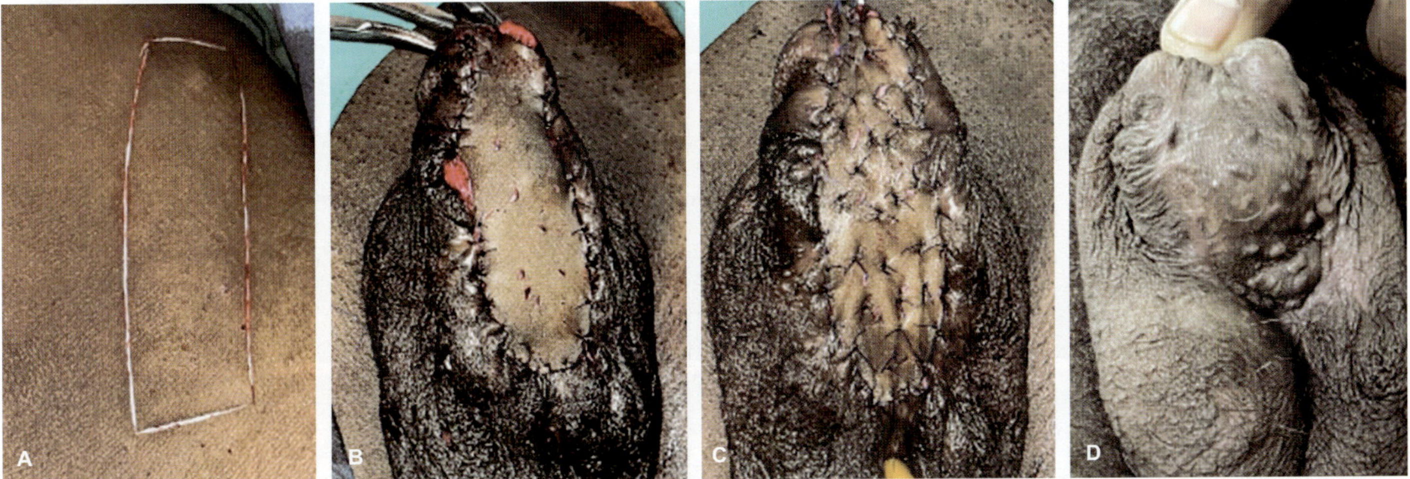

Fig. 9.17: Skin graft hypospadias cripple after failed buccal mucosa: (A) Groin skin flap marked; (B) Graft suture to ventral surface after correction of chordee; (C) Graft quilted and (D) Postoperative well taken up graft

penile skin flap, onlay flap) is available. But if tissue is not available then preferably two-stage urethroplasty should be planned. Bladder/buccal mucosal graft (Fig. 9.16), penile skin graft, non-hair bearing skin grafts can be used (Fig. 9.17).

3. Healthy tissue cover like dorsal, ventral and scrotal dartos/spongioplasty and tunica vaginalis flap.
4. Resurfacing of the skin: Primary skin closure, dorsal releasing incision, dorsal skin flap, scrotal flap and free skin graft, tissue expanders, and cecil culp staged repair.
5. Alternatively, penile skin graft, non-hair bearing skin grafts, buccal mucosal or bladder mucosal grafts are used to reconstruct the neo-urethra. In severe cases, cecil culp urethroplasty may be used where skin is unavailable to cover the penile shaft, and urethroplasty needs support.
6. If scrotoplasty has not been done earlier with hypospadias repair, it should be combine with the hypospadias repair.

24. How to tackle bifid scrotum or penoscrotal transposition?

Ans: Penoscrotal transposition and bifid scrotum is commonly seen in severe hypospadias. If it is not corrected in previous surgeries, then patients will be having penoscrotal transposition or bifid scrotum as it was seen in this case.

Repair may be staged or can be done in a single stage, provided the goals mentioned above are achieved. Scrotoplasty may be done in two or three stages in perineal hypospadias and in cases of bifid scrotum. The chordee correction in first stage is followed by urethroplasty or scrotoplasty in the second, and scrotoplasty or urethroplasty in the third stage. It is better to go for two-stage orthoplasty and/or scrotoplasty in the first stage, and urethroplasty glanuloplasty and scrotoplasty in the second stage. Prior reconstruction of transposition may give more satisfying results since the scrotum is placed in its proper anatomical position before urethroplasty. The penile shaft also becomes more prominent with an acceptable appearance cosmetically. The principle in all types of scrotoplasty is to preserve the blood supply and lymphatics of the penis to prevent complications like penile skin necrosis and lymphedema. The surgical technique includes rotation of the two scrotal flaps, join them in the midline, and then do skin closure vertically (Fig. 9.18). Complex surgical procedures require reoriention of the scrotum inferiorly with limited rotation flaps, inguinal based groin flaps and transposition of the penis superiorly in a planned two-stage approach.[11,12]

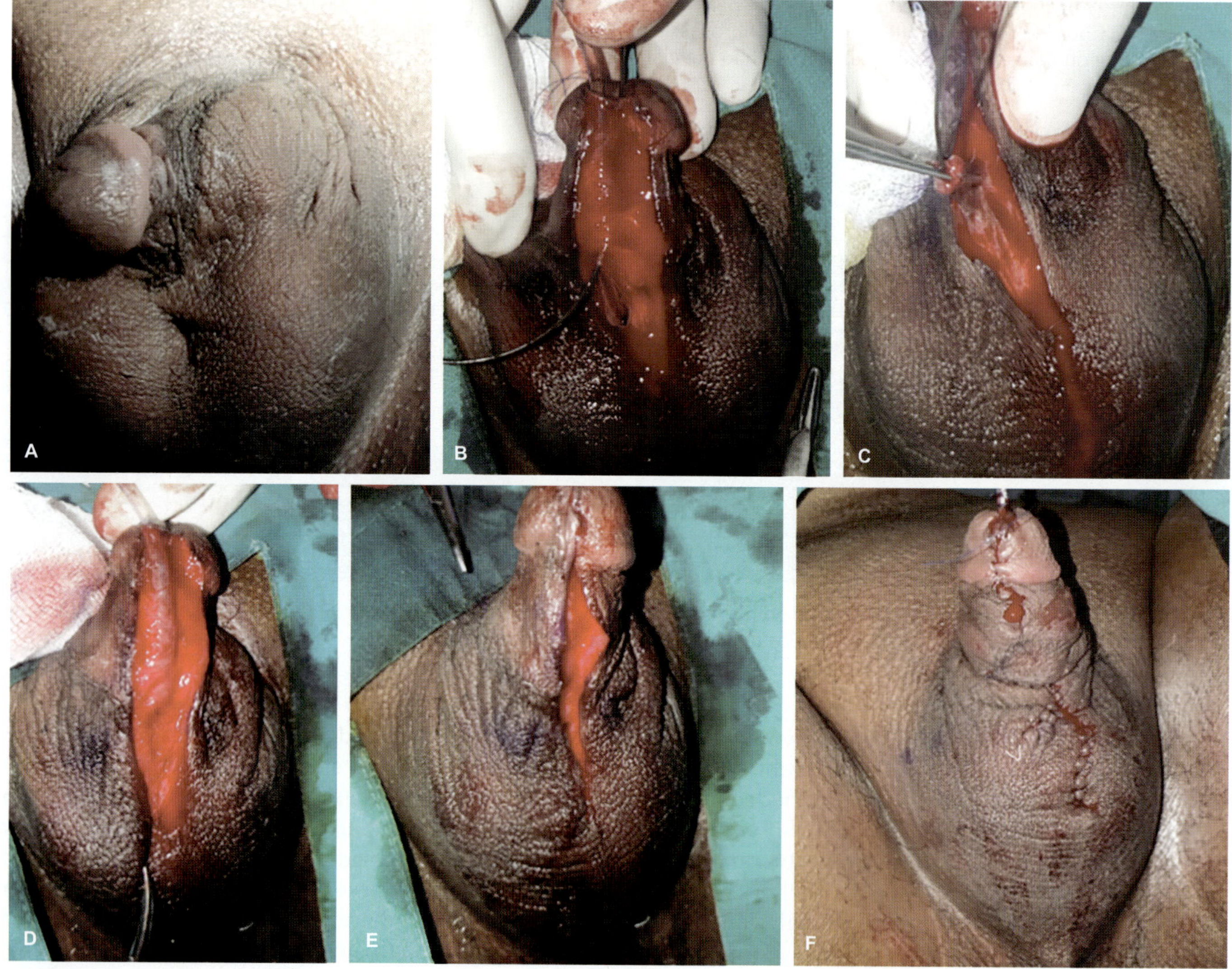

Fig. 9.18A to F: Fistula closure and scrotoplasty in hypospadias cripple: (A) Chordee, scrotal fistula bifid scrotum, rough skin ventrally and dorsally; (B) Partial penile degloving guidewire in fistula; (C) Mobilization of fistulous tract; (D) Fistula closure and dartos cover; (E) Glansplasty and (F) Z-plasty skin closure and scrotoplasty

SUMMARY

- All patients of severe hypospadias with or without UDT, with dimple in perineum, bifurcated median raphe and long ano-scrotal distance should be evaluated for DSD with MRI, genitogram and endoscopy.
- Residual chordee is managed by penile degloving, mobilization of urethral plate and spongiosum in previous failed TIPU, superficial corpotomy/dorsal plication in cases corporal disproportion. Corporoplasty is rarely needed.
- Penile torsion is managed by penile degloving, releasing the pedicle traction to mobilize it and final adjustment with counter traction by dartos or skin flap.
- An attempt of dilatation/VIU and urethroplasty may be tried but urethroplasty with flap or graft is preferred.
- Coronal, sub-coronal fistula is better managed by laying open the distal repair and redo TIPU or augmented TIPU with single or double dartos cover, simple fistula closed in two layers after excising the fistulous tract and trimming the margin cover with dartos single/double andor tunica vaginalis. Multiple fistulae are combined then onlay flap/replacement urethroplasty with tunica vaginalis cover. Two stage urethroplasty where adequate healthy tissue not available for reconstruction of urethra.
- Diverticula is to be managed by reduction urethroplasty with dartos pseudospongioplasty or tunica vaginalis cover with or without stricturoplasty.
- All patients with UDT are managed by repair of hypospadias with orchiopexy, orchidectomy in atrophic testis and excision of Mullerian duct remnant.
- Hypospadias cripple or multiple failed surgeries are managed by correction of chordee/torsion and urethroplasty with healthy tissue cover if tissue is available in single stage, otherwise correct chordee and put buccal mucosal graft and tubularize it in second stage.
- Scrotoplasty should be done all cases of failed hypospadias with bifid scrotum or penoscrotal trans position with the hypospadias repair or rarely as separate repair later on.

REFERENCES

1. Bhat AL. Management of hypospadias cripple. In Hypospadiology: Principles and Practices. Publishers Nature Springer Singapore Pte Ltd 2022,315–332.
2. Bhat AL. Late postoperative complication of hypospadias repair. In Hypospadiology: Principles and Practices. Publishers Nature Springer Singapore Pte Ltd 2022,295–313.
3. Bracka A (1995). Hypospadias repair: the two-stage alternative. British Journal of Urology 76 (6):31–41.
4. Shekhar A, Bhat AL. Management of Hypospadias in Patients with Disorders of Sexual Development. In Hypospadiology: Principles and Practices. Publishers Nature Springer Singapore Pte Ltd 2022,333–347.
5. Craig JR, Wallis C, Brant WO, Hotaling JM, Myers JB (2014). Management of adults with prior failed hypospadias surgery. Translational andrology and urology 3 (2):196.
6. Fam MM, Hanna MK (2017). Resurfacing the penis of complex hypospadias repair ("Hypospadias Cripples"). The Journal of Urology 197 (3 Part 2):859–864.
7. Bhat A, Singh V, Bhat M. Penile torsion. In surgical techniques in Pediatric and adult urology, Jaypee Brothers Medical Publishers New Delhi/London 1st edition 2020,207–222.
8. Sunay M, Dadalı M, Karabulut A, Emir L, Erol D (2007). Our 23-year experience in urethrocutaneous fistulas developing after hypospadias surgery. Urology 69 (2):366–368.
9. Vallasciani S, Berrettini A, Nanni L, Manzoni G, Marrocco G, Observational retrospective study on acquired megalourethra after primary proximal hypospadias repair and its recurrence after tapering. Journal of Pediatric Urology 2013,9(3):364–367.
10. Wiener JS, Sutherland RW, Roth DR, Gonzales ETJ Comparison of onlay and tubularized island flaps of inner preputial skin for the repair of proximal hypospadias. The Journal of Urology 1997158 (3):1172–1174.
11. Bhat A, Bhat M, Bhat A. Management of Penoscrotal transposition. In surgical techniques in Pediatric and adult urology, Jaypee Brothers Medical publishers New Delhi/ London 1st edition 2020,223–228.
12. Bhat AL. Management of Penoscrotal transposition with or without hypospadias. In Hypospadiology: Principles and Practices. Publishers Nature Springer Singapore Pte Ltd 2022, 349–362.

Chapter

10

Newborns with Exstrophy and Isolated Epispadias

• *Uday Sankar Chatterjee*

LEARNING OBJECTIVES

- Initial management
- Deformities in classic bladder exstrophy (CBE).
- Genitourinary system of CBE at birth.
- Principle of reconstruction.
- Expected final outcome.
- Mechanism of continence.
- Outlet sphincters.
- Embryology and genetic basis CBE.
- When to consider termination of pregnancy?
- Prenatal counseling.
- Why the Gordian knot has not yet been cut in management of CBE?

Case Scenario 1

Newborn with classic bladder exstrophy (CBE).

1. **What should be the initial management in these children?**
   Ans: At birth, umbilical plastic clamp might cause trauma to mucosa. So, it is to be substituted with silk suture knot. Bladder mucosa to be kept protected with thin plastic membrane (available as plastic gloves). Abdominal skin to be guarded from rash which might occur due to prolonged contact period of clothes soaked in urine. Exclusion of other anomalies, particularly cardiac, is mandatory with necessary investigations.
2. **What are the deformities seen in a case of CBE?**
   Ans: The rectus abdominis muscles get inserted at widely separated pubic bones resulting in divergent rectus abdominis muscles in the midline at lower abdominal wall. There are outward rotation and lateral displacement of innominate bones. As a consequence of this displacement, puborectalis, adductor longus, and other pelvic floor muscles are widely separated to get insertion at deviated pelvic bones. Thick bladder plate of CBE, five to six times thicker compared to normal newborn bladder, is exposed at lower abdominal wall and umbilical cord is attached at the midpoint of cephalad margin of CBE.
3. **What pathological changes are seen in the genitourinary system at birth?**
   Ans: Anterior corporal tissue is almost 50% shorter[1] at birth unlike normal neonates. Most children of CBE are born with normal kidneys. Density of the muscarinic cholinergic receptors in bladder plate of CBE is found to be normal. Type I collagen in the CBE is normal at initial closure. However, bladder wall thickness is five to six times unlike normal neonatal bladder; due to excess production of type III collagen[2] to cope with the pressure from abdominal cavity in absence of rectus abdominis muscle support at lower abdomen.
4. **What is the embryological basis of this anomaly?**
   Ans: Infraumbilical mesodermal ingrowth between the ectodermal and endodermal layers of thin cloacal membrane is necessary for the formation

of lower abdominal muscles and pelvic bones in the midline. Thus, the formation of bladder and urethra are protected. Absence of mesodermal support causes rupture of weak cloacal membrane resulting in CBE. The incidence of bladder exstrophy is estimated to be around one in 50,000 live births. Some authors[3] suggest a possible genetic basis for development of the CBE. Large doses of progesterone to mothers in first trimester may increase (~10-fold) the incidence of exstrophy. Similarly, it is observed that *in vitro* fertilization might also increase the incidence by 7.5-fold due to the effect of high doses of progesterone.

5. **Should be pregnancy be terminated after prenatal diagnosis of CBE?**

   Ans: Prenatal diagnosis of CBE is difficult with USG. Only 25% of CBE might be diagnosed prenatally.[4] In prenatal USG, both prune belly and exstrophy show deficiency in lower abdominal wall. But in prune belly, bladder and dilated upper tract is usually visible. MRI might increase the detection rate.

6. **How should we counsel the parents prenatally?**

   Ans: Compassionate, empathetic consolation and optimistic counselling would be necessary as because management of CBE has improved. Association or clubbing with the parents and patients having successful outcome in CBE would be very much helpful. Postnatal early consultation at tertiary centre is necessary; however, emergency reconstruction is not needed.

7. **What is the main goal of CBE management?**

   Ans: To achieve continence as well as protection of renal function.

8. **What are the principles of reconstruction in a case of CBE?**

   Ans: Reconstruction for CBE is not an emergency operation. However, full-term baby, body weight more than 3 kg, good bladder plate, child in anabolic state and absence of other serious anomalies; might be operated during newborn period. Otherwise, operative procedure is to be done at around three months of age. Bladder and urethral plate are to be reconfigured. Rectus abdominis should be brought at midline in between reconfigured bladder and abdominal wall to restore the mesodermal deficit. Osteotomy or muscle flaps are required to relocate rectus abdominis muscles in midline

9. **What is the expected final outcome?**

   Ans: Continent urethral void or with CIC (clean intermittent catheterisation) without renal damage is the expected outcome.

10. **What is the mechanism of continence in these children?**

    Ans: Adequate bladder capacity {(Age +2) × 30 ml}, optimum bladder pressure (DLPP < 40 cm of water) and synchronization of bladder contraction and relaxation of outlet sphincters are necessary for normal urethral void as well as to protect kidneys.

11. **Describe the neural control of sphincters.**

    Ans: Urethral intramural sphincters, i.e. rhabdo-sphincter and lisso-sphincter, supplied by sympathetic, parasympathetic and somatic pudendal nerves, are responsible for continence. Sympathetic neural supply keeps the slow twitch fibre of sphincters contracted for 24 hours. Parasympathetic relaxes those sphincters for micturition for a few minutes. Rhabdosphincter is basically a striated muscle, however, it has got ~ 70% slow twitch fibre like non-striated muscle and slow twitch fibre component is controlled by autonomic nerves. Pudendal nerve stimulation contracts fast twitch component of rhabdo-sphincter and fast twitch perineal muscles in emergency.[5]

12. **What is dreaded complication in achieving continence following reconstructive procedures?**

    Ans: Renal damage.

13. **Why is there VUR (vesico-ureteric reflux) and hydronephrosis following reconstructive surgery?**

    Ans: As per Laplace principle, following closure of thick and small bladder, there is increased bladder pressure.[6–9] The principle states that pressure produced within a closed sphere following contraction of wall, is inversely proportional to the volume of sphere. That means pressure within a thick and thimble bladder following reconfiguration of CBE will exert excessive pressure compared to normal bladder which is more capacious and has normal detrusor wall thickness. This increases pressure can lead to VUR or hydronephrosis.

14. **What are the consequences of excessive pressure in reconfigured bladder?**

    Ans: Excessive pressure created from the contraction force of thick walled small bladder[6,7] as per Laplace principle, might damage either the renal function or reconstructed continence mechanism or both. So a balance between achievement of continence and preservation of renal functions the most daunting challenge.[7]

15. **How to avoid the effect of high pressure from bladder?**

    Ans: It is suggested to vent out the pressure[8,9] that is produced following contraction of thick-walled small bladder following reconfiguration of CBE.

16. Is there any congenital defect at the uretero-vesical junction to cause VUR?

Ans: Although it was initially suspected, on later studies uretero-vesical junctions were found not to be defective to cause VUR.

17. Why single stage repair shifted to multistage procedure?

Ans: Outcome of single stage repair was a disaster due to excessive pressure in reconfigured bladder due to non-appreciation of Laplace principle. Incidence of kidney damage was ~ 90% and continence was very suboptimal, i.e. around 20%.[11] So, multistage procedure is preferred.

18. What are the main premises of multistage procedure, i.e. of MSRE (multistage repair of exstrophy)?

Ans: To keep bladder incontinent following initial repair, to allow the bladder to grow and allow the bladder to shred off its increased wall thickness as much as possible. So that damage of kidney function and widening of posterior urethra with sphincters or both would be averted. So, the outcome improved compared to single stage procedure.

19. Why the outcomes improve following MSRE?

Ans: In MSRE, there is no BNR (bladder neck reconstruction) in 1st stage procedure. Bladder neck is kept incontinent, possibly due to quasi appreciation of Laplace principle, to allow excessive pressure to be vented out. BNR was then recommended following increase in bladder capacity ~100 cc within 18 months. So, the bladder pressure during contraction would be less in comparison to the closed thick bladder with capacity ~5 cc done in single stage.

Nevertheless, following BNR, bladder compliance and normal stability would be lost in most[7] if the pressure is not kept in restrain in small bladder. So, normal or near normal capacity is essential, as early as possible, to prevent the generation of high pressure following contraction.

20. Is there any possibility for the "abnormal bladder" to achieve normal or near normal capacity following waiting for years?

Ans: Normal or near normal capacity is essential for urinary continence.[6,11–13] Some patients (~5%) may achieve normal capacity. However, most of reconfigured CBE grow from ~5 ml (neonatal) to ~ 150 ml, i.e. ~30 times, compared to normal bladder which grows from ~25 ml (neonatal) to ~400 ml, i.e. 16 times at adolescence as physiological capacity. However, we are expecting ~80 times growth of "abnormal bladder" to reach normal capacity for continence and to protect kidney.

21. Can we predict which CBE would achieve normal capacity?

Ans: No study is yet available.[13] However, in our personal observation, we found that if the capacity of reconfigured CBE grows more than 12 times in 12 months, there is a possibility to achieve normal capacity.

22. Are the urethral sphincters intramural (rhabdosphincter and lissosphincter) or extramural (puborectalis, levator ani group of pelvic floor muscles)?

Ans: Yes, urethral sphincters are intramural. rhabdosphincter and lissosphincter are situated at submucosa. Those are composed predominantly with slow twitch, and non-fatigable fibres. So they can keep the urethral lumen closed almost for 24 hours.

Previously it was presumed that urethral continence, for 24 hours, is maintained by pelvic and perineal striated muscles. Those are composed of fast twitch, fatigable fibres. As a result, it is not possible to maintain contraction for 24 hours with puborectalis, levator ani group of pelvic floor muscles. However, their contribution is very much needed in emergency situations in keeping the outlet closed voluntarily for a few minutes.

Kelly relied on the concept of extramural sphincters, i.e. puborectalis and levator ani group of muscles for continence. So, they did radical mobilisation of pelvic floor muscles around the reconfigured CBE.[14] Possibly, the mobilised pelvic floor muscles and soft tissues in midline supported the reconfigured tubular urethra and its intramural sphincters as reinforcement. So, there was some improvement in continence.

23. What is an exstrophy variant?

Ans: In CBE, defects are noted in skeletal, urinary, and genital system. In patients with exstrophy variants there are presence of wide pubic diastasis, wide separation of rectus abdominis, puborectalis, levator ani, etc, as similar as found in CBE. But patients with exstrophy variants are continent (Fig. 10.1) and have normal looking penis in spite of wide diastasis.

24. What have we learnt from exstrophy variants?

Ans: We appreciated the location of bona fide sphincters of continence. Normal urethral sphincters with slow twitch fibres are within urethra, i.e. intramural (Fig. 10.2) not in the muscles of pelvic floor with fast twitch fibre. Slow twitch fibres have got ability to keep the urethra closed for 24 hours. On the other hand, fast twitch can produce strong contraction for minutes.

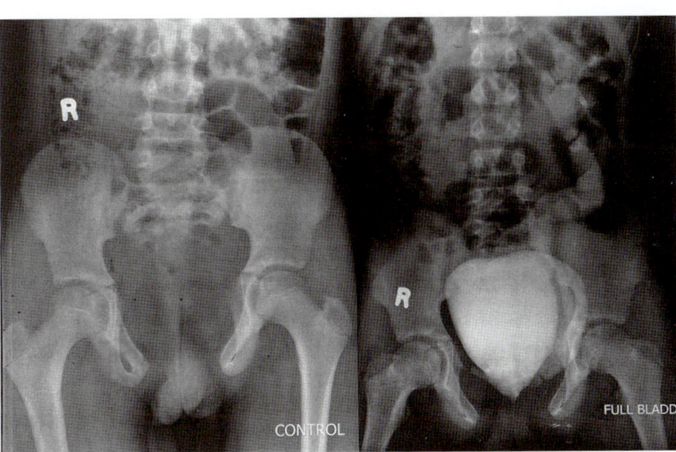

Fig. 10.1: MCU of continent pseudoexstrophy even with wide diastasis

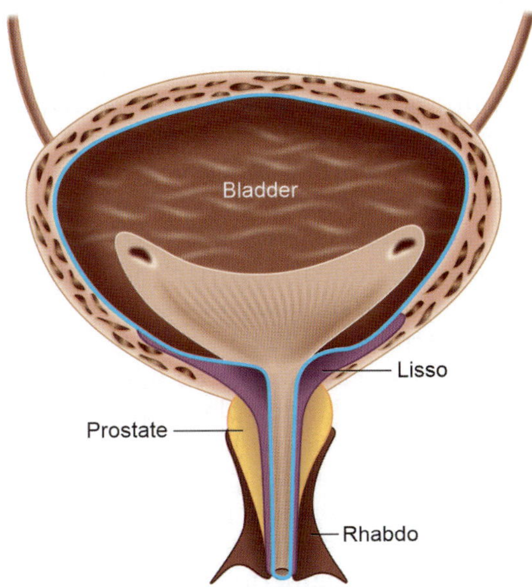

Fig. 10.2: Urethral intramural sphincters

25. Which one is responsible for urinary continence; particularly in male? Is it bladder neck or urethral sphincters?

Ans: Sphincter at bladder neck or lisso sphincter in male is mainly for antegrade ejaculation. However, lisso sphincter (Fig. 10.2) also helps rhabdo sphincter in urinary continence[3] in female as well as in male.

26. What should get higher consideration in creating continence mechanism? BNR or "reconfiguration of bladder neck" and reconfiguration of posterior urethral sphincter?

Ans: BNR means tightening of bladder neck. It might cause bladder outlet obstruction. But "reconfiguration" means merely closure of bladder neck and posterior urethral plate.[15] BNR might be a hindrance of natural urethral void.

27. Why Grady and Mitchell reconceptualised one stage procedure, i.e. complete primary repair of exstrophy (CPRE)?

Ans: Ellison *et al* and Grady realised the continence mechanism from exstrophy variants.[16] They realised that adequate bladder capacity is an essential factor for continence as well as to prevent VUR (vesicoureteric reflux), renal damage and damage of reconfigured bladder. However, they trusted on "abnormal bladder"[17,18] of CBE to pull off normal capacity following early CPRE and early bladder filling and cycling.[15] Grady realised that the urethral sphincters are intramural (Fig. 10.2) from their surveillance on exstrophy variants. That's why, Grady and Mitchell reconceptualised one stage procedure. So, they did CPRE without osteotomy and without re-implantation of ureters. However, afterwards they[19] realised osteotomy is necessary for low tension approximation of rectus abdominis particularly in wide pubic diastasis.

28. Why the CPRE failed to show significant outcome compared to MSRE?

Ans: Grady *et al* advanced the concept of intramural sphincters, necessity of normal bladder capacity for continence and for renal protection. However, they relied on "abnormal bladder" to grub up normal capacity! Their "reconfigured bladder" following CPRE suffered excessive bladder pressure that resulted in gradual breakdown of continence mechanism that decreased from 74%[19] to 42%.[16] Similarly, due to increased bladder pressure, 40% VUR[19] became 70% in next publication after 8 years.[16] So, bladder neck operation was necessary in 80%[16] in an attempt to regain continence. Their progressive concept was muddled due to the unawareness towards Laplace principle.

29. What are the harmful effects produced as per principle of Laplace principle?

Ans: Harmful effect as per Laplace principle was unknown to Grady (personal communication at USICON Agra 2010). Similarly, Laplace principle is unknown to many authors and common belief is that incontinent small and thick bladder might not create excessive pressure. However, that was overturned by Hollowell *et al*[7] with UDS. Bladder pressure was found to be as high as 55–165 cm of water even in incontinent patients following BNR without augmentation. Hollowell *et al* also found that increased DLPP (detrusor leak point pressure) is the primary risk factor for VUR, if DLPP is more than 30 cm of water.

30. Is osteotomy necessary for continence?

Ans: Previously it was believed that perineal and pelvic floor muscles (extramural sphincters)

are responsible for continence. Gradually the concept of sphincters shifted from extramural to intramural. Exstrophy variants, CPRE and other studies[5] showed urethral sphincters as intramural. Now it is appreciated that osteotomy has got no direct role in continence mechanism. Actually, main role of osteotomy is to bring rectus abdominis in midline without tension to prevent dehiscence of abdominal wall[20] which might invite collateral dehiscence of reconfigured bladder, bladder neck and posterior urethra. This newer information implies that the simpler osteotomy would be safe and easier to bring the rectus at midline. In this respect, POM[9] or bilateral pubic ramotomy[21] would meet the purpose. On the other hand, various types of iliac osteotomies are equally helpful but demand expertise; need fixator pins, external fixator bars, longer operative time and patients must remain in immobilisation for one month postoperatively.[20]

31. What should be the plan of management in these children with CBE?

Ans: Patients of CBE might be at risk of renal impairment subsequent to bladder outlet reconstruction or even with simple reconfiguration of CBE as explained above. So they need prior evaluation of renal status through USG renometry, DTPA renal scan for GFR (glomerular filtration rate) at the outset. Accordingly changes in those parameters, if present afterwards, following reconstruction would guide further management at follow-up.

Aim is to make the CBE patient continent for 24-hour like normal individual and continence might be either urethral or with CIC. At the same time we have to protect the GFR of kidneys from transmitted bladder pressure. For that we have to maintain DLPP below 40 cm of water and Pdet Qmax within normal range. So, that subsequent voluntary urethral voiding even with partial support of Valsalva manoeuvre (following augmentation) would not produce reflux and renal damage. In this respect bladder neck reconstruction better to be avoided as it might increase bladder outlet resistance[8] and might increase DLPP. So, it would be better to follow simple "reconfiguration" of bladder neck and posterior urethral plate, i.e. CPRE as described by Grady *et al.*[15] Along with CPRE, pubic osteotomy minimal or POM[9] and vesicostomy like cystostomy track, i.e. CT or a matured suprapubic track[8,9] to be kept to vent out bladder pressure till achievement of normal capacity of bladder or till augmentation. It would be justified to do augmentation, if the capacity of reconfigured CBE does not grow more than 12 times in 12 months. Osteotomy or muscle flap[22] is necessary to bring muscle at midline to preserve the reconfigured bladder and urethra.

Management algorithm:

- Clinical and per-operative assessment of bladder plate and intersymphyseal gap to be done to assess possibilities of bladder closure and for osteotomy. Bladder plate is to be pushed inside with lubricated gloved thumb. Bladder approximation would be possible if it allows half of thumb (~6–7 cc) inside. Apposition of pubic bones for neosymphysis following osteotomy would be easier provided intersymphyseal gap is ~3–4 cm. Final confirmation would be done under general anesthesia. However, gut preparation should be done beforehand. Sometimes bladder approximation might not be possible after separation of bladder plate. So primary augmentation might be necessary.
- Both ureteral osteum are to be identified (sufficient hydration and frusemide might be necessary) and to be catheterised with infant feeding tube (IFT) for easy identification during retrovesical dissection. IFTs should be transfixed near ureteric osteum with 5–0 catgut.
- Retroperitoneal approach is better avoided to minimise neuro-vascular injuries in reconstructing CBE.
- Peritoneal cavity is to be opened at cephalad portion of bladder plate and finger through peritoneal cavity to be placed in between the margins of bladder plate and rectus muscles. Separation of bladder plate from medial margins of rectus abdominis would be easier with monopolar diathermy under finger guidance from peritoneal cavity. Epidermal tissues to be kept away from bladder plate and at the same time migrated epidermal element in bladder mucosa, if present, to be excised to prevent excessive stone formation from the nidus of insoluble keratin[23] of epidermis.
- Downwards incision to be extended just beyond intra-symphyseal band (ISB) which is attached to medial ends of pubic bones and the posterior surface of vesicourethral plate of CBE. ISB is to be harvested by separating from medial end of pubic bones and this ISB would be wrapped over reconfigured neck and posterior urethra following CPRE to complete a circle of ISB around bladder neck to protect the reconfiguration from breakdown.
- Above incision to be extended to up to tip of glans along the lateral margins of urethral plate. Incision at the junction of inner and outer prepucial skin is essential to avail sufficient penile skin to cover the degloved phallus

following correction of dorsal chordee and urethroplasty.

- Posterior or prostatic urethral plate is to be separated from corpora cavernosa as described by Gearhart.[24] Following that bladder and urethral plates are reconfigured with interrupted stitches keeping a CT[9] created with a rectangular skin from abdominal wall at cephalad part of bladder plate (Fig. 10.3). Reconfiguration of urethra along with intramural sphincter is comparatively easier in female patients unlike male counterpart.
- Minimal osteotomy is done at the lateral margins of insertions of rectus abdominis and adductor longus[8] and two pieces of medial ends of pubic bones with insertions of above muscles are to be tied at midline (Fig. 10.3). This POM will bring the rectus abdominis in midline with minimal tension (Fig. 10.5) as well as the attached adductor longus would pull the bladder neck and posterior urethra downwards to place deeper in pelvis (Fig. 10.4) and would help in coaptation of urethral lumen created for eventual continence.[9]

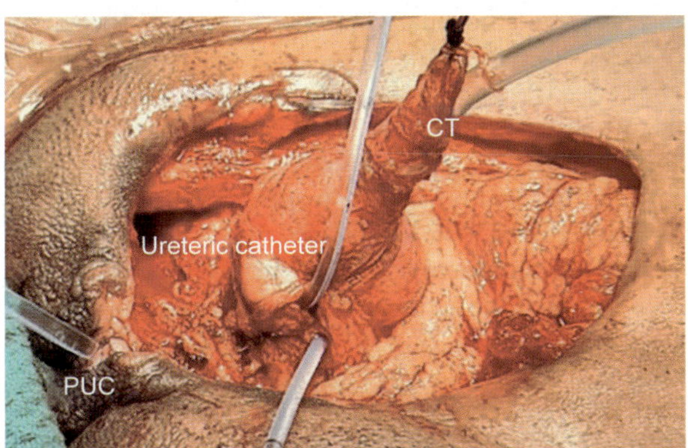

Fig. 10.3: Cystostomy tract or CT

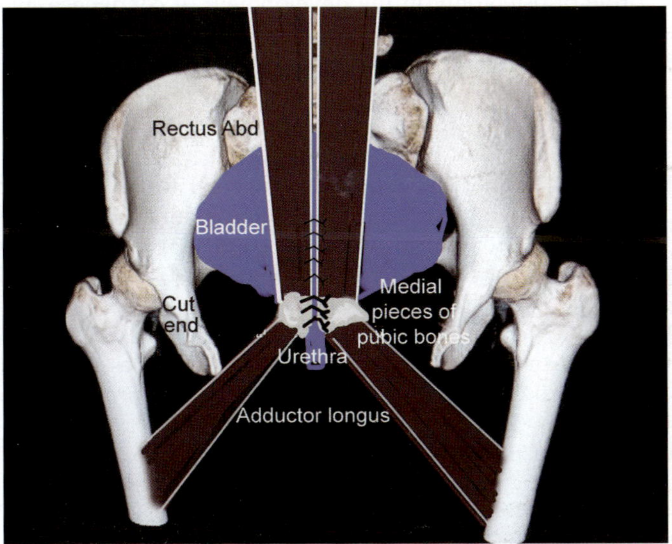

Fig. 10.4: Schematic pubic osteotomy minimal

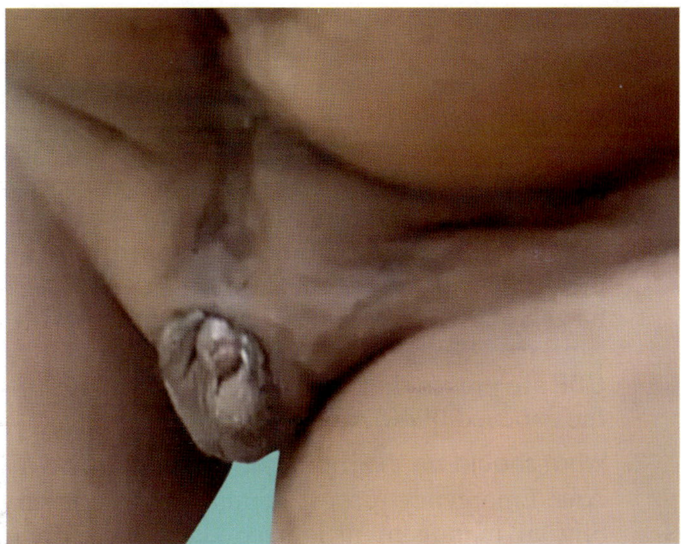

Fig. 10.5: Rectus abdominis muscle at midline following POM

- Rarely reconfiguration of CBE plate may not be possible due to thick wall of bladder plate found following separation of CBE plate; which was not anticipated clinically. In that situation, primary augmentation would be necessary.
- It is suggested to go for earlier augmentation to decrease the excessive pressure in system. Otherwise, expectant waiting might be done for years to allow natural bladder growth. During this waiting period bladder should be kept on suprapubic vent with CT[8] and UDS and DTPA renal scan would be necessary to monitor bladder pressure, DLPP and renal functions respectively. Suprapubic vent with CT will serve as a conduit for CIC as well as vent out excessive pressure in system following reconfiguration of CBE.
- Continence would be either with urethral void (Video 8) or through CIC void.
- DLPP should be below 40 cm of water to preserve renal functions which should be monitored with ACR (albumin creatinine ratio) and GFR.
- Video 8: Normal urethral void following augmentation and expulsion of mucus at the start of void.

Scan QR Code for Video on
Normal urethral void following augmentation and expulsion of mucus at the start of void

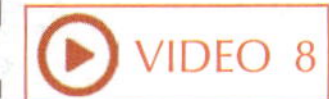

***Case Scenario* 2**

Newborn with an isolated epispadias.

1. What is isolated epispadias?

Ans: Incidence of isolated epispadias is around 1 in 1,00,000 in male population. In male 70%

of isolated epispadias is penopubic. Dorsal wall of the urethra is absent. So the wide glistening urethral plate on dorsum of phallus is exposed. Exposed urethral plate of epispadias may extend up to bladder neck and is then called penopubic or subsymphyseal epispadias. In subsymphyseal epispadias verumontanum would be visible on stretching the phallus and would indicate incontinence. Most of subsymphyseal epispadias have incontinence and inadequate bladder capacity. All the musculo-skeletal anomalies of CBE are present in isolated epispadias, excepting the exposed bladder plate.

2. **What should be the management of epispadias?**

   Ans: Emergency reconstruction is not necessary. Similar management is needed for incontinent peno-pubic epispadias as necessary for CBE. Otherwise, urethroplasty following dorsal chordee correction is done for continent epispadias, i.e. glandular and penile variety.

3. **What are the procedures for urethroplasty for epispadias?**

   Ans: Urethral plate with spongiosa is wider and resilient unlike urethral plate of hypospadias. Hence it is better not to incise the epispadiac urethral plate to correct dorsal chordee and to gain length. Separation of urethral plate with spongiosa from corpora cavernosa is possible from verumontenum to corona (partial disassembly) to get longer urethral plate to correct the chordee. In extreme situation, partially disassembled urethral plate with spongiosa might be detached at corona to create a penile epispadias for further reconstruction after six months. Assembling of both corpora at midline is done to relocate urethra at ventrum.

4. **What is new in this field?**

   Ans:
   - Appreciation of intramural urethral sphincters.
   - Minimal osteotomy.
   - Understanding of Laplace principle.
   - Venting out the pressure from reconfigured CBE.
   - Early augmentation.
   - Possibility of achievement of "Dry period" for 24 hours as normal children.

SUMMARY

- Management of CBE depends on detection and realisation of the effect of bladder pressure on kidney and on continence mechanism following reconfiguration of CBE; and finding out the causes. Appropriate evaluation and timely management would help to save renal function, bladder function and the continence. We hope this management algorithm would help to cut the *Gordian Knot.*

Section 2

REFERENCES

1. Perovic SV, Djinovic RP. New insight into surgical anatomy of epispadiac penis and its impact on repair, J Urol 2008; 179:689–95.
2. Peppas DS, Tchetgen MB, Lee BR, Jeffs RD, Gearhart JP. A quantitative histology of the bladder in various stages of reconstruction utilizing colormorphometry. In Gearhart JP, Mathews RI, editors: Exstrophy-epispadias complex: research concepts and clinical applications, New York, 1999, Plenum, p 41.
3. Ludwig M, Rushendorf F, Saar K, *et al.* Genome-wide linkage scan for bladder exstrophy-epispadias complex, Birth Defects Res A ClinMolTeratol 2009; 85:174–78.
4. Goyal A, Fishwick J, Hurrell R, *et al.* Antenatal diagnosis of bladder/cloacal exstrophy: challenges and possible solutions, J PediatrUrol 2012; 8:140.
5. Koraitim MM.The Male Urethral Sphincter Complex Revisited:An Anatomical Concept and its Physiological Correlate. J Urol 2008; 179: 1683–89.
6. Diamond DA, Bauer SB, Dinlenc C, *et al.* Normal urodynamics in patients with bladder exstrophy: are they achievable? J Urol 1999; 162:841.
7. Hollowell JG, Hill PD, Duffy PG, Ransley PG. Bladder function and dysfunction in exstrophy and epispadias. Lancet 1991; 338:926.
8. Chatterjee US. How we made exstrophy bladder continent and preserved the renal functions. J Indian AssocPediatrSurg 2022;27:605–9.
9. Chatterjee US. Pubic osteotomy minimal for abdominal wall closure in exstrophy bladder. J PediatrUrol 2020;16;394–96. doi.org/10.1016/j.jpurol.2020.05.003.
10. Lattimer JK, Smith MJV. Exstrophy Closure: a Followup on 70 Cases. J Urol 1966; 95: 354–59.
11. Ahmed S, Fouda-neel K, Borghol M. Continence after bladder neck repair in patients with bladder exstrophy and pubic diastasis. BJU 1996; 77: 896–99.
12. Heuser M, Zöller G, Seseke F, Zappel H, Ringert RH., *et al.* Bladder dysfunction in children with bilateral ectopic ureters. J PaediatrSurg 2002;37:E15.
13. Mathews R, Sponseller PD, Jeffs RD, Gearhart JP. Bladder neck reconstruction in classic bladder exstrophy: the role of osteotomy in the development of continence. BJU International 2000; 85: 498–500.
14. Kelly JH. Vesical exstrophy: repair using radical mobilisation of soft tissues. PediatrSurgInt 1995; 10: 298–304.
15. Grady RW, Mitchell ME. Complete primary repair of exstrophy. J Urol 1999; 162: 1415–20.
16. Ellison JS, Shnorhavorian M, Willihnganz-Lawson K, Grady R, Merguerian PA, A critical appraisal of continence in bladder exstrophy: long-term outcomes of the complete primary repair, Journal of Pediatric Urology 2016; 12: 205.e1–205.e7. doi: 10.1016/j.jpurol.2016.04.005.
17. Lee BR, Perlman EJ, Partin AW, Jeff RD, Gearhart JP. Evaluation of smooth muscle and collagen subtypes in normal newborns and those with bladder exstrophy. J urol 1996; 156: 2034–36.
18. Lais A, paolocci N, Ferro F, Bosman C, Boldrini R, Caino P. Morphometric analysis of smooth muscle in the exstrophy-epispadias complex. J Urol 1996; 156: 819–21.
19. Shnorhavorian M, Grady RW, Andersen A, Joyner BD, Mitchell ME. Long-term follow up of complete primary repair

of exstrophy: the Seattle experience. J Urol 2008;180:1615–9; discussion 9–20.

20. Wild AT, Sponseller PD, Stec AA, Gearhart JP. The role of osteotomy in surgical repair of bladder exstrophy. Seminars in Pediatric Surgery 2011; 20: 71–78).
21. Frey P, Cohen SJ. Anterior pelvic osteotomy. A new operative technique facilitating primary bladder exstrophy closure. Br J Urol 1989; 64:641–43.
22. Bhatnagar V, Mitra DK. Anterior abdominal wall closure in bladder exstrophy. PediatrSurgInt 1994; 9: 188–92.
23. Chatterjee US, Chatterjee I. Percutaneous cystolithotomy in augmented bladders. J Indian AssocPediatr 2021;26: 250–2.
24. Gearhart JP, Sciortino C, Ben-Chaim J, Peppas DS, Jeffs RD. The Cantwell-Ransleyepispadias repair in exstrophy and epispadias: lessons learned. Urology 1995; 46: 92–95.

Chapter

11

Wilms Tumor: Clinical Approach

• MS Ansari • Anwesa Chakraborty

LEARNING OBJECTIVES

- A comprehensive clinical approach to a case of renal mass in a child.
- How to extrapolate clinical history and findings to generate differential diagnosis and subsequently to reach to the most probable diagnosis?
- To differentiate masses of benign and malignant nature in paediatric age group.

INTRODUCTION

- Wilms' tumor (WT) is named after Carl Max Wilhelm Wilms, a German pathologist and surgeon. It is the most common primary malignant renal tumor of childhood and comprises 6% of all pediatric tumors.[1]
- Pediatric renal tumors include Wilms' tumor (WT), renal cell carcinoma (RCC), clear cell sarcoma of the kidney (CCSK), rhabdoid tumor of the kidney (RTK), congenital mesoblastic nephroma, cystic renal tumor, and angiomyolipoma.
- WT is by far the most common, accounting for approximately 91% of all renal tumors in childhood, whereas RCC comprises 5.9% of renal malignancies in children and adolescents.[1]
- Current treatment protocols for WT are developed by the Children's Oncology Group (COG), formerly this was done by the National Wilms' Tumor Study Group (NWTSG) in North America, and in Europe by the Socie´te´ Internationale d'Oncologie Pediatrique (SIOP).

Case Scenario

- 5-year-old well-preserved boy with painless gross hematuria and palpable nontender right side renal mass (Fig. 11.1).
- No H/O any other swellings in the body/bony pain/cough/haemoptysis/hypertension.
- Clinically not suggestive of any syndromic association.

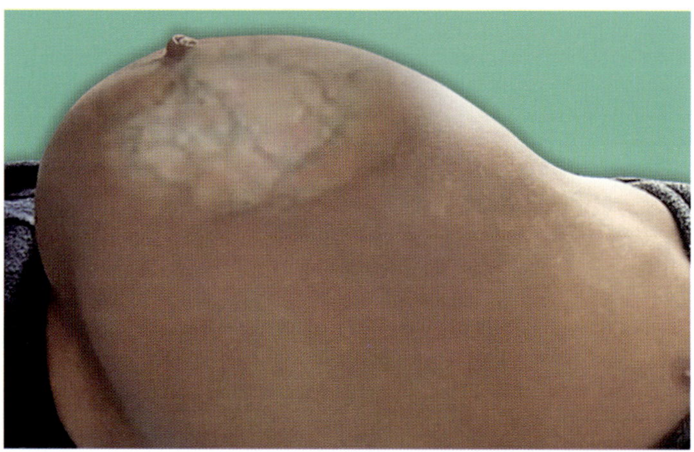

Fig. 11.1: Visible lump with prominent venous prominence

1. How do you examine a child with renal mass?

Ans:

- Child should be calm and quiet.
- Inspection of abdomen should follow a gentle palpation if the tumor is small.
- Palpation may be avoided in large tense masses as that may risk tumor rupture.
- Examine scrotum, phallus of the child for any abnormity (WAGR syndrome, vide infra).
- Examine extremities and eyes to rule out syndromic association.
- Evaluate for masses elsewhere, bony pain, lower limb weakness, fever, diarrhea (rule out neuroblastoma).

2. **What is your diagnosis?**
Ans: Right-sided renal mass, probably Wilms' tumor.

3. **What are your differential diagnoses?**
Ans:
A. Non-malignant
- Hydronephrosis
- Polycystic kidneys
- Mesoblastic nephroma (usually occur in infancy)
- Infective causes: Renal hydatid
- Arising from other organs—mesenteric cyst or intestinal duplication cyst
- Multicystic dysplastic kidney (rarely may present as large mass)

B. Malignant
- Wilms' tumor (age corroborates)
- Renal cell carcinoma (>9 years)
- Clear cell sarcoma of kidney (CCSK) (3%)—same age group as WT; early bone metastasis
- Rhabdoid tumor of kidney (RTK) (2%)—same age group as WT; early brain metastasis, dismal prognosis
- Neuroblastoma
- Primitive neuroectodermal tumors (PNET)
- Retroperitoneal rhabdomyosarcoma (RMS)
- Retroperitoneal germ cell tumor (GCT)
- Teratoma

4. **Why do you suspect WT in this patient?**
Ans:
- Age at presentation
- Well-preserved child
- Painless, palpable mass with hematuria

5. **What is the incidence and classical age group at presentation?**
Ans:
- Before the age of 15 years, Wilms tumor affects approximately one child per 10,000 children worldwide.[2]
- It forms 15% of all paediatric malignancies and is the commonest renal tumor of childhood worldwide.
- Median age at presentation is 3.5 years and there is no gender or side predilection.

6. **What are the known etiologies for WT?**
Ans:
- Mostly sporadic
- <10% from germline mutations:
  - WT1 (11p13) mutations
    WAGR complex: ***Wilms'*** tumor, aniridia, genitourinary anomalies and intellectual retardation
  - WT2 (11p15) LOH: Beckwith–Wiedemann syndrome, hemihypertrophy
- Other associated syndromes: Edward, Perlman, Klippel-Trenaunay-Weber, Sotos syndromes.

7. **What are the common clinical presentations of WT?**
Ans:
- Most common and classic—asymptomatic, smooth palpable flank mass in a well-preserved toddler
- Noticed incidentally or after a trivial trauma
- Abdominal pain or hematuria (may suggest extension into PCS)[3]
- UTI
- Varicocoele (left renal vein occluded by tumor ingrowth)
- Hypertension (25% due to increased Renin activity/renal vascular compression).

8. **What questions should be asked to rule out other differentials?**
Ans:
- Any lump noted on antenatal scans or lump noted since birth (?Hydronephrosis)
- If the lump is painful, associated bony pain or respiratory distress, anorexia, weight loss, or paraplegia, vomiting, diarrhoea, premature puberty (?Neuroblastoma).

9. **How will you proceed for work up in this child?**
Ans:
- Ultrasonography (USG) of whole abdomen with Doppler: It is ideally the first investigation; confirms vascular involvement like renal vein or IVC thrombus
- CECT abdomen and thorax (Fig. 11.2A and B) to confirm extent, resectability, unilateral or

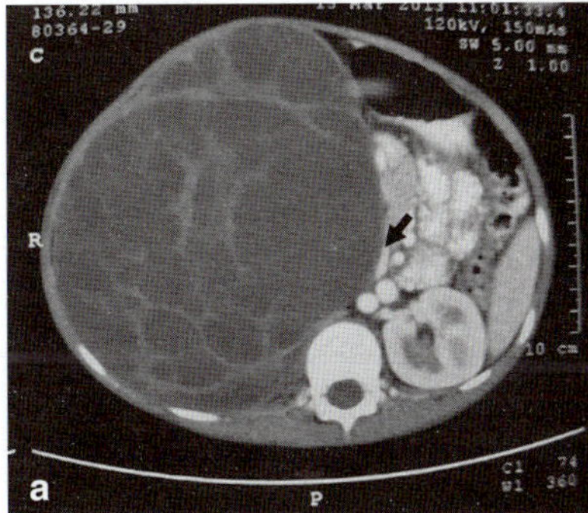

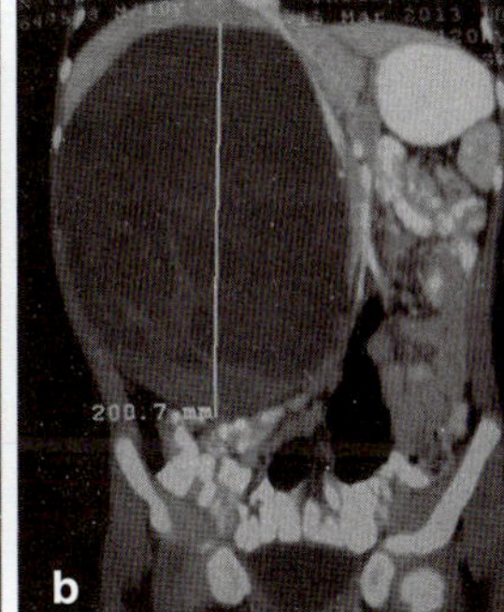

Fig. 11.2A and B: (A) Axial section CT scan: A large heterogeneous mass arising from the right kidney, replacing the most of the renal parenchyma and displacing the intrabdominal content anteromedially. The mass contains mixed solid and cystic areas. Renal vein appears to be compressed (arrow) and but clear of any filling defect along with IVC. No lymphadenopathy noted (B) Coronal section: A large heterogeneous mass arising from the right kidney, replacing the most of the renal parenchyma

bilateral, ureteric, vascular and lymph nodal involvement. Nearly 13% of WT have lung metastasis at diagnosis (Fig. 11.3).

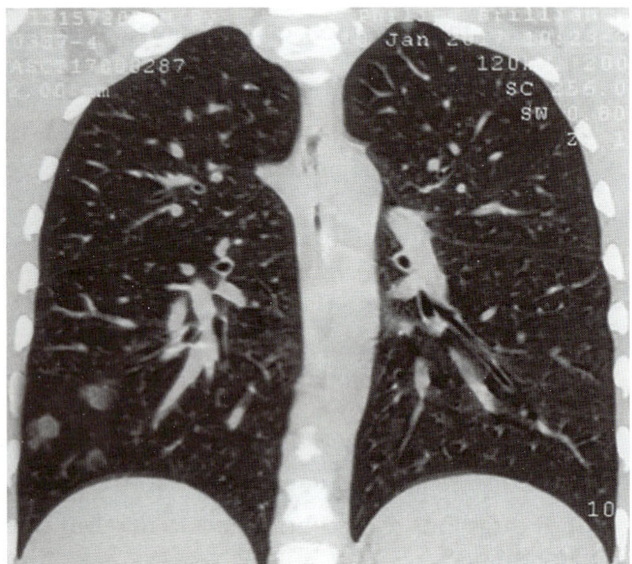

Fig. 11.3: CT chest showing right lung metastasis (arrows)

- Routine labs
- USG guided biopsy (if not resectable upfront, unusual age group)
- MRI abdomen (not mandatory)—better for assessing nephrogenic rests
- Cytogenetic study: Loss of heterozygosity (LOH) at 1p and 16q have high risk of recurrence and death (NWTS5) hence require more aggressive chemotherapy; TP53 mutations in WT are almost exclusively found in tumors with anaplastic histology
- 2D Echo (before starting chemotherapy with doxorubicin).

10. How do you determine its origin from kidney or differentiate it from neuroblastoma?

Ans:

- Neuroblastoma presents earlier, i.e. between 1–2 years
- Constitutional symptoms (weight loss, fever, poor appetite, tender bosselated mass) are common; baby is classically very sick, irritable and often presents with florid metastases.
- **Claw sign**: It refers to the finding "sharp angles on either side of the mass" formed by the normal renal parenchyma, confirming its origin from kidney. It is classical of Wilms tumor (Fig. 11.4).

11. What is the radiological feature to differentiate Wilms' tumor and neuroblastoma?

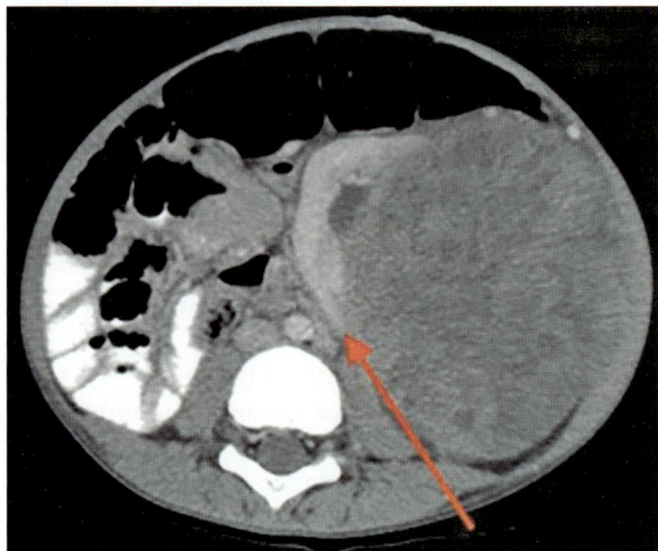

Fig. 11.4: Claw sign in CECT abdomen

Ans:

- Calcification less common (10%) in Wilms as compared to neuroblastoma (80–90%)
- WT may invade vascular structure, viz renal vein and IVC thrombus, while neuroblastoma encases vascular structure rather than invasion
- Lymph node involvement is less common in Wilms' tumor.

12. What are the histopathological types of WT?

Ans:

- Classically triphasic-blastemal (undifferentiated small blue cells), stromal (immature spindle cells), epithelial (abortive glomeruli and tubules)
- Biphasic or monophasic tumors—highly invasive
- Blastemal predominant—highly aggressive, presents at advanced stage
- Stromal predominant—resistant to chemotherapy.

13. What are nephrogenic rests or nephroblastomatosis?

Ans:

- Nephrogenic rests (NR) are "areas of metanephric (embryonal) tissue persisting after the 36th week of life." The presence of multiple or diffuse nephrogenic rests is termed nephroblastomatosis.[4]
- NRs maybe perilobar (subcapsular) or intralobar **based on location** or (1) incipient or dormant (2) hyperplastic (3) sclerosing **based on growth phase**
- Actively proliferating or hyperplastic rests can cause the greatest diagnostic challenge
- NR in resected WT signify high risk of metachronous contralateral tumor.

14. How do you stage Wilms tumor (Table 11.1)?

Ans:

- Two commonly used systems are Children Oncology Group (COG, American) and International Society of Paediatric Oncology (SIOP, European), National Wilms' tumor staging (NWTS)
- Both the stages are surgico-pathological.

TABLE 11.1: Comparison of NWTS and SIOP staging of Wilms' tumor

Stage	*NWTS*	*SIOP*
I	Tumor is limited to kidney Totally excised There is no tumoral involvement in surgical margin The vessels of renal sinus are not involved There is no tumoral rupture before or during removal	Tumor is limited to kidney No tumor cells at the surgical margin The vessels of renal sinus are not involved Intrarenal vessels may be involved
II	Tumor is outside the kidney Totally removed Local spillage and intrarenal vessels could be involved	Tumor extends outside of the kidney Totally resected but capsule, adjacent tissues, renal sinus and renal vessels can be involved
III	Intra-abdominal tumor Renal hilus, abdominal lymph nodes are involved Diffuse spillage Peritoneal involvement Thrombus in vena cava	Incomplete reasection Intra-abdominal lymph node involvement but renal hilus lymph node positivity makes it stage II Ureteral, peritoneal, and caval involvement preoperative or perioperative biopsy or rupture peritoneal metastates
IV	Hematogeneous or distant lymph node metastases	Hematogeneous and extra-abdominal lymph node metastases
V	Bilateral renal tumors	Bilateral renal tumors

15. What are the current treatment protocols to manage Wilms tumor (Flowchart 11.1)?

Ans:

- The *SIOP* recommends upfront chemotherapy to all patients, including stage I WT, except for children with less than 6 months of age.
- COG recommends upfront nephrectomy.

16. How will you manage this case?

Ans:

- CECT abdomen and thorax to look for resectability and metastases
- Doppler USG to rule out renal vein and IVC involvement
- Mass appears to be resectable (clear from parities, liver, no lymphadenopathy) and nonmetastatic
- Open Transperitoneal Radical Nephroureterectomy with Lymph Nodal Sampling (7 stations)
- Adjuvant chemo based on staging
  - Lung metastases are not a limitation to upfront nephrectomy unless decompensated by heavy tumor load

17. What will you do if the mass is not amenable to resection?

Ans:

- USG guided biopsy followed by neoadjuvant chemotherapy (NACT)
- NACT includes DD4A.
- Reimage with CECT abdomen and thorax and Doppler USG +/-rebiopsy to look for response to chemotherapy at 6 weeks and/or 12 weeks and plan radical nephrectomy whenever appears resectable.
- Subsequently complete 24 week adjuvant chemotherapy along with radiotherapy (RT) within 10 days of surgery.

Flowchart 11.1: Visible lump with prominent venous prominence

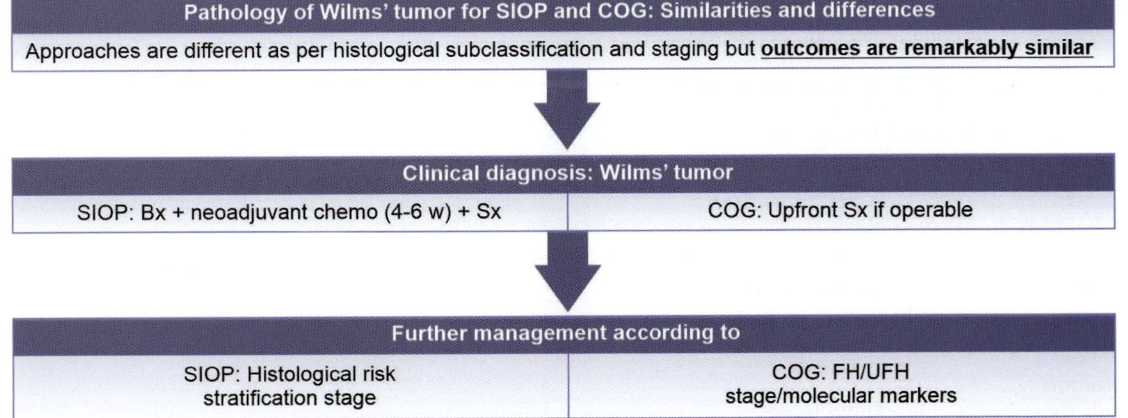

18. When will you prefer to go for neoadjuvant chemotherapy?

Ans: For COG protocols, neoadjuvant chemotherapy is recommended in cases considered as upfront inoperable, i.e.

- Tumor thrombus extending above the level of the hepatic veins,
- Gross involvement of contiguous structures whereby the only means of removing the tumor requires removal of the kidney (with exception of the adrenal gland),
- Bilateral WT
- Extensive pulmonary compromise from a compression by a massive tumor or
- Widespread metastatic disease and
- In large cystic/friable tumors where immediate nephrectomy may result in rupture and upstaging.

19. What are the surgical guidelines you will adhere to when operating on a WT?

Ans: Principles:

- Preferred surgical approach includes transabdominal/transperitoneal preferably through a Chevron or transverse incision (provides maximum exposure in a toddler)
- Gentle handling and enbloc removal without tumor rupture/spill
- Lymph nodal sampling (even if not enlarged) (minimum 7 stations: Paracaval supra-hilar and infra-hilar, paraaortic supra-hilar and infra-hilar, both iliac and 1 mesenteric lymph node)
- If extent of tumor into ureter, transect distal to same
- Removal of venous thrombus, if any, with cavotomy
- Biopsy any suspicious hepatic/peritoneal nodule.

20. What is the role of renal sparing surgery in Wilms' tumor?

Ans: Renal-sparing surgery (RSS) is recommended in children with bilateral WT, or those predisposed to develop bilateral tumors (syndromic) and in children with single/horseshoe kidney. It is currently not recommended in standard unilateral tumors.

21. What are the prognostic factors for Wilms' tumor (Table 11.2)?

Ans:

Prognostic Factors

- As per COG classification, WT is classified based on HPE as follows:
  Favourable histology (FH): 90%
  Unfavourable histology (UFH): 10%—presence of anaplasia
  - 3x nuclear diameter of adjacent cells
  - Hyperchromasia
  - Multipolar/polypoid mitotic figures
- Anaplasia is associated with chemoresistance and increased recurrence. It may be focal or diffuse
- The current prognostic factors used in COG trials for FH tumors are stage, age, tumor weight, response to therapy, and loss of heterozygosity at 1p and 16q.
- **Rapid response:** This is a prognostic category being evaluated in patients who have stage IV disease that is based on lung metastasis alone. The goal in these patients is to avoid lung radiation. Response to therapy is also being assessed in bilateral disease.

Table 11.2: Prognostic factors

Risk group	*Histological subtype after preoperative chemotherapy*	*Histological subtype after immediate nephrectomy*
	SIOP	*COG*
Low	Mesoblastic nephroma* Cystic partially differentiated nephroblastoma Completely necrotic nephroblastoma	
Intermediate (SIOP)/ favourable (COG)	Nephroblastoma: • Mixed subtype • Regressive subtype • Epithelial subtype • Stromal subtype • Focal anaplasia	Wilms' tumor—favourable histology (no evidence of any anaplasia)
High (SIOP)/ unfavourable (COG)	Diffuse anaplasia blastemal-type Wilms' tumor Blastemal-type Wilms tumor Clear-cell sarcoma of the kidney* Rhabdoid tumor of the kidney*	Diffuse and focal anaplasia

*Non-Wilms' tumors.
COG: Children's Oncology Group; SIOP: International Society fo Paediatric Oncology.

22. How do you manage pulmonary metastasis?

Ans:

- Patients with favourable histology with lung metastases and no other sites of distant spread or presence of 1p and 16q deletion undergo 6 weeks of actinomycin-D, doxorubicin, and vincristine (DD4A)
- If a complete response in the pulmonary nodules occur, then patients are not given whole lung irradiation
- This is supported by a European study which showed that whole lung irradiation may not be needed in many patients with pulmonary metastasis

23. What are the guidelines on post-operative chemotherapy?

Ans: Started as soon as ileus subsides after surgery, based on the post-operative histology as well as stage (Table 11.3).

TABLE 11.3: Post-operative chemotherapy regimen

Regimen name	*Regimen description*
Regimen EE-4A	Vincristine, dactinomycin × 18 weeks postnephrectomy
Regimen DD-4A	Vincristine, dactinomycin, doxorubicin ×24 weeks; baseline nephrectomy or biopsy with subsequent nephrectomy
Regimen I	Vincristine, doxorubicin, cyclophosphamide, etoposide ×24 weeks postnephrectomy
Regimen M	Vincristine, dactinomycin, doxorubicin, cyclophosphamide, and etoposide with subsequent radiation therapy

- Treatment on the current COG protocols for FH WT is determined by stage, histology, and LOH.
- Adjuvant chemotherapy is recommended for all tumor stages with the exception of children younger than 2 years of age with stage I disease and tumors with favourable histology weighing <550 g[5,6] NWTS 5 showed poor outcomes without chemo, so even in this group EE4A is added now (Table 11.4).

TABLE 11.4: Choice of post-operative chemotherapy regimen

FH	Stage I and II without LOH	Regimen EE-4A
FH	Stage III and IV without LOH	Regimen DD-4A
FH	Stage I or II LOH positive	Regimen DD-4A
FH	Stage III and IV LOH positive	Regimen M
UFH	Stage I focal or diffuse anaplasia	Regimen EE4A
UFH	Stage II to IV focal anaplasia	Regimen DD4A
UFH	Stage II to IV diffuse anaplastic WT	Regimen I

- Patients below 12 kg or with acute malnutrition should have a 2/3rd dose reduction of chemotherapeutic agents.
- Newborns and all infants younger than 12 months require a 50% reduction in chemotherapy dose.

24. How will you manage the recurrent disease?

Ans: Difficult condition to treat in children, survival is only ~50%.[7] Most recurrences happen by 18 months.

The tumor bed and/or the lungs are the two most frequent sites of recurrence.[8,9] The recurrence rate in patients with anaplastic histology is about 50% (Flowchart 11.2).

25. What are the recommendations for radiotherapy?

Ans: Ideally within 9–14 days of surgery unless medically contraindicated. RT is given to the flank.

Current Indications of Radiotherapy

- Stage II, III, IV with unfavourable histology
- Stage III and IV with favourable histology

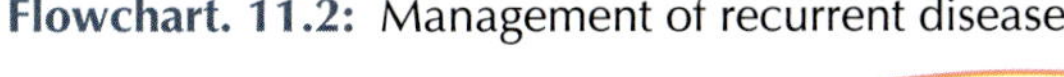

Flowchart. 11.2: Management of recurrent disease

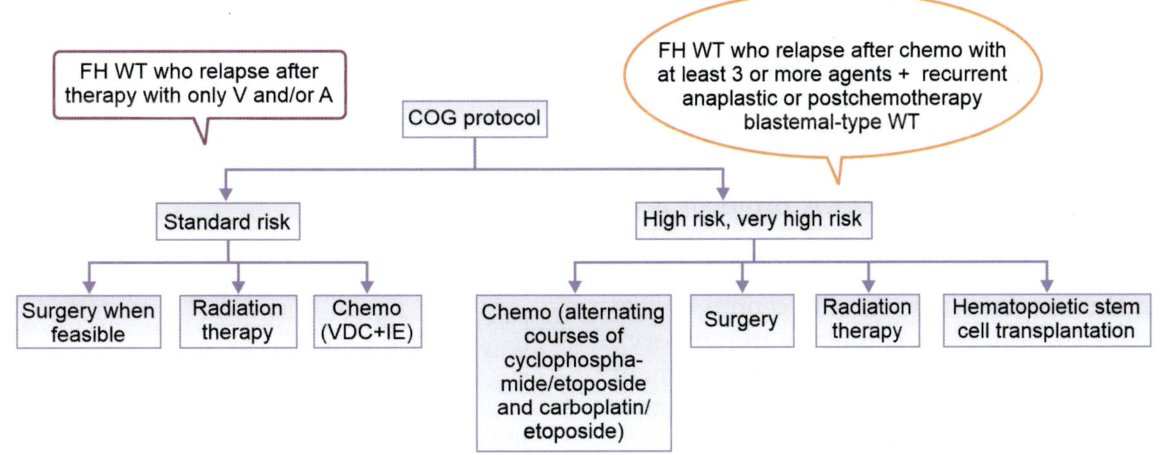

- Metastatic disease
  - Whole abdominal irradiation (WAI): Diffuse tumor spillage/intraperitoneal tumor rupture/peritoneal tumor seeding/hemorrhagic or cytology positive ascites.
  - Whole lung irradiation (WLI) is indicated for all patients with pulmonary lesions detected by CXR or CT scan except in rapid responders.

26. What long-term treatment effects will you be concerned about?

Ans:

- Cardiac: Acute cardiomyopathy (arrhythmias), subacute, chronic (decreased EF, CCF)—due to Doxorubicin (direct dose–response relationship—each 100 mg/m^2 of DOX exposure increased the relative risk of CHF by 3.3)[10] and lung irradiation.
- ~0.7% of patients with unilateral WT will develop renal failure (8 fold higher than that in the age-matched general population),[10] more common in bilateral and syndromic cases
- Recurrence/second malignancy (1.6% at 15 years from diagnosis)
- Fertility issues (due to cyclophosphamide/whole abdomen irradiation)

27. Which patients will you consider for surveillance?

Ans: Surveillance is recommended to continue until 5 years of age with renal US every 3 months in patients with predisposition due to *WT1* mutant syndromes, and until at least 7 years of age in Beckwith Wiedemann syndrome, isolated hemi-hypertrophy and in familial WT pedigrees.[11]

28. What do you know about the umbrella protocol?

Ans: The Renal Tumor Study Group of the International Society of Pediatric Oncology (SIOP–RTSG) has developed a new study protocol for pediatric renal tumors: The UMBRELLA SIOP–RTSG 2016 protocol (the UMBRELLA protocol).

Currently, the overall outcomes of patients with WT are excellent, but subgroups with poor prognosis and increased relapse rates require early identification to improve treatment stratification and ultimately reduction of the direct and late effects of chemotherapy (Fig. 11.5).

The aim of the UMBRELLA protocol is to collect all clinical, biological and outcomes data from children with primary renal tumors in a comprehensive data registry, with central review of diagnostics (radiology, pathology and surgery), standardized biobanking and precise treatment recommendations for the most common pediatric renal tumors (Flowchart 11.3).

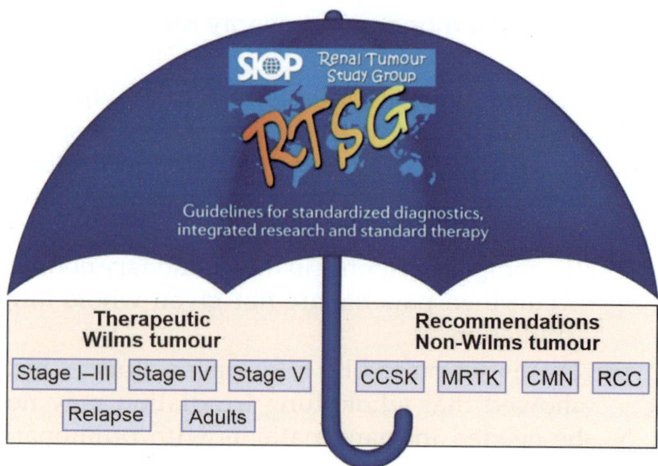

Fig. 11.5: Triphasic histology WT

Flowchart 11.3: Lymph nodal basin for sampling

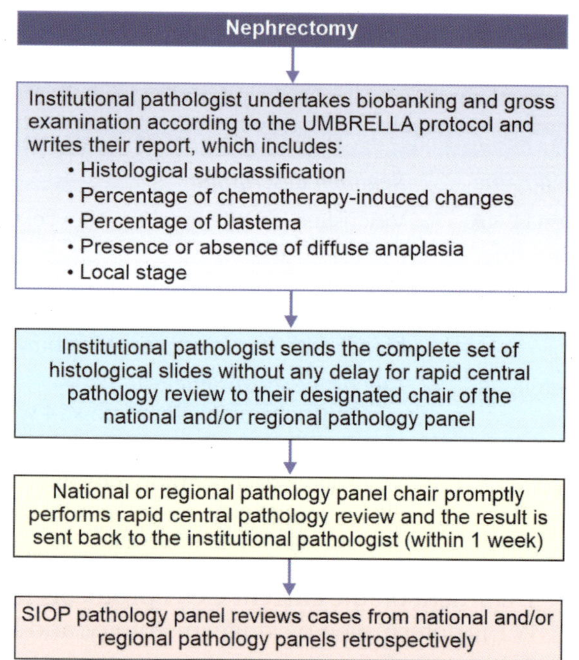

Molecular biology research within the protocol is primarily focused on the validation of the prognostic value of 1q gain, and TP53 mutations which might lead to a more personalized treatment approach. Consequently, short-term and long-term outcomes might be improved for all children with renal tumors by increasing survival, but also by reducing treatment in specific subgroups, resulting in diminished direct and late adverse effects.

REFERENCES

1. P.A. Pizzo, D.G. Poplack (Eds.), Principles and Practice of Paediatric Oncology (fifth ed.), Lippincott Williams and Wilkins, Philadelphia (2006), pp. 1–13.
2. Breslow N, Olshan A, Beckwith JB, Green DM. Epidemiology of Wilms tumor. Med Pediatr Oncol. 1993;21(3):172–81. doi: 10.1002/mpo.2950210305. PMID: 7680412.

3. Ritchey M, Daley S, Shamberger RC, Ehrlich P, Hamilton T, Haase G, Sawin R; National Wilms' Tumor Study Group. Ureteral extension in Wilms' tumor: a report from the National Wilms' Tumor Study Group (NWTSG). J Pediatr Surg. 2008 Sep;43(9):1625–9. doi: 10.1016/j.jpedsurg.2008.01.067. PMID: 18778996; PMCID: PMC2975738.
4. Beckwith JB. National Wilms Tumor Study: an update for pathologists. Pediatric and Developmental Pathology. 1998 Jan;1:79–84.
5. Dénes FT, Duarte RJ, Cristófani LM, *et al.* Pediatric genitourinary oncology. *Front Pediatr.* 2013;1:48. 10.3389/fped.2013.00048 [PMC free article] [PubMed] [CrossRef] [Google Scholar].
6. Lorenzo AJ, Romao RL: The Evolving Role of Minimally Invasive Surgery in Pediatric and Adolescent Uro-logic Oncology. *Urology.* 2016;91:180–9. 10.1016/j.urology.2015.12.023 [PubMed] [CrossRef] [Google Scholar].
7. Brok J, Treger TD, Gooskens SL, *et al.* Biology and treatment of renal tumors in childhood. *Eur J Cancer.* 2016;68:179–95. 10.1016/j.ejca.2016.09.005.
8. Malogolowkin M, Cotton CA, Green DM: Treatment of Wilms tumor relapsing after initial treatment with vincristine, actinomycin D, and doxorubicin. A report from the National Wilms Tumor Study Group. *Pediatr Blood Cancer.* 2008;50(2):236–41. 10.1002/pbc.21267.
9. Spreafico F, Pritchard Jones K, Malogolowkin MH, *et al.* Treatment of relapsed Wilms tumors: lessons learned. *Expert Rev Anticancer Ther.* 2009;9(12):1807–15. 10.1586/era.09.159.
10. Termuhlen AM, Tersak JM, Liu Q, *et al.* Twenty-five year follow-up of childhood Wilms tumor: a report from the Childhood Cancer Survivor Study. *Pediatr Blood Cancer.* 2011;57(7):1210–6. 10.1002/pbc.23090.
11. Scott RH, Rahman N: Genetic predisposition to Wilms tumor. In: Pritchard-Jones K, Dome JS (eds). *Renal Tumors of Childhood-Biology and Therapy* Berlin/Heidelberg, Germany: Springer-Verlag;2014:19–38. 10.1007/978-3-662-44003-2_2.

Chapter 12

Pediatric Renal Trauma

• *Priyank Yadav*

LEARNING OBJECTIVES

- Identify the clinical presentation of pediatric blunt renal trauma, including the risk factors.
- Explain the diagnostic tools and techniques used to evaluate and grade renal injuries in pediatric patients.
- Evaluate the appropriate management approach for different grades of renal injuries in pediatric patients, including conservative and surgical interventions.
- Analyze the potential complications of pediatric blunt renal trauma and the monitoring and follow-up measures needed to manage them.

INTRODUCTION

In pediatric trauma, the kidney is the most commonly injured organ of the urinary tract. Children are more susceptible to renal injuries than adults due to their anatomy and physiology. Blunt abdominal trauma is the most common cause of pediatric renal injuries. Clinical suspicion is important for prompt diagnosis, which includes flank bruising and pain, abdominal mass and distension, or fractured lower ribs. Urinalysis, hematocrit, and baseline creatinine levels are mandatorily performed for adequate diagnosis. Radiographic imaging is used to adequately stage the injury of the kidney and identify concomitant injuries to other organs. The American Association for the Surgery of Trauma (AAST) Organ Injury Scale (OIS) is used to grade renal injuries.[1] The vast majority of renal injuries can be treated conservatively, but hemodynamic instability requires operative intervention.[2] Conservative treatment is the preferred approach especially for those with lower grade injuries, consisting of bed rest, frequent vital sign evaluation, pain therapy, and intravenous fluid replacement.[3] Higher grade injuries are still a matter of debate, and close clinical observation with hemodynamic monitoring is recommended. Early complications of renal injuries include persistent bleeding, infection, perinephric abscess, sepsis, urinary fistula, urinary extravasation, and development of urinomas. Children with higher grade injuries have much greater risk of total loss of function. The risk of developing hypertension after pediatric higher grade renal trauma is low, but it is still advisable to repeatedly examine patients with high-grade injuries to rule out the development of hypertension.

Here, we will discuss the case of a 10-year-old boy who suffered from a right side high grade renal trauma and his management plan.

Case Scenario

The patient, a 10-year-old male with normal milestones and immunizations, had a history of blunt trauma to the abdomen in March 2017 after falling from a cycle after which he passed frank blood in urine. At the hospital, after hemodynamic stabilization, he underwent an ultrasonography that suggested a perinephric hematoma on the right side. Subsequently, a contrast enhanced CT scan was performed that revealed a complete transection in the middle of the right kidney, resulting in a 2.7 cm gap between the upper pole and the lower pole (Fig. 12.1). He had a large perinephric hematoma with leakage of contrast but was vitally stable.

1. **What do you think is the grade of renal injury? What should be the next plan of management?**

   Ans: Based on the evaluation, it seems that the patient has sustained a grade 4 renal injury. In such cases, the primary goal of management is

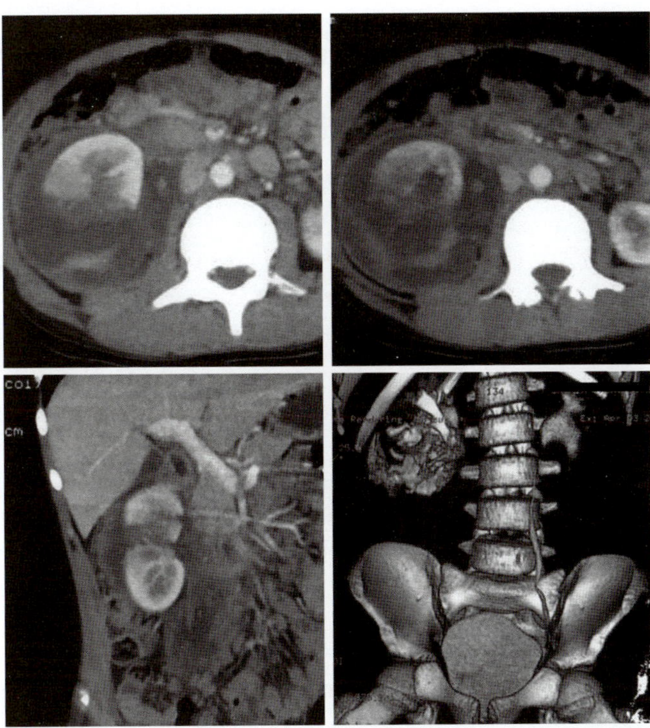

Fig. 12.1: Contrast enhanced CT scan of the child showing the extent of renal injury

to stabilize the patient and control bleeding. The treatment approach should include conservative management with close monitoring and follow-up imaging studies or surgical intervention, depending on the severity of the injury and the patient's clinical progress. Conservative management will involve bed rest, pain control, and close monitoring of vital signs and laboratory values (Flowchart. 12.1).

Clinical case: The injury was managed conservatively with strict bed rest as the patient remained hemodynamically stable. However, after eight days, a swelling was noted in the right flank, and an ultrasound showed a collection of 1L over the mid-pole of the right kidney.

2. **What should be done next?**

Ans: The presence of a collection over the kidney leading to flank swelling indicates bleeding or an extravasation of urine and may require intervention. The next step would be to perform a CT scan to evaluate the extent and size of the collection and to determine if it is causing any obstruction or compression of the adjacent structures. Depending

Flowchart 12.1: EAU treatment algorithm for renal trauma

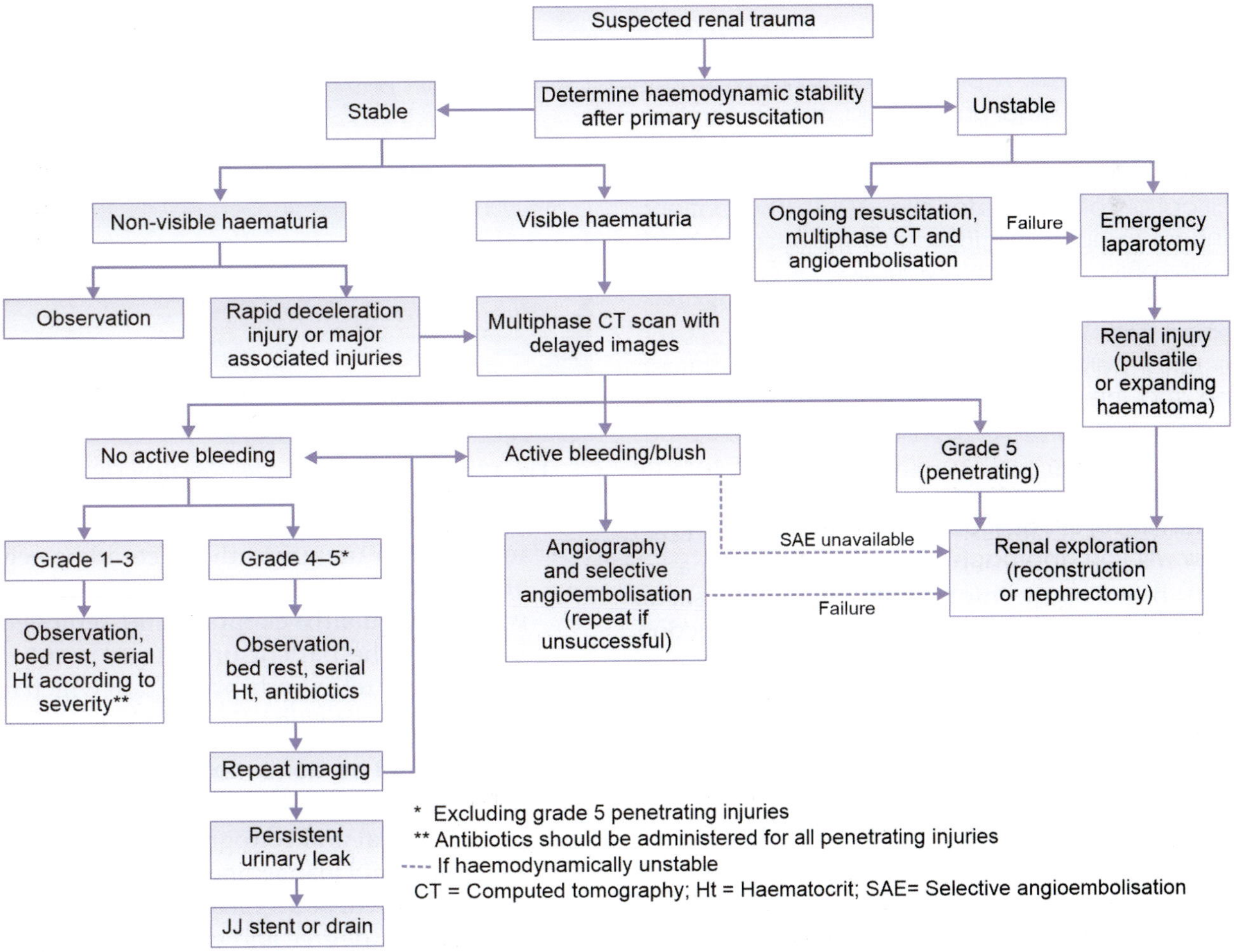

Suspected renal trauma
Determine haemodynamic stability after primary resuscitation
Stable
Unstable
Non-visible haematuria
Visible haematuria
Ongoing resuscitation, multiphase CT and angioembolisation
Failure
Emergency laparotomy
Observation
Rapid deceleration injury or major associated injuries
Multiphase CT scan with delayed images
Renal injury (pulsatile or expanding haematoma)
No active bleeding
Active bleeding/blush
Grade 5 (penetrating)
Grade 1–3
Grade 4–5*
Angiography and selective angioembolisation (repeat if unsuccessful)
SAE unavailable
Failure
Renal exploration (reconstruction or nephrectomy)
Observation, bed rest, serial Ht according to severity**
Observation, bed rest, serial Ht, antibiotics
Repeat imaging
Persistent urinary leak
JJ stent or drain

* Excluding grade 5 penetrating injuries
** Antibiotics should be administered for all penetrating injuries
---- If haemodynamically unstable
CT = Computed tomography; Ht = Haematocrit; SAE= Selective angioembolisation

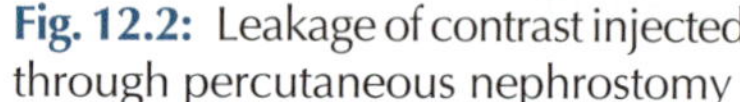

Fig. 12.2: Leakage of contrast injected through percutaneous nephrostomy

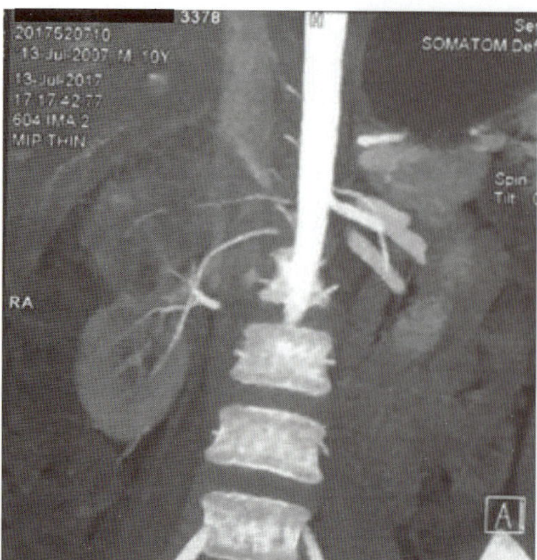

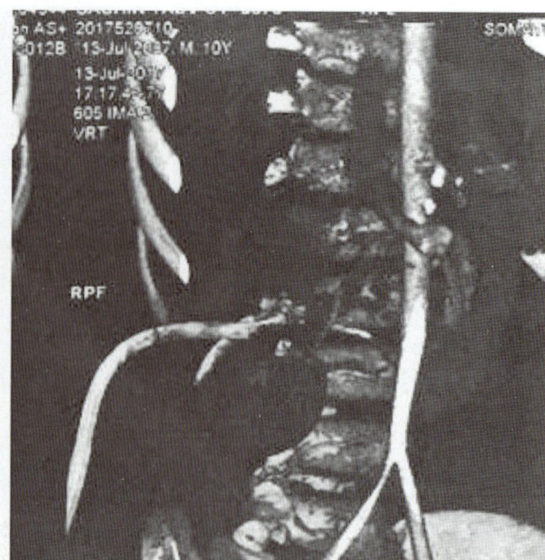

Fig. 12.3: CT angiography showing preservation of vascularity of the right kidney and nephrostomy *in situ*

on the findings, the patient may require a drainage procedure such as percutaneous nephrostomy or surgical exploration. It is important to monitor the patient's vital parameters and renal function closely and to manage any complications promptly.

Case Scenario *(Contd.)*

The patient underwent a CT urography that revealed urinary extravasation. A percutaneous nephrostomy (PCN) was inserted under anaesthesia, and on injecting the contrast, the collecting system was opacified along with leakage in the surrounding space without opacification of the ureter (Fig. 12.2). The patient continued to have the PCN until the resolution of the perinephric collection. Evaluation at one month showed that the blood supply to the right kidney was preserved (Fig. 12.3) and that the PCN was present in the renal pelvis. However, there was no contrast flowing into the right ureter. A nephrostogram was done subsequently, which confirmed UPJ obstruction (Fig. 12.4).

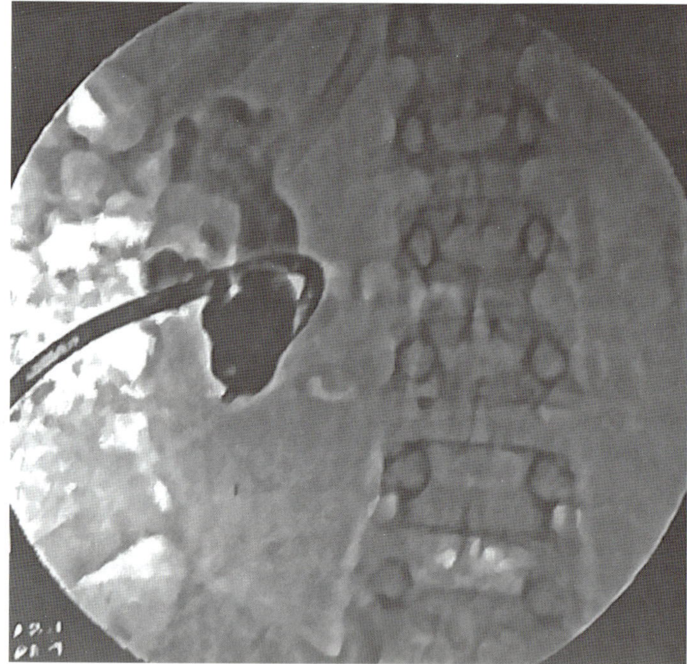

Fig. 12.4: Nephrostogram showing right UPJ obstruction

3. **What kind of UPJ obstruction does the patient have? How will you approach such a case?**

   Ans: Based on the information provided, it seems that the patient has a secondary UPJ obstruction, likely due to the injury and subsequent healing process. The extent of involvement can be determined by further evaluation, such as retrograde pyelography. Subsequent management will depend on the findings noted and may involve placement of a double J stent, if possible.[4]

   Clinical case: The boy underwent cystoscopy and retrograde pyelogram which revealed a short segment (1 cm) ureteric stricture through which, a 5-fr ureteric catheter could be negotiated and a double J stent could be placed. The PCN was subsequently clamped and removed. After 2 months, the patient underwent stent removal and another retrograde pyelogram which revealed persistent obstruction (Fig. 12.5).

4. **What should be done next?**

   Ans: Since persistent obstruction is noted after stent removal and retrograde pyelogram, further evaluation and management are required. The next step may involve a repeat retrograde pyelogram to assess the degree and extent of the obstruction.

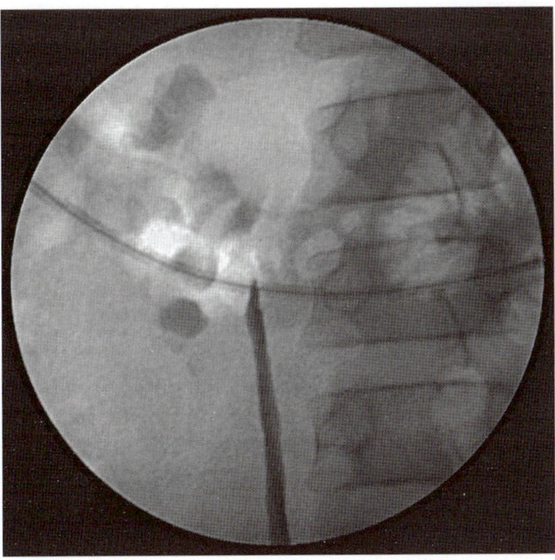

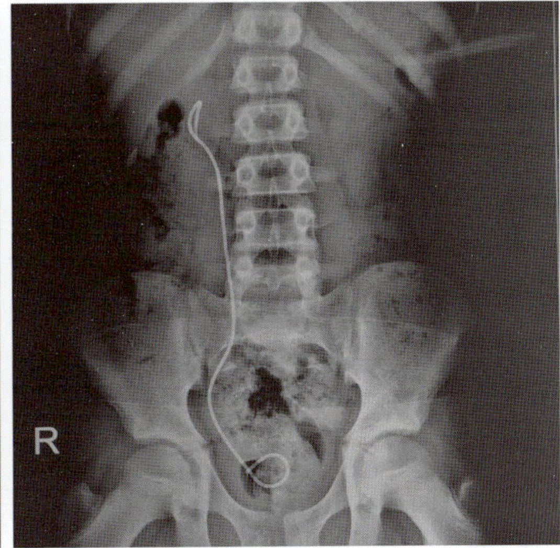

Fig. 12.5: Retrograde pyelogram showing recurrent UPJ obstruction and subsequent stent placement across the UPJ following balloon dilation

This patient has a history of perinephric urinoma so, he is expected to have a lot of fibrosis around the kidney and thus pyeloplasty may be technically challenging. Hence, less invasive techniques must be tried before resorting to that such as dilation of the stricture and upsizing of the stent.[5]

***Case Scenario** (Contd.)*

He underwent balloon dilatation and replacement of double J stent. After 3 months, the stent was removed and retrograde pyelogram showed adequate contrast drainage across the UPJ on delayed films.

5. **How is pediatric renal trauma different from the adult renal trauma?**

   Ans: Pediatric renal trauma is different from adult renal trauma in several ways. Children have more elastic and pliable tissue, which makes them more resilient to injury. However, when children do sustain renal trauma, they are more likely to have associated injuries due to their small size and the location of their kidneys. Children are more susceptible to renal injuries following blunt abdominal trauma than adults, possibly due to a decreased amount of perirenal fat, incompletely ossified lower ribs, weaker abdominal muscles and the relatively larger kidneys compared to the rest of the body.

6. **What are the urological indications to discontinue conservative treatment in a child with high grade renal trauma?**

   Ans: Conservative management in a child with high grade renal trauma must be discontinued if the patient shows signs of hemodynamic instability, persistent gross hematuria, expanding or pulsatile perirenal hematoma and urinary extravasation. The decision to discontinue conservative management and pursue surgical intervention should be based on a careful assessment of the patient's clinical status and imaging findings.

7. **Suppose this patient had renal trauma without secondary UPJ obstruction. How would you follow this patient in the clinic?**

   Ans: The follow-up plan in a child with grade 4 renal injury managed conservatively will depend on the clinical course and response to initial management. Generally, such a patient should have regular visits with a urologist to assess the recovery and monitor for any complications. An initial follow-up can be planned at 3 months with an ultrasonography. If there are no concerns, this patient can be followed annually with blood pressure checks for up to 3 years.

8. **Is there any role of subsequent imaging?**

   Ans: It is not necessary to perform routine follow-up imaging for grades 1–3 blunt renal injuries, and grade 4 renovascular injuries can be managed clinically without routine early follow-up imaging. For high-grade injuries (4 and 5), ultrasound is commonly used to assess for urinoma or perfusion deficits during follow-up, replacing DMSA scans. In cases when there is any indication of compromised renal function or hypertension, follow-up imaging through MAG3 renal scan or MRI may be necessary.[6]

9. **What are the long-term complications of high grade renal trauma in children?**

   Ans: There are several long-term complications of high grade renal trauma in children:

1. *Delayed bleeding:* Delayed bleeding can occur even after conservative management of renal trauma, which can lead to life-threatening hemorrhage. It may be due to a pseudoaneurysm which will require angioembolization or sometimes even nephrectomy.
2. *Renal Dysfunction:* Renal function may be compromised due to loss of renal tissue, which may lead to decreased kidney function over time.[7]
3. *Hypertension:* Hypertension may develop as a result of damage to the renal vasculature or loss of renal function.[8]
4. *Urolithiasis:* The incidence of recurrent urinary stones is increased in patients with renal trauma.
5. *Urinary tract infections:* Renal trauma can lead to scarring and obstruction of the urinary tract, which may increase the risk of urinary tract infections.
6. *Chronic pain:* Chronic pain in the affected flank may occur due to nerve damage or scar tissue formation.

SUMMARY

- The kidney is the most commonly injured organ of the urinary tract in pediatric trauma.
- Children are more susceptible to renal injuries than adults due to their lack of perirenal fat, incompletely ossified lower ribs, weaker abdominal muscles, and relatively larger kidneys.
- Pediatric blunt renal trauma should be suspected in all cases with severe injury and appropriate clinical findings, including flank bruising and pain, abdominal mass and distension, or fractured lower ribs.
- Hemodynamic instability requires immediate operative intervention, while the vast majority of renal injuries can be treated conservatively with bed rest, pain therapy, and intravenous fluid replacement.
- Diagnostic tools for pediatric blunt renal trauma include urinalysis, hematocrit, and baseline creatinine levels, as well as radiographic imaging such as ultrasound or CT scans to adequately stage the injury of the kidney, reveal pre-existing pathologies, and identify concomitant injuries to other organs.
- Early complications of renal injuries include persistent bleeding, infection, perinephric abscess, sepsis, urinary fistula, urinary extravasation, and development of urinomas.
- Children with grades II to IV injuries managed conservatively retain near-normal function, while those with grade V injuries have much greater risk of total loss of renal function.

REFERENCES

1. Buckley JC, McAninch JW. Revision of current American Association for the Surgery of Trauma Renal Injury grading system. J Trauma. 2011;70(1):35–37.
2. Henderson CG, Sedberry-Ross S, Pickard R, *et al.* Management of high grade renal trauma: 20-year experience at a pediatric level I trauma center. J Urol. 2007;178(1):246–250.
3. Jacobs MA, Hotaling JM, Mueller BA, Koyle M, Rivara F, Voelzke BB. Conservative management vs early surgery for high grade pediatric renal trauma-do nephrectomy rates differ? J Urol. 2012;187(5):1817–1822.
4. Matthews LA, Smith EM, Spirnak JP. Nonoperative treatment of major blunt renal lacerations with urinary extravasation. J Urol. 1997;157(6):2056–2058.
5. Shekar PA, Ansari MS, Yadav P, Srivastava A. "Functional outcome in pediatric grade IV renal injuries following blunt abdominal trauma salvaged with minimally invasive interventions". J Pediatr Urol. 2020;16(5):657.e1–657.e9.
6. Steinberger AE, Wilson NA, Fairfax C, Treon SJ, Herndon M, Levene TL, Keller MS. Implementation of a clinical guideline for nonoperative management of isolated blunt renal injury in children. Surg Open Sci. 2021 May 3;5:19–24.
7. Overs C, Teklali Y, Boillot B, *et al.* Evaluation of the management of severe trauma kidney injury and long-term renal function in children. J Trauma Acute Care Surg. 2018;84(6):951–955.
8. Monstrey SJ, Beerthuizen GI, vander Werken C, Debruyne FM, Goris RJ. Renal trauma and hypertension. J Trauma. 1989;29(1):65–70.

Chapter
13

Vesicoureteric Reflux (VUR)

• *Anil Takvani* • *Gyanendra Sharma*

LEARNING OBJECTIVES

- Diagnosis of urinary tract infection (UTI) in pediatric patients.
- How to diagnose vesico-ureteral reflux (VUR)?
- How does VUR harm the kidney?
- Risk stratification of VUR.
- Medical management of VUR.
- Surgical intervention in VUR—need and indications.

INTRODUCTION

VUR is a condition in which there is retrograde flow of urine to the upper tracts. It may be diagnosed following investigations done for an episode of urinary tract infection (UTI) or is detected following investigations done in a case of prenatally detected hydronephrosis. Often the presence of VUR is synonymous with occurrence of febrile UTI and renal scarring; but it must be understood that UTI and renal scarring can occur in the absence of VUR.[1]

VUR is due to incompetence of ureterovescial junction (UVJ) which normally prevents backflow of urine to the upper tracts during voiding. This incompetent UVJ can be due to improper insertion of ureter, short intravesical tunnel of the intramural ureter or also due to bladder dysfunction.

The management of VUR has undergone a sea change from the time that all children with VUR were advised surgical intervention to the present era where a more conservative approach is taken and surgical intervention is indicated only when conservative measures fail. This change has come about due to a better understanding of the pathophysiological factors causing renal damage in association with VUR.

This chapter aims to provide a standard approach for the diagnosis, management and follow-up of patients with VUR.

Case Scenario

A 3-year-old boy presented with complaints of fever for last 3 days. He has had episodes of fever in the last 12–18 months. On each of these occasions he was treated with antibiotics and antipyretics by the general practitioner. At present his dominant complaint was fever. The mother also noticed that he is passing urine more frequently and also complaints of pain while passing urine. She also noticed reddish colored urine on more than one occasion in the last 2 days.

On examination he has fever of 102°F. pulse rate of 126/min and BP of 80/50mm of Hg. Anthropometric measurement suggested that the child was small for his age which suggested failure to thrive. Per abdominal examination was normal and genital examination revealed phimosis.

1. What other history is important in this case?

Ans: The history is suggestive of a urinary tract pathology of infective nature. There is also history of episodes of fever in the past in the preverbal stage of the child which could have been due to the same etiological factor. Hence, the following history is important

- H/O hydronephrosis in the prenatal period
- H/O constipation
- H/O any voiding dysfunction like poor stream, intermittency, incontinence of urine and urgency–

prior to this episode when the child was apparently asymptomatic
- H/O difficulty in walking or any spine related problems or surgical interventions in the past
- H/O urological problems in his siblings
- Family H/O of any urological problems in parents in their childhood.

2. **How will you investigate this child?**

Ans: Considering his high grade fever in last 2 days it would be advisable to hospitalise the child. Biochemical evaluation in the form of complete blood count, urine routine, serum creatinine should be done. In this case it showed high total leucocyte count and presence of > 50–60 WBC/hpf in urinalysis. His urine was sent for C/S and ultrasonography of the abdomen was done which showed bilateral hydronephrosis with hydroureter. The child was started on broad spectrum antibiotics and later on culture specific antibiotics were given. His voiding cystourethrogram was done after 1 week which showed bilateral grade 4 VUR (Fig. 13.1).

3. **Why was this diagnosis not made earlier?**

Ans: The presentation of UTI in children is different from those in adults. In the preverbal stage the dominant symptom is presence of fever. As a rule any child presenting with fever of unknown origin and with a duration of 2–3 days should undergo a urine analysis to rule out infection. A child who can communicate can present with complaints of dysuria, haematuria. UTI presenting in the form of bowel disturbances, abdominal pain and vomiting is not uncommon in small children. Foul smelling urine noticed by the mother is another presentation of UTI in children.

In this case, this was the first time that a urine examination was done following an episode of fever which lead to the diagnosis of UTI.

4. **How common is VUR?**

Ans: About 1 in 3 children who have a UTI with a fever have VUR.[2] The number of children with VUR may be higher because some children with VUR who remain asymptomatic are never tested.

5. **Do all children with febrile UTI have VUR?**

Ans: VUR is one of the risk factors of development of febrile UTI but it is the not the only cause. It should be remembered as a risk factor which facilitates pyelonephritis

6. **Which children are at higher risk of having VUR?**

Ans: Generally, the younger the child, the more likely he or she will have reflux. VUR is more common in infants and children ages 2 and under, but it can also be present in older children and even adults.[3]

Children with abnormal kidney or the urinary tract are likely to have VUR. Girls are more likely than boys to have VUR.[3]

A child is more likely to have VUR if a brother, sister, or parent has had it. A little more than 1 in 4 siblings of children with VUR will have reflux. A little more than 1 in 3 children with a parent with VUR will have this condition.[3]

7. **What are the host risk factors for UTI in children?**

Ans:
- UTIs are more common in Caucasian girls compared with girls of other races
- Below the age of 1 year, UTI is more common in boys

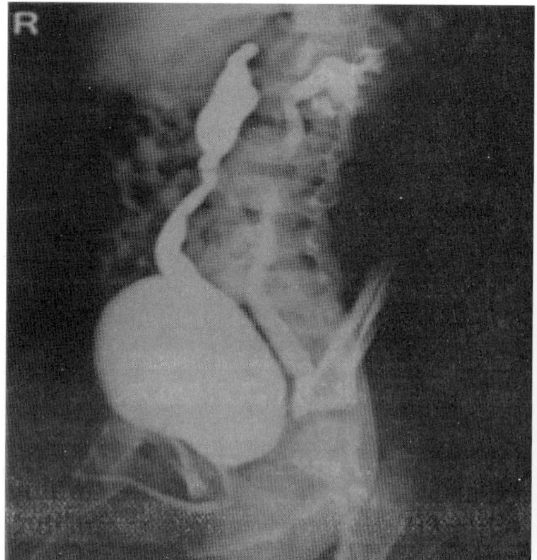

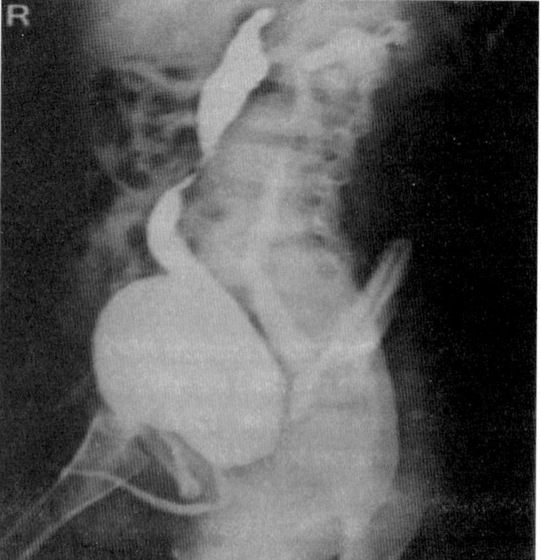

Fig. 13.1: Bilateral grade 4 VUR

Section 2

- After the age of 1 year UTI is more common in girls
- Some children are genetically more prone to develop UTI, though no specific gene has been identified
- Uncircumcised boys are at greater risk of developing UTI
- Children with anatomic abnormalities of the genitourinary tract and those with vesicoureteral reflux are at higher risk of developing UTI
- Children with bladder bowel dysfunction (BBD) are at increased risk of developing febrile UTI and also VUR.

8. What are the different ways in which urine sample can be collected in neonates, infants and non-toilet trained children?

Ans:

- Clean the genitalia and attach a plastic bag to it—high risk of contamination
- Clean catch midstream sample
- Catheterized sample
- Suprapubic aspiration—most sensitive but invasive.[4,5]

9. What is the two step approach in patients with suspected UTI?

Ans: A clean catch midstream sample is collected for analysis. If it is normal, then no further testing is done. However, if it shows evidence of infection or pyuria, then a catheterized or suprapubically aspirated urine sample is taken for culture and sensitivity.[4–6]

10. What is significant pyuria in children on urine microscopic analysis?

Ans: In children < 2 years of age the presence of > 10 WBC/hpf and in children > 2 years of age presence of > 5 WBC/hpf is considered significant.[7]

11. What is a positive urine culture in children?

Ans: There is no consensus on what constitutes a positive urine culture in children. The American Academy of Pediatrics suggests that a diagnosis of UTI should be made only if there is presence of pyuria along with a colony count of > 50000 cfu/ml in a catheterized sample or urine collected by suprapubic aspiration.The European Urology Association Guidelines have suggested the following criteria.[8]

- Midstream sample
  - Symptomatic patient with>10^4 cfu/ml
  - Asymptomatic patient with > 10^5 cfu/ml
- Urine collected after catheterization
  - > 1000–50000 cfu/ml
- Urine from suprapubic aspirate
  - Any number of cfu/ml (at least 10 identical colonies should be seen)

12. Why should a febrile UTI be diagnosed at the earliest?

Ans: Any delay in the diagnosis increases the risk of scarring. As per Ransley and Risdon's Big bang theory, the initial episode of pyelonephritis causes the maximum scarring and if further episodes of pyelonephritis do not occur, then the chances of further scarring are negligible.[9]

13. What are the causes of VUR?

Ans:

- Primary VUR
  - This occurs due to a congenital defect in the structure of the ureterovesical junction which leads to an altered length to diameter ratio of the intravesical segment of ureter (normal ratio is 5:1)
- Secondary VUR
  - Abnormal UVJ—diverticlum/duplication of ureter/ureterocele
  - Increased intravesical pressure
- Caused by bladder—neurogenic/non-neurogenic
- Caused by outlet
  - Mechanical—posterior urethral valves, stricture
  - Functional—neurogenic or non-neurogenic

14. What is the incidence of VUR in patients with UTI?

Ans: The incidence of VUR is higher if the age is < 2 years compared to those in their teens. The age wise incidence of VUR in patients of UTI is given in[10] Table 13.1.

TABLE 13.1: Incidence of VUR

Age	*Incidence*
< 2 years	38.6%
2–6 years	26.6%
7–11 years	19.7%
12–21 years	7.6%

15. What is the relation between number of episodes of febrile UTI and development of scarring?

Ans: More are the number of episodes of pyelonephritis, higher is the chances of scarring. The incidence of scarring with each episode of febrile UTI is depicted in[11] Table 13.2.

16. What are the risk factors for VUR-related scarring?

Ans:

Infections: An increased number of febrile UTIs increases the chances of scarring.

TABLE 13.2: Incidence of renal scarring following febrile UTI

Number of febrile UTI	*% of scar formation*
1	5
2	10
3	18
4	33
5	62

Age: Infants and toddlers are at higher risk of developing scarring following acute pyelonephritis.[12]

Grade of VUR: Higher the grade (dilating reflux), more the chances of recurrent PN and renal scarring.

BBD: The presence of bowel and bladder dysfunction can increase chances of breakthrough infections and similarly chances of renal scarring.

Presence of renal scars: It is suggestive of susceptibility of host tissues and virulence of infecting organism responsible for the scarring. These patients are susceptible to increased scar size or number of scars.[13]

17. **Which is the imaging investigation of choice for UTI and VUR?**

Ans:

Fluoroscopic VCUG is the imaging test of choice for detection of VUR as it gives:

- Exact grade of VUR
- Ureteral anatomy is seen
- Delineates the bladder outline, and bladder neck, estimate bladder capacity
- Urethral anatomy is depicted
- Postvoid residual urine can be seen

18. **What are various grades of reflux?**

Ans:

As per the International Grading System on a VCUG the reflux is graded as follows:[14]

- Grade 1: Reflux only into the non-dilated ureter.
- Grade 2: Reflux into the ureter and the renal pelvis without dilatation.
- Grade 3: Reflux with mildly dilated ureter and pyelocalyceal system.
- Grade 4: Reflux with the tortuous and moderately dilated ureter with blunting of renal fornices. The papillary impression is preserved.
- Grade 5: Reflux with the tortuous and severely dilated ureter, dilatation of pyelocalyces with loss of fornices, and papillary impression.

19. **What is the status of ultrasonography in evaluating patients with febrile UTI?**

Ans: Ultrasonography is the always to be done if a patient presents with febrile UTI. It can provide very useful information regarding renal size, echogenicity and scarring, dilatation of ureter, bladder morphology and presence of associated anomalies like vesical diverticulum, ureterocele, dilated posterior urethra etc[15] (Fig. 13.2). It is easily available, inexpensive and provides very

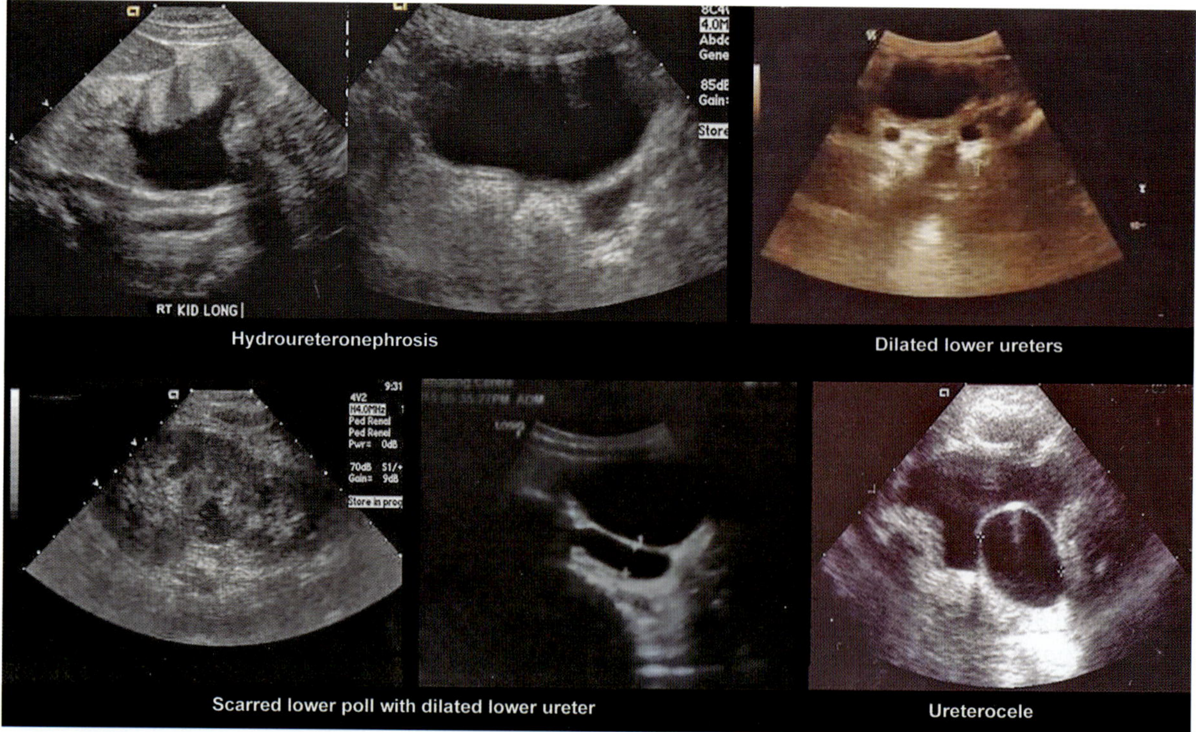

Fig. 13.2: Abnormalities on USG in patient with febrile UTI

useful indirect evidence regarding the presence of VUR.

20. What are the shortcomings of ultrasonography in the evaluation of patients with suspected VUR?

Ans:
- It carries a sensitivity of 40% and a specificity 76% for VUR
- Approximately 25% of the kidney with VUR are missed and they may have reflux of grade III or less.[16]
- Clinically significant VUR cannot be excluded even when ultrasonography is normal
- It is operator dependent
- It does not provide quantitative assessment of renal function.

21. What is direct radionuclide cystography (RNC) and what is its status in evaluating patients with VUR?

Ans: Direct RNC consists of filling the bladder with a radionuclide tracer and then using the gamma camera to diagnose the presence of VUR (Fig. 13.3).

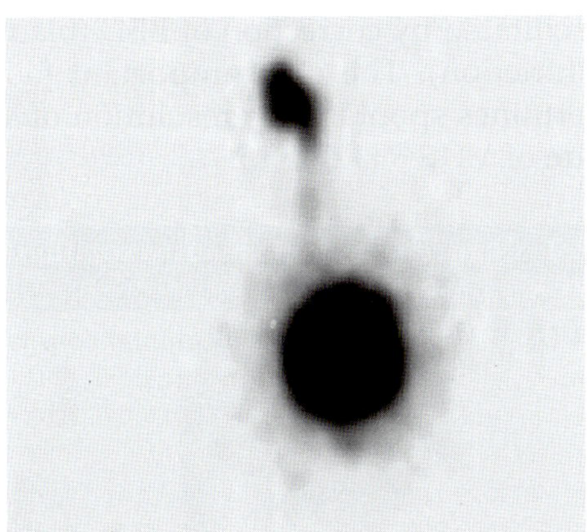

Fig. 13.3: Direct radionuclide cystography

It is indicated in the following scenarios
- Screening asymptomatic siblings or offspring,
- For follow-up examination of children with VUR
- For postoperative evaluation after ureteral reimplantation[17]

It has the following advantages
- It is more sensitive than VCUG to detect VUR
- It can depict as little as 1 mL of refluxed urine[17]
- Avoids radiation to gonads
- The radiation exposure is <1% compared to conventional fluoroscopic VCUG[18]

Its biggest drawback is its inability to delineate the anatomical details of the bladder and urethra and provide accurate grading of VUR.

22. What is the role of DMSA (dimercaptosuccinic acid) scan?

Ans: It is the gold standard for the functional assessment of the renal function. This radiotracer, when injected is picked up only by the proximal renal tubules and it binds there for several hours, hence it provides an excellent visualization of the renal cortex and its lesions[19] If it is done to diagnose presence of scars, then ideally it should be done 4–6 months after an episode of pyelonephritis.[20]

23. What are various lesions seen on DMSA scan in patients with VUR?

Ans: The various lesions seen on DMSA can be categorized into acquired and congenital lesions.

Acquired lesions: These are further divided into two categories:

1. Photopenic (less uptake) area without loss of renal contour, representative of acute pyelonephritis (Fig. 13.4).

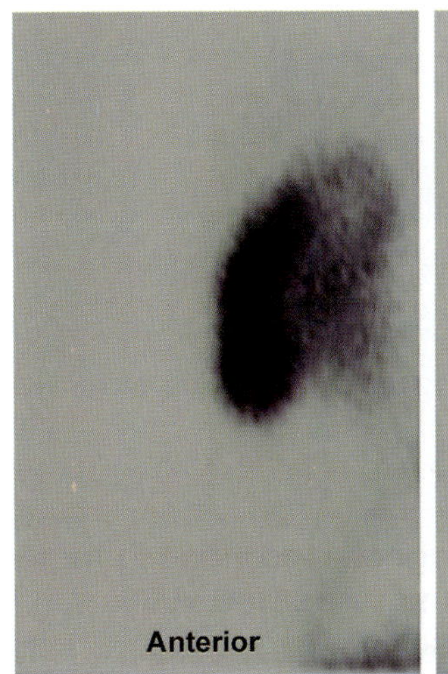

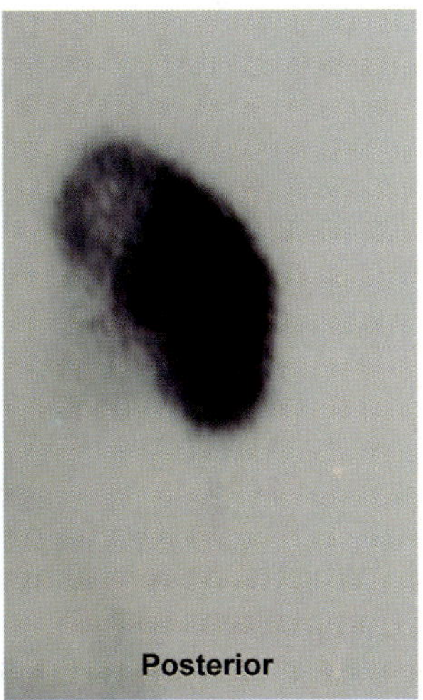

Fig. 13.4: DMSA scan showing photopenic areas

2. Absent or very less uptake with loss of contour represents post-pyelonephritis scar–These are most often at the poles but can be scattered and involve the renal cortex (Fig. 13.5). A DMSA scan has a 98% sensitivity and 92% specificity to detect a renal scar.[21]

Congenital: These are no uptake areas or global reduction of renal mass without loss of contour and without a history of pyelonephritis[22] (Fig. 13.6).

24. What is the role of Intravenous urography in patients with VUR?

Ans: In the modern evaluation of patients with febrile UTI and those with VUR, there is no role of doing intravenous urography.

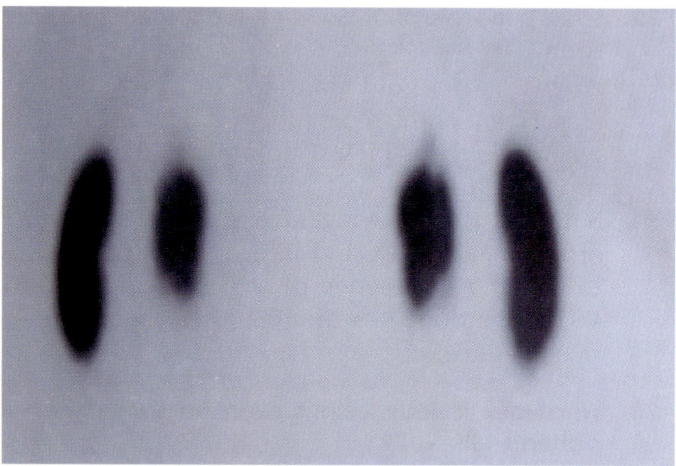

Fig. 13.5: DMSA scan showing loss of contour

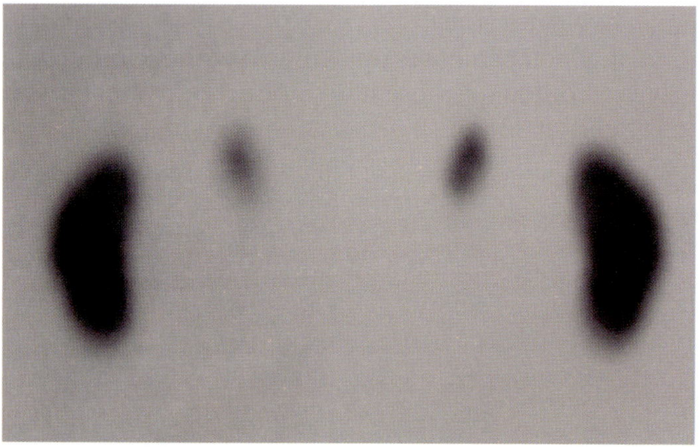

Fig. 13.6: DMSA scan showing global reduction of renal mass without loss of contour

25. What is the role of magnetic resonance urography in patients with UTI and suspected VUR?

Ans: Magnetic resonance urography (MRU) can provide both anatomic and functional data in one study. Congenital renal dysplasia can be differentiated from acquired renal damage on MRU.[23]

26. What do you mean by bottom-up and top-down approaches for evaluation for febrile UTI and VUR? What are pros and cons of each approach?

Ans: In the bottom-up approach, in a child with febrile UTI, initially a sonography is done followed by a VCUG while in a top-down approach initially a sonography and DMSA scan is done and if it is abnormal, then a VCUG is done.[24,25]

Advantages of bottom-up approach
- Highest sensitivity and specificity to diagnose VUR
- Lesser cost
- Ease of availability.

Drawbacks of bottom-up approach
- VCUG is a stressful study for the patient and family due to the need for catheterization.
- It identifies a population with VUR that may not be clinically significant

Advantages of top-down approach
- A negative DMSA precludes the need for a catheter, avoids VCUG in nearly 50% of patients
- A positive study identifies those patients who are most "at-risk" for subsequent renal scarring.

Disadvantages of top-down approach
- Misses 5–20% significant VUR
- More expensive
- Renogram is not easily available.

27. Does VUR resolve spontaneously?

Ans: Yes VUR can resolve spontaneously, especially in young patients and those with low grade VUR. The chances of spontaneous resolution of VUR are low in patients with high grade VUR. High grades of VUR is less likely to resolve spontaneously especially when diagnosed in older children after UTI. Importantly, spontaneous resolution of VUR is facilitated by correction of BBD (bladder bowel dysfunction). The most important factor which determines spontaneous resolution of VUR is the grade of VUR[26] (Table 13.3).

TABLE 13.3: Chances of spontaneous resolution as per the grade of VUR

Grade of VUR	*Chances of spontaneous resolution*
Grade I	72%
Grade 2	61%
Grade 3	49%
Grade 4/5	32%

28. What causes damage to the kidneys in VUR?

Ans: It is either infection whose passage to the kidney is facilitated by VUR (Big Bang Theory) or a high pressure reflux (Hammer Theory) which causes damage to the kidney. What needs to be emphasised is that sterile reflux, unless under high pressure, is unlikely to cause damage to the kidneys.

29. What is the basic principle of medical management of VUR?

Ans: The basic aim is to prevent damage to the kidneys which is achieved by preventing occurrence of infection and also by preventing high pressure reflux.

30. Does circumcision prevent UTI?

Ans: Yes, a systematic review and meta-analysis by Chan *et al* found that circumcised boys are at significantly lesser risk of developing any form of UTI.[27]

31. What is CAP?

Ans: This is continuous antibiotic prophylaxis. In this case an antibiotic is given at 1/4 to 1/2 of its therapeutic over long time preferably at night-time to prevent the occurrence of UTI.

32. What studies provide support to the concept of CAP?

Ans: Two important studies provide support to the practice of CAP to prevent occurrence of UTI.[28–30]

- Swedish reflux trial—it found that the incidence of recurrent UTI was 57% in those without CAP compared to 19% in those on antibiotic prophylaxis
- Randomized intervention for children with vesicoureteral reflux (RIVUR study)—it is the largest randomized placebo-controlled double blind multicenter study involving 607 children aged 2–72 months with Grade I–IV VUR. The important conclusions of this study are:
  - CAP reduces the risk of recurrent UTI by 50%.
  - CAP does not reduce the risk of renal scarring and its consequences
  - Children with BBD with VUR benefit by nearly 80%
  - Children who presented with febrile UTI benefitted by reduction in UTI by 60%

A reanalysis of the RIVUR study found that children who will benefit from CAP are those with BBD with any grade of VUR and those with grade IV VUR regardless of BBD.[30]

33. What are the drawbacks of keeping the patients on long-term CAP?

Ans: The most common problem is compliance in adhering to CAP. Besides this, the risk of developing antibiotic resistance, asthma and development of irritable bowel syndrome due to altered bacterial flora of the gut. Also, in developing countries CAP can significantly add to the cost of treatment.

34. Do all patients with VUR have the same risk of developing UTI?

Ans: No, as shown by the RIVUR study patients with high grade VUR and those with BBD are at higher risk of developing UTI. Hidas *et al* have categorized patients in low and high risk based on their risk of developing UTI[31] (Table 13.4).

Thus patients with high risk can be kept on CAP while antibiotic can be avoided in patients with low risk of developing UTI.

TABLE 13.4: Risk factors for developing UTI in children with VUR

Risk factor	*Low risk*	*High risk*
Age	5 years	<1 year
Gender	Male	Female
Race	Afro-American	Caucasian
Laterality	Unilateral	Bilateral
Grade of VUR	Grade I-II	Grade III-V
Scars	Absent	Present
BBD	Absent	Present
Presentation	Prenatal hydronephrosis	Multiple febrile UTIs

35. What is the relation between BBD and VUR?

Ans: VUR may be secondary to BBD and the treatment of BBD may help to correct VUR. At the same time, VUR may affect bladder dynamics which can lead to BBD. Patients with lower urinary tract dysfunction (LUTD) are at higher risk of developing UTI and renal scarring. Reflux with LUTD resolves faster after correction of LUTD.[32,33]

36. How should a child on CAP be monitored during follow-up?

Ans:

- Urine routine: Every month or whenever the child is sick
- USG: 6 monthly or yearly
- VCUG: If there are good chances of resolution, then after 1 year and if there are less chances of resolution of VUR, then after 2 years
- DMSA scan 2 yearly

It is important to look for weight gain, blood pressure monitoring on every follow-up.

37. What are indications for surgical Intervention in a patient with VUR?

- Breakthrough urinary tract infections in patient on CAP
- The progression or development of renal scarring in DMSA scan
- Non-resolving high-grade VUR (grade III–V VUR)
- Inability to maintain prophylaxis (treatment noncompliance)
- Parental preference

SUMMARY

- Rule out UTI in any child who presents with fever
- Diagnosis of UTI in a child is made using urine analysis and urine culture
- Imaging in a child with febrile UTI[20]
- Age < 1 year
  - USG
  - VCUG

  - DMSA scan—as they are at high risk of developing renal scars
- Age 1–5 years
  - USG and if it is abnormal, then VCUG and/or DMSA scan—either bottom-up or top-down approach
- Age> 5 years
  - Only USG
- VCUG/DMSA scan should be done selectively
- It may be difficult and risky to select patients who do not need CAP
- Initially manage all children presenting at age 1–5 years conservatively
- A safe approach would be to use CAP in most cases
- A practical approach would be to use CAP in all children with VUR till they are toilet trained and have NO LUTD.[34]

REFERENCES

1. Novak TE, Mathews R, Martz K, Neu A. Progression of chronic kidney disease in children with vesicoureteral reflux: the North American Pediatric Renal Trials Collaborative Studies Database. J Urol. 2009 Oct; 182(4 Suppl):1678–81. doi: 10.1016/j.juro.2009.02.085. Epub 2009 Aug 18. PMID: 19692051.
2. Litwin MS, Saigal CS, eds. Urologic diseases in America. National Institute of Diabetes and Digestive and Kidney Diseases website. www.niddk.nih.gov/about-niddk/strategic-plans-reports/urologic-diseases-in-america. Published 2012.
3. Management and screening of primary vesicoureteral reflux in children. American Urological Association website. www.auanet.org/guidelines-and-quality/guidelines/vesicoureteral-reflux-guideline External link. Published 2010. Validity confirmed 2017. Accessed June 4, 2018.
4. Kauffman JD, Danielson PD, Chandler NM. Risk factors and associated morbidity of urinary tract infections in pediatric surgical patients: A NSQIP pediatric analysis. J Pediatr Surg. 2020 Apr;55(4):715–720. doi: 10.1016/j.jpedsurg.2019.04.030.
5. Tosif S, Baker A, Oakley E, Donath S, Babl FE. Contamination rates of different urine collection methods for the diagnosis of urinary tract infections in young children: an observational cohort study. J Paediatr Child Health. 2012 Aug;48(8): 659–64.
6. Vaillancourt S, McGillivray D, Zhang X, Kramer MS. To clean or not to clean: effect on contamination rates in midstream urine collections in toilet-trained children. Pediatrics. 2007 Jun;119(6):e1288–93. doi: 10.1542/peds.2006–2392.
7. Bitsori M, Galanakis E. Pediatric urinary tract infections: diagnosis and treatment. Expert Rev Anti Infect Ther. 2012 Oct;10(10):1153–64.
8. Stein R, Dogan HS, Hoebeke P, Ko vara R, Nijman RJ, Radmayr C, Tekgül S; European Association of Urology; European Society for Pediatric Urology. Urinary tract infections in children: EAU/ESPU guidelines. Eur Urol. 2015 Mar;67(3):546–58. doi: 10.1016/j.eururo.2014.11.007
9. Ransley PG, Risdon RA. Reflux nephropathy: effects of antimicrobial therapy on the evolution of the early pyelonephritic scar. Kidney Int. 1981 Dec;20(6):733–42.
10. Chand DH, Rhoades T, Poe SA, Kraus S, Strife CF. Incidence and severity of vesicoureteral reflux in children related to age, gender, race and diagnosis. J Urol. 2003 Oct;170(4Pt2):1548–50.
11. Shaikh N, *et al.* Early antibiotic treatment for pediatric febrile urinary tract infection and renal scarring. *JAMA Pediatrics.* 2016 Sep 1; 170(9):848–54.
12. Capozza N, Gulia C, Heidari Bateni Z, Zangari A, Gigli S, Briganti V, Tursini S, Koh CJ, Gaffi M, Baldassarra S, Signore F, Porrello A, Piergentili R. Vesicoureteral reflux in infants: what do we know about the gender prevalence by age? Eur Rev Med Pharmacol Sci. 2017 Dec;21(23):5321–5329.
13. Prasad MM, Cheng EY. Imaging studies and biomarkers to detect clinically meaningful vesicoureteral reflux. *Investig Clin Urol.* 2017 Jun. 58 (Suppl 1):S23–S31.
14. Lebowitz RL, Olbing H, Parkkulainen KV, Smellie JM, Tamminen-Möbius TE. International system of radiographic grading of vesicoureteric reflux. International Reflux Study in Children. Pediatr Radiol. 1985;15(2):105–9.
15. Chang SJ, Tsai LP, Hsu CK, Yang SS. Elevated postvoid residual urine volume predicting recurrence of urinary tract infections in toilet-trained children. Pediatr Nephrol. 2015 Jul;30(7):1131–7.
16. Mathews R, Carpenter M, Chesney R, Hoberman A, Keren R, Mattoo T, Moxey-Mims M, Nyberg L, Greenfield S. Controversies in the management of vesicoureteral reflux: the rationale for the RIVUR study. J Pediatr Urol. 2009 Oct;5(5):336–41.
17. Unver T, Alpay H, Biyikli NK, Ones T. Comparison of direct radionuclide cystography and voiding cystourethrography in detecting vesicoureteral reflux. Pediatr Int. 2006 Jun;48(3): 287–91.
18. Ward VL, Strauss KJ, Barnewolt CE, Zurakowski D, Venkatakrishnan V, Fahey FH, Lebowitz RL, Taylor GA. Pediatric radiation exposure and effective dose reduction during voiding cystourethrography. Radiology. 2008 Dec; 249(3):1002–9.
19. A. Takvani, C. Gokani, P. Malaviya, Vesicoureteric reflux—a prospective study of 11 years, European Urology Supplements,Volume 14, Issue 2, 2015,Pages e505–e505a.
20. Ansari MS, Shekar PA, Singh C, Joshi SS. The Urological Society of India Guidelines for the management of pediatric urinary tract infection (Executive Summary). Indian J Urol. 2021 Jan-Mar;37(1):10–12.
21. Merrick MV, Notghi A, Chalmers N, *et al.* Long-term follow up to determine the prognostic value of imaging after urinary tract infections. Part 1: Reflux. *Arch Dis Child.* 1995;72(5): 388–92.
22. Wallin L, Bajc M. The significance of vesicoureteric reflux on kidney development assessed by dimercaptosuccinate renal scintigraphy. Br J Urol. 1994 Jun;73(6):607–11.
23. Morin CE, McBee MP, Trout AT, Reddy PP, Dillman JR. Use of MR Urography in Pediatric Patients. Curr Urol Rep. 2018 Sep 11;19(11):93.
24. Prasad MM, Cheng EY. Radiographic evaluation of children with febrile urinary tract infection: bottom-up, top-down, or none of the above? Adv Urol. 2012;2012:716739.
25. Abdelhalim A, Khoury AE. Critical appraisal of the top-down approach for vesicoureteral reflux. *Investig Clin Urol.* 2017 Jun. 58 (Suppl 1):S14–S22.
26. Estrada CR Jr, Passerotti CC, Graham DA, Peters CA, Bauer SB, Diamond DA, *et al.* Nomograms for predicting annual resolution rate of primary vesicoureteral reflux: results from 2,462 children. J Urol. 2009 Oct;182(4):1535–41.
27. Chan JY, Khondker A, Lee MJ, Kim JK, Chancy M, Chua ME, Santos JD, Brownrigg N, Richter J, Lorenzo AJ, Rickard M.

The role of circumcision in preventing urinary tract infections in children with antenatal hydronephrosis: Systematic review and meta-analysis. J Pediatr Urol. 2023 Aug 2:S1477–5131(23)00311-X.
28. Brandström P, Jodal U, Sillén U, Hansson S. The Swedish reflux trial: review of a randomized, controlled trial in children with dilating vesicoureteral reflux. J Pediatr Urol. 2011 Dec;7(6):594–600.
29. Carpenter MA, Hoberman A, Mattoo TK, Mathews R, Keren R, Chesney RW, Moxey-Mims M, Greenfield SP; RIVUR Trial Investigators. The RIVUR trial: profile and baseline clinical associations of children with vesicoureteral reflux. Pediatrics. 2013 Jul;132(1):e34–45. doi: 10.1542/peds.2012–2301.
30. Zhao B, Ivanova A, Shaikh N. Antimicrobial prophylaxis for vesicoureteral reflux: which subgroups of children benefit the most? Research Square. 2023 Aug 30:rs.3.rs-3286108.
31. Hidas G, Nam A, Soltani T, Pribish M, Watts B, Khoury AE. Primary vesico-ureteric reflux: The need for individualised risk stratification. Arab J Urol. 2013 Mar;11(1):8–12.
32. Koff, S.A., *et al.* The relationship among dysfunctional elimination syndromes, primary vesicoureteral reflux and urinary tract infections in children. J Urol, 1998. 160: 1019.
33. Meena, J., *et al.* Prevalence of Bladder and Bowel Dysfunction in Toilet-Trained Children With Urinary Tract Infection and/or Primary Vesicoureteral Reflux: A Systematic Review and Meta-Analysis. Front Pediatr, 2020. 8.
34. EAU Guidelines. Edn. presented at the EAU Annual Congress Milan 2023. ISBN 978-94-92671-19-6.

Chapter

14

Non-Palpable Testes in a 10-Year-Old Boy

• *Ulhas Sathaye*

LEARNING OBJECTIVES

Very often we come across older children with a non-palpable testis. Since these children have already passed the recommended age of treatment, there are doubts about the optimum line of treatment at this age.

This chapter aims:

- To analyze the cause of late presentation.
- Review the problem as a whole.
- Investigations for diagnosis.
- Points to be considered during counselling the parents.
- The best line of management at this age.

INTRODUCTION

The most common cause of a non-palpable testes in a 10-year-old is undescended testes. However, the other causes are retractile testes, sequelae of testicular torsion, testicular agenesis, trauma or infection. In the present time with awareness among healthcare professionals, these children are brought for evaluation and definitive treatment well in time by 6 months of age. Thus, though incidence of non-palpable testes at age 10 is rare it is still not infrequent.

This chapter will cover the topic as a whole, and guide for management options of all possible scenarios.

Case Scenario

A 10-year-old boy was brought to urology services by the parents with an absent testis on the left side. This was noted during a medical examination in the school. The boy was delivered at home by a midwife. The parents were unaware of this condition. On examination in the lying down position the left scrotum was empty. The testes was not palpable in the inguinal region. The right testes was palpable and was normal. His lab reports were normal. The parents have come for further management.

1. **What are the reasons of non-palpable testis in a 10-year-old boy?**

   Ans: Other than a congenital undescended testis (UDT), the other reasons for finding a non-palpable testis in a 10-year-old boy are: 1. Ascending or acquired UDT, 2. Parental delay mainly due to the fear of surgery in a child, 3. Late referrals because parents were wrongly advised to wait as their primary care provider felt the testis would descend eventually, 4. Iatrogenic (trapped following ipsilateral groin surgery), 5. Ignorance, 6. Unknown causes. There can even be an overlap of multiple reasons.[1]

2. **What is the etiology of UDT?**

   Ans: In the foetal period, both testes may not descend to the scrotum on time for various reasons, which can manifest as cryptorchidism at birth. Cryptorchidism may be closely related to genetics, hormone synthesis and secretion, premature delivery, pregnancy in older women, and the environment.

3. **What is the incidence of UDT?**

   Ans: The incidence of UDT is 30% in premature boys. It decreases to 3% in full term neonates. During the first months of life, testis may continue their normal descent process. Cryptorchidism occurs in 1–2% by 3-month of age[2] and decreases to 0.8–1.2% in boys at 1-year-old.[12]

4. What is the mechanism of descent of the testes?

Ans: There is a biphasic model for the explanation of testicular descent. The transabdominal phase and the inguinoscrotal phase. The first stage of testicular descent (transabdominal) occurs by the eighth gestational week. Between the eighth and fifteenth gestational weeks, the gubernaculum enlarges caudally, leading to the formation of the gubernacular bulb, whereas between the 10th to 15th gestational weeks, the cranial suspensory ligament (CSL) regresses. Regression of the CSL is a necessary step for testicular descent; however, regression of the CSL alone is not sufficient to initiate gonadal descent. This phase of testicular descent consists of the movement of the testes from their starting position on the posterior abdominal wall adjacent to the kidney down to the internal inguinal ring.

The second stage of testicular descent (inguino-scrotal) begins by the 26th gestational week. This stage is androgen-dependent and consists of the passage of the testes from the internal inguinal ring down into the scrotum. The inguinoscrotal stage of testicular descent has specific pre-requisite steps, includes the formation of the processus vaginalis, dilation of the inguinal canal by the gubernacular bulb, and abdominal pressure to push the testes through the inguinal canal. The contraction of the gubernaculum, along with intra-abdominal pressure, facilitates the movement of the testes through the inguinal canal into the scrotum.[16]

Another hypothesis for cryptorchidism is the inactivation of congenital hypogonadotropic hypogonadism (CHH) related genes.[10]

5. By what age should treatment be offered?

Ans: After the age of 6 months the testes cannot descend spontaneously and needs assistance either medical or surgical. Treatment should be preferably completed before the age of 18 months.

6. How is UDT diagnosed?

Ans: Locating the testes is important for optimum treatment. If the testis is palpable, there a very limited role of imaging. However, when the testis is not palpable, imaging should be done. The diagnostic tools available are ultrasonography, CT, MRI and laparoscopy. A CT scan is non-invasive but unreliable and carries the risk of radiation. MRI is sensitive in obese patients but requires anaesthesia. Hence, CT scans and MRI have their limitations in routine clinical practice. Sonography, though advocated by many for easy availability and repeatability does not have a good sensitivity. Hence examination under anaesthesia and laparoscopy have been adopted into routine practice.[2]

However, in expert hands, ultrasonography has a high positive predictive value for inguinally located testes (91%) and with a 78% of sensitivity. When ultrasound done by a paediatric expert locates a testis in an inguinal location, a primary inguinal exploration can be considered, preventing an unnecessary diagnostic laparoscopy.[14]

7. What is the best method of clinical examination in a child?

Ans: Testicular examination in infants and young children is performed using a two-handed technique in the frog legged position. Palpation should take place in anxiety-free and warm surroundings, since cold or anxiety can cause the cremasteric reflex to retract the testicle. One hand strokes from the anterior superior iliac spine along the inguinal canal towards the pubic bone, while the other hand attempts to palpate the testicle.[13]

8. What is the role of ultrasonography for diagnosis of UDT?

Ans: Ultrasound is the imaging modality most commonly used to evaluate boys with undescended testes. Ultrasound is non-invasive and does not use ionizing radiation, which makes it an attractive imaging option for children. However, the most important limitation of ultrasound is its inability to accurately localize undescended testes. Any diagnostic imaging should offer the theoretic possibility of sparing a child an operation if a non-palpable testis is confirmed to be absent with 100% certainty. For non-palpable testes, which is the clinical scenario for which ultrasound is most frequently ordered, the sensitivity and specificity of ultrasound is poor. Also, it was found that ultrasound falsely identified 10% of gubernacular structures as undescended testis. In a systemic review and meta-analysis, the sensitivity and specificity of ultrasound in correctly identifying a nonpalpable testis was 45% and 78%, respectively.[15] So, there is no role of ultrasound in the accurate diagnosis of a non-palpable testis.

9. Then, is there any role of ultrasound in undescended testis?

Ans: There is a definite role of USG after orchiopexy. It is to monitor testicular growth and function after surgery. Scrotal US can provide an accurate comparative assessment of the growth of testes before and after orchidopexy. It can also be used at follow-up of the operated testes because these testes are known to have a greater chance of malignancy.

10. What is the role of medical (hormonal) management?

Ans: The role of hormonal treatment for undescended testes is questionable. The treatment is with injections of hCG given in twice a week schedule. The dose should not exceed 15000 units for fear of early epiphyseal closure.[9] Inj. LHRH can also be used. Some studies have shown good results with the use of hormonal treatment.[2] Hormonal treatment may improve fertility indices and therefore serve as an additional tool to orchidopexy. It has been shown that men who were treated in childhood with LHRH analogues had better semen analyses compared with men who had childhood orchidopexy alone or placebo treatment. Elsherbeny *et al* analysed 75 boys with cryptorchidism who were treated with hCG. The results showed a low success rate of hCG in the treatment of cryptorchidism, which was attributed to the anatomical abnormality related to cryptorchidism.[10]

In conclusion, no guidelines recommend the use of hormone therapy to induce testicular descent in boys with cryptorchidism.

11. What is the risk of malignancy in UDT?

Ans: A meta-analysis of 21 controlled studies showed an increased odds ratio of 3.5 to 17.1 in men with a history of undescended testis.[13]

12. What is the risk of infertility in UDT?

Ans: Men with a history of undescended testis have a reduced probability of fertility with a low sperm count and generally poorer semen quality than men with normal testicular descent. This subfertility is not compensated by a normally descended contralateral testis. The probability of a fertility impairment is additionally increased in bilateral cryptorchidism and delayed treatment of the non-descended testicle.[13]

13. What are the various surgical techniques for a palpable testis?

Ans: For a palpable testis the surgery offered is either an inguinal or a prescrotal orchiopexy. The testis is placed in a subdartos pouch. A common technique of transparenchymal suture to fix the testis to the dartos has shown no benefit. If the testis cannot be brought to the scrotum without tension, a Prentiss maneuver (ligating and cutting the inferior epigastric vessels) can be added or a 2-stage procedure may be needed. To summarize, the various open surgical techniques are:

- Inguinal (Jones) approach orchiopexy.
- Prescrotal orchiopexy
- Two-stage Fowler-Stephens orchiopexy

14. What is a low intra-abdominal testis and a high intra-abdominal testis?

Ans: On laparoscopy, if the testis is within 2 cm of the internal ring, it is a low intra-abdominal testis. If the testis is >2 cm from the internal ring, it is called a high intra-abdominal testis.

15. What are the various surgical techniques/ approaches for an impalpable testis?

Ans: For non-palpable testis even when examined under anesthesia, the procedure of choice is laparoscopy. If the testis is low intra-abdominal, a single stage orchiopexy can be done. If high intra-abdominal, a two-stage laparoscopic orchiopexy may be required.

16. What are the types of two-stage laparoscopic techniques?

Ans:

- Shehata two-stage orchiopexy
- Two-stage Fowler-Stephens orchiopexy

17. What is Shehata's technique of two-stage laparoscopic orchiopexy?

Ans: In this technique the abdominal testis is mobilized and fixed to a point one inch above and medial to ASIS on the contralateral side at the level of the iliac crest. This elongates the pedicle of that testis. In the 2nd stage after 12 weeks, the testis is released from that point and placed in the ipsilateral scrotum.

18. What is Fowler-Stephens technique and its modification?

Ans: The Fowler-Stephens orchiopexy for a high intra-abdominal testis was originally a single stage procedure wherein the testicular vessels were tied off and the testis was brought to the scrotum with the vas and relying vasculature of the vas for its survival. The success rates of 33 to 90% (pooled success rate 78.7%, 749 testicles) have been reported. The modification is a two-stage procedure described first by Ransley in 1984. This is based on the principle that the vas deferens generally is sufficiently long to allow the IAT to reach the scrotum. If the main testicular vessels are tied off, then collateral blood flow through the deferential artery should increase gradually and support the IAT during the second step of a F-S orchiopexy. In this, the testicular artery and vein are tied off and 6 months later, a second-stage procedure is performed to transect the testicular vessels and mobilize the

IAT on its collateral blood supply. The deferential artery typically has excellent blood flow, and the testis generally reaches the scrotum.[17]

19. What is microvascular autotransplantation?

Ans: In this technique, the testicular artery and vein are divided high in the abdomen, and anastomosed to the inferior epigastric artery and vein.. The testicular artery is 0.5 to 1 mm in diameter and the inferior epigastric artery is 1 to 1.5 mm in diameter. The veins are a 1-to-1 match at 1 mm in diameter. The arterial anastomosis is performed with interrupted 10–or 11–0 nylon and the veins are anastomosed with 10–0 nylon. This is a technical feat, but should be considered if the surgical specialist has the available resources and there is a solitary intra-abdominal testis.

20. When is a testicular biopsy needed?

Ans: Doing a testicular biopsy during orchiopexy for determining the maturation status of the testicle is controversial and at present reserved for research purpose. A biopsy, however, is indicated if ovotestis (the simultaneous presence of testicular and ovarian tissue in one germ cell), dysgenesis, or tumour is suspected.[13]

21. What is acquired UDT?

Ans: This is the phenomenon of ascending testes in which the testes are present in the scrotum, but as the child grows, the vascular pedicle does not lengthen and hence the testis gets pulled into the inguinal canal to become acquired undescended testes. It has been postulated that absorption of the processus vaginalis peritoneum to form the parietal peritoneum causes cord traction leading to ascent of the testes.

22. What are the causes of bilateral non-palpable testis and what are the investigations required?

Ans: The various causes of bilateral non-palpable testis are DSD, bilateral anorchia or bilateral undescended testes. A chromosomal study along with imaging are indicated. If imaging is inconclusive, a laparoscopy will be indicated for diagnosis.

23. What is hCG challenge test?

Ans: In suspected anorchia, plasma testosterone levels are measured both before and after stimulation with inj hCG. If there is a rise in the serum testosterone level, it proves the presence of testes in the body[11] (Flowcharts 14.1 and 14.2).

SUMMARY

- Incidence of UDT is at birth is up to 3% and decreases to 1.2% at 1 year of age
- Spontaneous descent is unlikely after the age of 6 months
- Orchiopexy should be done preferably before the age of 18 months
- The various imaging modalities advocated are USG, CT scan and MRI
- CT and MRI have disadvantages and are not practical in routine practice
- Only a clinical examination and a laparoscopy are useful and diagnostic.
- Hormonal treatment is a first line of treatment in some European countries. The success rate is about 20% which does not compare to the success of surgery.
- WHO recommends Inj hCG and LhRH.
- Hormonal treatment given before or after orchiopexy improves the fertility rate in adult life.
- For non-palpable testis, a laparoscopic examination will decide the further management depending on the findings

Flowchart 14.1: Management algorithm for unilateral undescended testes

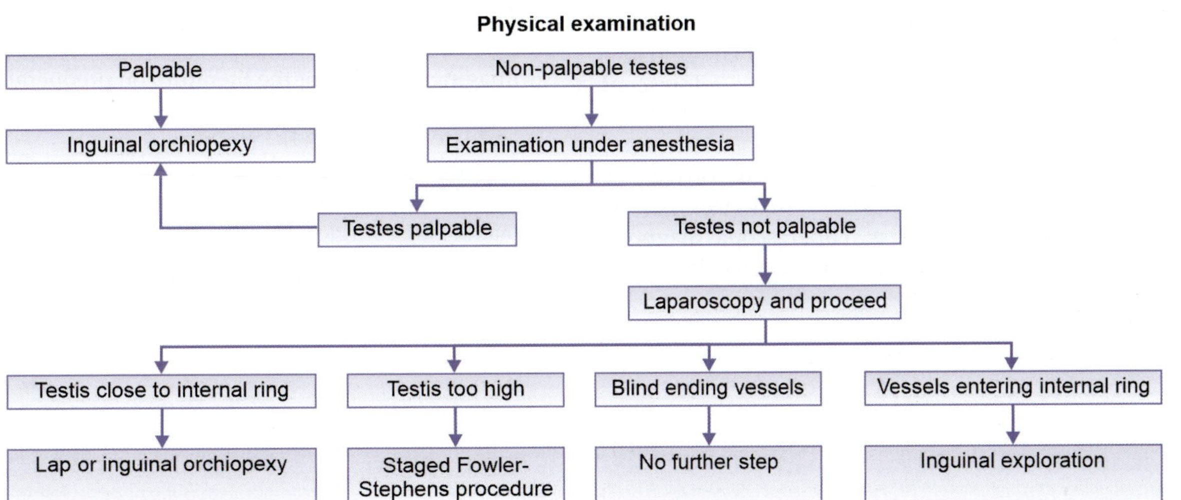

Flowchart 14.2: Algorithm for bilateral undescended testes

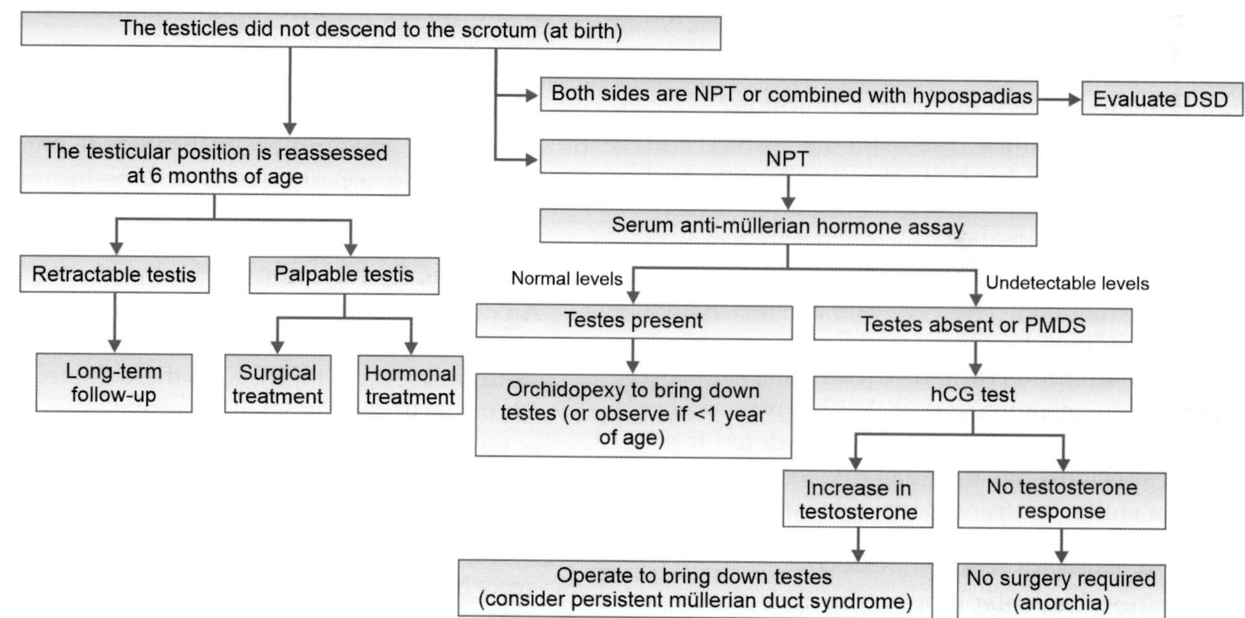

(*Courtesy:* Liu et el. Open controversies on the treatment of undescended testis: An update Frontiers in Paediatrics 2022 874995)

REFERENCES

1. Ahmet Guvena, Barry A. Koganb. Undescended testis in older boys: further evidence that ascending testes are common Journal of Pediatric Surgery (2008) 43, 1700–1704.
2. Hueih-Shing Hsu Management of boys with nonpalpable undescended testes Division of Urology, Department of Surgery, Lotung Pohai Hospital, Yilan, Taiwan Urological Science 23 (2012) 103e106.
3. WWM Hack, K Sijstermans, J van Dijk, L M van der Voort-Doedens, M E de Kok, M J Hobbelt-Stoker Prevalence of acquired undescended testis in 6-year, 9-year and 13-year-old Dutch schoolboys Arch Dis Child 2007 92, 17–20).
4. Shreyas K, Kirtikumar J. Rathod* and Arvind Sinha. Management of high inguinal undescended testis: a review of literature. Annals of Pediatric Surgery (2021) 17:42.
5. Jedrzejewski G, Wieczorek AP, Osemlak P, Nachulewicz P. The role of ultrasound in the management of undescended testes before and after orchidopexy - an update. Medicine. 2016;95(51):e5731.
6. S. Faisal Ahmed. John C. Achermann, Wiebke Arlt, Adam H. Balen, Gerry Conway, Zoe L. Edwards *et al* UK guidance on the initial evaluation of an infant or an adolescent with a suspected disorder of sex development Clinical Endocrinology (2011) 75, 12–26.
7. W Cheng, G H Mya, H Saing. Associated anomalies in patients with undescended testes J Trop Pediatric. 1996 Aug;42(4):204–6.
8. (Denes FT Saito FJ, Silva FA, *et al.* Laparoscopic diagnosis and treatment of nonpalpable testis. International Braz J Urol 2008;34:329–34; discussion 335).
9. Thomas F. Kolon Evaluation and Treatment of Cryptorchidism: AUA Guideline Journal of urology® Vol. 192, 337–345, August 2014.
10. Jie Liu *et al.* Open controversies on the treatment of undescended testes: An update. Frontiers in Paediatrics Volume 10 2022.
11. DB Grant *et al.* HCG stimulation test in children with abnormal sexual development Archives of Disease in Childhood, 1976, 51, 596.
12. Berkowitz GS, Lapinski RH, Dolgin SE, *et al.* Prevalence and natural history of cryptorchidism. Paediatrics 1993;92:44–9.
13. Michael J. Mathers, Herbert Sperling, Herbert Rübben, Stephan Roth. The Undescended Testis: Diagnosis, Treatment and Long-Term Consequences. Deutsches Ärzteblatt International Dtsch Arztebl Int 2009; 106(33): 527–32.
14. Ximena Sepúlveda1, Pedro-José López Egaña. Current management of non-palpable testes: a literature review and clinical result. Translational Paediatrics 2016;5(4):233–239.
15. Siobhán Hartigan1, Gregory E. Tasian Unnecessary diagnostic imaging: a review of the literature on preoperative imaging for boys with undescended testes. Translational Andrology and Urology 2014;3(4):359–364.
16. Owuraku A. Titi-Lartey; Yusuf S. Khan. Statpearls publishing. Embryology, Testicle Last Update: April 28, 2022.
17. Jack S. Elder. Surgical Management of the Undescended Testis: Recent Advances and Controversies. European J Pediatric Surgery 26(5) September 2016.

Section

3

Reconstructive Urology

Chapter

1

Diagnostic Evaluation of Male Urethral Stricture Disease

• *Sushil Shivlal Rathi* • *M. Gopichand*

LEARNING OBJECTIVES

To understand

- Clinical presentation, history, physical examination and role of IPSS score.
- Laboratory investigation—CBC, KFT, RBS, Urinalysis (+/– culture and sensitivity test).
- Role of uroflowmetry—indication, parameters, pattern and interpretation pertaining to stricture urethra.
- Role of ultrasonography KUB with postvoid residual (PVR) urine measurement.
- Role of radiological investigations in stricture urethra.
  - RUG, VCUG, RUG+VCUG
  - Sono-urethrography
  - MR urethrography
- Role of endoscopy.

SUMMARY

Urethral stricture is narrowing of anterior urethra due to fibrosis or scarring of urethral mucosa and surrounding spongiosum tissue (spongiofibrosis) and in posterior urethra, it is termed stenosis as there is absence of spongiosum.

Most common type of stricture is iatrogenic and site is bulbar urethra. Lichen sclerosis (LS) is the commonest cause of pan urethral stricture. Traumatic posterior urethral injury usually results in obliterative or near obliterative strictures with extensive fibrosis.

Decrease in the urethral lumen leads to obstructive voiding dysfunction which may cause deleterious effects on entire urinary tract, which substantially impacts the patient's quality of life.

A comprehensive diagnostic evaluation of stricture is necessary for prompt diagnosis and management which includes history, physical examination, urine analysis with urine culture if indicated, uroflowmetry, radiological assessment in terms of retrograde urethrography (RUG), voiding cystourethrography (VCUG), endoscopy and in more complex cases magnetic resonance urethrography (MRU), sonourethrogram (SUG) are indicated.

This topic aims to provide a practical summary outlining the diagnostic evaluation of the stricture urethra.

Case Scenario

A 65-year-old gentleman presented with inability to pass urine for the last 12 hours with severe discomfort and fullness in lower abdomen. He underwent TURP 3 years ago and was having obstructive LUTS for last one year. He has no h/o constipation, fever, trauma, or medication. His general examination is essentially normal; per abdominal examination revealed a palpable urinary bladder with normal genitalia. Anal tone and prostate are normal on digital rectal examination (DRE). A 14 Fr Foley catheter could not be passed per urethrally.

1. **What is your clinical diagnosis?**

   Ans: Clinical diagnosis is acute urinary retention with stricture urethra in operated case of trans-urethral resection of prostate (TURP).

2. **What are the other clinical presentations in patients of stricture urethra?**

   Ans: Other clinical presenting symptoms can be post-void dribble, dysuria, urinary frequency, urgency, incontinence, pain in lower abdomen and genitalia, UTI, hematuria, periurethral swellings, and pus discharge per urethra or perineum.[1]

3. **What important history will you ask in patients of stricture urethra and what is the role of international prostate symptoms score (IPSS)?**

   Ans: One should enquire about history regarding pus discharge through urethra, prior urethral instrumentation, transurethral surgery, circumcision, urethral or perineal trauma, hypospadias surgery, urethral dilatations, clean self- intermittent catheterisation (CSIC), and pelvic fracture with associated injuries. The sexual function is affected by the trauma and reconstructive surgery and it is essential to document sexual function before intervention. History of tobacco or betel leaves chewing should be documented. Assessment of general health status is important as it influences the choice between a palliative and a curative treatment. Any factor that impairs healing should be identified (i.e. diabetes mellitus, severe anemia, immunosuppression and smoking). Symptoms of renal impairment, history of pelvic radiation, and constipation should also be enquired.[2-4]

   Patient evaluation must include urethral stricture surgery patient related outcome measures (USS PROM) such as IPSS. In patients with urethral stricture, the highest scored questions are frequency and poor stream. Pre-operative documentation of IPSS score indicates degree of bother and allows comparison after corrective treatment.[2]

4. **What will you look for in physical examination of a patient of stricture urethra?**

   Ans: The abdomen is assessed for scars from previous surgery, and the presence of SPC should be noted. The genital examination should determine the size and location of the urethral meatus, changes of lichen sclerosus, chordee, prepuce, scars and urethro-cutaneous fistula. Urethra is palpated to check for induration. Testes, scrotum and perineum should be examined to rule out infective complications like epididymo-orchitis, periurethral or perineal abscess. The feasibility of giving lithotomy position is assessed in patients with pelvic fractures. The buccal and lingual mucosa is examined.

5. **What investigation will you consider in this case to confirm the diagnosis and how will you treat his retention?**

   Ans: Baseline investigations like complete blood count (CBC), kidney function test (KFT), serum electrolytes and coagulation profile, and ultrasonography of urinary tract with postvoid residue.

   I shall perform a suprapubic cystostomy (SPC) to relieve his retention of urine.

   Then, I would ask for further investigations to confirm my diagnosis like RUG (and VCUG, if needed.), urine analysis (and urine culture sensitivity, if needed).[2,5]

6. **Define and classify urethral strictures.**

   Ans: *Urethral stricture* is a scarring process that involves urothelium and surrounding corpus spongiosum resulting in the narrowing of urethral caliber. This may extend to the entire thickness of corpus spongiosum and sometimes extending into adjacent tissue (Fig 1.1).

   When the majority of the urethra is potentially "diseased" and the blood supply is compromised in other areas of the urethra, proximal or distal to the obvious stricture, it is referred to as urethral stricture disease.

   The corpus spongiosum covers only anterior urethra and its luminal narrowing, which would otherwise be called *anterior urethral stricture*, is referred to as *stricture* only. The posterior urethra is devoid of corpus spongiosum; hence, narrowing of posterior urethra is called *posterior urethral stenosis* instead of posterior urethral stricture and *posterior urethral Injury* when associated with pelvic fracture *(PFUI)*.[6–9]

   Male urethral strictures are classified according to stricture location and stricture tightness (Tables 1.1 and 1.2.).[1]

7. **What is etiology of stricture urethra?**

   Ans: Etiologically, anterior urethral strictures can be:

   1. Idiopathic (34%),
   2. Iatrogenic (32%),
   3. Inflammatory (20%) and
   4. Traumatic (14%).

   In India, urethral catheterization is a more common cause of stricture than transurethral surgery. Post-TURP strictures are thrice more common in the Indian population than in the West. Iatrogenic and idiopathic strictures are more common in the bulbar urethra and LS or hypospadias-associated strictures are at the meatus and may spread proximally.[9–11]

8. **What are the mechanisms of stricture formation?**

   Ans:

   A. Mechanisms of Iatrogenic Stricture Formation

   1. Instrument-related strictures

   When a rigid instrument is passed along the male urethra, a fulcrum is created at fixed points. Larger caliber instrument, longer procedure duration and inadequate lubrication results into pressure necrosis, scarring and stricture.[12]

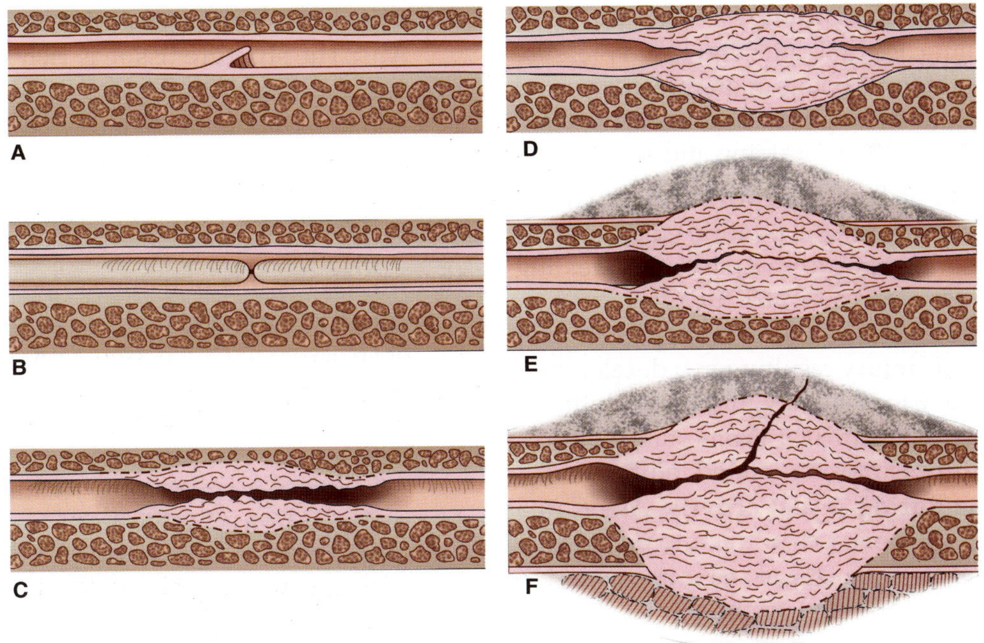

Fig. 1.1A to F: The anatomy of anterior urethral strictures: (A) Mucosal fold. (B) Iris constriction. (C) Full-thickness involvement with minimal fibrosis in the spongy tissue. (D) Full-thickness spongiofibrosis. (E) Inflammation and fibrosis involving tissues outside the corpus spongiosum. (F) Complex stricture complicated by a fistula. This can proceed to the formation of an abscess, or the fistula may open to the skin or the rectum[1]

TABLE 1.1: Male urethra stricture locations and anatomic landmarks for classification

Urethral segment		*Location—anatomic landmarks*
Anterior urethra	Meatal strictures	External urethral meatus; may extend into the fossa navicularis of the glans
	Penile strictures	Between fossa navicularis and bulbar urethra
	Bulbar strictures	Starting at the penoscrotal junction and ending at the level of the urogenital diaphragm
	Penobulbar strictures	From penile urethra into the bulbar segment (compromising long segments of urethra)
Posterior urethra	Membranous urethral stenosis	Segment traversing the urogenital diaphragm, from proximal bulbar to distal verumontanum
	Prostatic urethral stenosis	Segment through the prostatic gland, starting at the proximal membranous urethra and extending to the bladder neck
	Bladder neck stenosis	Junction between the prostatic urethra and the bladder, requiring that the prostatic gland is *in situ* (i.e. after TURP or simple prostatectomies)
	Vesicourethral anastomotic stenosis	Narrowing or obliteration at anastomotic site after radical prostatectomy

TABLE 1.2: EAU urethral stricture guidelines panel classification of male urethral stricture

Category	*Description*	*Urethral lumen (Fr)*	*Degree of obstruction*
0	Normal urethra on imaging techniques		
1	Subclinical strictures	Urethral narrowing but >16 Fr	Low
2	Low grade strictures	11–15 Fr	
3	High flow or flow significant strictures	4–10 Fr	High
4	Nearly obliterative strictures	1–3 Fr	
5	Obliterative strictures	No urethral lumen (0 Fr)	

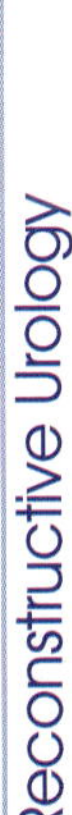

2. **Catheter-related strictures**
   Indwelling urethral catheters related pressure necrosis at fixed points of urethra, associated inflammatory response and superimposed infection results in scarring and stricture.[12]

B. Mechanisms of Traumatic Stricture Formation[9]

Any process that injures urethral epithelium or corpus spongiosum to the point that healing results in scar can cause stricture.

1. **Blunt trauma:** Direct blow in the perineum or fall astride injury resulting in a deceleration type injury to relatively immobile urethra.
2. **Penetrating injuries:** From stab wounds, firearms or explosion-related injuries.
3. **Trauma during sexual activity:** Associated with 10–20% of cases of fracture penis.
4. **Internal trauma:** Due to the introduction of foreign bodies in the urethra.

C. Mechanism of Development of Infective and Inflammatory Strictures[9]

The untreated gonorrheal infection spreads to surrounding corpus spongiosum resulting in venous thrombosis, tissue necrosis, scarring and stricture formation. The role of non-gonococcal urethritis in stricture formation is unclear.

Lichen sclerosus begins with inflammation of glans and meatal stenosis leading to high-pressure voiding, causing intravasation of urine into the glands of Litter, their inflammation and microabscesses. This results in spongiofibrosis and stricture formation.

D. Idiopathic Strictures

Bulbar urethral strictures are associated in some prepubertal and adolescent boys with idiopathic urethrorrhagia. Some of these may be related to unrecognised or repetitive perineal trauma.[9,13]

E. Congenital Urethral Stricture[9]

It can be a congenital narrowing of the bulbar urethra believed to be embryologically related to rupture of the cloacal membrane or urogenital diaphragm.

F. Mechanism of Injury to Posterior Urethra[14]

The membranous urethra is the least elastic portion of male urethra and is not protected by prostate or corpus spongiosum; hence it is susceptible to injury during high kinetic energy traumas. 70–75% of the lesions occur distal to the sphincter because proximal bulbar urethra is surrounded by only fat and loose connective tissue.

Posterior urethral stenosis can be caused by transurethral surgeries using different energy sources, radical prostatectomy and radiation therapy for carcinoma prostate.

9. What is pathogenesis of stricture urethra?

Ans: The stricture tissue is rich in myofibroblasts and multinucleated giant cells. The fibrous and non-compliant nature of the stricture is due to an increase in the amount of collagen, alteration in the ratio of various types of collagen and change in the concentration of elastic fibers.[9]

10. What is the role of ultrasonography?

Ans: USG of KUB provides information on signs of obstruction like increased PVR, increased bladder wall thickness, presence of diverticuli, calculi and upper tract changes. It estimates prostate volume, which can also contribute to obstructive LUTS. Amongst these parameters, bladder wall thickness is more specific for urethral obstruction.[2]

Its limitations are:

1. These signs are not specific for urethral stricture disease,
2. High intra- and interpersonal variation
3. Variation depending upon the bladder volume at the time of evaluation.[2]

11. What is the role of uroflowmetry in the diagnosis of stricture urethra?

Ans: Uroflowmetry is indicated in patients presenting with voiding difficulty (Fig. 1.2).

Decreased maximum flow rate with a prolonged plateau on uroflowmetry graph is characteristic of the constrictive obstruction caused by urethral stricture.

Uroflowmetry is used as

1. Screening tool for the detection of stricture
2. Monitoring patients and in the assessment of treatment response
3. A statistical model based on uroflowmetry parameters in predicting urethral stricture has sensitivity of 80–81% and specificity of 77–78%
4. Uroflowmetry is usually combined with USG estimation of PVR to identify patients with urinary retention who may require immediate bladder drainage.[1]

However, interpretation of flow patterns is not reliable and subjective.

12. Is there any role of urodynamic assessment in stricture urethra?

Ans: Urodynamic assessment is not indicated in the vast majority of patients.

It may help in surgical decision-making and patient counseling in patients with suspected bladder dysfunction. In patients with detrusor underactivity or an acontractile detrusor, it may predict need to perform CSIC post-operatively.

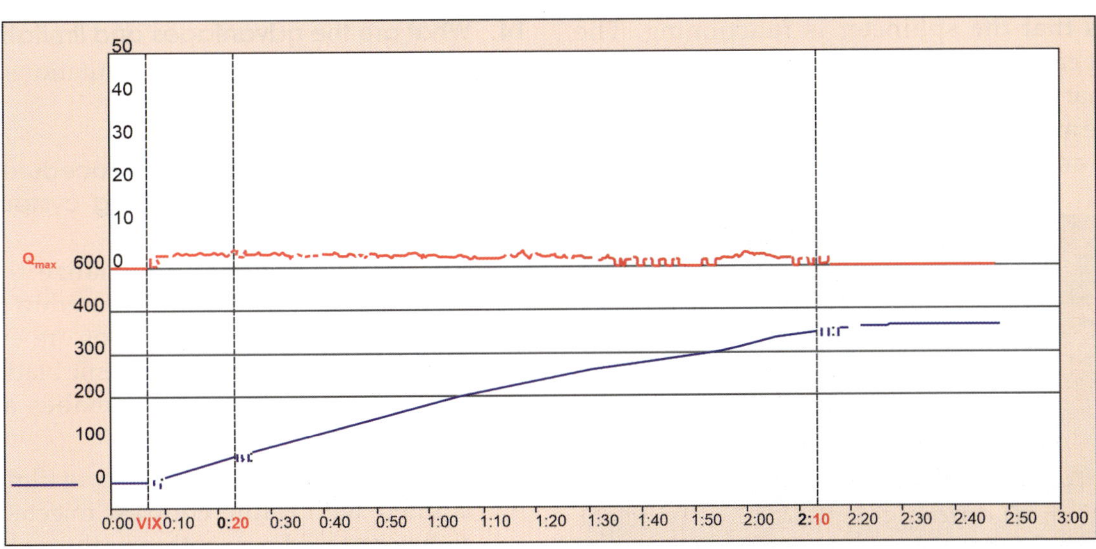

Fig. 1.2: Uroflow graph showing classic pattern of prolonged plateau-shaped graph with decreased maximum urinary flow (Q_{max})

Urethral closure pressure is lower in case of stricture due to the constrictive nature of the obstruction than benign enlarged prostate which will help in distinguishing one from another.[1]

13. What are the indications, types, procedure, limitations and interpretation of retrograde urethrography (RUG)?

Ans: RUG is the gold standard investigation for evaluation of anterior urethral stricture. It provides information about the stricture's number, location and length and helps in staging it. Other indications are pelvic trauma with suspected urethral injury, urethral diverticula, suspected urethral foreign bodies, urethral tumors and urethral fistula.[1,9]

Types of RUG: RUG can be dynamic (DRU) or static.

Procedure: The patient is positioned supine with 45° tilt to one side on the fluoroscopy table and the dependent thigh is flexed.

A scout film is taken to assess the position, exposure and rule out any radio-opaque urethral pathology like calculus. The dependent obturator fossa should not be seen.

A gentle stretch is given to the penis to straighten the urethra; after cleaning the glans, 15–20 ml of water-soluble contrast is injected slowly into the urethra through the meatus using a syringe attached to a Foley adapter. In case of meatal stenosis, adapter of ureteric catheter or plastic sheath of intravenous cannula can be used. Alternatively, a small-sized Foley catheter with inflation of its balloon in fossa navicularis can be used.[15] Manual compression, Brodny clamp, or Knutson clamp can be used to avoid spillage of contrast through the meatus.

Interpretation: On RUG, the normal urethra is divided into anterior and posterior urethra (Fig. 1.3). Anterior urethra is composed of **penile urethra**, which is smooth and uniform to the level of penoscrotal junction, where it transitions into wider **bulbar urethra**. The posterior urethra has two segments—membranous and prostatic urethra. **Membranous urethra** appears as a 1–2 cm long wisp of contrast extending to the verumontanum. The verumontanum marks the beginning of the **prostatic urethra** and is seen as a filling defect on RUG. The posterior urethra is coapted and narrow on RUG as the patient is not voiding and it also

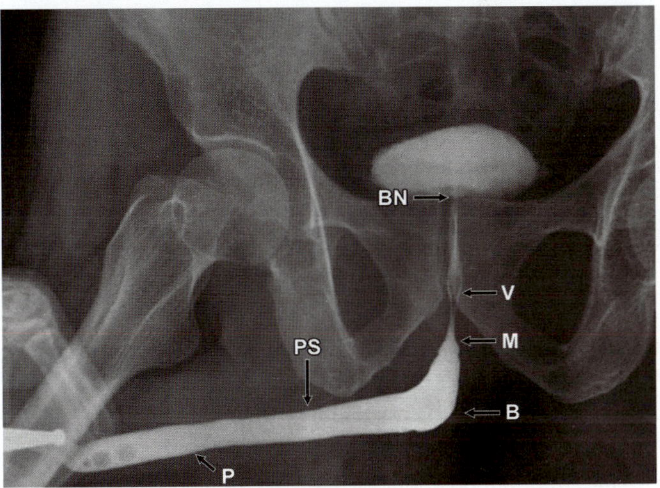

Fig. 1.3: Normal retrograde urethrogram (RUG)

Contrast can be seen jetting through the closed bladder neck (BN). The verumontanum (black arrow) is an ovoid filling defect in the prostatic urethra. The membranous urethra (white arrow) lies between the distal end of the verumontanum and the conical tip of the bulbous urethra. The mild angulation in the anterior urethra (open arrow) is the penoscrotal junction, dividing the bulbar and penile urethral segment

denotes that the sphincter is functioning. The contrast can be seen as a thin stream flowing into the urinary bladder.[15] RUG showing focal bulbar stricture and pan urethral stricture are depicted in Figs 1.4 and 1.5.

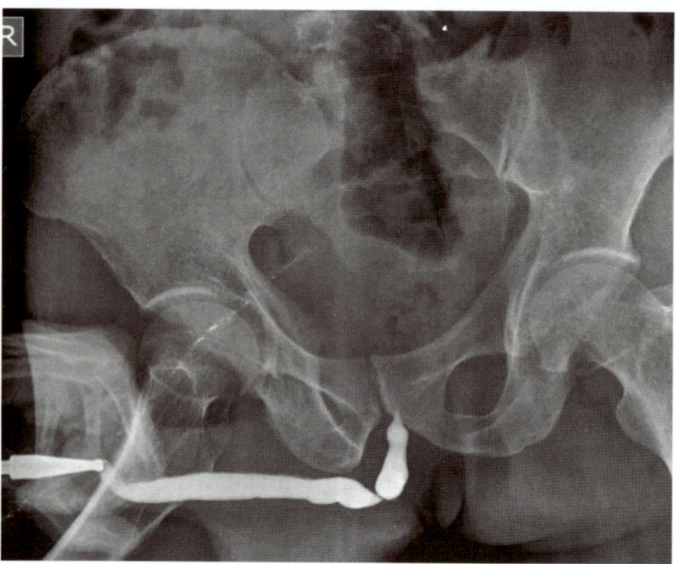

Fig. 1.4: RUG showing focal mid-bulbar urethral stricture

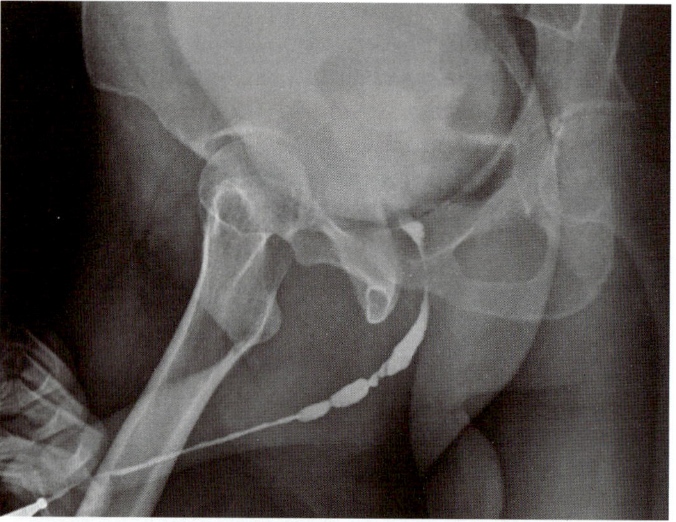

Fig. 1.5: RUG showing pan anterior urethral stricture

14. What are the advantages and limitations of RUG?

Ans: The advantages and limitations of RUG are mentioned in Table 1.3.[1,9,15]

15. What are the indications, procedure, limitations and interpretation of voiding cystourethrogram (VCUG)?

Ans: VCUG is done to visualize the posterior urethra and segment of the urethra proximal to the stricture. Other indications are evaluation of voiding dysfunction, neurogenic bladder, bladder diverticula, congenital anomalies and urinary incontinence.[1,9,15]

Procedure: After obtaining a scout film, the bladder is filled with dilute contrast injected through a catheter passed per urethra or through SPC, rarely can be done by injecting intravenous contrast. After removing per urethral catheter, films are obtained in antero-posterior and oblique positions (Fig. 1.6).

The distension of the bladder neck and prostatic urethra during voiding can provide a functional assessment of bladder neck and sphincter.

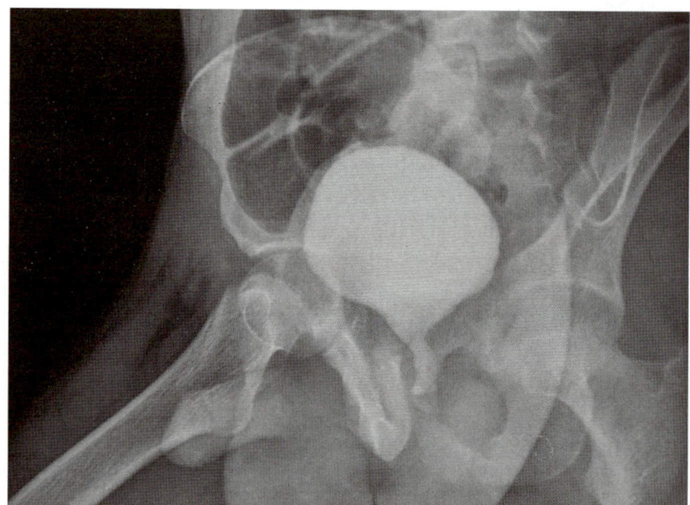

Fig. 1.6: VCUG in patient with PFUI

TABLE 1.3: Advantages and limitations of RUG

Advantages	*Limitations*
Readily available	Magnification artefacts, contrast hypersensitivity
Provides information about location, length and severity of stricture	Results affected by amount of penile stretch, degree of pelvic rotation and body habitus
Information of associated pathology	Limited assessment of meatal stenosis and fossa navicularis and posterior urethral stenosis
Can be combined with other modalities	Degree of spongiofibrosis cannot be assessed
High sensitivity and specificity	Limitations in completely obliterated urethral lumen, associated injuries, malignancy, fistulae, diverticuli.
Affordable	Two-dimensional assessment

Limitations: It needs catheter insertion, it does not optimally visualize anterior urethra, sometimes posterior urethra is not visualized if bladder neck does not open, filling of bladder may simulate bladder spasms, and sometimes it can precipitate autonomic dysreflexia in patients with spinal cord injury above T6 spinal level.

16. What are the indications and limitations of combined RUG + VCUG?

Ans:

Indications

- Obliterative strictures to assess length of stricture and status of proximal urethra
- Assessment of the gap in cases with PFUI to plan reconstruction (Fig. 1.7).[1]

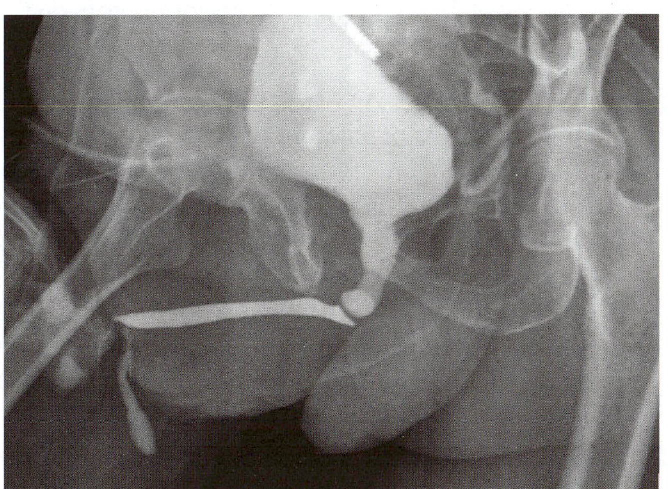

Fig. 1.7: RUG + VCUG showing pelvic fracture injury related stricture

Limitations

- It cannot visualize posterior urethra in cases where patient is unable to void
- Less accurate than MRU in estimation of stricture length.

Video 9: Demonstrating procedure to perform RUG, VCUG and combined RUG + VCUG:

Scan QR Code for Video on
How to perform RGU, VCUG and combined RGU + VCUG?

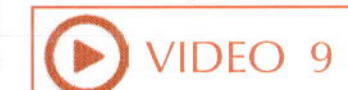

17. What is sonourethrogram and its role in stricture urethra?

Ans: Sonourethrography (SUG) provides a non-invasive three-dimensional assessment of location, length, and the degree of associated spongiofibrosis in urethral stricture (Figs 1.8 and 1.9). SUG is more accurate at diagnosing stricture presence and length compared to RUG.[1]

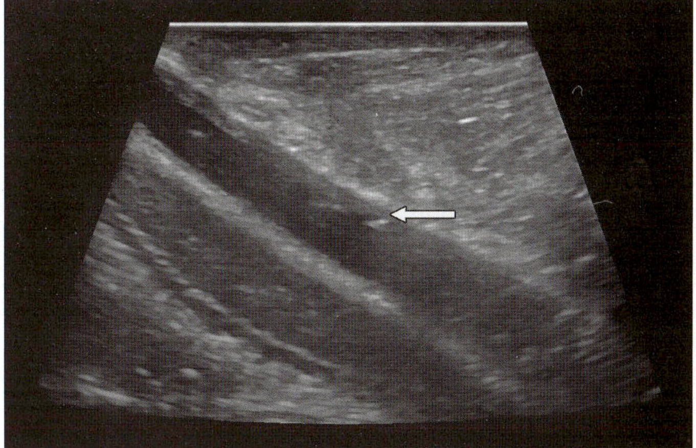

Fig. 1.8: SUG showing normal urethra

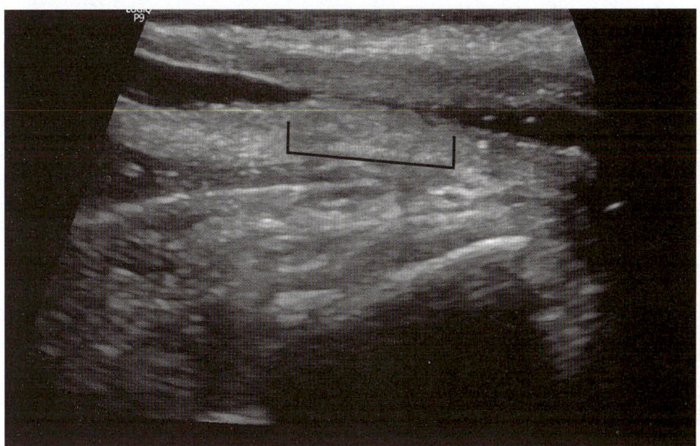

Fig. 1.9: SUG showing long segment urethral stricture

Advantages: It can be performed in the outpatient setting, provides information on the degree of spongiofibrosis, false passages, penile plaques, urethral neoplasms, urethral calculi and periurethral abscess and is relatively cheaper.

Limitations: Lower sensitivity for detecting strictures in the proximal urethra, operator dependence, needs specialized training, discomfort to patient and it is not performed commonly in clinical practice.[9]

18. What are the indications of MR urethrography?

Ans: MRU is done with retrograde injection of sterile lubricating jelly or saline through the meatus to visualize urethral strictures. Administration of an alpha-blocker on the day before MRU, can efficiently open the bladder neck.[16]

MRU is used to image PFUIs, posterior urethral stenosis and anterior urethral strictures and is also found to be more accurate at diagnosing associated pathologies, e.g. diverticula, tumors, fistulae, and stones.

It is as accurate as RUG at detecting stricture sites in anterior urethra and posterior urethral stenosis.[1]

The main advantages of MRU are greater anatomical details and help in diagnosing associated pathologies which is countered by the procedure's expense, greater complexity in interpreting images and not commonly used.[9,17]

19. What is the role of endoscopy in the evaluation of stricture urethra?

Ans: Smaller ureteroscope (6.4 Fr or 4.5 Fr) are used for cystourethroscopy as the caliber of most cystoscopes is larger than most symptomatic strictures.

Cystourethroscopy helps in

1. Accurate visual detection of a suspected stricture (Fig. 1.10)

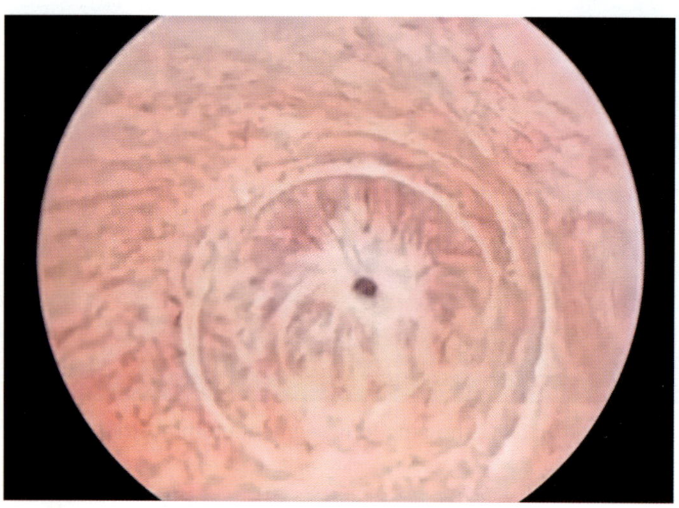

Fig. 1.10: Urethroscopy image showing pinpoint urethral stricture

2. To detect narrowing of the urethral lumen before changes in uroflowmetry and symptoms
3. To assess the presence of LS or other pathology
4. To assess the bladder before surgery and to rule out pathology like vesical calculus.
5. Retrograde urethroscopy combined with antegrade cystoscopy via the suprapubic tract may be used to evaluate PFUI and plan the surgical approach as it allows an assessment of the length of the defect, the competence of the bladder neck, the involvement of the bladder neck in scarring in addition to identifying the presence of bony spicules or other abnormalities (e.g. fistulae, stones).[1]

Scan QR Code for Video on **Endoscopic appearance of urethral stricture**

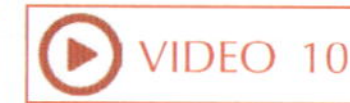

20. How will you assess stricture length and what is gapometry index?

Ans: Stricture length can be assessed by combined RUG + VCUG, SUG, MRU, or cystourethroscopy. Gapometry index is calculated by dividing length of urethral gap by length of bulbar urethra measured on urethrogram (RUG + VCUG) or MRU.[18]

21. How will you judge the need for pubectomy using radiological investigation?

Ans: Gapometry index lower than 0.35 predicts success of simple perineal repair, while longer gaps require more elaborate perineal or transpubic repair.[18]

On MRU, disruption at the prostate apex, greater urethral gap length, longer pubo-urethral stump length, and lower pubo-urethral stump angle are predictors of an elaborate approach needing pubectomy.[19]

22. What is the indication of the use of methylene blue in the diagnosis of stricture urethra?

Diluted methylene blue gently injected into the urethra via meatus before urethroplasty aids in delineating the urethral lumen and exact site of stricture that needs augmentation.

Methylene blue spongiography is a novel method in which methylene blue is injected in the spongiosa near stricture to assess presence of significant spongiofibrosis.[20]

23. What is the role of 3-D printing in the evaluation of stricture urethra?

Ans: For 3D printing models, contrast CT urethrography images are processed in standard 3D reconstruction software and a 3D printer is used to print the model.

It can be applied to PFUI to understand the anatomy of the posterior urethra, its distance from the rectum, length of gap, relation to the posterior urethra, direction of displacement of the urethra, need of pubectomy and as a patient education tool and training tool for urologists.[21]

The assessment protocol to evaluate the patient of suspected urethral stricture is depicted in Flowchart 1.1.

KEY POINTS

- Urethral stricture disease is more common than what people think;
- Consider it as a cause of progressive LUTS, LUTS not responding to alpha-blockers, obstructive LUTS in post-urethral instrumentation patients.
- Never forget to look for this in clinical examination—palpable bladder, any scar, meatal caliber, changes of LS, DRE.

(Contd.)

KEY POINTS (Contd.)

- Post-TURP strictures are thrice more common in Indian population than in the Western population. LS is the commonest cause of long-segment urethral strictures.
- USG KUB with PVR and uroflowmetry are commonly performed non-invasive tests for evaluation of urethral stricture.
- Bladder wall thickness is one of the important predictors of urethral stricture among all non-invasive tests.
- RUG is recommended as a reliable and accessible means to diagnose and stage urethral stricture.
- The combined RUG+VCUG allows precise assessment of location and length of stricture and helps in pre-operative staging of urethral stricture.
- VCUG helps in assessing bladder neck, posterior urethra and visualization of urethra proximal to stricture.
- In PFUI, a cystogram demonstrating an open bladder neck at rest may indicate a higher risk of incontinence once urethral patency is restored.
- SUG is more sensitive than RUG in the assessment of stricture length and degree of spongiofibrosis.
- MRU is helpful in complex cases like PFUI or luminal obliteration or when associated pathology is strongly suspected.
- Cystoscopy is the gold standard and most specific for the diagnosis of the stricture urethra and helps in staging of the urethral stricture.
- In PFUI, antegrade cystoscopy is a highly recommended staging modality to assess bladder neck and posterior urethra.

Flowchart 1.1: The assessment protocol to evaluate the patient of suspected urethral stricture

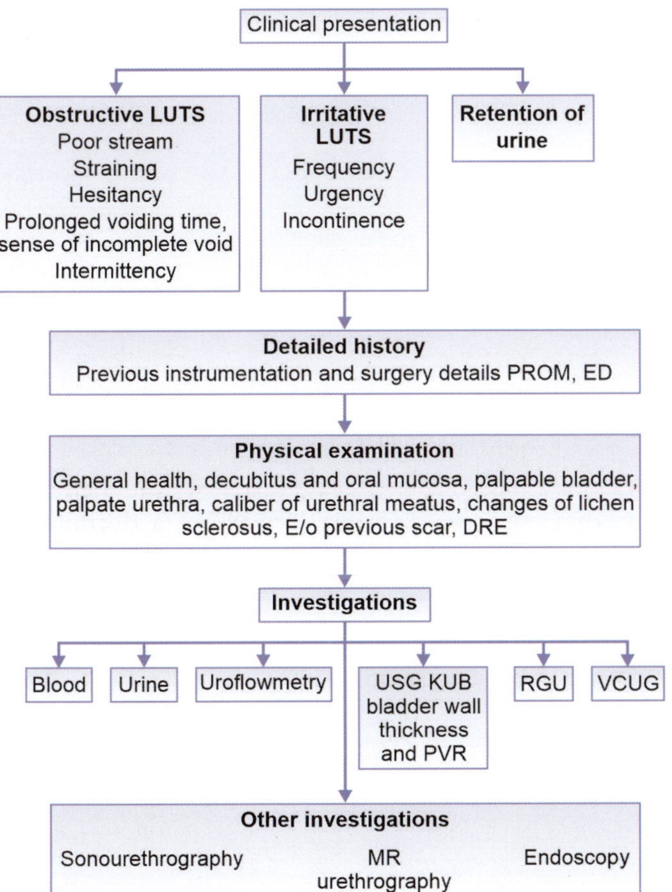

REFERENCES

1. Campos-JF, Osman NI, Greenwell T, Martins FE, *et al.* EAU Guidelines on Urethral Stricture Disease (Part 2): Diagnosis, Perioperative Management, and Follow-up in Males. Eur Urol. 2021; 80(2):201–212.
2. Krukowski J, Kału ny A, Kł cz J, Pi tkowska A, Matuszewski M. Evaluation of non-invasive tests as diagnostic tools in assessment of bladder outlet obstruction severity in men with anterior urethral stricture. Cent European J Urol. 2021;74(3):422–428.
3. Sinha RJ, Singh V, Sankhwar SN. Does tobacco consumption influence outcome of oral mucosa graft urethroplasty? Urol J. 2010 Winter;7(1):45–50.
4. Breyer BN, McAninch JW, Whitson JM, *et al.* Multivariate analysis of risk factors for long-term urethroplasty outcome. J Urol. 2010;183(2):613–617.
5. Ivaz S, Bugeja S, Andrich D, Urethral stricture disease in men, Trends in urology & Men's Health. 2015, 6. 21–24. 10.1002/tre.469.
6. Gerald H, Patrick C, Management of Urethral Stricture Disease, Urologic Clinics of North America, 15,1988, 277–289.
7. S.B. Brandes, Decision Making and Surgical Technique in urethroplasty, S.B Brandes, A.F. Morey (eds.), Advanced Male Urethral and Genital Reconstructive Surgery, 2nd edition,2014,1, 8.
8. Mundy AB, Andrich DE. Urethral Stricture, BJU Int 2010, 107:6–26
9. Latini *et al.* SIU/IUCD Consultation on Urethral Stricture: Epidemiology, Etiology, Anatomy & Nomenclature of Urethral Stenoses, Strictures & Pelvic Fracture Urethral Disruption Injuries. Urology 83 (Supplement 3A) 2014.
10. Kulkarni SB, Bhat A, Bhatyal HS, *et al.* The Urological Society of India Guidelines for the management of urethral stricture (Executive Summary). Indian J Urol. 2021 Jan-Mar;37(1):6–9.
11. Singh J, Priyadarshi V, Pandey P *et al.* Urethral Stricture Etiology Revisited: An Indian Scenario. UroToday International Journal, 2012, 020205. 1944–5792. 10.3834/uij.1944–5784.2013.02.05.
12. Dunnick NR, Sandler CM, Newhouse JH, Textbook of uroradiology, 5th Edition, Philadelphia, 2013, chapter 17, "Urethra and Penis", Page 341–342
13. Viers BR, Pagliara TJ, Rew CA at al, Characteristics of Idiopathic Urethral Strictures: A Link to Remote Perineal Trauma? Urology. 2017;110:228–233.
14. Laura GV and Reynaldo GG, 2021, Traumatic urethral injuries in: A clinical guide to urologic Emergencies (Editors- Hunter Wessels, Shigeo Horie, Reynaldo G. Gomez), 133
15. Gelman J, Furr J. Urethral Stricture Disease: Evaluation of the Male Urethra. J Endourol. 2020;34(S1):S2–S6.
16. Joshi PM, Desai DJ, Shah D, Joshi DP, Kulkarni SB. Magnetic resonance imaging procedure for pelvic fracture urethral injuries and recto urethral fistulas: a simplified protocol. Turk. J. Urol. 2021; 47: 35– 42
17. Horiguchi A, Edo H, Shinchi M *et al.* Role of magnetic resonance imaging in the management of male pelvic fracture urethral injury. Int J Urol. 2022 ;29(9):919–929
18. Koraitim MM, Gapometry and Anterior Urethrometry in the Repair of Posterior Urethral Defects, The Journal of Urology, 2008, 179:5, 1879–1881.
19. Horiguchi A, Edo H, Soga S *et al.* Pubourethral Stump Angle Measured on Preoperative Magnetic Resonance Imaging

Predicts Urethroplasty Type for Pelvic Fracture Urethral Injury Repair. Urology. 2018; 112:198–204.

20. Joshi P, Kaya C, Surana S *et al*. A novel method in decision making for the diagnosis of anterior urethral stricture: using methylene blue dye. Turk J Urol. 2017;43(4):502–506.
21. Joshi PM, Kulkarni SB. 3D printing of pelvic fracture urethral injuries-fusion of technology and urethroplasty. Turk J Urol. 2019, 14;46(1):76–79.

ABBREVIATIONS

LS : Lichen sclerosus
PROM : Patient reported outcome measures
IPSS : International prostate symptom score
USG : Ultrasonography
RUG : Retrograde urethrography
VCUG : Voiding cystourethrography
SUG : Sonourethrography
MRU : Magnetic resonance urethrography
LUTS : Lower urinary tract symptoms
H/O : History of
TURP : Trans urethral resection of prostate
DRE : Digital rectal examination
Fr : French
UTI : Urinary tract infection
CSIC : Clean self-intermittent catheterisation
SPC : Suprapubic cystostomy
KFT : Kidney function test
KUB : Kidney ureter bladder
PVR : Postvoid residue
PFUI : Pelvic fracture urethral injury
STD : Sexually transmitted disease
DRU : Dynamic retrograde urethrography
FOV : Field of view
3-D : 3-dimensional
CT : Computed tomography

Chapter
2

Surgical Management of Urinary Meatal Stenosis

• *Ashish Ramswarup Pardeshi* • *Vilas Sable*

LEARNING OBJECTIVES

- To diagnose urinary meatal stenosis at all age groups in men and women.
- To understand the relevance of clinical examination of the urinary meatus
- To plan the surgical approach to treat urinary meatal stenosis.
- To learn various surgical techniques to treat urinary meatal stenosis.

Case Scenario

A 38 years old diabetic gentleman, presented with a 4–5 months history of severe dysuria, straining to pass urine and prolonged urination time. He consulted a urologist and was prescribed medical therapy, but without much relief. He decided to take another opinion. This time the urologist examined the meatus carefully and found that he had a pin-hole meatus with changes of lichen sclerosis around it. The maximum flow rate on uroflowmetry was 3 ml/s and he took 98 secs to pass 190 ml of urine showing a flat graph. The diagnosis of urinary meatal stenosis was done.

INTRODUCTION

External urinary meatus is the window of modern endoscopic urology through which most of the therapeutic aims are achieved. Meatal stenosis is a common problem confronted by most urologists in both males and females, more often during any kind of endoscopic intervention. Being asymptomatic most of the times, meatal stenosis can seldom present as significant obstructive uropathy causing deranged kidney function and rarely renal failure.

Anatomy

In men the meatus opens as a vertical elliptical slit in the center of the glans. In women the external urinary meatus is a circular orifice between the clitoris and the introitus. It is engulfed with a rich mucosal fold around which might make its identification difficult. Histologically the distal urethra shows pseudo-stratified columnar epithelium which changes to stratified squamous epithelium at the meatus. Squamous cell carcinoma is a rare cause of meatal stenosis with urinary obstruction especially in patients with chronic balanitis xerotica obliterans (BXO).

1. **How do we classify urinary meatal stenosis?**

   Ans: Urinary meatal stenosis is classified as under:
   - **Sex:** Male/female
   - **Etiology:** Congenital/acquired
   - **Age:** Infants/young/elderly
   - **Severity:** Mild/moderate/severe

2. **What is the clinical pathogenesis of meatal stenosis?**

   Ans: With BXO/without BXO/infective: Meatal stenosis (MS) is the narrowing of the external urinary meatus and is defined as distortion of meatal shape and location forming a narrow pin-point opening oriented either to the dorsal or ventral aspect of the glans. Meatal stenosis should be considered in cases of reported urinary stream deviation in an upward direction resulting from a meatal baffle, narrow high velocity-stream, penile pain at the initiation of micturition, and the need to sit or stand back from the toilet bowel.

In Males

MS often presents after toilet training. Childhood meatal stenosis is usually caused due to mucosal adhesions caused due to irritation of the circumcised glans with the diaper and is termed "ammoniacal meatitis". Congenital meatal stenosis is rare and may be asymptomatic till the later age and is diagnosed on careful examination of the glans and corelating with the symptoms of unrelenting dysuria in the absence of other problems. Meatal stenosis severity grade is associated with narrow stream as reported by parent, prolonged urination, and upward deviation of urinary stream, with increasing severity with worsening stenosis. MS grade was also associated with significant worsening of uroflow measures: A lower Q_{max}, Q_{mean} and a longer time-to-Q_{max}. Postvoid residual volume was not significantly different between the different severity grades. [1] Although BXO in children is normally seen with a redundant prepuce, phimosis and balanitis, it has been suggested that BXO begins as a perimeatal process.

In the younger population meatal stenosis may be secondary to inflammatory urethritis caused due to sexually transmitted infections or allergic reactions.

Transurethral resection procedures and early balanitis xerotica obliterans (BXO) have been associated with isolated strictures of the meatus and fossa navicularis.

In patients with BXO who present early in the disease course with a meatal or fossa stricture, high intraurethral pressures appear to be generated during voiding, which leads to intravasation of urine into the glands of Littre. This intravasation may cause inflammation and micro-abscess formation, ultimately leading to a progressive and severe urethral stricture. One school of thought is that pan urethral stricture disease is avoided if early aggressive reconstruction is offered to these patients while the stricture process is confined to the meatus or distal fossa navicularis.[2]

3. What is the overall clinical impact of urinary meatal stenosis?

Ans: The cardinal symptoms of MS are narrow high-velocity stream, penile pain at the initiation of micturition; however, MS can be asymptomatic. Urinary tract infection (UTI), hematuria, incontinence, nocturnal enuresis, abdominal pain during and shortly after voiding, vesicoureteral reflux, hydronephrosis, and renal impairment, all are reported presentations of MS.[3]

4. How do we diagnose meatal stenosis?

Ans: Clinical examination is the key to diagnose meatal stenosis.

Diagnosis of meatal stenosis is usually based on a change in the elliptical shape of the meatal opening to a circular shape because of fibrosis or scarring, with visually apparent narrowing. There are, however, natural differences in meatal widths in different males, so a narrow meatus does not necessarily indicate functionally significant stenosis.[4]

Narrow-upward deflection of the urinary stream and dysuria are the most common presenting symptoms.[3]

Investigations

Uroflowmetry: It is an objective, simple, non-invasive and economic method to diagnose urinary meatal stenosis. However, results may be similar in other conditions causing bladder outlet obstruction, namely urethral stricture and prostatomegaly.

Ultrasound: Needed to confirm bladder status, presence of vesical calculi and backpressure changes in the upper tract.

Sono-urethrography may show presence of spongiofibrosis in the proximal part of the urethra.

Retrograde urethrography (RUG): RUG is needed in all cases of meatal stenosis associated with BXO and recurrent meatal stenosis after previous urethral surgery to rule out associated proximal urethral strictures. RUG may be difficult to perform in severe meatal stenosis and may require instillation of contrast with the help of an appropriate sized cannula.

5. Is there any grading system described for meatal stenosis?

Ans: Three grades were generated: Grade 0 (wide open meatus, visible mucosa), Grade 1 (minimal mucosa/fibrotic tissue visible), and Grade 2 (pinpoint meatus/no mucosa visible/large fibrotic layer).[5]

6. What is the role of dilatation in meatal stenosis?

Ans: Dilatation is the simplest and commonest method of treatment of moderate to severe meatal stenosis.

In males without BXO and moderate meatal stenosis the safest way for dilatation is by using a single step calibrated metal graded dilator. The dilator is well lubricated with xylocaine jelly and gradually advanced through the meatus till the desired calibration is achieved. It is of utmost importance to ensure that the patient has no penile urethral stricture by either doing a retrograde urethrography or by performing a urethroscopy with a 6 fr. ureteroscope prior to dilatation.

In cases of severe meatal stenosis passage of glidewire through the meatus into the urethra is necessary to avoid false passage and injury. Blind incision or dilatation should be avoided in any circumstance. Once the guidewire/glidewire is passed, serial dilatation is done by serial flexible Teflon dilators over the guidewire/glidewire. Forcible dilatation should be avoided and replaced with a gentle incision of the meatus ventrally over the guidewire/glidewire.

In males with BXO, severe meatal stenosis is the commonest presentation which may be associated with a proximal pan-urethral stricture or an isolated penile or bulbar urethral stricture. Hence meatal dilatation is not advisable in these patients as it may worsen the stenosis and the stricture. Meatotomy also may have disappointing results in these set of patients. The best option for these patients would be to do a staged repair by doing a ventral urethro-meatotomy as a first stage and later augmenting it dorsally with a buccal mucosal graft and a ventral urethral closure. Obstructive uropathy is reported as a rare complication of post-circumcision meatal stenosis (Fig. 2.1).

7. What are the options for surgical management of urinary meatal stenosis?

Ans: Various surgical methods have been described in the literature to treat meatal stenosis. The surgical methods range from meatal dilatation, simple meatotomy to use of grafts and flaps.

Meatotomy with meatoplasty: Meatotomy comprises a simple incisional extension of the meatus in a vertical fashion which can be done either dorsally or ventrally or sometimes both.

Ventral meatoplasty: Ventral meatoplasty is done by placing an incision on the ventral aspect of the meatus. One needs to follow the following steps for ventral meatoplasty.

1. Place a guidewire in severe stenosis or a metal dilator into the meatus before taking the incision. Placement of a metal dilator helps in hemostasis by pressure and helps the surgeon to evaluate the fibrotic scar while cutting over it.
2. Cut should be taken with a scalpel over the dilator. The proximal limit of the cut should be the end of the fibrotic scar felt while cutting against the dilator (Figs 2.2 to 2.5).
3. The inner mucosal edge is sutured to the outer glanular skin by interrupted absorbable sutures.
4. Silicon Foley catheter is placed for 2 days.
5. Topical antibiotic and steroid ointment are applied for 2 weeks to prevent adhesion and web formation.

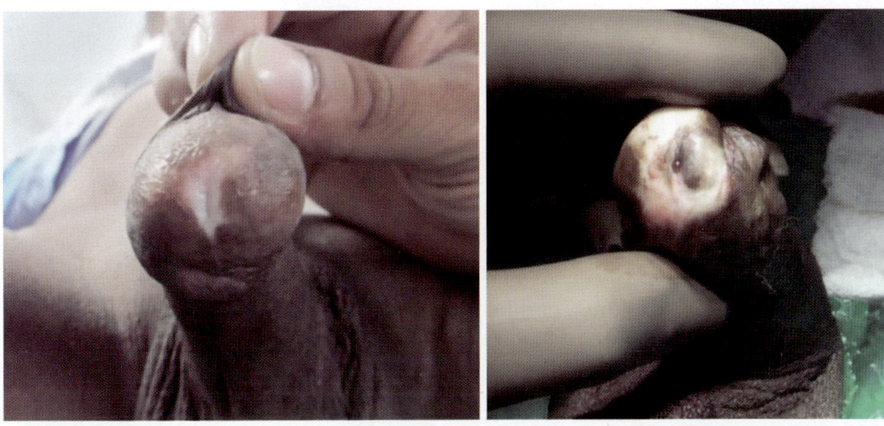

Fig. 2.1: BXO with moderate and severe meatal stenosis

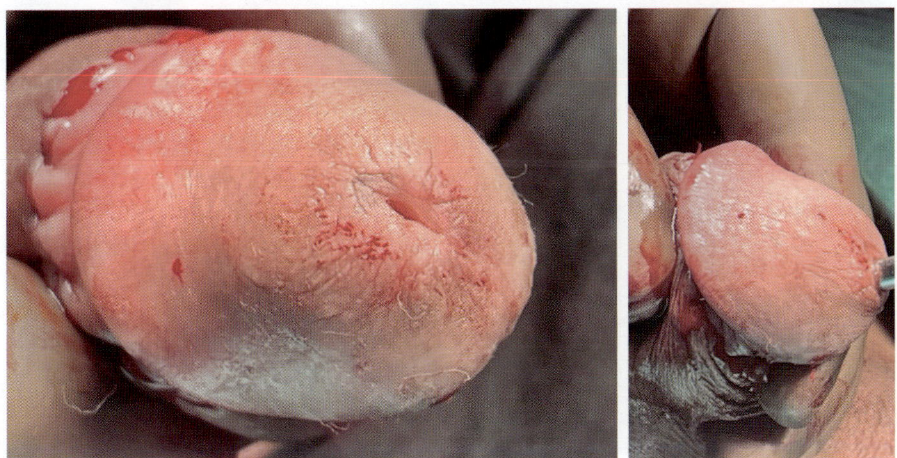

Fig. 2.2: Meatal stenosis calibrated to 6 Fr. dilator

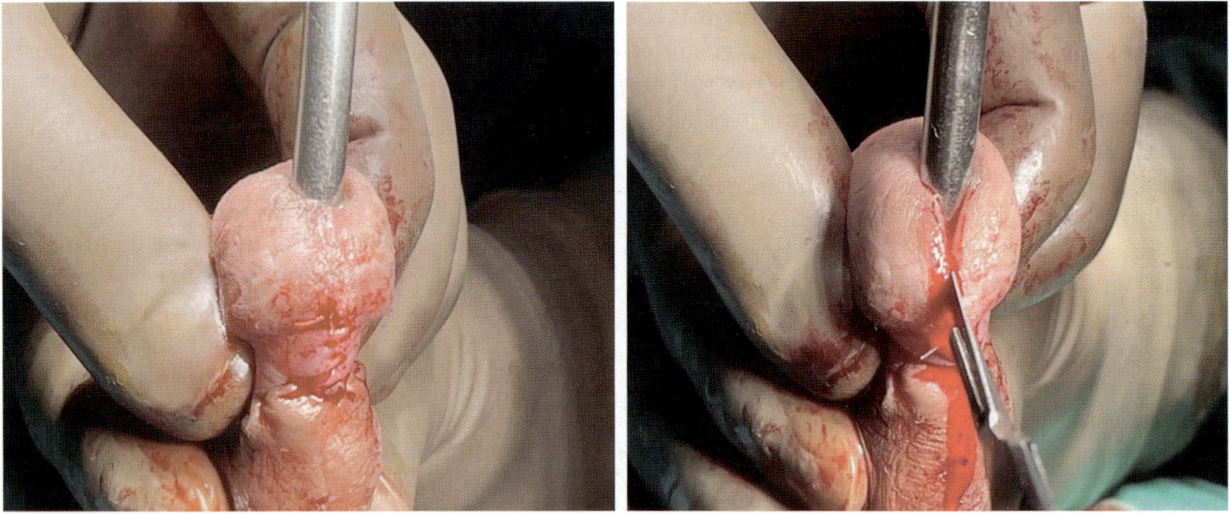

Fig. 2.3: Ventral meatotomy over metallic dilator

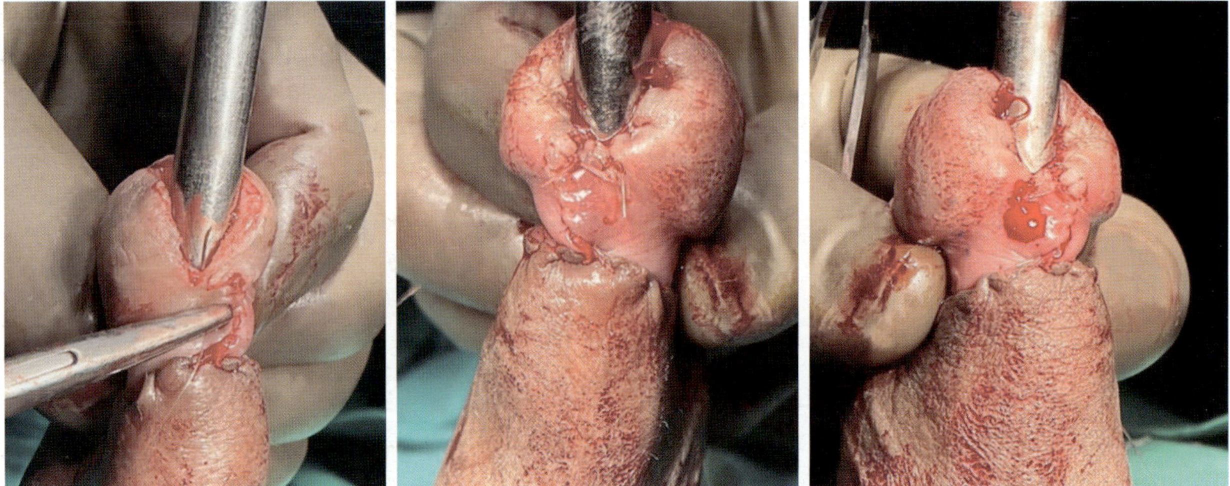

Fig. 2.4: Suturing of mucosa and skin over metallic dilator

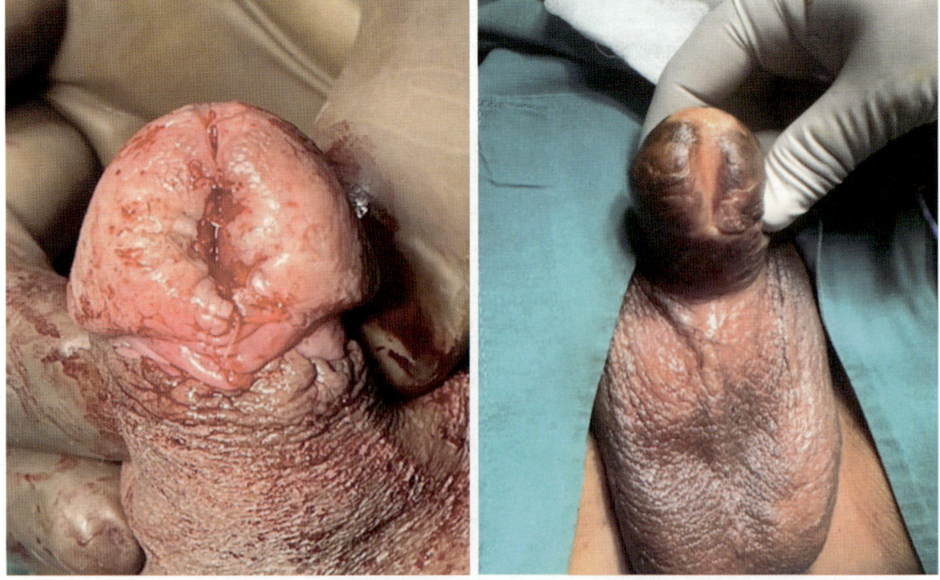

Fig. 2.5: Final result: Immediate and delayed

Dorsal meatoplasty: Dorsal meatoplasty is done by taking a "V"-shaped incision on the dorsal aspect of the meatus and extended vertically into the meatus to form a "Y". The "V-Y" plasty is achieved by approximating the corner of the "V" flap to the proximal end of the incision. Although easy to describe, this procedure can be challenging as incision on the dorsal aspect of glans can cause significant bleeding and cause difficulty in suturing. Formation of 'dog ears' can also be a challenge after dorsal meatoplasty. Functionally and cosmetically, dorsal meatoplasty is a less preferred operation.

Flap procedures: Meatal stenosis can sometimes be associated with an extension of narrowing up to the fossa naviculars. In such cases doing a mere meatoplasty will not help. Various flap procedures have been described in the past to repair these strictures which are not restricted to the meatus.

Y-V flap procedures: Flap procedures for repair of meatal stenosis extending as fossa navicularis strictures founded on the Y-V principle were described by Cohney and Blandy.

Cohney's procedure: Cohney's procedure uses a ventral transverse peninsula flap, usually with random vascularity. The flap is transposed and interdigitated into the meatotomy, creating a retrusive meatus with a 'dog ear' at the transposition site.

Blandy's modification of Cohney's procedure: Blandy's modification creates a vertical skin peninsula flap on the midline of the penile shaft that is usually elevated with random vascularity and advanced into the meatotomy. Although elevation with the fascial blood supply intact and elimination of the 'dog ear' are theoretic improvements over the Cohney procedure, the Blandy modification still leaves the patient with a coronal or distal shaft meatus.

Jordan's transverse ventral penile skin island flap: Jordan has described a procedure for reconstruction of the meatus and fossa navicularis, but can be used for distal penile strictures up to 4.5 cm in length.

Initially, a wide urethrostomy is created through the stenotic meatus and fossa down to the level of the normal urethra.

The technique then involves elevation of a transverse ventral penile skin island on a broad ventral dartos fascial pedicle. The skin island is transposed and inverted into the meatotomy defect.

Although the broad dartos pedicle allows vigorous mobilization of the ventral fascial pedicle, it requires more aggressive dissection of the lateral glans flaps to assure a tension-free ventral glans fusion.

8. What is the role of buccal mucosa graft in treatment of meatal stenosis?

Ans: Buccal mucosa graft has a unique role in meatal stenosis which presents as a part of a pan urethral stricture in BXO disease. In these patients the dorsal onlay buccal mucosa graft urethroplasty is done for the urethral repair. The same buccal graft is extended into the meatus by extending the dorsal urethrotomy into the meatus and fixing the graft dorsally (Fig. 2.6).

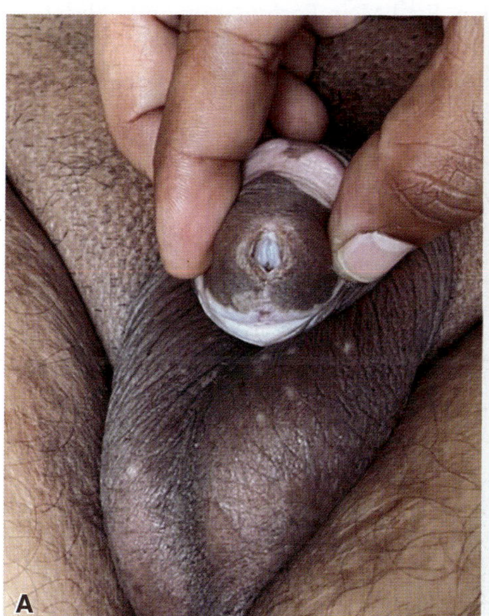

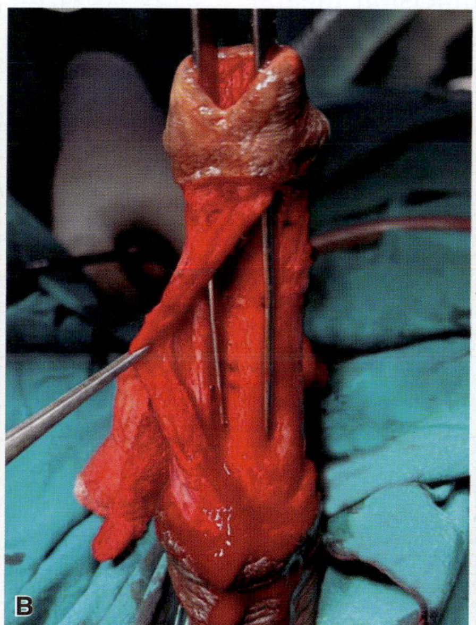

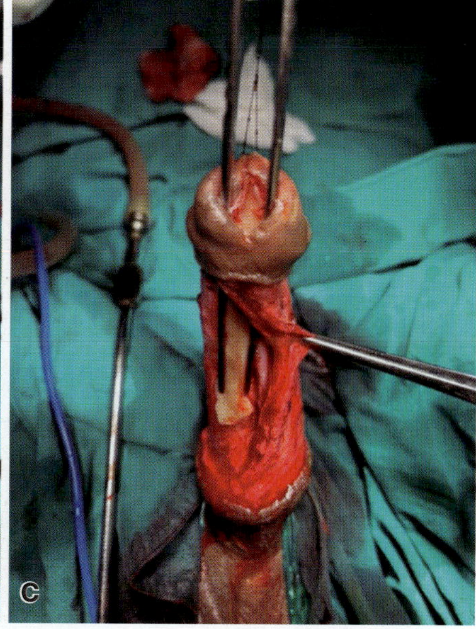

Fig. 2.6: (A) BXO with meatal stenosis (B) Dorsal urethro-meatotomy through penile degloving (C) Dorsal onlay buccal graft from meatus to proximal part of urethra

Female Meatal Stenosis

Female meatal stenosis is usually a problem of post-menopausal women. BXO with meatal stenosis is an unusual presentation in women of all age groups. Women with meatal stenosis are asymptomatic most of the time and usually present with complications like secondary bladder calculi, febrile urinary tract infection, bilateral obstructive uropathy or acute urinary retention. Meatal stenosis is encountered in most post-menopausal women either during catheterization or during an endoscopic procedure.

Treatment options for female meatal stenosis depends on severity of the stenosis and presence of proximal urethral stricture. Meatal dilatation is the safest and durable mode of treatment of mild to moderate meatal stenosis not associated with proximal urethral stenosis. Meatal dilatation is best done with a single step metallic calibrated dilator up to 24 Fr.

In cases of severe meatal stenosis where the orifice is difficult to identify, glidewire placement is imperative before dilatation. Blind dilatation can cause false passages, bladder injury or torrential bleeding and hematoma formation.

Relation with Circumcision

Meatal stenosis (MS) is one of the late and potential complications of male circumcision that occurs in 5–20% of boys circumcised during infancy or childhood.[2]

It should be noted that being uncircumcised can increase MS risk because of the higher risk of penile inflammatory conditions, especially lichen sclerosus, and from urinary tract infections, each of which is more common in uncircumcised males, especially when the uncircumcised male is elderly[4] (Flowchart 2.1).

One of the reasons for post-circumcision meatal stenosis may be an injury to the frenular artery[3] or excessive use of cautery causing tissue destruction is also associated with meatal stenosis post-circumcision.

There was a significant association between type of circumcision and MS (P = 0.04) while the association between the person who did the circumcision and MS was not statistically significant (P = 0.07).[3]

The cautery heat can cause an uncontrolled vascular and tissue damage resulting in various degrees of burn, edema, ischemic damage to penile tissue, and later MS and scar formation around the glans penis. Chemical and diaper use may not be responsible for MS post-neonatal circumcision as it is absent in boys with the hooded prepuce.

KEY POINTS

- Rule out proximal urethral stricture before surgery for meatus
- Ventral meatotomy over a rigid metal dilator is an easy surgical approach for treatment of meatal stenosis
- Meatal stenosis associated with fossa navicularis strictures should be treated with an only graft urethra-meatoplasty.
- Cautery use should be done with caution especially in pediatric age group.
- Meatal stenosis associated with lichen sclerosus should be treated primarily by surgery avoiding dilatation.

REFERENCES

1. Matan Mekayten, Eyal. Meir, Is there a correlation between meatal stenosis severity, lower urinary tract symptoms and uroflowmetry? J Pediatric Urol. 2022 Jun;18(3):342.e1-342.e6
2. Jordan, Schrieter. Urethral Reconstructive Surgery, Hypospadias Repair, Chapter 6 2006, 36–37.
3. Ammar Fadil Abid , Naser Sabah Hussein. Meatal stenosis post-traditional neonatal circumcision-cross-sectional study, Urol Ann 2021;13:62–66.
4. Morris BJ, Moreton S, Krieger JN. Meatal stenosis: getting the diagnosis right, Res Rep Urol. 2018; 10:237–239
5. Matan Mekayten, Eyal Meir. Formulation and validation of meatal stenosis grading. system; J Pediatr Urol 2020;16: 205.

Flowchart 2.1: Algorithm for management of meatal stenosis

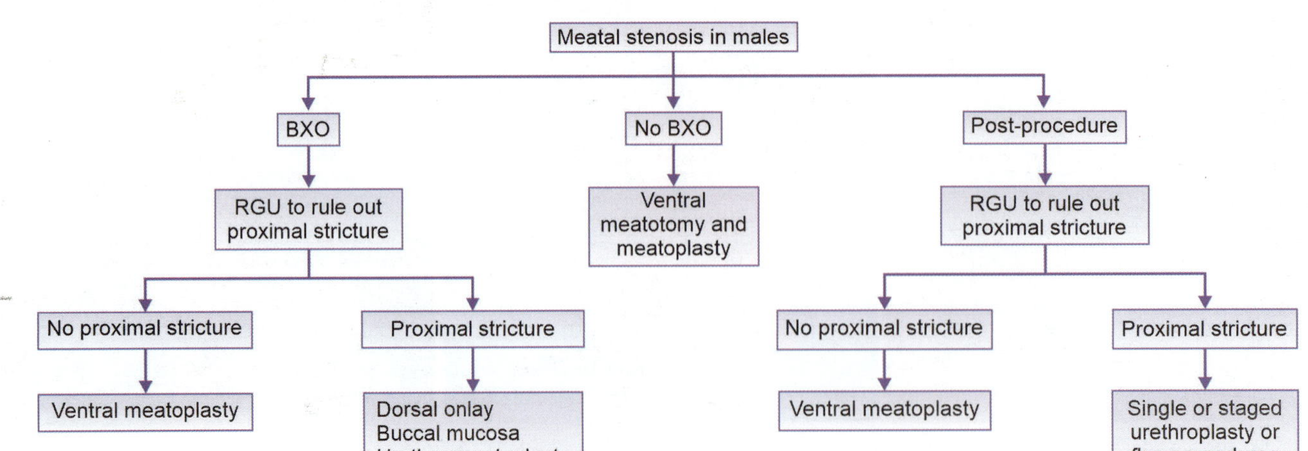

Chapter

3

Penile Urethral Stricture: Surgical Management

• *Hemant Goel* • *Umesh Sharma*

LEARNING OBJECTIVES

- To understand the anatomy of the anterior urethra and the potential sites of penile urethral strictures.
- To understand the etiological factors that can lead to penile urethral strictures.
- To understand the clinical presentation of penile urethral strictures.
- To understand the diagnostic workup for penile urethral strictures.
- To understand the various treatment options for penile urethral strictures, including urethral dilation, direct vision internal urethrotomy, urethroplasty, and tissue engineering approaches.
- To understand the potential complications of penile urethral stricture, such as recurrence, incontinence, and erectile dysfunction.
- To understand the importance of follow-up care and long-term monitoring for patients with penile urethral strictures.

INTRODUCTION

The anatomy of the penile urethra presents additional challenges when compared to other urethral segments during open stricture surgery particularly because of its unsuitability for excision and primary anastomosis and its relatively deficient corpus spongiosum. The spongiosum is concentrically located around the urethra in the distal pendulous urethra. In the bulbar urethra, it becomes eccentrically located with a larger component on the ventral surface while it is absent in posterior urethra. The most common cause of penile urethral strictures is trauma to the urethra, such as from a previous surgery, injury or infection. Other causes may include untreated sexually transmitted infections, chronic inflammation, or congenital abnormalities. The male urethra is supplied proximally by the bulbar arteries, which are branches of the penile artery, whereas the distal urethra is perfused by retrograde flow from the dorsal penile artery.

Spongiofibrosis refers to the deposition of collagen and fibrous tissue deep to the urethral mucosa in an injured area. In urethral strictures, spongiofibrosis can be more extensive than mucosal involvement, rendering the effective stricture length longer than that seen on imaging or endoscopic studies.

Case Scenario

A 24-year-old gentleman presents to urology OPD with a history of poor stream and straining for the past 2 years. Patient also has frequency (10 to 12 times per day) and urgency. Initially patient had mild symptoms with IPSS score of 8 now progressed to severe symptoms with IPSS score of 25. Patient had two episodes of culture proven UTI from the past 6 months, taken antibiotics appropriately. He has undergone DVIU one year back, following which was symptomatically better for 3 months and now in view of acute retention with failed Foley's insertion, SPC was inserted 4 months before.

Patient has no history of periorbital/ pedal edema, flank pain or fever at present. He denies any history of sexually transmitted infections or recent trauma to the genital area. Patient is moderately built and nourished. On local examination, the patient is circumcised, external urethral meatus is normal, BXO is present, no fistula, urethral thickenings or induration absent (Fig. 3.1). 16 Fr SPC present 4 cm above the pubic symphysis in midline. Patient has normal DRE and systemic examination.

After obtaining sterile urine culture he underwent RUG/ VCUG (Figs 3.2 and 3.3).

Fig. 3.1: Male patient with lichen sclerosus

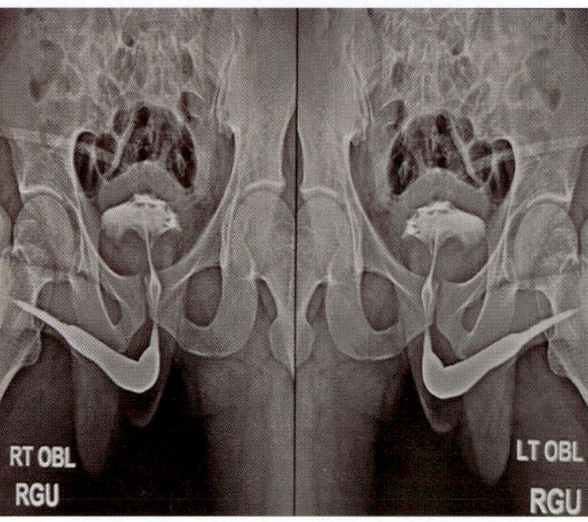

Fig. 3.2: RUG showing penile stricture

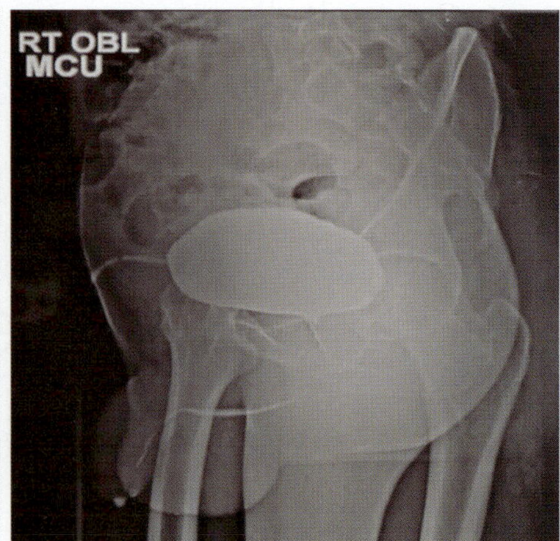

Fig. 3.3: Penile stricture

1. **What are penile urethral strictures?**

   Ans: These are located in the segment between the fossa navicularis and the bulbar urethra. Externally, the penile urethra begins approximately at the balano-preputial sulcus and continues to the penoscrotal junction. The whole penile urethral segment lies in the groove ventral to corpora cavernosa and is surrounded by a thin layer of corpus spongiosum (EUA 2023).

2. **How common is penile urethral stricture?**

   Ans: Urethral stricture is a common disease encountered by urologists world over, with an estimated prevalence in the United Kingdom of 10/100,000 men during youth, increasing to about 40/100,000 by age 65 years and to more than 100/100,000 thereafter. Still higher rates were reported from the United States.[1,2] The incidence of urethral stricture in India is unknown but it is estimated to comprise about 10% of the practice of urologists.[1]

3. **Describe the surgical anatomy of penile urethra.**

   Ans: The penile (or pendulous) urethra is the distal part of the male anterior urethra. It is about 15 cm in length and extends from the external meatus, the narrowest part of the urethra (21, 27 F), to the penoscrotal junction where the bulbar segment starts. The penile urethra presents important anatomical differences compared with the bulbar segment.[9] It is surrounded by the thinnest part of the corpus spongiosum in the penile shaft, meaning that it does not provide the best vascular support for a graft.

   The glans penis, which is the expanded distal end of the corpus spongiosum, surrounds the navicular fossa. On the contrary, this rich glanular blood supply provides an ideal vascular bed for successful graft take. The urethra and the spongiosum are covered by the anterior extension of Buck's fascia, and a layer of dartos areolar tissue (continuation of Colles' fascia) that provides blood supply to the penile shaft skin. This dartos tissue is also very well vascularised, making it an ideal graft bed or a pedicle for skin grafts.

4. **Why are there limited surgical options for penile urethral stricture?**

   Ans: Unlike the bulbar urethra, which can be mobilised proximally and distally to allow excision of a stricture and a tension free primary anastomosis, this is not possible in the penile urethra due to the risk of loss of length and curvature during erection. This means that reconstructive techniques in the penile urethra are limited to augmentation or substitution using free grafts or flaps which in themselves may also result in chordee if used incorrectly. Moreover, pendulous strictures usually tend to be longer (in some series nearly twice as long) than in the bulbar urethra.[3]

5. **What is the etiology of penile urethral stricture?**

   Ans: The aetiology of penile urethral stricture is multifactorial, and can result from a variety of causes. The following are some of the most common etiological factors:[4]

   1. **Trauma:** Penile urethral stricture can occur as a result of trauma to the penis, such as a pelvic fracture or a straddle injury.
   2. **Infection:** Inflammatory conditions such as urethritis and sexually transmitted infections (STIs) can lead to urethral inflammation and scarring, which can eventually result in urethral stricture.
   3. **Inflammatory disorders:** Certain inflammatory disorders, such as Lichen sclerosus en atrophicus or balanitis xerotica obliterans (**BXO**) can cause chronic inflammation and scarring of the penile urethra, leading to the development of strictures.

4. **Congenital anomalies:** Some individuals may be born with a narrow urethra which can predispose them to developing urethral strictures later in life.
5. **Iatrogenic causes:** Urethral instrumentation, such as catheterization or endoscopic procedures, can cause damage to the urethra, leading to the formation of strictures.
6. **Radiation therapy:** Pelvic radiation therapy for prostate cancer or other pelvic malignancies can cause scarring and narrowing of the penile urethra.
7. **Idiopathic:** In some cases, the cause of penile urethral stricture may not be readily identifiable, and may be classified as idiopathic.

Inflammatory stricture refers to a post-infectious inflammatory reaction and accounts for about 15% of urethral strictures in the industrialised world.[5–7] This aetiology is more common in the non-industrialized world.

Traumatic injury accounts for approximately 19% of urethral stricture or stenosis. The most frequently injured segment of the anterior urethra is the bulbar urethra. The penile urethra is rarely injured, due to the mobility of the penis, but may be damaged at the time of penile fracture in 3–20% of cases.[8]

6. Explain the pathophysiology of BXO related strictures.

Ans: The commonest identifiable cause of penile strictures in young and middle-aged adults is lichen sclerosus (LS) or BXO. The pathophysiology of BXO-related strictures is thought to involve several mechanisms:

1. **Chronic inflammation:** BXO is characterised by chronic inflammation of the skin of the penis, which can spread to involve the underlying tissue, including the urethra. The inflammation can cause scarring and fibrosis, leading to narrowing of the urethral lumen and eventual development of a stricture.
2. **Autoimmunity:** BXO is thought to be an autoimmune disorder, in which the body's immune system attacks its own tissues. In BXO, the immune system attacks the skin of the penis, leading to inflammation and fibrosis.
3. **Ischemia:** BXO can cause narrowing and occlusion of the blood vessels that supply the penis and urethra, leading to ischemia (lack of blood flow) and tissue damage. This ischemia can contribute to the development of urethral strictures.
4. **Mechanical damage:** The chronic inflammation and fibrosis associated with BXO can cause physical compression and distortion of the urethra, leading to mechanical damage and eventual formation of strictures.

This atrophic fibrosis can extend proximally, affecting the fossa navicularis and penile urethra, which may be associated with palpable thickening at the level of the strictures. The progression of a distal stricture proximally is related to metaplastic changes due to chronic distension and extravasation of urine with subsequent inflammation of the periurethral glands as a result of pressure during voiding. This may be reversible if the obstruction is relieved early.

7. How do you diagnose or investigate penile urethral stricture?

Ans: Recent consensus panel recommended dynamic retrograde urethrogram (RUG) as a reliable method to stage and diagnose urethral stricture or stenosis with a sensitivity of 75–100% and a specificity of 72–97%.[9] Urethral ultrasonography has greater sensitivity in the evaluation of stricture length, diameter, and degree of spongiofibrosis compared to RUG; however, this is recommended as an adjunct study to RUG.

Voiding cystourethrogram is recommended as an adjunct study to evaluate the bladder neck and posterior urethra, especially in the setting of posterior urethral stenosis with obliteration of the urethral lumen.

Cystoscopy is recommended as the most specific test to diagnose a urethral stricture and adjunct test for staging.

MRI commonly used for posterior urethral stricture and complex anterior urethral stricture (with diverticula/fistula), associated pathologies which may alter patient management.

8. What is the advantage of sono-urethrogram (SUG) over RUG in penile urethral strictures?

Ans: It is more accurate at diagnosing stricture presence compared to RUG.[10] Sono-urethrography was also found to more accurately estimate stricture length (94% correlation with intraoperative findings) than RUG (59% correlation with intraoperative findings) ($p < 0.001$).[11] Advantages of SUG are that it can be performed in the outpatient setting, provides information on the degree of spongiofibrosis and its relatively low cost.[12]

The clinical relevance of assessing the degree of spongiofibrosis pre-operatively remains to be established.

9. What is the role of SPC in penile urethral stricture?

Ans:
- If urinary retention
- Ensure adequate resolution of acute urethral inflammation and allows narrowed areas to declare themselves, i.e. urethral rest.

10. What are management options for penile urethral stricture?

Ans: The management options for penile urethral strictures depend on the severity and location of the stricture, as well as the patient's overall health and preferences.

1. **Urethral dilation:** This involves passing a series of progressively larger dilators through the urethra to stretch the narrowed segment of the urethra. This is a minimally invasive procedure that can be done in an outpatient setting, but the results are often temporary, and strictures can recur.
2. **Direct vision internal urethrotomy (DVIU)**: There is no role of DVIU in penile urethra
3. **Urethroplasty**: This is a surgical procedure that involves excising the narrowed segment of the urethra and reconstructing it using a tissue graft, such as skin, bladder, or buccal mucosa. It has a higher success rate and lower recurrence rate than dilation or DVIU.
4. **Tissue engineering approaches**: Researchers are developing new techniques for tissue engineering that involve growing new tissue in the laboratory and implanting it into the urethra to replace the narrowed segment. These approaches are still experimental and not widely available.
5. **Placement of a urethral stent**: Stents are used less frequently for penile urethral strictures because of a higher risk of complications such as stent migration, infection, and erosion.

   Stricture aetiology is one of the most important factors determining the choice of management strategy. In LS related strictures the use of mucosal grafts (usually oral but bladder or rectal also possible) is recommended since LS is a skin condition and any skin used for reconstruction is either already, or has the potential to become involved by the disease process.[11] On the other hand, genital skin is suitable for use as a flap or graft for reconstructing the urethra in selected patients with previous hypospadias surgery or instrumentation related strictures.

11. What are the available urethroplasty options for penile urethral stricture and its patency rates?

Ans: Stricture-free rates for single-stage penile augmentation urethroplasties range from 70–100% for dorsal oral mucosal graft (OMG) augmentation, 67–100% for penile skin flap (PSF) augmentation, 55–92.6% for ventral OMG augmentation and 62–78% for dorsal SG (skin graft) augmentation. Overall stricture-free rates for staged OMG penile augmentation urethroplasties range from 70 to 100% (EAU 2023).

12. What are the treatment options using graft and which grafts are used for penile urethra?

Ans:
1. Dorsally placed buccal mucosal flap (BARBAGLI)
2. Ventrally placed dorsal buccal mucosal graft: Dorsal inlay (ASOPA)
3. Penile invagination and one-sided dissection for Dorsal onlay BMG graft urethroplasty (KULKARNI)

Graft used are: BMG, inner prepuce, bladder mucosa, tunica vaginalis, etc

Staged penile urethral stricture repair (Johanson two-stage urethroplasty)

13. What are the possible flap options available for penile urethral stricture?

Ans:
1. Distal penile circular fasciocutaneous flap (McAninch)
2. Longitudinal ventral penile skin flap with a lateral pedicle (Orandi)
3. Longitudinal Ventral penile skin flap with a ventral pedicle (Turner-Warwick).

14. Are flaps better than grafts for penile urethra?

Ans: Flaps are typically used in cases where there is a short or localised stricture and there is adequate tissue available for reconstruction. Flaps have a robust blood supply, which can improve healing and reduce the risk of complications such as graft failure or infection.

On the other hand, grafts are typically used in cases where the stricture is longer or more diffuse and there is inadequate tissue available for reconstruction using flaps. However, grafts have a higher risk of complications, including graft contracture, graft failure, and infection especially for longer or more complex stricture.[13]

15. What are the newer modality treatment options available for penile stricture?

Ans: Urethral stents, aim to oppose wound contraction after DVIU. Stent insertion is a short procedure (<60 minutes) that can be done under local or spinal anaesthesia as "day care" surgery.

Drug (paclitaxel)-coated balloon dilatation is associated with higher anatomic patency rates (at six months) and lower risk of retreatment (at one year) as compared to standard dilatation/DVIU in patients with short (< 3 cm), bulbar strictures that underwent at least two prior failed endoscopic treatments. But, the above treatment in penile urethral strictures needs further studies.

Tissue engineering: Autologous cells were seeded on the luminal (urothelial cells) and outer surface (muscle cells) of a tubularized polyglycolic acid mesh scaffold to mimic histologic composition of urethra. These constructs were used as urethral replacement grafts[14] with a variable success rate of 60–70%.[15]

Local injection of **platelet-rich plasma (PRP)** is postulated to work by delivering growth factors and cytokines that recruit healer cells and enhance recovery process at the injection site.[16] This has been used in combination with other treatments like DVIU to decrease the recurrence rate.

16. How do you manage recalcitrant strictures in old age?

Ans: For most recalcitrant strictures after multiple failures and sparse remaining urethral plate extraordinary measures may not be justified and there may be a role for definitive perineal urethrostomy.

KEY POINTS

- Primary anastomosis, is not possible in the penile urethra due to the risk of loss of length and curvature during erection.
- Recent consensus panel recommends dynamic retrograde urethrogram (RUG) as a reliable method to stage and diagnose urethral stricture.
- Ensure adequate resolution of acute urethral inflammation and allows narrowed areas to declare themselves, i.e. URETHRAL REST.
- There is no role of DVIU in penile urethra.
- Overall stricture-free rates for staged OMG penile augmentation urethroplasties range from 70 to 100%.

REFERENCES

1. Kulkarni SB, Joshi PM, Venkatesan K. Management of panurethral stricture disease in India. J Urol. 2012;188:824–30.
2. Wessells, H., & McAninch, J. W. Use of Free Grafts in Urethral Stricture Reconstruction. The Journal of Urology.1996;155, 1912–15.
3. Fenton AS, Morey AF, Aviles R, Garcia CR. Anterior urethral strictures: etiology and characteristics. Urology. 2005;65: 1055–58.
4. Barbagli G, Palminteri E, Guazzoni G, Montorsi F, Turini D. Anterior urethral strictures. J Urol. 1996;156:73–7.
5. Angermeier KW, Rourke KF, Dubey D, Forsyth RJ, Gonzalez CM. SIU/ICUD consultation on urethral strictures: Evaluation and follow-up. Urology 2014;83:S8–17.
6. Gupta N, Dubey D, Mandhani A, Srivastava A, Kapoor R, Kumar A. Urethral stricture assessment: A prospective study evaluating urethral ultrasonography and conventional radiological studies. BJU Int 2006;98:149–53.
7. Osman NI, Hillary C, Bullock AJ, MacNeil S, Chapple CR. Tissue engineered buccal mucosa for urethroplasty: Progress and future directions. Adv Drug Deliv Rev 2015;82–83:69–76.
8. Smith TG 3rd. Current management of urethral stricture disease. Indian J Urol. 2016 Jan-Mar;32(1):27–33.
9. Gallentine ML, Morey AF. Imaging of the male urethra for stricture disease. Urol Clin North Am 2002;29:361–72.
10. Berna-Mestre, J.D., *et al.* Optimisation of sonourethrography: the clamp method. Eur Radiol, 2018. 28: 1961.
11. Kalabhavi S., *et al.* Role of Sonourethrogram in Evaluation of Anterior Urethral Stricture and its Correlation with Retrograde Urethrogram and Intraoperative Findings-A Prospective Study. J Clin Diag Res, 2018; 12: 1.
12. Bryk, D.J., *et al.* Outpatient Ultrasound Urethrogram for Assessment of Anterior Urethral Stricture: Early Experience. Urology. 2016; 93: 203.
13. Palminteri E, Berdondini E, Fusco F, De Nunzio C, Giannitsas K, vartolomei MD, *et al.* Contemporary urethral stricture management in adult patients. BJU Int.2021;127:256–70.
14. Raya-Rivera A., Esquiliano D.R., Yoo J.J., Lopez-Bayghen E., Soker S., Atala A. Tissue-Engineered Autologous Urethras for Patients Who Need Reconstruction: An Observational Study. *Lancet.* 2011;377:1175–82.
15. El-Kassaby A., AbouShwareb T., Atala A. Randomized Comparative Study between Buccal Mucosal and Acellular Bladder Matrix Grafts in Complex Anterior Urethral Strictures. *J.Urol.* 2008;179:1432–36.
16. Rezaei M, Badiei R, Badiei R. The effect of platelet-rich plasma injection on post-internal urethrotomy stricture recurrence. World J Urol. 2019;37:1959–64.

Chapter

4

Panurethral Strictures

• Pankaj M Joshi • Sanjay B. Kulkarni

LEARNING OBJECTIVES

- To understand the definition of panurethra stricture.
- To understand the physiopathology of lichen sclerosus.
- To understand the investigations for panurethra stricture.
- To understand the tips and tricks for urethroplasty in panurethra stricture.

INTRODUCTION

Panurethral strictures refer to obstruction from the meatus to the bulbo-membranous junction, sparing the membranous urethra or when multiple segments are compromised with a stricture length longer than 10 cm.[1,2] The most common cause of panurethra stricture is lichen sclerosus, although iatrogenic factors are increasing in the last decade with the advent of endourological procedures.[3,4] The incidence of urethra stricture is unknown but it compromises about 10% of the practice of urologist in India and has a prevalence of more than 100/10,000 in men older than 65 years in United Kingdom.[5]

In the past, multistage urethroplasty was used to repair panurethra strictures. However, contemporary approaches now enable a single-stage procedure using the one-sided dissection Kulkarni technique. Conversely, in cases where a compromised urethral plate is present, a staged urethroplasty is recommended. Urethroplasty for panurethra stricture has success rate of 90% for primary cases and 57.8% for redo cases.[6]

Case Scenario

A 46-year-old male patient complaints of poor flow in the last 3 years, associated with dysuria and incomplete bladder emptying. KUB ultrasound was performed showing increased bladder wall thickness and post-void residual volume of 250 ml. Uroflowmetry was done, showing a flattened curve with a Q_{max} of 6 ml/s. Retrograde urethrogram was performed showing a stricture form the meatus to the proximal bulbar urethra.

1. What is lichen sclerosus?

Ans: Lichen sclerosus (LS) is an inflammatory condition, a lymphocyte-mediated process that affects the genital skin and the urethra.[6] The epidermis and dermis are affected, in the compromised area, the skin becomes thickened and appears white, this is the typical finding in physical examination for patients with LS.[7] Nowadays it is believed that LS has an autoimmune etiology, with findings of immune dysregulation being common. Patients with LS have extracellular matrix protein 1 auto-antibodies, and some have an association with HLA subtypes.[6] LS also has an increased incidence of other autoimmune disease, like vitiligo, alopecia arreata and thyroid disease. When LS is present, it involves the foreskin/glans and in severe cases the urethra, this is secondary to the spongiofibrosis that might extend to the urethra.[6–8]

2. Which investigations are needed for panurethra stricture?

Ans: Pre-operative assessment includes ultrasound examinations to assess renal health and rule out hydronephrosis. Uroflowmetry is conducted as a fundamental baseline test. Urethrograms and voiding cystourethrogrphy are performed before the procedure.

The day of surgery urethroscopy and cystoscopy is performed with small caliber scopes, usually we use 4.5 Fr, 6.5 Fr ureteroscopes or a 7 Fr min-inephroscope. It is important to assess for bladder stones as these patients have chronic urinary stasis.

Surgical Steps of Urethroplasty for Panurethra Stricture

Methylene blue is used to stain the strictured urethra, aiding in the identification of the lumen. A midline perineal incision is made, exposing the bulbospongiosus muscle. In the lower half, the muscle wraps around the bulbar urethra, while in the upper half, a sleeve of muscle extends to the corpora, this upper portion is known as the bulbocavernosus part (Fig. 4.1). Only this section of the muscle is incised to gain access to the dorsal wall of the urethra. This technique is referred to as muscle-preserving urethroplasty.

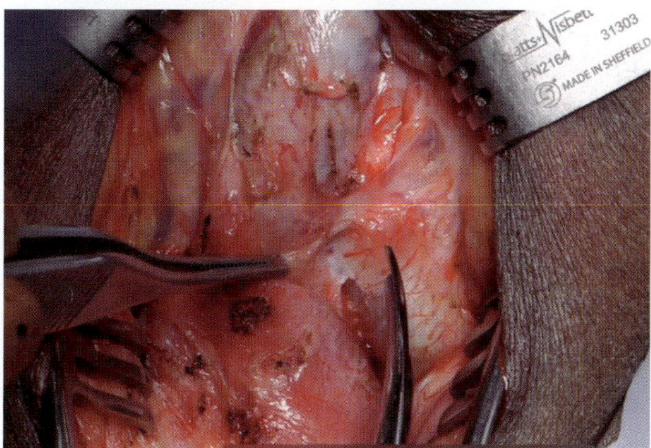

Fig. 4.1: Bulbocavernosus muscle

Penile invagination: The key to invaginating the penis is to incise the fascia above the urethra. Normally, a right-handed surgeon employs their left hand to push the penis down into the perineum, and the dissection is carried out on the left side of the urethra (Fig. 4.2). Through this pushing technique and dissection, the penis can be successfully invaginated.

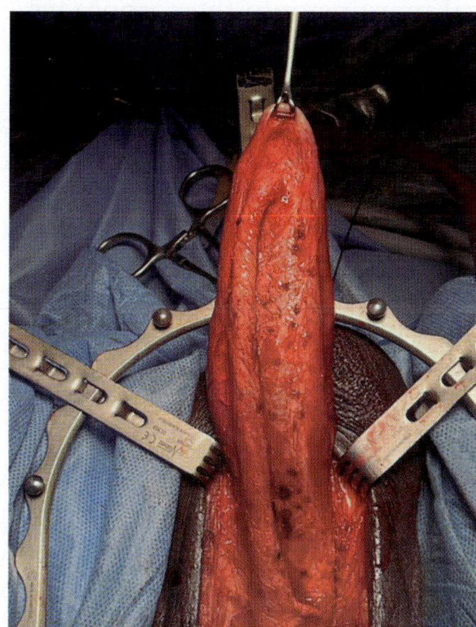

Fig. 4.2: Penile invagination and one-sided dissection of anterior urethra

Urethral dissection: The urethra is dissected from the underlying corpora, following a technique similar to dorsal onlay (Fig. 4.2). Care must be taken to avoid entering the intercrural plane. The urethra is rotated along its long axis without complete circumferential mobilization. The neurovascular supply from the right side is preserved intact.

Urethral incision: A dorsal incision is made across the full length of the urethra. Proximally, the incision extends beyond the stricture to ensure a healthy, pink, and supple urethral lumen (Fig. 4.3). A broad DeBakey's forceps is utilized to gently retract the urethra intraluminally. Distally, dissection is carried out up to the fossa navicularis. The penis is then repositioned to the pubic region, and a small DeBakey's forceps is inserted into the meatus. A wide dorsal meatotomy is performed (Fig. 4.4). This meatotomy should align with the dorsal incision in the urethral plate.

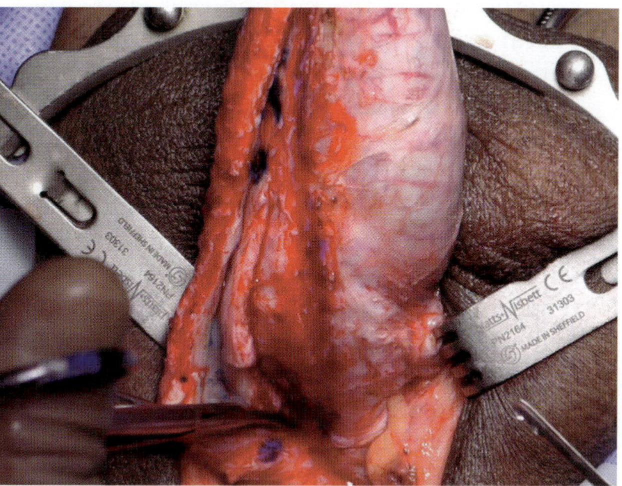

Fig. 4.3: One-sided dissection of anterior urethra

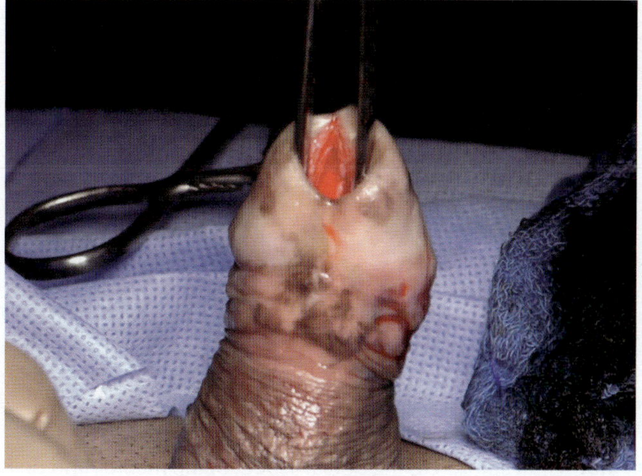

Fig. 4.4: Dorsal meatotomy

3. **When to take a buccal mucosa graft (BMG)?**

Ans: Most cases of panurethra stricture have LS, an inflammatory condition of the skin as mentioned previously. To ensure a higher success rate, it is advisable to perform a BMG urethroplasty in these patients. Urethroplasty for panurethra strictures requires two long buccal grafts each measuring 1.5 cm in width. It is routine in our practice to give nasal intubation for these patients to facilitate the harvesting the graft from both cheeks. Occasionally, a third graft may be necessary, which can be harvested from the undersurface of the tongue.

We prefer to keep the graft area open and discourage the use of lip grafts. Lip grafts have a higher incidence of cosmetic disability when compared to cheek grafts. Despite what the literature might suggest, the use of lip grafts has been largely abandoned in the majority of high-volume centers.

Graft placement: The first buccal graft is sutured to the dorsal apex of the meatus, then pushed into the penile urethra, spread, and fixed to the corpora cavernosa over the midline (Fig. 4.5). Another buccal graft is applied to the corpora cavernosa opposite the bulbar urethra. Continuous upward traction is applied to the inverted penis while applying the penile graft to prevent chordee. It is important to apply traction on the penis and not on the grafts themselves. The grafts, each measuring 1.5 cm in width, are spread and fixed with quilting sutures, usually 3 rows of quilting are done (Fig. 4.6). The margin of the buccal graft is sutured to the patient's right side of the urethral plate, and a 14 or 16 Fr silicone catheter is inserted. The full length of the urethra is rotated back to its original position over the graft (Fig. 4.7). Continuous 4–0 polyglactin sutures are used to stabilize the urethral margins onto the corpora cavernosa on the left side.

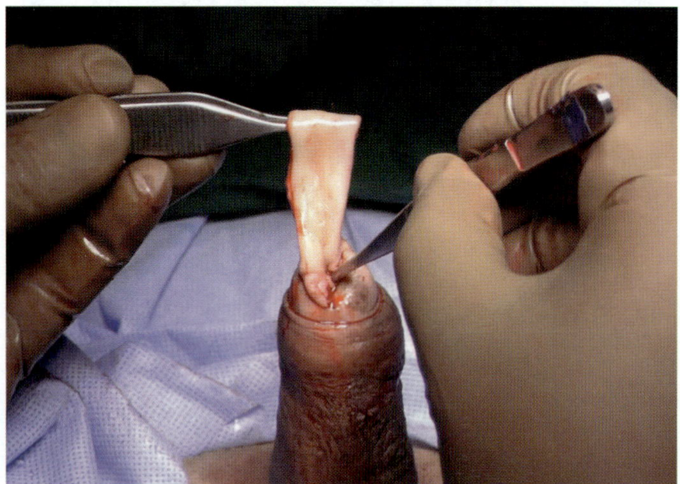

Fig. 4.5: Graft sutured to the dorsal aspect of the meatus and being pushed into the urethra through the meatus

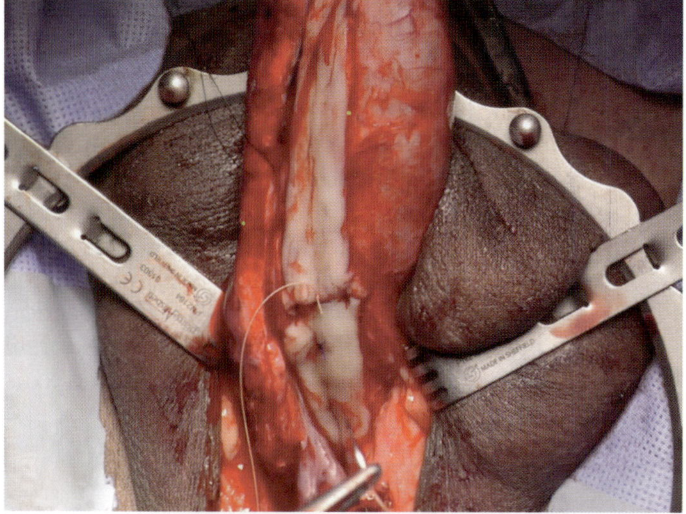

Fig. 4.6: Quilted grafts

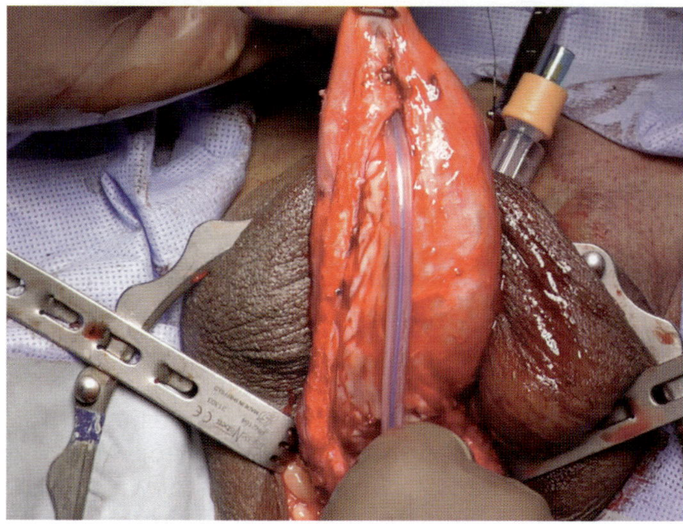

Fig. 4.7: Closure of urethra

At the end of the procedure, the graft is completely covered by the urethra and muscle. Colles' fascia, perineal fat, and skin are closed with interrupted absorbable sutures.

4. **When to use a preputial graft?**

Ans: Spiral preputial grafts are specifically employed in patients without lichen sclerosus. A spiral preputial mucocutaneous graft is derived from a 5 cm wide preputial skin, harvested in a helicoidal shape, and can extend up to 20 cm in length. Two circumferential lines are drawn on the preputial skin to create the spiral graft. The first line is positioned 5 mm below the coronal sulcus on the inner preputial mucosa, while the second line is marked 5 cm proximally on the outer preputial skin with the prepuce retracted.

Two circumferential incisions are made along these lines (Figs 4.8 and 4.9).

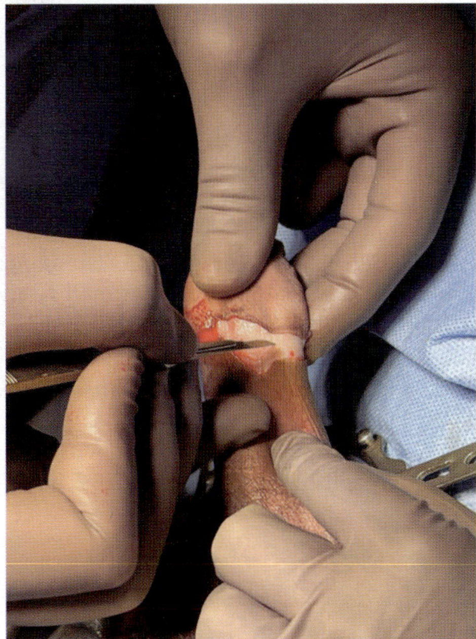

Fig. 4.8: Circum-coronal incision

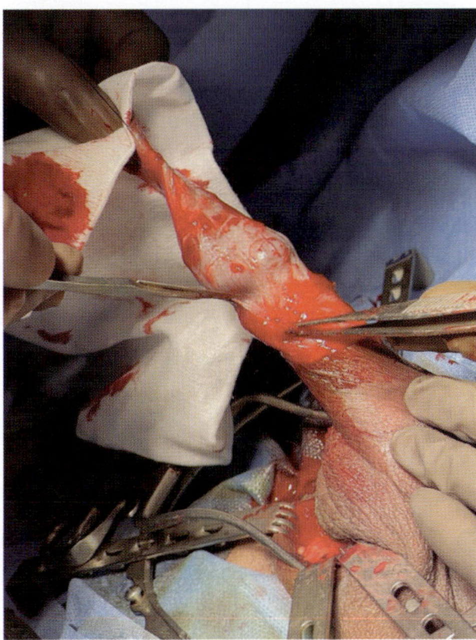

Fig. 4.9: Circumcision using sleeve technique for harvesting of the spiral graft

The incisions are deepened to the level of the dartos fascia. Starting from the proximal incision on the outer preputial skin, the preputial mucocutaneous graft is separated from its dartos using a 15-blade scalpel, with careful preservation of the dartos fascia. Penile traction is applied to facilitate dissection, ensuring the blade remains tangent to the dartos fascia. When the dissection reaches the distal circumferential mark on the inner preputial mucosa, the second incision on the distal line is made, resulting in the harvest of a cylinder of preputial skin. To aid in harvesting the spiral preputial graft, the preputial skin cylinder is placed around a 30 cc syringe (Fig. 4.10). Using a plastic scale arranged in a spiral fashion over the preputial cylinder, a 2 cm wide graft is obtained. With a 5 cm long cylinder, it is straightforward to achieve a spiral graft approximately 15–20 cm in length (Fig. 4.11).[1]

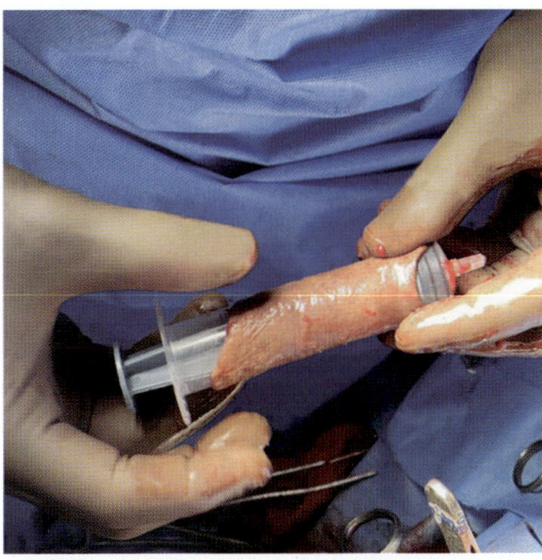

Fig. 4.10: Spreading the prepuce on a syringe to make a spiral graft

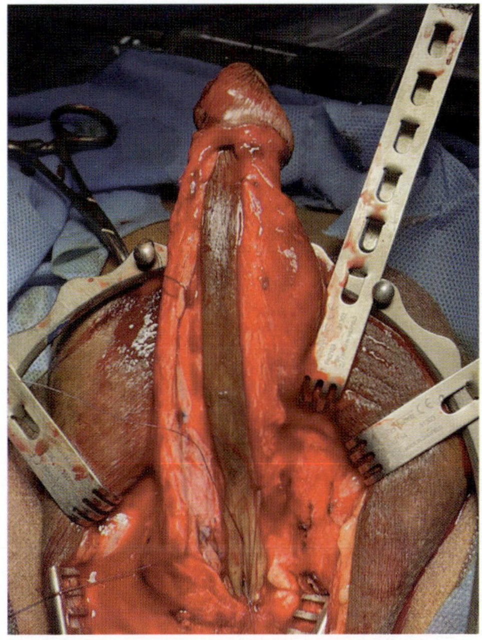

Fig. 4.11: Length of the preputial spiral graft covers the entire anterior urethra

SUMMARY

- The most common cause of panurethra stricture is LS.
- LS is an autoimmune disease that affects foreskin/ glans and urethra.

- One-stage urethroplasty is the gold standard for treating panurethra strictures with a high success rate.
- BMG urethroplasty must be done for patients with LS.
- Only use preputial spiral graft in patient without LS.
- The success rate of one-stage urethroplasty for panurethra stricture is 90%.

REFERENCES

1. Kulkarni SB, Joshi PM, Basile G, Bandini M. Novel single-stage preputial spiral graft for panurethral stricture: a step-by-step description of the technique. World J Urol [Internet]. 2023;41(9):2459–63. Available from: https://doi.org/10.1007/s00345-023-04514-9.
2. Kulkarni S, Kulkarni J, Surana S, Joshi PM. Management of panurethral strictures. Urol Clin North Am [Internet]. 2017;44(1):67–75. Available from: http://dx.doi.org/10.1016/j.ucl.2016.08.011.
3. Kulkarni S, Joshi P, Surana S, Hamouda A. Management of panurethral strictures. African J Urol [Internet]. 2016;22(1):33–9. Available from: http://dx.doi.org/10.1016/j.afju.2016.01.001.
4. Chodisetti S, Boddepalli Y, Kota M. Repair of panurethral stricture: Proximal ventral and distal dorsal onlay technique of buccal mucosal graft urethroplasty. Arab J Urol [Internet]. 2018;16(2):211–6. Available from: https://doi.org/10.1016/j.aju.2017.11.007.
5. Kulkarni SB, Joshi PM, Venkatesan K. Management of panurethral stricture disease in India. J Urol [Internet]. 2012;188(3):824–30. Available from: http://dx.doi.org/10.1016/j.juro.2012.05.020.
6. Belsante MJ, Selph JP, Peterson AC. The contemporary management of urethral strictures in men resulting from lichen sclerosus. Transl Androl Urol. 2015;4(1):22–8.
7. Mangera A, Osman N, Chapple C. Recent advances in understanding urethral lichen sclerosus. F1000Research. 2016;5:22–5.
8. Desai D. Panurethral Strictures: A Review of Management Options. Urol Nephrol Open Access J. 2017;4(6):204–7.

Chapter

5

Management of Bulbar Urethral Stricture: Excision and Anastomosis

• *Ajit Sawant* • *Prakash Pawar*

LEARNING OBJECTIVES

- To understand the stricture disease including the aetiology, classification and clinical evaluation.
- To understand the evaluation protocol in such cases.
- To understand the role of EPA in cases of bulbar urethral stricture.
- To understand the operative steps and post-operative care and follow-up in such cases.

INTRODUCTION

Urethra is defined as a fibromuscular conduit which transports urine from bladder and semen from ejaculatory ducts to exterior.

Urethral stricture is defined as narrowed segment of the anterior urethra due to process of fibrosis and cicatrisation of urethral mucosa and surrounding spongiosus tissue (spongiofibrosis).[1,2]

Bulbar Urethra

Bulbar urethra extends from urogenital diaphragm till penoscrotal junction.

This urethra is surrounded by bulbospongiosus muscle (Fig. 5.1).

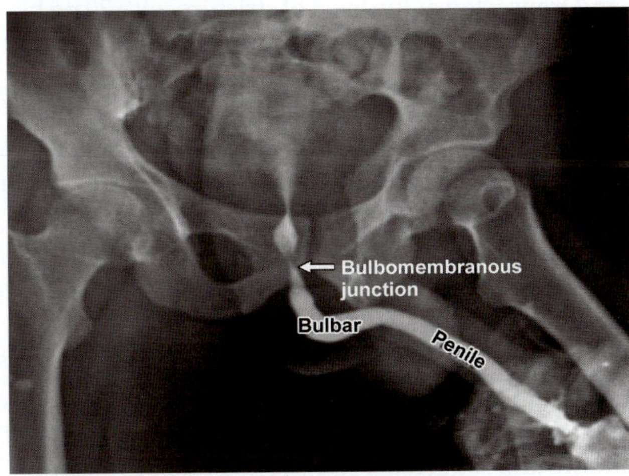

Fig. 5.1: Retrograde urethrogram

Etiology of Stricture

Latini *et al* 2014 proposed a broad categorisation of urethral stricture disease into iatrogenic, traumatic, inflammatory and idiopathic causes. A recent meta-analysis of aetiology found that most common causes are idiopathic (33%) and iatrogenic (33%), followed by post-traumatic (19%) and inflammatory (15%).

1. **Idiopathic:** Idiopathic urethrorrhagia that causes denuded epithelium with acute haemorrhage and neutrophilic infiltration with microcalcification is the histopathology of stricture.
2. **Iatrogenic:** Both diagnostic and therapeutic procedures like ureteroscopy, TURP, TURBT, etc. can cause strictures.
3. **Trauma:** Bulbar strictures are caused because of fall astride injuries.
4. **Inflammatory:** Gonococcus, chlamydia, urea plasma are the common organisms involved but the strictures due to these organisms has gone down due to decrease in STD rates.

   Lichen sclerosus is the most common inflammatory condition these days associated with stricture.
5. **Congenital:** When there is no identifiable cause, the stricture is termed congenital.

Stricture Classification (Table 5.1)

1. **Bulbar strictures:** The bulbar urethra is subdivided into proximal and distal part. The proximal bulbar urethra is defined as the segment within 5 cm of membranous urethra; the urethra lies eccentrically

in this part with abundant ventral spongiosus tissue. The distal bulbar urethra is defined as the adjoining segment extending to the penoscrotal junction.[3]

2. **According to stricture tightness:** Definition of high grade and low grade stricture remains debatable.[4–6] The urethral plate less than 3 mm is considered high grade or tight stricture.[7]

TABLE 5.1: Classification for urethral stricture

Category	*Presentation*	*Lumen in Fr*	*Degree*
0	Normal	-	-
1	Subclinical	Narrowing but >16	Low
2	Low grade	11–15	Low
3	High grade	4–10	High
4	Near obliterative	1–3	High
5	Obliterative	0 (no lumen)	High

Clinical Presentation

In a retrospective analysis, LUTS were the most common presentation (54.3%) followed by acute urinary retention (22.3%), UTI (6.1%) and difficult catheterisation (4.8%).[8]

Weak stream was reported as the most common LUTS (49%) followed by incomplete emptying (27%) and urinary frequency (20%).[9]

Diagnostic Evaluation

For treatment plan to be established length, location, depth and density have to be defined (Flowchart 5.1).

Excision and primary anastomosis (EPA) in bulbar strictures

Indication: Straddle injuries causing short segment bulbar strictures amenable to the repair

Principle: Complete excision of the diseased segment with wide oblique anastomosis till 26 Fr after spatulation of both proximal and distal end.

Position: High extended lithotomy position with patient's leg resting on Allen's stirrup. Padding of pressure points done. Operative time is to be kept to minimal to avoid complications of lithotomy position.

Operative Steps

1. Incision: Vertical midline along the perineal raphe from base of scrotum to 1–2 cm above anal verge.
2. Skin, subcutaneous tissue, Colles fascia incised in midline and self-retaining retractor applied.
3. Bulbospongiosus identified and divided with scissors in midline exposing the urethra (Fig. 5.2).
4. 12–14 Fr soft urethral catheter is passed till level of stricture and distal limit of stricture is marked.
5. Urethral mobilisation: Urethra mobilised sharply, laterally and dorsally for 2–3 cm distal and proximal to the stricture segment.

Flowchart 5.1: Management of patient with LUTS

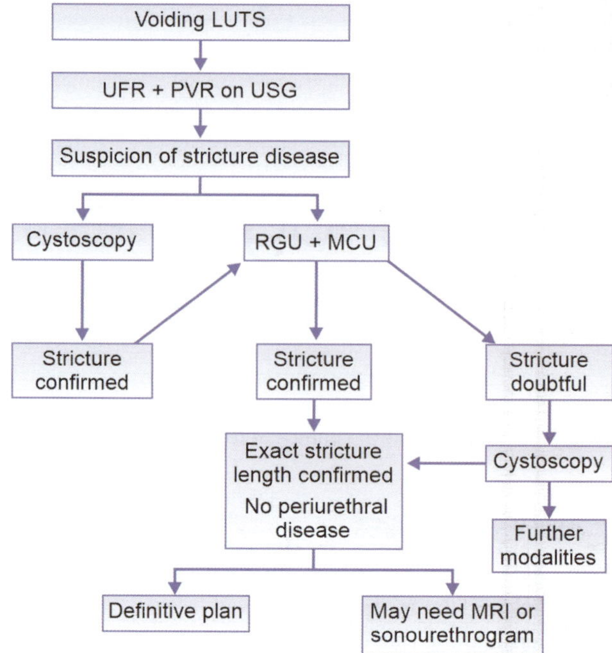

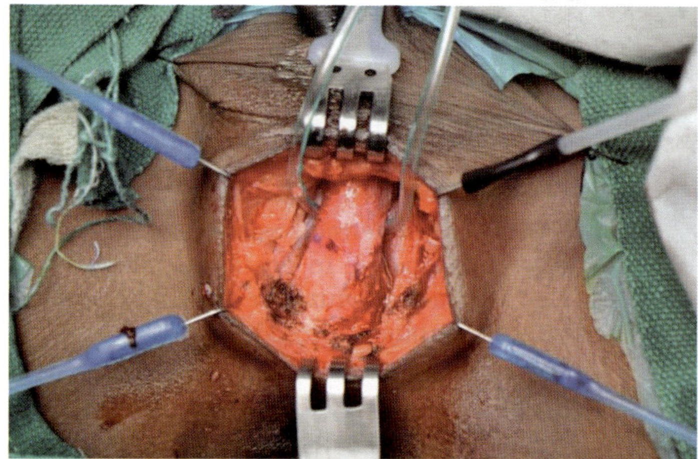

Fig. 5.2: Vertical perineal incision opened in layers

6. **Transection:** Urethra stabilised with vascular forcep and transected at the level of stricture with 20 no blade. Progressive excision is done proximally till normal urethra identified. This is aided by flow of urine or methylene blue injected suprapubically (Fig. 5.3).
7. **Spatulation:** Proximal dorsal and distal ventral spatulation performed. Check scopy done to confirm normal urethral passage.
8. **Anastomosis:** Around 6 to 8 circumferential sutures with polyglactin 4–0 or 5–0 over 16 Fr all silicon catheter is done (Fig. 5.4).
9. **Closure:** After haemostasis, closure done in layers.

Patency: International Consultation on Urological Diseases (ICUD) performed an extensive review of the literature and reported a composite patency rate of 93.8% for EPA.[10]

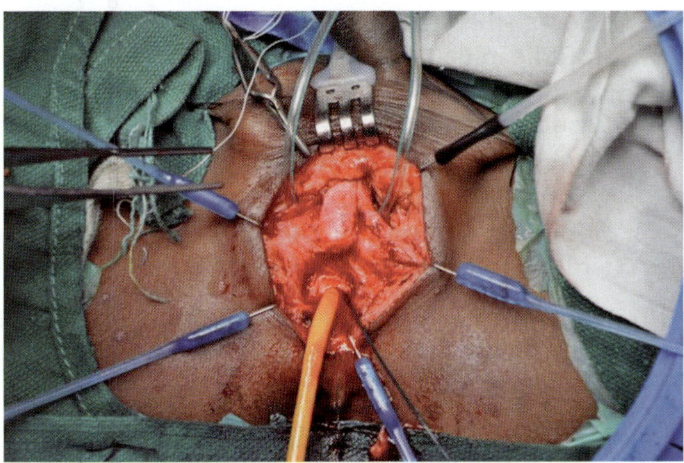

Fig. 5.3: Transection of urethra at the level of stricture

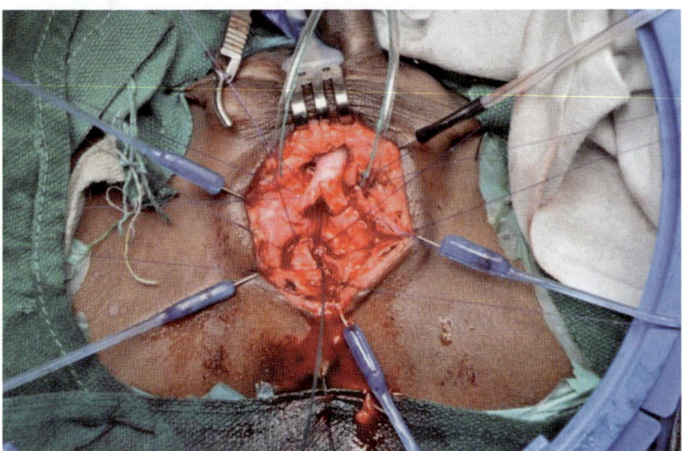

Fig. 5.4: EPA of urethra after spatulation 8 4-0 vicryl sutures

Anatomical definition of failure: Inability to pass 16 Fr catheter after the procedure.

Complications: Hematoma, neuralgia, infections, erectile dysfunction, chordee, cold glans, decreased glandular tumescence.

Case Scenario

40 years old male

Presented with palpable bladder for which SPC was inserted due to failed catheterization.

Patient had significant voiding symptoms which he developed poststraddle injury.

1. **What are the significant points to assess in history taking?**

   Ans:

   - Past history: Co-morbidities
   - Addictions: Smoking and tobacco chewing
   - Performance status
   - Sexual function

2. **What are the most common presentations in such cases?**

   Ans:

   - LUTS (54.3%)
   - Acute urinary retention (22.3%)
   - UTI (6.1%) and
   - Difficult catheterisation (4.8%).

   Weak stream was reported as the most common LUTS (49%) followed by incomplete emptying (27%) and urinary frequency (20%)

3. **What are the points not to be missed on physical examination?**

   Ans:

   - Per abdomen for palpable bladder and SPC site for location and skin health.
   - Local examination: To rule out LS; and urethral palpation to access grade of induration.
   - Examination of oral cavity (to check for oral hygiene if need arises for BMG).
   - Hip mobility.
   - BMI.

4. **Which validate PROM (patient related outcome measure) is used to access symptom severity and impact on QOL in stricture disease?**

   Ans: ICIQ-MLUTS

5. **What is the differential diagnosis in a young male presenting with LUTS?**

   Ans:

   - BOO secondary to urethral stricture disease
   - Neurogenic bladder
   - Bladder stone

6. **How do proceed with diagnostic evaluation?**

   Ans: Follow the same diagnostic Flowchart 5.1 as explained.

7. **Is urine analysis important component of the workup?**

   Ans: Urine analysis is not indicated if patient is already on a catheter. Urine culture and sensitivity is must in all cases as bacteriuria has to be treated before providing any definitive intervention in cases of stricture disease.

8. **What is sensitivity and specificity of UFR and MCU/RUG?**

   Ans:

TABLE 5.2: Sensitivity and specificity of RUG/VCUG

	UFR	*RUG/VCUG*
Sensitivity	80–81%	91%
Specificity	77–78%	72%

9. How is RUG performed? Describe the RUG findings in the image of the above patient.

Ans:

- Position: Supine with 45-degree oblique
  - Lower hip flexed at 90 degrees
  - Upper leg straight. The above positioning avoids bony margins overlapping the image
  - 10–12 Fr Foley's with 2 cc balloon inflated in fossa navicularis
  - Stretch the penis and instill the dye
- **Contrast used:** Diatrizoate meglumine
  - Iothalamate meglumine
  - 20 ml of 60% dilution needed

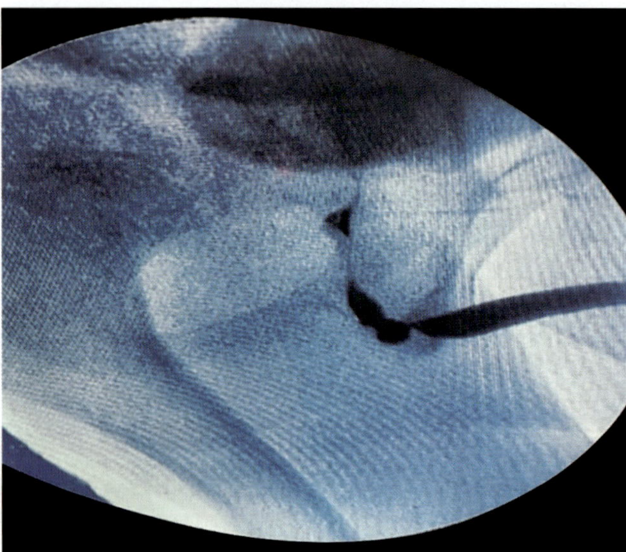

Fig. 5.5: Urethrogram showing bulbar stricture

Describe the anterior urethra on an RUG image. Comment on the view, status of penile urethra, bulbar urethra, the site of the stricture, the length of stricture and whether the dye reaches the bladder.

10. Why is cysto-urethroscopy important in such cases?

Ans: Urethroscopy helps to determine the condition of the urethra distal and proximal to the stricture.

Cystoscopy is important to rule out associated bladder pathology.

11. What is the role of MR urethrography and sono-urethrogram?

Ans: Though usually not done, MRI has a role in evaluating nature of the stricture and spongiofibrosis.

Sono-urethrogram also helps to determine the degree of spongiofibrosis at the stricture segment.

12. What are the indications of EPA in bulbar strictures? What is the principle behind anastomosis?

Ans: The indications must be clear and patients must be strictly selected to comply with these criteria; the stricture must be <2 cm long, post straddle injury and in the bulbous urethra. Longer strictures, and those in the pendulous urethra, are unsuitable for this procedure because it may cause excessive shortening leading to ventral curvature of the penis.

Principle: Excision of complete spongiofibrosis with wide, spatulated tension free anastomosis.

13. What are the techniques used for delineation of stricture segment intra-operatively in any case of stricture repair?

Ans:

- Urethro-cystoscopy
- Methylene blue
- Bouginage

14. At what dilution should methylene blue be used?

Ans: 1: 2

15. How to do spatulation? How to confirm adequate spatulation?

Ans: A wide spatulated anastomosis is important for success of the surgery. Ideal spatulation is done at 12 o'clock at the proximal end and 6 o'clock at the distal end.

Adequate spatulation is confirmed by passing a dilator or doing a scopy after spatulation.

16. What is the ideal suture material used?

Ans: Ideal suture is a monofilament absorbable 4–0 or 5–0.

Routinely used is polydioxanone or polyglycolic acid.

17. What is the post-operative management?

Ans: Foley's catheter is kept for 2–3 weeks. A pericatheterogram is indicated before catheter removal only if leak is suspected. Patient is given a voiding trial after catheter removal and regular follow-up done.

18. How to follow-up this patient after EPA?

Ans: Follow-up strategies after urethral stricture treatment include non-invasive (symptom assessment, urinary flow study) and invasive methods (retrograde urethrography, urethral calibration/bouginage and urethrocystoscopy).

Urinary flow rate measurement is often used as an objective test. The presence of a urethral stricture is suggested by a peak urinary flow rate (Q_{max}) <15 ml/s and a uroflow tracing which is flat and box-shaped. If flow max descends 10 ml/sec from the new baseline (3 months value), significant worsening of PROM values, if clinically indicated.

Using a combination of the American Urological Association Symptom Severity Index (AUA-SSI) and Q_{max} may avoid invasive testing.

There is no consensus about the optimal intervals and duration of follow-up. Since most stricture recurrence occurs in the first 12 months after treatment, 3–4 monthly follow-up for 24 months and then yearly till 5 years seems reasonable.

19. What is the definition of success after urethroplasty?

Ans: A successful urethroplasty has been variably defined as absence of need for retreatment functional success is measured by lack of voiding symptoms or strong force of stream, and anatomical success on cystoscopy or urethrography. There is a lack of universal agreement on the definition of success after urethroplasty.

1. Symptom free period
2. Absence of retreatment
3. Anatomical absence of stricture-cystoscopy or urethrogram

    Cystoscopy is an excellent option for an objective, reproducible, research-based definition of success.

    Success by uroflow: Q_{max} >15 ml/second

20. What is Jordan's technique?

Ans: Jordan's technique is the vessel sparing technique used in EPA. The vessel spared is bulbar artery which is a branch of common penile artery.

SUMMARY

- Defining the stricture length, location, depth and density is important before planning any reconstructive procedure in bulbar urethral stricture.
- Only strictures caused by straddle injury are amenable to EPA.
- A good wide spatulated, tension free anastomosis is must for the success of repair.
- A definitive follow-up protocol is necessary to check for recurrence.

REFERENCES

1. Mundy AR, Andrich DE. Urethral trauma. Part I: introduction, history, anatomy, pathology, assessment and emergency management. BJU international. 2011 ;108:310–27.
2. Latini JM, McAninch JW, Brandes SB, Chung JY, Rosenstein D. SIU/ICUD consultation on urethral strictures: epidemiology, etiology, anatomy, and nomenclature of urethral stenoses, strictures, and pelvic fracture urethral disruption injuries. Urology. 2014;83:S1–7.
3. Terlecki RP, Steele MC, Valadez C, Morey AF. Grafts are unnecessary for proximal bulbar reconstruction. The Journal of urology. 2010;184:2395–9.
4. Baradaran N, Fergus KB, Moses RA, Patel DP, Gaither TW, Voelzke BB, Smith TG, Erickson BA, Elliott SP, Alsikafi NF, Vanni AJ. Clinical significance of cystoscopic urethral stricture recurrence after anterior urethroplasty: a multi-institution analysis from Trauma and Urologic Reconstructive Network of Surgeons (TURNS). World Journal of Urology. 2019;37: 2763–8.
5. Purohit RS, Golan R, Copeli F, Weinberger J, Benedon M, Mekel G, Blaivas JG. Natural history of low-stage urethral strictures. Urology. 2017;108:180–3.
6. Erickson BA, Elliott SP, Voelzke BB, Myers JB, Broghammer JA, Smith III TG, McClung CD, Alsikafi NF, Brant WO. Multi-institutional 1-year bulbar urethroplasty outcomes using a standardized prospective cystoscopic follow-up protocol. Urology. 2014;84:213–7.
7. Palminteri E, Lumen N, Berdondini E, Di Pierro GB, Cucchiarale G, Tenti G, De Nunzio C. Two-sided dorsal plus ventral oral graft bulbar urethroplasty: long-term results and predictive factors. Urology. 2015 ;85:942–7.
8. Rourke K, Hickle J. The clinical spectrum of the presenting signs and symptoms of anterior urethral stricture: detailed analysis of a single institutional cohort. Urology. 2012; 79:1163–7.
9. Nuss GR, Granieri MA, Zhao LC, Thum DJ, Gonzalez CM. Presenting symptoms of anterior urethral stricture disease: a disease specific, patient reported questionnaire to measure outcomes. The Journal of Urology. 2012;187:559–62.
10. Morey AF, Watkin N, Shenfeld O, Eltahawy E, Giudice C. SIU/ICUD consultation on urethral strictures: anterior urethra–primary anastomosis. Urology. 2014 ;83:S23–6.

Chapter

6

Complete Bulbar Urethral Necrosis

• Pankaj M Joshi

LEARNING OBJECTIVES

- To understand the definition of bulbar necrosis.
- To understand the necessary Investigations for suspected bulbar necrosis.
- To understand the management options for bulbar necrosis.
- To understand the strategies to prevent bulbar necrosis.

INTRODUCTION

Pelvic fracture urethral injury (PFUI) occurs in 10% of those who suffer from pelvic fractures.[1] Urethroplasty involving anastomosis remains the benchmark for addressing PFUI (pelvic fracture urethral injury). The preferred surgical technique is the progressive perineal approach, with the transabdominal approach employed when necessary. Bulbar urethral ischemic necrosis (BUN) is an iatrogenic condition arising from unsuccessful prior PFUI repairs. Historically, it was characterized as a "long gap" or deemed "irreparable following unsuccessful interventions."[2,3] Turner-Warwick defined spongionecrosis of the bulbar urethra in 1986.[4]

Case Scenario

A 33-year-old male patient suffered a road traffic accident 2 years ago, he had PFUI at that time, and developed a urethral stricture due to trauma.

The initial management included suprapubic catheter insertion and patient stabilization. Subsequently, after 6 months, the patient underwent anastomotic urethroplasty. After the urethroplasty, he passed urine for one month and then developed poor flow and urine retention. Repeat investigation revealed a long gap between the bulbar urethra and the membranous urethra. This was classified as bulbar urethral necrosis.

1. What are the anatomical considerations in defining bulbar necrosis?

Ans: The urethra is categorized into the anterior and posterior sections. Additionally, the anterior urethra is further divided into the penile and bulbar urethra, with the bulbar urethra spanning from the penoscrotal junction to the membranous urethra.

The bulbar urethra can be segmented into distal, mid, and proximal sections. Notably, the proximal and mid portions exhibit distinctive characteristics, with a more pronounced development of spongy tissue in this area. Additionally, they are enveloped by the bulbospongiosus muscle. The proximal two-thirds of this muscle encircle the urethra in a circumferential manner, while the distal one-third surrounds the corpus cavernosum at the base of the penis alongside the bulbospongiosus-cavernous muscle.[5]

The antegrade blood supply to the urethra originates from both the bulbar arteries and cavernosal arteries. Conversely, the retrograde blood supply is sourced from the dorsal penile artery. Lateral blood supply to the urethra is provided by the circumflex vessels, all of which are branches stemming from the internal pudendal artery, itself a branch of the anterior division of the internal iliac artery.

2. What is the pathophysiology of bulbar necrosis?

Ans: Bulbar urethral ischemic necrosis (BUIN) denotes the loss of an extensive segment or the entire bulbar urethra due to inadequate blood supply. The term bulbar urethral ischemic stenosis is used to describe an almost obliterated ischemic stricture in the bulbar urethra. Anastomotic urethroplasty implies mobilization of the distal urethra and, consequently, the sacrifice of the lateral circumflex vessels. After transecting the urethra within the scar tissue, the bulbourethral vessels are divided, and the urethral blood supply becomes dependent on retrograde flow, particularly via the dorsal penile vessels.

Individuals who undergo crural separation and inferior pubectomy, and subsequently experience impaired retrograde flow or damage to the dorsal penile vessels, face an elevated risk of developing BUIN.[6]

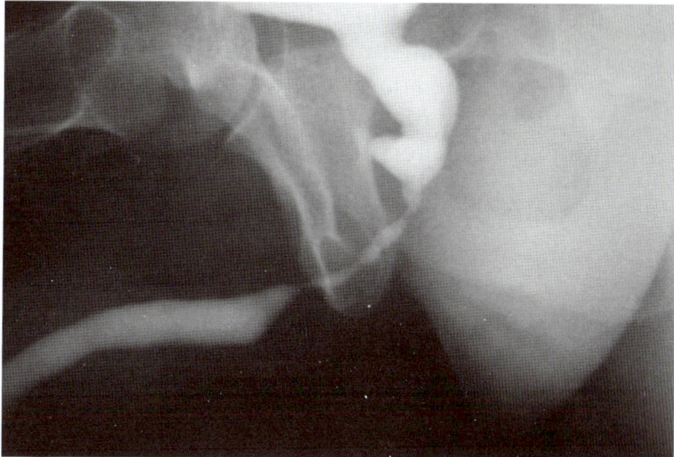

Fig. 6.1: RUG and VCUG suggestive of bulbar urethral stenosis

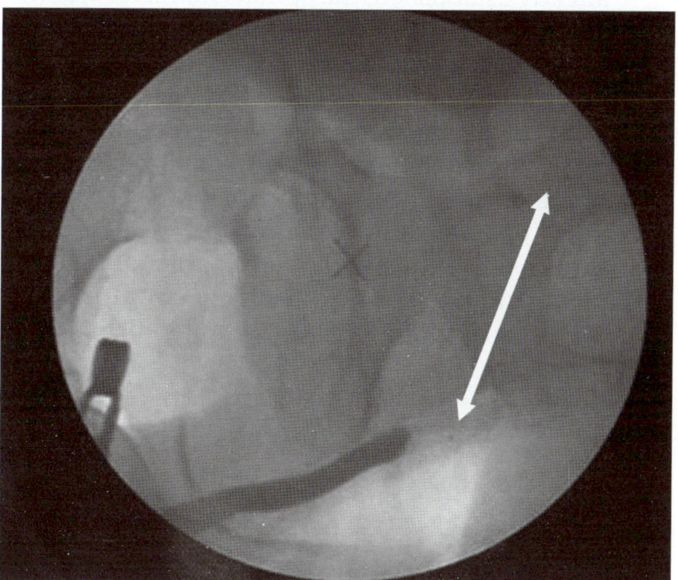

Fig. 6.2: RUG and VCUG depicting bulbar urethral ischemic necrosis (BUIN)

3. **What are the causes of bulbar necrosis?**

Ans: Turner-Warwick (1986) described the causes of spongionecrosis.[4]

1. Over-mobilization of the distal urethra
2. Hypospadias
3. Extensive spongiofibrosis resulting from multiple earlier surgeries.

Improper pubectomy can also lead to bulbar urethral necrosis. In the midline, there is the dorsal penile vein. Lateral to the dorsal penile vein are the two dorsal penile arteries. While performing an inferior pubectomy, it is essential to raise the periosteum. The best way to raise the periosteum is by making a midline incision and then performing lateral periosteal elevation. If you make an inverted U on the periosteum of the inferior pubic bone using an electrocautery, it can cause damage to the dorsal penile arteries, which are lateral to the vein. Improper pubectomy can also injure the dorsal penile arteries, compromising retrograde blood flow and leading to bulbar urethral necrosis.

4. **How to identify bulbar necrosis?**

Ans: According to Kulkarni *et al.* the length of penile urethra should be equal to the length of bulbar urethra. The midpoint of anterior urethra is the penoscrotal junction. When you find a smaller bulbar urethra as compared to penile urethra this is defined as bulbar urethral necrosis. Occasionally there can be a bulbar segment which is narrowed, and this is called bulbar urethral stenosis. (Figs 6.1 and 6.2).

5. **How does penile Doppler help in identifying risk of bulbar necrosis?**

Ans: Preoperative penile Doppler is performed by injection of papaverine into the corpora. We measure the velocities in the cavernosa artery as well as dorsal panel arteries. In anastomotic urethroplasty after transection of urethra the retrograde blood flow is dependent on the dorsal arteries. Any injury to the arteries on one side or either side at the time of accident or damage to the internal pudendal artery can increase the risk of bulbar necrosis. This can be identified preoperatively by performing penile Doppler. All patients who underwent PFUI repair at our institution received a penile Doppler examination before the repair. The assessed parameters included peak systolic velocity (PSV), end-diastolic velocity (EDV), and resistance index for both cavernosal and dorsal penile arteries, both before and after the administration of intracavernosal PGE1. Patients with a PSV greater than 35 cm/sec were considered to exhibit a normal arterial response, while those with a PSV less than 25 cm/sec were deemed to have severe arterial insufficiency. In cases of severe arterial insufficiency, we recommend penile revascularization as a procedure, involving microvascular anastomosis between the inferior epigastric artery and dorsal penile vessels prior to PFUI repair, to prevent bulbar urethral ischemia.[7–10] A high level of suspicion is crucial for diagnosing bulbar urethral ischemia. Radiographic examinations such as retrograde urethrogram (RUG) and micturating cystourethrogram (VCUG) would reveal a long-segment bulbar stenosis. In cases of necrosis, there might be a complete lack of visualization of the bulbar urethra.

6. What are the treatment options of bulbar urethral necrosis?

Ans: In cases where bulbar urethral ischemia is already established, the options for reconstruction become limited. These patients constitute a complex subset that necessitates care at a high-volume specialized centers. The initial assessment should focus on determining the type and extent of the injury, evaluating the prior number and type of repairs, and conducting a preoperative assessment of both antegrade and retrograde blood flow to the urethra, which is of paramount importance. We present our management algorithms (Flowchart 6.1) for bulbar urethral ischemia.[7]

Flowchart 6.1: Our algorithm for managing bulbar urethral ischemia

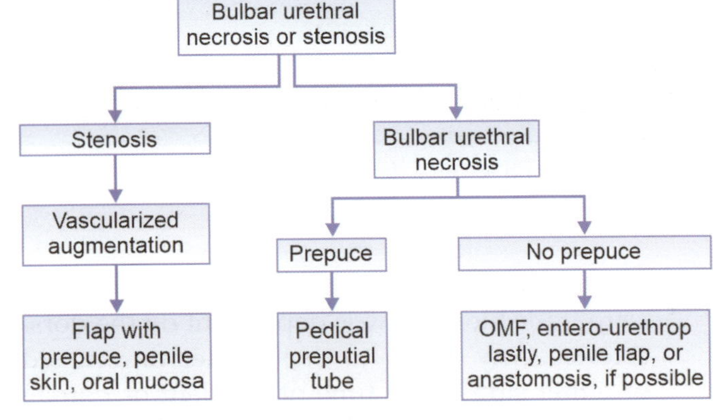

The most common surgery performed for bulbar necrosis is a pedicle preputial tube.

In cases of bulbar urethral ischemic necrosis (BUIN), it is crucial to preoperatively determine whether the patient is circumcised. For non-circumcised patients, our preferred approach involves using a pedicled preputial tube for repair. This technique involves two parallel circumcision incisions. The outer circumcision is deep to the skin and superficial to the dartos fascia, advancing forward to the base of the penis. The inner circumcision is performed deep to the dartos and superficial to Buck's fascia. Mobilizing the entire prepuce based on the dartos pedicle, this dartos derives its blood supply dorsally. The skin and dartos are split ventrally to the penoscrotal junction, and the prepuce is channeled into the perineum on a vascularized dartos flap. The inner prepuce is tabularized and used to bridge the substantial gap between the anterior and posterior urethra. The outer prepuce is sacrificed. This technique can be done using distal penile skin in cases where the prepuce is not available[11] (Fig. 6.3).

BUIN in patients who are circumcised poses a particular challenge. The alternative options for repair include:[12–15]

1. Oral mucosal flap (OMF): A 7 × 3 cm buccal mucosal graft is placed and quilted on the dartos at the midline scrotal septum. After a few weeks, the graft derives its blood supply from the underlying dartos and can be mobilized on the dartos pedicle, transposed to the perineum, and can be used as an onlay flap or tabularised for repair (Fig. 6.4).
2. Scrotal drop back (Turner-Warwick).
3. Pedicled penile skin flap (O flap and McAninch flap): Patients with exceptionally long obliterative ischemic segments that cannot be bridged by pedicled preputial or penile skin flaps

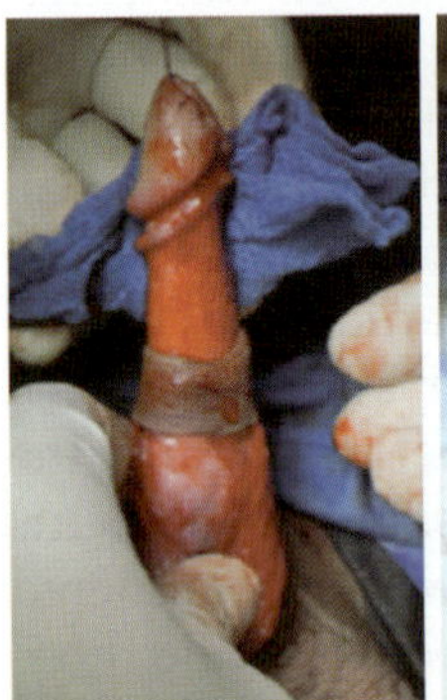
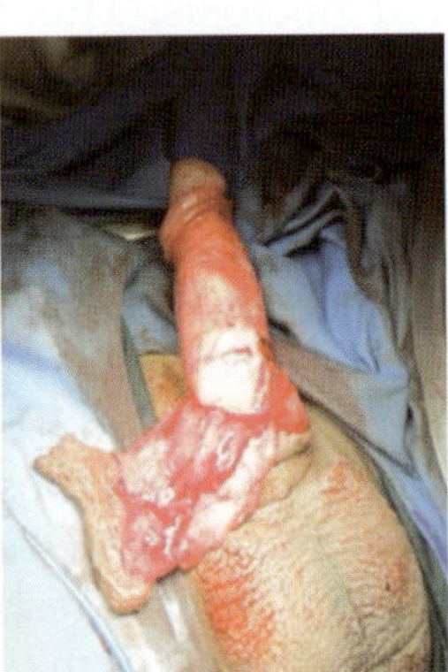
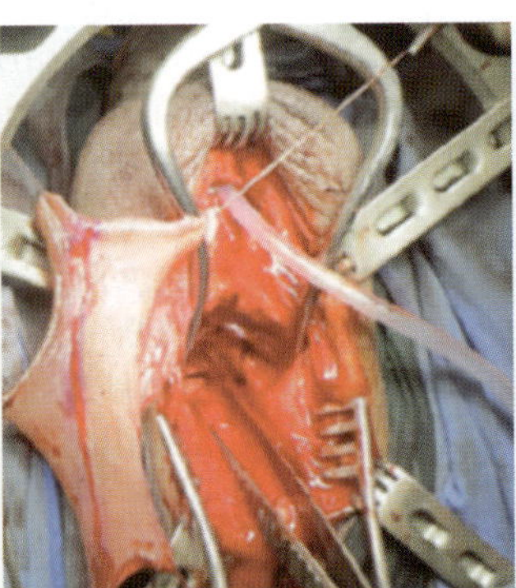
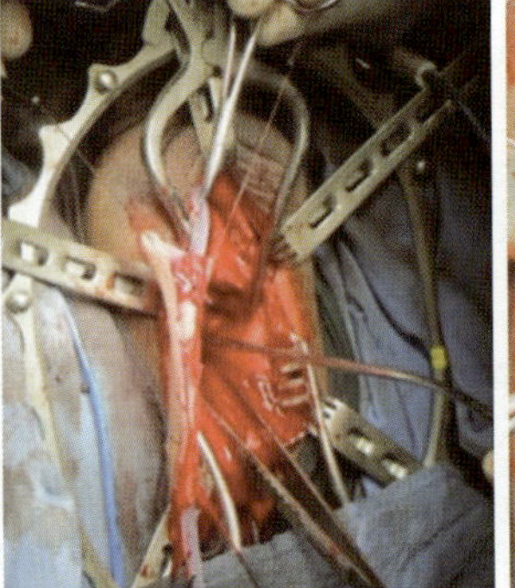
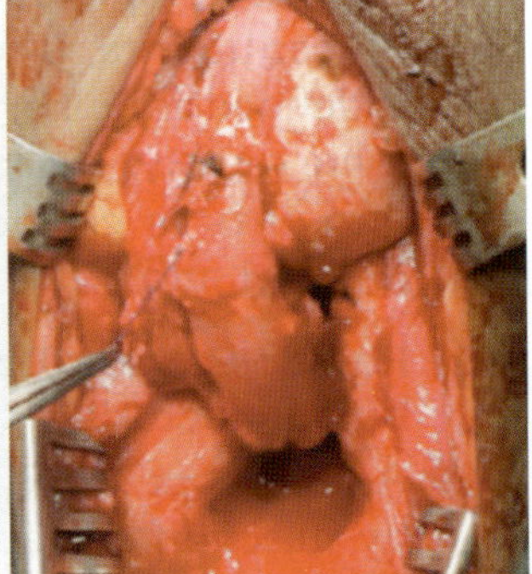

Fig. 6.3: Pedicled preputial tube urethroplasty

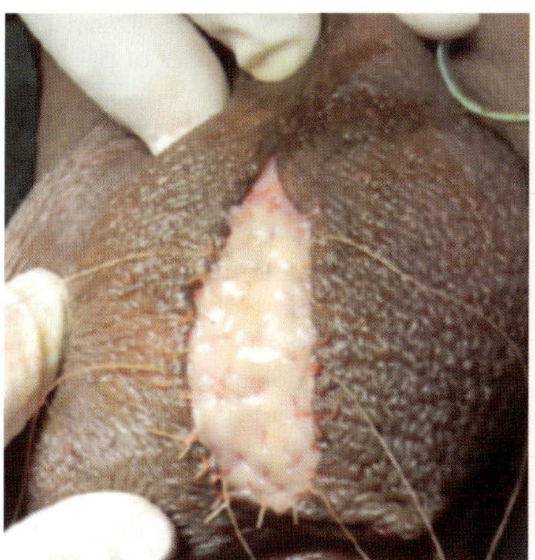

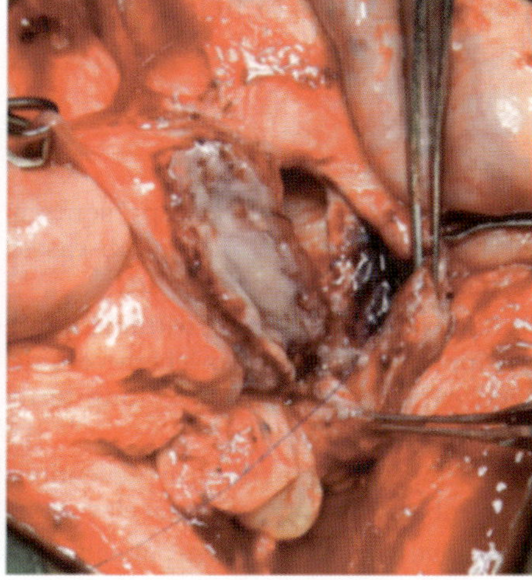

Fig. 6.4: Oral mucosal flap

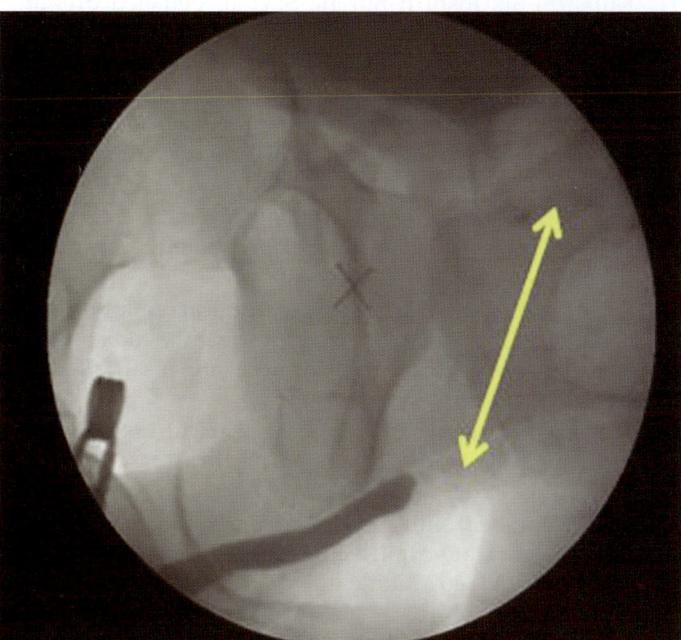

Fig. 6.5: RUG showing a long obliterative segment

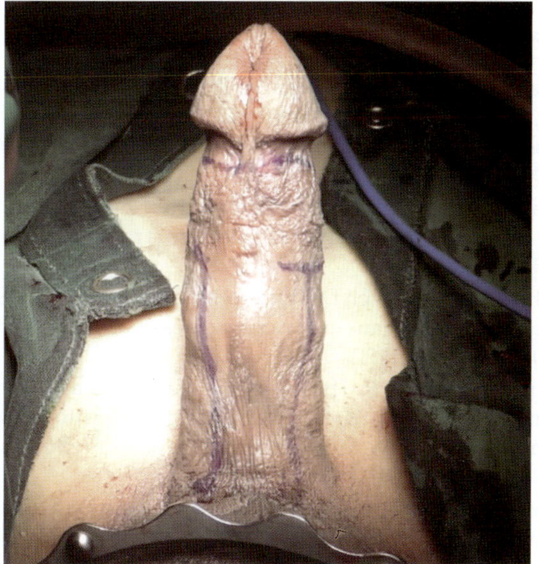

Fig. 6.6: "Q" flap marking

(Fig. 6.5). In these cases, the "Q" flap provides with excellent results (Fig. 6.6).

4. Enterourethroplasty: Described by Mundy and Andrich using sigmoid colon. (Fig. 6.7).
5. Use of buccal mucosa graft dorsally and flap externally. This can be performed provided inferior pubectomy is not required. An intact corpora cavernosa positioned in the midline is repaired to quilt the mucosal graft.
6. Pedicled anterolateral thigh flap for reconstruction of urethral defects.
7. Forearm flap with microvascular anastomosis to the inferior epigastric artery.
8. Dorsal BMG with ventral BMG over gracilis flap can also be considered.

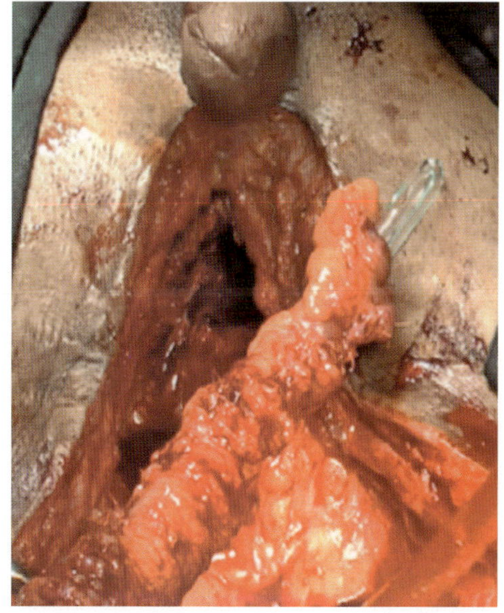

Fig. 6.7: Enterourethroplasty using sigmoid colon

In a large series of 172 cases of BUIN, the best results were achieved using a pedicled preputial tube.[16]

SUMMARY

- Bulbar urethral ischemic necrosis (BUIN) represents a challenging subset within the spectrum of urethral diseases, emphasizing the importance of prevention over cure.
- Reconstructive interventions for BUIN are constrained and necessitate a meticulous approach, preferably in a high-volume center with specialized expertise, to optimize long-term outcomes.
- Preservation of the dorsal penile arteries is critical in prevention, and this involves proper pubectomy and periosteal elevation.
- Staged surgeries are ineffective in managing these patients, and a more favorable approach involves a single-stage procedure utilizing a pedicled flap sourced from either the prepuce or penile skin.

REFERENCES

1. Demetriades D, Karaiskakis M, Toutouzas K, Alo K, Velmahos G, Chan L. Pelvic fractures epidemiology and predictors of associated abdominal injuries and Outcomes. J Am Coll Surg. 2002;195(1):10.
2. Barbagli G. History and evolution of transpubic urethroplasty: a lesson for young urologists in training. Eur Urol. 2007;52:1290–1292.
3. Mundy AR, Andrich DE. Entero-urethroplasty for the salvage of bulbo-membranous stricture disease or trauma. BJU Int. 2010;105:1716–1720.
4. Turner-Warwick R. The principles of urethral reconstruction. In: Rob C, Smith R, Scott McDougal W, editors. Rob and Smith's Operative Surgery, Urology. London: Butterworths; 1986. p. 480–519.
5. Joshi P, Kaya C, Kulkami S. Approach to bulbar urethral strictures: Which technique and when? Turk J Urol. 2016;42(2):53–59. DOI: 10.5152/tid.2016.12989.
6. Kulkarni SB, Surana S, Desai DJ, *et al.* Management of complex and redo cases of pelvic fracture urethral injuries. Asian Journal of Urology. 2018. Available at: https://doi.org/10.1016/j.ajur.2018.02.005.
7. Kulkarni SB, Joshi PM, Hunter C, *et al.* Complex posterior urethral injury. Am J Urol. 2015;13:43–52.
8. Rosen RC, Riley A, Wagner G, *et al.* The international index of erectile function (IIEF): a multidimensional scale for assessment of erectile dysfunction. Urology. 1997 Jun;49(6):822–830.
9. Guan Y, Wendong S, Zhao S, *et al.* The vascular and neurogenic factors associated with erectile dysfunction in patients after pelvic fractures. Int Braz J Urol. 2015 Sep-Oct;41(5): 959–966.
10. Zackerman JM, McCammon KA, Tisdale BE, *et al.* Outcome of penile revascularization for arteriogenic erectile dysfunction after pelvic fracture urethral injuries. Urology. 2012 Dec;80(6):1369–1373. Doi: 10.1016/j.urology.2012.07.059.
11. Kulkarni SB, Joshi P, Surana S, *et al.* Pedicled preputial tube urethroplasty for bulbar urethral necrosis after failed anastomotic urethroplasty for pelvic fractures urethral distraction defects. Eur Urol Suppl. 2018;17(2):e1937.
12. Mundy AR, Andrich DE. Entero-urethroplasty for the salvage of bulbo-membranous stricture disease or trauma. BJU Int. 2010;105:1716–1720.
13. Zhe Y, Yangqun L, Yong T, Muxin Z, Wen C, Ning M, *et al.* The pedicled anterolateral thigh flap for penile reconstruction. Chin J Plast Surg. 2015;11:406–410.
14. Chauhan A, Sham E, Chee J. Microsurgical urethroplasty for complex bulbar urethral strictures using the radial forearm free flap prelaminated with buccal mucosa. J Reconstr Microsurg. 2016;32:378–385.
15. Nikolavsky D. Prelaminated gracilis flap with buccal mucosal graft for salvage of devastated urethra. Case Rep Urol. 2015;2015:490518.
16. Joshi P and Kulkami. Pedicled preputial tube urethroplasty for long gaps after failed urethroplasty for PFUDD. BJUI Knowledge Video Module. August 2018.

Chapter

7

Post-TURP Urethral Stricture

• *Rishi Grover* • *Bhavatej Enganti*

LEARNING OBJECTIVES

- To understand the etiopathogenesis of post-TURP urethral strictures.
- To discuss the clinical presentation and evaluation of such strictures.
- To understand the management of such strictures keeping in mind various factors like the general health of the patient, the location and extent of the stricture, availability of necessary surgical expertise and experience, and the patient's expectations with regards to the surgical outcomes.
- To discuss the outcomes of the various management options.

INTRODUCTION

Urethral stricture is a complication which generally manifests a few months after transurethral resection of the prostate (TURP) and can occur in any part of the urethra. There are various etiological factors, some of which are preventable. Depending upon factors like the patient's general health, the location, length and density of the stricture and the patient's expectations from the proposed treatment, various endoscopic and open surgical procedures have been described for the treatment of such strictures.

Case Scenario

A 65-year-old male presented with acute urinary retention. Catheterization was unsuccessful and a suprapubic catheter (SPC) was placed. He had a complaint of poor urinary stream for the last one to two months. Seven months prior, he had undergone TURP for benign prostatic hyperplasia with refractory urinary retention. Postoperatively he had an initial improvement in the urine stream. He had no known medical illness. General and systemic examination was unremarkable and the focused neurological examination was normal. Laboratory parameters were within normal limits. Ultrasound of the kidneys, ureters and urinary bladder showed a small residual prostate and no hydronephrosis. The combined retrograde urethrogram and voiding cystourethrogram (VCUG) is shown in Fig. 7.1.

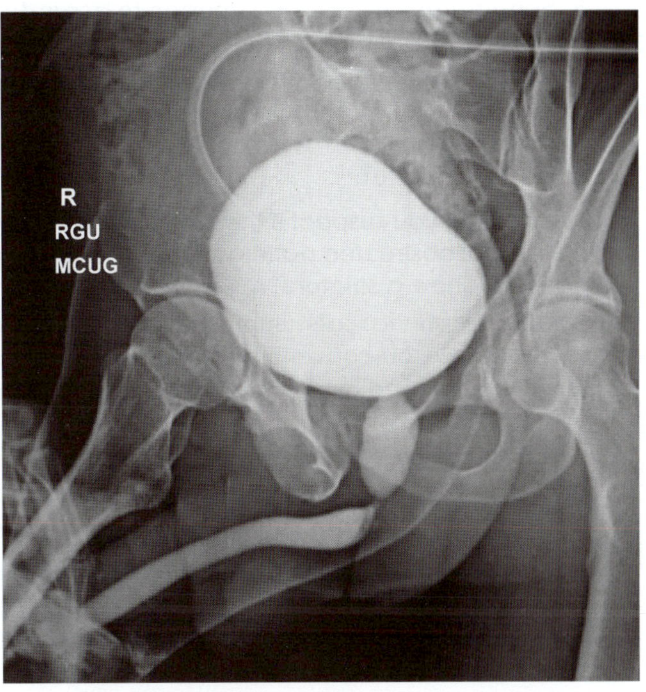

Fig. 7.1: Urethrogram: Proximal bulbar stricture

1. **What is your clinical diagnosis and why?**

   Ans: The patient may be suffering from either urethral stricture or bladder neck contracture because of the history of decreased urinary stream which developed a few months after he underwent TURP and the failed attempt at catheterization.

2. **How will you evaluate patients presenting with a poor urinary stream after TURP and which investigations will you do for confirmation of the diagnosis?**

Ans: The following investigations are required:

1. Laboratory investigations, urinalysis and urine cultures.
2. Ultrasound imaging may reveal high post-void residual urine, and in delayed cases, hydroureteronephrosis.
3. Uroflowmetry will show poor flow rates and a classical box pattern may be observed.
4. A properly done retrograde urethrogram is generally conclusive and should delineate the length and caliber of the stricture. If the patient happens to have an indwelling suprapubic catheter, then a voiding cystourethrogram may help to assess the proximal extent of the stricture and should be done. A combined retrograde and voiding study may correctly delineate the exact length and caliber of the stricture segment.
5. Urethrocystoscopy is preferred by some for diagnosis and evaluation of post-TURP strictures.[1] However, endoscopy will only confirm the presence of a stricture and its distal extent. It will not be able to assess the proximal extent of the stricture.
6. Sonourethrograms are superior to ascending urethrogram in the identification of spongiofibrosis, diameter and length of the stricture.[2] Sonourethrogram and MRI are not widely or routinely used in the routine evaluation of urethral strictures.

3. **What would you suspect if the uroflowmetry shows a classical obstructed pattern but the urethrogram does not show a stricture?**

Ans: Fossa navicularis (submeatal) strictures are easily missed on conventional urethrograms and may be diagnosed by palpation of local induration or by meatal calibration (especially when the urethrogram does not reveal a stricture more proximally). A bladder neck stenosis or contracture is another possibility to be considered in this scenario.

4. **How and when do patients present with stricture after undergoing TURP?**

Ans: Patients typically present with poor urinary stream 2 to 3 months or later, after surgery. Patients may occasionally present with urinary retention. If catheterization has been attempted, then urethral bleeding is common. Superadded infection may cause dysuria, frequency, urgency and urge incontinence. Examination is generally unremarkable but may reveal prostatic or epididymal tenderness. Submeatal induration may be palpable in cases with submeatal strictures.

5. **What else would you suspect in a patient who presents with poor urinary stream or retention within a few days or a few weeks after TURP?**

Ans: In patients presenting with poor urinary stream or high postvoid residual urine soon after surgery, pre-existing detrusor underactivity should be kept in mind. Occasionally, residual apical tissue may also present similarly.

6. **What are the common locations for post-TURP strictures?**

Ans: The common sites of post-TURP urethral strictures are the meatus, the fossa navicularis or sub-meatal region, the penoscrotal junction, the distal and mid-bulbous regions, and the proximal bulbous urethra, just distal to the urethral sphincter (often erroneously referred to as membranous urethral strictures).[3,4]

7. **What is the incidence of urethral stricture or bladder neck stenosis after TURP?**

Ans: Urethral strictures occur in 2.8–9.8% cases and bladder neck stenosis in 0.3–9.2% cases post-TURP.[5]

8. **Enlist the probable causes and factors which predispose to the development of post-TURP strictures.**

Ans: The probable causes may be broadly classified into patient related factors and technique or technology related factors (Table 7.1).

TABLE 7.1: Etiology of TURP strictures

Patient related	*Technique related*
For stricture	**Size of sheath**
Age	Mechanical trauma to the urethral mucosa
Pre-operative urinary tract infection (UTI)	Type and amount of jelly or lubricant use
Post-operative urinary tract infection	Lower temperature of the irrigation fluid
Pre-existing meatal stenosis	Prolonged resection time
For bladder neck stenosis	Electrical leak from resecting system
Smaller prostate gland	Duration of post-operative catheter
Severe storage symptoms pre-operatively	Monopolar versus bipolar versus laser type of energy source
Chronic prostatitis	

9. **Discuss the mechanism of stricture formation according to different etiologies and predisposing factors.**

Ans:

Age: Older age at the time of surgery is associated with a lower stricture rate, probably due to the decreased tissue response to inflammatory and traumatic stimuli.[6]

Pre-operative infection: Pre-operative UTI and prostatitis which are inadequately treated, increases the risk of urethral stricture after TURP.[7,8]

Post-operative infection: Post-operative UTI strongly predisposes to development of urethral strictures.[6]

Pre-existing meatal stenosis: Pre-existing meatal stenosis or a small caliber meatus which needs dilatation for introducing the resectoscope, predisposes to formation of urethral strictures.[9]

Pre-operative symptoms and prostate size: Small prostatic adenoma with severe storage symptoms and chronic prostatitis are associated with a higher risk of bladder neck contracture after TURP.[10–12]

Sheath size: Use of instruments which are relatively larger for the meatus and urethra are another cause of stricture formation.[13,14] Indian urologists often opine that Western instruments are too large for Indian urethra. Studies have shown that Indian men have a shorter urethral and penile length compared to men from Western countries. However, there is currently no comprehensive global data available on the urethral caliber.[15,16]

Mechanical urethral mucosal damage

The possible mechanisms are:

1. Compression injury to proximal bulbous urethra and penoscrotal junction by the resectoscope sheath.[17,18]
2. Mucosal damage due to axial and rotational movements of the resectoscope.[19,20]
3. Urethral mucosal damage due to mechanical stress induces inflammation and ischemia. This leads to subepithelial fibrosis and subsequently strictures.[21]

Jelly/lubricant used: If the jelly or lubricant used has a lower conductivity than that of the urethral mucosa, any leaking current may pass from the surface of the sheath to the surrounding urethra.[22]

Temperature of irrigation fluid: Colder irrigation fluids may lead to the constriction of blood vessels in the urethra with a higher risk of urethral stricture formation.[13,14]

Resection time: Large prostate volume and prolonged resection time increases the risk of developing urethral stricture, probably due to increased exposure of the urethra to electrical energy and more frequent instrument sheath movements, leading to greater manipulation and trauma to the urethra.[23,24]

Electric current leakage: A short circuit between the active electrode and the metal sheath can lead to electrothermal injury to the urethral mucosa. The current leak may occur due to

1. Broken electrode loops
2. Insulation defects on the sheath
3. Trapped carbonized resected materials on the loop, which can cause direct contact between the resection loop and the metallic sheath.[22]

Post-operative catheter duration: Prolonged post-operative catheterization time increases the risk of stricture formation.[25, 26]

Monopolar TURP vs Bipolar TURP vs Laser Prostatectomy: Initial studies had shown a higher urethral stricture rate in the TURis compared with monopolar TURP in patients with a prostate volume >70 ml.[24]

However, contemporary data shows that there is no difference in the stricture rates after monopolar or bipolar TURP or laser prostatectomy.[9, 27–29]

10. What are the stricture and patient related factors which will guide in deciding the management plan?

Ans: To plan treatment, it is important to determine the location, length, depth, and density of the stricture (spongiofibrosis).

Management of post-TURP urethral strictures would depend upon the age and general condition of the patient, existing comorbidities, location and extent of the stricture, availability of suitable grafts or flaps and importantly, the patient's preference and expectations from the planned procedure.

11. Enlist the treatment options depending upon the location of the stricture.

Ans: The management options according to the location of the stricture are given in Table 7.2.

TABLE 7.2: Management options

	Location	*Options*
1	Meatal/submeatal stenosis	Dilatation Ventral/dorsal meatotomy OTIS urethrotomy Meatoplasty Augmentation urethroplasty (graft/flap)
2	Pendulous urethral stricture	Dilatation Substitution, augmentation urethroplasty Johanson stage 1 urethroplasty
3	Bulbous urethral stricture	
3a	Short bulbous stricture	Visual internal urethrotomy End to end anastomosis Augmentation urethroplasty
3b	Long bulbous stricture	Substitution/augmentation urethroplasty Perineal urethrostomy

(Contd.)

TABLE 7.2: Management options *(Contd.)*		
3c	Proximal bulbous/ Bulbomembranous stricture	Dilatation Visual internal urethrotomy Augmentation urethroplasty (ventral approach)
4	Long/complex strictures	Dilatation Substitution urethroplasty Perineal urethrostomy Indwelling SPC

12. Discuss in detail the advantages, disadvantages and surgical outcomes of each treatment option which is available for managing post-TURP strictures.

Ans:

Meatal/sub-meatal strictures: Very small mucosal stricture can be managed with **meatal dilatation** alone, however, this is unusual. Dilatation, at best, is a temporary solution with very high re-stricture rate. Some patients, especially those with advanced age and with multiple comorbidities may not want an elaborate reconstructive procedure and may opt for regular dilatation (either self-dilatation or at a hospital).

A **ventral meatotomy** has a low failure rate but it would result in hypospadias. For patients who do not mind the cosmetic outcome and want a procedure with a low complication rate, a ventral meatotomy is a good option.

A **dorsal meatotomy** leaves the external meatus intact but may cause bleeding and has a high restenosis rate.

A **meatoplasty** gives a functional outcome like a meatotomy, but with a slightly better cosmetic outcome. There are various techniques described, but a local flap meatoplasty is commonly performed and is a technically straightforward procedure.[30]

For patients who do not want regular dilatation, do not accept hypospadias and are fastidious about cosmetic outcome; substitution urethroplasty is the preferred option. Substitution of the urethra can be performed by various techniques like ventral graft, dorsal graft,[31] circular grafts,[32] transmeatal (incision less) ventral onlay graft[33] or combined techniques. A local skin flap like a Jordan flap may also be used for reconstruction.[34]

Pendulous urethral strictures: The pendulous urethra is not a good site for conventional internal urethrotomy due to the thin corpus spongiosum dorsally which predisposes to cavernosal injuries and near certain recurrence of the stricture. **Visual internal urethrotomy is not recommended for pendulous urethral strictures and should not be offered as a treatment option for the same.**

Short pendulous urethral strictures are not amenable to resection and end to end anastomosis due to the high risk of ventral chordee during penile tumescence.

Some patients may opt for regular dilatation alone.

For patients with dense, small caliber, distal penile strictures who want a procedure with a low complication rate and do not mind a proximal penile meatus, a Johanson stage 1 urethroplasty is a good procedure followed by the option of a second stage procedure if and when the patient desires.

In most patients, a substitution urethroplasty can be done with good outcomes. Buccal mucosa is the graft of choice. Inner prepucial skin and distal penile skin grafts can also be considered. In patients with lichen sclerosus, who are chronic tobacco chewers, the oral mucosa and genital skin cannot be utilized. In such cases, extra genital skin from the upper thigh or the lower abdomen may be harvested for grafting.[35]

Bulbous urethral strictures

Short bulbous urethral strictures may be offered visual internal urethrotomy. Short annular strictures have a good long-term response to endoscopic treatment. However, long strictures with dense spongiofibrosis are prone to early recurrence.

Non-transecting anastomotic urethroplasty can be offered for dense, but short strictures, with favorable results.

Resection with end to end anastomosis has also been described, but postoperative erectile dysfunction is a potentially troublesome complication.[36] However, some experts strongly recommend avoiding excision and anastomosis due to concerns about pre-existing tissue ischemia. They opine that transection of the corpus spongiosum aggravates the local ischemia and thus leads to failure of the procedure. Instead they prefer substitution urethroplasty, which has a standard success rate of about 80% (which is similar to those reported for urethroplasty done for other etiologies).[37]

Long bulbous strictures are best treated with substitution urethroplasty with buccal mucosal graft being the tissue of choice.

For patients who are unwilling for, or not ideal candidates for reconstruction, a permanent perineal urethrostomy is an effective compromise solution.

Complex strictures: Long, dense strictures with obliterative segments may require complex reconstructive techniques like double face grafts, flaps and occasionally a combination of flaps and grafts.[38]

Proximal bulbous strictures (commonly referred to as bulbomembranous strictures) which are close to the sphincter respond well to ventral onlay graft urethroplasty with minimal risk of urinary incontinence.[39]

The striated urinary sphincter has an omega (Ω) shaped anatomy. The bulk of the muscle fibers are present in a sheet-like arrangement at the 12 o'clock position. They wrap around the urethra superiorly and extend down on both sides. However, the muscle fibers do not meet inferiorly and are deficient around the 6 o'clock region.[40] Due to this arrangement, the dorsal approach carries a risk of injury to the sphincteric fibers and may result in urinary incontinence. At the same time, the chances of sphincteric injury are negligible even with a deep incision into the urethral mucosa at 6 o'clock position. In case of long strictures extending close to the striated sphincter, a dorsal graft in the pendulous and distal bulbous region combined with a ventral graft for the proximal bulbous region gives satisfactory results while avoiding the risk of urinary incontinence.[37]

Such complicated reconstructive procedures are best performed by expert surgeons. If such expertise is not available or if the patient is not medically fit or unwilling for such extensive reconstruction, then a perineal urethrostomy is a reasonable solution with favorable long-term outcomes.

For obliterative urethral strictures involving the proximal bulbous or bulbomembranous region, urinary incontinence is a concern following major reconstruction. In such patients, often a visual internal urethrotomy (the so called core-through or cut-to-light) followed by regular, intermittent self-catheterization is often the most practical solution.[37]

There may be some patients who have multiple comorbidities or may have developed some debilitating medical problem after the primary TURP. Additionally, patients with poor general health, malnourishment or moribund status may not be suitable candidates for any form of surgery. There may also be situations where multiple procedures have failed and further attempts at complex surgery may not be prudent. In such cases, avoiding heroic surgeries and instead opting for an indwelling suprapubic catheter may be the most appropriate alternative. Although this may not be an ideal treatment, it is often appropriate when no other procedure is feasible or advisable.

Case management and outcome: The patient initially opted for endoscopic treatment and a visual internal urethrotomy was done. However, he developed recurrence of stricture within 4 months and subsequently underwent a double-faced buccal graft urethroplasty after which he had no recurrence till his last follow-up at 4 years.

SUMMARY

- The incidence of urethral strictures post-TURP is approximately 10%
- Patients commonly present after 3 to 6 months after the primary surgery.
- Retrograde urethrograms are diagnostic in most patients.
- Meatal and submeatal stenosis can be managed with meatotomy or a variety of flap or graft procedures.
- Pendulous urethral strictures are not amenable to endoscopic treatment or anastomotic repair and generally require substitution urethroplasty or staged procedures.
- Short bulbous urethral strictures may be managed with internal urethrotomy, non-transecting anastomosis or substitution urethroplasty depending upon the location and degree of local fibrosis.
- Long bulbous urethral strictures mostly need substitution urethroplasty.
- Proximal bulbous (bulbomembranous) strictures respond well to ventral graft urethroplasty with minimal risk of incontinence.
- Long and complex strictures may require technically demanding techniques like double face grafts, flap and graft combinations or sometimes staged repairs.
- A perineal urethrostomy, if acceptable to the patient, is often a practical solution where complicated procedures are not feasible or not advisable.

REFERENCES

1. Nasra WA, Ahmed MA, Visoky A, Huckim M, Elias MD, Katz I. The importance of cystoscopy in diagnosis and treatment of urethral stricture following transurethral prostatectomy. Isr Med Assoc J. 2020;22:241–3.
2. Ravikumar BR, Tejus C, Madappa KM, Prashant D, Dhayanand GS. A comparative study of ascending urethrogram and sono-urethrogram in the evaluation of stricture urethra. Int Braz J Urol. 2015;41:388–92.
3. Blandy HP, Notley RG, Reynard JM. In: Transurethral Resection. London, England: Taylor & Francis; 2005. p. 183–96.
4. Sekar H, Palaniyandi V, Krishnamoorthy S, Kumaresan N. Post-transurethral resection of prostate urethral strictures: Are they often underreported? A single-center retrospective observational cohort study. Urol Ann. 2021;13:329–35.
5. Rassweiler J, Teber D, Kuntz R, Hofmann R. Complications of transurethral resection of the prostate (TURP)-incidence, management, and prevention. Eur Urol. 2006;50:969–80.
6. Balbay MD, Ergen A, Sahin A, Lekili M, Ulucay S, Karaa ao lu E. Development of urethral stricture after transurethral prostatectomy: a retrospective study. Int Urol Nephrol. 1992;24:49–53.
7. Latini JM, McAninch JW, Brandes SB, Chung JY, Rosenstein D. SIU/ICUD Consultation On Urethral Strictures: Epidemiology,

etiology, anatomy, and nomenclature of urethral stenosis, strictures, and pelvic fracture urethral disruption injuries. Urology. 2014;83:S1-7.

8. Doluoglu OG, Gokkaya CS, Aktas BK, Oztekin CV, Bulut S, Memis A, *et al.* Impact of asymptomatic prostatitis on re-operations due to urethral stricture or bladder neck contracture developed after TUR-P. Int Urol Nephrol. 2012;44:1085–90.
9. Mannem SR, Mallikarjuna C, Bhavatej E, Taif NBM, Ravichander O, Syed MG. Incidence of urethral stricture following bipolar transurethral resection of prostate: A single-center study. Indian J Urol. 2022;38:146–50.
10. Tao H, Jiang YY, Jun Q, Ding X, Jian DL, Jie D, *et al.* Analysis of risk factors leading to postoperative urethral stricture and bladder neck contracture following transurethral resection of prostate. Int Braz J Urol. 2016;42:302–11.
11. Abbosov SA, Sorokin NI, Kadrev AV, Shomarufov AB, Nesterova OY, Akilov FA, *et al.* Predictors of bladder neck contracture after transurethral procedure on the prostate. Urologiia. 2021 ;5:73–77.
12. Chen Y-H, Li X-D, Ke Z-B, Chen J-Y, Lin T, Lin T-T, *et al.* Risk factors for the postoperative bladder neck contracture in patients with small-volume prostatic hyperplasia. Asian J Surg. 2023;46:373–9.
13. Park JK, Lee SK, Han SH, Kim SD, Choi KS, Kim MK. Is warm temperature necessary to prevent urethral stricture in combined transurethral resection and vaporization of prostate? Urology. 2009;74:125–9.
14. Jaffe JS, McCullough TC, Harkaway RC, Ginsberg PC. Effects of irrigation fluid temperature on core body temperature during transurethral resection of the prostate. Urology. 2001;57:1078–81.
15. Krishnamoorthy V, Joshi PB. Length of urethra in the Indian adult male population. Indian J Urol. 2012;28:297–9.
16. Grover RA, Vaidya H, Rajatiya H, Moitra M. A Study Of The Urethral And Stretched Penile Lengths In The Adult, Indian, Male Population. Journal Of Indian Medical Association. 121:64–6.
17. Mamoulakis C, Skolarikos A, Schulze M, Scoffone CM, Rassweiler JJ, Alivizatos G, *et al.* Results from an international multicentre double-blind randomized controlled trial on the perioperative efficacy and safety of bipolar vs monopolar transurethral resection of the prostate. BJU Int. 2012;109:240–8.
18. Mamoulakis C, Trompetter M, de la Rosette J. Bipolar transurethral resection of the prostate: the 'golden standard' reclaims its leading position. Curr Opin Urol. 2009;19:26–32.
19. Günes M, Keles MO, Kaya C, Koca O, Sertkaya Z, Akyüz M, *et al.* Does resectoscope size play a role in formation of urethral stricture following transurethral prostate resection? Int Braz J Urol. 2015;41:744–9.
20. Michielsen DPJ, Coomans D. Urethral strictures and bipolar transurethral resection in saline of the prostate: Fact or fiction? J Endourol. 2010;24:1333–7.
21. Mundy AR, Andrich DE. Urethral strictures: Urethral strictures. BJU Int. 2011;107:6–26.
22. Faul P, Schlenker B, Gratzke C, Stief CG, Reich O, Hahn RG. Clinical and technical aspects of bipolar transurethral prostate resection. Scand J Urol Nephrol. 2008;42:318–23.
23. Tan GH, Shah SA, Ali NM, Goh EH, Singam P, Ho CC, *et al.* Urethral strictures after bipolar transurethral resection of prostate may be linked to slow resection rate. Investig. Clin. Urol. 2017;58:186–91.
24. Komura K, Inamoto T, Takai T, Uchimoto T, Saito K, Tanda N, *et al.* Incidence of urethral stricture after bipolar transurethral resection of the prostate using TURis: Results from a randomised trial. BJU Int. 2015;115:644–52.
25. Hammarsten J, Lindqvist K, Sunzel H. Urethral strictures following transurethral resection of the prostate. The role of the catheter. Br J Urol. 1989;63:397–400.
26. Afandiyev F, Ugurlu O. Factors predicting the development of urethral stricture after bipolar transurethral resection of the prostate. Rev Assoc Med Bras. 2022;68:50–5.
27. Tang Y, Li J, Pu C, Bai Y, Yuan H, Wei Q, *et al.* Bipolar transurethral resection versus monopolar transurethral resection for benign prostatic hypertrophy: a systematic review and meta-analysis. J Endourol. 2014;28:1107–14.
28. Kumar BN, Srivastava A, Sinha T. Urethral stricture after bipolar transurethral resection of prostate–truth vs hype: A randomized controlled trial. Indian J Urol 2019;35:41–7.
29. Yan P, Cui Y, Huang Y, Che X, Zhou Z, Feng F. Intraoperative and postoperative outcomes of thulium laser enucleation versus bipolar resection in the transurethral treatment of benign prostatic hyperplasia: a meta-analysis. Lasers Med Sci. 2022;37:2517–25.
30. Blandy JP, Tresiddek GC. Meatoplasty. Br J Urol. 1967;39:633–4.
31. Farrell MR, Campbell JG, Zhang L, Nowicki S, Vanni AJ. Transurethral reconstruction of fossa navicularis strictures with dorsal inlay buccal mucosa graft urethroplasty. World J Urol. 2022;40:1523–8.
32. Önol Y, Önol FF, Gümü E, Topakta R, Erdem MR. Reconstruction of distal urethral strictures confined to the glans with circular buccal mucosa graft. Urology. 2012;79:1158–62.
33. Nikolavsky D, Abouelleil M, Daneshvar M. Transurethral ventral buccal mucosa graft inlay urethroplasty for reconstruction of fossa navicularis and distal urethral strictures: Surgical technique and preliminary results. Int Urol Nephrol. 2016;48:1823–9.
34. Tonkin JB, Jordan GH. Management of distal anterior urethral strictures. Nat Rev Urol. 2009;6:533–8.
35. Wang JW, Man LB. Transurethral resection of the prostate stricture management. Asian J Androl. 2020;22:140.
36. Barbagli G, Guazzoni G, Lazzeri M. One-stage bulbar urethroplasty: Retrospective analysis of the results in 375 patients. Eur Urol. 2008;53:828–33.
37. Kulkarni SB, Joglekar O, Alkandari M, Joshi PM. Management of Post TURP Strictures. World J Urol. 2018;37:589–94.
38. Kore RN. Management of urethral strictures and stenosis caused by the endo-urological treatment of benign prostatic hyperplasia—a single-center experience. Asian J Urol. 2023;10:137–43.
39. Barbagli G, Kulkarni SB, Joshi PM, Nikolavsky D, Montorsi F, Sansalone S, *et al.* Repair of sphincter urethral strictures preserving urinary continence: Surgical technique and outcomes. World J Urol. 2019;37:2473–9.
40. Strasser H, Klima G, Poisel S, Horninger W, Bartsch G. Anatomy and innervation of the rhabdosphincter of the male urethra. Prostate. 1996;28:24–31.

Chapter

8

Pelvic Fracture Urethral Injury: Acute Management

• *Dhananjay Vinayak Selukar* • *Sadashiv Bhole*

LEARNING OBJECTIVES

- To understand the history, clinical presentation and physical examination in a patient with PFUI.
- To understand the primary assessment of patients with PFUI.
- To understand the diagnostic evaluation of PFUI.
- To understand the treatment options available for PFUI as a primary management.
- To understand the outcomes and follow-up of various treatment options available during the acute management.

INTRODUCTION

High-velocity blunt injuries, often linked to the disruption of the pelvic ring and unstable pelvic fractures, can lead to injury in the posterior urethra, termed pelvic fracture urethral injury (PFUI). Contrary to earlier belief, PFUI is now recognized as a partial or complete disruption of the urethra rather than a complete defect. The current incidence of PFUI is estimated to be between 5% and 25%, commonly resulting from blunt trauma in motor vehicle accidents, with less frequent occurrences due to falls from height, industrial accidents, and similar incidents.

In the setting of severe multi-trauma, along with primary and secondary survey for assessment of general condition, associated injuries and hemodynamic status of patient, pelvic fracture urethral injury (PFUI) should be suspected in patients who present with symptoms such as blood at the meatus and/or difficulty in voiding. When the patient is stable, retrograde urethrography is recommended to confirm the presence of urethral injury. This diagnostic procedure is crucial in assessing and delineating the extent of the urethral injury in order to guide appropriate management. If patient is unstable assessment of urethral injury is often postponed as it is not considered immediately life-threatening but should not be forgotten.

Management of PFUI is a source of significant debate as there are various management options described which includes primary surgical repair, delayed primary repair, primary open realignment (POR), and primary endoscopic realignment (PER), suprapubic cystostomy (SPC) with delayed endoscopic management or delayed urethroplasty (DU). Immediate suprapubic catheter placement (SPC) with planned delayed reconstruction is the standard of care.

Case Scenario

35 years old male patient was brought by relatives to casualty with history of fall from height. He had inability to pass urine, blood at meatus and difficulty in walking. He had no history of any head injury, chest trauma, ENT bleed or loss of consciousness. His general examination was normal and he was hemodynamically stable.

Abdominal examination showed palpable bladder with tenderness in suprapubic area. His genital examination was normal except blood at meatus and had high riding prostate on digital rectal examination. His emergency retrograde urethrography suggested a complete urethral injury with extravasation of contrast (Fig. 8.1) for which he underwent emergency sonography guided suprapubic catheter (SPC) placement.

1. **What is your clinical diagnosis and why?**

   Ans: Clinical diagnosis is pelvic fracture urethral injury (PFUI) because patient has history of fall from height with difficulty in walking which can be due to pelvic fracture. He has inability to pass

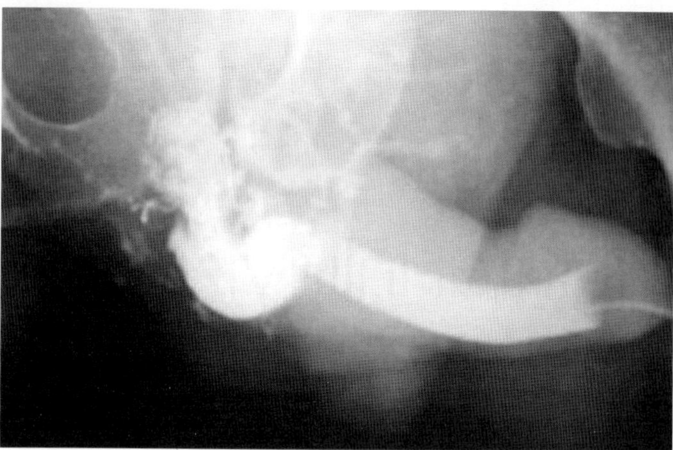

Fig. 8.1: Retrograde urethrogram in a patient with pelvic fracture showing complete disruption of posterior urethra with contrast extravasation

urine and palpable urinary bladder which suggest urethral injury. He has blood at meatus and high riding prostate which is classical finding in PFUI.[1]

2. **How will you do the primary assessment of this patient?**

Ans: There are two important assessments of the patient with trauma in emergency room:

- Primary survey
- Secondary survey

They both represent the overarching and sequential aspect of casualty assessment. Using these two assessments, one can identify whether a person is in a life-threatening situation.

Primary survey: The primary survey in emergency situations aims to assist first responders in identifying immediate threats to life. Immediate life threats often revolve around the patient's responsiveness, airway, and breathing, which are critical factors in determining the further course of treatment.

The widely used mnemonic for the primary survey is 'DRABC,' which represents Danger, Responsiveness, Airway, Breathing, and Circulation. This order of priority ensures that the most critical steps are taken care in a systematic and logical sequence, addressing the immediate and life-threatening aspects of the situation.

Secondary survey: The secondary survey should commence after the primary survey is completed completed and immediate immediate life-threats are identified and managed. This entails a comprehensive head-to-toe examination, and as part of urological assessment, a digital rectal examination should be conducted. In the context of potential urethral injury, specific indicators such as a high-riding prostate, the presence of blood at the urethral meatus, and an inability to void should be carefully noted. These signs can suggest the possibility of urethral trauma and contribute to a more accurate diagnosis and appropriate management.[2,3] The presence of perineal hematoma and edema should also prompt suspicion of potential pelvic injuries. To assess the pelvis, an anteroposterior compression test is employed. Pelvic instability, indicated by any movement during the test, suggests a pelvic fracture. It is important to note that any compressive force causing pelvic movement can disrupt hemostasis, so such force is typically limited to a single attempt to avoid exacerbating potential injuries. This evaluation is crucial in identifying and addressing pelvic trauma in a timely and appropriate manner.[4,5]

3. **What is the incidence of PFUI?**

Ans: Pelvic fracture urethral injuries (PFUI) occur in about 10% of male patients with pelvic fracture. PFUI in women is rare (<1%) because of shortened urethral length, mobility, and lack of attachments to the pubic symphysis.[6]

4. **What is the etiopathogenesis of PFUI?**

Ans: Pelvic fracture urethral injuries are usually caused by motor vehicular accidents (68–84%), or fall from height (6–25%). The type of pelvic fracture as a risk factor for urethral injury is influenced by the number of broken pubic rami and the involvement or non-involvement of the posterior pelvic arch with fractures of the anterior arch.[7,8]

Urethral injury in male patients typically results from a force causing soft tissue disruption, with the urethra and bladder neck less commonly torn directly by sharp edges of bone fragments. Major forces causing pelvic fractures lead to compression of the pelvis and the squeezing of its soft contents, including the bladder and prostate. Due to the fixed attachment of the membranous urethra to the tough perineal membrane, firmly connected to the pubic arch, and the loose attachment of the bladder and prostatic base to the bony pelvis, the squeezed prostate tends to move upward. This sudden and severe stretch–strain on the membranous urethra can lead to partial or complete disruption, particularly at the fixed and vulnerable bulbomembranous junction.

In cases of partial rupture, the membranous urethra is still stretched, and extravasation is usually localized to the urogenital diaphragm. In complete rupture, the proximal urethral end retracts upward while the distal end remains fixed to the perineal membrane, resulting in extravasation in the pelvis. Following complete rupture, the prostate is displaced upward, causing a loss of alignment of the urethra. This displacement also disrupts the periprostatic venous plexus, leading to a large hematoma that often displaces the prostate gland upward and posteriorly.[7,8]

5. **Describe the procedure and role of emergency retrograde urethrography (RUG) in assessment of PFUI.**

Ans: For performing RUG, patients should be placed in an oblique or lateral decubitus position, and it is preferable to perform the study under fluorography. Using sterile techniques, the glans penis is cleansed with antiseptic solutions. A small-bore urethral catheter of 16 Fr is placed unlubricated 1 cm into the fossa navicularis, and the balloon is filled with 3 ml of water to achieve a snug fit. Other devices for RUG include a suction catheter, a cone-tipped catheter, or a Brodney's clamp; 25 ml of diluted contrast medium is instilled gently by a 60 ml catheter-tip syringe, and the films are captured.

Because the anterior urethra is distended during the RUG, this examination is most useful for evaluation of the anterior segment. The site, and severity of urethral injury can be well delineated. Depending on the urethrographic appearance urethral injuries can be classified as per Colapinto and McCallum; or the Goldman classification system.[9]

6. **How will you classify and grade these injuries?**

Ans: Colapinto and McCallum[10] classified posterior urethral injuries into three categories based on radiological findings from retrograde urethrography:

Type 1: The membranous urethra is stretched but not severed.

Type 2: The membranous urethra is ruptured above the urogenital diaphragm, the contrast material extravasates into the pelvic extra peritoneal space above the urogenital diaphragm.

Type 3: The membranous urethra is ruptured and the injury extends into the bulbous urethra due to a tear in the urogenital diaphragm. Contrast material leaks above and below the urogenital diaphragm.

Goldman *et al*[11] proposed an extended classification of urethral injuries based on the anatomical description of traumatic urethral injuries:

Type 1: Posterior urethra is stretched but still intact (Colapinto-McCallum type 1).

Type 2: Partial or complete pure posterior urethral injury with tear of the membranous urethra while the urogenital diaphragm is intact. Contrast medium extravasates only above the urogenital diaphragm (Colapinto-McCallum type 2).

Type 3: Partial or complete anterior and posterior urethral injury with disruption of the urogenital diaphragm; contrast agent leaks above and below the urogenital diaphragm (Colapinto-McCallum type 3).

Type 4: Bladder neck injury extending into the urethra. The extravasation of contrast medium is around the bladder neck.

Type 5: Bladder base injury with periurethral extravasation similar to posterior urethral injury.

Type 6: Partial or complete isolated anterior urethral injury.

Thus, the classification of Goldman *et al* has retained the Colapinto-McCallum classification but with the addition of the injuries to the bladder neck, bladder base and anterior urethra, attempting to include all possible urethral injuries, bladder injuries and bladder neck injuries.

7. **What are the classifications of pelvic fracture?**

Ans: The three commonly used orthopaedic pelvic fracture classifications are: Young-Burgess, Tile and AO/ OTA. These systems is based upon mechanism of injury and associated injuries.

Tile classification[12] is commonly used and is as follows and shown in Fig. 8.2.

Type A:

Stable (posterior arch intact)

- A1: Avulsion injury
- A2: Iliac-wing or anterior-arch fracture due to a direct blow
- A3: Transverse sacrococcygeal fracture

Type B

Partially stable (incomplete disruption of the posterior arch)

- B1: Open-book injury (external rotation)
- B2: Lateral-compression injury (internal rotation)
  - B2-1: Ipsilateral anterior and posterior injuries
  - B2-2: Contralateral (bucket-handle) injuries
- B3: Bilateral

Type C

Unstable (complete disruption of the posterior arch)

- C1: Unilateral
  - C1-1: Iliac fracture
  - C1-2: Sacroiliac fracture—dislocation
  - C1-3: Sacral fracture
- C2: Bilateral, with one side type B, one side type C
- C3: Bilateral

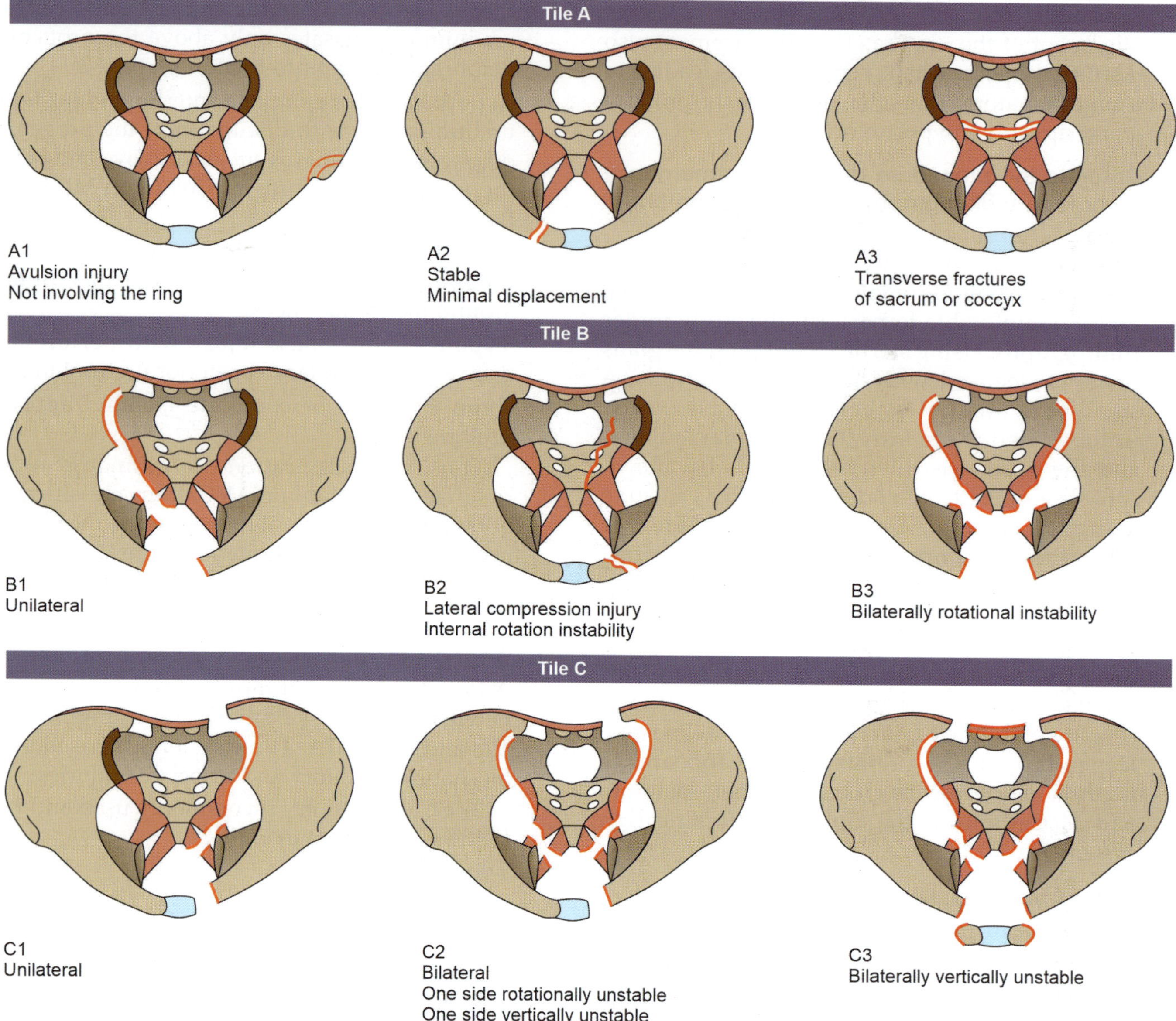

Fig. 8.2: Tile classification of pelvic fractures

8. What is clinical presentation of PFUI and triad of urethral injury?

Ans: Patient presents with history of some form of injury like road traffic accident or fall from height with impact to pelvic region with inability to pass urine, pain in lower abdomen, palpable urinary bladder and blood at the meatus. These are called **triad of urethral injury**.[13] Other classic findings, such as a "high-riding" prostate or a "butterfly" perineal hematoma, may frequently be absent or difficult to detect. Urethral disruption is often first detected when a urethral catheter cannot be placed by the trauma team or when it is misplaced into a pelvic hematoma.

Although rarer than in male counterparts, female patients also may develop proximal urethral avulsion injuries. They present with vulvar edema and blood at the vaginal introitus, indicating the need for careful vaginal examination in all female patients with pelvic fracture.

9. What is mechanism of the PFUI in pediatric and female patients?

Ans: In children, PFUI is less common but is more likely to extend proximally to the bladder neck because of the rudimentary nature of the prostate, the fragile tissues of an immature pelvic structure, and the relative intra-abdominal position of the bladder.[14]

The true incidence of female urethral injuries is not well established. Pelvic fracture urethral injuries are generally less common in females.

This lower incidence is likely influenced by factors such as the flexibility provided by the vagina and the inherent elasticity of the female urethra in adults. The female anatomy, with its unique characteristics, contributes to a lower frequency of urethral injuries compared to males, particularly in the context of pelvic fractures.[15]

10. What is the role of RUG and VCUG in diagnosis of PFUI?

Ans: The RUG has good utility among trauma patients and is easily performed at the bedside. On stout film of RUG, any pelvic fracture can be appreciated if present. A retrograde urethrogram is highly sensitive in detecting urethral injuries but falls short in identifying the precise location of the injury and is somewhat operator-dependent.[16–18] To address the time sensitivity often associated with trauma patients, the retrograde urethrogram (RUG) is considered the primary and most effective modality for evaluating individuals with concerning findings of urethral injury. This diagnostic test is readily available in locations equipped with radiology capabilities and can be promptly performed in the radiology department. The RUGs utility in early diagnosis is crucial, and when used in conjunction with additional studies, it facilitates early management of urethral injuries. This approach ensures timely assessment and intervention for better patient outcomes.

Voiding cystourethrography (VCUG) is the most appropriate way to evaluate the posterior part of the male urethra and injuries to the female urethra. VCUG shows posterior urethra, and hence proximal extent of urethral injury. It also shows bladder capacity, bladder contour and bladder neck status.[19]

11. What is the role of computed tomography and magnetic resonance imaging in management of PFUI?

Ans: Computed tomography (CT) is the investigation of choice to assess intra-abdominal urinary system including kidney, ureter and bladder. Any other intra-abdominal injury can be appreciated on CT. It does not replace the need for a retrograde urethrogram as CT fails to adequately evaluate the urethra.[20]

Magnetic resonance imaging (MRI) has been employed to define the length of the defect and to determine the extent and direction of urethral distraction and the extent of prostatic displacement, and it may help in planning the surgical approach. some authorities have advocated its use among children with a urethral injury where advanced imaging is warranted.[21]

12. What are the primary options available for management of this case?

Ans: Various management options available are: Treatment algorithm: Acute management of PFUI is shown in Flowchart 8.1.

- Primary open realignment (POR)
- Primary endoscopic realignment (PER)
- Primary surgical (open) repair
- Delayed primary repair
- Delayed repair with SPC (deferred urethroplasty)

13. What is primary realignment?

Ans: Primary open realignment (POR) was initially described in 1934 by Ormond and Cothran, and later in 1961 by Wilkinson, as a treatment for acute urethral injuries. Various techniques, including interlocking urethral sounds, retrograde catheter placement under direct vision, and combined anterograde/retrograde catheters, have been described for the purpose of re-establishing early urethral realignment. POR is a method employed to promptly address acute urethral injuries and restore proper alignment, aiming to improve outcomes for the affected individuals.[20–25]

In today's era, urethral realignment is performed by endoscopic guidance with rigid or flexible cystoscopy. This is called primary endoscopic realignment (PER). The process typically involves the use of two cystoscopes—one inserted anterograde through the suprapubic tract and the other inserted retrograde through the external meatus. A wire, passed through the anterograde scope, is grasped with forceps via the retrograde scope and externalized through the urethral meatus. Subsequently, the wire serves as a guide for the placement of a Foley catheter, which is left in place for a duration typically ranging from 4 to 6 weeks. This technique, combining anterograde and retrograde approaches, is utilized in primary open realignment to facilitate the proper realignment of the urethra and promote healing.[26–28]

The advantage of primary realignment is that the patients are more likely to have a shorter stricture (<2 cm), than those managed solely with SPC diversion. Even if urethral stenosis occurs after catheter removal, it can be managed endoscopically or by urethroplasty.[29]

However, due to high rates of complications in some studies, namely high restenosis rate (14–66%), erectile dysfunction (14–62.5%), and incontinence (4–25%) primary realignment is not preferred.[30]

14. What is primary repair?

Ans: Young originally described primary surgical (open) repair of PFUI in 1929.[31] The rationale

Flowchart 8.1: Steps of acute management in PFUI

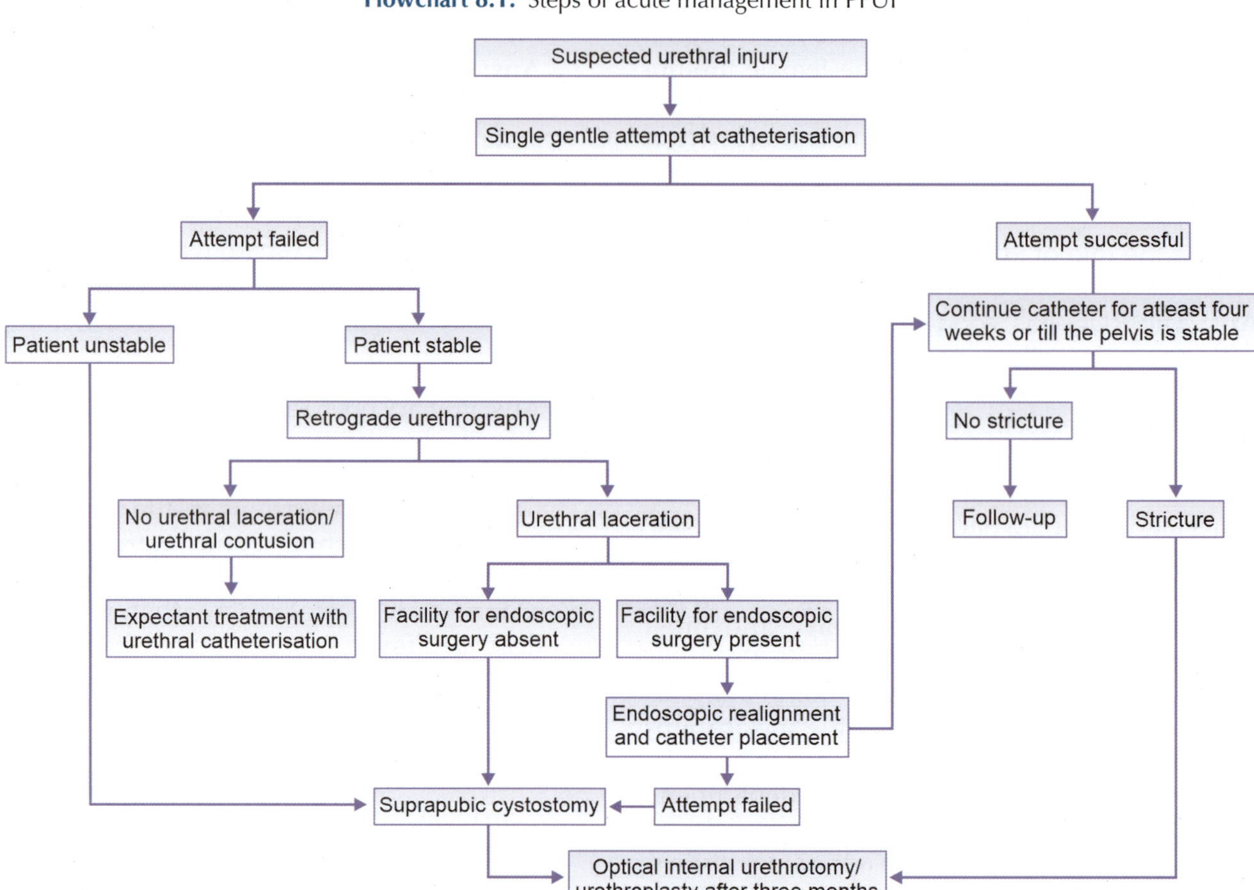

behind primary open realignment is to evacuate the pelvic hematoma and achieve a watertight repair of the urethra. This approach aims to prevent urine extravasation and subsequent infection. However, it is important to note that primary open realignment is associated with significant intraoperative blood loss, often exceeding 3 liters, and a prolonged hospital stay, typically extending beyond 28 days. Despite its potential benefits in preventing complications, the procedure is associated with challenges and outcomes need to be carefully considered in the overall management of urethral injuries.[31–33]

This approach has high complication rates like restenosis (54%), erectile dysfunction (23%) and urinary incontinence (14%). It is now rarely used unless there is a simultaneous bladder neck or rectal injury requiring definitive reconstruction or diverting sigmoid colostomy.[34]

Delayed primary repair was described by **Mundy** in 1991. The principle underlying delayed primary repair in the context of a severe urethral injury is based on the understanding that the recovery from such an injury is likely to be slow. The rationale is that conservative treatment may result in the formation of a long stricture, making subsequent surgery more challenging with limited success. In delayed primary repair, bulboprostatic anastomosis is typically performed 7–10 days after the injury. This timing allows for the evacuation of the hematoma and brings the ends of the urethra together once acute bleeding has ceased, and the patient is stable from their other injuries. The primary aim is not to prevent a stricture but to ensure that if a stricture does develop, it would be more easily treatable.[35]

15. How will you proceed with this patient?

Ans: Single attempt of gentle catheterization can be done as there is no evidence that a gentle attempt of PUC can convert an incomplete transaction into complete one. If urethral catheterization fails, then suprapubic catheter insertion (SPC) under local or regional anesthesia should be performed.

The insertion of an SPC can be performed using either an open or percutaneous technique. In the open cystostomy technique, a small transverse incision is made, typically about 2 fingerbreadths above the pubic symphysis. The rectus fascia is opened, providing access to the preperitoneal space. The bladder is identified, and stay sutures

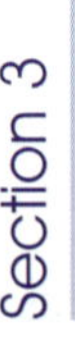

are placed on either side of the intended cystostomy site. A small incision is made in the bladder, and the drainage tube is inserted. The tube is then secured to the bladder using an absorbable suture. The fascial layers and skin are closed around the tube, and the tube is finally secured to the skin. This method is used for establishing suprapubic drainage when needed.[36]

The percutaneous technique is more commonly used. Distention of the urinary bladder is necessary for this approach. In an area, roughly 2 fingerbreadths above the pubis, a small incision is given, confirmed with needle aspiration of urine and SPC trocar is inserted. Alternatively, this can also be done by Seldinger technique.[36]

16. **What is the appropriate period to perform delayed reconstruction after PFUI? Why?**

Ans: After a period of three months, when scar tissue at the urethral disruption site has stabilized, it becomes safe to undertake posterior urethroplasty. This, however, is contingent upon the stabilization of any associated injuries and the patient being ambulatory. It is advisable to maintain suprapubic cystostomy drainage until all associated injuries have healed and the patient can be properly positioned for the reconstructive procedure. This approach ensures that the patient is in optimal condition for the reconstructive surgery and helps mitigate potential complications.[37,38]

SUMMARY

- Urethral distraction injuries typically occur as a consequence of blunt pelvic trauma and are observed in approximately 10% of pelvic fracture injuries. In many cases, the injury does not involve the total distraction of the entire circumference of the urethra; instead, a strip of epithelium may be left behind.
- This type of injury requires careful assessment and management to address the extent of the damage and ensure appropriate treatment.
- The early use of aligning catheters is a topic of debate. However, a consensus among most clinicians is that, at the very least, the aligning catheter facilitates subsequent reconstruction. At best, it often results in a situation where the patient has an endoscopically manageable stenosis. The decision to use aligning catheters is likely to be influenced by various factors, including the specific characteristics of the urethral injury, the patient's overall health, and the potential benefits and risks associated with this intervention.
- The anatomical status must be assessed. Contrast-enhanced studies along with endoscopy and selective MRI are useful.
- Prompt suprapubic catheter drainage is recommended as an initial management of PFUI.
- Primary realignment may be performed in stable patients, close follow-up is essential because of the high rate of stricture formation.
- Posterior urethroplasty by excision and primary anastomosis is the treatment of choice for urethral distraction injuries.

REFERENCES

1. Brandes S. Initial management of anterior and posterior urethral injuries. Urol Clin North Am 2006;33:87–5.
2. Coccolini F, Stahel PF, Montori G, Biffl W, Horer TM, Catena F, *et al.* Pelvic trauma: WSES classification and guidelines. World J Emerg Surg. 2017;12:5.
3. Ingram MD, Watson SG, Skippage PL, Patel U. Urethral injuries after pelvic trauma: evaluation with urethrography. Radiographics. 2008;28:1631–43.
4. Coughenour J. Initial Evaluation and Management of the Injured Patient. Mo Med. 2018;115:429–33.
5. Geeraerts T, Chhor V, Cheisson G, Martin L, Bessoud B, Ozanne A, Duranteau J. Clinical review: initial management of blunt pelvic trauma patients with haemodynamic instability. Crit Care. 2007;11:204.
6. Johnsen NV, Dmochowski RR, Young JB, Guillamondegui OD. Epidemiology of blunt lower urinary tract trauma with and without pelvic fracture. Urology 2017; 102: 234–9.
7. Koraitim MM. Pelvic fracture urethral injuries: the unresolved controversy. J Urol 1999;161:1433.
8. Koraitim MM, Marzouk ME, Atta MA, Orabi SS. Risk factors and mechanism of urethral injury in pelvic fractures. Brit J Urol 1996;71:876.
9. Kirshy DM, *et al.* Autourethrography. Radiology. 1991;180:443–5.
10. SM Colapinto, R.M. McCallum Injury to the male posterior urethra in fractured pelvis: a new classification J. Urol., 118;1977: 575–80.
11. S.M. Goldman, C.M. Sandler, J.N. Corriere Jr, E.J. McGuire Blunt urethral trauma: a unified, anatomical mechanical classification. J. Urol. 157;1997: 85–9.
12. Tile M. Pelvic ring fractures: should they be fixed? J Bone Joint Surg Br. 1988;70:1–12.
13. Singh L, Sharma PK. Managing urethral injuries in suburban India-general surgeon's perspective. Med J Armed Forces India. 2012;68:159–64.
14. Al-Rifaei MA, Gaafar S, Abdel-Rahman M: Management of posterior urethral strictures secondary to pelvic fractures in children, J Urol 1991;145:353–56.
15. Venn SN, Greenwell TJ, Mundy AR. Pelvic fracture injuries of the female urethra. BJU Int.1991;83:626–30.
16. Mundy AR, Andrich DE. Urethral trauma. Part II: Types of injury and their management. BJU Int. 2011;108:630–50.
17. Chapple C, Barbagli G, Jordan G, Mundy AR, Rodrigues-Netto N, Pansadoro V, McAninch JW. Consensus statement on urethral trauma. BJU Int. 2004 ;93:1195–202.
18. Mundy AR, Andrich DE. Urethral trauma. Part II: Types of injury and their management. *BJU Int*. 2011;108:630–50.
19. Ormond JK, Cothran RM. A simple method of treating complete severance of the urethra complicating fracture of the pelvis. JAMA 1934;102:2180–1.
20. Wilkinson FO. Rupture of the posterior urethra with a review of twelve cases. Lancet 1961;1:1125–9.
21. Webster GD, Mathes GL, Selli C. Prostatomembranous urethral injuries: a review of the literature and a rational approach to their management. J Urol 1983;130:898–902.
22. Elliott DS, Barrett DM. Long-term follow-up and evaluation of primary realignment of posterior urethral disruptions. J Urol 1997;157:814–6.
23. DeWeerd JH. Immediate realignment of posterior urethral injury. Urol Clin North Am 1977;4:75–80.

24. Follis HW, Koch MO, McDougal WS. Immediate management of prostatomembranous urethral disruptions. J Urol 1992;147:1259–62.
25. Gheiler EL, Frontera JR. Immediate primary realignment of prostatomembranous urethral disruptions using endourological techniques. Urology 1997;49:596–9.
26. Herschorn S, Thijssen A, Radmoski S. The value of immediate or early catheterisation of the traumatised posterior urethra. J Urol1 1992;148:1428–31.
27. Kielb SJ, Voeltz ZL, Wolf JJ. Evaluation and management of traumatic posterior urethral disruption with flexible cystourethroscopy. J Trauma 2001;50:36–40.
28. Koraitim MM. Effect of early realignment on length and delayed repair of postpelvic fracture urethral injury. Urology 2012;79:912–5.
29. Dixon AN, Webb JC, Wenzel JL, Wolf JS Jr, Osterberg EC. Current management of pelvic fracture urethral injuries: to realign or not? Transl Androl Urol 2018;7:593–602.
30. Young HH. Treatment of complete rupture of the posterior urethra, recent or ancient, by anastomosis. J Urol 1929;21: 417–50.
31. Trafford HS. Traumatic rupture of the posterior urethra; with a review of thirty-two civilian cases. Br J Urol 1955;27:165–71.
32. Simpson-Smith A. A Traumatic rupture of the urethra: eight personal cases and a review of 381 recorded ruptures. Br J Surg 1936;24:309–32.
33. Pierce JMJ. Management of dismemberment of the prostatic-membranous urethra and ensuing stricture disease. J Urol 1972;107:259–64.
34. Mundy AR. The role of delayed primary repair in the acute management of pelvic fracture injuries of the urethra. Br J Urol 1991;68:273–6.
35. Ghaffary C, Yohannes A, Villanueva C, Leslie SW. A practical approach to difficult urinary catheterizations. Curr Urol Rep. 2013;14:565–79.
36. Gelman J. Tips for successful open surgical reconstruction of posterior urethral disruption injuries. Urol. Clin. North Am. 2013; 40: 381–92.
37. Wessells H, Angermeier KW, Elliott S *et al.* Male urethral stricture: American Urological Association Guideline. J. Urol. 2017; 197: 182–90.47.
38. Koraitim MM. Optimising the outcome after anastomotic posterior urethroplasty. Arab. J. Urol. 2015; 13: 27–31.

Chapter 9

Surgical Reconstruction of Pelvic Fracture Urethral Injury

• Sanjay B Kulkarni • Pankaj M Joshi

LEARNING OBJECTIVES

- To understand the etiology of pelvic fracture urethral injury (PFUI).
- To understand the investigations needed for PFUI.
- To understand the tips and tricks of anastomotic urethroplasty.

INTRODUCTION

The incidence of posterior urethral injury varies from 3 to 9.9% of pelvic fractures.[1,2] The mean age of presentation is 33 years in the majority of series reported.[3–5] Other less common causes are described like gunshot injuries and explosive blasts.[6] Female urethral injuries due to pelvic fracture are very rare, 0.7% reported in large series.[7]

Case Scenario

A 28-year-old male patient was driving a bicycle. He was hit by a truck from behind. The lower half of the body came under the rear tyre of the truck. There was a crush injury of the pelvis followed by unconsciousness. He was taken to the hospital where his hemodynamic condition was stabilised. On investigation, it was found that he had retention of urine. An attempt at urethral catheterization failed. The catheterization was abandoned and a suprapubic catheter was inserted. About 800 ml of urine was drained. After stabilization he was then taken for endoscopic realignment. Endoscopic realignment was unsuccessful. After 3 months of recovery from the rest of the injuries, he presented to a urologist for management of pelvic fracture urethral injury.

1. **What is the etiopathogenesis of PFUI?**

   Ans: Different mechanisms of urethral injury have been proposed, these include crush, laceration, avulsion and distraction. The pubic ramus and ischium can act as "switch-blade" and lacerate or disrupt the urethra. Other explanations propose a shearing force which leads to disruption of the membranous urethra from the apex of the prostate.[8]

   At present, we know that these injuries occur distal to the striated sphincter in the majority of cases (70 to 75%)[9,10] demonstrated urodynamically[11] cystoscopically,[12] and surgically.[13]

   The etiology, severity and management of posterior urethral injury varies according to the demographic location. In developed countries, the most common etiology is motor vehicle accidents. Morey *et al* reported that 40% of injuries were associated with a car to pedestrian trauma while car to motorcycle and falling down and crash injuries accounted for 26% each.[14]

   In developing countries, pedestrian (35%), motorcycle (26.5%) and bicycle (12.8%) accidents are more common. Nevertheless, the severity and complexity of these injuries increases in the developing countries and seems to be linked to the initial management. In developing countries, the primary treatment is provided by the general surgeon in comparison with developed countries where the urologists manage the case.[15]

   Other less common causes are gunshot injuries and explosive blasts.[16]

2. **What is the preoperative evaluation of PFUI?**

   Ans: Imaging

   The most widespread and gold standard diagnostic method for PFUI is the combined dynamic retrograde urethrography (RUG) and voiding cystourethrography (VCUG), these assess the continuity of urethra, site, severity and length of urethral injury, bladder neck competence (open or closed) and the state of the bladder (capacity, vesicoureteric reflux, stones, diverticulum, fistula).

3. **What are the classifications of PFUI based on imaging?**

Ans: Colapinto and McCallum classified posterior urethral injuries in three types[17]

Type 1. The prostate or the urogenital diaphragm is dislocated, causing elongation and tension of the bulbomembranous urethra. There may be urethral contusion or laceration.

Type 2. The membranous urethra is ruptured above the urogenital diaphragm, with or without prostatic injury. The bulbar urethra is intact. The rupture may be partial or complete.

Type 3. The membranous urethra is disrupted both above and below the urogenital diaphragm. The rupture is usually complete and may be associated with rupture of the urogenital diaphragm and rupture of the bulbar urethra.

Recently Goldman *et al* proposed a new anatomical classification to compare the treatment options and outcomes of each kind of injury.[18]

Goldman classification

I. Posterior urethra stretched but intact.
II. Tear of the prostatomembranous urethra above the urogenital diaphragm.
III. Partial or complete tear of both anterior and posterior urethra with disruption of the urogenital diaphragm.
IV. Bladder injury extending into the urethra, injury of the bladder base with periurethral extravasation simulating posterior urethral injury.
V. partial or complete pure anterior urethral injury.

4. **What is the role of penile Doppler in PFUI?**

Ans: Penile duplex Doppler ultrasound has documented that among patients with PFUI, 48.7% have arterial ED, 14.6% venous leak and 36.5% have non-vascular ED most likely due to neurogenic etiology.[19]

A multivariate analysis documented that diastasis of the pubic symphysis, lateral prostatic displacement, and a long urethral gap at surgery are predictors of ED.[20]

Doppler duplex penile ultrasound with intracavernous injection (0.1 ml Trimix) is suggested in patients with any degree of preoperative erectile dysfunction. Systolic velocity < 25 ml/sec, rise time >80 msec, or both suggest arteriogenic ED. Jordan G *et al* reported high risk of ischemic bulbar necrosis after urethral reconstruction in these patients so they suggest primary penile revascularization prior to definitive urethroplasty helps improve the quality of erections and outcomes in urethroplasty.[21]

Please read details of penile Doppler in Chapter 6 on bulbar necrosis.

5. **What are the operative steps of anastomotic urethroplasty?**

Ans:

Position and preparation

Simple lithotomy position is needed, this is enough to give an adequate exposure. Some surgeons prefer exaggerated lithotomy, but the risk of neurovascular complications increases. The patient should have antithrombotic stockings and intermittent pneumatic compression leggings. Allen yellofin stirrups are the best for any kind of perineal surgery.

6. **What are the steps of progressive perineal approach?**

Step 1: Bulbar urethral mobilization
Step 2: Crural separation
Step 3: Inferior pubectomy
Step 4: Supracrural rerouting
Step 5: Abdominoperineal approach
Step 6: Abdominoperineal approach with omental wrap.

Surgical Approach

A midline perineal incision (Fig. 9.1), is made along the line of the raphe. The incision is deepened through the subcutaneous tissue and Colles' fascia until the bulbospongiosus muscle (Fig. 9.2). The bulbospongiosus muscle is then incised in midline (Fig. 9.3).

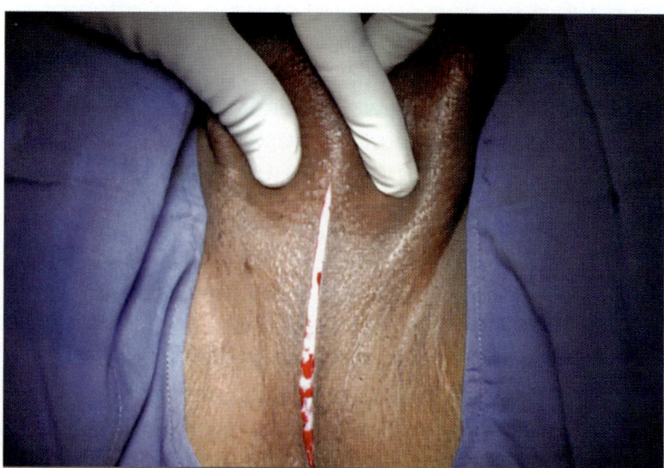

Fig. 9.1: Midline perineal incision

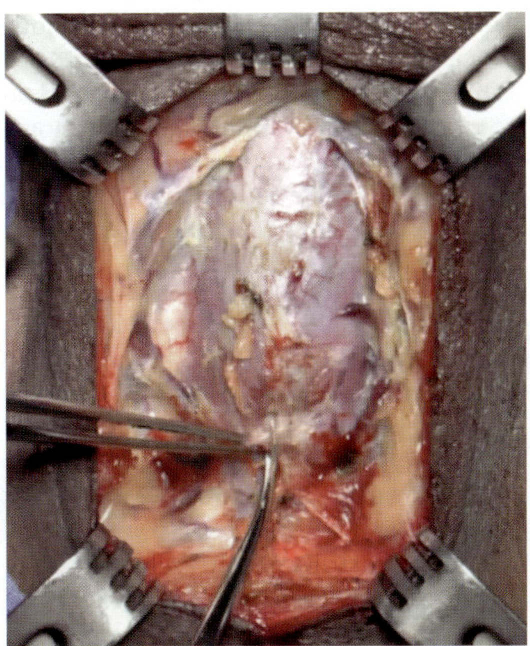

Fig. 9.2: Exposure of the bulbar urethra

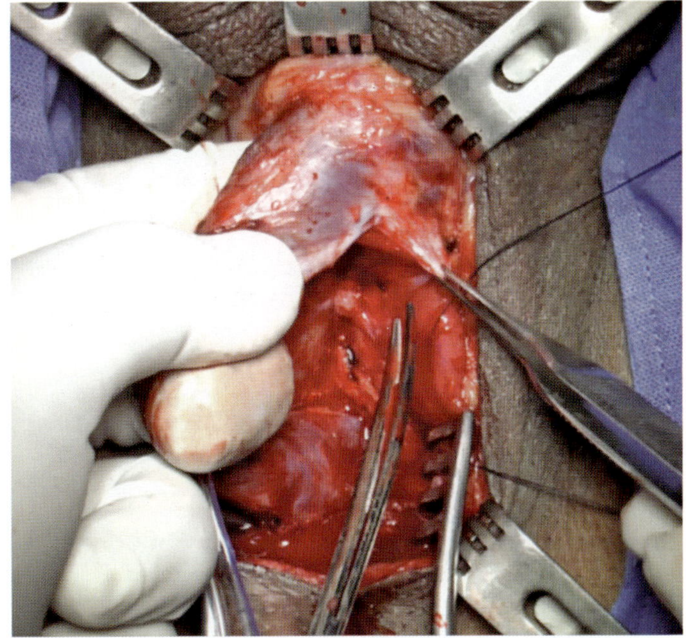

Fig. 9.4: Mobilization of the urethra proximal and distally

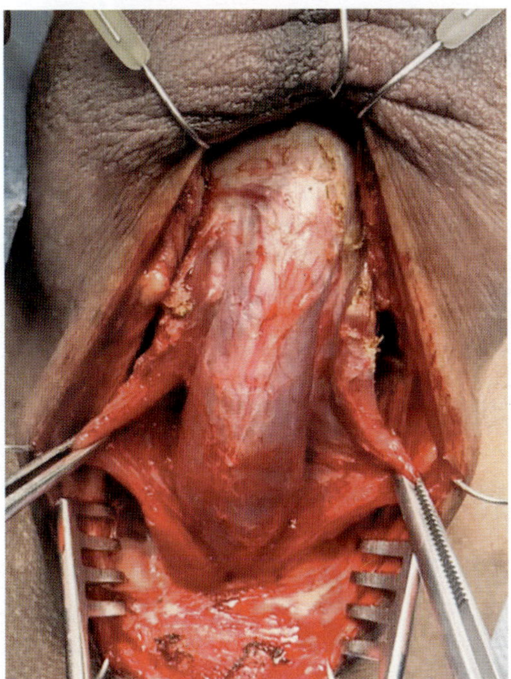

Fig. 9.3: Detaching of the bulbospongiosum muscle

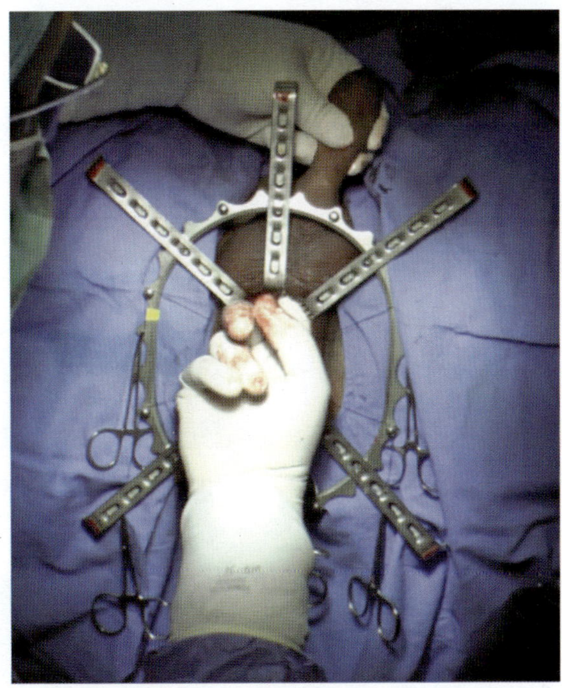

Fig. 9.5: Mobilization until penoscrotal junction

The proximal bulbar urethra is separated posteriorly from the perineal body (Fig. 9.4). The bulbar urethra should now be completely dissected until the peno-bulbar junction (Fig. 9.5). The remaining postero-lateral attachments are the points where the bulbar arteries enter into the corpus spongiosum on either side. In cases of pelvic fracture urethral injuries, they will need to be ligated and divided.

14 Fr blunt tip catheter or metal sound is then passed carefully down the urethra to the site of the obstruction. The urethra is then transected through the site of obliteration (Fig. 9.6). The scarred tissue is removed until healthy mucosa and spongy bleeding tissue is seen (Fig. 9.7).

The bulbourethral arteries tend to bleed at this point of surgery. The hemostasis can be achieved by 5 minutes compression with a gauze (Fig. 9.8).

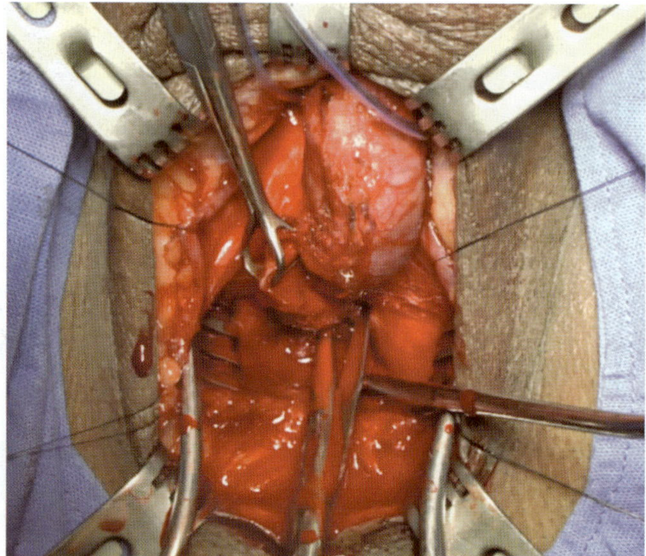

Fig. 9.6: Transection of the urethra in the scarred proximal urethra

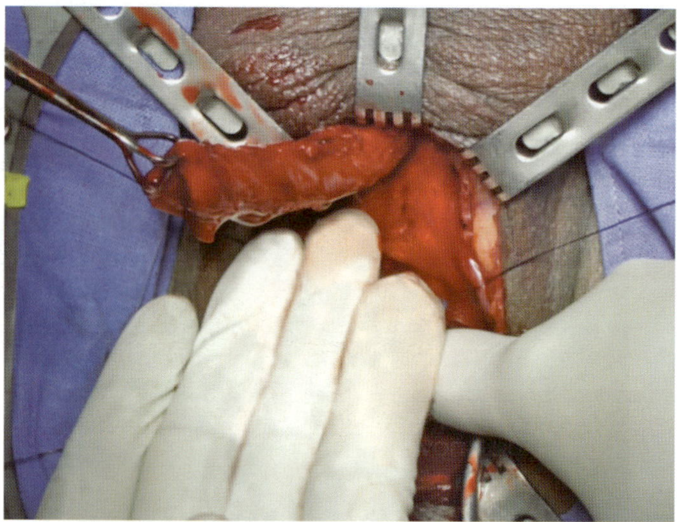

Fig. 9.7: Removed scarred tissue until spongy healthy bleeding and healthy mucosa is found

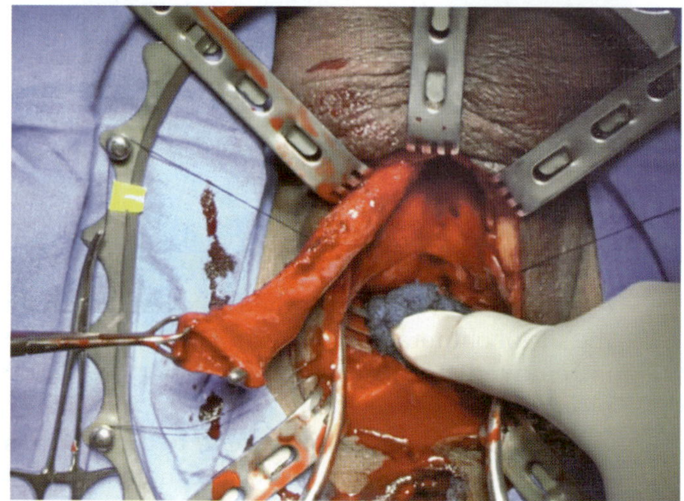

Fig. 9.8: Compression for bleeding control

Then the bulbar arteries can be ligated, fulgurated with cautery or bipolar forceps (Fig. 9.9).

The next step is the most critical and complex step of the surgery. Optimal scar excision is done between 9 and 3 o'clock. Posterior urethra is incised on a metal sound passed through suprapubic tract (Fig. 9.10).

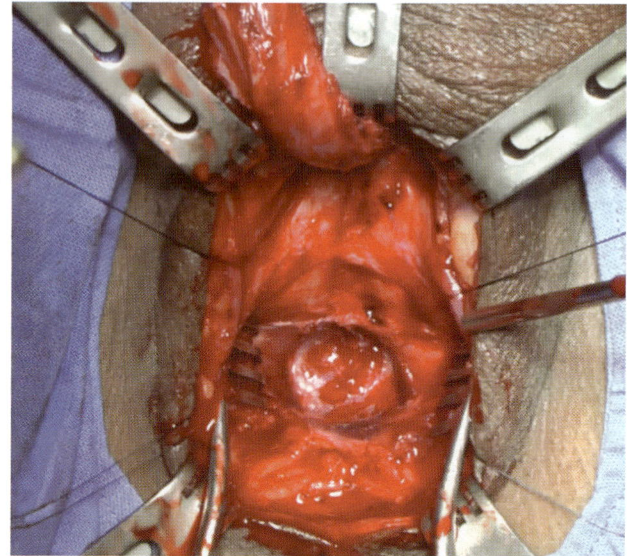

Fig. 9.9: Control of the bleeding

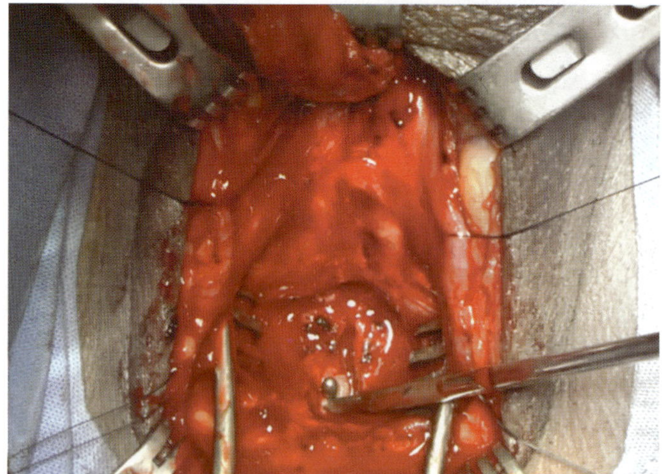

Fig. 9.10: Cutting in the tip of the metal sound

Other technique is called Hosseini technique. This involves use of a flexible cystoscope. The scope is passed through the bladder neck and the tip of the cystoscope is placed at the obliterated part of the proximal urethra. Then a needle is passed through the fibrotic tissue of the perineum until it reaches the proximal healthy urethra under direct endoscopic vision. A guidewire can be passed through the needle (Figs 9.11 and 9.12). The scar tissue is cut until the proximal healthy

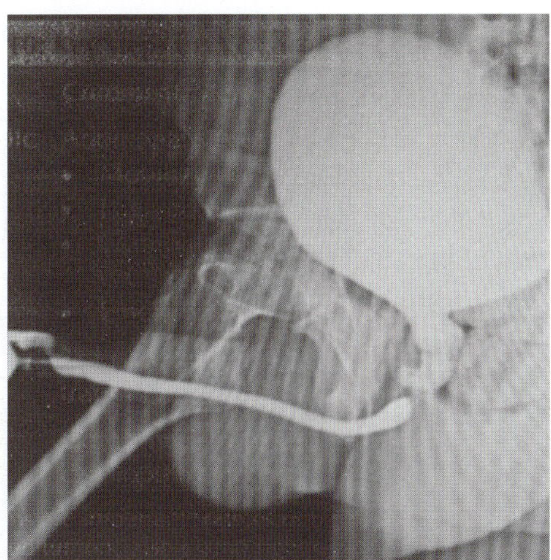

Fig. 9.11: Failed anastomosis trough a false passage

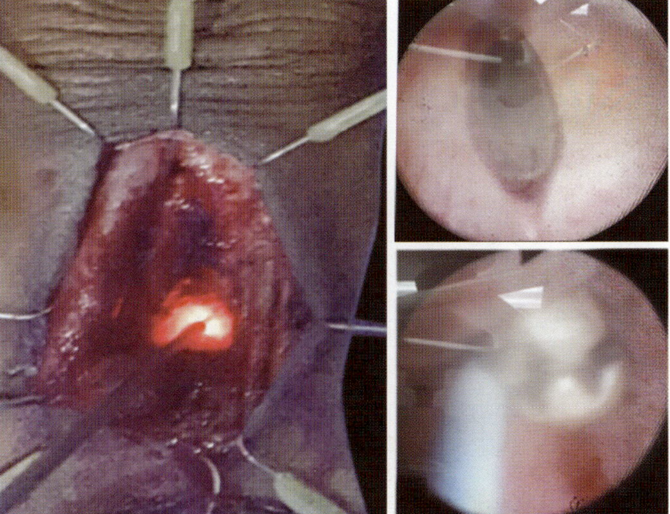

Fig. 9.12: Hosseini technique

urethra is found. This technique has two main advantages, we can avoid false passages and this helps in determining the abnormal placement of the proximal end of the urethra and its deviation on the rectum, lateral displacements and "S" shape deformity behind the pubis.[22]

The margins of the proximal urethra are then visualised (Fig. 9.13). Posterior urethra should appear pink and supple (Fig. 9.14).

The distal urethra is now spatulated 1 to 1.5 cm dorsally (Fig. 9.15).

Six 4/0 Vycril or polyglactin sutures are placed at 11, 1, 3, 9, 5 and 7 o' clock positions.

Then a 14 Fr or 16 Fr silicone Foley urethral catheter is placed and the sutures are tied in the parachute style (Fig. 9.16).

7. **How to perform crural separation?**[23]

Ans: The two cura are convex cylinders which are attached to each other in the midline. Crural

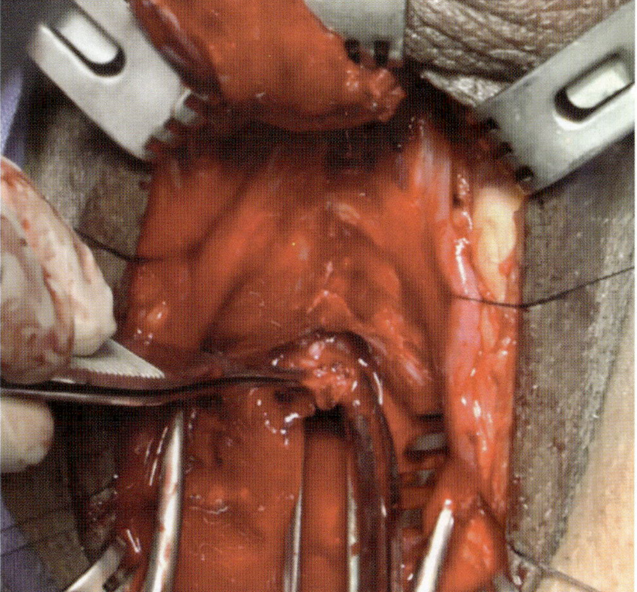

Fig. 9.13: Wide scared tissue removal

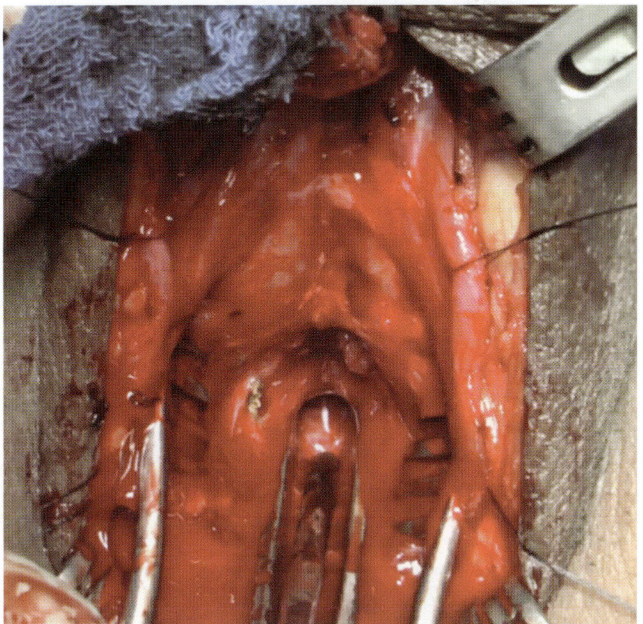

Fig. 9.14: Appearance of proximal healthy urethra

separation should be performed by sharp dissection using a knife or a scissor. A small incision is made in between the space of the two corpora.The incision is then carefully deepened. A mastoid forceps applied in the reverse manner helps in retraction of the corpora. Gentle dissection will expose the deep dorsal vein. Usual about 2 to 3 cm of crural separation is needed (Figs 9.17 and 9.18). This vein can be ligated or separated from the midline to preserve it. At the end of this maneuver, the urethra can lie within the inter-crural plane and tension on the anastomosis is reduced.

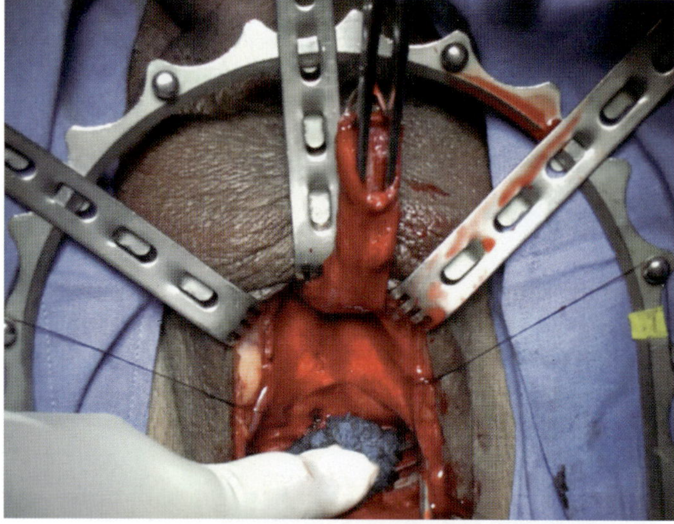

Fig. 9.15: Spatulated urethra

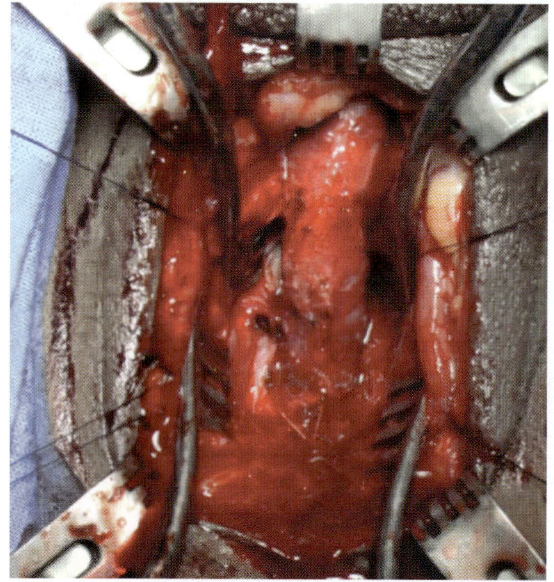

Fig. 9.16: Parachute style final anastomosis

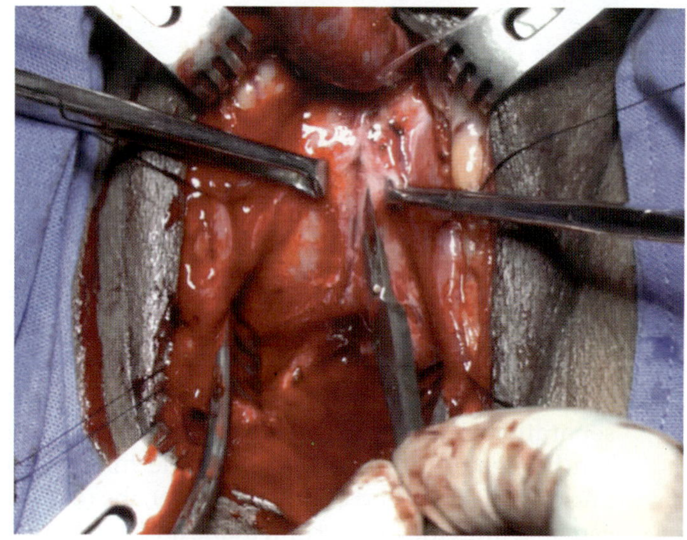

Fig. 9.17: Crural separation

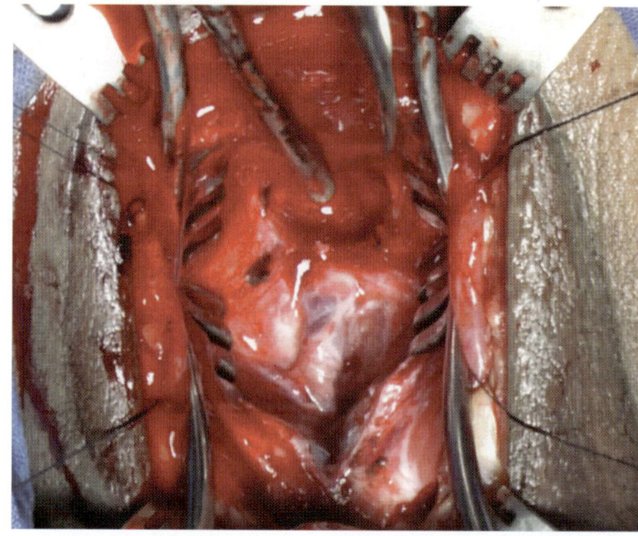

Fig. 9.18: Deep dorsal vein of the penis (arrow) during crural separation

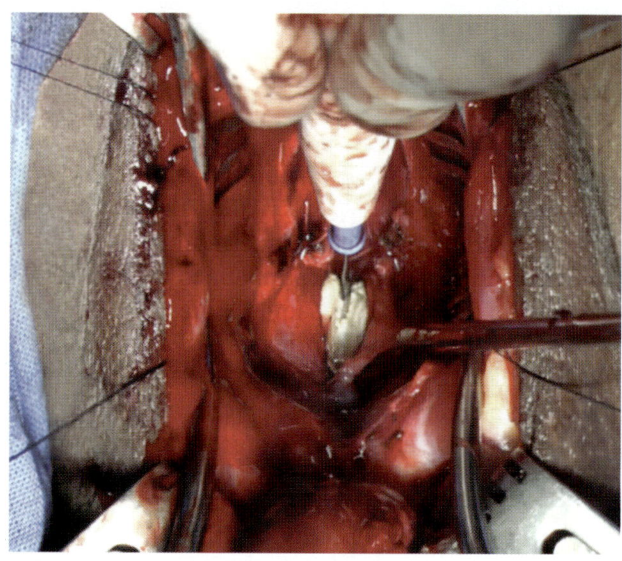

Fig. 9.19: Diathermy midline incision of the periosteum

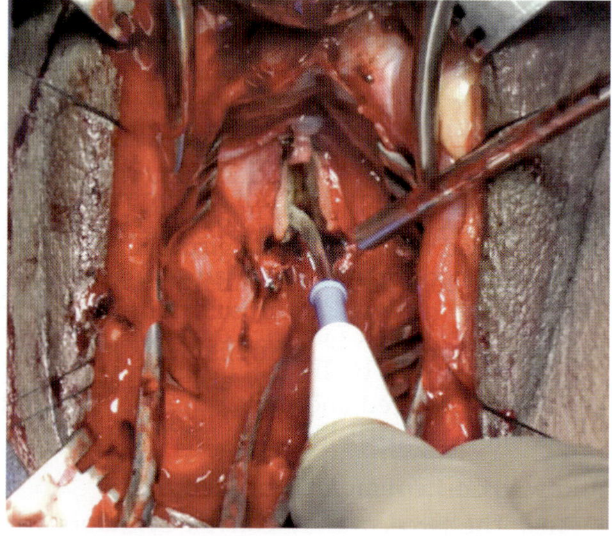

Fig. 9.20: Lateral detachment of the periosteum

8. **How to perform inferior pubectomy?**

A midline incision is made on the periosteum using an electrocautery. The incision on the periosteum is then extended laterally. To do this maneuver the tip of the cautery forceps is bent about 90 degrees. On exposing the periosteum the anterior and inferior bone of the pubis is exposed. The initial part of the pubectomy is superficial and wedge shaped. To perform deeper pubectomy the angle of the gauge to the pubic bone can be made horizontal (Figs 9.19 to 9.22).

9. **How to perform supracrural rerouting?**

Ans: In supracrural rerouting we take the urethra on the left side of the crura and perform direct anastomosis between the anterior and posterior ends. To perform this maneuver both the crura are identified. Lateral dissection is done in between the crura and the pubic bone. For a right-handed surgeon it is easier to do this section on the left side of the patient. After creating a space between the corpora and the pubic bone, an artery forceps is passed and the space is widened and some amount of pubectomy may be required so as to prevent obstruction to the urethra. This step of supracrural routing should rarely be done. The reason is, in case the patient needs a redo surgery, it would be very difficult to dissect the urethra between the superolateral and the posterolateral components. Theoretically it can also pose a risk while performing a penile prosthesis after supracrural rerouting.

10. **What is transpubic urethroplasty or abdominal perineal urethroplasty?**

Ans: Occasionally the gap in between the anterior and posterior urethra is too long and cannot be bridged through a perineal anastomosis. In those cases we require an abdomino-perineal reconstruction. This was first described by Waterhouse and then perfected by Turner-Warwick. This includes an initial surgery which is done through the perineal approach, the bulbar urethra is mobilised and transacted. Crural separation is performed and inferior pubectomy is performed. Then a midline abdominal incision is made. Appropriate amount of superior and posterior pubectomy is performed to reach the scar above the prostate. The scar above the prostate is then excised. A window is created in between the perineum and the abdomen. In the initial part of the description of abdominoperineal approach the entire pubic bone was removed. This led to waddling gait and formation of hernia. In the new modified technique we do not reset the anterior part of pubic bone. The arc is kept intact. Just a wedge superior and posterior pubectomy is performed. Once an abdominoperineal window is created, the scar is excised. We can then identify the posterior urethra through a dilator passed through the suprapubic track. The anastomosis is then done between the anterior and posterior urethra.

SUMMARY

- Anastomotic urethroplasty is the standard of care for management of pelvic fracture urethral injury
- The steps of anastomotic urethroplasty have been explained in details in the chapter
- Optimal scar excision and crural separation and inferior pubectomy are key steps for success of anastomotic urethroplasty.
- Abdomino-perineal approach is occasionally required in management of pelvic fracture urethral injury.
- The success rate of anastomotic urethroplasty should be above 90%.

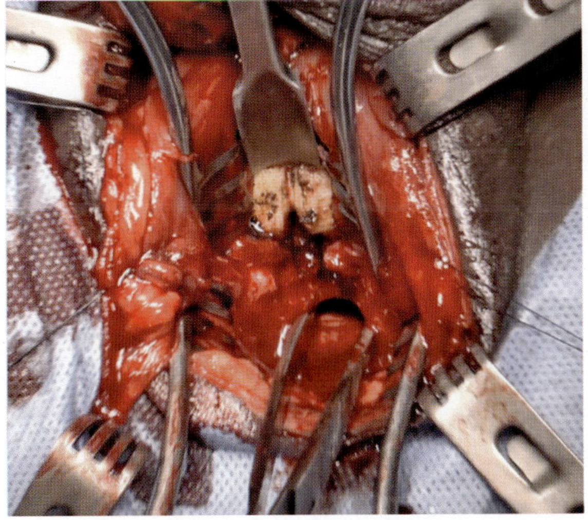

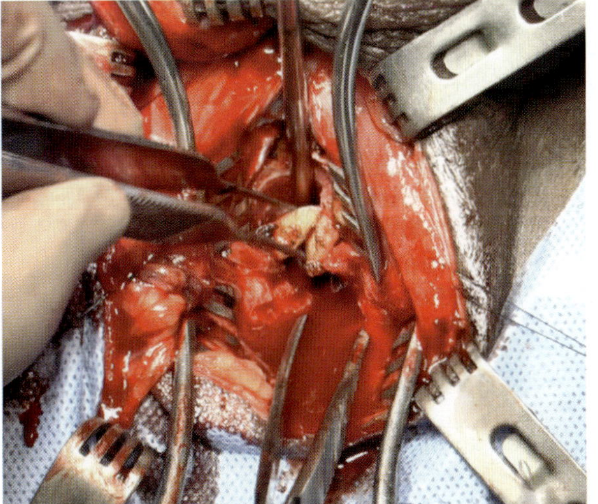

Figs 9.21 and 9.22: Inferior pubectomy

REFERENCES

1. J.M. Latini, J.W. McAninch, S.B. Brandes, J.Y. Chung, D. Rosenstein SIU/ICUD consultation on urethral strictures: epidemiology, etiology, anatomy, and nomenclature of urethral stenoses, strictures, and pelvic fracture urethral disruption injuries Urology, 83 (Suppl. 3) (2014), pp. S1-S7
2. Demetriades D, Karaiskakis M, Toutouzas K, Alo K, Velmahos G, Chan L. Pelvic fractures: epidemiology and predictors of associated abdominal injuries and outcomes. J Am Coll Surg 2002; 195:1–10.
3. Palmer, J.K., Benson, G.S. and Corriere, J N., Jr.: Diagnosis and initial management of urological injuries associated with 200 consecutive pelvic fractures. J Urol 1983, 130: 712.
4. Fallon, B, Wendt, J.C and Hawtrey, C.E: Urological injury and assessment in patients with fractured pelvis. J Urol., 1984, 131. 712.
5. Kulkarni SB, Barbagli G, Kulkarni JS, Romano G and Lazzeri M. J Urol, 2010. 183, 1049–54.
6. Tausch T J, Calvalcanti A G, Soderdahl D W, Favorito L, Rabelo P and Morey A F. Gunshot Wound Injuries of the Prostate and posterior urethra: Reconstructive Armamentarium. J Urol. 2007, 178, 1346–48.
7. Rosenberg S, Joshi P, Laerence A, Surana S, Alhajeri F and Kulkarni S B. Management of female urethral trauma. J Urol, 2014. 191 (suppl 4),pp. 129.
8. Clark SS, Prudencio RF. Lower urinary tract injuries associated with pelvic fractures. Surg Clinics North Am. 1972;52: 183–20
9. Mouraviev VB and Santucci RA: Cadaveric anatomy of pelvic fracture urethral distraction injury: most injuries are distal to the external urinary sphincter. J Urol 2005; 173: 86 9.
10. Andrich, D. E. and Mundy, A. R.: The nature of urethral injury in cases of pelvic fracture urethral trauma. J Urol, 2001. 165: 1492–5.
11. Whitson JM, Mc Aninch JW, Tanagho EA, Metro JM and Rahman NU. Mechanism of continence after repair of posterior urethral disruption: Evidence of Rhabdosphincter activity. J Urol2008; 179: 1035–1039.
12. Andrich, D. E. and Mundy, A. R.: The nature of urethral injury in cases of pelvic fracture urethral trauma. J Urol, 2001. 165: 1492–5
13. Mundy, A. R.: The role of delayed primary repair in the acute management of pelvic fracture injuries of the urethra. Br J Urol, 1991. 68 (3): 273–6.
14. Morey AF, McAninch JW. Reconstruction of posterior urethral disruption injuries: outcome analysis in 82 patients. J Urol 1997; 157:506–10.
15. Kulkarni SB, Barbagli G, Kulkarni JS, Romano G and Lazzeri M. J Urol, 2010. 183, 1049–54.
16. Tausch T J, Calvalcanti A G, Soderdahl D W, Favorito L, Rabelo P and Morey A F. Gunshot Wound Injuries of the Prostate and posterior urethra: Reconstructive Armamentarium. J Urol. 2007, 178, 1346–4
17. Colapinto V, MacCallum RM. Injury to the male posterior urethra in fractured pelvis, a new classification. J Urol 1977; 18: 575.
18. Goldman SM, Sandler CM, Corriere JN, McGuire EJ. Blunt urethral trauma a unified, anatomical mechanical classification. J Urol 1997; 157: 85–9.
19. Fu Q, Sun X, Tang C, Cui R and Chen L. J Sex Med. 2012, 9. 282–87.
20. Koraitim MM. Predictors of erectile dysfunction post pelvic fracture urethral injuries: a multivariate analysis. Urology. 2013, 81. 1081–85.
21. Zukerman J, Mc Cammon K, Tisdale B, Colen T, Urosjie T, McAdams P, Jordan G. Urology 2012, 80,6. 1369–74.
22. Hosseini SJ, Kaviani A, Jabbari M, Hosseini MM, Haji-Mohammadmehdi-Arab A, Simaei NR. Diagnostic application of flexible cystoscope in pelvic fracture urethral distraction defects. J Urol. 2006;3: 204–7.
23. Joshi P, Desai D, Surana S, Orabi H, Kulkarni SB. PD 29–11 Magnetic Resonance Imaging (MRI) in pelvic fracture imaging injuries to evaluate urethral gap: a new point of technique. 2017; 197 (4) suppl. e 576–77.

Chapter

10

Perineal Urethrostomy for Urethral Stricture

• Shailesh Shah • Utsav Shah

LEARNING OBJECTIVES

- To understand the indications of perineal urethrostomy.
- To learn the various techniques of perineal urethrostomy.
- To understand the complications and overall management.
- To enlighten the reader about urinary function and the quality of life post-perineal urethrostomy.

INTRODUCTION

Perineal urethrostomy is a technique of creation of a urethral opening in the perineum for expulsion of urine and semen. The patient needs to sit and void after undergoing this procedure. This procedure is often undertaken for complex, recurrent anterior urethral strictures either as a first step of a staged procedure or as a definitive procedure. It is beneficial to patients who want a single stage repair in a complex stricture and offers good voiding as well as sexual quality of life.

Case Scenario

A 79-year-old gentleman from rural background, a devoted Muslim, uncontrolled diabetic, hypertensive with a history of tobacco chewing since the past 52 years came with complaints of difficulty in passing urine since 12 years. He has undergone buccal mucosal graft urethroplasty 10 years ago followed by DVIU 3 times and multiple episodes of urethral dilatation every 3–6 months. Clinical examination revealed BXO changes over glans with induration along the entire penile urethra. An ascending urethrogram (AUG) revealed penile urethral stricture with a poorly distensible urethra and a normal bulbar and posterior urethra. The patient expresses a preference for a single-stage repair, emphasizing the desire for an approach that boasts a high success rate.

1. **What is the next step for this patient?**

   Ans: In order to provide this patient long-term success, it is imperative that he undergoes a definitive surgical repair which is long lasting. It should be borne in mind that he has previously undergone anterior urethroplasty which subsequently failed.

2. **What are the usual reasons or scenarios where an anterior urethroplasty might fail?**

   Ans: Anterior urethroplasty failure requiring a repeat procedure is associated with longer strictures, prior urethroplasty, failed hypospadias and lichen sclerosus.[1,2]

3. **What would be the surgical approach in this case?**

   Ans: This patient desires a permanent cure with an approach which has the least chance of recurrent stricture. A urethroplasty in this case would expose the patient to up to a 50% chance of failure considering his lichen sclerosis, past history of failed urethroplasty and long stricture length.[3] In such a case, a perineal urethrostomy is a good option.[4]

4. **How does perineal urethrostomy affect patient's quality of life?**

   Ans: Perineal urethrostomy has been reported to be a satisfactory solution especially in the elderly who are fine with expulsion of urine and semen from a perineal opening.[4] In a comprehensive evaluation comparing functional and quality of life outcomes, including sexual function, between anterior urethroplasty and perineal urethrostomy in men with extended urethral stricture disease, it was observed that perineal urethrostomy resulted in enhanced urinary function without any adverse impact on sexual function.[5]

5. What are the pre-requisites for a perineal urethrostomy?

Ans:

- A preoperative sterile urine culture is mandatory
- A healthy perineum and perineal skin
- Consideration of perineal urethrostomy should include assessing the patient's acceptance of certain aspects, such as the necessity to sit while urinating and the inability to inseminate into the vagina.

6. Briefly describe the various techniques for creating a perineal urethrostomy.

Ans:

1. **Percutaneous endoscopically guided perineal urethrostomy:** The resectoscope is inserted antegrade via the SPC tract in the bulbar urethra and is pressed against the perineum. A small incision is made in the area over the tip of the resectoscope, allowing the scope to be advanced through the incision. Subsequently, a larger sheath is placed over the resectoscope sheath. The larger sheath is then slowly withdrawn while visually hugging the dorsal aspect of the urethra. Care is taken to redirect it into the proximal urethra and then advance it into the bladder. A Foley catheter is positioned over a guidewire, and no suturing is required.[6]

   This procedure is largely condemned due to high re-stenosis rates and should be avoided.
2. **The end urethral stump perineal urethrostomy:** A sound is passed through a pre-placed suprapubic catheter (SPC), and pressure is applied from inside the urethra onto the perineal region. The urethra is then opened vertically over the sound, and after spatulation, its edges are sutured to the perineal skin.
3. **The grooved sound technique:** A grooved sound is passed through the penile external urethral meatus and maneuvered up to the prostatic urethra. The perineal skin is then incised vertically while palpating until the groove of the sound is felt. The urethra is stabilized between the fingers, and after the urethra is opened, the edge of the urethral mucosa is grasped and sutured to the skin with absorbable suture.[7]
4. **The "7-flap" perineal urethrostomy:** In this technique, a number '7'-shaped perineal skin flap is utilized to create a urethrostomy.[8] This method enables the formation of a flap that can be customized precisely to the required length, addressing challenges in obese patients during the execution of a posterior-based flap urethroplasty.
5. **The posterior flap-based perineal urethrostomy with preservation of dorsal plate (described by Johanson and modified by Blandy):**[4]
   After creating an inverted U-shaped perineal incision, the bulbar urethra is completely mobilized and ventrally opened. The apex of the inverted U-incision is then re-approximated to the edge of the urethra using interrupted absorbable sutures. It is hypothesized that leaving the dorsal plate intact promotes the continuation of retrograde blood flow to the urethra. This preservation of blood flow theoretically enhances the vascular supply to the reconstructed area, reducing the risk of subsequent restenosis (Fig. 10.1).

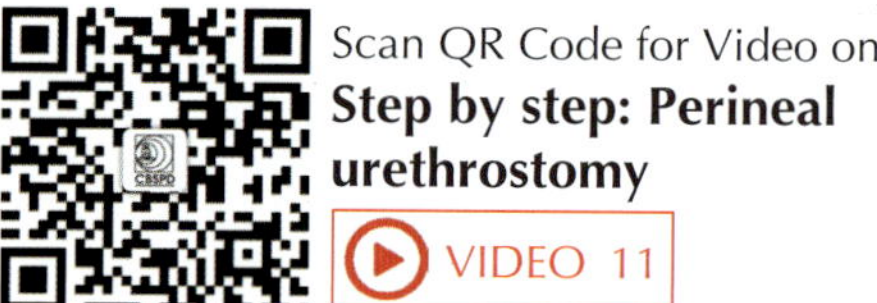

7. What are the common complications after perineal urethrostomy?

Ans: The most concerning complication associated with perineal urethrostomy is the recurrence of stenosis, even after the creation of a perineal urethrostomy with a wide base and caliber.[9] Other complications include postoperative bleeding and infections. Lithotomy position related neuropathy, hip and back pain and rarely deep vein thrombosis are encountered.

8. How to deal with stenosis of perineal urethrostomy?

Ans: To start, patients can be managed with self-calibration, which is a convenient and well-tolerated method through the perineal urethrostomy, effectively bypassing the majority of the urethral stricture disease.

However, if the stenosis is severe or unrelenting, definitive repair is an option. Definitive treatment of recalcitrant perineal urethrostomy is challenging especially in patients with lichen sclerosus. A technique of placing buccal mucosae at 4, 7 and 12 o' clock positions in a stenotic perineal urethrostomy has been described with excellent results.[10]

9. How does perineal urethrostomy affect the patient's sexual function?

Ans: Unlike urethroplasty in complex strictures after which erections might be affected due to extensive dissection and mobilization, perineal urethrostomy does not lead to erectile dysfunction.

Patients need to be counselled about ejaculation through the perineal opening during intercourse or masturbation. A questionnaire based assessment of sexual function following perineal urethrostomy revealed that almost 82% of patients had no problems with their partner with regard to sexual activity or any psychological problem.[4]

10. Which group of patients generally select perineal urethrostomy?

Ans: Perineal urethrostomy has often been cited as a technique not offering permanent cure and hence should be chosen wisely.[11] However, it has been seen that the idea of using perineal urethrostomy only as the 'last resort' leads to dissatisfaction by the patients who complain why they were not given this option earlier.[12]

In India, patients who generally opt for perineal urethrostomy are:

- Those who have no issues in urinating in a sitting position
- Patients who are not concerned about expulsion of semen through the perineal opening
- Patients with complex strictures (with or without previously failed surgeries) who wish to have a successful surgical result in a single stage. (It should be noted that perineal urethrostomy done in a patient who has undergone previous urethral repairs might have a bulbar urethra with a poor blood supply; thus reducing success rates in such cases of perineal urethrostomy.)
- Patients who live in a rural area with limited access to urological help and those who are financially challenged.

Often, when perineal urethrostomy is performed in a staged setting (Johanson stage 1), many patients do not return to get operated for stage 2 in view of excellent first stage results.[13] This might probably be a result of patients' concerns about undergoing a secondary procedure to close the urethrostomy, particularly for erect voiding. The realization of the potential for recurrent stricture in the reconstructed urethra may contribute to this anxiety.[14]

KEY POINTS

- Perineal urethrostomy offers an option in complex, recalcitrant and recurrent penile urethral stricture cases where patients are tired of repeated procedures and want a definitive repair in single stage.
- Before embarking upon perineal urethrostomy, it is important to ensure a sterile urine culture alongwith the patient's acceptability regarding the need to sit and void.
- A good vascular flap-based technique of creating a perineal urethrostomy reduces the risk of stenosis.
- Perineal urethrostomy stands as a viable option, providing comparable, if not superior, urinary function without compromising sexual well-being in comparison to urethroplasty for long and complex anterior urethral strictures.

REFERENCES

1. Palminteri E, Brandes SB and Djordjevic M: Urethral reconstruction in lichen sclerosus. Curr Opin Urol 2012; 22: 478.
2. Kulkarni S, Kulkarni J, Surana S *et al*. Management of panurethral stricture. Urol Clin North Am 2017; 44: 67.
3. Lumen N, Beysens M, Van Praet C, Decaestecker K, Spinoit A-F, Hoebeke P, *et al.* Perineal urethrostomy: Surgical and functional evaluation of two techniques. BioMed Research International. 2015;2015:1–6.
4. Barbagli G, De AM, Romano G, Lazzeri M. Clinical outcome and quality of life assessment in patients treated with perineal urethrostomy for anterior urethral stricture disease. J Urol. 2009;182(2):548–57.
5. Murphy GP, Fergus KB, Gaither TW, Baradaran N, Voelzke BB, Myers JB, *et al.* Urinary and sexual function after perineal urethrostomy for urethral stricture disease: An analysis from the turns. Journal of Urology. 2019;201(5):956–61.
6. Sokoloff MH, Michel K, Smith RB. Complications of transurethral resection of the prostate. In: Taneja SS, Smith RB, Ehrlich RM, editors. Complications of urologic surgery: prevention and management. 3rd ed. Philadelphia: W.B. Saunders Company; 2001. p. 229–43.
7. Clark PB. Non-continent urinary diversion: perineal urethrostomy. In: Hinmnan F, editor. Atlas of urologic surgery. 2nd ed. Philadelphia: W. B. Saunders Company; 1998. p. 623–76.
8. French D, Hudak SJ, Morey AF. The "7-flap" perineal urethrostomy. Urology. 2011;77(6):1487–9.
9. Peterson AC. Perineal urethrostomy. Advanced Male Urethral and Genital Reconstructive Surgery. 2013;:457–68.
10. Kamat N. Perineal urethrostomy stenosis repair with buccal mucosa: description of technique and report of four cases. Urology. 2008;72(5):1153–5
11. Kulkarni SB. Perineal urethrostomy: Useless and use less!! International Journal of Reconstructive Urology. 2023;1(1):2.
12. Jackson MJ, Sciberras J, Mangera A, Brett A, Watkin N, N'Dow JMO, *et al.* Defining a patient-reported outcome measure for urethral stricture surgery. European Urology. 2011;60(1):60–8.
13. Singhal A, Arya MC, Vasudeo V, Shyoran Y, Gandhi A, Maan R, *et al.* Perineal urethrostomy: A single-stage viable option for complex anterior urethral strictures. Urology Annals. 2021;13(2):142.
14. Yadav P, Danish N, Sureka SS, Rustagi S, Kapoor R, Srivastava A, *et al.* Permanent perineal urethrostomy for anterior urethral strictures: A critical appraisal of long-term outcomes and erectile function. Türk Üroloji Dergisi/Turkish Journal of Urology. 2021;47(2):158–63.

Chapter 11

Redo Urethroplasty

• Gaurang Shah • PVLN Murthy

LEARNING OBJECTIVES

- To understand the evaluation and the etiopathogenesis of the failure of primary urethroplasty.
- To understand how to overcome challenges associated with redo urethroplasty.
- To understand the important investigations required before proceeding with redo surgery.
- To understand the algorithmic approach to a patient with recurrent urethral stricture and failed urethroplasty.
- To understand the tips and tricks to ensure good vascularity and maintain a tension free anastomosis so as to improve success rate of redo urethroplasty.
- To understand the various graft options and surgeries for redo urethroplasty.
- To understand the difficulties associated with redo urethroplasty in pediatric age group.
- To assess outcome and follow-up of redo urethroplasty.

INTRODUCTION

Surgery for stricture urethra is very challenging and hence many surgeons opt for the simpler endourological approach to treat them by doing direct vision internal urethrotomy (DVIU). Amongst proximal and distal urethral strictures, pelvic fracture urethral distraction defects (PFUDD) may be considered to be surgically one of the most difficult procedures performed by the treating urologist. Anastomotic urethroplasty is the established surgical procedure for the treatment of PFUDD.

Progressive perineal anastomotic repair of PFUDD is well established. But redo surgery after the failure of primary repair is extremely difficult.

The associated loss of tissue, impaired vascularity, fibrosis with loss of planes, proximity to rectum, limited space to operate and demanding on-table decisions regarding the reconstructive procedure further adds to the complexity of the surgical procedure.

Before doing a redo urethroplasty, it is very important to know the details about the previous surgery and the post-operative course.

The help of an experienced surgeon improves the surgical outcomes.

Urethral strictures can be extremely treacherous and can make the patient incapacitated as it can lead to infertility, impotence and incontinence.

Case Scenario

A 6-year-old boy had met with a road traffic accident with pelvic fracture and urethral distraction defect (PFUDD) and left femur fracture with shortened left lower limb. Suprapubic catheterization was done in emergency with stabilization of the femur. Six months later after work up (Fig. 11.1), he was operated for progressive perineal urethroplasty.

Thereafter, the patient was adequately passing urine per urethra for 15 days after which he developed difficulty in passing urine and went into retention. PUC could not be negotiated and hence, SPC was reinserted. Patient was evaluated with RUG and VCUG which showed complete bulbar urethral necrosis (Figs 11.2 and 11.3). He was treated by redo urethroplasty using a penile circular fasciocutaneous flap over 8 Fr Foley's catheter.

1. **What is the definition of recurrent urethral stricture?**

   Ans: Failure after primary urethroplasty should be suspected when patient has recurrent urinary symptoms, Q_{max} on uroflowmetry is <15 ml/s and there is recurrence of stricture on imaging which usually requires additional intervention after the primary urethroplasty which may include dilatations, urethrotomies or redo urethroplasty.[1–3]

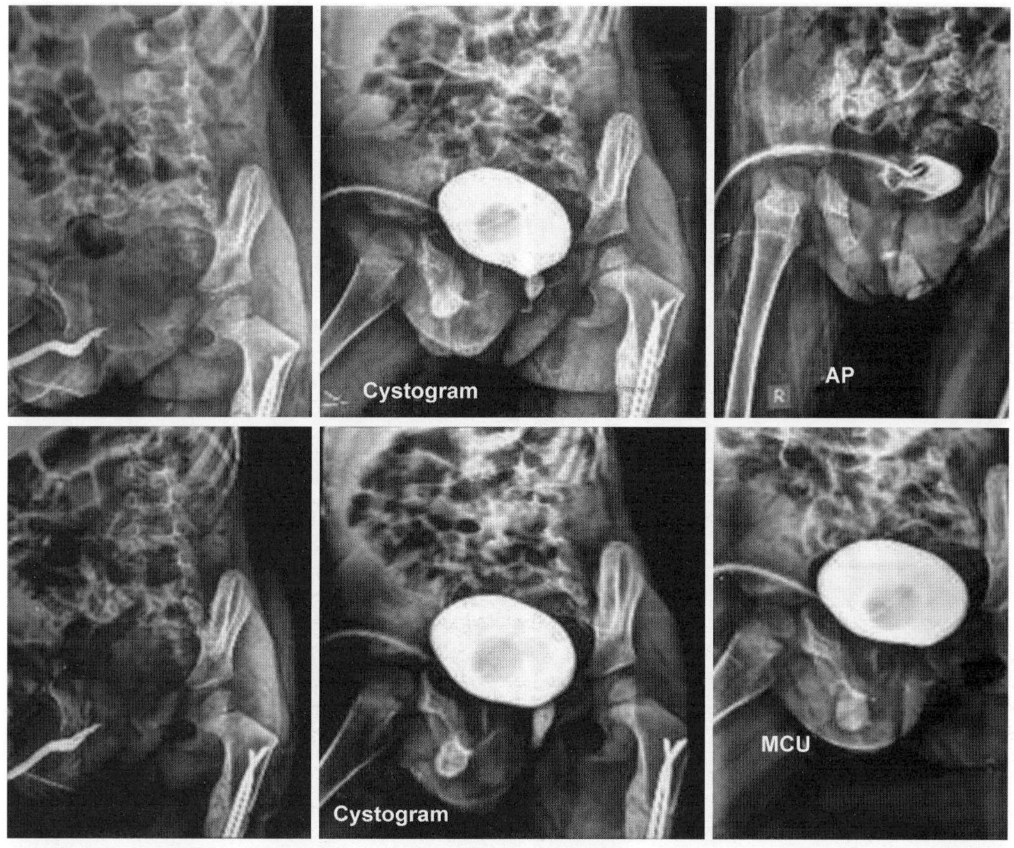

Fig. 11.1: ASU (ascending cystourethrogram) and VCUG (voiding cystourethrogram) prior to first urethroplasty

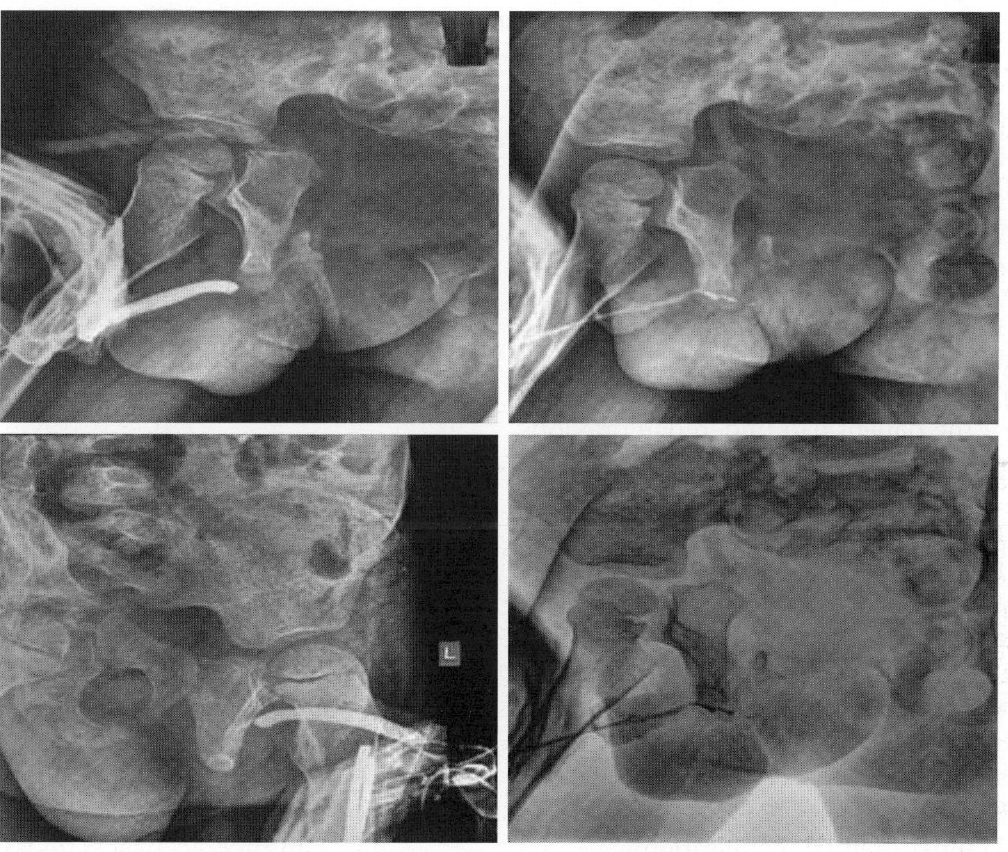

Fig. 11.2: RUG prior to redo urethroplasty

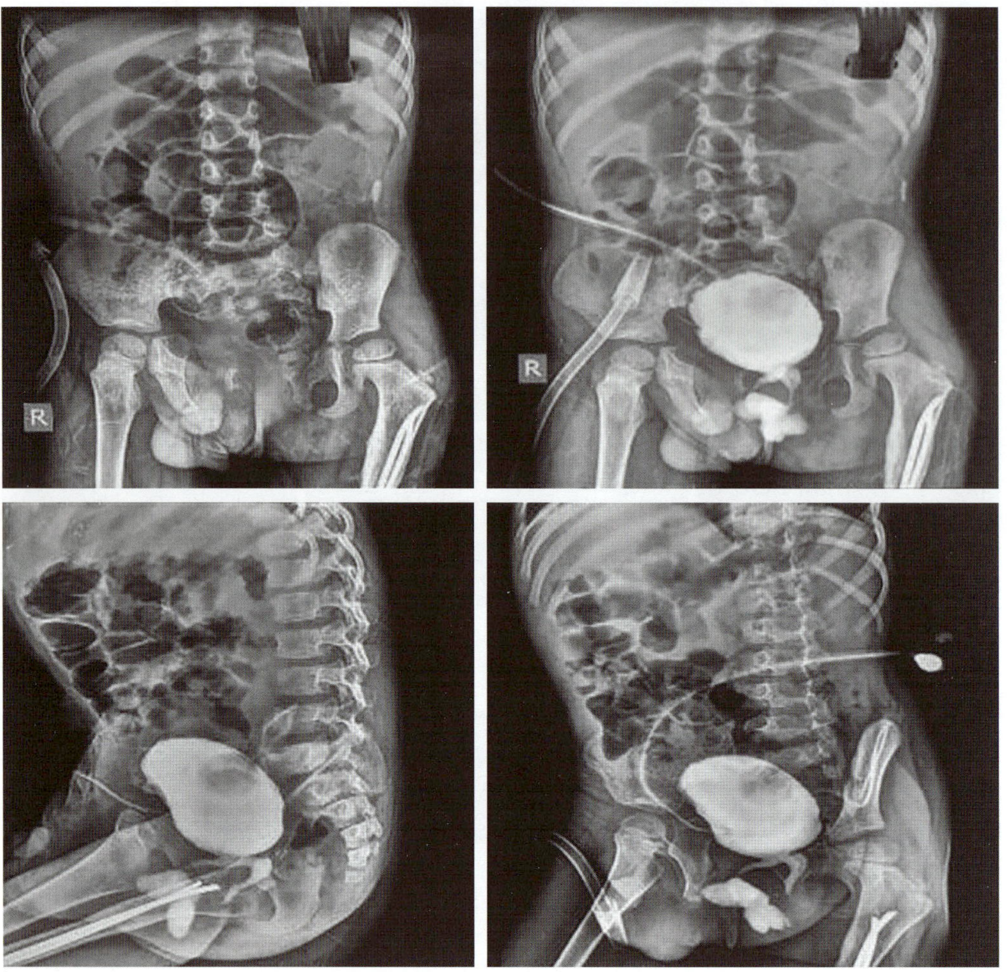

Fig. 11.3: VCUG prior to redo urethroplasty

2. What is the incidence and etiopathogenesis of recurrence of stricture after urethroplasty?

Ans: Incidence of urethral stricture recurrence ranges between 2 and 36.4% with 75% occurring within the first 6 months after surgery.[4]

- Prior manipulation—failure rate doubled from 14.3% for patients without any prior manipulation to 27.6% for those with multiple dilations and an even greater failure rate (31.6%) if the patient had undergone previous urethroplasty.
- Urinary infection—patients with preoperative urinary tract infection had twice as many failures (28.6%) as were noted in those with sterile urine (14.5%).[5]
- Technical factors as follows:
  - Inadequate excision of scar tissue or anastomosis to avascular fibrotic apex with unhealthy adherent mucosa.
  - Anastomosis to false passage.
  - Anastomosis under tension due to inadequate distal bulbar urethral mobilisation.[5–7]

3. How will you evaluate the patient of failed primary urethroplasty?

Ans:

- Detailed history
- Thorough clinical examination
- USG KUB with PVR
- Uroflowmetry
- **Retrograde urethrography (RUG) and voiding cystourethrography (VCUG)** are still the most commonly used diagnostic tools.

  The advantages are that it instantly diagnoses the location, number and length of the strictures and also enables diagnosis of urethral wall damage, fistula or false passage.

  The disadvantages are that it does not provide assessment of pathologies that extend beyond the urethral lumen.[8]
- **Sonourethrography:** Benefits are that it allows assessment of the bulbar urethra stricture length more accurately than RUG and it helps to detects periurethral spongiofibrosis.[9] It also has a higher accuracy for strictures arising

from traumatic catheterizations and idiopathic stenosis compared to VCUG. The technique is straightforward, readily available and cost effective.

The drawbacks are that it has a lower accuracy in evaluation of post-traumatic strictures which are usually located in the bulbar urethra, often difficult or impossible to be depicted by SUG, especially in obese patients. It is a highly subjective study and it is relatively easy to over-diagnose a urethral stricture if the ultrasound probe is used with too much pressure on the urethra during the test. Also the assessment of multiple or long strictures is limited because of small field-of-view.[10]

- **Rigid and flexible suprapubic cystoscopy:** It is very useful for diagnosis of bladder neck false passages, which are mainly caused by previous manipulations. It helps in evaluation of proximal urethral length and fistula, especially when the proximal urethra is not visualized on voiding cystography. It helps in assessment of cases in which there is serious damage resulting in severe deformation of the pelvis and posterior urethra. It also allows accurate determination of the severe proximal deviation of the urethral end and helps us do an exact and sighted opening of the posterior urethra in such cases.[11]
- **Urethro-cystoscopy:** Direct visual assessment of the appearance along the length of the urethra up to the beginning of the stricture and a direct visual assessment of the calibre of the distal aspect of the stricture.[11]
- **Magnetic resonance urethrography [MRU]:** It provides excellent soft tissue contrast, and depicts the urethra and periurethral structures without exposure to radiation. MRU is also reported to show particular effectiveness in diagnosing strictures that occur after pelvic injuries, providing additional information about the prostatic apex displacement.[12]

4. How will you approach a case of recurrent urethral stricture?

Ans: The algorithm is given in Flowchart 11.1[13]

Internal urethrotomy has long been recognized as a temporizing measure for urethral stricture disease with a low success rate and a decreasing success rate with repeat procedures.[14]

Urethroplasty is the gold standard treatment with better success rate and cost effectiveness.[4,15]

5. How will you assess stricture length and what is meant by gapometery index?

Ans: Preoperative voiding cystourethrogam (VCUG) and retrograde urethrogram (RUG) films can be used to assess length of stricture and to calculate the gapometry index.

Gapometry index (G/U index) is defined as the length of urethral gap divided by the bulbar urethral length.[16]

Flowchart 11.1: Algorithm for management of redo strictures

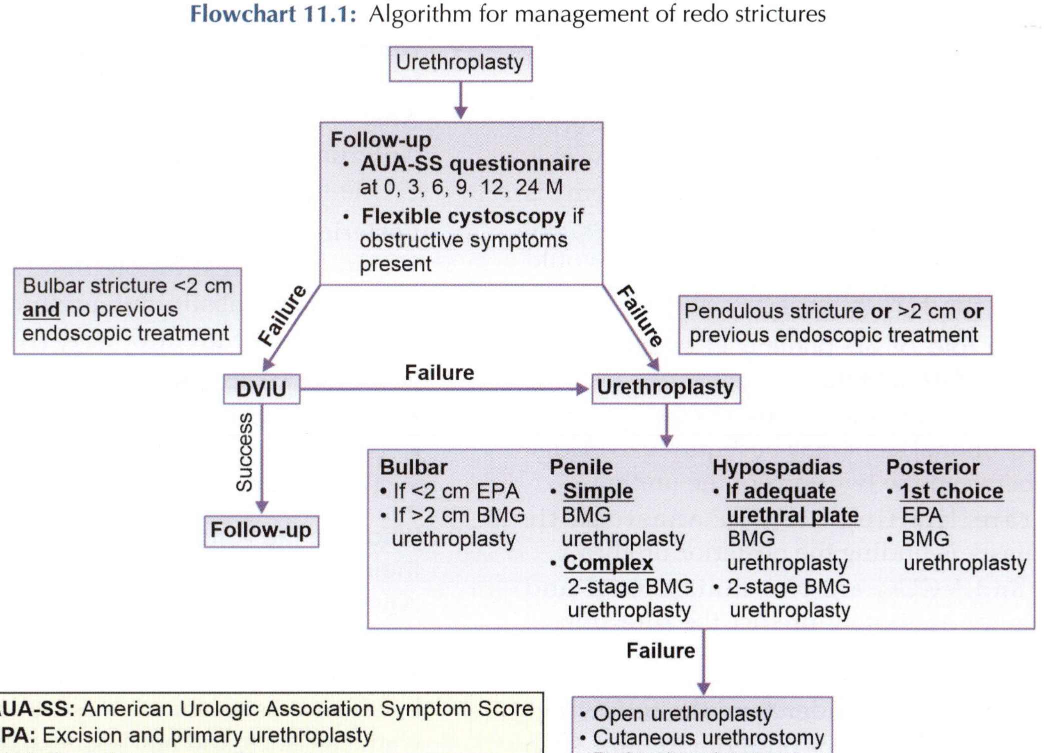

$$\text{Index of elastic lengthening} = \frac{\text{Bulboprostatic urethral gap}}{\text{Length of bulbar urethra}}$$

< 0.35 simple perineal operation.

>0.35 elaborated perineal or transpubic procedure.

Magnetic resonance urethrography (MRU) is done with the penis in a flaccid state. A catheter with attached syringe filled with 10–20 ml of sterile lubricating anesthetic gel is introduced into the urethral meatus and gel is infused to distend the urethra sufficiently. Multiplanar images are obtained to outline the entire length of the urethra.

Total stricture length is measured with inclusion of tapered segments on either side of the tight stricture. Spongiofibrosis is depicted on T1- and T2-weighted images as hypointense areas distinguishable from normal spongy tissue. Contrast-enhanced MRI may have an advantage in cases of extensive tumors and inflammation involving the urethra and periurethral tissues.[12]

6. How will you judge need of pubectomy using radiological investigation?

Ans: Conventional assessments include RUG and VCUG. However, the accuracy of these assessments is limited when the urethral gap of the bladder neck is not open, there is prostatic displacement on the horizontal or vertical axis, and when the condition is complicated, e.g. fistula, diverticula, or false passages.

MRI has been used in complex PFUI cases to overcome these limitations.

A horizontal line is drawn from the lower edge of the pubic bone anteriorly to the rectum, posteriorly in the sagittal image. If the tip of the posterior urethra (membranous urethra) is seen below this horizontal line, the need for inferior pubectomy is low, but if the tip is above this horizontal line, the risk is high. A high-lying posterior urethra would indicate the need for a transpubic approach.[17]

7. What is the role of 3D printing in evaluation of recurrent stricture urethra?

Ans: The most unpredictable part of the operation is what additional steps may be required to bridge the gap between the two ends of the urethra.

The rate limiting step in anastomotic urethroplasty is finding the posterior urethra.

RUG and VCUG are two dimensional and hence cannot accurately predict the direction of the posterior urethra.

3D printing can help understand the following:

- Complex anatomy of the posterior urethra, such as re-redo PFUI, bulbar necrosis, rectourethral fistula, young girls with urethrovaginal fistula, bladder neck injury, and double block.
- Its distance from the rectum,
- Length of the urethral gap,
- Relation to the posterior urethra,
- Direction of displacement of the urethra,
- Would inferior pubectomy be required or not.

The shortcomings of this technology is that it may not be easily available, and the model is scaled to 80% size for faster availability. True depiction would be to print 100% original size of the patient.[18]

8. What is the use of methylene blue in diagnosis of stricture urethra and assessment of severity of spongiofibrosis?

Ans: Principle: The healthy urothelium is waterproof and not permeable to fluids. Nonetheless, the stricture causes gaps in between the cells. This allows for staining of the abnormal epithelium.

Advantages: It allows us to assess the length of urethra that merits augmentation. The graft should extend both proximally and distally beyond the length of the stricture. The recurrence after urethroplasty can be associated with inadequate placement of the graft.

Many strictures are almost obliterative and guidewire or narrow ureteral catheter may not pass across the stricture. Thus, we may not precisely incise urethral lumen due to near obliterative nature of stricture, and this may lead to a false passage. MB stains urethra precisely and serves as an exact guide for making the incision.[19]

9. What are the various surgical procedures available for recurrent urethral stricture?

Ans:

Anterior urethral strictures:

- One-stage substitution urethroplasty.

Posterior urethral strictures:

- One-stage substitution urethroplasty.
- Two-stage substitution urethroplasty.
- Anastomotic urethroplasty (AU).

Pan-urethral strictures:

- One-stage substitution urethroplasty.
- Two-stage substitution urethroplasty.
- Anastomotic urethroplasty (AU).[13]

10. What are the various types of grafts available and their role in redo urethroplasty?

Ans:

Buccal mucosa graft (BMG): Initially described by Humby, it has become an ideal urethral substitute because of ease of harvest, surgical handling characteristics, and hairlessness, compatibility in a wet environment, and its early in-growth and graft survival. Standard BMG bulbar urethroplasties have a success rate approaching 92%.

Most commonly it is used for ventral onlay buccal urethroplasty for bulbar stricture. It is also used to augment an inadequate urethral plate during first stage Johanson urethroplasty in penile urethral stricture.[20–23]

Patients who consume tobacco and have poor oral hygiene should be warned regarding poorer outcomes after BMG urethroplasty.[24]

Potential buccal harvest site complications include haemorrhage, pain, facial swelling, and damage to Stensen's duct, lip paraesthesia, and restriction in mouth opening.

Perineal complications like wounds infections, hematomas, skin anaesthesia/paraesthesia, urinary fistula, and graft contracture and graft failure can rarely occur.[23,25]

Lingual mucosa graft (LMG): LMG has the same biological properties and functional results as that of BMG. It has the added benefit of being useful in panurethral strictures when BMG is insufficient. Furthermore, oral complications are temporary and minimally disabling.

However, the tissue is fragile and maybe difficult to manage by inexperienced surgeons.[26]

Inner preputial skin graft (IPG): IPG has the advantage of being in use for a longer time, available locally, lower donor site morbidity, can be harvested under same regional anaesthesia of urethroplasty and morbidity of general anaesthesia can be avoided in high-risk patients.

Donor site edema may occur which usually resolves spontaneously but may require circumcision.[27]

Other options for grafts are: Fasciocutaneous graft, penile island flap, penile skin graft, free patch, forearm free flap, tunica vaginalis graft, scrotal skin graft, post-auricular skin graft, and mesh.[13]

11. Describe the steps of redo urethroplasty done for this representative case.

Ans:

- Patient was put in lithotomy position.
- Suprapubic and per-urethral cystoscopy was done.
- A dilator was inserted via the suprapubic tract and placed into proximal urethra (Fig. 11.4).
- Dilator was felt abutting anterior rectal wall.
- Midline perineal incision was taken.
- The distal urethra was dissected up until the stricture and disconnected.
- It was noted that the distal urethra was anastomosed to a false passage near the bladder neck during previous urethroplasty.

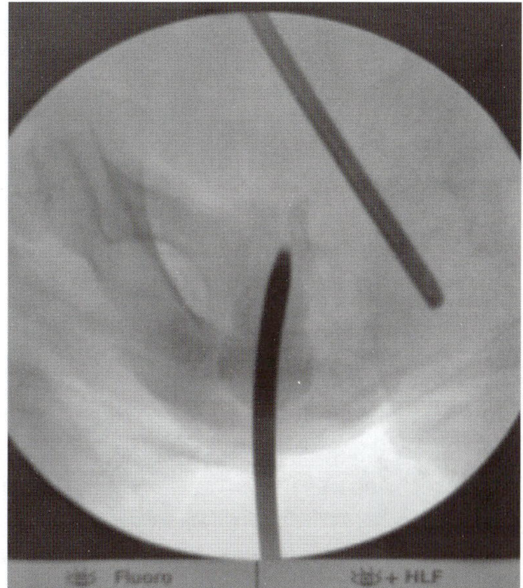

Fig. 11.4: Intra-operative oblique fluoroscopy

- The distal part of the proximal urethra was dissected and separated from the rectum and guidewire inserted (Fig. 11.5). Suprapubic cystoscopy done and proximal urethra delineated (Fig. 11.6).
- The defect was calculated to be approximately 6 cm in length and fibrotic tissue was excised (Fig. 11.7).
- Since patient was circumcised, a penile circular fasciocutaneous flap was harvested with the width calculated over 8 Fr Foley's catheter (Figs 11.8 to 11.10).

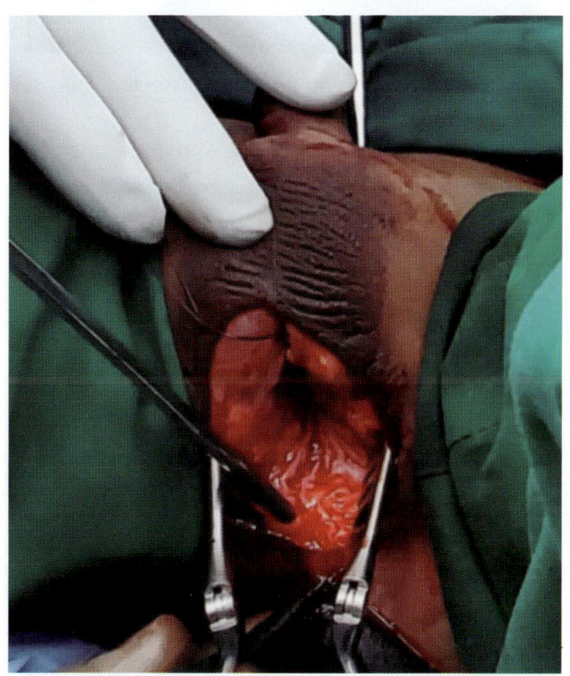
Fig. 11.5: Perineal incision taken and distal urethra dissected. Guidewire passed

Fig. 11.6: Suprapubic cystoscopy done to visualise proximal urethra

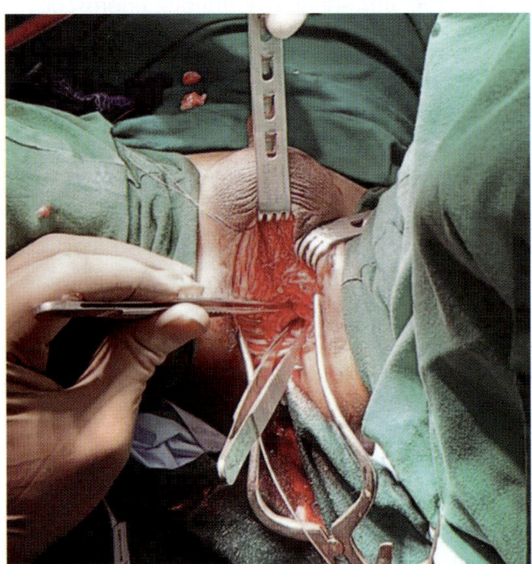

Fig. 11.7: Proximal membranous urethra dissected. Fibroses tissue removed. (Pieces seen on abdomen)

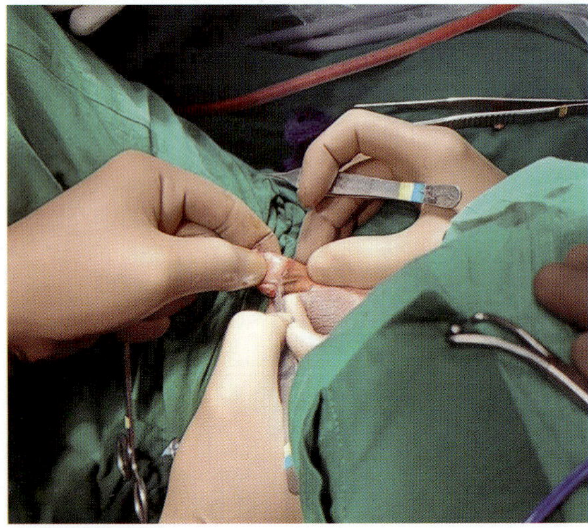

Fig. 11.8: Circumferential incision taken over penis and pedicle graft created

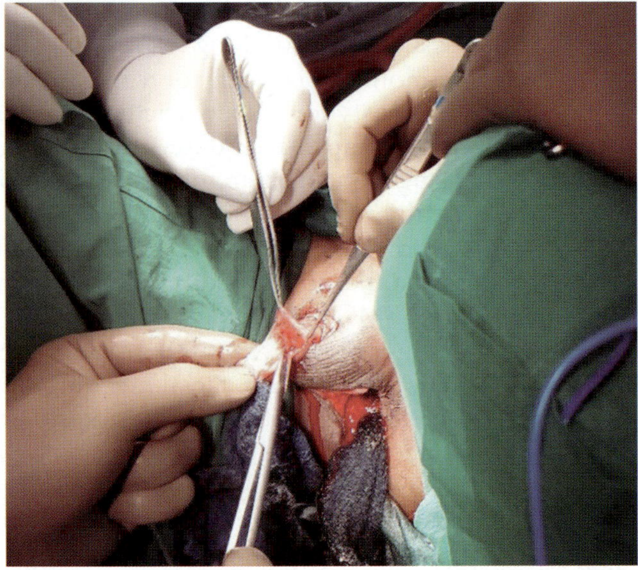

Fig. 11.9: Development of pedicle graft

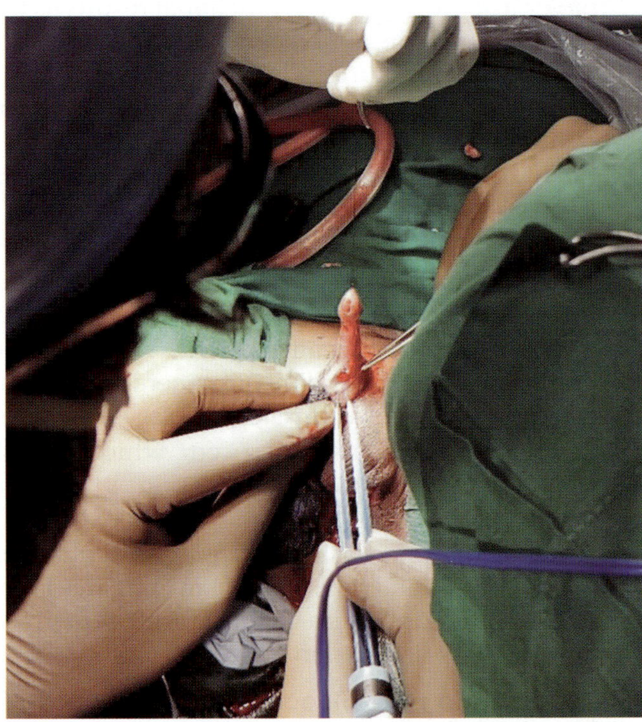

Fig. 11.10: Graft completely created

- The graft was transpositioned through a penoscrotal incision (Fig. 11.11).
- The flap was placed dorsally between the two ends of the urethra and posterior anastomosis was done to proximal and distal urethra with 4'O PDS continuous sutures.
- An 8 Fr Foley catheter was placed into the bladder and then the flap was tubularized over it and remaining anastomosis was completed proximally and distally (Figs 11.12 and 11.13).
- The incision was closed in layers.

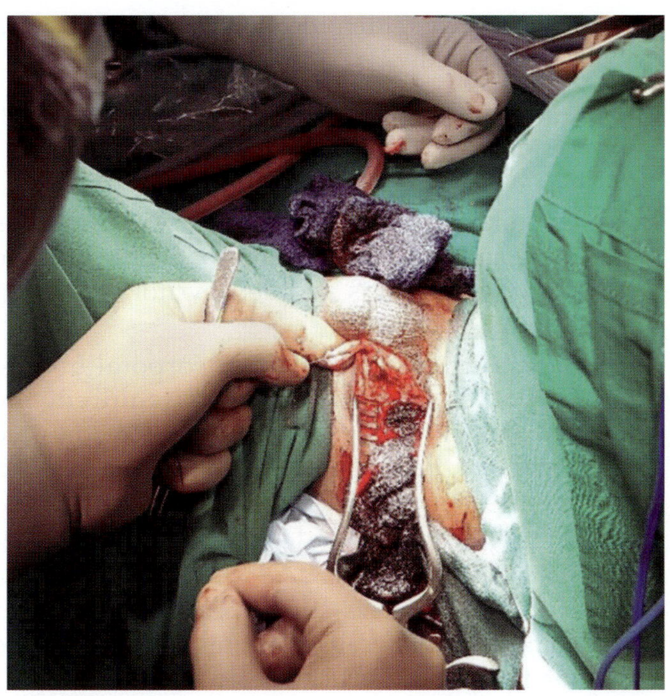

Fig. 11.11: Brought in perineal wound from peno-scrotal junction

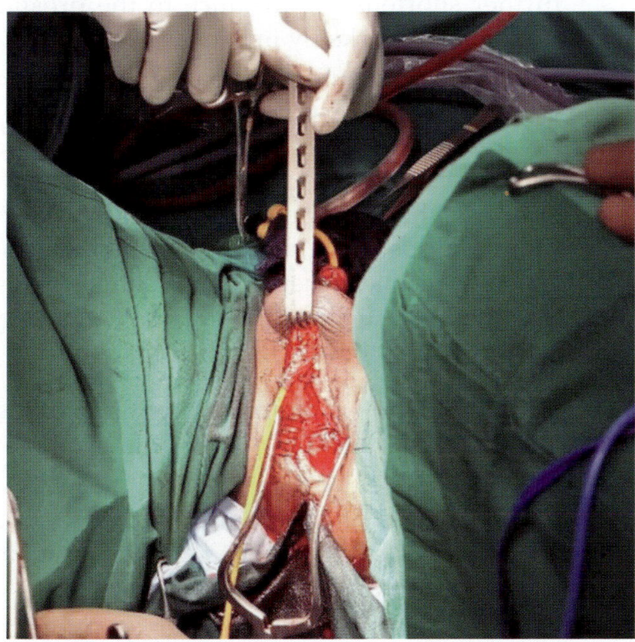

Fig. 11.12: Tubularization of graft started over 8 Fr Foley's catheter

12. How will you assess the primary and secondary outcome of various redo-urethroplasty techniques used?

Ans: Overall success rates of redo-urethroplasty range between 67 and 92%.[28]

Excision and primary anastomotic urethroplasty has a success rate of 58–100%.

Success rates vary according to the site of the stricture: Bulbar (58–100%) and posterior (69–100%) recurrent strictures.

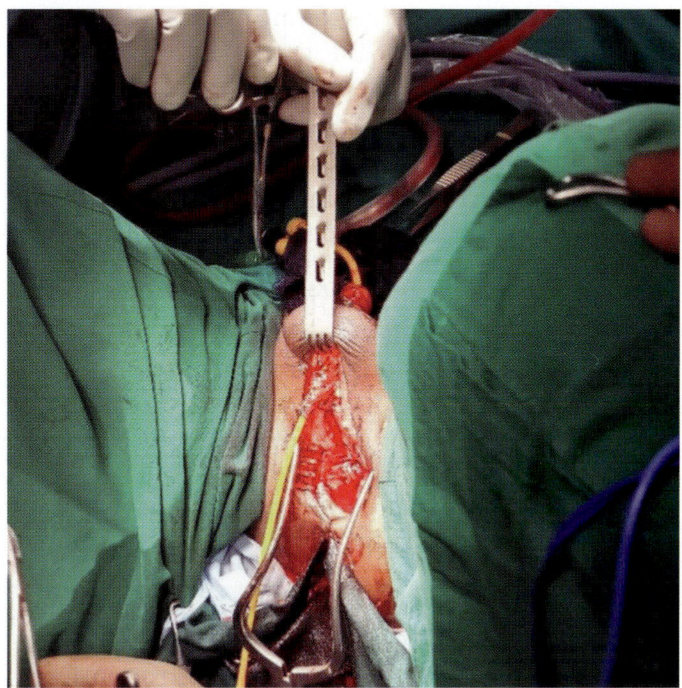

Fig. 11.13: Tubularization of graft completed

One-stage substitution urethroplasty has a success rate ranging from 18% to 100% (maximum evidence for BMG) with the best outcomes reported for bulbar (58–100%) and hypospadias-related (78.6–82%) strictures. For two-stage substitution urethroplasty, the success rates reported are between 20% and 100%, with the best evidence related to hypospadias-related and posterior urethral strictures.[13]

Success criteria are defined as re-establishment of a homogenous urethral calibre, no further urethral dilatations, internal urethrotomies or additional surgical procedures needed and maximum urine flow rate (Q_{max}) of >15 ml/s on UFM or normal RUG or urethroscopy.[29,30]

Failure of urethroplasty is defined as need for stricture retreatment, anatomical recurrence on cystoscopy, peak flow rate <15 ml/second, weak stream on questionnaire and failure by any of these measures.[31]

13. What are the post-operative complications of redo urethroplasty?

Ans: Common complications seen after redo urethroplasty are altered glans sensitivity (24.2%), UTI (36.1%), chordee (14.3%), post-void dribbling (12%), urge incontinence (16.2%), stress incontinence (10.8%), hematoma, abscess and wound infection (9.52%), urethrocutaneous fistula (5.88%), epididymo-orchitis (4.76%), iatrogenic hypospadias meatus in 4.76%, erectile dysfunction (2.94%) and diverticulum (2.94%).

Chronic leg pain is seen in 5% and foot neuralgia in 4.76% patients due to prolonged lithotomy position or pubectomy.[13]

14. What are the challenges encountered during redo urethroplasty and PFUDD management in children?

Ans: Recurrent urethral stricture disease after urethroplasty creates reconstructive challenges that are not present with initial repair. Patients with urethroplasty failure typically have:

- Less healthy tissue to use for reconstruction leading to tension at anastomotic site.
- They may have denser, more extensive scarring which can lead to graft necrosis due to inadequate blood supply.
- Surrounding tissue for flaps may have already been used and the penile blood supply may be altered.
- May have an underlying etiology that predisposes to failure, such as prior hypospadias repair, pelvic radiation history and lichen sclerosis.
- Proximity and adhesions to the rectum.
- In PFUDD-narrow space, displaced bone fragment and shorter posterior urethra leads to difficulty in anastomosis.[32,33]

In children, restricted surgical access to reach a high lying proximal urethral end, long distraction defects, simultaneous bladder neck and membranous urethral lesions and small urethral calibre makes the management more challenging.[29]

15. What are the tips and tricks used to avoid further failure while doing redo urethroplasty?

Ans: Adequate excision of scar tissue and anastomosis to healthy pliable tissue.

A tension-free urethral anastomosis is crucial for a successful result. This can be achieved through the perineum by liberal circumferential mobilization of the anterior urethra as far as the penoscrotal junction, but overextensive mobilization should be avoided because of the risk of proximal ischemia and chordee. The main blood supply of the bulbar spongy tissue is derived from the posterior bulbar arteries, which are necessarily divided during proximal urethral transection. However, the retrograde blood flow is usually sufficient for vascularization and hence it should not be compromised.

Pubectomy should be carried out in cases where gap between the two ends is very large to obtain a tension free anastomosis. Preoperative radiological assessment of urethral gap is a very useful measure to plan surgery.

Prevent anastomosis to false tract by calibration of the proximal urethra with catheter, adequate mobilisation and identification of healthy mucosa circumferentially.[5,7,17]

16. What are the methods of achieving extra length of distal urethra for a tension free anastomosis?

Ans:

- Circumferential mobilization of the urethra is done as far as the suspensory ligament of the penis. Chordee is avoided by not dissecting beyond this point.
- Separation of the proximal corporal bodies: If further urethral length is required, the proximal 4 to 5 cm of the corporal bodies are separated, beginning at the level of the crus and progressing distally. The urethra is then routed between the separated bodies, thus shortening the distance.
- If the anastomosis still appeared to be under some tension because of a high-lying prostate inferior pubectomy can be done.
- Routing the mobilized urethra between the separated corpora and through the bony defect further shortens the distance to the prostatic urethra and markedly improves access.
- Urethral ends should be prepared by spatulation to achieve an anastomosis of at least 40 F in calibre, and the anastomosis can be performed with interrupted 3 or 4-zero polyglycolic acid sutures. The anastomosis is facilitated by a long nasal speculum, and the verumontanum is generally visible in the floor assures anastomosis to the prostatic urethra. Intraoperative endoscopy can also be performed for confirmation.[29]

17. What is the follow-up protocol after urethroplasty in children and adults?

Ans: Follow-up protocol:

- Clinical visits and retrograde urethrograms 1 month after DAU, repeated at 1, 3, 5, 7, 10 and 15 years thereafter.
- Patients with incontinence after urethroplasty need to undergo video urodynamic studies.
- Erectile dysfunction can be identified in older children who can give information of their ability to have erections.[28]

In adults

Multitier follow-up approach using questionnaires (study-specific questionnaires or AUA symptom score) or uroflowmetry as an initial screening tool.

The cut-off point of maximum urinary flow triggering secondary investigations is 12 ml/s.

Cystoscopy or urethrography are only conducted if obstructive symptoms are present.[13, 34]

17. **What is the role of tissue engineering in urethroplasty?**
Ans: Tissue-engineered oral mucosa has been successfully used.
- It could be potentially useful for very long strictures.
- Long-term success rates of tissue engineering is only 20%.
- Patients with longer strictures, penile or distal urethral strictures, and extensive periurethral spongiofibrosis typically do not respond well to repeated incisions.
- Tissue engineering of autologous tissue is expensive.
- A great deal of work would be necessary to develop an appropriate matrix.
- At present, there is no effective and validated tissue engineering solution for the management of urethral stricture disease.[35]

SUMMARY

- Meticulous dissection and complete removal of fibrous tissue is imperative.
- Graft with adequate blood supply should be harvested.
- Wide calibre and tension free anastomosis to supple proximal urethra is the key to success.
- In children delicate handling of tissues is mandatory.

REFERENCES

1. Bello J. Impact of preoperative patient characteristics on posturethroplasty recurrence: the significance of stricture length and prior treatments. Niger J Surg. 2016;22(2):86–89.
2. Meeks JJ, Erickson BA, Granieri MA, Gonzalez CM. Stricture recurrence after urethroplasty: a systematic review. J Urol. 2009;182(4):1266–1270.
3. Kinnaird AS, Levine MA, Ambati D, Zorn JD, Rourke KF. Stricture length and etiology as preoperative independent predictors of recurrence after urethroplasty: a multivariate analysis of 604 urethroplasties. Can Urol Assoc J. 2014;8 (5–6):296–300.
4. Ofoha CG, Ramyil VM, Dakum NK, Shu'aibu SI, Akpayak IC, Magnus FE, Swem U, Oshagbemi A, Osunaiye O, Akhaine J. Predictors of urethral stricture recurrence following urethroplasty: a retrospective review at the Jos University Teaching Hospital, Nigeria. Pan Afr Med J. 2019 Apr 18;32:190.
5. Koraitim MM. Failed posterior urethroplasty: lessons learned. Urology. 2003 Oct;62(4):719–22.
6. McCammon KA, Zuckerman JM, Jordan GH. Surgery of the penis and urethra. In: Alan J wein, Louis R kavoussi, Alan W partin, Craig A peters, editors. Campbell-Walsh Urology. 11th ed. Philadelphia: Elsevier; 2016; 907–945.
7. Levine MA, Kinnaird AS, Rourke KF. Revision urethroplasty success is comparable to primary urethroplasty: A comparative analysis. J Urol. 2016;84(4):2014; 928–933.
8. Peskar DB, Perovi AV. Comparison of radiographic and sonographic urethrography for assessing urethral strictures. Eur Radiol. 2004;14:137–144.
9. McAninch JW, Laing FC, Jeffrey RB., Jr Sonourethrography in the evaluation of urethral strictures: a preliminary report. J Urol. 1988;139:294–297.
10. Krukowski J, Kału ny A, Kł cz J, Matuszewski M. Comparison between cystourethrography and sonourethrography in preoperative diagnostic management of patients with anterior urethral strictures. Med Ultrason. 2018;20:436–440.
11. Xu Li Ying Long Sa Yue Min Xu Qiang Fu Jiong Zhang. Flexible Cystoscope for Evaluating Pelvic Fracture Urethral Distraction Defects. Urol Int 2012;89:402–407.
12. Frankiewicz M, Markiet K, Krukowski J, Szurowska E, Matuszewski M. MRI in patients with urethral stricture: a systematic review. Diagn Interv Radiol. 2021 Jan;27(1):134–146.
13. Jasionowska S, Brunckhorst O, Rees RW, Muneer A, Ahmed K. Redo-urethroplasty for the management of recurrent urethral strictures in males: a systematic review. World J Urol. 2019 Sep;37(9):1801–1815.
14. Santucci R, Eisenberg L. Urethrotomy has a much lower success rate than previously reported. J Urol. 2010; 183:1859.
15. Otele, Willy H. *et al.* Efficacy of revision urethroplasty in the treatment of recurrent urethral strictures at a tertiary hospital (Kenyatta National Hospital–KNH), in Nairobi Kenya: 2015–2018. *Bali Medical Journal*. 2020;9(1): 67–76.
16. Sekhon V, Kudchadkar SJ, Raj A, Ansari MS. Radiographic gapometry score: A simple predictor for surgical approach in pediatric traumatic posterior urethral strictures. J Pediatr Urol. 2017 Dec;13(6):624.e1–624.e5.
17. Joshi PM, Desai DJ, Shah D, Joshi DP, Kulkarni SB. Magnetic resonance imaging procedure for pelvic fracture urethral injuries and recto urethral fistulas: A simplified protocol. Turk J Urol. 2021 Jan;47(1):35–42.
18. Joshi PM, Kulkarni SB. 3D printing of pelvic fracture urethral injuries-fusion of technology and urethroplasty. Turk J Urol. 2019 Nov 14;46(1):76–79.
19. Joshi P, Kaya C, Surana S, Desai DJ, Orabi H, Iyer S, Kulkarni SB. A novel method in decision making for the diagnosis of anterior urethral stricture: using methylene blue dye. Turk J Urol. 2017 Dec;43(4):502–506.
20. Humby G. A one-stage operation for hyposadius repair. Br J Surg 1941;29:84–92.
21. Bhargava S, Chapple CR. Buccal mucosal urethroplasty: Is it the new gold standard? BJU Int 2004;93:1191–3.
22. Morey AF, McAninch JW. When and how to use buccal mucosal grafts in adult bulbar urethroplasty. Urology 1996;48:194–8.
23. Zimmerman WB, Santucci RA. Buccal mucosa urethroplasty for adult urethral strictures. Indian J Urol. 2011 Jul;27(3):364–70.
24. Sinha RJ, Singh V, Sankhwar SN, Dalela D. Donor site morbidity in oral mucosa graft urethroplasty: implications of tobacco consumption. BMC Urol. 2009 Sep 21;9:15.
25. Spilotros M, Sihra N, Malde S, Pakzad MH, Hamid R, Ockrim JL, Greenwell TJ. Buccal mucosal graft urethroplasty in men-risk factors for recurrence and complications: a third referral centre experience in anterior urethroplasty using buccal mucosal graft. Transl Androl Urol. 2017 Jun;6(3):510–516.
26. Abrate A, Gregori A, Simonato A. Lingual mucosal graft urethroplasty 12 years later: Systematic review and meta-analysis. Asian J Urol. 2019 Jul;6(3):230–241.
27. Tyagi S, Parmar K, Sharma A, Devana S, Kumar S, Singh SK, Bora G, Mavuduru RM. Dorsolateral inner preputial graft urethroplasty for anterior urethral strictures: long-term

outcomes from a single tertiary care centre. World J Urol. 2021 Sep;39(9):3549–3554.

28. Rosenbaum C, Schmid M, Ludwig T et al. (2016) Redo buccal mucosa graft urethroplasty: success rate, oral morbidity and functional outcomes. BJU Int 118(5):797–803.
29. Podesta M, Podesta M Jr. Delayed surgical repair of posttraumatic posterior urethral distraction defects in children and adolescents: long-term results. J Pediatr Urol. 2015 Apr;11(2):67.e1–6.
30. Faridi MS, Sharma V , Sharma AK , Yadav R. Tunica albuginea versus buccal mucosa graft urethroplasty for anterior urethral stricture: A prospective randomised pilot study. Asian J. Urol. 2023 April;10(2):189–194.
31. Anderson KT, Vanni AJ, Erickson BA, Myers JB, Voelzke B, Breyer BN, Broghammer JA, Buckley JC, Zhao LC, Smith TG 3rd, Alsikafi NF, Rourke KF, Elliott SP. Defining Success after Anterior Urethroplasty: An Argument for a Universal Definition and Surveillance Protocol. J Urol. 2022 Jul;208(1):135–143.
32. Blaschko SD, McAninch JW, Myers JB, Schlomer BJ, Breyer BN. Repeat urethroplasty after failed urethral reconstruction: outcome analysis of 130 patients. J Urol. 2012 Dec;188(6):2260–4.
33. Webster GD, Ramon J. Repair of pelvic fracture posterior urethral defects using an elaborated perineal approach: experience with 74 cases. J Urol. 1991 Apr;145(4):744–8.
34. Kulkarni S, Barbagli G, Joshi P et al. (2015) Laparoscopic omentoplasty to support anastomotic urethroplasty in complex and redo pelvic fracture urethral defects. Urology 85(5):1200–1205.
35. Chapple C. Tissue engineering of the urethra: where are we in 2019? World J Urol. 2020 Sep;38(9):2101–2105.

Chapter 12

Male Urethral Diverticulum: Surgical Reconstruction

• Rajiv Kore • Rishikesh Kore

LEARNING OBJECTIVES

- To know the approach to diagnose male UD and their classification.
- To allude to the investigations for conclusive diagnosis.
- To understand etiopathogenesis and the mechanisms involved in different types of male UD.
- To learn about the management principles and the steps of repair.
- To educate regarding complications of treatment, follow up and comparative outcome of different modalities of treatment.

INTRODUCTION

The male urethral diverticulum (UD) is defined as a saccular dilatation extending from and contiguous with the true urethral lumen. The UD is relatively common in females, but it has a very low incidence in males. The prevalence is not even estimated for males. There are two types of UD. The first is congenital, and the other is acquired. The latter is more common. The typical clinical presentation is postvoid dribbling or urinary incontinence. Other common presenting features are recurrent urinary tract infection (UTI), weak stream, poor bladder emptying, penile-penoscrotal-perineal mass, urethro-cutaneous fistula, and urethral calculus. The consequences of a UD in a male are often related to inadequate drainage leading to nidus for urinary stasis with its resultant effects of UTI, calculi formation, urinary leakage, incontinence, or a palpable ventral penile mass.[1] The common investigation is ultrasound. Additionally, a retrograde and antegrade urethrogram are done to define the UD more precisely. The diagnosis is simple in relatively straightforward cases, but in complex scenarios, especially in congenital varieties where there is no visible mass, the investigations aid the diagnosis. A high index of suspicion is necessary to detect a greater number of cases in the right patient population . The management of urethral diverticulum depends on type, size, symptoms and complication of diverticulum. The treatment plan consists of the options of conservative, endoscopic and reconstructive procedures. It is always prudent to leave alone asymptomatic inconspicuous diverticulum without any complication. Others do require intervention that ranges from simple excision to complex diversion.

Case Scenario

A 63-year-old male, non-diabetic, presented with a history of painless swelling at the peno-scrotal junction (Fig. 12.1). The swelling first appeared three months after he had trans-urethral resection of his prostate (TURP), which was done a year ago. Since then, the lump had been progressively increasing in size. It used to bulge even more during voiding. He complained that he leaked urine through his urethra when this lump was manually compressed. He denied any history of direct trauma. He neither had fever nor any history of recurrent urinary tract infection. He stated that he had a decent urinary stream and was able to empty his bladder completely. There was no history of haematuria. His past medical history was unremarkable.

General examination revealed an averagely built and nourished man. He was afebrile. Local clinical examination revealed a soft, globular mass of 5.1 × 4.3 × 3.3 cm at the peno-scrotal junction. The mass was nontender and extended from the upper ventral scrotum to the lower ventral shaft. A light pressure on this mass resulted in urinary leak through the meatus, however, there was no purulent discharge or any evidence of a fistula.

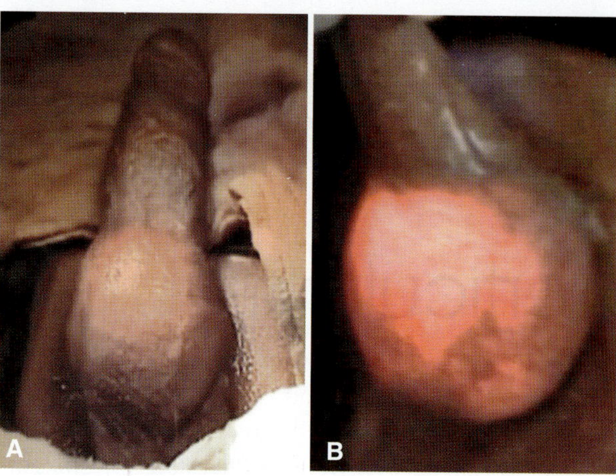

Fig. 12.1: (A) Urethral diverticulum; (B) Diverticulum seen illuminated during cystosocpy

1. **What is your clinical diagnosis?**
   Ans: The clinical history of the mass arising at the penoscrotal junction after TURP points to this operation as the causative etiology. The lump is progressively increasing in size. Clinical examination shows a soft and cystic mass that is located adjacent to the urethra. The urinary leak through the urethra with manual pressure clinches the diagnosis of UD.

2. **What investigation will you do to confirm your diagnosis?**
   Ans: It is relatively straightforward to detect a large penoscrotal diverticulum on clinical examination. However, more challenging diverticula to evaluate clinically are those that appear as scrotal masses, those that are deeply lodged, or those that have a modest size. The initial investigation is ultrasound. It verifies the diagnosis, evaluates the neck size, and measures the dimensions. A retrograde urethrogram is another investigation that will confirm the contiguity of the sacculated dilatation with the urethral lumen (Fig. 12.2). Male UD seldom requires magnetic resonance imaging (MRI), which is in fact the gold standard test for female urethral diverticulum.[2] The final diagnosis is confirmed by cysto-urethroscopy, which can be performed at the time of the reconstructive treatment. (refer to Video II)

3. **What are the different types of UD and which is the commonest among them?**
   Ans: There are two types. 1. Congenital; and 2. Acquired. Two-thirds UDs are acquired, and one-third is congenital. The congenital variety is again classified as saccular (true neck) or tubular (diffuse, located in the bulbar urethra), the former being more prevalent.[3]

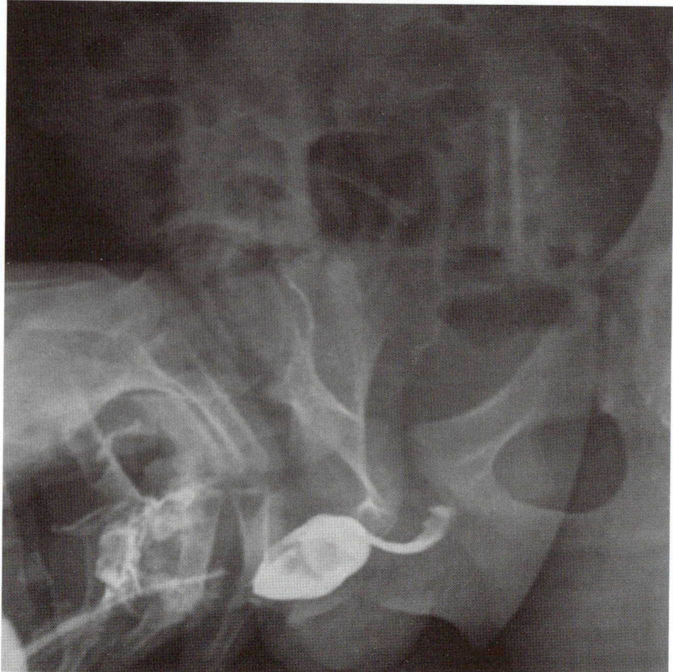

Fig. 12.2: Urethrogram showing urethral diverticulum

4. **What is the etiopathogenesis of congenital UD?**
   Ans: The congenital UD is usually associated with congenital anterior urethral valves,[4] and the exact etiologic mechanism has not been ascertained. Proposed theoretical explanations are a failed attempt at urethral duplication, an anomaly of the developing urethra resulting in excessive tissue growth, failure of alignment between the proximal and distal urethra, a permanent valve or flap mechanism, and a cystic dilation of periurethral glands (Cowper's gland).[5] These congenital UDs contain all the layers of the urethral wall that is lined by epithelium.

5. **What is the etiopathogenesis of acquired UD?**
   Ans: Acquired UD can develop due to an indwelling urethral catheter[6] or previous surgery. It can result from trauma, stricture, and infection.[7] It can also develop after surgical treatment of hypospadias or urethral strictures, transurethral prostatectomy or bladder procedures, and implant surgeries or their complications.[8]

   There are three mechanisms described for the development of acquired diverticulum. One mechanism is due to increased urethral pressure as a result of obstruction causing herniation of the urethral epithelium. This is seen in patients undergoing complex procedures for urethral stricture, hypospadias, and trauma.[9] The second mechanism is a result of constant pressure on the penoscrotal junction, leading to ischemic urethral fibrosis and scar formation. Typically, this is observed in patients with long standing indwelling catheters.[10] The third mechanism involves anorectal malformation repair. As more urine fills in the part that is herniated, the UD develops. This type of UD occurs in 12% to 18% of cases.[11,12]

6. **What is the clinical presentation of UD?**

Ans: The commonest presenting feature is postvoid dribbling, which the patient typically perceives as urinary incontinence. Other common presenting features are a penile-penoscrotal-perineal mass, a recurrent UTI, a weak stream, poor bladder emptying, urethro-cutaneous fistula, and a urethral calculus.

7. **What are the treatment options available and what are the surgical principles for the treatment of UD?**

Ans: The options are as follows:

I. Conservative (non-operative) Treatment

Patients having smaller size UD with a wider neck that can be emptied successfully with manual compression are treated conservatively. Patients with a UD and recurrent UTIs in the absence of urethral obstruction, however, responding to prophylactic antibiotics subsequently, without UTI recurrence, are selectively treated conservatively.

II. Endoscopic deroofing of UD (*See* video 12)

Scan QR Code for Video on
Endoscopic deroofing of a congenital penile diverticulum

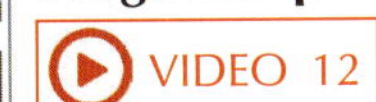

Trans-urethral deroofing may be considered as a primary approach in some patients having small UD with narrow neck and with good integrity of surrounding spongiosum and intact supportive tissue.[13] This integrity is evidenced by the lack of bulge of UD. In other words, the endoscopic treatment is possible only for those UD that are contained within the intact corpus spongiosum. Despite it being a minimally invasive and technically easier approach, the recurrence rate of UD and possibility of developing urethro-cutaneous fistula make it an inferior option.[8] In a series of 22 patients by Cinman and Breyer, none was considered for this approach.[14] It is observed that a large, poorly draining cavity is likely to remain, leading to recurrence. When the UD is too thick for adequate incision, this approach is not advisable.[15] Scar tissue formation and subsequent urethral strictures are additional potential consequences after the endoscopic approach.

III. Surgical reconstruction (*See* video 13)

Scan QR Code for Video on
Diverticulectomy and repair of post-TURP penoscrotal diverticulum

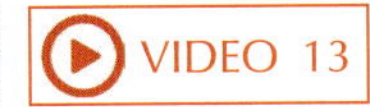

The most common indications for reconstruction are recurrent UTI with or without purulent collection in the diverticulum, urethral obstruction due to stricture, stone in the diverticulum, and an associated urethro-cutaneous fistula. Some patients would demand correction of UD for cosmetic reasons, even though they are able to empty it effortlessly and may not have any complications arising from UD. The diverticulum is dissected from the surrounding fascial covering. It is excised, leaving behind adequate wall to use for the repair. This repair is performed with absorbable suture material over a catheter. It is ensured that the lumen of the urethra is sufficient to allow for possible contraction. Overlying fascia is closed to support the repair. Skin closure is done, observing the principle of non-overlapping suture lines.

The procedure is covered with prophylactic antibiotics. All the reconstructive procedures should be done over a silicone catheter of appropriate size for the age. The catheter is removed after 3 to 4 weeks after confirmation of integrity with a urethrogram.

IV. Urinary diversion

In a more complex situation like the neurogenic bladder associated with a large UD, it is logical to do urinary diversion.[14] This would provide treatment for the source of urinary stasis and potential infection, namely the UD and the neurogenic bladder requiring clean intermittent catheterization (CIC). Reconstructing the urethra with UD in this setting would still require CIC, which could traumatize and compromise healing. This would then cause false passages and a recurrence of UD. These reasons would substantiate the decision of supra-vesical (ileal conduit) urinary diversion in these cases. Another reason to consider diversion in UD is non-reconstructable urethra due to multiple surgeries, anatomical abnormalities. The preferred approach would be an infra-vesical diversion, such as a perineal urethrostomy, if the posterior urethra is healthy.

8. What procedure will you do for this case?

Ans: The patient has a large penoscrotal diverticulum. It is an acquired diverticulum in an adult and has developed after transurethral instrumentation. It will have a thin wall with no covering of spongiosa. It is symptomatic and progressively enlarging. It has the potential to get infected. Moreover, there is also a possibility of forming a urethro-cutaneous fistula. Considering all these clinical features and the symptomatic nature of this UD, reconstruction with excision and repair appears to be appropriate.

9. What steps will you take during the procedure for this case?

Ans: Initial confirmation of the diagnosis is done with urethrocystoscopy, which shows the diverticulum glowing with endoscopic light. A longitudinal incision is made ventrally on the diverticulum. Adequate amount of normal saline is instilled subcutaneously, and hydrodissection is done. The cystic mass is then dissected circumferentially and excised. The diverticular wall is used as a flap to close the urethra over a silicon catheter. Ventral dartos fascia is then used to cover the underlying suture-line of urethral closure. The skin closure is then done, avoiding overlapping suture lines.

10. What are the complications of various treatment options and procedure used for this case?

Ans: A congenital variety or a small symptomatic UD is treated endoscopically, where deroofing is done. In some of these cases, the spongiosa or the fascial coverings are not strong enough and can be easily perforated, converting the diverticulum into a urethro-cutaneous fistula. Occasionally, while deroofing, a new urethral stricture may be formed due to fibrosis. Inadequate deroofing also leads to recurrence. The acquired type, on the other hand, is prone to urethro-cutaneous fistula, infection, wound sepsis, and wound dehiscence. Excessive trimming of the diverticular wall will lead to urethral stricture. Occasionally, epididymo-orchitis can ensue in all the treatment options. The overall complication rate is 9–42%.[14,16]

11. How will you follow-up such cases post-operatively?

Ans: In both varieties of UD, the patient needs early and long-term follow-up. In the early follow-up local wound and catheter care are essential. In the long-term follow-up patient needs urine analysis, uroflowmetry, ultrasound for residual urine, and local examination at regular intervals. Invasive investigations such as urethrogram and urethro-cystoscopy are rarely needed and are done for appropriate indications such as recurrence or new onset stricture formation.

Comparative outcome of each procedure used

Due to the small number of cases that are reported, there is no case series that compares the outcomes of each management approach head-to-head. In the anecdotal case reports, each clinician has dealt with the UD on its own merits. The endoscopic approach is considered inferior due

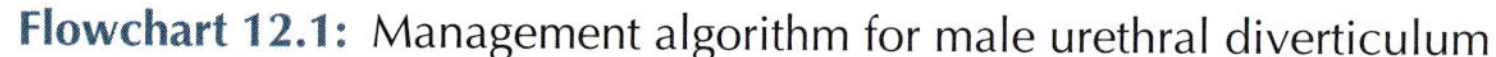

Flowchart 12.1: Management algorithm for male urethral diverticulum

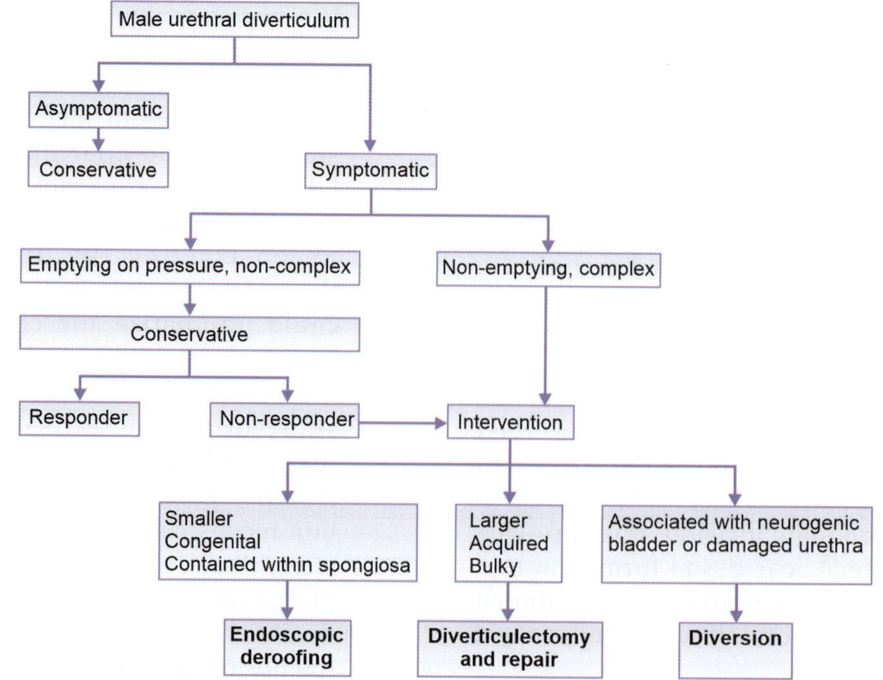

to possible complications such as recurrence, urethro-cutaneous fistula, urethral fibrosis, and stricture formation. Diverticulectomy with repair, on the other hand, is a more definitive option with acceptable perioperative complications and better long-term success. The approach of urinary diversion is rarely required, but it is the only option with a good outcome. Overall success in the case series available in the literature is 91–92%.[14,16]

KEY POINTS

- Male UD is rare.
- The acquired variety is more common than the congenital variety.
- High index of suspicion is needed, however, they can be evaluated with basic investigations.
- Non-operative treatment of self-milking should be considered primarily.
- Reconstructive procedure of excision and repair is more effective compared to endoscopic deroofing sometimes performed for smaller congenital UD.
- In complex situations of neurogenic bladder needing CIC and in case of end stage urethra urinary diversion may be considered.

REFERENCES

1. De Filippo RE, Kurzrock EA, Stein JP, Skinner DG. A giant urethral diverticulum presenting as a scrotal mass in an adult male. BJU Int. 1999;83:522–3.
2. Greenwell TJ, Spilotros M. Urethral diverticula in women. Nat Rev Urol 2015;12:671–80.
3. Bote SM, Gite VA, Siddiqui AK, Patil SR, Nikose JV. Acquired male urethral diverticulum: Report of two cases. Arch Int Surg 2016;6:54–6.
4. Firlit CF. Urethral abnormalities. Urol Clin North Am. 1978;5:31–55.
5. Rawat J, Khan TR, Singh S, Maletha M, Kureel S. Congenital anterior urethral valves and diverticula: diagnosis and management in six cases. Afr J Paediatr Surg.2009;6:102–5.
6. Stephan-Carlier A, Facione J, Gervaise A, Chapus JJ, Lagauche D. A 24-year-old patient with paraplegia and acquired urethral diverticulum: a case report. Ann Phys Rehabil Med. 2011;54:48–52.
7. Ho CH, Yu HJ, Huang KH. Scrotal mass with bladder outlet obstruction. Urology. 2008;72:66–7.
8. Peralta JP, Reis M, Rabaça C, Sismeiro A. Acquired male urethral diverticulum: a complication following artificial urethral sphincter implantation. BMJ Case Rep. 2013;bcr2013201542.
9. Allen D, Mishra V, Pepper W, Shah S, Motiwala H. A single-center experience of symptomatic male urethral diverticula. Urology. 2007;70:650–3.
10. Ortlip SA, Gonzalez R, Williams RD. Diverticula of the male urethra. J Urol. 1980 ;124:350–5.
11. Alam S, Lawal TA, Peña A, Sheldon C, Levitt MA. Acquired posterior urethral diverticulum following surgery for anorectal malformations. J Pediatr Surg. 2011 ;46:1231–5.
12. Hong AR, Acuña MF, Peña A, Chaves L, Rodriguez G. Urologic injuries associated with repair of anorectal malformations in male patients. J Pediatr Surg. 2002 ;37:339–44.
13. Quoraishi SH, Khan F, Besarani D, Patil K. Congenital anterior urethral diverticulum in a male teenager: a case report and review of the literature. Case Rep Urol. 2011;2011:738638.
14. Cinman NM, McAninch JW, Glass AS, Zaid UB, Breyer BN. Acquired male urethral diverticula: presentation, diagnosis and management. J Urol. 2012;188:1204–8.
15. Labanaris AP, Zugor V, Witt JH, Nützel R, Kühn R. Urethral diverticulum with massive lithiasis presenting as a scrotal mass. Urol Int. 2011;87:481–3.
16. Alphs HH, Meeks JJ, Casey JT, Gonzalez CM. Surgical reconstruction of the male urethral diverticulum. Urology. 2010;76:471–5.

Chapter

13

Bladder Trauma

• Sudheer K Devana • Shrawan K Singh

LEARNING OBJECTIVES

- To understand the initial evaluation of blunt trauma abdomen with suspected bladder trauma.
- To understand when and how to perform imaging evaluation for bladder trauma.
- To understand the indications for immediate surgical intervention for bladder trauma.
- To understand the delayed complications of bladder trauma.
- To understand the management of gunshot and penetrating bladder trauma.

INTRODUCTION

Bladder injury following blunt abdominal trauma is one of the most common urological emergencies being managed by urologists. Bladder injury is commonly associated with pelvic fracture and sometimes urethral disruption, vaginal and rectal injuries can also be there. Detailed history and clinical examination are a very important part of initial management. Imaging in the form of contrast enhanced computed tomography scan (CECT) of abdomen with delayed excretory films or CT cystography can characterize the type of bladder injury. Conservative bladder drainage with perurethral catheter or immediate surgical repair of bladder injury are the management options. This chapter gives an overview of approach to management of a suspected case of bladder injury following trauma. Additional note on penetrating and gunshot injuries of bladder and delayed complications of bladder injury are also mentioned.

Case Scenario

A 35-year-old male presented to emergency with history of blunt trauma abdomen due to a road traffic accident while riding a motorcycle. On examination, he was conscious but irritable due to severe pain. His pulse rate was 130/min and blood pressure was 80/60 mm Hg. He was immediately resuscitated with intravenous fluids and his blood pressure improved to 110/80 mm Hg. Severe tenderness was noted in the region of pelvis (pelvic compression test was positive) with ecchymosis of the skin over suprapubic region. His abdomen was diffusely distended and per urethral catheter was placed which revealed gross hematuria.

1. **What are the various causes for bladder trauma or injury?**

   Ans: Bladder is the most commonly injured organ in the lower urinary tract following blunt abdominal trauma secondary to road traffic accidents (deceleration injury), fall from height, runover by a vehicle or assault in the form of direct blow to the lower abdomen. Bladder injury secondary to blunt trauma abdomen is frequently not isolated and is associated with other organ injuries. Bladder is well protected in the pelvis by the surrounding pelvic bone and hence it is frequently associated with pelvic fracture (83–95%). If the injury is severe enough other associated injuries like injuries involving the urethra (4–15%), rectum, vagina and perineal tear can also be there.[1] Penetrating injuries in the region of lower abdomen, pelvis and buttocks can lead to bladder injury, however, they are very rare. Gunshot injuries are also a rare cause for bladder injury if the trajectory of the bullet passes through the bladder. Bladder injury frequently occurs secondary to iatrogenic trauma during any pelvic surgery. For example, most commonly during gynecological procedures like laparoscopic or open hysterectomy, caesarean section, surgical management of placenta accreta, percreta and endometriosis. Surgeries related to rectal cancer like abdominoperineal resection or low anterior resection and excision of tumors located in the rectovesical pouch can be associated with iatrogenic bladder injury. Bladder injury can also occur during surgical procedures done for treating stress urinary incontinence like sling procedures done or cystocele repair. Bladder perforation can occur during endoscopic procedures like transurethral resection of bladder tumor (TURBT) or transurethral resection of prostate (TURP). During TURBT the reported incidence of bladder perforation is 0.4% to 58.3%.

2. How will you evaluate a suspected case of bladder trauma secondary to abdominal trauma?

Ans: Evaluation starts with detailed history and clinical examination. History taking involves enquiry into the mode of accident like road traffic accident, runover by a vehicle or fall from height. Gross hematuria is the most common presentation (77–100%) in cases of suspected bladder trauma. Severe bladder injury is unlikely if a patient passes clear urine after blunt trauma abdomen. Very rarely there can be a patient with bladder injury who had microscopic hematuria (<5%). Patients may not have the sensation of bladder fullness and they might not pass urine after injury particularly when intraperitoneal bladder rupture is present. Such patients have abdominal distension due to urinary ascites and can also have decreased urine output. Urinary ascites can also lead to increased blood urea nitrogen and serum creatinine levels due to peritoneal absorption of urine. A palpable bladder rules out the presence of a severe bladder injury but there can be associated pelvic fracture urethral injury (PFUI). Presence of blood at the urethral meatus is a sign of associated urethral injury or PFUI.[2] In patients with extraperitoneal bladder rupture, urine can extravasate into the subcutaneous planes of lower abdomen, scrotum, penis, perineum and also the upper part of thighs leading to swelling in the above-mentioned areas. Severe tenderness in the suprapubic region and pelvis can be there due to associated pelvic fracture. Presence of ecchymoses in the lower abdomen can be a sign of pelvic hematoma.

Perineal examination can show associated other injuries like perineal tear, rectal injury and vaginal injury particularly in females. In females traumatic vesicovaginal fistula or PFUI or traumatic rectovaginal fistula can be there. Hence examination of rectum and vagina should always be done in patients presenting with blunt trauma abdomen. Presence of crepitus in the region of the lower abdomen or upper part of thigh is sometimes the only sign of occult rectal injury.

Gunshot and penetrating pelvic injury patients should be examined particularly looking into entry and exit wounds carefully whether the trajectory of the injured weapon passed through the bladder region.

3. What are the indications of cystography in a blunt trauma abdomen patient?

Ans: The indications can be categorized into absolute and relative indications according to AUA urotrauma guidelines[3,4]

- Absolute indications
  - Presence of gross hematuria with pelvic fracture
- Relative indications
  - Presence of gross hematuria without pelvic fracture
  - Presence of microscopic hematuria with pelvic fracture[5]

4. What radiological imaging is needed to detect a suspected bladder injury?

Ans: Bladder injury following blunt trauma is frequently associated with other abdominal organ injuries. Initially in any trauma patient at bed side, FAST (focused assessment with sonography for trauma) is done to look for evidence of fluid collection in the abdomen. After that further imaging in the form of CECT abdomen is done particularly in a hemodynamically stable trauma patient when FAST is positive or history and examination is suggestive of abdominal organ injury.[6–9] Bladder injury secondary to blunt trauma abdomen is conventionally categorized into intraperitoneal or extraperitoneal bladder rupture. 60% of bladder injuries are intraperitoneal, 30% are extraperitoneal and 10% are both. In suspected cases of bladder injury, CECT abdomen with delayed excretory films can depict bladder injury whether it is an intraperitoneal or extraperitoneal. It is very important to clamp the per urethral catheter during CECT abdomen to detect bladder rupture. In patients with extraperitoneal bladder rupture the contrast gets collected in the extraperitoneal space and it can extend into the retroperitoneal space as well (Fig. 13.2). In patients with intraperitoneal bladder rupture the contrast gets collected in the peritoneal cavity outlining the small bowel loops as shown in Fig. 13.1. Sometimes an occult bladder injury can be missed by CECT imaging where antegrade filling of contrast material into bladder is followed.[10]

Fig. 13.1: (A) Delayed films of CECT scan of a patient with blunt trauma abdomen showing contrast extravasation from bladder into the peritoneal cavity suggestive of intraperitoneal bladder rupture; (B) The contrast was seen extravasating from the dome of the bladder outlining the small bowel loops.

Retrograde cystogram with adequate bladder distension (around 350 ml) diagnoses bladder injury better than antegrade cystogram. Retrospective study by Wirth *et al* have shown that inadequate bladder distension during CT cystogram can miss bladder injury in 11% of cases.[11] Both cytogram and CT cystogram have shown to have comparable sensitivity and specificity in diagnosing bladder injury.[12,13] In patients with suspected isolated bladder injury (gross hematuria with pelvic fracture), retrograde cystography can be performed to detect bladder injury. An extraperitoneal bladder rupture characteristically shows a dense flame-shaped contrast extravasation on retrograde cystogram. Depending on the severity of bladder injury the contrast can extend into the retroperitoneum, scrotum, penis, anterior abdominal wall and thigh (Fig. 13.2).[14] Stress cystogram is done to detect occult bladder injuries. A CT cystogram can also be done to detect bladder injury which has the added advantage of locating the exact site of contrast leak from the bladder and also pelvic fracture can be seen clearly.[15–17] In females' opacification of vagina with contrast suggests an associated traumatic vaginal tear along with bladder rupture (Fig.13.3).

Fig. 13.2: (A) Coronal view of CECT scan of a patient with extraperitoneal bladder rupture showing characteristic flame shaped extravasation of contrast into the perivesical space; (B) The contrast extravasation was seen extending high up even into the left retroperitoneal space (shown by arrows). The associated pelvic fracture can also be noticed on right side (black arrow)

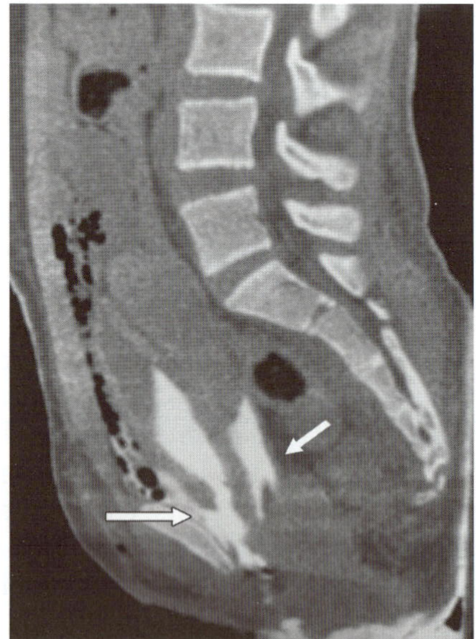

Fig. 13.3: CECT scan of a 14-year-old female showing contrast leak from anterior bladder wall close to bladder neck (big arrow) and also contrast opacification of vagina (small arrow) suggestive of combined bladder and vaginal injury following blunt trauma abdomen

5. How do we grade the severity of bladder injury following trauma?

Ans: American Association for the Surgery of Trauma have graded the severity of bladder injury as depicted in Table 13.1.[18]

TABLE 13.1: Classification of bladder injury	
Grade	*Description of injury*
1	Haematoma, partial thickness laceration
2	Extraperitoneal bladder wall laceration <2 cm
3	Extraperitoneal bladder (>2 cm) or intraperitoneal (<2 cm) bladder laceration
4	Intraperitoneal bladder wall laceration >2 cm
	Intraperitoneal or extraperitoneal bladder wall laceration extending into the bladder neck or ureteric orifice

6. How to treat a patient with bladder trauma? What are the indications of conservative or immediate surgical repair following bladder trauma?

Ans: Any patient of blunt trauma abdomen with gross hematuria should first be evaluated for airway, breathing and circulation. If hemodynamically unstable, then he should be first resuscitated by giving intravenous fluids including blood and blood products. If the patient is still unstable after adequate resuscitation, then he has to be rushed to operation theatre for immediate surgical exploration. Intraoperatively if there is suspicion of bladder injury based on the presence of urinary ascites, then bladder integrity should be checked on table by filling bladder with saline via per-urethral catheter. A bladder rupture (either intra or extraperitoneal) if found intraoperatively should be repaired immediately. Unnecessary dissection of a pelvic hematoma secondary to pelvic fracture should not be done. In case of unstable pelvic fracture with hemodynamic instability, an orthopedic consultation for open reduction with internal fixation of pelvic bone can be sought. If there is no urinary ascites, then gross hematuria could be due to renal trauma. Renal trauma patients are mostly managed conservatively and the retroperitoneum should not be disturbed by unnecessary exploration. Other causes for hemodynamic instability should be looked into like an associated liver or splenic injury. In the event of persistent hemodynamic instability and the presence of an expanding retroperitoneal hematoma, the retroperitoneum be explored.

After initial fluid resuscitation if the patient is hemodynamically stable, then imaging in the form of CECT abdomen with delayed excretory films or a CT cystogram is performed to first differentiate whether we are dealing with intraperitoneal or extraperitoneal bladder rupture. An uncomplicated extraperitoneal bladder rupture is generally managed conservatively with bladder drainage by placing a wide bore per-urethral catheter for a period of 2–3 weeks.[19] Sometimes a patient with intraperitoneal bladder rupture if not taken up for surgical exploration due to any reason, a percutaneous abdominal drain can be placed to drain urinary ascites which relieves abdominal distension and prevents occurrence of infection or paralytic ileus.

Indications for immediate surgical repair of bladder injury[20]

1. Intraperitoneal bladder rupture
2. Penetrating/gunshot bladder injury
3. Bladder rupture with
   a. Associated bladder neck injury
   b. Associated vaginal or rectal injury
   c. Pelvic fracture requiring open reduction and internal fixation
   d. When there is concern for contamination with urine of pelvic hardware placed for stabilizing pelvic fracture
   e. Bony spicule or fragment impinging onto the site of bladder injury
   f. Other abdominal organ injury needing emergency exploration
   g. Associated PFUI with failure to catheterize perurethrally

Exploration via a lower midline laparotomy incision with presence of urinary ascites confirms the diagnosis of intraperitoneal bladder rupture. Dome of the bladder is the most common site of intraperitoneal bladder rupture. Retrograde filling of bladder with saline also confirms the site of bladder rupture. Sometimes bladder rupture at multiple sites can be there, hence the surgeon should spend time in examining the bladder thoroughly. Always the integrity of the bladder neck and involvement of both ureteric orifices should be checked. In case of associated PFUI the per-urethral catheter can be railroaded into the bladder over a guidewire. The retropubic pelvic hematoma should not be disturbed in cases of pelvic fracture. Bladder rupture is repaired in two layers using absorbable sutures over a perurethral catheter (Fig. 13.4). Laparoscopic management

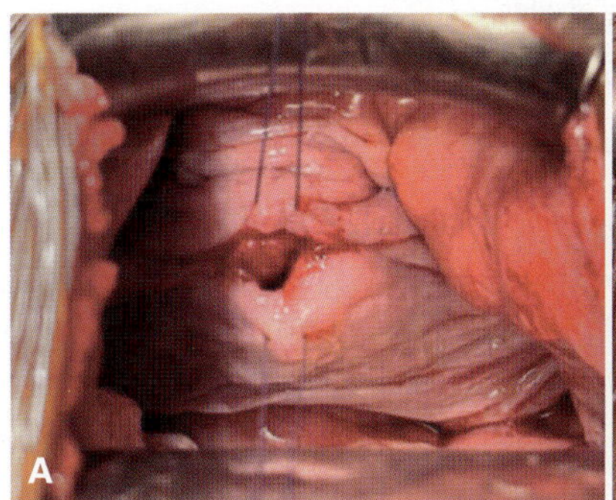

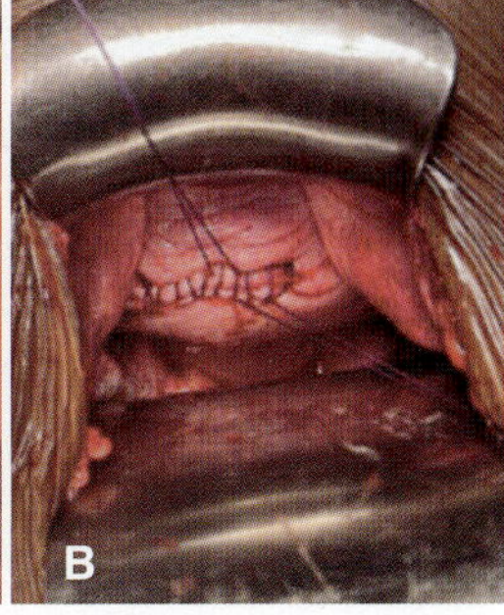

Fig. 13.4: (A) Intraoperative picture showing intraperitoneal rupture of 2–3 cm in the region of dome of bladder following blunt trauma abdomen; (B) Bladder repaired using absorbable suture in a continuous fashion

of intraperitoneal bladder rupture following blunt abdominal trauma has been described in hemodynamically stable patients with no associated other organ injury. It has the advantage of faster recovery and better cosmetic results.[21] Suprapubic catheter is not generally needed and can only be considered in special situations like a gunshot injury or multiple bladder injuries. Studies have shown that there is no added advantage of placing suprapubic catheter in addition to a perurethral catheter.[22] Associated vaginal and perineal tears should be repaired simultaneously. In cases of associated rectal injury, a temporary diversion colostomy is performed. Bladder neck injury if found should also be repaired over a Foley's catheter. If a bony spicule or a broken bony fragment is impinging onto the bladder wall, it should be removed. Flowchart 13.1 depicts evaluation and management of a case of blunt trauma abdomen with gross hematuria.

Iatrogenic bladder injuries during any pelvic abdominal surgery most commonly during gynecological surgeries like hysterectomy, caesarean section should be repaired immediately similar to intraperitoneal bladder rupture following blunt trauma abdomen.[23] Bladder injury which occurred during endoscopic procedures like TURBT or TURP is generally detected by finding interruption of detrusor muscle at the site of resection with presence of perivesical fat or a dark area seen in between detrusor muscle fibers which is suggestive of free perforation. Bladder injury following endoscopic surgery can be missed and detected in the postoperative period because of abdominal distension due to fluid accumulation in the intra- or extraperitoneal space. There is no consensus on the management of bladder perforation which occurred during endoscopic procedures. If detected intraoperatively, the procedure is abandoned by doing prompt hemostasis and draining the bladder by placing a catheter. Another percutaneous drain is placed to drain the fluid collected in the abdomen. If detected in the postoperative period, then also it is managed with placement of an extra or intraperitoneal drain with or without ultrasound guidance based on the site of fluid collection. The percutaneous drain is removed once the output is minimal.

Immediate open exploration and repair of free perforation of bladder during TURBT has also been described. Thorough lavage of abdomen in such cases is needed to reduce the possibility of tumors cell implantation in the peritoneal cavity.[24]

7. What is follow-up care and outcome in bladder trauma patients?

Ans: A check cystogram is generally performed after 2–3 weeks of perurethral catheter drainage

Flowchart 13.1: Evaluation and management of a case of blunt trauma abdomen with gross hematuria with or without pelvic fracture

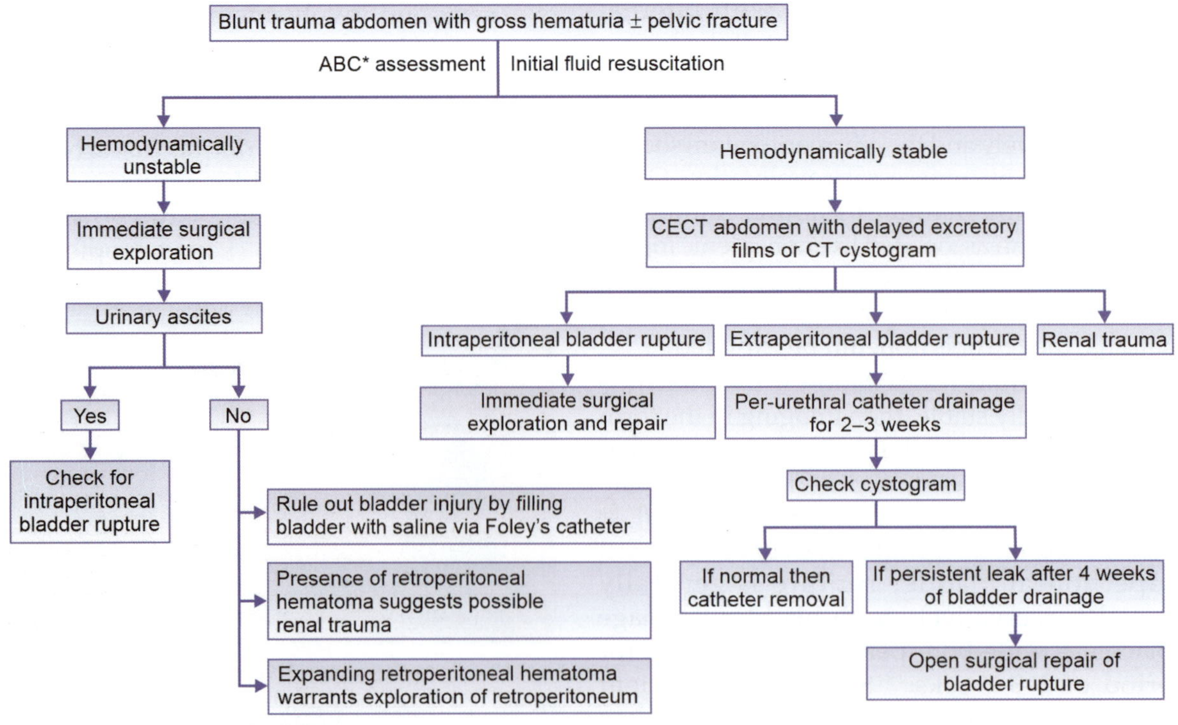

Section 3

in cases of extraperitoneal bladder rupture or intraperitoneal bladder rupture repair.[25] In the absence of contrast leak on check cystogram the perurethral catheter is removed. It is important to remember that an extraperitoneal bladder rupture which failed to heal even after 4 weeks of per urethral catheter drainage needs open surgical repair. Mortality following bladder trauma largely depends on the clinical state of the patient at initial presentation following trauma (presence of hemorrhagic shock, low Glasgow Coma Scale score) and associated other organ injuries. The mortality rate following bladder trauma in various published series ranged from 0 to 34%.[26]

8. What are the delayed complications of bladder injury?

Ans: Delayed bladder repair or a missed bladder injury or improperly repaired bladder rupture can lead to some delayed complications like sepsis, peritonitis, ileus, abscess formation and vesicocutaneous fistula formation. Vesicocutaneous fistula can form anywhere in the region of perineum, thigh or buttock.[27,28] Such fistulas can heal conservatively by catheter drainage of bladder or might need complex surgical repair.

9. How are penetrating or gunshot wounds of bladder managed?

Ans: These injuries are managed with immediate surgical exploration and repair as they are associated with increased risk of deep-seated infection. Bladder is opened at the site of injury and the entire bladder lumen is examined from within. Entry and exit wounds in the bladder should be carefully examined and devitalized edges of the wound are freshened and then repaired. Associated bladder neck injury if present should be repaired. Adequate bladder drainage is ensured by placement of perurethral and also suprapubic catheter in these patients. Placement of bilateral external ureteric splints and keeping the bladder completely dry will helpful in patients with extensive gunshot bladder injuries. Associated rectal injuries should also be repaired and it is prudent to place an omental interposition flap in between the suture lines to prevent future formation of rectovesical fistula.[29] Culhane *et al* have suggested that minimally invasive management by observation, catheter drainage or use of endoscopy like cystoscopy is also a safe option in selected cases of penetrating bladder trauma.[30]

KEY POINTS

- Bladder injury following blunt abdominal trauma is frequently associated with pelvic fracture.
- Gross hematuria is seen in almost all cases of bladder injury following trauma.
- Initial evaluation of hemodynamic status, other associated organ injuries specifically pelvic fracture and urethral injury should also be looked into.
- CT cystogram or CECT abdomen with delayed excretory films can identify the type of bladder rupture following trauma.
- Uncomplicated extraperitoneal bladder rupture is generally managed conservatively with perurethral catheter drainage for 2–3 weeks.
- Intraperitoneal bladder rupture needs immediate surgical repair.
- Missed bladder injury or improperly repaired bladder injury can lead to delayed complications like sepsis, peritonitis, ileus, abscess formation and vesicocutaneous fistula formation.
- Morbidity and mortality following bladder trauma is dependent on clinical state of initial presentation following trauma and associated other organ injuries.

REFERENCES

1. Hochberg E, Stone NN. Bladder rupture associated with pelvic fracture due to blunt trauma. Urology. 1993; 41:531.
2. Hsieh CH, Chen RJ, Fang JF, *et al.* Diagnosis and management of bladder injury by trauma surgeons. Am J Surg. 2002; 184:143.
3. Morey AF, Brandes S, Dugi DD, *et al.* Urotrauma: AUA guideline. J Urol 2014; 192:327–35.
4. Morey AF, Broghammer JA, Hollowell CMP *et al.* Urotrauma Guideline 2020: AUA Guideline. J Urol. 2021;205(1):30–35.
5. Brewer ME, Wilmoth RJ, Enderson BL, *et al.* Prospective comparison of microscopic and gross hematuria as predictors of bladder injury in blunt trauma. Urology. 2007; 69:1086.
6. Mokoena T, Naidu AG. Diagnostic difficulties in patients with a ruptured bladder. Br J Surg. 1995; 82:69.
7. Avey G, Blackmore CC, Wessells H, *et al.* Radiographic and clinical predictors of bladder rupture in blunt trauma patients with pelvic fracture. Acad Radiol. 2006; 13:573.
8. Morgan DE, Nallamala LK, Kenney PJ, *et al.* CT cystography: radiographic and clinical predictors of bladder rupture. AJR Am J Roentgenol. 2000; 174:89.
9. Ishak C, Kanth N. Bladder trauma: multidetector computed tomography cystography. Emerg Radiol. 2011;18(4):321–7.
10. Haas CA, Brown SL, Spirnak JP. Limitations of routine spiral computerized tomography in the evaluation of bladder trauma. J Urol. 1999; 162:51.
11. Wirth GJ, Peter R, Poletti PA, Iselin CE. Advances in the management of blunt traumatic bladder rupture: experience with 36 cases. BJU Int. 2010;106(9):1344–9.
12. Peng MY, Parisky YR, Cornwell EE III, *et al.* CT cystography versus conventional cystography in evaluation of bladder injury. AJR Am J Roentgenol. 1999; 173:1269.
13. Quagliano PV, Delair SM, Malhotra AK. Diagnosis of blunt bladder injury: A prospective comparative study of computed tomography cystography and conventional retrograde cystography. J Trauma. 2006; 61:410.
14. Mathew JE, Chaudhary K, Devana SK, Sharma AP. High rising flames: a sign of complex extraperitoneal bladder rupture. Ann R Coll Surg Engl. 2022;104(2): e35–e36.

15. Fouladi DF, Shayesteh S, Fishman EK, Chu LC. Imaging of urinary bladder injury: the role of CT cystography. Emerg Radiol. 2020;27(1):87–95.
16. Haroon SA, Rahimi H, Merritt A, Baghdanian A, Baghdanian A, LeBedis CA. Computed tomography (CT) in the evaluation of bladder and ureteral trauma: indications, technique, and diagnosis. Abdom Radiol. 2019;44(12):3962–3977.
17. Deck AJ, Shaves S, Talner L, Porter JR. Computerized tomography cystography for the diagnosis of traumatic bladder rupture. J Urol. 2000;164(1):43–6.
18. Lumen N, Kuehhas FE, Djakovic N *et al.* Review of the current management of lower urinary tract injuries by the EAU Trauma Guidelines Panel. Eur Urol. 2015;67(5):925–9.
19. Anderson RE, Keihani S, Moses RA *et al.* Current Management of Extraperitoneal Bladder Injuries: Results from the Multi-Institutional Genito-Urinary Trauma Study (MiGUTS). J Urol. 2020;204(3):538–544.
20. Gomez RG, Ceballos L, Coburn M, *et al.* Consensus statement on bladder injuries. BJU Int 2004;94(1):27–32.
21. Kim FJ, Chammas MF, Gewehr EV, *et al.* Laparoscopic management of intraperitoneal bladder rupture secondary to blunt abdominal trauma using intracorporeal single layer suturing technique. J Trauma. 2008; 65:234–236.
22. Alli MO, Singh B, Moodley J, *et al.* Prospective evaluation of combined suprapubic and urethral catheterization to urethral drainage alone for intraperitoneal bladder injuries. J Trauma. 2003; 55:1152.
23. Patel UJ, Heisler CA. Urinary Tract Injury During Gynecologic Surgery: Prevention, Recognition, and Management. Obstet Gynecol Clin North Am. 2021;48(3):535–556.
24. Lonati C, Esperto F, Scarpa RM *et al.* Bladder perforation during transurethral resection of the bladder: a comprehensive algorithm for diagnosis, management and follow-up. Minerva Urol Nephrol. 2022;74(5):570–580.
25. Inaba K, McKenney M, Munera F, *et al.* Cystogram follow-up in the management of traumatic bladder disruption. J Trauma. 2006; 60:23.
26. Phillips B, Holzmer S, Turco L, Mirzaie M *et al.* Trauma to the bladder and ureter: a review of diagnosis, management, and prognosis. Eur J Trauma Emerg Surg. 2017;43(6):763–773.
27. Banihani MN, Al-Azab RS, Waqfi NR *et al.* Vesicocutaneous fistula presenting as a thigh abscess. Singapore Med J. 2009;50(9): e336–7.
28. Albay C, Güleç MA. Urine in the thigh, an extraordinary complication of pelvic fracture: Vesicocutaneous fistula. Acta Orthop Traumatol Turc. 2021;55(1):80–83.
29. Hornez E, Monchal T, Boddaert G *et al.* Penetrating pelvic trauma: Initial assessment and surgical management in emergency. J Visc Surg. 2016; 153:79–90.
30. Culhane J, Syed JR, Siddiqui S. Minimally invasive management versus open surgery in the treatment of penetrating bladder injuries: a retrospective cohort study. BMC Urol. 2021;21(1):138.

Chapter 14

Urethral Injury with Penile Fracture

• *Martand G Patil* • *Tarun Jain*

LEARNING OBJECTIVES

- To understand the anatomy of penis.
- To understand the causes and presentation of urethral injury in cases of penile fracture.
- To understand the role of investigations.
- To understand the treatment options available.
- To understand the long-term complications and outcomes of fracture penis with concomitant urethral injury.

INTRODUCTION

Urethral rupture associated with fracture penis is very rare condition. It can be partial or complete and the incidence varies from 1% to 38%.

Patients of urethral injury associated with fracture penis usually presents with blood at meatus, hematuria and urinary retention but the absence of these findings does not exclude urethral injury. Diagnosis of fracture penis is clinical and patients usually present with history of crackling sound, swelling and ecchymosis of the penis which is followed by immediate detumescence.

History, clinical examination, retrograde urethrography (RUG), ultrasound (USG), flexible cystoscopy and if required magnetic resonance imaging (MRI) will help in diagnosis of urethral injury associated with fracture penis.

When urethral injury is suspected to be associated with fracture penis, surgical intervention is always required with objective of preserving sexual potency and normal micturition function.

Case Scenario

A 28-year-old male came to emergency room with history of trauma to penis during sexual intercourse with swollen penis and mild pain. He gave history of hearing crackling sound which was followed by detumescence. He had not passed urine for the last 3 hours since injury. He was recently married and did not have any previous medical or surgical illness, urinary complaints, or erectile dysfunction.

On examination, he had blood at meatus, swelling and the penile discoloration (Fig. 14.1) with palpable bladder with lower abdominal tenderness. Diagnosis of fracture penis and urethral injury was confirmed on RUG as it showed extravasation of contrast. Doppler ultrasound showed a breach in continuity of tunica albuginea with a surrounding hematoma. He underwent exploration with circumcising incision with two-layer repair of tunical breach on the dorsolateral aspect of left corpora (Fig. 14.2). Closure of urethral injury (Fig. 14.3) over 14 Fr silicon catheter was also performed.

Post-operative course of patient was uneventful with asymptomatic, normal uroflowmetry with insignificant postvoid residue on ultrasonography and no erectile dysfunction at 1 year follow-up.

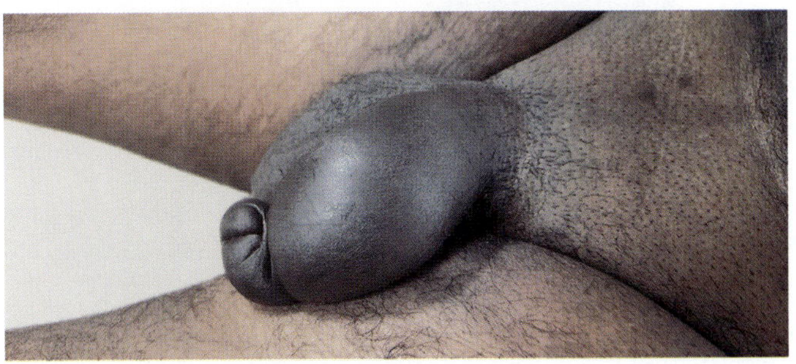

Fig. 14.1: Penile fracture

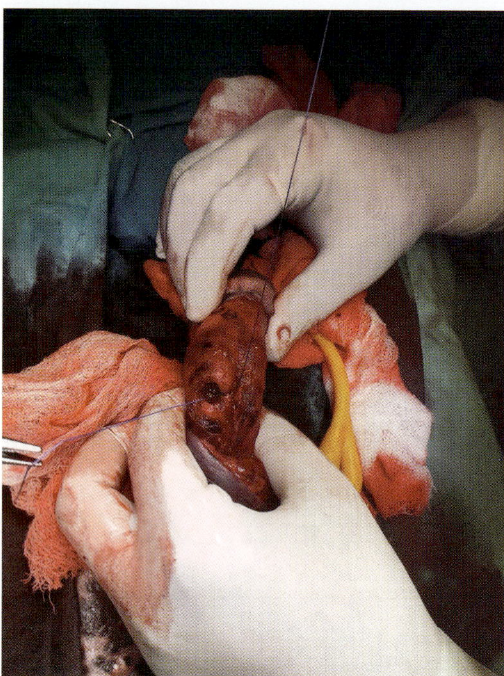

Fig. 14.2: Exposed penis with tunical defect

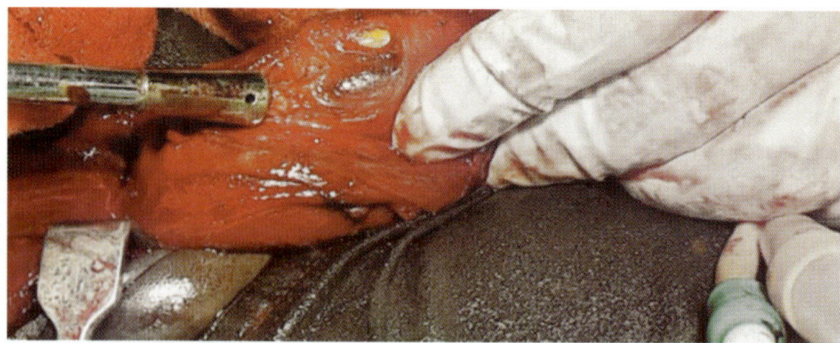

Fig. 14.3A: Closure of tunical defect and urethral injury

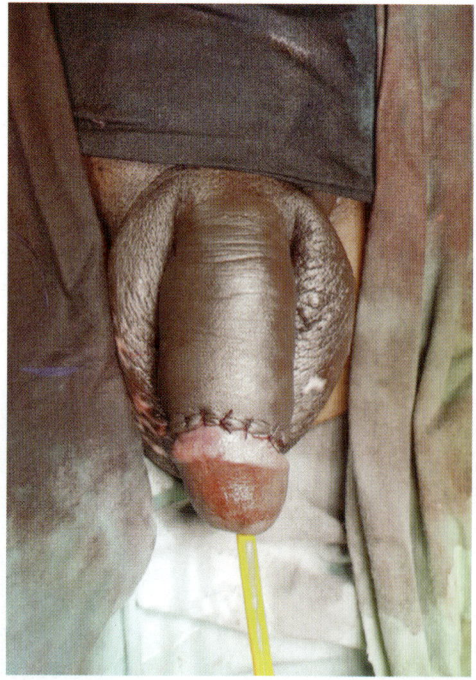

Fig. 14.3B: Closure of circumcision incision

1. **What is a penile fracture?**

   Ans: Penile fracture is caused due to trauma to erect penis causing a breach in the tunica albugenia of the corpora cavernosa.[1] It may be associated with or without urethral injury.

2. **What are the causes of penile fracture?**

   Ans: Penile fracture is most commonly caused when during the process of sexual intercourse the penis slips out of the vagina and buckles between the perineum of the partner and the pubis of the patient.[2–4] Other causes include intercourse in abnormal positions, rolling over the bed on erect penis, forceful bending to achieve detumescence (taghaandan), masturbation, anal intercourse, fall on erect penis.[2]

   Tunica albuginea is made of two layers. The inner circular and outer longitudinal is composed of collagen and elastin. It is the outer layer which is responsible for its strength.[5]

3. **Why does penile fracture occur in an erect penis and not a flaccid penis?**

   Ans: During erection there is engorgement of the erectile tissues of penis. There are three erectile tissues in penis. Two cavernosal bodies and one spongiosal body which has urethra in it. During erection the tunica stretches and forms a non-compliant rigid covering over the cavernosal tissues. It is this non-compliant tunica seen in an erect penis that fractures when it comes under stress due to trauma and tears causing a fracture. In a flaccid penis the tunica is not under stress and compliant and hence does not tear/fracture due to its elasticity. The tensile strength of the tunica albuginea can resist tearing until the intracavernous pressure exceeds 1500 mm Hg.[6] It is when this pressure is exceeded that the tunica ruptures resulting in penile fracture. Also the thickness of tunica reduces from 2 mm in a flaccid penis to 0.25 mm in erect penis due to the stretch during erection,[6] hence it ruptures more easily during erect penis rather than a flaccid penis.

4. **What has been observed in the histology study of tunica albugenia in cases of penile fracture?**

   Ans: Histology of tunica albuginea in 83% of patients had fibrosclerosis and 50% patients had cellular infiltrate consisting of lymphocytes and histiocytes.[7]

5. **How does a patient with penile fracture present?**

   Ans: Patient is generally a young male (most common age group is 25–35 years. with a mean age of 27.8 years.) complaining of trauma during sexual intercourse wherein he classically hears a popping sound followed by rapid detumenscence.[8] This is followed by swelling due to hematoma in the subcutaneous tissue resulting in an eggplant deformity. There may be associated bleeding per meatus.[9]

6. **When will you suspect a urethral injury in a patient of penile fracture?**

Ans: Blood at meatus indicates there is associated urethral injury. The patient may complain of difficulty to pass urine and many a times there is urinary retention. The injury can be of various grade. It can range from just mild contusion to complete urethral disruption.

Grade 1: Contusion with intact spongiosa.

Grade 2: Partial transection of urethra

Grade 3: Complete transection of urethra.

7. **What are clinical findings to be elicited in the patient?**

Ans: The penis is deviated opposite to the site of tear and there is discoloration and swelling of the skin due to underlying hematoma. On palpation, we might be able to feel the defect in the corpora. In fracture penis pain is not a classical finding. On squeezing the urethra if there is blood at the meatus, we should suspect urethral injury.[10] However, presence or absence of blood at meatus may not be consistent with concomitant urethral injury.[11]

8. **What is the role of imaging to diagnose urethral injury in a patient of penile fracture?**

Ans: A clinical suspicion and examination remain the mainstay. Color Doppler ultrasound, RUG, MRI and cystoscopy are the options available.

Color Doppler ultrasound: Although easily available and can be done bedside. It can diagnose the presence of hematoma and breach of corpora cavernosa with high accuracy. It can miss urethral injury.

RUG: Whenever urethral injury is suspected, an RUG can be done as it will demonstrate a leak of the contrast. It will help us to know the site of urethral injury and also help us demonstrate continuity of urethra or complete transection.[11]

MRI: Although MRI has high sensitivity for diagnosing cavernosal injury with the site and degree of injury. It has low accuracy to diagnose urethral injury.[12] The sensitivity and specificity for cavernosal injury was 100% and 77.8% respectively. However, MRI had inferior results for diagnosing urethral injury with a sensitivity and specificity of 60% and 78.3%.[12]

Cystoscopy: Flexible cystoscopy at the time or before the surgery to treat penile fracture can help in diagnosing urethral injury with good accuracy without delaying the procedure. However, its availability can be a concern.

9. **What are the types of penile fracture?**

Ans:

- Fracture with breach in single cavernosa
- Fracture with breach in both the cavernosa
- Fracture with breach in spongiosa with or without urethral injury
- Complex injury with degloving of penis/ injury to crus.

10. **What are the treatment options available?**

Ans:

- Urethral catheterization
- Suprapubic—cystostomy.
- Primary repair

For partial rupture of urethra all above have been tried with variable outcomes. However, majority of the reports suggest excellent results with primary repair.[13, 14]

For complete transection of urethra, surgical correction provides the only possible chance of cure. The timing of the surgery is of paramount importance. Earlier the better with better sexual outcomes.[15]

11. **What are the steps of the surgery?**

Ans: Degloving of penis with circum-coronal incision.

Thorough wash is given with debridement of necrotic tissue.

The site of injury is identified.

- The cavernosa is sutured with non-absorbable suture.
- Urethral injury can be repaired with absorbable suture.

Primary closure of urethra.

- If partial transection is there it can be closed over a Foley's with interrupted absorbable sutures.
- If complete transection is there, the urethra may have to be mobilized proximally and distally to achieve a tension free anastomosis.

Primary closure with graft augmentation is needed for patients with complete transection in whom tension free repair cannot be achieved. Graft can be used to bridge the defect and achieve a tension free anastomosis. Graft is placed on the corporal body and quilted and urethroplasty performed on lines of ventral onlay repair. Buccal graft and preputial graft are the options available. Pedicled prepucial graft is another option.

Staged repair would be performed in cases in which a tension free repair is not possible. Here staged Johansson's repair can be done.

12. What are the complications of surgery?

Ans: Immediate complications:[14]

1. Edema of the penis specially the prepuce
2. Wound infection
3. Abscess formation
4. Injury to neurovascular bundle in the Buck's fascia.
5. Fistula formation.

Delayed complications:[14]

1. Penile curvature.
2. Erectile dysfunction.
3. Urethral stricture.
4. Urethral fistula.
5. Urethral diverticulum with or without calculi in it.

13. How to manage urethral stricture in patients of penile fracture?

Ans: Treatment is on lines with management anterior urethral stricture. A staged or primary augmentation urethroplasty based on RUG findings can be planned.

KEY POINTS

- Penile fracture with urethral involvement is an uncommon urological emergency.
- History and clinical examination are the most important parts of diagnosis.
- Urethral injury should be suspected in the presence urethral bleeding, hematuria or urinary retention.
- Urgent urethral reconstruction is mandatory to produces satisfactory results with low levels of complications.

REFERENCES

1. Falcone M, Garaffa G, Castiglione F, Ralph DJ. Current Management of Penile Fracture: An Up-to-Date Systematic Review. Sex Med Rev. 2018;6(2):253–260.
2. Barros R, Schulze L, Ornellas AA, Koifman L, Favorito LA. Relationship between sexual position and severity of penile fracture. Int J Impot Res. 2017 Sep;29(5):207–209.
3. Ory J, Bailly G. Management of penile fracture. Can Urol Assoc J. 2019;13(6 Suppl4):S72–S74.
4. Gulmi FA. Penile Fracture. Rev Urol. 2018;20(1):41–42.
5. Mirzazadeh M, Fallahkarkan M, Hosseini J. Penile fracture epidemiology, diagnosis and management in Iran: a narrative review. *Transl Androl Urol.* 2017;6(2):158–166.
6. Yogi P, Sapkota S, Shiwakoti S, Dongol UMS, Paudyal P, Karki A. Penile Fracture: A Case Report. JNMA J Nepal Med Assoc. 2022;60(254):895–897.
7. De Rose AF, Giglio M, Carmignani G. Traumatic rupture of the corpora cavernosa: new physiopathologic acquisitions. Urology. 2001;57(2):319–322.
8. Lee SH, Bak CW, Choi MH, Lee HS, Lee MS, Yoon SJ. Trauma to male genital organs: a 10-year review of 156 patients, including 118 treated by surgery. BJU Int. 2008;101(2):211–215.
9. Mirzazadeh M, Fallahkarkan M, Hosseini J. Penile fracture epidemiology, diagnosis and management in Iran: a narrative review. Transl Androl Urol. 2017;6(2):158–166.
10. Barros R, Ribeiro JGA, da Silva HAM, de Sá FR, Fosse AM Júnior, Favorito LA. Urethral injury in penile fracture: a narrative review. Int Braz J Urol. 2020;46(2):152–157.
11. Mydlo JH, Hayyeri M, Macchia RJ. Urethrography and cavernosography imaging in a small series of penile fractures: a comparison with surgical findings. Urology. 1998;51(4):616–619.
12. Sokolakis I, Schubert T, Oelschlaeger M, *et al.* The Role of Magnetic Resonance Imaging in the Diagnosis of Penile Fracture in Real-Life Emergency Settings: Comparative Analysis with Intraoperative Findings. J Urol. 2019;202(3):552–557.
13. Fergany AF, Angermeier KW, Montague DK. Review of Cleveland Clinic experience with penile fracture. Urology. 1999;54(2):352–355.
14. Jack GS, Garraway I, Reznichek R, Rajfer J. Current treatment options for penile fractures. Rev Urol. 2004;6(3):114–120.
15. Naraynsingh V, Raju GC. Fracture of the penis. Br J Surg. 1985;72(4):305–306.

Chapter 15

Surgical Reconstruction in Thimble Bladder

• Ganesh Gopalakrishnan • Suresh K Bhagat

LEARNING OBJECTIVES

- To define thimble bladder and give simple concepts to identify it.
- To describe the management of such pathology.

SUMMARY

The thimble bladder is a low-capacity bladder of about 20 to 50 ml in volume. Its clinical presentation can include LUTS, hydronephrosis, or even renal failure. Multiple surgical treatments are available for this condition, all of which are based on augmenting bladder capacity.

INTRODUCTION

There are no clearcut bladder volumes which decide if a bladder is actually thimble; nevertheless, bladder volumes between 20 and 50 ml have been considered to qualify for the term "thimble bladder".[1,2]

In many situations it is the symptom(s) and not the actual bladder volume which could dictate the future course of action. A clear distinction needs to be made between the conscious bladder capacity and that which is determined under anaesthesia at physiological pressures. A bladder whose conscious and unconscious capacities are equal is deemed as "fixed" and will require surgical correction if low.

In this context a voiding diary is one of the most reliable clinical tools for assessing the conscious bladder capacity and helps in deciding further course of action.

In certain inflammatory conditions, the conscious capacity may be lower than that found under anaesthesia; urinary bladders that fall into this category could improve and hence one should not rush into offering surgical correction.

Disruption of apical layer of urothelium by factors causing inflammation is an important initiating event in the pathogenesis of thimble bladder.

Subsequently there is a loss of viscoelastic property and compliance, leaving a small capacity causing intolerable storage symptoms like frequency, urgency, nocturia, pain and haematuria requiring treatment.

The International Continence Society has not yet defined inflammatory contracted bladder and there are no guidelines specifying the capacity of bladder.

Thimble bladder can be either due to tuberculous or nontuberculous conditions.

Nontuberculous conditions like radiation, neurogenic vesical dysfunction, post-intravesical BCG or mitomycin therapy, prior cyclophosphamide therapy, severe form of interstitial cystitis and schistosomiasis are among the common causes of a thimble bladder. A diligent effort to establish the cause of contracted bladder must be made.

This would be testing urine for AFB—both culture and the geneXpert test. At times bladder biopsy and sending the tissue obtained for analysis will help.

As a general rule of thumb, if the bladder is contracted due to tuberculosis, then the upper tracts are likely to be involved.

There are a variety of reconstructive procedures for thimble bladder. There are different bowel segments from stomach to sigmoid colon, which have been used for bladder reconstruction.

The most important investigation that needs to be done before undertaking surgery to increase bladder capacity using bowel segments is the GFR.

A value below 40 ml/min is considered undesirable for augmentation cystoplasty.

The choice of bowel segment for reconstruction is purely a surgeon's preference. However, individual experience, mobility of the bowel segment and length of mesentery are important considerations. Inflammatory bowel conditions are contraindication to augmentation.

While preservation of natural voiding should be the goal, this may not be possible in every patient and hence counselling for carrying out clean intermittent self-catheterisation after surgery needs to be done.

Complications like metabolic acidosis, hour glass anastomotic contracture, mucus production, infection, stone disease and haematuria dysuria syndrome should be kept in mind.

In this chapter we will focus on all the details about various types of surgical procedures to correct the thimble bladder, their complications with illustrated cases.

Case Scenario

A 32-year-old male presented with severe storage LUTS (increased frequency every 10–15 minutes, urgency, dysuria and urge incontinence), recurrent low-grade fever with loss appetite for last 6 months. He had received ATT for pulmonary TB 10 years ago. On evaluation, serum creatinine was 3.2 mg%, USG: B/L moderate hydroureteronephrosis and very small capacity bladder, VCUG showed small capacity bladder with left side grade IV and right side grade 1 reflux as shown in Fig. 15.1.

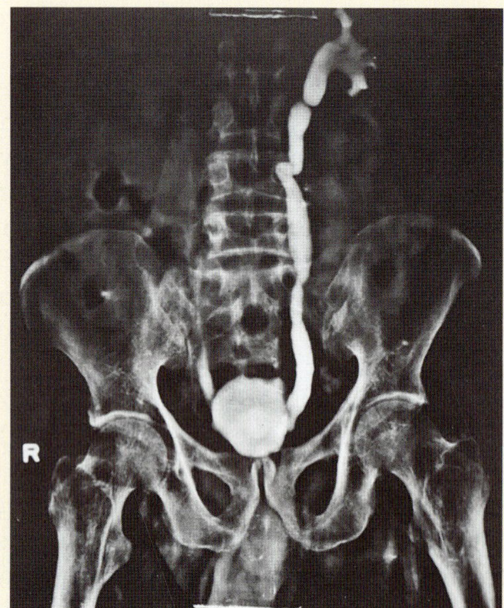

Fig. 15.1: Vesicoureteric reflux on the left side grade IV and right side grade I reflux

1. **What is your clinical diagnosis?**

   Ans: GUTB with thimble bladder and renal failure.

2. **What is incidence and etiopathogenesis of thimble bladder?**

   Ans: Urinary bladder is involved in about one-third cases of GUTB. Disruption of apical layer of urothelium by factors causing inflammation is an important initiating event and eventually mural fibrosis results in thimble bladder. Subsequently there is a loss of viscoelastic property and compliance, leaving a small capacity.

3. **What are the clinical presentation of thimble bladder?**

   Ans: Storage LUTS (frequency, urgency, dysuria, incontinence), upper tract dilation, renal failure.

4. **How will you evaluate the patient of thimble bladder?**

   Ans: Renal biochemistry, routine and culture sensitivity urine, urine for AFB smear and culture, urine for geneXpert, CT urogram (if creatinine is normal), VCUG.

5. **How will you manage this patient?**

   Ans: Bilateral US guided percutaneous nephrostomy and start ATT.

6. **What is the treatment schedule in GUTB with normal GFR and reduced GFR?**

   Ans: The initial phase should consist of two months of isoniazid (H), rifampicin (R), pyrazinamide (Z), and ethambutol (E). The continuation phase should consist of three drugs (isoniazid, rifampicin and ethambutol) given for at least four months in patients with normal GFR and about 50% reduction in dose of ethambutol and pyrazinamide in patients with reduced GFR.

7. **What are the issues related to bowel augmentation in this man with reduced GFR?**

   Ans: Worsening of renal failure and metabolic acidosis hence bone related events.

8. **Serum creatinine came down to normal after 6 weeks, VCUG showed a small contracted bladder and bilateral VUR, now what is the next line of management?**

   Ans: Augmentation ileocystoplasty

9. **What are the aims of surgical reconstruction for thimble bladder?**

   Ans: To increase the bladder capacity to enable the patient to retain urine for a reasonable period of time.

   To restore the function as a low-pressure (less than 30 cm of water) reservoir during storage and to enable the patient to void naturally.

   Prevention of incontinence and infection that may jeopardize upper urinary tract integrity.

10. How to sort out poor quality of life due to frequency—what surgical procedures are applicable?

Ans: To increase the bladder capacity following surgical procedures are applicable: Ileocystoplasty, caecocystoplasty, ileocaeco cystoplasty, colocystoplasty, gastrocystoplasty, jejunocystoplasty, orthotopic neobladder. Small bowel segment specially ileum is the most commonly utilized bowel segment for bladder augmentation,[4] but the use of caecum,[5] sigmoid[6] and stomach is also described.

11. In case we do a standard bowel augmentation, what is the likely outcome over time?

Ans: Recurrent UTI, calculus formation, mucus production, slowly progressive renal dysfunction, malignancy and bone related issues.

12. What are the technical difficulty with bowel augmentation with very small bladder? How to overcome?

Ans: Hourglass contracture which can be overcome by making stellate-shaped incision over bladder for wide anastomosis.

13. Describe the steps of augmentation ileocystoplasty. What are its complications?

Ans: Augmentation cystoplasty in humans was first described in the late nineteenth century by von Mikulicz.[3]

Prof. Antoni was the first person to introduce ileocystoplasty for augmenting the thimble bladder.[8] The ileum is an excellent segment to enlarge the capacity of thimble bladder. The results of augmentation ileocystoplasty are excellent in thimble bladder but with possible risk of renal function impairment due to urinary infection, urolithiasis, VUR and stenosis of various anastomoses.

A segment of ileum at least 15 to 20 cm proximal to the ileocecal valve should be selected. The isolated segment should be 20 to 40 cm in length, depending on patient size, native bladder capacity, and the desired final capacity. With short ureters, an extra tail of isoperistaltic ileum can be useful to reach the foreshortened ureters. The segment to be used should have an adequate mesentery to reach the native bladder without tension. The continuity of ileum is restored with running absorbable sutures.

The harvested ileal segment is irrigated clear with normal saline and opened on its antimesenteric border. The ileum is reconfigured into shape to achieve low pressure reservoir. The anastomosis of the reconfigured ileum to native bivalved bladder is easy when started posteriorly.

The anastomosis is usually done in a single layer fashion, always using absorbable suture and inverting the mucosa to the lumen.

Non-absorbable sutures should never be used for any cystoplasty because they serve as a nidus for stone formation. A suprapubic tube is brought through the native bladder when possible and secured. The anterior aspect of the anastomosis is then completed. A drain is placed near the bladder and brought out of the pelvis through a separate stab incision. It should be removed promptly if not draining urine.

Complications: Early complications are pulmonary embolism, myocardial infarction, progressive azotemia, urinary and intestinal fistulas, sepsis, contracture of vesicointestinal anastomosis, ischemic fibrosis of intestinal patch and wound dehiscence. Chronic exposure of enteric mucosa with urine leads to increased mucus production with stone formation and infection, spontaneous perforation, metabolic disturbance, growth retardation and malignant metaplasia. Progressive azotemia, renal stones, small intestinal obstruction, ureter stricture and osteitis pubis constitute the majority of the late complications.

14. What are the indications, steps of procedure and complication of various types of surgical reconstruction used for thimble bladder?

Ans:

Caecocystoplasty

Couvelaire was the first to advocate caecocystoplsty in 1950.[9] The favourable factors for the caecum for augmentation include protection afforded by ileocaecal valve, easy mobility requiring no refashioning and its rich blood supply.

It has been suggested that native bladder wall should be preserved as much as possible which makes anastomosis easier and allows the patients to void better.

Added advantage of caecum for augmenting the small contracted bladder, is that it generates adequate voiding pressure and might help patients void normally.

Complications: Ileocecal valve removal may significantly decrease intestinal transit time and thus causes diarrhoea. Ileocecal valve loss can also allow bacterial backflow into the ileum, and the organisms may interfere with fat and vitamin B_{12} metabolism. Terminal ileum is the sole site of vitamin B_{12} absorption. Removal of the distal ileum from the gastrointestinal tract may therefore result in vitamin B_{12} deficiency and megaloblastic anaemia.

No case of significant electrolyte imbalance is encountered. Common complications are enuresis, external urinary fistula, wound disruption, incisional hernia, bladder outlet obstruction (BOO), intestinal obstruction from adhesions and contraction of cystoplasty anastomosis.

Ileocaecocystoplasty

Indications: Ileocaecal segment is well suited in patients with severely contracted and diseased bladder in which supratrigonal cystectomy in contemplated. An antireflux ureteroileal anastomosis to the ileal part of ileocaecal segment better protects the upper tracts from back pressure and ascending pyelonephritis.

Factors favouring ileocaecal segment for augmentation cystoplasty are good blood supply, ileal segment can be exteriorized without disturbing ureteroileal anastomosis in case failed reconstruction, ileal segment can be used for ureteral replacement.

The ileocecal segment is isolated, irrigated clear with normal saline and opened on its antimesenteric border through the ileocecal valve for its entire length. The continuity of gut is maintained by ileo-ascending colon anastomosis.

In the typical ileocecal augmentation, the ileal and caecal segments are of equivalent length so that the borders of the open segment can be anastomosed and then folded on themselves to form a cup cystoplasty. The anastomosis of the reconfigured segments to the widely opened bivalved bladder is done in one-layer with absorbable suture. The mesenteric window is closed, and a suprapubic tube is placed through the native bladder and secured through the abdominal wall.

Complications: Same as seen in cecocystoplasty

Colocystoplasty:

Indications: Colonic segment is reserved for the more severely diseased and contracted bladder. Leomone was the first surgeon to use sigmoid colon for augmentation cystoplasty and reported it in 1912.[10]

Colon is usually used for more severe disease and contracted bladder. Because of the strong unit contractions of the sigmoid, it is imperative to detubularize and reconfigure the segment to provide maximum compliance and disruption of contractions.

About 15–20 cm of sigmoid colon is identified and mobilized. After identification of its blood supply, the surgeon must ensure that the segment can reach the bladder without tension. The bowel segment is divided between clamps, and a colocolostomy is performed. Detubularization and reconfiguration is done in a fashion determined by the surgeon's preference. The sigmoid patch is anastomosed to the bivalved bladder in a manner similar to that previously described for ileocystoplasty.

Complications: Chronic cystitis, persistent dysuria and frequency, along with electrolyte imbalance and metabolic disturbances.

15. Is augmentation procedures possible if the GFR is low?

Ans:

Gastrocystoplasty

Indication: The main indication of gastrocystoplasty are impaired renal function and metabolic acidosis, and insufficient large and small bowel. Decreased mucus production is a major advantage.[11]

Two techniques of gastrocystoplasty have been described.

Leong and Ong (1972) described the use of the entire antrum with a small rim of body for gastric replacement. With this technique, the left gastroepiploic artery is used as vascular pedicle. Continuity of the upper gastrointestinal tract restored by Billroth I gastroduodenostomy.

A wedge-shaped segment of body based on the midportion of the greater curvature may also be used but contains higher concentration of acid producing cells. The right or the left gastroepiploic artery may be used as vascular pedicle. The segment used may be 10 to 20 cm in length along the greater curvature depending on patient age, size and needed volume. The incision into stomach is stopped just short of the lesser curvature to avoid injury to the branches of the vagus nerve controlling gastric emptying.

When compared with intestinal bladder augmentation, augmentation gastrocystplasty has many advantages including fewer contractions, less mucus production, non-absorption of urinary electrolytes and fewer histological changes suggestive of malignancy. The technical ease of ureteral reimplantation makes the procedure suited for a severely contracted bladder due to TB with concomitant ureteral structural and renal function impairment.[12] However, use of the pedunculated wedge in reconstruction leads to transposition of more cell mass to the neobladder making urine more acidic (>3.0 pH). Also, on removal of the parietal mass from the stomach, gastric activity is reduced to a level insufficient to suppress the release of gastrin leading to severe metabolic alkalosis, harmful aciduria and hypergastrinemia. Hence antral gastrocytoplasty may be considered a better orthotopic cystoplasty wherein a simpler detubularized version proves beneficial to dampen the forceful peristaltic antral contractions compared to the more difficult muscular tunnel.[13] A further modification of the original antral technique uses the body of stomach[14] wherein the body acts as a barrier to the absorption of urinary salts and actually secretes acid.

Complications: Hematuria-Dysuria syndrome. It is imperative to achieve reliable urinary continence in patients undergoing gastrocystoplasty because urinary leakage may result in the exposure of the skin to gastric secretions. Hypersecretion of acid after meals is usually due to a portion of antrum inadvertently included in the augmentation.

Orthotopic Neobladder

Indication:

Although augmentation cystoplasty is an accepted method of surgical reconstruction for thimble bladder, but it may not provide symptomatic relief in severely contracted bladder with LUTS and suprapubic pain. Additionally, there is a risk of stricture at anastomotic site and developing an hourglass contracture. Hence thimble bladder is best managed by orthotopic neobladder.[15]

In this reconstructive procedure all diseased and fibrosed tissue of bladder is removed and anastomosis of the neobladder is done with prostatic urethra. In case of associated advanced prostatic tuberculosis, nerve sparing cystoprostatectomy is done and anastomosis is performed with membranous urethra.

Complications: Hypercontinence, with incomplete evacuation, nocturnal enuresis and stress incontinence, in addition to various metabolic complications of using bowel segments.

Jejunum

The jejunum has the largest diameter of the small bowel and longest mesentery. The jejunum is rarely used and should be employed under rare circumstances in which there are no other acceptable segment available for use, like extensive radiation that involves the ileum, those with severe adhesions of the ileum and absence of large bowel, and those who have an absent colon with inflammatory disease of distal small bowel.

The contraindications to its use are severe bowel nutritional disorders and presence of another acceptable segment. Jejunum is not used because of severe electrolytes abnormalities like hyperkalemia, hyponatremia, hypochloremia, azotemia and metabolic acidosis. These electrolytes abnormalities result in lethargy, nausea, vomiting, dehydration, muscular weakness and an elevated temperature. Problem is often associated with significant hypovolemia. If the abnormalities are allowed to persist, the patient may become moribund and finally die. The jejunal syndrome is treated by administering normal saline. Hyperkalemia may be treated judiciously with hydrochlorthiazide.

16. Discuss the complications of augmentation cystoplasty and their management in general.

Ans: Following are the main complications

Hyperchloremic metabolic acidosis: Clinical features are fatigue, weakness, anorexia, and polydipsia. Such complications may be debilitating to the patient if not recognized and treated in time, can result in bone demineralization and hence osteoporosis. Best diagnosed by arterial blood gas analysis. Treated by oral bicarbonate therapy.

In severe cases of acidosis, chloride transport can be blocked with chlorpromazine and nicotinic acid.

Hyponatremic, hypochloremic and hyperkalemic metabolic acidosis if jejunal segment is used for augmentation cystoplasty.

Hypokalemic and hypochloremic alkalosis: In some patients with gastrocystoplasty during an acute gastrointestinal illness with dehydration.

Mucus: Routine use of daily bladder irrigations with normal saline would reduce the mucus plugs and may minimize UTI and stone formation.

Recurrent urinary tract infection: Bacteriuria is common after augmentation cystoplasty particularly in patients who need CIC. Bacteriuria should be treated in presence of significant symptoms such as incontinence and suprapubic pain, haematuria, foul smelling urine and remarkably increased mucus production.

Bacteriuria should be treated if urine cultures shows urea-splitting organism that may lead to stone formation.

Hepatic encephalopathy

Urinary ammonium excreted by kidneys is reabsorbed by the intestinal segment, returned to the liver through portal circulation, and then metabolized to urea through ornithine cycle. In liver dysfunction the metabolic reserve may exceed and lead to ammoniagenic encephalopathy and coma.

Systemic bacteraemia and urinary tract infections with urea-splitting organisms can impair the hepatic metabolism and cause hyperammonemia syndrome, even with normal hepatic function.

Delayed Spontaneous Bladder Perforation

Patients with spontaneous perforation after augmentation cystoplasty are typically ill with abdominal pain, distention, and fever. Sepsis is common. Nausea, decreased urine output, and shoulder pain from diaphragmatic irritation have also been noted. Patients with neurogenic dysfunction often have impaired lower abdominal sensation and are seen later in the course of the illness; severe sepsis and death have occurred. Patients with perforation after gastrocystoplasty often seek care promptly because of acid irritation. A high index of suspicion for perforation is necessary. Contrast cystography is diagnostic in most cases.

Etiology: The cause of delayed perforations within a bowel segment is unknown. It has been suggested that some perforations may be secondary to traumatic catheterization.[16,17] It seems unlikely that catheterization trauma is the lone cause in most patients. The location of the perforations has been variable among patients and even in a single patient may have multiple perforations. Perforations have occurred in patients after augmentation who did not catheterize at all. Other authors have suggested that trauma to the bowel because of fixed adhesions resulting in sheering forces with emptying and filling may result in perforation.[16] Transmural infection of the bladder wall has also been proposed as a cause.

Histologic examination of areas of perforation has noted necrosis, vascular congestion, haemorrhage, and hemosiderin deposition compatible with chronic bowel wall ischemia.[18] Chronic overdistention of the bladder may result in such ischemia. High outflow resistance may maintain the bladder pressure rather than allowing urinary leakage and venting of the pressure, potentially increasing ischemia.[19] However, once bowel is reconfigured, it may be more prone to ischemia if high pressure does persist. Failure to perform CIC on a regular basis when needed to empty may exacerbate such issues.

Incidence: Delayed perforations more commonly occur within the bowel segment and represent a problem with long-term storage of urine within an intestinal segment. With inconsistent differences across multiple large series, it is unlikely that any given enteric segment is at significantly increased risk for perforation and that multiple factors influence the risk for the complication. A recent analysis of morbidity in patients undergoing augmentation cystoplasty using the pediatric health information system database showed that the risk of perforation was doubled in those who had bladder outlet procedures.[19]

Treatment: The standard treatment of spontaneous perforation of the augmented bladder is immediate surgical repair. Although conservative management including catheter drainage, antibiotics, and serial abdominal examinations can be successful in the absence of clinical deterioration, severe peritonitis, and extensive extravasation. Increasing sepsis and death of the patient may result from a delay in diagnosis or treatment.

Tumour formation: Filmer and Spencer[20] identified 14 patients who have developed adenocarcinoma in an augmented bladder, and several more have been reported since then; 9 of those tumors occurred after ileocystoplasty and 5 after colocystoplasty.

Patients undergoing augmentation cystoplasty should be made aware of a potential increased risk for tumour development. Yearly surveillance of the augmented bladder with cystoscopy is important. Transitional cell carcinoma, hyperplasia, and dysplasia have also been noted near the anastomosis.

17. If ileal conduit is being considered due to reduced GFR, what is to be done to the bladder if left *in situ* to avoid the risk of pyocystis?

Ans: Ileovesicostomy should be considered as a fall back procedure in case of reduced GFR and morbidity associated with cystectomy of the diseased bladder. Retaining a diseased bladder and diverting urine runs the significant risk of pyocystis.

18. What would you do with urinary bladder in case of female? Is there a risk of pyocystitis in such cases?

Ans: If bladder is retained, then one should consider doing vaginocystostomy (Spence procedure) because there is a risk of pyocystitis.

19. How will you manage large bladder stone in post-augmentation cystoplasty patient with bilateral hydroureteronephrosis with serum creatinine 2.4 mg%?

Ans: Bladder drainage with a bigger size urethral catheter and start culture specific antibiotic. The stone can be later removed when he is stable either by open cystolithotomy of via a percutaneous approach. The risk of sepsis and the time to fragment this size of stone could lead to serious consequences especially sepsis and if the procedure is done endoscopically, then due diligence should be given to the above factors before embarking on treatment.

20. What advice will you give to the patient at discharge?

Ans: Regular CIC, low dose antibiotic prophylaxis, and regular follow-up.

21. A post-sigmoid cystoplasty patient presents to the emergency department with history of fatigue, weakness, anorexia and polydipsia. On clinical examination there was a suprapubic lump. How will you manage?

Ans: USG is needed initially to confirm that the suprapubic lump is the bladder and also to assess for hydroureteronephrosis. Indwelling urethral catheterisation and to send CBC, creatinine, electrolytes and ABG.

22. What is your probable diagnosis?

Ans: Hyperchloremic metabolic acidosis.

23. What next?

Ans: Correction of metabolic acidosis by intravenous soda bicarbonate.

24. What advice will you give at discharge?

Ans: Teach CIC, put him on regular oral sodium bicarbonate tablets, regular follow-up in OPD with renal biochemistry at 6 months.

KEY POINTS

- Surgical reconstruction of urinary bladder has a very important role in the management of thimble bladder.
- It is not the volume of the thimble bladder which matters but the bothersome symptoms that matters.
- The goal of treatment in thimble bladder is to provide better quality of life to the patient, stable renal function and prevention of upper tract damage.
- However, these reconstructive procedures require stringent long-term follow-up for evaluation and management of metabolic complications, UTI and renal failure.

REFERENCES

1. Tuberculosis and Parasitic Infections of the Genitourinary Tract. Alica H. Chang, Brian G. Blackburn, Michael Hsieh. Campbell's Urology; 12th Edition Vol 2 Chapter 60, Page 1309.
2. Krotoszyner M. The cystoscopic diagnosis of contracted bladder. J Am Med Assoc 1917;LXVIII:687–91.
3. Von Mikulicz J. Zur operation der angebarenen blaben Spalte. Zentralbl Chir 1889;20:641–3
4. Biers SM, Venn SN, Greenwell TJ. The past, present and future of augmentation cystoplasty. BJU Int. 2012;109:1280–93.
5. Vajda P, Pinter AB, Harangi F, Farkas A, Vastyan AM, Oberritter Z. Metabolic findings after colocystoplasty in children. Urology 2003;62(3):542–6.
6. Yuan L, Xu Q, Liao LM, Ma LL, Wang L, Wang Y *et al.* Comparison of bowel function pre and post-sigmoid augmentation cystoplasty in spinal cord injury patients. Zhonghua Yi Xue Za Zhi 2012; 92(12): 842–4
7. Bramble FJ. The treatment of adult enuresis and urge incontinence by enterocystoplasty. Br J Urol 1982; 54(6): 693–6.
8. Jurasz A. Operacja wytwareza percherza. Polski Przeglad Chirurgiczny 1928;7:453–454
9. Couvelaire R. The "little bladder" of genitourinary tuberculosis; classification, site and variants of bladder-intestine transplants. J. Urol 1950;56:381–434.
10. Leomine G, J. Urology 1913;4:367–72.
11. Adams MC, Mitchel ME, Rink RC. Gastrocystoplasy: An alternative solution to the problem of urological reconstruction in severely compromised patient. J. Urol 1988; 140:1152–61.
12. Shamsa A. Gastric neobladder for treatment of tubercular cystitis. J Urol. 1998;159:202.
13. Leong CH. Use of stomach for bladder replacement in urinary diversion. Am Roy Coll Surg Eng. 1971;60:283–8.
14. Adams MC, Mitchell ME, Rink RC. Gastrocystoplasty: An alternative solution to the problem of urological reconstruction in severely compromised patient. J Urol.1988;140:1152–61.
15. Hemal AK, Aron M. Orthotopic neobladder in management of tubercular thimble bladders: Initial experience and long term results. Urology. 1999; 53:298–301.
16. Elder JS *et al.* Perforation of the augmented bladder in patients undergoing clean intermittent catheterisation. J Urol 1988; 140:1159.
17. Rushton HG *et al.* Delayed bladder rupture after augmentation enterocystoplasty. J Urol 1988;140:344.
18. Crane JM *et al.* Ischemic necrosis; A hypothesis to explain the pathogenesis of spontaneously ruptured enterocystoplasty. J Urol 1991; 146:141–44.
19. Urinary Tract Reconstruction in Children. John C. Thomas *et al.* Campbell's Urology; 12th Edition Volume 1, Chapter 129, Page 700.
20. Filmer RB, Spencer JR: Malignancies in bladder augmentations and intestinal conduit. J Urol1990; 143: 671.

Chapter

16

Non-Transecting Anastomotic Urethroplasty in Bulbar Urethral Stricture

• *Venkat Arjunrao Gite*

LEARNING OBJECTIVES

To understand the

- Anatomical basis for NTBU.
- Clinical and diagnostic evaluation of bulbar urethral stricture.
- Selection of patient, approach and type of NTBU.
- Principle and steps of various NTBU techniques.
- Outcome and follow-up of various NTBU techniques.
- Advantages of non-transecting over transecting urethroplasty technique.

INTRODUCTION

Bulbar urethra is the most common site of anterior urethral stricture, about 40% are idiopathic, particularly in the developed world, generally short, sometimes only a membrane and associated with less than 10% degree of fibrosis.

Usually they are amenable to endoscopic management but if it fails, the best form of urethroplasty is excision of the strictured urethral segment (spongiofibrosis and surrounding corpus spongiosum) in which large amount of normal tissue is excised including segment of bulbar arteries and tension-free end-to-end anastomosis of the healthy spatulated edges (EPA).

Penile complications especially reduced glans sensation, penile shortening, sexual dysfunction and erectile dysfunction were reported in transecting urethroplasty for short bulbar stricture.

Every surgeon should attempt to reduce iatrogenic damage to surrounding structure and their vasculature during their surgical intervention.

Dorsal aspect of the bulbomembranous urethra has concave configuration when it curves around the point of fusion of the corporal bodies and is devoid of corpus spongiosum. This provides anatomical basis for the non-transecting bulbar urethroplasty (NTBU) which results into preservation of sexual function and proximal blood supply of the urethra.

The primary aim of non-transecting techniques for bulbar urethroplasty is to replicate functional outcomes of transecting technique while limiting the surgical trauma and morbidity. All aspects of results after urethral surgery should be developed using Validated Patient-Reported Outcome Measures (PROM).

Case Scenario

A 32-year-old man presented with a history of difficulty while passing urine and poor flow since 1 year. He had persistent voiding symptoms despite one attempt at direct visual internal urethrotomy (DVIU) in recent past. Ultrasonography reported normal upper tract and significant PVR and thickened bladder wall of 7 mm. Laboratory parameters were within normal limits. Uroflowmetry revealed maximum flow rate (Q_{max}) of 7 ml/sec and average flow rate was 3 ml/sec for 255 ml voided volume with voiding time 69 sec (Fig. 16.1). Retrograde urethrogram (RUG) and voiding cystourethrogram (VCUG) showed a short segmental bulbar urethral stricture as shown in Fig. 16.2A and B.

1. **What are the points would you like to note on clinical examination of such patient?**

   Ans: The abdomen should be examined for the presence of a palpable bladder, location of any suprapubic tube to assess its potential utility for

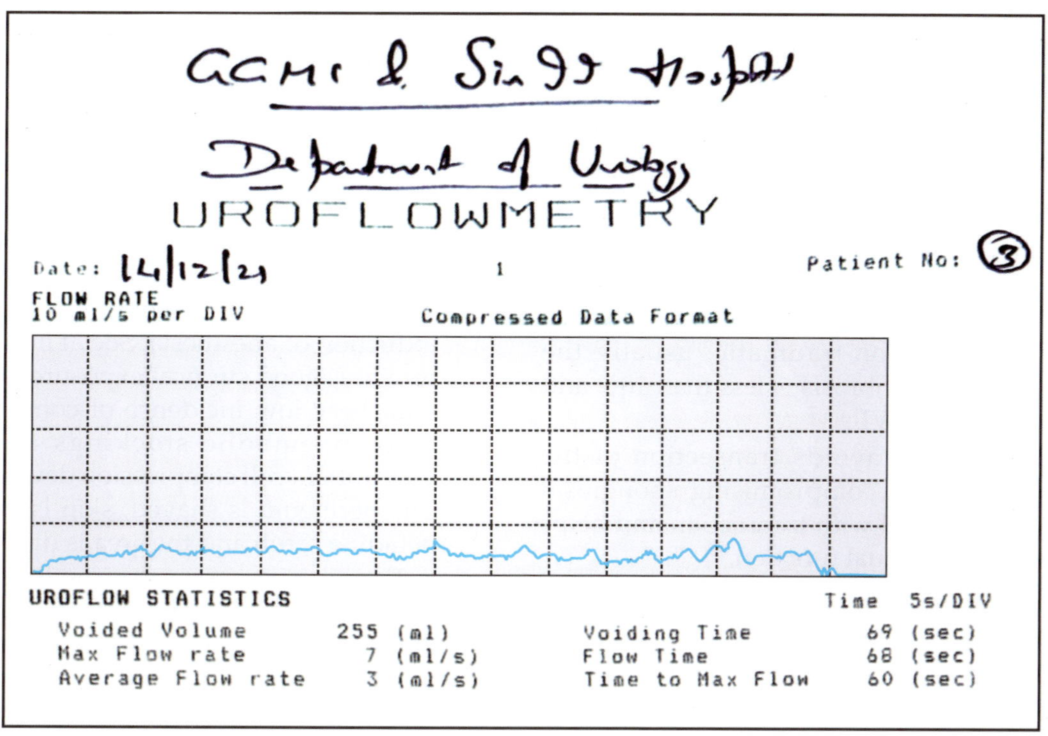

Fig. 16.1: Preoperative uroflowmetry of a representative case

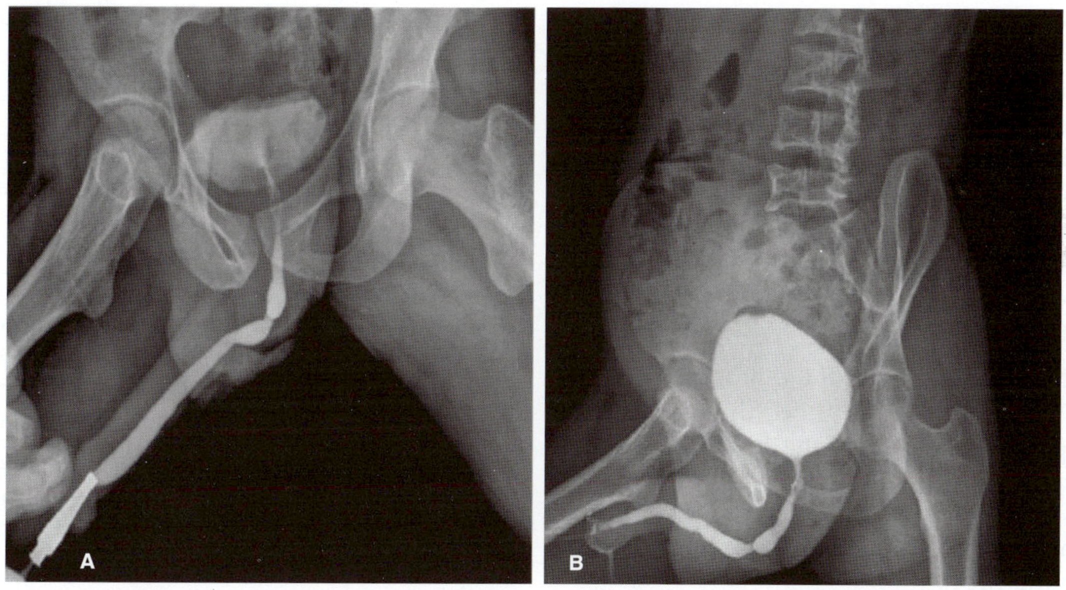

Fig. 16.2A and B: RUG and VCUG in representative case showing short segment mid-bulbar stricture

antegrade cystoscopy or the placement of a sound to facilitate repair.

Examination of the genitalia: To note the presence of foreskin, the position and size of the meatus, lichen sclerosis atrophicus changes on glans or prepuce. Thickening or induration along the urethra on palpation. Testis—to look for signs of epididymo-orchitis and sinuses and fistulas in scrotum and perineum. The oral cavity should be examined for the suitability of oral mucosa.[1,2]

2. **Which are the basic and radiological investigation you will consider in this patient and why?**

Ans: Complete blood count (CBC), urine analysis, urine culture to rule out infection, renal function test and random blood sugar.

Ultrasonography abdomen and pelvis to assess the upper tract, bladder wall thickness, post-void residual (PVR) urine and to rule out other associated pathology.

RUG to assess site, number and length of stricture in the anterior urethra. VCUG to assess the posterior urethra and bladder and to rule out reflux and RUG+VCUG to assess the stricture length.

Duplex ultrasound can be used to assess the amount of spongiofibrosis.[3–5]

3. **What is your surgical plan in this patient and why?**

Ans: Non-transecting anastomotic bulbar urethroplasty (NTABU) is preferred in this case because stricture is short, non-traumatic, usually the associated degree of fibrosis is less than 10% and is refractory to one DVIU.[6,7]

NTBU technique avoids transection of the corpus spongiosum, compromising spongiosal blood flow associated with transection and helps in preservation of sexual function.[4,8]

4. **What are the indications for non-transecting urethroplasty?**

Ans: Indications are:

1. Short membrane-like strictures.[12]
2. Non-traumatic small segment bulbar urethral stricture but less than 2 cm.[10,11]
3. Post-transurethral resection of prostate bulbar stricture.[10]
4. Bulbar urethral stricture with compromised vascular supply to distal urethra such as the elderly, those with vascular disease, hypospadias, previous urethroplasty and candidates for artificial urinary sphincter implantation who may be at increased risk of ischemic erosion.[4]
5. Failure after DVIU.[13]
6. Non-traumatic long bulbar strictures not amenable for excision or NTABU.

5. **Why not transecting type of urethroplasty?**

Ans: When strictures are short, the best form of urethroplasty is excision of the strictured urethral segment (spongiofibrosis and surrounding corpus spongiosum) and tension-free end-to-end anastomosis of the healthy spatulated edges (transecting EPA).

But transecting EPA is associated with vascular damage to the urethra, more penile complications especially reduced glans sensations, penile shortening, and curvature during erection if longer segments are excised, and increased sexual dysfunction which are related to both neural and vascular disruptions associated with mobilization and transection of the bulbar urethra.[4–8]

NTBU is preferred as it is highly successful, has proven efficacy and safety of the technique, and results are comparable with traditional transecting anastomosis for short bulbar urethral strictures in appropriately selected patients.[9]

6. **What are the indications of preoperative placement of the suprapubic catheter (SPC)?**

Ans: SPC should be considered when patient has retention of urine, obliterative stricture with significant PVR, back pressure changes in the upper tracts, and cases where urethral rest is indicated.

7. **What are the general steps of non-transecting urethroplasty?**

Ans: Prophylactic antibiotics are administered at induction of anesthesia. Social lithotomy position provides good surgical exposure of the perineum with very low incidence of complications. Antithromboembolic stockings and pneumatic intermittent calf compression devices are a routine. The perineum is shaved, skin is 'prepped' using betadine scrub and the area is draped.

Endoscopic assessment of urethra is done with 6 Fr ureteroscope and a hydrophilic guidewire is advanced through the stricture, which is extremely helpful to facilitate identification of the urethral lumen during stricturotomy when the stricture is extremely tight.

A midline perineal incision is made from perineo-scrotal junction to about 1 cm above the anal verge. Incision is deepened down through the subcutaneous tissue and Colles' fascia to expose the bulbospongiosus muscle. Plane between this and the underlying bulbar urethra is easily created by opening Gallaudet's fascia. The bulbospongiosus muscle is divided in the midline and retracted.

As per the intraoperative finding and approach, the decided procedure specific steps should be performed.

Perineal wound is closed in layers over a corrugated drain and pressure dressing is applied to the perineum which is removed on the day following surgery. Patient is discharged as per institutional protocol and clinical condition.[4,10]

8. **What is the role of endoscopic assessment and methylene blue test in management of stricture urethra?**

Ans: Cystourethroscopy is performed intraoperatively with a 6 Fr ureteroscope to assess the tissue quality, location, calibre, and visual characteristics of the stricture. It also provides insight into other associated pathologies such as, urethral and bladder neoplasms and stones.[3–5]

Instillation of a diluted 50:50 saline and methylene blue through urethral meatus helps in identifying the normal urethra (true lumen) as methylene blue stains the abnormal urethra.[10]

9. **How the concept of non-transecting urethroplasty evolved?**

Ans: The concept of non-transecting anastomotic urethroplasty was introduced by Jorden *et al* in

2007. Jordan et al and Bugeja et al described a dorsal approach, sparing vessels and spongiosum in the hope of decrease in the surgical side effects.[6]

Transection of the urethra for short bulbar strictures was originally challenged at the 2009 American Urological Association meeting.[4] Heineke-Mikulicz (HM) technique was first described by Lumen *et al* in 2010, for very short stricture less than 1 cm, not too narrow lumen, without underlying spongiofibrosis.[3]

The dorsal approach was first reported by Andrich *et al* in 2012.[4]

10. Which approach would you prefer in this case and why?

Ans: Types of approaches used are dorsal and ventral but dorsal approach is preferred in this case because:

1. Dorsal approach is carried out through the thinnest part of the spongiosum.[11]
2. Through dorsal approach, length of the stricture and degree of spongiofibrosis can be accurately assessed.
3. It provides chance to carry out any of the procedures without any vascular compromise to the urethra.[5]

11. What is anatomical basis for nontransecting urethroplasty?

Ans: Anatomical basis for the non-transecting techniques are:

1. 25% intrinsic elasticity and straightening of the curve of bulbar urethra provides sufficient length to allow closure of a longitudinal stricturotomy in horizontal plane without tension and avoids shortening and helps in mobilization of bulbar urethra.[3]
2. The dorsal aspect of the bulbomembranous urethra is concave in configuration and devoid of corpus spongiosum, hence dorsal stricturotomy is performed in a relatively avascular plane preserving the spongiosal blood flow ventrally.[4]
3. Non-transecting anastomotic technique would provoke some urethral shortening, so it is not indicated in penile urethral strictures.[3]

12. What are the steps pertaining to dorsal nontransecting urethroplasty?

Ans: Bulbar urethra is mobilized dorsally off the tunica albuginea of the corpora cavernosa by dividing Buck's fascia on either side and is mobilised from the distal margin of the bulbospongiosus muscle to the perineal membrane. No need to mobilize the bulb of the corpus spongiosum from its attachment to the perineal body, thus preserving the main bulbar arteries.

One-sided dissection to access the dorsal urethra in most cases in an efforts to minimize trauma to the local tissues, and to maintain future surgical options.

The level of the stricture is determined by sounding the urethra with a 16 Fr catheter or metal dilator and palpating the point at which it cannot be advanced any further. A dorsal stricturotomy is made by cutting down onto a catheter in the urethra at the stricture site and stay sutures positioned.

Stay stitches are used to facilitate visualization and rotation of the urethra into the surgical field. At this time, the full length of stricture and degree of spongiofibrosis is determined, which will dictate the surgical technique.[5] A gorget facilitates extension of the stricturotomy into healthy urethra on either side of the stricture (Fig. 16.3A and B).

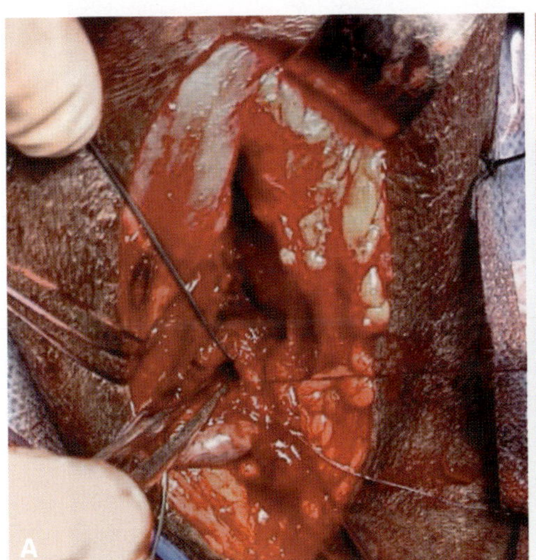

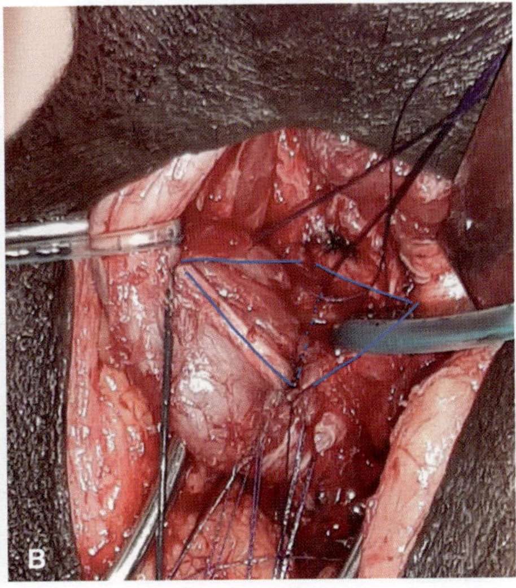

Fig. 16.3A and B: (A) Intraoperative picture of non-transecting urethroplasty showing wide open proximal end of urethra; (B) Intraoperative picture of dorsal non-transecting anastomotic urethroplasty (bold line shows edges of dorsal urethrotomy, dotted line shows post-stricture excision anastomosis of normal ventral mucosa

As per the intraoperative findings, type of NTBU selected and is performed over 14 Fr or 16 Fr silicone Foley catheter.

13. What are the steps pertaining to ventral nontransecting urethroplasty?

Ans: A ventral midline urethrotomy is made and extended to assure a good caliber lumen both distally and proximally. The mucosal scar tissue is marked and a mucosectomy is performed, preserving the spongiosum. Bring the distal and proximal edges of healthy mucosa together without tension with a 5/0 absorbable suture (Fig. 16.4A and B). Spongioplasty done with a 4/0 absorbable suture.

Ventral stricturotomy is closed over a 14/16 Fr catheter, in a HM fashion.[6] Perineal wound is closed in layers over a corrugated drain.

14. What are the different types and principles of non-transecting urethroplasty?

Ans: Following are the types of nontransecting urethroplasty:

1. *HM-type stricturoplasty:* Short membrane-like strictures (one or two millimeters) in whom no or very little tissue is excised through dorsal approach, mucosal margins on either side of this are sutured and the longitudinal stricturotomy is closed transversely.

   Conversion to other nontransecting technique should be considered, if closure over 16 Fr is not possible.[3,4]

2. Non-transecting excision of the stricture and mucosal anastomosis, as described by Mundy *et al* (NTABU)

   The stricture up to 2 cm with good urethral mobility and elasticity having moderate underlying fibrosis is amenable for NTABU.[4,5] The scarred epithelium with the surrounding spongiofibrosis is excised leaving the healthy underlying spongiosum intact. The mucosal edges on either side of the excised segment are then sutured to each other bring these two edges together in a tension-free manner (Fig. 16.5).

   Longitudinal dorsal stricturotomy is then closed transversely.

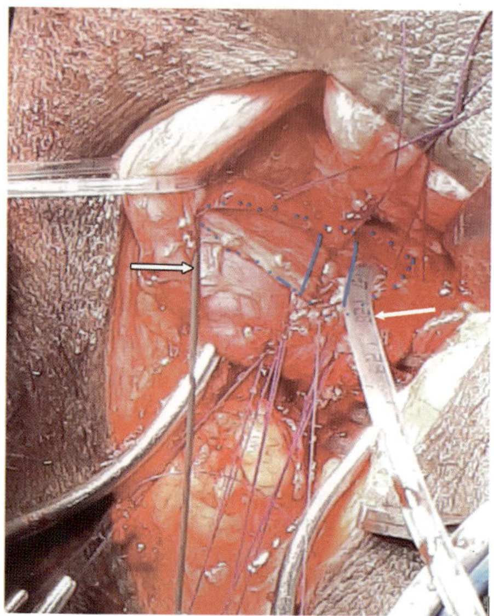

Fig. 16.5: Intraoperative picture of dorsal nontransecting anastomotic urethroplasty (dotted line shows edges of dorsal urethrotomy, small arrow—guidewire in distal urethra,long arrow—cathater in proximal uretha, in between two horizontal bold lines—post-stricture excision anastomosis of normal ventral mucosa)

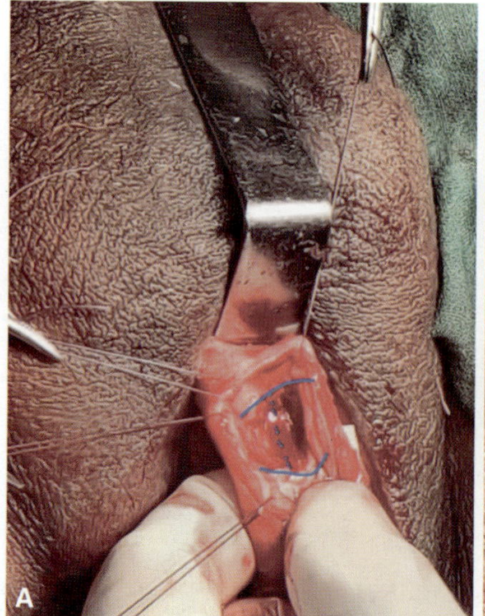

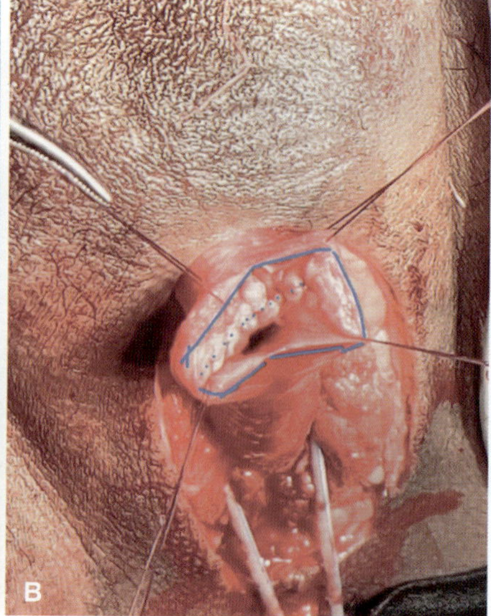

Fig. 16.4A and B: (A) Ventral non-transecting urethroplasty (Dotted line: Post-excision of stricture (mucosectomy) sparing the dorsal spongiosus tissue. Bold line: Dorsal normal mucosal edges); (B) Ventral non-transecting urethroplasty—transverse suture of the dorsal healthy mucosa (shown as dotted line and bold line indicates edges of urethra)

3a. Augmented non-transecting anastomotic bulbar urethroplasty (ANTABU)

Strictures too long for a NTABU should be considered for ANTABU.

Length and width of dorsal urethral opening is measured and graft is harvested, defattened, meshed and quilted to corporal bodies.[3,4] (Fig. 16.6A and B).

3b. ANTABU technique is also considered in the patients having long bulbar stricture with focal areas of urethral stenosis.

Focal area having significant spongiofibrosis may be excised in the non-transecting fashion and the urethral plate reconstituted ventrally by a mucosa-to-mucosa anastomosis.

The dorsal stricturotomy is then augmented with buccal mucosal graft[4] (Fig. 16.6A and B).

15. How will you decide which type of non-transecting technique to be performed?

Ans:

1. Decision on the type of NTBU to be performed is made after dorsal stricturotomy which will be influenced by degree of spongiofibrosis and length of a stricture (usually underestimated on pre-operative fluoroscopic assessment).
2. If the stricture is longer than anticipated, then need to convert from a non-transecting anastomotic bulbar urethroplasty to a dorsal augmentation urethroplasty which is also non-transecting.[4]
3. Types of NTBU as per the length of the stricture and size of lumen
   a. Non-traumatic, short (<2 cm) but non-obliterative (>4 Fr) stricture: NTABU.
   b. Non-traumatic longer (>2 cm) but non-obliterative (>4 Fr) stricture—non-transecting techniques using onlay buccal mucosa graft.
   c. One-sided dorsal graft if the stricture lumen is >4 Fr and a two-sided (ventral and dorsal) graft if lumen < 4 Fr[5] (Fig. 16.7).

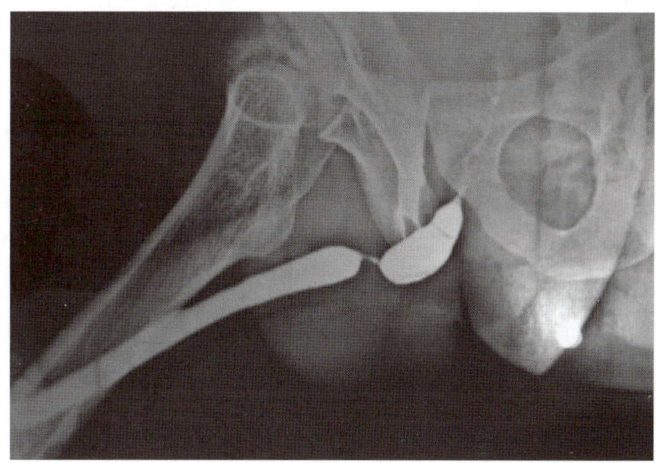

Fig. 16.7: RUG: Near obliterative stricture in distal bulbar urethra

16. What are the principles of non-transecting bulbar urethroplasty?

Fig. 16.8: QR code: PROM[15]

Ans: Most strictures are short, without gross spongiofibrosis, occur in the proximal bulbar

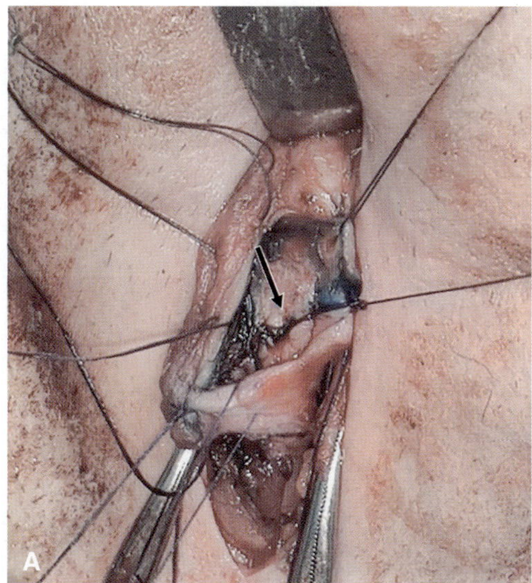

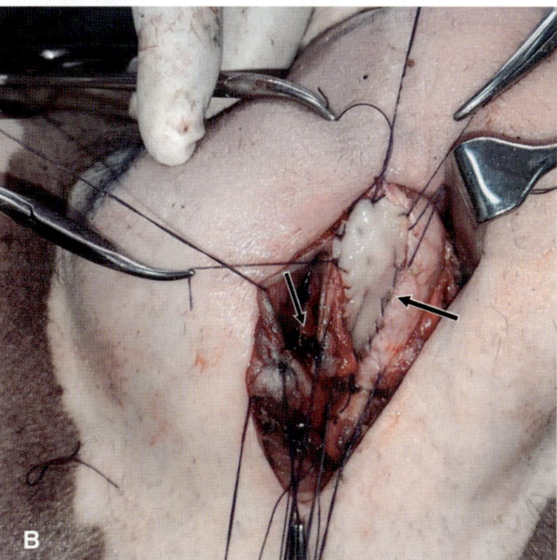

Fig. 16.6A and B: (A) Dorsal non-transecting urethroplasty—arrow indicates post-stricture excision ventral mucosal anastomosis; (B) Dorsal non-transecting augmentation urethroplasty—post-stricture excision ventral mucosal anastomosis and dorsal BMG augmentation

urethra and are amenable to local excision with an aim to achieve immediate and long-term results with less morbidity with minimal operative trauma.

Dorsal approach is preferred as bulbar urethra can be stretched and has less vascular supply to the dorsal aspect. Ventral approach is used for short (<1 cm), not too narrow or fibrotic stricture at the mid or distal bulbar urethra.

In both the approaches it is possible to excise spongiofibrosis with preservation of spongiosal blood supply without injury to the bulbar arteries.[3,7,14]

17. What are the outcomes of nontransecting bulbar urethroplasty?

Ans: Parameters for satisfactory outcomes are significant improvement in PROM, normal range uroflowmetry and radiologically normal caliber urethra.

Failure is defined as the need for any intervention, including urethral dilatation.[10] Subjective failure is a failure to achieve an improvement in PROM and objective failure is inadequate flow rate or decreased urethral caliber.

They usually have buckling of ventral aspect of urethra as a result of longitudinal shortening of dorsal aspect of urethra produced by stricturoplasty.[7]

Different types of non-transecting and transecting urethroplasty have comparable success rates (93.8%).[5,16,17] Reported objective, subjective and overall success rate of NTABU is 97.7%, 95.3% and 96.5% respectively at one year follow-up.[4,5,13]

18. What are the complication following non-transecting urethroplasty?

Ans: Complications after nontransecting urethroplasty are:

1. Post-micturition dribble (PMD)-common after non-transecting urethroplasty and highest in ANTABU. Reported incidence was 15.4% without significant bother and negative impact on the outcomes.[3]
2. Recurrent stricture incidence (2.3%)—most stricture recurrences become clinically apparent within the first one to two years.[4,5,13]
3. Erectile dysfunction (ED): ED has not been reported post-stricturoplasty but observed in non-transecting EPA and ANTABU (long-term ED occurred in 2.4%).[3] Incidence of new onset ED was 6.5% which is usually transient and resolves within one year.[4]
4. Sexual dysfunction risk associated with NTABU is less compared to the transecting technique.[18] Immediate or long-term ejaculatory disturbances, ED, or diminished penile sensitivity in sexually active patients are not reported in ventral non-transecting urethroplasty.[14]

19. How will you follow-up the case of nontransecting urethroplasty?

Ans: Peri-catheter urethrogram is not routinely performed, although subjective complexity of the case increases the need for a peri-catheter RUG in occasional cases. It is performed three to four weeks later and if this shows no leak the catheter is removed. If a leak is demonstrated then catheter is kept in place for another week to two weeks and a peri-catheter urethrogram is repeated. There is no role of continuing catheter more than six weeks.[4,10]

Clinical and radiological follow-up is performed at one and three months, and every 3 monthly thereafter for the first 1 year and then yearly for 5 years after the surgery. At each visit the patient undergoes uroflowmetry and bladder ultrasonography for PVR[10] (Fig. 16.9A to C).

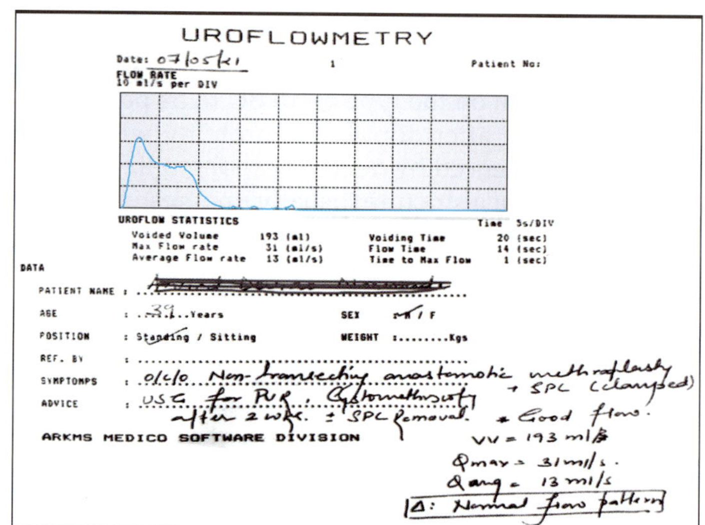

Fig. 16.9A: Normal uroflow pattern post-nontransecting anastomotic urethroplasty

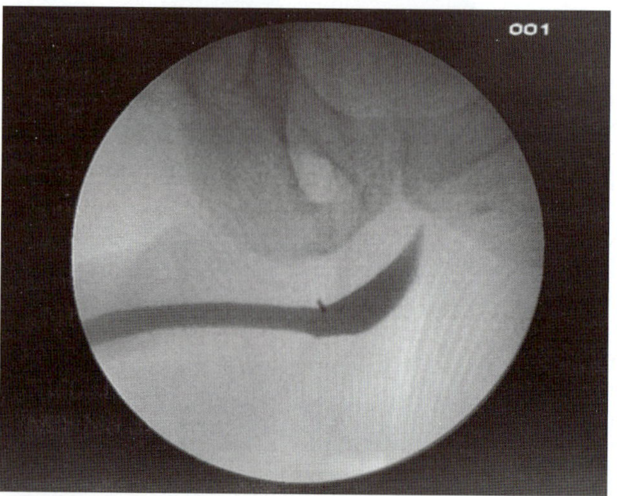

Fig. 16.9B: Normal RUG post-nontransecting anastomotic urethroplasty in representative case

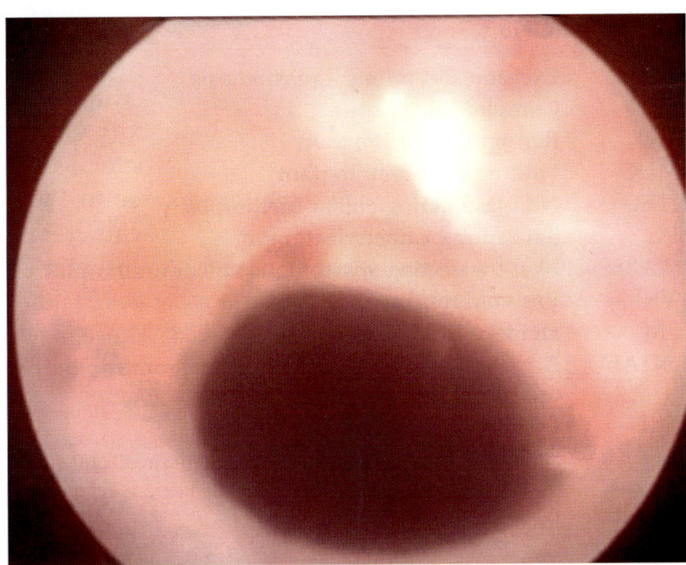

Fig. 16.9C: Post-nontransecting urethroplasty—endoscopic view of anastomotic site

Indication for intervention-flow rate less than 15 ml/s, clinically symptomatic and radiologically proven stricture recurrence.[19]

20. What are the benefits of non-transecting urethroplasty?

Ans: Benefits of NTBU are

1. NTABU avoids donor site morbidity associated with harvesting a buccal graft and PMD following augmentation bulbar urethroplasty.[4]
2. Sparing of ventral spongiosus tissue, preservation of blood supply to remaining spongiosal tissue and bulbourethral artery is advantageous in case of redo urethroplasty and in elderly patients with cardiovascular comorbidity which helps in reducing the risk of subsequent ischemic spongiofibrosis and stricture formation.[3]
3. NTBU is safe without a substantial learning curve.[20]

KEY POINTS

- NTBU is efficient, highly successful and an excellent alternative to transecting EPA for short non-traumatic bulbar strictures in appropriately selected patients.
- Non-transecting excision of spongiofibrosis with preservation of well vascularized underlying spongiosum provides improved sexual outcomes with similar patency rates.[4,5]
- The ventral NTBU approach is a feasible and reproducible technique with a significant increase in Q_{max} and improvement in PROM without decrease in erectile function.[6]
- In obliterative inflammatory urethral strictures, non-transecting bilayer substitution urethroplasty is safe and has better short-term outcomes.[19]
- Several urethroplasty centers have shifted from classical transecting to nontransecting approaches.[3,9]

REFERENCES

1. Gelman J, Wisenbaugh ES. Posterior Urethral Strictures. Adv Urol.2015;2015:628107.
2. Potts BA, Belsante MJ, Peterson AC. Intraurethral Steroids are a Safe and Effective Treatment for Stricture Disease in Patients with Biopsy Proven Lichen Sclerosus. J Urol.2016;195:1790–6.
3. Waterloos M, Verla W, Oosterlinck W, Lumen N. Role of non-transecting anastomotic urethroplasty for bulbar urethral strictures. In: Martins F, Kulkarni S, Köhler T, editors. Textbook of male genitourethral reconstruction. Cham: Springer; 2019;151–61.
4. Bugeja S, Andrich DE, Mundy AR. Non-transecting bulbar urethroplasty. Transl Androl Urol. 2015;4:41–50.
5. Coddington N, Higgins M, Mian A, Flynn B. Non-Transecting Urethroplasty for Bulbar Urethral Strictures-Narrative Review and Treatment Algorithm. J Clin Med. 2022;11:7033.
6. Morán E, Sáez Moreno I, Bonillo MA, Dagá O, Martínez-Cuenca E, Arlandis S, Broseta E. Ventral Approach for the Non-transecting Bulbar Urethroplasty. Urology. 2021;152:197–98.
7. Mundy, A.R., Andrich, D.E. Non-transecting Bulbar Urethroplasty. In: Brandes, S., Morey, A. (eds) Advanced Male Urethral and Genital Reconstructive Surgery. Current Clinical Urology. Humana Press, New York, NY. 2014;531–41.
8. Nilsen OJ, Holm HV, Ekerhult TO, Lindqvist K, Grabowska B, Persson B, *et al.* To Transect or Not Transect: Results from the Scandinavian Urethroplasty Study, A Multicentre Randomised Study of Bulbar Urethroplasty Comparing Excision and Primary Anastomosis Versus Buccal Mucosal Grafting. Eur Urol. 2022;81:375–82.
9. Virasoro R, DeLong JM. Non-transecting bulbar urethroplasty is favored over transecting techniques. World J Urol. 2020;38:3013–18.
10. Joshi P, Kaya C, Kulkarni S. Approach to bulbar urethral strictures: Which technique and when? Turk J Urol. 2016;42:53–9.
11. S. Bugeja, S. Ivaz, A.V. Frost, D.E. Andrich, A.R. Mundy. Non-transecting bulbar urethroplasty using buccal mucosa, Afr J Urol. 2016;22:47–53.
12. Behnam Nabavizadeh, Benjamin N. Breyer, German Patino. The Urethroplasty Evolution and Rise of the Non-transecting Techniques for Bulbar Urethral Strictures Editorial Colombian Urology Journal. 2021;30:003–004.
13. Mummalaneni Sitaram, Suraj Jayadeva Reddy, Arun Chawla, Jean J.M.C.H de la Rosette', Pilar Laguna, Sunil Pillai *et al.* 'Comparison of Patient Reported Outcome Measures for Direct Visual Internal Urethrotomy and Non-Transecting Urethroplasty for Short Bulbar Stricture'. 2021, available at Research Square.[https://doi.org/10.21203/rs.3.rs-659152/v1].
14. Lumen N, Hoebeke P, Oosterlinck W. Ventral longitudinal stricturotomy and transversal closure: the Heineke-Mikulicz principle in urethroplasty. Urology. 2010;76:1478–82.
15. Jackson MJ, Sciberras J, Mangera A, Brett A, Watkin N, N'dow JM, *et al.* Defining a patient-reported outcome measure for urethral stricture surgery. Eur Urol. 2011;60:60–8.
16. Barbagli G, Sansalone S, Romano G, Lazzeri M. Bulbar urethroplasty: transecting vs. nontransecting techniques. *Curr Opin Urol.* 2012;22:474–77.

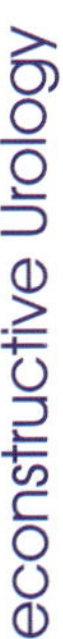

17. Yılmaz M , Kokurcan A, Uysal F, Özenç G, Yalçınkaya F. Non-transecting urethroplasty in patients with bulbar urethral strictures shorter than three centimeters. Scand J Urol. 2023;57:97–101.
18. Chapman DW, Cotter K, Johnsen NV, Patel S, Kinnaird A, Erickson BA etal. Nontransecting Techniques Reduce Sexual Dysfunction after Anastomotic Bulbar Urethroplasty: Results of a Multi-Institutional Comparative Analysis. J Urol. 2019;201:364–70.
19. Rajaian S, Murugavaithianathan P, Krishnamurthy K, Murugasen L. Non Transecting Dorsal Onlay and Ventral Inlay Buccal Mucosal Substitution Urethroplasty for Obliterative Bulbar Urethral Strictures. Urol Int. 2019;103:454–58.
20. Lumen N, Poelaert F, Oosterlinck W, Lambert E, Decaestecker K, Tailly T, *et al.* Nontransecting Anastomotic Repair in Urethral Reconstruction: Surgical and Functional Outcomes. J Urol. 2016;196:1679–84.

ABBREVIATIONS

EPA : Excision and primary anastomosis
CBC : Complete blood count
RUG : Retrograde urethrogram
VCUG : Voiding cystourethrogram
NTBU : Non-transecting bulbar urethroplasty
SPC : Suprapubic catheterization
NTABU : Non-transecting anastomotic bulbar urethroplasty
PVR : Postvoid residue
H M : Heineke-Mikulicz
ANTABU : Augmented non-transecting anastomotic bulbar urethroplasty
DVIU : Direct visual internal urethrotomy
PROM : Patient reported outcomes measure questionnaire
PMD : Post-micturition dribbling
ED : Erectile dysfunction

Chapter

17

Surgical Management of Ureteric Injury

• *Shivam Priyadarshi* • *Somendra Bansal*

LEARNING OBJECTIVES

- To understand the incidence and etiopathogenesis of ureteric injury
- To understand the evaluation for a patient with suspected ureteric injury.
- To understand the emergency management of ureteric injury.
- To understand special situations like ureteral injury occurring during vascular surgery.
- To understand the management of the ureteric injuries based on the site of injury.

INTRODUCTION

Ureteric injury (UI) can be either traumatic or iatrogenic. Iatrogenic ureteric injury (IUI) is the most common cause of UI and accounts for almost three-fourths of cases. Surgical management of UI will depend upon its severity, extent and site of ureteric involvement. It includes from simple stenting to auto-transplantation or nephrectomy.

Case Scenario

A 48 years old female had undergone abdominal hysterectomy 2 days ago. The patient is unwell and complaining of left flank pain and fever and a urological injury is suspected by the gynaecology team.

1. **What would be the initial steps in this patient?**

   Ans: This is a urological emergency keeping in mind that urological complication in a gynaecological surgery can occur. Take a proper history, perform a physical examination and carry out necessary investigations.

   Ask the operating surgeons regarding indication of surgery (benign or malignant aetiology), any difficulty encountered at the time of surgery (excessive bleeding, adhesions or long duration of surgery), past medical history of endometriosis or previous abdominal surgery or any previous radiotherapy treatment.

2. **On assessment patient is stable but febrile, with tenderness in the left flank and excessive clear fluid from the drain. What investigations are needed in this situation?**

   Ans: Complete blood count, urine microscopy and culture, drain fluid creatinine (suggesting urine in drain if the creatinine level >300 umol/L in a patient with normal serum creatinine), ultrasound to look for any collection or hydronephrosis and finally CT urography to confirm any ureteric or bladder injury.

3. **What are the types and mechanism of ureteric injuries and their aetiology?**

   Ans: Ureteric injuries can be traumatic and iatrogenic. Ureteral trauma is very rare and accounts for 1–2.5% of urinary tract trauma. Penetrating trauma, mostly by gunshot wounds, is the commonest form (60 to 77%) in most modern series.[1,2] About one-third of cases of external trauma to the ureters are caused by blunt trauma, mostly road traffic accidents.[2,3] The proximal ureter is most commonly involved.[4] Traumatic ureteral injury is highly associated with concomitant injuries to surrounding structures due to close associations. In blunt injury such as road traffic accidents, deceleration can result in avulsion of the ureter at the ureteropelvic junction (UPJ) or distally along the ureter.[5] Bowel and vascular injuries are commonly associated with penetrating injury, whereas bony pelvic fracture is associated with blunt ureteral injury.

Iatrogenic ureteral injuries can occur during various abdominopelvic and retroperitoneal surgical procedures as well as during endoscopic manipulation, or lithotripsy for ureteral calculi. Most of the ureteral injuries occur during gynaecologic procedures (55%), followed by urologic procedures (25%), colorectal operations (15%), and vascular surgery like aortic aneurysm repair (5%). Majority of these injuries occur in the distal ureter.[2, 3]

4. How do ureteric injuries present?

Ans:

- Prolonged paralytic ileus (due to urinoma)
- Prolonged postoperative fever or overt urinary sepsis
- Persistent drainage of fluid from drains or abdominal wound or the vagina (send drain fluid for creatinine level)
- Flank pain if the ureter has been ligated
- Abdominal mass representing a urinoma or a hydronephrotic kidney
- Vague abdominal pain
- It is important to note that the absence of hematuria does not exclude ureteral injury as it is present in less than one half of patients with a ureteric injury.[6]

5. How do missed ureteric injuries present?

Ans: Missed ureteric injuries present with delayed urine leak causing urinary ascites, urinoma, ileus, periurethral abscess, sepsis, ureteral fistula (uretero-vaginal fistula), or ureteral stricture and potential loss of ipsilateral kidney. As per literature 38% of ureteral injuries are initially missed.[4] The majority of missed ureteric injuries are located in the proximal ureter, a region with less accessibility, particularly in the setting of retroperitoneal hematoma, and therefore with less likelihood of being explored.

6. What are the investigations to diagnose the ureteral injury?

Ans: In hemodynamically stable patients, the diagnosis of ureteral injury is typically made using contrast-enhanced computed tomography (CT) scan of the abdomen and pelvis with delayed urographic images. Identification of ureteral injuries requires a delay of 5 to 10 minutes after the administration of intravenous (IV) contrast to allow contrast to reach the ureters.[7] Findings suggestive of ureteral injury are no visualization of the ureter, contrast extravasation from the ureter, ipsilateral hydroureteronephrosis, and poor renal excretion localized to one side. To reduce radiation exposure during repeat CT imaging, delayed phase imaging can be performed with a low-dose protocol and increased axial image slice thickness (5 mm). If suspicion remains high in the setting of a negative CT scan, then cystoscopy and retrograde pyelography is recommended.

In the operating room (e.g. trauma patients requiring laparotomy, suspected intraoperative injury), direct inspection of the ureters is the most sensitive method to assess for ureteral injury. Intravenous dyes (e.g. methylene blue, indigo carmine) can be used to aid the assessment by looking for dye leakage along the course of the ureter.

7. What is the grading system for the ureteric injury?

Ans: The American Association for the Surgery of Trauma (AAST) grading system for ureteral injury relies on visual inspection of the injury to make a diagnosis since injury grades are difficult to assess using imaging alone. Rather than stratifying ureteral injuries by grade, most surgeons distinguish them based upon location of ureteral injury (upper, mid, lower), mechanism of injury (blunt versus penetrating), and severity of injury (complete versus partial transection) as these categories guide the type of surgical management necessary for repair (Table 17.1).

TABLE 17.1: American Association for the Surgery of Trauma (AAST) organ injury severity scale for the ureter

*Grade**	*Type*	*Description*
I	Hematoma	Contusion or hematoma without devascularisation
II	Laceration	<50% transection
III	Laceration	≥50% transection
IV	Laceration	Complete transection with <2 cm devascularisation
V	Laceration	Avulsion with >2 cm devascularisation

*Advance one grade for bilateral up to grade III

8. How are ureteric injuries treated?

Ans: Ureteral injuries identified intraoperatively should generally be repaired surgically, unless there is a complex injury, or other severe concomitant injuries limiting allowable repair time.[8] If the injury cannot be managed adequately in the acute setting, ureteral ligation and the kidney drainage postoperatively through a percutaneous nephrostomy with definitive reconstruction at a later date or a single J stent placed up to the renal pelvis, secured to the ureter and brought out through the flank are the management options.[9]

For uncomplicated incomplete ureteral injury, retrograde ureteral stenting can be attempted. This is also an option for limited blunt ureteral contusion (e.g. periureteral contusion from gunshot blast) and some partial penetrating ureteral injuries depending on the degree of surrounding tissue damage. However, when tissue viability is questionable, excision and ureteral reconstruction are strongly recommended.

The blast effect from penetrating gunshot injuries can cause tissue ischemia and lead to delayed necrosis. Thus, adequate debridement and reconstruction is recommended at the time of laparotomy, depending on the extent of ureteral tissue involvement. The ureter should be debrided and repaired using a spatulated tension-free anastomosis.

Intraoperative iatrogenic ureteral injuries, if recognized during the procedure, should be repaired in that setting. Ureteral injuries identified in the postoperative period require a delayed operative repair.

Iatrogenic injuries that occur during endoscopic procedures can initially be managed with a ureteral stent. Endoscopic realignment utilizing one or more stents for complete ureteral transections has been described for immediate postoperative and delayed injury cases.[10]

If placement of a ureteral stent is not possible or if stent placement fails to adequately divert the urine, then a percutaneous nephrostomy tube should be placed. If there is a large urinoma, a periureteral drain can be placed in the urinoma. Delayed ureteral reconstruction is often necessary.

If the ureter is inadvertently ligated, the suture should be removed and the ureter observed for viability. If vascular compromise is observed, the injured ureter should be resected and an ureteroureterostomy performed. Treatment of ureteric injury is shown in the algorithm (Flowchart 17.1A and B).

9. When to repair the ureteric injury?

Ans: Generally best time to repair the ureter is as soon as the injury has been diagnosed. Definitive repair may be delayed if the patient is unstable or there is evidence of active infection at the site of proposed ureteric repair.

If the injury is recognized late and there are complications (e.g, abscess, urinary infection, and urinary fistula) that would interfere with ureteral healing, proximal urinary drainage by a percutaneous nephrostomy is performed.

10. How is the lower ureteric injury treated?

Ans: Transection injuries are repaired by a primary ureteroureterostomy, ureteral re-implant, with or

Flowchart 17.1A: Treatment algorithm of ureteric injury

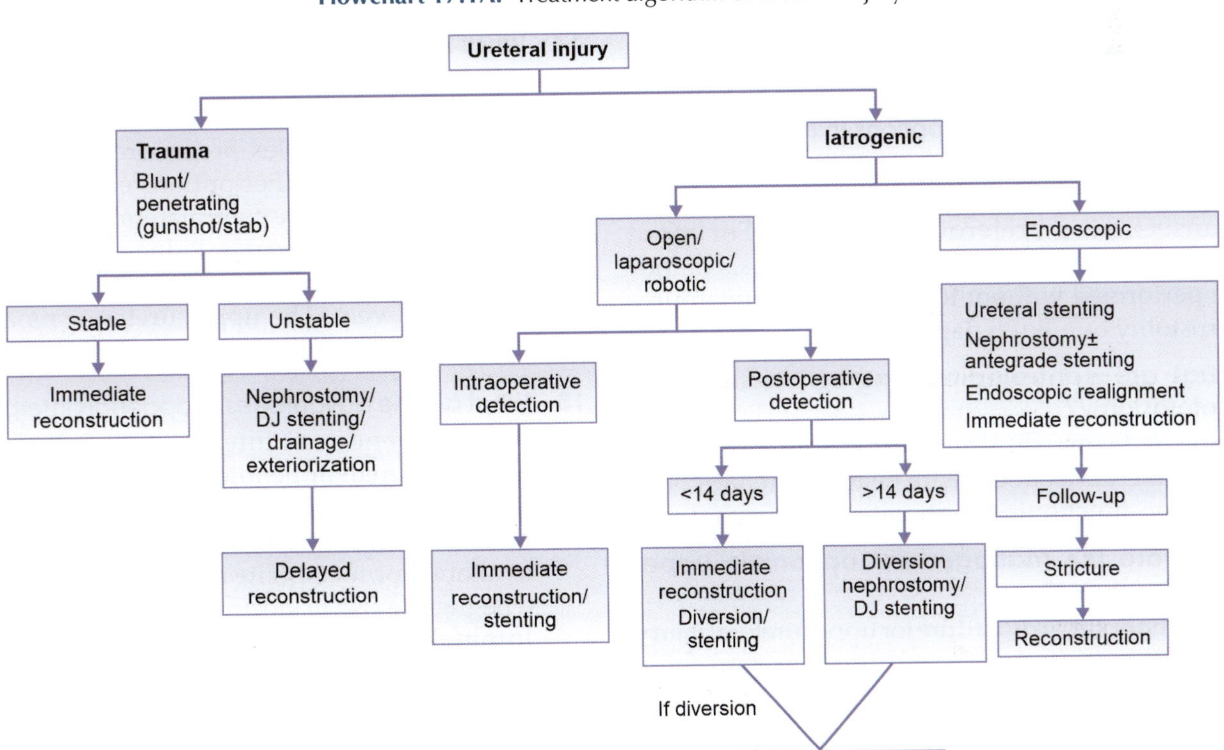

Flowchart 17.1B: Treatment algorithm of ureteric injury

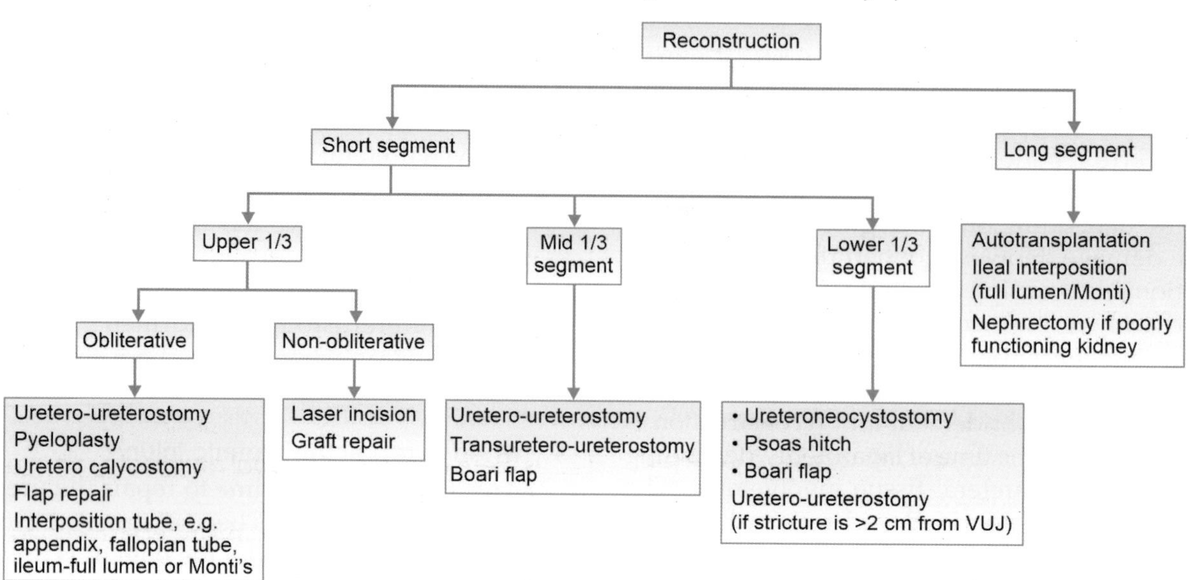

without psoas hitch, depending on the severity of the injury and approximity to the ureterovesical junction. If the ureteral injury is approximately 3 to 4 cm proximal to the ureterovesical junction, a primary ureteral anastomosis can be performed.

When the ureteral injury is within the distal 2 cm from the ureterovesical junction, a primary ureteral repair is difficult. In these settings, a ureteroneocystostomy (ureteral reimplant) is usually preferred.

The psoas hitch ureteral reimplantation is the best approach when a primary ureteroureterostomy or ureteroneocystostomy cannot be performed without tension.

11. What are the treatment options in middle ureteric injuries?

Ans: The optimal repair for a mid-ureteral transection is ureteroureterostomy. For more extensive injuries, or when an anastomosis cannot be performed without tension, a transureteroureterostomy or a Boari flap is used.

12. What are contraindications of transuretero-ureterostomy?

Ans: A transureteroureterostomy cannot be performed in a patient with history of renal stones or a non-functioning contralateral kidney.

13. What are the management options in upper ureteric injuries?

Ans: The optimal procedure for upper ureteral injury repair is ureteroureterostomy, pyeloureterostomy or ureterocalycostomy, if sufficient length can be mobilized for a primary repair without tension. This can be facilitated by mobilization of the kidney with fixation to the psoas tendon (nephropexy) to provide for a tension free anastomosis. Mobilization of the left kidney can provide up to 4 cm of length, but mobilization of the right kidney does not add much length to the right ureter, as the right kidney is limited by a short right renal vein. When sufficient length cannot be mobilized, the options include ileal or appendiceal interposition graft, auto-transplantation, or a nephrectomy. In most settings of an upper ureteral injury, the Boari flap is technically difficult.

14. What is auto-transplantation?

Ans: It involves moving the injured ureter and ipsilateral kidney to an ectopic site (e.g. iliac fossa). It is a complex procedure and should not be undertaken if other options exist. It is usually considered when the contralateral kidney is absent or poorly functioning. The kidney is harvested with maximal vessel length for anastomoses to the iliac artery and vein. The upper ureter or renal pelvis can be directly anastomosed to the bladder.

15. What are the advantages of appendix interposition?

Ans: Appendiceal interposition is technically easy and small appendiceal calibre matches with that of the ureter (Figs 17.1 and 17.2). Another advantage is its decreased mucosal surface area available for metabolite absorption that results in a negligible risk of electrolyte disorders. The small luminal diameter of the appendix restricts the tendency to dilate with the passage of time, and together its intrinsic peristalsis leads to a minimal risk of urinary stasis and reflux. The length of the appendix is finite, replacing approximately 3 cm

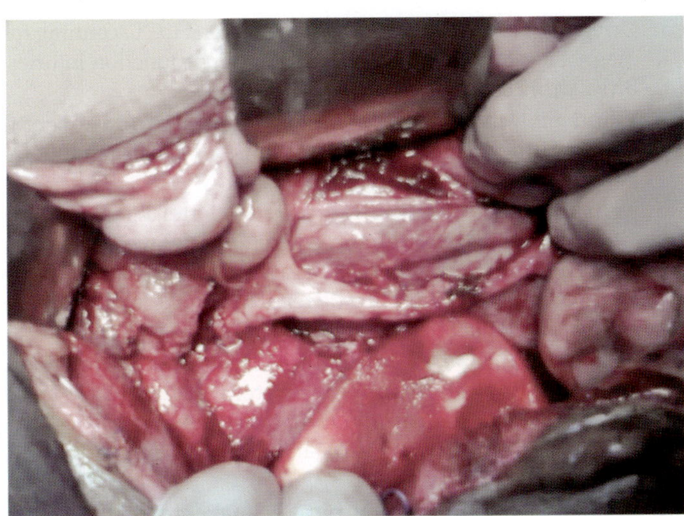

Fig. 17.1: Appendix detached with its vascular pedicle

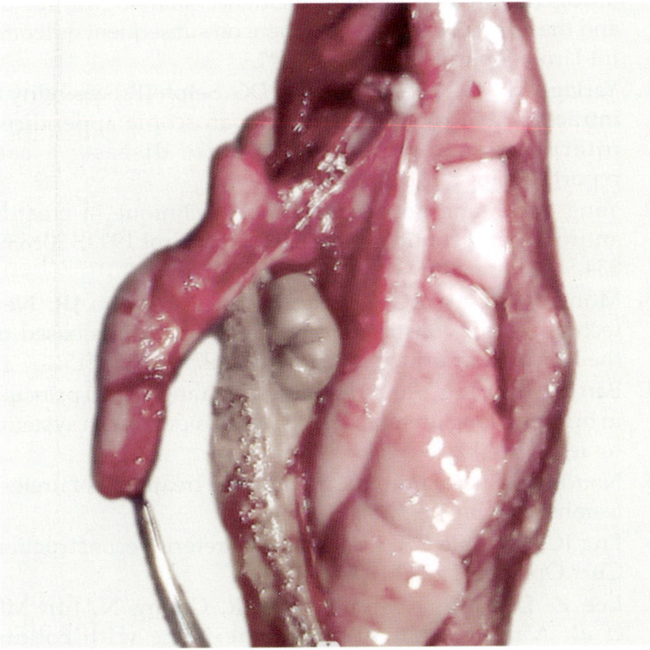

Fig. 17.2: Appendix with its pedicle used as interposition tube in a case of obliterative right upper ureteric stricture by the author

ureteral defects on average, and usually it fails to bridge long-segment strictures or a left-sided injury.[11]

Appendix could also be used as an onlay flap by detubularising the appendix on its antimesenteric border on a non-obliterative ureteral stricture by incising it anteriorly and covering with appendiceal flap.

16. What is Yang-Monti ileal ureter procedure?

Ans: The Yang-Monti procedure allows the reconfiguration of short ileal segment into a long tube of small diameter by converting the circular ileal configuration into longitudinal axis. It also effectively overcomes the drawbacks of simple ileal ureter.[12–14] A conspicuously short ileal segment is required. An ileal segment can bridge approximately threefold length of ureteral defects after reconfiguration, and its diameter is close to that of the ureter. It provides active antegrade propulsion for urinary drainage, mimicking the function of a native ureter, whereas intact or tailored ileal ureters showed irregular peristalsis that failed to propagate urine forward. The possibility of excessive mucus production and metabolic acidosis is almost absent because of the reduction of surface area with secretive and absorptive characteristics.

17. Is there any role of buccal mucosal graft in ureteric injury repair?

Ans: The use of BMG in ureteral reconstruction was first described in 1999 when Nuade described his experience over six years in six patients with complex ureteral strictures with excellent results.[15] The use of BMG in upper tract ureteral reconstruction provides an additional tool in the arsenal of reconstructive urologists when approaching complex ureteral strictures from various modes of injury.

18. When is nephrectomy performed in a case of ureteric injury?

Ans: A nephrectomy should only be used in rare settings. When a normal contralateral kidney is present, a simple nephrectomy can be considered as an expeditious option to an extensive upper ureteral repair, or poorly functioning kidney or when ureteral injury occurs during procedures using prosthetic grafts. Nephrectomy eliminates the risk of ureteral leak from an anastomosis and, as an independent procedure, is associated with low mortality.

19. Is there a role of laparoscopic or robotic ureteric reconstruction?

Laparoscopic and robotic ureteral repair is technically feasible and is an alternative to open repair for ureteric stricture. Most cases and series involve ureteroneocystostomy with psoas hitch ureteral implantation either by an extravesical or intravesical or extravesical cystoscopy-assisted techniques.[16]

The collaborative of reconstructive robotic ureteral surgery (CORRUS) has published a study of 54 patients with robotic ureteroplasty using buccal mucosal grafts describing a 87% success rate at a median follow-up of 27.5 months. The surgical technique consists of incising the stenotic segment longitudinally and putting a 10–18 mm wide buccal mucosal graft as an onlay. Neovascularisation to

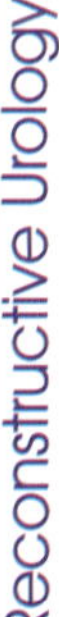

the graft is provided by an omental wrap. In case of obliterative segment an augmented anastomotic approach is used by excising the obliterative segment with ureterostomy made on the same side of the proximal and distal ureteral segments. A posterior plate of anastomosed native ureter is then covered with a buccal onlay graft.[17]

SUMMARY

- Iatrogenic ureteric injury accounts for the majority of ureteric injuries (UI).
- In recent years there has been an increase in the ureteric injuries following endoscopic intervention.
- To avoid this surge in endoscopic ureteric injuries, safe ureteroscopy practice should be followed including using sound technique, limiting ureteroscopy time, using safety wires, scoping over guidewires, proper use of laser and staging the procedure in case of ureteral injury.
- Diagnosis of UI could be either intraoperative recognition or by imaging in delayed cases.
- Intraoperative iatrogenic ureteral injuries, if recognized during the operation, should be repaired immediately. Ureteral injuries identified in the postoperative period require a delayed operative repair.
- Surgical management of UI will depend upon its severity, extent and site of ureter involvement. It includes from simple stenting to auto-transplantation or nephrectomy.

REFERENCES

1. Elliott SP, McAninch JW. Ureteral injuries: external and iatrogenic. Urol Clin North Am 2006;33:55–66.
2. McGeady JB, Breyer BN. Current epidemiology of genitourinary trauma. Urol Clin North Am 2013;40:323–334.
3. Phillips B, Holzmer S, Turco L, Mirzaie M, Mause E, Mause A, *et al.* Trauma to the bladder and ureter: a review of diagnosis, management, and prognosis. Eur J Trauma Emerg Surg 2017;43:763–773.
4. Clement ND, Tennant C, Muwanga C. Polytrauma in the elderly: predictors of the cause and time of death. Scand J Trauma Resusc Emerg Med 2010;18:26–32.
5. Ortega SJ, Netto FS, Hamilton P, Chu P, Tien H. CT scanning for diagnosing blunt ureteral and ureteropelvic junction injuries. BMC Urol 2008;8:3.
6. Elliott SP, McAninch JW. Ureteral injuries from external violence: the 25-year experience at San Francisco General Hospital. J Urol 2003; 170:1213–1216.
7. Keihani S, Putbrese BE, Rogers DM, Patel DP, Stoddard GJ, Hotaling JM, *et al.* Optimal timing of delayed excretory phase computed tomography scan for diagnosis of urinary extravasation after high-grade renal trauma. J Trauma Acute Care Surg 2019;86:274–281.
8. Best CD, Petrone P, Buscarini M, Demiray S, Kuncir E, Kimbrell B, *et al.* Traumatic ureteral injuries: a single institution experience validating the American Association for the Surgery of Trauma-Organ Injury Scale grading scale. J Urol 2005;173:1202–1205.
9. Zinman LN, Vanni AJ. Surgical Management of Urologic Trauma and Iatrogenic Injuries. Surg Clin North Am 2016;96:425–439.
10. Al-Awadi K, Kehinde EO, Al-Hunayan A, Al-Khayat A. Iatrogenic ureteric injuries: incidence, aetiological factors and the effect of early management on subsequent outcome. Int Urol Nephrol 2005;37:235–241.
11. Yarlagadda VK, Nix JW, Benson DG, Selph JP. Feasibility of intracorporeal robotic-assisted laparoscopic appendiceal interposition for ureteral stricture disease: a case report. Urology 2017;109:201–205.
12. Yang WH. Yang needle tunnelling technique in creating antireflux and continent mechanisms. J Urol 1993;150: 830–834.
13. Monti PR, Lara RC, Dutra MA, de Carvalho JR. New techniques for construction of efferent conduits based on the Mitrofanoff principle. Urology 1997; 49:112–115.
14. Bao JS, He Q, Li Y, Shi W, Wu G, Yue Z. Yang-Monti principle in bridging long ureteral defects: cases report and a systemic review. Urol J 2017;14:4055–4061.
15. Naude JH. Buccal mucosal grafts in the treatment of ureteric lesions. *BJU Int* 1999;83:751–754.
16. Png JC, Chapple CR. Principles of ureteric reconstruction. Curr Opin Urol 2000;10:207–212.
17. Lee Z, Lee MS, Koster H, Lee R, Cheng N, Jun MS, *et al.* A multi-institutional experience with robotic ureteroplasty with buccal mucosa graft: an updated analysis of intermediate-term outcomes. *Urology.* 2021;147:306.

Section

4

Female Urology

Chapter 1

Uncomplicated Stress Urinary Incontinence (SUI) in a Female

• *Sameer Trivedi*

LEARNING OBJECTIVES

- To identify the type of incontinence from the symptoms.
- To develop a clear understanding of the risk factors involved in the etiology of SUI.
- To review the initial assessment of women with uncomplicated SUI.
- To review the role of urodynamic studies in evaluation of uncomplicated SUI.
- To offer clear and simple guidance on management of women with uncomplicated SUI.
- To understand the role of education, behavioural, and lifestyle modification in management of SUI.
- To discuss the choice of optimal surgical procedure for uncomplicated SUI.
- To review the existing surgical procedures for SUI, viz colposuspension, PVS and MUS in terms of outcomes, risks and PROMs.

INTRODUCTION

This chapter highlights the identification and diagnosis of uncomplicated stress urinary incontinence in females and addresses key aspects in evaluation and management including role of urodynamics, importance of conservative treatment and choice of appropriate surgical management.

Case Scenario

A 43-year-old fit female office worker presents with worsening complaints of urinary leakage when coughing, sneezing and lifting heavy items. She has to change pads two to three times in a day. She does not have any voiding difficulty, urgency, frequency or burning during micturition. The patient's quality of life is affected by the episodes of urinary leakage and has disturbed her occupational and social life. She has a history of two full-term vaginal deliveries 15 and 18 years back with normal perinatal course. There are no comorbidities or history of any surgical procedures. The patient is a non-smoker, does not have constipation and is not on any medications.

On examination, the patient is of average build (BMI 23.5) with normal general and systemic examination. On pelvic examination, vagina is capacious with healthy, pink mucosa, no apparent pelvic organ prolapse and normal pelvic muscle tone. The focussed neurological examination is normal and cough test reveals presence of SUI.

History taking—pointers

- Ascertain type of incontinence i.e. stress, urge or mixed*
- Concomitant LUTS
- Bowel dysfunction (constipation and faecal leakage).
- Assess severity of SUI using questionnaires like ICIQ-SF
- Quantifying leakage based on daily use of pads—number, type and degree of wetness
- Impact on QOL and degree of bother*
- Prior treatments (surgical and non-surgical) received
- Patient's wishes and expectations about future treatment.
- Obstetrics and gynaecology history—number and details of pregnancies (vaginal delivery or LSCS), menopausal status, history of hysterectomy, intake of hormonal agents
- History of dyspareunia, vaginal irritation or dryness.
- Detailed past medical and surgical history especially DM, neurological disorders and prior pelvic surgery or radiation
- History of smoking and a complete drug history, particularly drugs like diuretics, anticholinergics and anti-psychotics.
- Bladder diary (2–3 days)—daily fluid intake, drinking habits, frequency, maximum voided volume, nocturnal/global polyuria and incontinence episodes.*

* (USI Urinary Incontinence Guidelines Panel Recommendation)[1]

Components of physical examination

- Informed verbal consent
- Presence of a female nurse or relative.
- General examination with emphasis on BMI
- Per abdominal examination—focus on a palpable bladder
- Detailed pelvic examination—inspection of introitus and vagina to assess tissue state (well oestrogenised or atrophic), assess vaginal grip, exclude any vaginal, cervical or adnexal masses.
- Cough test—lithotomy or standing position, ask the patient to cough or perform a Valsalva manoeuvre. (ICS cough test—supine/lithotomy position with 200–400 ml fluid in the bladder and performing one to four coughs).[4] EAU recommends a standing cough test.[3]
- Pelvic floor muscle tone assessment using Oxford grading system.

Modified Oxford grading scale for pelvic floor muscles	
0	No muscle activity
1	Minor muscle "flicker"
2	Weak muscle activity without a circular contraction
3	Moderate muscle contraction
4	Good muscle contraction
5	Strong muscle contraction

- Per speculum examination using a warmed lubricated Sim's speculum for cystocele, enterocele and rectocele.
- Focussed neurological examination to check perineal sensation and anal tone.
- Tests like Q-tip, Bonney's and Marshall tests no longer recommended.

1. **What should be the next step in assessment and what investigations should be performed?**
   Ans: As per the recommendations of USI Urinary Incontinence Guidelines Panel, a basic urinalysis should be performed to look for presence of infection or microscopic haematuria.[1] A urine culture should be obtained in case of suspected UTI. Estimation of postvoid residual urinary volume should be performed by an ultrasound. There is no evidence to suggest routine use of cystoscopy in evaluation of SUI. Further investigations depend on causative factors in the history.

2. **What is the role of pad test in the evaluation of SUI?**
   Ans: A pad test quantifies urinary leakage by weighing a pad before and after provocation testing. Short-term pad tests are usually performed over 1 hour while longer term pad tests last for 24 hours. In a 1-hour test, the patient is asked to consume around 500 mL of water or non-saline based liquid and execute a sequence of exercises over the next 1 hour, while the 24-hour test is a more physiological test where the patient continues normal daily routine including activities which provoke urinary leakage. An increase in pad-weight of up to approximately 1.4 g for the 1-hour pad test and up to 8 g for the 24-hour pad test is considered normal (1 g pad weight = 1 mL of urine). While pad testing is not recommended in the routine assessment of women with urinary incontinence according to the USI and NICE guidelines, EAU guidelines recommend a standardised pad test to quantify SUI.[1–3]

3. **What is uncomplicated SUI?**
   Ans: USI Guidelines panel defines uncomplicated stress UI as that which occurs in an adult woman under 65 years with a history of stress-induced leak without urgency or voiding symptoms who has not undergone pelvic surgery or radiation therapy. The uncomplicated patient has demonstrable stress UI with urethral hypermobility, no pelvic organ prolapse beyond the introitus, low postvoid residual urine and a normal uroflow.[1]

4. **What is the role of urodynamics (UDS) in evaluation of SUI?**
   Ans: Role of urodynamic studies in evaluation of SUI is controversial. The current consensus is that UDS is not indicated for diagnosis of straightforward 'pure' SUI or prior to starting conservative treatments for patients with uncomplicated SUI. A few studies have indicated a favourable impact of performing urodynamics prior to invasive treatment in uncomplicated SUI.[5] However, a growing body of evidence as well as recommendations of USI Urinary Incontinence Guidelines Panel suggest that UDS can be omitted in patients with uncomplicated stress urinary incontinence being considered for invasive therapies.[1]

   Urodynamic parameters like VLPP (Valsalva leak point pressure) and UPP (urethral pressure profile) to differentiate urethral hypermobility from intrinsic sphincter deficiency are no longer recommended for assessing severity of incontinence. Evidence about their predictive value for outcomes of surgical procedures is unclear. They are cumbersome to perform and have standardisation difficulties.[3]

   In patients with complicated SUI (mixed symptoms, prior failed incontinence surgery, suspicion of neuropathic bladder or voiding dysfunction), urodynamic evaluation should be performed before considering any invasive therapy. Multichannel urodynamics are strongly recommended in this setting. Video-urodynamics, wherever available, has certain ostensible advantages over conventional urodynamic techniques like real-time evaluation of urethral hypermobility with better assessment of bladder neck descent and urethra as well as superior quantification of anterior wall prolapse. However, combining a conventional urodynamics with voiding cystourethrogram is sufficiently informative about the underlying abnormalities in majority of cases.

5. **Are there clinical methods of assessing urethral function without resorting to urodynamics?**

   Ans: Clinical measures of urethral function include the empty bladder supine stress test which is used for making a diagnosis of intrinsic sphincter deficiency and visual demonstration of urethral mobility. A fixed urethra such as following pelvic radiation or repeated surgeries is a marker for a particularly difficult class of patient[1] (describe bladder supine test).

6. **A diagnosis of uncomplicated stress incontinence is made in this 43-year-old woman. Is there any role of education, behavioural, and lifestyle modification for SUI?**

   Ans: All patients should be counselled and educated about the pelvic anatomy, voiding function and pathophysiology of stress urinary incontinence. Lifestyle changes and behavioural modifications like weight loss, avoidance of sedentary lifestyle, treatment of constipation, cessation of smoking, dietary and fluid advice are an essential component of the management protocol.[1,3]

7. **What is the role of pelvic floor muscle training (PFMT) and biofeedback in treatment of uncomplicated SUI?**

   Ans: PFMT is widely used to enhance pelvic floor function by narrowing the levator hiatus, increasing muscle strength and urethral closure pressure, and lifting of the bladder neck and rectum, thus improving urethral stability and preventing occurrence of SUI.[6] There is plenty of evidence regarding utility of PFMT in treatment of SUI/MUI including well-designed RCTs and Cochrane reviews with reported subjective cure rates of 30–40% and objective cure rates approaching 50%.[7] However, it is important to remember that up to 50% of women cannot identify pelvic floor muscles correctly. Hence, there is a demonstrable benefit of high-intensity, supervised PFMT regimens over unsupervised PFMTs.[2] PFMT has very low incidence of adverse effects. The purported benefits of adding biofeedback or pelvic floor muscle stimulation to PFMT have not been substantiated and USI guidelines panel does not recommend routine use of biofeedback, vaginal cones, pessaries or pelvic floor stimulation.[1]

8. **What is the role of medical therapy and evidence to support its use in management of uncomplicated SUI?**

   Ans: Role of medical therapy in treating SUI is limited and debatable. Oestrogen replacement therapy for SUI has been tried using oral, transdermal and vaginal routes of administration in post-menopausal atrophic vaginitis associated with SUI. It reportedly improves urethral mucosal coaptation and has a positive impact on the tone of connective tissue. However, systemic administration of oestrogen preparations is associated with an increased risk of thromboembolism, endometrial hypertrophy, and breast cancer. The adverse effects of topical application include vaginal burn, itching, and spotting. There is no consensus about the ideal regimen and duration of treatment and the long-term implications. A Cochrane review reported short-term improvement in SUI symptoms.[8]

   Duloxetine inhibits the presynaptic reuptake of serotonin and noradrenaline (NE) at the spinal cord level (Onuf's nucleus). This results in an increased concentration of 5-HT and NE which stimulates 5-HT and NE receptors localised on the pudendal motor neurons, thus augmenting the resting tone and contraction strength of the urethral striated sphincter. Many reports suggest that Duloxetine improves SUI in some patients with associated improvement in quality of life.[9] Duloxetine is not recommended as a first-line treatment for most women with predominant SUI but may be considered as second-line therapy in patients not responding to conservative therapy and not fit/willing for invasive treatments. However, the patients need to be counselled about the adverse effects like nausea and vomiting, dryness of mouth, constipation, behavioural changes, dizziness, insomnia, somnolence and rarely suicidal tendencies.

9. **How would you plan surgical therapy for SUI?**

   Ans: Cases being considered for invasive therapy for SUI should be discussed in a multidisciplinary team meeting comprising a urologist/urogynaecologist, a specialist nurse, a specialist physiotherapist, a subspecialist with interest in functional bowel problems and a member of the geriatric team for women with functional impairment. The factors taken in consideration while deciding the choice of therapy include patient's age, lifestyle, preference and expectations, past management, co-morbidities, available treatment options and expertise, proportional involvement of urethral hypermobility and ISD, likelihood of impaired detrusor contractility and the need for concomitant genital prolapse repair, hysterectomy or fistulae.

10. What surgical procedures would you offer for treatment of uncomplicated SUI in this patient?

Ans: The surgical procedures for correction of SUI can be classified into:

1. Periurethral support procedures (supportive)
   - Suspension procedures
   - Mid-urethral sling (MUS)
   - Autologous sling
2. Sphincter augmentation procedures designed to augment urethral closure mechanism (occlusive)
   - Bulking agents
   - Pubovaginal sling
   - Artificial sphincter—reserved for selected cases of complicated SUI

Suspension procedures are designed to attach the periurethral support tissues to fixed structures causing re-elevation of the bladder neck into the abdominal pressure zone, thus preventing descent and providing equal transmission of intra-abdominal pressure to the bladder neck. Open Burch colposuspension has been considered the gold-standard among suspension procedures with a reported long-term efficacy of 85–90%.[10] It involves approximation of paravaginal tissues to iliopectineal line (ligament of Cooper) by typically using 2–4 sutures on each side.

Backplate procedures are intended to restore firm tissue, support tissue behind the urethra to thwart descent of bladder neck and urethra and enable closure of urethra during raised intra-abdominal pressure. These procedures include various slings or tapes which may be biological (autologous rectus fascia/fascia lata) or synthetic (polypropylene or Dacron). They may be classified as mid-urethral or bladder neck slings depending on the site of placement, or as retropubic (TVT) or trans-obturator (TOT) depending on the route of placement.

11. How would you choose surgical procedure for uncomplicated SUI?

Ans: Mid-urethral slings, autologous slings and colposuspensions are typically indicated in patients having a predominant urethral hypermobility rather than ISD.

In patients with uncomplicated SUI, synthetic mid-urethral tapes usually constitute the first line treatment. Choice of approach for mid-urethral sling (TVT vs TOT) is largely dictated by personal preferences and individual choices.

Current data indicates that MUS and pubovaginal slings have similar success rates in short-term, whereas MUS have a better success rate than Burch colposuspension.[11]

Pubovaginal slings have a higher 5-year satisfaction rate than Burch colposuspension and similar short-term outcomes as mid-urethral slings. However, this procedure may have an additional donor site morbidity which should be counselled to the patient.

Colposuspension (open or laparoscopic) can be offered as the initial surgical treatment to a young woman with uncomplicated SUI due to significant urethral hypermobility, on account of high long-term cure rates and the recent concerns about the long-term complications of synthetic mesh procedures.

Autologous pubovaginal slings have been traditionally reserved for patients having SUI with significant ISD component, presence of erosion, fistula or tissue loss, and prior failed mid-urethral sling surgery.

Injection of periurethral bulking agents can be considered in symptomatic patients with mild to moderate SUI having high risk for major surgery, elderly or frail patients not suitable for surgical intervention, previous multiple failed procedures and individual patient preferences. They should be counselled that the overall success rate is between 50% and 70%, effects are not long lasting, repeat injections may be needed to achieve desired outcomes, and overall efficacy is inferior to that of MUS or autologous slings.

12. How would you counsel the patient regarding pros and cons of different procedures for uncomplicated SUI?

Ans: Various studies including meta-analyses and systematic reviews have compared the short-term and long-term objective and subjective outcomes along with complications of various procedures.[11,12] (Table 1.1).

13. What are the parameters used to evaluate outcomes following surgery for SUI and what is the role of patient reported outcome measures (PROMs)?

Ans: Traditional methods of outcome assessment include continence rates, complications, and QoL measures pertaining to overall well-being, sexual function and urinary continence. However, there is a growing realization, especially after the "mesh controversy", that the outcome assessment should also include uniform and consistent PROMs. Unfulfilled expectations are key to patient dissatisfaction after surgery. The existing PROMs include Patient Global Impression of Improvement [PGI-I], Urinary Distress Inventory-Short Form [UDI-6], International Consultation on Incontinence Questionnaire, Urinary Incontinence-Short Form [ICIQ-SF], and Incontinence Impact Questionnaire-short form [IIQ-7]).

TABLE 1.1: Comparison of outcomes and complications of surgical procedures for uncomplicated SUI

	TOT	*TVT*	*Open colposuspension*	*Lap Colposuspension*	*Autologous sling*
SUCRA rating for cure*	64.1%	89.1%	76.7%	48.9%	89.4%
SUCRA rating for improvement*	76%	97%	63.8%	45.8%	67.7%
Rate of repeat surgery for SUI (at 5 years)	9.4%	1.5%	11.9%	Not available	1.8%
Bladder/urethral perforation	0.2–0.7%	3.6–10.1%	1.5–2.8%	2.1%	2.3–5.2%
Voiding difficulty including urinary retention	2.4–3.7%	2.7–10.2%	7.8%	6.32%	7.5–15.4%
Groin pain	6.3–6.5%	1.3–1.5%	1.1%	Not available	0.34%
Suprapubic pain	1.2%	4.0%	0%	Not available	0%
Persistent pain/discomfort	4.93%	5.09%	0.15%	Not available	7.0%
Tape/mesh erosion/extrusion/exposure	2.2–3.7%	1.4–2.1%	0.0	0.0	0.17%
De novo urgency or UI	5.3–9.2%	6.9–9.5%	4.3–11%	8.38%	8.6%
Wound infection	0.74%	0.75%	7.0%	Not available	2.6%

*SUCRA: Surface under cumulative ranking curves (Based on ESTER systematic review)[11]

KEY POINTS

- Diagnosis of SUI based on history and examination.
- SUI classified as complicated and uncomplicated based on associated risk factors.
- Urodynamic studies not required in evaluation of uncomplicated SUI.
- Patient education, PFMT, behavioural, and lifestyle modification important in management of SUI.
- Pharmacotherapy for uncomplicated SUI has a limited role in selected patients.
- Surgical therapy cornerstone of management for uncomplicated SUI.
- Surgical options for uncomplicated SUI include Burch colposuspension (open or lap), mid-urethral slings (TVT or TOT), autologous pubo-vaginal slings, bulking agents (selected cases).
- Prior to planning surgery, consider patient's age, lifestyle, preference and expectations, past management, co-morbidities, available treatment options and expertise, proportional involvement of urethral hypermobility and ISD, likelihood of impaired detrusor contractility and the need for concomitant genital prolapse repair, hysterectomy or fistulae.
- Assessment of procedure outcomes must include PROMs.

SUMMARY

- The chapter aims to provide evaluation and management of a case of uncomplicated SUI. While the evaluation is straightforward without too many controversies, the management has multiple options and issues of clinician's discretion in choosing appropriate therapy. Efforts have been made to provide the readers with best available evidence and make an informed decision.

REFERENCES

1. Sinha S, Agarwal MM, Vasudeva P, Khattar N, Madduri VKS, Yande S, Sarkar K, Patel A, Vaze A, Raina S, Jain A, Gupta M, Mishra N. The Urological Society of India Guidelines for the Evaluation and Management of Nonneurogenic Urinary Incontinence in Adults (Executive Summary). Indian J Urol. 2019 Jul-Sep;35(3):185–188.
2. NICE Guidance-Urinary incontinence and pelvic organ prolapse in women: management: © NICE (2019) Urinary incontinence and pelvic organ prolapse in women: management. BJU Int. 2019 May;123(5):777–803.
3. Nambiar, Arjun K. *et al.* European Association of Urology Guidelines on the Diagnosis and Management of Female Non-neurogenic Lower Urinary Tract Symptoms. Part 1: Diagnostics, Overactive Bladder, Stress Urinary Incontinence, and Mixed Urinary Incontinence. European Urology, Volume 82, Issue 1, 49–59, February 22, 2022.
4. Guralnick, M.L., *et al.* ICS Educational Module: Cough stress test in the evaluation of female urinary incontinence: Introducing the ICS-Uniform Cough Stress Test. Neurourol Urodyn, 2018. 37: 1849.
5. Agarwal A, Rathi S, Patnaik P, Shaw D, Jain M, Trivedi S, *et al.* Does preoperative urodynamic testing improve surgical outcomes in patients undergoing the transobturator tape procedure for stress urinary incontinence? A prospective randomized trial. Korean J Urol 2014;55:821–7.
6. Zubieta, M., *et al.* Influence of voluntary pelvic floor muscle contraction and pelvic floor muscle training on urethral closure pressures: a systematic literature review. Int Urogynecol J, 2016. 27: 687.
7. Dumoulin, C., *et al.* Pelvic floor muscle training versus no treatment, or inactive control treatments, for urinary incontinence in women. Cochrane Database Syst Rev, 2018. 10: CD005654.
8. Cody, J.D., *et al.* Oestrogen therapy for urinary incontinence in post-menopausal women. Cochrane Database Syst Rev, 2012. 10: CD001405.
9. Li, J., *et al.* The role of duloxetine in stress urinary incontinence: a systematic review and metaanalysis. Int Urol Nephrol, 2013. 45: 679.
10. Lapitan, M.C., *et al.* Open retropubic colposuspension for urinary incontinence in women. Cochrane Database Syst Rev, 2016. 2: CD002912.
11. Brazzelli, M., *et al.* Surgical treatments for women with stress urinary incontinence: ESTER systematic review and economic evaluation. Health Technol Assess,2019.23:1.
12. Wu JM. Stress incontinence in women. New England Journal of Medicine. 2021 Jun 24;384(25):2428–36.

Chapter

2

Overactive Bladder in a Female

• *Shirish Yande*

LEARNING OBJECTIVES

To understand:
Definition and prevalence of overactive bladder.
Differential diagnosis of overactive bladder
Etiopathogenesis of overactive bladder
Clinical evaluation and diagnostic algorithm of overactive bladder.
Management of overactive bladder
Refractory overactive bladder; its evaluation and management options

Case Scenario

A 68-year-old woman was referred to the department of urology by her family practitioner for symptoms suggestive of recurrent urinary tract infections for the past 7 years. Besides, she had increased urinary frequency (every half an hour) day and night associated with urgency and occasional incontinence. She also complained of poor urinary stream and sense of incomplete evacuation for all this period. Her symptoms were getting worse for the past two months. She is a known hypertensive (on beta blockers) and had laparoscopic hysterectomy in the year 2006. She was also a patient of "arthritis" for the past 17 years. Bladder diary (over 24 hours) showed small volume voids (50 ml to 130 ml every half an hour) on a single 24-hour sample sheet (This was thought to be representative) (Fig. 2.1).

USG showed normal kidneys and bladder with normal contours. Prevoid volume was 140 ml and postvoid was 27 ml. A urine culture was obtained at this stage. Urine did not grow any organisms.

Bladder Diary
(before treatment)

दिनांक 05

वेळ	किती लघवी झाली	संवेदना	
		घाईची लागली	वेदना
5:30 Am	180 mL	✓	
8:15 Am	130 mL	✓	
8:30 Am	30 mL	✓	
9:15 Am	50 mL	✓	
9:40 Am	90 mL	✓	
9:55 Am	100 mL	✓	
10:05 Am	90 mL	✓	
10:40 Am	90 mL	✓	
11:10 Am	50 mL	✓	
11:55 Am	70 mL	✓	
12:15 Pm	60 mL	✓	
1:25 Pm	80 mL	✓	
1:40 Pm	80 mL	✓	
1:50 Pm	110 mL	✓	
2:00 Pm	100 mL	✓	
2:05 Pm	100 mL	✓	
2:15 Pm	140 mL	✓	
2:20 Pm	110 mL	✓	
2:30 Pm	110 mL	✓	
2:45 Pm	90 mL	✓	

Fig. 2.1: Bladder diary before treatment

1. **How was the initial approach to management in this case?**
   Ans: She was advised about importance of fluid management. Pelvic floor muscle training (PFMT) was explained verbally and the contraction of anal sphincter was confirmed by digital examination. She was given a booklet, explaining the process of pelvic floor muscle contraction, including the frequency and duration of contractions of the pelvic floor muscles.

2. **What medications were recommended in this scenario?**

Ans: At this point she was prescribed Tab. Mirabegron 50 mg daily for a period of three weeks. She reported three weeks later with "slight improvement in her symptoms" but remained dissatisfied with the overall outcome. Subsequently Solifenacin was added (Mirabegron 50 mg + Solifenacin 5 mg daily) for three more weeks. The patient remained grossly symptomatic at the end of this treatment, nocturnal frequency being her main concern.

3. **Is there an alternative drug strategy to antimuscarinics and beta agonists?**

Ans: Yes, apart from the drugs which have direct action on the bladder, synthetic antidiuretic hormone preparations (desmopressin) and anxiolytics (Amitriptyline) may offer relief of bothersome symptoms in OAB. Our patient in question was offered Desmopressin 100 µg along with Tab. Amitriptyline 10 mg both at bedtime for a period of two weeks.

Although she had no untoward effects, she remained symptomatic and felt that the symptom of incontinence became even worse intermittently. There was no pain reported.

4. **What is refractory overactive bladder?**

Ans: An overactive bladder symptom complex can be labelled "refractory" where there is no satisfactory response to physical measures and an adequate standard pharmacotherapy of three months' duration, where a bladder diary has proven unsatisfactory outcome to these measures.[2]

In view of intractable symptoms, repeat bladder diary was requested.

This revealed no real improvement in frequency and incontinence episodes. Indeed, her repeat chart showed a slight worsening of incontinence episodes (Fig. 2.2). At this stage this case was labelled as one of "refractory overactive bladder" and more invasive measures were considered to control her symptoms.

Urodynamics was therefore scheduled at this stage. This was considered complying with recommendations of USI guidelines for urinary incontinence in adults.[2]

5. **At what stage is urodynamic investigation performed? What should we expect in the Urodynamic evaluation in this case?**

Ans: Urodynamic investigation is indicated in a case of OAB, before an invasive management is proposed.

Urodynamic investigation is expected to give the following information:

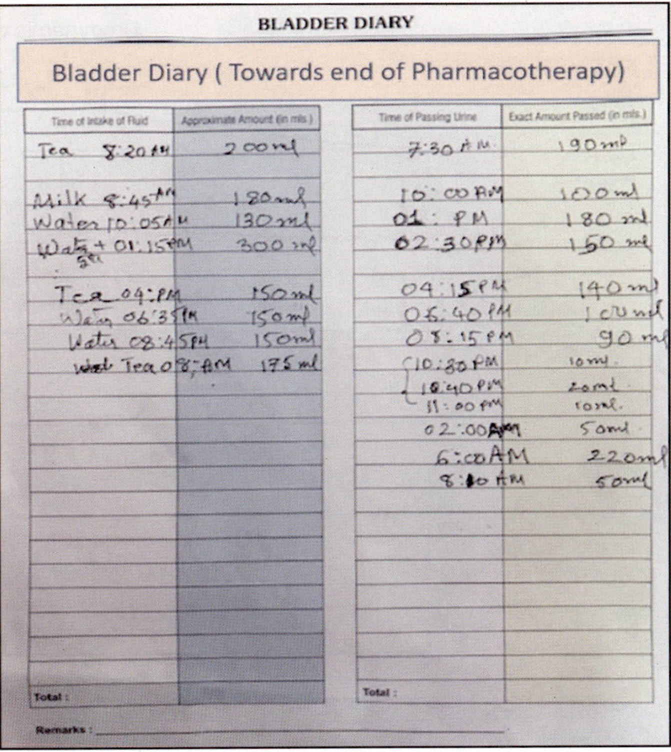

BLADDER DIARY

Bladder Diary (Towards end of Pharmacotherapy)

Time of Intake of Fluid	Approximate Amount (in mls.)
Tea 8:20 AM	200 ml
Milk 8:45 AM	180 ml
Water 10:05 AM	130 ml
Water + Tea 01:15 PM	300 ml
Tea 04: PM	150 ml
Water 06:35 PM	150 ml
Water 08:45 PM	150 ml
Tea 08: AM	175 ml
Total :	

Time of Passing Urine	Exact Amount Passed (in mls.)
7:30 AM	190 ml
10:00 AM	100 ml
01: PM	180 ml
02:30 PM	150 ml
04:15 PM	140 ml
06:40 PM	100 ml
08:15 PM	90 ml
10:30 PM	10 ml
10:40 PM	20 ml
11:00 PM	10 ml
02:00 AM	50 ml
6:00 AM	220 ml
8:10 AM	50 ml
Total :	

Remarks :

Fig. 2.2: Bladder diary after treatment

1. It confirms the presence as well as severity of detrusor overactivity (which reproduces the symptom of urgency with/without incontinence).
2. It may also help to exclude other unrelated conditions which may produce the symptoms of OAB. These are bladder outlet obstruction, detrusor underactivity and a sphincter dysfunction. It may also raise the suspicion of a neurogenic dysfunction.

URODYNAMICS

Filling cystometry was performed using 6 F double lumen catheter. Filling was performed in sitting position with the infusion rate of 40 ml per min after emptying the bladder. Storage phase showed detrusor overactivity from the beginning of the filling phase. Involuntary contractions ranged from 16 to 21 cm H_2O associated with urgency and pericatheter leakage. Bladder proprioception was abnormal with early sensations (Fig. 2.3). End fill pressure was 8 cm H_2O and detrusor compliance was normal. Capacity was 120 ml. Of note, in such situations, reducing the filling rate can help get a more representative filling phase assessment. Voiding pressure flow study showed an unobstructed outlet with normal flow and voiding detrusor pressure with negligible residual.

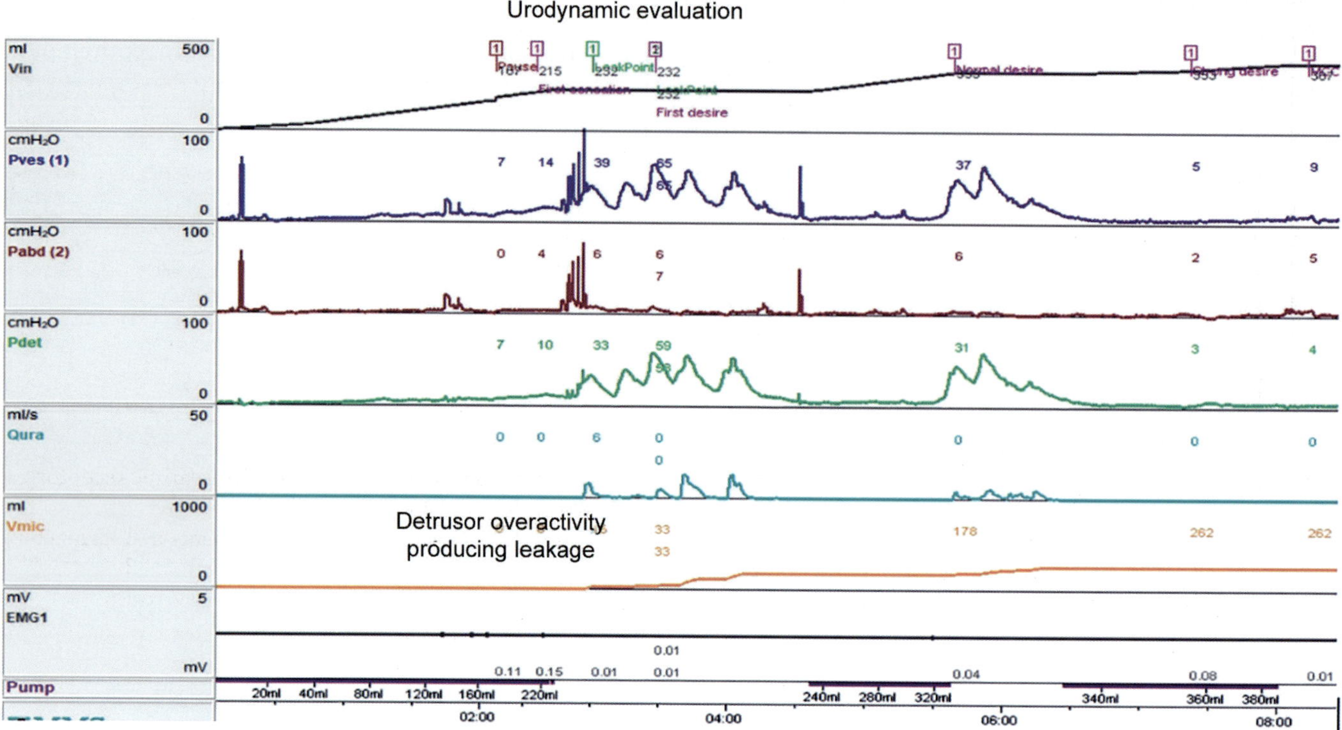

Fig. 2.3: Urodynamic trace of storage phase showing detrusor overactivity producing urine leak

6. **How does this information change your plan of further action?**

   Ans: With the confirmation of underlying the diagnosis, one can proceed to offer more invasive measures such as intra-detrusor injection of botulinum toxin or sacral nerve stimulation (neuromodulation).

7. **What treatment option was chosen in this case?**

   Ans: Her urodynamics evaluation was consistent with refractory OAB. Hence, she was advised intra-detrusor injection of botulinum toxin.

   She was administered intra-detrusor injection of botulinum toxin under spinal anaesthesia. 100 IU of botulinum toxin A (diluted with 20 ml of normal saline) was injected submucosally at 20 sites in the bladder under spinal anaesthesia. A Foley urethral catheter was left indwelling overnight.

8. **What was the response?**

   Ans: The patient reported progressive improvement in her symptoms from day 5 of the injection. At three months (till the time of reporting the case) she remains almost completely asymptomatic with acceptably normal urinary frequency, only mild urgency and no incontinence episodes.

SUMMARY

- The term "overactive bladder" is a symptom complex and is not to be confused with the term "detrusor overactivity", which is a urodynamic observation.
- Bladder diary offers the most objective tool for quantification of patient's symptoms as well as helps to assess response to therapy.
- Routine cystoscopic evaluation is not recommended in initial evaluation of urinary incontinence in women.[2]
- Overactive bladder symptoms can be called refractory when there is no satisfactory response to physical measures and the drug therapy (including a combination of antimuscarinic and beta agonists) for a period of 12 weeks. USI Guidelines also recommend that the unsatisfactory response should be objectively demonstrated using a bladder diary.[2]
- Invasive urodynamic testing is indicated in overactive bladder only after fair trial to physical measures and pharmacotherapy of sufficient duration. It aims to identify intractable detrusor overactivity or any other factors which may be responsible for persistence of the patient's symptoms.
- Intradetrusor injection of botulinum toxin A is considered as the first invasive option in the Indian scenario.
- Sacral nerve stimulation (neuromodulation) is a viable alternative,[10] although device care, possible need for revisions, and cost seem to have limited its use in India.
- Patients who persist with intractable symptoms after the above measures should be considered for augmentation cystoplasty with or without Intermittent Self Catheterisation Program.[3]

Challenges

- Despite such an exhaustive work on this bothersome urinary symptom complex, a number of lacunae still remain in the understanding and management of overactive bladder disease.
- The definition is still unclear and does not underline any particular disease process.

- Behavioural therapy and lifestyle modifications demand a high patient motivation.
- Drug therapy continues to have untoward effects in the long-term, leading to inconsistent patient compliance.[8]
- Refractory overactive bladder remains a challenge and demands invasive treatment options, which offer either short-lived efficacy or threaten to have serious morbidity in the long-term.
- With a higher aging population in our society and with a higher prevalence with advancing age, the quantum of overactive bladder patients threatens to be high and is increasing rapidly.

REFERENCES

1. Stewart WF, Van Rooyen JB, Cundiff GW *et al.* Prevalence and burden of overactive bladder in the United States. World J. Urol. 2003;20(6):327–36.
2. Sinha S, Agarwal MM, Vasudeva P, Kha]ar N, Madduri VKS, Yande S, *et al.* The Urological Society of India Guidelines for the Evaluation and Management of Nonneurogenic Urinary Incontinence in Adults (Executive Summary). Indian J Urol. 2019;35(3):185–8.
3. Gross M, Boone TB, Appell RA. Surgical management of overactive bladder. Curr Urol Rep 2002; 3:388–95.
4. Abrams P, Cardozo L, Fall M, *et al.* The standardisation of terminology in lower urinary tract function: report from the standardisation subcommittee of the International Continence Society. Urology. 2003; 61(1):37–49.
5. Brading AF. A myogenic basis for the overactive bladder. Urology 50(Suppl. 6A), S57–S67; discussion S68–S73 (1997).
6. Roe B, Ostaszkiewicz J, Milne J, and Wallace S. Systemic reviews of bladder training and voiding programmes in adults: a synopsis of findings from data analysis and outcomes using metastudy techniques. J. Adv. Nurs. 2007; 57:15–31.
7. Lekskulchai O, Dietz HP. Detrusor wall thickness as a test for detrusor overactivity in women. Ultrasound Obstet. Gynecol. 2008; 32:535–39.
8. Scarpero HM, Dmochowski RR. Muscarinic receptors: what we know. Curr Urol Rep. 2003;4(6):421–28.
9. Chapple C, Gormley EA. Developments in pharmacological therapy for the overactive bladder. BJU Int 2006; 98:78–87.
10. Leng WW, Morrisroe SN. Sacral nerve stimulation for the overactive bladder. Urol Clin North Am 2006;33: 491–501.

Chapter 3

Post-SUI Surgery Urinary Retention

• Nikhil Khattar

LEARNING OBJECTIVES

- Urinary retention is a cardinal complication that can complicate surgery for stress urinary incontinence.
- Retention resolves on its own in most cases but when it extends beyond a week, a decision needs to be taken whether or not to intervene.
- Sling release or loosening can be offered only early in the postoperative course. Beyond two or three weeks, fibrosis might prevent success.
- When performed correctly, sling release is unlikely to lead to a recurrence of incontinence.
- Patients are typically advised to self-catheterize while awaiting resolution. Beyond three weeks sling transection is typically required. This most often relieves retention but with recurrence of incontinence in approximately 25–50%.
- More delayed intervention can necessitate a formal urethrolysis heralded by a lack of springback of the cut edges of the transected sling.
- Women who achieve spontaneous voiding after prolonged retention might continue to remain in obstruction with consequent risk. Storage symptoms can dominate and mislead the clinician.
- Retention due to overcorrection of incontinence as well as literature on the standardisation of sling-tensioning are discussed with tips on avoiding this complication.

Case Scenario

"Re-catheterise her. Reassure her that there is no need to worry as it can happen at times because of inflammation, we can give her another voiding trial after 2 days". I disconnected the line.

The patient in question was a 55-year-old female with uncomplicated stress incontinence without any previous voiding symptoms in whom I had performed a tension free vaginal tape on the previous morning. I was not worried because post-operative retention is common after sling surgery and women most often resume voiding when the pain subsides.

1. **Should one be worried of every retention occurring in the post-operative period after sling surgery?**

   Ans: Retention after SUI surgery is one of the most common complications. The exact incidence may be unknown but according to an estimate it may approach up to 20% after sling surgery. And it is known to resolve in most, bringing the need for re-operations to around 6%.[1] Several non-technical factors can contribute to early retention after a sling surgery, namely pain, anaesthesia related side effects, local hematoma, fecal impaction, etc.[2]

2. **Do all types of sling procedures predispose to retention? Are there differences between retropubic and transobturator routes?**

   Ans: The rates are higher for pubovaginal slings than in mid-urethral synthetic slings. Amongst mid-urethral slings, retropubic tapes have slightly higher rates of retentive complications as compared to trans-obturator tapes. Going further, in each of these approaches, the rates are higher for retropubic tapes if the approach is top-down (towards vagina) and in contrast higher for trans-obturator tapes if the approach is inside-out (away from vagina).[3]

Case Scenario *(Contd.)*

Two days later after making sure that she was pain free, afebrile and had evacuated her bowel well in morning, she was given a repeat voiding trial which again failed.

I revisited her preoperative details again. She did not have any history suggestive of urgency or urge incontinence, there was no associated pelvic organ prolapse, she had a demonstrable stress urinary incontinence and had a hypermobile urethra on examination. Her voiding diary had good functional bladder capacity but she used to void frequently to remain dry and used a couple of pads every day. Her uroflowmetry showed a good peak and nice curve.

Preoperative urodynamics demonstrated a capacity of 320 cc with normal compliance and no detrusor overactivity with demonstrable leak on Valsalva after 100 cc. Abdominal leak point pressure of 40 cm H_2O. Voiding phase demonstrated a good flow with Q_{max} of 25 ml/s with Pdet@Q_{max} of 17 cm H_2O and no straining.

I was sure of my precautions taken during the surgery, namely a catheter in the urethra and an instrument between the sling and the urethra while tensioning the sling.

I reassured her and taught clean intermittent self-catheterisation (CISC) so that she had repeated opportunity to try voiding on her own. We decided to review in another three days.

3. **Was there any predisposing factor for retention in this lady, which was omitted during evaluation?**

   Ans: The patient had all parameters satisfying the uncomplicated SUI definition in USI guidelines 2019.[4]

   Patients with pre-existing voiding dysfunction or Valsalva voiders are known to have a predilection for retention but none of that was present in this case.

4. **Being an uncomplicated case, how do you justify getting a urodynamics in this patient?**

   Ans: This lady had severe degree of incontinence and abdominal leak point pressures of 40 cm H_2O hinted towards a component of intrinsic sphincter deficiency. Presence of demonstrable urethral hypermobility prompted me to chose a mid-urethral sling but out of the two routes retropubic route was chosen because of low ALPP as retropubic slings provide better chances of success in such cases.

   Moreover, she had now persistent retention, a baseline preoperative urodynamics was reassuring that I had not missed any subtle voiding dysfunction.

5. **What could have lead to, now seemingly, a tight sling?**

   Ans: Overcorrection mostly results after a relatively difficult plastic sheath removal which stretches the tape even if there is an instrument separating the urethra and the tape, and leaves the urethra compressed after instrument removal.[5]

Case Scenario *(Contd.)*

Nothing improved in further waiting and now I had to take a call on either leaving her like that and waiting for spontaneous, to do something about it right then.

6. **Why is this time point of 1 week important in decision making?**

   Ans: Non-resolving retention at one week after sling surgery is an important juncture as the outcomes may differ with the approach one chooses. Urethral dilatation comes up as an instinctive solution but has long been tried and given up following poor results.[6] In the early phase before the tissue ingrowth happens over the mesh, a mobilisation of the sling is possible to create further space between the urethra and the sling. On the other hand, if one chooses to wait, more than half of the patients would start voiding by 6 weeks. However, beyond two weeks, tissue ingrowth over the mesh incorporates the mesh in the tissues and it would not be possible to pull the sling out and release the tension, should the retention remain unrelieved. In this phase a sling transection or a sling lysis is required with a higher chance of recurrence of incontinence.

   While this would mean a visit to the operation theatre again, but would most likely relieve the retention with a minimal risk to the continence already achieved.

7. **Do the two approaches, i.e. taking patient early for sling mobilisation vs keeping the patient waiting on CISC and delayed sling transection, if required (thereby avoiding intervention in nearly half), have similar outcomes as regards to continence?**

   Ans: In one of the earlier experiences in tape mobilisation after sling surgery (TVT), Nguyen reported successful resumption of voiding in 10 patients when mobilisation was done between days 3 and 10 after sling placement. The overall success and satisfaction scores were not different from the rest 153 immediate voiders after sling surgery at one year of follow-up in this report.[5]

   Glavind and Glavind encountered postoperative prolonged retention 1–2 weeks in 10 of their 143 patients after TVT. Five underwent tape mobilisation within 3 weeks resulting is resumption of voiding without recurrence of stress incontinence, two required tape transection at 5 and 7 months resulting in free voiding but both developed incontinence. Three patients continued CISC for 6 and 9 months with gradually decreasing residuals but all had a restricted flow and required to double void and one also developed urge incontinence.[7]

A large retrospective study from Norway collected data from female incontinence registry to compare outcomes of CISC, sling mobilisation and sling transection in cases of urinary retention after sling surgery. Out of 18772 women undergoing sling surgery between 1998 and 2013, urinary retention (defined by need for any of the above three interventions) developed in 585 (3.1%). Median follow-up was 9 months. IC was required in 328 patients (62 later underwent sling transection), sling mobilisation in 136 patients (14 later required sling transection) and direct sling transection in 121 patients (probably they were not in retention and required transection for voiding dysfunction). Overall, 197 women required sling transection at a median time of 24.5 weeks between surgery and transection. All those women who never required sling transection after their initial retention (whether they initially required CISC or sling mobilisation) had no difference in their subjective or objective postoperative outcomes. On the contrary, all those women requiring sling transection (whether primarily or after failure to void after a period of CISC or sling mobilisation) were significantly less satisfied and had significantly higher incidence of recurrent stress incontinence (25%). On subgroup analysis of women who never required transection, i.e. all those who resumed voiding either after a period of CISC or after sling mobilisation, women who underwent upfront tape mobilisation were 'very satisfied' more often. Also, the need for sling transection was higher in women who chose CISC vs sling mobilisation (19% vs 10%). The study concluded sling mobilisation to be superior to CISC or sling transection.[8]

Regarding the ability to address our question, this study has two drawbacks: Firstly, it considers all women who underwent tape transection as retention which means they were either on an indwelling catheter or they were voiding but having significant obstructive symptoms. I would exclude the subgroup who were not in retention and got the tape transected for voiding dysfunction. Secondly, it does not give details and differences in outcome of those women who had to undergo sling transection after failing their first choice treatment of either CISC or sling mobilisation.

A prospective study addresses decision making at this juncture. Thirty-one of 687 women continued to be in retention >7 days after a midurethral sling surgery (4.5%). Out of these 31 women, 10 chose early sling mobilisation while the remaining 21 chose to be on CISC to wait for spontaneous voiding. Out of these 21 women, 11 required sling lysis at different time points after surgery (9 within 2 months, 1 within 6 months and 1 beyond 6 months). Of the early mobilisation group, 8 of 10 women were relieved of retention and resumed voiding without developing SUI after single attempt at mobilisation, whereas two required a second release with similar outcome. Of the sling lysis group, seven patients developed recurrence of SUI within 6 months and one continued to require CISC even after sling lysis.[9]

Case Scenario *(Contd.)*

The above discussion based on contemporary evidence along with discussion with my senior colleagues was convincing enough for me to take her up for sling mobilisation which was done on 8th postoperative day. Under general anaesthesia, I reopened the vaginal incision, carefully identified and looped the sling with an infant feeding tube and gave controlled tug till I could mobilise the sling to create an additional 5 mm–1 cm space between the urethra and the sling. She started voiding well and maintained her continence after the sling release.

8. How can tensioning be better standardised to prevent overcorrections?

Ans: To find the most reproducible method of sling tensioning, MUST (Mid Urethral Sling Tensioning) trial randomised between the use of a Mayo scissors as a separator vs holding two fixed points on the tape 1.4 cm apart with a Babcock clamp while tensioning the sling. In this multi-centre prospective study, 318 women undergoing TVT were randomised equally to both groups. The postoperative retention, need for self-catheterisation, was significantly less in Babkock group. Need for surgical sling release was 12 vs 0 in favour of Babcock clamp technique. Incidentally, vaginal mesh erosion were also higher in Babcock group.[10]

9. Do all the patients who start voiding after a prolonged retention become free from all concerns?

Ans: Although most of the cases of early postoperative urinary retention start voiding in first few days after sling surgery, ***but an even more***

careful monitoring of these patients is required in the course because, now dry after months or years of their incontinence, they may not be forthcoming in reporting their voiding symptoms. An insignificant postvoid residue and lack of new onset symptoms of overactivity is generally sufficient to let them "off the hook". Presentation of postsling surgery bladder outlet obstruction is generally subtle and a thorough work up with a video urodynamics or VCUG with urodynamics should be undertaken if any suspicion remains.

10. What is urethrolysis and what is its role in postsling obstruction?

Ans: Urethrolysis is reserved for even more delayed presentations or unfavorable outcome after a prolonged hopeful wait on CISC. Beyond 3 months, generally the mesh incorporation in the fibrotic process is complete and on division of sling there is no sagging of the urethra or recoil of the sling. In such cases, the entire part of circumference of urethra in contact with the sling needs to be made free of the mesh and fibrosis. Freeing of urethra is achieved transvaginally in most cases, whereas a suprapubic or retropubic route is reserved for select cases. Procedure is challenging and demanding but results are generally gratifying.[2]

KEY POINTS

- Urinary retention is a common complication after sling surgery which resolves spontaneously in most cases.
- If retention does not resolve after one week, sling release should be offered.
- It is not unwise to perform a preoperative urodynamic study in an uncomplicated SUI patient if the facility is available.
- Sling release intends to increase the suburethral space between the sling and urethra by 5 mm to 1 cm.
- It does not result in incontinence in most cases.
- A second release may be required in some cases.
- Late sling transection, if required, may lead to recurrence of incontinence in approximately 25–50% cases.
- Placement of Babcock clamp to hold a portion of sling should be preferred over keeping a Mayo scissors under the urethra while tensioning the sling.

REFERENCES

1. Malacarne DR, Nitti VW. Post-Sling Urinary Retention in Women. Curr Urol Rep. 2016 Nov;17(11):83.
2. Sinha S, Bladder Outlet Obstruction after Sling Surgery for Stress Urinary Incontinence. N. Khattar *et al.* (eds.), Female Bladder Outlet Obstruction and Urethral Reconstruction, Springer 2021
3. Ford AA, Rogerson L, Cody JD, Aluko P, Ogah JA. Mid-urethral sling operations for stress urinary incontinence in women. Cochrane Database Syst Rev. 2017 Jul 31;7(7):CD006375.
4. Sinha S *et al.* The Urological Society of India Guidelines for the Evaluation and Management of Nonneurogenic Urinary Incontinence in Adults (Executive Summary). Indian J Urol. 2019 Jul-Sep;35(3):185–188.
5. Nguyen JN. Tape mobilization for urinary retention after tension-free vaginal tape procedures. Urology. 2005 Sep;66(3):523–6.
6. Sokol AI, Jelovsek JE, Walters MD, Paraiso MF, Barber MD. Incidence and predictors of prolonged urinary retention after TVT with and without concurrent prolapse surgery. Am J Obstet Gynecol. 2005 May;192(5):1537–43.
7. Glavind K, Glavind E. Treatment of prolonged voiding dysfunction after tension-free vaginal tape procedure. Acta Obstet Gynecol Scand. 2007;86(3):357–60.
8. Moksnes LR, Svenningsen R, Schiøtz HA, Moe K, Staff AC, Kulseng-Hanssen S. Sling mobilization in the management of urinary retention after mid-urethral sling surgery. Neurourol Urodyn. 2017 Apr;36(4):1091–1096.
9. Brennand EA, Tang S, Birch C, Robert M, Kim-Fine S. Early voiding dysfunction after midurethral sling surgery: comparison of two management approaches. Int Urogynecol J. 2017 Oct;28(10):1515–1526.
10. Brennand *et al.* Two Intraoperative Techniques for Midurethral Sling Tensioning: A Randomized Controlled Trial. Obstet Gynecol. 2020 Sep;136(3):471–481.

Chapter

4

Anterior Compartment Prolapse with Occult SUI

• T Srikala Prasad

LEARNING OBJECTIVES

- Pelvic organ prolapse (POP) and stress urinary incontinence (SUI) seem to co-exist in 54% of women.[1] Both are associated with multiparity, aging, postmenopausal status, obesity, and conditions resulting in increased intra-abdominal pressure like weightlifting, chronic cough, and constipation.
- Anterior compartment prolapse or cystocele occurs when there is a pathological descent of the anterior vaginal wall along with the overlying bladder base. Three distinct defects can result in anterior vaginal wall prolapse.
- The midline cystocele also known as distension cystocele is due to overstretching and attenuation of the anterior vaginal wall. There will be a loss of vaginal rugosities in the anterior vaginal wall.
- The lateral cystocele, a displacement cystocele occurs as a result of the pathological detachment of the anterolateral wall supports from the lateral attachment, the arcus tendineus fascia pelvis (ATFP), or the white line. The presence of paravaginal defect can be assessed during surgery when the anterior vaginal wall is reflected from the underlying bladder wall up to the inferior pubic rami on both sides. In patients having a paravaginal defect due to complete detachment, this dissection will lead directly into the retropubic space and the retropubic fat will be visualized.
- A transverse defect occurs when the pubocervical fascia separates from its insertion around the cervix or the apex. Anterior vaginal wall prolapse can be associated with an enterocele in a post-hysterectomy patient.[2]
- Women with anterior compartment prolapse may not manifest SUI because of kinking of the urethra. If SUI can be demonstrated after prolapse reduction techniques in a patient in whom SUI was not earlier demonstrable, it is called occult SUI. This is seen in up to 30% of cases.[3] These women need to be counseled regarding the pros and cons of doing a concomitant anti-incontinence surgery.

Case Scenario

Mrs X, a 62-year-old, diabetic, hypertensive, multiparous, postmenopausal lady comes with complaints of mass descending per vaginum for the past two years. She also complained of increased urinary frequency and burning micturition. The frequency is 10–12 times in the day and 3 times during the night with urgency. Clinical examination reveals a stage III anterior vaginal wall prolapse and a stage I descent of the cervix. Point C was –2. Point Ba was +2. There was a loss of vaginal rugosities and examination revealed a midline defect. A cough stress test after prolapse reduction with a pessary revealed SUI. The cervix was looking healthy. The uterus was retroverted, normal sized and the adnexa was normal. The vaginal wall showed atrophic changes.

1. How would you evaluate a lady with LUTS along with a history suggestive of prolapse?

Ans: A good history taking will help differentiate the causes of incontinence (SUI vs UUI vs MUI).

Assess for obstructive voiding symptoms which could be present because of the descent of the bladder below the urethra resulting in urethral compression. Such patients help themselves by re-positioning the prolapsed bladder. Rarely voiding LUTS could be because of detrusor underactivity. Also, assess for the presence of any urinary incontinence and resulting bother, usage of diapers, or any lifestyle changes because of the urinary leak. Storage LUTS in women with prolapse could be due to incomplete emptying and increased residual urine. This stasis also predisposes to infections and stone formation.

Assess other storage symptoms like urgency, nocturia, or continuous leakage. Other relevant history as per Table 4.1 could further be important in such a case.

TABLE 4.1: Other history
• General history of comorbidities including DM, HTN, neurological disorders, etc.
• Obstetric history (LSCS or vaginal delivery), past surgical history (anti-incontinence surgery, POP surgery, radical pelvic surgery), and history of prior radiotherapy.
• History of recurrent UTI and any condition that affects the urinary tract is ascertained.
• History of smoking as stopping smoking reduce cough and is a health benefit.
• The medication list also has to be scrutinized.
• Other causes of incontinence like fistulae, malignancy, neurogenic causes, and radiation are excluded.
• Constipation can be both a cause and effect of POP. The effects of POP on sexual function also need to be ascertained and documented. We need to know how bothersome the complaints are.

Examination of the patient should be roughly as per Table 4.2. Efforts should always be made to reveal an occult SUI after the reduction of prolapse either manually or with a pessary.

2. **What other investigations will you do?**

Ans: Apart from a urinalysis, an ultrasound with PVR is most often required. While there is no clear evidence to support a specific cut-off value for PVR, large residuals or low void% might indicate the need for further evaluation.

As per USI guidelines, urodynamics (UDS) should not be performed if only conservative management is planned. In women with uncomplicated stress incontinence (implying prolapse is not beyond the introitus), UDS is not required. Most such women will not present for prolapse surgery. However, in women with higher stage prolapse with demonstrable urinary incontinence, UDS is indicated if stress incontinence surgery is being contemplated.

Several methods of prolapse reduction have been used during UDS such as manual reduction, packing, pessary, sponge stick or split speculum. Each method yields a slightly different outcome in terms of identification of occult stress incontinence or the presence of voiding dysfunction. Each method also has a variable effect of biasing the UDS findings. However, one or the other method of prolapse reduction must be used and the UDS is best performed both with prolapse unreduced as well as following reduction.

Pre-operative UDS can also help evaluate the underlying diagnosis behind voiding dysfunction. The demonstration of improved voiding parameters on prolapse reduction can reassure the surgeon

TABLE 4.2: Examination

Examination	*Comments*
A complete general and focused urological, gynaecological, and neurological examination is done	
Abdomen examination	Look for distended bladder, mass lesions, scars of previous surgery, etc
Genitourinary examination	Assessment of estrogenic status, urethral diverticulum, vaginal capacity, POP, pelvic mass, vaginal mass, and fistula. The pelvic floor strength is also assessed. A video on POP-Q is embedded.
Focused neurological examination	Assess sensation and bulbocavernosus reflex (BCR). Up to 30% of women may have a negative BCR and yet be neurologically normal.[5]
Cough stress test (CST)	**CST** is done when the patient has a comfortably full bladder. She is examined in the dorsal lithotomy position and asked to cough. Patients who suffer from SUI will leak urine simultaneously with the cough. If the patient leaks large quantities of urine a little later, it is due to a cough-associated detrusor overactivity (CADO) and is treated like an overactive bladder (OAB). In case the cough stress test is negative, the test is repeated with the patient in a standing position and with the legs apart, ensuring that the bladder is filled to around 300 ml.
Supine empty stress test	The patient is asked to cough on a near-empty bladder (less than 100 ml). If they do not leak, the chances of having intrinsic sphincter deficiency (ISD) are low. Patients who leak even on an empty bladder may have increased failure rates with trans-obturator tape and will require surgeries like a pubovaginal sling.
Test for urethral hypermobility	**SUI** occurs primarily because of urethral hypermobility and intrinsic sphincter deficiency. Urethral hypermobility is when the urethra is displaced ≥30 degrees from the horizontal when the patient is in supine lithotomy during straining and can be assessed using the Q-tip test. In those with fixed urethra, mid-urethral slings may have more failure rate, and a pubovaginal sling would be a better choice.

that voiding LUTS are likely to improve following surgery although the converse is not necessarily true.

Indications for cystoscopy are a few (Table 4.3). Some cases may require referral to a specialist (Table 4.4). Uncomplicated patients will not require additional testing. Additional imaging may be required for women with complicated SUI like patients with previous sling or mesh. CT or MRI may be needed for women with pain, previous mesh, or haematuria.

TABLE 4.3: Cystoscopy indications
• Storage voiding symptoms refractory to first- and second-line treatments
• Bladder pain
• Recurrent cystitis
• Hematuria
• Pelvic mass
• Patients with previous incontinence surgery or POP surgery with mesh

TABLE 4.4: Red Flags in Incontinence (require further evaluation or specialist referral)
• Microscopic or gross hematuria
• Rectal or pelvic mass
• Palpable bladder
• Failure of initial therapies or failed previous surgeries
• New onset enuresis
• Continuous leakage suggestive of fistula
• Suspected neurological cause

This patient has urgency in addition to occult SUI and anterior vaginal wall prolapse beyond the hymen and a significant PVR and hence will need UDS prior to surgery.

3. **What is the conservative line of management available for this patient?**

Ans: Behavioral Treatments

It is recommended as the first-line therapy and includes patient education along with other components such as a bladder diary, supervised pelvic floor muscle training (PFMT), stress management strategies, biofeedback, electrical stimulation, and lifestyle modification.

Weight reduction: Obesity is the most clearly established risk factor for UI with obese women having 2 times the risk of UI. Weight reduction of even a moderate amount improves symptoms of UI.

Supervised PFMT is recommended as a first-line conservative treatment for women of all ages with SUI, UUI, or MUI. In women not needing a vaginal pessary or surgical surgery for POP, PFMT offers potential relief from LUTS.[4]

Pessaries are useful in the management of POP in pregnant, puerperal women and patients who do not desire surgical treatment and can help alleviate stress/urge urinary incontinence and other symptoms of urogenital prolapse.[3] Serious complications are seen following unsupervised long-term usage of pessaries.

Topical estrogen in the form of estriol, conjugated estrogens applied twice weekly helps relieve the symptoms of vulvovaginal atrophy (VVA).

4. **What is the role of medical line of management?**

Ans:

Duloxetine

Duloxetine is a selective serotonin-norepinephrine reuptake inhibitor (SSNRI) commonly used as an antidepressant. Studies reveal high rates of drug discontinuation due to adverse effects like nausea, vomiting, constipation, dry mouth, giddiness, insomnia, and fatigue.[6,7]

Suicidal tendencies were one of the major concerns. An SR published in a psychiatry journal concluded that there was substantial evidence to support the efficacy, safety, and tolerability of Duloxetine in the treatment of SUI. Mild to moderate side effects were seen which diminished with continued treatment.[8] The drug must be slowly tapered and withdrawn to minimize the side effects.

5. **Can you give us an update on recent treatment modalities?**

Ans:

Platelet-rich plasma therapy (PRP) in SUI

Autologous PRP obtained from the blood of the patient injected into the urethral sphincter could enhance sphincter muscle bulk resulting in improved outcomes in SUI patients.[9] Such treatment can be done for patients who failed initial conservative treatment only in a clinical trial setting until definite evidence is available.

Stem cell therapy in SUI

Stem cells have the ability of self-renewal as well as differentiation into specialized cells and they possibly can help in tissue regeneration and healing and are hence used to potentially repair injured or damaged urethral sphincter in an attempt to treat SUI.[10] Until we have definitive evidence, such treatment should only be done in the setting of a clinical trial.

Vaginal laser therapy in SUI

Some studies have reported that vaginal laser treatment appears to be a safe, effective, well-tolerated minimally invasive modality of treatment. However, RCT with control as a sham has not shown that CO_2 laser is better than sham treatment.[11] The USI guidelines have a 'strong' recommendation against the use of lasers for SUI outside of a research setting.[4]

6. Discuss the management of anterior compartment prolapse.

This patient has a stage III anterior compartment prolapse (Point Ba is +2). She seems to have a midline cystocele as evidenced by loss of rugosities. She complained of mass descending per vaginum and also has increased urinary frequency. Midline cystocele repair is done by plication of the layers of the vaginal muscularis and the adventitia overlying the bladder (pubocervical fascia) by taking rows of imbricating sutures with 2-0 delayed absorbable sutures. The redundant vaginal wall is trimmed and approximated.[2]

The patient gets good relief from storage symptoms like increased urinary frequency and urgency. Her voiding is also improved.

7. Discuss the arguments with regard to simultaneous SUI surgery or delayed SUI surgery and the outcomes.

Ans: Women with POP and occult are at risk of developing post-operative SUI. However, women might not develop overt SUI after POP surgery alone with 75% of women in one study showing continence.[12] The most important risk factors for *de novo* incontinence after POP surgeries were found to be positive pessary testing, older age, and low MUCP $\leq$ 60 cm H_2O. The patients who will benefit most from concomitant POP and SUI surgery are women who present with POP and overt SUI which this patient did not have.[12]

Women need to be informed of the increased risk of adverse events with combined prolapse and anti-urinary incontinence surgeries especially in a setting of occult SUI where the woman is not have urinary symptoms pre-operatively.[3] Women with *de novo* voiding dysfunction following prophylactic surgery are less likely to accept the complication. In general, in most settings it is probably wiser to avoid performing a combined surgery for occult stress incontinence in women undergoing POP surgery and to counsel carefully if the woman chooses to do so.

SUMMARY

- While women with occult SUI are at risk of postoperative overt SUI following POP surgery alone, this risk is not universal.
- Concomitant POP and SUI surgery carries higher risk of adverse events than isolated POP surgery.
- Concomitant POP and SUI surgery should be undertaken only after proper explanation of risks vs benefits of this procedure.

REFERENCES

1. Wong JWH, Ramm O. Urinary Incontinence and Pelvic Organ Prolapse. Clin Obstet Gynecol. 2021 Jun 1;64(2):314–320. doi: 10.1097/GRF.0000000000000615. PMID: 33859096.
2. Karram, M.M (2021). Atlas of Pelvic Anatomy and Gynecologic Surgery (5th Ed., pp.623).Elsevier.
3. Harding CK, Lapitan MC, Arlandis S, *et al.* Non-neurogenic Female LUTS. European Association of Urology Guidelines. 2023. Available at: https://uroweb.org/guideline/non-neurogenic-female-luts, accessed May 1, 2023.
4. Sinha S, Agarwal MM, Vasudeva P, Khattar N, Madduri VKS, Yande S, Sarkar K, Patel A, Vaze A, Raina S, Jain A, Gupta M, Mishra N. The Urological Society of India Guidelines for the Evaluation and Management of Nonneurogenic Urinary Incontinence in Adults (Executive Summary). Indian J Urol. 2019; 35: 185–188.
5. Tunn R, Baessler K, Knüpfer S, Hampel C. Urinary Incontinence and Pelvic Organ Prolapse in Women. DtschArztebl Int. 2023 Feb 3;120(5):71–80. doi: 10.3238/arztebl.m2022.0406. PMID: 36647585; PMCID: PMC10080228.
6. Bump, R.C., *et al.* Long-term efficacy of duloxetine in women with stress urinary incontinence. BJU. Int, 2008. 102: 214. https://www.ncbi.nlm.nih.gov/pubmed/18422764. DOI: 10.1111/j.1464–410X.2008.07577.x.
7. Vella, M., *et al.* Duloxetine 1 year on: the long-term outcome of a cohort of women prescribed duloxetine. Int Urogynecol J Pelvic Floor Dysfunct, 2008. 19: 961. https://www.ncbi.nlm.nih.gov/pubmed/18231697.DOI: 10.1007/s00192-008–0564–4.
8. Rodrigues-Amorim, D., *et al.* A Sytematic Review of Efficacy, Safety and Tolerability of Duloxetine.Front. Psychiatry, 2020. 11. https://doi.org/10.3389/fpsyt.2020.554899. DOI:10.3389/fpsyt.2020.554899.
9. Jiang, Y-H., *et al.* Therapeutic Efficacy of Urethral Sphincter Injections of Platelet-Rich Plasma for Treatment of Stress Urinary Incontinence due to Intrinsic Sphincter Deficiency: A Proof-of-Concept Clinical Trial. Int Neurourol J. 2021. 25(1):51–58. DOI: 10.5213/inj.2040272.136.
10. Gill, B.C., *et al.* Stem Cells for Urinary Incontinence: Functional Differentiation or Cytokine Effects? Urology, 2018. 117: 9–17. doi: 10.1016/j.urology.2018.01.002.
11. Alexander JW, Karjalainen P, Ow LL, *et al.* CO_2 surgical laser for treatment of stress urinary incontinence in women: a randomized controlled trial. Am J Obstet Gynecol. 2022;227(3):473.e1–473.e12. doi:10.1016/j.ajog.2022.05.054.
12. Pecchio S, Novara L, Sgro LG, Rapetti G, Fuso L, Menato G, Biglia N. Concomitant stress urinary incontinence and pelvic organ prolapse surgery: Opportunity or overtreatment? Eur J Obstet Gynecol Reprod Biol. 2020 Jul;250:36–40. doi: 10.1016/j.ejogrb.2020.04.057. Epub 2020 May 1. PMID: 32387890.

Chapter

5

Vault Prolapse with Voiding Dysfunction

• *N Rajamaheswari* • *Harini Sivamani*

LEARNING OBJECTIVES

- Vaginal cuff scar that remains after a hysterectomy is referred to as the vaginal vault. The descent of the vaginal cuff scar (apex of the vagina) through the vaginal introitus is described as post-hysterectomy vaginal vault prolapse (PHVP)[1] or vault prolapse (VP).
- Vaginal vault prolapse is defined as the descent of the vaginal cuff below a point that is 2 cm less than the total vaginal length above the plane of the hymen.[2]
- Failure to reattach the structures that support the upper vagina and uterus to the vault at the time of hysterectomy or weakening of these supports over time results in vault prolapse. The vaginal apex (cuff scar) corresponds to point C on the Pelvic Organ Prolapse Quantification (POP-Q). (Figs 5.1 to 5.3).

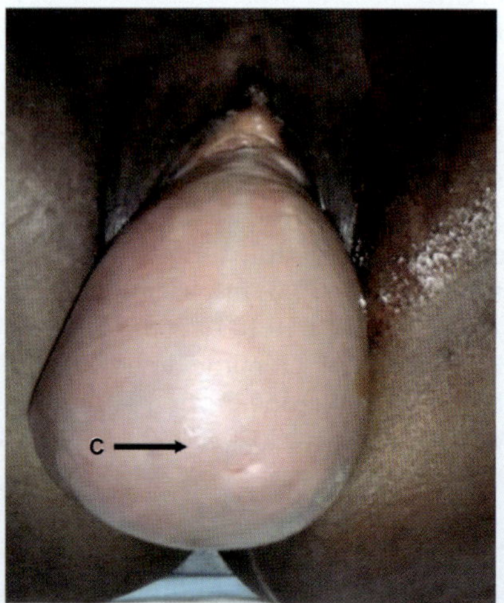

Fig. 5.1: Vault prolapse with C point [arrow indicates point C (vaginal apex or cuff scar)]

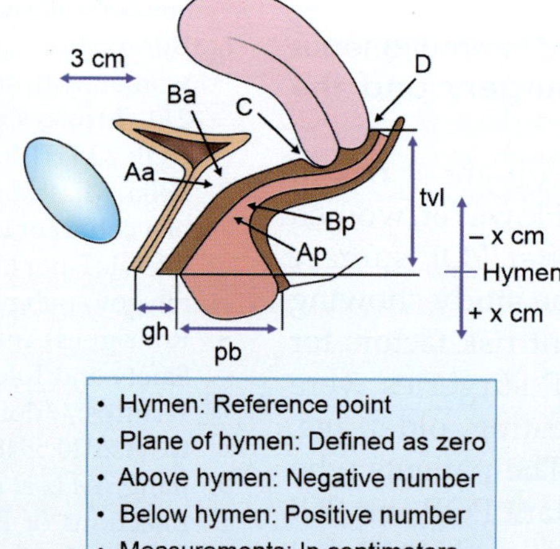

Fig. 5.2: Pelvic organ prolapse quantification (POP-Q)

Anterior wall **Aa**	Anterior wall **Ba**	Cervix or cuff **C**
Genital hiatus **gh**	Perineal body **pb**	Total vaginal length **tvl**
Posterior wall **Ap**	Posterior wall **Bp**	Posterior fornix **D**

Fig. 5.3: Pelvic organ prolapse quantification grid

- Vault prolapse has been reported among 0.2–43% of women[3,4] but the frequency of vault prolapse requiring surgery is only 6% to 8%.[5] Vault prolapse has been reported to follow in 11.6% of hysterectomies performed for uterovaginal prolapse (pelvic organ prolapse) and in 1.8% for other benign diseases.[6]
- Several factors can predispose to a vault prolapse. This includes a history of childbirth trauma, multiparity, delivery of a large baby, forceps delivery, advanced age, post-menopausal status, Asian ethnicity, obesity, previous prolapse surgery, connective tissue disorder, increased intra-abdominal pressure related to chronic cough, or constipation.
- In cases of stage III or IV vault prolapse with enterocele, cystocele, or rectocele, symptoms due to prolapse of the vault, bladder, bowel, and sexual dysfunction are inevitable. Vault prolapse *per se* results in symptoms of the bulge in the vagina, pressure in the pelvis, bleeding, discharge, and low backache.
- Associated cystocele and rectocele with its anatomical distortion results in hesitancy, poor stream, straining to void/defecate, incomplete emptying of bladder/bowel, splinting/digitation to complete micturition or defecation.
- Detailed history and systematic clinical examination including pelvic examination, basic neurological evaluation, assessment for urinary incontinence, bladder outlet obstruction, and fecal incontinence are necessary.

- Pessary offers temporary symptomatic relief.[7] Appropriate for elderly, frail, bedridden women who are unfit for reconstructive surgeries. Surgical repair and reconstruction only can provide a definitive remedy. The aim of surgical repair and reconstruction is to relieve prolapse symptoms and restore vaginal, bladder, and bowel function. Reconstruction should restore normal vaginal axis and length.
- Defect in level I support (uterosacral and cardinal ligament complex) results in the descent of the vault with or without enterocele. Mostly VP will be accompanied by level II anterior and posterior defects resulting in cystocele and rectocele. Associated level III anterior defect leads to SUI and posterior defect results in a deficient perineal body and enlarged hiatus (Figs 5.4 and 5.5).

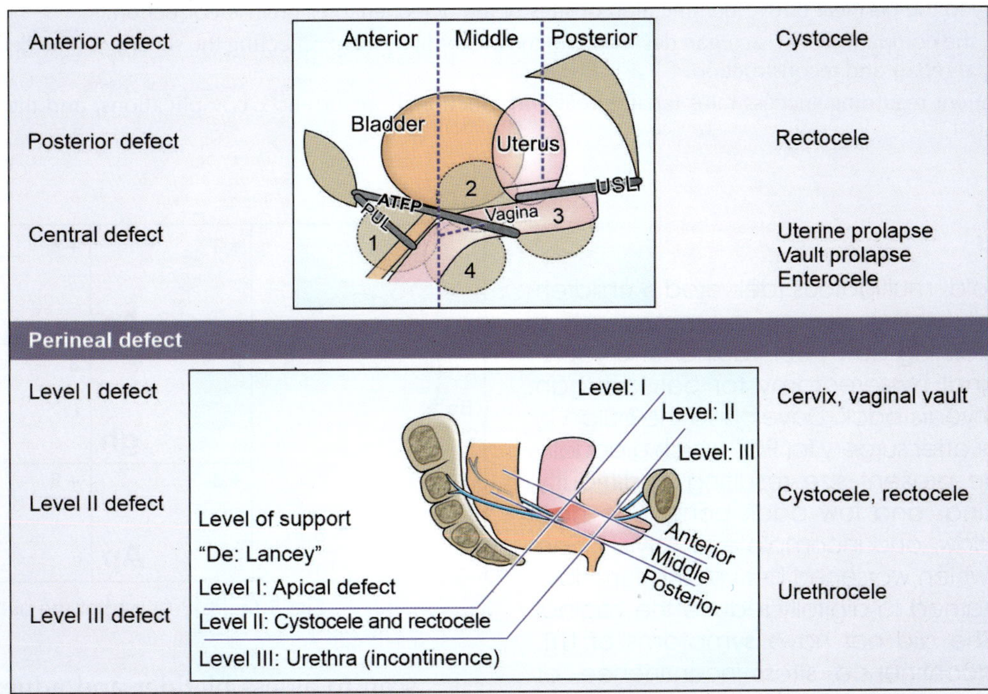

Fig. 5.4: Classification of POP

Stage 0	No prolapse
Stage I	Inside vagina
Stage II	Up to hymenal ring
Stage III	Beyond hymenal ring
Stage IV	Complete eversion

Hymenal remnants
Stage 0
Stage I
Stage II
Stage III
Stage IV

Fig. 5.5: Stages of POP

The effect of compression of the baby's head (circles) during the process of vaginal delivery resulting in damage to the pelvic floor at different levels is shown:
1. Stress incontinence, 2. Cystocoele (Anterior vaginal wall descent), 3. Uterine/apical prolapse, 4. Rectocoele (posterior vaginal wall descent).
ATFP- Arcus Tendinous Fascia Pelvis, USL- Uterosacral Ligament.
Picture Courtesy: Petros P. The integral system. Cent European J Urol. 2011;64(3):110-9.

- **Level I defect demands suspension of the vault to one of the following structures:**
  a. Anterior longitudinal ligament of sacrum S1 or S2 (Sacrocolpopexy: SCP)
  b. Uterosacral ligament (High uterosacral ligament Suspension: HUSLS)
  c. Sacrospinous ligament (Sacrospinous ligament suspension: SSLS)
  d. Ileococcygeous fascia (Ileococcygeous pexy)

- **Level II anterior defect correction involves:**
  a. Reattaching the pubocervical fascia (PCF) to the vault restores the transverse attachment of the trapezoid configuration of PCF.
  b. Midline plication of PCF corrects the central defect.
  c. Reattaching PCF to the white line corrects paravaginal defect and is effectively accomplished by robotic or laparoscopic techniques.
- Level II posterior defect requires reattaching the rectovaginal fascia (RVF) laterally to the iliococcygeal fascia, proximally to the vault, and distally to the perineal body. Identification of sites of the defect enables precise correction.
- The defect level, the compartment-wise organ descent, and the extent of descent reflecting the severity of the defect will determine the type of surgical repair and reconstruction.
- Informing the patient regarding success rates (anatomical and functional), recurrence, complications, and the impact on sexual function is essential.

Case Scenario

Mrs. X, 50 years old, multiparous (delivered 6 children vaginally), sexually active woman, presented with a history of mass coming down per vagina for 3 years. Underwent vaginal hysterectomy for pelvic organ prolapse (POP) 4 years back. Developed the bulge in her vagina 1 year after surgery for POP which gradually increased to the present size resulting in difficulty in voiding, walking, and low back ache. She had hesitancy, poor flow, and incomplete emptying. She strained to void which worsened her voiding function. Over time she learned to digitally reduce the vaginal mass to void. She did not have symptoms of UTI, urgency, urge incontinence, stress incontinence, or increased frequency. She had constipation and used to strain to defecate. She refrained from sexual intercourse because of the vaginal mass.

Examination revealed a well-built woman with a BMI of 29 kg/m^2, general and other systemic examinations were normal.

Pelvic examination revealed, a huge reducible mass protruding through the vagina. The vaginal mucosa was pink and smooth without any ulceration or discharge. The mass appeared to be dumbbell-shaped suggesting the descent of the bladder (cystocele) and intestines (enterocele). There was complete eventration of the vaginal vault. A cough stress test (CST) with the mass reduced revealed SUI (occult). No associated urethral or rectal prolapse was seen. The anal tone was normal. POP-Q staging of the multilevel vault prolapse was done.

Video 14, (Fig. 5.6). https://youtu.be/n2bTkXJ-9gk

1. **How will you evaluate the case further?**

   Ans: Urine analysis, blood biochemistry, renal function tests, ultrasound imaging of the KUB area to assess the upper urinary tract, and pelvic scan to assess bladder and adnexa. Haematuria, urolithiasis, or abnormal ultrasound KUB results require CT imaging. Transperineal ultrasound or MR imaging is beneficial in the early stages of VP and valuable in confirming levator muscle trauma, and avulsions.

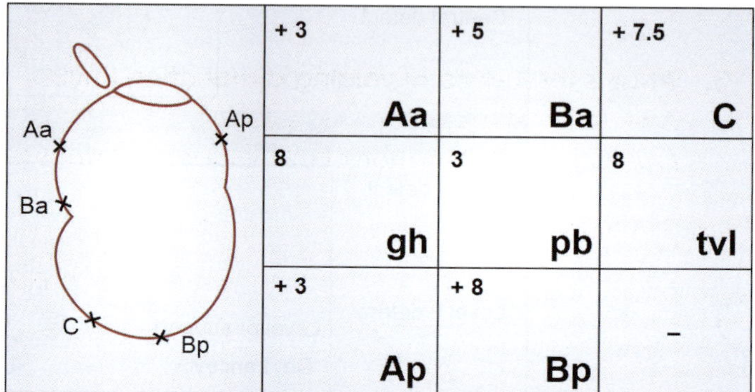

Fig. 5.6: POP-Q grid of the patient

   Uroflowmetry: Voided 180 ml, maximum flow rate 8 ml/sec (poor flow), voiding time 80 sec (prolonged) with intermittent flow pattern (straining), and postvoid residual urine (PVR) of 110 ml.

2. **What is the role of urodynamic evaluation in cases of VP?**

   Ans: Green top guidelines do not recommend routine pre-operative urodynamic assessment for women with VP.[8]

   However, the presence of LUTS (filling and voiding) especially frequency, urgency, urinary incontinence (stress incontinence overt or occult, urge incontinence) along with significant PVR demand full urodynamic workup.

   Cystometry and pressure flow study should be done after reducing the prolapse with a pessary or a vaginal plug.

   Cystometry identifies the reason for urinary incontinence and differentiates SUI from detrusor overactivity. The plan for concomitant surgical correction of SUI demands pre-operative confirmation of urodynamic SUI. A pressure flow study confirms the cause of voiding dysfunction and differentiates bladder outlet obstruction from detrusor underactivity.

In this patient, cystometry did not reveal detrusor overactivity.

Cough stress test (CST) during cystometry confirmed urodynamic SUI with 350 ml. Does this make sense?

Pressure flow revealed uninterrupted flow with a maximum flow of 14 ml/sec, voiding detrusor pressure of 40 cm of water, and PVR of 60 ml. The pressure flow study had ruled out detrusor underactivity and abdominal leak point pressure (ALPP) was 90 cm of water.

3. **What is the cause of voiding dysfunction in VP?**

Ans: It may be due to:

a. Anatomical distortion of the bladder and urethra associated with or without bladder outlet obstruction (BOO)
b. Detrusor underactivity

Stage IV vault prolapse with cystocele causes significant anatomical distortion of the bladder and urethra resulting in voiding dysfunction. Reducing the mass with a pessary will improve her flow indicating that the surgical repair will correct anatomical distortion of the bladder outlet and urethra and relieve her voiding dysfunction.

4. **Is there a need for a video urodynamic study for this patient?**

Ans: No. All relevant information is available with a basic urodynamic study (uroflowmetry, cystometry, and pressure flow study).

5. **Is pre-operative cystoscopy essential for a patient with VP?**

Ans: The presence of LUTS (filling and voiding), recurrent UTI, haematuria, and suspected stone in the lower urinary tract requires cystoscopy.

Combining cystoscopy and examination on the table (EOT) under local anesthesia is advantageous.

Patulous external meatus, failure of closure of bladder neck during cystoscopy, and nonmobile urethra suggest SUI due to intrinsic sphincter deficiency (ISD).

EOT permits assessment of the vaginal mobility, length, perineal body, the strength of pelvic floor muscles, perineal deficiency, and prominence of ischial spines which will be beneficial in planning the surgical repair.

6. **What is the comprehensive clinical diagnosis of this patient?**

Ans: It is a multilevel VP involving all three levels (I, II and III). Level I stage IV—vault prolapse with enterocele, Level II—cystocele and rectocele, and Level III SUI [urethral hypermobility (HM)].

7. **Is there a role for pessary in this patient?**

Ans: Pessary will be beneficial only as a diagnostic tool in this patient and not as a therapeutic option. Pessary usage in stage III/IV vault prolapse offers only temporary symptomatic relief[7] with a high spontaneous expulsion rate. However, stage IV vault prolapse in this medically fit patient with significant voiding dysfunction demands surgical repair and reconstruction.

8. **What are the surgical options for this patient?**

Ans:

Abdominal procedures

- Abdominal sacrocolpopexy (ASCP)
- Laparoscopic or robotic sacrocolpopexy
- Along with Halban or Moschowitz procedure (corrects enterocele) and Burch colposuspension (corrects SUI).

Vaginal procedures

- High uterosacral ligament suspension: HUSLS
- Sacrospinous ligament suspension: SSLS
- Along with cystocele, rectocele repair, and a mid-urethral sling to correct SUI.

9. **What is the ideal vault suspension surgical technique for this patient?**

Ans: Sacrocolpopexy (SCP).

SCP corrects Level I and Level II anterior and posterior defects using monofilament, macroporous, polypropylene "Y"-shaped mesh (Fig. 5.7).

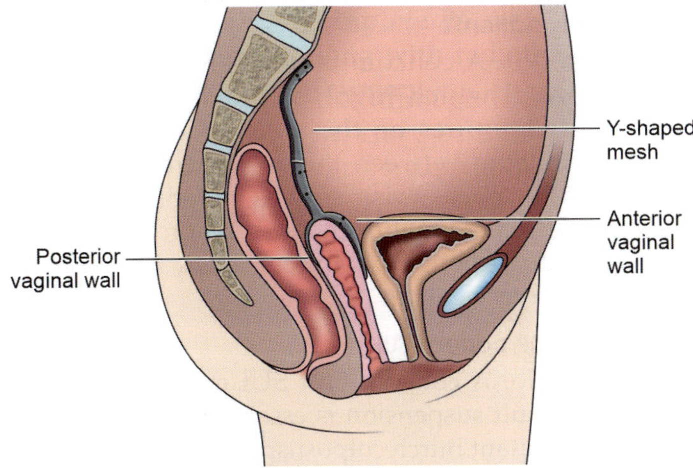

Fig. 5.7: Sacrocolpopexy

10. **What are the essential surgical steps of SCP?**

Ans: SCP involves the suspension of the vault to the anterior longitudinal ligament of the sacrum (S1 or S2) with a permanent Y-shaped mesh (macroporous, monofilament, polypropylene). The junction of the inverted Y-shaped mesh is attached to the vault to correct the level I defect. Fixing the remaining two mesh arms to the anterior and posterior vaginal walls respectively corrects the level II anterior and posterior defect. Injuries to the intestines, bladder, and vagina are likely.

Posterior peritoneum over sacral promontory incised (safeguarding right ureter and iliac vessels) and anterior longitudinal ligament over S1 and S2 vertebra exposed.

The vertical part of Y mesh was brought to the presacral area through a tunnel created under the posterior peritoneum and the mesh is fixed to the anterior longitudinal ligament over S1 or S2 without tension. After fixing the mesh, the vault, and presacral area peritonealised.

11. **Why SCP is considered as the gold standard surgical correction for stage III or IV vault prolapse?**

Ans: SCP has a high success rate,[9] restores normal vaginal axis, and effectively corrects level I, level II anterior (cystocele), and posterior (rectocele) defects. All three techniques (abdominal, laparoscopic, and robotic) accomplish a similar success rate.

12. **What are the demerits of SCP?**

Ans: Abdominal SCP needs laparotomy.

Laparoscopic and robotic SCP requires special equipment and expertise.

Postoperative mesh exposure, mesh extrusion, infection, and lumbosacral discitis can occur irrespective of the technique of SCP.

13. **Is it possible to correct the enterocele by SCP alone in this patient?**

Ans: No. A concomitant enterocele repair is essential which involves placing successive sagittal sutures on the anterior and posterior peritoneum between the uterosacral ligaments (USL) or purse string sutures including anterior, posterior peritoneum and USL. Approximation of the sutures obliterates the cul-de-sac and corrects the enterocele.

14. **Can SCP correct SUI?**

Ans: No. A concomitant SUI correction along with vault suspension is essential. In this case, a concomitant Burch colposuspension is justified as she has urethral hypermobility. The presence of ISD requires a pubovaginal sling.

15. **What are the vaginal vault suspension procedures available for this patient?**

Ans: High uterosacral ligament suspension or sacrospinous ligament suspension can be considered which corrects level I defect. However, level II anterior, posterior defect, and level III anterior defect (SUI) repair should be combined with vault suspension.

Though vaginal procedures have many advantages, the chances of recurrence are higher with vaginal techniques compared to abdominal suspension procedures (SCP).

16. **What is the surgical principle of vaginal high uterosacral ligament suspension?**

Ans: Vaginally, the vault is suspended to the intermediate part of the uterosacral ligament on either side by the intraperitoneal approach. If adhesions prevent entry into the peritoneal cavity, an extraperitoneal approach can be used.

17. **Should cystocele, and rectocele repair be combined with HUSLS?**

Ans: Yes.

The two pairs of suspension sutures placed cephalad on the USL are passed through PCF anteriorly and RVF posteriorly. Distal suspension suture on the USL is passed anteriorly through the PCF and anterior vaginal wall. The same suture is passed posteriorly through RVF and the posterior vaginal wall. Approximation of these sutures accomplishes anchoring the vaginal vault to the USL along with PCF and RVF. Though PCF and RVF are attached to the vault by this step, midline plication of PCF is also combined, and finally, approximation of superficial perineal muscles is carried out as part of pelvic floor repair.

18. **Why HUSLS is preferred over other vaginal suspension procedures in this patient?**

Ans:

- Restores normal vaginal axis and length
- Permits concomitant cystocele, rectocele repair, and mid-urethral sling
- Usage of autologous USL avoids mesh-related complications
- 80–98% success rate.[10,11]

Identifying the USL to place the suspension sutures precisely and avoiding ureters that run lateral to the USL is crucial. Pre-operative cystoscopy to confirm ureteral patency is essential.

19. **Can SSLS, cystocele, rectocele repair, and mid-urethral sling be considered?**

Ans: Yes, it can be considered. However, it distorts the vaginal axis and is associated with recurrence[12] as high as 37% particularly in the anterior compartment. SSLS corrects advanced stages (III/IV) of VP but corrects only level I defect. Hence level II and III defects correction should be combined with SSLS. Vault is suspended to autologous sacrospinous ligament, hence mesh-related complications are avoided. Mostly unilateral suspension is sufficient.

Possible complications are hemorrhage, rectal injury, pudendal nerve/sciatic nerve injury, and gluteal pain.

OPTIMAL TRIAL[13] compared HUSLS vs SSLS (concomitant mid-urethral sling) for PHVP with SUI and reported similar anatomical, functional, and adverse event outcomes with both procedures.

20. Can obliterative surgeries like colpocleisis be considered for this patient?

Ans: No. It is reserved only for women who are sexually inactive and unfit for long reconstructive surgeries.

21. How to prevent recurrent vault prolapse?

- Selection of appropriate suspension technique and approach.
- Addressing coexisting enterocele, cystocele, and rectocele.
- Correcting defects at all levels without creating a new defect following the correction.
- The presence of level II and III posterior defects requires fixing the distal edge of the posterior arm of the inverted Y mesh to the perineal body during SCP to address the deficiency in RVF and perineum.
- Vaginal correction of large levator hiatal defects will be beneficial in minimizing the recurrence further.

Preventing recurrent vault prolapse is crucial as surgical repair of recurrent vault descent could be challenging.

SUMMARY

- Symptomatic and advanced stages of vault prolapse demand vault suspension as surgical correction.
- SCP offers superior outcomes and is the procedure of choice for young, healthy patients having stage III /IV vault prolapse
- SCP corrects level I and II anterior (cystocele) and posterior (rectocele) defects. Co-existing enterocele, and SUI warrant concomitant repair.
- Correction of defects in all 3 levels is essential.
- HUSLS is superior to other vaginal suspension procedures.
- All vaginal suspension procedures require a concomitant repair of cystocele, rectocele and SUI.

REFERENCES

1. Haylen BT, de Ridder D, Freeman RM, Swift SE, Berghmans B, Lee J, *et al*. An International Urogynecological Association (IUGA)/International Continence Society (ICS) joint report on the terminology for female pelvic floor dysfunction. Int Urogynecol J. 2010 Jan;21(1):5–26. doi 10.1007/s00192–009–0976–9. Epub 2009 Nov 25. PMID: 19937315.
2. Abrams P, Cardozo L, Fall M, Griffiths D, Rosier P, Ulmsten U, *et al.*; Standardisation Sub-Committee of the International Continence Society. The standardization of terminology in lower urinary tract function: report from the standardization sub-committee of the International Continence Society. Urology. 2003 Jan;61(1):37–49. doi: 10.1016/s0090–4295(02)02243–4. PMID: 12559262.
3. Symmonds RE, Pratt JH. Vaginal prolapse following hysterectomy. Am J Obstet Gynecol. 1960 May;79:899–909. doi: 10.1016/0002–9378(60)90684–0. PMID: 13836216.
4. Barrington JW, Edwards G. Posthysterectomy vault prolapse. Int Urogynecol J Pelvic Floor Dysfunct. 2000;11(4):241–5. doi 10.1007/s001920070033. PMID: 11005477.
5. Aigmueller T, Dungl A, Hinterholzer S, Geiss I, Riss P. An estimation of the frequency of surgery for post-hysterectomy vault prolapse. Int Urogynecol J. 2010 Mar;21(3):299–302. doi 10.1007/s00192–009–1033–4. PMID: 19936593.
6. Marchionni M, Bracco GL, Checcucci V, Carabaneanu A, Coccia EM, Mecacci F, Scarselli G. True incidence of vaginal vault prolapse. Thirteen years of experience. J Reprod Med. 1999 Aug;44(8):679–84. PMID: 10483537.
7. National Institute for Health and Clinical Excellence. Infracoccygeal sacropexy using mesh for vaginal vault prolapse repair. NICE interventional procedure guidance 281. Manchester: NICE; 2009.
8. Green-top Guideline No. 46. Post-Hysterectomy Vaginal Vault Prolapse. RCOG/BSUG Joint Guideline I July 2015.
9. Rondini C, Braun H, Alvarez J, Urzúa MJ, Villegas R, Wenzel C, Descouvieres C. High uterosacral vault suspension vs Sacrocolpopexy for treating apical defects: a randomized controlled trial with twelve months follow-up. Int Urogynecol J. 2015 Aug;26(8):1131–8. doi 10.1007/s00192–015–2666–0. Epub 2015 Apr 25. PMID: 25910610.
10. Shull BL, Bachofen C, Coates KW, Kuehl TJ. A transvaginal approach to repair of apical and other associated sites of pelvic organ prolapse with uterosacral ligaments. Am J Obstet Gynecol. 2000 Dec;183(6):1365–73; discussion 1373–4. doi 10.1067/mob.2000.110910. PMID: 11120498.
11. Margulies RU, Rogers MA, Morgan DM. Outcomes of transvaginal uterosacral ligament suspension: systematic review and meta-analysis. Am J Obstet Gynecol. 2010 Feb;202(2):124–34. doi: 10.1016/j.ajog.2009.07.052. PMID: 20113690.
12. Paraiso MF, Ballard LA, Walters MD, Lee JC, Mitchinson AR. Pelvic support defects and visceral and sexual function in women treated with sacrospinous ligament suspension and pelvic reconstruction. Am J Obstet Gynecol. 1996 Dec;175(6):1423–30; discussion 1430–1. doi: 10.1016/s0002–9378(96)70085–6. PMID: 8987920.
13. Barber MD, Brubaker L, Burgio KL, Richter HE, Nygaard I, Weidner AC, *et al*; Eunice Kennedy Shriver National Institute of Child Health and Human Development Pelvic Floor Disorders Network. Comparison of 2 transvaginal surgical approaches and perioperative behavioral therapy for apical vaginal prolapse: the OPTIMAL randomized trial. JAMA. 2014 Mar 12;311(10):1023–34. doi: 10.1001/jama.2014.1719. Erratum in: JAMA. 2015 Jun 9;313(22):2287. PMID: 24618964; PMCID: PMC4083455.

Chapter

6

Nocturia

• Arabind Panda • Ahsan Ahmad

LEARNING OBJECTIVES

- Nocturia is defined as waking up to void during the main sleep period. It should be preceded and followed by sleep or the intent to sleep.[1]
- It is highly prevalent and causes significant reduction in the quality of life. It has been liked to early mortality due to the reduction in the quality and duration of sleep.[2]
- The pathophysiology is varied, it is symptom complex and not a disease *per se*.
- It is important to consider underlying conditions including hypertension, diabetes mellitus, cardiac disease, obstructive sleep apnea, dependent edema during its evaluation.[3]
- A through history, clinical examination and accurate bladder diary are essential components of the evaluation.
- Quality of life questionnaires should be used in the evaluation and follow-up of nocturia whenever possible.
- The causes of nocturia are varied. They include among others:
  a. Reduced nocturnal bladder capacity.
  b. Global polyuria
  c. Nocturnal polyuria
- Management strategies must be tailored according to the etiology.
- It may include behavioral modification, to pharmacological agents, and occasionally surgery.
- Its multifactorial etiology means that a single treatment modality will not give optimal results.

Case Scenario 1

A 64-year-old man presents to you with predominantly storage lower urinary tract symptoms (LUTS). He complains of frequency, occasional urgency and need to get up 3–4 times to pass urine at night. He has no significant voiding LUTS. He has had type 2 diabetes mellitus for the past 3 years, with poor control. The physical examination was essentially unremarkable. Digital rectal examination reveals a normal anal tone with a 20 ml benign prostate. The glycosylated haemoglobin is 8.5%. The renal function parameters and urine microscopic is normal. The uroflowmetry shows a Q_{max} of 14 ml/sec with a postvoid residue of 40 ml for a voided volume of 200 ml. He is specially bothered that he has to get up frequently at night. He drinks approximately around 2 and ½ liters of fluids daily. His bowel habits are normal. The ultrasound KUB shows normal sized kidneys, no hydronephrosis. The bladder wall is normal with a postvoid residual urine of 40 ml. The prostate size is 22 ml without a significant median lobe. He has no history of haematuria. He has occasional constipation, but generally has normal bowel habits.

1. **How will you evaluate this patient?**

   Ans: It is imperative to have objective criteria to evaluate and document the storage LUTs (frequency, urgency and nocturia). This also helps in the objective assessment of the response to treatment. The international Prostate Symptom Score (IPSS) is a validated, patient reported questionnaire (that may also be administered by the care giver). More specific patient reported measures will be the nocturia score and the bladder dairy.

   It is essential to request a bladder diary for all patients. It objectively reflects the intake and the output of the patient (Table 6.1).

The maximum voided volume (MVV) is a rough estimate of the bladder capacity at that point in time. Primary polydipsia and nocturnal polyuria will also be identified by the bladder diary. The cause of nocturia is usually directed by the bladder diary (Table 6.1).

TABLE 6.1: Causes of nocturia—bladder diary suggested diagnosis

Nocturnal polyuria	Pedal edema Obstructive sleep apnea syndrome Glycosuria Cardiac dysfunction Behavioral (too much intake in the evening) Hypertension
Low bladder capacity (nocturnal or global)	Urinary tuberculosis or other causes of small capacity bladder Bladder outlet obstruction Lower urinary tract cancer Neurogenic bladder with detrusor overactivity Nocturnal detrusor overactivity
Pseudo-frequency	Highpost void residual urine
Global polyuria	Diabetes mellitus Primary polydipsia Diabetes insipidus

2. **How should you proceed after this?**

   Ans: The patient has type 2 diabetes mellitus which is likely uncontrolled. Fasting and postprandial blood sugar will allow optimum management of the blood sugars. The osmotic diuresis that accompanies the glucosuria aggravates the nocturia and may occasionally be its cause. Treatment of the deranged sugar itself can significantly improve the nocturia.

3. **What is the pattern that is likely to be seen in this patient in the bladder diary?**

   Ans: He likely to have global polyuria. It is defined as a 24-h urine output > 40 ml/kg.[3]

4. **After treating the DM-2, his nocturia improved to 2 times/ night. What is the advice you will give him now? The bladder diary shows a MVV of 300 ml.**

   Ans: Modification of fluid intake with reduction of fluids to *as needed basis* and generally less than 2 litres/day. Excess water intake after 6 pm is to be discouraged.

   An alpha-1 receptor antagonist can be started, preferably Silodosin or Tamsulosin. These drugs have a documented effect in the treatment of LUTS, including nocturia.[4] When symptoms are secondary to bladder outlet obstruction, both alpha blockers and transurethral resection of the prostate (TURP) have been shown to decrease nocturia episodes in 17.9% and 32.2% of patients, respectively.[4]

   The mechanism may have to do with the reduction in outlet resistance or its effect on the central nervous system relevant for micturition control. There is no role of combination therapy with the prostate size of less than 25 ml.

5. **Is there any role of antimuscarinic or beta-3 agonist drugs for nocturia?**

   Ans: Both classes of drugs have a role in overactive bladder related nocturia. They do not reduce the number of nocturnal voids but reduce the associated urgency. There is no convincing role in patients who do not have bladder overactivity or have nocturnal polyuria.

Case Scenario 2

Mrs. P, 65-year-old female, hypertensive, well-controlled with Amlodepine 5 mg once a day, presents with increased frequency of urine at night. She voids only 3–4 times during the day and 4 times at night. She has no urgency during the day, there is urgency at night. On examination, she has atrophic vaginitis. The rest of the physical examination is unremarkable except for significant pedal edema.

The blood investigations and urine microscopic examination is normal. She drinks approximately around 2 liters of fluids daily. Her bowel habits are normal. The ultrasound KUB shows normal sized kidneys with no hydronephrosis. The bladder wall thickness is normal with a postvoid residual urine of 10 ml. The uroflowmetery-Q_{max} of 22 ml/sec, for a voided volume of 250 ml.

1. **What will be the next step in your evaluation?**

   Ans:

   1. She needs a bladder diary to document the intake, the output, frequency, maximal voided volume and any urge leaks.
   2. The bladder diary shows an intake of 2200 ml and a total output of 1800 ml of which 900 ml is between 10 pm and 6 am.

2. **How will you distinguish pure nocturnal frequency from nocturnal polyuria?**

   Ans: Nocturnal polyuria (NP) is defined as increased urine production rate only at night, with a normal 24-hr urine output.[4]

   It is said to be present when the nocturnal urine volume exceeds 20% of 24-h urine volume in younger patients, or 33% of 24-h urine volume in people aged over 65 years. An alternative definition of nocturnal polyuria is a nocturnal urine production greater than 90 ml/hour in the night.[4]

The causes of nocturnal polyuria are varied. It ranges from blunting in production of arginine vasopressin (AVP), excess production of atrial natriuretic peptide (ANP), peripheral edema (which gets mobilized into the blood stream when supine at night), increased nighttime fluid intake, and as an adverse effect of certain medications such as diuretics. Since the causes of NP are varied and often overlapping, the treatment needs to be multifactorial and depends on the etiology.[3]

3. **How will you treat nocturnal polyuria?**

Ans: The causes are varied, the treatment will depend on the cause. The treatment will generally be multifactorial. Behavioral modifications include evening fluid restriction, compression stockings for patients with peripheral edema, optimizing sleep hygiene.

Adjustment of hypertension medications, including adding a mild diuretic, e.g. hydrochlorothiazide 12.5 mg once daily in the mid-afternoon, and elimination of medications that can potentially contribute to nocturnal polyuria,[5] e.g. calcium channel blockers causing pedal edema. Comorbid conditions including peripheral edema, obstructive sleep apnea (OSA), diabetes mellitus, congestive heart failure, and hypertension are important causes of nocturnal polyuria.[6]

Nocturnal polyuria secondary to OSA can be caused by increases in atrial natriuretic peptide due to increased right atrial pressures, which in turn results in increased sodium and water excretion. A significant decrease in the number of night urination episodes has been attributable to treatment of OSA with continuous positive airway pressure (CPAP).[4]

Hypertension (HTN) has also been linked to nocturnal polyuria. A recent cross-sectional study conducted amongst black men aged 35–49 years old found uncontrolled hypertension to be an independent determinant of nocturia. Blunting of nocturnal blood pressure dipping amongst hypertensives often results in "pressure natriuresis" with increased urine output during hours of sleep; this is known as nondipping hypertension.[4]

4. **What are the pharmacological interventions that are possible?**

Ans: Desmopressin is the drug of choice when NP is likely due to nocturnal production of ANP. Desmopressin is a synthetic analogue of antidiuretic hormone (ADH) and it binds to V2 receptors in the renal collecting duct and stimulates water reabsorption. Close monitoring of serum sodium levels after initiation of desmopressin therapy is recommended. Administration of 50 µg of desmopressin melt for males and 25 µg for females will significantly reduce the number of nightly voids. Women are more sensitive to the effect of desmopressin compared to men as the gene for the vasopressin V2 receptor is located on the X chromosome. The major adverse effect is hyponatremia which occurs in a small but significant number of patients.[5]

Case Scenario 3

A 32 years old male patient presented with increased frequency of micturition both during day and night and urgency for the last two years. Initially he used to void 8–10 times during daytime and 3–4 times during night which gradually progressed to 15–20 times during daytime and 8–10 times during night. He had no history of any obstructive lower urinary tract symptoms and hematuria. He had no significant past medical or surgical history. On clinical examination, pallor was present. Rest examination findings were unremarkable. His frequency volume chart revealed average voided urinary volume in the range of 50–100 ml. His uroflowmetery showed low voided volume. His urine examination suggested sterile pyuria. His Hb was 6.8 g/dl and serum creatinine was 3.5 mg/dl. His USG abdomen was suggestive of right-sided atrophic kidney along with left-sided hydroureteronephrosis. The MCU showed a small bladder with secondary reflux. DMSA scan showed a non-functioning right kidney.

The urine smear was positive for acid-fast bacilli. The GeneXpert was positive for *Mycobacteria tuberculosis* without rifampicin resistance. A left DJ stent was placed and he was started on anti-tubercular therapy (Fig. 6.1).

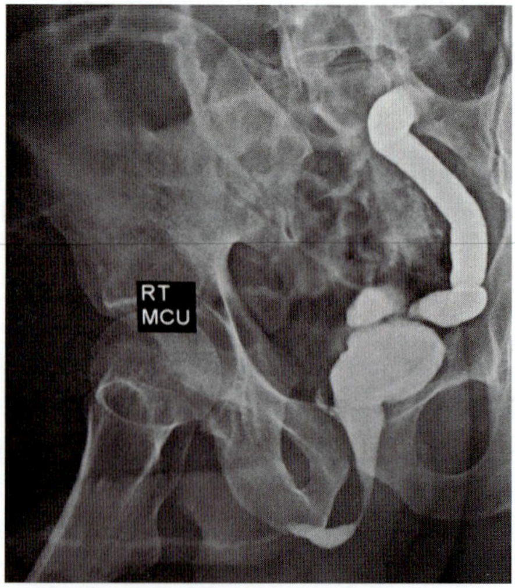

Fig. 6.1: MCU suggestive of small capacity bladder and left-sided reflux

1. **What is the difference between true nocturia and the nocturia in this patient?**

   Ans: The frequency and nocturia in this patient is due to the global reduction in bladder capacity due to the tubercular cystitis. It must be differentiated from the nocturia that occurs due to the over production of urine. The treatment of the early tubercular cystitis can in many cases result in improvement of the bladder capacity.

   Follow-up to detect fibrosis and subsequent obstruction of the ureters is important.

2. **What is the plan for management?**

   Ans: The management of the primary condition is primary. After diagnosis, double J stenting on the left side with antitubercular therapy (ATT) should be started. The nocturia can worsen with subsequent contraction of the bladder secondary to antitubercular therapy. Depending on the final state of the urinary tract and the creatinine, further reconstruction can be planned after treatment with ATT.

SUMMARY

- Nocturia is usually multifactorial.
- It is imperative to evaluate carefully to detect most or all the factors that are responsible.
- The bladder diary plays a critical role in diagnosis and management.
- There is no standard treatment. Management must be tailored to the individual patient.
- Fluid restriction, pharmacotherapy, specific treatment for certain conditions and occasionally reconstructive surgery may be required.

REFERENCES

1. ICS [Internet]. [cited 2023 Jul 21]. Nocturia. Available from: https://www.ics.org/committees/standardisation/terminologydiscussions/nocturia.
2. C. Madhu, Coyne K, Hashim H, Chapple C, Milsom I, Kopp Z. Nocturia: risk factors and associated comorbidities; findings from the EpiLUTS study. Int J Clin Pract. 2015 Dec;69(12):1508–16.
3. Gordon DJ, Emeruwa CJ, Weiss JP. Management Strategies for Nocturia. Curr Urol Rep. 2019 Nov 9;20(11):75.
4. Weiss JP, Wein AJ, van Kerrebroeck P, Dmochowski R, Fitzgerald M, Tikkinen KAO, et al. Nocturia: new directions. Neurourol Urodyn. 2011 Jun;30(5):700–3.
5. Andersson KE, Van Kerrebroeck P. Pharmacotherapy for Nocturia. Curr Urol Rep. 2018 Feb 9;19(1):8.
6. Lombardo R, Tubaro A, Burkhard F. Nocturia: The Complex Role of the Heart, Kidneys, and Bladder. Eur Urol Focus. 2020 May 15;6(3):534–6.

Chapter

7

Neurogenic LUTS in a Girl with Anorectal Malformation

• *Ashwin Shekar P*

LEARNING OBJECTIVES

- Neurogenic bladder occurs in many patients who are born with anorectal malformations (ARM).
- Bladder dysfunction causes significant urological morbidity in the pediatric population, resulting in renal damage from recurrent urinary tract infections and urinary incontinence, both of which can cause profound morbidity and disability.[1,2]
- Recurrent urinary tract infection may be overlooked or attributed to coexisting vesicoureteric reflux or renal anomalies, which are prevalent in a high proportion of these children.
- Consequently, detecting bladder dysfunction at an early age is essential in avoiding deterioration in renal function.
- The role of the urologist is to ensure that renal and bladder functions are appropriately investigated and managed during childhood.[3]
- Having a urologist's involvement in the collaborative center caring for these patients affords focused attention on bladder and kidney management in the effort to minimize potential long-term problems.
- It is critical to have urologic involvement in the care of patients with ARM, especially those with bladder involvement, as onset of chronic kidney disease can significantly decrease their life expectancy, with end stage renal disease rates reported as high as 6.4% in complex ARM subtypes.[3]

Case Scenario

A 4-year-old female presented with continuous incontinence of urine since birth for which she was on diapers. She had been evaluated for ambiguous genitalia outside for an enlarged clitoris and her karyotype was 46 XX with normal serum hormones. She was born out of a non-consanguineous marriage and had achieved normal milestones. She gave no history of constipation. On examination, she had continuous urine leakage from a single opening in the perineum which was close to the anal opening along with an enlarged clitoris (Fig. 7.1). There was no palpable mass in abdomen.

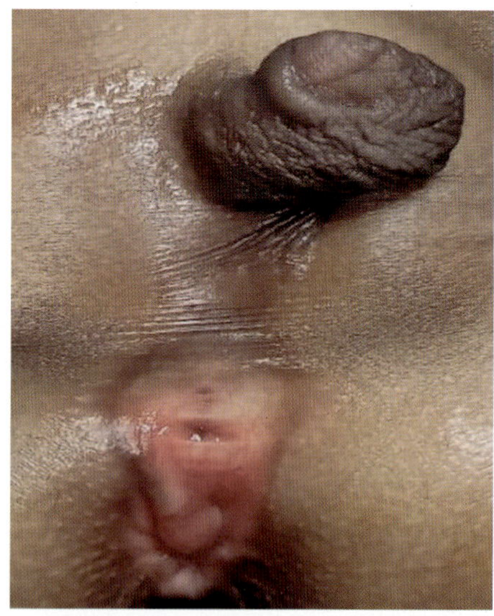

Fig. 7.1: Clinical picture showing single urogenital opening placed posteriorly close to rectum suggestive of posterior cloaca

1. What are the salient points in past history with regards to genitourinary system that have to be asked in a child with anorectal malformation (ARM)?

Ans: Some of the important points in history that have to be elicited in history in these children are

- History of present urinary complaints like incontinence, recurrent UTI, recurrent epididymo-orchitis in boys.
- History of constipation /encopresis
- History of any neurological deficit in lower limbs due to spinal pathology
- History of any previous intervention to the urinary tract like a vesicostomy

- If the child is on clean intermittent catheterisation (CIC), check CIC diary to see for compliance and CIC volumes
- Details of their previous intervention for anorectal malformation including type of surgery, age of intervention, previous urinary symptoms before and after surgery for ARM, any worsening of symptoms since surgery.

2. What are the important physical findings that have be noted in a child with ARM with respect to genitourinary system?

Ans: Examination of such children should include

- Examination of abdomen for any palpable mass or presence of vesicostomy or colostomy
- Examination of external genitalia for associated anomalies
- Perineal examination to check for scars of previous surgery
- Focused neurological examination including anal tone, perianal sensation
- Examination of back to see for scars for previous surgery, spinal anomalies

3. What are the chances of bladder bowel dysfunction in children with ARM?

Ans: Bowel dysfunction is seen in most children with ARMs and is strongly related to associated anomalies commonly found in these patients. Negative predictors for improvement in bowel function during growing up are spinal cord malformation, neurogenic bladder dysfunction and complex type of fistula malformation.[4]

4. What is the etiology of lower urinary tract dysfunction in ARM and cloacal anomalies?

Ans: There are two common ways in which children with ARM can have bladder involvement. First, it can be iatrogenic due to injury to the innervation of the bladder during surgery.[5] Another reason is the presence of associated spinal cord abnormalities like hemivertebra, sacral agenesis, tethered cord and myelomeningocele which has been reported to occur in 26% to 60% of these patients.[6,7] Sometimes, such dysfunction can happen *de novo* without any evidence of spinal anomaly also.[7,8]

5. What is the initial urological workup in a child with ARM?

Ans:

- **Clinical workup including** physical anthropometrics, BP measurement, bladder diary or CIC diary
- **Biochemical workup includes**
  - Serum creatinine, eGFR estimation
  - Urine examination for pyuria, albuminuria
- **Diagnostic radiologic work-up includes**
  - Abdominal ultrasound to see for upper urinary tracts, bladder thickness, postvoid residual urine, any hydrocolpos.
  - X-ray of lumbosacral spine to see for vertebral anomalies
  - **VCUG** in selected patients based on distal ureteric dilatation or HN (distal ureteric dilatation on ultrasound, hydronephrosis)
  - **Spinal ultrasound** (in very young children) or **MRI spine** (older children)
  - **Genitogram** to see for level of confluence
- **Examination under anaesthesia with urethrocystoscopy**—to see for common channel length, site of confluence, urethra length, bladder status

6. What is the incidence of urological anomalies in children with ARM? Is there a relationship between type of ARM and presence of other urological anomalies? What are the common urological anomalies associated with anorectal malformation?

Ans: The reported incidence of urologic anomalies in patients with ARM varies considerably but is estimated to occur in as many as one half of patients in large cohorts.[9] Also, more complex ARM subtypes are associated with a higher rate of associated urologic anomalies. Common urological anomalies associated with ARM include hydronephrosis, vesicoureteral reflux (VUR), solitary kidney, renal ascent anomalies (ectopic or pelvic), renal fusion anomalies (horseshoe or cross fused kidney), duplex kidney, hypospadias and undescended testicle.

7. Is a preoperative urodynamic study needed in all children undergoing definitive ARM surgery?

Ans: A preoperative urodynamic study can be a useful baseline tool to know the present condition of the bladder with respect to storage pressures and compliance and also to assess the changes in the bladder dynamics following surgery. However, it is necessary to perform urodynamic studies in the first week of life in all children who have sacral agenesis.[6,7,10] This is required to assess and define the type of lower urinary tract dysfunction and to start the appropriate treatment regimen, which includes CIC in the majority of cases.

***Case Scenario** (Contd.)*

Her serum creatinine was found to be elevated 1.1 with estimated eGFR of around 35 ml/min/m.[2] Ultrasound screening of abdomen revealed bilateral hydroureteronephrosis (left > right) with thickened bladder wall and high PVR (Fig. 7.2). Spine imaging was normal. A voiding cystourethrogram (VCUG)

(Contd.)

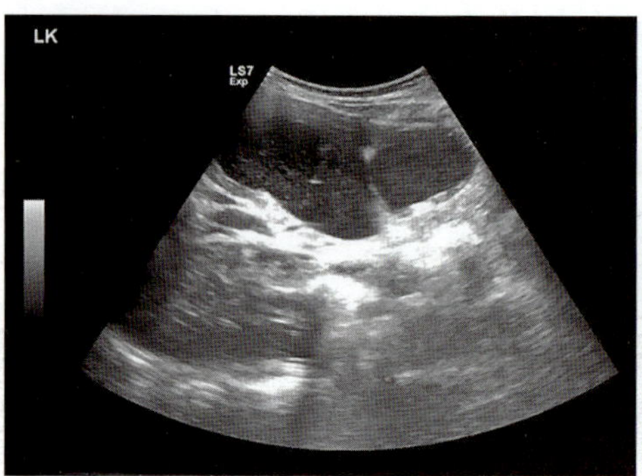

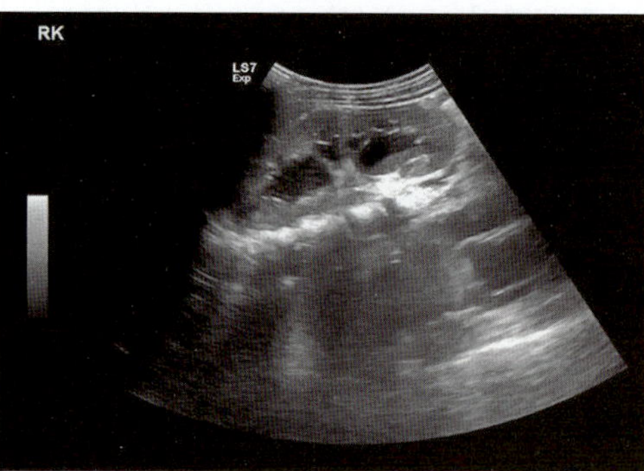

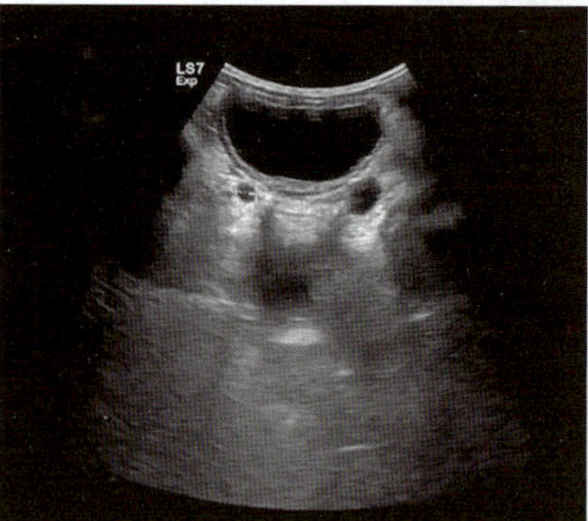

Fig 7.2: Ultrasound picture showing bilateral hydroureteronephrosis with thickened bladder wall and increased postvoid residual urine

***Case Scenario** (Contd.)*

showed grossly trabeculated bladder with 85 ml capacity and on voiding there was extreme dilatation of urethra suggestive of distal obstruction (Fig. 7.3). On examination, under anaesthesia revealed a stenotic urethral opening into the anterior wall of vagina suggestive of a low confluence urogenital sinus which was placed close to the rectum. The findings pointed to a diagnosis of a posterior cloaca. Scopy of the bladder through the stenotic urethra showed a grossly trabeculated thickened bladder with laterally placed U/O. Diagnostic laparoscopy revealed normal Mullerian structures that ruled out DSD. In view of her elevated creatinine, a suprapubic catheter was placed for urinary diversion.

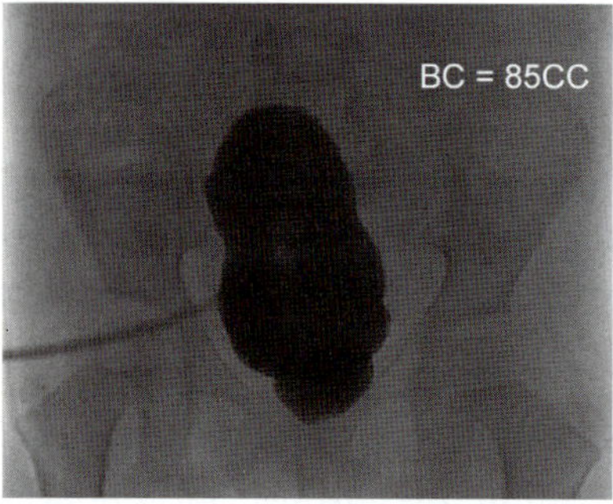

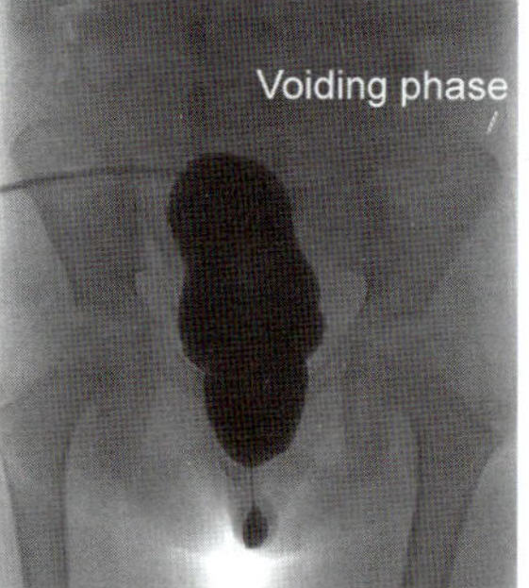

Fig 7.3: VCUG picture showing grossly trabeculated bladder with dilatation of urethra during voiding

8. What are the indications and options for preoperative urinary diversion in children with ARM?

Very young children, children with elevated creatinine or in sepsis may need preoperative urinary diversion for stabilisation before proceeding for definitive repair. This is usually combined with a diverting colostomy in these children.[11] In these situations a vesicostomy or an ureterostomy is usually preferred. Care must be taken the place the stomas in the abdomen so that application of a colostomy appliance is not hindered by the urinary diversion. In older children, a suprapubic catheter can also be considered for temporary urinary diversion.

***Case Scenario** (Contd.)*

Following normalisation of serum creatinine and upper tracts, the child underwent partial urogenital mobilisation (PUM) with anterior sagittal anorectoplasty and feminising genitoplasty (Fig. 7.4). A diverting loop sigmoid colostomy was also done to prevent wound infection or disruption. The perurethral catheter was removed at 4 weeks and a VCUG was done. The VCUG showed a grossly trabeculated bladder with bilateral grade 4 VUR and the child failed to void in the study (Fig. 7.5). An urodynamic study showed a poorly compliant bladder with occasional detrusor overactivity. She was started on anticholinergics and she was also started on a regime of laxatives to avoid constipation. The parents of the girl were taught 2 hourly CIC through the reconstructed urethra along with overnight indwelling catheterisation which they were able to do with ease. The diverting colostomy was closed after 6 weeks after ensuring complete wound healing and stabilisation of CIC schedule.

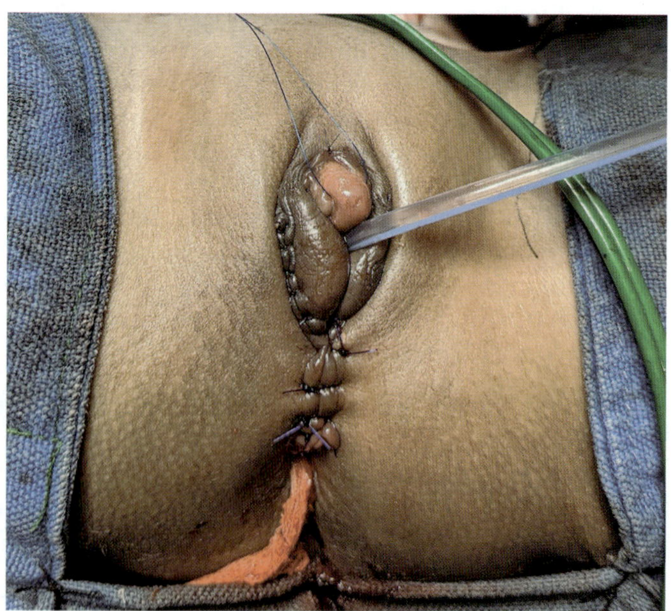

Fig. 7.4: Intraoperative picture following anterior sagittal Anorectoplasty and partial urogenital sinus mobilisation with feminising genitoplasty

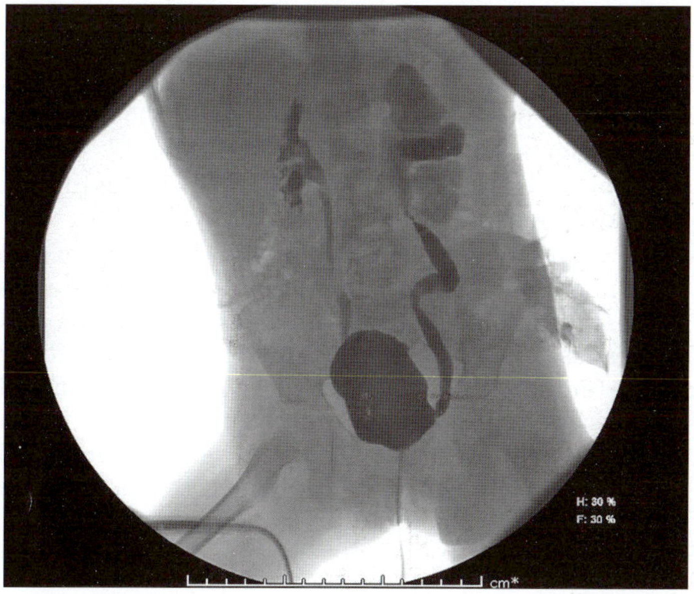

Fig. 7.5: Post-operative VCUG showing trabeculated bladder with bilateral grade IV vesicoureteral reflux (patient unable to void)

9. **Does surgery for ARM lead to LUTD in all cases?**

Ans: The effect of operative repair on bladder function seems to depend on the type of malformation and how much dissection is required close to pelvic nerve plexuses lying within the endopelvic fascia on the anterior surface of the rectum. Denervation of the lower urinary tract has been observed following posterior sagittal anorectoplasty (PSARP) and with other techniques used to reconstruct ARM and its incidence ranges from 5 to 10%.[3,5] In contrast, the incidence of neurogenic bladder is much greater in patients with a cloacal anomaly who undergo reconstruction using PSARP and total urogenital mobilization, with 50% showing deterioration in bladder function.[1,2] This change was more commonly noted when the length of the common channel was greater than 3 cm.

10. **What are the points to be taken into account while considering CIC in children with ARM?**

Unlike patients with spina bifida, ARM patients are usually sensate and therefore introducing CIC in the older patients can be difficult. Early institution of CIC regimen allows the child and the parents to become accustomed to the daily routine of CIC.[5,6] Furthermore, because urinary retention can develop after reconstruction of an ARM, it is suggested that CIC be continued until a postoperative urodynamic study has shown that it is safe to discontinue it. For those that are unable to perform CIC per urethra then creation of a continent catheterizable channel (Mitrofanoff or Monti) is necessary.

11. **What are the common urodynamic findings seen in children following ARM repair?**

Ans: The type of urodynamic findings in children with ARM depends on the presence or absence of associated spinal anomalies and the meticulousness of the surgical repair. Different urodynamic patterns ranging from typical UMN pattern (detrusor overactivity, poor compliance with dyssynergia between external urethral sphincter and detrusor, elevated leak point pressures during filling phase) to LMN type pattern (large capacity, atonic bladder) or mixed pattern have been observed in these children emphasizing the need for an individualized approach to each child.

12. **What is the follow-up protocol in these children?**

Ans: Monitoring at outpatient visits

- Take a urological history at outpatient visits including whether the child has had urinary tract infections and the development or loss of urinary continence
- Annual renal tract ultrasound (more frequent if hydronephrosis or scarring)
- Annual renal blood work including cystatin C and eGFR
- Screening questions about symptoms of tethered cord

Consider urodynamics if there are infections, worsening hydronephrosis, renal scarring or poor renal growth on renal ultrasound or in presence of symptoms of tethered cord.[6,7,10]

Case Scenario *(Contd.)*

She returned after 6 months of good compliance with CIC and anticholinergics and did not have any intervening episodes of UTI or leak. Ultrasound revealed good reduction in dilatation of upper tracts and her creatine was normal for her age. The parents were counselled that compliance with her medication and CIC schedule is likely the reason for this improvement but if symptoms return or her upper tracts worsen, she may need further escalation in therapy.

13. **How do we identify worsening clinical status with respect to the urinary tract in these children during follow-up and how to manage it?**

Ans: Worsening bladder function in these children like in all case of neurogenic bladder is based on clinical, radiological and urodynamic parameters.

- Development of new symptoms or worsening of previous symptoms like urine leakage, recurrent UTI
- Rise in serum creatinine and deterioration in GFR
- Increasing upper tract dilatation in imaging

- Video urodynamic showing decreased bladder capacity with poor compliance with high detrusor leak point pressure and decreased average filling pressures.

14. What are the management options in children who have worsening renal function or upper tracts during follow-up?

Ans: First and foremost in management of these children is checking for compliance with medications and CIC using CIC diary and ensuring compliance

In situations where clinical deterioration has happened in spite of good compliance, then escalation of therapy may be needed in the form of

- Increasing dose of anticholinergic medications
- Change in anticholinergics or addition of newer β3 agonists like mirabegron
- Botulinum toxin injection into the bladder
- Surgical augmentation of bladder using bowel
- For those children who have urinary incontinence due to detrusor overactivity, sacral nerve stimulation appears to be a promising therapy.[12]

15. What are the factors influencing long-term urinary outcomes in children with ARM?

Ans: There are 4 main factors that influence long-term urinary outcomes:

1. The presence of intrinsic kidney or bladder anomalies at birth
2. The presence of sacral anomalies
3. The effect of the operative intervention to correct the ARM
4. The effect of spinal cord tethering causing bladder dysfunction which may change over time.[3]

16. What are the continence rates in children with history of ARM surgery?

Ans: Achievement of urinary continence is strongly related to the underlying anorectal malformation. Many complex ARMs require further urologic reconstructive surgery to achieve continence. The rate of urinary incontinence varies greatly in the literature depending on the severity of the original ARM and on the definitions used to describe continence. Overall incontinence rates in the literature vary from 10% up to 25%.[1–3] The rate of incontinence in girls born with a cloacal anomaly can approach 60–70%.

17. What are the chances of CKD in children with ARM? What are the challenges in management of CKD in this cohort of patients?

With regards to long-term renal function, the type and complexity of malformation and presence of associated urinary tract anomalies significantly affects the risk of developing end stage renal failure.[11] In a longitudinal study of cloaca patients up to 50% were found to have CKD and 11% progressed to end stage renal failure.[1–3,13] The presence of a solitary kidney also increases the risk of progressing to renal failure.

The management of chronic renal failure and end-stage disease in children with ARM raises specific challenges too. Peritoneal dialysis and subsequent renal transplantation can be technically demanding due to the previous abdominal operations. In addition, those patients who go on to renal transplantation need specific attention to the neuropathic bladder, which could continue to damage the new kidney.

SUMMARY

- Neurogenic LUTD is a common finding in children with ARM.
- The etiology can be iatrogenic due to surgery or due to associated spinal anomalies.
- Some children can have *de novo* neurovesical dysfunction even without surgery or associated anomalies.
- Diagnostic workup include biochemical investigation for serum creatinine, eGFR and radiological imaging in the form of ultrasound, VCUG.
- Evaluation of the spine using ultrasound in young children and MRI in older children is crucial in all these children.
- Urodynamic study is a crucial part of diagnostic workup with common findings include hyperreflexic bladder or an underactive bladder.
- Initial management should be conservative in the form of CIC with or without anticholinergics therapy.
- In patients not compliant to CIC, option of CIC through Mitrofanoff can be discussed with parents.
- In patients not responding to conservative measures, options include botulinum injection or surgical measures like augmentation cystoplasty.
- Long-term continence outcomes depend on complexity of underlying anorectal malformation.
- Long-term renal function needs to be monitored as many children can develop CKD due to recurrent infections and associated anomalies.

REFERENCES

1. Levitt MA, Pena A. Anorectal malformations. Orphanet J Rare Dis. 2007; 26:33.
2. Harris KT, Wilcox DT. Management of the urological tract in children with anorectal malformations-a contemporary review. Ther Adv Urol. 2023 Mar 21; 15:17562872231161468.
3. Skerritt C, DaJusta DG, Fuchs ME, Pohl H, Gomez-Lobo V, Hewitt G. Long-term urologic and gynecologic follow-up and the importance of collaboration for patients with anorectal malformations. Semin Pediatr Surg. 2020 Dec;29(6):150987.
4. Borg HC, Holmdahl G, Gustavsson K, Doroszkiewicz M, Sillén U. Longitudinal study of bowel function in children with anorectal malformations. J Pediatr Surg. 2013

Mar;48(3):597–606. doi: 10.1016/j.jpedsurg.2012.10.056. PMID: 23480919.

5. Versteegh HP, Wolffenbuttel KP, Sloots CEJ, *et al.* Effects of reconstructive surgery on bladder function in patients with anorectal malformations. J Urol. 2014;192(6):1789–1793.
6. Boemers TM, Beek FJ, van Gool JD, de Jong TP, Bax KM. Urologic problems in anorectal malformations. Part 1: Urodynamic findings and significance of sacral anomalies. J Pediatr Surg. 1996 Mar;31(3):407–10.
7. Boemers TM, de Jong TP, van Gool JD, Bax KM. Urologic problems in anorectal malformations. Part 2: functional urologic sequelae. J Pediatr Surg. 1996 May;31(5):634–7.
8. Sheldon C, Cormier M, Crone K, Wacksman J. Occult neurovesical dysfunction in children with imperforate anus and its variants. J Pediatr Surg. 1991; 26:49–54.
9. Fuchs ME, Halleran DR, Bourgeois T, Sebastião Y, Weaver L, Farrell N, Vilanova-Sánchez A, Gasior A, Halaweish I, Jayanthi VR, Wood RJ, Dajusta DG. Correlation of anorectal malformation complexity and associated urologic abnormalities. J Pediatr Surg. 2021 Nov;56(11):1988–1992.
10. Mosiello G, Capitanucci ML, Gatti C, Adorisio O, Lucchetti MC, Silveri M, Schingo PS, De Gennaro M. How to investigate neurovesical dysfunction in children with anorectal malformations. J Urol. 2003 Oct;170(4 Pt 2):1610–3.
11. VanderBrink BA, Reddy PP. Early urologic considerations in patients with persistent cloaca. Semin Pediatr Surg. 2016 Apr;25(2):82–9.
12. Dewberry L, Trecartin A, Peña A, Pierre MS, Bischoff A. Systematic review: sacral nerve stimulation in the treatment of constipation and fecal incontinence in children with emphasis in anorectal malformation. Pediatr Surg Int. 2019 Sep;35(9):1009–1012.
13. Chong C, Hamza Y, Tan YW, Paul A, Garriboli M, Wright AJ, Olsburgh J, Taylor C, Sinha MD, Mishra P, Taghizadeh A. Long-term urology outcomes of anorectal malformation. J Pediatr Urol. 2022 Apr;18(2):150.e1–150.e6.

Chapter

8

Spina Bifida with Hydronephrosis Refractory Storage

• Pawan Vasudeva

LEARNING OBJECTIVES

- Spina bifida (SB) is a congenital malformation in which the spinal column is split as a result of failed closure of the embryonic neural tube. SB occulta, closed spinal dysraphism, meningocele and myelomeningocele are the various types of spina bifida.
- Vast majority of newborns with SB have essentially normal kidneys at birth, with no clinically significant findings on baseline imaging.[1]
- Since SB is one of the common paediatric causes of high risk neurogenic bladder, where damage to the kidneys can start soon after birth, the EAU/ESPU guidelines on neurogenic bladder recommend a proactive approach (wherein invasive interventions like urodynamics and clean intermittent catheterisation (CIC) are initiated before the onset of renal abnormalities) over the expectant approach where invasive interventions and drugs are started after abnormalities are identified.[2]
- Initial management of high-risk neurogenic bladder involves instituting CIC and oral drug therapy (antimuscarinics and/or mirabegron)
- The goals of management of a high risk neurogenic bladder include: (a) To ensure a safe, low pressure adequate capacity bladder for storage, (b) continence, (c) emptying at low pressure (usually by CIC) and (d) no recurrent infections, among others.
- Close follow-up of SB patients with neurogenic bladder is essential as urodynamic patterns may change over time, e.g. during periods of physical growth spurts.
- In patients in whom the bladder is unsafe for storage despite oral drug therapy (antimuscarinics and mirabegron) and CIC, intradetrusor Botulinum toxin A should be strongly considered.
- For those refractory to even botulinum toxin A injection, augmentation cystoplasty may be required to ensure a low-pressure adequate capacity reservoir that protect the kidneys and allows for the patient to be continent.

Case Scenario

A 11-year-old male presented with continuous dribbling of urine since birth, both daytime and nighttime along with fecal incontinence. He had been diagnosed with a lumbar myelomeningocele at age 10 when he underwent a neurosurgical procedure for the same. Post-surgery, the fecal incontinence improved. For his urinary complaints he was advised CIC 4 hourly and a combination of Solifenacin 5 mg and Mirabegron 50 mg. Despite adhering to timely CIC and oral drug therapy, troublesome incontinence persisted for which he presented to the urology unit. There was no history of any urinary tract infections. Examination revealed a scar over the lumbar region. Anal tone was lax and BCR was absent. Higher functions and hand dexterity were normal.

1. How would you approach this patient

a. Is there a role of bladder diary?

Ans: Bladder diary (Intermittent catheterisation diary in this case) forms an integral part of evaluation and must be done in all such patients. His catheterization volumes were between 80 and 120 ml and there were multiple leaks in between.

b. Is there a role of baseline blood chemistry and urine examination?

Ans: Yes. Baseline blood investigations and urine examination are in order (urine exam as he would be subsequently undergoing a urodynamic study. Otherwise, routine urine examination in neurogenic bladder patients on CIC and otherwise asymptomatic is not recommended). His creatinine was 0.6 mg/dl and his urine was normal.

c. **Is there a role of an ultrasound KUB region?**

Ans: Upper tract assessment is paramount in these patients and ultrasound should be done upfront. He had left gross hydroureter-onephrosis with thinned out parenchyma. Right kidney was normal. Bladder was thickened.

To note that ultrasound cannot be a substitute for invasive urodynamics as high-risk neurogenic bladder may be missed in nearly 20% of patients if only ultrasound was to be done.[3] On the other hand, urodynamics alone is not enough to draw conclusions with regard to safety.

d. **Is there a role of invasive testing?**

Ans: Invasive urodynamics should be done in all patients with high risk neurogenic bladder at baseline. Ideally a videourodynamics should be performed. In case of non-availability, a invasive urodynamics can be combined with a micturating cystourethrogram. The micturating cystourethrogram of this patient showed a left grade V reflux and a fir tree-like trabeculated bladder typically seen in neurogenic bladders (Fig. 8.1). Invasive urodynamics revealed high amplitude compound detrusor overactivity (staring at about 90 cc filling) with poor compliance with multiple leaks (Fig. 8.2).

e. **Is there any role of renal scan?**

Ans: A nuclear renogram, usually DTPA scan, should be done to document baseline renal function. The renal scan of this patient showed a left kidney GFR of 7 ml/min and the right kidney GFR of 73 ml/min (Fig. 8.3).

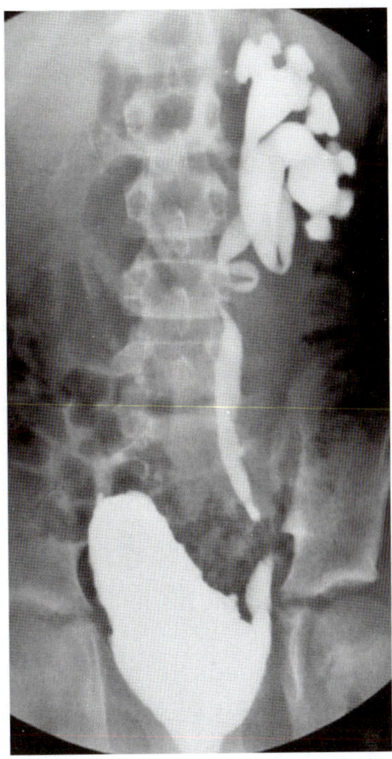

Fig. 8.1: Micturating cystourethrogram

2. **What is the diagnosis for this patient? What needs to be addressed?**

Ans:

a. *Diagnosis:* He has a neurogenic bladder (consequent to a lumbar myelomeningocele) wherein the filling phase reveals a high pressure, low capacity bladder that is unsafe for storage.

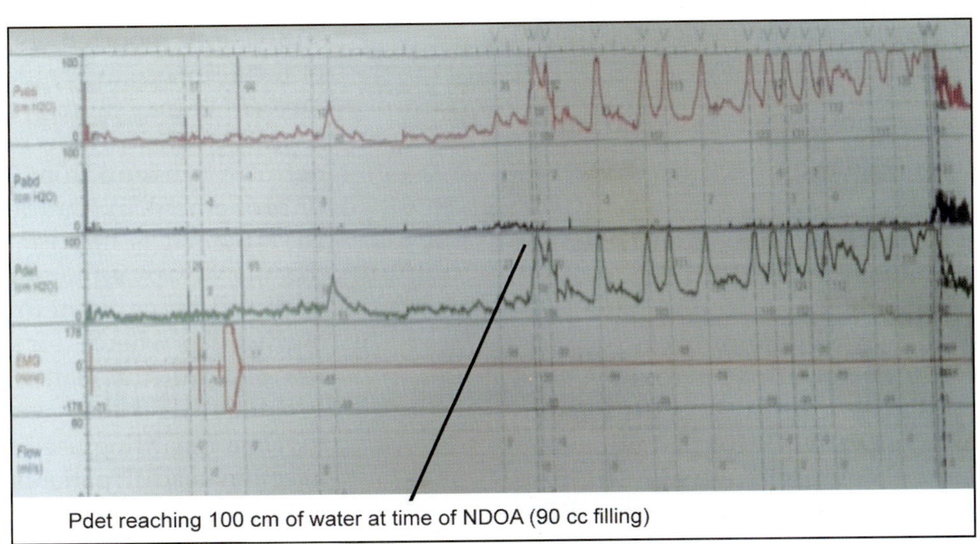

Fig. 8.2: Urodynamic study

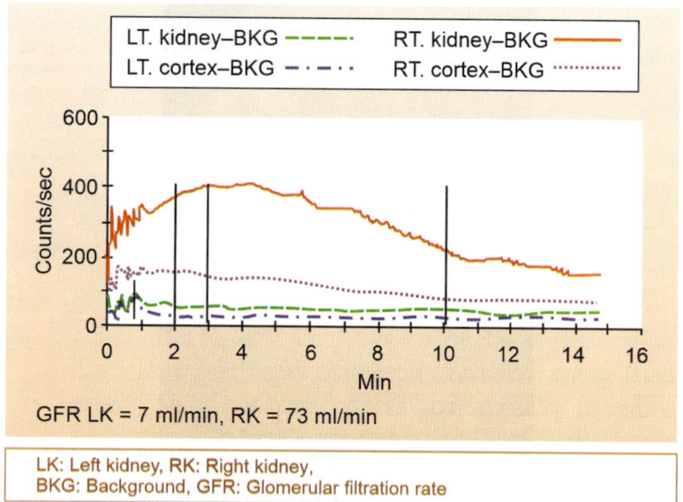

Fig. 8.3: DTPA scan

Consequent to that his left kidney has become non-functioning.

b. His bladder needs to be made into a low-pressure reservoir of adequate capacity. That should help protect the kidneys from further damage (in this case the remaining functional kidney) and and also help in continence. Intermittent catheterisation will continue as before. Since this patient is "refractory" to the first-line therapies, he is now a candidate for more aggressive therapies.

The term "refractory storage", although awaits a consensus definition, logically refers to: (a) Patients with neurogenic bladder in whom antimuscarinics and possibly mirabegron have been used (also in combination) for a reasonable period of say 3 month, (b) Other confounding factors like constipation, non-adherence to CIC have been addressed and (c) In spite of the above adequate urine storage at low intravesical pressure is not achieved. This could lead to socially unacceptable incontinence, risk to the upper tracts, recurrent UTIs, etc.

3. What are the treatment options for this patient?

i. Intradetrusor Botulinum toxin for Refractory Storage

a. Which of the botulinum toxin types are approved for this indication?

Ans: While almost all studies have published on two botulinum toxin preparations, i.e. Onabotulinum toxin A and Abobotulinum toxin A, it is the Onabotulinum toxin A (Botox®) which has been more comprehensively studied. Onabotulinum toxin A received FDA approved for adult patients with refractory neurogenic detrusor overactivity in 2011 and for paediatric patients (age >5 years) with refractory neurogenic detrusor overactivity in 2021. The two preparations should not be used interchangeably, either in terms of predicting outcome or in determining doses to be used.[4]

b. What dosage to inject and how to inject?

Ans: The FDA registration studies demonstrated a similar efficacy and adverse event profile for 200 units and 300 units onabotulinum toxin A, suggesting a plateau in the efficacy of the toxin. Hence providing for the best benefit/risk ratio, 200 units of onabotulinum toxin A is recommended for adult neurogenic detrusor overactivity.[5,6] In the pivotal studies, injections were given as 1 ml (~6.7 Units) injections across 30 sites into the detrusor, sparing the trigone. However, there is some data now that trigone including onabotulinum toxin A injections has superior efficacy and similar safety profile when compared to trigone sparing injections.[7] There is a large variance in the number of sites and the volume that has been injected by various authors. The effect of these variables on outcomes, if any, has not been well studies.

For paediatric patients, the recommended dose is also 200 U, but not to exceed 6 U/kg.[8]

c. Is it an effective treatment in the SB sub-population?

Ans: A systematic review looked at the efficacy of intradetrusor botulinum toxin in spina bifida patients refractory to antimuscarinics. The review, which included 12 published series (n = 293 patients, all <18 years), reported complete resolution of incontinence in 32–100% of patients, an increase in maximum cystometric capacity from 27 to 162%, a decrease in maximum detrusor pressure from 32 to 54% and an improvement in bladder compliance of 28–176%.[9] It is important to underscore that the therapy is more effective in patients with evidence of neurogenic detrusor overactivity, whereas for those with isolated low bladder compliance without detrusor overactivity, results have been poor.[9,10]

Data regarding use of botulinum toxin injection in adult patients with spina bifida is limited. In a multicenter retrospective chart review of 125 patients who underwent a total of 561 intradetrusor botulinum toxin injections, resolution of urinary incontinence was seen in 73.5% of the patients with significant improvements in the maximum cystometric capacity, maximum detrusor pressure and compliance. Like in the paediatric population, effectiveness was much lower in spina bifida patients who had poor bladder compliance.[11]

d. How long does the effect last and are repeat injections effective?

Ans: The mean duration of efficacy of a single injection is 6–16 months and efficacy is sustained over repeat treatment sessions.[4,12] A caution in this regard has to be exercised as there is no way to know as to when the effect has started waning and hence the patient must be monitored for any reappearance of symptoms. Monitoring of patients with unsafe storage without accompanying symptoms can be challenging and might necessitate urodynamics. There is lack of good evidence with regard to these issues.

e. What are the possible side effects?

Ans: The treatment is overall safe. Significant increase in PVR in patients not on intermittent catheterisation, an increased risk of UTI, hematuria, constipation and flu like symptoms are some of the concerns that should be discussed with the patient. Generalized paraparesis is extremely rare (0.005%) with Onabotulinum toxin A. In the event of it happening, the effect resolves spontaneously after 4–6 weeks.[4]

ii. Augmentation cystoplasty for refractory storage

a. What are the types of augmentation cystoplasty?

Ans: Augmentation cystoplasty may be refer to: (i) Autoaugmentation (vesicomyotomy) (ii) Ureterocystoplasty (iii) Enterocystoplasty (ileocystoplasty (ileum) or colocystoplasty (sigmoid colon) (iv) Gastrocystoplasty (stomach) (v) Seromuscular augmentation and (vi) Tissue engineering cystoplasty.

b. Which augmentation cystoplasty is most commonly done?

Ans: The most commonly used technique remains augmentation with a detubularised patch of ileum (ileocystoplasty).[13]

c. How effective is augmentation cystoplasty?

Ans: In a systematic review that looked at long-term effectiveness in patients undergoing bladder augmentation (most having undergone ileocystoplasty), the authors reported that no patient had deterioration in renal function postoperatively, 87% were completely continent, average bladder capacity increased from 169 to 559 ml, detrusor pressure at maximum capacity decreased from 65 to 19 cm of water and that the quality of life significantly improved. They concluded that augmentation cystoplasty was a highly effective procedure for protecting the upper tracts.[14]

d. What are the possible side effects?

Ans: Bladder augmentation is associated with a relatively high morbidity both in the short and the long-term. Long-term complications include bladder perforation (2%), mucus retention (13%), metabolic abnormalities (3%), bowel dysfunction (15%), and stone formation (10%). While there is consensus that augmented bladders (where intestine/stomach has been used) have a higher risk of developing tumours than the matched population, the risk has not yet been defined.[14]

e. What are the concerns with augmentation when renal function is significantly reduced?

Ans: When renal function is significantly compromised, augmentation with ileum may worsen the existing metabolic acidosis, even though there are some studies which have shown that an ileum patch is feasible in patients with advanced chronic kidney disease (stage 3-4).[15] Stomach can be a valuable alternative in the select group of neurogenic bladder patients with chronic kidney disease and significant metabolic acidosis in whom an augmentation cystoplasty is otherwise indicated.[16]

f. How to sequence augmentation cystoplasty vis-à-vis intradetrusor botulinum toxin A injection?

Ans: In general, augmentation cystoplasty is a bigger surgical intervention and an irreversible procedure when compared to botulinum toxin. While it may be more effective than botulinum toxin injection, the probability of major complications is also more. Bigger the intervention, bigger is the probability of major complications.

It should only be considered in patients after failed botulinum toxin treatment or in those not willing/not suitable for botulinum toxin. The ability to do clean intermittent catheterisation is a prerequisite that must be explained to the patient during counselling.

Our patient received 200 units of botulinum toxin without much benefit and subsequently underwent an open left nephroureterectomy with clam ileocystoplasty. Post-procedure he continues to be on intermittent catheterisation, is continent and urodynamics revealed a low pressure good capacity reservoir.

SUMMARY

- Onabotulinum Toxin A intradetrusor injection is an effective treatment for spina bifida patients with refractory neurogenic detrusor overactivity and is recommended at a dosage of 200 units (not more than 6 U/kg in paediatric patients). Patients who have isolated poor compliance without obvious detrusor contractions are poor responders.
- In patients refractory to /unsuitable for botulinum toxin injection, augmentation cystoplasty may be considered. Detailed patient counselling and the ability to do CIC is a prerequisite.
- Invasive treatments are not benign. Bigger the intervention, the bigger is the probability of major complications.

REFERENCES

1. Tanaka ST, Paramsothy P, Thibadeau J, Wiener JS, Joseph DB, Cheng EY, Tu D, Austin C, Koh CJ, Wallis MC, Walker WO, Smith KA, Routh JC, Baum MA. Baseline Urinary Tract Imaging in Infants Enrolled in the UMPIRE Protocol for Children with Spina Bifida. J Urol. 2019 Jun;201(6):1193–1198.
2. Stein R, Bogaert G, Dogan HS, Hoen L, Kocvara R, Nijman RJM, Quadackers JSLT, Rawashdeh YF, Silay MS, Tekgul S, Radmayr C. EAU/ESPU guidelines on the management of neurogenic bladder in children and adolescent part I diagnostics and conservative treatment. Neurourol Urodyn. 2020 Jan;39(1):45–57.
3. Bawa M, Dash V, Kalavant A, Mahajan JK, Rao KLN. Is urodynamic evaluation a must in all operated cases of open neural tube defects. J Pediatr Urol. 2017 Dec;13(6):614.e1–614.e4.
4. Mangera A, Andersson KE, Apostolidis A, Chapple C, Dasgupta P, Giannantoni A, Gravas S, Madersbacher S. Contemporary management of lower urinary tract disease with botulinum toxin A: a systematic review of botox (onabotulinumtoxinA) and dysport (abobotulinumtoxinA). Eur Urol. 2011 Oct;60(4):784–95.
5. Cruz F, Herschorn S, Aliotta P, Brin M, Thompson C, Lam W, *et al.* Efficacy and safety of onabotulinumtoxinA in patients with urinary incontinence due to neurogenic detrusor overactivity: a randomised, double-blind, placebo-controlled trial. Eur Urol. 2011;60(4):742–50.
6. Ginsberg D, Gousse A, Keppenne V, Sievert KD, Thompson C, Lam W, *et al.* Phase 3 efficacy and tolerability study of onabotulinumtoxinA for urinary incontinence from neurogenic detrusor overactivity. J Urol. 2012;187(6): 2131–9.
7. Hui C, Keji X, Chonghe J, Ping T, Rubiao O, Jianweng Z, Xiangrong D, Liling Z, Maping H, Qingqing L, Qiuling L, Jiebing H, Tanghai H. Combined detrusor-trigone BTX-A injections for urinary incontinence secondary to neurogenic detrusor overactivity. Spinal Cord. 2016 Jan;54(1):46–50.
8. Austin PF, Franco I, Dobremez E, Kroll P, Titanji W, Geib T, Jenkins B, Hoebeke PB. OnabotulinumtoxinA for the treatment of neurogenic detrusor overactivity in children. Neurourol Urodyn. 2021 Jan;40(1):493–501.
9. Hascoet J, Manunta A, Brochard C, Arnaud A, Damphousse M, Menard H, Kerdraon J, Journel H, Bonan I, Odent S, Fremond B, Siproudhis L, Gamé X, Peyronnet B; French Referral Network of Spina Bifida. Outcomes of intradetrusor injections of botulinum toxin in patients with spina bifida: A systematic review. Neurourol Urodyn. 2017 Mar;36(3):557–564.
10. Danacioglu YO, Keser F, Ersoz C, Polat S, Avci AE, Kalkan S, Silay MS. Factors predicting the success of intradetrusor onabotulinum toxin-A treatment in children with neurogenic bladders due to myelomeningocele: The outcomes of a large cohort. J Pediatr Urol. 2021 Aug;17(4):520.e1–520.e7.
11. Peyronnet B, Even A, Capon G, De Seze M, Hascoet J, Biardeau X, Baron M, Perrouin-Verbe MA, Boutin JM, Saussine C, Phé V, Lenormand L, Chartier-Kastler E, Cornu JN, Karsenty G, Manunta A, Schurch B, Denys P, Amarenco G, Game X; GENULF and the AFU Committee of NeuroUrology. Intradetrusor Injections of Botulinum Toxin A in Adults with Spinal Dysraphism. J Urol. 2018 Oct;200(4):875–880.
12. Rovner E, Kohan A, Chartier-Kastler E, Jünemann KP, Del Popolo G, Herschorn S, Joshi M, Magyar A, Nitti V. Long-Term Efficacy and Safety of OnabotulinumtoxinA in Patients with Neurogenic Detrusor Overactivity Who Completed 4 Years of Treatment. J Urol. 2016 Sep;196(3):801–8.
13. Biers SM, Venn SN, Greenwell TJ. The past, present and future of augmentation cystoplasty. BJU Int. 2012 May; 109(9):1280–93.
14. Hoen L', Ecclestone H, Blok BFM, Karsenty G, Phé V, Bossier R, Groen J, Castro-Diaz D, Padilla Fernández B, Del Popolo G, Musco S, Pannek J, Kessler TM, Gross T, Schneider MP, Hamid R. Long-term effectiveness and complication rates of bladder augmentation in patients with neurogenic bladder dysfunction: A systematic review. Neurourol Urodyn. 2017 Sep;36(7):1685–1702.
15. Sinha S, Shah M. Augmentation cystoplasty in children with stages III and IV chronic kidney disease secondary to neurogenic bladder. Asian J Urol. 2022 Jul;9(3):313–317.
16. Vasudeva, P. (2023). Gastrocystoplasty. In: Liao, L., Madersbacher, H. (eds) Handbook of Neurourology. Springer, Singapore. https://doi.org/10.1007/978-981-16-7939-1-91-1.

Chapter

9

Spinal Cord Injury (Cervical) in Male

• *Vineet Narang*

LEARNING OBJECTIVES

- NLUTD (neurogenic lower urinary tract dysfunction) refers to abnormal function of either the bladder, bladder neck, and/or its sphincters related to a neurologic disorder.[1] Earlier the word "neurogenic bladder" was used to describe this condition. With the understanding this is not just an issue confined to the bladder, NLUTD is the preferred terminology now.
- Most patients with spinal cord injury develop neurogenic bladder dysfunction, which represents one of the most devastating sequelae for patients' quality of life and might lead to complications such as recurrent urinary tract infections (UTIs), urethral strictures, calculus disease, hydronephrosis, and renal failure.[2] Neuro-urological management aims to preserve or improve upper urinary tract function, control UTIs, and maintain a low-pressure bladder that is both continent and capable of emptying completely.
- The initial urological management is indwelling catheter during the stage of spinal shock. After medical stabilisation Intermittent catheterisation (IC) is initiated.[3]
- Intermittent catheterization (IC) can be sterile or clean. Various types of catheters single use/reuse, hydrophilic/ non-hydrophilic, latex or non-latex can be used. The risk of UTI remains the same irrespective of the method of CIC and type of catheter.
- Nocturnal polyuria occurs in more than 60% of SCI (spinal cord injured) patients regardless of their age, level of lesion and completeness of the lesion. It is associated with nocturnal enuresis and high-volume IC amounts in the first morning.Continuous Nocturnal drainage decreases incidence of AD (autonomic dysreflexia) and decreases episodes of UTI and incontinence.[4]
- Video-urodynamics is the combination of cystometry and pressure-flow study (when spontaneous voiding is possible) with imaging. It is the gold standard for urodynamic investigation in neuro-urological disorders especially in patients with SCI.[5]
- DSD (detrusor sphincter dyssynergia) is the contraction of the sphincter during voiding which can result in dangerously high pressures within the bladder leading to complications like vesicoureteral reflux, hydronephrosis, pyelonephritis, urosepsis, and renal dysfunction.[6]
- Autonomic dysreflexia (AD) is a potentially life-threatening complication of spinal cord injury above T6 level. It is caused by an unopposed sympathetic nervous system response to noxious stimulation below the level of the injury. There is vasodilation above the level of injury and vasoconstriction below the level of injury.[7]
- Spinal cord injury causes a high-risk NLUTD and requires close follow-up with: Annual focused history, physical exam, and symptom assessment, annual renal function and upper tract imaging and multichannel urodynamic studies.[8]

Case Scenario

A 25-year-old male sustained a road traffic accident in January 2018. He was diagnosed as having a fracture dislocation C4–C5 vertebrae for which he underwent surgical fixation. Following surgery, his neurological assessment revealed quadriplegia with ASIA-A impairment (complete injury, no motor or sensory function). He was kept on indwelling catheter for 2 weeks and after medical stabilisation intermittent catheterisation (IC) was initiated (Fig. 9.1).

1. What is the initial neuro-urological management of these patients?

Ans: The initial management is indwelling catheter during the stage of spinal shock. Early initiation of IC is the rule. Once the patient is medically stable and can regulate the own fluid intake, intermittent catheterization may be considered. Patients with adequate hand function should try to learn how to do intermittent catheterization themselves and those without adequate hand function may still

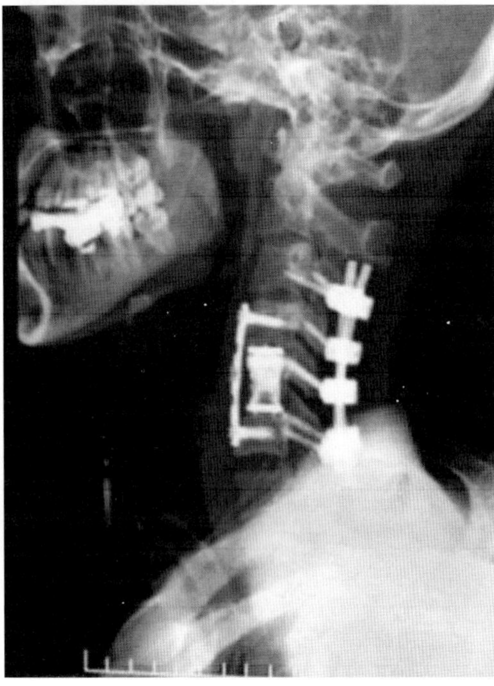

Fig. 9.1: Post-fixation cervical spine X-ray

be able to do intermittent catheterization with appropriate caregiver or nursing support.

Our patient was also started on intermittent catheterisation 2 weeks after injury.

2. What does the Initial evaluation of these patients include?

Ans: The initial assessment of these patients includes history, examination, urine analysis, renal function assessment and imaging.

History

- Mechanism of injury, the level and completeness of the injury, associated urologically relevant injuries (pelvic fracture and urethral injuries)
- Past urological history, a transurethral resection of the prostate (where the loss of the bladder neck sphincter can result in stress urinary incontinence or a significant stone surgery)
- History of bowel and sexual function
- Motor abilities, cognitive function, and support systems.

Examination

- General physical examination of the patient with particular attention to body habitus, such as obesity, should be carried out, as it could affect the ability to self-catheterize or the placement of a suprapubic catheter.
- Assessment of hand function (for example, watching how a patient can handle a pen, or rip a piece of paper) for self-IC
- Focused neurological examination; Included in this is an assessment of anal tone, perianal sensation, and the bulbocavernosus reflex.

Urine analysis: To rule out UTI or haematuria

Renal function: Kidney function test for assessment of renal function

Imaging: Ultrasound of the kidneys to look for any hydronephrosis, stone, etc.

Bladder diary is a simple, non-invasive, and inexpensive method of collecting objective information about catheterization habits and fluid intake and is a very useful tool for managing incontinence and UTI in spinal cord injured patients.

Our patient had tetraplegia with poor hand function and was not able to do self-CIC, his wife was doing the IC. He had normal urine analysis, normal renal blood chemistry and normal upper tracts on ultrasound.

3. What are the techniques of IC (intermittent catheterisation) and types of catheters used?

Ans: IC can be either sterile technique or clean technique.

The sterile technique is used in hospitals, uses genital disinfection/sterile gloves and sterile catheter, whereas in the clean technique (CIC) the user touches the catheter with clean hands. The clean technique is preferred.

The risks of UTI is similar in both methods.[9]

Various types of catheter can be used for IC: Latex vs non-latex, hydrophilic vs non-hydrophilic, multiple use versus single catheter and anti-bacterial catheters.

The usual size of catheter ranges from 12 to 16 Fr. The risk of UTI is similar irrespective of type of catheter used.

Long-term IC by a caregiver may often be necessitated in patients with cervical spinal injury due to impairment of hand function. This is associated with additional challenges. It is impractical to use the services of a healthcare professional because this is seldom a long-term solution. In the fortuitous circumstances that there is a family member who is willing, able and motivated, long-term IC by a caregiver should be encouraged. One must always be mindful of additional responsibilities that might fall upon able-bodied family members and a private discussion with the concerned member is recommended.

Our patient was on clean IC 4-hourly by a caregiver using a non-latex catheter which was being reused. IC volume was ~200 ml. He was having a multiple incontinence episodes.

4. **The patient is keen to discontinue IC and void spontaneously. Is this advisable?**

 Ans: Crede and Valsalva should be avoided as primary methods of bladder emptying in SCI individuals because it is usually inefficient at emptying the bladder, can result in high intravesical pressure leading to vesicoureteral reflux, hydronephrosis, and renal insufficiency. Other consequences could be abdominal muscle strain, hernia, pelvic organ prolapse, or haemorrhoids. Patient who are on reflex voiding need urodynamics to ensure a low pressure bladder.

 Meanwhile our patient continued to have leaks and wanted to be shifted to indwelling catheter.

5. **When is an indwelling catheter acceptable? Is it better to offer a suprapubic catheter or a urethral catheter?**

 Ans: Whenever possible, IC remains the treatment of choice. However, patients with poor hand skills, tetraplegics, female patients, patients with cognitive impairment, and those who have limited assistance from a caregiver, may require an indwelling catheter. The options include transurethral indwelling catheterization and suprapubic catheterisation. Transurethral indwelling catheterisation carries >5-fold increase risk of recurrent UTIs when compared to suprapubic catheterisation (SPC) and CIC.[10]

 Suprapubic catheterisation may be offered to the following subset of patients.

 - Urethral abnormalities, such as stricture, false passages, urethral fistula.
 - Recurrent urethral catheter obstruction.
 - Difficulty with urethral catheter insertion.
 - Perineal skin breakdown due to urine leakage secondary to urethral incompetence.
 - Psychological considerations, such as body image or personal
 - A desire to improve sexual genital function.

 Our patient opted for a suprapubic catheter.

6. **What is nocturnal polyuria? What is the role of continuous nocturnal drainage in patients with high cord SCI?**

 Ans: Majority of patients with SCI have nocturnal polyuria. It is associated with nocturnal enuresis and high volume of morning IC. In such situations, nocturnal bladder drainage might be necessary. The IC catheter used at night is strapped to the thigh and attached to a collection bag to facilitate continuous nocturnal drainage to keep the bladder empty. Continuous nocturnal drainage decreases incidence of AD and decreases episodes of UTI and incontinence[4] (Fig. 9.2).

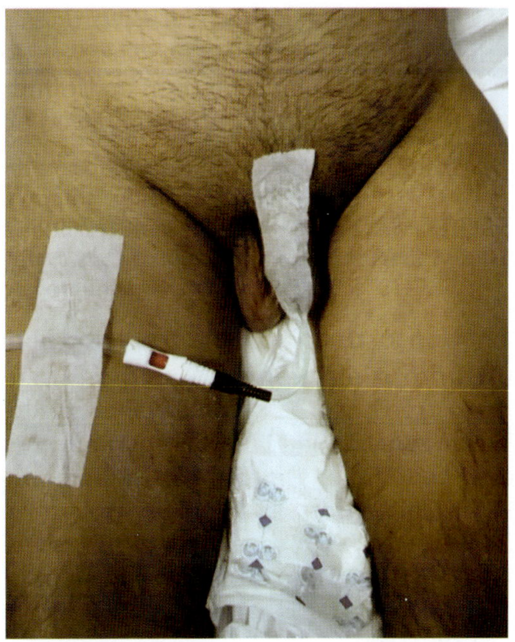

Fig. 9.2: Nelaton catheter strapped to the thigh at night to provide continuous nocturnal drainage

7. **What is the role of urodynamics in neurogenic bladder? When is the ideal time and method to perform it?**

 Ans: Urodynamic investigation is the gold standard to evaluate lower urinary tract function in patients with SCI. Complete neuro-urological assessment including urodynamic investigation is strongly recommended in all acute SCI patients.[5] The ideal time to do a urodynamic is at three months, after the phase of spinal shock is over. However, many patients show early unfavourable urodynamic parameters within the first 40 days after SCI warranting timely urodynamics to optimise patient-tailored therapy.[11]

 Video-urodynamics is the combination of cystometry and pressure-flow study (when spontaneous voiding is possible) with imaging. It is the gold standard for urodynamic investigation in neuro-urological disorders especially in patients with SCI. However, non-video urodynamics is an acceptable option when fluoroscopy is not available. It is preferable to get an MCU done in conjunction with the urodynamics in such situations.

 Urodynamics in our patient (at 2 months after injury) revealed multiple neurogenic detrusor overactivity with low compliance and maximum cystometric capacity (MCC) of 180 ml.

8. **What are unfavourable features on urodynamic and why do we need to know these?**

 Ans: Unfavourable urodynamic parameters include high maximum detrusor pressure [Pdet]

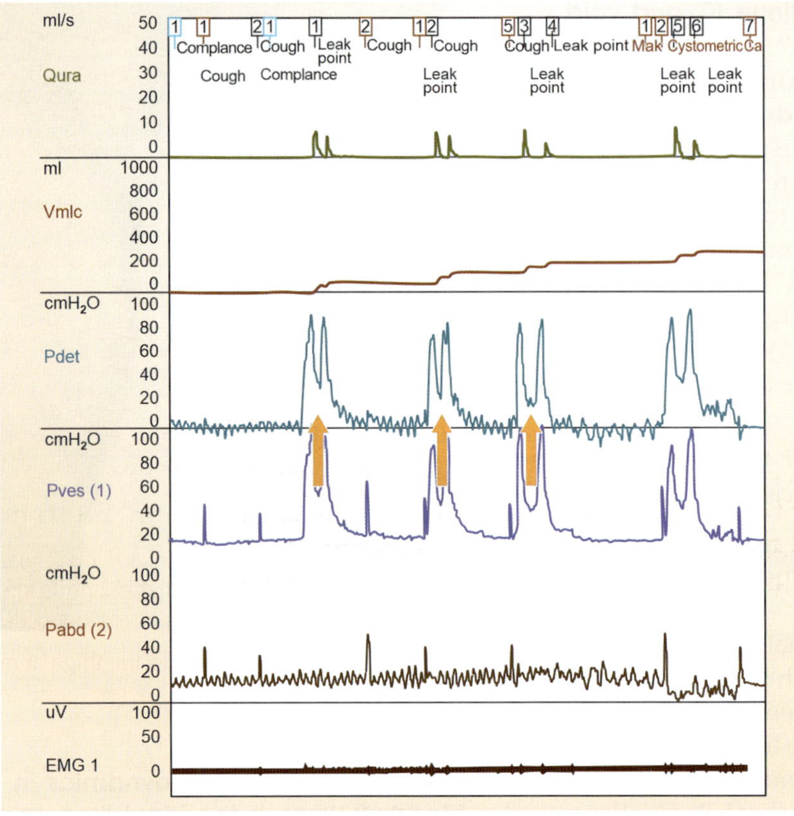

- Multiple NDO
- Maximum detrusor pressure of 90 cm H_2O
- Decreased compliance
- MCC = 180 ml

Fig. 9.3: Urodynamic at 2 months after spinal cord injury showing multiple neurogenic detrusor contractions

during the storage phase [> 40 cm H_2O], low-compliance bladder [< 20 ml/cm H_2O], detrusor overactivity, DSD, and vesico-uretero-renal reflux.[3]

These patients have high risk of upper tract deterioration and follow-up urodynamics should be considered 1–3 months after initiation of therapy to assess the efficacy of the treatment.

Our patient had unfavourable findings on urodynamics. This re-affirmed the high-risk nature of his nLUTD

9. What is DSD (detrusor sphincter dyssynergia)?

Ans: Normal (synergistic) micturition is initiated by increase in detrusor pressure and relaxation of urethral sphincter. If there is simultaneous contraction of sphincter and detrusor without any synergy, it is called DSD.

DSD may be defined on urethral pressure measurement as an acute urethral pressure rise >20 cmH_2O within 30 seconds prior to or during a voluntary or involuntary detrusor contraction.[6] It can be of three types:

Type 1: Increasing sphincter activity during detrusor contraction which then ceases and detrusor pressure decreases to allow urination;

Type 2: Clonic contractions intermittently during voiding causing intermittent urinary stream

Type 3: Continuous sphincter activity during detrusor contraction resulting in inability to void per urethra.

The usual cause is a supra-sacral spinal cord injury or multiple sclerosis.

It may cause complications like reflux, hydronephrosis, pyelonephritis, urosepsis, renal stones and renal dysfunction and also may contribute to difficult intermittent catheterization.

The treatment of DSD includes pharmacological agents like alpha blockers and muscle relaxants like baclofen. Intermittent catheterisation, indwelling catheterisation, urethral stents and intra-sphincteric botulinum toxin.

Surgical external sphincterotomy may be used as a reserve procedure and carries a high revision rate.

Rarely, augmentation cystoplasty or urinary diversion might be necessary.

10. What is autonomic dysreflexia (AD)?

Ans: AD is a potentially life-threatening complication of spinal cord injury above T6 level.It is caused by an unopposed sympathetic nervous system response to noxious stimulation below the level of the injury. There is vasodilation above the level of injury and vasoconstriction below the level of injury.[7]

Clinical features include

- Hypertension: Greater than 20 mmHg above baseline
- Severe bilateral pounding headache
- Diaphoresis or flushing above the level of the spinal cord lesion
- Visual changes or disturbances
- Bradycardia or tachycardia (bradycardia at onset, tachycardia follow)
- Pallor or gooseflesh below the level of the spinal cord lesion
- Respiratory distress or bronchospasms
- Anxiety (apprehension, fear of death is common)

Most common cause is bladder distension and UTI. Other causes include constipation, fissure, haemorrhoids, pressure sore, burn, tight clothes and ingrowing toe nail.

Treatment includes

- Make the patient sit upright
- Loose or remove any tight clothing
- Monitor BP every 2–5 minutes
- Check for bladder distension/blocked catheter and decompress bladder
- Remove faecal mass per rectum
- If systolic BP > 150 mm of Hg, then 10 mg Nifedipine sublingual or GTN (Glycerltrinitrate) spray

Preventive measures include bladder care: Prevent bladder distension and UTI.

Bowel care: Prevent faecal impaction by good bowel management program and skin and soft tissue care.

Our patient had multiple episodes of headache with goosebumps below the level of injury and was found to have an ingrowing toenail as the culprit.

11. What are the aims and management strategies for such patients with NLUTD?

Ans: The aims of management are to preserve or improve upper urinary tract function, control UTIs, and maintain a low-pressure bladder that is both continent and capable of emptying completely. The methods include bladder drainage by intermittent catheterisation or indwelling catheter.

Oral antimuscarinics (tolterodine, darifenacin, solifenacin) and mirabegron with dose-escalation are the first-line pharmacological treatment for patients with NLUTD in order to improve NDO, decrease urinary incontinence, and lower detrusor pressures. Combining antimuscarinics may be beneficial for patients who are refractory to dose escalation antimuscarinic monotherapy.[2] The response rate to oral antimuscarinics is 30–40%.[12] In whom antimuscarinic drugs have proved to be ineffective or poorly tolerated or patients with unfavourable urodynamic findings consider intravesical botulinum toxin 200 vs 300 units.[13]

12. How do you follow-up such patients?

Ans: SCI patients are considered to be having moderate to high risk NLUTD and require annual focused history, physical exam, and symptom assessment.

Annual renal function assessment and annual upper tract imaging. Annual urodynamic studies preferably with fluoroscopy should be done.[8]

13. What is asymptomatic bacteriuria and its significance?

Ans: CA-ASB (catheter associated asymptomatic bacteriuria) in patients with indwelling urethral, indwelling suprapubic, or intermittent catheterisation is defined by the presence of ≥105 cfu/ml of ≥1 bacterial species in a single catheter urine specimen in a patient without symptoms compatible with UTI.[14] First and foremost, catheter-associated ASB should not be screened for, unless there is suspicion of a UTI except in pregnant patients and patients undergoing urological procedures where mucosal bleeding is likely to be encountered. Do not treat asymptomatic bacteriuria except in pregnant women and patients undergoing urological intervention.

SUMMARY

- Urologists must be aware of the terminology of NLUTD and its significance.
- The method of CIC and type of catheter of IC does not affect rates of UTI in SCI patients.
- Urologist should be aware of the occurrence of Nocturnal polyuria in SCI and its sequalae along with management strategies.
- Video-urodynamics is the gold standard to evaluate lower urinary tract function in patients with SCI and should be done in all cases.
- Urologist must be aware of the entity autonomic dysreflexia, its causes and management.
- SCI patients require lifelong urological follow-up on an annual basis to prevent harmful sequalae.
- Asymptomatic bacteriuria should not be screened or treated for in SCI patients on IC unless they are undergoing any urological intervention.

REFERENCES

1. Stohrer M., Blok B., Castro-Diaz D., Chartier-Kastler E., del Popolo G., Kramer G., Pannek J., Radziszewski P., Wyndaele J.J. EAU guidelines on neurogenic lower urinary

tract dysfunction. *Eur. Urol.* 2009;56:81–88. doi: 10.1016/j.eururo.2009.04.028

2. Groen J, Pannek J, Castro Diaz D, Del Popolo G, Gross T, Hamid R, Karsenty G, Kessler TM, Schneider M, t Hoen L, Blok B (2016) Summary of European Association of Urology (EAU) Guidelines on Neuro-Urology. Eur Urol 69(2):324–333.
3. Welk B, Schneider MP, Thavaseelan J, Traini LR, Curt A, Kessler TM. Early urological care of patients with spinal cord injury. World J Urol. 2018 Oct;36(10):1537–1544. doi: 10.1007/s00345–018–2367–7. Epub 2018 Jun 9. PMID: 29948046.
4. Evaluation of the occurrence and diagnose definitions for nocturnal polyuria in spinal cord injured patients during rehabilitation. European Journal of Physical and Rehabilitation Medicine 2019 February;55(1):40–6
5. Panicker JN, Fowler CJ, Kessler TM (2015) Lower urinary tract dysfunction in the neurological patient: clinical assessment and management. Lancet Neurol 14(7):720–732.
6. Stoffel JT. Detrusor sphincter dyssynergia: a review of physiology, diagnosis, and treatment strategies. Transl Androl Urol. 2016 Feb;5(1):127–35. doi: 10.3978/j.issn.2223–4683.2016.01.08. PMID: 26904418; PMCID: PMC4739973.
7. Cowan H, Lakra C, Desai M. Autonomic dysreflexia in spinal cord injury *BMJ* 2020; 371 :m3596 doi:10.1136/bmj.m3596
8. Ginsberg DA, Boone TB, Cameron AP, Gousse A, Kaufman MR, Keays E, Kennelly MJ, Lemack GE, Rovner ES, Souter LH, Yang CC, Kraus SR. The AUA/SUFU Guideline on Adult Neurogenic Lower Urinary Tract Dysfunction: Diagnosis and Evaluation. J Urol. 2021 Nov;206(5):1097–1105.
9. Kiddoo, D., Sawatzky, B., Bascu,., & Moore, K. N. (2015). Randomized Crossover Trial of Single Use Hydrophilic Coated vs Multiple Use Polyvinylchloride Catheters for Intermittent Catheterization to Determine Incidence of Urinary Infection. The Journal of Urology, 194(1), 174–179.
10. Kavanagh A, Baverstock R, Campeau L, Carlson K, Cox A, Hickling D, Nadeau G, Stothers L, Welk B. Canadian Urological Association guideline: Diagnosis, management, and surveillance of neurogenic lower urinary tract dysfunction-Full text. Can Urol Assoc J. 2019 Jun;13(6):E157–E176.
11. Bywater M, Tornic J, Mehnert U, Kessler TM. Detrusor Acontractility after Acute Spinal Cord Injury-Myth or Reality? J Urol. 2018 Jun;199(6):1565–1570.
12. Madersbacher H, Murtz G, Stohrer M. Neurogenic detrusor overactivity in adults: A review on efficacy, tolerability, and safety of oral anti-muscarinics. Spinal Cord 2013;51:432–41.
13. Urologic Management of the Spinal Cord Injured Patient. A Joint SIU-ICUD International Consultation", Buenos Aires, Argentina, October 22, 2016.
14. Hooton TM, Bradley SF, Cardenas DD, *et al.* Diagnosis, prevention, and treatment of catheter-associated urinary tract infection in adults: 2009 International Clinical Practice Guidelines from the Infectious Diseases Society of America. Clin Infect Dis 2010;50:625–63.

Chapter
10

Initial Evaluation and Approach to Male LUTS

• *Joy Narayan Chakraborty*

LEARNING OBJECTIVES

- In most men, LUTS are primarily a quality-of-life problem rather than a health hazard.
- A stepwise approach to LUTS must include detailed evaluation to exclude confounding conditions or absolute indications requiring interventions.
- Patient reported outcome measures are useful in objectively assessing symptoms and quantifying them.
- A three day comprehensive bladder diary is very useful in assessing symptoms especially for men with storage LUTS. A uroflow and postvoid residual urine (PVR) measurement on ultrasonography are useful adjuncts.
- Perception of the patient is an important consideration in decision with regard to therapy. Advice must be offered taking into account concerns with regard to adverse effects that patients might have.
- As a general guideline, watchful waiting with lifestyle advice will be provided when symptoms are mild to moderate with minimal bother. For men with voiding LUTS, alpha-adrenegic blockers are the first choice in case of moderate to severe symptoms. In addition, 5α-reductase inhibitors (5-ARIs) can be added for prostates > 40 g.
- Antimuscarinics or beta-3 adrenergic agonists can be used in patients with bothersome storage LUTS.
- Tadalafil can relieve symptoms only in moderate to severe LUTS with or without erectile dysfunction.
- Surgery is typically effective in relieving symptoms in most men with refractory voiding symptoms. Surgical procedures need to be chosen based on considerations for patient co-morbidity, prostate size, patient expectations of adverse effects, availability of equipment, and skill of the urologist.
- Some men with may choose to undergo minimally invasive therapies suited to smaller glands and have a lower long-term efficacy. Enucleation procedures are usually reserved for men with larger prostates >80 g.

Case Scenario

A 54-year-old male IT professional presents with LUTS with predominantly voiding symptoms for six months. His IPPS score is 12 (predominantly voiding) [moderate], bother score is 3 (Mixed: Equally satisfied and dissatisfied), and the IIEF-5 score is 23 (normal). DRE reveals Grade I prostate with benign feeling. USG shows a 25 g prostate, no median lobe and a PVR of 45 ml. Urinalysis is normal. Uroflowmetry: Q_{max} 10 ml/s with a steady uninterrupted but slow flow. His PSA (after counselling) is 1.8 ng/ml, creatinine 0.87 mg/dl, and IIEF-5 score: 23. He has no comorbid conditions and is otherwise normal.

1. **What is your provisional diagnosis? Can you define the terms like LUTS, BPE, BOO and BPH?**

   Ans: Based on these findings, he has voiding dysfunction suggestive of bladder outlet obstruction.

The **International Continence Society** (*ICS Glossary on https://www.ics.org/glossary*) defines the following relevant terms:

Lower urinary tract symptoms (LUTS): A symptom related to the lower urinary tract.

Benign prostatic enlargement (BPE): A term describing increased volume of the prostate gland usually secondary to BPH.

Benign prostatic obstruction (BPO): A term used to describe bladder outlet obstruction (BOO) secondary to BPE and, therefore, usually due to BPH. BOO is an urodynamic entity and can only be diagnosed via pressure-flow studies.

Bladder outlet obstruction (BOO): A diagnosis based on urodynamic investigations, generally with relevant symptoms and signs, manifest by an abnormally slow urine flow rate, with evidence of abnormally high detrusor voiding pressures and abnormally slow urine flow during pressure-flow studies, with or without a high PVR *(modified).*

Benign prostatic hyperplasia (BPH): A term that is used exclusively to describe the histologic changes related to benign prostatic growth.

2. **Should ultrasonography and renal function tests be routinely used in all LUTS cases? What is the significance of PVR, and how would you measure it?**

Ans: The role of ultrasonography in LUTS is mainly to assess PVR and void%. Men with LUTS are not at increased risk for upper tract malignancy or other abnormalities compared to the overall population, so ultrasonography of the kidneys is not indicated unless there is: Large PVR, hematuria, or a history of urolithiasis. The incidence of renal dysfunction in male LUTS is only 11%. Thus, serum creatinine and eGFR are indicated when there is: Hydronephrosis, urinary retention and prior comorbidities like diabetes, hypertension or renal insufficiency.[1] However, in India, ultrasonography is usually performed by a radiologist with a standard full-function machine and it is reasonable to examine the kidneys. A high PVR is more closely associated with poor detrusor function rather than BOO. While there are no precise cutoffs, PVR has the following relevance:

- Higher PVR is associated with a greater chance of symptomatic progression and need for invasive therapy.
- PVR (along with serum creatinine) is useful as a safety measure—watchful waiting might not be appropriate in a patient with > 300 ml PVR.
- PVR is neither a strong predictor of future AUR nor a predictor of symptomatic outcomes from TURP.
- Otherwise, in general, elevated PVR is not a contraindication to watchful waiting or medical therapy.[2–4]

On a bladder scan, PVR can be calculated using the formula: Bladder volume (ml) = Bladder height (cm) × width (cm) × depth (cm) × 0.7.

3. **What are the shortcomings of the IPSS? Is it specific to BPH? How does AUA scoring differs from IPSS? Can you name some questionnaires other than IPSS and AUA? Alongside IPSS scoring, is it important to assess baseline sexual function?**

Ans: IPSS questionnaire has seven (7) symptom domains and one quality of life (QOL) domain, each domain has 5 points (total: 35 points) and one (1) QOL domain. The categorization is done as: Mild (0–7), Moderate (8–19) and Severe (20–35). QOL score is expressed separately. In contrast, AUA does not have any QOL domain. Other similar questionnaires are the Danish prostatic symptom score (DAN-PSS), Bristol male LUTS score, the international consultation on incontinence questionnaire for male LUTS (ICIQ-MLUTS) and the visual symptom score (VSS).

Limitations of IPSS are: (a) Storage[3] and voiding scores[4] are not distinctly categorized (b) LUTS questionnaire is non-specific to male-LUTS only (c) The score does not clarify precisely which symptom is bothersome to the patient (d) Urgency incontinence does not figure in the score although, when present, it is highly bothersome.

Also, it is preferable to assess baseline sexual health (for instance, by using the IIEF-5 questionnaire) before treating male LUTS since there is an association between sexual health and LUTS and there is an impact of all forms of treatment on sexual function.

4. **Is the PSA test mandatory before treating LUTS?**

Ans: PSA estimation is not mandatory for BPH treatment; however, it can be indicated in the following situations (after discussing with the patient): (a) To assist in the decision-making process (baseline PSA has an excellent predictive value for prostate volume and prostatic growth as well as the risk of AUR and BOO-related surgery) (b) An abnormal DRE (when the diagnosis of cancer prostate will change the management) and (c) If the patient is concerned about prostate cancer[1] (d) The patient has high-risk factors for developing prostate cancer.

5. **Would you like to do UDS in this case?**

Ans: UDS is not necessary in this case. In general, urodynamics is advised before prostate surgery in the following group of patients:

a. Men who have had previous unsuccessful (invasive) treatment for LUTS.
b. Patients who cannot void >150 ml for a valid uroflow trace
c. When considering surgery in men with bothersome, predominantly voiding LUTS with
   i. a PVR >300 ml
   ii. age >80 years and <50 years.
d. Men with relatively higher flow rates (>10 ml/s) with bothersome voiding symptoms
e. Concomitant neurological conditions such as Parkinsonism
f. Dominant storage symptoms[1]

6. **What treatment option would you offer this patient at this point? Do you think this patient has the potential for disease progression?**

Ans: As this patient has only moderate symptoms (IPSS 12) with fewer bothersome symptoms,[3] watchful waiting with behavioural and dietary modifications is reasonable. It includes patient education, reassurance (that cancer is not a cause of the urinary symptoms), periodic monitoring and lifestyle advice. The 5-year treatment failure rate is 20%, and 80% of patients remain clinically stable.

He has predictive factors [PSA value >1.4 and IPSS >7] for BPH progression.

In general, the predictors of BPH-progression are: Age > 60, Prostate volume > 30 ml., PSA > 1.4, IPSS > 7, Q_{max} < 12 ml/s and PVR > 50 ml/s[2].

The Olmsted County study revealed a symptom score deterioration of 0.18/year, with the fastest rate of deterioration observed in the 60–69 age group. There is a gradual increase in urinary symptoms with age, with a prevalence of 13% of men aged 40–49, rising to 28% of men over 70. PLESS study (placebo arm) also showed a decreased flow rate over four years, 7% AUR and 45% needed TURP. In MTOPS (placebo arm) study, only 17% of patients show clinical progression.[3]

7. **How would you monitor this patient and assess whether BPH progresses clinically?**

Ans: I would monitor him periodically at six weeks, and then every 6–12 months using IPPS-score, uroflow and PVR, and will look for the clinical indicators of progression, which are: IPSS > 4 points increase (on two occasions within four weeks), AUR, recurrent UTI, renal insufficiency (> 50% rise in baseline creatinine or > 1.5 mg/dl) and incontinence.[2]

8. **This patient returned after six months with increasing voiding difficulty. IPSS is now 18, bother score 5, Q_{max} 13 ml/s, IIEF-5 score 23 and a PVR of 50 ml. What treatment would you offer now?**

Ans: In addition to patient education and lifestyle advice, I would offer medical management (Alpha blocker: Alfuzosin). Alpha-1 Blockers are the first-line treatment for male LUTS because of their rapid onset of action, good efficacy, and low rate and severity of adverse events. Among the Alpha-1 blockers, Tamsulosin and Silodosin are more associated with ejaculatory disorder (EjD) than Alfuzosin or Doxazocin. As the patient is younger, I would prefer Alfuzosin.

9. **What is your opinion regarding combination therapy with 5-ARI for this patient?**

Ans: Combination therapy with 5-ARI is not indicated here, as his prostate is small (<40 g) with moderate symptoms only. However, 5-ARI is beneficial when prostate size is >40 g. It is slow acting (it takes 3–6 months to start work).

5-ARIs reduce the prostatic volume by 25%, improves symptom score by 1.6 points, and, to some extent, improve flow rate by 2 ml/s. Combination therapy reduces the risk of clinical progression by two-thirds (66%) and reduces the relative risk of AUR by 68%, and the need for surgery by 64% at four years[2,4,5] It is important to exclude prostate cancer and document a baseline serum PSA before initiating therapy.

10. **Do you think he will benefit from tadalafil? Does Q_{max} increase with the use of PDEI-5?**

Ans: Suitable candidates for PDEI-5 are: Younger men with low BMI and more severe LUTS. Our index patient has an IIEF score of 23 (normal sexual function). Although tadalafil is not indicated for improving erectile function, tadalafil has been shown to independently improve LUTS without improving Q_{max}.[6] However, most clinicians would choose to use the drug when there is concomitant LUTS and erectile dysfunction.

11. **This patient returned after another eight months. Although there is some improvement in flow rate (Q_{max} 13.5 ml/s), he has developed storage symptoms (daytime frequency of 10 and nocturia of 3 times) with a PVR is 70 ml. What can you offer him? Any additional drugs?**

Ans: Yes, at this point, I would like to add anti-muscarinics. Options for antimuscarinics are Tolterodine ER,[7] Solifenacin [M2 and M3 selective],[8] or Darifenacin [M3 selective]. Antimuscarinics considerably help reduce the storage symptoms; however, they can increase PVR, although there is no evidence of AUR. Hence it should be avoided when the baseline PVR is >150 ml. Also, regular vigilance for worsening IPSS, Q_{max} and PVR is crucial while on antimuscarinics.[9]

Alternatively, a beta-3 agonist (mirabegron) can be given.[10] Mirabegron improves storage LUTS and has a better patient tolerance. However, untreated hypertension or hypersensitivity to mirabegron is its contraindication. Mirabegron does not adversely affect voiding urodynamic parameters and the small increase in PVR seen in systematic review is not clinically relevant.

It is reasonable to start with one drug for improving storage symptoms and add a second class of mediation in case symptoms fail to improve. This strategy is preferable to enhance the dose of antimuscarinics.[11]

12. **This patient returned after 18 months with increasing voiding difficulty. IPSS is 24, bother score 6 and Q_{max} 9.5 ml/s. Prostate size is 30 g with 100 ml**

PVR, no middle lobe. The patient is now visibly upset with his flow. What will you offer him now?

Ans: I would counsel him in favour of surgical intervention as his symptom score, and PVR is rising with a reduced Q_{max} despite continuing medical management.

13. **Flexible cystoscopy shows high bladder neck with bladder trabeculations, Grade I prostate, and no middle lobe. Which surgical technique would you like to choose and why?**

Ans: Options for surgical management for him are: TUIP (transurethral incision of the prostate) or prostatic urethral lift (PUL): **The MIST of choice in this situation is iTIND**. As the prostatic volume is small, a monopolar TUIP (transurethral incision of the prostate) after proper patient counselling is reasonable. One must counsel the patient regarding risks of EjD and ED, which are 40% and 14%, respectively. For men concerned with loss of ejaculation, an ejaculation-sparing technique can be offered.

Another option for men who want to preserve ejaculation is UroLIFT. This is indicated only if the gland shows enlargement. It is effective in: (a) Relieving symptoms, (b) ejaculation and continence preserving, (c) no sexual dysfunction and (d) but has a higher surgical re-treatment rate as compared with conventional surgery. UroLIFT is easy to apply, with rapid onset of action without post-procedure catheterisation. It is preferable when the prostate volume is <80 g without any middle lobe.

Rezum™ is a minimally invasive water therapy for benign prostate enlargement. It utilizes conductive heat transfer that exploits the thermodynamic properties of water. The system comprises the radiofrequency generator and single use transurethral delivery system. The system is approved by FDA. The advantages are that it can be performed under sedation only, as a day case procedure, there are no reports of *de novo* sexual dysfunction, can be done in an obstructing median lobe. Results show sustained improvement in IPSS, QOL

iTIND™, a device from Olympus™. The principle on which it works considers the prostatic obstruction as a structural obstruction and works to reshape the prostate. The device is placed in the urethra in a folded configuration . During the 5 to 7 days that it is inserted it reshapes the urethra. Between the 5th and 7th day the device is removed. The advantage of iTND is that it can act as a bridge in young patient sexually active requiring treatment and not responding to medical management.

A flexible cystoscopy is not ordinarily necessary but might be useful in select situations for excluding confounding diagnoses or in case minimally invasive surgical therapies are being considered.

SUMMARY

- The most critical domain in IPSS scoring is the QOL score which is closely reflects the patient's bother and might indicated the need for invasive interventions.
- Alpha-blockers do not reduce the long-term risk of AUR or the need for surgery. There is a little evidence to show that any one alpha adrenergic blocker is more effective than the others.
- 5-ARI improves IPSS and improves Q_{max} but the effects take several months. Also, it reduces prostatic volume and the risk of AUR and BPH-related surgery.
- Do not prescribe antimuscarinics when PVR>150 ml.
- Mirabegron has a better tolerance profile than antimuscarinics.

REFERENCES

1. EAU Guidelines. Edn. presented at the EAU Annual Congress Milan March 2023. ISBN 978-94-92671-*19-6*. [http://uroweb.org/guidelines/compilations-of-all-guidelines/]
2. Marberger M. The MTOPS Study: New findings, new insights, and clinical implications for the management of BPH. European urology supplements. 2006 Jun 1;5(9):628–33.
3. Fitzpatrick JM. The natural history of benign prostatic hyperplasia. BJU international. 2006 Apr;97:3–6.
4. Roehrborn CG, *et al.* The effects of combination therapy with dutasteride and tamsulosin on clinical outcomes in men with symptomatic benign prostatic hyperplasia: 4-year results from the CombAT study. European urology. 2010 Jan 1;57(1):123–31.
5. Roehrborn CG. BPH progression: concept and key learning from MTOPS, ALTESS, COMBAT, and ALF-ONE. BJU Int, 2008. 101 Suppl 3: 17.
6. Gacci M, *et al* A systematic review and meta-analysis on the use of phosphodiesterase 5 inhibitors alone or in combination with alpha-blockers for lower urinary tract symptoms due to benign prostatic hyperplasia. Eur Urol, 2012. 61: 994.
7. Kaplan SA, *et al.* Extended-release tolterodine with or without tamsulosin in men with lower urinary tract symptoms and overactive bladder: effects on urinary symptoms assessed by the International Prostate Symptom Score. BJU international. 2008 Nov;102(9):1133–9.
8. Abrams P, *et al.* Combination treatment with mirabegron and solifenacin in patients with overactive bladder: exploratory responder analyses of efficacy and evaluation of patient-reported outcomes from a randomised, double-blind, factorial, dose-ranging, Phase II study (SYMPHONY). World J Urol, 2017. 35: 827.
9. Chapple C, *et al.* Fesoterodine clinical efficacy and safety for the treatment of overactive bladder in relation to patient profiles: a systematic review. Curr Med Res Opin, 2015. 31: 1201.
10. Kakizaki H, *et al.* Mirabegron add-on therapy to tamsulosin for the treatment of overactive bladder in men with lower urinary tract symptoms: a randomised, placebo-controlled study (MATCH). European Urology Focus. 2020 Jul 15;6(4):729–37.
11. Drake MJ, *et al.* Efficacy and Safety of Mirabegron Add-on Therapy to Solifenacin in Incontinent Overactive Bladder Patients with an Inadequate Response to Initial 4-Week Solifenacin Monotherapy: A Randomised Double-blind Multicentre Phase 3B Study (BESIDE). Eur Urol, 2016.70: 136.

Chapter

11

Surgical Management of Patients with Large Benign Prostatic Enlargement (>80 gm) Refractory to Medical Management

• Rohit Sethi • Nitin Kekre

LEARNING OBJECTIVES

- Evaluation of LUTS with emphasis on the role of proper history, physical examination and assessment of prostate volume.
- Role of basic investigations like ultrasonography and uroflowmetry and pressure flow studies.
- Management issues with regards to large prostate gland.
- Treatment options for large prostate gland with their pros and cons.
- Role of emerging future technologies.

Case Scenario

66 years old gentleman presented with complains of poor flow, straining, frequency, nocturia (2–3 times) and incomplete emptying for 2 years. On digital rectal examination, his anal tone was normal, he had grade 3 clinically benign enlarged prostate. His IPSS score was 24/35 and QOL score was 5. His flowmetry report was 7/320/100. He was on combination therapy for 2 years with minimal symptomatic benefit.

1. **How would you evaluate this patient?**

   Ans: A **complete medical history** should be elicited with special emphasis on patient symptoms, bother, previous treatment, retention episodes (if any) with volume drained on catheterisation, urethral instrumentation, patient's comorbid illness (medications including antiplatelets/ anticoagulants or any recent prescriptions which can precipitate retention), sexual history, fluid intake and his overall fitness and health.

   Physical examination including digital rectal examination and focussed neurological examination should be performed. It is important to note that DRE estimation of prostate volume is not accurate, more so in larger glands.

   Laboratory investigations including **urinalysis** (to look for haematuria, pyuria to rule out infection and glucosuria), **renal function test** and **blood glucose estimation. Uroflowmetry with postvoid residue** assessment should be performed in all cases. **Serum PSA** estimation as a proxy for prostate volume may be performed.

   Imaging with ultrasonography should be performed to look for upper tracts (especially in cases with high PVR and increased creatinine). **Ultrasound estimation of prostate volume** and presence of intravesical protrusion is helpful in planning treatment. Intravesical **prostatic protrusion more than 10 mm** correlates with urodynamically proven bladder outlet obstruction.[1] It also predicts poor outcomes with medical therapy.[1] Increased bladder wall thickness is associated with urodynamically confirmed BOO.[2] Prostate volume can be assessed with abdominal or transrectal ultrasonography or cross-sectional imaging techniques such as computed tomography (CT) or magnetic resonance imaging (MRI). Most common modality for assessment of prostate size in routine clinical practice is transabdominal ultrasound. Apart from the fact that any **ultrasound is operator dependent**, it is important to remember that transabdominal ultrasound overestimates gland size by over 50%[12]. Transrectal ultrasound assessment is more accurate but uncomfortable and is not performed routinely. **Assessment of prostate volume and presence or absence of median lobe is essential** to best select the surgical procedure for management. It has direct relationship with the outcome, durability, and risk of surgical procedures (Fig. 11.1).

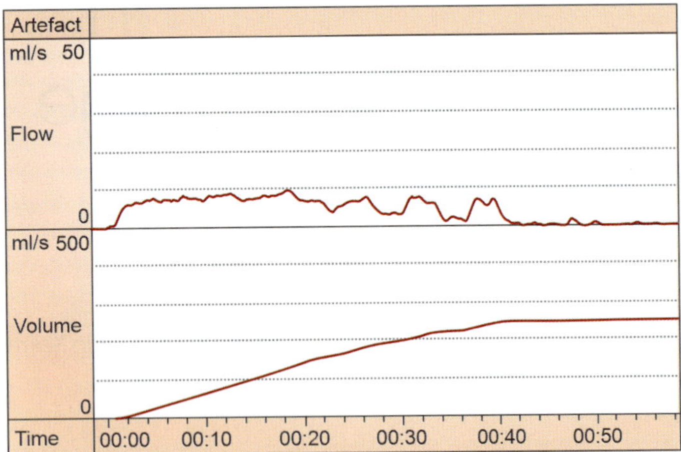

Fig. 11.1: Uroflowmetry showed Q_{max} of 7 ml/sec, voided volume of 320 ml and postvoid residue of 100 cc

2. **What is the definition of large prostate?**

   Ans: A large prostate is arbitrarily defined as a prostate size of more than 80 g or 80 cc on transabdominal ultrasound imaging as per EAU guidelines and size cut-off taken as per clinical trials.

3. **What is the role of pressure flow studies in evaluation of BPO?**

   Ans: Pressure flow studies are not routinely recommended prior to surgical intervention, but should be considered when there is a doubt regarding diagnosis of bladder outlet obstruction. As per EAU guidelines, it **should be performed in following situations:**[17]
   - Voided volume less than 150 ml
   - Q_{max} more than 15 ml/sec
   - Age less than 50 or more than 80 years
   - Persistent postvoid residue over 300 ml
   - History of previous surgical treatment

   It can also be performed in patients with long-standing diabetes with peripheral neuropathy, history of stroke or intermittent straining pattern of uroflowmetry.

4. **How would you counsel the patient regarding surgical treatment?**

   Ans: Patient **should be counselled thoroughly** regarding various **surgical alternatives**, their expected outcomes and specific side effect profile, more so regarding sexual side effects. **Most surgical procedures cause ejaculatory dysfunction**. Libido and Erectile function are usually not affected unless present prior to surgical intervention.[3] **The patients desirous of preserving ejaculatory function may be offered either water vapor thermal therapy or prostatic urethral lift.**

5. **What are the various surgical approaches for management of BPO?**

   Ans: The treatment approach would depend on the availability of newer technology and expertise, presence of large median lobe, patient on anticoagulants, concurrent vesical stone and patient's attitude towards potential sexual side effects.[4] Surgeon's own experience, preference and cost of treatment would also play a major role in treatment selection.

   Various surgical approaches can be classified as:
   - Resection: Monopolar or bipolar TURP, thulium vaporesection
   - Enucleation: LASER enucleation (holmium, thulium, TFL and diode), bipolar transurethral enucleation, open prostatectomy, minimally invasive laparoscopic or robotic assisted simple prostatectomy
   - Vaporisation: Transurethral bipolar vaporisation of prostate, green light LASER vaporisation of prostate

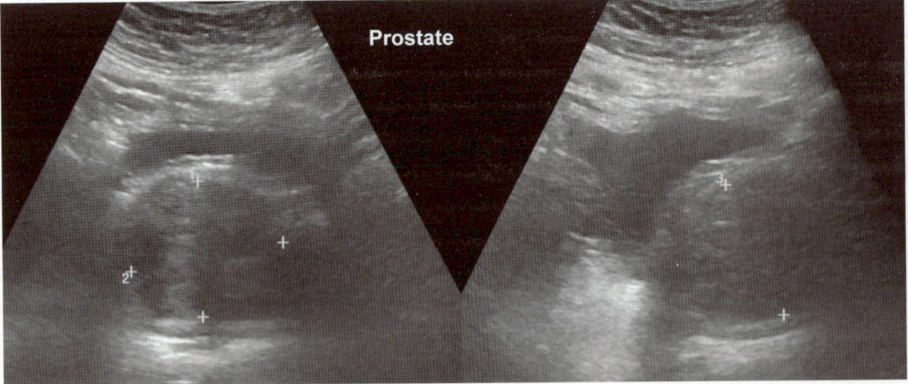

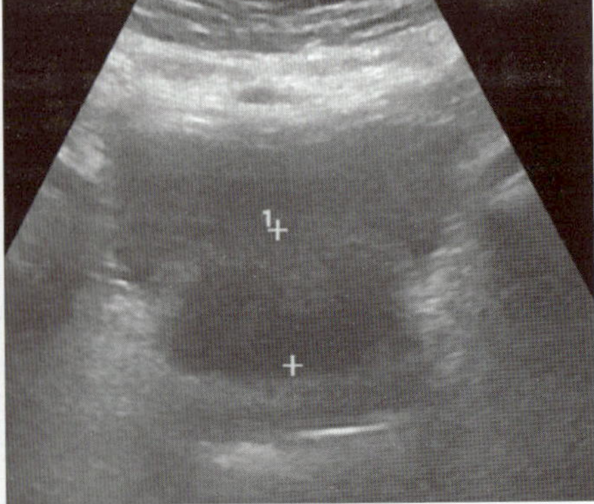

Fig. 11.2: Ultrasonography showed enlarged prostate of 120 cc volume with intravesical prostatic protrusion of about 2 cm and thickened and irregular bladder wall

- Alternative ablative techniques: Aquablation, convective water vapour energy ablation (Rezum) and prostatic artery embolization.
- Non-ablative techniques: Prostatic urethral lift, intraprostatic injections, iTIND.

6. **What are the problems with monopolar TURP in surgical management of larger prostates?**

Ans: Monopolar TURP (M-TURP) has long been a gold standard technique for the surgical management of LUTS/BPO with proven track record. However, M-TURP has major limitations in larger glands (>80 cc) due to increased risks of dilutional hyponatremia, excessive blood loss and increased perioperative morbidity. Outcome depends upon surgeon's skill, experience and resection speed. Hence, **M-TURP is not a preferable approach for treatment of patients with larger glands**. In situations where other modalities/expertise is not available, a staged M-TURP can be an option. Many a times patient can have a successful outcome even with hemi-TURP. Most of these limitations can be overcome with use of bipolar saline TURP.

7. **What are the preferred surgical treatment modalities for larger glands?**

Ans: Preferred surgical treatment for patients with gland size **more than 80 ml are HOLEP, Bipolar enucleation and Open prostatectomy** (EAU guidelines 2023). Other alternative treatments include LASER vaporisation, Thulium enucleation and bipolar TURP.[5]

8. **What is the status of HOLEP in large prostates?**

Ans: Holmium LASER energy creates a vaporization bubble that destructs prostatic tissue with minimal deep tissue penetration. Enucleation is carried out along the surgical capsule. The enucleated prostatic adenoma is then morcellated and removed.

HOLEP is a size independent option and has outcomes equivalent to TURP and open prostatectomy.[6,7] But has **advantage of shorter indwelling catheter time, hospital stay** and fewer perioperative bleeding related complications.[7] It can be safely performed on patients on anticoagulants and antiplatelets.[4]

The **main limitations are increased cost, longer operative time** and higher incidence of transient stress urinary incontinence.[6] It has a steep learning curve and is available only in select centres.

9. **Is Bipolar enucleation a good alternative?**

Ans: Obstructive adenoma is enucleated endoscopically using bipolar technology. The enucleated gland is either removed by morcellation or resection.

A RCT evaluating BPEP vs. B-TURP in prostate volume > 80 ml reported that BPEP had comparable outcomes with respect to reduction in IPSS, improvement in Q_{max} and reduction in PVR. It showed longer operative time, shorter catheterisation and hospitalisation time with no differences in blood transfusion, urethral stricture and UI rates at 24 months follow-up.[8]

An RCT comparing HoLEP vs. bipolar transurethral enucleation reported no significant difference in IPSS, QoL score, PVR, and Q_{max} at one month, three-, and twelve months follow-up.[9]

10. **What are the advantages and disadvantages of open prostatectomy?**

Ans: Obstructive adenomas are enucleated using the index finger, approaching from within the bladder (Freyer procedure) or through the anterior prostatic capsule (Millin procedure). **It is used for substantially enlarged glands, preferably for over 150 g.**

A systematic review and meta-analysis of RCTs comparing transurethral enucleation of prostate (TUEP) and transvesical open prostatectomy (OP) showed equivalent clinical outcomes at 1, 3, 6 months and 1 year follow-up. Perioperative outcomes including hemoglobin level drop, catheter period, irrigation length and hospital stay favoured TUEP, while operative time and resected prostate weight favoured OP. There was significantly less blood transfusion with TUEP.[10]

Open prostatectomy is the most invasive surgical method, but it is an effective and durable procedure for the treatment of LUTS/BPO. In the absence of an endourological armamentarium including a holmium laser or a bipolar system and with appropriate patient consent, OP is a reasonable surgical treatment of choice for men with prostates >100 ml.

11. **What is the role of minimally invasive simple prostatectomy?**

Ans: Minimally invasive simple prostatectomy (MISP) including laparoscopic simple prostatectomy and robotic assisted simple prostatectomy have shown similar functional outcomes when compared with open prostatectomy with shorter hospital stay, blood loss and transfusion rates and longer operative duration.[11] Most studies on MISP are of retrospective nature. The literature lacks good quality evidence but it is a reasonable option in experienced hands.

12. **What are the newer emerging treatment modalities?**

Ans: Newer treatment options like **Prostalift, Rezum, Aquablation, iTIND and prostatic artery**

embolization are emerging and require good quality RCTs to define their role in management of large prostates.

13. **What is the role of prostatic artery embolization?**
Ans: The role of prostatic artery embolization in management of BPO is evolving. Studies with 1 year and 2 years follow-up have shown significant clinical improvement in patient reported outcomes like IPSS, QoL, flow rate, postvoid residual urine and prostate volume.[14] However, in comparison to TURP the reported clinical outcomes were inferior with increased retreatment rate.[15] PAE may be a safe and effective treatment option in patients who are not fit for surgery or not desirous of surgical treatment.

14. **What is the role of aquablation?**
Ans: Aquablation is a novel, minimally invasive treatment that uses high speed water jet for prostate ablation using image guidance and robotics using the Aquabeam system (PROCEPT BioRobotics). A multicentre international prospective trial (Water II) in treatment in men with prostate volume of 80–150 cc showed effective clinical outcomes which were sustained at 3 years follow-up with low retreatment rates.[16]

KEY POINTS

- A complete history with physical examination with focussed neurological examination are essential for evaluation of such a patient.
- Intravesical prostatic protrusion of more 10 mm correlates with urodynamically proven obstruction.
- As per EAU guidelines a large prostate is arbitrarily defined as a prostate measuring larger than 80 cc.
- Preferred surgical treatment for patients with gland size **more than 80 ml are HoLEP and bipolar enucleation. Open/robotic/laparoscopic simple prostatectomy are options where expertise are available.**
- Newer treatment options like **Prostalift, Rezum, Aquablation, iTIND and prostatic artery embolization** are emerging technologies and require good quality RCTs to establish their role.

SUMMARY

- Evaluation of LUTS includes complete medical history, physical examination and laboratory investigations including urinalysis, renal function tests, blood glucose estimation, uroflowmetry with postvoid residue assessment and imaging with ultrasonography to assess bladder wall thickness, prostate volume and presence of intravesical protrusion.
- Ultrasonography is operator dependent and transabdominal ultrasound overestimates gland size by over 50%.[12] Transrectal ultrasound assessment is more accurate.
- Factors predicting poor outcome with medical management are: Prostate volume more than 40 ml,[13] serum PSA more than 1.4 ng/ml,[13] significant intravesical prostatic protrusion[1] and increased bladder wall thickness.[2]
- Intravesical prostatic protrusion more than 10 mm correlates with urodynamically proven bladder outlet obstruction.[1]
- Assessment of prostate volume and presence or absence of median lobe is essential to select the appropriate surgical procedure.
- Pressure flow studies are not routinely recommended prior to surgical intervention, but should be performed when there is doubt regarding diagnosis of bladder outlet obstruction.
- A large prostate is arbitrarily defined as a prostate size of more than 80 g or 80 cc on ultrasound imaging as per EAU guidelines.[5]
- Limitations of monopolar TURP in surgical management of large prostate are: Increased risks of dilutional hyponatremia, excessive blood loss, increased perioperative morbidity and outcome dependent upon surgeon's skill, experience and resection speed. Hence, M-TURP is not a preferrable approach for treatment of patients with larger glands.
- Preferred surgical treatment for patients with gland size more than 80 ml are: HoLEP, bipolar enucleation and open prostatectomy. Other alternative treatments include LASER vaporisation, thulium enucleation and TURP.[5] Minimally invasive simple prostatectomy (MISP) including laparoscopic simple prostatectomy and robotic assisted simple prostatectomy are reasonable treatment options in experienced hands.
- Prostalift, Rezum, Aquablation, iTIND and prostatic artery embolization are emerging new technologies and require good quality RCTs to define their role.

REFERENCES

1. Keqin Z, *et al.* Clinical significance of intravesical prostatic protrusion in patients with benign prostatic enlargement. Urology. 2007; 70(6) : 1096.
2. Bright E, Oelke M, Tubaro A, Abrams P. Ultrasound estimated bladder weight and bladder wall thickness–Useful non-invasive methods for assessing the lower urinary tract? J Urol. 2010; 184(5) : 1847. Epub 2010 Sep 17.
3. Mishriki SF, Grimsley SJS, Lam T, Nabi G, Cohen NP. TURP and Sex : Patient and partner prospective 12 years follow up study. BJUI; 28 June 2011.
4. Lerner LB, McVary KT, Barry MJ *et al.* Management of lower urinary tract symptoms attributed to benign prostatic hyperplasia: AUA guidelines part II – Surgical evaluation and treatment. J Urol 2021: 206(4) : 818. Epub 2021 Aug 13.
5. EAU guidelines. Edn. Presented at EAU annual Congress Milan 2023. ISBN 978-94-92671-19-6.
6. Kuntz RM, Ahyai S, Lehrich K, Fayed A. Transurethral Holmium LASER enucleation of prostate versus transurethral electrocautery resection of prostate : A randomized prospective trial in 200 patients. J Urol 2004; 172(3): 1012.
7. Kuntz RM, Lehrich K, Ahyai SA. Holmium laser enucleation of prostate versus open prostatectomy for prostates greated than 100 grams : 5 year follow up results of a Randomized clinical trial. Eur Urol. 2008; 53(1):160. Epub 2007 Aug 28.
8. Samir M., *et al.* Two year follow up in Bipolar transurethral enucleation and resection of prostate in comparison with Bipolar transurethral resection of prostate in treatment of large prostates. Randomized Controlled trial. Urology 2019. 133:192.

9. Higazy A. *et al.* Holmium laser enucleation of prostate versus bipolar transurethral enucleation of prostate in management of Benign prostatic hyperplasia. A RCT. Int J Urol, 2021.28:333.
10. Lin Y, *et al.* Transurethral enucleation of prostate versus transvesical open prostatectomy for large benign prostatic hyperplasia. A systematic review and Meta analysis of RCTs. World J Urol, 2016. 34:1207.
11. Li J, *et al.* Comparison between Minimally invasive Simple prostatectomy and open simple prostatectomy for large prostates : A systematic review and meta analysis of comparative trials. J Endourol, 2019.33:767.
12. Stravodimos KG, Petrolekas A, Kapetanakis T, Vourekas S, Koritsiadis G, Adamakis I, Mitropoulos D, Constantinides C. TRUS versus transabdominal ultrasound as a predictor of enucleated adenoma weight in patients with BPH: a tool for standard preoperative work-up? Int Urol Nephrol. 2009 Dec;41(4):767–71. Epub 2009 Apr 7.
13. Roehrborn CG, Boyle P, Bergner D, Gray T, Gittelman M, Shown T, Melman A, Bracken RB, deVere White R, Taylor A, Wang D, Waldstreicher J. Serum prostate-specific antigen and prostate volume predict long-term changes in symptoms and flow rate: results of a four-year, randomized trial comparing finasteride versus placebo. PLESS Study Group. Urology. 1999 Oct;54(4):662–9.
14. Somwaru, A.S., Metting, S., Flisnik, L.M. *et al.* Prostate artery embolization has long term efficacy for treatment of severe lower urinary tract symptoms from giant prostatic hyperplasia. *BMC Urol* 20, 153 (2020).
15. Dominic A, Müllhaupt G, Hechelhammer L, Markart S, Güsewell S, *et al.* Prostatic Artery Embolisation Versus Transurethral Resection of the Prostate for Benign Prostatic Hyperplasia: 2-yr Outcomes of a Randomised, Open-label, Single-centre Trial, European Urology, Volume 80, Issue 1, 2021, Pages 34–42.
16. Assad A, Nguyen D, Barber N, Bidair M, Gilling P, Anderson P, Badlani G, Humphreys M, Kaplan S, Kaufman R, So A, Paterson R, Desai M, Roehrborn C, Chughtai B, Zorn KC, Elterman D, Bhojani N, WATER vs WATER II 3-Year Update: Comparing Aquablation Therapy for Benign Prostatic Hyperplasia in 30–80 cc and 80–150 cc Prostates, Urology, Volume 165, 2022, Pages 268–274.
17. Gratzke C. *et al.* (2015). EAU guidelines on the assessment of non-neurogenic male lower urinary tract symptoms including benign prostatic obstruction. Eur. Urol. 67(6) : 1099–1109.

Chapter 12

Parkinsonism with Male LUTS

• *Sanjay Sinha*

LEARNING OBJECTIVES

- Parkinson's disease (PD) is a common degenerative neuro-urological condition chiefly affecting dopamine pathways in the substantia nigra, that can cause or complicate the presence of lower urinary tract symptoms (LUTS) in the elderly male. The classical triad of clinical features includes skeletal muscle rigidity, tremors and bradykinesia. These symptoms are often referred to as Parkinsonism.
- Several allied conditions can mimic the condition and often appear under an umbrella of the term 'Parkinsonism'. The precise underlying diagnosis can have profound implications for the outcome of urological treatments and interventions.
- LUTS can be the primary presenting feature of PD-like conditions such as MSA. Hence, it is imperative that the urologist should be able to identify the potential presence of this condition and seek a neurological consultation before offering surgical intervention.
- Patients with PD typically develop LUTS years after the onset of PD. Storage symptoms tend to be dominant with some patients experiencing difficulty in voiding. Urodynamics typically shows neurogenic detrusor overactivity. While some patients may show an impaired relaxation of the striated sphincter (bradykinesia) genuine dyssynergia has not been demonstrated.
- Patients with MSA develop LUTS early in the course of disease and often present with LUTS. Common symptoms include storage symptoms, voiding difficulty and urinary retention. Urodynamics typically shows neurogenic detrusor overactivity and inappropriate bladder neck relaxation during filling, with detrusor sphincter dyssynergia during voiding.
- Conservative management is the first option in a setting of LUTS with PD. Standard medication for storage symptoms includes beta-3 and (cautious use of) antimuscarinics. Alpha-adrenergic blockers are the mainstay for voiding LUTS. Patients with a large prostate or PSA≥1.4ng/ml can be offered a 5ARI after excluding the possibility of a neoplasm as per guidelines.[1,2]
- Differentiating the underlying diagnosis and the precise lower urinary tract dysfunction on the basis of clinical evaluation alone can be challenging. Hence, surgery should ordinarily be offered only following urodynamics evaluation. Video-urodynamics is the preferred method of evaluation.
- Men with PD who have video-urodynamics confirmed obstruction at the bladder neck or prostate can undergo surgery for the prostate or bladder neck with the expectation of a satisfactory outcome. Men with MSA who show a dyssynergic outlet should not be offered surgery and should be managed by intermittent catheterization or an indwelling catheter (suprapubic when appropriate).

Case Scenario

A 73-year-old male presented with refractory LUTS both storage and voiding for the last 1 year. He has urinary frequency, urgency, occasional urgency incontinence, voiding difficulty and nocturia, 3 times a night. He has mild constipation but evacuates daily with the help of a laxative. Digital rectal examination shows normal perineal sensation, absent cremasteric reflex, normal anal tone with mild reduction in bulbocavernosal reflex. Overall, focused neuro-urological examination is age-appropriate. Prostate gland is about 35 g in size consistent with benign enlargement. He is not diabetic or hypertensive and has normal blood chemistry and urine examination. He has been seen by the physician and is on treatment for Parkinson's disease for the last 4 months. He underwent an ultrasound scan that showed prevoid bladder volume 190 ml, postvoid residual (PVR) 70 ml, prostate 42 g, and no hydronephrosis. He has been taking silodosin 8mg at night for the past 6 months but continues to have bothersome symptoms. A uroflow test done on presentation showed sustained flow with maximum flow rate 9ml per second, voided volume 130 ml with 40ml PVR.

1. **How would you approach evaluation of his LUTS?**

   Ans: It is crucial to determine what symptoms are bothering the patient.[3,4] This can be determined by careful questioning but is best confirmed by use of a patient reported outcome measure such as IPSS score. Specifically, it is important to determine whether he is more bothered by storage LUTS or voiding LUTS. In general, urgency and urgency incontinence (when present) tend to be bothersome for patients. Drawbacks of the IPSS scoring system are lack of a question with regard to urgency incontinence and lack of information with regard to the bother from individual symptoms. The 'International Consultation on Incontinence Male LUTS' scoring addresses these issues and is validated. There are also translations for this questionnaire available in most Indian languages.[3] He needs a bladder diary to document baseline symptoms and check for overhydration as well as nocturnal polyuria. The PD symptoms, severity, course of illness, physical limitations or cognitive dysfunction, and therapy must be assessed.

This patient has an **IPSS score of 22 (severe) with dominant storage symptoms**. Voiding sub-score is 9, while storage sub-score is 13. **Quality of life score is 5** (unhappy). His PD symptoms are mild. He has slow but independent ambulation and has mild cognitive dysfunction. He can take care of himself. ICI mLUTS questionnaire of the patient can also be mentioned and the difference b/w IPSS and ICI score be briefly demonstrated.

2. **What medication would you recommend for his bothersome urgency?**

   Ans: Both antimuscarinics and beta-3 agonists are recommended options. However, given his voiding symptoms and neurological condition, and the small possibility of aggravation by antimuscarinics, hence mirabegron is perhaps the better choice. In case he has adverse events with mirabegron, solifenacin, darifenacin and trospium are the antimuscarinics least likely to cause neuro-cognitive deterioration. He must continue his lifestyle changes, bladder training and bowel care.[4,5]

3. **How does PD impact LUTS in the elderly male?**

   Ans: Parkinson's disease is an idiopathic neurodegenerative disorder primarily impacting the dopamine pathways in the substantia nigra as well as other locations. Reduction in dopaminergic activity is associated with the clinical features of Parkinsonism. The classical triad of presenting features is rigidity of the skeletal muscles, tremor and bradykinesia. Several conditions can present with features of Parkinsonism including multisystem atrophy (MSA), progressive supranuclear palsy and Lewy body dementia. LUTS is noted in one-third to two-thirds of patients and includes nocturia, urinary frequency, urgency and urgency urinary incontinence. These four symptoms account for half to three quarters of patients. Voiding difficulty is less common. Symptoms of PD can overlap regular LUTS in the elderly male owing to problems related to the bladder or prostate. Non-urological symptoms can complicate the presentation of LUTS including conversion of urgency into urgency incontinence in patients with limited mobility.[6–8]

4. **What would you recommend for LUTS that remains refractory despite silodosin 8 mg, solifenacin 5 mg, and mirabegron 50 mg in this patient?**

   Ans: He needs a re-evaluation of bladder diary, uroflow, PVR, and desire for further escalation. Therapies for PD such as deep brain stimulation can improve urinary symptoms while drugs such as bromocriptine might exacerbate them. Further improvements in LUTS are likely to only come from invasive urological therapies. Invasive urodynamics is recommended in this setting prior to urological intervention.[5,7,9]

5. **What are the typical urodynamics findings in PD?**

   Ans: Patients with PD classically show (neurogenic) detrusor overactivity (45–93%) during filling cystometry. This is associated with early sensations and reduced bladder capacity (46%).[6] Voiding phase abnormality is less common. Detrusor underactivity, acontractility and combined detrusor overactivity with underactivity have been noted in 40%, 16% and 9%, respectively.[6]

6. **What is the key differential diagnosis?**

   Ans: PD is characterized by resting tremor, an asymmetry of neurological findings and good response to levodopa therapy. It is crucial to exclude MSA as a differential diagnosis. MSA is another neuro-degenerative condition with symptoms of parkinsonism along with autonomic failure and cerebellar ataxia. There is diffuse gliosis and cellular destruction. There is involvement of the parasympathetic pathways and Onuf's nucleus. MSA has a different clinical course, is less responsive to medication, and seldom responds to surgery. Identifying MSA can help avoid prostate surgery which almost invariably fails.[7]

7. **How does the presentation of MSA differ from PD?**

   Ans: Patients with MSA typically present with LUTS early in the course of disease (Table 12.1). More importantly, in some patients, LUTS can be the first presenting feature. This implies that the urologist must be able to spot a possible MSA even before other clinicians or the patient is able to identify it. Similarly, erectile dysfunction occurs along with or even before neurological symptoms. Urinary incontinence is more common and patients are more likely to have high PVR. In contrast, the PVR is typically <100ml in PD.[6,7] In this patient, the early presentation of LUTS and presence of voiding difficulty are red flags raising the possibility of MSA.

TABLE 12.1: Differentiating the underlying cause of Parkinsonism symptoms

	Parkinson's disease	Multisystem atrophy
Onset of LUTS	Average 5 years	Early; Often present with LUTS
Erectile dysfunction	Late	Early
Urinary incontinence	Less common	Often at onset
Elevated PVR	Uncommon	Common
Urinary retention	Rare	Common
Detrusor overactivity	More pronounced	Less dominant
Open bladder neck	Unusual	Common
Detrusor sphincter dyssynergia	Rare. Some have bradykinesia	Common
Outcome of prostate surgery	Usually benefit (caution)	Rarely benefit

8. **Can urodynamics help differentiate PD from MSA?**

Ans: Urodynamics can be very helpful. Specifically, video-urodynamics in MSA can show diagnostic features including an open bladder neck during filling and classical detrusor sphincter dyssynergia during voiding. Electromyography may show features of sphincter denervation. In contrast, patients with PD do not show classical dyssynergia. They may show delayed relaxation of the sphincter, termed 'bradykinesia of the sphincter'. Sphincter bradykinesia is a component of the global bradykinesia of striated muscles. This can be suspected on clinical examination by asking the patient to contract the sphincter during digital rectal examination. Patients often show a delayed and slow contraction. On video-urodynamics, the sphincter opening is delayed during the voiding phase and coincides with a drop in voiding pressure and improvement in flow.[7,8] Other options for diagnosing dyssynergia include use of sphincter electromyography or a stand-alone micturating cystourethrogram. The former is particularly prone to artifacts and should be interpreted cautiously.[10]

Video-urodynamics in this patient showed reduced capacity (180 ml) with early sensations and neurogenic detrusor overactivity incontinence (Fig. 12.1). Capacity was noted to be reduced across all cycles of testing. Voiding pressure flow

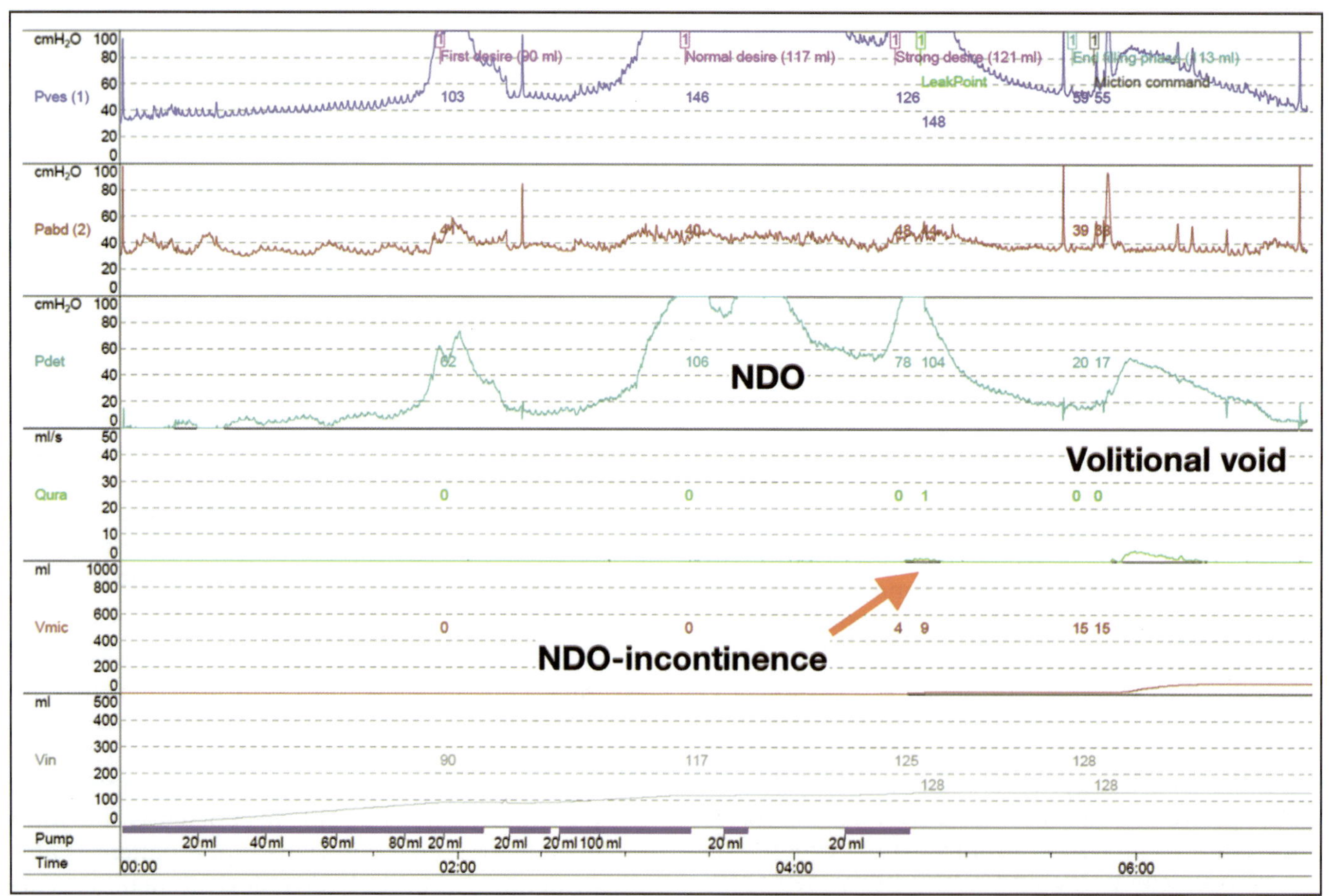

Fig. 12.1: Urodynamic study showing markedly reduced capacity (180 ml) with neurogenic detrusor overactivity (NDO) and NDO-incontinence. The patient produced a volitional contraction at instruction to void. There was obstruction with underactivity (see text)

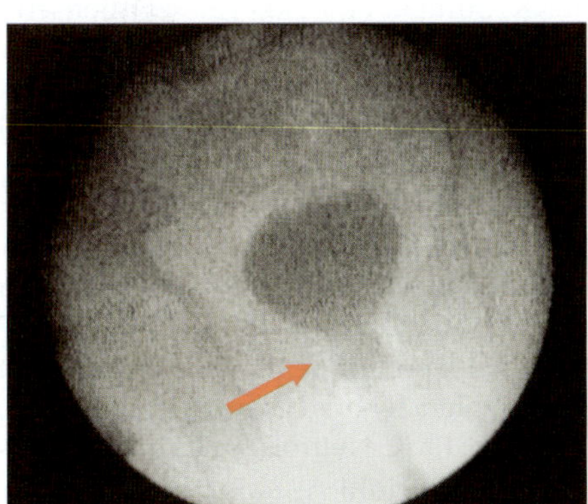

Dilated prostatic urethra during voiding (red arrow)

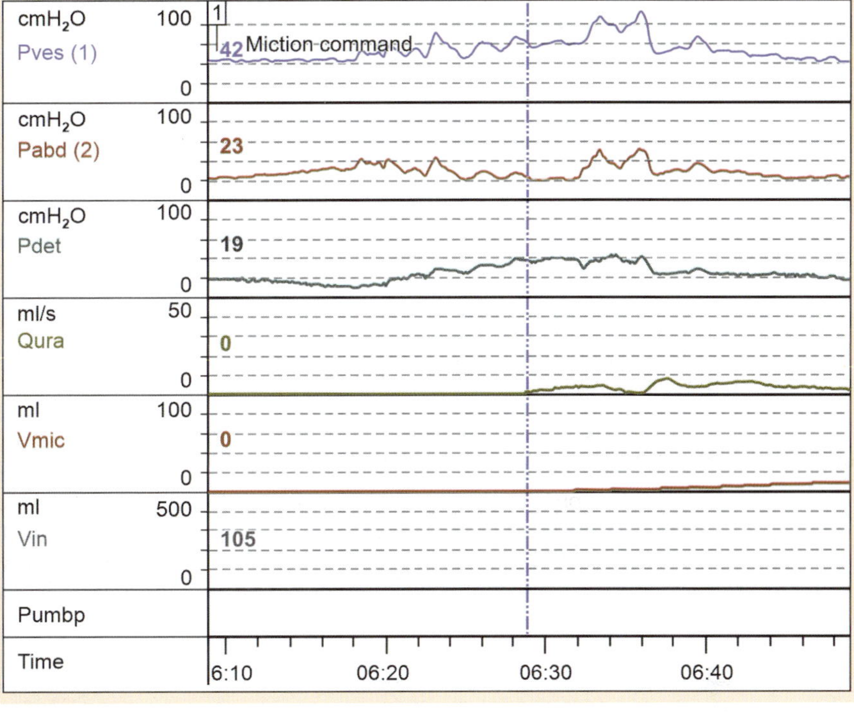

Fig. 12.2: Video-urodynamics showing grossly dilated prostatic urethra (Red arrow) during the entire voiding phase. This (repeat) cycle showed less prominent phasic contractions during storage, similar low capacity, and confirmed the voiding phase findings of the first cycle of testing.

showed detrusor underactivity (ICS-DCI 74) with bladder outlet obstruction (ICS-BOOI 46). Video-urodynamics showed grossly dilated prostatic urethra **all through the voiding phase** consistent with genuine detrusor sphincter dyssynergia (Fig. 12.2, Video 15 link in **QR code**). Stand alone MCU may erroneously show unrelaxed bradykinesic sphincter as DSD (which would later relax).

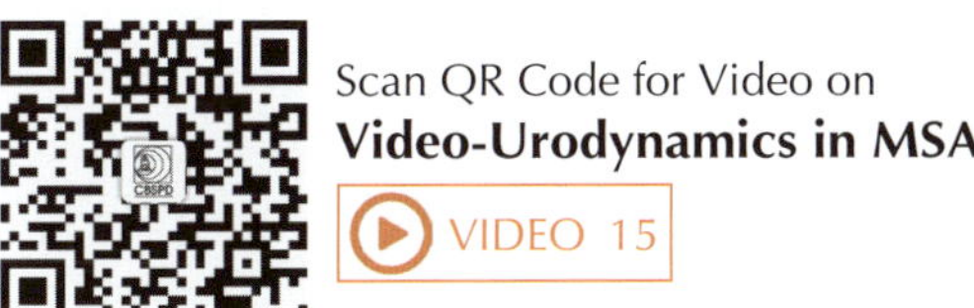

Scan QR Code for Video on **Video-Urodynamics in MSA**

VIDEO 15

9. What is your diagnosis?

Ans: The clinical features and video-urodynamics are consistent with multisystem atrophy rather than Parkinson's disease. From a urologist's perspective, the presentation of LUTS almost at the onset of neurological symptoms is an important clue. The video-urodynamics findings are diagnostic of MSA in this setting.[7,11,12]

10. What is your treatment plan?

Ans: The patient has refractory storage LUTS despite combined drug therapy for neurogenic detrusor overactivity. He also has voiding LUTS with detrusor sphincter dyssynergia. He is markedly bothered and is otherwise in good health with adequate hand function and cognition for intermittent catheterization.

He was initiated on **Intermittent Self Catheterization and underwent intra-detrusor injection of Onabotulinum Toxin A 200 units** with resolution of symptoms. His CISC diary record shows satisfactory ability to store urine. Urinary incontinence episodes are reduced to an average of 1 per day and his quality of life is markedly improved.

SUMMARY

- Urologists must search for clues to parkinsonism in elderly men who present with LUTS.
- Urological evaluation plays a role in making the correct neurological diagnosis.
- The diagnosis of parkinsonism encompasses a group of heterogenous conditions with implications for urological care
- Urological symptoms often mirror the course of parkinsonism
- Initial care is along standard lines for men with LUTS.
- Men with refractory LUTS and parkinsonism should undergo urodynamics prior to invasive treatments or prostate surgery. When available, videourodynamics is preferable.
- Surgery is often successful in men with Parkinson's disease but almost invariably fails in men with multisystem atrophy.

REFERENCES

1. Sabnis RB, Mulawkar PM, Joshi RN. The Urological Society of India guidelines on management of benign prostatic hyperplasia/benign prostatic obstruction (Executive summary). Indian J Urol. 2021;37(3):210–3.

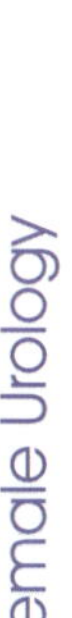

2. Cornu JN, Gravas S, Gacci M, Gratzke C, Herrmann TRW, Mamoulakis C, Rieken M, Speakman MJ, Tikkinen KAO. Non-neurogenic Male LUTS. European Association of Urology Guidelines. [Internet]. EAU Guidelines Office, Arnhem, The Netherlands.; 2022 [cited 2022 Aug 22]. Available from: https://uroweb.org/guideline/treatment-of-non-neurogenic-male-luts/
3. Sinha S, Agarwal MM, Vasudeva P, Khattar N, Madduri VKS, Yande S, *et al*. The Urological Society of India Guidelines for the Evaluation and Management of Nonneurogenic Urinary Incontinence in Adults (Executive Summary). Indian J Urol. 2019;35(3):185–8.
4. Ginsberg DA, Boone TB, Cameron AP, Gousse A, Kaufman MR, Keays E, *et al*. The AUA/SUFU Guideline on Adult Neurogenic Lower Urinary Tract Dysfunction: Diagnosis and Evaluation. J Urol. 2021 Nov;206(5):1097–105.
5. Blok B, Pannek J, Castro-Diaz G, Del Popolo G, Groen, J, Hamid R, *et al*. Neuro-Urology. European Association of Urology Guidelines [Internet]. EAU Guidelines Office, Arnhem, The Netherlands.; 2023 [cited 2023 Apr 14]. Available from: https://uroweb.org/guideline/neuro-urology/
6. Sakakibara R, Hattori T, Uchiyama T, Yamanishi T. Videourodynamic and sphincter motor unit potential analyses in Parkinson's disease and multiple system atrophy. J Neurol Neurosurg Psychiatry. 2001 Nov;71(5):600–6.
7. Brucker BM, Kalra S. Parkinson's Disease and Its Effect on the Lower Urinary Tract: Evaluation of Complications and Treatment Strategies. Urol Clin North Am. 2017 Aug;44(3):415–28.
8. Sakakibara R, Panicker J, Finazzi-Agro E, Iacovelli V, Bruschini H, The Parkinson's Disease Subcomittee TNPC in TICS. A guideline for the management of bladder dysfunction in Parkinson's disease and other gait disorders. Neurourology and Urodynamics. 2016;35(5):551–63.
9. Winge K, Nielsen KK, Stimpel H, Lokkegaard A, Jensen SR, Werdelin L. Lower urinary tract symptoms and bladder control in advanced Parkinson's disease: effects of deep brain stimulation in the subthalamic nucleus. Mov Disord. 2007 Jan 15;22(2):220–5.
10. Kirby AC, Nager CW, Litman HJ, Fitzgerald MP, Kraus S, Norton P, *et al*. Perineal surface electromyography does not typically demonstrate expected relaxation during normal voiding. Neurourol Urodyn. 2011 Nov;30(8):1591–6.
11. Xing T, Ou T, Ma J. Evaluation of neurogenic bladder outlet obstruction mimicking sphincter bradykinesia in male patients with Parkinson's disease. BMC Neurol. 2021;21(1):125.
12. Eschlbock S, Krismer F, Fanciulli A, Kaindlstorfer C, Seppi K, Kiechl S, *et al*. Urodynamic Evaluation in Multiple System Atrophy: A Retrospective Cohort Study. Mov Disord Clin Pract. 2021;8(7):1052–60.

Chapter 13

Lower Urinary Tract Symptoms in a Young Male (<40 years)

• Venkatesh Krishnamoorthy

LEARNING OBJECTIVES

- Lower urinary tract symptoms are not an uncommon complaint in young adult men, significantly impacting the quality of life (QoL), with the need for prolonged medical care.
- The term "Lower Urinary Tract Symptoms" (LUTS), was adopted in the mid 1990s, representing a paradigm shift from the word prostatism, which 'assigned' the diagnosis for these symptoms. This change in the terminology has come about with a better understanding of the lower urinary tract, as a single functional unit, and the multifactorial etiology.
- It is now well known that many of these LUTS, have very little to do with the prostate. LUTS is known to have a similar prevalence in age-matched women. The fact that LUTS is not significantly affected by gender, underscores the possibility, that the symptoms in both young men and women have similar etiologies like functional bladder neck obstruction and dysfunctional voiding.
- The incidence of LUTS in men aged 18–29 years was 2% (IPSS >7). It was 12% in men aged 40–49 years.[1] In another study, a survey of younger men for LUTS, reported an IPSS ≥7 in 5% of men in their 20s. This rose to 15% among those in their 40s.[2]
- There is reasonable evidence now, establishing a relationship between increased LUTS and metabolic disorders such as diabetes, hypertension, obesity, alcohol consumption, poor physical exercise, etc.[3]

Case Scenario

DS, a 33-year-old male presented with hesitancy to void, poor urine stream, prolonged voiding time, and pain during voiding, for the past several months. He has no history of catheterisation, urethral trauma or urethral discharge. He has no constipation and bowel movements are normal.

His urine frequency is 6–7/1–0. His fluid intake is around 2–3 litres per day. His IPSS score is 18.

1. **What is the differential diagnosis for LUTS in males under 40 years of age? Are there any pointers to diagnosis in history and examination?**

   Ans: Unlike in older men the etiology is more varied in young men. Anatomical obstruction due to urethral stricture is more common. Functional causes include primary bladder neck obstruction (PBNO), dysfunctional voiding (DV), and underactive bladder. LUTS may be caused or complicated by mental health problems, metabolic conditions or endocrine disorders such as polyuria. Concomitant medication history is important since many drugs such as antiepileptics, anxiolytics or antidepressants are associated with LUTS.

   Even though a precise diagnosis is not possible by history alone, a detailed medical history should be taken. This is to identify likely contributory causes, relevant co-morbidities, current medications, lifestyle habits, including emotional and psychological factors.[4]

2. **Is the use of symptoms score questionnaires of help in the management?**

   Ans: Worldwide, guidelines recommend the use of validated symptoms score questionnaires, for the quantitative assessment of LUTS.[5,6] These have now become a routine part of the evaluation. They help to quantify LUTS, to both assess the severity, and also to monitor patient related outcome measures (PROM), with the various treatments offered.

   These questionnaires are not disease or pathology specific. However, since the ultimate goal is relief of symptoms, to that extent, these symptoms scores are of great use. While questionnaires are not validated specifically for younger men or the Indian population, it is reasonable to use them.

Of the several questionnaires the ones commonly used are International Prostate Symptoms Score (IPSS), and International Consultation on Incontinence Questionnaire (ICIQ-mLUTS).[7,8] The IPSS does not include symptoms of urge incontinence or pain in its 8-item questionnaire. While the former is validated only for men >40 years, the latter can be used across all age groups. Symptom scoring helps in establishing a uniform standard of comparison for symptom assessment, and later, treatment response.

Physical examination was entirely normal. The prostate was flat, benign, with no tenderness. The rectum was empty.

3. **What is considered important in the physical examination?**

Ans: Physical examination is an important part of evaluation for LUTS. It must include examination of the perineum, rectal examination, prostate evaluation, observation of any fecal impaction, and a focused neuro-urological examination. The latter includes perianal sensations, cremasteric reflex, anal tone, bulbocaversonal reflex and lower limb function.

4. **How important is the use of a frequency–volume chart or bladder diary?**

Ans: These are an important part of evaluation and are integral to the diagnosis of the various contributory causes to LUTS. These charts initially started off as only frequency–volume charts (FVCs), but to obtain more information, have expanded to becoming a full-fledged bladder diary. Though there is agreement on the usefulness of the FVCs, the structure, its content, and the duration of charting have not been standardized. However, it is very easy to add information on waking and sleep timings, fluid intake, urgency and incontinence episodes, and symptoms such as burning and pain during voiding, to transform it to a comprehensive bladder diary.[9,10]

5. **What about a urine examination?**

Ans: Urine analysis should be done in every initial assessment for LUTS. It is inexpensive, and adds value when it reports the presence of microscopic hematuria, presence of nitrites and leukocyte esterase.[11]

6. **Is it necessary to perform tests of renal function?**

Ans: Renal function testing is commonly done, though it appears that renal function has no bearing on LUTS. Conditions like diabetes mellitus may be a contributory factor to both deteriorating renal function as well as LUTS.[12,13] The risk of developing *de novo* renal failure in men with LUTS is insignificant (<1%). However, the recommendation to do a renal functional assessment remains.

7. **What about obtaining a prostate-specific antigen (PSA)?[14,15]**

Ans: Unless there is a strong family history of related malignancies, there is no validity in doing PSA testing in a young male with LUTS. In some situations use of PSA testing might help identify prostatitis in a young male.

8. **How useful is assessment of prostate?**

Ans: Currently, the transrectal ultrasound is the most frequently used method to assess prostatic volume. Certainly, it is more accurate than the DRE. Magnetic Resonance Imaging (MRI) is even more accurate.[16,17] It is arguable whether increasing precision in measurement of prostate size adds substantially to outcomes. However, prostate configuration, such as intravesical prostatic protrusion (IPP) has been noted to be useful at predicting bladder outlet obstruction. IPP is more relevant to an older age group with prostatomegaly, which is seldom noted in men under 40 years of age.

9. **What is the role for measuring postvoid residual (PVR)?**

Ans: PVR by itself cannot differentiate between obstructed and non-obstructed patients, and there is no agreed-upon standard definition of what exactly constitutes an elevated PVR. However, the measurement of PVR can aid in treatment decisions as well follow-up.

10. **Is uroflowmetry useful?**

Ans: Even though uroflowmetry cannot specifically diagnose outflow obstruction from bladder underactivity, it has value in identifying disorders of voiding, and by comparing to pre-therapy recordings, is especially useful for monitoring treatment outcomes, and correlating symptoms with objective findings.[18,19] In clinical practice, uroflowmetry is often the first investigation to objectively document a poor flow. *He underwent a uroflowmetry* (Fig. 13.1).

11. **Is urotherapy a good initial treatment in younger men with poor flow?**

Ans: As behavioral modifications are non-invasive and non-pharmacological, it may be worth a try especially if urethral stricture is low on the suspicion list. This includes pelvic floor muscle training, timed voiding, avoidance of constipation, behavioral modifications regarding fluid and

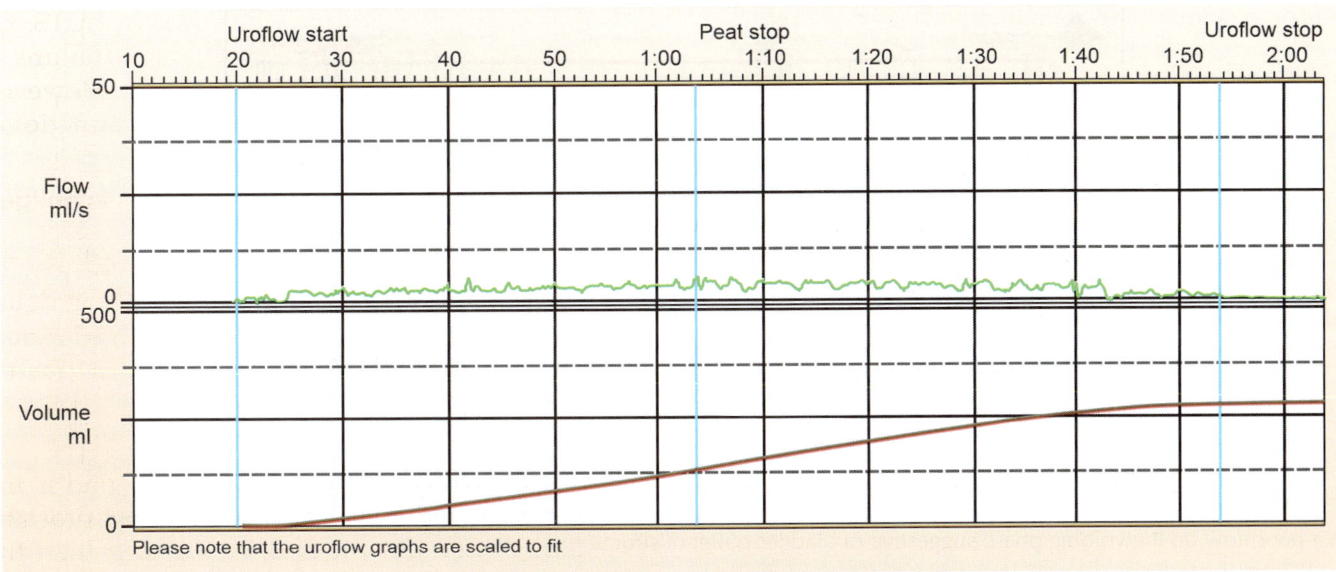

Uroflow summary

			Dev (male)
Maximum flow:	5.8	ml/s	– 64%
Average flow:	3.0	ml/s	– 73%
Voiding time:	1:33.9	sec	– 289%
Flow time:	1:31.9	sec	
Time to peak flow:	43.6	sec	– 292%
Voided volume:	276.6	ml	
Flow at 2 seconds:	0.8	ml/s	
Acceleration:	0.1	ml/s/s	
Residual volume:	________	ml	

Fig. 13.1: Uroflowmetry showing slow and prolonged flow

caffeine intake and a voiding diary. These measures may be especially useful in symptoms resulting from pelvic floor disorders or overactive bladder.[20]

With urotherapy, timed voiding, and advice to "sit, relax and let the urine flow out", his symptoms did not improve.

His urine stream, however, continued to remain poor along with recurrent urinary tract infection. He then underwent a RGU and VCUG (Figs 13.2A and B), which revealed poor bladder neck opening. *We followed this with a urodynamic study (Fig. 13.3) which revealed very high voiding pressures,*

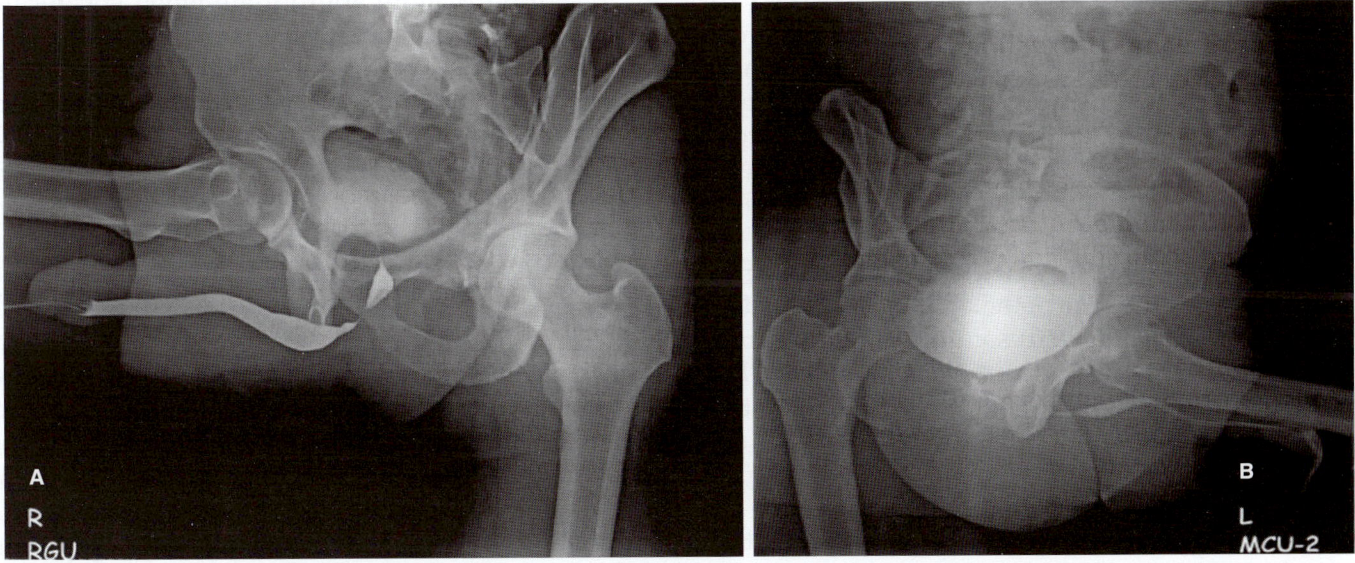

Fig. 13.2A and B: A. Retrograde urethrogram confirming absence of stricture; B. Voiding cystourethrogram showing poor bladder neck opening

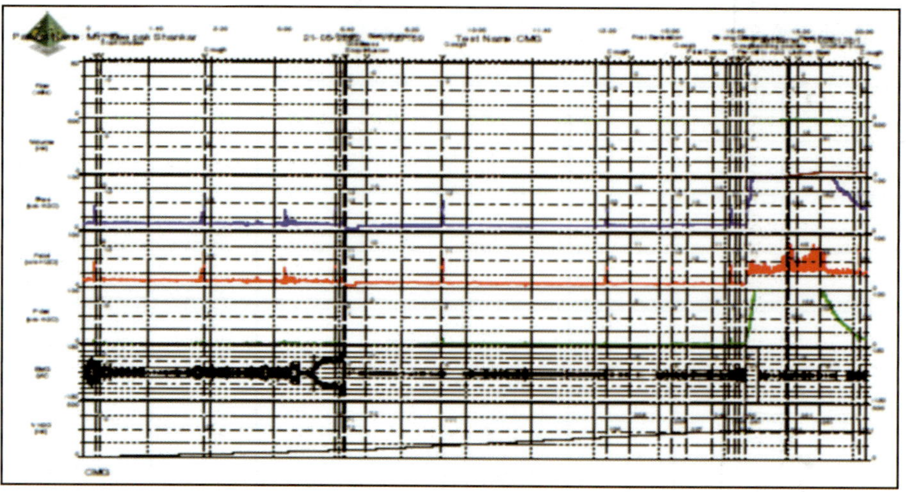

Fig. 13.3: Urodynamic study showing stable bladder with normal compliance on filling phase and a very strong detrusor contraction with a poor flow on the voiding phase suggestive of bladder outlet obstruction

with a poor stream, indicating bladder outlet obstruction.

12. What is the role of voiding cystography, cystoscopy and urodynamics in young men with LUTS?

Contrary to elder men where VCUG is not a routine in evaluation of LUTS, in younger men it gives valuable information and should be ordered in conjunction with a retrograde urethrogram. Apart from completing the roadmap for stricture evaluation, the information on voiding study becomes even more valuable if stricture not detected as now the level of obstruction whether at bladder neck (PBNO) or at the level of sphincter (DV or pelvic floor relaxation disorders) is pointed out. Also, it may be useful for detection of vesicoureteric reflux, bladder diverticula and other urethral pathologies.

Urethrocystoscopy should be reserved for specific indications such as gross hematuria, strong suspicion for urethral stricture, bladder cancer, etc., and when definitive endoscopic treatment is planned.[21,22] However, if an office cystoscopy with a flexible cystoscope has already excluded a stricture, a videourodynamic study can complete the desired information.

Urodynamic study helps in identification of the various bladder pathologies such as bladder outlet obstruction, detrusor overactivity, detrusor underactivity and impaired compliance. While urodynamics is an important tool, it must be utilized selectively, when the initial lifestyle changes, behavioural therapy and pharmacological management has not helped This is due to the invasive nature of the test, and a small percentage of morbidity associated. Videourodynamics is particularly useful in young males and can enhance the diagnostic certainty of dysfunctional voiding or PBNO.

Patient underwent a bladder neck incision. The bladder was trabeculated with saccules, with florid prominent submucosal vessels around the bladder base. BNI was done at the 6 o'clock position.

13. What is the difference between a BNI and TUIP? What are the considerations before performing a bladder neck incision in young men?

Ans: Essentially for men procedure wise both the terms are same but transurethral incision of the prostate (TUIP) is more appropriate when we are dealing with a provisional diagnosis of BPH where it is the endoscopic procedure of choice for prostates less than 30 gm. It is also preferred for young, sexually active men. Bladder neck incision (BNI) or transurethral incision of bladder neck (TUIBN) is more appropriate when specifically dealing with bladder neck pathologies like PBNO (both male and female), neurogenic bladder neck dysfunctions or post-TURP bladder neck contractures.

The potential for causing ejaculatory disturbances makes BNI a challenge both to offer and to accept in cases of young men. Classical TUIP type incision at 5 and 7 o' clock results in retrograde ejaculation in a significant number of patients (18.2%).[23] Cryopreservation of semen before the surgery is a recommended practice if the patient has not completed their family. Unilateral incision helps reducing the incidence of retrograde ejaculation.

Currently to preserve antegrade ejaculation, an ejaculation sparing technique is advisable. This is achieved by preserving the supramontanal tissue (about 1 cm), typically with no detrimental effect on surgical success. This modified incision can preserve ejaculation in a high proportion of patients.[24] The efficacy of modified TUIBN is close to 85%.

He has had complete resolution of his symptoms following the procedure: Post-BNI uroflowmetry (Fig. 13.4).

KEY POINTS

- Unlike in older men the etiology of LUTS does not revolve around prostate in young men. Anatomical obstruction due to urethral stricture is more common. Functional causes include primary bladder neck obstruction (PBNO), dysfunctional voiding (DV), and underactive bladder.
- Apart from a detailed history and examination, a uroflowmetry and ICIQ-mLUTS questionnaire would be useful for evaluation.
- Voiding cystogram gives valuable information especially if stricture is unlikely cause of LUTS in this age group.
- Videourodynamics is particularly useful in young males and can enhance the diagnostic certainty of dysfunctional voiding or PBNO.
- Urethrocysoscopy should be reserved for specific indications such as gross hematuria, strong suspicion for urethral stricture, bladder cancer, etc.
- Behavioral therapy including pelvic floor muscle training, timed voiding, avoidance of constipation, behavioral modifications regarding fluid and caffeine intake and a voiding diary may be a good starting point if stricture is ruled out or is lower on the suspicion list.
- Modified TUIP/BNI in men with PBNO (a relatively common cause of functional obstruction in young men) can help relieve symptoms along with preservation of ejaculation.

REFERENCES

1. Mueller ER, Latini J, Lux M, *et al.* International Prostate Symptoms Scores in young asymptomatic American men. BJU Int. 2005; 95 (4): 554–556.
2. Moon TD, Hagen L, Heisey DM, Urinary symptomatology in younger men. Urology. 1997; 50(5):700–703.
3. Male Lower Urinary Tract symptoms (LUTS): C. Chappel & P. Abrams; 2012; Page 42.
4. EAU 2022 guidelines.
5. Novara G, *et al.* Critical Review of Guidelines for BPH Diagnosis and Treatment Strategy. Eur Urol Suppl 2006. 4: 418.
6. Bosch J, *et al.* Etiology, Patient Assessment and Predicting Outcome from Therapy. International Consultation on Urological Diseases Male LUTS Guideline 2013.
7. Barry MJ, *et al.* The American Urological Association symptom index for benign prostatic hyperplasia. The Measurement Committee of the American Urological Association. J Urol, 1992;148:1549.

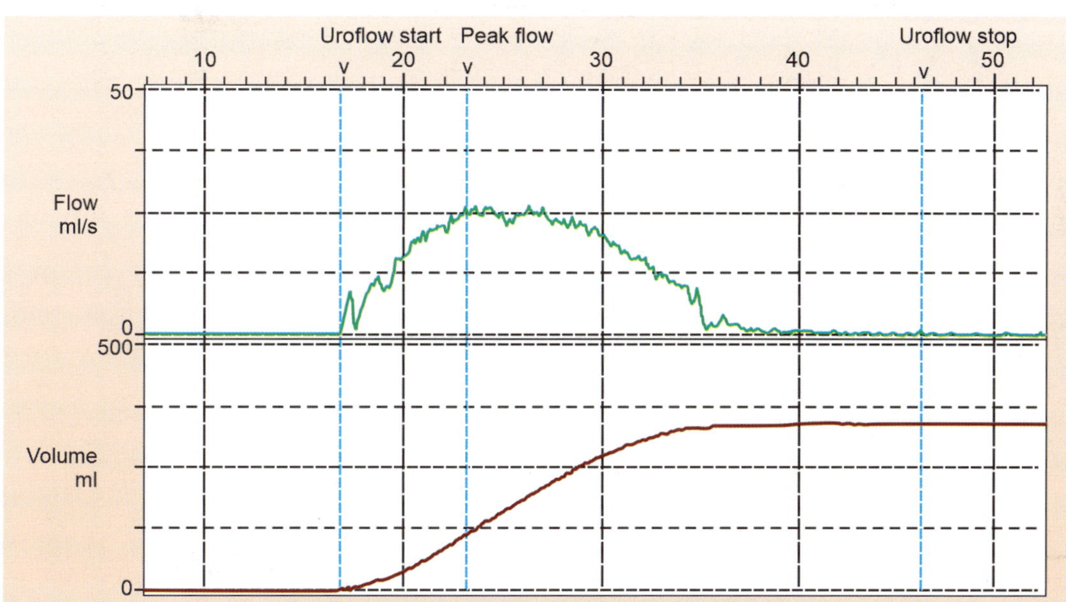

Uroflow summary

			Dev (male)
Maximum flow:	26.2	ml/s	45%
Average flow:	14.1	ml/s	8%
Voiding time:	29.6	sec	– 13%
Flow time:	23.7	sec	
Time to peak flow:	6.3	sec	45%
Voided volume:	335.9	ml	
Flow at 2 seconds:	9.4	ml/s	
Acceleration:	3.9	ml/s/s	
Residual volume:	5	ml	

Fig. 13.4: Follow-up uroflowmetry post-bladder neck incision

8. Donovan JL, *et al.* Scoring the short form ICSmaleSF questionnaire. International Continence Society. J Urol, 2000. 164: 1948.
9. de la Rosette J. Alivizatos G. Madersbacher S, *et al.* European Association of Urology. Guidelines on benign prostatic hyperplasia 2006.
10. National Institute of Health and Clinical Excellence. NICE clinical guideline 97: The management of lower urinary tract symptoms in men. 2010.
11. Khasriya R, Khan S, Lunawat R, *et al.* The inadequacy of urinary dipstick and microscopy as surrogate makers of urinary tract infection in urological outpatients with lower urinary tract symptoms without acute frequency and dysuria. J Urol. 2010;183(5):1843–1847.
12. Rule AD, Jacobson DJ, Roberts RO, *et al.* The association between benign prostatic hyperplasia and chronic kidney disease in community-dwelling men. Kidney Int. 2005; 67(6):2376–2382.
13. McConnell JD, Roehrborn CG, Bautista OM, *et al.* Long-term effects of Doxazosin, Finasteride, and combination therapy on the clinical progression of benign prostatic hyperplasia. N Eng J Med. 2003; 349(25);2387–2398.
14. Andriole GL, Grawford ED, Grubb RL 3rd, *et al.* Prostate cancer screening in the randomised prostate, lung, colorectal, and ovarian cancer screening trial; mortality results after 13 years of follow-up. J Natl Cancer Inst. 2012;104(2):125–132.
15. Schroder FH, Hugosson J. Roobol MJ, *et al.* Prostate-cancer mortality at 11 years of follow-up. N. Eng J Med. 2012;366(11):981–990.
16. Loeb S, Han M, Roehl KA, *et al.* Accuracy of prostate weight estimation by digital rectal examination versus transrectal ultrasonography. J Urol. 2005;173(1):63–65.
17. al-Rimawi M, Griffiths DJ, Boake RC, *et al.* Transrectal ultrasound versus magnetic resonance imaging in the estimation of prostate volume. Br J Urol.1994;74(5):596–600.
18. Siroky MB, *et al.* The flow rate nomogram: I. Development. J Urol, 1979. 122: 665.
19. Siroky MB, *et al.* The flow rate nomogram: II. Clinical correlation. J Urol, 1980. 123: 208.
20. Beland L, Martin C, Han JS. Lower Urinary Tract Symptoms in Young Men-Causes and Management. Curr Urol Rep. 2022 Feb;23(2):29–37. doi: 10.1007/s11934–022–01087–9.
21. National Institute of Health and Clinical Excellence. The management of lower urinary tract symptoms in men: Methods, evidence & guidance. 2010.
22. Lucas MG, Bosch RJ, Burkhard FC, *et al.* EAU guidelines on assessment and nonsurgical management of urinary incontinence. Eur Urol. 2012.
23. Mardersbacher S, Marberger M. Is Transurethral Resection of the Prostate still justified: BJU Int. 1999; 83(3): 227–237.
24. Yang SS-D, Tsai Y-C, Chen J-J, Peng C-H, Hsieh J-H & Wang, CC (2008). Modified Transurethral Incision of the Bladder Neck Treating Primary Bladder Neck Obstruction in Young Men: A Method to Improve Voiding Function and to Preserve Antegrade Ejaculation. Urologia Internationalis, 80(1), 26–30. doi:10.1159/000111725.

Chapter 14

Voiding Difficulty in a Middle-aged Female

• *Mayank Mohan Agarwal*

LEARNING OBJECTIVES

- **Components of initial assessment before starting treatment**
  - **A detailed history** is essential—current symptoms and their bother, associated symptoms (particularly constipation and pelvic pain), neurological conditions (known or suspected), prior pelvic surgery/radiation, medications. Employing symptom—scores and proforma-based history taking are encouraged.
  - **A comprehensive clinical examination** is mandatory—abdominal examination (particularly masses, palpable bladder), introital, vaginal, bimanual examination, focused neurological examination of S2–S4 nerve segments, pelvic strength and responsiveness.
  - **Uroflowmetry with postvoid residual (PVR) urine**—an intelligent interpretation of flow–volume relations has in principle 2 components: (1) Numerical—most notably Q_{max}, Q_{ave}, voided volume, PVR. Flow–volume indices (VQI) defined as Q/√(V-V+PVR). (2) Graphical flow pattern, positioning of patient's flow volume on Flow-volume nomogram. For Caucasian population: Liverpool nomogram. For Indian population, we prefer to use PGIMER nomograms.
  - **Urine analysis**—many symptoms of voiding dysfunctions overlap with that of urinary tract infection (UTI). Moreover, UTI can result from voiding dysfunction, particularly in presence of large PVR or urinary incontinence.
- **Multichannel urodynamics (UDS)**—timing of UDS is a shared decision between patient and clinician. In low-risk patients, treatment can be initiated empirically and UDS reserved for treatment failure. Conversely, in high-risk patients (e.g. recurrent UTI, chronic retention, upper tract changes) UDS is preferred early in the course. Main differential diagnoses are bladder neck obstruction, detrusor underactivity and pelvic floor dysfunction. In want of standardized pressure flow criteria for bladder outlet obstruction and detrusor underactivity, radio-fluoroscopy is often required for diagnosis and localization of obstruction (either video-UDS or separately done voiding cystourethrography).
- **Initial treatment:** After ruling out various anatomical and neurological causes of voiding dysfunction (VD), clinician can proceed with the following treatment–
  - ***Alpha-blockers***—tamsulosin is the most studied agent in women with VD. It has been found to reduce pressure throughout the urethral length. In view of lower density of alpha-1 receptors in female urethra the clinical effects in women are modest, compared to men in whom the effects are marked. Although silodosin has not been studied in women, it is used widely clinically.
  - ***Skeletal muscle relaxants (SMR)***—there are no site-specific SMRs since there are no site-specific skeletal muscle receptors in pelvic floor. Baclofen is commonly used centrally acting $GABA_A$ receptor agonist for PFD in men and women. Tizanidine is a centrally acting alpha-2 agonist which has only be studied in children with PFD.
  - ***Pelvic floor relaxation exercises***—these have established role in PFD in children. The available data on adults also favors its use. It is an essential conservative measure for PFD with VD as well as constipation.
  - ***Treatment of constipation***—high fiber diet, pelvic floor relaxation and laxatives form the first line treatment for constipation in this scenario. Polyethylene glycol 3350 has an excellent safety record and therefore a safe first choice. Clinician must be able to identify high-risk situations e.g. weight loss, hematochezia, melena, cramping, refractory constipation.
- **Treatment options in refractory cases:**
  - **Bladder-neck incision (BNI)**—for refractory urodynamic BNO. Several techniques are described, 10 and 2 o'clock incisions, 5 and 7 o'clock incisions and 3—6—9— and 12 o'clock incisions. Resection between 5 and 7 o'clock is also described. Major adverse effects are rare, notably vesicovaginal fistula and stress urinary incontinence.
  - **Onabotulinum toxin infiltration into external sphincter (BTX)**—for women with unequivocal PFD and those with unspecified DU (e.g. post radical hysterectomy) infiltration of 100 units of BTX has been found to be effective in 56% women with DU and 74% with PFD. Notably, in a randomized study even saline infiltration without BTX was found to lead to significant improvement.
  - **Sacral neuromodulation**—neuromodulation acts on the basic pathophysiology of PFD, i.e. disturbances in primary and secondary urethra-to-bladder and bladder-to-urethra reflexes. Success rates of 65–78% have been reported in patients with idiopathic retention. These success rates were sustained even after 10 years of follow-up. However, apart from high cost, significant revision rates (30–50%) are a concern.

Case Scenario

A 38-year-old woman with no medical comorbidity, presented with bladder and bowel symptoms for 5 years-difficulty in urination, straining, incomplete voiding, increased frequency (due to persistence of urine sensation), straining for defecation, hard stools, frequency 2–4/d for completion. Her American Urological Association (IPSS/AUA) symptom score was 22/35 with quality-of-life (QOL) score 4/6. She is a mother of 2, both normal vaginal deliveries. Her periods were normal with no dysmenorrhea. No significant surgical/medication history. Examination–overweight (BMI 32 kg/m^2). No vaginal prolapse, no stress incontinence, pelvic floor strength 4/6. Urethral caliber 20 fr easy. PVR 200 ml.

1. **What are the Important points to ask in history?**

   Ans: Voiding dysfunction (VD)/bladder bowel dysfunction (BBD) is a functional problem of pelvic floor muscles. It is paramount to ask for present symptoms as well as medical-comorbidities, psychological disturbance, triggers, medications/substance-abuse, prior surgery/intervention/radiation (particularly those affecting pelvic floor structure or function) and child-birth. There are some neurological conditions where LUTS are an early presentation. An alert clinician should look for potential features of a possible occult neuropathy. For example, sudden severe storage or voiding symptoms or dysuria in absence of urinary tract infection (UTI), altered/decreased bladder sensations, enuresis, accidental voiding in socially inappropriate situation, stress incontinence (SUI) in a nullipara, etc. Further clue may be provided by alteration in gait, speech, vision or comprehension. Although constipation is a common problem as such, its co-presence should prompt clinician to carefully assess for occult neuropathy.[1]

2. **Is there a role for symptom-scores and proforma for assessment?**

   Ans: Though not mandatory, employing symptom scores for urinary and defecatory dysfunction help in standardizing clinical assessment as well as for collecting data for research. ICIQ-FLUTS score can be used for all-encompassing LUTS and impact of each symptom[2] [ICIQ-FLUTS LF | ICIQ]. Alternatively, AUA symptom score can be used for quick assessment.[3] Similarly, Cleveland-clinic constipation chart is an easy-to-use tool and urologists are encouraged to employ in their functional urology practice.[4] Furthermore, taking proforma-based history/examination go a long way for a comprehensive initial assessment to avoid accidental omissions.

3. **What are the important elements for physical examination? What is focused neurological examination?**

   Ans: Along with a detailed history, importance of a comprehensive physical examination cannot be overemphasized for making initial impressions of the diagnosis. Elements of pelvic examination are as under:

   - ***Introitus***—lesions, cleanliness, discharge
   - ***Vagina***—urethral meatus, prolapse (as per POP-Q standards), stress incontinence, cervix (tenderness/discharge/mass). Pelvic floor tenderness is commonly assessed on a 5-point scale (0: No pain; 1: Comfortable pressure; 2: Uncomfortable pressure, slight pain; 3: Moderate pain, intensifies with muscle contraction; 4: Severe pain, patient unable to contract).
   - ***Pelvic-floor***—sensation, strength and responsiveness, bulbocavernosus reflex (BCR). Tenderness along bladder, pelvic floor, elsewhere. Elicitation of BCR signify intactness of S2–4 reflex-pathway and voluntary pelvic-floor contraction–relaxation cerebral connectivity, in addition. Modified Oxford-scale is commonly used for basic assessment of strength and responsiveness of PFM contraction on a scale of 0 to 5.[5] Laycock and Jerwood's[6] PERFECT scheme (**P**ressure, equivalent of Oxford scale, **E**ndurance, **R**epetitions, **F**ast contractions, **E**very **C**ontraction **T**imed) can be utilized if physician chooses to train the patient's pelvic floor.
   - ***Urethral calibration***—is selectively employed for urethral-stricture screening, when index of suspicion is high. However, caliber defining stricture urethra is not clear in women. Kalra *et al*[7] found that a successful calibration with 14 Fr catheter would not rule out stricture in women. Given normal caliber of urethra being 22–26 Fr, a successful calibration with 18–20 Fr catheter without resistance is considered acceptable among functional urologists (unpublished).

4. **Can you initiate treatment purely based only on clinical history and examination?**

   Ans: Clinician should not make conclusions based solely on history and examination in women. In a retrospective clinicourodynamic analysis of 1605 women HC Kuo[8] concluded that differential diagnosis of VD was not possible solely on symptoms. Lowenstein *et al*[9] found poor correlation between elevated postvoid residual urine and obstructive voiding symptoms. Therefore, clinicians should base their diagnosis on history, examination as well as investigations.

Case Scenario *(Contd.)*

Uroflowmetry revealed maximum flow-rate (Q_{max}) of 7.2 ml/sec, average flow-rate (Q_{ave}) 4.1 ml/sec, voided-volume (VV) 335 ml and postvoid residue (PVR) 180 ml (Fig. 14.1). Uroflowmetry pattern was combined staccato-intermittent. Ultrasound revealed no hydronephrosis, normal bladder-wall thickness 3 mm (BWT) and PVR 250 ml. Urine routine did not reveal any evidence of bacteriuria/pyuria.

5. **What are initial investigations required before initiating treatment?**

   Ans: Uroflowmetry with PVR, urine-analysis with/without ultrasound of kidney-ureter-bladder are minimum investigations required before initiating treatment.

6. **What information do you get with uroflowmetry?**

   Ans: Uroflowmetry with PVR is cornerstone for initial screening for voiding dysfunction. Numerical (Q_{max}, Q_{ave}, VV, PVR) as well as graphical information (flow pattern) is obtained. A careful and intelligent interpretation is required.

   a. **What uroflowmetry values are abnormal?**

   Ans: Q_{max} of <15 ml/sec for VV of 150 ml with/without a PVR 50 ml is considered abnormal. Since uroflow-rate is dependent on bladder volume (BV), inspired by von Garrelts' formulae of corrected-Q_{max} we conceptualized volume-normalized Q_{max} and Q_{ave} indices (VQI = Q/ (VV+PVR)) and found a VQI_{max} <1 and/or VQI_{ave} <0.6 sensitive (90.5% and 95.4%, respectively) and specific (88.9%) indicators of voiding dysfunction. Flow-volume (VQ) nomograms are graphical representation of these indices. Position of patient's flow volume relation on the nomogram suggests voiding dysfunction. Liverpool nomogram is commonly used across the globe for this purpose. We found Caucasian nomograms relatively nonspecific for Indian population and constructed-validated PGIMER-nomogram in north Indian population (PGIMER abbreviation of my *alma mater* Postgraduate Institute of Medical Education and Research, Chandigarh). In index case VQI_{max} 0.31 and positioning of VQ point way below 5th percentile on PGIMER nomogram is highly indicative of voiding dysfunction.

   b. **Can uroflowmetry pattern indicate towards the diagnosis?**

   Ans: Some patterns point towards a diagnosis, for example, ***plateau***—urethral stricture, ***staccato with/without intermittent***—pelvic-floor dysfunction (PFD), **tower**—overactive-bladder/stress-incontinence. However, there is significant overlap among patterns; moreover, suboptimal interobserver variability in defining a pattern. In index case, combined staccato–interrupted pattern was found which indicated towards PFD.

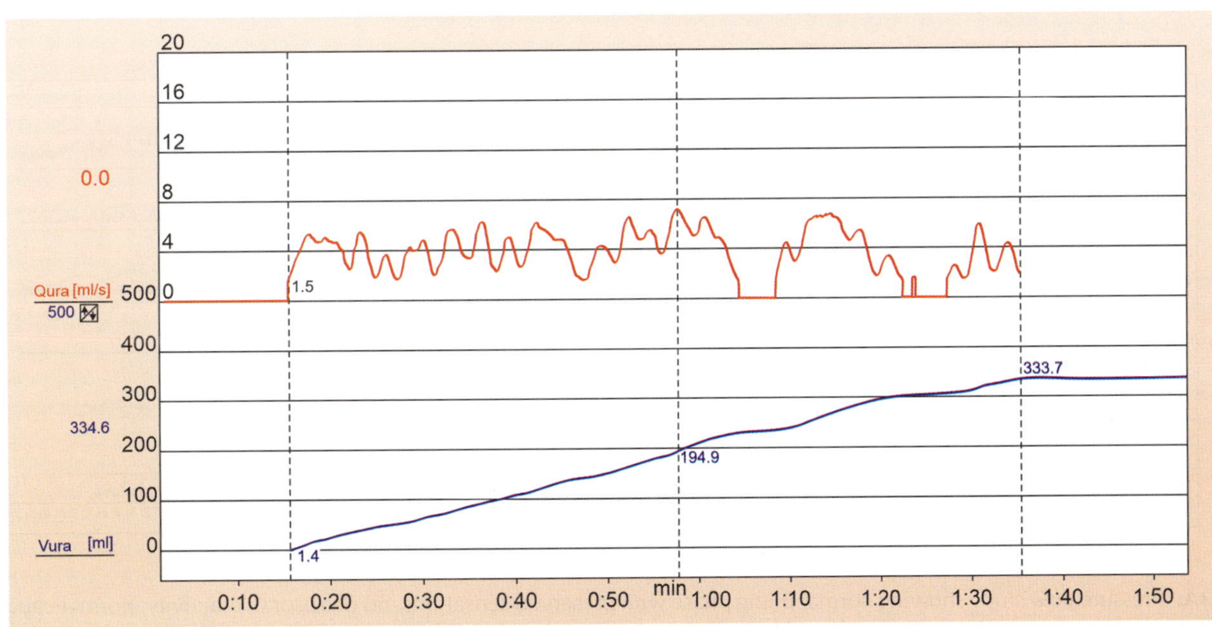

Fig. 14.1: Pre-treatment uroflowmetry of index patient showing mixed intermittency and staccato pattern. Q_{max} 7.2 ml/sec, voided volume 335 ml, PVR 180 ml. VQI_{max} 0.32.

Case Scenario *(Contd.)*

She was initiated on tamsulosin 0.4 mg once daily with 3 times daily postvoid self-catheterisation, polyglycol, high-fiber diet and was taught pelvic-relaxation exercises. There was improvement in clinical symptoms with residual AUA score being 15/35 and QOL 3/6. Her PVR reduced to <100 ml and she stopped doing CIC. Uroflowmetry showed some improvement (Q_{max} 9.9 ml/sec, Q_{ave} 5.1ml/sec, voided volume 326ml and PVR 50 ml. VQlm 0.55. (Fig. 14.2).

In view of persistence of bothersome residual LUTS, urodynamics (UDS) with dynamic voiding cystourethrography (VCUG) was performed which revealed features of pelvic floor dysfunction with resulting secondary detrusor underactivity (DU) (Figs 14.3A and B).

7. When should one perform urodynamics during evaluation of such a patient?

Ans: Timing of urodynamics is an individualized shared decision between clinician and patient.

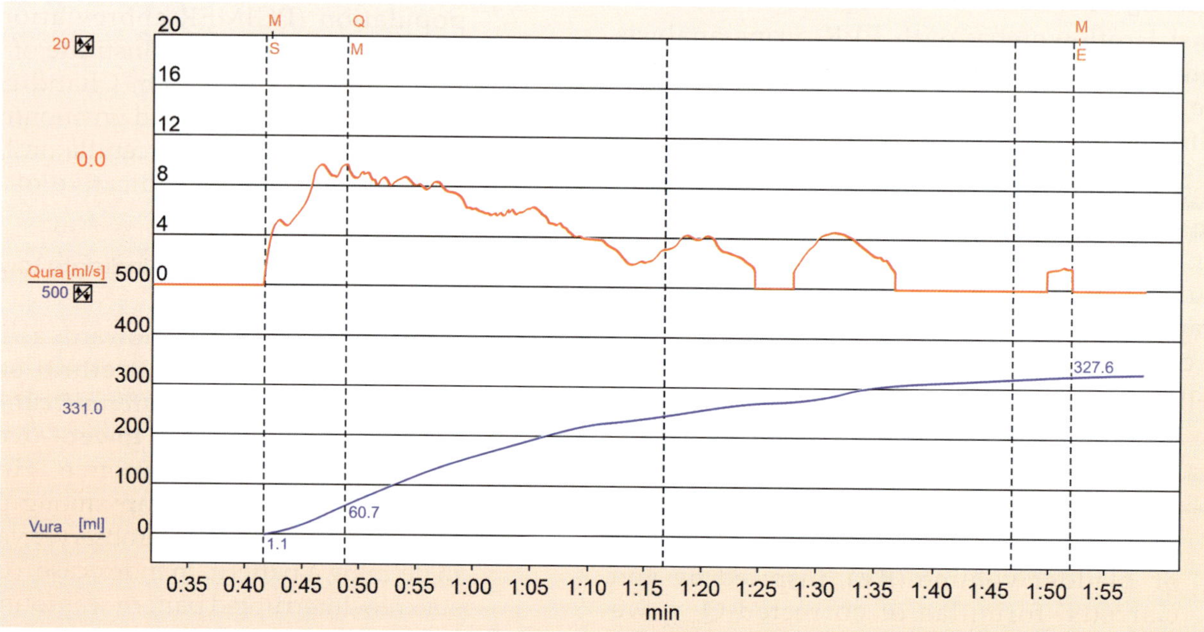

Fig. 14.2: Uroflowmetry of index patient after initial treatment showing improvement in flow pattern as well as in VQI. Q_{max} 9.9 ml/sec, voided volume 326 ml and PVR 50 ml. VQI_{max} 0.51 (an improvement of 59%).

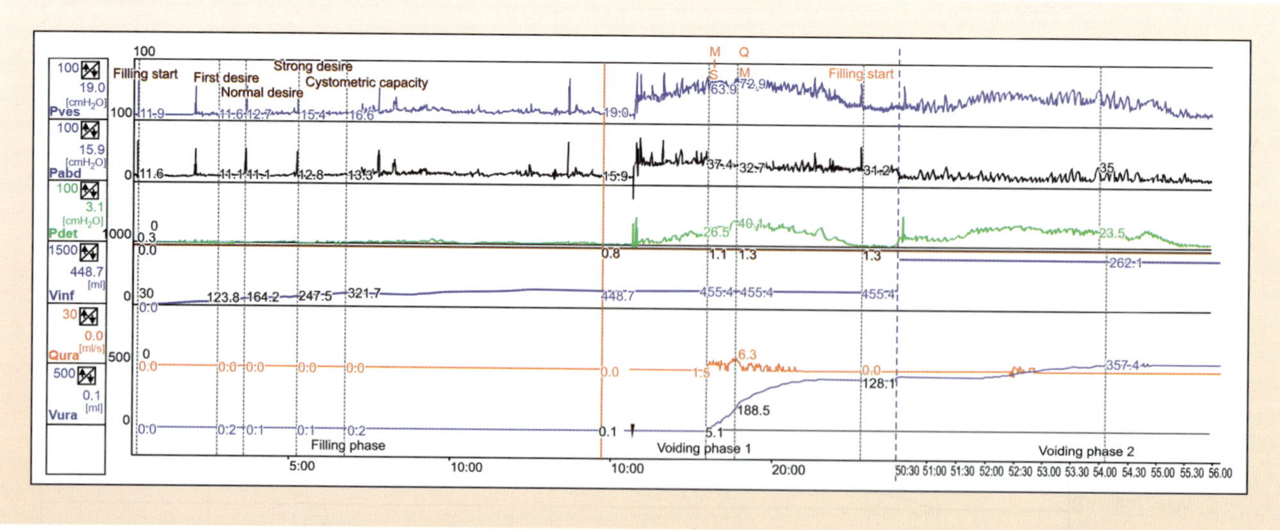

Fig. 14.3A: Pressure flow study showing normal filling phase with preserved sensations, no detrusor overactivity, normal capacity (strong desire at 455 ml) and compliance (100 ml/cm H_2O). Voiding phase revealed PdetQmax of 40 cmH_2O, Qmax 6 ml/sec, PVR 10%. Detrusor pattern—irregular bell in first cycle and plateau in second cycle. Grenwell Solomon BOOI = 26 clearly suggestive of bladder outlet obstruction.

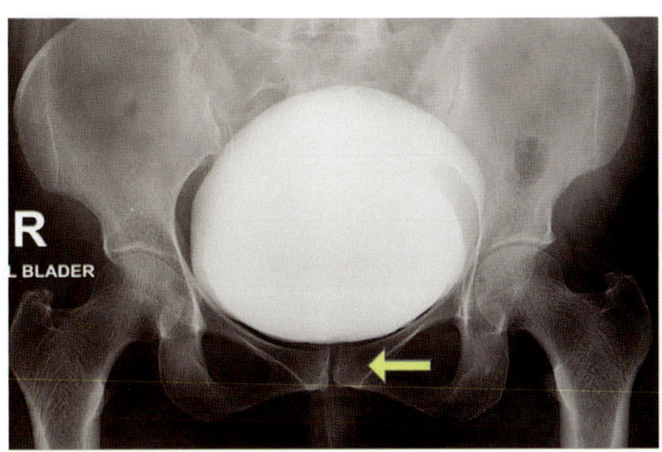

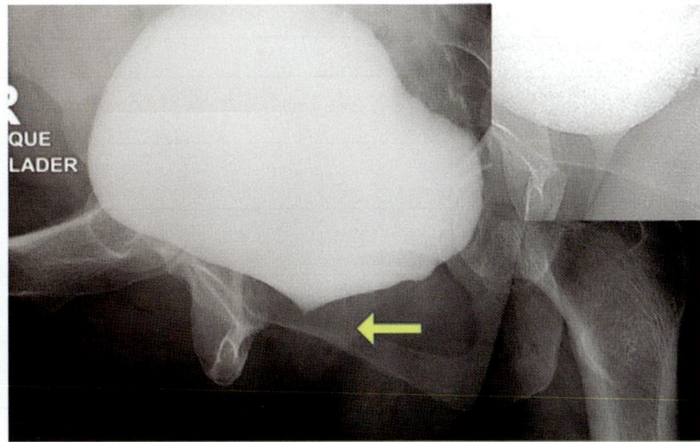

Fig. 14.3B: Static cystographic image of full bladder showing normal capacity bladder with mild irregularity of outline. Voiding cystographic image showing smooth tapering at midurethra level s/o nonrelaxing external sphincter

One may get urodynamics done during initial evaluation only, or may empirically try alpha blockers, treat constipation and teach pelvic-floor relaxation exercises and order urodynamics if faced with suboptimal response. Timing is not clear even in the most comprehensive European Association of Urology (EAU) and British Association of Urological Surgeons (BAUS) guidelines.[10,11] Nevertheless, it is clear that urodynamics is essential for diagnosis of voiding dysfunction; main differential diagnoses being DU, bladder neck obstruction (BNO) and PFD.

8. What urodynamic tests are required?

Ans: Urodynamic definitions of bladder-outlet obstruction (BOO) and DU are still not standardized in women. Therefore, diagnosis and localization of obstruction often requires radio-fluoroscopic assistance. This could be performed simultaneously with urodynamics (i.e. videourodynamics) or as a closely followed separate study (VCUG).

9. How does one define BOO and DU in women?

Ans: Pressure and flow cutoffs have been variable across studies: $PdetQ_{max}$ ranging from 20–50 cm H_2O with Q_{max} 12–15 ml/sec. The most comprehensive and validated criteria have been published by Solomon *et al* from a cohort of 647 women with VD. The authors found that cutoff-values of 0, 5 and 18 from formula [$PdetQ_{max}$–2.2 XQ_{max}] were predictive of BOO in 10%, 50% and 90%, respectively.[12] This is quite similar to BOO-index [$PdetQ_{max}$–2XQ_{max}] in men where cutoffs of 20 and 40 are used. We found plateau-pattern of detrusor contraction as a useful surrogate of PFD as a cause of BOO.[13]

Defining DU is even more intriguing and descriptive. The International Continence Society defines DUA as "a contraction of reduced strength and/or duration, resulting in prolonged bladder emptying and/or a failure to achieve complete bladder emptying within a normal time-span". No numerical values were defined. There have been several attempts: Projected isovolumetric pressure-1 defined as [$Pdet.Q_{max}$ + Q_{max}][14] and the 'k' value on Valentini-Besson-Nelson (VBN) nomogram[15] are the most notable numerical representations of detrusor-contractility and most differentiative of normal from DUA (PIP1 41.6±10.3 vs 23.7±9.9 and k value 0.43±0.22 vs. 0.04±0.17, respectively).[16]

In the index case, Greenwell-Solomon value of 26 was highly predictive of BOO and presence of plateau detrusor pattern along with non-relaxing pelvic floor on VCUG indicated dysfunctional voiding as the location of obstruction. A PIP1 value of 46 was indicative of normal detrusor contractility.

Case Scenario *(Contd.)*

After making urodynamic diagnosis of dysfunctional voiding, tizanidine 2 mg three times daily was added to her current treatment regimen. Her symptoms were significantly improved, IPSS score being improved to 8/35 and QOL to 2/6. Uroflowmetry also showed further improvement: Q_{max} 13.9 ml/sec, Q_{ave} 8.1ml/sec, VV 456 ml and PVR 20 ml VQlm = 0.63 (Fig. 14.4).

10. What is the role of alpha-blockers in VD in women?

Ans: Alpha-blockers are often prescribed as first-line for VD in women. Tamsulosin is the most commonly studied pharmaceutical agent, followed by terazosin. There are no studies on silodosin. Small studies on alfuzosin found

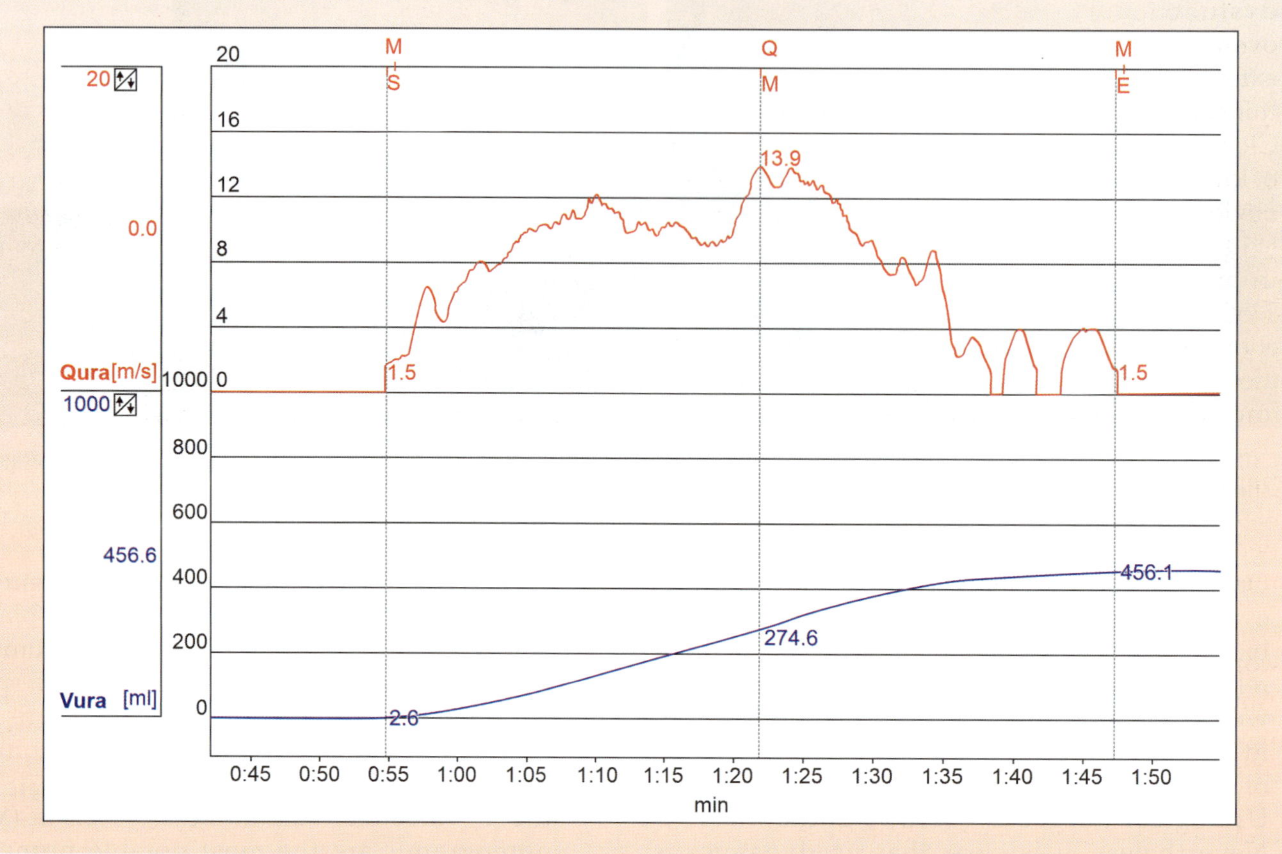

Fig. 14.4: Follow-up uroflowmetry after addition of tizanidine, showing further improvement in flow pattern and VQI. Q_{max} 13.9 ml/sec, voided volume 456 ml and PVR 20 ml. VQI_{max} 0.63 (a further improvement of 23.5%)

only equivocal results. A meta-analysis of six randomized studies (tamsulosin vs. placebo, vs prazosin) found tamsulosin to improve IPSS (–4.08, 95% CI–5.92 to-2.23) and QOL (–2.1, 95% CI–2.67 to –1.71) compared to placebo.[17] Improvement in urodynamic parameters was not found to be very significant. These improvements are not to the extent of that found in men with bladder neck obstruction or prostatomegaly.[18] This can be attributed to lower density of –1A adrenergic receptors in women compared to men. Nevertheless, alpha blockers do reduce urethral pressure along the entire length of female urethra and therefore should be considered.[19]

11. Is there a role of PDE-5 inhibitors in women with VD?

Ans: Tadalafil, a phosphodiesterase-5 inhibitor, is well established in combination with alpha-1 blockers for treatment of voiding dysfunction in men.[20,21] However, situation in women is far from established. A study of 24 healthy volunteers, Christoffersen *et al* found single dose tadalafil 40 mg to reduce urethral closure pressure.[22] In a randomized study with Fowler's syndrome, Datta *et al* found sildenafil (100 mg/day) not to be superior to placebo.[23] At present, PDE-5 inhibitors is not recommended in women with VD outside clinical trial or off-label use.

12. Are Skeletal-muscle relaxants (SMR) useful in women with PFD?

Ans: SMRs are a heterogenous group of medications which are used for neurogenic/non-neurogenic spastic muscular conditions with or without pain. Role of SMRs in the management of DV is plausible; however, there is no agent with site-specific (in this case, pelvic floor) action. Baclofen, a centrally acting agonist of $GABA_B$ receptors, is the most studied SMR for PFD. In a randomized study on 60 female participants with DV, Xu *et al* found significant reduction in number of voids and EMG activity with baclofen 10 mg thrice daily.[24] Tizanidine is centrally acting alpha-2 adrenergic receptor agonist which has been used for myofascial pain syndromes since 90s. In a randomized study, El-Hefnawy *et al* found tizanidine to be more efficacious than doxazosin in children with DV.[25]

13. What is the importance of evaluation of constipation in women with VD?

Ans: VD and defecatory-dysfunction often co-exist. Constipation coexists more often with dysfunctional voiding and encopresis, with overactive bladder symptoms.[26,27] Although, most extensively studied in children and adolescents, this coexistence is not uncommon in adults too.[28,29] Close physical proximity and shared innervation of lower urinary tract and rectum-anal complex are obvious reasons for this association. It is paramount to identify and treat co-existing defecatory disorder in any patient with VD. Polyethylene glycol 3350 along with high fiber diet is a common first choice in view of its excellent safety and efficacy record.[30] Prosecretory agents, colonic stimulants and serotonergic agent may judiciously be used.[31] However, it is recommended to refer a patient of refractory constipation or that with alarm features (e.g. unexplained loss of weight, hematochezia, melena, excessive cramping) to a medical gastroenterologist.

14. What are the other conservative measures for women with DV ?

Ans: Pelvic-floor muscle training (PFMT) with/without biofeedback has been extensively studied in children with VD. The available data favors supervised PFMT relaxation in adults. Biofeedback and stimulation therapies are often employed when the patient is unable to perform PFMT properly. In a prospective study of 48 women Lazaros *et al* found supervised PFMT for 6 months led to reduction in urinary-tract infection episodes and PVR.[32] In another prospective study of 60 women with functional BOO (site not mentioned) Koh *et al* found both alfuzosin and magnetic stimulation effective in improving Q_{max}, bladder capacity, AUA score and QOL.[33]

15. What are the interventional options for VD in women?

Ans: Bladder-neck incision (BNI)—for refractory urodynamic BNO. Several techniques are described, 10 and 2 o'clock incisions, 5 and 7 o'clock incisions and 3, 6, 9 and 12 o'clock incisions. Resection between 5 and 7 o'clock is also described. In the largest series of 84 women with BNO, Zhang *et al* reported excellent outcomes in terms of improvement in IPSS (22.9 to 7.9) and uroflow rates (Q_{max} 9.75 to 18.79 ml/sec). Three patients developed vesicovaginal fistula in 5 and 7 o' clock technique and 4 developed stress-incontinence.[34]

Onabotulinum toxin infiltration into external sphincter (BTX)–for women with unequivocal PFD and those with unspecified DU (e.g. post radical hysterectomy). In a large series of 138 women, Kao *et al*[35] reported excellent to marked improvement in 56% women with DU and 74% with PFD. Interestingly, in a small RCT of 62 women with DU and PFD, Jiang *et al*[36] found similar success rate with botulinum toxin as well as saline injection. Repeated injection of BTX offered greater therapeutic response.

Sacral neuromodulation—neuromodulation is the only therapy affecting the basic pathophysiology of PFD, i.e. disturbances in primary and secondary urethra-to-bladder and bladder-to-urethra reflexes. At different frequencies, pulse-width and amplitudes it has been found effective in storage as well as voiding dysfunction. Success rates of 65–78% have been reported in patients with idiopathic retention.[37,38] These success rates were sustained even after 10 years of follow-up. However, apart from high cost, significant revision rates (30–50%) are a concern.

SUMMARY

- A detailed history and physical examination including focused neurological assessment is paramount initial step in evaluation of voiding dysfunction. Most clinical errors happen at this step.
- A baseline uroflowmetry with ultrasound assessment of post-void residual urine and urine analysis are basic minimum investigations for making initial impression since it is not uncommon to find discrepancy in clinical findings and uroflowmetry.
- Alpha blocker (tamsulosin or silodosin), pelvic floor training, treatment of constipation with or without CIC (if PVR is 'high') is an effective initial treatment strategy.
- Urodynamics with fluoroscopy (videourodynamics or pressure–flow study with separately done VCUG) should be reserved for women who are refractory to initial treatment or who initially present with high risk features (most remarkably upper tract changes).
- Once diagnosis of dysfunctional voiding is made of urodynamics, one may consider adding skeletal muscle relaxants (baclofen, tizanidine) to initial treatment outlined above.
- Intradetrusor onabotulinum toxin injection and sacral neuromodulation are next-line invasive interventions for women refractory to the previously outlined treatment.
- One must understand the current limitations of lack of high level of scientific evidence for treatment of voiding dysfunction in women and appropriately discuss with the patient.

REFERENCES

1. Roy HA, Nettleton J, Blain C, Dalton C, Farhan B, Fernandes A, *et al.* Assessment of patients with lower urinary tract symptoms where an undiagnosed neurological disease is suspected: A report from an International Continence Society consensus working group. Neurourol Urodyn. 2020; 39:2535–43.
2. Brookes ST, Donovan JL, Wright M, Jackson S, Abrams P. A scored form of the Bristol Female Lower Urinary Tract Symptoms questionnaire: Data from a randomized controlled trial of surgery for women with stress incontinence. Am J Obstet Gynecol 2004;191:73–82.

3. Barry MJ, Fowler FJ, O'Leary MP, Bruskewitz RC, Holtgrewe HL, Mebust WK, *et al.* The American Urological Association Symptom Index for Benign Prostatic Hyperplasia. J Urol 199;148:1549–57.
4. Agachan F, Chen T, Pfeifer J, Reissman P, Wexner SD. A constipation scoring system to simplify evaluation and management of constipated patients. Dis Colon Rectum 1996;39:681–5.
5. Da Roza T, Mascarenhas T, Araujo M, Trindade V, Jorge RN. Oxford Grading Scale vs manometer for assessment of pelvic floor strength in nulliparous sports students. Physiotherapy (United Kingdom) 2013;99:207–11.
6. Laycock J, Jerwood D. Pelvic floor muscle assessment: The PERFECT scheme. Physiotherapy. 2001;87:631–42.
7. Kalra S, Gupta P, Dorairajan LN, Ramanitharan M, Sreenivasan SK, Hota S. Does successful urethral calibration rule out significant female urethral stenosis? confronting the confounder-an outcome analysis of successfully treated female urethral strictures. International braz j urol. 2021;47:829–40.
8. Kuo HC. Clinical symptoms are not reliable in the diagnosis of lower urinary tract dysfunction in women. Journal of the Formosan Medical Association. 2012;111:386–91.
9. Lowenstein L, Anderson C, Kenton K, Dooley Y, Brubaker L. Obstructive voiding symptoms are not predictive of elevated postvoid residual urine volumes. Int Urogynecol J 2008;19:801–4.
10. Harding CK, Lapitan MC, Arlandis S, *et al.* EAU guidelines on non-neurogenic female lower urinary tract symptoms. European Association of Urology. 2022.
11. Biers SM, Harding C, Belal M, Thiruchelvam N, Hamid R, Sahai A, *et al.* British Association of Urological Surgeons (BAUS) consensus document: Management of female voiding dysfunction. BJU Int. 2022;129:151–9.
12. Solomon E, Yasmin H, Duffy M, Rashid T, Akinluyi E, Greenwell TJ. Developing and validating a new nomogram for diagnosing bladder outlet obstruction in women. Neurourol Urodyn. 2018;37:368–78.
13. Agarwal MM, Sharma S, Jain S, Prasad D, Bhaskar V, Gupta S, *et al.* Can urodynamic diagnosis of dysfunctional voiding/external sphincter nonrelaxation be made on two-channel pressure-flow study without video-urodynamics, electromyography, or urethral pressure profilometry? Plateau detrusor pattern in perspective. Neurourol Urodyn 2022;41:935–44.
14. Thai LT, Bergmann MA, Griffiths D, Resnick NM. Stop test or pressure-flow study? Measuring detrusor contractility in older females. Neurourol Urodyn 2004;23:184–9.
15. Valentini FA, Marti BG, Nelson PP, Zimmern PE, Robain G. Usefulness of an algebraic fitting of nomograms allowing evaluation detrusor contractility in women. Progrès en Urologie. 2017;27:261–6.
16. Valentini FA, Marti BG, Robain G, Zimern PE, Nelson PP. Comparison of indices allowing an evaluation of detrusor contractility in women. Progrès en Urologie. 2020;30:396–401.
17. Zhang HL, Huang ZG, Qiu Y, Cheng X, Zou XQ, Liu TT. Tamsulosin for treatment of lower urinary tract symptoms in women: a systematic review and meta-analysis. Int J Impot Res;29:148–56.
18. Zhou Z, Cui Y, Wu J, Ding R, Cai T, Gao Z. Meta-analysis of the efficacy and safety of combination of tamsulosin plus dutasteride compared with tamsulosin monotherapy in treating benign prostatic hyperplasia. BMC Urol 2019;19:1–12.
19. Reitz A, Haferkamp A, Kyburz T, Knapp PA, Wefer B, Schurch B. The effect of tamsulosin on the resting tone and the contractile behaviour of the female urethra: A functional urodynamic study in healthy women. Eur Urol 2004; 46:235–40.
20. Pattanaik S, Mavuduru RS, Panda A, Mathew JL, Agarwal MM, Hwang EC, *et al.* Phosphodiesterase inhibitors for lower urinary tract symptoms consistent with benign prostatic hyperplasia. Cochrane Database of Systematic Reviews. 2018;11:CD010060.
21. Zhou R, Che X, Zhou Z, Ma Y. A Systematic Review and Meta-Analysis of the Efficacy and Safety of Tamsulosin Plus Tadalafil Compared With Tamsulosin Alone in Treating Males With Lower Urinary Tract Symptoms Secondary to Benign Prostrate Hyperplasia. Am J Mens Health 2023;17:15579883231155096.
22. Christoffersen T, Riis T, Kornholt J, Sonne DP, Klarskov N. The effect of single-dose tadalafil on urethral pressure and voiding parameters: a double-blind, randomized, placebo-controlled, crossover study in healthy women. Neurourol Urodyn 2022;2:100193.
23. Datta SN, Kavia RBC, Gonzales G, Fowler CJ. Results of Double-Blind Placebo-Controlled Crossover Study of Sildenafil Citrate (Viagra) in Women Suffering from Obstructed Voiding or Retention Associated with the Primary Disorder of Sphincter Relaxation (Fowler's Syndrome). Eur Urol. 2007;51:489–97.
24. Xu D, Qu C, Meng H, Ren J, Zhu Y, Min Z, *et al.* Dysfunctional voiding confirmed by transdermal perineal electromyography, and its effective treatment with baclofen in women with lower urinary tract symptoms: A randomized double-blind placebo-controlled crossover trial. BJU Int 2007;100:588–92.
25. El-Hefnawy AS, Helmy T, El-Assmy MM, Sarhan O, Hafez AT, Dawaba M. Doxazosin Versus Tizanidine for Treatment of Dysfunctional Voiding in Children: A Prospective Randomized Open-labeled Trial. Urology 2012;79:428–33.
26. Combs AJ, Van Batavia JP, Chan J, Glassberg KI. Dysfunctional Elimination Syndromes—How Closely Linked are Constipation and Encopresis with Specific Lower Urinary Tract Conditions? J Urol 2013;190:1015–20.
27. Halachmi S, Farhat WA. The impact of constipation on the urinary tract system. Int J Adolesc Med Health 2008;20:17–22.
28. White BA, Linder BJ, Szarka LA, Prichard DO. Urinary Symptoms and Bladder Voiding Dysfunction Are Common in Young Men with Defecatory Disorders: A Retrospective Evaluation. Dig Dis Sci 2022;67:3036–44.
29. Klingele CJ, Lightner DJ, Fletcher JG, Gebhart JB, Bharucha AE. Dysfunctional urinary voiding in women with functional defecatory disorders. Neurogastroenterology & Motility 2010;22:1094–e284.
30. Erickson BA, Austin JC, Cooper CS, Boyt MA. Polyethylene Glycol 3350 for Constipation in Children With Dysfunctional Elimination. J Urol 2003;170:1518–20.
31. Camilleri M, Ford AC, Mawe GM, Dinning PG, Rao SS, Chey WD, *et al.* Chronic constipation. Nature Reviews Disease Primers 2017;3:1–19.

32. Lazaros T, Ioannis T, Vasileios S, Christina P, Michael S. The effect of pelvic floor muscle training in women with functional bladder outlet obstruction. Arch Gynecol Obstet 2023;1:1–6.

33. Koh JS, Kim SJ, Kim HS, Kim JC. Comparison of alpha-blocker, extracorporeal magnetic stimulation alone and in combination in the management of female bladder outlet obstruction. Int Urogynecol J 2011;22:849–54.

34. Zhang P, Wu ZJ, Xu L, Yang Y, Zhang N, Zhang XD. Bladder neck incision for female bladder neck obstruction: long-term outcomes. Urology 2014;83:762–7.

35. Kao YL, Ou YC, Tsai KJ, Kuo HC. Predictive Factors for a Successful Treatment Outcome in Patients with Different Voiding Dysfunction Subtypes Who Received Urethral Sphincter Botulinum Injection. Toxins 2022;14:877.

36. Jiang YH, Wang CC, Kuo HC. Onabotulinumtoxin a urethral sphincter injection as treatment for non-neurogenic voiding dysfunction-A randomized, double-blind, placebo-controlled study. Sci Rep 2016;6:38905.

37. Elneil S. Urinary retention in women and sacral neuromodulation. Int Urogynecol J 2010;21(SUPPL. 2):475–83.

38. El-Azab AS, Siegel SW. Sacral neuromodulation for female pelvic floor disorders. Arab J Urol 2019;17:14–22.

Chapter 15

Voiding Dysfunction: Female Urethral Stricture Disease

• *Ankur Mittal* • *Deepak Kumar*

LEARNING OBJECTIVES

- Bladder outlet obstruction in females is a challenging scenario which can occur due to functional and anatomical causes. Functional obstruction is more commonly seen than anatomical obstruction. Careful evaluation and precise diagnosis are important for the best outcomes.
- Uroflowmetry and PVR are important screening tools for patients having voiding LUTS. Calibration can help to identify the narrowing in the urethra.
- Proximal urethral dilatation and sudden tapering of the urethra on VCUG is suggestive of bladder outlet obstruction but it does not rule out functional causes.
- Cystourethroscopy helps in the identification and localization of urethral stricture. VUDS with EMG helps to rule out functional causes of bladder outlet obstruction.
- MRI is not routinely used in evaluation of urethral stricture disease, however, it may help to identify the rare causes of BOO including urethral malignancy, urethral diverticulum, and cervical malignancy.
- Urethral dilatation is recommended in newly diagnosed female urethral stricture disease. The success rate is significantly low in recurrent FUS.
- Augmentation urethroplasty is the definitive management of female urethral stricture disease. Meatoplasty has a good outcome in patients having meatal stenosis only.
- Grafts and flaps both have been used in female urethroplasty and have shown good outcomes. Local tissues for graft (vaginal mucosa or labial mucosa) have shown the equivalent results to buccal mucosa graft.

Case Scenario

A 37-year-old female gravida 1 para 1, no comorbidities presented with a 2 years history of bothersome lower urinary symptoms including frequency, urgency, weak urinary stream, nocturia 2–3 times per night and hesitancy. She noted her symptoms started shortly after the delivery of her child which was full-term normal vaginal delivery. She had a history of urethral dilatation one year back. Her symptoms improved after dilatation but again symptoms recurred after three months.

1. **How will you evaluate this patient?**

   Ans: Comprehensive history and physical examination are essential parts of the assessment of any patient. A detailed history of initiation and progression of lower urinary tract symptoms should be taken. History of other associated symptoms including suprapubic pain, any urethral or vaginal discharge, history of incontinence and flank pain should be taken.

   A detailed history should also include menstrual history, obstetric history, history of any previous surgery, history of urethral dilatation, and history of previous vaginal delivery.

   The examination should include a detailed pelvic examination to assess the external urethral meatus, palpation of the anterior vaginal wall for any fibrosis, and assessment for prolapse, masses, scars and vulval dermatological disorders such as lichen sclerosis, lichen planus or age-related atrophy.[1]

   Adjuncts to history and examination include uroflowmetry and PVR measurement.

   Ultrasonography for evaluation of upper tracts can be advised if there is doubt of upper tract changes or any lesion in the upper tract and/or in the urinary bladder. Routine blood investigations should be advised if surgical intervention is planned. Urine routine examination and urine culture and sensitivity should be advised in patients presenting with lower urinary tract symptoms to rule out underlying urinary tract infections.

Urethroscopy and voiding cystourethrography are the two most frequent diagnostic tests used in patients having suspected bladder outlet obstruction. Voiding cystourethrography(VCUG) and/or videourodynamics (VUDS) will help in the diagnosis of BOO.[2]

This index patient had history of normal vaginal delivery and no other significant history. Examination findings revealed normal external urethral meatus, supple urethra on palpation and healthy vaginal mucosa. Patient had no pelvic organ prolapse, and no local dermatological disease.

Role of uroflowmetry in evaluation of this patient

Although there are no specific cutoff values for uroflowmetry and PVR volumes, a plateau curve, flow rates less than 12 to 15 ml/s, and postvoid residuals > 100, may suggest obstruction.[3] Staccato pattern of voiding is more suggestive of dysfunctional voiding. Fractionated flow can be suggestive of detrusor underactivity.

Index patient: Uroflowmetry showed low maximum flow rate with plateau curve with high postvoid residue is suggestive of bladder outlet obstruction (Fiq. 15.1).

Role of calibration in evaluation of this patient

Urethral calibration can help to assess for definite narrowing in the female urethra. But the successful calibration does not rule out obstruction or stricture.[4]

Index patient: On calibration, 16 to 12 F catheter could not be negotiated beyond 0.5 cm, however, 10 F could be negotiated.

Role of VCUG in evaluation of this patient

VCUG helps in the identification of BOO. Ballooning of the proximal urethra and sudden tapering of flow is suggestive of BOO. Although it does not differentiate between anatomical and functional causes of BOO. Bladder trabeculations and diverticula, and the presence of vesicourethral reflux (VUR) can be other associated findings on VCUG.

Index patient: VCUG showed significant dilatation of proximal urethra. Bladder showed regular outline, normal capacity and no VUR (Fig. 15.2).

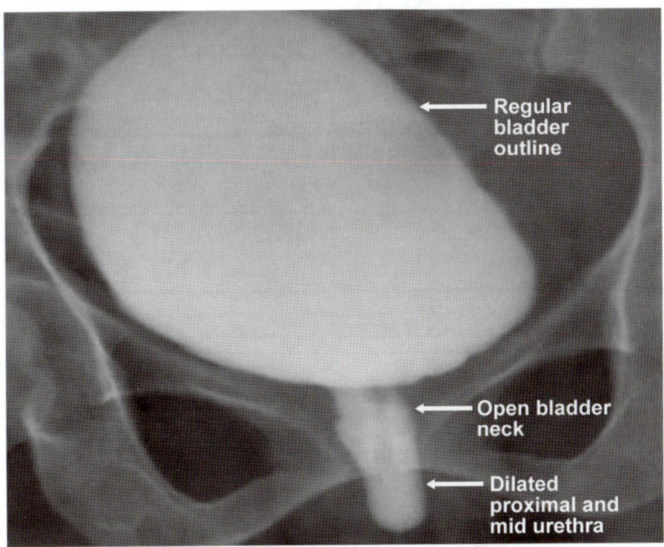

Fig. 15.2: Voiding cystourethrogram

Role of VUDS in evaluation of this patient

VUDS with EMG can help to rule out functional obstruction. Sporadic increase and decrease in

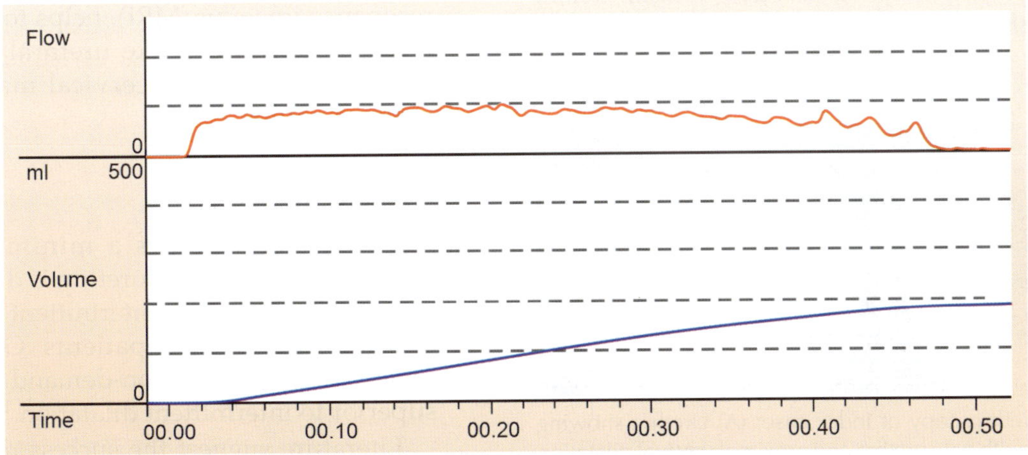

Fig. 15.1: Uroflowmetry curve

EMG activity can suggest dysfunctional voiding.[5] Urethral pressure profilometry also can help to rule out dysfunctional voiding. Plateau detrusor pressure during voiding is more suggestive of dysfunctional voiding in females.[6]

Index patient: Urodynamics showed high pressure low flow voiding with normal EMG activity (Fig. 15.3).

As most of the investigations were suggestive of urethral stricture disease, cystourethroscopy was done to confirm the diagnosis and to see the extent of urethral stricture.

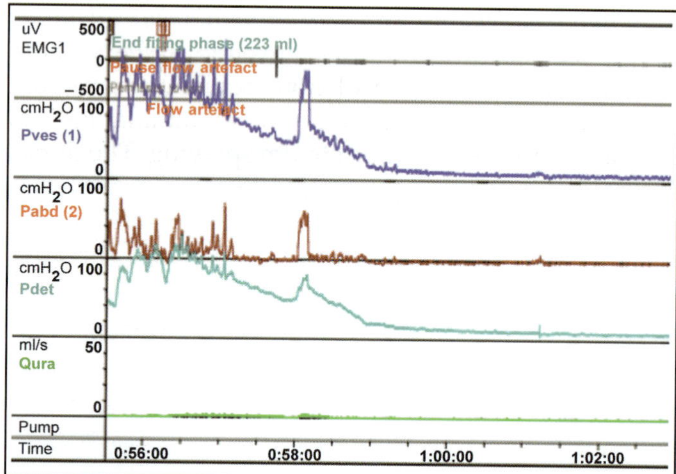

Fig. 15.3: Voiding phase of urodynamics of index case

Role of cystourethroscopy in evaluation of this patient

Cystourethroscopy allows the localization of urethral stricture specifically the distal extent of urethral stricture. Urethroscopy findings of pale or whitish discolouration urethra and luminal narrowing are suggestive of urethral stricture. Cystourethroscopy also helps to rule out other functional causes of urethral stricture.[7]

Index patient: Cystourethroscopy with 8 French Ureteroscope showed scarred narrowing in distal urethra (.5 cm) with proximal dilatation and trabeculations in bladder (Figs 15.4 A and B).

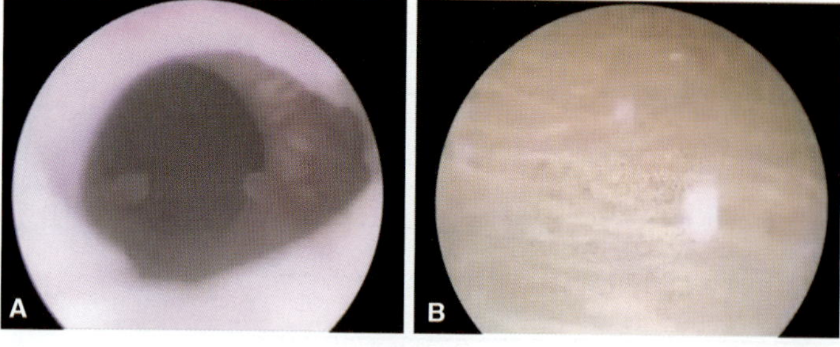

Figs 15.4: Cystourethroscopy of index case: (A) Urethra showing urethral narrowing with pale urethra and proximal urethral dilatation (B) Trabeculations in the bladder wall

Based on the above-mentioned findings (low maximum flow rate, and plateau pattern on uroflowmetry, dilated proximal urethra and distal urethral narrowing on VCUG, pale white narrowing in the distal urethra, dilated proximal urethra and bladder trabeculations on cystourethroscopy, and high pressure low flow with normal EMG on urodynamics), index patient was diagnosed as female urethral stricture disease.

2. **What is female urethral stricture disease?**

   Ans: Bladder outlet obstruction (BOO) is a challenging scenario that includes functional and anatomical causes. A thorough evaluation is needed to avoid misdiagnosis of functional causes as anatomical ones. Female urethral stricture disease is responsible for around 4–18% of cases of bladder outlet obstruction.

   Most widely accepted definition of female urethral stricture (FUS) "fixed anatomical narrowing" causing reduced urethral calibre, varying between <10 Fr and <20 Fr, with the majority of series defined <14 Fr as diagnostic, for urethral stricture disease. It can be diagnosed on calibration, endoscopy or on radiography.[8,9] Urodynamics findings of high pressure and low flow can adjunct the diagnosis of female urethral stricture disease.

3. **What are the causes of female urethral stricture?**

   Ans: The aetiology of FUS is mainly idiopathic (48.5%), followed by iatrogenic (24.1%) and traumatic (16.4%) causes.[10–12] In cases with iatrogenic aetiology, difficult or traumatic catheterisation with subsequent fibrosis, vaginal surgery, urethral surgery, repair of urethral diverticula, prior urethral dilations, and anti-incontinence procedures are responsible for stricture development in the majority of patients.

Role of MRI in the diagnosis of female urethral stricture disease

Three-dimensional imaging, such as magnetic resonance imaging (MRI), helps to identify other rare causes of BOO like urethral diverticulum, urethral malignancy, cervical malignancy and urethral polyps.[13,14]

Treatment Options

Urethral dilatation

Urethral dilatation is a minimally invasive technique in which the urethra is dilated between 24 F and 41 F.[15,16] Self-intermittent dilatation was also advised in some patients. One systematic review suggested that on-demand dilatation was superior to intermittent dilatation.[17]

Literature suggest the success rate of UD was 49% at a mean follow-up of 32 months and in patients who underwent previous instrumentation it was significantly low in comparison to patients with no such history (26.6% vs 75.1%).[17]

Role of meatoplasty

Meatal stenosis in females is a rare entity. Meatoplasty has an excellent success rate and minimal complications. Meatoplasty is the first line of management in patients having short-segment meatal stenosis.[18]

Role of urethrotomy

Data are scarce on the use and outcome of urethrotomy in female urethral stricture patients. One study, where urethrotomy used in management of BOO, suggested symptomatic improvement in 80% of patients.[19]

Role of urethroplasty

Definitive repair with urethroplasty is a recommended option both in patients with primary stricture disease as well as recurrence after urethral dilatation. Repeat dilatation is associated with a low success rate and repeat dilatation can make a complex scar which can make definitive repair difficult.[20]

Augmentation urethroplasty is the most common technique used in the female urethral reconstruction. Augmentation urethroplasty is done mainly by ventral (posterior) and dorsal (anterior) approach. Grafts and flaps both have shown good outcomes.

Index patient was diagnosed as a case of female urethral stricture disease and had history of previous urethral dilatation. Patient was managed with dorsal onlay vaginal mucosa graft urethroplasty.

Role of grafts in female urethroplasty and its outcome

Graft augmentation has gained popularity in both males and females. Grafts can be harvested from oral mucosa (buccal or labial) or local tissue (vaginal or labial). All grafts have shown similar success rates.[17] A healthy vaginal graft can be harvested easily and without the need for general anaesthesia. The vaginal mucosa is moist, elastic and hairless so it is suitable for augmentation urethroplasty.[21] Labial grafts also show comparable results to vaginal grafts. Local grafts are not suitable in cases of lichen sclerosis, vaginal fibrosis or any other local dermatological disease.

Oral mucosa has also gained significant popularity because of its versatility. It is easy to harvest, easy to handle, and has good graft uptake and minimal contracture making these grafts an ideal substitute for urethroplasties.[22] Although Buccal mucosa graft is versatile, there is minimal risk of injury of parotid ducts mental nerve, and neurosensory complications. This risk can be avoided by using a lingual graft.

Dorsal (anterior) vs ventral (posterior) onlay urethroplasty

There is debate regarding the dorsal vs ventral approach. Ventral graft placement relies on the presumption that ventral dissection is easier than dorsal dissection and it has a lesser effect on sexual function because the dissection plane is away from the dorsal neurovascular bundle. However, no study documented a change in sexual function after the dorsal approach of urethroplasty.

The dorsal approach is presumed to have better mechanical and vascular support to the graft and helps to prevent sacculation and maintain urethral angulation—avoiding stream splaying. The dorsal approach has a lower risk of diverticula formation and fistula formation. The ventral wall is spared in the dorsal approach for future incontinence procedures.

Both approaches can be used with a comparable success rate and minimal complications.

The index case underwent dorsal onlay vaginal graft urethroplasty. Click on QR code to see the video or visit link (https://youtu.be/VQW3d55oLdQ)

Scan QR Code for Video on
Dorsal onlay vaginal mucosal graft urethroplasty
VIDEO 16

Role of flaps in female urethroplasty and its outcome

Vaginal and labial flaps are commonly used flaps in urethroplasty. Vaginal flaps, being well-vascularized and freely mobile, yield good results with the lowest morbidity to the vaginal wall.[38] Many techniques of vaginal flap urethroplasty have been described in the literature. Vaginal flap urethroplasty can be done using a U- or C-shaped inlay flap and also using ventral, dorsal, or lateral approaches.[23,24]

Role of meatal sparing urethroplasty in the management of female urethral stricture disease

The meatal sparing technique has been explained in both the dorsal onlay and ventral onlay techniques. The main advantage of the meatal sparing technique is the preservation of natural urine flow patterns in patients. Another advantage of the ventral technique is to minimise the risk of hypospadias meatus[25,26] (Figs 15.5A–E).

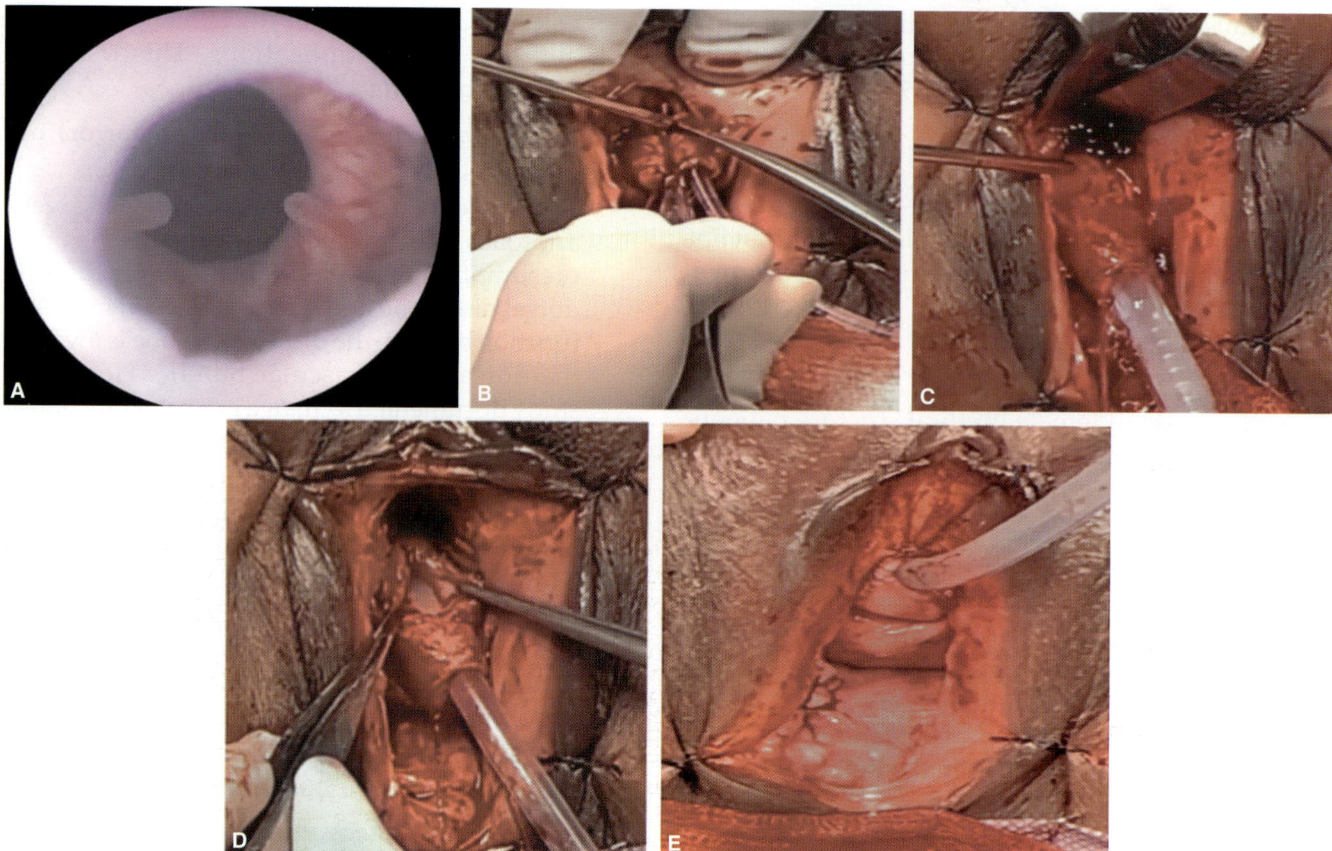

Fig. 15.5An to E: Dorsal onlay meatal sparing vaginal graft urethroplasty: (A) Urethral stricture seen on urethroscopy (B) Suprameatal semilunar incision (C) Plane made dorsally over urethra (D) Slitting the urethra dorsally over the stricture segment to safeguard the meatus (E) Graft placed dorsally and final image showing wide open urethra

Future Directions

Diagnostic criteria for female urethral stricture are not well defined. Dynamic voiding transvaginal ultrasonography may have some role in diagnosis as it shows the dynamic delineation of the urethra as it distends with urine.[27]

In the future, new techniques like genetic tissue engineering and drug-coated balloon dilatation can have some role in the management of female urethral stricture disease.

SUMMARY

- All efforts should be made to differentiate the anatomical cause from the functional cause of bladder outlet obstruction as the management of both entities is different.
- Urodynamics can help in the differentiation of functional cause from anatomical cause in bladder outlet obstruction.
- Modality of treatment should be opted after share decision-making. The patient should be explained about the possible need for repeated visits after minimal invasive techniques (especially in developing countries).

REFERENCES

1. Agochukwu-Mmonu N, Srirangapatanam S, Cohen A, *et al.* Female Urethral Strictures: Review of Diagnosis, Etiology, and Management. Curr Urol Rep. 2019 Nov 8;20(11):74. doi: 10.1007/s11934-019-0933-1. PMID: 31705324.
2. Hsiao SM, Lin HH, Kuo HC. Videourodynamic Studies of Women with Voiding Dysfunction. Sci Rep. 2017 Jul 28;7(1):6845. doi: 10.1038/s41598-017-07163-2. PMID: 28754926; PMCID: PMC5533800.
3. Groutz A, Blaivas JG, Chaikin DC. Bladder outlet obstruction in women: definition and characteristics. Neurourol Urodyn. 2000;19(3):213–20. doi: 10.1002/(sici)1520-6777(2000)19:3<213::aid-nau2>3.0.co;2-u. PMID: 10797578.
4. Kalra S, Gupta P, Dorairajan LN, *et al.* Does successful urethral calibration rule out significant female urethral stenosis? confronting the confounder-an outcome analysis of successfully treated female urethral strictures. Int Braz J Urol. 2021;47(4):829–840. doi:10.1590/S1677-5538.IBJU.2020.0857.
5. Sinha S. Dysfunctional voiding: A review of the terminology, presentation, evaluation and management in children and adults. Indian J Urol. 2011 Oct;27(4):437–47. doi: 10.4103/0970-1591.91429. PMID: 22279306; PMCID: PMC3263208.
6. Agarwal MM, Jain S, Mavuduru R, *et al.* Plateau pattern of detrusor contraction: A surrogate indicator of presence of external sphincter dysfunction during micturitional phase of urodynamic study. Indian J Urol. 2016 Apr-Jun;32(2):137–40. doi: 10.4103/0970-1591.174777. PMID: 27127357; PMCID: PMC4831503.
7. Mukhtar BMB, Spilotros M, Malde S, *et al.* Ventral-onlay buccal mucosa graft substitution urethroplasty for urethral

stricture in women. BJU Int. 2017 Nov;120(5):710–716. doi: 10.1111/bju.13970. Epub 2017 Aug 20. PMID: 28749039.

8. Osman NI, Mangera A, Chapple CR. A systematic review of surgical techniques used in the treatment of female urethral stricture. Eur Urol. 2013 Dec;64(6):965–73. doi: 10.1016/j.eururo.2013.07.038. Epub 2013 Aug 3. PMID: 23937829.
9. Smith AL, Ferlise VJ, Rovner ES. Female urethral strictures: successful management with long-term clean intermittent catheterization after urethral dilatation. BJU Int. 2006 Jul;98(1): 96–9. doi: 10.1111/j.1464–410X.2006.06206.x. PMID: 16831151.
10. Rijal A, Little B, McPhee S, *et al.* Bladder outflow problems in females. Nepal Med Coll J. 2013 Mar;15(1):46–9. PMID: 24592794.
11. Spilotros M, Malde S, Solomon E, *et al.* Female urethral stricture: a contemporary series. World J Urol. 2017 Jun;35(6):991–995. doi: 10.1007/s00345–016–1947–7. Epub 2016 Oct 4. PMID: 27704202.
12. Tao, T.T.X., *et al.* Novel surgical technique for female distal urethral stricture disease: an evaluation of efficacy and safety compared with urethral dilatation. Int J Clin Exp Med, 2018. 11: 12002.
13. Elsayes KM, Mukundan G, Narra VR, *et al.* Endovaginal magnetic resonance imaging of the female urethra. J Comput Assist Tomogr. 2006 Jan-Feb;30(1):1–6. doi: 10.1097/01.rct.0000187420.61062.f9. PMID: 16365564.
14. Theisen KM, Kadow BT, Rusilko PJ. Three-Dimensional Imaging of Urethral Stricture Disease and Urethral Pathology for Operative Planning. Curr Urol Rep. 2016 Aug;17(8):54. doi: 10.1007/s11934–016–0616–0. PMID: 27278565.
15. Popat S, Zimmern PE. Long-term management of luminal urethral stricture in women. Int Urogynecol J. 2016 Nov;27(11):1735–1741. doi: 10.1007/s00192–016–3006–8. Epub 2016 Mar 30. PMID: 27026141.
16. Romman AN, Alhalabi F, Zimmern PE. Distal intramural urethral pathology in women. J Urol. 2012 Oct;188(4):1218–23. doi: 10.1016/j.juro.2012.06.016. Epub 2012 Aug 16. PMID: 22902013.
17. Sarin I, Narain TA, Panwar VK, *et al.* Deciphering the enigma of female urethral strictures: A systematic review and meta-analysis of management modalities. Neurourol Urodyn. 2021 Jan;40(1):65–79. doi: 10.1002/nau.24584. Epub 2020 Dec 8. PMID: 33617047.
18. Heising J, Seiferth J. Die Meatusstenose des Mädchens--Klinik und Therapie [Meatus stenosis of girls--clinical demonstration and therapy (author's transl)]. Urologe A. 1978 Sep;17(5):292–5. German. PMID: 706007.
19. Massey JA, Abrams PH. Obstructed voiding in the female. Br J Urol. 1988 Jan;61(1):36–9. doi: 10.1111/j.1464–410x.1988.tb09158.x. PMID: 3342298.
20. Rehder P, Glodny B, Pichler R, *et al.* Dorsal urethroplasty with labia minora skin graft for female urethral strictures. BJU Int. 2010 Oct;106(8):1211–4. doi: 10.1111/j.1464–410X.2010.09240.x. PMID: 20230383.
21. Petrou SP, Rogers AE, Parker AS, *et al.* Dorsal vaginal graft urethroplasty for female urethral stricture disease. BJU Int. 2012 Dec;110(11 Pt C):E1090–5. doi: 10.1111/j.1464–410X.2012.11233.x. Epub 2012 May 17. PMID: 22594612.
22. Sharma GK, Pandey A, Bansal H, *et al.* Dorsal onlay lingual mucosal graft urethroplasty for urethral strictures in women. BJU Int. 2010 May;105(9):1309–12. doi: 10.1111/j.1464–410X.2009.08951.x. Epub 2009 Oct 28. PMID: 19874307.
23. Ackerman AL, Blaivas J, Anger JT. Female Urethral Reconstruction. Curr Bladder Dysfunct Rep. 2010 Dec;5(4):225–232. doi: 10.1007/s11884–010–0071–6. Epub 2010 Oct 19. PMID: 21475706; PMCID: PMC3061629.
24. Simonato A, Varca V, Esposito M, *et al.* Vaginal flap urethroplasty for wide female stricture disease. J Urol. 2010 Oct;184(4):1381–5. doi: 10.1016/j.juro.2010.06.042. Epub 2010 Aug 19. PMID: 20727538.
25. Katiyar, V.K., Sood, R., Singla, A. *et al.* Urethral meatus preserving ventral onlay augmentation urethroplasty for female urethral stricture: our technique with initial experience. Afr J Urol **27**, 127 (2021). doi.org/10.1186/s12301–021–00231–0.
26. Mittal A, Bahuguna G, Sarin I, Narain TA, *et al.* Meatal-sparing dorsal onlay vaginal graft urethroplasty: widening the surgical horizons of female urethral stricture. Int Urogynecol J. 2021 Mar;32(3):737–739. doi: 10.1007/s00192–020–04524–w. Epub 2020 Sep 14. PMID: 32926293.
27. Bhatt S, Goel M, Gupta A, *et al.* Diagnosis of Urethral Stricture on Dynamic Voiding Transvaginal Sonourethrography: A Case Report. Journal of Diagnostic Medical Sonography. 2017;33(2):140–143. doi 10.1177/8756479316688435.

Chapter

16

Bladder Pain Syndrome: Non-Hunner's Lesion

• *Anita Patel*

LEARNING OBJECTIVES

- Primary **BPS** is defined by the International Continence Society (ICS) as 'persistent or recurrent chronic pelvic pain, pressure or discomfort perceived to be related to the urinary bladder accompanied by at least one other urinary symptom such as an urgent need to void or urinary frequency'[1] Often under-reported, and seen more commonly in women, the prevalence in USA is 3.3 to 7.9 million women 18 years old or older.[2] The various aetio-pathology theories are presence of trans mural bladder wall inflammation, bladder biopsy showing mast cells, depletion of GAG [glycosa amino glycans] layer in the bladder mucosa making bladder more vulnerable to microbiological or chemical irritation, etc. The disease almost never leads to major renal damage or cancer.
- Pain in lower abdomen and/or urethra, perineum and pelvic floor relieved by voiding is the most frequent reason for seeking medical advice. Diurnal urinary frequency is commonly associated with the pain, +/-urgency but "urge incontinence' is rarely seen in a typical case. Typically patients "tend to void to avoid pain".[3] The diagnosis is essentially clinical but challenging due to heterogeneity of symptoms and its overlap with many other urological conditions with similar symptoms. Pain may be associated with negative cognitive, behavioural, sexual or emotional consequences and may be associated with symptoms of sexual dysfunction. The symptoms are known to have waxing and waning pattern and may be closely linked with mental stress.
- **Differential diagnoses** clinically include OAB and other painful conditions such as vulvodynia (pain in vulva with/ without any LUTS) or prostatodynia in a male.
- **Clinical examination** is usually normal but special note should be made of any obvious signs such as supra-pubic tenderness, any local inflammation in introitus, vulva [women] or penis and scrotum [men]. A detailed PV [women] and PR [men] examination should be done to confirm intact local neurology and to look for any vaginal atrophy or pelvic organ prolapse [women] and prostatic enlargement and tenderness [men]. Any painful trigger painful points should be noted.
- The clinical diagnosis should be supported by a **bladder diary.** Small frequent voided volumes day and night is a common pattern seen in BPS patients, however, some patients may void normal volumes also.
- **Investigations** should include routine **urine analysis**, [usually normal but rarely there may be microscopic hematuria], and a bladder **sonography** to see pre- and postvoid volumes. This usually shows small pre-void volume and variable postvoid residue.. Any **microscopic hematuria** or persistent **pyuria** merits further evaluation. **Urodynamic study** is rarely indicated but can help in ruling out other conditions such as OAB and bladder outlet obstruction. UDS may show small capacity normally compliant painful bladder, sometimes with overactivity and these patients often fail to void during the test especially with indwelling urethral pressure line.
- **Treatment** essentially involves giving symptomatic relief but it starts with **general counselling** and reassurance. **Avoidance of triggers** such as excess coffee or tea or spice consumption, ensuring adequate water consumption to keep urine dilute and observing timed voiding helps in early cases. **Pain management** medications range from simple **paracetamol** to antispasmodics, Amitryptilene and **Pregebalin** to opioid painkillers. Bladder relaxants such as Flavoxate, **antimuscarinics** such as Solifenacin and **beta-3 agonists** such as Mirabegron may also help in cases with pain + frequency as the main presentation. Patients with pain induced reflex pelvic muscle contraction/spams, may benefit from biofeedback and pelvic floor relaxation techniques as well as alpha blockers. Oral supplement of **sodium pentosan polysulfate** can help in recreating the GAG layer and is useful in 50% of cases after 4–6 months treatment. Patients with nocturia as main bothersome complaint may benefit from **ADH supplement**. There is literature evidence showing response to Cimetidine, and oral cyclosporine, the latter needs careful monitoring.[4]
- **Cystoscopy under sedation** is done when standard conservative measures fail; primarily **to rule out any other serious cause** such as carcinoma *in situ*. Bladder capacity, any mucosal ulcers and **glomerulations** [not diagnostic] on distension with bleeding during decompression are noted.[5] Patients having a typical **Hunner's ulcer** [more diagnostic of BPS][5] on cystoscopy belong to a different clinical category and merit different Rx. Under same anaesthesia, cystodistension can be done.
- **Post-cystoscopy** intravesical instillations can be offered with various combinations of Heparin, local anaesthetic agent and steroid, and DMSO.[6]
- **Botulinum toxin** injection [100 units] can be used at the time of scopy. This has variable response and should be offered after careful counselling.[7]

- Patients refractory to these may need **Neuromodulation or epidural pain block**, again with an unpredictable treatment response. Needless to say this should be the last resort and should be offered only after careful counselling. Very rarely patients might need an augementation cystoplasty or cystectomy but this may not rid them of their pelvic pain![8] In the rare event that augmentation cystoplasty is performed, a supratrigonal cystectomy has been suggested. This approach minimizes the scope of reconstruction but leaves behind the trigone which might be important in the causation of pain. However removal of the entire bladder including trigone might still leave the patient with phantom pain akin to pain associated with an amputated limb. Hence, careful counselling is recommended.

Case Scenario

Mrs PA, a 42-year-old lady presented with storage LUTS with day frequency of 1–2 hourly, nocturia of 4 times with pain on full bladder relieved by voiding since 3 years. There was no incontinence. Her urine flow was satisfactory but she described difficulty initiating voiding if she held urine for too long. There were no comorbidities. She had normal menstruation and had had 1 FTND 12 years ago. She passed motion once a day. She was a marketing professional and her job involved a lot of travel. There was a fear of not finding toilet facility when she needed to and she preferred voiding at slightest desire to do so. She consumed 8 cups of black coffee daily. She described her QOL as terrible. Her clinical examination revealed a lady with BMI of 24, normal general and abdominal exam, normal urethral meatus, no pelvic organ prolapse but she described severe pain during a vaginal exam. Vagina was moist and pelvic muscle contraction strength was normal. A rectal exam was normal.

1. **What is your clinical diagnosis? Is there a differential diagnosis? How would you evaluate this lady?**

   Ans: The most likely clinical diagnosis here is bladder pain syndrome though patients with OAB might have similar presentation. Pain is the main differentiating feature. The initial evaluation will involve routine tests such as urine analysis, a bladder diary and pre- and postvoid sonography. Urine analysis is usually normal but microscopic hematuria might be present and if yes, it will need further evaluation with upper tract sono and a cytology. A bladder diary will be extremely useful, and apart from showing fixed small volume frequent voids diurnally, it can rule out polyuria as these patients might drink excess water to keep their urine dilute. Any triggers for her symptoms will be specifically looked for. Bladder ultrasonography with small pre- and variable postvoid volume will usually give a clue. Leading questions to rule out any mental stress will help as BPS patients may have psychological, emotions and sexual dysfunction.

   A screening uroflowmetry is advisable. This can help direct search for an organic cause such as stricture. There is also a link between chronic pelvic pain, bladder pain, overactive pelvic floor and dysfunctional voiding. Abnormalities in uroflow might offer a clue.

   Bladder diary revealed diurnal volumes of 120 to 160 ml per void, 1–2 hourly, nocturia 4 times with max night voided volume of 200 ml. Total 24-hour volume was 1600 to 2000 millilitres. Urine routine showed microscopic hematuria [2 reports] and sterile culture. Bladder sono showed pre-void 140 ml with 30 ml PVR. Routine blood tests, renal sonography and urine cytology were normal. Though she described her QOL as terrible, her LUTS was the main stress. She was dependent on coffee to keep her alert

2. **What will be your initial treatment approach?**

   Ans: Initial treatment will involve counselling, allaying any fears regarding the seriousness of the diagnosis, reducing her coffee intake and adjusting her overall liquid intake especially when she has to be out due to her profession. Early dinner and stopping liquid consumption 3 hours before bedtime will help in reducing her nocturia. She can be encouraged to follow a fixed routine and to add meditation and relaxation technique to her day. As regards pain, simple paracetamol at 500 or 650 mg twice daily along with mild bladder relaxants such as Flavoxate can give considerable symptoms relief. If frequency is still bothersome, bladder relaxants such as Solifenacin [5 mg] or Mirabegron [50 mg] can be added.

   She was started on Paracetamol 650 mg in the morning and Solifenacin 5 mg after lunch. Her employer was requested to shift her responsibility from outdoor marketing to indoor desk job. She reduced her coffee intake to 3 cups daily and also added 30 minutes of meditation to her routine. She had significant benefit in her symptoms and she appeared happy at 3 month follow-up. However, at follow-up after a year, her symptoms reappeared and excruciating pain was the biggest bother. Repeat treatment with earlier painkillers did not help and she had to take a break from her work due to pain. Repeat bladder diary revealed volumes hovering at 100–120 ml per void and routine tests were again normal.

3. **What would be your approach? Will you add another painkiller? What is the role of pentosan polysulfate in BPS?**

Ans: Trying a different painkiller such as Pregabalin 75 mg twice daily might help when simple analgesics have failed. Patients need to be counselled regarding possible drowsiness. Oral Pentosan polysulfate can be added. However, this needs to be used for minimum 3–6 months and should be administered on empty stomach three times a day making patient compliance a bit tricky. Other management tools such as counselling need to be continued forever.

She started Pregabalin at 75 mg night-time dose. This helped her sleep better in addition to pain contol. Pentosan polysulfate was also added though she could take it twice daily. She also started formal counselling sessions to help her deal with the pain and loss of her job. At this stage she specifically asked if any surgical and permanent solution was available.

4. **How does cystoscopy help? What is the role of cystodistension? Is the management different if a Hunner's ulcer is noted?**

Ans: A cystoscopy is carried out for persistent symptoms, despite standard conservative treatment. Apart from ruling out other conditions such as carcinoma *in situ*, it might show classic glomerulations on distending the bladder with bleeding during decompression. **Cystoscopy** is best done **under Sedation or GA** as these patients find any urethral manipulations painful. It may show a Hunner's ulcer [a stellate mucosal superficial ulcerative lesion. The management of this is discussed in another chapter in this book.] Simultaneously cysto-distension with saline with irrigation column at 20 min is excessive period for hydrodistension. even ref 6 does not support this. we should change this at low pressure (< 80 cm H_2O) and short duration (<5 minutes) hydrodistension can give short-term benefit.[6]

The patient underwent a cystoscopy and cystodistension which gave her relief for 4 weeks. She refused a repeat cystoscopy!

5. **What is the role of intravescical instillation therapy?**

Intravescical instillations of alkalinised Lidocaine with heparin, or hyaluronic acid, or DMSO, or Pentosan polysulfate at varying dose, instilled weekly for 6 weeks followed by monthly instillations are known to give short-term symptom relief in up to 70% of patients. The mechanism of action is believed to be local anaesthetic effect or by replenishing or repairing GAG layer. Pain, UTI and irritation are minor side effects. Opacification of lens is a peculiar side effect of DMSO though described in animals.[6]

Patient was offered instillations but gave it up after 4 weeks due to catheter-induced pain. She also joined a support group due to persistent symptoms, left her job and reported severe insomnia due to pain and frequency. By now she wished to have her bladder removed and also decided to try alternative therapy with meditation and acupressure!!

6. **What will you offer her now? Can anything be done?**

Ans: A review can be done with pain and QOL score as well as repeat bladder diary. Intradetrusor botulinum toxin is a distinct option, with injection of 100 units [non-trigone sparing] is reported to be equally efficacious.[7] Patient should be taught CIC and counselled about temporary benefit. Neuro-modulation can also be offered though with very careful counselling due to its unpredictable success rate. Unfortunately major surgery such as augmentation or simple cystectomy also may not give symptom relief![8]

KEY POINTS

- Bladder pain syndrome is a clinical diagnosis, and careful history along with a bladder diary usually leads to the diagnosis.
- Standard investigations are usually normal and help in ruling out other conditions such as OAB.
- Initial treatment involves pain control, counselling and lifestyle changes. The disease may have a waxing and waning pattern with exacerbation during stressful conditions.
- Bladder relaxants and pentosan sulphate show variable response.
- Cystoscopy is useful in ruling out other diseases and may show glomerulations or Hunner's ulcer. Intravescical instillation of DMSO, heparin, lignocaine, hyaluronic acid can give short-term relief.
- Refractory cases might need intradetrusor botulinum toxin and neuromodulation.
- Major surgeries such as augmentation or simple cystectomy are best avoided and can only be undertaken as the last resort after thorough patient counselling.

REFERENCES

1. How can we improve the diagnosis and management of bladder pain syndrome? Part 1: ICI-RS 2018. Vik Khullar, *et al.* Neurourology and Urodynamics/ Vol 38 issue S5/ p 566–570
2. Berry SH, Elliott MN, Suttorp M, *et al.* Prevalence of symptoms of bladder pain syndrome/interstitial cystitis among adult females in the United States. *The Journal of Urology.* 2011;**186**(2):540–544.
3. Hanno PM, Erickson D, Moldwin R, Faraday MM, American Urological Association Diagnosis and treatment of interstitial cystitis/bladder pain syndrome: AUA guideline amendment. *The Journal of Urology* . 2015;**193**(5):1545–1553.

4. Juliebø-Jones P, Hjelle KM, Mohn J, Gudbrandsdottir G, Roth I, Chaudhry AA, Bergesen AK, Beisland C. Management of Bladder Pain Syndrome (BPS): A Practical Guide. Adv Urol. 2022 Jan 10;2022:7149467.
5. Wennevik GE, Meijlink JM, Hanno P, Nordling J. The role of glomerulations in bladder pain syndrome: a review. *The Journal of Urology*. 2016;195(1):19–25.
6. Jones P, Hjelle KM, Mohn J, *et al*. Current status of intravesical therapies for bladder pain syndrome (BPS): a narrative review of emerging evidence. *Urology*. 2021;**156**:e48–e57.
7. Kuo H-C, Jiang Y-H, Tsai Y-C, Kuo Y-C. Intravesical botulinum toxin-A injections reduce bladder pain of interstitial cystitis/bladder pain syndrome refractory to conventional treatment-a prospective, multicenter, randomized, double-blind, placebo-controlled clinical trial. *Neurourology and Urodynamics*. 2016;**35**(5):609–614.
8. Osman NI, Bratt DG, Downey AP, Esperto F, Inman RD, Chapple CR. A systematic review of surgical interventions for the treatment of bladder pain syndrome/interstitial cystitis. *European Urology Focus*. 2021;**7**(4):877–885.

Chapter

17

Bladder Pain Syndrome: Hunner Lesion

• *Rajesh Taneja*

LEARNING OBJECTIVES

- Interstitial cystitis (IC) was first used to describe an unusual type of inflammation of bladder by Skene in 1887.[1] Later it was described as an ulcer at the dome in 1915 by Hunner.[2] Messing and Stamey, described an inflammatory condition of the bladder with glomerulations on second distension in a bladder with reduced capacity but without the typical Hunner's lesion.[3] These were termed non-classic IC. NIDDK (National Institute of Diabetes and Digestive and Kidney diseases) in 1987 developed inclusion criteria for Interstitial cystitis for research purposes, which were modified in 1990.[4,5] These included nonspecific glomerulations as inclusion criteria.
- European Society for Study of Interstitial Cystitis (ESSIC) defined the 'Bladder Pain Syndrome' (BPS) to include patients clinically having bladder pain or discomfort with urinary symptoms[6,7] and re-named Hunner's 'ulcers' as Hunner's lesions (HL), stating that these were lesions which disrupt on bladder filling. They also described the multiple superficial cracks in the bladder on distension and terming them nonspecific as these were found in asymptomatic patients.
- PBS is recognized as a clinical syndrome characterized by bladder related pain, with or without the presence of erstwhile inflammatory disease of bladder involving all layers (pan cystitis) and Hunner's lesions (HL) on cystoscopy.
- Several publications suggesting that Hunner's lesion is a separate disease entity.[8,9]
- HL is a circumscript hyperemic stellate patch with almost parallel radiating blood vessels towards a pale center with a fibrin deposit.[10] This may crack upon distension and start to ooze blood. The superficial cracks on overdistention not associated with signs of inflammation as hyperemia are nonspecific and should not be confused with Hunner's lesion. Hydrodistension may also result in multiple petechial hemorrhages over the mobile portion of bladder. These are termed glomerulations and not specific to interstitial cystitis as they may be encountered even in asymptomatic patients, radiation cystitis and tubercular cystitis. Profuse bleeding without typical circumscript lesion should not be termed Hunner's lesion.
- Prevalence of Hunner's lesion is highly variable ranging from 3.5 to 56%[9] In a recent publication from India, the prevalence of HL has been reported to be 23%.[11]
- Histopathological examination of Hunner's lesion reveals inflammatory exudate in lamina propria with intense infiltration of neutrophils lymphocytes, plasma cells, macrophages, mast cells and lymphoid aggregates.[12] Mast cells infiltration in the detrusor is often associated with Hunner's lesion.
- Clinical scoring system should be used for these patients in order to objectively evaluate the response to treatment. In addition, scores also serve as a useful biofeedback.[13]

ESSIC Definition of Bladder Pain Syndrome[7]

BPS would be diagnosed on the basis of chronic pelvic pain, pressure, or discomfort perceived to be related to the urinary bladder accompanied by at least one other urinary symptom such as persistent urge to void or urinary frequency. Confusable diseases as the cause of the symptoms must be excluded (see Table 17.1).

TABLE 17.1: Confusable diseases for bladder pain syndrome (ESSIC)[7]

- Carcinoma and carcinoma *in situ*
- Infection with
  - Common intestinal bacteria
  - *Chlamydia trachomatis, Ureaplasma urealyticum*
  - *Mycoplasma hominis, Mycoplasma genitalium*

(Contd.)

TABLE 17.1: Confusable diseases for bladder pain syndrome (ESSIC)[7] *(Contd.)*

- *Corynebacterium urealyticum*, Candida species
- *Mycobacterium tuberculosis*
- Herpes simplex and human papillomavirus

- Radiation
- Chemotherapy, including immunotherapy with cyclophosphamide Anti-inflammatory therapy with tiaprofenic acid.
- Bladder-neck obstruction and neurogenic outlet obstruction Bladder stone
- Lower ureteric stone
- Urethral diverticulum
- Urogenital prolapse
- Endometriosis
- Vaginal candidiasis
- Cervical, uterine, and ovarian cancer incomplete bladder emptying (retention): Overactive bladder.
- Prostate cancer
- Benign prostatic obstruction, chronic bacterial prostatitis, chronic non-bacterial prostatitis
- Pudendal nerve entrapment
- Pelvic floor muscle-related pain

Case Scenario

A forty-five years old lady presented with increased frequency of urination which gradually progressed over last two years. Upon filling of bladder, there is an intense discomfort which rapidly translates into pain in suprapubic area, vulva and anal canal. During the day she passes urine almost every 20–30 minutes. She is typically woken up from sleep every 30–45 minutes with intense pain which reduces to some extent.

1. **How would you proceed with the history?**

   Ans:

   A. Ask the following questions:

   1. Are there aggravating or relieving factors?
   2. Is there any difficulty in initiating the stream to pass urine?
   3. Is there any pin prick sensation?
   4. Is there any relation to posture?
   5. Any vaginal discharge?
   6. History of treatment for infertility?
   7. What is the relationship with menstrual cycle?
   8. Is there dyspareunia? If so, superficial or deep?
   9. Are there any leakages of urine?
   10. Is there any history of allergies?
   11. Are there any associated co-morbidities like migraine, fibromyalgia, chronic fatigue syndrome, Jorgen's syndrome, IBS?
   12. Does any specific dietary item causes flare of symptoms?
   13. Are there any exacerbations during stress?

B. What would you like to focus during examination?

1. General physical examination to look for evident signs of anxiety and/or depression.
2. Abdominal examination for any scars in lower abdomen from previous surgeries
3. Local examination for vaginal discharge, excoriations, abrasions, cervical erosions
4. Digital pelvic examination for ant fornicial tenderness or pelvic mass/nodules
5. Pelvic floor examination for any fibromuscular bands.
6. Focused neurological examination.

C. What investigations would you like to ask for?

1. Frequency volume chart. Presence of functional bladder capacity less than 350 cc is more likely to be associated with presence of HL.[14]
2. Urine routine examination for presence of pus cells, leucocyte esterase or nitrite, which exclude the diagnosis of BPS/IC. If any of these is present, a sample of urine needs microbiological investigation for causative microbe, beginning from aerobic culture.
3. Ultrasound KUB with residual urine to exclude a bladder pathology like stone or inflammatory/neoplastic mass in bladder and any upper tract pathology likely to be associated with and causing bladder symptoms.
4. In case of doubt if the pain is coming from bladder or surrounding pelvic organs, intravesical Lignocaine test may be done, which is an office procedure.

D. Cystoscopy under anesthesia[15]

1. Cystoscopy should be done early in the course of disease for excluding serious pathology like malignancy and tuberculosis besides other confusable disorders like cystitis cystica.
2. Early cystoscopy also helps in phenotyping and identifying the presence of Hunner's lesion leading to appropriate and effective treatment.
3. Cystoscopy done with local anesthesia may not allow proper examination as bladder distension is certain to cause pain and prevent complete evaluation and any therapeutic procedure.
4. Cystoscopy should be done under general anesthesia as it reduces the patients' discomfort, allows for the detailed evaluation

of the bladder, assessment of anesthetic bladder capacity, hydrodistension and ablation of Hunner's lesion should there be one.

5. Bladder biopsy is indicated in case there is any suspicious lesion or for research purposes and must be done after hydrodistension.

Case Scenario *(Contd.)*

The patient was indeed anxious and depressed. She had an otherwise unremarkable abdomen except deep tenderness in hypogastrium. The vagina was clean, and anterior fornix was tender. No mass or nodule was felt and there were no palpable myofascial bands.

Frequency volume chart suggested a maximal functional volume of 190 ml, that too post-midnight and the most frequent value of voided volume was 80 ml. Urine test was unremarkable and ultrasound revealed partly filled urinary bladder which was emptying completely without any concomitant upper tract pathology.

After due institutional procedure, patient underwent cystoscopy under general anesthesia. The bladder had three confluent Hunner's lesion on the anterior wall. Hydrodistension was carried out with irrigant height of 80 cm from pubic symphysis for 2 minutes after reaching maximum bladder capacity under anesthesia which was 400 ml. Deflation of bladder under vision revealed oozing of blood from the ruptured Hunner's lesions and glomerulations from the anterior bladder wall. Hunner's lesions were fulgurated using ball electrode TURP working element. Bladder was drained over night with 18 F three-way catheter with slow irrigation which was stopped after 4 hours.

A solution of hydrocortisone (200 mg) and heparin (25000 IU) in 40 ml of normal saline was left in bladder before removing the catheter subsequent morning.

Management of Hunner's Lesion

A. Education of the patient and family It is extremely important to spend time with the patient and immediate family to educate them that the patient is suffering from real disease, and this is not something which is only in her mind.

B. As per the histopathological morphology, Hunner's lesion is evidently a result of inflammatory process.[16] Hence the treatment is directed towards reducing inflammation:

1. Reduction of inflammatory process can be done by using hydroxyzine, which is expected to stabilize the mast cells in the final pathogenetic mechanism.[17] The most common adverse effect of hydroxyzine is sedation, which must be brought to the notice of patient at the time of counselling.
2. Up to 67% percent of patients with HL have been found to have history of allergic background.[11] Such patients may be advised anti-histamines in addition to hydroxyzine.
3. Intravesical steroids have been used as a follow-up of ablation of Hunner's. lesion.[18]

C. Treatment directed towards promoting healing. The glycosamine glycan (GAG) layer is the protective barrier which has been found to be deficient in cases of HL. GAG layer replenishment has been shown to aid in healing of bladder urothelium and reversing the pain and unpleasant sensation arising from bladder.[19]

1. Oral pentosan polysulphate (PPS). This is a plant product which has close molecular resemblance to naturally occurring GAG constituents. (T) Food in stomach interferes with the absorption of drug taken orally. After oral administration with optimal conditions of absorption, almost 6% of ingested dose is excreted in urine and reaches bladder. This is expected to fill the gaps in the damaged GAG layer coating of urothelium, preventing noxious urinary constituents to get in touch with urothelium and deeper layers of bladder. This prevents triggering of pain fibers originating from the that healing takes. The oral dose is 100 mg three times a day to be taken one hour prior to food and nothing to eat two hours prior to the oral dose. The clinical response is slow to develop over next 10–12 weeks. It is important to wait for three months before concluding the lack of clinical response. The most important adverse effects are gastrointestinal upset, alopecia, and rectal bleeding. It has a weak heparin like action and any concomitant antiplatelet/anticoagulant therapy is to be continued with caution.
2. Intravesical instillation of GAG analogues has been found to be clinically effective in reducing symptoms. While hyaluronic acid and chondroitin sulphate have been shown individually and in combination to improve the symptoms due to BPS, these agents are not available in India at the time of writing this piece.[19]
3. Intravesical heparin has been used with good results.[20] various regimes are available including heparin as ingredient of intravesical cocktail for BPS/IC.
4. Intravesical pentosan polysulphate has been used in past with some encouraging results.[19]

However, stabilizing the solution with acceptable shelf life is a challenge. Recently it has been approved by the DCGI (Drug controller general of India). Intravesical use of PPS solution can cause pain and therefore it is important to use alkalized lidocaine prior to instillation of PPS. The available solution is 200 mg in 30 ml vial.

D. Treatment of pain
Pain must be respected.
1. Non-steroidal anti-inflammatory drugs are effective, but the effect is short lived and prolonged treatment must be avoided to prevent renal injury and other side effects.
2. Amitriptyline has been found to effective in some series.[21] Being a neuromodulator, it may reduce the pain by blocking the neuronal pathways. Since many patients have neuropathic inflammation, this further adds up to the beneficial effects of amitriptyline. The most common adverse effect of amitriptyline is sedation. One can start with 10 mg at bedtime and slowly progress to 25 mg two twice a day depending upon the response and tolerability. It has been found that cumulative effect of amitriptyline over a period of time even on a lower dose may be efficacious enough. Nortriptyline has similar effect but better adverse effect profile.
3. Gabapentinoid drugs include Gabapentin and pregabalin. These are considered as effective medication for neuropathic pain and may be tried for control of pain in these patients, either alone or in combination with nortriptyline.
4. Opioids may be needed in severe cases, and these have to be handled by pain therapist.

E. Dietary modification. It is quite well known that certain dietary ingredients are known to cause flare of symptoms. This occurs as the GAG layer is defective and there is an increased permeability of substances from the urine into the bladder wall. Spices, as most of them are acidic in nature, get accentuated in acidic medium. Therefore, urinary alkalizers help in reducing the symptoms to some extent. Besides pH, there may be other determinants in the urine which might be secondary to metabolites of certain food items which might be responsible for flare of bladder symptoms. Patients tend to learn on their own to avoids certain food items. They should be counselled to take bland diet for a couple of weeks and slowly introduce the items suspected to cause flare of symptoms. This method of dietary exclusion can lead to individualize the diet sheet for a given patient. Help can be sought from internet-based BPS/ IC sites and patient support groups. Indian diet book for BPS/ IC patients is also available for starters.[22]

F. Physiotherapy. In various series, it has been found that sizable percentage of BPS/IC patients, up to 87% in some series, may be suffering from overactive pelvic floor causing a sort of dysfunction. [23] These patients may be benefited by pelvic floor relaxation exercise. These patients may also be helped by skeletal muscle relaxants like valium suppositories.

SUMMARY

- Bladder pain syndrome is clinical pain syndrome, used for all bladder pain with lower tract symptoms in the absence of known etiology.
- Interstitial cystitis is an organic disease of bladder with feature of pan cystitis with or without presence of Hunner's lesions.
- Treatment of Hunner's lesions is multi-modal and needs continual follow-up.

REFERENCES

1. Skene A. Diseases of bladder and urethra in women. New York (NY): Wm Wood; 1887.
2. Hunner GL. A rare type of bladder ulcer in women; report of cases. Boston Med Surg J. 1915;172(18):660–664.
3. Messing EM, Stamey TA. Interstitial cystitis: early diagnosis, path-ology and treatment. Urology. 1978;12(4):381–392.
4. Wein A, Hanno P, Gillenwater J. Interstitial cystitis: an introduction to the problem. Interstitial cystitis. London: Springer-Verlag. 1990. p. 3–15.
5. Hanno P, Levin RM, Monson FC, *et al* Diagnosis of Interstitial cystitis. J Urol. 1990;143(2):278–281.
6. Nordling J, Anjum F, Bade J, *et al* Primary evaluation of patients suspected of having interstitial cystitis (IC). Eur Urol. 2004; 45(5): 662–669.
7. van de Merwe JP, Nordling J, Bouchelouche P, *et al* Diagnostic criteria, classification, and nomenclature for painful bladder syn-drome/interstitial cystitis: an ESSIC proposal. Eur Urol. 2008;53(1): 60–67.
8. Magnus Fall, Jørgen Nordling, Mauro Cervigni, Paulo Dinis Oliveira, Jennifer Fariello, Philip Hanno, Christina Kåbjörn-Gustafsson, Yr Logadottir, Jane Meijlink, Nagendra Mishra, Robert Moldwin, Loredana Nasta, Jorgen Quaghebeur, Vicki Ratner, Jukka Sairanen, Rajesh Taneja, Hikaru Tomoe, Tomohiro Ueda, Gjertrud Wennevik, Kristene Whitmore, Jean Jacques Wyndaele & Andrew Zaitcev (2020): Hunner lesion disease differs in diagnosis, treatment and outcome from bladder pain syndrome: an ESSIC working group report, Scandinavian Journal of Urology, DOI: 10.1080/21681805.2020.1730948.
9. Whitmore, K.E., Fall, M., Sengiku, A., Tomoe, H., Logadottir, Y. and Kim, Y.H. (2019), Hunner lesion versus non-Hunner lesion interstitial cystitis/bladder pain syndrome. Int. J. Urol., 26: 26–34.
10. Fall M, Baranowski AP, Fowler CJ, *et al* EAU guidelines on chronic pelvic pain. Eur Urol. 2004;46(6):681–689.
11. Taneja R, Chugh DK. Clinical phenotyping linked treatment strategies in patients with bladder pain syndrome. Urol Nephrol Open Access J. 2020;8(4):93–97. DOI: 10.15406/unoaj.2020.08.00283.
12. Johansson SL, Fall M. Clinical features and spectrum of light microscopic changes in interstitial cystitis. J Urol. 1990;143(6): 1118–1124.

13. Taneja R, Massand S. A modified clinical scoring system for bladder pain syndrome: Long term experience. Int J Urol. 2019 Jun;26 Suppl 1:61–67. doi: 10.1111/iju.13977. PMID: 31144746.
14. Quaghebeur J, Wyndaele JJ. Bladder pain syndrome (BPS): symptom differences between type 3C BPS and non-type 3C BPS. Scand J Urol. 2015;49(4):319–320.
15. Taneja R, Pandey S, Priyadarshi S, Goel A, Jain A, Sharma R, Purohit N, Bandukwalla V, Tanvir, Ragavan M, Agrawal A, Shah A, Girn Z, Ajwani V, Mete U. Diagnostic and therapeutic cystoscopy in bladder pain syndrome/interstitial cystitis: systematic review of literature and consensus on methodology. Int Urogynecol J. 2023 Jan 28. doi: 10.1007/s00192–023–05449–w.
16. Vera PL, Preston DM, Moldwin RM, *et al* Elevated urine levels of macrophage migration inhibitory factor in inflammatory bladder conditions: a potential biomarker for a subgroup of interstitial cystitis/bladder pain syndrome patients. Urology. 2018;116: 55–
17. Theoharides TC, Sant GR. Hydroxyzine therapy for interstitial cystitis. *Urology*. 1997;49(5A Suppl):108–110.
18. Rajesh Taneja and Kailash K. Jawade (2007) A rational combination of intravesical and systemic agents for the treatment of interstitial cystitis, Scandinavian Journal of Urology and Nephrology, 41:6, 511–515, DOI: 10.1080/00365590701435918.
19. Wyndaele JJJ, Riedl C, Taneja R, Lovász S, Ueda T, Cervigni M. GAG replenishment therapy for bladder pain syndrome/interstitial cystitis. Neurourol Urodyn. 2019;38(2):535–44. https://doi.org/10. 1002/nau.23900.
20. Taneja R. Current status of oral pentosan polysulphate in bladder pain syndrome/interstitial cystitis. Int Urogynecol J. 2021 May;32(5):1107–1115. doi: 10.1007/s00192–020–04517–9. Epub 2020 Sep 7. PMID: 32894327.
21. Van Ophoven A, Pokupic S, Heinecke A, *et al* A prospective, randomized, placebo controlled, double-blind study of amitriptyline for the treatment of interstitial cystitis. *J Urol.* 2004;172(2):533–536.
22. Rahnama'i MS, Javan A, Vyas N, Lovasz S, Singh N, Cervigni M, Pandey S, Wyndaele JJ, Taneja R. Bladder Pain Syndrome and Interstitial Cystitis Beyond Horizon: Reports from the Global Interstitial Cystitis/Bladder Pain Society (GIBS) Meeting 2019 Mumbai-India. Anesth Pain Med. 2020 May 12;10(3):e101848. doi: 10.5812/aapm.101848. PMID: 32944561; PMCID: PMC7472163.
23. Gupta P, Gaines N, Sirls LT, *et al* A multidisciplinary approach to the evaluation and management of interstitial cystitis/bladder pain syndrome: an ideal model of care. *Transl Androl Urol*. 2015;4(6):611–619.

Chapter

18

Post-Hysterectomy Vesicovaginal Fistula

• *Divakar Dalela*

LEARNING OBJECTIVES

- Post-hysterectomy vesicovaginal fistula (PH-VVF) occurs in 0.1 to 0.2% patients following hysterectomy.[1]
- A combination of risk factors include those related to the patient's bodily habitus, the disease or indication of hysterectomy, to the surgeon's experience, or the technique used. (Table 18.1).

TABLE 18.1: Risk factors for occurrence of post-hysterectomy VVF

Patient related factors	***Disease related factors***		***Surgeon related factors***	
Obesity Previous pelvic surgery	A	Diseases that induce severe fibrosis	A	Technique
		• Endometriosis • Previous radition • Multiple LSCS		• Surgery without good exposure • Excessive diathemy usage
	B	Diseases that distort anatomy	B	Surgeon's experience
		• Large/multiple fibroids		• Limited experience, e.g. in laparoscopic surgery • Overconfidence
	C	Cervical fibroids Diseases that infiltrate bladder		
		• CA Cx		

- The most patients typically present with continuous urinary leakage per vaginum after 7 to 10 days of hysterectomy typically despite a catheter. Minute fistulae can cause a slow vaginal pooling of urine that might mimic stress urinary incontinence. A small fistula with an oblique tract might leak only after bladder gets filled up to a certain volume. This can present as urinary frequency as an 'avoidance' behaviour. However, in most patients, incontinence is total. If the patient has concurrent involvement of ureteric office or lower ureter, she may also have ipsilateral flank pain with or without fever.
- Good clinical examination in lithotomy position in good light in operation theatre will easily reveal the leakage per vagina through a small hole in the vault or anterior wall of vagina. In cases of doubt, bladder can be filled with methylene blue solution.
- The most valuable test is cystoscopy with vaginoscopy which reveals the location and size of fistula as well as the degree of necrosis and inflammation on the edges of the fistula. The status of both the ureteric orifices and the urinary efflux coming out of them must also be take a note of.
- It is important to perform a screening ultrasonography of the upper tracts to look for hydronephrosis that might offer a clue to concomitant ureteric injury. CT urography is the most accurate method of excluding concurrent ureterovaginal fistula. In some patients an MRI of pelvis may also be done to understand the degree of tissue damage and resultant fibrosis in vesico-vaginal septum. Digital intravenous urogram is less commonly in use.
- The overall objective of the investigative evaluation is to first ascertain the patient's fitness for surgery and more importantly to grade the surgical complexities of the VVF[2] as per the diagram given in Fig. 18.1.
- Prompt catheterization with small balloon fill and antimuscarinics for 4–8 weeks can rarely allow spontaneous healing in women a small fistula who achieve dryness with the catheter.

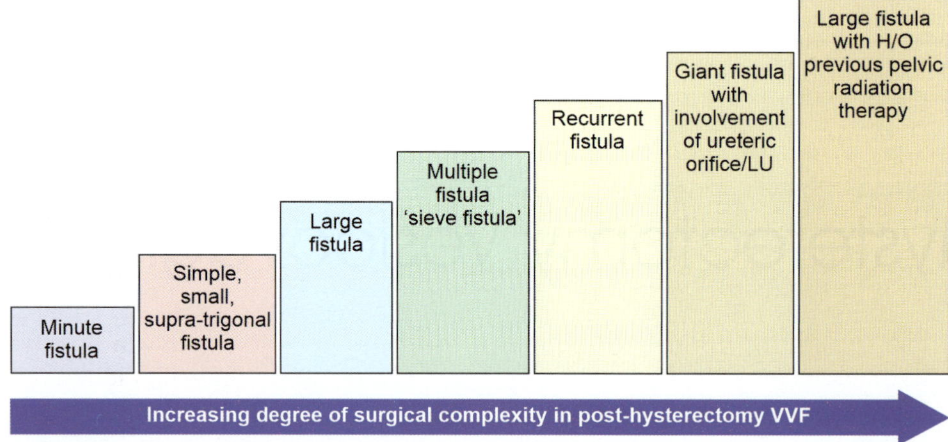

Fig. 18.1: Complexity grades in PH-VVF

- The persistent fistula or large/giant fistula from the beginning, require surgical reconstruction. If the vaginal access is roomy, a vaginal re-construction with a without without Martius or peritoneal flap can be undertaken but if vagina is narrow or scarred, a modified O'Connors repair is an effective method with good results.
- With the current level of advancements in surgical technique, intraoperative illumination and sutures, the standard O'Connors procedure is not required. Instead, the modifications suggested by us offer many advantages and should be practised.[3] Apart from the short cystotomy incision, the major modification is in the technique of suturing the bladder wherein more detrusor muscle and less mucosa is taken to attain a single layer, robust closure. We call this technique as continuous pyramidal suture technique.[4]
- If patient has ureteric involvement, concurrent reimplantation surgery may also be required. The algorithm given in Fig. 18.2 explains this in details.

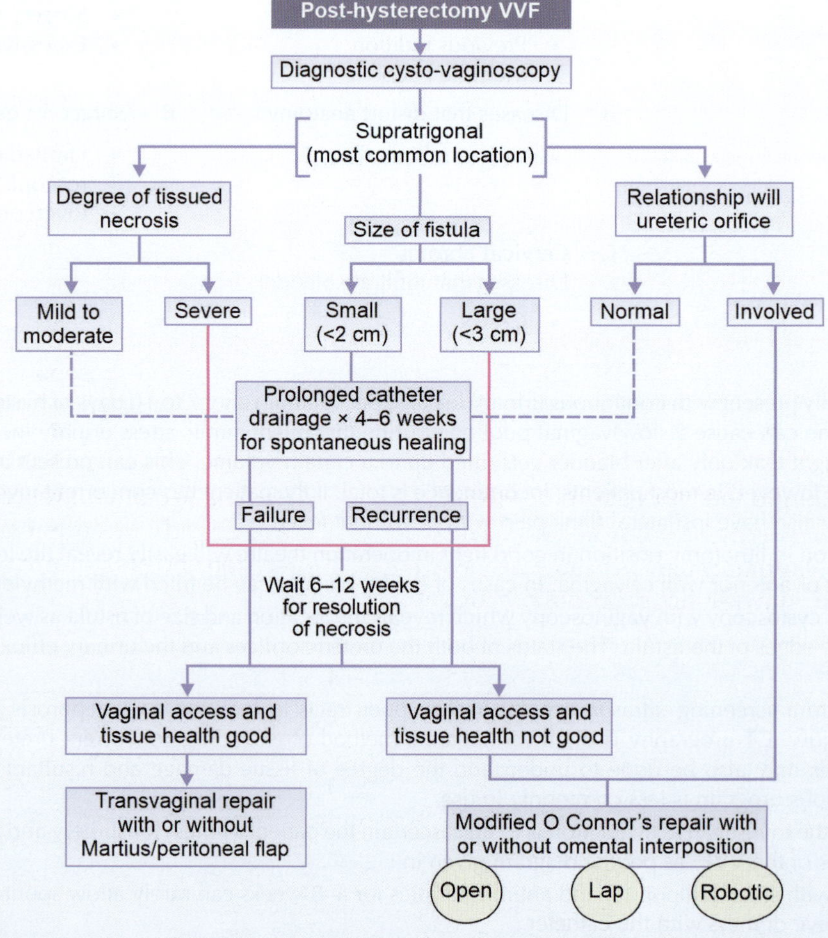

Fig. 18.2: Algorithm for management of PH-VVF

Case Scenario

A 52 years obese lady presented on urethral catheter on account of a large supra-trigonal trigonal post-hysterectomy, VVF. The cysto-vaginoscopic examination showed extensive necrosis on going on edges of the fistula, so patient waited for six more weeks. The repeat clinical and cysto-vaginoscopic evaluation showed absence of tissue reaction/necrosis and a three finger wide supratrigonal fistula. A modified O'Connors repair[3] was done.

1. **What was the complexity in this case?**

   Ans: The main complexity of the case was the large size and proximity of ureteric orifices to the edges of fistula. In such case, if a midline vertical closure of bladder is attempted, it requires a wider lateral mobilisation of bladder edges risking injury to lower ureters. If somehow closure is done, both the ureteric orifices are dragged medially and a continuous traction strain is maintained on the bladder edges. This may result in higher failure rate. Therefore, a bladder rotation flap technique as shown in Fig. 18.3 was utilised. The rotational advancement of bladder flap maintains the position of ureteric orifices at their place and achieve sound bladder closure without the need for major mobilisation of bladder edges and compromising the bladder capacity.

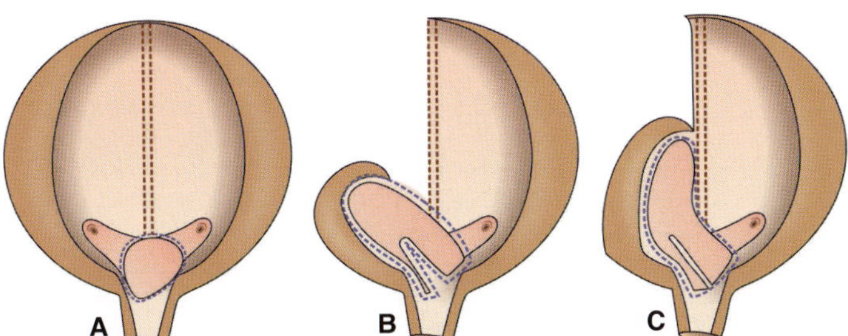

Fig. 18.3: Use of bladder rotation flap to repair a large PH-VVF

2. **What factors influence the approach to repair?**

   Ans: Vaginal repair is the default option at most centers globally. Vaginal repair is associated with lower morbidity, shorter hospital stay, quicker return to work, and lower cost. Hence, for most patients with uncomplicated fistulae, the vaginal approach is preferred. Abdominal approach may be necessitated by a large fisula, high and inaccessible location especially if the vagina is narrow, a history of radiation, failed transvaginal approach, the need for bladder augmentation or ureteric reimplantation as well as problems with patient positioning. Some of these problems can be circumvented with additional techniques such as an episiotomy or use of balloon catheter traction to bring the fistula down. Surgeon comfort and expertise is crucial. Ultimately, the first surgery carries the best chance for success.

3. **When should an omental flap interposition be used?**

   Ans: In a rather straightforward case omental interposition is not needed. But if the tissue and the bladder edges are not found healthy or the repair has been rather complex, as in recurrent cases, the omentum flap should be interposed. If the healthy omentum is not available, a paravesical pad of fat covered with peritoneum can be mobilised and used as tissue interposition to support the healing.

4. **When should an additional suprapubic catheter be used?**

   Ans: In most patients only a F 18 or 20 catheter is adequate to drain the bladder but if the repair is complex as in patients of recurrent VVF, a suprapubic catheter may be placed in addition to a urethral catheter. The reason to avoid suprapubic catheter in all patients is that the two Foley balloons inside bladder lumen may give rise to greater post-operative bladder spasms, which may have adverse effect on the bladder healing because of repeated spasm induced traction on suture lines. However, this decision should best be left on the operator.

5. **What should be the duration of post-operative indwelling catheterisation?**

   Ans: If the operator feels that his bladder closure has been sound, water tight (as shall be feasible with the use of our continuous, pyramidal suturing technique) and the tissue conditions were good, the catheter can be removed after seven days. If the situation is different, a longer duration of catheterization may be required.

6. **What are the current advancements in the management of such a case?**

   Ans: The use of laparoscopic or robotic technique is a major advancement as it enhances the surgical precision and also shortens post-operative recovery time.

SUMMARY

- Proper evaluation and understanding of the morbid anatomy of a case of post-hysterectomy VVF is crucial for its management.
- The surgical approach should be selected on the basis of the morbid anatomy as well as the experience of the operator.
- Irrespective of the approach used, major emphasis is required on good mobilisation of the edges of fistula and sound, tension-less closure.
- The additional use of tissue interposition techniques improves the success.

REFERENCES

1. Hilton P & Cromwell D. (2012). The risk of vesicovaginal and urethrovaginal fistula after hysterectomy performed in the English National Health Service-a retrospective cohort study examining patterns of care between 2000 and 2008. BJOG: An International Journal of Obstetrics & Gynaecology, 119(12), 1447–1454. doi:10.1111/j.1471–0528.2012.03474.x
2. Bhandari M and Dalela D. Complexities of vesico-vaginal fistula. (Editorial) Arch Esp De Urol.1994; 47(3): 303–306.
3. Dalela D, Ranjan P, Sankhwar PL, Shankhwar SN, Naja V, Goel A, Supratrigonal VVF Repair by modified O'Connor's Technique: An experience of 26 Cases. European Urology 2006; 49 551–556.
4. "Continuous pyramidal suture: A new technique to ensure robust single layered closure of bladder for VVF repair" (Poster) 9th Asian Congress of Urology, Urological Society of India held at New Delhi on 2nd–5th October, 2008.

Chapter

19

Post-Radiation Vesicovaginal Fistula

• *Rishi Nayyar* • *Lovekesh Kumar*

LEARNING OBJECTIVES

- Radiation fistulae should be regarded as complex and are best handled by an experienced surgeon.
- Radiation fistulae often have a delayed presentation and may continue to evolve. Timing the surgery after most of this evolution is apparently complete, typically at least 6–12 months, is important to ensure success.
- Assessment must include a search for any recurrence of the original neoplasm. This includes multiple focal biopsies per-vaginally or cystoscopically from any suspicious areas and use of appropriate imaging.
- Most centers use vaginal approach in the majority of cases. The surgeon's comfort and experience with the approach and such cases is paramount for good results.
- While vascularized tissue interposition is often used, it is not mandatory.
- A success rate of 60–65% is expected.

Case Scenario

A 55-year-old post-menopausal lady, P3L3 was referred from gynae-oncology with diagnosis of non-keratinizing squamous cell cervical cancer stage IVA with bladder and vaginal wall invasion. She was given chemotherapy (Paclitaxel + Carboplatin) for 5 cycles followed by 20 Gy radiotherapy in 5 fractionated doses over 5 days to the pelvis. After 2nd cycle chemotherapy she developed continuous total urine leak per vaginum. After completion of chemotherapy and radiotherapy, she was put on Tab Geftinib and had complete resolution of the mass.

General examination: Average built and nutrition, no pallor.

Per-vaginal and per-speculum examination: A large juxta-cervical vesio-vaginal fistula (VVF) was noted in upper anterior vaginal wall with anterior bladder wall mucosa protruding through the defect. Cervix was palpable and os normal. All fornices were obliterated due to previous tumor and scarring with no active inflammation, ulceration or discharge. Rest of vaginal mucosa was normal, allowing 3 fingers with ease and depth of 10 cm.

Per-rectum examination: Anal tone, mucosa, bilateral parametrium and rectovaginal septum were normal with no mass, induration or tenderness.

Cystoscopy and vaginoscopy (after oral phenazopyridine): 5 × 5 cm VVF was confirmed, extending from bladder neck to anterior vaginal fornix. Bilateral ureteric orifices were 1–1.5 cm away from the fistula edge with some radiation-induced changes (mucosal atrophy, ulceration, capillary glomerulations and bleed). Cervix was atrophic with obliteration of fornices and hyperemic patches on posterior lip.

1. **What is the incidence of radiation cystitis and VVF after pelvic radiotherapy?**

   Ans: Incidence of VVF after pelvic radiotherapy is very low, being <0.5–1% in most series.[1] Other genito-urinary complications are more common. According to the Radiation Therapy Oncology Group (RTOG)/European Organisation for Research and Treatment of Cancer (EORTC) morbidity scoring criteria, Grade 1–2 genitourinary complications occur in 7–9.8% while grade 3-4 complications occur in 1.3–14.5% patients after 3 years (late complications) of radiotherapy.

2. **When does VVF occur after pelvic radiotherapy?**
   Ans: VVF can present any time during or after radiotherapy ranging up to several years. However, most cases present 1.5–2 years after radiotherapy.[1]

3. **How does a VVF form after pelvic radiotherapy?**
   Ans: Fibrosis and obliterative arteritis due to ionizing radiation lead to relative ischemia, necrosis and atrophy of tissues. Typically a pure radiation-induced fistula is preceded by symptoms of radiation-induced cystitis and/or vaginitis or proctitis. Fever, vaginal bleed and hematuria may be present just before manifestation of urine leak. A cystoscopy done to assess for hematuria or radiation cystitis may itself be the precipitating factor for development of a VVF.[2]

4. **What are the risk factors for development of VVF after pelvic radiotherapy?**
   Ans: Radiation related risk factors for development of VVF include high radiation dose and prolonged therapy.[3] In one study, more than 86% of the females who developed fistula had received a cumulative radiation dose of 40–60 Gy.[4] Other factors predisposing to VVF include previous pelvic or vaginal surgery, direct bladder infiltration at diagnosis, smoking, infection and use of bevacizumab.[5]

5. **What special considerations are important when clinically evaluating cases of radiation VVF?**
   Ans: Apart from VVF, it is important to be aware about the risk of associated malignancy as well as the impact of radiation on healing capacity of local tissues. One should assess for any residual or recurrent disease in the cervix or edges of the VVF by taking multiple punch biopsies. Examination and imaging to rule out any disease in parametrium, recto-vaginal septum and pelvic lymph nodes is also important. A persistent or recurrent disease at any of these sites has a direct bearing on management. Treatment of a recurrent disease would always take precedence over fistula repair. Limited longevity of the patient, poor tissue healing and need for additional definitive therapy must be weighed against improved quality of life and extent of reconstruction needed before any attempt at repair is considered. Assessment of anaemia and nutritional status are additional important factors.

6. **How to assess for local recurrence and tissue healing/vascularity before VVF repair?**
   Ans: Multiple focal biopsies should be taken per-vaginally or cystoscopically from any suspicious areas.[4] Axial imaging in the form of CT or MRI or PET-CT should also be done prior to considering fistula repair. Tissue healing and local vascularity are difficult to quantify before surgery. However, earlier concept of excision of fibrotic non-bleeding edges for routine VVF is no-longer practised.

7. **When should a post-radiation VVF be repaired?**
   Ans: Repair should not be done immediately when a radiation fistula manifests itself, even if it manifests late after radiotherapy. Repair should be attempted only after acute phase has settled. Generally, 6–12 months rest phase is allowed before considering any surgical repair.[4]

8. **What additional factors are clinically important and could impact decision of repair or type of repair?**
   Ans: Bladder compliance and capacity; vaginal tissue pliability and scarring, and; number of previous failed repairs are important considerations for any radiation associated VVF, beside routine evaluation for characteristics of the fistula. Fistula may be blocked with Foley's catheter to assess bladder capacity. For patients who do not allow examination because of pain due to radiation changes, a separate session of examination under anaesthesia should be considered to decide a surgical road map.

9. **Should hysterectomy be a part of fistula repair in these cases?**
   Ans: A large percentage of radiation VVFs happen in cases of carcinoma cervix. Locally advanced cases are mostly treated with concurrent chemo-radiotherapy with no defined role for adjuvant hysterectomy as per guidelines because of the associated risks of surgery in an irradiated pelvis, like fistula, bladder injury and vaginal cuff dehiscence with no demonstrable benefit of overall survival till date.[6]

10. **Should interposition tissue always be used for repair of radiation VVF?**
    Ans: Recurrent, large or fistulas associated with extreme fibrosis and loss of elasticity of tissues should be repaired using a vascularised interposition tissue like Martius' flap. However, not all radiation VVF require interposition. One large study used it in only 41% of their vaginal radiation VVF repairs.[4] A peritoneal or omental flap are also good options with minimal donor site morbidity, wherever available and feasible.

11. **What is the success rate for repair of radiation-induce VVF?**
    Ans: A success rate of 60–65% is expected in cases where an attempt at closure is made.[7] The

success rate is 40% in those with spontaneous fistulae compared with 100% in those in whom VVF is precipitated after some additional surgery post-radiation. However, a large percentage of radiation VVFs receive urinary diversion rather than an attempt at repair. Therefore, overall success is even lower. The success rate based upon the patient profile must be discussed with the patient and caregivers before mutually deciding upon a surgical repair or diversion.

12. **Are any adjuncts available that may help improve results of surgery for radiation VVF?**

   Ans: Apart from interposition tissue, there are no reliable adjuncts to improve success of surgery. Hyperbaric oxygen therapy,[8] dehydrated amniotic allograft[9] and intra-venous platelet rich plasma[10] have been used anecdotally with questionable results.

13. **How are radiation fistulas classified?**

   Ans: All radiation fistulas should be considered as complex fistulas, irrespective of site and size of fistula. Goh or Waldjik's classification were developed primarily for obstetric/iatrogenic causes of VVF. Whether these classifications are applicable to predict success of repair for other etiologies remains unknown.[11]

14. **Which approach (trans-vaginal or abdominal) should be used for treating radiation VVFs?**

   Ans: Most centers use vaginal approach in the majority of cases. Pushkar *et al* used vaginal approach in 97.2% of their primary repair cases of radiation VVF.[4] The surgeon's comfort and experience with the approach and such cases is paramount for good results. Although there are reports of successful repair of radiation fistula using laparoscopic or robotic approach.[9] it must be borne be mind that adjacent bowel and bladder may also have been exposed to radiation.

15. **What are the salvage surgical options for failed radiation VVF repair?**

   Ans: Majority of primary cases are repaired using standard Latzko, Raz or O'Connor repair techniques. However, for more complex or failed cases particularly the ones who are highly motivated for attempt at tissue repair, other reported options include gracilis myocutaneous flap, pedicled labial flap, combined gastric and omental flap and rectus abdominis myofascial flap.[12,13] All these repairs are based on bringing in some vascularised tissue flaps to create a wall between bladder and the vagina.

16. **What is the role of bladder augmentation for radiation VVF repair?**

   Ans: Bladder augmentation may become necessary in cases with very small bladder capacity.[14] However, use of bowel in such cases should be limited in light of possibility of radiation exposure to bowel as well. A peritonealised rectus abdominis muscle flap based on inferior epigastric artery provides another option in these rare cases providing both interposition as well as augmentation without use of bowel.[15]

17. **What are the other non-surgical options beside VVF repair to improve quality of life in these cases?**

   Ans: Non-surgical interventions (largely directed at reducing impact of urine leak on skin and foul odour) are equally important particularly while waiting for surgery. Local hygiene, lifestyle management, psychological motivational therapies, catheter insertion, zinc oxide creams, diapers, urinary diversion, etc are other options to mitigate the impact of VVF on these patients' overall health.

Final management of the case

The patient was asked to wait for at least 1 year after completion of chemo-radiotherapy, after which multiple fistula edge biopsies were taken to rule out active malignancy. A PET scan was also conducted to rule out residual disease. Finally, transvaginal repair with Martius flap interposition was done. (Video 1, Fig. 19.1). Catheter was removed after 3 weeks with a successful outcome. She continues to be in follow-up with the gynae-onco team.

Video 1. Cystoscopy was done with 19 Fr, 30° cystoscope. Urethra was normal. Fistula started at bladder neck itself and was large not allowing the bladder to distend for assessment. Vagina was packed with a mop to reduce irrigant leak after which scopy was continued.

https://drive.google.com/file/d/1SJ5s-xDQrOILgs7WteBPW93spRV4L4xh/view?usp=drive_web

SUMMARY

- Radiation induces vesio-vaginal fistula (VVF) by obliterative arteritis, tissue ischemia and fibrosis
- Repair should not be attempted during the acute phase of radiation cystitis
- Evaluation for recurrence of tumor, tumor biology and follow-up are equally important as management of fistula
- Bladder capacity and compliance are important assessments in every case of radiation VVF
- Vascularised tissue interposition is a good clinical practice in every case of radiation VVF repair
- Success rate of radiation VVF repair is much poorer than other more common causes of VVF

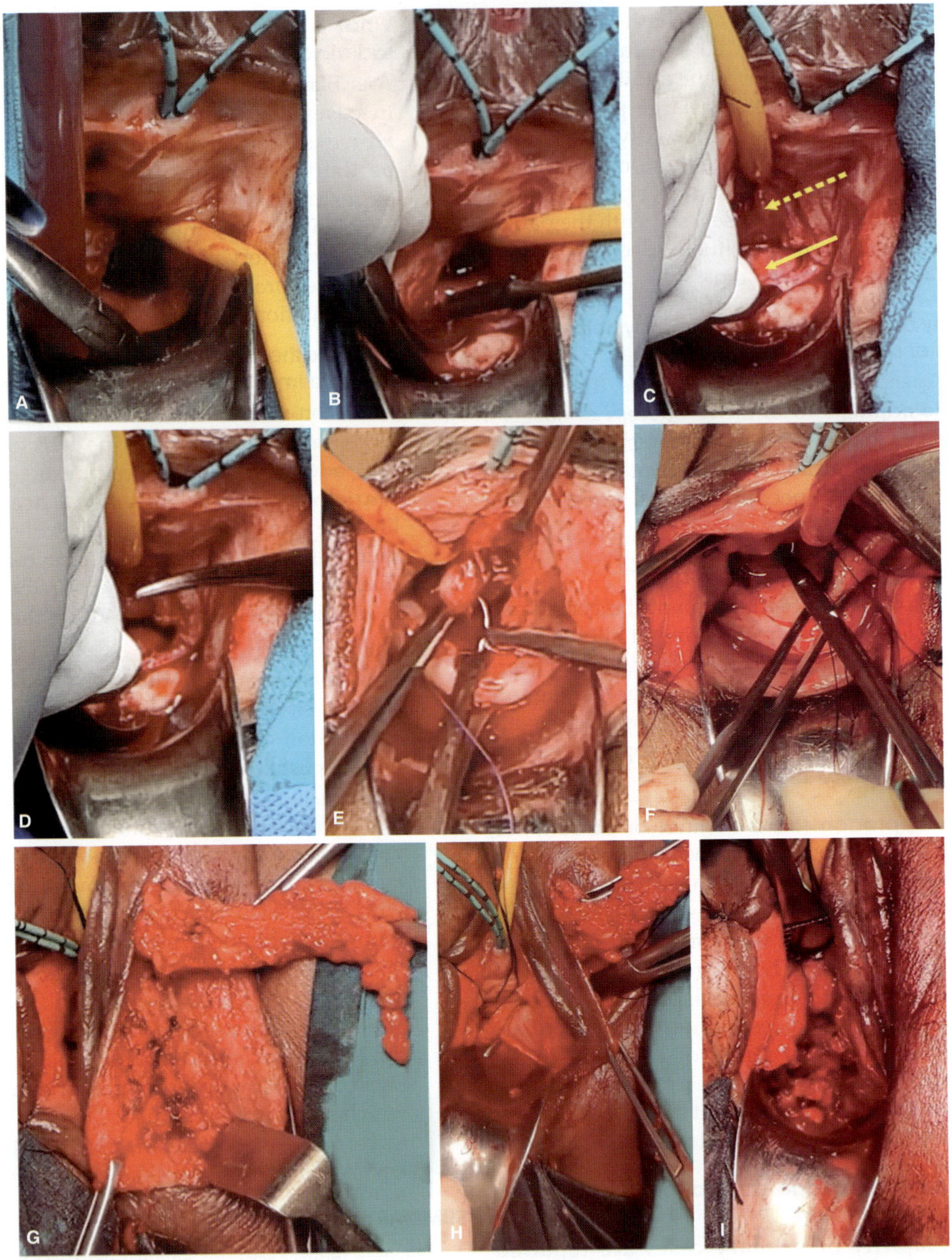

Fig. 19.1A to L: (A) Bilateral access catheters were placed in ureters and 18 Fr Foley's catheter placed through fistula with 35 cc balloon. Cervix was held with volsellum. (B)The fistula margins were circumscribed (2–3 mm from the edge of fistula) and vaginal flaps dissected away from underlying bladder wall using a right-angled forceps and Metzenbaum scissors. Wide mobilization of vaginal flaps was achieved all around except the cervix margin. Mobilization should be adequate enough to bring the edges of bladder as well as vaginal side of fistula close enough for tension free repair. (C,D) Lower segment cervix is visible after dissection (bold arrow). Corresponding mobilized edges of fistula on bladder side can be seen (dashed arrow). Sufficient mobilization to allow for easy approximation of fistula edges was ensured before starting closure. (E) The bladder side of fistula was closed using 3'0 polyglactin sutures with reverse needle hold inverting the small rim of vaginal mucosa around the fistula into the bladder. Methylene blue dye test was done to confirm a water-tight closure. (F) Four sutures were pre-placed about 5–6 mm away from closed fistula edges to be used subsequently for holding the interposition flap in place. (G) Harvested Martius' flap from left labia based on anterior pedicle. (H) Creation of tunnel underneath the vagina wide enough to accommodate the thickness of the flap. Tip of the right angled forceps can be seen projecting from the tunnel near the fistula (I) Martius' flap was transposed and fixed at four corners using pre-placed sutures. *(Contd.)*

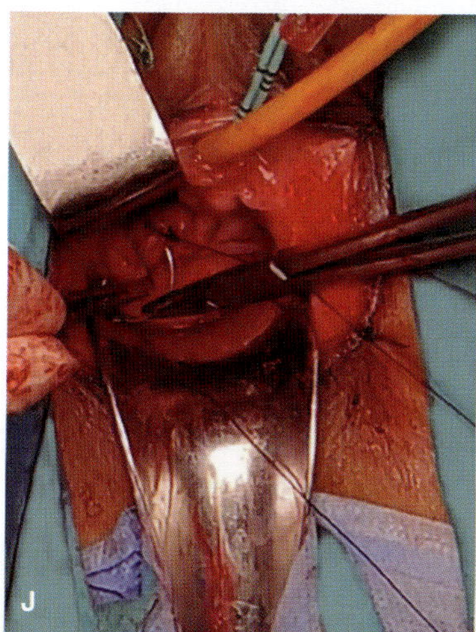

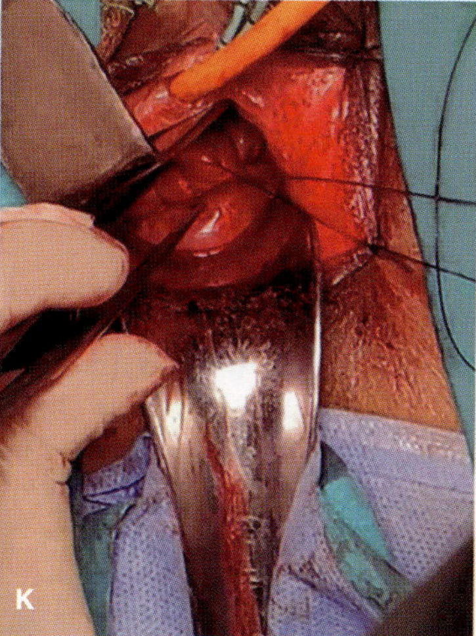

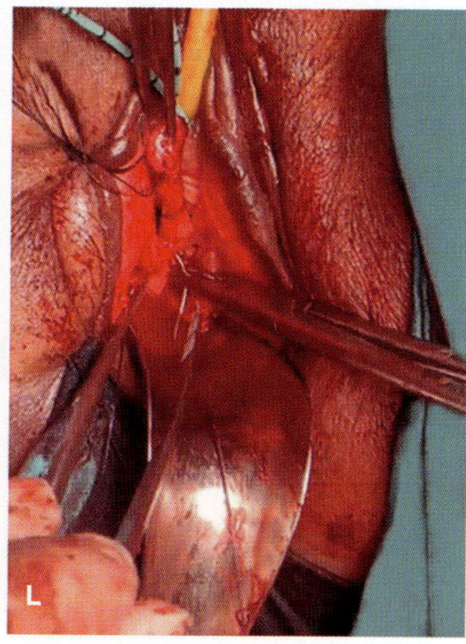

Fig. 19.1A to L: (J,K) Vaginal flaps were first closed on to cervix from either side using 2′0 polyglactin. (L) Closure was then continued vertically to close the vaginal defect. All sutures were taken with reverse-needle orientation on a long needle holder using back-hand throws.

REFERENCES

1. Chorbi n'ska J, Krajewski W, Zdrojowy R. Urological complications after radiation therapy-nothing ventured, nothing gained: a Narrative Review. Transl Cancer Res. 2021 Feb;10(2):1096–1118.
2. Radswiki T, Amer M, Worsley C, *et al.* Urinary bladder trauma. Reference article, Radiopaedia.org (Accessed on 28 Mar 2024) https://doi.org/10.53347/rID–12756
3. Spampinato S, Fokdal LU, Pötter R, Haie-Meder C, Lindegaard JC, Schmid MP, Sturdza A, Jürgenliemk-Schulz IM, Mahantshetty U, Segedin B, Bruheim K, Hoskin P, Rai B, Huang F, Cooper R, van der Steen-Banasik E, Van Limbergen E, Sundset M, Westerveld H, Nout RA, Jensen NBK, Kirisits C, Kirchheiner K, Tanderup K; EMBRACE Collaborative Group. Risk factors and dose-effects for bladder fistula, bleeding and cystitis after radiotherapy with imaged-guided adaptive brachytherapy for cervical cancer: An EMBRACE analysis. Radiother Oncol. 2021 May;158:312–320.
4. Pushkar DY, Dyakov VV, Kasyan GR. Management of radiation-induced vesicovaginal fistula. Eur Urol. 2009 Jan;55(1):131–7.
5. Kim N, Choi SH, Chang JS, Kim YT, Kim SW, Kim GM, Kim YB. Use of bevacizumab before or after radiotherapy increases the risk of fistula formation in patients with cervical cancer. Int J Gynecol Cancer. 2021 Jan;31(1):59–65.
6. Kokka F, Bryant A, Brockbank E, Powell M, Oram D. Hysterectomy with radiotherapy or chemotherapy or both for women with locally advanced cervical cancer. Cochrane Database Syst Rev. 2015:CD010260.
7. Toia B, Pakzad M, Hamid R, Greenwell T, Ockrim J. Surgical outcomes of vesicovaginal fistulae in patients with previous pelvic radiotherapy. Int Urogynecol J. 2020 Jul;31(7):1381–1385.
8. McGlynn J, Heyboer M. Successful treatment of radiation-induced vaginal soft tissue radionecrosis with HBO2. Undersea Hyperb Med. 2023 First Quarter;50(1):9–15.
9. Price DT, Price TC. Robotic repair of a vesicovaginal fistula in an irradiated field using a dehydrated amniotic allo-graft as an interposition patch. J Robot Surg. 2016 Mar;10(1):77–80.
10. Kołody n'ska A, Streit-Cie kiewicz D, Kot A, Kuliniec I, Futyma K. Radiation-Induced Recurrent Vesicovaginal Fistula-Treatment with Adjuvant Platelet-Rich Plasma Injection and Martius Flap Placement-Case Report and Review of Literature. Int J Environ Res Public Health. 2021 May 3;18(9):4867.
11. Beardmore-Gray A, Pakzad M, Hamid R, Ockrim J, Greenwell T. Does the Goh classification predict the outcome of vesico-vaginal fistula repair in the developed world? Int Urogynecol J. 2017 Jun;28(6):937–940.
12. Fujiwara K, Koshima I, Tanaka K, Moriguchi T, Kohno I. Radiation-induced vesico-vaginal fistula successfully repaired using a gracilismyocutaneous flap. Int J Clin Oncol. 2000;5, 341–344.
13. Bissada SA, Bissada NK. Repair of active radiation-induced vesico-vaginal fistula using combined gastricand omental segments based on the gastroepiploic vessels. ObstetGynecol1990;75:727–33.
14. Hsu TH, Rackley RR, Abdelmalak JB, Madjar S, Vasavada SP. Novel technique for combined repair of postirradiation vesicovaginal fistula and augmentation ileocystoplasty. Urology. 2002 Apr;59(4):597–9.
15. Viennas LK, Alonso AM, Salama V. Repair of radiation-induced vesicovaginal fistula with a rectus abdominis myocutaneous flap. PlastReconstr Surg. 1995 Nov;96(6):1435–7.

Chapter
20

Urethral Diverticulum

• Vijay Madduri

LEARNING OBJECTIVES

- Urethral diverticulum (UD) is an important cause of recurrent urinary tract infections (UTIs). A high index of suspicion is required for the diagnosis of UD.
- Classically, it is said that UD presents with the triad of dysuria, dyspareunia and postvoid dribbling of urine. However, the most common presenting complaints in the order of frequency are: Recurrent UTI (70%), Stress urinary incontinence: 60%, Dyspareunia: 60%, Vaginal mass: 52%.
- UD is thought to arise from obstructed and infected periurethral glands. Such glands form cysts, which rupture into the urethra, forming a diverticulum.
- UD must be differentiated from other genital swellings in the female, e.g. Bartholin cyst and Gartner duct cyst.
- The most important diagnostic tests for UDS are voiding cystourethrogram (VCUG), magnetic resonance imaging (MRI) and urethroscopy.
- The recommended treatment of UD is transvaginal excision of UD and closure of urethra.

Case Scenario

A 35-year-old female with no comorbidities presents with recurrent UTI for the past 2 years. She has been evaluated multiple times and treated with culture sensitive antibiotics. She also complains of dyspareunia and occasional urinary incontinence on cough and sneeze. There are no voiding lower urinary tract symptoms (LUTS). She has had a full-term vaginal delivery 7 years ago. On examination, there is a tender suburethral mass palpable on vaginal examination. Purulent material was seen on expressing the mass. There is demonstrable urine leak on cough. She underwent a voiding cystourethrogram (VCUG) which showed a diverticulum in the distal half of the uretha on left side. She underwent an MRI which showed a diverticulum arising from the left lateral wall of the distal one-third of urethra. She underwent cystoscopy which revealed a small opening in the distal third of the urethra at 4 o' clock position. A urodynamic study was performed which was consistent with the diagnosis of Stress Urinary Incontinence (SUI) with no component of urgency incontinence, and a normal pressure flow study. Once the diagnosis of UD with SUI was confirmed, she underwent diverticulectomy and autologous pubovaginal sling for SUI. Her symptoms were relieved after the surgical procedure.

1. **What are the most common presenting complaints of urethral diverticulum (UD)?**

   Ans: The most common presenting complaints are:[1]
   - Recurrent UTI: 70%
   - Stress urinary incontinence: 60%
   - Dyspareunia: 60%
   - Vaginal mass: 52%

   The presentation is varied and a high index of suspicion is required, especially in cases of recurrent UTIs.

2. **What conditions can mimic the symptoms of UD?**

   Ans: The following can mimic symptoms of UD: Recurrent UTI, interstitial cystitis, bladder tumor, etc.

3. **What are the 3Ds of UD?**

   Ans: Dysuria, dyspareunia and postvoid dribbling of urine are classically described as the 3Ds of UD.

4. **What are the physical findings of a UD?**

Ans: A mass is usually felt on palpation of anterior vaginal wall. Tenderness is usually present. Urine/pus may be expressed from external urinary meatus on compressing the mass.If a mass or stone is formed inside the diverticulum then it may be hard to palpation.[2] Stress incontinence may be elicited on cough/Valsalva maneuver. Urethral hypermobility may be demonstrated. Rarely, large diverticulae may cause bladder outlet obstruction and acute urinary retention.[3]

5. **How does UD form?**

Ans: UD is a localized outpouching of the urethra into the anterior vaginal wall. Urinary infection may lead to infection of periurethral glands and obstruction of their ducts. This causes the periurethral glands to dilate, forming suburethral cysts. These cysts rupture into the urethra, forming a diverticulum. Urine starts to pool in these diverticulae giving rise to repeated bouts of infection.[4]

6. **Which type of malignancy, is found in association with UD?**

Ans: Adenocarcinoma is the most common type of malignancy associated with UD.[5]

7. **From where does the UD arise?**

Ans: It usually arises in the mid or distal urethra.

8. **What are the differentials to be considered? How do you differentiate UD from Gartner duct cyst and Bartholin cyst?**

Ans: The following are the differential diagnoses of an anterior vaginal wall mass:

- Skene gland abscess
- Bartholin cyst
- Gartner duct cyst
- Ureterocele
- Vaginal leiomyoma

Gartner duct is the vestigial remnant of mesonephric (Wolffian) duct in females. It occurs in relation to the lateral walls of the vagina. UD is usually palpated on the anterior vaginal wall.

Bartholin cysts are formed by the cystic dilation of the greater vestibular glands (of Bartholin). They occur in relation to the labia minora, whereas UD is usually palpated as a mass in the anterior vaginal wall.

9. **What is the most common test for UD?**

Ans: The most common test for UD is the voiding cystourethrography. Test should be performed with patient in oblique position under antibiotic cover.

10. **Which phase of MRI is used?**

Ans: T2 weighted images are used. Urine inside the diverticulum is seen as a bright signal on T2 weighted images. (Ref: "The axial plane by T2-weighted MRI of normal fetal abdomen at the level of gallbladder usually shows bright signals from both gallbladder and renal pelvis as a result of bile liquid and urine. Thus, indirect mark of renal agenesis is the absence of renal pelvic urine signals in T2-weighted MRI."[12]

11. **What are the advantages of MRI over VCUG?**

Ans: Reconstructed images can give an idea of the 3D anatomy of the diverticulum which is greatly helpful in intraoperative decision making. The ostium may also be seen.[6]

12. **Which catheter is used for urethrography and what is the role of positive pressure urethrography?**

Ans: Madduri catheter is used for urethrography (also known as positive pressure urethrography, in contradistinction to VCUG).[7] It has a balloon and a retention plug. The balloon occludes the bladder neck and the retention plug occludes the external urinary meatus. Contrast injected into the urethra and the diverticulum is delineated. This is particularly valuable in cases where VCUG has failed to show a diverticulum (Fig. 20.1).

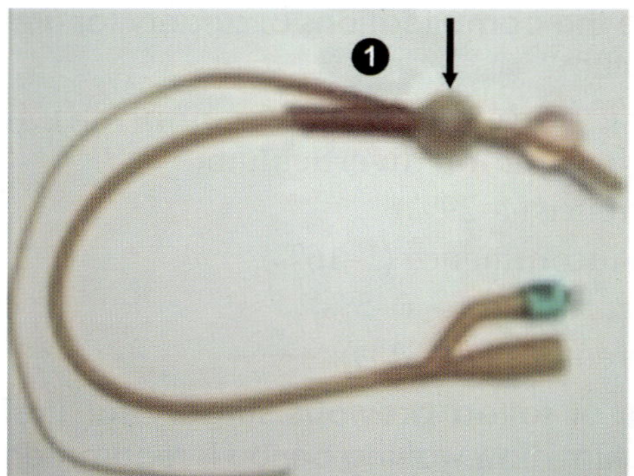

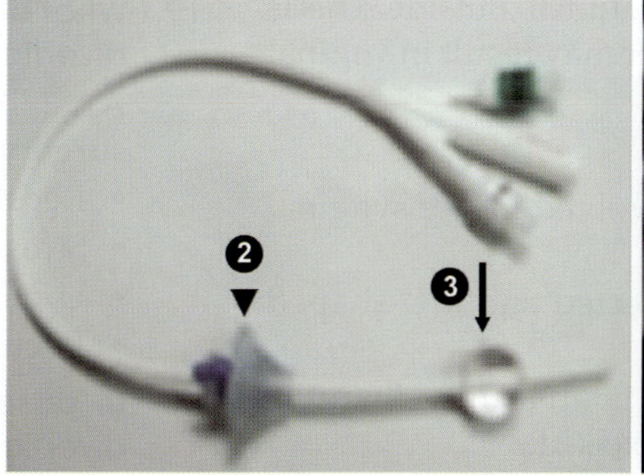

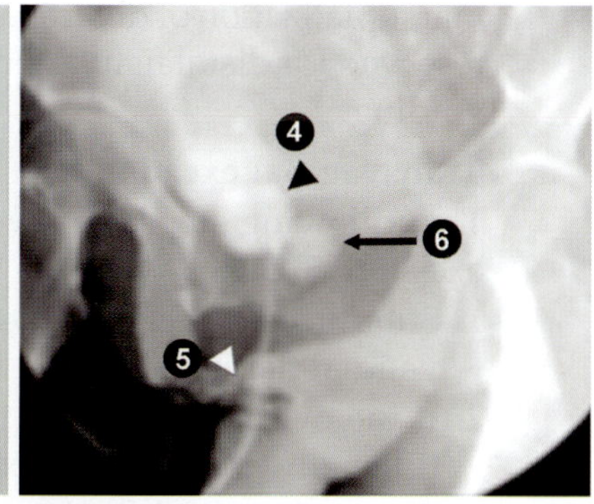

Fig. 20.1: 1. Second (proximal) balloon. 2. Retention plug at the urethral meatus prevents the backflow of contrast agent. 3. Silicone balloon occludes the bladder neck. 4. Double-balloon urethrogram obtained with a Madduri catheter shows the urethral lumen is occluded distally by the second balloon. 5. Proximal retention plug. 6. Diverticulum with posterior extension

13. What are the precautions to be followed during urethroscopy for UD?

Ans: Cystoscope sheath with a short beak is used. Traditional cystoscope sheath contains a large beak which leads to loss of irrigation fluid proximal to the catheter and poor distension of the urethra. A zero degree lens should be used. If short beaked cystoscope is not available, then visual internal urethrotomy (VIU) sheath may be used. Confirmation may be obtained by pressing the mass in anterior vagina and observing efflux in the urethra.

14. What are the indications of surgery?

Ans: The following are the indications of surgery: UTI, pain, dyspareunia, postvoid dribbling, malignancy and calculus.

15. What are the surgical methods for treating urethral diverticula and what is the preferred procedure?

Ans: The following are the surgical methods for treating UD:[8]

- Transurethral saucerisation (TS)
- Marsupialisation into anterior vaginal wall[9]
- Excision of diverticulum

Of all the three, the recommended treatment is excision of diverticulum.[10,11]

16. What are the surgical steps?

Ans: Before any surgery, urine culture must be obtained and if it shows growth of bacteria, the appropriate culture specific antibiotic should be started and continued for at least a week.

Transurethral saucerization: In this, the narrow neck of UD is converted into wide neck by transurethral resection. It is reserved for distal fistulas.

Marsupialisation: This involves creation of hypospadiac meatus, made by incising the anterior wall of vagina across the urethral meatus and distal urethra up to the diverticulum. This leads to receding of the meatus proximally along with marsupialization of diverticulum to outside. This is reserved for distal fistulas. It may result in vaginal voiding.

Transvaginal excision

The following steps are involved in transvaginal excision of UD:

1. Submucosal saline is injected and a U-shaped vaginal flap is raised.
2. If the overlying mucosa is unhealthy, then the unhealthy part may be excised.
3. The periurethral fascia underlying the vaginal musoca (i.e. overlying the diverticulum) is identified and incised.
4. The diverticular wall is gently grasped with a babcock forcep and traction applied. Dissection is continued all around till the diverticular neck is reached.
5. The diverticular wall is incised and inspected for communication with the urethra and other associated abnormalities. The diverticulum is excised flush with the urethral wall.
6. The urethra is closed with 4–0 poliglecaprone or polyglactin suture in a continuous longitudinal fashion, incorporating both the mucosa and the muscularis.
7. The periurethral tissue is closed horizontally over the urethra.
8. The vagina is closed with 3–0 polyglactin. If needed a labial fat pad (Martius flap) may be interposed between the urethra and vagina. Also, an autologous fascial sling, if required to treat SUI, may be interposed before vaginal closure.
9. An overnight vaginal pack is placed which is removed the next day. The patient is started on oral anticholinergics if required to prevent bladder spasms.
10. The perurethral catheter is kept for 3 weeks. Usually a VCUG is not required before catheter removal except in the case of difficult reconstructions.

(Steps have been shortened)

17. How to treat SUI coexisting with urethral diverticulum?

Ans: Autologous fascial pubovaginal sling is used to treat SUI coexisting with a urethral diverticulum.[11]

18. In how many layers should the repair of diverticulum be done?

Ans: Repair should be done in a minimum of three layers (urethral wall, periurethral tissue and vagina). In case of complex reconstructions or tenuous repairs, a labial fat pad (Martius flap) may interposed before vaginal closure.

19. What are the complications of surgery for urethral diverticulum?

Ans: The following are the complications of surgery for urethral diverticulum:

- Recurrence (1–29%)
- Stress incontinence (1–16%)
- Urethral stricture (0–5%)
- Recurrent UTI (0–31%)

20. In cases of failed previous surgery for urethral diverticulum, how waiting period is recommended before embarking on redo repair?

Ans: A minimum waiting period of three months is recommended before redo surgery

Video link: https://www.ncbi.nlm.nih.gov/pmc/articles/PMC4300579/bin/IJU-31-75-v001.flv

Courtesy: Sanjay Sinha,[1] Rooma Sinha. Excision of urethral diverticulum in a 24-year-old woman. Indian J Urol.2015 Jan-Mar;31(1):75–6.

SUMMARY

- Urethral diverticulum (UD) most commonly presents as recurrent UTI. The 3 Ds of UD are postvoid dribbling, dysuria and dyspareunia.
- A high index of suspicion is required for diagnosis.
- VCUG, MRI and urethroscopy are appropriate for evaluation and planning management.
- Urethroscopy should be performed with a short beaked sheath and 0 degree lens. Alternatively, a visual internal urethrotome (VIU) sheath may be used.
- Urethral diverticulum is best treated by excision.
- Closure should be performed in multiple layers with labial fat pad interposition (if required).

REFERENCES

1. Baradaran N, Chiles LR, Freilich DA, Rames RA, Cox L, Rovner ES. Female Urethral Diverticula in the Contemporary Era: Is the Classic Triad of the "3Ds" Still Relevant? Urology. 2016 Aug;94:53–6.
2. Cameron AP. Urethral diverticulum in the female: a meta-analysis of modern series. Minerva Ginecol. 2016 Apr;68(2):186–210.
3. Larkin GL, Weber JE. Giant urethral calculus: A rare cause of acute urinary retention. J Emerg Med. 1996 Nov; 14(6):707–9.
4. Magann EF, Newton LS, Barr SA. Urethral Diverticulum Presenting as a Large Vaginal Mass Complicating Pregnancy and Delivery. Am J Case Rep. 2017 Oct 13;18:1095–8.
5. Kim TH, Kim SY, Moon KC, Lee J, Cho JY, Kim SH. Clear Cell Adenocarcinoma of the Urethra in Women: Distinctive MRI Findings for Differentiation From Nonadenocarcinoma and Non-Clear Cell Adenocarcinoma of the Urethra. Am J Roentgenol. 2017 Apr;208(4):805–11.
6. Dwarkasing RS, Dinkelaar W, Hop WCJ, Steensma AB, Dohle GR, Krestin GP. MRI Evaluation of Urethral Diverticula and Differential Diagnosis in Symptomatic Women. Am J Roentgenol. 2011 Sep;197(3):676–82.
7. Méndez-Probs, Razvi H. Fundamentals of instrumentation and urinary tract drainage. In: Campbell-Walsh Urology. 10th ed. Philadelphia: Saunders; 2012. p. 177–89.
8. Bodner-Adler B, Halpern K, Hanzal E. Surgical management of urethral diverticula in women: a systematic review. Int Urogynecology J. 2016 Jul;27(7):993–1001.
9. Spence HM, Duckett JW. Diverticulum of The Female Urethra: Clinical Aspects and Presentation of a Simple Operative Technique for Cure. J Urol. 1970 Sep;104(3):432–7.
10. El-Nashar SA, Singh R, Bacon MM, Kim-Fine S, Occhino JA, Gebhart JB, *et al* Female Urethral Diverticulum: Presentation, Diagnosis, and Predictors of Outcomes After Surgery. Female Pelvic Med Reconstr Surg. 2016;22(6):447–52.
11. Crescenze IM, Goldman HB. Female Urethral Diverticulum: Current Diagnosis and Management. Curr Urol Rep. 2015 Oct;16(10):71.
12. J Poutamo[1], R Vanninen, K Partanen, P Kirkinen. Diagnosing fetal urinary tract abnormalities: benefits of MRI compared to ultrasonographyActa Obstet Gynecol Scand. 2000 Jan;79(1):65–71.
13. Agwu NP, Umar AM, Oyibo UE. Review article: Urethral catheters and catheterization techniques. Niger J Med 2022;31:497–508.

Section

5

Andrology

Chapter

1

Unconsummated Marriage

• *Gautam Banga* • *Mohsin Quadri*

LEARNING OBJECTIVES

- To identify a case of unconsummated marriage (UC).
- To differentiate between male and female causes of UC.
- To strategize treatment in liaison with the treating gynaecologist.

INTRODUCTION

Unconsummated marriages (UC) are on the rise. It could be due to male or female factors or both. Male factor is usually erectile dysfunction which may be primary ED leading to UC or UC due to vaginismus leading to secondary ED. This involves careful discussion with both partners and the treating gynaecologist, gaining confidence of the couple and directing appropriate counselling and management of the underlying factors.

Case Scenario

Couple married for two years, husband 30 years old and wife 28 years old. Referred by a gynaecologist colleague after female evaluation which seems to be normal for male evaluation and management. They strongly desire to have a child and there is pressure from their relatives for the same. On history taking he has good morning erections but somehow loses erection while he tries to penetrate and revealed to be an unconsummated marriage. His physical, hormonal examination and semen analysis were normal.

1. **What is an non-consummated marriage?**

   Ans: Non-consummated marriage (UCM) is a condition where a heterosexual couple is unable to perform vaginal penetration and intercourse since getting married.[1] It is common in the first few nights of marriage, the penetrative vaginal intercourse may not be successful.[2] The other factors to consider are privacy for the couple to perform and absence of any other pressure.[3]

2. **What are causes and factors related to unconsummated marriage?**

   Ans: Common causes of unconsummated marriage:

   Both male and female sexual dysfunctions can contribute to unconsummated marriages/relationships.

   a. **Vaginismus:** This is a situation in which the pelvic floor muscles of the female partner contract involuntarily at the start of penetration. This contraction makes the vagina tighter and narrower, making penetration (such as with a penis, finger, or gynecologist's speculum) becomes extremely difficult or impossible. [Note: Vaginismus is now placed under genito-pelvic pain/penetration disorder (GPPPD).]
   b. **Erectile dysfunction (ED):** The male partner is unable to initiate or maintain an erection which is sufficient for penetration. ED may have physical or psychological causes.
   c. **Severe premature ejaculation (PE):** This is a situation where a man ejaculates before vaginal penetration.

   Couples can have difficulties consummating their relationships for a variety of reasons.

   1. **Anxiety:** Couples who have a little or no sexual experience may feel anxious about their first

intercourse. They may not know what to expect or worry about their performance.

2. **Insufficient sex education:** Partners may be unfamiliar with sexual anatomy and the sexual response cycle, especially if they have never been in sexual situations before.
3. **Fear of pain:** People may expect intercourse to be painful. For some, this fear may be the result of insufficient education. Hearing stories about painful first intercourse experiences can add to apprehension, too.
4. **Taboos or negative feelings about sex:** People who have grown up believing that sex is "bad" or "dirty" may have trouble consummating their relationships.
5. **Societal pressure:** In some cultures, couples are expected to consummate their marriages within a certain period of time, and families might require proof that consummation has taken place. In others, couples may feel they are supposed to have sex within a certain time frame, regardless of whether they feel ready to do so.
6. **A sexual secret:** People may have an undisclosed sexual orientation or preference.

3. What are the relationships between the average delay for medical consultation in various causes that leads to unconsummated marriage?

Ans: Non-consummated marriages are due to female factors such as vaginal tightness or male factors such as ED or severe PE.[7] As shown in Table 1.1, women take a long time to come for a consultation, while men with ED or PE reach the doctor early.[4]

4. Elaborate the range of manifestations in both the partners involved in an unconsummated marriage?

Ans: Spectrum of unconsummated marriage: In men, ED could be organic, psychogenic or mixed and due to penile curvatures.[2,9] In women, vaginal tightness may happen due to mechanical factors like thick or septate hymen and inflammation in the vulva or vestibule or psychogenic causes like anxiety, fear of pain on penetration, fear of pregnancy, phobias, aversions or previous bitter experiences.[11]

5. How to manage this current case scenario effectively?

Ans: Both partners may have a poor idea of male and female genital anatomy and physiology. Their knowledge of sexual positions and techniques should be explored and accordingly counselling has to be planned.

Background

Background of the present situation is very important in UC marriage. Both partners were educated, husband being an accountant and wife was a homemaker. It was a traditional arranged marriage, they had a private bedroom, and they were staying away from parents and had not disclosed their problem to their respective families.

Detailed history and basic examination

Failure of vaginal penetration was due to the male partner's inability to maintain erections till penetration; early morning erections were normal. They were otherwise compatible, with normal sex drive. Physical examination, hormonal evaluation and semen analysis found to be normal. A multi-disciplinary team approach is necessary for further evaluation and management. The team includes a sex therapist (psychologist), gynaecologist, uro-andrologist and trained nurses are part and parcel for effective management in such cases. Whenever necessary, the history should date back to childhood to identify unpleasurable experiences.

6. What is vaginismus in detail, how to diagnose, various scoring methods and how to treat this?

Ans: A subset of the GPPPD, it is characterised as an inability to penetrate the vagina for placing

TABLE 1.1: Causes and duration of UC marriage

Author	*Duration average (min-max)*	*Main etiology referred*	*Nation of study population*
Blazer[4]	8 years (1 to 21 years)	Bride's fear of pain in the initial coitus	United States
Bramley *et al*[5]	4.2 years	Vaginismus	England and Wales
Ozdemir *et al*[6]	2.8 years (no data)	Vaginismus	Turkey
Zargooshi[7]	137 days (1 day 8 years)	Vaginismus	Iran
Fageeh[8]	1 year (60 days 5 years)	Vaginismus	Saudi Arabia
Ghanem *et al*[9]	4 days to 3 years	Psychogenic ED and vaginismus	Egypt
Raham *et al*[10]	46 days (10–84)	Penile curvature	Egypt
Shamloul[2]	180 days (60–270)	Psychogenic ED	Egypt
Michetti *et al*[3]	5.2 years (1 to 18 years)	Psychogenic ED, severe PE and vaginismus	Italy

tampons, performing digital gynecologic pelvic examination or trying serial vaginal dilators.

Sexual intercourse is painful or often impossible.[13] GPPPD combines dyspareunia and vaginismus into a single entity.[14] Vaginismus can be primary or secondary. In primary type, the woman has never had a non-painful intercourse, and in secondary type, the woman has had earlier non-painful sexual intercourse and starts reporting pain later.[12]

Evaluation and diagnosis of vaginismus is based on history. Pain and anxiety scores can be measured for inserting cotton-tipped applicator, tampon, dilator, finger, gynecological examination and intercourse. Lamont-Pacik classification helps the women to score by herself based on experience of penetrative intercourse (Table 1.2 and 1.3).[16,17]

The mainstay of treatment for vaginismus treatments include counselling, reassurance and providing confidence to the woman. It involves education about vaginal and pelvic anatomy, gradually try self-insertion of fingers, performing Kegel's exercises, slowly introducing vaginal dilators, generous use of lubricants, initiating psychotherapy including cognitive behavioural therapy, and relationship and sex counselling and medications.[15]

7. **Does vaginismus lead to erectile dysfunction in a male partner?**

   Ans: The vaginal musculature is usually under the woman's control, which can strongly contract during sexual intercourse before penetration, making it almost impossible.[13,18] Repeated attempts of failure of penetration due to vaginismus or anxiety about the female partner's condition can be one of the reasons for erectile dysfunction in the man, even if he had good erectile function to start with.[19]

8. **What are the psychological factors involved in an unconsummated couple?**

   Ans: This is a multidimensional disorder.[20] The factors which lead to non-consummation are fear of penetration, stress of erection, poor interpersonal relationship, depression, lack of self-esteem, impaired quality of life and sexual dis-satisfaction.

9. **What are the treatment steps in non-consummated marriage?**

   Ans: Treatment is planned based on which symptom started first; whether erectile dysfunction is primary or secondary to either vaginal tightness or other conditions in the male or due to indifference between the couple.

TABLE 1.2: Pacik penetration questionnaire: History

After answering yes or no, please rate each of the following items with pain scores (1 = Okay no pain, 5 = Moderately uncomfortable, 10 = impossible or extremely painful, N/A—not applicable, no experience) and **anxiety scores** 1–10 (1 = none, 5 = moderate, 10 = severe, N/A). ***This is an important part of your evaluation.***

	Pain score	Anxiety score	
1. Insertion of tampons:	Yes	No	
2. Insertion of Q-Tip:	Yes	No	
3. Insertion of finger:	Yes	No	
4. GYN exams:	Yes	No	
5. Use of dilators:	Yes	No	
6. Intercourse:	Yes	No	
6A. Tip only?	Yes	No	
6B. Partial?	Yes	No	
6C. Full?	Yes	No	
6D. Age first attempted intercourse?			
6E. Age first **aware** of problems with any penetration?	**Details:**		
7. Anal intercourse:	Yes	No	Not applicable

Source: Pacik patient questionnaire

TABLE 1.3: Pacik penetration questionnaire: Clinical examination

Lamont grade 1:	Patient is able to relax for pelvic exam
Lamont grade 2:	Patient is unable to relax for pelvic exam
Lamont grade 3:	Buttocks lift off table, early retreat. Toes curl upward
Lamont grade 4:	Generalized retreat: Buttocks lift, thighs close, patient retreats
Pacik grade 5:	Generalized retreat as in Lamont level 4 plus visceral reaction which may result in any one or more of the following: Palpitations, hyperventilation, sweating, severe trembling, uncontrollable shaking, screaming, hysteria, wanting to jump off the table, a feeling of going unconscious, nausea, vomiting and even a desire to attack the doctor.

Note: It is difficult to examine women who are Lamont levels 3 and 4, Pacik level 5.

The next step is to identify if it is psychogenic predominant or organic predominant ED. It is also essential to identify the level of stress caused by this problem and overall stress levels in the man. It could be possible that a stressful mind is the predisposing factor for the entire problem.

The next step is to also identify if it is erectile dysfunction or severe premature ejaculation where there is inability to control ejaculation till the moment of penetration.

10. What are the treatment options available?

Ans: The treatment is multimodal. It involves evaluation and medical management of ED, assessment of comorbid conditions and their control and lifestyle changes and resurrection from addictions, if any. The treatment should simultaneously address concerns of vaginismus in the female partner. Assuming that there is no vaginismus, there should be a stepwise plan for management of ED.

The first step includes evaluation, medical management with medicines, psychosocial assessment and treatment of underlying psychogenic component, and counselling the female partner. This should also include sex education in the form of explaining the role of foreplay, partner expectations and vaginal containment. This should be closely followed up with cognitive behavioral therapy and systematic desensitization. Multiple sessions in a motivated couple are the key elements to success. Prognosis is guarded in patients presenting late after marriage with lack of motivation or with the sole motive being fertility.

If there is no significant improvement, the further treatment is based on the office erection assessment. In case there is poor response to office sildenafil test or the man is unable to perform the test for various reasons, then a low dose diagnostic intracavernosal injection test with bimix would provide a pathway for management. If there has been no significant improvement with medicines and psychotherapy, then it is possible to attempt self-intracavernosal injections which should involve both partners in the treatment. Initial success with a prolonged erection with vaginal intromission and completion of intercourse can be a huge boost for both the partners and can lead to removal of a major psychological barrier and gain in confidence. Further success without needing intracavernosal injections is possible as the anxiety abates.

In case this fails or there is hesitation, inability to perform or poor compliance, a discussion about penile prosthesis is valid especially if the marriage is on the cusp. The diagnosis of organic causes, arteriogenic (or vasculogenic ED) or venous leak can be made only after failure to attain satisfactory erections with moderate to high doses of bimix (at least 0.5 ml) although severe psychogenic ED can also respond to these doses occasionally. Hence, if there has been no significant improvement with medical management despite having a good response on intracavernosal injection testing, the most likely cause would be severe psychogenic ED, then there should be a detailed discussion with both partners about the role of the surgery. Prosthesis placement for organic causes and particularly psychogenic cases should be done only after appropriate counselling and discussion about the procedure and its expected results.

11. What are the goals of treatment in UC?

Ans:

- Identifying the cause and which partner is more involved
- Establishing a pathway for treatment
- Allaying fears and confusion in the patients' mind
- Reassurance and psychotherapy
- Discussing the concerns which arise during treatment
- Giving importance to both partners' desire, expectations and concerns
- Addressing fertility issues based on societal, familial, personal pressure and female partner fertility potential

12. What are various options for fertility in an unconsummated couple?

Ans: The reported incidence is about 5% in couples presenting with infertility. There is a raising trend in metropolitan cities due to stress and lifestyle. Many of them choose assisted reproduction either because of lack of interest, lack of proper guidance or frustration and also due to declining fertility potentials. Shyness to visit the doctor or openly discuss about their problems is a major hurdle.

The options include home intravaginal insemination, intrauterine insemination and *in vitro* fertilisation. This decision is based on two factors: First is duration of married life, female factor and male factor problems and second is pressure to have a conception at the earliest. It has been shown that whenever the fertility part has been taken care of, the male partner and also the female partner reaches a state of relaxed mind and treatments aimed at erectile dysfunction work better.

13. How one can achieve success in managing such cases?

Ans: The important components of treatment include both partners understanding the genital anatomy and physiology, clarifying their doubts and concerns, learning about foreplay and exploring their body and cognitive behavioral therapy. Male partner after office erection assessment can be initiated on low dose PDE5 inhibitors (tadalafil 5 mg) along with good counselling to encounter performance anxiety during early part and regular assessment of couple's satisfaction toward their performance. Success can be achieved over a period of 3–6 months with a multi-disciplinary team approach, even though it can take longer in some couples. Time should not be considered as a limiting factor in treatment.

Take home messages:

- UC marriage can be multifactorial
- It requires careful couple assessment to identify the etiology
- Treatment involves both partners and counselling
- Erectile function assessment and treatment based on response can result in successful outcomes
- Vaginismus is an important cause and has to be evaluated and managed by a specialist for best results

REFERENCES

1. Usta MF, Erdo ru T, Tefekli A, Köksal T, Yücel B, *et al.* (2001) Honeymoon impotence: psychogenic or organic in origin? Urology 57(4): 758–762.
2. Shamloul R (2006) Management of honeymoon impotence. J Sex Med 3(2): 361–366.
3. Michetti PM, Silvaggi M, Fabrizi A, Tartaglia N, Rossi R, *et al.* (2014) Unconsummated marriage: can it still be considered a consequence of vaginismus? Int J Impot Res 26(1): 28–30.
4. Blazer JA (1964) Married virgins-Studies of unconsummated marriages. Journal of Marriage Family 26: 213–214.
5. Bramley HM, Brown J, Draper KC, Kilvington J (1983) Non-consummation of marriage treated by members of the Institute of Psychosocial Medicine: a prospective study. Br J Obstet Gynaecol 90(10): 908–913.
6. Ozdemir O, Simsek F, Ozkardes S, Incesu C, Karakoc B (2008) The Uncosummated marriage: its frequency and clinical characteristics in a sexual dysfunction clinic. J Sex Marital Ther 34(3): 268–279.
7. Zargooshi J (2008) Male sexual dysfunction in unconsummated marriage: long-term outcome in 417 patients. J Sex Med 5(12): 28952903.
8. Fageeh WM (2011) Different treatment modalities for refractory vaginismus in Western Saudi Arabia. J Sex Med 8(6): 1735–1739.
9. Ghanem H, El-Dakhly M, Shamloul R (2008) Alternate-day tadalafil in the management of honeymoon impotence. J Sex Med 5(6): 1451–1454.
10. Zahran AR, Abdeldaeim HM, Fouda K, Elgebaly OF(2012) Congenital penile curvature presenting as unconsummated marriage. Repair by 16-dot plication with subjectively reported patient and partner satisfaction. Arab J Urol 10(4): 429–433.
11. Chakrabarti N, Sinha V. Marriage consummated after 22 years: a case report. Journal of Sex &Marital Therapy. 2002;284:301–304. PubMed.
12. Crowley T, Goldmeier D, Hiller J. Diagnosing and managing vaginismus. BMJ (Clinical Research ed) 2009;338:b2284.
13. American Psychiatric Association. 5th ed. American Psychiatric Association; Washington, DC: 2013. Diagnostic and statistical manual of mental disorders.
14. Binik Y.M. The DSM diagnostic criteria for vaginismus. Arch Sex Behav. 2010;39:278–291.
15. Pacik P.T. Understanding and treating vaginismus: a multimodal approach. Int Urogynecol J. 2014;25:1613–1620.
16. Pacik P.T. Vaginismus: review of current concepts and treatment using Botox injections, bupivacaine injections, and progressive dilation with the patient under anesthesia. Aesthetic Plast Surg. 2011;35:1160–1164.
17. Lamont J.A. Vaginismus. Am J Obstet Gynecol. 1978;131: 633–636.
18. Butcher J. ABC of Sexual Health: Female Sexual Problems II: Sexual Pain and Sexual Fears. BMJ. 1999;318:110–2.
19. Kaplan HS. The New Sex Therapy: Active Treatment of Sexual Dysfunctions. 1th edition. New York: Routledge; 1974.
20. Bokaie M, Khalesi ZB, Yasini-Ardekani SM. Diagnosis and treatment of unconsummated marriage in an Iranian couple. Afr Health Sci. 2017;17(3):632–6.

Premarital Anxiety

• Prabhakar Srinivasan

LEARNING OBJECTIVES

- To understand premarital anxiety and the causes.
- To learn evaluation of premarital anxiety.
- To provide effective treatment options to men with premarital anxiety.

INTRODUCTION

The incidence of premarital anxiety is gradually increasing due to multiple factors. It is important for the urologist to understand the etiopathogenesis and treat these men. It is essential to differentiate between psychogenic and organic etiology and provide the best management plan to the patient to reduce his anxiety and have a successful outcome after marriage. This involves not only medical treatment, but also inculcate lifestyle changes and adequate appropriate counseling to men with anxiety about erections especially when they have failed sexual intercourse.

ED in young men less than 40 years of age has been reported to be of non-organic/psychogenic origin (80–85%). It could be organic in 15–20% of these young males and this is the role of the andrologist to differentiate these two components. With increasing prevalence of metabolic disorders like diabetes mellitus, hypertension, dyslipidemia, and lifestyle related issues like smoking, alcohol, substance abuse and stress in the younger population, a focused history, physical examination and basic lab profile should be done in this subset of individuals.

Case Scenario

A 25-year-old unmarried male had a recent encounter with a new partner where he could not achieve and sustain a good erection. After this he had 2 more failed attempts with the same partner. He presented to the andrologist and expressed his stress about the next time they have an opportunity will he succeed in satisfying his partner. He, however, mentions he had good erections and successful intercourse with one previous partner. He also feels that he has reduced morning erections.

1. How to approach this patient?

Ans: The approach starts with detailed history, approaching the patient with empathy and aimed at gaining the patient's trust.[1] It is important to keenly listen to the patient with interest and care. History includes how the problem started, its duration, severity and aims at picking up the root cause of the problem. Stressors, previous or present relationships which might potentially act as etiology, and overall mental well-being should be assessed. It is possible to categorize ED into psychogenic, organic, or mixed, at the end of a good history.

2. What is the goal of evaluation in this patient?

Ans:

- Aim of the evaluation is to identify the cause and to try and differentiate between the types of ED—psychogenic versus organic.
- If the onset of ED is sudden, with preserved erectile function till recently, especially coupled with new or past stress or psychological issues, it is more possible to be psychogenic in nature. A prolonged onset of the problem, with reduced erections for quite some time and good libido mean that the problem be organic in etiology.[2]

- In a young male with situational ED, if the history reveals he can have spontaneous and early morning erections, during masturbation and watching or reading erotic content, it is most likely that the patient is having psychogenic ED.[3]

3. **How to differentiate psychogenic from organic ED on history?**

   Ans: Table 2.1 depicts how to differentiate psychogenic from organic etiology in detail.

4. **What are the factors which can be contributory to premarital psychogenic ED?**

   Ans: Lots of concerns about one's erections, expectations after watching erotic content, lack of sex education, family pressures, interpersonal and premarital/relationship conflicts are the most common factors which may predispose to premarital psychogenic ED. On deeper interrogation, a feeling of insecurity during childhood, a sense of guilt about childhood sexual experiences, partner expectations and concerns over sexual experience or phallus length, prior or current psychiatric conditions or medicines, drug abuse or childhood sexual abuse can play a major role in precipitating and maintaining the psychogenic component of ED.

5. **What are the psychiatric conditions associated with psychogenic ED?**
   - Among psychiatric conditions, depression has been shown to have a significant association of severe ED; it seems to be bidirectional relationship where depression can be the cause or effect of ED.[4]
   - Anxiety is one of the leading causes of ED. Whenever a man is constantly worried and anxious about the quality of his erections and performance or gets distracted during the act, ED worsens.[5–8]

6. **What are the non-psychological predictors or factors associated with premarital ED?**

   Ans:
   - The most important factors which have a bearing in ED include unhealthy and stressful lifestyle, substance abuse or recreational drug abuse, obesity and sometimes over-indulgence in physical fitness.[9]
   - Cognitive behavioral factors include negative thoughts, difficulty to adapt to situations and negative beliefs about erections. These can finally result in an anticipated failure and augments performance anxiety, leading to significant premarital ED.[9–10]
   - Men keep high hopes and thoughts about their appetite for sex and their insistence on satisfying their partners. A man counts his physical strength on his ability to maintain erections till his partner is satisfied and feels that strong erections mean strong physique.[10]
   - Failure to perform, especially in an individual who is vulnerable to performance anxiety, in the premarital setting, creates a vicious cycle during every encounter. A distraction during performance and unable to concentrate, can worsen ED.[11–12] Drugs such as SSRI (selective serotonin reuptake inhibitors), benzodiazepines, etc., which are frequently used in premarital anxiety, can cause worsening of erectile function, delayed ejaculation and anorgasmia in some men.[13–14]
   - A good relationship with the partner is an important prerequisite for good erections. Women report a reduced desire, arousal and orgasm when the male partner has ED; these improve with better erections after using PDE5 inhibitors, as confirmed by randomized trials. Cognitive behavioral therapy has also been showed to improve the efficacy of PDE5 inhibitors.

7. **What are the diagnostic tools in this case?**
   - No biomarkers for non-organic ED
   - A thorough sexual history
   - Baseline tests to rule out an organic pathology—fasting lipid profile, glycosylated hemoglobin, hormonal profile (total testosterone, preferably between 7 and 11 AM ± estradiol, prolactin)

TABLE 2.1. Differentiating psychogenic and organic ED on history

Characteristic	*Psychogenic > Organic*	*Organic >> Psychogenic*
Onset	Sudden	Slow
Occurrence	On some occasions	On most occasions
Nature or problem	Erratic	Continuous
Non-coital erections	Generally good	Generally reduced
Early morning erections	Generally good	Generally reduced
Psychosexual problems	Often precede ED	Often new onset
Partner issues	More significant	Less significant

- Office sildenafil test/ low dose intracavernosal injection test with bimix (papaverine and chlorpromazine) or alprostadil
- NPT (nocturnal penile tumescence)

8. What is the plan of management in these situations?

Ans:

- Detailed history helps in planning the treatment. Sociocultural and religious attributes, medical and associated conditions including psychologic problems and prescription/nonprescription medications and substance abuse should be taken into consideration while planning treatment.
- Every effort be made to differentiate organic and psychosexual dysfunctions. Treatment includes medications as per the office erection assessment and psychotherapy.

9. What are the available psychotherapy modalities?

Ans:

- Individual psychotherapy: This is analytically oriented; fetches good results. Combined sex therapy and psychoanalytically oriented psychotherapy helps resolution of the sexual problem with relearning of sexual satisfaction.
  - Therapist is not alone; rather a team is involved.
  - Psychotherapy sessions are interactive, including discussion on sexual functioning
  - Duration of therapy is short and behavior oriented. Practice sessions with specific exercises are assigned for the couple to practice at home.
  - Relaxation exercises are useful adjuncts particularly in anxiety associated sexual impairment.
- Cognitive Behavioral Therapy (CBT): This form of therapy is specific to modify redundant thoughts and depression/ anxiety.
  - Combining cognitive and behavioral procedures with techniques such as sensate focus and sexual skills training.
  - Systematic desensitization especially in erectile and ejaculatory dysfunction.
  - Assertiveness training in conjunction with sex therapy in order to help patients express their sexual desires and needs as well as disagreement about certain requests viewed by them as unreasonable.

10. What is the role of medical management?

Ans: Medical therapy may not result in a complete recovery; however, 30–35% of men may not fully respond to PDE5 inhibitors.[15] CBT can salvage these men and ED can improve with medical therapy.[15]

11. What is the plan of management of the index case?

Ans:

- The fact that this patient has had successful intercouse with a previous partner suggests psychogenic ED is a more likely possibility. Failure with a new partner appears to be situational resulting in anxiety, depression and low self-esteem.
- The main focus is on evaluating his erection with office sildenafil or low dose diagnostic intracavernosal injection of vasoactive drug, to confirm the diagnosis. This also can be reassuring to the patient that he has the potential to produce a good ereciton.
- This followed by psychological counselling sessions would be more helpful to resolve his problem and improve self-esteem.
- Short course daily low dose tadalafil can help.
- If the response to PDE5i is not satisfactory despite counseling sessions, the patient could be counseled about self-ICI especially if he would like to perform sexual intercourse. Self-ICI can be used as first line therapy in such individuals to restore confidence and early switch over to oral PDE5i and gradual weaning.
- Sexual counselling including behavioral and cognitive therapy to reduce severity of depression and anxiety and build confidence and regain self-esteem.
- Partner involvement in the treatment whenever possible would improve the overall success of the treatment.

KEY POINTS

- Premarital anxiety is an important problem in young men especially with ED.
- The etiology may be organic or psychogenic. It is essential for the urologist to identify the etiology.
- Not only medical management, the treatment is centered around lifestyle and behavioral changes.
- A successful treatment can improve the self-esteem and boost the confidence of the male.
- Partner counseling whenever possible can improve treatment outcomes.

REFERENCES

1. Lue T. Campbell-Walsh Urology. Physiology of Erection and Pathophysiology of ED. Ch. 23. Philadelphia: Elsevier Inc.; 2011.
2. Ralph D, McNicholas T. UK management guidelines for erectile dysfunction. Br Med J 2000; 321: 499–503.

3. Med J 2000; 321: 499–503. 13 Corona G, Petrone L, Mannucci E, Mansani R, Balercia G, *et al.* Difficulties in achieving vs maintaining erection: organic, psychogenic and relational determinants. Int J Impot Res 2005; 17: 252–8.
4. McCabe MP, Althof SE. A systematic review of the psychosocial outcomes associated with erectile dysfunction: Does the impact of erectile dysfunction extend beyond a man's inability to have sex? J Sex Med 2014;11:347–63.
5. McCabe MP, Connaughton C. Psychosocial factors associated with male sexual difficulties. J Sex Res 2013;51:31–42.
6. Jern P, Gunst A, Sandnabba K, *et al.* Are early and current erectile problems associated with anxiety and depression in young men? A retrospective self-report study. J Sex Marital Ther 2012;38:349–64.
7. Yafi FA, Jenkins L, Albersen M, *et al.* Erectile dysfunction. Nat Rev Dis Primers 2016;2:16003.
8. Hale VE, Strassberg DS. The role of anxiety on sexual arousal. Arch Sex Behav 1990;19:569–81.
9. Akre C, Berchtold A, Gmel G, *et al.* The evolution of sexual dysfunction in young men aged 18–25 years. J Adolesc Health 2014;55:736–43.
10. Nobre PJ, Pinto-Gouveia J. Cognitions, emotions, and sexual response: analysis of the relationship among automatic thoughts, emotional responses, and sexual arousal. Arch Sex Behav 2008;37:652–661.
11. Nobre PJ. Psychological determinants of erectile dysfunction: testing a cognitive-emotional model. J Sex Med 2010;7 (4 PART 1):1429–1437.
12. Banner LL, Anderson RU. Integrated sildenafil and cognitive behavior sex therapy for psychogenic erectile dysfunction: a pilot study. J Sex Med 2007;4(4 Pt 2):1117–1125.
13. Boddi V, Castellini G, Casale H, *et al.* An integrated approach with vardenafil orodispersible tablet and cognitive behavioral sex therapy for treatment of erectile dysfunction; a randomized controlled pilot study. Andrology 2015;3: 909–918.
14. Objectification, restrained eating, and math performance. J Pers Soc Psychol 1998;75:269–84.
15. McMahon CN, Smith CJ, Shabsigh R. Treating erectile dysfunction when PDE5 inhibitors fail. BMJ. 2006;332(7541):589–592. doi:10.1136/bmj.332.7541.589.

Chapter 3

Acquired Premature Ejaculation

• Puvai Murugan P

LEARNING OBJECTIVES

- Differentiate between various types of premature ejaculation.
- Evaluation of patient with acquired premature ejaculation.
- Treatment options for acquired premature ejaculation.

INTRODUCTION

Acquired premature ejaculation (PE) is characterised by inability to control ejaculation, associated with bother and the ejaculation latency is reduced when compared to previous sexual experiences.[1]

The various types include lifelong PE where symptoms exist from the time of the man's first sexual encounter and acquired PE where symptoms start after a period of normal intravaginal ejaculatory latency time (IELT).[6] In natural variable PE, the patient has shorter ejaculatory latency, which is inconsistent and associated with a sense of reduced ejaculation control. In subjective PE, though the actual intravaginal ejaculation latency is longer (at least >5 min), the subject perceives it as reduced IELT (Flowchart 3.1).

Flowchart 3.1: Classification of premature ejaculation

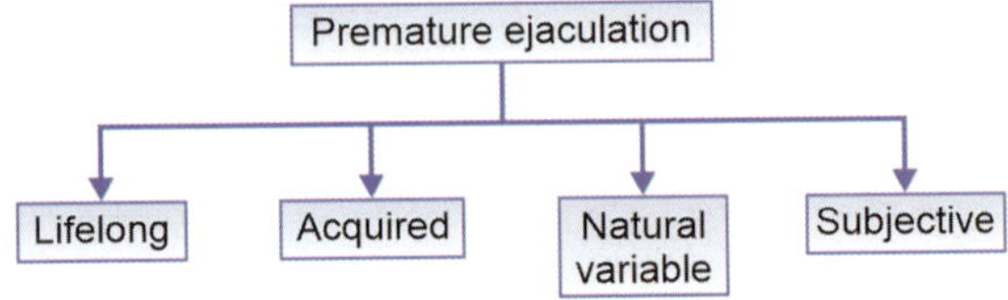

Case Scenario

A 45-year-old male married for 10 years with 2 children, reports to the andrologist in a very soft tone that he previously used to last very long for 8–10 minutes and his wife used to be happy and now he ejaculates in 1–2 minutes and his partner has told him to get this problem treated.

His erections are normal, but he ejaculates early.

When they do intercourse twice in quick succession, the 2nd time it lasts for 2–3 minutes but still the partner is not satisfied.

He is a non-diabetic, has no thyroid ailments, no other co-morbidities.

He does give a history that 2 years back he had frequency, urgency, and burning which was treated with one-month medications and occasionally still he does experience pain in the perineal area during urination.

1. **What are the causes of acquired PE?**

Ans: Acquired PE is seen in ~4% of sexually active men.[2] Various factors such as psycho-relational, endocrinological, urological, and associated sexual disorders have been attributed to cause acquired PE.

Anxiety, alexithymia, sadistic or narcissistic behavior, and social phobia are some of the psycho-relational factors attributed to acquired PE but conclusive evidence is lacking. Reduced desire, ED, PE and female sexual dysfunction have been found to coexist.

Hyperthyroidism, hypoprolactinaemia, and high testosterone levels are some of the endocrine abnormalities found in patients with PE but the causal relationship can be only established in hyperthyroidism. Treatment of hyperthyroidism leads to prolongation of latency time (Table 3.1).[3]

PE is associated with acute and chronic inflammation of prostate (chronic prostatitis), prostatodynia, or chronic pelvic pain syndrome (CPPS); these men often complaint of painful ejaculation. Though there is no evidence, varicocoele and circumcision have been attributed as for acquired PE.[4,5]

TABLE: 3.1. Etiological causes of acquired premature ejaculation[2–5]

Acquired PE	*Strong correlation*	*Weak correlation*
Urological condition	Chronic prostatitis CPPS Acute prostatitis	Circumcision Varicocoele
Endocrine condition	Hyperthyroidism	Hypoprolactinemia High testosterone levels
Sexual disorders	Hypoactive sexual desire Erectile dysfunction Female partner Sexual dysfunction	
Psycho-relational disorders	Alexithymia	Anxiety Sadistic or narcissistic behaviour Social phobia

2. **How does chronic prostatitis cause PE?**

Ans:

Chronic prostatitis and PE

The prevalence of PE in CPPS is around 40%.[6] It has been postulated that there is altered sensation due to prostatic inflammation.[2] Prolonged antibiotics, especially based on cultures improved IELT in up to 84% of men with CPPS.[7] The other useful drugs are SSRIs, PDE5 inhibitors, alpha-1 blockers, anti-inflammatory drugs, and 5-alpha reductase inhibitors.

3. **What is the management of the index case?**

Ans: This patient has acquired PE secondary to probable CPPS.

He needs further evaluation in the form of a per rectal examination to look for status of the prostate gland, a prostatic massage sample for culture and sensitivity to look for specific infection, microscopy of prostatic massage secretions to characterize prostatitis and an abdominal ultrasound to assess the prostate volume and post-void residual urine measurement (Flowchart 3.2).

Flowchart 3.2: Algorithm for premature ejaculation

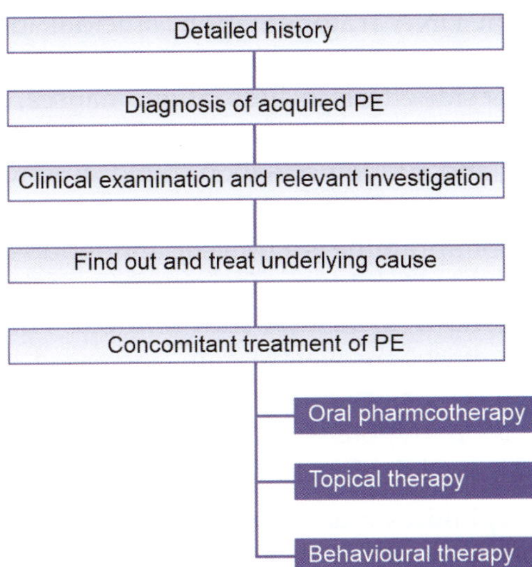

4. **What is the strategy to treat his PE?**

Ans: He needs a multi-pronged strategy to deal with his PE. The first step would be the treatment of his underlying chronic prostatitis. Based on the culture and sensitivity report, the patient needs to be started on a long course of antibiotics, alpha-blockers, and anti-inflammatory drugs. Further, based on the motivational status of the patient and his partner they can be offered a combination of cognitive behavioral therapy (CBT) and oral pharmacotherapy.

The first line of oral pharmacotherapy would be either on-demand dapoxetine or a daily dose of paroxetine. A decision to use either of them can be reached after discussing with the patient about their preference for on-demand or daily dose therapy and their side effects.

A review of the patient and his partner after 2–3 weeks regarding his progress and modification of his treatment modalities can be planned at that time.

5. **What are the oral pharmacotherapeutic agents available for the management of PE?**

Ans: Drug therapy for PE has been described in the previous chapter.

SSRI

Dapoxetine is a short-acting SSRI.[8] Dapoxetine has rapid absorption and elimination (peak concentration 1–2 h after oral intake), and is suitable for on-demand PE treatment.[8] It causes a 2.5–3 times additional improvement in IELT over the baseline. Paroxetine, a long-acting SSRI, has good oral bioavailability (peak concentration: 4–8 hours after oral intake; elimination t ½: 21 h) Paroxetine causes 8.8 times better improvement in IELT and gives the strongest ejaculation delay.[9] Used at a dose of 10–40 mg once daily or on-demand (3–6 h before intercourse), the effect starts in 5–10 days but full therapeutic effect is usually reached at 2–3 weeks. Weight gain is a serious side effect. Other important side effects are abnormal sperm DNA fragmentation, suicidal ideations, hypomania and agitation and upper GI bleeds.[10] Minor side effects include fatigue, nausea, diarrhea and sweating. Patients may develop addiction to the drug and sudden cessation/rapid dose reduction may result in SSRI withdrawal syndrome.

Clomipramine is a tricyclic antidepressant, and acts as an inhibitor of serotonin uptake. It has been shown to increase IELT fourfold.[11] Important side effects are weight gain, increased appetite, sedation, dry mouth, urinary retention, blurring of vision, hypotension, restlessness, perspiration, and sexual dysfunction.[12,13]

Phosphodiesterase Type 5 Inhibitors

The clear role of PDE5i in PE is not clear.[16] By increasing cGMP and nitric oxide activity in the medial preoptic area, PDE5i reduce the sympathetic tone and may delay ejaculation. Also, PDE5i's may delay ejaculation by relaxing smooth muscles in vas deferens, seminal vesicles, prostate, and urethra by the same mechanism.[14]

The combination of PDE5i and SSRI have shown to improve IELT better than either drug alone.[16] EAU guidelines recommend the combined use of PDE5i in the treatment of PE, either alone or in combination with SSRIs (Flowchart 3.3).[15]

6. What are the topical agents available for the management of PE?

Ans:

Topical therapies

Topical anesthetics have been shown to improve IELT by reducing glans sensitivity.[17,18] This has been described in the previous chapter.

7. Describe the behavioral therapy used in the management of PE.

Ans:

Behavioral therapies

CBT for PE is aimed at improving the skill set of men to delay ejaculation by improving self-confidence, reducing anxiety associated with performance and have a broader idea of sex.[19] CBT also relies on removing barriers such as interpersonal issues or personal issues that may precipitated, maintain or are the consequence of the PE for the man or the couple, on a whole.[20] CBT for PE revolves around stop-start (Semans; 1956) and squeeze technique (Masters and Johnson; 1970).[21]

Squeeze technique

Patient is instructed to hold the penis with thumb and index finger at the "points of no return" for a few seconds. This pressure over the glans penis leads to contraction of bulbospongiousus muscle (bulbospongiosus reflex) resulting in reduced ejaculatory urgency, a reduced desire to ejaculate and reduced penile erection. This also results in sustained pelvic floor muscle contractions (internal squeeze) of the pelvic floor muscles.[22] Pelvic floor therapy can be of great benefit in men with PE and especially in pelvic floor dysfunction.[23]

Start/stop technique

Partner stimulates the penis until the male feels that he is about to ejaculate. Partner stops the stimulation at this point and the male waits for the sensation to pass. This cycle is repeated again till the "point of no return." This can result in prolonging sexual activity. This technique can be then practiced during penetrative intercourse.

Flowchart 3.3: Pharmacotherapy of premature ejaculation

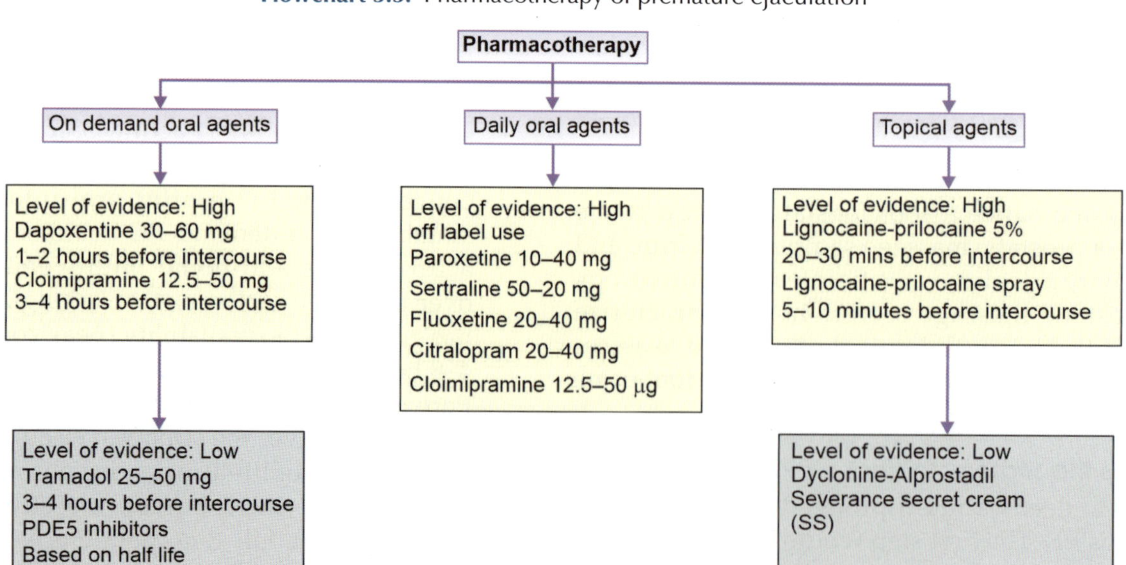

8. What are the options for the treatment of refractory PE?

Ans: All options need to be proved by well-designed randomized controlled trials. Their use is not supported by guidelines yet.

1. Botulinum toxin A injection[24–27]
2. Glans penis augmentation with hyaluronic acid

   Hyaluronic acid provides a bulky barrier and may reduce the sensitivity of glans penis to tactile stimuli. Potential major complications such as necrosis or fibrosis of the glans, limit the common use of this technique.[28]
3. Selective resection of the dorsal penile nerves (SRDN)

   This method has been proposed as a strategy to cure PE. Selective resection of the dorsal penile nerves (SRDN) has shown promising results on Phase 2 trials, however, is not recommended because it is irreversible and invasive. [1,15, 29,30]
4. Neuromuscular electrical stimulation

   There is increased EMG activity in pelvic floor muscles (bulbospongiosus and ischiocavernosus) during ejaculation.[31] The contractility of perineal muscles can improve following physio-kinesiotherapy and electrostimulation and patients are taught to recognise the closing strength of external urethral sphincter by biofeedback.[32] This is cumbersome and time taking but has good results. Further refinements in devices could improve patient acceptability.[33]
5. Transcutaneous posterior tibial nerve stimulation.

   Posterior tibial nerve stimulation may inhibit emission (Emission: T12–L1—sympathetic) and ejaculation (Expulsion: S2–S4—parasympathetic).[34,35]

   Preliminary results of phase II trials are contradictory.

9. What are the investigational drugs for the treatment of PE?

Ans:

1. Oxytocin receptor antagonists: GSK557296
2. 5-HT1A receptor antagonist: GSK958108
3. New SSRI: DA-8031
4. Modafinil

SUMMARY

- Premature ejaculation can be lifelong, acquired, natural variable or subjective types
- Acquired PE is characterised by reduced control over ejaculation, which is different from previous normal sexual experiences and is associated with bother and stress.
- Acute and chronic prostatitis, hyperthyroidism, and other sexual dysfunction in self and partner are some of the common causes of acquired PE.
- Treatment of acquired PE is multimodal, i.e., treatment of the underlying cause, behavioral therapy with or without concomitant oral or topical pharmacotherapy for PE.
- Some of the invasive methods of treatment of PE have shown promising results but their use in routine clinical practice would need further large-scale studies.

REFERENCES

1. Shindel AW, Althof SE, Carrier S et al: Disorders of Ejaculation: An AUA/SMSNA Guideline. J Urol 2022.
2. McMahon CG, Jannini EA, Serefoglu EC, Hellstrom WJ. The pathophysiology of acquired premature ejaculation. Transl Androl Urol. 2016 Aug;5(4):434–49.
3. Carani C, Isidori AM, Granata A, *et al.* Multicenter study on the prevalence of sexual symptoms in male hypo- and hyperthyroid patients. J Clin Endocrinol Metab 2005; 90:6472–9.
4. Morris BJ, Krieger JN. Does male circumcision affect sexual function, sensitivity, or satisfaction?-a systematic review. J Sex Med 2013 Nov;10(11):2644–57.
5. Tian Y, Liu W, Wang JZ, *et al.* Effects of circumcision on male sexual functions: a systematic review and meta-analysis. Asian J Androl 2013;15:662–6.
6. Li HJ, Kang DY. Prevalence of sexual dysfunction in men with chronic prostatitis/chronic pelvic pain syndrome: a meta-analysis. World J Urol. 2016 Jul;34(7):1009–17.
7. El-Nashaar A, Shamloul R. Antibiotic treatment can delay ejaculation in patients with premature ejaculation and chronic bacterial prostatitis. J Sex Med. 2007 Mar;4(2):491–6.
8. Pryor JL, Althof SE, Steidle C, Rosen RC, Hellstrom WJG, Shabsigh R, *et al.* Efficacy and tolerability of dapoxetine in treatment of premature ejaculation: an integrated analysis of two double-blind, randomised controlled trials. Lancet. 2006 Sep 9;368(9539):929–37.
9. Waldinger MD, Zwinderman AH, Schweitzer DH, Olivier B. Relevance of methodological design for the interpretation of efficacy of drug treatment of premature ejaculation: a systematic review and meta-analysis. Int J Impot Res. 2004 Aug;16(4):369–81.
10. Tanrikut C., Feldman A. S., Altemus M., Paduch D. A., Schlegel P. N.. Adverse effect of paroxetine on sperm. Fertil. Steril. 2010; Aug 94(3):1021–1026.
11. Waldinger, M. D., Zwinderman, A. H. & Olivier, B.On-demand treatment of premature ejaculation with clomipramine and paroxetine: a randomized, double-blind fixed-dose study with stopwatch assessment. Eur. Urol.2004; 46, 510–515.
12. Hollander E, Kaplan A, Allen A, Cartwright C. Pharmacotherapy for obsessive-compulsive disorder. Psychiatr Clin North Am. 2000 Sep;23(3):643–56.
13. Dold M, Aigner M, Lanzenberger R, Kasper S. Antipsychotic augmentation of serotonin reuptake inhibitors in treatment-resistant obsessive-compulsive disorder: a meta-analysis of double-blind, randomized, placebo-controlled trials. Int J Neuropsychopharmacol. 2013 Apr;16(3):557–74.
14. Dayer, P., Desmeules, J. & Collart, L. Pharmacologyof tramadol. Drugs. 1997; 53 (Suppl. 2), 18–24.
15. Salonia, A. *et al.* European Association of Urology guidelines on sexual and reproductive health—2021update: male

sexual dysfunction. Eur. Urol. https://doi.org/10.1016/j.eururo.2021.06.007.

16. Chen, J., Keren-Paz, G., Bar-Yosef, Y. & Matzkin, H.The role of phosphodiesterase type 5 inhibitors in the management of premature ejaculation: a critical analysis of basic science and clinical data. Eur. Urol. 2007;52:1331–1339.
17. Sahin H, Bircan MK. Re: efficacy of prilocaine-lidocaine cream in the treatment of premature ejaculation. J Urol. 1996;156(5):1783–1784.
18. Dinsmore WW, Hackett G, Goldmeier D, *et al.* Topical eutectic mixture for premature ejaculation (TEMPE): a novel aerosol-delivery form of lidocaine-prilocaine for treating premature ejaculation. BJU Int. 2007;99(2):369–375.
19. Melnik T, Althof S, Atallah AN, dos Santos Puga ME, Glina S, Riera R. Psychosocial interventions for premature ejaculation. Cochrane Database of Systematic Reviews 2011: CD008195.
20. Semans JH. Premature ejaculation: a new approach. South Med J. 1956;49(4):353–358.
21. Masters WM, Johnson VE. Human sexual inadequacy. Boston, MA: Little, Brown; 1970.
22. Siegel AL. Pelvic floor muscle training in males: practical applications. Urology 2014; 84: 1–7.
23. Pastore AL, Palleschi G, Leto A, Pacini L, Iori F, Leonardo C, *et al.* A prospective randomized study to compare pelvic floor rehabilitation and dapoxetine for treatment of lifelong premature ejaculation. Int J Androl 2012; 35: 528–533.
24. Gerstenberg, T. C., Levin, R. J. & Wagner, G.Erection and ejaculation in man. Assessment of the electromyographic activity of the bulbocavernosus and ischiocavernosus muscles. Br. J. Urol.1990; 65, 395–402.
25. Serefoglu, E. C. *et al.* Effect of botulinum-A toxin injection into bulbospongiosus muscle on ejaculation latency in male rats. J. Sex. Med.2014; 11, 1657–1663.
26. Aoki, K. R. J. Pharmacology and immunology of botulinum toxin serotypes. J. Neurol.2001; 248 (Suppl. 1),3–10.
27. Chermansky, C. J. & Chancellor, M. B. Use of botulinum toxin in urologic diseases. Urology.2016;91, 21–32.
28. Moon du, G., Kwak, T. I. & Kim, J. J. Glans penis augmentation using hyaluronic acid gel as an injectable filler. World J. Mens. Health.2015:33, 50–61.
29. Zhang, G. X., Yu, L. P., Bai, W. J. & Wang, X. F.Selective resection of dorsal nerves of penis for premature ejaculation. Int. J. Androl.2012: 35, 873–879.
30. Althof, S. E. *et al.* An update of the International Society of Sexual Medicine's Guidelines for the diagnosis and treatment of premature ejaculation(PE). Sex. Med.2014; 2, 60–90.
31. Pischedda, A., Fusco, F., Curreli, A., Grimaldi, G. & Farina, F. P. Pelvic floor and sexual male dysfunction. Arch. Ital. Urol. Nefrol. Androl. 2013;85, 1–7.
32. Pastore, A. L. *et al.* Pelvic muscle floor rehabilitation as a therapeutic option in lifelong premature ejaculation: long-term outcomes. Asian J. Androl.2018;20, 572–575.
33. Gul M, Bocu K, Serefoglu EC. Current and emerging treatment options for premature ejaculation. Nat Rev Urol. 2022 Nov;19(11):659–680.
34. Giuliano, F. Neurophysiology of erection and ejaculation. J. Sex. Med.2011; 8 (Suppl. 4):310–315.
35. Puppo, V. & Puppo, G. Comprehensive review of the anatomy and physiology of male ejaculation: premature ejaculation is not a disease. Clin. Anat. 2016;29,111–119.

Lifelong Premature Ejaculation

• Arun Karthik P

LEARNING OBJECTIVES

- Understanding evaluation of a patient presenting with premature ejaculation.
- Treatment modalities for PE.
- Comprehensive management of PE.

INTRODUCTION

Lifelong premature ejaculation (PE) is a condition where the intravaginal ejaculation latency time (IELT) is always very less or from the beginning of sexual life. This is associated with issues in arousal, erection, detumescence and lead to interpersonal relationships. This chapter aims to summarize the pathophysiology of PE and approach to lifelong PE.

Case Scenario

A 29-year-old male, divorced due to severe premature ejaculation; plans for another marriage. He visits the andrologist and asks whether he can marry again or will he be able to satisfy his new partner.

1. **What is the definition of premature ejaculation (PE)?**

   Ans: In 2014, the ISSM PE Guidelines Committee introduced a unified (for both lifelong and acquired subtypes of PE) definition of PE[1] that states.

   "PE is a male sexual dysfunction characterized by:

   - Ejaculation which always or nearly always occurs prior to or within about one minute of vaginal penetration from the first sexual experience (lifelong premature ejaculation), OR, a clinically significant reduction in intravaginal ejaculatory latency time (IELT), often to about 3 minutes or less (acquired premature ejaculation), and
   - The inability to delay ejaculation on all or nearly all vaginal penetrations, and negative personal consequences, such as distress, bother, frustration and/or the avoidance of sexual intimacy.

   In 2013, the DSM-5 adopted the ISSM definition of lifelong premature ejaculation. It included the requirement that the dysfunction occur in 75–100% of encounters and needs to be present for 6 months.[2] "

With this background,

On enquiry about his past marriage he tells he used to ejaculate initially with few strokes only and then his partner would not be satisfied and with time the dominating partner warned him that if he did not solve the issue she would leave him, post which on subsequent attempts he used to ejaculate even on one stroke and then he developed problems with erection too.

Eventually the marriage ended and now he is looking to remarry.

He does not have any comorbidities and did not have any partners before marriage. On masturbation currently he gets good erection but he feels he ejaculates very quickly sometimes even at the thought.

2. **Explain the pathophysiology of lifelong PE.**

   Ans: Lifelong PE is probably familial or genetic; this is due to reduced central 5-HT neurotransmission, higher 5-HT1A (5-hydroxy tryptamine) receptors and a reduced function of 5-HT2C receptors.[3,4] The pathophysiology of lifelong PE is not only related to the serotonergic system but is supposed to be a complex interplay of central and peripheral serotonergic, dopaminergic, oxytocinergic, endocrinological, genetic and epigenetic factors or threshold of penile vibration.[5–7] Men with lifelong PE have more dorsal penile nerves which cause an increased sensitivity.

3. **What are the psychological factors in lifelong PE?**

Ans: Psychological factors include performance anxiety, previous life events and vulnerabilities in childhood and adolescence.[4,8] An anxiety about performance or anticipation of quick ejaculation is very important association with lifelong PE and this can distract the patient from maintaining an erection or ejaculation.[9] It has been also shown that men who had nervousness and anxiety during early sexual experiences, became accustomed to PE.[10,11]

4. **How do you approach this gentleman with lifelong PE?**

Ans: This involves detailed history about his problem, his erections, during the previous marital life and presently with masturbation and any other previous sexual encounters. It is important to assess during the history how much impact it does have on the overall quality of life of the man. It is also essential to check for etiological factors for secondary PE such as erectile dysfunction (ED), dysuria or pain during ejaculation, lower urinary tract symptoms and local anatomical problems like phimosis or balanoposthitis. Basic evaluation includes assessment of erections, screening for diabetes mellitus and genitourinary infection/inflammation.

Considering that the erections are EHS 4 and he does not have any other medical illness, this patient appears to be having lifelong PE.

5. **What are the treatment options for this patient?**

Ans: The options for PE include medical, behavioral therapy and treatment of associated medical conditions along with physical exercises aimed at improving the pelvic floor tone. This also includes treatment for associated erectile dysfunction, prostatitis or local penile problems.

6. **What are the oral medications for management of PE?**

Ans: Oral medications include selective serotonin reuptake inhibitors (SSRI) [paroxetine, sertraline, fluoxetine or citalopram] and tricyclic antidepressant (TCA) [clomipramine] form the mainstay treatment options for PE.

7. **How is clomipramine used?**

Ans: Clomipramine used as continuous or on-demand dose can prolong IELT.[12,13] Continuous dosing has been shown to be efficient based in a meta-analysis and also that results are comparable to SSRI.[12]

8. **How do SSRI and TCA drugs act?**

Ans: TCA inhibits noradrenaline and serotonin reuptake. SSRI blocks reuptake of serotonin in the synaptic cleft of central serotonergic neurons by 5-HT transporters. This leads to greater 5-HT microneuronal transmission and stimulation of postsynaptic membrane serotonin receptors.

9. **What are the doses of these drugs?**

Ans: The commonly used drug dosages are paroxetine at 10–40 mg, clomipramine at 12.5–50 mg and fluoxetine at 20–40 mg.[14-20]

10. **What are the side effects associated with these drugs?**

Ans: Side effects include sexual and non-sexual; these drugs can reduce libido, or lead to anorgasmia and erectile dysfunction.[21] The specific non-sexual side effects include reduced sleep, tiredness, loss of appetite and sometimes SSRI can affect sperm motility.[22,23] It is important to exercise caution in PE in <18 years or depression.

11. **How is dapoxetine different?**

Ans: Dapoxetine (30–60 mg) is a novel SSRI, has quick onset of action, short t½, suitable for on-demand use and has least drug interactions.[24–26]

12. **Is tramadol effective in PE?**

Ans: Tramadol is a centrally acting analgesic. It acts on µ-opioid receptor and inhibits serotonin and noradrenaline reuptake.[27] At 25–100 mg doses, it can increase IELT by 2.4–12.6-fold.[28,29] Dose dependent negative consequences include sleepiness, itching, giddiness, dryness of mouth, nausea and vomiting, and risk of addiction.[28,29]

13. **What is the role of phosphodiesterase inhibitors in PE?**

Ans: It is useful for concomitant ED. The temporal relationship may not be known in some men. Sildenafil has been reported to work independent of SSRI to improve IELT, but robust evidence lacks.[30]

14. **What is the role of topical agents in management of PE?**

Ans: Topical anesthetics act by reducing glans hypersensitivity.[31] Topical sprays or creams are lignocaine based.[32] Application of eutectic mixture of local anesthetic (2.5% lidocaine and 5% prilocaine), 20 minutes before sex can be effective (RCT).[33] Spray formulation with 7.5 mg lidocaine and 2.5 mg of prilocaine may improve

IELT by 6-fold,.[34] There is no much reported hypoesthesia in the female partners, but some report of burning.[34–36]

15. **What are the behavioral therapies suggested for management of PE?**
Ans: This is described in much detail in the next chapter.[37,38] Kegel pelvic floor exercises and pelvic muscle physiotherapy have been shown benefit.[40-43] Behavioral techniques include sensate focus, alternative sexual positions, adjusting the time gap between episodes, and performing longer foreplay.

16. **Are there any surgical or experimental therapies available for the management of PE?**
Ans: Treatment options like ablation and dorsal penile neuromodulation are not recommended.[44,45] Newer options include unilateral or bilateral, cryoablation or radiofrequency ablation and selective resection of dorsal nerve of penis (SRDN).[45,46] Though not recommended, augmentation of glans penis with hyaluronic acid has been shown to improve IELT by 2.4–4.5 times and can work for 4-5 years. [47–49] Botulinum toxin has been tried in rats.[50,51]

17. **What is the role of intracavernosal injections (ICI) in management of PE?**
Ans: There is limited evidence.[52] ICI may be of particularly useful in patients with severe PE with ejaculation without intromission and may help in vaginal containment even after ejaculation. This can help in positive reinforcement especially in the initial phases of treatment of severe psychogenic PE.

18. **What are the psychological interventions for lifelong PE?**
Ans: Psychological interventions include steps to improve patient confidence, giving necessary space for the couple to explore solutions based on facts and providing hope to improve outcomes.[53–56]

Cognitive behavioral therapy includes identification and clarifying misconceptions, desensitization of focus from PE (sensate focus), improving self-reinforcement and bringing the couple as a single unit into the treatment.[57,58]

19. **What are the options for treatment of refractory PE?**
Ans: Combination of drug therapy and cognitive behavioral therapy performed by a dedicated and trained team provides the best solution for PE.[59,60]

20. **What is the plan of management of this index case?**
Ans: This patient needs to be started on tirated daily dosing of SSRI such as clomipramine from 10 mg onwards. Addition of PDE5 inhibitors may help in case of weak erections during evaluation. It is important to combine medical with behavioural and psychotherapy. Physical techniques help him to relieve anxiety and depression and improve his confidence. He shall need continuous training to master certain sexual skills to delay ejaculation time and the challenge is because he is presently single.

21. **When can the patient proceed for next marriage?**
Ans: The patient should be provided with a realistic review of this disorder. The patient should be explained the success rates of multimodal combination treatment as mentioned and that a vast majority usually overcome lifelong PE. Once the patient is able to halt his race to ejaculation during self-pleasure or masturbation and is reasonably confident, he can proceed for his next marriage.

KEY POINTS

- Lifelong premature ejaculation is a difficult condition to treat.
- Treatment depends upon the expectation of the partners.
- A significant part of the treatment is contributed by cognitive behavioral therapy and making the man (and his partner) understand the condition.
- Medical therapy may benefit the patient, when combined with cognitive behavioral therapy.
- Evaluation involves detailed history, assessment of erection and routine tests as indicated.

REFERENCES

1. Althof SE, McMahon CG, Waldinger MD, *et al.* An Update of the International Society of Sexual Medicine's Guidelines for the Diagnosis and Treatment of Premature Ejaculation (PE). Sex Med 2014;2:60–90.
2. American Psychiatric Association. Diagnostic and statistical manual of mental disorders: DSM-5™. 5th ed. Arlington, VA: American Psychiatric Publishing, 2013.
3. Waldinger MD, Berendsen HH, Blok BF, *et al.* Premature ejaculation and serotonergic antidepressants-induced delayed ejaculation: the involvement of the serotonergic system. Behav Brain Res 1998;92:111–8.
4. Waldinger MD, Rietschel M, Nöthen MM, *et al.* Familial occurrence of primary premature ejaculation. Psychiatr Genet 1998;8:37–40.
5. Waldinger MD. The pathophysiology of lifelong premature ejaculation. Transl Androl Urol 2016;5(4):424–433.
6. Zhu L, Mi Y, You X, Wu S, Shao H, *et al.* A meta-analysis of the effects of the 5-hydroxytryptamine transporter gene-linked promoter region polymorphism on susceptibility to lifelong premature ejaculation. PLoS One 2013; 8: e54994.
7. Guo L, Liu Y, Wang X, Yuan M, Yu Y, *et al.* Significance of penile hypersensitivity in premature ejaculation. Sci Rep 2017; 7: 104–41.

8. Hartmann U. [Psychological stress factors in erectile dysfunctions. Causal models and empirical results]. Urologe A 1998; 37: 487–94.
9. Zilbergeld B. The new male sexuality. New York: Random House Publishing Group; 2013. p432.
10. Masters WM, Johnson VE. Human sexual response. Boston: Little, Brown; 1966. p. 366.
11. Masters W, Johnson V. Human sexual response. Boston: Little Brown; 1970. p386.
12. Waldinger MD, Zwinderman AH, Schweitzer DH, Olivier B. Relevance of methodological design for the interpretation of efficacy of drug treatment of premature ejaculation: a systematic review and meta-analysis. Int J Impot Res. 2004;16:369–381.20.
13. Waldinger MD, Zwinderman AH, Olivier B. On-demand treatment of premature ejaculation with clomipramine and paroxetine: A randomized, double-blind fixed-dose study with stop-watch assessment. Eur Urol. 2004;46:510–515.
14. Althof S *et al.* A double-blind crossover trial of clomipramine for rapid ejaculation in 15 couples. Journal of Clinical Psychiatry. 1995;56(9):402–7.
15. Atmaca M *et al.* The efficacy of citalopram in the treatment of premature ejaculation: a placebo-controlled study. Int J Impot Res. 2002;14(6):502–5.
16. Goodman RE. An assessment of clomipramine (Anafranil) in the treatment of premature ejaculation. J Int Med Res.1980;8 Suppl 3:53–9.
17. McMahon CG. Treatment of premature ejaculation with sertraline hydrochloride: a single-blind placebo-controlled crossover study. J Urol. 1998;159(6):1935–8.
18. Waldinger MD *et al.* Paroxetine treatment of premature ejaculation: a double-blind, randomized, placebo-controlled study. Am J Psychiatry. 1994;151(9):1377–9.
19. Kara H *et al.* The efficacy of fluoxetine in the treatment of premature ejaculation: a double-blind placebo-controlled study. J Urol. 1996;156(5):1631–2.
20. Waldinger MD *et al.* Relevance of methodological design for the interpretation of efficacy of drug treatment of premature ejaculation: a systematic review and meta-analysis. Int J Impot Res. 2004;16(4):369–81.
21. Hellstrom WJG. Emerging treatments for premature ejaculation: focus on dapoxetine. Neuropsychiatr Dis Treat. 2009;5:37–46.
22. Sadeghi-Nejad H, Watson W. Premature ejaculation: current medical treatment and new directions. J Sex Med. 2008;5:1037–1050.
23. Tanrikut C, Feldman AS, Altemus M, Paduch DA, Schlegel PN. Adverse effect of paroxetine on sperm. Fertil Steril 2010;94:1021–6.
24. Hellstrom WJ, Althof S, Gittelman M, Streidle C, Ho KF, Kell S, Nilson-Beijber A. Dapoxetine for the treatment of men with premature ejaculation (PE): Dose-finding analysis. J Urol 2005;173:238. abstract 877.
25. McMahon C, Kim S, Park N, Chang C, Rivas D, Tesfaye F, Rothman M, Aquilina J. Treatment of premature ejaculation in the Asia-Pacific region: Results from a phase III double-blind, parallel-group study of dapoxetine. J Sex Med 2009;7:256–68.
26. Dresser MJ, Desai D, Gidwani S, Seftel AD, Modi NB. Dapoxetine, a novel treatment for premature ejaculation, does not have pharmacokinetic interactions with phosphodiesterase-5 inhibitors. Int J Impot Res 2006;18:104–10.
27. Olivier JD *et al.* Tramadol: Effects on sexual behavior in male rats are mainly caused by its 5-HT reuptake blocking effects. Neuropharmacology. 2016;116: 50–8.
28. Eassa BI, El-Shazly MA. Safety and efficacy of tramadol hydrochloride on treatment of premature ejaculation. Asian J Androl. 2013;15(1):138–42.
29. Bar-Or D *et al.*; Tramadol ODT Study Group. A randomized double-blind, placebo-controlled multicenter study to evaluate the efficacy and safety of two doses of the tramadol orally disintegrating tablet for the treatment of premature ejaculation within less than 2 minutes. Eur Urol. 2012;61(4):736–43.
30. Wang WF, Wang Y, Minhas S, Ralph DJ. Can sildenafil treat primary premature ejaculation? A prospective clinical study. Int J Urol. 2007;14:331–335.
31. Xin ZC *et al.* Somatosensory evoked potentials in patients with primary premature ejaculation. J Urol. 1997;158(2): 451–5.
32. Morales A *et al.* A review of the current status of topical treatments for premature ejaculation. BJU Int. 2007;100(3): 493–501.
33. Atikeler MK *et al.* Optimum usage of prilocaine-lidocaine cream in premature ejaculation. Andrologia. 2002;34(6): 356–9.
34. Dinsmore WW *et al.* Topical eutectic mixture for premature ejaculation (TEMPE): a novel aerosol-delivery form of lidocaine-prilocaine for treating premature ejaculation. BJU Int. 2007;99(2):369–75.
35. Dinsmore WW, Wyllie MG. PSD502 improves ejaculatory latency, control and sexual satisfaction when applied topically 5 min before intercourse in men with premature ejaculation: results of a phase III, multicentre, double-blind, placebo controlled study. B J U Int. 2009;103:940–94.
36. Gurkan L, Oommen M, Hellstrom WJG. Premature ejaculation: current and future treatments. Asian J Androl. 2008;10(1):102–109.
37. Semans J. Premature ejaculation; a new approach. South Med J. 1956;49:353–358.
38. Masters W, Johnson V. Human Sexual Inadequacy. Boston, MA: Little Brown and Company; 1970.
39. Hawton K. Treatment of sexual dysfunctions by sex therapy and other approaches. Br J Psychiatry. 1995;167(3):307–14.
40. Segraves RT, Saran A, Segraves K, Maguire E. Clomipramine versus placebo in the treatment of premature ejaculation: a pilot study. J Sex Marital Ther. 1993 Fall;19(3):198–200.
41. Myers C, Smith M. Pelvic floor muscle training improves erectile dysfunction and premature ejaculation: a systematic review. Physiotherapy. 2019 Jun;105(2):235–243. [PubMed].
42. Jiang M, Yan G, Deng H, Liang H, Lin Y, Zhang X. The efficacy of regular penis-root masturbation, versus Kegel exercise in the treatment of primary premature ejaculation: A quasi-randomised controlled trial. Andrologia. 2020 Feb;52(1):e13473. [PubMed].
43. Yaacov D, Nelinger G, Kalichman L. The Effect of Pelvic Floor Rehabilitation on Males with Sexual Dysfunction: A Narrative Review. Sex Med Rev. 2022 Jan;10(1):162–167.
44. David Prologo J, Snyder LL, Cherullo E, Passalacqua M, Pirasteh A, Corn D. Percutaneous CT-guided cryoablation of the dorsal penile nerve for treatment of symptomatic premature ejaculation. J Vasc Interv Radiol 2013;24:214–9.
45. Basal S, Goktas S, Ergin A, Yildirim I, Atim A, Tahmaz L, Dayanc M. A novel treatment modality in patients with premature ejaculation resistant to conventional methods:

The neuromodulation of dorsal penile nerves by pulsed radiofrequency. J Androl 2010;31:126–30.

46. Shi WG, Wang XJ, Liang XQ, Liu ZQ, Huang MJ, Li SQ *et al.* (2008) Selective resection of the branches of the two dorsal penile nerves for primary premature ejaculation. Zhonghua Nan Ke Xue 14, 436–438.
47. Wein A, Kavoussi L, Partin A, *et al.* Campbell-Walsh Urology (eleventh Ed.). Elsevier, 2016:692–700.
48. Kwak T.I., Jin M.H., Kim J.J. Long-term effects of glans penis augmentation using injectable hyaluronic acid gel for premature ejaculation. Int J Impot Res. 2008;20:425–428.
49. Kim J.J., Kwak T.I., Jeon B.G. Effects of glans penis augmentation using hyaluronic acid gel for.
50. Serefoglu EC, Silay MS. Botulinum toxin-A injection may be beneficial in the treatment of life-long premature ejaculation. Med Hypotheses. 2010;74(1): 83–4.
51. Serefoglu ECHW, Lesker GF, Grissom EM, Sikka SC, Dohanich GP, Hellstrom WJG. Effect of botulinum—A toxin injection into Bulbospongiosus muscle on ejaculatory latency time in male rats. In: Goldstein I, ed. World meeting on sexual medicine. Chicago: Wiley-Blackwell; 2012:331.
52. Fein RL. Intracavernous medication for treatment of premature ejaculation. Urology 1990;35:301–3.
53. Althof SE. Psychological treatment strategies for rapid ejaculation: rationale, practical aspects, and outcome. World J Urol 2005;23:89–92.
54. Althof SE. Psychological approaches to the treatment of rapid ejaculation. The Journal of Men's Health & Gender 2006;3:180–6.
55. Althof SE. Treatment of Premature Ejaculation: Psychotherapy, Pharmacotherapy, and Combined Therapy. Binik YM, Hall KS. Principles and Practice of Sex Therapy, Fifth Edition. New York: Guilford Press, 2014:112–37.
56. Donahey KM, Miller SD. What works in sex therapy: a common factors perspective. In: Klein-platz PJ. editor. New directions in sex therapy: innovations and alternatives. Philadelphia: Bruner Routledge, 2001:210–33.
57. Beck JG, Barlow DH. Current conceptualizations of sexual dysfunction: A review and an alternative perspective. Clinical Psychology Review. 1984;4(4):363–78.
58. Jannini EA, Lenzi A. Epidemiology of premature ejaculation. Current opinion in urology. 2005;15(6):399–403
59. Althof S. The psychology of premature ejaculation: therapies and consequences. J Sex Med. 2006;3 Suppl 4:324–31.
60. Perelman MA. A new combination treatment for premature ejaculation: a sex therapist's perspective. J Sex Med. 2006;3:1004–12.

Chapter
5

Anejaculation

• Deepak Gupte • Vijayant Govinda Gupta

LEARNING OBJECTIVES

- Understand the physiology and causes of anejaculation.
- Differentiating different types of anejaculation.
- Diagnosis and evaluation in a patient of anejaculation.
- Vibrator therapy for anorgasmic anejaculation.

INTRODUCTION

Anejaculation is a condition characterized by the inability to ejaculate during sexual intercourse or masturbation. It is a relatively rare condition that affects approximately 1–5% of men. Anejaculation can be a result of a variety of factors, including physical, psychological, and pharmacological causes. This chapter will discuss the various causes of anejaculation, the diagnosis and evaluation of patients with anejaculation, and the management and treatment options available for this condition.

Case Scenario

A 32-year-old male and 30-year-old female married for 1 year present with the complaint that the male partner is unable to ejaculate even after 20–30 minutes of sexual activity. He has not been able to ejaculate even once after marriage. Now the couple wants to conceive.

He has no co-morbidities.

His serum prolactin levels are normal.

He has occasionally nocturnal discharge of semen.

Management

The management of a 32-year-old male with anejaculation involves a comprehensive assessment to determine the underlying cause of the condition and to develop an appropriate treatment plan. The following are the steps and algorithm for managing a patient with anejaculation:[1]

Step 1: Assessment

A detailed medical and sexual history is important to identify any underlying medical conditions, medications, or psychological factors that may be contributing to anejaculation. Physical examination, including genital examination, would also be necessary. Diagnostic tests, such as hormone levels, or imaging studies, may be ordered to rule out any underlying medical conditions.

Step 2: Treatment of underlying medical conditions

If an underlying medical condition is identified, such as a prostate disorder, it should be treated accordingly. Medications that may be contributing to anejaculation should also be reviewed and changed, if necessary.

Step 3: Behavioral therapy

Behavioral therapy, including desensitization techniques and relaxation exercises, may be effective in treating anejaculation. Patients may be referred to a sex therapist or counselor for this type of treatment.

Step 4: Pharmacological therapy

Pharmacological therapy may be considered if behavioral therapy is not effective. Medications, such as dopamine agonists or alpha adrenergic agonists, may be prescribed to help stimulate ejaculation.

Step 5: Surgical intervention

Surgical intervention may be necessary in rare cases of anatomic abnormalities, such as a blocked ejaculatory duct. Surgery may be performed to remove any obstruction or to repair any abnormalities.

Algorithm for the management of anejaculation:

1. Assess the patient's medical and sexual history, as well as any underlying medical conditions.
2. Conduct a physical examination, including genital examination.
3. Order diagnostic tests, such as semen analysis or hormone levels, to rule out any underlying medical conditions.
4. Treat any underlying medical conditions or medications that may be contributing to anejaculation.
5. Consider behavioral therapy, such as desensitization techniques and relaxation exercises.
6. In rare cases of anatomic abnormalities, surgical intervention may be necessary.
7. Regular follow-up should be scheduled to assess treatment efficacy and adjust treatment, if necessary.

Overall, the management of anejaculation requires a comprehensive and individualized approach that addresses any underlying medical, psychological, or behavioral factors. A multidisciplinary team approach, including a urologist, sex therapist or counselor, and primary care physician, may be necessary for optimal management of this condition.

Physiology of Ejaculation[2]

Ejaculation is a complex physiological process that involves the coordinated contraction of various muscles and nerves. It is an essential process for sexual reproduction, as it allows for the delivery of sperm to the female reproductive tract. In this article, we will discuss the physiology of ejaculation in detail.

The process of ejaculation is initiated by sexual stimulation, which triggers the activation of the sympathetic nervous system. This, in turn, leads to the contraction of the smooth muscles in the walls of the seminal vesicles, vas deferens, and prostate gland. The contractions of these muscles propel the semen towards the base of the penis, where it is stored in the urethral bulb. The process of semen emission is mediated by the sympathetic nervous system and involves the contraction of the smooth muscle cells in the vas deferens, seminal vesicles, and prostate gland (phase 1). The contraction of bladder neck simultaneously thus results in the accumulation of semen in the prostatic urethra (phase 2).

Once a sufficient amount of semen has accumulated in the urethral bulb, the muscles surrounding the bulb begin to contract rhythmically. These contractions are known as the rhythmic contractions of the bulbocavernosus muscle, and they play a crucial role in the expulsion of semen from the body (phase 3). The rhythmic contractions of the bulbocavernosus muscle generate pressure within the urethra, which propels the semen out of the body in a series of spurts. The process of semen expulsion is mediated by the somatic nervous system and involves the rhythmic contraction of the bulbocavernosus and ischiocavernosus muscles.

The contractions of the bulbocavernosus muscle are controlled by the somatic nervous system, specifically the pudendal nerve. This nerve originates in the spinal cord and travels to the perineum, where it branches out to supply the muscles of the pelvic floor. When the pudendal nerve is stimulated, it activates the contraction of the bulbocavernosus muscle, leading to the expulsion of semen. The pudendal nerve also plays a role in the sensation of orgasm and ejaculation.

The process of ejaculation is regulated by a complex interplay of neurotransmitters and hormones. Dopamine, a neurotransmitter that plays a role in reward and pleasure, has been shown to increase sexual arousal and facilitate ejaculation. In contrast, serotonin, another neurotransmitter, has been shown to inhibit ejaculation. This suggests that the balance between dopamine and serotonin may play a role in the regulation of ejaculation. Understanding the physiology of ejaculation is essential for the diagnosis and treatment of sexual dysfunction

1. **What are the types of anejaculation?**

Ans: Anejaculation can be classified into two types. The two types of anejaculation are as follows:

Retrograde anejaculation (orgasmic anejaculation): In this type of anejaculation, the ejaculate is propelled backward into the bladder instead of being expelled through the penis during ejaculation. This happens because the bladder neck muscles fail to close during ejaculation, causing the semen to enter the bladder. Retrograde anejaculation can be caused by various factors, such as nerve damage, medication side effects, or previous surgery on the bladder or prostate.

Dry anejaculation: In this type of anejaculation, no semen is ejaculated from the ejaculatory ducts during sexual activity or masturbation, but the orgasmic sensation may or may not be present. This type of anejaculation is often caused by damage or disruption to the nerve pathways responsible for the ejaculation process. It can also occur as a result of certain medications, radiation therapy, or surgical procedures.

Anorgasmic anejaculation, which is common form of anejaculation seen in practice can be situational or global. Situational is because of certain situations which give rise to anxiety and inability to reach a level of arousal for ejaculation (periovulatory, partner specific, situation specific) or global anejaculation which is a from of delayed ejaculation where longer or stronger stimulation is required wherein the patient has never experienced orgasm or experiences only with prolonged stimulation.

It is important to differentiate between the two types of anejaculation as the treatment options can vary.

Retrograde ejaculation can often be managed by treating the underlying cause or with medication to close the bladder neck during ejaculation. Anorgasmic anejaculation, on the other hand, may require more extensive evaluation and treatment, such as penile vibratory stimulation or electroejaculation.

2. **What is the relationship between anejaculation and anorgasmia?**

Ans: These are two sexual dysfunctions that are often confused with each other. While both conditions can occur in men, anorgasmia can also affect women. Although anejaculation and anorgasmia can have overlapping symptoms, they are distinct conditions with different causes and treatments.

Anejaculation is the inability to ejaculate during sexual activity or masturbation, despite normal sexual stimulation. This can be caused by various factors, such as nerve damage, medication side effects, or previous surgery on the bladder or prostate.

Anorgasmia, on the other hand, is the inability to achieve an orgasm, despite normal sexual stimulation. This condition can be caused by various factors such as psychological issues, medication side effects, hormonal imbalances, or nerve damage. Anorgasmia can also be classified as primary or secondary, depending on whether the individual has never experienced an orgasm or has lost the ability to achieve an orgasm after previously being able to.

While anejaculation and anorgasmia can both be distressing for individuals and their partners, there are several key differences between the two conditions. For example, anorgasmia may still result in ejaculation for men, while anejaculation does not. Additionally, anejaculation is typically more closely associated with physical causes, such as nerve damage, while anorgasmia is often more closely associated with psychological causes, such as stress or anxiety.

3. **How the treatment of anorgasmia and anejaculation differs?**

Ans: The treatment options for anejaculation and anorgasmia can also differ. For anejaculation, treatment options may include medication or other therapies to help stimulate the ejaculatory reflex or other physical interventions, such as penile vibratory stimulation or electroejaculation. For anorgasmia, treatment may involve addressing underlying psychological factors, such as therapy or counseling, or changes in medication or hormone levels.

4. **What are the causes of anejaculation?[3]**

Ans: Anejaculation can be caused by a variety of factors, including physical, psychological, and pharmacological causes.

Physical Causes

- *Spinal cord injury:* Anejaculation is a common complication of spinal cord injury, particularly injuries above the level of T10.
- *Pelvic surgery:* Pelvic surgery, particularly radical prostatectomy, can result in anejaculation due to damage to the nerves and muscles involved in ejaculation.
- *Diabetes:* Diabetes can cause damage to the nerves and blood vessels that are involved in the process of ejaculation.
- *Multiple sclerosis:* Multiple sclerosis can cause damage to the nerves that are involved in the process of ejaculation.
- *Retroperitoneal lymph node dissection:* Anejaculation is a common complication of retroperitoneal lymph node dissection, particularly when the dissection involves the sympathetic nerves that are involved in the process of ejaculation.
- *Medications:* Certain medications, such as alpha-blockers, can interfere with the process of ejaculation.

Psychological Causes

- *Anxiety:* Anxiety can interfere with the process of ejaculation by causing the sympathetic nervous system to be activated, which can inhibit the process of ejaculation.
- *Depression:* Depression can interfere with the process of ejaculation by causing a decrease in libido and an inhibition of the sympathetic nervous system.
- *Stress:* Stress can interfere with the process of ejaculation by causing the sympathetic nervous system to be activated, which can inhibit the process of ejaculation.
- *Relationship problems:* Relationship problems can interfere with the process of ejaculation by causing anxiety, stress, and depression.

5. **How will you evaluate a case of anejaculation?**

The evaluation and diagnosis of anejaculation require a thorough medical history and physical examination. The medical history should include questions about the onset and duration of the anejaculation and whether the patient ejaculates on self stimulation. Enquiry into any associated symptoms, and any medications that the patient is taking should be done. The physical examination should include a genital examination to assess for any abnormalities, such as varicocele or hypospadias. The presence of retrograde ejaculation should also be assessed by examining the urine for the presence of sperm.

6. **What other diagnostic tests may be used to evaluate anejaculation?**

Ans:

- *Ultrasound:* An ultrasound can be used to evaluate the anatomy of the prostate gland, seminal vesicles, and ejaculatory ducts.
- *Electromyography (EMG):* Electromyography can be used to evaluate the function of the pelvic floor muscles and the muscles involved.
- *Magnetic resonance imaging (MRI):* An MRI can be used to evaluate the anatomy of the spinal cord and the nerves involved in ejaculation.

7. **What are the treatment options for anejaculation?**

The treatment of anejaculation depends on the underlying cause of the condition. Treatment options include the following.

Behavioral therapy: Behavioral therapy is a non-invasive and effective treatment option for anejaculation, a condition characterized by the inability to ejaculate. Behavioral therapy involves the use of specific techniques to help patients learn how to achieve ejaculation through a process of desensitization.

The desensitization process involves gradually exposing the patient to increasing levels of stimulation, allowing them to become more comfortable with sexual activity and eventually reach a point where they are able to achieve ejaculation. This may involve the use of masturbation or sexual activity with a partner, and may also involve the use of visual aids, such as erotic images or videos.

In addition to desensitization techniques, behavioral therapy for anejaculation may also involve the use of relaxation techniques, such as deep breathing or progressive muscle relaxation, to help patients reduce anxiety and stress related to sexual activity. Education about sexual anatomy and the physiology of ejaculation may also be provided to help patients better understand their bodies and the processes involved in achieving ejaculation.

Overall, behavioral therapy for anejaculation is a safe and effective treatment option that can help patients achieve ejaculation and improve their sexual functioning and satisfaction. It is important for patients to work with a trained therapist who can provide individualized treatment and support throughout the therapy process.

Pharmacological therapy: Medications such as sympathomimetics, cholinergic agents, and dopamine agonists can be used to stimulate ejaculation in patients with anejaculation. However, these medications may have significant side effects and are not always effective.[4]

Electroejaculation is a technique used to induce ejaculation in men with anejaculation or other conditions that prevent them from ejaculating normally. The procedure involves the use of an electric probe that is inserted into the rectum to stimulate the nerves that control ejaculation.

Electroejaculation can be an effective way to obtain semen for use in assisted reproductive techniques, such as *in vitro* fertilization (IVF) with intracytoplasmic sperm injection (ICSI). It may also be used to diagnose the underlying cause of anejaculation or to evaluate the function of the seminal vesicles, prostate gland, and other structures involved in the ejaculatory process.

Electroejaculation is typically performed under anesthesia or sedation to minimize discomfort and ensure safety. The procedure can be performed in a hospital, clinic, or fertility center by a qualified healthcare professional, such as a urologist, and typically takes about 30 minutes to complete.

While electroejaculation can be an effective treatment for anejaculation, it is generally reserved for cases where other treatments, such as behavioral therapy or pharmacological therapy, have been unsuccessful. Electroejaculation may also be associated with some risks, including rectal bleeding, infection, and nerve damage, although these complications are rare.

8. **What are the principles for vibratory stimulation?**

Ans: Vibration stimulation therapy is a non-invasive technique used to induce ejaculation in patients with anejaculation. This technique involves the use of a vibrating device that is applied to the penis to stimulate ejaculation. Vibration stimulation therapy is typically used in patients with spinal cord injuries or other neurogenic causes of anejaculation.

The use of vibration stimulation therapy to treat anejaculation was first reported in the 1970s.[5] Since then, several studies have reported its efficacy in inducing ejaculation in patients with anejaculation. A study published in the Journal of Urology reported a success rate of 70% in inducing ejaculation in patients with spinal cord injuries using a vibrating device.[6] Another study published in the Journal of Sexual Medicine reported a success rate of 60% in inducing ejaculation in patients with anejaculation due to multiple sclerosis.[7]

Vibration stimulation therapy is a non-invasive technique that can be performed at home by patients or their partners. The device used for vibration stimulation therapy is typically a handheld device that delivers a high-frequency vibration to the penis. The device is applied to the glans penis and shaft for 5–10 minutes before sexual activity. The vibration stimulates the nerve fibers in the penis and can induce ejaculation in patients with anorgasmic anejaculation.

Vibration stimulation therapy has several advantages over other treatments for anejaculation. It is non-invasive and can be performed at home, making it more convenient for patients. It also has fewer side effects compared to pharmacological therapies, which can cause significant side effects such as nausea, vomiting, and dizziness. Vibration stimulation therapy has been reported to have minimal side effects, with the most common side effect being mild penile discomfort.

Despite its efficacy and advantages, vibration stimulation therapy may not be effective in all patients with anejaculation. The success rate of vibration stimulation therapy varies depending on the underlying cause of anejaculation. Patients with complete spinal cord injuries or other severe neurogenic causes of anejaculation may not respond to vibration stimulation therapy. In such cases, other treatments such as electroejaculation or surgical interventions (surgical sperm retrieval) may be necessary.

In conclusion, vibration stimulation therapy is a non-invasive technique that can induce ejaculation in patients with anejaculation. It has several advantages over other treatments for anejaculation and is well tolerated by patients. However, its efficacy may be limited in patients with severe neurogenic causes of anejaculation. Patients with anejaculation should consult their healthcare provider to determine the most appropriate treatment for their condition.

Surgical intervention: Surgical intervention may be necessary in patients with anatomic abnormalities that are causing anejaculation, such as obstruction of the ejaculatory ducts or retrograde ejaculation. Surgery may also be necessary in patients who have had pelvic surgery that has damaged the nerves and muscles involved in ejaculation. Surgical sperm retrieval could be the last resort option for fertility, followed by IVF/ICSI.

Conclusion

Anejaculation is a relatively rare condition that can be caused by a variety of factors, including physical, psychological, and pharmacological causes. The evaluation and diagnosis of anejaculation require a thorough medical history and physical examination, as well as diagnostic tests such as semen analysis, ultrasound, EMG, and MRI. Treatment options for anejaculation include pharmacological therapy, electroejaculation, vibratory stimulation, and surgical intervention. The choice of treatment depends on the underlying cause of the condition and the individual needs of the patient.

KEY POINTS

- Anejaculation is a rare condition and requires detailed assessment.
- A careful history is essential to guide the evaluation.
- Differentiating between the types of anejaculation has prognostic significance and treatment implications.
- Apart from medical therapy, penile vibrostimulation provides benefit to men with anejaculation.
- Urologist should know how to titrate the treatment and manage infertility.

REFERENCES

1. McMahon CG. Physiology of ejaculation. In: Mulcahy JJ, editor. Male Sexual Function: A Guide to Clinical Management. 2nd ed. Totowa, NJ: Humana Press; 2004. p. 33–48.
2. Melman A, Gingell C, Moreland RB. Physiology of penile erection and pathophysiology of erectile dysfunction. Urol Clin North Am. 1998 Nov;25(4):209–17.
3. Dell'Atti L, Galosi AB. Ejaculatory disorders: pathophysiology and management. Nat Rev Urol. 2016 Aug;13(8):466–80. doi: 10.1038/nrurol.2016.124. Epub 2016 Jun 28. PMID: 27349906.
4. Brackett NL, Lynne CM. The management of ejaculatory dysfunction. Nat Clin Pract Urol. 2005 Mar;2(3):114–22. doi: 10.1038/ncpuro0117. PMID: 16474832.
5. Wyllie M. The use of a vibrator in the treatment of male sexual dysfunction. Br J Psychiatry. 1978;133:123–125.
6. Brackett NL, Ferrell SM, Aballa TC, Amador MJ, Padron OF, Lynne CM. An analysis of 653 trials of penile vibratory stimulation in men with spinal cord injury. J Urol. 1998; 159(6):1931–1934.
7. Esmailzadeh S, Maleknejad P, Moghadam KG. Penile vibratory stimulation in multiple sclerosis patients with and without sexual disorder. J Sex Med. 2010;7(1 Pt 1):271–276.

Chapter

6

Peyronie's Disease

• *Sanjay Pandey* • *Krishna Mohan Boopathy Vijayaraghavan*

LEARNING OBJECTIVES

- Define and understand the etio-pathogenesis of Peyronie's disease.
- Salient points about clinical examination, pre-operative assessment counselling and expectation management.
- Have an overview of the management of Peyronie's disease, surgical procedures routinely done in current practice and its complications.

INTRODUCTION

Peyronie's disease (PD) is characterised by an abnormality of shaft of the penis due to fibrous, firm to hard scar in the tunica albuginea.[1]

Case Scenario

A 45-year-old diabetic male with 60-degree dorsal curvature for 14 months, with dense plaque 2 × 2 cm, on the dorsal surface, with well-maintained erections.

On office sildenafil test, stretched penile length of convex border of penis is 13 cm and concave border is 11 cm.

1. **What is the prevalence?**

   Ans: It affects 3–9% of men especially in 40–60 years age group. The prevalence is more in diabetic men and those with erectile dysfunction (ED).[1,2]

2. **What is the etiology?**

   Though idiopathic, it is proposed that PD is due to abnormal wound healing which occurs after trivial trauma in genetically predisposed males. Fibrosis and inflammation set in after microvascular injury and bleeding following repeated sexual intercourse.[2,3]

3. **What is the pathogenesis of this condition?**

   Plaque formation occurs over the tunica albuginea, resulting in penile curvature because fibrosed penile tissue cannot lengthen fully on the side of the plaque (Fig. 6.1). Fibrosis is due to abnormal excess of connective tissue caused by randomly proliferating collagen fibers. This disease is characterized by an active phase and a quiescent or stable phase.[2,3]

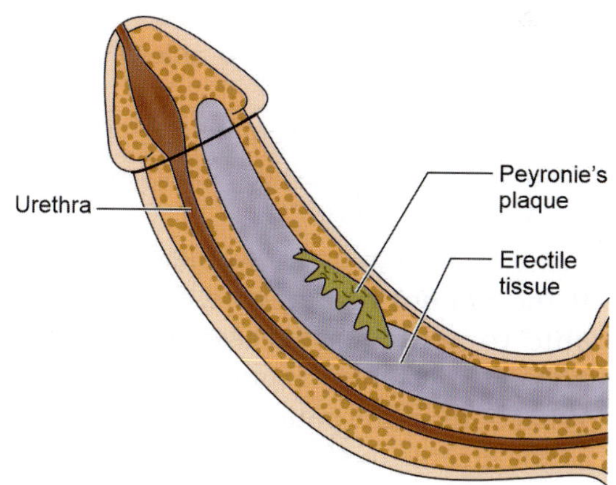

Fig. 6.1: Peyronie's disease

4. **What is the clinical presentation?**

   Ans: They usually present with one or combination of the following
   - Painful erections,
   - Plaque leading to curvature of penis,
   - Erectile dysfunction (40%),
   - Shortening, indentation, hour-glass deformity

5. **What are the clinical phases of Peyronie disease?**

Ans:

- Active (1–6 months) or inflammatory phase:
  - Painful erections and evolving penile deformity
  - Medical therapy with pain management is the ideal treatment option in active phase.
- Quiescent or stable phase (9–18 months)
  - Burnt out disease
  - Inflammation and pain settle
  - Deformity stabilizes
  - Ideally suited for surgical management.

Over a period of 18 months, 40% of PD progress, 47% of PD are stable and 13% of PD will improve.[2–5]

6. **What are the associated conditions with Peyronie disease?**

Ans: Common comorbidities associated with Peyronie's disease are diabetes mellitus (30%), Dupuytren's contracture (25%), plantar fascial contracture, tympanosclerosis, erectile dysfunction, dyslipidemia, hypertension, low testosterone, arterial disease.[2,5]

7. **What are the essential points in history taking in a patient with PD?**

Ans: Take a full medical history including history about patient's erectile function. Psychological evaluation of the patient, his confidence-morale and also assessment of patient expectations are also essential before going ahead with the treatment.[2,6]

Important questions to be asked as a part of history:

- Can the patient still achieve penetrative sexual intercourse? (if there is need for surgical correction)
- Overall duration of PD
- Does the patient have erectile dysfunction?
- If the patient has erectile dysfunction, is he able to achieve successful erections with phosphodiesterase-5 inhibitors (PDE 5)?
- What bothers the patient the most the curvature or the erectile dysfunction?

8. **How would you examine a patient with Peyronie's disease?**

Ans:

- Location, size and number of plaques
- Measurements:
  a. Self-photographs (erect penile self-photograph)
  b. Stretched penile length is important to help advice the patient
  c. Angulation-curvature: Goniometer
- Outpatient office sildenafil test or intra-cavernosal injections to assess degree of ED and degree of penile curvature
- Any complex deformities like hour-glass, waist deformity.[1,2,6]

Present case scenario clinical examination findings:

- A 45-year-old diabetic male
- A 60-degree dorsal curvature (moderate) for 14 months
- Single dense plaque 2 × 2 cm, on the dorsal surface
- Well-maintained erections on office sildenafil test
- Stretched penile length of convex border of penis is 13 cm and concave border is 11 cm.

9. **Does the patient require any further investigations?**

Ans: No further investigation is required in the above patient.

10. **What is the role of penile duplex in this patient?**

Ans: In a patient with erectile dysfunction with vascular abnormalities a penile ultrasound with Doppler is useful. In patients with extensive cavernosal fibrosis and complex deformities a preoperative contrast enhanced magnetic resonance penile imaging with intra-cavernosal injection is useful for preoperative surgical planning of correction and when considering penile prosthesis.[6,7]

11. **How will you manage this patient?**

Ans: This patient is in the stable phase, a single dense dorsally located plaque, with a moderate dorsal penile curvature, with no erectile dysfunction and no significant shortening. This patient is ideally suited for plication procedure—Nesbitt's procedure or 16-dot plication procedure. While considering above, will counsel him towards realistic expectations over one or more counselling sessions thus allaying anxiety.

12. **What are the different methods of plication?**

Ans: Nesbitt's plication procedure: Circumcoronal incision and degloving of penis, followed by artificial erection (Gittes technique) with intra-cavernosal saline injection (or papaverine) is used to assess curvature. A small ellipse of tunical tissue is excised at equal levels on the convex side of the penis opposite to the maximal deformity, in individual corpora or in the midline after urethral mobilization. Roughly, 1 mm of tunical tissue has to be excised for every 10° of penile curvature. Defect is closed with 4–0 inverting PDS sutures (Fig. 6.2). The success rates are 88–94%.[4,8,9]

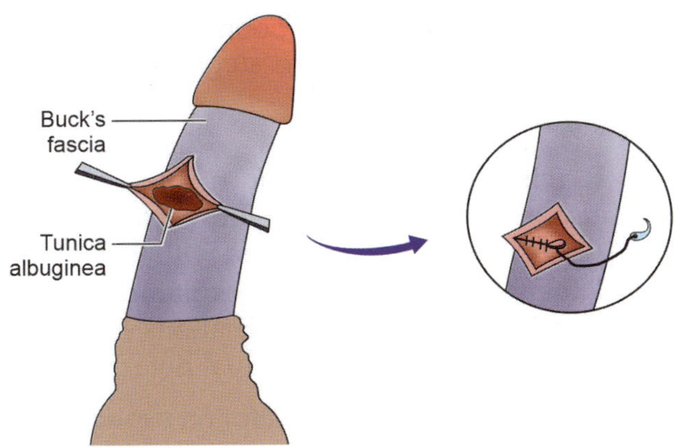

Fig. 6.2: Nesbitt's plication for Peyronie disease with curvature

Simple plication procedure: This involves placement of sutures opposite to the maximal deformity to straighten the penis. Many modifications have been developed for plication without excision including multiple parallel plication such as 16 dot plication technique (Baskin and Lue, 1998) (Fig. 6.3).[1,8–10]

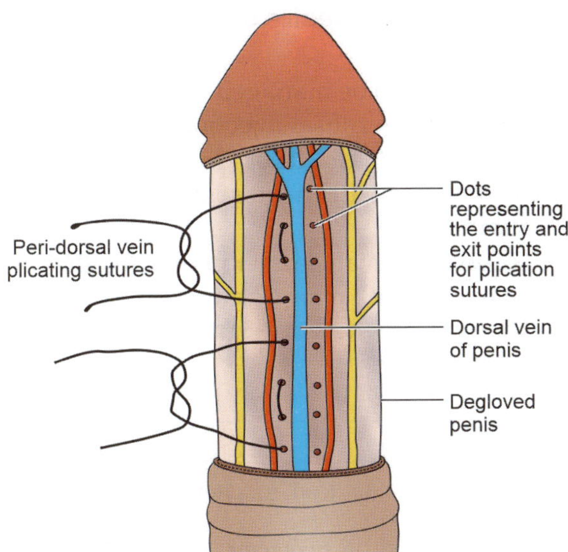

Fig. 6.3: 16-dot repair of ventral curvature. Peri-dorsal vein sutures without dissection of neurovascular bundles

Lemberger/Yachia technique:
This involves making a vertical tunical incision over the corpora, opposite the plaque with maximal convexity and horizontal suture closure, similar to Heineke-Mikulicz repair is done.[1,8,9]

13. What are the factors for assessment before plication?

Ans:

- Location, size and number of plaques
- Pre-operative stretched penile length measurement is important to help advice the patient about expected penile shortening
- Pre-operative erectile function—to assess degree of ED and curvature
- Look for complex deformities like hour-glass, waist deformity using diagnostic intracavernosal injection testing in case of doubts
- Assessment and counseling regarding patient expectations is also essential before going ahead with the plication.[11–14]

14. How do you manage ventral curvature?

Ans:

- The incidence of ventral curvatures is less commoner in Peyronie's disease
- Shortening the dorsal aspect of the corpora cavernosa by plication or lengthening the ventral aspect by patching the tunica albuginea with several types of tissue, all the principles and factors for assessment before plication in dorsal curvatures also apply for ventral curvatures.[15–17]
- Dissection and raising of neurovascular bundle (NVB) to facilitate plication (Nesbitt's procedure) can be done by one of the two techniques:
- Medial or lateral dissection techniques
  - Lateral dissection:
    - Mobilise NVB at 5 and 7 o'clock by longitudinal incisions over the Buck's fascia lying above urethra
    - Diamond-shaped tunica excised symmetrically
  - Medial dissection:
    - Open Buck's fascia dorsally and remove deep dorsal vein at its most prominent part of curvature
    - Dissect NVB only 0.5 cm from each side in a medial-to-lateral direction
    - Single or multiple diamond-shaped tunica excised from inter-cavernous septum.
    - Residual defect is closed transversely with non-absorbable inverting sutures to bury the knots under the tunica and second layer using absorbable sutures.[15–17]
    - Plication without mobilisation of NVB can be done by 16-dot repair with peri-dorsal vein sutures (Fig. 6.3).[8–10]

15. What is the role of circumcision?

Ans:

- A circumcision is indicated in patients with associated phimosis, grossly redundant prepuce or history of previous penile surgery.[1,2] It is performed routinely by some surgeons to avoid postoperative wound edema and wound related complications. This should be discussed with the patient preoperatively.

16. What are the incisions known to be chosen for Peyronie's disease repairs?

Ans:

- Circum-coronal:
  - More commonly applied is the circum-coronal (circumcision) with degloving incision to be able to reach most of the plaques and allowing on table pre-operative and post-operative assessment of correction
- Ventral raphe
- Dorsal penile inversion
- Peno-scrotal

17. What are the management options for severe curvature?

Ans:

- The main aim in surgical correction of severe curvature > 60° and hinge deformity is to minimise loss of penile length
- This can be achieved by incision and grafting (Lue procedure) of plaque.[18–21]

18. What are the salient features of plaque incision and grafting?

Ans:

- Plaque incision and graft placement lengthen the affected side.
- Various grafts are available in India, the most common is the Biocor (Bovine pericardium) graft and others are saphenous vein patch and pelvicol (porcine dermal collagen). Newer grafts include tachosil (collagen fleece).
- Success rates are 75–96%.
- Complications include ED (0–25%), penile shortening (0–20%), bleeding, infection, residual deformity and penile numbness.[18–23]

19. What are the postoperative complications of plication for penile curvature?[1,24,25]

TABLE: 6.1: Postoperative complications after plication

Complication	*Incidence (%)*
Objective shortening	18–41
Subjective shortening	50–75
Shortening affecting intercourse	5–11.9
Recurrence of curvature requiring reoperation	0–20
Worsening of ED	0–6
Palpable knots	50–100
Knots interfering with coitus	0–10
Glans and penile hypoesthesia due to neuropraxia/neurovascular injury; more common in diabetic	6–75

20. Explain the preoperative counselling and expectant management before surgical correction of penile curvatures.

Ans:

- Psychological evaluation of the patient and also assessment of patient expectations is also essential before going ahead with the treatment.
- Patient should be clearly explained about the details of surgery, its complications, loss of penile length and chance of residual deformity.[26,27]

21. What are the penile rehabilitation aspects in post-Peyronie's disease repair?

Ans: Layers of integuments have a propensity to tighten, fibrose in the recovery periods over next few months, post-repair techniques giving a subjective penile shortening. Penile rehabilitation techniques starting at 3–4 weeks and continued into healthy sexual possibles are:

1. Penile stretching devices
2. Vacuum erection devices (VED)
3. Low dose sildenafil/tadalafil

22. How to manage erectile dysfunction in this patient?

Ans:

- Mild ED can be managed with PDE-5 inhibitors or intra-cavernosal injections
- Penile prosthesis is kept for men with moderate and severe ED not responding to PDE-5 inhibitors
- Residual curvature after penile prosthesis can be managed with manual modelling and if this fails then plaque incision + grafting is the treatment of choice.[2,6,7]

KEY POINTS

- Peyronie disease can lead to pain, curvature or erectile dysfunction
- Treatment is based on symptoms, quality of erections and progression of disease
- Surgical treatment should be planned after adequate counselling and the patient has understood the treatment
- The common operations for curvature are plication and incision and grafting, when the erectile function is preserved.
- Surgical treatment is done after plaque has stabilised.

SUMMARY

- The most essential part of pathogenesis is that it has two phases: An active phase and a quiescent or stable phase.
- Take a full medical and sexual history including history about patient's erectile function, as 40% of patients have concomitant erectile dysfunction. Psychological evaluation of the patient and also assessment of patient expectations is also essential before going ahead with the treatment.
- The clinical examination includes location, size and number of plaques, stretched penile length, outpatient office sildenafil test

or intra-cavernosal injections can be used to assess the degree of curvature and also associated erectile dysfunction.

- Treatment is based on the degree of erectile dysfunction; The decision for upfront penile prosthesis is based on the severity of ED. In men with good erections, plication procedures (<60° curvature) and plaque incision and grafting (>60° curvature) can be done.

REFERENCES

1. Mobley EM, Fuchs ME, Myers JB, Brant WO. Update on plication procedures for Peyronie's disease and other penile deformities. Ther Adv Urol. 2012 Dec;4(6):335–46.
2. David Ralph, MD, Nestor Gonzalez-Cadavid, PhD, Vincenzo Mirone, MD, Sava Perovic, MD, Michael Sohn, MD, Mustafa Usta, MD, Laurence Levine, MD, The Management of Peyronie's Disease: Evidence-based 2010 Guidelines, *The Journal of Sexual Medicine*, Volume 7, Issue 7, July 2010, Pages 2359–2374.
3. Akin-Olugbade Y, Mulhall J.P. (2007) The medical management of Peyronie's disease. *Nat Clin Pract Urol* 4: 95–103.
4. Andrews HO, Al-Akraa M., Pryor J.P., Ralph D.J. (2001) The Nesbit operation for Peyronie's disease: an analysis of the failures. *Br J Urol Int* 87: 658–660.
5. Bacal V, Rumhor J, Sturm R, Lipshutz LI, Schumacher M, Grober E.D. (2009) Correlation of degree of penile curvature between patient estimates and objective measures among men with Peyronie's disease. *J Sex Med* 6: 862–865.
6. El Sakka AI. Prevalence of Peyronie's disease among patients with erectile dysfunction. *Eur Urol* 2006;49:564–569.
7. Rahman NU, Carrion RE, Bochinski D, Lue TF. Combined penile plication surgery and insertion of penile prosthesis for severe penile curvature and erectile dysfunction. *J Urol* 2004; 171: 2346–2349.
8. Essed E., Schröder FH. New surgical treatment for Peyronie disease. *Urology* 1985;25:582–587.
9. Geertsen UA, Brok KE, Andersen B, Nielsen HV. Peyronie curvature treated by plication of the penile fasciae. *Br J Urol* 1996;77:733–735.
10. Gholami SS, Lue TF. Correction of penile curvature using the 16-dot plication technique: a review of 13 patients. *J Urol* 2002; 167: 2066–2069.
11. Greenfield JM, Lucas S, Levine LA. Factors affecting the loss of length associated with tunica albuginea plication for correction of penile curvature. *J Urol* 2006;175:238–241.
12. Hseih JT, Liu SP, Chen Y, Chang HC, Yu HJ, Chen CH. Correction of congenital penile curvature using modified tunical plication with absorbable sutures: the long-term outcome and patient satisfaction. *Eur Urol* 2007;52:261–266.
13. Kadioglu A, Küçükdurmaz F, Sanli O. Current status of the surgical management of Peyronie's disease. Nat Rev Urol 2001;8:95–106.
14. Kadioglu A, Oktar T, Kandirali E, Kendirci M, Sanli O, Ozsoy C. Incidentally diagnosed Peyronie's disease in men presenting with erectile dysfunction. *Int J Impot Res* 2004;16: 540–543.
15. Baskin LS, Duckett JW. Dorsal tunica albuginea plication for hypospadias curvature. *J Urol* 1994;151:1668–1671.
16. Baskin LS, Lue TF. The correction of congenital penile curvature in young men. *Br J Urol* 1998;81:895–899.
17. Brant WO, Mobley EM, Taylor MB, Myers JB. Emergent repair of congenital penile curvature for unconsummated marriage. *J Sex Med* 2011;9:34.
18. Langston JP, Carson CC. Peyronie's disease: plication or grafting. *Urol Clin North Am* 2011;38:207–216.
19. Perovic SV, Djinovic RP. Current surgical management of severe Peyronie's disease. *Arch Esp Urol* 2010;63:755–770.
20. Taylor FL, Levine LA. Surgical correction of Peyronie's disease via tunica albuginea plication or partial plaque excision with pericardial graft: long-term follow up. *J Sex Med* 2008;5: 2221–2228.
21. Pryor JP, Fitzpatrick JM. A new approach to the correction of penile deformity in Peyronie's disease. *J Urol* 1979;122: 622–623.
22. Tornehl CK, Carson CC. Surgical alternatives for treating Peyronie's disease. *Br J Urol Int* 2004;94:774–783.
23. Taylor FL, Levine LA. Surgical correction of Peyronie's disease via tunica albuginea plication or partial plaque excision with pericardial graft: long-term follow up. *J Sex Med* 2008;5: 2221–2228.
24. Leonardo C, De Nunzio C, Michetti P, Tartaglia N, Tubaro A, De Dominicis C, *et al.* Plication corporoplasty versus Nesbit operation for the correction of congenital penile curvature. A long-ter follow-up. *Int Urol Nephrol* 2012;44:55–60.
25. Syed AH, Abbasi Z, Hargreave TB. Nesbit procedure for disabling Peyronie's curvature: a median follow-up of 84 months. *Urology* 2003;60:999–1003.
26. Tal R, Nabulsi O, Nelson CJ, Mulhall JP. The psychosocial impact of penile reconstructive surgery for congenital penile deviation. *J Sex Med* 2010;7:121–128.
27. Van Der Horst C, Martinez Portillo FJ, Seif C, Alken P, Juenemann KP. Treatment of penile curvature with Essed-Schröder tunical plication: aspects of quality of life from the patients' perspective. *Br J Urol Int* 2004;93:105–108.

Chapter

7

Retrograde Ejaculation

• *Debabrat Kumar Sabat*

LEARNING OBJECTIVES

- Diagnosis should be considered in patients with low volume ejaculate.
- The presence of other comorbidities needs to be considered and adequately treated.
- Retrograde ejaculation is potentially a correctable aetiology of infertility.

INTRODUCTION

Retrograde ejaculation (RE) is defined as complete or partial absence of semen expulsion. As semen passes backward into the bladder, semen volume is low. The orgasm may be normal or reduced. Presence of 10–15 sperms (>1 million sperms in sample) in each high-power field of centrifuged post-orgasmic urine clinches the diagnosis of retrograde ejaculation.[1,2]

Case Scenario

A 27-year-old male who is a known case of type 1 DM with diabetic nephropathy has ED and reduced ejaculate volume. He is married for 3 years and expresses his desire to conceive with his wife in the near future.

1. **What is the diagnosis?**

   Ans: The most likely diagnosis is retrograde ejaculation (RE) because of low ejaculate volume, type 1 diabetes mellitus with neuropathy. The other differentials could be erectile dysfunction, an anatomic or functional obstruction in the ejaculatory passage or seminal vesicle hypoplasia. Another close differential is orgasmic anejaculation and this depends on the amount of semen ejaculated during coitus or masturbation. Anejaculation has been separately discussed in another chapter. This topic focusses on RE.

2. **What are the causes of reduced ejaculate volume?**

   Ans:
   - Improper sample collection
   - Spillage
   - Inappropriate surroundings
   - Erectile dysfunction
   - Retrograde ejaculation (RE)
   - Reduced semen production

3. **What should one understand about the physiology of ejaculation with respect to RE?**

   Ans: Ejaculation comprises two phases: Emission and expulsion.

   Emission

   Emission is controlled by sympathetic nervous system (T10-L2). Emission involves closure of bladder neck, followed by deposition of secretions from seminal vesicle, prostatic, vas deferens, and Cowper's glands into the prostatic urethra.[5]

   Expulsion

   Expulsion is due to coordinated rhythmic contraction of bladder neck, external urethral sphincter, urethra, bulbospongiosus muscle and pelvic striated muscles to propel the semen through the urethra and out the meatus.

   This reflex arc includes sensory input through perineal branch of the pudendal nerve which synapse on the pudendal motor neurons in the nucleus of Onuf and to spinal interneurons communicating with the thoracolumbar spinal cord (T10-L2) to trigger emission. Efferents travel via the perineal nerve to bulbospongiosus muscle leading to ejaculation.[6]

   RE occurs due to disruption of the reflex arc that affects bladder neck contraction.

4. **What are the points on history?**

Ans: The evaluation is aimed at differentiating this ejaculatory dysfunction from erectile dysfunction or concurrent presence of both conditions. Men with RE have reduced ejaculate volume or dry orgasm. They may give history of passing cloudy urine, which gives idea of mixing of semen and urine.[2]

The following important questions as given in Table 7.1 help in differentiating organic from functional causes of ejaculatory dysfunction.

TABLE 7.1: Important questions for differentiating organic and functional causes
When did you first masturbate? When did you ejaculate for the first time?
Do you get nocturnal emissions?
How long does it take to ejaculate?
Do you have an orgasm at ejaculation?
Which is impossible? Ejaculations during masturbation or intravaginal ejaculation or both?
How about the volume and color of semen?
Is the urine cloudy immediately after ejaculation?
Is the erection sufficient?
Any history of surgery? (Especially pelvic, retroperitoneal, and nervous system surgery)
Are you on any regular medications? (Especially alpha receptor antagonists, psychotropic drugs such as SSRI, etc.)

5. **What are the points to be focused on examination?**

Ans: This aims to identify the cause. Examine the genitalia for obvious abnormalities like phimosis, meatal stenosis, testicular volume, vas deferens and epididymis. A rectal exam to look for prostate issues and a focused neurologic exam are important to complete.

6. **How is the diagnosis of RE established?**

Ans: Semen analysis: A low volume ejaculate (<1.5 ml) termed hypospermia in the appropriate clinical situation as in our case, should indicate the possibility of RE.[3,4]

Post–orgasmic urine examination: In case of low volume ejaculate or drops of semen being submitted for examination, request the patient to collect post-orgasmic (or termed post-ejaculatory urine) for sperms. Visualization of 10–15 sperms per high-power field.[1] The presence of fructose in urine also indicates the presence of semen in urine.[18]

7. **Why does RE happen in diabetic men?**

Ans: It has been reported that up to 32% of diabetic men could have RE.[7] The mechanism of RE in diabetic men is impaired bladder neck contraction due to autonomic neuropathy damaging sympathetic output.

RE is an etiology for 0.3–2% of male infertility cases.[17]

8. **What are the treatment goals in RE?**

Ans: Several methods exist to retrieve sperm from urine for infertility treatment.

- Improving antegrade ejaculation rates and try for natural conception.
- Sperm collection for performing assisted reproductive techniques.

9. **What is the medical management of RE?**

Ans: Sympathomimetic drugs facilitate bladder neck contraction during the expulsion, which could be effective in up to 28% patients.[8]

Antimuscarinics, including brompheniramine maleate and imipramine, can be used along with sympathomimetics (Efficacy: Antimuscarinics 22%; Antimuscarinics + sympathomimetics 39%) (Table 7.2).[8]

10. **What is the surgical treatment for RE?**

Ans: It is a specific situation where the bladder neck is anatomically incompetent. Bladder neck reconstruction can be done by:

- V-Y plasty (Abrahams).[11]
- Bladder neck (Young Dees) reconstruction (Middleton and Urry).[12]
- Collagen injection into the bladder neck.[13]

11. **What are the methods of sperm retrieval in RE?**

Ans: Electroejaculation, penile vibratory stimulation or surgical sperm retrieval.

TABLE 7.2: Common pharmacologic treatments for retrograde ejaculation[9]

Medication	*Class*	*Dose/frequency*	*Efficacy (%)*	*Side effects*
Pseudoephedrine	Alpha agonist	60 mg QID or 120 mg BD	30	Hypertension, abdominal pain, nausea/ vomiting
Brompheniramine	Anti-histamine	16–24 mg daily	38	Anticholinergic side effects
Imipramine	Tricyclic antidepressant	25 mg twice daily	65	Anticholinergic side effects including cardiac dysrhythmias
Ephedrine	Indirect adrenergic agonist	50–100 mg per day	20	Tachycardia, hypertension, nausea, headache

Centrifugation and resuspension: Since acidic pH leads to loss of sperm motility, increased fluid intake with alkalinization (sodium bicarbonate or acetazolamide or potassium citrate) can help. Sperm wash medium is instilled into bladder and post-orgasmic urine is collected by voiding or catheter.[19] This sample is centrifuged and processed. It can be used for assisted reproduction with around 15% success rates based on sperm quality.[8]

Hotchkiss method: Bladder is emptied using a catheter and Ringer's lactate is instilled, similar to sperm wash medium as mentioned above.[10] The pregnancy rates reported are up to 24% per cycle.[8]

Ejaculation on a full bladder: Rarely used; sample is collected after ejaculating on full bladder; this semen is suspended in Baker's buffer.[8,14,15]

Electroejaculation (EEJ): Retrograde and antegrade ejaculate are collected, following instillation of Earle's medium into the bladder after catheterization. EEJ is performed under anesthesia with a rectal probe. This sample can be used for IVF or ICSI, with a maximum success rate of up to 50%.[16]

Penile vibrostimulation (PVS): PVS is more often used in anejaculation. Here, a penile vibrator is placed in the peri frenular region of the glans penis for at least 30 minutes in single or multiple sessions, until antegrade ejaculation occurs. It is an office-based procedure and is usually well tolerated. It is usually safe. PVS can be dangerous in specific situations of SCI above T6 level, with risk for autonomic dysreflexia.[20] These men should have an intact reflex arc. It has been reported to up to 88% successful in spinal cord lesions above T10 and as low as 15% in men with lesions above T10 level.[21,22]

Surgical sperm retrieval: The semen quality in men with SCI is usually poor. Surgical sperm retrieval in the form of needle testicular sperm aspiration or epididymal sperm aspiration provide better quality sperms and ICSI has a better success.

KEY POINTS

- Diagnosis of retrograde ejaculation is based on history and testing a post-ejaculation urine sample for sperms.
- The management includes treatment of the primary problem such as diabetes mellitus, erectile dysfunction and hormonal imbalance, if any.
- A careful detailed history and counseling helps the patient and the urologist understand the plan of treatment.
- Clinical examination, hormonal evaluation and semen analysis can guide in the appropriate management of infertility. This helps to decide between sperms retrieved from urinary bladder and IUI or testicular sperm aspiration and ICSI.

REFERENCES

1. McMahon CG. Disorders of Male Orgasm and Ejaculation. In: Wein AJ, Kavoussi LR, Partin AW, *et al*. eds. Campbell-Walsh Urology. Philadelphia: Elsevier, 2016;692–708. [Google Scholar].
2. Fedder J, Kaspersen MD, Brandslund I, *et al*. Retrograde ejaculation and sexual dysfunction in men with diabetes mellitus: a prospective, controlled study. *Andrology* 2013;1:602–6. 10.1111/j.2047–2927.2013.00083.x [PubMed] [CrossRef] [Google Scholar].
3. Cooper TG, Noonan E, von Eckardstein S, *et al*. World Health Organization reference values for human semen characteristics. *Hum Reprod Update* 2010;16:231–45. 10.1093/humupd/dmp048 [PubMed] [CrossRef] [Google Scholar].
4. Robin G, Marcelli F, Mitchell V, *et al*. Why and how to assess hypospermia? *Gynecol Obstet Fertil* 2008;36:1035–42. 10.1016/j.gyobfe.2008.04.021 [PubMed] [CrossRef] [Google Scholar].
5. Revenig L, Leung A, Hasio W. Ejaculatory physiology and pathophysiology: assessment and treatment in male infertility. Transl Androl Urol. 2014 Mar; 3(1): 41–49.
6. Wieder JA, Brackett NL, Lynne CM, *et al*. Anesthetic block of the dorsal penile nerve inhibits vibratory-induced ejaculation in men with spinal cord injuries. *Urology* 2000;55:915–7. [PubMed] [Google Scholar].
7. Dunsmuir WD, Holmes SA. The etiology and management of erectile, ejaculatory, and fertility problems in men with diabetes mellitus. *Diabet Med* 1996;13:700–8. [PubMed] [Google Scholar].
8. Jefferys A, Siassakos D, Wardle P. The management of retrograde ejaculation: a systematic review and update. *Fertil Steril* 2012;97:306–12. [PubMed] [Google Scholar].
9. Kamischke A, Nieschlag E. Update on medical treatment of ejaculatory disorders. *Int J Androl* 2002;25:333–44. [PubMed] [Google Scholar].
10. Hotchkiss RS, Pinto AB, Kleegman S. Artificial insemination with semen recovered from the bladder. *Fertil Steril* 1954;6:37–42. 10.1016/S0015–0282(16)31863–5 [PubMed] [CrossRef] [Google Scholar].
11. Abrahams JI, Solish GI, Boorjian P, *et al*. The surgical correction of retrograde ejaculation. *J Urol* 1975;114:888–90. [PubMed] [Google Scholar].
12. Middleton RG, Urry RL. The Young-Dees operation for the correction of retrograde ejaculation. *J Urol* 1986;136:1208–9. [PubMed] [Google Scholar].
13. Reynolds JC, McCall A, Kim ED, *et al*. Bladder neck collagen injection restores antegrade ejaculation after bladder neck surgery. *J Urol.* 1998;159:1303. 10.1016/S0022–5347(01)63592–4 [PubMed] [CrossRef] [Google Scholar].
14. Templeton A, Mortimer D. Successful circumvention of retrograde ejaculation in an infertile diabetic man. Case report. *Br J Obstet Gynaecol* 1982;89:1064–5. 10.1111/j.1471–0528.1982.tb04668.x [PubMed] [CrossRef] [Google Scholar].
15. Crich JP, Jequier AM. Infertility in men with retrograde ejaculation: the action of urine on sperm motility, and a simple method for achieving antegrade ejaculation. *Fertil Steril* 1978;30:572–6. 10.1016/S0015–0282(16)43640-X [PubMed] [CrossRef] [Google Scholar].
16. Jefferys A, Dimitrios S, Wardle P. The management of retrograde ejaculation: a systematic review and update. Department of Women's Health, Southmead Hospital, Bristol, United Kingdom.vol.97 no. 2/february 2012.

17. Yavetz H, Yogev L, Hauser R, Lessing JB, Paz G, Homonnai ZT. Retrograde ejaculation. *Hum Reprod.* 1994;9:381–386. [PubMed] [Google Scholar].
18. Cruz N, Porst H. In: *The ESSM syllabus of sexual medicine.* Porst H, Reisman Y, editors. Amsterdam: Medix Publishers BV; 2012. Ejaculatory and orgasmic disorders other than premature ejaculation; pp. 737–790.
19. Mehta A, Sigman M. Management of the dry ejaculate: a systematic review of aspermia and retrograde ejaculation. *Fertil Steril.* 2015;104:1074–1081.
20. Ohl DA, Quallich SA, Sønksen J, Brackett NL, Lynne CM. Anejaculation and retrograde ejaculation. Urol Clin North Am 2008; 35: 211–20.
21. Brown R, Stolzenhein G, Engel S, Macefield VG. Cutaneous vasoconstriction as a measure of incipient autonomic dysreflexia during penile vibratory stimulation in spinal cord injury. Spinal Cord 2009; 47: 538–44.
22. Kafetsoulis A, Brackett NL, Ibrahim E, Attia GR, Lynne CM. Current trends in the treatment of infertility in men with spinal cord injury. Fert Steril 2006; 86: 781–9.

Chapter

8

Penile Fracture

• *Ashish Sabharwal* • *Shivakumar V*

LEARNING OBJECTIVES

- Identification and diagnosis of penile fracture.
- Treatment of penile fracture.
- Long-term prognosis of penile fracture in terms of erectile function.

INTRODUCTION

Penile fracture is a rare but serious urological emergency that occurs when the erect penis is forcefully bent or twisted, resulting in a tear in the tunica albuginea, the tough fibrous covering of the cavernous tissue. Despite the name, there is no actual bone in the penis, so the term " penile fracture" is misnomer.[1,2]

However, the injury can cause severe pain, swelling, and deformity of the penis in the acute phase and difficulty in achieving or maintaining an erection if left untreated as the corporal integrity is compromised. If left untreated, it can also lead to penile curvature.

Penile fractures are relatively rare, with an estimated incidence of 1 in 175,000 men per year in the United States. However, the actual incidence may be higher due to underreporting and misdiagnosis.

Penile fractures most commonly occur during sexual intercourse, particularly when there is vigorous or rough thrusting, or when the penis slips out and hits the perineum, pubic bone, or partner's body. Other causes of penile fracture include masturbation, penile trauma, falls, sports injuries, and penile manipulation during medical procedures.

Case Scenario

A 32-year-old male married to a 22-year-old female, experienced a cracking sound while having intercourse in the women on top position, after which the penis detumesced suddenly and then he presented to the emergency room with pain and swelling over the penis. He did not complain of hematuria.

1. **What is the outline of management?**

   Ans: This patient's presentation is highly suspicious of penile fracture with low suspicion of urethral injury as he does not complain of hematuria.

   Patient might require emergency exploration to repair the injury to the tunica albuginea. Sometimes a similar presentation can be without a penile fracture due to rupture of the superficial penile veins.

2. **What are the investigations to confirm the diagnosis?**

   Ans: Investigations to confirm our diagnosis would include an ultrasound of the penis, which will confirm the presence of a defect in the tunica and its size. It will also provide us with the information whether the defect is proximal, midshaft or distal and will help in lateralising the injury. In the hands of an experienced ultrasonologist, ultrasound is very sensitive in picking up defects although small defects may be missed. MRI if available is another non-invasive and accurate method to establish the diagnosis. These investigations provide confirmation of diagnosis for medicolegal purposes and also help in selecting the approach. Final decision depends on clinical correlation of signs and imaging findings.

3. **How to proceed with treatment?**

Ans: Once the fracture is confirmed, then the patient is counselled and taken up for emergency surgical exploration to repair the defect in the tunica albuginea.

4. **What factors increase the chances of penile fracture?**

Ans: Some factors that may increase the chances of penile fracture include:

1. Intense or vigorous sexual activity: Penile fracture is more likely to occur during rough or aggressive sexual activity, particularly when there is a lot of force or pressure on the penis. The penis slips out of vagina and strikes the pubic bone or perineum.[3]
2. During the practice known as 'taghaandan,' in which the erect penis is pushed down to achieve detumescence, resulting in a click.[4]
3. Incorrect positioning: Certain sexual positions, such as the woman on top or doggy style, may increase the risk of penile fracture due to the angle and positioning of the penis.
4. Penile curvature: the penis may be more susceptible to trauma during sexual activity due to buckling of penis during intercourse.

5. **What are the typical symptoms of penile fracture?**

Ans:

1. A popping sound or sensation: A penile fracture often occurs during sexual intercourse or masturbation when the penis is forcefully bent or twisted. This can cause a popping sound or sensation, followed by pain, rapid detumescence of penis and discoloration and swelling.
2. Swelling: The penis may become swollen and discoloured due to bleeding and bruising. If the bucks fascia is intact swelling is limited to skin and tunica, resulting in eggplant deformity. If Buck's fascia is disrupted, the hematoma may extend into the scrotum, perineum and suprapubic regions.
3. Blood in urine or difficulty urinating: Penile fracture can cause damage to the urethra, making it difficult or painful to urinate.[5]

6. **How to examine this patient and what are the physical findings to elicit?**

Ans: Physical examination: The doctor will examine the penis, looking for signs of swelling, bruising, and deformity. They will also check for any signs of bleeding or discharge from the urethra. The doctor may gently squeeze the penis to check for any areas of tenderness or pain.

A palpable tunical defect and hematoma with a 'rolling sign' are usually considered pathognomonic features for this condition.[6]

7. **What is the role of imaging in the diagnosis of penile fracture?**

Ans: Ultrasound is the most commonly used imaging modality for the evaluation of penile fractures in the emergency department.[7] It is non-invasive, readily available, and provides excellent visualization of the penis. Ultrasound can detect the presence of a hematoma or disruption of the tunica albuginea, which is the fibrous tissue surrounding the corpora cavernosa, and is the site of injury in penile fractures.

In some cases, magnetic resonance imaging (MRI)[8] may be used to evaluate penile fractures, particularly in cases where the diagnosis is unclear or the extent of the injury is not clear on ultrasound. MRI can provide more detailed information about the extent of the injury, including involvement of the urethra or other surrounding structures. However, MRI is not as readily available as ultrasound and may not be the first choice for imaging in the emergency department.

In summary, ultrasound is the most commonly used imaging modality for the evaluation of penile fractures in the emergency department. MRI may be used in some cases where the diagnosis is unclear or the extent of the injury is not clear on ultrasound. Prompt diagnosis and treatment of penile fractures are crucial to ensure optimal outcomes for patients.

8. **What is the protocol for conservative management of penile fracture?**

Ans: This involves non-surgical treatment with bed rest, pressure dressings, catheterization, and ice packs for 24–48 hours in addition to antibiotics, fibrinolysis, oestrogens and diazepam for suppressing erection.[9,10]

9. **When to consider conservative management of penile fracture?**

Ans:

1. Small or partial tears of the tunica albuginea.
2. No evidence of urethral injury.
3. No significant penile deviation or curvature and pain
4. Stable and small hematoma.

10. **What is the prognosis of conservative management?**

Ans: Prognosis of conservative management of penile fracture is good if the above criteria are met, and there is no associated urethral injury or significant penile deviation.

11. What is the course of men undergoing conservative treatment?

Ans: Most patients will experience resolution of symptoms within 4–6 weeks of conservative management, with no long-term sequel. However, ten to thirty percent of patients receiving such conservative management developed impaired erections, permanent deformity, or suboptimal coitus.[11] Therefore, it is important to monitor patients closely during conservative management and consider surgical intervention if symptoms persist or worsen.

12. What approaches can be used for surgical management of penile fracture?

Ans:

1. Circumcoronal repair: In this approach, an incision is made in the circumcoronal skin of the penis 1 cm below the glans, penis is degloved and the tunica albuginia is exposed. The torn or ruptured tissue is then repaired with absorbable sutures. This distal circumcising (degloving) incision is appropriate in most cases, as advocated by Zargooshi,[4] Miller and McAninch.[12]
2. Limited dorsal slit: This approach involves making a small incision in the skin of the penis along the top or side to expose the tunica albuginea. The torn tissue is repaired with sutures and the incision is closed with sutures. This approach is less invasive and may be used for less severe injuries like localized haematomas or palpable tunical defects.[5]
3. Penoscrotal approach: In this approach, an incision is made in the skin between the penis and scrotum to access the tunica albuginea. The torn tissue is repaired with absorbable sutures, and the incision is closed with sutures. This approach provides good access to the injury site and is often used for more complex injuries.[13]
4. Artificial erection-assisted repair: In this approach, an artificial erection is induced using medication (intracavernosal papaverine or alprostadil) to identify the location of the injury. The torn tissue is then repaired with sutures and the erection is allowed to subside before the incision is closed with sutures. This approach may be used for injuries that are difficult to identify or repair.[14]

The choice of approach depends on the extent and location of the injury, as well as the surgeon's experience and preference. It is important to seek prompt medical attention for penile fracture to prevent long-term complications.

13. What are the steps of repair of penile fracture, especially in the emergency situation?

Ans: The repair procedure typically involves the following steps:

1. Anesthesia: The patient is given general or regional anesthesia to ensure pain-free surgery.
2. Exposure: The penile shaft is exposed by making a circumcoronal degloving incision in the skin.
3. Hemostasis: The bleeding vessels are identified and cauterized to achieve hemostasis.
4. Exploration: The Buck's fascia is opened and the underlying tunica albuginea are explored to identify the site and extent of the fracture. Most common sites of fracture are ventral or ventrolateral aspect, over the right corpora and the proximal 3rd of the shaft.
5. Repair: The ruptured tunica albuginea is repaired with absorbable sutures in an interrupted pattern. The suture material used for penile fracture repair is typically absorbable. Commonly used suture materials include 2–0 polyglactin (e.g. Vicryl) and polyglycolic acid (e.g. Dexon).
6. Closure: The skin is closed with 3-0 monocryl.

14. Can a circumcision be done at the time of repair of penile fracture?

Ans: Yes, we should do circumcision and penile fracture repair at the same time specially when the approach is circumcoronal. Because if we do not do circumcision at the same time, there is high incidence of foreskin oedema and at risk for ischemia in the immediate post-operative period, because wide mobilization of the foreskin.[15]

Usually a limited circumcision at the conclusion of the repair procedure is enough.

15. How does one counsel a patient regrading follow-up and recovery of erections post-penile fracture repair?

Ans: Postoperative counselling and management of erections after penile fracture are critical components of the patient's recovery process.[16]

Patients should follow the surgeon's recommendations carefully and attend all follow-up appointments to ensure proper healing and minimize the risk of complications.

16. What are the postoperative recommendations?

Ans:

- Sexual abstinence: The patient should avoid sexual activity for at least six to eight weeks after surgery to allow for proper healing of the penile tissue.

- Elevation of the penis: Keeping the penis elevated for the first few days after surgery can help reduce swelling and pain.
- Pain management: Pain management is crucial after penile fracture repair surgery. The surgeon may prescribe pain medication or recommend over-the-counter pain relief medication.
- Management of erections: Erections may occur naturally or through sexual stimulation during the postoperative period. However, the patient must avoid any vigorous penile manipulation or sexual activity during this time. Erections may cause pain or damage to the surgical site, which can delay healing. Application of crepe bandage to the penis at night time keeps the penis stabilised during erections at night avoiding reinjury or twisting at night.

The surgeon may schedule follow-up appointments to monitor the patient's recovery and check for any signs of complications.

17. What additional treatment is done in these men during follow-up?

Ans: *Psychological counselling:* Penile fracture can be a traumatic experience for the patient and may cause psychological distress. Psychological counselling may help the patient cope with the emotional effects of the injury and recovery process.[16]

Sexual rehabilitation: Usually sexual activity can start without any problem. In some cases, patients may experience erectile dysfunction or difficulty achieving and maintaining an erection after surgery. So we recommend penile rehabilitation in these patients by prescribing tadalafil 5 mg daily for 3 months and the vacuum therapy system temporarily in the recovery period.[16]

18. What is the prognosis for erectile function post-repair after penile fracture?

Ans: The prognosis for erections post-repair after a penile fracture can vary depending on the severity of the injury and the success of the repair surgery. However, in general, studies have shown that most men who undergo timely and appropriate surgical repair for penile fracture can achieve satisfactory erections following the procedure.

Immediate surgical reconstruction results in faster recovery, decreased morbidity, lower complication rates, and a lower incidence of penile curvatures.

A retrospective analysis of conservative treatment showed an unacceptable rate of immediate and late complications, such as persisting hematoma, infections and abscesses, deformity of the penis, pulsatile diverticulum, fistula, ED and decrease in turgidity.[17]

It is important to note that complications such as erectile dysfunction and curvature of the penis (known as Peyronie's disease) can occur following penile fracture repair, specially if treatment is delayed. Regular follow-up can help to monitor for any potential issues and ensure optimal recovery.

19. How to manage a concomitant urethral injury?

Ans: The association of urethra rupture ranges from 1% to 38% in different literature. An associated urethral injury should be suspected if there is blood at meatus, microscopic, or gross hematuria, with or without voiding difficulty.[18] Diagnosis of penile fracture is mainly clinical, although there may be an absence of typical signs and symptoms. Associated urethral injuries may or may not present with haematuria and at times can pose a challenge to complete diagnosis. Therefore, an adequate history and good physical examination are cornerstones of the diagnosis of penile injury complex.

Management of concomitant urethral injury depends on the severity and extent of the injury, as well as the patient's overall health and any associated injuries. Here are some general guidelines:

1. **Initial evaluation:** The patient should undergo a thorough evaluation to determine the extent and severity of the urethral injury, as well as any associated injuries. This may include a physical exam, urethrogram, and urine tests.

   Retrograde urethrogram is helpful in confirming the presence of a urethral injury. However, urethrography may give false negative results and is not recommended in routine practice.[19,20] The cause for false negative urethrography is assumed to be the presence of overlying hematoma at the site of injury which masks the defect.
2. **Urinary diversion:** If the urethral injury is severe, a urinary catheter or suprapubic tube may be placed to divert urine away from the injured area.
3. **Surgical repair:** Depending on the extent of the injury, surgical repair of the urethra may be necessary. Partial urethral injury may be over sewn over catheter with 3–0 or 4–0 absorbable sutures. Complete urethral injuries: One must avoid contact between the severed corpus spongiosum and corporal tissue to obviate the risk of postoperative impotence as a consequence of spongio-cavernosal fistula. The repair should involve complete evacuation of the hematoma, debridement of the margins, watertight closure of the tunica and spongiosum separately and wrapping of

the urethral anastomotic site with a sub-dartos vascularised flap to prevent fistula formation in case of overlapping suture lines.[18]

4. **Antibiotics:** Patients with urethral injuries are at risk for developing urinary tract infections, so antibiotics should be prescribed for 2 weeks to prevent infection.
5. **Follow-up:** Patients should undergo regular follow-up exams to monitor their progress and ensure that the urethral injury has healed properly.

KEY POINTS

- Penile fracture is an andrological emergency and produces considerable anxiety.
- A careful clinical examination can clinch the diagnosis; additional imaging is required in doubtful cases.
- Exploration and repair is the treatment of choice for documented penile fracture.

SUMMARY

- Penile fracture is urological emergency.
- Diagnosis is established by typical history, physical examination, and a penile ultrasound in the emergency department.
- Treatment of choice is emergency surgical repair.
- Postoperative counselling and management of erections after penile fracture are critical components of the patient's recovery process.
- The association of urethra rupture ranges from 1 to 38%. A urethral injury should always be evaluated and treated concomitantly with penile fracture repair if it is present.

REFERENCES

1. Agarwal MM, Singh SK, Sharma DK, Ranjan P, Kumar S, Chandramohan V, *et al*. Fracture of the penis: a radiological or clinical diagnosis? A case series and literature review. Can J Urol. 2009; 16:4568–4575.
2. Malis J, Zur K. Der fractura penis. Arch Klin Chir. 1924; 129:651.
3. Galanakis I, Adamos K, Spyropoulos E, Mavrikos S (2018) Delayed successful surgical repair of penile fracture: a case report. Curr Urol 12:111–112.
4. Zargooshi J. Penile fracture in Kermanshah, Iran: report of 172 cases. J Urol. 2000; 164:364–366.
5. Jack GS, Garraway I, Reznichek R, Rajfer J. Current treatment options for penile fractures Rev Urol. 2004;6:114–20.
6. Walton JK. Fracture of the penis with laceration of the urethra. Br J Urol. 1979; 51:308–309.
7. Koga S, Saito Y, Arakaki Y, Nakamura N, Matsuoka M, Saita H, *et al*. Sonography in fracture of the penis. Br J Urol. 1993; 72:228–229.
8. Abolyosr A, Moneim AE, Abdelatif AM, Abdalla MA, Imam HM. The management of penile fracture based on clinical and magnetic resonance imaging findings. BJU Int. 2005; 96:373–377.
9. Farah RN, Stiles R, Jr., Cerny JC. Surgical treatment of deformity and coital difficulty in healed traumatic rupture of the corpora cavernosa. *Journal of Urology*. 1978;120(1):118–120.
10. Jallu A, Wani NA, Rashid PA. Fracture of the penis. *Journal of Urology*. 1980;123(2):285–286.
11. Ozen HA, Erkan I, Alkibay T, Kendi S, Remzi D. Fracture of the penis and long-term results of surgical treatment. *British Journal of Urology*. 1986;58(5):551–552.
12. Miller S, McAninch JW. Penile fracture and soft tissue injury. In: McAninch JW, editor. Traumatic and reconstructive urology. Philadelphia: W.B. Saunders;1996. p. 693–698.
13. Joshi BM, Ranjan SK, Jain M, Kumar A.Penile Fracture with Urethral Rupture: The Feasibility of Repair through Penoscrotal Approach. J Emerg Trauma Shock. 2022 Jul–Sep; 15(3): 149–151.
14. Basal S, Can U, Akan S. Artificial erection-assisted repair of penile fracture: long-term outcome and patient satisfaction. Int J Impot Res. 2017; 29(5): 208–212.
15. Morey AF, Dugi DD 3rd. Genital and lower urinary tract trauma. In: Wein AJ, Kavoussi LR, Partin AW, Novick AC, editors. Campbell-Walsh urology. 10th ed. Philadelphia: Elsevier-Saunders, Co.;2012. p. 2507. p. 2520.
16. A. Zaidi *et al*. Psychological distress and sexual dysfunction following penile fracture: A systematic review and meta-analysis" Sex Med Rev. 2021.
17. Thompson RF. Rupture of the penis. *J Urol*. 1954;71:226.
18. Amit A, Arun K, Bharat B, Navin R, Sameer T, Shankar DU. Penile fracture and associated urethral injury: Experience at a tertiary care hospital. *Can Urol Assoc J*. 2013;7:E168–70.
19. Jack GS, Garraway I, Reznichek R, *et al*. Current Treatment Options for Penile Fractures. *Rev Urol*. 2004;6:114–20.
20. Mydlo JH, Hayyeri M, Macchia RJ. Urethrography and cavernosography imaging in a small series of penile fractures: a comparison with surgical finding. *Urology*. 1998;51:616–9.

Chapter

9

Priapism

• *Vineet Malhotra* • *Nilanjan Mitra*

LEARNING OBJECTIVES

- Pathophysiology and types of priapism.
- Emergency management of priapism.
- Shunts and role of early prosthesis for priapism.

INTRODUCTION

Priapism is an andrological emergency and needs to be addressed at the earliest while ascertaining the cause. The prognosis is directly related to the time of initiating treatment from the time of diagnosis. Aspiration or slow continuous drainage with or without alpha adrenergic, if done in a timely manner can lead to detumescence and complete recovery. In case of prolonged erections shunt surgeries present a traditional solution with immediate prosthesis being studied recently to avoid difficult inevitable prosthesis surgeries later albeit at higher rate of complications.

Case Scenario

A 22 years old male presented in emergency room with prolonged erection since last 24 hours with pain in the penis. He had regular normal erections in the past, though he had never performed intercourse. He has no significant medical or surgical past history or history of injury. He tried to do masturbation 24 hours back and since then he is having this condition. On examination, general survey was normal, local examination showed rigid erected penis with dusky discoloration of the glans, which is soft.

1. **What is priapism?**

   Ans: Priapism is a disorder in which the penis maintains a full or partial erection that continues more than 4 hours beyond sexual stimulation and orgasm or is unrelated to sexual stimulation.

2. **How to classify priapism?**

   Ans:
   - Ischemic priapism (veno-occlusive, low-flow)
   - Stuttering priapism (intermittent, recurrent ischemic priapism)
   - Nonischemic priapism (arterial, high flow)

3. **What is the pathophysiology of ischemic priapism?**

   Ans: Ischemic priapism is a persistent erection marked by rigidity of the corpora cavernosa and a little or no cavernous arterial inflow. In ischemic priapism there are time-dependent changes in the corporal metabolic environment with progressive hypoxia, hypercarbia, and acidosis. The **patient typically reports penile pain after 6 to 8 hours,** and the examination reveals a rigid erection. The condition is analogous to a muscle compartment syndrome, with initial occlusion of venous outflow and subsequent cessation of arterial inflows. Well-documented histologic changes occur within the corporal smooth muscle as a consequence of prolonged ischemia. **Interventions beyond 36 hours of onset may help relieve erection and pain but have no benefit in preserving potency.**[1]

   Ischemic priapism is an emergency.[2] When left untreated, resolution may take days to weeks, and severe corporal fibrosis and erectile dysfunction (ED) invariably result.

4. **What is the pathophysiology of stuttering priapism?**

   Stuttering priapism is characterized by a pattern of recurrence. The term has historically described recurrent unwanted and painful erections in men with sickle cell disease (SCD), Any patient who has experienced an episode of ischemic priapism is also at risk for stuttering priapism.[3]

5. What is the pathophysiology of nonischemic priapism?

Ans: Nonischemic priapism is a persistent erection caused by unregulated cavernous arterial inflow. Typically, **the corpora are tumescent but not rigid and the penis is not painful**. A history of blunt trauma to the perineum or an iatrogenic needle injury is common. Whatever the mechanism of injury, the result is a disruption of the cavernous arterial anatomy creating an arteriolar-sinusoidal fistula. The cavernous environment does not become ischemic and cavernous blood gases do not show hypoxia, hypercarbia, or acidosis. This type of priapism, once properly diagnosed, does not require emergent intervention although delayed treatment may be necessary if it does not resolve on conservative management. Normal erectile function has been reported after recovery from the initial event. [4]

6. What are the causes of ischemic priapism?[5]

Ans:

1. Hematologic dyscrasias: Sickle cell disease, thalassemia, leukemia, multiple myeloma, fat embolism. Sickle cell hemoglobinopathy accounts for at least one-third of all cases of priapism. The lifetime probability of a man with SCD developing ischemic priapism ranges from 29% to 42%.
2. Drugs:
   a. Adrenergic receptor antagonists: Prazosin, terazosin, doxazosin, tamsulosin
   b. Attention-deficit/hyperactivity disorder agents: Methylphenidates, atomoxetine
   c. Recreational drugs: Alcohol, cocaine (intranasal and topical), crack cocaine, marijuana, synthetic cannabinoids
   d. Hormones: Gonadotropin-releasing hormone, testosterone
   e. Vasoactive erectile agents: Papaverine, phentolamine, prostaglandin E1, oral phosphodiesterase type 5 inhibitors, combination intracavernous therapy
3. Infectious (toxin-mediated) causes: Scorpion sting, spider bite, rabies, malaria
4. Metabolic conditions: Amyloidosis, Fabry disease, gout
5. Neoplastic causes (metastatic or regional infiltration): Prostate, urethra, testis, bladder, rectum, lung, kidney.
6. Neurogenic conditions: Syphilis, spinal cord injury, cauda equina compression, autonomic neuropathy.

7. SCD and Priapism: Why so prevalent?

Ans: Sickle cell hemoglobinopathy accounts for at least one-third of all cases of priapism. Mechanisms of SCD-associated priapism may involve derangements of several signalling pathways in the penis,[11] resulting in disinhibited vasorelaxation of the cavernous smooth muscle by NOS and Rho-associated protein kinase (ROCK) signalling, and increased oxidative stress associated with nicotinamide adenine dinucleotide phosphate (NADPH) oxidase-mediated signalling.[12]

Contrary to traditional belief, maintenance of physiological testosterone levels does not cause priapism, but rather preserves penile homeostasis and promotes normal erectile function. Testosterone deficiency is considered a controversial risk factor: It is prevalent in patients with SCD, but recent evidence indicates that it is not a risk factor *per se* for priapism.[13]

8. What history will you take from the patient?

Ans:

- Duration of erection
- Presence of pain
- Previous episodes of priapism and method of treatment
- Baseline erectile function
- Use of any erectogenic therapies (prescription and nutritional supplements)
- Medications and recreational drugs
- Sickle cell disease, hemoglobinopathies, hypercoagulable states
- Trauma to the pelvis, perineum, or penis

9. What will you look for in physical examination?

Ans: Inspection and palpation of the penis are recommended to determine the extent and degree of tumescence and rigidity; the involvement of the cavernous bodies; the presence of pain; and the evidence of trauma to the perineum.

In ischemic priapism the corporal bodies will be completely rigid; the glans penis and corpus spongiosum are not.

Examination of the abdomen, testicles, perineum, rectum, and prostate may help identify a primary cancer leading to priapism. Malignant infiltration of the penis causes indurated nodules within or replacing corporal tissue.

In nonischaemic priapism the corpora will be tumescent but not completely rigid. In children and adults with HFP, depending on the location of trauma and time since the traumatic event, there may be residual bruising at the perineum from straddle injury (Table 9.1).

10. What are the laboratory investigations to be done?

Ans: Complete blood count (CBC), platelet count, coagulation profile, hemoglobin electrophoresis, reticulocyte count, lactate dehydrogenase.

A **corporal blood gas analysis** by aspiration is recommended in the emergency evaluation of priapism. The corporal blood aspirate differentiates ischemic from nonischemic priapism. Aspiration may be diagnostic and therapeutic. Visual inspection of the color and consistency of an initial penile aspirate will reveal dark deoxygenated blood with a "crankcase oil" appearance in ischemic priapism. The initial corporal aspirate may be sent for blood gas testing to document pH, PO_2, and PCO_2 (Table 9.2).

Aspirated corporal blood gas in non-ischemic priapism: pH = 7.4 (or >7.2), pO_2 >90 mmHg, and pCO_2 <40 mmHg.

Penile Imaging

Colour Doppler USG of the penis and perineum is recommended as an adjunct to the corporal aspirate in differentiating ischemic from nonischaemic priapism. Patients with prolonged ischemic priapism will have no blood flow in the cavernous arteries; the return of the cavernous artery waveform will accompany successful detumescence. Patients with nonischemic priapism have normal to high blood flow velocities detectable in the cavernous arteries; an effort should be made to localize the characteristic blush of color emanating from the disrupted cavernous artery or arteriole.[14]

Examination of the entire penile shaft and perineum is recommended; this can be done with the patient supine but frog-legged.

Penile arteriography should be reserved for the management of HFP, when embolization is planned.[15]

Magnetic resonance imaging (MRI) or magnetic resonance angiography (MRA) can be used to evaluate for:[16]

i. Imaging of a well-established arteriolar-sinusoidal fistula
ii. To demonstrate the presence and extent of tissue thrombus and corporal smooth muscle infarction
iii. To detect corporal malignancy or metastasis
iv. To predict the viability of corpora tissue after prolonged or repeated episodes of priapism before going for prosthesis.

Differential diagnosis of priapism

D/D: "Sleep-related painful erections" is a rare condition that is somewhat similar to priapism. It is defined as frequent awakenings due to penile pain during REM sleep from nocturnal erections resulting in severe sleep disruptions. The duration of the erections is insufficient to qualify these episodes as priapism as they typically remain rigid for only 15 to 60 minutes. Daytime, normal sexual

TABLE 9.1: Key findings in priapism

Findings	*Ischemic priapism*	*Nonischemic priapism*
Perineal trauma	Seldom	Usually
Hematologic abnormalities	Usually	Seldom
Recent intracorporal injection	Sometimes	Sometimes
Corpora cavernosa fully rigid	Usually	Seldom
Penile pain	Usually	Seldom
Abnormal penile blood gas	Usually	Seldom
Cavernous inflow (on Doppler)	Seldom	Usually

Modified from Montague DK, Jarow J, Broderick GA, et al.: American Urological Association guideline on the management of priapism. J Urol 170:1318–1324, 2003.

TABLE 9.2: Typical blood gas values

Source	*pO_2 (mm Hg)*	*pCO_2 (mm Hg)*	*pH*
Normal arterial blood (room air)	>90	<40	7.40
Normal mixed venous blood (room air)	40	50	7.35
Ischemic priapism (first corporal aspirate)	<30	>60	<7.25

Modified from Montague DK, Jarow J, Broderick GA, et al.: American Urological Association guideline on the management of priapism. J Urol 170:1318–1324, 2003.

activities are completely unaffected. Testosterone levels and libido are also normal, and there is no evidence of hematological disorders, which are common in stuttering priapism. The cause is unknown, although hypertonicity of the pelvic floor muscles has been implicated, and physical therapy appears to be helpful in some cases. The most effective treatment is baclofen. Surgical interventions and penile prostheses are ineffective for relieving pain in this condition.

Differentiation between different types of priapism is given in Flowchart 9.1[27]

11. What is the medical management of Priapism?

Ans: The initial approach to ischemic priapism is to treat it as a true emergency.

Any priapism episode lasting >4 hours requires early intervention to decrease the likelihood of irreversible corporal damage and future erectile dysfunction.

PDE 5 inhibitor therapy has also been advocated by a few studies, where the epiosodes of stuttering priapism are redcued with this otherwise erectogenic agent.

Ketoconazole and Baclofen are other drugs advocated for the use. Ketoconazole 200 mg three times a day for 6–8 weeks has found to be beneficial in a few studies.[8–10]

Oral therapies such as **etilefrine, pseudoephedrine, metaraminol, phenylpropanolamine,** and **terbutaline** may be tried while awaiting for OT but has not shown sufficient efficacy with failure rates of 75%. Sustained activity increasing flow to lower limb and diverting blood from the penis can be occasionally successful.

12. What is the emergency management of priapism?

Ans: Aspiration and normal saline irrigation are recommended as the initial medical therapy under dorsal penile block. Aspiration is generally done using a large diameter needle, butterfly, or angiocath (19 gauge or larger) at either the 2 o'clock or 10 o'clock position on the penis near the base while milking the shaft. About 20 ml to 30 ml should be aspirated, and the color of the blood should be noted. This process leads to a marked decrease in the intracavernous pressure, relieves pain, and resuscitates the corporal environment, removing anoxic, acidotic, and hypercarbic blood. **Aspiration alone is only effective in about one-third of patients.** It must be combined with other treatments, such as irrigation with normal saline or diluted sympathomimetic agents, to achieve successful, prolonged detumescence. **Aspiration with cold normal saline irrigation** has been reported to successfully achieve detumescence in 66% of cases. The same needle can be used for blood gas determinations, aspiration, irrigation, and sympathomimetic drug instillation. While only one needle is required, some recommend two to facilitate the irrigation process. Typically, after several rounds of aspiration and normal saline irrigation, oxygenated blood with a bright red color is usually observed. This reoxygenation of the corpora greatly enhances the smooth muscle contractile response to sympathomimetic injections.[17]

Intracavernosal drug therapy is generally the next step in priapism treatment. Phenylephrine is the most recommended preferred first-line agent due to its efficacy and superior safety profile.[18] The recommended injectable diluted concentration is from 100 to 500 μg/ml. A 1 ml injection of the diluted phenylephrine solution should be injected every 3 to 5 minutes for up to about 1 hour or until full detumescence.[6]

The American Urological Association Guidelines on priapism recommends an intra-

Flowchart 9.1: Priapism

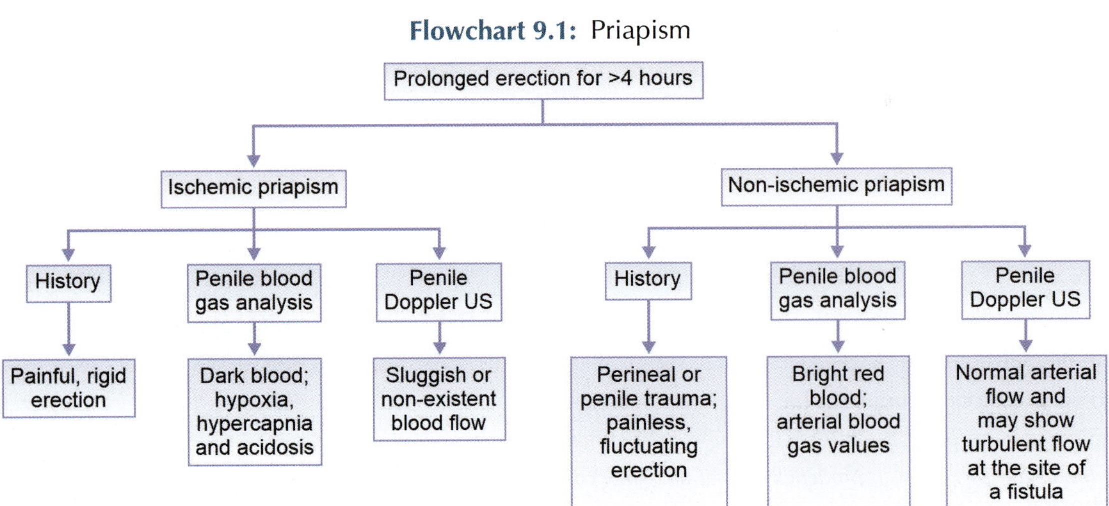

cavernosal injection of 0.5 to 1 ml of a diluted phenylephrine concentration of 100 to 500 µg/ml every 5 minutes for a total of up to 3 injections. Prepare a 10 ml syringe of normal saline with *200 µg/ml* of phenylephrine. **(Dilution formula is 1 ml of 10 mg phenylephrine diluted in 49 ml of normal saline)**. Inject 1 ml every 5 minutes and 5 injections has been found to be safe in most healthy individuals.[7] Pinch the penis at its base by thumb and index finger, inject distal to it, wait for 5 minutes before next dose and aspirate in between to take out the deoxygenated blood. Possible side effects include cardiac palpitations, dizziness, and headache. **The reported success rate of diluted phenylephrine injections alone is 58%, but this increases to 81% when combined with aspiration and irrigation.**[19]

Other potential sympathomimetic drugs for injection include etilephrine, ephedrine, norepinephrine, and epinephrine. All patients receiving intracorporal sympathomimetic agents should be monitored for arrhythmias and elevated blood pressure. If completed within 12 hours of priapism onset, some studies have reported a near 100% success in achieving detumescence with this therapy.

Flowchart 9.2: Algorithm for managing ischemic priapism

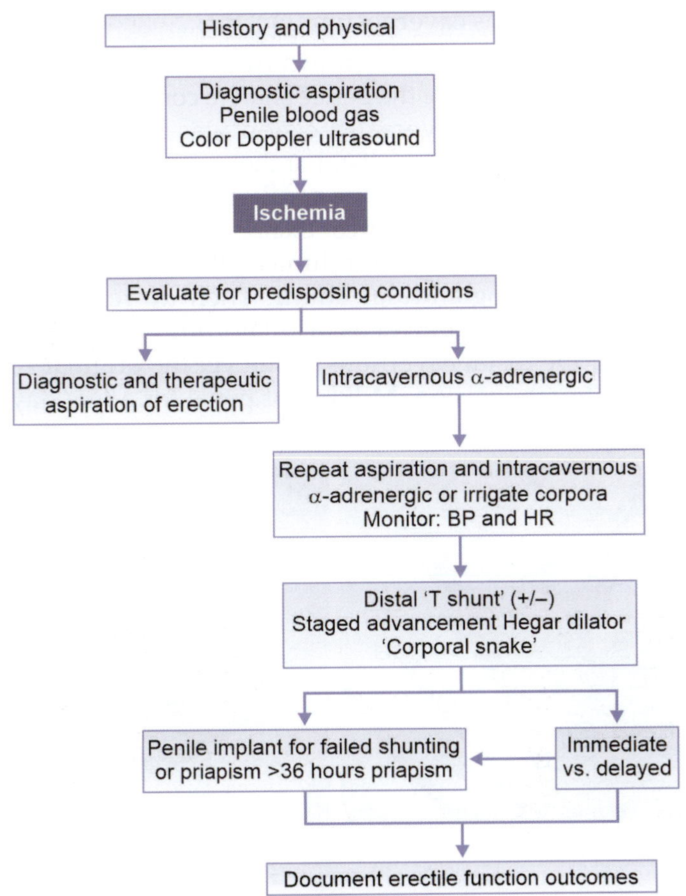

Flowchart 9.3: Algorithm for the management of priapism[28]

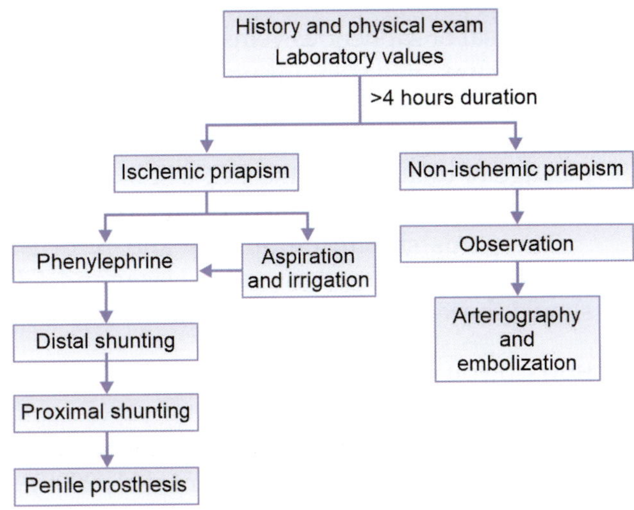

13. What is the surgical management of ischemic priapism.

Ans: Surgical interventions include penile shunt surgery and penile implant insertion for refractory or delayed ischemic priapism (Flowcharts 9.2 and 9.3).[20]

Indication: Surgical management of ischemic priapism is indicated after repeated penile aspirations and injections of sympathomimetics have failed after 1 hour of trial or if such an attempt has resulted in a significant cardiovascular side effect. Early surgical intervention may be preferable in patients with malignant or poorly controlled hypertension or for men who are using MAO inhibitor medications contraindicating adrenergic therapies.

Safety measures: A comprehensive discussion and documentation that includes baseline erectile function, duration of priapism, risks and benefits of the surgery, and ED and requirement of prosthesis in future should be held with the patient or guardian and an informed consent form signed by the patient or guardian.

14. What is the objective of shunt operations?

Ans: The International Society for Sexual Medicine Standards Committee (expert opinion) stated that shunting is to be considered for ischemic priapism events lasting 72 hours or less. Consideration should be given to foregoing a shunt in priapism events lasting longer, in particular when cavernous thrombosis is evident and no blood can be aspirated from the corporal bodies.[20]

The objective of shunt surgery is reoxygenation of the cavernous smooth muscle. The shared principle of shunt procedures is to re-establish corporal inflow by relieving venous outflow obstruction;

this requires creation of a fistula between the CC and glans penis, CC and corpus spongiosum, or CC and dorsal or saphenous veins.[21]

Although distal shunting can be performed with penile block and sedation in the emergency department, open shunting, especially that requiring passage of dilators into the CC, will likely require general anaesthesia and an operating room suite.

The penis should detumesce and refill with sequential compression and release; and CDU should show resumption of cavernous artery inflow.

15. How do you classify shunts for priapism?

Ans:

- Percutaneous distal shunts—Ebbehoj (1974), Winter (1976), or T shunt (Brant *et al.*, 2009)
- Open distal shunt—Al-Ghorab (1983) or corporal snake (Burnett and Pierorazio, 2009)
- Combined T shunt and corporal snake maneuver—Zacharakis *et al.* (2014)
- Open proximal shunt—Quackles (1964) or Sacher *et al.* (1972)
- Saphenous vein—Grayhack *et al.* (1964)
- Deep dorsal vein shunt—Barry (1976)

16. What are the distal shunts available?

Ans: A distal cavernoglanular shunt should be the first choice of shunting procedures because it is technically easier to perform than proximal shunting. Percutaneous distal shunting is less invasive than open distal shunting and can be performed with local anaesthetic in the emergency department.

Glans-Corpora Cavernosa Shunt (Winter)[22]

After LA, aspirate one corpus cavernosum with a large-bore needle passed through the glans (to avoid a hematoma of the shaft) in the midline and irrigate with saline solution through one corpus. Insert a biopsy needle (Tru-Cut) through the glans in the midline dorsal to the meatus. Pass the obturator through the septum to enter the right corpus cavernosum. Push the sheath home; rotate the needle 360 degrees and withdraw the needle. Repeat the manoeuvre to obtain two cores from the septum between the glans and the corpora on each side. Close the puncture site with a figure eight 3–0 CCG suture. Have the patient squeeze the penis every few minutes to keep it empty for the next 12 hours (Fig. 9.1).

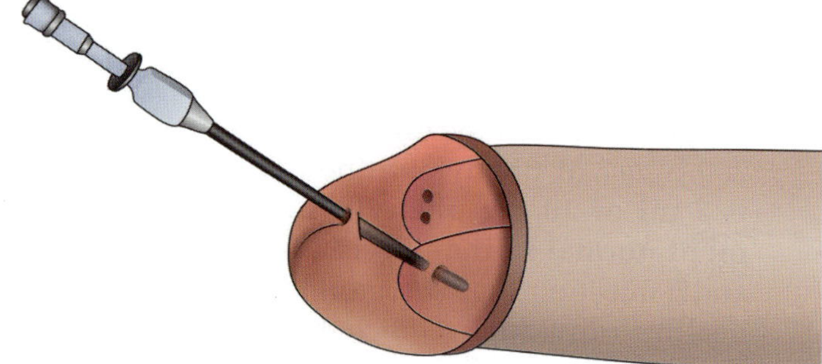

Fig. 9.1: Corpora glanular shunt

T Shunt

The most recently described distal shunt creates a T-shaped shunt between the CC and glans penis.[23]

In T shunting a No. 10 blade is placed vertically through the glans 4 mm away from the meatus; the blade pierces through the glans to the CC and is rotated 90 degrees away from the urethra and removed. Deoxygenated blood is milked out of the wound. The glans is then sutured with absorbable suture. Patient can be discharged home if the penis remains flaccid for 15 minutes. If erection returns or persists, a second T shunt is recommended on the opposite side of the meatus. When ischemic priapism has been present for more than 36 hours, immediate placement of bilateral T shunts is recommended, with passage of 20-Fr dilators into the fistula tract and well into the CC down to the crus. This technique is more traumatic and requires general anaesthesia.

In *Ebbehoj percutaneous cavernoglanular shunt*, a No. 11 blade leaves a straight incision into the glans and corpus cavernosum (Fig. 9.2).

Al-Ghorab shunt: A tourniquet is placed at the proximal end of the penile shaft to control bleeding. A 2 cm transversal incision was made on the penile glans, 1 cm distal of the coronal sulcus. The cavernous tissue at the penile glans was retracted, fixed with 2–0 sutures. Excise two 5 mm circular cone segments of the tunica albuginea to create a corporoglandular shunt. Then do retrograde insertion of a 7/8 Hegar dilator into the opening of the distal cavernous tissue via the original Al-Ghorab incision. Milking of penis for a few days

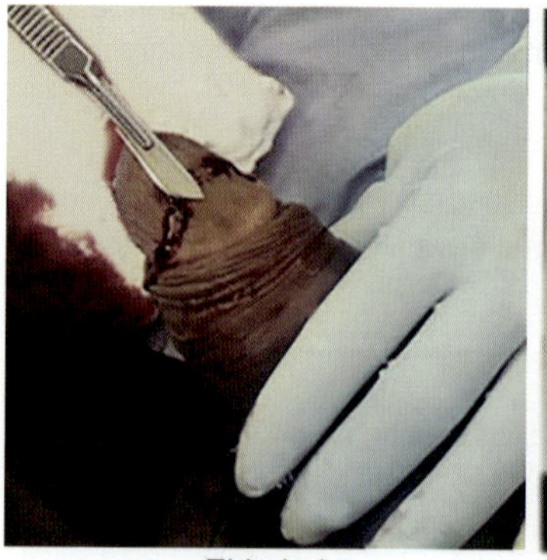

Ebbehoj

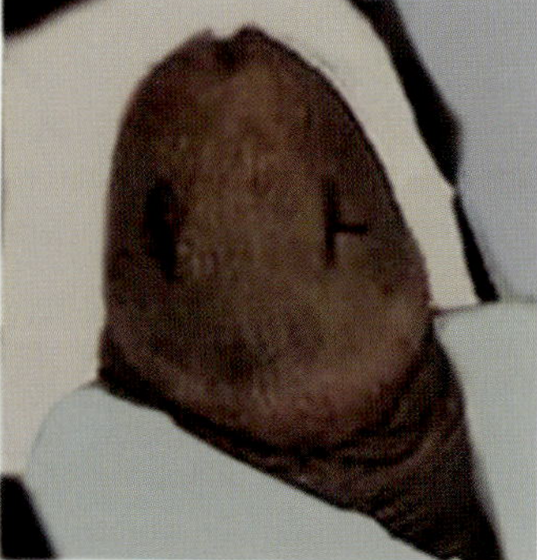

T shunt

Fig. 9.2: Ebbehoj and T shunt

for the blood to flow across the shunt is mandatory to avoid closure of shunt (Fig. 9.3).

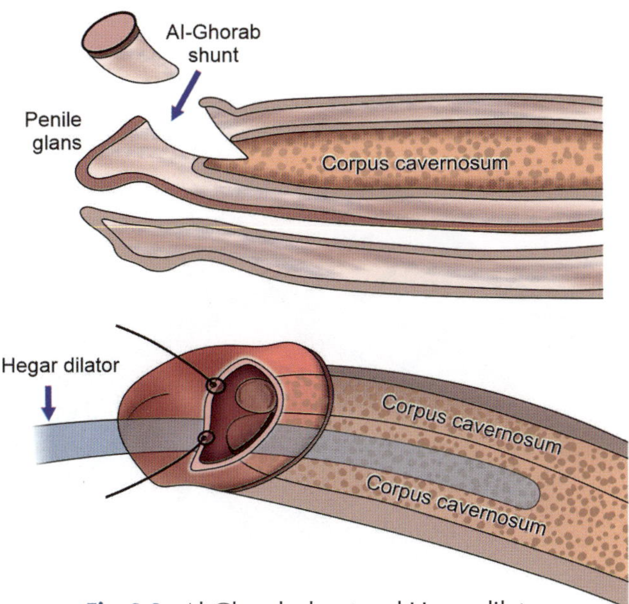

Fig. 9.3: Al-Ghorab shunt and Hegar dilator

Corporal Snake

It is a modification of the Al-Ghorab corporoglanular shunt (Burnett and Pierorazio (2009)).[24] Rather than excising a wedge of tunica and underlying CC muscle, a 7/8 Hegar dilator is advanced through each of the tunica windows proximally several centimetres to release blood and thrombus. The penis is made flaccid by repeated manual compression and release; the glans skin is then approximated with 4–0 chromic sutures.

17. What are the proximal shunts available?[25]

Cavernosospongiosum Shunt (Quackels)

After failure of distal shunts, a shunt more proximally has to be made where the circulation is better. 18 F 5 ml balloon catheter is placed in the bladder. Skin of the penis is incised vertically on the undersurface 1 cm off the midline, just distal to the penoscrotal junction (Fig. 9.4).

Instead of placing the incision on the shaft, it may be made more posteriorly where the substance of the corpus spongiosum is greater. Buck's fascia is incised and mobilized 3 cm of both cavernous bodies to create a groove between the corpus cavernosum and the corpus spongiosum. Walls of these structures are sutured together with a running 5–0 PDS. An ellipse 1 cm long has to be created from both structures. The spongy tissue of the corpus cavernosum is thin and the urethra is easily entered. The two structures are anastomosed with running 5–0 PDS, beginning at both ends of the defect. Close the subcutaneous tissues and skin. If detumescence is not satisfactory, repeat the procedure at a different level on the other side.

Cavernososaphenous Shunt (Grayhack)

Skin of the penis is incised at the base and the tunica albuginea of the corpus cavernosum is exposed. The femoral artery is palpated, and an oblique incision is made over it 3 or 4 cm below the inguinal ligament. The saphenous vein is exposed for a distance of 10 to 12 cm. The vein is divided distally so that it is long enough to reach the penis, and the distal end is tied with 3–0 PDS (Fig. 9.5).

The skin with the index finger is burrowed to join the two incisions (Fig. 9.6).

An ellipse of tunica albuginea about 1 cm long has to be excised. A needle is inserted through the glans, and thoroughly irrigated the corpora cavernosa to obtain a flow of bright red blood (Fig. 9.7).

A clamp is inserted through the skin tunnel and the vein is drawn into the penile wound. The vein is cut obliquely and spatulated. A 5–0 prolene

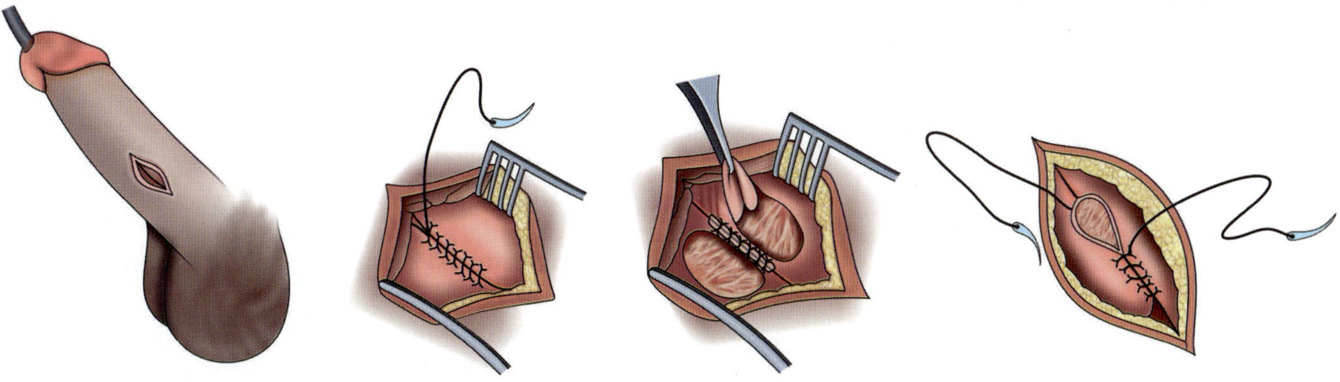

Fig. 9.4: Cavernosospongiosum shunt (Quackels)

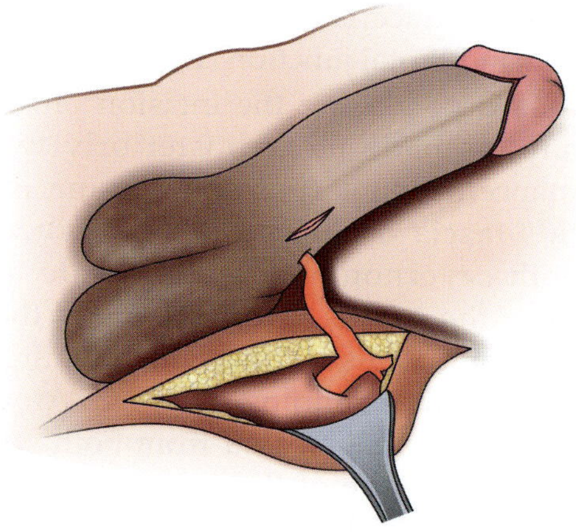

Fig. 9.5: Cavernososaphenous shunt

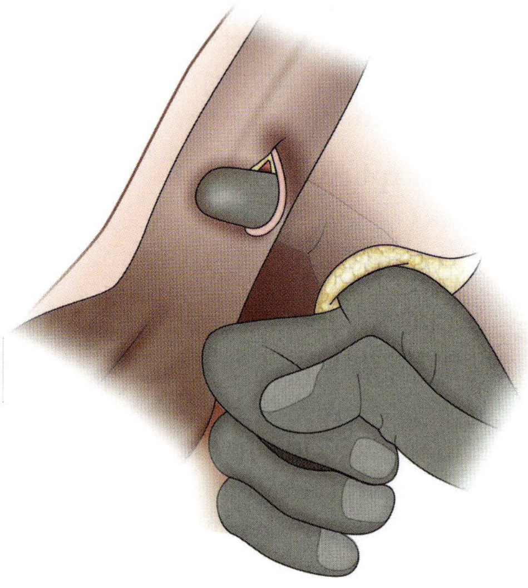

Fig. 9.6: Creating space for dorsal vein shunt

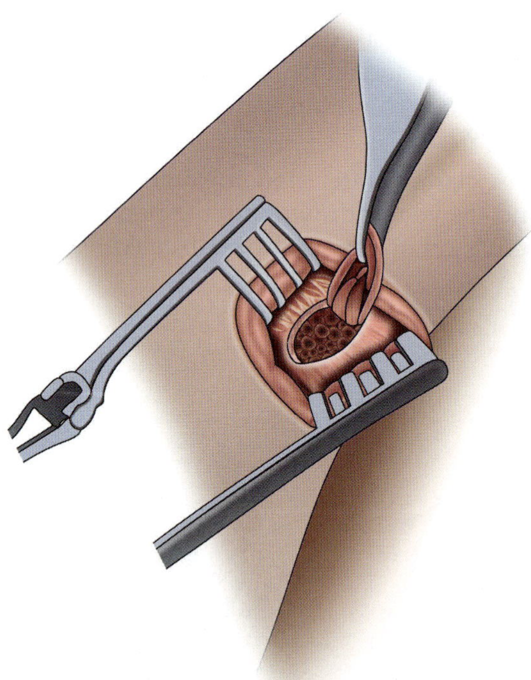

Fig. 9.7: Incision on tunica albuginea of one corpus

is placed and tied at each end of the cavernous defect, leaving the ends long. The back walls are sutured together, then the front walls are completed (Fig. 9.8).

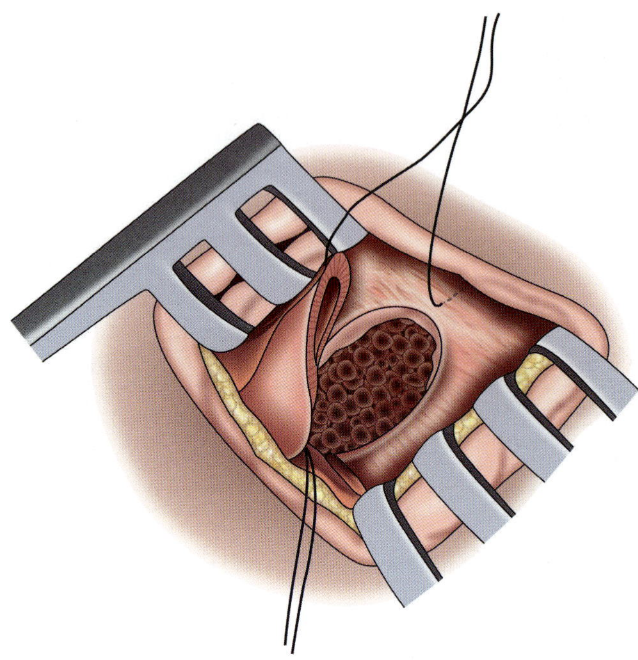

Fig. 9.8: The saphenous vein being sutured to the corpora cavernosa

The subcutaneous tissues are closed with 4–0 PDS and the skin incisions with 4–0 subcuticular PDS. A dry dressing is applied. The steps are proceeded with intermittent squeezing as previously described (Fig. 9.9).

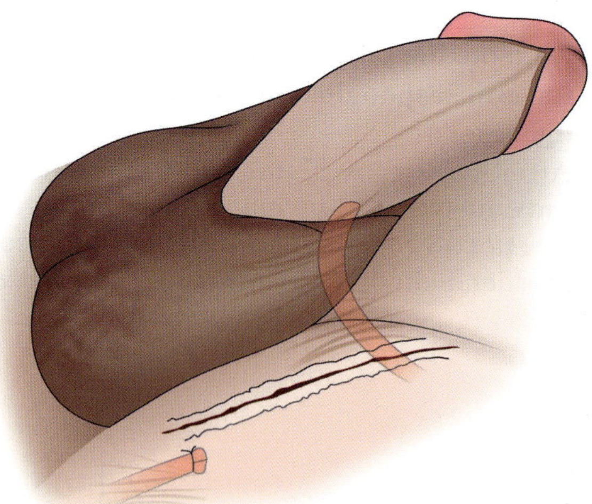

Fig. 9.9: The proximal end of the saphenous vein is tunneled and sutured to the corporal incision

Cavernous Vein: Dorsal Vein Shunt (Barry)

A circumcising incision is made and the penis is degloved. In midshaft, the superficial fascia is opened and Buck's fascia is incised. The dorsal

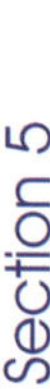

vein is dissected from its bed, taking care not to injure the dorsal artery or nerves. It is tied distally with an PDS. An incision is made in the tunica albuginea of one corpus opposite the proximal end of the vein, and the vein is anastomosed to the corpus end to side with a running 7–0 prolene. The penile skin is replaced and sutured at the corona. A compression dressing is never placed (Fig. 9.10).

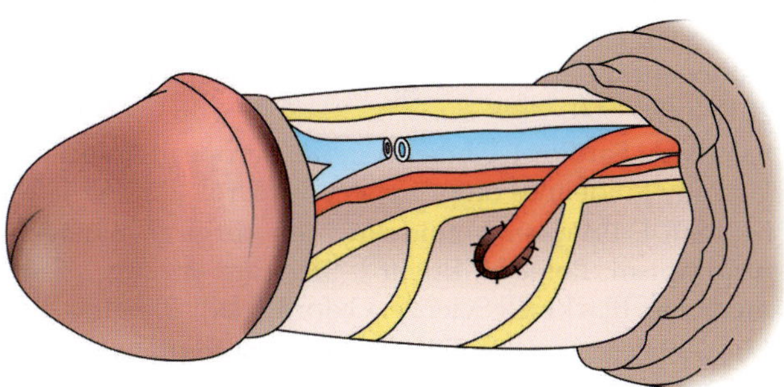

Fig. 9.10: Cavernous vein: Dorsal vein shunt

18. What are the complications of shunt surgery?

Ans:

- Penile edema
- Hematoma
- Infection
- Conversion of low-flow to high-flow (iatrogenic laceration of a cavernous artery)
- Urethral fistula
- Penile necrosis
- Pulmonary embolism
- Shunt failures

Distal shunt failures may be the consequence of inadequate size and/or formation of a clot at the site. Shunts cut through the collagen-rich tunica albuginea; collagen-activated platelets and fibrin form as a reaction to surgical injury and will work to seal off the shunt. Premature thrombosis of the site could lead to shunt failure.[26]

19. How to avoid distal shunt failure?

Ans:

1. Compressive penile dressings should be avoided;
2. The patient should periodically squeeze and release the distal penis to "milk" the shunt maintaining patency;
3. Anticoagulation should be considered with shunting. Some regimens include preoperative aspirin 325 mg coupled with subcutaneous heparin 5000 units and postoperative aspirin 81 mg daily for 2 weeks.

20. When to consider immediate implantation of penile prosthesis?

Ans:

- The natural history of untreated ischemic priapism or priapism refractory to interventions is severe fibrosis, penile length loss, and complete ED.
- Some have recommended performing an immediate penile prosthesis procedure in the acute management of ischemic priapism in patients in whom sympathomimetic intracavernous therapies and shunt surgery have both failed.
- Advantages to immediate implantation:
  i. Corporal fibrosis is not yet established
  ii. Penile length may be preserved
  iii. Technically easier implant insertion
- The exact time point at which prosthetic insertion becomes a reasonable option for managing ischemic priapism is unclear.
- Compared with prosthesis insertion in a typical patient with ED, there are significantly higher rates of complications noted in priapism cases: Infection, urethral injury, device migration, device erosion, and need for revision surgeries.
- The surgeon must be familiar with the additional technical concerns posed by weaknesses in the tunica albuginea in the region of prior shunts.
- Penile prosthesis should be considered in the following circumstances:
  a. Aspiration and sympathomimetic ICI have failed
  b. Distal and proximal shunting procedures have failed
  c. Ischemia has been present for longer than 36 hours
- MRI before surgery or corporal biopsy at the time of implant should be considered to document corporal smooth muscle necrosis for medicolegal purposes.[27]

KEY POINTS

- Priapism is an andrological emergency and needs urgent treatment.
- Evaluation in the emergency room can include blood gas analysis and color Doppler, especially in recurrent cases or following trauma, respectively; slow continuous external drainage is the treatment of choice.
- It is essential to drain completely and look for fresh blood before using a vasoconstrictor agent.
- Etiological assessment is done post-drainage and prophylaxis is essential in stuttering priapism.
- Surgical management is dependent upon the timing of presentation and severity of corporal damage.

REFERENCES

1. Bennett N, Mulhall J. Sickle cell disease status and outcomes of African American men presenting with priapism. J Sex Med. 2008;5(5):1244–1250.
2. Spycher MA, Hauri D. The ultrastructure of the erectile tissue in priapism. J Urol. 1986;135:142–147.
3. Hoeh MP, Levine LA. Management of recurrent ischemic priapism 2014: a complex condition with devastating consequences. Sex Med Rev. 2015;3(1):24–35.
4. Bertolotto M, Ciampalini S, Martingano P, *et al*. High flow priapism complicating ischemic priapism following iatrogenic laceration of the dorsal artery during a Winter procedure. J Clin Ultrasound. 2009;37(1):61–64.
5. Modified from Lue TF: Physiology of penile erection and pathophysiology of erectile dysfunction and priapism. In Walsh PC, Retik AB, Vaughan ED, *et al*., editors: Campbell's urology, Philadelphia, 2002, Saunders, pp 1610–1696.
6. Muneer A, Minhas S, Freeman A, *et al*. Investigating the effects of high-dose phenylephrine in the management of prolonged ischaemic priapism. J Sex Med. 2008;5:2152–2159.
7. Munnarriz R, Wen CC, McAuley I, *et al*. Management of ischemic priapism with high-dose intracavernosal phenylephrine: from bench to bedside. J Sex Med. 2006; 3:918–922.
8. Bivalacqua TJ, Musicki B, Champion HC, *et al*. Phosphodiesterase type 5 inhibitor therapy for priapism. Carson CC, Kirby RS, Goldstein I, *et al*. Textbook of erectile dysfunction. 2nd ed. Informa Healthcare: London; 2009:428–433.
9. Champion HC, Bivalacqua TF, Takimoto E, *et al*. Phosphodiesterase-5A dysregulation in penile erectile tissue is a mechanism of priapism. Proc Natl Acad Sci USA. 2005;102:1661–1666.
10. Anele UA, Morrison BF, Burnett AL. Molecular pathophysiology of priapism: emerging targets. Curr Drug Targets. 2015;16(5):474–483.
11. Kuypers FA. Hemoglobin s polymerization and red cell membrane changes. Hematol Oncol Clin North Am. 2014;28(2):155–179.
12. Aliyu ZY, Kato GJ, Taylor J, *et al*. Sickle cell disease and pulmonary hypertension in Africa: a global perspective and review of epidemiology, pathophysiology, and management. Am J Hematol. 2008;83:63–70.
13. Kato GJ. Priapism in sickle-cell disease: a hematologist's perspective. J Sex Med. 2012;9:70–78.
14. Broderick GA, Lue TF. Evaluation and nonsurgical management of erectile dysfunction and priapism. Walsh PC, Retik AB, Vaughan ED, *et al*. Campbell's urology. Saunders:Philadelphia; 2002:1619–1671.
15. McMahon CG. High flow priapism due to an arterial-sinusoidal fistula complicating initial veno-occlusive priapism. Int J Impot Res. 2002;14:195–196.
16. Kirkham A, Illing RO, Minahas S, *et al*. MR imaging of nonmalignant penile lesions. Radiographics. 2008;28:837–853.
17. Montague DK, Jarow J, Broderick GA, *et al*. American Urological Association guideline on the management of priapism. J Urol. 2003;170:1318–1324.
18. Broderick GA, Kadioglu A, Bivalacqua TJ, *et al*. Priapism: pathogenesis, epidemiology, and management. J Sex Med. 2010;7:476–500.
19. Salonia A, Eardley I, Giuliano F, *et al*. European Association of Urology guidelines on priapism. Eur Urol. 2014;65:480–489.
20. Mulhall J. Priapism—guidelines for surgical management of priapism. Porst H, Buvat J. Standard practice of sexual medicine. Blackwell Science: Oxford (UK); 2006:180–190.
21. Lue TF, Pescatori ES. Distal cavernosum-glans shunts for ischemic priapism. J Sex Med. 2006;3:749–752.
22. Brady Urological Institute. From Burnett AL, Pierorazio PM: Corporal "snake" maneuver: corporoglanular shunt surgical modification for ischemic priapism. J Sex Med 6:1171–1176, 2009.
23. Brant WO, Garcia MM, Bella AJ, *et al*. T-shaped shunt and intracavernous tunneling for prolonged ischemic priapism. J Urol. 2009;181:1699–1705.
24. Burnett AL, Pierorazio P. Corporal "snake" maneuver: corporoglanular shunt surgical modification for ischemic priapism. J Sex Med. 2009;6:1171–1176.
25. Atlas of Urologic Surgery, Second Edition, Frank Hinman, Jr., MD, FACS, FAAP, FRCS ENG (HON)
26. Mistry NA, Tadros NN, Hedges JC. Conversion of low-flow priapism to high-flow state using t-shunt with tunneling. Case Rep Urol. 2017;2017:7394185.
27. Priapism; Gregory A. Broderick MD; Campbell-Walsh-Wein Urology; 12th edition.
28. Montague DK, Jarow J, Broderick GA, et al. Members of the Erectile Dysfunction Guideline Update Panel; American Urological Association. American Urological Association guideline on the management of priapism. J Urol 2003;170:1318–1324.

Chapter

10

Andropause

• *Vinay Chougule* • *Priyank Kothari*

LEARNING OBJECTIVES

- Definition of adult onset hypogonadism (andropause).
- Evaluation of patient with suspected adult onset hypogonadism.
- Management of patient with andropause.
- Caveats to testosterone replacement therapy.

INTRODUCTION

Progressive reduction in testosterone levels associated with aging is called andropause, male climacteric or androgen deficiency in aging male (ADAM) or partial androgen deficiency in aging male (PADAM). In fact, andropause is male age-relative hypogonadism, which unlike menopause, is not always accompanied by symptoms.

Case Scenario

A 65-year-old male complains of decreased libido, less frequent morning erections, irritability, mood swings, loss of libido and generalized absence of energy in daily life. He also complaints of interpersonal conflicts. His clinical examination is normal and total serum testosterone (morning sample) -160 ng/dl (270 to 1070 ng/dl). Clinical examination shows normal genitalia, normal prostate and neurological examination. He does not have any comorbid condition.

1. What is the diagnosis?

Ans: This could be a case of ADAM. The close differential could be erectile dysfunction and depression.

2. What are symptoms of andropause?

Ans: Clinical manifestations of ADAM are slow onset and gradually progressive. This picture can mimic consequences of aging:

1. Reduced libido, erectile dysfunction (ED), particularly nocturnal.
2. Mood swings, depression, anger.[1]
3. Reduced lean body mass and muscle mass.[2]
4. Reduced body hair and skin changes.
5. Osteoporosis.[3]
6. Deposition of visceral fat.

3. What is pathophysiology of andropause?

Ans: Mean androgen levels decline at approximately 1% per year after the age of 50 years. Also, elevated sex hormone-binding globulin (SHBG) levels lead to a further decrease in bioavailable and free testosterone levels. With age, the circadian rhythm flattens and the testosterone levels are steadily low over the 24-hour cycle.[4] The response of target organs such as prostate, brain, bone, and muscle, are dampened with age. By 50 years age, dehydroepiandrosterone (DHEA) levels decrease to less than 30% of that in men younger than 30 years.[5]

4. What should be the plan of treatment?

Ans: After taking detailed history including stressors, relationship with wife, overall mental status and effort tolerance, routine blood investigations such as complete blood count, serum creatinine, glycosylated hemoglobin, lipid profile, serum total testosterone and prostate specific antigen can be done. A digital rectal examination (DRE) should be done to assess the prostate gland. After establishing the diagnosis, we can initiate testosterone replacement therapy after risk assessment and counseling.

5. **How to evaluate patient of andropause?**

Ans: It is difficult to detect adult onset (or late onset) hypogonadism just based on clinical symptoms. Serum total testosterone levels (preferably on two occasions at least one month apart, between 8 to 10 AM, in same laboratory ideally by gas chromatography/mass spectrometry) should be done to confirm hypogonadism.

6. **What is free testosterone?**

Ans: Testosterone and dihydrotestosterone (DHT) are bound to albumin (low affinity, high binding) and SHBG (high affinity, low binding). Around 1.5–2% of serum testosterone is free and believed to represent bio-active component of testosterone. The measurement of SHBG and free testosterone is valuable for assessment of androgenization. It has specific utility when there is a discrepancy in clinical symptoms and testosterone levels or associated conditions which can affect SHBG levels like cirrhosis, obesity, etc (Flowchart 10.1).[5]

Flowchart 10.1: Algorithm for adult hypogonadism

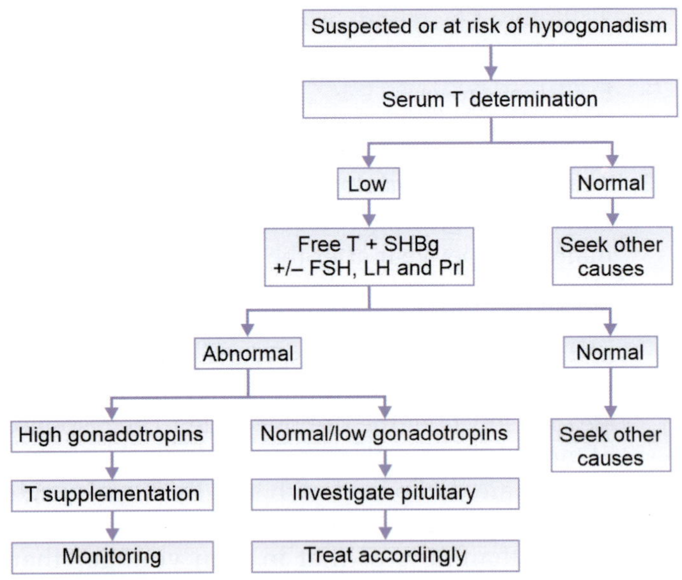

7. **What are the available options for testosterone replacement therapy (TRT) in India?**

Ans: TRT can be oral capsules, gel formulation or injections.

Oral Preparations

Testosterone undecanoate (capsules 40 mg) can be started at 120–160 mg daily for a period of 2 to 3 weeks and maintenance at 40–120 mg per day titrated based on clinical effect and side effects. There may be unpredictable serum levels of testosterone due to rapid hepatic metabolism (absolute bioavailability: 6.83 +/– 3.32%).[6] Testosterone undecanoate (single orally effective formulation) is not hepatotoxic; works better with meals as it is lipid soluble. Used at a dose of 120 to 200 mg in 3 divided doses, oral TRT not a preferred modality.

Gel Preparations

Single application (preferably morning) of transdermal testosterone gel (1%; 5 gram sachet) results in continuous delivery (for 24 hours). This is applied on intact, clean, dry, non-hairy skin of the shoulders, upper arms and/or abdomen. Measure testosterone levels after ~14 days and the dose can be increased to 7.5 or 10 gm.

Intramuscular Injections

Monthly Preparations

A combination of testosterone esters (propionate, decanoate, phenylproprionate and isocaproate) is available and the total dosage per ml is 250 mg. Maximum concentration after these intramuscular injections is attained at 72 hours and starts diminishing during next 10–14 days.[5] It is recommended that starting dose should be 250 mg deep intramuscular injection 4 weekly which can be increased to 250 mg once every 2 weeks depending on the total testosterone levels 2 weeks after the injection. Supra physiological levels can cause breast tenderness and gynecomastia. These injections may lead to significant mood swings, libido and sexual function.

Depot Preparations

The recommended dose is 1000 mg (4 ml) of testosterone undecanoate injected every 10–14 weeks, deeply into gluteal muscle. Testosterone level should be measured at 6 weeks and then one week prior to next scheduled dosage. Depending on clinical symptoms and serum testosterone level the interval can vary from 8–12 weeks. The aim should be to have total testosterone between 400 and 600 ng/dl, without fluctuation in symptoms.

Precautions

Pretreatment screening for prostate cancer by DRE and PSA is mandatory. TRT is contraindicated in severe cardiac, hepatic or renal insufficiency and heart failure. It should be used with caution in patient with epilepsy and migraine. Pre-existing sleep apnea may worsen. Concurrent use of drugs such as rifampicin, barbiturates, carbamazepine, dichloralphenazone, phenylbutazone, phenytoin or primidone may decrease the effect of testosterone.[7]

8. How to monitor a patient on TRT?

Ans: Hematocrit, PSA and DRE for prostate at 3 monthly intervals are important during follow-up. Patients should be counseled about advantages and disadvantages of each preparation and TRT should be started according to his informed choice.

Men who are stable may subsequently be followed annually. Tests include hemogram, LFT, lipid profile, PSA and serum calcium. Bone mineral density assessment can also be performed to document baseline values. Patients who have high hematocrit (>52%) will need phlebotomy and dose titration. Higher testosterone levels are associated with erythrocytosis and rise in hematocrit and blood viscosity.

9. Does TRT initiate BPH or prostate cancer?

Ans: Evidence suggests that TRT given in hypogonadal men increases the prostate volume, especially in the central zone, for sub-normal to normal values compared with age-matched normal men.[7]

10. What are the effects of TRT on the existing prostate cancer?

Ans: Documented prostate cancer in an absolute contraindication to testosterone therapy.

KEY POINTS

- Testosterone therapy for hypogonadism is based on clinical symptoms and lab values.
- Before starting testosterone, perform a thorough evaluation of symptoms, comorbid conditions including cardiac assessment.
- Assess if testosterone replacement would benefit the patient.
- Initiate lifestyle changes alongside testosterone replacement.
- Monitor for side effects and improvement in levels and symptomatic improvement to decide if replacement benefits patient.

SUMMARY

- Diagnosis of andropause or adult onset hypogonadism is based on clinical picture and testosterone levels.
- It is essential to evaluate for other causes and then decide if testosterone treatment would benefit the patient.
- Lifestyle changes and optimization of comorbidities is also important.
- Follow-up with DRE, PSA and hematocrit is important while on testosterone replacement.
- Treatment of erectile dysfunction involves standard treatment such as PDE5 inhibitors.
- Testosterone replacement can only potentiate and not replace PDE5 inhibitor therapy.

REFERENCES

1. Burris AS, Banks SM, Carter CS, *et al.* A long-term prospective study of the physiological and behavioral effect of hormone replacement in untreated hypogonadal me. J Androl, 1992; **13:** 297.
2. Urban RJ, Bondeburg YH, Gilkisonm C, *et al.* Testosterone administration to elderly men increases skeletal muscle strength and protein synthesis. Am. J Physiol, 1995; **269:** E820.
3. Abu EO, Horner A, Kusec V, *et al.* The localization of androgen receptors in human bone. J Clin Endocrinol Metab, 1997;**82:** 3493.
4. Plymate SR, Tenover JS and Bremner WJ. Circadian variation in testosterone, Sex hormone-binding globulin bound testosterone in healthy young and elderly men. J. Androl, 1989; **10:** 366.
5. Tenovar JL. Testosterone and the aging male. J Androl 1997; **18:** 103.
6. Täuber U, Schröder K, Düsterberg B, Matthes H. Absolute bioavailability of testosterone after oral administration of testosterone-undecanoate and testosterone. Eur J Drug Metab Pharmacokinet. 1986 Apr-Jun;11(2):145–9. doi: 10.1007/BF03189840. PMID: 3770015.
7. Bhasin S. Androgen treatment of hypogonadal men. J Clin Endocrinol Metab, 1992;**74:**1221.

Chapter

11

Post-Radical Prostatectomy Erectile Dysfunction

• Rohan Batra • Ashwin Mallya

LEARNING OBJECTIVES

- Understanding the pathophysiology of erectile dysfunction associated with radical pelvic uro-oncologic surgery (neurogenic and vasculogenic).
- Understanding different modes and sequence for treatment of erectile dysfunction post-radical prostatectomy (PDE5i, ICIVAD, vacuum devices, prosthesis).
- Understand the basics of penile prosthesis, their indications and contraindications in such patients.

Case Scenario

A 67-year-old male underwent robotic assisted radical prostatectomy (RARP) 1 year back, presents with erectile dysfunction and he does not get natural erections. He has been on daily tadalafil 5 mg for the past one year. There was only mild improvement in the tumescence with the treatment and good rigid erections were not achieved. He enquires about intrapenile injections, chances for further recovery and the possible need for prosthesis.

1. **How to initiate the management in this patient?**

   Ans: This gentleman has undergone robotic assisted radical prostatectomy (RARP). His evaluation should ideally start from preoperative interview and documentation of erectile dysfunction (ED), best done by using IIEF-5/SHIM scores. A thorough examination of penis should be done and any fibrosis should be documented. Comorbidities like diabetes mellitus, spinal cord surgery, etc. should be noted.

2. **What is the etiopathogenesis of post-RP erectile dysfunction?**

   Ans: The basic pathophysiology involves disruption of the normal mechanism of erection. The cavernous nerves which produce nitric oxide, and blood vessels (neurogenic and vasculogenic component) are in very close proximity of the prostate and run along the prostate bilaterally. During sexual stimulation, the neurotransmitters which cause relaxation of the smooth muscles of the blood vessels to the erectile tissue are released by the cavernous nerve terminals. These provide parasympathetic supply to the corpora cavernosa and form a dense network known as pelvic plexus.

   In the non-nerve sparing radical prostatectomy, the cavernous nerves are disrupted which provide para-sympathetic innervation to the corpora cavernosa which leads to inability to achieve erection due to failure of smooth muscle relaxation (neurogenic ED). In nerve sparing radical prostatectomy, ED is because of traction injury and diathermy damage to the periprostatic neurovascular bundles which causes neuropraxia, and hence ED. Because of the denervation of corpora, the penile hypoxia is there and it results into collage accumulation and smooth muscle apoptosis which leads to cavernosal fibrosis. Also, injury to the arteries like accessory pudendal artery leads to penile hypoxia which leads to cavernosal fibrosis (arteriogenic)[1–3] (Flowchart 11.1).

3. **How is the recovery of erectile function post-RP?**

   Ans: Current studies report a postoperative erectile dysfunction rate of 19–78% and this variation is due to discrepancy in defining ED and ranges

Flowchart 11.1: Pathogenesis of erectile dysfunction in radical prostatectomy

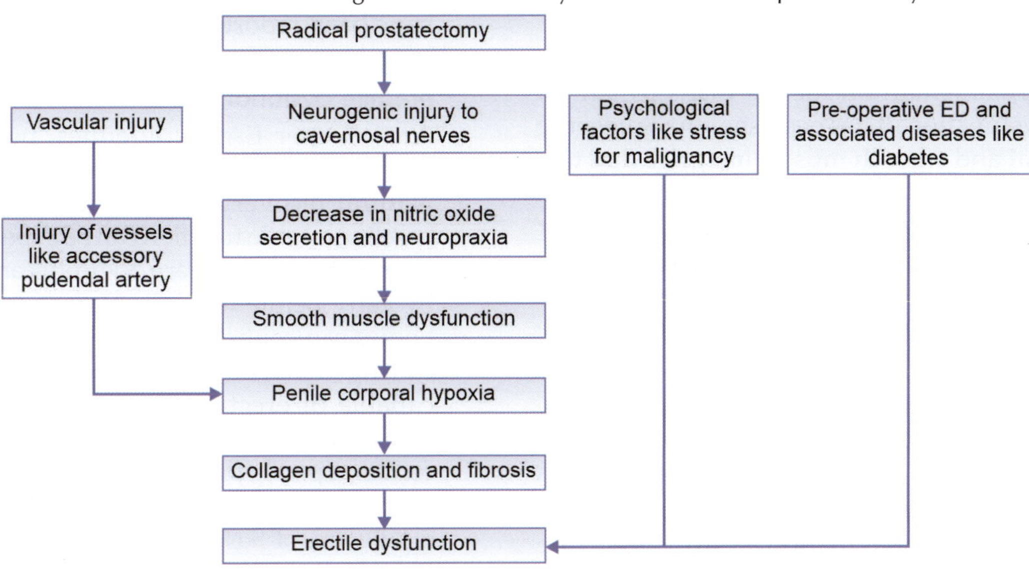

from 78–87% at 2–15 years post-RP.[4,5] The erectile function returns in about 20–30% patients but it can take two or more years.[6]

4. **What is penile rehabilitation?**

Ans: Counseling men about the expected perioperative erectile dysfunction, length and girth changes, different sensation of orgasm and dry ejaculate go a long way in improving functional outcomes. It is also important to have penile rehabilitation to maintain the penile length and girth.

Penile rehabilitation is the protocol which aims in reducing the hypoxia to the penile corpora and irreversible structural changes in the cavernosal smooth muscle, maintains penile length and helps in delivery of treatment aimed at enhancing erectile function. This therapy is planned at a stage where erectile function is not the primary concern but is essential to be inculcated as part of the overall management of PCa.

5. **What is the role of low dose Tadalafil?**

Ans: Daily dose of phosphodiesterase inhibitors (PDE-5i) is considered safe and efficacious, especially after nerve sparing RP.[7] Sildenafil is identified to be more efficient but with slightly higher adverse effects. Low-dose tadalafil typically is 5 mg once daily and has a better side effect profile. This has been shown to be effective in achieving drug-assisted EF among men with ED following nerve sparing RP.[8] It has been shown to protect against both length loss and structural cavernosal changes after NSRP.[9] Tadalafil is better than placebo.[10]

6. **What is the next step?**

Ans: The next step is intracavernosal injections (ICI) that involves the injection of vasoactive medication directly into the erectile tissue of the penis. This is used when there is inadequate response to PDE5i. ICI for penile rehabilitation has shown very good results in terms of erectile function recovery, but has a high drop-out rate, up to 11% after twice weekly low dose alprostadil due to pain.[11] ICI also has shown better response rates than placebo.[12] Injection of bimix (containing papverine and phentolamine/chlorpromazine) can circumvent the pain associated with alprostadil injection and improve adherence rates.

The timing of ICI is still debatable. The neuropraxia after RP can improve even after 2 years but the effects of penile fibrosis can set in due to reduced blood flowing into the penis. The advantages of early ICI include resumption of erections and satisfaction and penile length preservation. However, ICI therapy does come with some risks and potential side effects. The most common side effect is pain or discomfort at the injection site, which can usually be managed with proper injection technique. Other potential side effects include penile fibrosis due to ICI. Corporal fibrosis might also adversely affect the penile prosthesis outcomes at least in some men but, the amount of fibrosis induced that can affect prosthesis outcomes is observed after a prolonged period of usage of 5–10 years.

The timing of ICI should probably be early in men undergoing a more extensive procedure, requiring adjuvant therapy in the form of hormonal or radiation therapy, preoperative ED and young men.

7. **What is the role of vacuum erection device in post-RP ED?**

Ans: Vacuum erection device (VED) therapy is another armamentarium for the management of erectile dysfunction. It has been shown to preserve endothelial and smooth muscle integrity due to a transient increase in arterial flow and oxygenation in the corpora cavernosa. Use of VED alone or in combination with PDE5i can provide variable results.[13,14] This can help in avoiding penile length loss and may reduce corporal fibrosis due to hypoxia.

8. **What are the measures during radical prostatectomy to minimize the chances of ED?**

Ans: During RP, in addition to direct injury to the nerves there can be neuropraxia caused by traction, compression and coagulation.[1] Care should be taken during periprostatic dissection. Sparse use of diathermy especially beginning lateral to the seminal vesicles and along the prostatic tissue as well as decreased traction of the neural tissue can be useful.

Nerve sparing techniques have been postulated to improve potency rates following RP. Tewari *et al* propose a 4 degree NS approach. In grade I the dissection plane runs between the pseudo capsule and the periprostatic veins. Moving laterally from veins to the levator fascia, grades 2, 3 and 4 can be achieved with progressively less NS to non-NS approach.[15] In addition, preservation of the accessory pudendal arteries which could be present in up to 75% of men has been proposed as a method of preserving penile arterial sufficiency.[1]

Autologous sural and genitofemoral nerve interposition graft placed during RP and dehydrated human amnion chorion membrane allograft nerve wrap around neurovascular bundle have been reported.[16,17]

9. **What is the role of penile prosthesis in post-RP erectile dysfunction?**

Ans: As per EAU guidelines, penile prosthesis is a third line option in the management of ED.[16] Natural recovery post-RP in patients with good baseline erectile function can be expected to occur till 24 months post-surgery. Rigidity can be maximized by early penile rehabilitation so that the corporal bodies can continue to get fresh oxygenated blood during the recovery phase and continue to be capable of erections once nerves regenerate. In case penile rehabilitation does not achieve desired results, a penile prosthesis is warranted. The patient and partner satisfaction in this group of patients is upward of 90%. Simultaneous penile prosthesis have been placed following laparoscopic RP with satisfactory results in well-selected and motivated patients.[18] However, this is not standard practice. Despite the beneficial effect of penile prosthesis, it is grossly under-utilized in the post RP setting. Various studies have shown utilization in the range of 0.8–1.9% in the post-RP setting. Some other studies show post-RP prosthesis contributing about 22% of the total prosthesis cases performed internationally.[19]

10. **What are the types of penile prostheses available?**

Ans: The implants are summarized in Table 11 1. Broadly the prosthesis available are of two types, inflatable and malleable. Inflatable implants are supposed to closely replicate natural erection and are easier to conceal.

11. **What are the factors to be considered during patient selection?**

Ans: Ziegelmann *et al* discuss patient non-psychological and psychological factors in the

TABLE 11.1: Types of prosthesis available

Prosthesis type	*Models*	*Advantages*	*Disadvantages*
Malleable	Boston scientific Tactra AMS Spectra Shah prosthesis Zephyr ZSI 100 Coloplast genesis	Easier to place Less expensive	Permanently rigid Has to be positioned
Two pieces inflatable	AMS Ambicor	Not permanently rigid. Has a reservoir at the posterior aspect of the cylinders and a pump (no separate reservoir)	Increased chance of mechanical failure.
Three pieces inflatable (prosthesis, pump and reservoir)	AMS 700 CX AMS 700 CXR, LGX Rigicon Infla 10X Coloplast Titan Zephyr ZSI 475	More natural erection and flaccidity Less chance of pain and erosion	Difficult to implant Mechanical failure (average life of 10–15 years)

satisfaction rates after penile prosthesis. Among non-psychological factors the salient ones are severity of underlying condition, prior surgeries in the area and local treatments, comorbid conditions or medications that may impair healing, drug and alcohol use. Among psychological factors, the salient ones are availability of an understanding partner, unrealistic expectations, revision surgery, denial and feeling of entitlement.[20] A detailed informed consent is a must when considering penile prosthesis surgery. Chances of wound infection, mechanical failure, revision surgery, removal of infected prosthesis, permanent dependence on penile prosthesis should be explained in detail.

12. What are the techniques used and steps involved?

Ans: The main techniques utilized include a penoscrotal approach or an infrapubic approach. The broad steps are

a. *Preoperative preparation*: Antibiotics such as Vancomycin and Gentamicin 1 hour prior to the procedure. Shaving and skin prep (chlorhexidine/alcohol × 5 min) are done.
b. *Position and incision*: Supine with pubic symphysis at point of flexion so that table tilt elevates the pubic rami up allowing more proximal crural exposure. Foley catheter insertion is done. Frog leg position is preferred especially for inflatable prosthesis for proximal access to the corpora.
c. *Placement of the penile cylinders*: Initial dissection and exposure of the corporal bodies, corporotomy, dilatation and corporal sizing, followed by priming and testing if inflatable, before placement of cylinders and corporotomy closure.
d. *Placement of penile pump*: This is made into a scrotal pouch.
e. *Placement of reservoir*: Space of Retzius or in a pre-peritoneal space/ectopic; 60–100 ml reservoirs are available.
f. Wound closure and post-operative care; catheter removal on 1st postoperative day.
g. Pump cycling can be started at 2–4 weeks once patient is comfortable.

13. What are the contraindications for penile prosthesis surgery?

Ans: Active infection, particularly urinary tract or genital infection. Unresolved problems of elevated residual urine volume or bladder outlet obstruction, patients not willing for device revision surgery, poorly controlled diabetes and immunosuppressive therapies, low motivation and unrealistic expectations are the most important contraindications.[21,22]

14. What are the complications of penile prosthesis surgery?

Ans: Complications during the surgery:[23,24]

1. During corporal dilatation: (a) Corporal cross over and crural perforation; (b) Urethral injury
2. During reservoir placement: (a) Vascular injury (b) bowel injury (c) bladder injury

Complications after the surgery: 1. Infection of prosthesis 2. Mechanical failure 3. Corporal erosion 4. Glans necrosis and deformity 5. Reservoir herniation 6. Scrotal hematoma

Conclusions

Erectile dysfunction post-RP is psychologically very disturbing for the patient and his confidence. Penile rehabilitation is a patient-centric approach with all the available therapies to be used as complementary approaches rather than a singular approach. Again, the therapies have to be used in accordance with the approach to patient's quality of life. Penile rehabilitation and sustenance of erectile function completes the trifecta of radical prostatectomy, that is, oncology control, incontinence control and erectile function control. If the medical therapy fails, then the patient has to be counselled for penile prosthesis. Various types of prosthesis are available that suits all the patients. The quality of life is significantly enhanced if patient is treated in correct manner.

SUMMARY

- The pathophysiology of erectile dysfunction post-radical prostatectomy is a combination of neurogenic and vasculogenic components.
- The maximal recovery of erectile function post-radical prostatectomy may take up to 2 years
- Penile rehabilitation should be started early to prevent cavernosal fibrosis.
- Treatment of erectile dysfunction should be offered to all the patients to improve their quality of life.
- Penile prosthesis surgery is a feasible and acceptable modality of treatment in patients who do not improve after 2 years of their surgery.

REFERENCES

1. Capogrosso P, Salonia A, Briganti A, Montorsi F. Postprostatectomy erectile dysfunction: a review. The world journal of men's health. 2016 Aug;34(2):73–88.
2. Blecher G, Almekaty K, Kalejaiye O, Minhas S. Does penile rehabilitation have a role in the treatment of erectile dysfunction following radical prostatectomy?. F1000Research. 2017;6.
3. Emanu, Jessica C; Avildsen, Isabelle K; Nelson, Christian J. (2016). Erectile dysfunction after radical prostatectomy. Current Opinion in Supportive and Palliative Care, 10(1), 102–107. doi:10.1097/spc.0000000000000195

4. Salonia A, Adaikan G, Buvat J, *et al.* Sexual Rehabilitation After Treatment For Prostate Cancer-Part 2: Recommendations From the Fourth International Consultation for Sexual Medicine (ICSM 2015). J Sex Med. 2017;14(3):297–315.
5. Resnick MJ, Koyama T, Fan KH, *et al.* Long-term functional outcomes after treatment for localized prostate cancer. N Engl J Med. 2013;368(5):436–445.
6. Rabbani F, Schiff J, Piecuch M, *et al.* Time course of recovery of erectile function after radical retropubic prostatectomy: does anyone recover after 2 years?. J Sex Med. 2010;7(12):3984–3990.
7. Montorsi F, Brock G, Stolzenburg JU, *et al.* Effects of tadalafil treatment on erectile function recovery following bilateral nerve-sparing radical prostatectomy: a randomised placebo-controlled study (REACTT). Eur Urol. 2014;65(3):587–596.
8. Brock G, Montorsi F, Costa P, *et al.* Effect of Tadalafil Once Daily on Penile Length Loss and Morning Erections in Patients After Bilateral Nerve-sparing Radical Prostatectomy: Results From a Randomized Controlled Trial. Urology. 2015;85(5):1090–1096.
9. Sari Motlagh R, Abufaraj M, Yang L, *et al.* Penile Rehabilitation Strategy after Nerve Sparing Radical Prostatectomy: A Systematic Review and Network Meta-Analysis of Randomized Trials. J Urol. 2021;205(4):1018–1030.
10. Mulhall JP, Bivalacqua TJ, Becher EF. Standard operating procedure for the preservation of erectile function outcomes after radical prostatectomy. J Sex Med. 2013;10(1):195–203.
11. Qiu S, Tang Z, Deng L, *et al.* Comparisons of regular and on-demand regimen of PED5-Is in the treatment of ED after nerve-sparing radical prostatectomy for Prostate Cancer. Sci Rep. 2016;6:32853. Published 2016 Sep 9.
12. Yiou R, Cunin P, de la Taille A, *et al.* Sexual rehabilitation and penile pain associated with intracavernous alprostadil after radical prostatectomy. J Sex Med. 2011;8(2):575–582.
13. Raina R, Agarwal A, Ausmundson S, *et al.* Early use of vacuum constriction device following radical prostatectomy facilitates early sexual activity and potentially earlier return of erectile function. Int J Impot Res. 2006;18(1):77–81.
14. Basal S, Wambi C, Acikel C, Gupta M, Badani K. Optimal strategy for penile rehabilitation after robot-assisted radical prostatectomy based on preoperative erectile function. BJU Int. 2013;111(4):658–665.
15. Tewari AK, Srivastava A, Huang MW *et al.* Anatomical grades of nerve sparing: a risk stratified approach to neural-hammock sparing during RARP. BJU Int.2011 Sep; 108: 984–92.
16. Castiglione F, Ralph DJ, Muneer A. Surgical techniques for managing post-prostatectomy ED. Curr Urol Rep. 2017 Sep 30; 18(11):90.
17. Patel VR, Samavedi S, Bates AS *et al.* Human Amnion/chorion membrane Allograft Nerve Wrap around the Prostatic NVB accelerates early return to continence and apotency following RARP: Propensity score matched analysis. Eur Urol.2015 Jun ;67(6):977–980
18. Mondaini N, Cai T, Sarti E *et al.* A case series of patients who underwent Laparoscopic Extraperitoneal Radical prostatectomy with simultaneous implant of a penile prosthesis: focus on penile length preservation. World J Men's health.2018 May; 36(2): 132–138
19. Baas W, O'Connor B, Welliver C *et al.* World wide trends in penile implantation surgery: data from over 63000 implants. Transl Androl Urol.2020 Feb; 9(1): 31–37.
20. Ziegelmann M, Koehler TS, Bailey GC *et al.* Surgical patient selection and counseling. Transl Androl Urol. 2017 Aug;6(4): 609–19.
21. Cavayero CT, McIntosh GV. Penile prosthesis implantation. 2022 Sep 26. In:stat pearls (Internet). Treasure Island (FL): StatPearls Publishing; 2023 Jan
22. Bettocchi C, Palumbo F, Spilotros M *et al.* Penile Prosthesis. Ther adv Urol.2010 Feb; 2(1):35–40.
23. Bennett N, Huang IS. Inflatable penile prosthesis in the Radical prostatectomy patient: a review. F1000 Res.2018 Jun 19; 7:770.
24. Cayetano-Alcatraz AA, Yassin M, Desai A *et al.* Penile implant surgery-managing complications. Fac Rev. 2021 Sep 24; 10:73.

Male Infertility

Chapter

1

Oligospermia

• *Arun Kumar K*

LEARNING OBJECTIVES

- Define and identify causes of low sperm counts.
- Application of existing treatment options to improve sperm parameters.
- To pick up early referral points for assisted reproductive techniques.

INTRODUCTION

Oligozoospermia refers to a sperm concentration below the 5th centile (16 million/ml); in at least 2 semen samples obtained four weeks apart[1]. It is usually associated with reduced sperm motility and sperm morphology reflecting both quantitative and qualitative defects in sperm production. Most commonly in around 60–75% of cases there is no clear etiology (idiopathic).[2]

Case Scenario

A 34-year-old male and a 25-year-old lady married for 4 years, presenting with primary infertility; semen analysis shows 10 million sperms per ml, 30% progressive motility and 3% normal forms. How to approach this couple? Clinical examination is normal.

1. **What is the diagnosis?**

   Ans: As per the WHO 2021 sixth edition manual the above patient has a count below 5th centile (16 million) and borderline progressive motility (30%). The morphology is near normal (>4%). European Andrology Association recommends at least 2 semen analysis over 2–3 months to define OAT.[3]

2. **What is the importance of HPG axis in spermatogenesis?**

   Ans: Spermatogenesis requires an intact hypothalamo-pituitary-gonadal axis and feedback mechanisms. Due to pulsatile GnRH release from the hypothalamus, anterior pituitary secretes luteinizing (LH) and follicle stimulating (FSH) hormones.[4] Drugs like glucocorticoids, opiates, antidepressants, SSRI, antipsychotics. Androgens and anabolic steroids can have long lasting effect on spermatogenesis.[5,6]

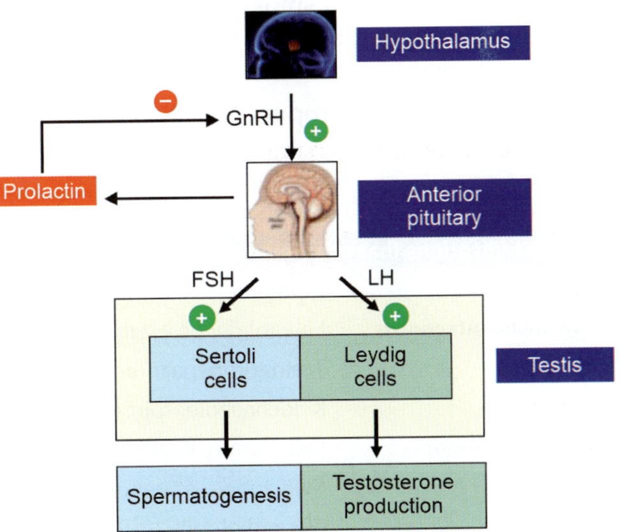

Fig. 1.1: HPG axis

3. **What are the causes of low sperm count?**

   Ans: A meta-analysis of over 13000 men demonstrated that obese and overweight states was associated with elevated risk of oligozoospermia.[7] Obesity increases the leptin and insulin resistance which downregulates GnRH secretion. Adiposity

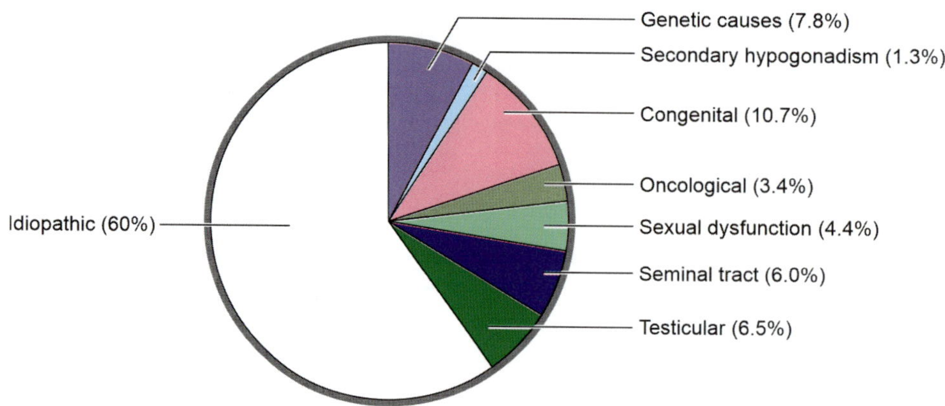

Fig. 1.2: Causes of low sperm count[2]

increases the peripheral aromatase activity exacerbating androgen deficiency including an epigenetic impact.[8,9]

4. **How will you classify oligospermia?**

   Ans: Oligozoospermia can be classified as mild (10–15 million sperms/ml), moderate (5–10 million sperm/ml), severe (<5 million).[10]

5. **What are the points to be noted in the clinical history?**

   Ans: The history focuses on important aspects such as:[11]
   - Childhood genital surgeries/development/testicular infection or swelling
   - Prior fertility attempts/drug therapy
   - Comorbidities
   - Addictions such as smoking, ethanol, tobacco and recreational drugs
   - Specific drugs

6. **How do medications impact fertility?**

   Ans: Medications which impact fertility are given in Table 1.1.

7. **What are the findings to be noted on clinical examination?**

   Ans:
   - Look for secondary sexual characters (Tanner stage) and body mass index
   - Assess the volume and consistency of testis and epididymis
   - Look for bilateral vas, and notice if it is absent, beaded or thickened
   - Examine for varicocele

   Males with OATS have an increased risk for testicular cancer.[12]

8. **How do you clinically assess the testicular volume?**

   Ans: Prader orchidometer is used to assess volume though orchidometer over-estimates volume measured on ultrasound by 2–3 ml. [13] Longitudinal axis of testis (4.6 cm) is usually used as a parameter.

9. **Is scrotal ultrasound required for this patient?**

   Ans: The EAA guidelines recommend USG scrotum for all patients (low quality evidence) to exclude

TABLE 1.1: Medications that can suppress fertility[5,6]

Medication class	*Examples*	*Mechanism*
GnRH agonists/antagonists	Leuprolide, goserelin	Suppression of gonadotropins
Androgens	Testosterone, nandrolone	Suppression of gonadotropins
Anti-androgens	Ketoconazole, spironolactone, flutamide	Inhibits biosynthesis of testosterone or its binding
5α reductase inhibitors	Dutasteride, finasteride	Inhibition of DHT synthesis from testosterone
Opiates	Methadone, morphine	Suppresses gonadotropins
Oestrogens	Oestradiol, oils	Suppresses gonadotropins
Antipsychotics	Risperidone, chlorpromazine	Hyperprolactinemia suppresses gonadotropins
Alpha blockers	Silodosin, tamsulosin	Retrograde ejaculation
Steroids	Dexamethasone, prednisolone	Suppresses gonadotropin secretion and hypothalamus
Cannabinoids	Tetrahydrocannabinol	Anti-motility effect
Antidepressants	Citalopram	Directly affects spermatogenesis
Chemotherapy	Cisplatin, cyclophosphamide, vinblastine, methotrexate	Directly affects spermatogenesis

testicular cancer/microlithiasis; confirm a clinical varicocele and when genital tract obstruction is suspected. However, the AUA/ASRM suggested scrotal USG only when clinical examination is difficult obese or previously operated cases.[14]

The next step in evaluation will be to do a serum hormonal assay.

10. What is indication for hormone testing?

Ans: Follicle stimulating hormone (FSH), total testosterone (7–11 AM), luteinizing hormone (LH) and estradiol in men with oligospermia (EAA/AUA/ASRM).

Sperm concentration <10 million per ml, impaired libido, erectile dysfunction or atrophic testis are indications for.[15] FSH is an important factor which shows the level of testicular failure leading to oligospermia, guided by the other hormone levels as given below.[16] A lower normal or lower testosterone level, along with elevated estradiol levels can guide the treatment plan.

11. What are the reference values of hormones routinely prescribed in low sperm counts?

Ans:

TABLE 1.2: Reference values for reproductive hormones (values here are representative and vary markedly depending on the assay used

Hormone	*Values*	*Units*
LH	2–8	IU/L
FSH	2–8	IU/L
Testosterone, total	300	ng/dl
Estradiol	20–45	pg/ml
Prolactin	<15	ng/ml

12. Is there a cut-off value of FSH to suggest primary testicular cause?

Ans: FSH >7.6 suggests spermatogenic failure.[16] The value has to be interpreted in accordance with the reference range for the assay used. Another study by Jensen *et al.* suggests that FSH >10 IU/ml has 85% predictive power to detect count <20 million/ml.[17]

13. When is prolactin indicated?

Ans: Prolactin levels should be checked in cases of hypogonadotropic hypogonadism. Thyroid evaluation is not usually done.[18] Prolactin is performed in men with total testosterone <200 ng/dl, impaired libido or those with headache or visual disturbances. Hyperprolactinemia (1.5 times normal value) independently suppresses the HPG axis.[15]

Let us assume that our index case has normal values of FSH/LH/testosterone (LH: 4.5 IU/L; FSH 5.6 IU/L; Testosterone, total 321 ng/dl; estradiol 33 pg/ml)

14. When is genetic testing indicated in oligospermia?

Ans: Genetic testing is indicated when sperm densities are less than 5 million/ml.[16]

15. What are the usual genetic tests for oligospermia?

Ans: In case of men with <5 million per ml, karyotyping should be done and also for Y chromosome should be screened for microdeletions.[16]

16. How to proceed in case of pyospermia?

Ans: If there are plenty of round cells in semen with symptoms of genital infection appropriate antibiotics are needed.[19] This is separately dealt with in subsequent topics.

17. When do you suspect partial obstruction of distal seminal tract in oligospermic individuals?

Ans: Men with OATS and reduced semen volume (not related to hypogonadism or absent vas) and/or significant semen parameter problems, an acidic pH or low fructose should be investigated with transrectal USG. Intraprostatic cyst; Wolffian (communicating) or Mullerian (non-communicating) but compressing ejaculatory duct (ED) or ED stenosis can give rise to obstruction.[20]

Assuming that hormones, semen leucocytes are all normal and patient BMI is 24 kg/m^2, which probably qualifies for idiopathic oligospermia, the routine management is to initiate on antioxidants and non-medical therapy.

18. What is the role of supplements in oligospermia?

Ans:

- Vitamin supplements have weak or anecdotal evidential support but nevertheless appealing as they do no harm, less expensive and the doctor does something while the sperm counts improve spontaneously.[21]

19. What are the non-medical treatment aspects for oligospermia?

Ans:

- Lifestyle changes
  - Healthy balanced diet
  - Good sleep
  - Regular resistance and/or high intensity exercise
- There are no well-powered studies for role of heat, type of underwear.[22]

20. What are the lifestyle and environmental changes recommended in present case?

Ans: There is low quality evidence linking diet, smoking to sperm motility and morphology with poor ART results. Similarly, stress is linked to decreased progressive motility, while cell phones have no impact. Finasteride at doses <1 mg/day for hair loss treatment is not harmful. Lead, heavy metals, agricultural pesticides, oil and natural gas extraction industries affects sperm production.[23] Phthalates are solvents used in personal care products/enteric coated medications which may impact motility and concentration of sperms.[24]

21. What are the antioxidants used in treatment of OAT?

Ans: Zinc, folic acid, vitamins C and E, co-enzyme Q10, selenium, carnitine, N-acetyl cysteine are commonly used. Showell *et al.* in a Cochrane review of 48 RCTs of 4179 sub-fertile men concluded that a low-quality evidence of increased pregnancy rates exists.[25]

As the couple age is < 35 years and provided the female partner has no adverse factors, we can recommend a trial of medical therapy with antioxidants, vitamins in this patient.

As our patient had almost normal hormonal evaluation, can we start him on clomiphene citrate along with antioxidants/vitamin supplements over 2–3 months before re-assessment. The role of clomiphene citrate is more so in patients with lower FSH and low normal testosterone.

22. What is the role of antiestrogens in OAT?

Ans: Though not FDA approved the selective estrogen receptor modulator clomiphene blocks estrogen feedback in pituitary, thereby increasing FSH/LH levels. A recent meta-analysis of all studies suggested that 50 mg doses may improve concentration motility and spontaneous pregnancy rate.[26] Another recent systematic review published in 2019 comparing clomiphene or tamoxifen 20 mg to placebo or no treatment suggested improvement in gonadotropin/testosterone levels along with the morphology and pregnancy rates.[27] We conclude that clomiphene or tamoxifen can be prescribed in idiopathic infertility with low FSH levels and low normal testosterone levels.

23. What is the role of gonadotropins in oligospermia?

Ans: They are mainly indicated in those with hypogonadotrophic hypogonandism.

24. What is TE ratio?

Ans: Ratio of serum testosterone in ng/ml to estradiol level in pg/ml, values should be > 10: 1 If ratio < 10:1, especially in an obese individual, then anastrazole 1 mg per day or letrozole 2.5–5 mg per day is indicated.[28]

25. What is the role of aromatase inhibitors?

Aromatase inhibitors; letrozole 2.5–5 mg or anastrozole 1mg block the enzyme aromatase that converts testosterone to estradiol. As a result, the negative feedback on pituitary is removed and FSH increases. Also, intra-testicular and serum levels of testosterone increase. In obese individuals aromatase expression is greater exacerbating testosterone deficiency.[28]

26. Is there a role of routine application of newer sperm function tests in this patient?

Ans: The role of seminal oxidative stress and sperm DNA fragmentation is yet to be applied on large scale setting. Studies have suggested a decreased abstinence may limit sperm DNA damage.[29]

27. What is the importance of sperm DNA fragmentation in these patients?

Ans: According to AUA/ASRM guidelines, no prospective data is available on its impact on clinical management. DNA fragmentation index can be done in the semen analysis with cut-off values <15%: Normal; 15–30%: Moderate damage may need ART;>30%: Poor fertility potential proceed with testis-ICSI (values vary as per the assay used). It is indicated when planning for ART, whether to consider ART vs natural conception or when IUI is considered to measure success.[30]

28. How does reactive oxygen species (ROS) affect sperms?

Ans: In about 50% of male infertility, an imbalance between oxidative stress and the antioxidant capacity is found in semen. ROS causes damage to membranes of sperm. This leads to lipid peroxidation which affects motility and acrosome reaction. They also lead to DNA fragmentation.[31]

Advanced sperm function tests are discussed in detail in further cases. As patient did not have significant improvement the couple was considered for ART.

29. When is early assisted reproduction considered in low sperm counts?

Ans: Assisted reproduction (ART) may be required if there are adverse female factors (age 35; Tubal block) or advanced paternal age/genetic defects, failure of medical therapy, couples seeking immediate results; with IUI being the initial therapy. ART particularly ICSI is a powerful tool as it bypasses the need for thorough male partner evaluation albeit with risks to female partner.[32]

30. What is the role of injectable FSH in this case?

Ans: Although indicated only in hypogonadotrophic hypogonadism—treatment with 150 IU twice a weekly over a period of 12 weeks resulted in better sperm concentration and also pregnancy rates.[33] A sub-group meta-analysis from this study showed resultant overall OR was 4.5 (CI 2.17 to 9.33 $p < 0.001$). FSH showed beneficial effects of FSH on live birth and pregnancy.[34] Limitation of FSH therapy is that it is not FDA approved and costly; response depends on FSH receptor polymorphisms.[35]

31. Is there a benefit of hCG injection in this case?

Ans: For men with infertility and low gonadotrophin levels it is primarily indicated. It is less expensive and in adults can be used without adding FSH too. Improvement in sperm output is noted after 3–6 months therapy at doses 1000–2500U/2–3 times a week.[36]

32. What is the success rate for IUI for this patient?

Ans: IUI processes semen by washing and involves injecting this low volume sample into the uterine cavity at the time of ovulation with or without ovarian stimulation. For IUI a minimum of 3–5 million motile sperms per ejaculate are needed.[37] During processing 50% of sperms do not survive, so at least 5–10 million sperms must be there in the sample. Men with low TMSC <5 million after processing have lower pregnancy rates.[37]

33. What is the role of IVF in this case scenario?

Ans: The likelihood of natural conception depends on the severity of oligospermia, duration of frequent timed sexual activity, partners age and reproductive status. The outcome of ICSI in oligospermia depends on female partner age. This in turn has an impact on oocyte and embryo quality. If the woman is < 35 years there is 20% success rate per cycle and 70% cumulative pregnancy rate.[38] There are methods to select individual sperms in oligospermia using morphology, electrophoresis and binding of sperm to zona.

KEY POINTS

- Oligospermia is characterised by a variety of factors including hormonal imbalance and genetic causes
- Evaluation includes physical examination and hormonal panel
- Medical treatment includes antioxidants, hormonal manipulation if reports suggest and lifestyle changes
- Assisted reproduction is considered if adequate improvement is not possible with conservative treatment and there is no surgical cause.

SUMMARY

- Oligozoospermia (<16 million per ml) is diagnosed based on multiple semen analysis and is followed by etiology assessment. History, hormones, look for varicocele and drugs causing infertility are important. There is no routine role for ultrasound or routine sperm function tests.
- Treatment of cause such as hormonal problems, varicocele or male accessory gland infection can help in improvement of sperm parameters along with empiric antioxidants.
- There is no role for empiric antiestrogen or hormonal therapy.
- In case there is no improvement with lifestyle changes and empiric medical therapy, one has to proceed for assisted reproduction.
- Treatment should involve evaluation of female partner and prior treatment failures.

REFERENCES

1. Agarwal, A.; Mulgund, A.; Hamada, A.; Chyatte, M.R. A unique view on male infertility around the globe. Reprod. Biol. Endocrinol.2015, 13, 37.

Flowchart 1.1: Evaluation of oligospermia[39]

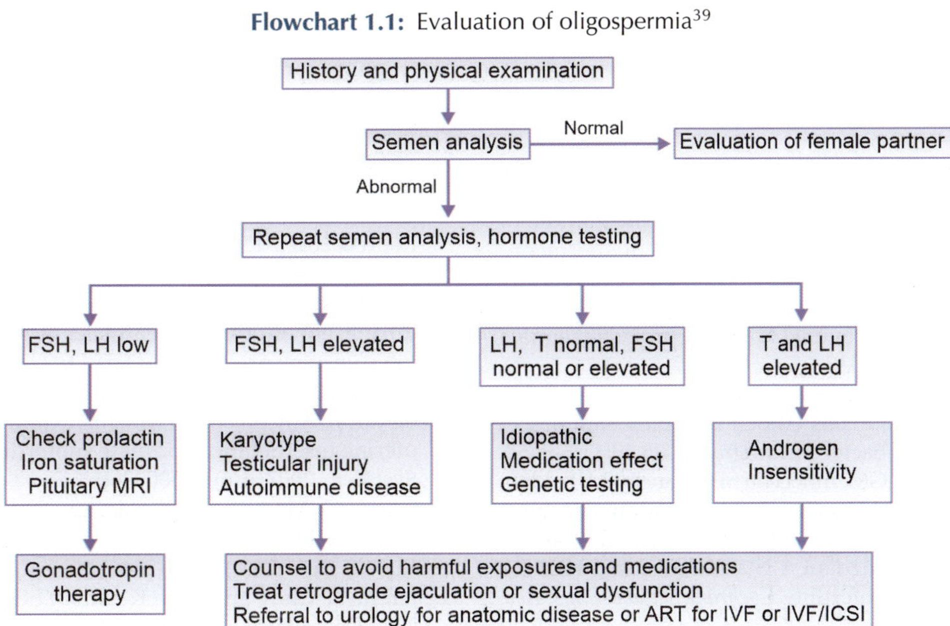

2. Punab M, Poolamets O, Paju P, *et al.* Causes of male infertility in 1737 patients. *Hum Reprod.* 2017;32(1):18–31.
3. Francavilla F, Barbonetti A, Necozione S, Santucci R, Cordeschi G, Macerola B & Francavilla S.Within-subject variation of seminal parameters in men with infertile marriages. Int J Androl 2007;30, 174–181.
4. Anawalt BD, Braunstein GD. Testes. In: Gardner DG, Shoback D, eds. *Greenspan's Basic and Clinical Endocrinology.* 10th ed. New York, NY: McGraw-Hill Education; 2017.
5. Antony T, Alzaharani SY, El-Ghaiesh SH. Opioid-induced hypogonadism: pathophysiology, clinical and therapeutics review. *Clin Exp Pharmacol Physiol.* 2020;47(5):741–750.
6. de Ronde W, Smit DL. Anabolic androgenic steroid abuse in young males. *Endocr Connect.* 2020;9(4): R102–R111.
7. Levine H, Jorgensen N, Martino-Andrade A, *et al.* Temporal trends in sperm count: a systematic review and meta-regression analysis. *Hum Reprod Update.* 2017;23(6):646–659.
8. Fernandez CJ, Chacko EC, Pappachan JM. Male obesity-related secondary hypogonadism–pathophysiology, clinical implications, and management. *Eur Endocrinol.* 2019;15(2): 83–90.
9. Kasman AM, Zhang CA, Li S, Stevenson DK, Shaw GM, Eisenberg ML. Association of preconception paternal health on perinatal outcomes: analysis of U.S. claims data. *Fertil Steril.* 2020;113(5):947–954.
10. Shaw W, Padubidri V, Daftary S, Howkins J, Bourne G. Infertility and sterility. In: *Shaw's Textbook of Gynaecology.* 16th ed. New Delhi, India: Elsevier; 2015:237–262.
11. Overhoff S, Dahm C, Rivero MA, Ferreira U, Schirren C. Andrological findings in hemicastration, lack of a testis, and reduced testicular volume. *Andrologia.* 1989;21(5):490–497.
12. Hanson HA, Anderson RE, Aston KI, Carrell DT, Smith KR & Hotaling JM Subfertility increases risk of testicular cancer: evidence from population-based semen samples. Fertil Steril 2016;105, 322–328. e321.
13. Behre HM, Nashan D and Nieschlag E. Objective measurement of testicular volume by ultrasonography: evaluation of the technique and comparison with orchidometer estimates. Int J Androl 1989;12, 395–403.
14. Lotti F and Maggi M: Ultrasound of the male genital tract in relation to male reproductive health. Hum Reprod Update 2015; **21:** 56.
15. Ventimiglia E, Capogrosso P, Boeri L *et al.* Validation of the American society for reproductive medicine guidelines/ recommendations in white European men presenting for couple's infertility. Fertil Steril 2016;**106:** 1076.
16. Oates R: Evaluation of the azoospermic male. Asian J Androl 2012; **14:** 82.
17. Jensen TK, Andersson AM, Hjollund NH, Scheike T, Kolstad H, Giwercman A, Henriksen TB, Ernst E, Bonde JP, Olsen A & McNeilly A (1997) Inhibin B as a serum marker of spermatogenesis: correlation to differences in spermconcentration and follicle-stimulating hormone levels. A study of 349 Danishmen. J Clin EndocrinolMetab 82, 4059–4063.
18. Samperi I, Lithgow K, Karavitaki N. Hyperprolactinaemia. *J Clin Med.* 2019;8(12): E2203.
19. Lackner J, Schatzl G, Horvath S, Kratzik C, Marberger M. Value of counting white blood cells (WBC) in semen samples to predict the presence of bacteria. *Eur Urol.* 2006;49(1):148–52.
20. Lotti F, Corona G, Colpi GM, Innocenti SD, Mancini M, Baldi E, Noci I, Forti G & Maggi M. Seminal vesicles ultrasound features in a cohort of infertility patients. Hum Reprod 2012; 27, 974–982.
21. Showell MG, Brown J, Yazdani A, Stankiewicz MT, Hart RJ. Antioxidants for male subfertility. *Cochrane Database Syst Rev.* 2011;1:CD007411.
22. Wise LA, Cramer DW, Hornstein MD, Ashby RK & Missmer SA. Physical activity and semen quality among men attending an infertility clinic. Fertil Steril 2011; 95, 1025–1030.
23. Martenies SE and Perry MJ: Environmental and occupational pesticide exposure and human sperm parameters: A systematic review. Toxicology 2013; **307:** 66.
24. Zota AR, Calafat AM and Woodruff TJ: Temporal trends in phthalate exposures: Findings from the national health and nutrition examination survey, 2001–2010. Environ Health Perspect 2014; **122:** 235.
25. Showell MG, Mackenzie-Proctor R & Brown J. Antioxidants for male subfertility. Cochrane Database Syst Rev, 2014 CD007411.
26. Chua ME, Escusa KG, Luna S, Tapia LC, Dofitas B & Morales M. Revisiting oestrogen antagonists (clomiphene or tamoxifen) as medical empiric therapy for idiopathic male infertility: a metaanalysis. Andrology 2013; 1, 749–757.
27. Cannarella R, Condorelli RA, Mongioì LM, Barbagallo F, Calogero AE, La Vignera S. Effects of the selective estrogen receptor modulators for the treatment of male infertility: a systematic review and meta-analysis. *Expert Opin Pharmacother.* 2019;20(12):1517–1525.
28. Shoshany O, Abhyankar N, Mufarreh N, Daniel G, Niederberger C. Outcomes of anastrozole in oligozoospermic hypoandrogenic subfertile men. *Fertil Steril.* 2017;107(3):589–594.
29. Ayad BM, Horst GV and Plessis SSD: Revisiting the relationship between the ejaculatory abstinence period and semen characteristics. Int J Fertil Steril 2018; **11:** 238.
30. Dong J, Lv Y, Zhu G *et al.* Effect of sperm DNA fragmentation on the clinical outcomes of two assisted reproduction methods: Ivf and icsi. Int J Clin Exp Med 2017; **10:** 11812.
31. Agarwal, A.; Finelli, R.; Selvam, M.K.P.; Leisegang, K.; Majzoub, A.; Tadros, N.; Ko, E.; Parekh, N.; Henkel, R.; Durairajanayagam, D.; *et al.* A Global Survey of Reproductive Specialists to Determine the Clinical Utility of Oxidative Stress Testing and Antioxidant Use in Male Infertility. World J. Men's Health **2021**, 39, 470–488.
32. Verpoest W, Tournaye H. ICSI: hype or hazard? *HumFertil (Camb).*2006;9:81–92.
33. Santi D, Granata ARM and Simoni M: Fsh treatment of male idiopathic infertility improves pregnancy rate: A meta-analysis. Endocr Connect 2015; **4:** R46.
34. Attia AM, Abou-Setta AM & Al-Inany HG (2013) Gonadotrophins for idiopathic male factor subfertility. Cochrane Database Syst Re, CD005071.
35. Simoni M, Santi D & Negri L. Treatment with human, recombinant FSH improves sperm DNA fragmentation in idiopathic infertile men depending on the FSH receptor polymorphism p. N680S: a pharmacogenetic study. Hum Reprod 2016;31, 1960–1969.
36. Liu PY, Baker HW, Jayadev V, Zacharin M, Conway AJ, Handelsman DJ. Induction of spermatogenesis and fertility during gonadotropin treatment of gonadotropin-deficient infertile men: predictors of fertility outcome. *J Clin Endocrinol Metab.* 2009;94(3):801–808.
37. Bensdorp AJ, Cohlen BJ, Heineman MJ, Vandekerckhove P. Intrauterine insemination for male subfertility. *Cochrane Database Syst Rev.* 2007; 4(4):CD000360.
38. Gnoth C, Maxrath B, Skonieczny T, Friol K, Godehardt E, Tigges J. Final ART success rates: a 10 years survey. *Hum Reprod.* 2011;26(8):2239–2246.
39. Jeremy T Choy and John K Amory.J Clin Endocrinol Metab. 2020 Dec; 105(12): e4194–e4207.

Chapter

2

Asthenozoospermia

• Guru Balaji Shanmugham • Sanjay Prakash J

LEARNING OBJECTIVES

- To assess the etiology of asthenospermia.
- To formulate the management and decide regarding surgical management.
- To proceed with assisted reproduction techniques after reasonable attempt to improve sperm parameters.

INTRODUCTION

Asthenozoospermia is pathological state where the progressive motility of sperm is defective. Although it commonly occurs in combination with abnormality of counts and morphology, the incidence of isolated asthenozoospermia itself is 18–20%. This chapter discusses the various etiological factors, algorithmic management and the fertility outcomes.

Case Scenario

A 36-year-old obese IT professional with diabetes mellitus for 4 years, and wife 26-year-old, married for 5 years, primary infertility; SA shows 16 million sperm per ml; 10% PR and 3% normal forms. How to approach this situation?

1. **What is the definition of asthenozoospermia as per the WHO 6th manual of semenology?**

   Ans:

   - According to the WHO 5th manual, asthenozoospermia refers to percentage of progressively motile (PR) spermatozoa less than 32%, which is below the lower reference limit (5th percentile).[1] But the 6th manual has removed the term asthenozoospermia has revised PR to 30% and also has introduced the concept of "decision limits". The latest edition has explained that the reference thresholds alone are meaningless and multiparametric interpretation is necessary to establish the diagnosis of male infertility. The lower 5th percentile of data may not be representative of fertile versus infertile men.[2] However, guidelines bodies like EAU, still consider the usage of removed nomenclatures still clinically relevant in practice.[3] For practical purposes PR less than 30% can be considered as asthenozoospermia.

2. **What are the causes of asthenozoospermia?**

   Ans:

   - There are many causes for asthenozoospermia. Usually multiple causes co-exist. Hence eliciting a proper and detailed history is indispensable. The various causes are enlisted in Table 2.1.[4–12]

TABLE 2.1: Etiology of asthenozoospermia

Common causes
1. Lifestyle—tobacco chewing and smoking, moderate to heavy alcohol consumption, caffeine, drugs of abuse usage, obesity, metabolic syndrome, advance age.
2. Diet—prepared meat, fatty dairy products, excess coffee, aerated and non-aerated sweet drinks
3. Mental stress, sleep disorders
4. Hormonal imbalance—hypogonadism (primary and secondary), T:E ratio reversal (<10:1), hyperprolactinemia
5. Environmental—radiation, occupational exposure (e.g. pesticides, excess heat), radiofrequency electromagnetic fields (RF-EMF), e.g. excess mobile phones, laptop exposure
6. Iatrogenic—anti-androgens, steroids, radiotherapy, and chemotherapy (especially alkylating agents)

(Contd.)

TABLE 2.1: Etiology of asthenozoospermia *(Contd.)*
7. Varicocele
8. Genitourinary infections, STI (Claymdia trachomatis)
9. Sample collection errors—prolonged abstinence, lubricant use, contamination of sample with antiseptic solution, soap or water
10. Trauma
11. Idiopathic
Uncommon Causes
1. Genetic—immotile cilia syndrome, cystic fibrosis, PCKD, rare mutations (AKAP3, AKAP4, AXDN1, DNAH1, 2, 6, 8, etc.)
2. Acute systemic illness
3. Antisperm antibodies
4. Testicular malignancy, GCNIS
PCKD: Polycystic kidney disease, T:E: Testosterone: Estradiol, RF-EMF: Radiofrequency electromagnetic field, STI: Sexually transmitted infection, GCNIS: Gonadal cell neoplasia-*in-situ*

3. How do you approach a patient with asthenozoospermia?

Ans:

- Evaluation of asthenozoospermia starts with detailed history of both the partners, focussed examination of the male reproduction and first line investigations include a semen analysis and hormonal profile. It is ideal to perform two semen analysis 2–4 weeks apart to confirm the diagnosis. Ancillary tests can be ordered based on specific history and examination findings. Doppler ultrasound of scrotum is indicated in specific circumstances such as doubtful clinical varicocele, tight scrotum precluding examination, obese men or previous scrotal surgery including varicocele repair. Table 2.2 enlists the salient features in evaluation of asthenozoospermia[3,12–14] and Flowchart 2.1 depicts algorithmic approach to asthenozoospermia.

TABLE 2.2: Evaluation of asthenozoospermia
A. Medical history
1. Patient and partner's age
2. Duration of marriage
3. Since when trying for a child
4. Any h/o horomonal constraception
5. Any clinical/biochemical pregnancies, abortions, IUI/IVF attempts
6. Any ED, frequency of intercourse
7. Past history—medical (recurrent chest infections, tuberculosis, etc) and surgical (UDT with orchidopexy, torsion testis, etc)
8. Drug history
9. Personal history: Habits, occupation
10. Partner history: Menstrual history, any previous evaluations
B. Examination
i. General—assessment of secondary sexual characters, gynecomastia ii. Local a. Testis—size, volume, texture and consistency b. Cord—presence/absence of vas, varicocele c. Epididymis—full/fat d. Penis—any abnormalities
C. Investigations
i. Semen analysis (1–2 days abstinence) ii. Hormone profile: FSH, LH, total testosterone, E2 iii. Scrotal Doppler: Testicular size assessment, epididymal head size, varicocele
D. Ancillary investigations
i. DFI, ROS ii. Prolactin, 17-OHP iii. TRUS—if infective etiology is suspected, to assess SV and prostate iv. MRI pelvis and scrotum—if scrotal Doppler is difficult (obesity), TRUS equivocal or patient uncooperative for TRUS v. Semen C/S, gene Xpert TB semen—clinical suspicion of GUTB vi. Urine R/E, urine C/S, USG KUB—to investigate for UTI
IUI: Intrauterine insemination, IVF: In-vitro fertilization, ED: Erectile dysfunction, UDT: Undescended testis, DFI: DNA fragmentation index, ROS: Reactive oxygen species, FSH: Follicular stimulating hormone, LH: Luteinizing hormone, E2: Estradiol, 17-OHP-17 Hydroxyprogesterone, TRUS: Transrectal ultrasound, TB: Tuberculosis

4. What is the management of isolated asthenozoospermia and what is the duration of treatment?

Ans: There are multiple facets in management of asthenozoospermia. They are being enlisted below and discussed in detail.

a. Ensure proper semen sample collection:

- Ensure ideal abstinence time is minimum 2 days and maximum 7 days for the first sample, and instruct for shorter abstinence time (1–2 days) for the 2nd sample.
- Ensure no lubricant use/condom collection, contamination or antiseptic solution and soap
- Examination time—ideal is 30 minutes and maximum is 60 minutes.
- Viscous sample—start testing if liquefies in 30 minutes; else leave at 37 °C (incubator) for 30 minutes, and then investigations should be started. Warm the sample to 37 °C as the motile spermatozoa is temperature dependent. Viscosity can be broken manually by repeated aspiration or adding bromhelain to the sample.[1,14]

Flowchart 2.1: Algorithmic approach to asthenozoospermia

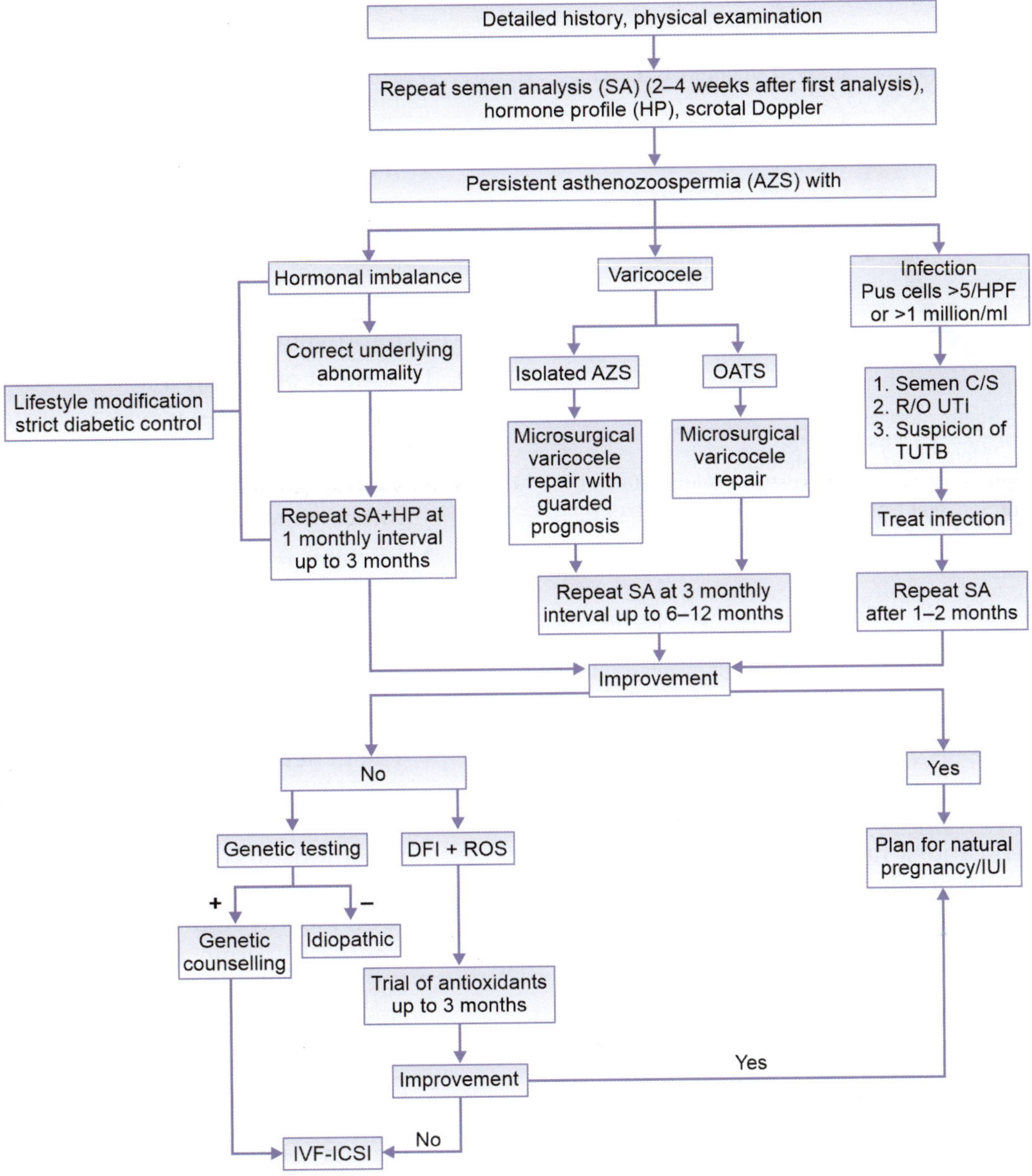

b. Lifestyle modification:

- Regular exercise and avoidance of sedentary lifestyle
- Management of obesity and metabolic syndrome
- Stress management (yoga and medications) and sleep disorders correction
- Diet: Fruits, vegetables, poultry, fish, cereals and low-fat dairy products
- Occupation related modification—prevention of excess genital heat exposure, reduction of Radio-frequency electromagnetic field exposure
- Adhering to a good lifestyle, not only overall improves the semen parameters by 10–15% but also improves the response to specific treatment.[9–11,15,16]

c. Role of antioxidants:

- The routinely used antioxidant combinations include vitamin A, vitamin C, vitamin E, carnitine, N-acetyl cysteine, coenzyme Q10 and lycopene, along with zinc, selenium, and folic acid (Fig. 2.1), however, there is no evidence of advantage in prescribing multiple antioxidants over single antioxidant
- The commercially available preparations include combinations in varying doses and are prescribed either as once daily or twice daily dosing as there is no specific consensus on dosage.
- There are variable reports regarding sperms parameters improvement and pregnancy outcomes in the literature

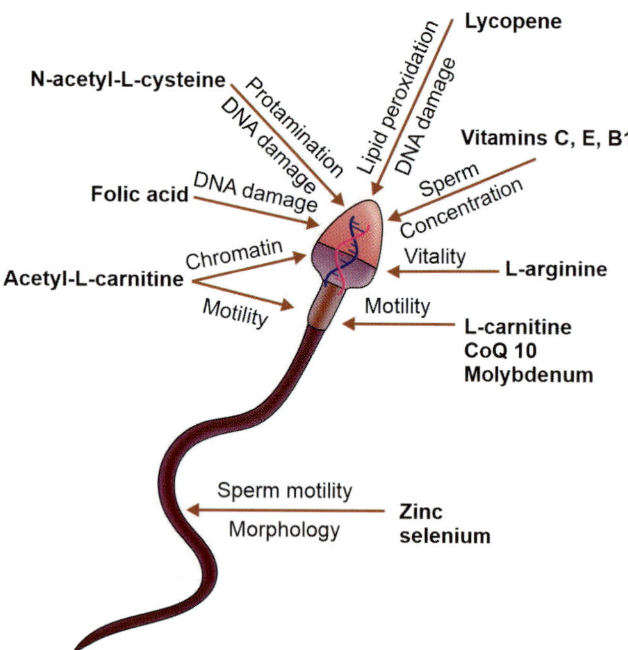

Fig. 2.1: Role of antioxidants in different parts of the sperms

- Studies have used them for different durations, from 1 to 12 months as primary treatment and adjunct post-varicocele repair.
- 10–15% improvement has been documented
- The medications have to be prescribed for a minimum of 3 months (at least 1 spermatogenesis cycle) for any improvement.
- Beyond 3 months if no improvement is there, continuing medications may not be beneficial.[17–19]

d. Role of varicocele repair (VR):

- As per AUA/ASRM and EAU guidelines, varicocele repair is recommended when there is infertility associated with at least single sperm parameter abnormality or oligoasthenoteratozoospermia (OATS). Guarded prognosis has to be discussed if it is isolated asthenozoospermia. It takes a 3–6 months (1–2 spermatogenesis cycles) for the improvement to reflect on the sperm parameters.[3,13,20]
- Factors such as grade of varicocele (higher grades have better outcomes), testicular volume (low volume has lesser chances of improvement), semen parameters (severe abnormalities may not show significant improvement), hormonal levels (preoperative elevated FSH and LH will have poor outcomes), prognostic biomarkers, duration of infertility, and the couple's age decide success of VR.[21,22]
- VR before proceeding to IVF-ICSI is controversial. Meta-analysis by Esteves et al, and Kirby et al, have reported improved clinical pregnancies and live birth rates. Hence, some couples may benefit from having VR before IVF-ICSI.[23,24]
- It is increasingly becoming a routine practice to perform DNA fragmentation index (DFI), reactive oxygen species (ROS) before a varicocele repair for recurrent pregnancy loss and a repeat after 3 months to look for improvement in DFI, ROS.[25]

e. Treatment of infections:

- Antibiotics to 3–4 weeks according to semen C/S antibiogram
- Repeat semen analysis after 6–8 weeks for improvement
- In case of genitourinary tuberculosis, treatment with antituberculous treatment for 6–9 months, with prior cryopreservation is essential due to chances of epididymal fibrosis.[28,26]

f. Role of genetic testing:

- The genetic etiology of asthenozoospermia is heterogenous. The incidence of MMAF is <10%. Genetic counselling (both genetic mutations and PGT) can help in reducing risk of transmission of genetic defects by ICSI. However, in routine practice it is not frequently done as it is time consuming, costs involved and lower incidence. It should be a joint decision of the clinician and the couple.[27]
- Primary ciliary dyskinesia (PCD)– suspected in patients with normozoospermia/oligozoospermia, severe/absolute asthenozoospermia with acceptable morphology/teratozoospermia and vitality, normal hormone profile and h/o recurrent chest infections. Pregnancy can be achieved by IVF-ICSI using ejaculate sperm or testicular sperms in azoospermia (rarely).[28]

5. What are the genetic and flagellar defects in asthenozoospermia?

Ans:

- Flagella, the structure responsible for sperm motility, contains axonemal and peri-axonemal structures (Fig. 2.2). Based on the peri-axonemal structures, there are four regions in the sperm flagellum-connecting piece, midpiece, principal piece, and end piece.[6,17,29,30,31]
- AZS can be isolated (no other major health complications. Multiple morphological

Section 5

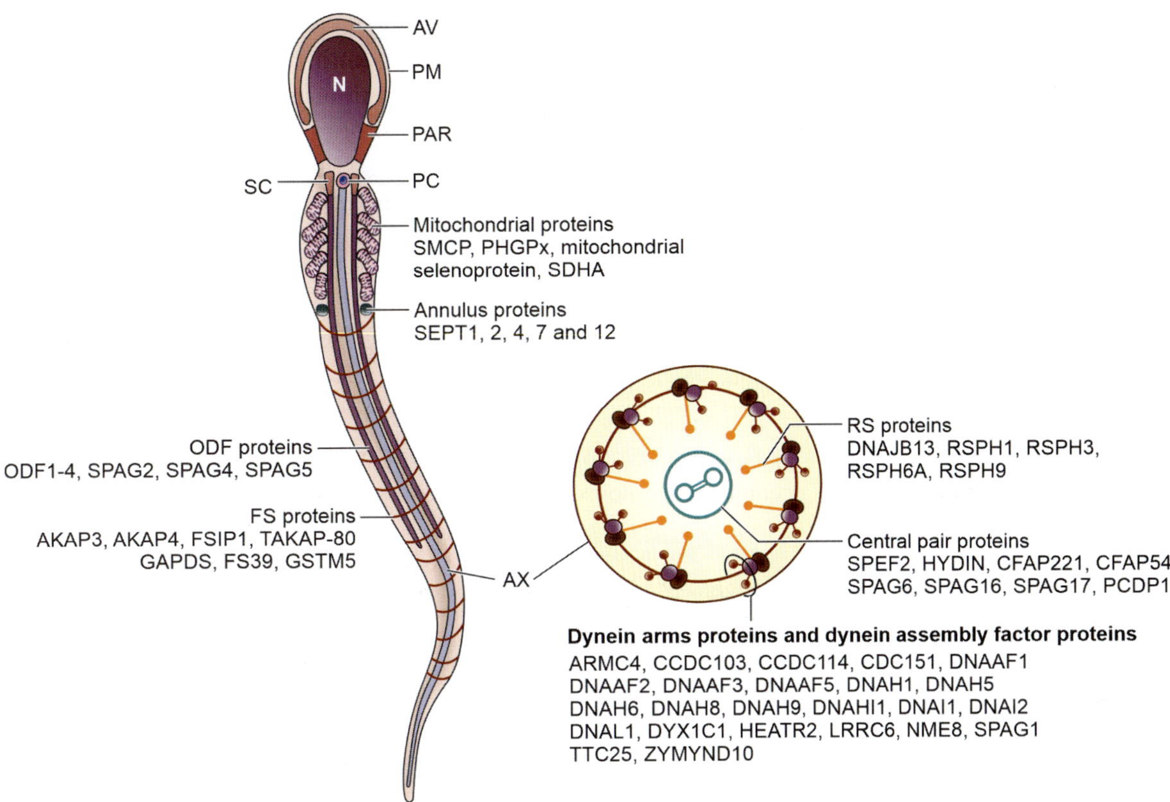

Fig. 2.2: Structure of sperm flagella and significant genes modulating their function (Adopted from Pereira R, Sousa M. Morphological and Molecular Bases of Male Infertility: A Closer Look at Sperm Flagellum. Genes (Basel). 2023 Feb 1;14(2):383. doi: 10.3390/genes14020383. PMID: 36833310; PMCID: PMC9956255)

abnormalities of the sperm flagella (MMAF)) and a syndromic form of AZS characterized by several concurrent clinical symptoms with varied phenotypic expressivity. Table 2.3 summarises the various genetic defects associated with AZS.[27]

TABLE 2.3: Genetic defects associated with AZS and their significance

Isolated AZS (MMAF: Multiple morphological abnormalities of sperm flagella)		
Structural defects	***Function***	***Gene mutation***
Outer dynein arms (ODAs) and inner dynein arms (IDAs)	Maintaining flagellum/ciliary beat frequency and normal waveform	DNAHl, DNAH2, DNAH6, DNAH8, DNAH17, CFAP70, CFAP43 and CFAP44
Radial spokes and central pair complex (CPC)	Beating of flagella/cilia by regulating the activity of the dyneins	CFAP251, CFAP91, CFAP65, CFAP58, and SPEF2
FS (fibrous sheath)-related protein		AKAP3, AKAP4, FSIP2
Centrosome-related proteins		CEP135 and DZIPl
Axoneme, mid-piece of flagellum	FT complexes, protein degradation, and undefined sperm localization	TTC21A, TTC29, CFAP69, QRICH2, AK7, and ARMC2,
Energy supply and signalling pathways		
FS related	Harbours the majority of glycolytic enzymes and signalling molecules that are essential for energy production for sperm motility using glycolysis	AKAP3, AKAP4, FSIP2
Annulus related	Functions as a morphological organizer, guiding flagellum assembly, as well as a diffusion barrier in mature sperm	Septin family (septins 1, 4, 6, 7 and 12), SLC26A8, CYP24A1, DNAJB13

(Contd.)

TABLE 2.3: Genetic defects associated with AZS and their significance *(Contd.)*

Sperm mitochondria	Oxidative phosphorylation (energy production), oxidative metabolism, free radical generation	Mitochondrial DNA (mtDNA) 4977bp deletion, COIII, ND4
Soluble adenylyl cyclase (sAC)	cAMP/PRKA (protein kinase-A) pathways—cAMP dependant phosphorylation of agellar proteins, including axonemal dynein, essential step in the initiation and maintenance of sperm motility	ADCY10 gene
CatSper channels	cAMP-stimulated rise in intracellular sperm calcium which plays a central role in sperm motility and fertilization	CATSPER 1,2,E
SYNDROMIC		
Primary ciliary dyskinesia	Defects in dynein arms, formation of the central pair complex and radial spokes	DNAAFI,2,3,4,5,6, ZMYND10, LRRC6, C11orf70, TTC12, DNAHS,9, DNAIl,2, CCDC39, CCDC40, RSPH1,3,4A,9, SPAG6, HYDIN, DNAJB13, GAS2L2
ADPCKD	Arrangement of axonemal structures in flagellum	PKDI or PKD 2
Retinal Ciliopathy	Arrangement of axonemal structures in flagellum	TILLS, ARL2BP

6. How to specifically evaluate and manage the given case scenario?

Ans: Specific management is described in Flowchart 2.2.

7. How to differentiate between asthenozoospermia and necrozoospermia?

Ans: As per the WHO 5th manual, necrozoospermia (NZS) is defined as low percentage of live (<58%), and high percentage of immotile spermatozoa in the ejaculate. Testing for necrozoospermia is done if motility is less than 40%.[1] As aforementioned, the 6th edition of the WHO manual has removed the standards suggests that it is not necessary to assess vitality when at least 40% of spermatozoa are motile and the normal vitality has been revised to 54%.[2] Despite the prevailing confusions in definitions, for practical purposes testing for NZS is done when motility is ≤ 40%.[32] The incidence is about 0.2–0.4% of male infertility cases. The causes are mostly the same as aforementioned but its impact is more severe to cause necrozoospermia.[33] Absolute asthenozoospermia, denied as 100% immotile sperms, has to be differentiated from NZS, where although sperms are live but are immotile.[33,34] Management of NZS and absolute AZS is described in Flowchart 2.3.

8. What is the approach for assisted reproduction in patients of asthenozoospermia?

Ans:

- The chance of natural pregnancy decreases proportionally with the severity of AZS.
- But through assisted reproduction (ART) the couples can have their own child.
- By estimating the total motile sperm count [TMSC = (Sperm Density × Ejaculate Volume × Total Motility) ÷ 100], which serves as a better predictor of outcomes of ART). IUI should be considered for TMSC at least 5 million in the ejaculate; IVF-ICSI if TMSC <2 million and IVF if TMSC is 2 to 5 millions motile sperm.
- In case of IUI, the post-wash sperm motility carries more significance for improved outcomes.
- ICSI is the only way forward for these couples with asthenospermia.[27,29,35–38]

9. How to counsel the patients with asthenozoospermia regarding approach to fertility and pregnancy?

Ans:

- If the couples wish to conceive naturally or by IUI, has no problem waiting for minimum 3–6 months, specific treatment for asthenozoospermia can be started.
- But if the couples are already exhausted of previous investigations and treatments and if the male partner's parameters are adequate for IVF-ICSI, then the couple should be counselled directly for IVF-ICSI.
- The chances of natural conception with isolated asthenozoospermia or in combination with other pathological parameters is less
- The outcomes in terms of fertilization and pregnancy rates are better with IUI and IVF-ICSI depending on the severity of asthenozoospermia[27]

Flowchart 2.2: Specific management of the mentioned case

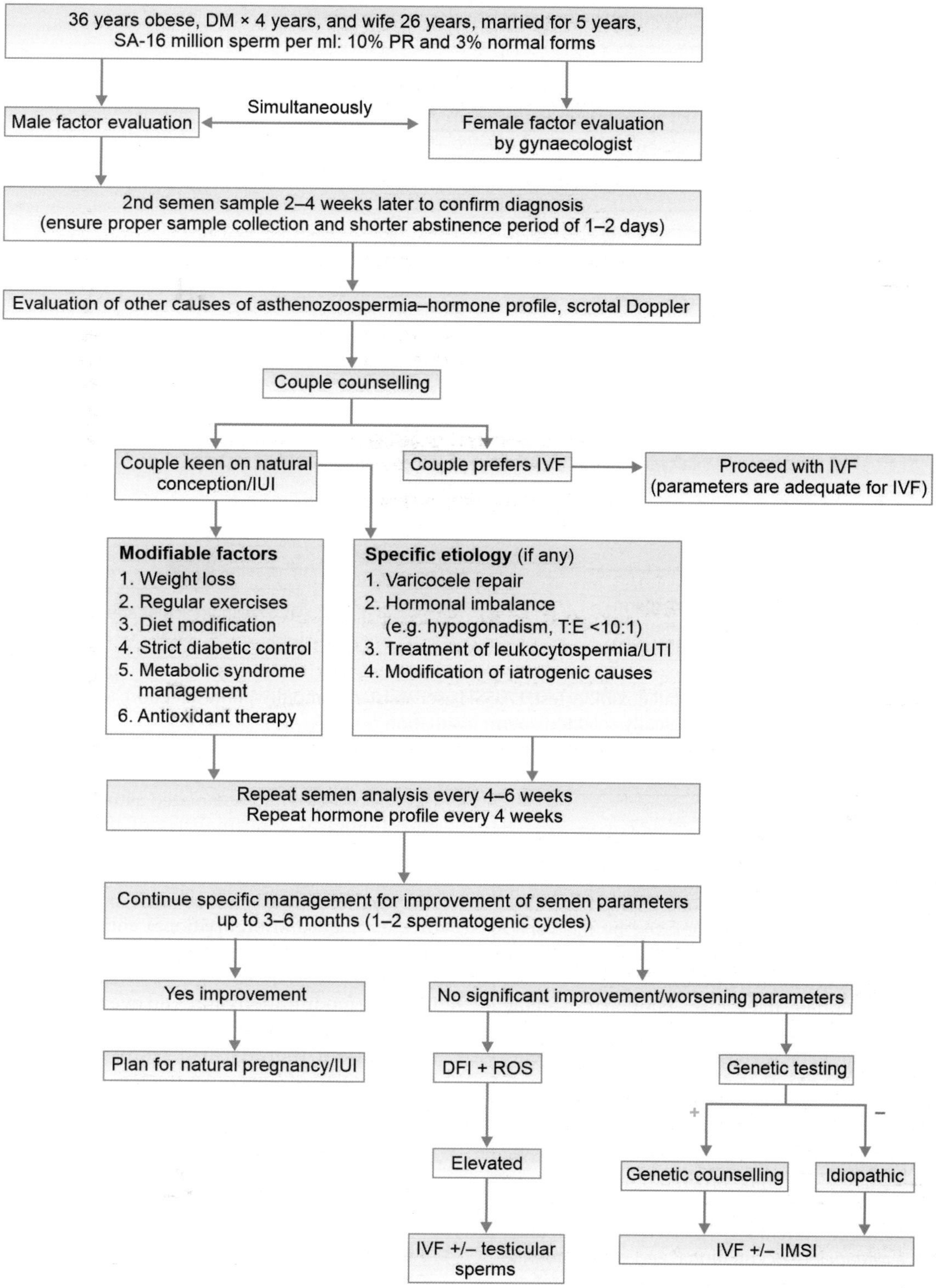

- Counsel regarding the correctable factors, probability of improvement in parameters with duration and outcomes in terms of fertilization and pregnancy rates
- With regards to genetic testing and preimplantation genetic testing (PGT), although the incidence is low, there is a chance of inheritance by the offspring, and considering the cost and time involved, it should be a combined decision of the clinician and the couples
- Encourage for a healthy lifestyle and occupational modification
- Simultaneous evaluation of the female partner and decision of waiting for a natural pregnancy/ART should be a collective decision considering the female parameters

Flowchart 2.3: Management of necrozoospermia/absolute asthenozoospermia

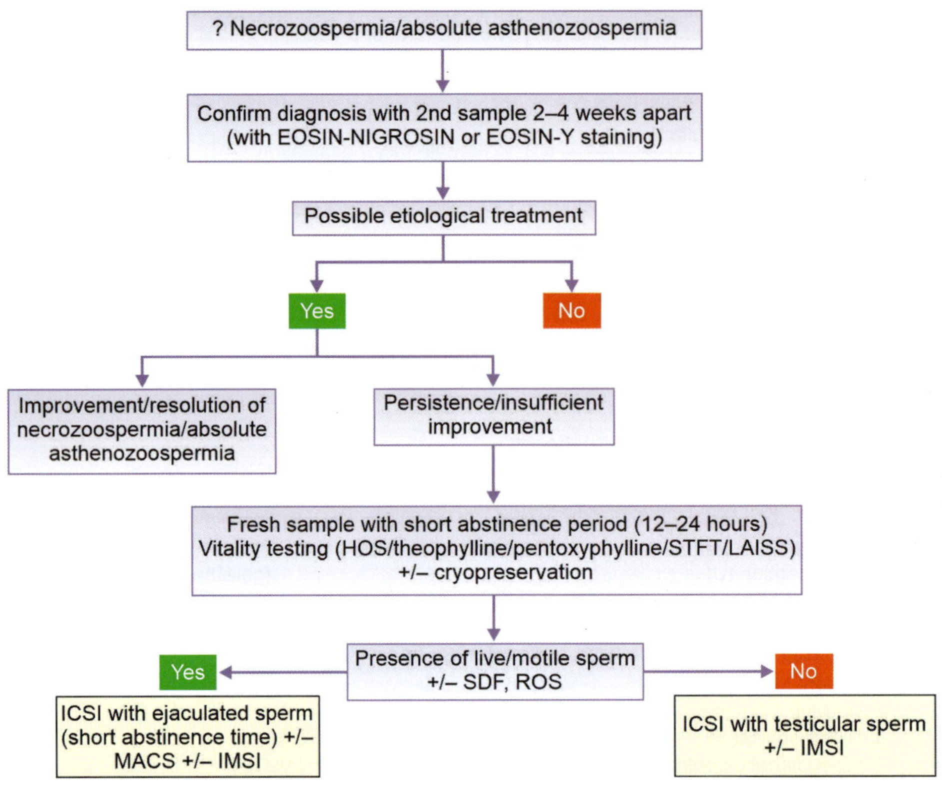

HOS: Hypoosmotic swelling test, STFT: Sperm tail flexibility test, LAISS: Laser assisted immotile sperm selection, MACS: Magnetic–activated cell sorting, IMSI: Intracytoplasmic morphologically selected sperm instillation

KEY POINTS

- Asthenozoospermia, as per WHO 5th manual, defined as percentage of progressively motile (PR) spermatozoa below the lower reference limit (5th percentile) which is 32%. Although the terminology has been removed by the WHO 6th manual, guideline committees like EAU continue to use these terminologies for practical purposes.
- Causes are multifactorial—infections, hormonal, sample collection errors, lifestyle, environmental and occupational factors, varicocele, iatrogenic, acute systemic illness, genetic, etc.
- Evaluation includes complete detailed history, focussed clinical examination of reproductive organs, investigations including semen analysis, hormonal profile and scrotal Doppler and ancillary tests can be ordered based on clinical suspicion.
- Management strategy includes lifestyle modification including diet, avoidance of occupational and environmental hazards, specific treatment of infections, varicocele repair, hormonal regulation.

SUMMARY

- Asthenozoospermia usually presents in combination with oligozoospermia with pathological morphology
- Causes are multifactorial—infections, hormonal, sample collection errors, lifestyle, environmental and occupational factors, varicocele, iatrogenic, acute systemic illness, genetic, etc.
- Genetic causes could be isolated asthenozoospermia (multiple morphological abnormalities of the flagella; MMAF) and syndromic association like primary ciliary dyskinesia and Kartagener's syndrome
- Management strategy includes lifestyle modification including diet, avoidance of occupational and environmental hazards, specific treatment of infections, varicocele repair, hormonal regulation.
- Lifestyle modification causes an overall 10–15% improvement of semen parameters
- Antioxidant therapy also results in an overall 10–15% improvement of semen parameters but has to be taken for at least 3 months
- Genetic testing for gene defects and preimplantation genetic testing has to be a shared decision between the couple and the treating clinician

REFERENCES

1. World Health Organization. WHO laboratory manual for the examination and processing of human semen. 5th ed. Geneva: WHO; 2010.
2. World Health Organization. WHO laboratory manual for the examination and processing of human semen. 6th ed. Geneva: WHO; 2021.
3. *EAU Guidelines. Edn. presented at the EAU Annual Congress Milan 2023. ISBN 978- 94-92671-19-6. ISBN 978-94-92671-19-6.*
4. Okonofua FE, Ntoimo LFC, Omonkhua A, Ayodeji O, Olafusi C, Unuabonah E, *et al.* Causes and Risk Factors for Male

Infertility: A Scoping Review of Published Studies. Int J Gen Med. 2022;15:5985–97.

5. Shah KM, Gamit KG, Raval MA, Vyas NY. Male infertility: A scoping review of prevalence, causes and treatments. Vol. 10, Asian Pacific Journal of Reproduction. Wolters Kluwer Medknow Publications; 2021. p. 195–202.
6. Pereira R, Sousa M. Morphological and Molecular Bases of Male Infertility: A Closer Look at Sperm Flagellum. Genes (Basel). 2023 Feb 1;14(2).
7. Seckin S, Ramadan H, Mouanness M, Gidon A, Thornton M, Merhi Z. A Case of Asthenozoospermia Following COVID-19 Infection. Reprod Sci. 2022 Sep;29(9):2703–5.
8. Ortega C, Verheyen G, Raick D, Camus M, Devroey P, Tournaye H. Absolute asthenozoospermia and ICSI: what are the options? Hum Reprod Update [Internet]. 2011 Sep [cited 2023 Apr 17];17(5):684–92. Available from: https://pubmed.ncbi.nlm.nih.gov/21816768/
9. Balawender K, Orkisz S. The impact of selected modifiable lifestyle factors on male fertility in the modern world. Cent European J Urol. 2020;73(4):1–6.
10. Durairajanayagam D. Lifestyle causes of male infertility. Arab J Urol. 2018 Mar;16(1):10–20.
11. Kumar N, Singh AK. Impact of environmental factors on human semen quality and male fertility: a narrative review. Vol. 34, Environmental Sciences Europe. Springer Science and Business Media Deutschland GmbH; 2022.
12. Agarwal A, Baskaran S, Parekh N, Cho CL, Henkel R, Vij S, *et al.* Male infertility. Lancet. 2021 Jan 23;397(10271):319–33.
13. Schlegel PN, Sigman M, Collura B, De Jonge CJ, Eisenberg ML, Lamb DJ, *et al.* Diagnosis and treatment of infertility in men: AUA/ASRM guideline part I. Fertil Steril. 2021 Jan 1;115(1):54–61.
14. Katz DJ, Teloken P, Shoshany O. Male infertility-The other side of the equation. Aust Fam Physician. 2017 Sep;46(9):641–6.
15. Montano L, Ceretti E, Donato F, Bergamo P, Zani C, Viola GCV, *et al.* Effects of a Lifestyle Change Intervention on Semen Quality in Healthy Young Men Living in Highly Polluted Areas in Italy: The FASt Randomized Controlled Trial. Eur Urol Focus [Internet]. 2022 Jan 1 [cited 2023 Apr 17];8(1):351–9. Available from: https://pubmed.ncbi.nlm.nih.gov/33579652/
16. Emokpae MA, Brown SI. Effects of lifestyle factors on fertility: practical recommendations for modification. Reproduction and fertility. 2021 Jan;2(1):R13–26.
17. Shahrokhi SZ, Salehi P, Alyasin A, Taghiyar S, Deemeh MR. Asthenozoospermia: Cellular and molecular contributing factors and treatment strategies. Andrologia. 2020 Mar;52(2):e13463.
18. Agarwal A, Leisegang K, Majzoub A, Henkel R, Finelli R, Panner Selvam MK, *et al.* Utility of Antioxidants in the Treatment of Male Infertility: Clinical Guidelines Based on a Systematic Review and Analysis of Evidence. World J Mens Health. 2021 Apr;39(2):233–90.
19. Wei G, Zhou Z, Cui Y, Huang Y, Wan Z, Che X, *et al.* A Meta-Analysis of the Efficacy of L-Carnitine/L-Acetyl-Carnitine or N-Acetyl-Cysteine in Men With Idiopathic Asthenozoospermia. Am J Mens Health. 2021;15(2):15579883211011372.
20. Machen GL, Johnson D, Nissen MA, Naber E, Sandlow JI. Time to improvement of semen parameters after microscopic varicocelectomy: When it occurs and its effects on fertility. Andrologia. 2020 Mar;52(2):e13500.
21. Agarwal A, Finelli R, Durairajanayagam D, Leisegang K, Henkel R, Salvio G, *et al.* Comprehensive Analysis of Global Research on Human Varicocele: A Scientometric Approach. World J Mens Health. 2022 Oct;40(4):636–52.
22. Agarwal A, Cannarella R, Saleh R, Boitrelle F, Gül M, Toprak T, *et al.* Impact of Varicocele Repair on Semen Parameters in Infertile Men: A Systematic Review and Meta-Analysis. World Journal of Men's Health. 2022;40.
23. Esteves SC, Roque M, Agarwal A. Outcome of assisted reproductive technology in men with treated and untreated varicocele: systematic review and meta-analysis. Asian J Androl [Internet]. 2016 Mar 1 [cited 2023 Apr 17];18(2):254. Available from: /pmc/articles/PMC4770495/
24. Kirby EW, Wiener LE, Rajanahally S, Crowell K, Coward RM. Undergoing varicocele repair before assisted reproduction improves pregnancy rate and live birth rate in azoospermic and oligospermic men with a varicocele: a systematic review and meta-analysis. Fertil Steril [Internet]. 2016 Nov 1 [cited 2023 Apr 17];106(6):1338–43. Available from: https://pubmed.ncbi.nlm.nih.gov/27526630/
25. Wood GJA, Cardoso JPG, Paluello DV, Nunes TF, Cocuzza M. Varicocele-Associated Infertility and the Role of Oxidative Stress on Sperm DNA Fragmentation. Frontiers in Reproductive Health. 2021 Oct 29;3:71.
26. Olooto WE. Infertility in male; risk factors, causes and management-A review serum concentrations of ghrelin, leptin and lipid profile in type 2 diabetes mellitus view project.
27. Wang WL, Tu CF, Tan YQ. Insight on multiple morphological abnormalities of sperm flagella in male infertility: what is new? Asian J Androl. 2020;22(3):236–45.
28. Newman L, Chopra J, Dossett C, Shepherd E, Bercusson A, Carroll M, *et al.* The impact of primary ciliary dyskinesia on female and male fertility: a narrative review. Hum Reprod Update. 2023 Jan 31;
29. Tu C, Wang W, Hu T, Lu G, Lin G, Tan YQ. Genetic underpinnings of asthenozoospermia. Best Pract Res Clin Endocrinol Metab. 2020 Dec;34(6):101472.
30. Abd Elrahman MM, El Makawy AI, Hassanane MS, Alam SS, Hassan NHA, Amer MK. Assessment of correlation between asthenozoospermia and mitochondrial DNA mutations in Egyptian infertile men. J Genet Eng Biotechnol. 2021 Jan 18;19(1):11.
31. Li L, Chen S. Screening, identification and interaction analysis of key MicroRNAs and genes in Asthenozoospermia. Int J Med Sci. 2021;18(7):1670–9.
32. Agarwal A, Sharma RK, Gupta S, Boitrelle F, Finelli R, Parekh N, *et al.* Sperm Vitality and Necrozoospermia: Diagnosis, Management, and Results of a Global Survey of Clinical Practice. World J Mens Health. 2022 Apr;40(2):228–42.
33. Boursier A, Dumont A, Boitrelle F, Prasivoravong J, Lefebvre-Khalil V, Robin G, *et al.* Necrozoospermia: The tree that hides the forest. Andrology. 2022 May;10(4):642–59.
34. Máté G, Balló A, Márk L, Czétány P, Szántó Á, Török A. Magnetic-Activated Cell Sorting as a Method to Improve Necrozoospermia-Related Asthenozoospermic Samples. J Clin Med. 2022 May 21;11(10).
35. Chen T, Fan D, Wang X, Mao C, Chu Y, Zhang H, *et al.* ICSI outcomes for infertile men with severe or complete asthenozoospermia. Basic Clin Androl. 2022 Apr 5;32(1):6.

36. Dcunha R, Hussein RS, Ananda H, Kumari S, Adiga SK, Kannan N, *et al.* Current Insights and Latest Updates in Sperm Motility and Associated Applications in Assisted Reproduction. Reprod Sci. 2022 Jan;29(1):7–25.
37. Hajder M, Hajder E, Husic A. The Effects of Total Motile Sperm Count on Spontaneous Pregnancy Rate and Pregnancy After IUI Treatment in Couples with Male Factor and Unexplained Infertility. Med Arch. 2016 Feb;70(1):39–43.
38. Turhan N, Pekel A, Ayrim A, Bayrak Ö. ICSI outcome in severely oligoasthenozoospermic patients and its relationship to prewash progressive sperm motility. Turk J Med Sci. 2011;41(6):995–9.

Chapter

3

Oligoasthenoteratozoospermia

• Vinod KV

LEARNING OBJECTIVES

- To understand the morphology of a normal sperm.
- To understand the significance of teratospermia in fertility evaluation.
- To understand the etiology and causative factors for teratospermia.
- To understand the different types of teratospermia.
- To understand the management of the patients with teratospermia.

INTRODUCTION

Morphological features of sperms are yet another important microscopic parameter considered as the indicator of fertility potential of the male partner. Defining the 'normal' sperm is tricky as the semen may have a mix of morphologically normal and abnormal sperms.[1]

The criteria for defining the normal sperm were developed from evaluating the morphology of spermatozoa recovered from the endocervical mucus and from the surface of zona pellucida since they can be considered potentially fertilizing spermatozoa. The sperms can be evaluated by examining the stained semen smears. The techniques of preparing and staining the slides are standardized by WHO for uniformity and included in the manual.[1]

TERATOSPERMIA—IMPACT ON FERTILITY OUTCOME

Sperm morphology assessment has only limited value in predicting spontaneous pregnancy and ART outcomes. Patients with very low levels of normal sperms or completely abnormal sperms have also shown natural conception. At the same time, patients with normal sperms above the reference limits have shown poor outcome in fertilization, natural conception or ART. Even in patients with severe teratospermia, option of IUI or natural conception can be offered if the female partner is normal and there are no other seminal abnormalities.[2]

The various indices are also not helpful in distinguishing fertile couple from infertile couples.

Morphological assessment provides information about the functional state of testicles and epididymis.[1]

Case Scenario

A 28-year-old male is married to his 24-year-old wife for 6 years; SA shows 100 million sperms per ml, 34% PR and 0% normal forms; wife is normal on evaluation; how to proceed?

1. **What is teratospermia?**

   Ans: Teratospermia is defined as reduced percentage of morphologically normal sperms in the ejaculate below the accepted reference limits. When reporting results, the reference criteria should be specified.[3] Kruger et al in 1986 had found that normal forms above or equal to 14% had a significantly better outcome of pregnancy and fertilization rate.[4] Later WHO has changed the reference limit, and in the WHO 5th manual, the lower reference limit was considered as <4%. WHO 6th manual has not mentioned any reference limit.[1]

2. **What are the causes for teratospermia?**

   Ans: Teratospermia is due to defective spermatogenesis and sometimes due to epididymal pathologies. Morphologically abnormal spermatozoa show lower fertilizing potential. They are associated with increased DNA fragmentation or other DNA abnormalities, immature chromatin, structural chromosomal aberrations, and aneuploidy. Coiled tails may indicate epididymal dysfunction. Excess residual cytoplasm is due to a defective spermiation process.[1]

3. **What are the types of teratospermia?**

Ans: There are two types of teratospermia. Ejaculate with spermatozoa showing more than one type of morphological abnormality is called polymorphic teratozoospermia. This is the more common type of tetratospermia. On the otherh and, in monomorphic teratospermia all the sperms have a single abnormality. Two forms of monomorphic teratospermia are recognized: Macrozoospermia (sperms with large irregular head and multiple flagella) and globozoospermia (round heads). Globozoospermia lacks acrosome. These sperms lack fertilization capacity and show poor results even with ICSI.[5]

4. **What is the most important information needed from the semen analysis for planning further management?**

The given semen analysis report comments about the sperm concentration and the motility as above reference limits (WHO 5th manual). There is severe teratospermia with no normal forms. It is essential to know whether the teratospermia is monomorphic or polymorphic. Morphological abnormalities need to be reported separately for head, neck and midpiece, tail (principal piece) and excess residual cytoplasm. Usually the abnormalities are mixed or polymorphic. Occasionally, there can be a single defect seen in all sperms: Monomorphic. The common forms are the globozoospermia and macrozoospermia. Absent heads are seen as pin heads or free tails. The monomorphic forms have very poor fertilization outcome. In polymorphic types also, the percentage of round heads and pinheads carry poor outcome. Knowledge about the details of the abnormalities in morphology and their percentage is essential in counselling and planning further management.

5. **How will you assess the quality of semen analysis report?**

Ans: Semen analysis need to be reported by a laboratory personnel trained in processing and examination of semen as per WHO standards. The quality of slide preparation and the proper staining techniques need to be adhered to. A minimum of two hundred sperms needs to be examined for preparing the report. Defect in head, neck and tail has to be reported separately along with presence of excess residual cytoplasm. Many sperms have multiple abnormalities.

6. **What are causative factors for teratospermia?**

Ans: Testicular and epididymal pathologies can produce teratozoospermia. Defects in spermatogenesis can produce abnormal morphological features. Drugs, smoking, environmental toxins, and chemicals are known to produce defects in spermatogenesis. Chromosomal and genetic defects can contribute to defective spermatogenesis.

To understand teratospermia, one should know the morphological features of normal sperms.

7. **What are the most important features of a normal sperm?**

Ans: Morphological features of normal sperms[1]

Head

Head should be smooth and oval. The acrosomal region should extend over 40–70% of the head. The acrosomal region should not contain large vacuoles or more than two small vacuoles. The vacuoles should not occupy more than one-fifth of the head. No vacuoles should be present in the postacrosomal region. Length of sperm head: 4.1 µm (3.7–4.7 µm); Width: 2.8 µm (2.5–3.2 µm); Ratio of length to width: 1.5 (1.3–1.8).

- **Midpiece:** Midpiece is regular and thin with length equal to the head: 4 µm (3.3–5.2 µm) and width: 0.6 µm (0.5–0.7 µm). Major axis of midpiece and that of sperm head should be aligned.
- **Principal piece (tail):** Tail is around ten times the length of sperm head –45 µm. The principal piece should have a uniform caliber throughout its length. It should be thinner than midpiece.
- **Cytoplasmic residue:** Cytoplasmic droplets less than one-third the size of normal sperm head are normal. Usually they are not seen since the slides are air dried.

8. **What morphological abnormalities constitute teratospermia?**

Ans: Morphological abnormalities of sperm: During morphology assessment we need to assess the proportion of 'normal' spermatozoa and evaluate the defects in the head, midpiece and principal piece along with the presence of excess residual cytoplasm. Morphological abnormalities are usually mixed. Normal cytoplasm is not seen when the slides are prepared for evaluating morphology since they are air dried. But excess cytoplasm can be seen in the slides.

Abnormalities of head

- Round (length–width ratio < 1.5) or elongated head (ratio >2) (tapered)
- Large or small acrosome (> 70% or < 40%)
- Vacuoles in post-acrosomal area or more than one-fifth of the head area
- Abnormal shapes—amorphous or pyriform
- Double heads

Abnormalities of midpiece

- Irregular, thick or thin
- Sharply bent
- Angled insertion

Abnormalities of principal piece or tail

- Coiled
- Short
- Multiple tails
- Sharp bents
- Irregular width

Excess cytoplasmic residue

Residual cytoplasm exceeds one-third of sperm head size

Other specific sperm defects

Failure of the development of the acrosome produces round head defect or globozoospermia and absent head produce pinhead defect (free tails). They are usually reported separately.

9. How is teratospermia reporting done?

Ans: Percentage of normal forms is reported after examining 200 sperms. The percentage should be reported to the nearest whole number.

10. What are the morphological indices which can be used to quantify teratospermia?

Ans: Teratozoospermia index (TZI) is the sum of all abnormalities divided by the number of abnormal spermatozoa. This index should always be between 1 and 4. An abnormal sperm can have 1–4 abnormalities (one each for head, midpiece, principal piece and excess residual cytoplasm). This ratio should be expressed till two decimal places[6] (Menkveld 2001 criteria).

Multiple anomalies index (MAI) is similar to TZI. But all the abnormalities in the head, midpiece and principal defects are scored (excess residual cytoplasm is not included). The total number of anomalies are divided by the number of abnormal sperms as in TZI. The morphology criteria used for this analysis are different (David's morphological classification modified by Auger and Eustache 2000).[7]

Sperm deformity index (SDI): Number of defects divided by the number of spermatozoa both normal and abnormal. Here multiple head anomalies are counted different but only one each for midpiece and principal piece defect.

11. What are the tests to be done in a case of teratospermia?

Ans: Confirmation of semen analysis report from a standardized laboratory is the most important step considering the wide variability of reporting of the sperm morphology. Identification of the type of the morphological defect may guide in choosing the appropriate treatment (Agarwal). A detailed clinical evaluation of the patient helps in identifying the modifiable factors predisposing to the semen abnormality including sperm morphology. Genetic evaluation, DNA fragmentation, advanced sperm function tests are limited to research settings rather than clinical management.

12. What is the role of DNA fragmentation tests in teratospermia?

Ans: Teratospermia patients show increased DNA fragmentation when compared with individuals having normal fertility.[5]

13. What are the genetic causes of severe teratospermia? What is the indication for genetic evaluation in a case for teratospermia?

Ans: Globozoospermia may be associated with DPY19L2 mutation. Pinhead abnormality may be due to the mutation in the Sad1 and UNC84 domain containing 5 (SUN5) gene (Yassine). Presently, the detection of the genetic defect associated with teratospermia is limited to research settings and not helpful in clinical practice.

14. How to manage the index case?

Ans: Presence of severe teratospermia is a poor prognostic factor for fertilization outcome. Lifestyle modifications, avoidance or limitation of the exposure to environmental toxins and antioxidant supplementation may help the patient. Vitamin E, N-acetyl cysteine, lycopene, zinc and selenium may be helpful in improving sperm morphology.[8]

This patient has isolated teratozoospermia without compromise in the total sperm count or motility. Female factors are also normal. Female partner is only 24 years old. There is an option of trying for natural conception or IUI. Many studies have shown positive results for live birth rate in patients with severe teratospermia having 0–1% normal forms.[2] But these options should be considered for a limited time frame after which the option of IVF/ICSI should be considered. Increase in age of the female factors may compromise the results as years pass by.

Proposed management algorithm for a patient presenting with tetratozoospermia. Sperm concentration and motility reference range according to the WHO 5th edition

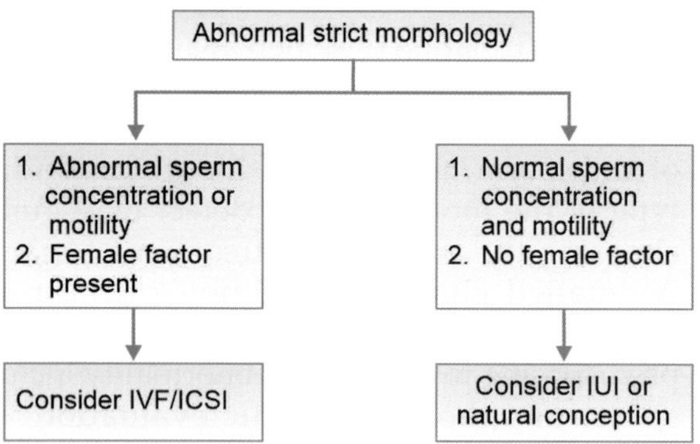

15. What are the pitfalls in the assessment of teratospermia?

Ans: Morphological assessment of sperms has a lot of challenges. Subjective assessment of the morphology of sperms can result in intra- and inter-observer variability. Experience of the technician, staining methods and availability of good equipment can affect the quality of the result. To reduce the variability in results, morphological assessment needs to be standardized.

WHO has put forth clear guidelines for standardizing the technique of morphological assessment. Microscope with ocular micrometer is essential to categorize sperms as normal or abnormal as per strict criteria. Papanicolaou staining is the best staining method for morphological assessment. Diff-Quick also can be used. Strict quality checking and audit are essential for improving the reliability of the report. Under reporting and over reporting of abnormal sperms are highly probable if good quality checking and internal audit are not maintained.[9]

16. What is the role of CASA in morphological assessment?

Ans: Main issue of morphological assessment in the inter- and intra-observer variability in making the assessment. Use of computer assisted morphometric assessment can address these deficiencies. But the lack of standardization of CASA algorithms and approaches is a significant barrier to this application. This also requires extensive quality control to ensure accuracy. For these reasons, this technology has not become widely accepted for morphological assessment.[10]

Role of higher magnification in treatment of teratospermia

Severely teratospermic patients may need ICSI. Selection of best available sperms plays an important role in improving outcomes. Morphological details of sperms are difficult to be identified in unstained preparations. This becomes challenging in the setting of severe teratospermia.

Morphology of motile sperms can be examined without staining under high magnification (6000 x) using an inverted light microscope with high power differential interference contrast (Motile Sperm Organelle Morphology Examination: MSOME). Intracytoplasmic morphologically selected sperm injection (IMSI) is devised by Integrating MSOME technique into the ICSI procedure. Best available sperm can be selected by observing the ultrastructural details of the sperm.

Clinical utility of IMSI procedure is doubtful as there is no strong evidence of positive outcome. But this technique may be useful In selected patients.[11]

SUMMARY

- The techniques of preparing and staining the slides for morphological assessment of sperms are standardized by WHO for uniformity and included in the manual.
- Sperm morphology assessment has only limited value in predicting spontaneous pregnancy and ART outcomes.
- Teratospermia is due to defective spermatogenesis and sometimes due to epididymal pathologies.
- There are two types of teratospermia: Polymorphic teratozoospermia and monomorphic teratospermia
- Percentage of normal forms are reported after examining 200 sperms.
- Teratozoospermia Index (TZI), Multiple Anomalies Index (MAI), Sperm Deformity Index (SDI) are the indices used to quantify the morphological abnormalities.
- Routine evaluation of DNA fragmentation or genetic evaluation may not be helpful in management of the patient.
- CASA has not become widely accepted for morphological assessment.
- Clinical utility of IMSI procedure in teratospermia is doubtful as there is no strong evidence of positive outcome.
- Lifestyle modifications, avoidance or limitation of the exposure to environmental toxins and antioxidant supplementation may help the patient. Vitamin E, N-acetyl cysteine, lycopene, zinc and selenium may be helpful in improving sperm morphology. Option of IUI may also be considered, for selected cases, for a limited time frame after which the option of IVF/ICSI should be considered.

REFERENCES

1. World Health Organization. Examination and processing of human semen [Internet]. Vol. Edition, V, World Health. 2010. 286 p. Available from: http://whqlibdoc.who.int/publications/2010/9789241547789_eng.pdf.
2. Shabtaie SA, Gerkowicz SA, Kohn TP, Ramasamy R. Role of Abnormal Sperm Morphology in Predicting Pregnancy Outcomes. Curr Urol Rep. 2016 Sep;17(9):67.

3. Zegers-Hochschild F, Adamson GD, De Mouzon J, Ishihara O, Mansour R, Nygren K, et al. International Committee for Monitoring Assisted Reproductive Technology (ICMART) and the World Health Organization (WHO) revised glossary of ART terminology, 2009*. Fertil Steril. 2009 Nov;92(5):1520–4.
4. Kruger TF, Menkveld R, Stander FSH, Lombard CJ, Van Der Merwe JP, Van Zyl JA, et al. Sperm morphologic features as a prognostic factor in *in vitro* fertilization. Fertil Steril. 1986 Dec;46(6):1118–23.
5. De Braekeleer M, Nguyen MH, Morel F, Perrin A. Genetic aspects of monomorphic teratozoospermia: a review. J Assist Reprod Genet. 2015 Apr;32(4):615–23.
6. Menkveld R. Semen parameters, including WHO and strict criteria morphology, in a fertile and subfertile population: an effort towards standardization of in-vivo thresholds. Hum Reprod. 2001 Jun 1;16(6):1165–71.
7. Auger J, Eustache F, Andersen AG, Irvine DS, Jørgensen N, Skakkebæk NE, et al. Sperm morphological defects related to environment, lifestyle and medical history of 1001 male partners of pregnant women from four European cities. Hum Reprod. 2001 Dec;16(12):2710–7.
8. Agarwal A, Sharma R, Gupta S, Finelli R, Parekh N, Panner Selvam MK, et al. Sperm Morphology Assessment in the Era of Intracytoplasmic Sperm Injection: Reliable Results Require Focus on Standardization, Quality Control, and Training. World J Mens Health. 2022;40(3):347.
9. Yassine S, Escoffier J, Martinez G, Coutton C, Karaouzène T, Zouari R, et al. Dpy19l2-deficient globozoospermic sperm display altered genome packaging and DNA damage that compromises the initiation of embryo development. MHR Basic Sci Reprod Med. 2015 Feb;21(2):169–85.
10. Majzoub A, Agarwal A. Systematic review of antioxidant types and doses in male infertility: Benefits on semen parameters, advanced sperm function, assisted reproduction and live-birth rate. Arab J Urol. 2018;16(1):113–24.
11. Agarwal A, Sharma R, Gupta S, Finelli R, Parekh N, Selvam MKP, et al. Sperm morphology assessment in the era of intracytoplasmic sperm injection: Reliable results require focus on standardization, quality control, and training. World J Mens Health. 2021;39(3):347–60.
12. Baldi E, Gallagher MT, Krasnyak S, Kirkman-Brown J, Apolikhin O, Barratt CLR, et al. Extended semen examinations in the sixth edition of the WHO Laboratory Manual for the Examination and Processing of Human Semen: contributing to the understanding of the function of the male reproductive system. Fertil Steril. 2022;117(2):252–7.
13. Karabulut S, Aksunger O, Korkmaz O, Eren Gozel H, Keskin I. Intracytoplasmic morphologically selected sperm injection, but for whom? Zygote. 2019;27(5):299–304.

Notes

Chapter

4

Varicocele

• Praveen Joshi • Sitaram Mummalaneni

LEARNING OBJECTIVES

- To understand the detrimental effects of varicocele on male infertility.
- To be able to decide when to perform varicocele repair in men with infertility.
- Understanding and mastering the right technique for varicocele repair.

INTRODUCTION

Varicocele is characterised by dilation and tortuosity of pampiniform plexus.[1,2] Varicoceles can lead to oligo-asthenoteratospermia, raised sperm DNA fragmentation and Leydig cell dysfunction.[3] The greatest challenge is to decide which couple will benefit from varicocele repair (VR) in terms of pregnancy and live birth rates.[4]

Case Scenario

A 30-year-old male, wife 31-year-old, married for 4 years; Semen analysis shows sperm count of 8 million per ml, 24% PR and 2% normal forms; wife has irregular cycles (repeated SA show OATS), AMH is 1.8 and husband has left clinical grade 3 varicocele? How to evaluate and decide the treatment in this couple?

1. **What are the causes of varicocele?**

   Ans: It is multifactorial. The longer left testicular vein (8–10 cm) perpendicularly enters the left renal vein and hence left-sided varicocele is more common.[5] Bilateral abnormal venous reflux is seen in ~80% patient with clinically unilateral varicocele and hence unilateral varicoceles may lead to bilateral testicular dysfunction.[6] Since internal spermatic veins lack functional valves, blood can flow in reverse direction.[7,8] The "nutcracker phenomenon" is a very rare cause; left renal vein is compressed between the superior mesenteric artery and aorta causing partial obstruction of left spermatic vein.[9]

2. **Discuss about the pathophysiology of varicocele and its effect on fertility.**

   Ans: Oxidative stress (OS) is caused by a disturbance in balance between reactive oxygen species (ROS) and antioxidants.

   - OS can harm germ cells directly[10]
   - Induce apoptosis in mature spermatozoa.[11]
   - Impair sperm concentration, motility, morphology and DNA fragmentation

   OS is worsened due to hyperthermia in scrotum, venous reflux, testicular hypoxia and cadmium accumulation.[12–20] This reflux impairs spermatogenesis, intratesticular testosterone levels and Sertoli cell function.[9,13,14] Type-B spermatogonia and developing sperms are more vulnerable to heat.[15,16,21–24] Cadmium accumulation triggers apoptosis through the induction of Fas ligand and generation of ROS.[25,26]

   The possible reasons for linking varicocele with infertility are:

   1. Varicoceles are more common in infertile men
   2. Varicoceles are associated with reduced testis volume and OATS
   3. Surgical repair of clinical varicoceles leads to improvement in sperm parameters

   But it is still unclear the reasons why about two-thirds of men with varicocele retain their fertility and why fertility potential is not always improved after surgical varicocele repair.[27,28]

3. **How to examine for a varicocele?**

Ans: A "clinically palpable" varicocele is significant. Patient should be examined in upright and recumbent positions, and Valsalva manoeuvre should be performed for grading varicocele.

4. **Discuss the clinical and radiological classification of varicocele and their correlation.**

Ans: The clinical classification was proposed by Dubin and Amelar. The WHO classification, expanded this with the addition of "sub-clinical varicocele".[30,31] Varicocele identified only on colour Doppler ultrasound (US) is termed "subclinical." According to ESUR-SPIWG, a maximum diameter of 3 mm is considered diagnostic for a varicocele and with the patient standing, during Valsalva manoeuvre, reflux > 2 seconds is considered abnormal.[32,33] The EAA US consortium defined "severe" varicocele as vein dilation > 3 mm, with continuous venous reflux at rest, consistent with grade 4 and 5 varicoceles (Sarteschi/Liguori classification).[34] Table 4.1 gives a correlation between clinical and sonological grading of varicocele.

5. **Is it mandatory to perform US during evaluation of varicocele?**

Ans: US is not routinely done as the clinic-radiological correlation of severity is poor.[35]

6. **Why is it deemed unnecessary to routinely perform US for evaluation of varicocele?**

Ans: As per consensus, US over diagnoses subclinical varicoceles resulting into unnecessary surgeries and/or confusion about outcomes after treatment of 'Clinical grade-I' varicoceles.[36] Till these problems are overcome, clinical examination stays the "Gold Standard."

7. **When is US useful during the evaluation of varicocele?**

Ans: When clinical examination is inconclusive in low-grade varicocele or difficult in prior scrotal surgeries, hydroceles, tight scrotum or obesity, US is useful. US detects contralateral subclinical varicocele. In these men with unilateral clinical varicocele and contralateral subclinical varicocele (US detected) with abnormal semen parameters, the option of bilateral varicocele repair needs to be contemplated. Ultrasound can also be useful to quantify reflux in a clinically grade 1 and 2 varicocele, where the decision to operate depends on the degree of reflux on Doppler.

8. **Mention the indications for varicocele repair and predictors of improvement.**

Ans: According to the AUA Best Practice Statement on indications for treatment of a varicocele.[37–39]

- Palpable varicocele
- Proven infertility
- Normal or potentially correctable female factor
- Abnormal semen parameters or sperm function tests
- Adult male with palpable varicocele and abnormal semen analysis not currently attempting to achieve conception, but with desire to preserve fertility.

TABLE 4.1: Clinical and radiological classification of varicocele and their compatibility

Ultrasound classification[34]	Grade I: Inguinal reflux only during Valsalva in not enlarged vessels	Grade 2: Supra-testicular varicosities with reflux only during Valsalva	Grade 3: Peri-testicular reflux only during Valsalva in enlarged vessels. Visible but not dilated vessels when supine. Enlarged when standing	Grade 4: Enlarged vessels in supine and standing position, with increasing caliber during Valsalva. Reflux at rest, increasing during Valsalva. Possible testicular hypothrophy	Grade 5: Enlarged vessels in supine and standing position, with caliber not increasing with Valsalva. Reflux at rest, not increasing during Valsalva. Testicular hypothrophy. Intratesticular varices may be present
Clinical classification[30]	Subclinical: Seen on imaging but no varicocele on examination		Grade 1: Small, palpable with Valsalva	Grade 2: Moderate, Palpable when standing without Valsalva	Grade 3: Large, easily visible
Correlation of US and clinical classification[35]	Grade 1 and 2 in ultrasonographic grading is most compatible with grade 0 (sub-clinical) in clinical evaluation		Grade 3 in US correlates with grade 1 in clinical grading	Grade 4 in US correlates with grade 2 in clinical grading	Grade 5 in ultrasonography correlates with grade 3 in clinical grading

9. Is there a relation between size of varicocele and fertility outcomes?

Ans: Surgical repair of larger varicoceles has a better improvement in seminal parameters and higher natural pregnancy rates.[40,41]

10. How is FSH useful in deciding prognosis?

Ans: Though relationship of FSH with VR is controversial, men with normal preoperative FSH values. Lower preoperative FSH (< 7 IU/L) has a better outcome.[42–44] Hormonal evaluation forms an integral part of evaluation of infertile men with varicocele. Table 4.2 depicts prognostic factors for VR and chose candidates for early ART.

TABLE 4.2 : Preoperative predictors of varicocele repair outcomes[38,39]

Good prognosis	*Poor prognosis*
Large varicocele (grade III)	Subclinical varicocele
Bilateral Large varicocele (grade III)	Presence of Y chromosome microdeletion
Normal serum FSH	Testicular atrophy
Total motile sperm count $>5 \times 10^6$	FSH: Above normal

11. Discuss surgical approaches to varicocele repair (VR).

Ans: All internal and external spermatic and cremasteric veins should be ligated ideally; spermatic arteries and lymphatics are preserved; this gives the lowest complication rate and significant improvements in fertility (Table 4.3).

Microsurgical VR is gold standard procedure because optical magnification is supposed to result in least complications, recurrence, pain and best success rates; along with shorter postoperative recovery.[46,47] Microsurgical VR is performed by subinguinal or inguinal approach. The subinguinal incision obviates the need for opening any fascial layer, which helps in faster recovery but subinguinal approach is usually associated with higher number of arteries and internal spermatic veins with a smaller diameter and can be challenging.[48]

A magnification of 6–10x is well suited for external and internal spermatic fascia opening and 20x magnification for inspection of spermatic cord; in at least half of the pateints, the testicular artery is seen adhered to the under surface of a large vein.[49]

A 3 mm intraoperative microvascular Doppler is useful in differentiating vascular structures and its systematic use allows for identification and preservation of more arterial branches and ligation of more internal spermatic veins. Papaverine irrigation can be used as an additional technique for identification of arteries.[50] Once identified, the testicular artery is dissected free and isolated with a vascular loop. Veins are dissected free of lymphatics, ligated with 3-0 or 4-0 silk and divided. The vas deferens and associated vasal vessels need to be preserved. It is not routinely necessary to deliver the testis for collaterals and gubernacular vessels.

12. Outline the management of given case scenario (index case of OATS + VARICOCELE).

Ans: Algorithm to manage an index case is depicted in Flowchart 4.1.[40,51]

13. What are the female factors to be remembered during decision for VR?

Ans: Couples with advanced female partner age (>35 years) or low ovarian reserve (AMH <1 ng/ml) should be aware of the time delay associated with a VR and that this could result in an unfavourable situation. These couples should be counselled and should consider opting for ART early or consider VR as a simultaneous procedure to improve semen quality for future attempts.

14. What is the role of sperm DNA fragmentation (DFI) and varicocele?

Ans: Sperm parameters may not completely reflect sperm DNA integrity.[52] Impaired sperm DNA

TABLE 4.3 : Effects of the various treatment options for VR[45]

Technique	*Internal spermatic vein ligation (%)*	*External spermatic vein ligation (%)*	*Failure or recurrence rate (%)*	*Hydrocele rate (%)*	*Spontaneous pregnancy rate (%)*
Retroperitonal ligation	Yes	No	12.6	7.5	37
Inguinal	Yes	Yes	9.6	5.3	26
Microsurgical subinguinal	Yes	Yes	1.2	0.6	41
Laparoscopic	Yes	No	8.4	6.7	26
Embolisation	Yes	No	7.4	0.0	36

Flowchart 4.1: Case management—algorithm

Clinical varicocele with abnormal semen parameters

Normal female factor or potentially treatable female factor (AMH 1.5–2.5, usually indicates good ovarian reserve)

↓

Discuss varicocele repair with couple
Prefer sub-inguinal microscopic varicocele repair
Keep patient on oral antioxidants for 3 months
Follow-up with semen analysis 3 monthly, improvement in sperm parameter usually noted by 3–6 months

→ Not willing → ART-ICSI

↓

Improvement in semen analysis—natural conception/IUI

→ No improvement in semen analysis → ART-ICSI

Presence of uncorrectable female factor → ART-ICSI

Contraindications for varicocele repair?

- No concrete contraindications
- But consider ART or simultaneous varicocele repair with ART in:
  - Advanced maternal age >35 and poor ovarian reserve
  - Subclinical varicocele and normal semen parameters
  - Extreme OAT (<100,000/ml)
  - FSH above normal
  - Testicular atrophy

integrity is detrimental for ART outcomes.[53,54] Hence, conventional semen parameters are now making way to the OS and DFI of the sperms tests.[55] It is thought that elevated testis temperature and the ROS are potential causes for sperm DNA damage.[56] Literature including EAU guidelines suggest that VR is being practiced to reduce SDF and improve ART outcomes; recommending VR for men with raised SDF and failed ART after extensive counselling.[57,58]

15. How to do counselling of the couple, if the female partner is normal?

Ans:

- The couple must be explained the severity of sperm damage. In men with mild variations of semen parameters or low grade varicocele, trial of antioxidants and attempting for natural conception can be considered. In moderate to severe OAT, especially with a large grade varicocele, the possibility of varicocele repair must be explored.
- The following factors must prompt towards surgical correction:
  - Sperm factor abnormalities
  - Previous failed ART especially ICSI
  - Recurrent early pregnancy loss
  - High DFI and/or ROS is an upcoming indication for VR.
- If the couple are keen on ICSI/IVF due to severe OAT, they must be explained about reduction in sperm defect score after VR. Fertilization, clinical pregnancy and live birth rates after ICSI were significantly higher in men post-VR. Chances of blastocyst formation will be < 20% in cases with varicocele and up to about 80% in cases with varicocele repair and VR can give the couple higher chances for conception.[59]

If the male hormonal balance suggests testicular failure, the couple must be explained the seriousness of early testicular damage and shift of severe OAT to azoospermia. This may need early ART.

16. How to counsel the couple in the presence of concomitant female factor as well?

Ans: If female factor is abnormal, such as, PCOS/premature ovarian failure/age/endometriosis/uterine factors, then it is important to determine which partner has worse parameters.

- If male factor is mild, early ART as deemed by female partner factors may be suggested with empiric antioxidants
- If male factor is severely compromised, then it may be a difficult situation to prioritize as to whether male factor can be improved and then ART can be planned or couple should go for ICSI upfront due to shortage of time. Such decisions have to be done with couple involvement in the decision.

However, some studies have not shown significant difference in the outcomes and are not in favour of the varicocele repair. Reduction in sperm concentrations post-VR could be due to spontaneous decline or undetected testicular artery damage.[40] There is the need to perform preoperative sperm cryopreservation. Improvement in sperm parameters should be expected within 1–2 spermatogenic cycles, that is within 3 to 6 months. This may be longer in men with severe OAT.

17. What is the role of varicocele repair in NOA?

Ans: Varicocele in seen in 5–10% of men with NOA.[60] Post-VR, up to 40% men may have appearance of a few sperms in the ejaculate.[61–63] Even in men with persistent azoospermia post-VR, surgical sperm retrieval rates (60.8% *vs* 38.46%, $P = 0.01$) are better.[64]

Despite this, VR in NOA is controversial because of the following factors:

- Improvement is seen but ICSI is still needed.[65]
- Despite improvement, in up to 55.5%, men again develop NOA one year after VR.[66]
- Upfront microdissection testicular sperm extraction is more cost effective than VR followed by microTESE.[67–69]

The EAU does not take a stand for or against the routine varicocelectomy in NOA as the evidence is of low quality, but suggests to treat the possible cause of azoospermia prior to the sperm retrieval. AUA and ASRM do not favour the varicocelectomy prior to the microTESE for sperm retrieval.

Men with large varicoceles, reasonable sized testes and normal FSH, no genetic or known causes for testicular failure, the risks and benefits of VR must be discussed fully with the patient.[40,70–72]

KEY POINTS

- Varicocele is the most common surgically correctable cause of male infertility.
- Varicocele affects sperm parameters and increases oxidative stress.
- VR in a clinical varicocele has shown significant improvement in pregnancy rates.
- Microsurgical varicocelectomy is considered the gold standard due to high precision and least complications.
- Female factors must be taken into account before finalising the treatment.

SUMMARY

- Varicocele is a common cause and amenable to surgical correction. The most important idea of evaluation is to assess if varicocele is the cause of infertility and can it improve sperm parameters and thereby male fertility status. It is essential to understand the pathophysiology of symptoms/sperm abnormalities before treating varicocele. The clinician should be able to weigh the female factors, previous treatments and sperm parameters, with inputs of newer sperm function tests, clinical and radiological grade of varicocele and finalise the treatment.

REFERENCES

1. Su JS, Farber NJ, Vij SC. Pathophysiology and treatment options of varicocele: an overview. Andrologia. 2021 Feb;53(1):e13576.
2. Alsaikhan B, Alrabeeah K, Delouya G, Zini A. Epidemiology of varicocele. Asian journal of andrology. 2016 Mar;18(2):179.
3. Damsgaard J, Joensen UN, Carlsen E, Erenpreiss J, Jensen MB, Matulevicius V, Zilaitiene B, Olesen IA, Perheentupa A, Punab M, Salzbrunn A. Varicocele is associated with impaired semen quality and reproductive hormone levels: a study of 7035 healthy young men from six European countries. European urology. 2016 Dec 1;70(6):1019–29.
4. Persad E, O'Loughlin CA, Kaur S, Wagner G, Matyas N, Hassler-Di Fratta MR, Nussbaumer-Streit B. Surgical or radiological treatment for varicoceles in subfertile men. Cochrane Database of Systematic Reviews. 2021(4).
5. Hamada A, Esteves SC, Agarwal A. Varicocele and male infertility: current concepts, controversies and consensus.
6. Gat Y, Bachar GN, Zukerman Z, Belenky A, Gornish M. Varicocele: a bilateral disease. Fertility and sterility. 2004 Feb 1;81(2):424–9.
7. Sofikitis N, Dritsas K, Miyagawa I, Koutselinis A. Anatomical characteristics of the left testicular venous system in man. Archives of andrology. 1993 Jan 1;30(2):79–85.
8. Braedel HU, Steffens J, Ziegler M, Polsky MS, Platt ML. A possible ontogenic etiology for idiopathic left varicocele. The Journal of urology. 1994 Jan 1;151(1):62–6.
9. Naughton CK, Nangia AK, Agarwal A. Varicocele and male infertility: part II: pathophysiology of varicoceles in male infertility. Human reproduction update. 2001 Sep 1;7(5): 473–81.
10. Romeo C, Santoro G. Free radicals in adolescent varicocele testis. Oxidative Medicine and Cellular Longevity. 2014 Dec 14;2014.
11. Agarwal A, Sekhon LH. Oxidative stress and antioxidants for idiopathic oligoasthenoteratospermia: Is it justified?. Indian journal of urology: IJU: Journal of the Urological Society of India. 2011 Jan;27(1):74.
12. Agarwal A, Sharma RK, Sharma R, Assidi M, Abuzenadah AM, Alshahrani S, Durairajanayagam D, Sabanegh E. Characterizing semen parameters and their association with reactive oxygen species in infertile men. Reproductive Biology and Endocrinology. 2014 Dec;12(1):1–9.
13. Rajfer J, Turner TT, Rivera F, Howards SS, Sikka SC. Inhibition of testicular testosterone biosynthesis following experimental varicocele in rats. Biology of Reproduction. 1987 May 1;36(4):933–7.
14. Sofikitis N, Miyagawa I. Effects of surgical repair of experimental left varicocele on testicular temperature, spermatogenesis, sperm maturation, endocrine function, and fertility in rabbits. Archives of andrology. 1992 Jan 1;29(2):163–75.
15. Ko, E. Y., Sabanegh, E. S., & Agarwal, A. (2014). Male infertility testing: Reactive oxygen species and antioxidant capacity. Fertility and Sterility, 102(6), 1518–1527.
16. Tawadrous GA, Aziz AA, Mostafa T. Seminal soluble fas relationship with oxidative stress in infertile men with varicocele. Urology. 2013 Oct 1;82(4):820–3.
17. Comhaire F, Kunnen M. Selective retrograde venography of the internal spermatic vein: a conclusive approach to the diagnosis of varicocele. Andrologia. 1976 Jan 3;8(1):11–24.
18. Cohen MS, Plaine L, Brown JS. The role of internal spermatic vein plasma catecholamine determinations in subfertile men with varicoceles. Fertility and Sterility. 1975 Dec 1;26(12): 1243–9.
19. Sofikitis N, Miyagawa I. Left adrenalectomy in varicocelized rats does not inhibit the development of varicocele-related physiologic alterations. International journal of fertility and menopausal studies. 1993 Jul 1;38(4):250–5.
20. Ito H, Fuse H, Minagawa H, Kawamura K, Murakami M, Shimazaki J. Internal spermatic vein prostaglandins in varicocele patients. Fertility and Sterility. 1982 Feb 1;37(2): 218–22.
21. Gat Y, Zukerman Z, Chakraborty J, Gornish M. Varicocele, hypoxia and male infertility. Fluid Mechanics analysis of

the impaired testicular venous drainage system. Human Reproduction. 2005 Sep 1;20(9):2614–9.

22. Cho CL, Esteves SC, Agarwal A. Novel insights into the pathophysiology of varicocele and its association with reactive oxygen species and sperm DNA fragmentation. Asian Journal of Andrology. 2016 Mar;18(2):186.
23. Masson P, Brannigan RE. The varicocele. Urologic Clinics. 2014 Feb 1;41(1):129–44.
24. Ozturk U, Kefeli M, Asci R, Akpolat I, Buyukalpelli R, Sarikaya S. The effects of experimental left varicocele on the epididymis. Systems Biology in Reproductive Medicine. 2008 Jan 1;54(4–5):177–84.
25. Benoff SH, Millan C, Hurley IR, Napolitano B, Marmar JL. Bilateral increased apoptosis and bilateral accumulation of cadmium in infertile men with left varicocele. Human Reproduction. 2004 Mar 1;19(3):616–27.
26. Liu J, Qian SY, Guo Q, Jiang J, Waalkes MP, Mason RP, Kadiiska MB. Cadmium generates reactive oxygen-and carbon-centered radical species in rats: insights from in vivo spin-trapping studies. Free Radical Biology and Medicine. 2008 Aug 15;45(4):475–81.
27. Evers JL, Collins JA. Assessment of efficacy of varicocele repair for male subfertility: a systematic review. The Lancet. 2003 May 31;361(9372):1849–52.
28. Nieschlag E, Hertle L, Fischedick A, Abshagen K, Behre HM. Update on treatment of varicocele: counselling as effective as occlusion of the vena spermatica. Human Reproduction (Oxford, England). 1998 Aug 1;13(8):2147–50.
29. Redmon JB, Carey P, Pryor JL. Varicocele–the most common cause of male factor infertility?. Human reproduction update. 2002 Jan 1;8(1):53–8.
30. Dubin L, Amelar RD. Varicocele size and results of varicocelectomy in selected subfertile men with varicocele. Fertility and sterility. 1970 Aug 1;21(8):606–9.
31. Niederberger C. WHO manual for the standardized investigation, diagnosis and management of the infertile male. Urology. 2001 Jan 1;57(1):208.
32. Bertolotto M, Freeman S, Richenberg J, Belfield J, Dogra V, Huang DY, Lotti F, Markiet K, Nikolic O, Ramanathan S, Ramchandani P. Ultrasound evaluation of varicoceles: systematic literature review and rationale of the ESUR-SPIWG Guidelines and Recommendations. Journal of Ultrasound. 2020 Dec;23:487–507.
33. Freeman, S., Bertolotto, M., Richenberg, J., Belfield, J., Dogra, V., Huang, D.Y., Lotti, F., Markiet, K., Nikolic, O., Ramanathan, S. and Ramchandani, P., 2020. Ultrasound evaluation of varicoceles: guidelines and recommendations of the European Society of Urogenital Radiology Scrotal and Penile Imaging Working Group (ESUR-SPIWG) for detection, classification, and grading. *European radiology*, *30*, pp.11–25.
34. Sarteschi M. Lo studio del varicocele con eco-color-Doppler. G It Ultrason. 1993;4:43–9.
35. Foroughi AA, Yazdanpanah E, Nazeri M, Eghbali T, Arasteh P, Ariafar A. Clinical grading and color Doppler ultrasonography-based grading of varicocele: how compatible are the two grading systems?. World Journal of Urology. 2019 Jul 1;37:1461–5.
36. Grasso M, Lania C, Blanco S, Confalonieri S, Grasso AA. Efficacy of spermatic vein ligation in patients affected by high grade left varicocele. International braz j urol. 2014 Jan;40:62–6.
37. Schlegel PN, Sigman M, Collura B, De Jonge CJ, Eisenberg ML, Lamb DJ, Mulhall JP, Niederberger C, Sandlow JI, Sokol RZ, Spandorfer SD. Diagnosis and treatment of infertility in men: AUA/ASRM guideline part I. The Journal of urology. 2021 Jan;205(1):36–43.
38. Kamal KM, Jarvi K, Zini A. Microsurgical varicocelectomy in the era of assisted reproductive technology: influence of initial semen quality on pregnancy rates. Fertility and sterility. 2001 May 1;75(5):1013–6.
39. Cocuzza M, Cocuzza MA, Bragais FM, Agarwal A. The role of varicocele repair in the new era of assisted reproductive technology. Clinics. 2008 Jun 1;63(3):395–404.
40. Shah R, Agarwal A, Kavoussi P, Rambhatla A, Saleh R, Cannarella R, Harraz AM, Boitrelle F, Kuroda S, Hamoda TA, Zini A. Consensus and diversity in the management of varicocele for male infertility: results of a global practice survey and comparison with guidelines and recommendations.
41. Asafu-Adjei D, Judge C, Deibert CM, Li G, Stember D, Stahl PJ. Systematic review of the impact of varicocele grade on response to surgical management. The Journal of urology. 2020 Jan;203(1):48–56.
42. Pasqualotto FF, Lucon AM, de Góes PM, Sobreiro BP, Hallak J, Pasqualotto EB, Arap S. Semen profile, testicular volume, and hormonal levels in infertile patients with varicoceles compared with fertile men with and without varicoceles. Fertility and sterility. 2005 Jan 1;83(1):74–7.
43. Ok F, Erdogan O, Durmus E. Can preoperative gonadotropin and testosterone levels predict the success of varicocelectomy?. Andrologia. 2020 Dec;52(11):e13887.
44. Madhusoodanan V, Blachman-Braun R, Patel P, Ji L, Masterson TA, Owyong M, Greer A, Ramasamy R. Preoperative follicle-stimulating hormone: A factor associated with semen parameter improvement after microscopic subinguinal varicocelectomy. Canadian Urological Association Journal. 2020 Jan;14(1):E27.
45. Lundy SD, Sabanegh Jr ES. Varicocele management for infertility and pain: a systematic review. Arab journal of urology. 2018 Mar 1;16(1):157–70.
46. Mehta A, Goldstein M. Microsurgical varicocelectomy: a review. Asian Journal of Andrology. 2013 Jan;15(1):56.
47. Jungwirth A, Gögüs C, Hauser G, Gomahr A, Schmeller N, Aulitzky W, Frick J. Clinical outcome of microsurgical subinguinal varicocelectomy in infertile men. Andrologia. 2001 Mar 3;33(2):71–4.
48. Çayan S, Shavakhabov S, Kadio lu A. Treatment of palpable varicocele in infertile men: a meta analysis to define the best technique. Journal of andrology. 2009 Jan 2;30(1):33–40.
49. Beck EM, Schlegel PN, Goldstein M. Intraoperative varicocele anatomy: a macroscopic and microscopic study. The Journal of urology. 1992 Oct 1;148(4):1190–4.
50. Tatem AJ, Brannigan RE. The role of microsurgical varicocelectomy in treating male infertility. Translational andrology and urology. 2017 Aug;6(4):722.
51. Colpi GM, Francavilla S, Haidl G, Link K, Behre HM, Goulis DG, Krausz C, Giwercman A. European Academy of Andrology guideline Management of oligo-astheno-teratozoospermia. Andrology. 2018 Jul;6(4):513–24.
52. Agarwal A, Allamaneni SS. Sperm DNA damage assessment: a test whose time has come. Fertility and sterility. 2005 Oct 1;84(4):850–3.
53. Guzick DS, Overstreet JW, Factor-Litvak P, Brazil CK, Nakajima ST, Coutifaris C, Carson SA, Cisneros P, Steinkampf

MP, Hill JA, Xu D. Sperm morphology, motility, and concentration in fertile and infertile men. New England Journal of Medicine. 2001 Nov 8;345(19):1388–93.

54. Simon L, Emery BR, Carrell DT. diagnosis and impact of sperm DNA alterations in assisted reproduction. Best Practice & Research Clinical Obstetrics & Gynaecology. 2017 Oct 1;44:38–56.
55. Agarwal A, Majzoub A, Esteves SC, Ko E, Ramasamy R, Zini A. Clinical utility of sperm DNA fragmentation testing: practice recommendations based on clinical scenarios. Translational andrology and urology. 2016 Dec;5(6):935.
56. Saleh RA, Agarwal A, Sharma RK, Said TM, Sikka SC, Thomas Jr AJ. Evaluation of nuclear DNA damage in spermatozoa from infertile men with varicocele. Fertility and sterility. 2003 Dec 1;80(6):1431–6.
57. Roque M, Esteves SC. Effect of varicocele repair on sperm DNA fragmentation: a review. International urology and nephrology. 2018 Apr;50(4):583–603.
58. Kadioglu TC, Aliyev E, Celtik M. Microscopic varicocelectomy significantly decreases the sperm DNA fragmentation index in patients with infertility. BioMed Research International. 2014 Oct;2014.
59. Neto FT, Roque M, Esteves SC. Effect of varicocelectomy on sperm deoxyribonucleic acid fragmentation rates in infertile men with clinical varicocele: a systematic review and meta-analysis. Fertility and Sterility. 2021 Sep 1;116(3):696–712.
60. Qiu D, Shi Q, Pan L. Efficacy of varicocelectomy for sperm DNA integrity improvement: A meta-analysis. Andrologia. 2021 Feb;53(1):e13885.
61. M. Smit, J. C. Romijn, M. F. Wildhagen, J. L. M. Veldhoven, R. F. A. Weber, and G. R. Dohle, "Decreased sperm DNA fragmentation after surgical varicocelectomy is associated with increased pregnancy rate," Journal of Urology, vol. 183, no. 1, pp. 270–274, 2010
62. C Esteves S, T Schneider D. Male infertility and assisted reproductive technology: lessons from the IVF. The Open Reproductive Science Journal. 2011 Sep 23;3(1).
63. Matthews GJ, Matthews ED, Goldstein M. Induction of spermatogenesis and achievement of pregnancy after microsurgical varicocelectomy in men with azoospermia and severe oligoasthenospermia. Fertility and sterility. 1998 Jul 1;70(1):71–5.
64. Elzanaty S. Varicocele repair in non-obstructive azoospermic men: diagnostic value of testicular biopsy–a meta-analysis. Scandinavian journal of urology. 2014 Dec 1;48(6):494–8.
65. Weedin JW, Khera M, Lipshultz LI. Varicocele repair in patients with nonobstructive azoospermia: a meta-analysis. The Journal of urology. 2010 Jun 1;183(6):2309–15.
66. Esteves SC, Miyaoka R, Roque M, Agarwal A. Outcome of varicocele repair in men with nonobstructive azoospermia: systematic review and meta-analysis. Asian Journal of Andrology. 2016 Mar;18(2):246.
67. Haydardedeoglu B, Turunc T, Kilicdag EB, Gul U, Bagis T. The effect of prior varicocelectomy in patients with nonobstructive azoospermia on intracytoplasmic sperm injection outcomes: a retrospective pilot study. Urology. 2010 Jan 1;75(1):83–6.
68. Abdel-Meguid TA. Predictors of sperm recovery and azoospermia relapse in men with nonobstructive azoospermia after varicocele repair. The Journal of urology. 2012 Jan 1;187(1):222–6.
69. Pasqualotto FF, Sobreiro BP, Hallak J, Pasqualotto EB, Lucon AM. Induction of spermatogenesis in azoospermic men after varicocelectomy repair: an update. Fertility and sterility. 2006 Mar 1;85(3):635–9.
70. Schlegel PN, Kaufmann J. Role of varicocelectomy in men with nonobstructive azoospermia. Fertility and sterility. 2004 Jun 1;81(6):1585–8.
71. Althakafi SA, Mustafa OM, Seyam RM, Al-Hathal N, Kattan S. Serum testosterone levels and other determinants of sperm retrieval in microdissection testicular sperm extraction. Translational andrology and urology. 2017 Apr;6(2):282.
72. Lee R, Li PS, Goldstein M, Schattman G, Schlegel PN. A decision analysis of treatments for nonobstructive azoospermia associated with varicocele. Fertility and sterility. 2009 Jul 1;92(1):188–96.

Chapter

5

Non-Obstructive Azoospermia

• Sathish Babu Pigilam • Vilvapathy Senguttuvan Karthikeyan

LEARNING OBJECTIVES

- To differentiate between non-obstructive and obstructive azoospermia.
- To confidently decide about surgical sperm retrieval options and plan the management.
- To be able to liaise with the reproductive medicine team to plan the management.

INTRODUCTION

Non-obstructive azoospermia is a severe form of spermatogenic failure. The diagnosis is based on clinical examination including testis volume, FSH levels and normal semen volume and pH. Management includes appropriate genetic evaluation and surgical sperm retrieval. Treatment involves female partner evaluation, assessment of oocyte reserve, discussion of the options of donor sperm assisted reproduction and own sperm ICSI, their outcomes, success rates, cost and a final of adoption. Treatment should be planned in liaison with the reproductive medicine team for optimal outcomes.

Case Scenario

A 34-year-old male, wife 29-year-old are married for 2 years; SA shows volume 2 ml, Fructose + Azoospermia, FSH 15.1, clinical exam shows bilateral 12 cc testes; how to proceed?

1. **What is the diagnosis?**

   Ans: This couple has primary infertility due to azoospermia; probably non-obstructive azoospermia (NOA) with primary testicular failure.

2. **How to arrive at a diagnosis of NOA in this patient?**

   Ans: Semen analysis shows normal volume azoospermia. With an elevated follicle stimulating hormone (FSH) values, this is suggestive of primary testicular failure. Cut-off FSH >7.6 IU/L is suggestive of defective spermatogenesis especially in the presence of NOA. The other important clinical examination points include androgenization and testis volume. If the long axis of the testis is <4.6 cm, it is suggestive of defective spermatogenesis.[1]

3. **What other hormone tests are required?**

   Ans: The other hormones usually done are total testosterone and it may be reduced, in up to 30% men with NOA.[7–9] In men with low testosterone (<300 ng/dl) estradiol is also done. Luteinizing hormone (LH) can guide in treatment as well. Evaluation starts from clinical examination where body mass index (BMI), testis volume and palpable vas are important.

4. **What should be the approach to evaluation of NOA?**

   Ans: A correct definition of the type of the associated hypogonadism (i.e. hypogonadotropic hypogonadism vs hypergonadotropic vs eugonadotropic hypogondism) is relevant to differentiate diagnostic and therapeutic approaches to the patient.[10]

5. **What is the incidence of azoospermia?**

   Ans: Azoospermia affects approximately 15% of infertile couples and is the most severe from of male infertility.[1]

6. **What are the causes of NOA?**

   Ans: Non-obstructive azoospermia causes can be either pre-testicular (endocrinal) or testicular (testicular failure).

7. What are the pre-testicular causes of NOA?

Ans: Pre-testicular causes are due to hypothalamic and pituitary malfunction, which may be congenital hypogonadotrophic hypogonadism. Kallman syndrome is one of the commonest causes; Isolated LH or FSH deficiency, Prader-Willi syndrome, Bardet-Biedel syndrome and cerebellar ataxia are other causes. Acquired causes include pituitary tumors or infarcts, post-radiation, blood dyscrasias like hemochromatosis and sickle cell anemia.

Exogenous administration of testosterone or its synthetic derivatives induces feedback inhibition on the hypothalamic-pituitary axis resulting in reduction of FSH and LH synthesis and consequently a decrease in intratesticular testosterone levels. Infertility after anabolic androgenic steroids can present as azoospermia or oligozoospermia.[2,3] Hyperprolactinemia will lead to inhibition of testosterone production either directly at testicular level or through inhibition of pituitary gonadotropins causing NOA.

8. What are the testicular causes of NOA?

Ans: Testicular causes of NOA are idiopathic in 49–93% of cases.[4] Genetic abnormalities may account for up to 21%; most common is Klinefelter syndrome followed by chromosomal translocations and Y chromosome microdeletions. Bilateral testicular injury due to inflammation, orchitis, torsion and infarction will lead to NOA. Exposure to gonadotoxins especially chemotherapy and radiotherapy, bilateral undescended testis, renal and liver failure may also present as NOA.[5,6]

9. Is there a role of ultrasound testis?

Ans: Testicular ultrasound assessment is rarely indicated; it may show signs of testicular dysgenesis (non-homogenous testicular architecture/microcalcification) and testicular tumors. Testicular volume may be predictor of spermatogenic function and is usually, but not invariably, low in patients with NOA.[11]

10. What are the genetic tests for NOA?

Ans: Karyotyping and screening for Y-chromosome microdeletions are very essential for NOA work up.

Karyotyping is done to detect chromosomal abnormalities which can be numerical (e.g., trisomy) or structural (e.g., inversions or translocations), which can be seen in up to 5.8% (sex chromosomal 4.2%; autosomal 1.5%).[12] Klinefelter's syndrome is the most common sex chromosomal abnormality. Microdissection testicular sperm extraction (microtese) in these patients results in sperm retrieval rates ranging from 30 to 70%.[13,14]

Y chromosome microdeletion is seen in 13% of NOA cases. It has three regions; AZF-a and AZF-b have almost 0% chance to find sperm in testis while sperm could be retrieved by TESE in up to 70% of AZF-c deletion.

11. What is the plan of management in this couple?

Ans: This patient has NOA with spermatogenic failure considering normovolemic ejaculate, elevated FSH and relatively smaller testis (12 cc).

12. Is there any role for prior hormonal therapy prior to sperm retrieval and effect of exogenous testosterone therapy?

Ans: In men with hypogonadotropic hypogonadism, the best prognosis with appearance of sperm in semen and spontaneous pregnancy is high. This is covered in the chapter on hypogonadotropic hypogonadism.[15,16]

It has been shown that azoospermic patients with elevated gonadotropin levels that administration of hCG and/or FSH can lead to so called "Gonadotropins reset" with a reduction in FSH concentrations and improvement in Sertoli cell function.[17]

Hormonal therapy has been proposed to increase the change of sperm retrieval at salvage surgery after previously failed cTESE or mTESE. Retrospective data have shown that treatment with hCG and human menopausal gonadotropin (HMG)/recombinant FSH could lead to 10–15% successful retrieval at salvage mTESE.[18,19]

13. What would be the role of surgery in case the patient has a palpable varicocele with NOA?

Ans: NOA in association with varicocele is estimated to range between approximately 4–14%. Varicocele repair in azoospermic men have also increased the success rates of assisted reproductive techniques such as intracytoplasmic sperm injection (ICSI) by providing motile sperm for sperm ejaculate or for testicular sperm extraction (TESE). A larger varicocele with reasonable sized ipsilateral testis, FSH levels and at least hypospermatogenesis on testis biopsy has a better success chance with varicocelectomy.[20-23]

14. What would be the preferred sperm retrieval approach for this couple?

Ans: Micro dissection TESE is the technique of choice for retrieving sperm in patients with NOA and should be offered, if it is available. A single session surgical sperm retrieval is proposed to have the best success rate with least invasiveness; testicular sperm aspiration, followed by testicular mapping and microTESE (Table 5.1).

TABLE 5.1: Conventional vs micro TESE

S. No	Description	Conventional TESE	MicroTESE
1	Success of retrieval	45%	62%
2	Advantages	Less cost Availability No need of microsurgical skills	Lower incidence of hematoma Lower incidence of testis atrophy

15. What factors can predict sperm retrieval rates in this case?

Ans: No definitive factors have been demonstrated to predict sperm retrieval.[24]

Hormonal levels, including FSH, LH, inhibin B and AMH have been variably correlated with sperm retrieval and in a recent study, the size of seminiferous tubules assessed with pre-operative USG has been linked to higher success.[25–28] There is good correlation between histology found at testicular biopsy and the likelihood of successful surgical sperm retrieval.

16. What is the role of a diagnostic testicular biopsy?

Ans: A formal diagnostic biopsy is not recommended as it causes scarring and fibrosis as a result of devascularization.[29–32] It is also recommended to perform testicular biopsy only when sperm cryopreservation is available.

17. What factors denote successful outcome for this couple if they choose to proceed with micro TESE and ICSI?

Ans: Success in NOA is about finding sperms during the sperm retrieval, ability to identify morphologically good sperms for ICSI and then embryo quality.

18. Which is better: Fresh sperm or frozen sperm for ICSI?

Ans: Fresh testicular sperm has high viability approaching 90% despite its low motility, whereas only 33% of testicular samples from men with NOA show documentable viability after freeze-thaw.[24] The outcomes of fresh and frozen sperm ICSI have been shown to be similar.

19. What is the best time to perform a surgical sperm retrieval?

Ans: As the outcomes of fresh and frozen sperm ICSI are almost similar, the timing of surgical sperm retrieval does not matter. In India, especially in case of NOA, it is preferable to perform surgical sperm retrieval on the day of oocyte pick up (OPU).

20. What is the counseling done to couples with NOA?

Ans: The counseling for NOA involves the discussion about genetics and its transmissibility to offspring. It also revolves around the success at the time of sperm retrieval. In case the sperm retrieval done on the day of OPU is negative, then the couple should have the options discussed about donor sperm, oocyte cryopreservation and its implications.

21. What are the chances that a redo microTESE would succeed if first time SSR fails?

Ans: The chances that redo microTESE after a well-performed bilateral microTESE would succeed are less; however, in couples who desperately prefer salvage microTESE, there is a role of empiric gonadotropins.

KEY POINTS

- Non-obstructive azoospermia is diagnosed by clinical exam, semen analysis and hormonal evaluation.
- A sound knowledge to differentiate between obstructive and non-obstructive azoospermia is important to deliver the best care.
- Appropriate genetic evaluation and counseling is required before treatment.
- Andrologist should have a clear knowledge and confidence to counsel the couple and liaise with the reproductive medicine team and embryologist to provide the best solution.
- Surgical sperm retrieval should be planned; single stage sperm retrieval including testicular sperm aspiration to microdissection testicular sperm extraction should be kept in mind during treatment planning.

REFERENCES

1. Schoor RA, Elhanbly S, Niederberger CS, Ross LS. The role of testicular biopsy in the modern management of male infertility. *J Urol.* 2002;167(1):197–200.
2. Jarow JP, Espeland MA, Lipschlutz LI. Evaluation of the azoospermic patient J urol. 1989; 142:62.
3. Sjoqvist F, Garle M, Rane A. Use of doping agents, particularly anabolic steroids in sports and in society.
4. Grokett BH, Ahmad N, Warren DW. The effects of anabolic steroid (oxandralone) on reproductive development in the male rat. Acta Endocrinol. 1992; 126(2): 173–
5. Jarvi K, Lo K, Fisher A, Grantmyre J, Zini A, Chow A, Mak V. CUA guideline: The workup of azoospermic males. Can Urol Assoc J. 2010; 4(3): 163–7
6. Male infertility best practice policy committee of the American society for reproductive medicine. Report on evaluation of the azoospermic male. Fertil Steril 2006; 86 (Suppl 1): S210–5

7. Esteves S. Clinical management of infertile male with non-obstructive azoospermia. Asian J androl. 2015; 17:459–70.
8. Capogrosso, P., *et al*. Erectile Recovery After Radical Pelvic Surgery: Methodological Challenges and Recommendations for Data Reporting. J Sex Med, 2019.
9. Bobjer, J., *et al*. High prevalence of androgen deficiency and abnormal lipid profile in infertile men with nonobstructive azoospermia. Int J Androl, 2012. 35: 688.
10. Patel, D.P., *et al*. Sperm concentration is poorly associated with hypoandrogenism in infertile men. Urology, 2015. 85: 1062.
11. Ventimiglia, E., *et al*. Primary, secondary and compensated hypogonadism: a novel risk stratification for infertile men. Andrology, 2017. 5: 505.
12. Lotti, F., *et al*. Ultrasound of the male genital tract in relation to male reproductive health. Hum Reprod Update, 2015. 21: 56.
13. Johnson, M.D. Genetic risks of intracytoplasmic sperm injection in the treatment of male infertility: recommendations for genetic counseling and screening. Fertil Steril, 1998. 70: 397.
14. Palermo GD, Schlegel PN, Sills ES, Veeck LL, Zaninovic N, Menendez S, Rosenwaks Z. Births after intracytoplasmic injection of sperm obtained by testicular extraction from men with nonmosaic Klinefelter's syndrome. N Engl J Med. 1998; 338:588–90.
15. Ramasamy R, Ricci JA, Palermo GD, Gosden LV, Rosenwaks Z, Schlegel PN. Successful fertility treatment for Klinefelter's syndrome. J Urol. 2009;182:1108–13.
16. Pitteloud N, Hayes FJ Dwyer A, Boepple PA, Lee H, Crowley WF Jr. Predivtors of outcome of long term GrnRH therapy in men with idiopathic hypogonadotropic hypogonadism. J Clin Endocrinol Metab. 2002;87(9)4128–36.
17. Sykiotis GP, Hoang XH, Avbelj M, Hayes FJ, Thambundit A, Dwyer A, *et al*. Congenital idiopathic hypogonadotropic hypogonadism: evidence of defects in the hypothalamus, pituitary and testes. J Clin Endocrinol Metab. 2010;95(6): 3019–27.
18. Foresta, C., *et al*. Suppression of the high endogenous levels of plasma FSH in infertile men are associated with improved Sertoli cell function as reflected by elevated levels of plasma inhibin B. Hum Reprod, 2004. 19: 1431.
19. Shinjo, E., *et al*. The effect of human chorionic gonadotropin-based hormonal therapy on intratesticular testosterone levels and spermatogonial DNA synthesis in men with non-obstructive azoospermia. Andrology, 2013. 1: 929.
20. Shiraishi, K., *et al*. Salvage hormonal therapy after failed microdissection testicular sperm extraction: A multi-institutional prospective study. Int J Urol, 2016. 23: 496.
21. Czaplicki M, Bablok L, Janczewski Z. Varicocelectomy in patients with azoospermia. Arch Androl, 1979; 3:51–5.
22. Kadioglu A, Tefekli A, Cayan S, Kandrali E, Erdemir F, Tellaloglu S. Microsurgical inguinal varicocele repair in azoospermic men. Urology. 2001;57:328–33.
23. Schlegel PN, Kaufmann J. Role of varicocelectomy in men with Non-Obstructive Azoospermia. Fertil Steril. 2004;81: 1585–8.
24. Cakan M, Altug U. Induction of spermatogenesis by inguinal varicocele repair in azoospermic men. Arch Androl. 2004;50:145–50.
25. Schlegel PN, Liotta D, Hariprashad J, Veeck LL. Fresh testicular sperm for men with nonobstructive azoospermia works best for ICSI. Urology. 2004;641069–71.
26. Bernie, A.M., *et al*. Comparison of microdissection testicular sperm extraction, conventional testicular sperm extraction, and testicular sperm aspiration for nonobstructive azoospermia: a systematic review and meta-analysis. Fertil Steril, 2015. 104: 1099.
27. Nariyoshi, S., *et al*. Ultrasonographically determined size of seminiferous tubules predicts sperm retrieval by microdissection testicular sperm extraction in men with nonobstructive azoospermia. Fertil Steril, 2020. 113: 97.
28. Cocci, A., *et al*. Effectiveness of highly purified urofollitropin treatment in patients with idiopathic azoospermia before testicular sperm extraction. Urol J, 2018. 85: 19.
29. Cissen, M., *et al*. Prediction model for obtaining spermatozoa with testicular sperm extraction in men with non-obstructive azoospermia. Hum Reprod, 2016. 31: 1934.
30. Alfano, M., *et al*. Anti-Mullerian Hormone-to-Testosterone Ratio is Predictive of Positive Sperm Retrieval in Men with Idiopathic Non-Obstructive Azoospermia. Sci Rep, 2017. 7: 17638.
31. Abdel Raheem, A., *et al*. Testicular histopathology as a predictor of a positive sperm retrieval in men with non-obstructive azoospermia. BJU Int, 2013. 111: 492.
32. Caroppo, E., *et al*. Testicular histology may predict the successful sperm retrieval in patients with non-obstructive azoospermia undergoing conventional TESE: a diagnostic accuracy study. J Assist Reprod Genet, 2017. 34: 149. 1954.

Failed IVF

• *Raghavender Kosgi*

LEARNING OBJECTIVES

- To know the definition of recurrent ART failure.
- To know common causes of recurrent ART failure.
- To know how to evaluate couple with recurrent ART failure.
- To understand management of index case.

INTRODUCTION

Fertilization is a process in which sperm fuses with a mature acolyte to form an embryo. ART is useful when couples are unable to conceive due to maternal or paternal factors or both or sometimes in unexplained infertility. Despite technological advances and standard protocols, fertilization failure during ART is common. The etiology of multiple failed *in-vitro* fertilization (IVF) cycles is unfortunately elusive. Failure of IVF is a frustrating condition for both patients and treating clinicians. It causes a lot of physical, emotional, financial and social trauma to the couple. The urologists treating male infertility should have a sound idea of ART failure and its evaluation. This chapter is to provide an overview of recurrent ART failure from both male and female perspective.

Case Scenario

A 39-year-old male, 38-year-old wife; Married for 10 years

Male examination: Normal (no varicocele)

Semen analysis shows sperm concentration of 14 million per ml; semen volume 2 ml total sperm count per ejaculate 28 million; 24% progressive motility; 2% normal forms; Primary infertility; Failed 3 IUI, 2 IVF-ICSI.

Female evaluation shows anti-Mullerian Hormone (AMH): 2.1 IU/L; Antral follicle count (AFC): 5 on each side; How to proceed?

1. What is the diagnosis? Mention stepwise management of index case.

Ans: Above case capsule shows recurrent failure of assisted reproduction techniques (ART) in an older couple.

Stepwise Management of Index Case:

Male management:

a. In the above case scenario male partner is suffering from oligo-astheno-teratozoospermia (OAT). Physical examination is normal.
b. History should focus on consanguinity, congenital malformations in the family, infertility in siblings.
c. As a first step we have to cross verify previous evaluation of the male. We have to confirm abnormal semen analysis (SA) with repeat assay from standard laboratory after one month gap. It is common in my practice to see substandard semen analysis reports from various labs.
d. Hormonal evaluation: Follicle stimulating hormone (FSH), luteinizing hormone (LH), total testosterone (TT) and estradiol (E2) should be assessed.
e. Asymptomatic/symptomatic genital and urinary tract infections and sexually transmitted infections (STI) should be ruled out.
f. Advanced sperm function tests like DNA fragmentation index (DFI), if available, oxidative stress tests [ORP (oxidation reduction potential) estimation by Myoxis device] can be ordered.

g. Whole exome genome sequencing can be done in research institutes to explore and identify novel mutations.
h. Genetic counselling for the couple is mandatory for any abnormal genetic report
i. Based on the hormone values empirical medical therapy (injection FSH or clomiphene, if it is low or normal, injection hCG (human chorionic gonadotrpin) if testosterone is low or aromatase inhibitors, if low T: E ratio (<10:1) can be opted.
j. Antioxidants can be tried on empirical basis for at least two spermatogenic cycles, if not tried before.
k. Infections should be treated accordingly.
l. Patients with idiopathic high DNA fragmentation index can be treated with lifestyle modifications, balanced diet, regular meditation, exercise, smoking cessation, alcohol reduction, etc.
m. Patients with persistent high DFI can proceed with testicular sperm extraction (TESA) and ICSI. Testicular sperm may have less fragmented DNA than the ejaculate sperm.
n. Insufficient evidence to recommend one treatment over the other for couples suffering from recurrent ART failure.

Female management: Index patient is elderly lady. Her AMH value and astral follicle count is normal. She will be evaluated and treated accordingly by female fertility specialist. The above case scenario highlights the importance of the multidisciplinary, coordinated approach by female reproductive specialist, urologist and embryologist. Comprehensive management of recurrent ART failure in female is beyond the scope of this chapter.

2. What are the common female factors for ART failure?

Ans: The most common reasons for failed IVF are poor embryo quality and defects in endometrial receptivity.

3. What are the risk factors for recurrent implantation failure?

Ans:

Advanced maternal age

Maternal age plays an important role in embryo quality. There is a higher incidence of aneuploidy and reduced pregnancy rates with advancing maternal age, as also highlighted by European Society of Human Reproduction and Embryology (ESHRE). Maternal age over 40 years is a risk factor for recurrent pregnancy loss (RPL).[1–3]

Obesity

Causes of obesity such as unhealthy eating habits, endocrine abnormalities, genetic predispositions and sedentary lifestyles contribute to infertility and poorer ART outcomes. Obese women suffer from poor embryo quality, fewer oocytes and an increased incidence of miscarriages. Higher rates of implantation failure, pregnancy loss is noted, when body mass index (BMI) increases from 25 to 40 kg/m^2.[4,5]

Smoking

Smoking leads to significantly increased risk of miscarriage for each pregnancy as compared to non-smoking patients undergoing ART.[6]

4. What is a clinical pregnancy?

Ans: Clinical pregnancy as determined by ultrasound examination with evidence of a gestational sac or by histopathological examination (ASRM practice committee).[7]

5. What is a biochemical pregnancy?

Ans: Biochemical pregnancy is defined as detection of human chorionic gonadotrpin (hCG) in blood or urine without subsequent clinical signs of pregnancy.[8] Coolum defines biochemical pregnancy when two or more increased values of hCG can be measured, yet there can be no evidence of gestational sac detected on transvaginal ultrasound 2 weeks later.[9]

6. Define pregnancy loss (miscarriage).

Ans: Spontaneous loss of pregnancy before fetus reaches viability, i.e. from conception to until 24 weeks of gestation.

7. What is the difference between biochemical and implantation failure? Explain.

Ans: Implantation failure is defined as failure to show quantifiable signs of implantation such as increased levels of hCG, and those who have increased hCG production without later ultrasound evidence of a gestational sac.[1] Biochemical pregnancy is defined only based on the increased levels of blood or urine hCG, whereas implantation failure is defined based on the absence of gestational sac on ultrasound after embryo transfer in IVF-ICSI (*in-vitro* fertilisation—intracytoplasmic sperm injection) or natural conception. Implantation is a process by which embryo will attach and integrate with uterine endometrium. Failure of this process is called implantation failure.

8. What is recurrent IVF failure?

Ans: Recurrent IVF failure is commonly defined as failure to achieve a pregnancy following 2–6 IVF cycles, in which more than 10 high-grade embryos were transferred into the uterus.[10]

Failure of implantation in at least 3 fresh *in-vitro* fertilisation-embryo transfer (IVF-ET) cycles and/or failure of implantation following the transfer of 10 or more embryos.[11,12]

9. What is recurrent implantation failure (RIF)?

Ans: RIF is the failure of clinical pregnancy after 4 good quality embryo transfers, with at least three fresh or frozen IVF cycles, and in women under the age of 40 years.[1]

10. What is recurrent pregnancy loss (RPL)?

Ans: RPL is the loss of two or more consecutive clinical pregnancies until 20 weeks gestation-according to ASRM.[7] Two or more pregnancy losses until 24 weeks' gestation (including chemical pregnancy) is another definition for RPL as per ESHRE. The prevalence of RPL is about 1–2% of women.[13]

11. What is recurrent early pregnancy loss (REPL)?

Ans: REPL is defined as loss of 2 or more pregnancies before 10 weeks of gestational age.[14]

12. What are the female risk factors for recurrent pregnancy loss?

Ans:

i. Maternal age above 40 years
ii. Smoking
iii. Obesity or underweight
iv. Excessive alcohol consumption
v. Antiphospholipid syndrome
vi. Stress
vii. Occupational and environmental exposure to hazardous chemicals
viii. Chronic endometritis
ix. Excessive caffeine intake
x. Excessive radiation exposure

13 What are the investigations required to evaluate RPL in female?

Ans: RPL evaluation is difficult, expensive and may be confusing. It involves multiple tests and includes evaluation of anatomy, hormones and genetics.

i. Karyotyping
ii. Thyroid profile
iii. Serum prolactin
iv. Antiphospholipid antibodies screening (Lupus anticoagulant, anticardiolipin antibody (ACA) testing
v. Antinuclear antibody testing (ANA)
vi. Beta-2-Glycoprotein I (B2GPI) screening
vii. Assessment of uterine anatomy (transvaginal 3D ultrasound/Hysteroscopy/son hysterography/Hysterosalpingogram (HSG))
viii. Karyotyping of the products of conception (POC)
ix. Array CGH (comparative genomic hybridisation) of the POC (product of conception)
x. Next generation genome sequencing (NGS)
xi. Whole genome sequencing (WGS)
xii. Whole exome sequencing (WES)
xiii. Hereditary thrombophilia screening in high-risk patients for thrombophilia (Factor V Leiden mutation: Prothrombin mutation—MTHFR mutation—protein C, protein S and antithrombin deficiency)
xiv. NK cell testing

14. What are the male factors responsible for recurrent pregnancy loss?

1. Advanced paternal age >45 years[15]
2. Excessive alcohol consumption
3. Smoking
4. Increased sperm DFI
5. Karyotype abnormalities (e.g. sperm aneuploidy)
6. Yq microdeletions
7. Occupational and environmental exposure to hazardous chemicals
8. Obesity

15. What are the investigations required to evaluate RPL in male?

Ans:

1. Sperm DNA fragmentation
2. Karyotyping
3. Oxidative stress testing

16. What are the lifestyle modifications to reduce the risk of RPL?

Ans:

i. Smoking cessation
ii. Maintain normal BMI (neither obesity nor underweight)
iii. Reduce caffeine intake
iv. Regular exercise
v. Avoid or limit alcohol consumption
vi. Avoid radiation exposure

17. What is unexplained male infertility?

Ans: Unexplained male infertility diagnosis is reserved for men with normal semen parameters and without physical as well as endocrine abnormalities.

18. What is idiopathic male infertility?

Ans: Male infertility with abnormal semen parameters, without known aetiology is known as idiopathic male infertility.

19. What are the therapeutic interventions are considered to reduce male factors influence on RPL?

Ans:

i. Stop smoking
ii. Maintain normal BMI (neither obesity nor underweight)
iii. Reduce caffeine intake
iv. Regular exercise
v. Avoid or limit alcohol consumption
vi. Avoid radiation exposure
vii. Varicocele ligation
viii. Sperm selection methods [Physiological intracytoplasmic sperm injection (PICSI), microfluidics, magnetic-activated cell sorting (MACS), intracytoplasmic morphologically selected sperm injection (IMSI)]

20. What are the available interventions for couples with RPL due to genetic abnormalities?

Ans:

i. Preimplantation genetic testing (PGT) for unexplained RPL
ii. Preimplantation genetic testing (PGT) for known genetic problems
   a. PGT for monogenic/single gene defects (PGT-M)
   b. PGT for chromosomal structural rearrangements (PGT-SR)
iii. Genetic counselling is mandatory for all the couple with genetic abnormalities

21. What are the treatment options available for unexplained RPL?

Ans:

i. Intravenous immunoglobulin therapy (IVIG) for suspected immunological or inflammatory diseases
ii. Vaginal progesterone therapy
iii. Folic acid supplementation is beneficial but may prevent RPL
iv. Multivitamin supplementation
v. Antioxidants

KEY POINTS

- Failed IVF/ICSI is an important subset of patients which the uro-andrologist will face in practice.
- Male factor may be the reason for failure, especially if IVF/ICSI was done for male factor infertility.
- Identifying the cause is the most important logical step before proceeding for another IVF/ICSI.
- Identifying modifiable risk factors such as varicocele may improve IVF outcomes.
- Sperm function tests are increasingly being used by female fertility experts and urologist has to understand the implications of these tests.

SUMMARY

- Despite technological advances and standard protocols, fertilization failure during ART is common. The etiology of multiple failed *in-vitro* fertilization (IVF) cycles is unfortunately elusive. Failure of IVF is a frustrating condition for both patients and treating clinicians. It causes a lot of physical, emotional, financial and social trauma to the couple. Comprehensive evaluation of couple by team of female reproductive specialist, urologist, embryologist and geneticist is needed for better outcomes.

REFERENCES

1. Coughlan C, *et al*. Recurrent implantation failure: definition and management. Report Biomed Online. 2014;28(1):14–38.
2. Zeyneloglu HB, Onalan G. Remedies for recurrent implantation failure.Semin Reprod Med. 2014;32(4):297–305.
3. Zeadna A, *et al*. A comparison of biochemical pregnancy rates betweenwomen who underwent IVF and fertile controls who conceivedspontaneously. Hum Reprod. 2015;30(4):783–8.
4. Orvieto R, *et al*. The influence of body mass index on in vitro fertilizationoutcome. Int J Gynaecol Obstet. 2009;104(1):53–5.
5. Moragianni VA, Jones SM, Ryley DA. The effect of body mass index on theoutcomes of first assisted reproductive technology cycles. Fertil Steril. 2012;98(1):102–8.
6. Waylen AL, *et al*. Effects of cigarette smoking upon clinical outcomes ofassisted reproduction: a meta-analysis. Hum Reprod Update. 2009;15(1):31–44.
7. Practice Committee of the American Society for Reproductive Medicine.Evaluation and treatment of recurrent pregnancy loss: a committee opinion. Fertil Steril. 2012;98(5):1103–11.
8. Maesawa Y, *et al*. History of biochemical pregnancy was associated with the subsequent reproductive failure among women with recurrent spontaneous abortion. Gynecol Endocrinol. 2015;31(4):306–8.
9. Coulam CB, Roussev R. Chemical pregnancies: immunologic and ultrasonographic studies. Am J Reprod Immunol. 2002;48(5):323–8.
10. Tan BK, Vandekerckhove P, Kennedy R, Keay SD. Investigation and current management of recurrent IVF treatment failure in the UK. *BJOG*. 2005;112:773–780
11. Raziel A, Friedler S, Schachter M, Kasterstein E, Strassburger D, Ron-El R. Increased frequency of female partner chromosomal abnormalities in patients with high-order implantation failure after in vitro fertilization. Fertil Steril. 2002;/78:/515_8.
12. Stern C, Chamley L, Norris H, Hale L, Baker HWG.A randomized, double-blind, placebo-controlled trial of heparin and aspirin for women with in vitro fertilization implantation failure and antiphospholipid or antinuclear antibodies. Fertil Steril. 2003;/80:/376_83.
13. Group, E.E.P.G.D. Recurrent Pregnancy Loss: European Society of HumanReproduction and Embryology; 2017.
14. Kolte AM, Olsen LR, Mikkelsen EM, Christiansen OB, Nielsen HS. Depression and emotional stress is highly prevalent among women with recurrent pregnancy loss. *Human reproduction (Oxford, England)* 2015b;30: 777–782.
15. Du Plessis SS, Cabler S, McAlister DA, Sabanegh E, Agarwal A. The effect of obesity on sperm disorders and male infertility. *Nat Rev Urol*2010;7: 153–161.

Chapter 7

Male Accessory Gland Infection and Infertility

• Ashit Shah • Shiv Charan Navriya

LEARNING OBJECTIVES

- To understand the definition and criteria of MAGI.
- To understand the concept of Infertility due to MAGI and its pathophysiology.
- To understand the evaluation of Infertile patients with MAGI.
- To understand the causative organisms and management principles of MAGI.
- To understand the fertility outcomes after treatment of MAGI.

INTRODUCTION

Male accessory gland infection (MAGI), considered to be the third (6–10%) most important cause of infertility, happens due to inflammatory response and accumulation of ROS and cytokines. MAGI is associated with impaired spermatogenesis, defective sperms, abnormal semen parameters, reduced secretory capacity of accessory glands and obstruction of ducts.

Case Scenario

A 31-year-old male, wife 26 years; married for 3 years; primary infertility; SA 17 million per ml, 28% PR and 2% normal forms, PC 8–10; semen culture shows Klebsiella; How to manage his seminal infection and infertility?

1. **What is the definition of MAGI?**

   Ans: MAGI (male accessory gland infection) is defined as a group of infection/inflammation of one or more sites of male accessory reproductive glands such as Cowper's glands (bulbourethral glands), seminal vesicles and the prostate.[1] In many published reports, epididymitis and orchitis are also included in the term 'MAGI'[3–5] (Fig. 7.1).

2. **Explain the pathophysiology of MAGI.**

   Ans: Inflammation of the male accessory glands leads to a sequence of changes (Flowchart 7.1).

   Inflammation and obstruction have been proposed as mechanisms causing loss of male accessory gland function.[3,5,6]

3. **What are the different organisms involved in MAGI?**

   Ans: The most prevalent sexually transmitted pathogens are: *Ureaplasma urealyticum, Chlamydia trachomatis, Neisseria gonorrhoeae, Mycoplasma genitalium* and *Mycoplasma hominis*. Another common pathogen is *Escherichia coli*, which particularly results in prostatitis and epididymo-orchitis in 65% to 80% of patients.[7]

4. **How you will assess the functional loss of an accessory gland due to MAGI?**

   Ans: Accessory glands secretions can be measured in the seminal plasma to assess the function of the gland.[7]

   Seminal vesicles: Ascorbic acid, fructose, bicarbonate and prostaglandins

   Epididymis: L-carnitine, neutral glucosidase and glyceryl phosphoryl choline

   Prostate: Seminal plasma c-glutamyl transpeptidase, pH, zinc, citric acid, and acid phosphatase.[7]

5. **What is the difference between infection and inflammation in MAGI?**

   Ans: Infection is the invasion of tissues with disease-causing agents. This incites an inflam-

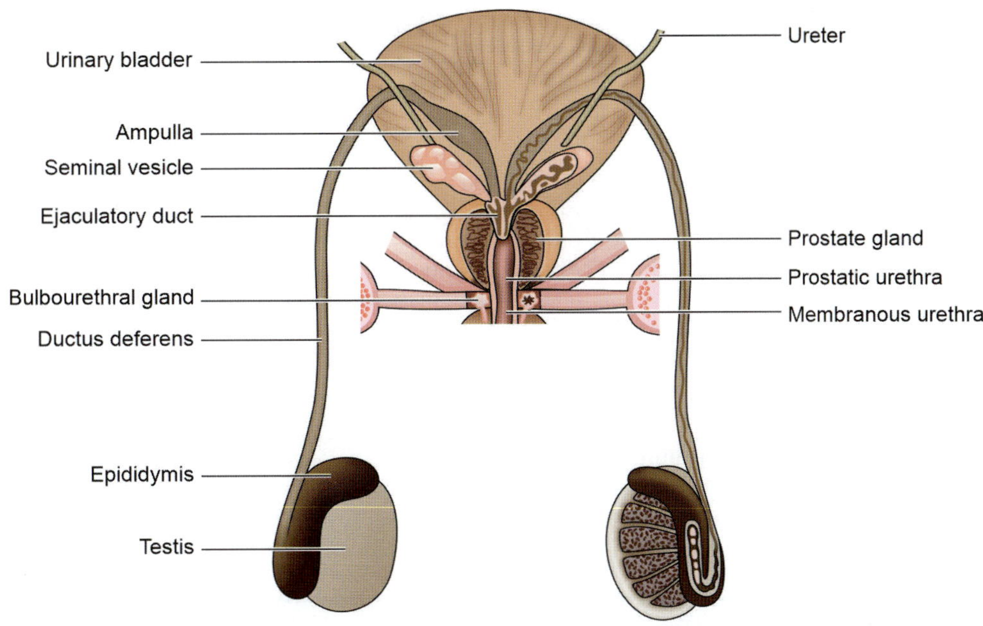

Fig. 7.1: Male accessory glands

Flowchart 7.1: Pathophysiology of MAGI[3,5]

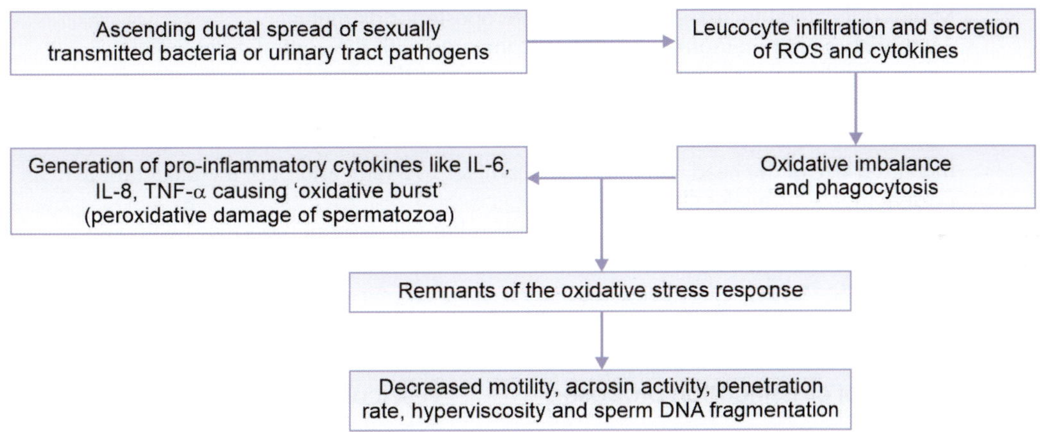

matory response from the host. Infections are commonly due to microbes such as bacteria, viruses or fungi rarely.[8] Non-infectious inflammation can also occur. Leukocytospermia may be seen in infection or inflammation of the male accessory sex glands.

6. **What are the possible ways by which MAGI can affect fertility potential?**

   Ans:
   - Direct action of the microorganisms on sperm function
   - Release of cytokines and ROS causing damage to sperm function
   - Decreased secretions of the accessory glands
   - Obstruction of seminal tract outflow
   - Disturbance of the local immunoregulation leads to formation of anti-sperm antibodies[3,5]

7. **Why chronic epididymitis is a major problem in infertile male?**

   Ans: Chronic epididymitis is one of spectrums of MAGI, having more influence on semen parameters and male infertility than infection of the seminal vesicle or prostate. The diagnosis of chronic epididymitis is very difficult owing to its asymptomatic presentation and lack of local signs on examination.[5]

8. **How to diagnose MAGI?**

   Ans: MAGI should be diagnosed by a combination of clinical history, physical examination signs, and testing of urine and semen (Tables 7.1 and 7.2).

TABLE 7.1: WHO diagnostic criteria[2]

Oligo/asthenospermia and/or teratozoospermia +			
Factor	***A***	***B***	***C***
Description	***Clinical*** History of: 1. Urinary tract infection 2. Epididymitis 3. Sexually transmitted infection Physical signs: 1. Tender thick epididymis 2. Tender vas deferens 3. Abnormal digital rectal examination (DRE)	***Prostatic fluid*** 1. Abnormal expressed prostatic secretion (EPS) 2. Abnormal voided urine after prostate massage (VB3)*	***Semen*** 1. $\geq 1 \times 10^6$ leukocytes/ml 2. Semen culture with significant growth of pathogenic bacteria 3. Abnormal semen appearance 4. Increased semen viscosity (hyper-viscosity) 5. Increased pH abnormal biochemistry of the seminal plasma
Positive diagnosis criteria	Any one factor A plus one feature from factor B or C	Any one factor B plus one feature from factor A or C	Any two factor C features or one factor C feature plus one feature from either factor A or factor B

TABLE 7.2: Ultrasonography criteria to evaluate the inflammatory involvement of each male accessory gland[9,10]

Gland	***Ultrasonographic abnormalities (presence of at least two of the following)***
Prostatitis	Asymmetry of the gland volume Areas of hypoechogenicity Areas of hyperechogenicity Dilatation of periprostatic venous plexus
Vesiculitis	Mono- or bilateral increased (>14 mm) anteroposterior diameter Asymmetry >2.5 mm (normal 7–14 mm) compared with the contralateral vesicle Mono- or bilateral reduced (<7 mm) anteroposterior diameter Thickened and/or calcified glandular epithelium Polycyclic areas separated by hyperechoic septa in one or both vesicles
Epididymitis	Increased size of the head (craniocaudal diameter >12 mm) and/or of the tail (craniocaudal diameter >6 mm) present mono- or bilaterally Presence of multiple microcysts in the head and/or tail, present mono- or bilaterally Mono or bilateral hypo- or hyperechogenicity Large mono- or bilateral hydrocele

9. What are different types of classification proposed for MAGI?

Ans: *Microbiological criteria:* (a) Microbial (bacterial) and (b) Inflammatory (abacterial)

USG criteria: (a) Uncomplicated (prostatitis) and (b) Complicated (prostato-vesiculitis and prostato-vesiculo-epididymitis), and depending on their extension, into unilateral or bilateral forms.

Pathological criteria: (a) Hypertrophic-congestive (HCUF) and (b) Fibro-sclerotic forms (FSUF)

National Institutes of Health (NIH) developed a classification of prostatitis[1,3,4,11] (Table 7.3).

TABLE 7.3: NIH classification and definition of the categories of prostatitis[11]

NIH classification	***Class***	***Definition***
Category I	Acute bacterial prostatitis	Acute infection of the prostate gland
Category II	Chronic bacterial prostatitis	Recurrent infection of the prostate
Category III	Chronic abacterial prostatitis/CPPS	No demonstrable infection
Category III A	Inflammatory CPPS	White blood cells in semen/EPS/VB-3 sample
Category IIIB	Noninflammatory CPPS	No white blood cells in semen/EPS/VB3*
Category IV	Asymptomatic inflammatory prostatitis	No subjective symptoms, detected either by prostate biopsy or the presence of white blood cells in EPS/ semen

*VB3 = voided urine sample after prostatic massage

10. How to interpret leucocytospermia?

Ans: Leukocytospermia (LCS) is characterised by finding >1 × 10^6/ml peroxidase positive leukocytes in semen. Initially, semen analysis is performed to estimate round cells on wet preparation. These round cells in the semen could be leukocytes, immature germ cells, large anucleate residual cytoplasm, epithelial cells or *Trichomonas vaginalis*. Testing for WBC is indictated in case of 5 round cells/high power field (≥1 × 10^6/ml).[12] Semen sample is examined using a phase-contrast microscope with a green filter.

11. Enumerate the indications and ideal method for semen culture.

Ans: Leukocytospermia does not predict semen infection. EAU and AUA guidelines recommend performing a semen culture when the seminal leucocyte concentration is 1 × 10^6/ml.[12,13]

Ideal method of semen culture: Sample should be collected avoiding any external bacterial contamination. The WHO guidelines recommend washing of hands and penis with soap and urinating before collection of semen sample while others advise shower followed by antibacterial skin preparation by hand, perineal and penile wash with 10% povidone-iodine and 4% chlorhexidine.[12,13]

USG guided prostatic massage can be done over the area of acinar ectasia to collect the representative sample. Expressed prostate secretions (EPS) and/or post-prostatic massage urine sample can also be obtained to diagnose chronic prostatitis.

12. What are the different methods of quantification of white blood cell in semen?

Ans:

1. Immunochemistry: Gold standard, uses antibodies against CD45 or CD53 and can detect lymphocytes, granulocytes, and macrophages concurrently.
2. Seminal granulocyte elastase test
3. Peroxidase tests (conventional): (A) Ortho-toluidine test (B) Endtz test.

13. What are the management strategies for MAGI with infertility?

Ans: Treatment is tailored according to the type of MAGI.[3,12]

Targets of therapy

- Eradication of microorganisms
- Normalization of inflammatory process

Treatment should be individualised and includes—antibiotics, alpha blockers in prostatitis with LUTS, steroids, anti-inflammatory compounds (NSAIDs), antioxidant therapy for at least one month and frequent ejaculation.

Sequential treatment with antibiotics (based on cultures), anti-inflammatory agents and antioxidant therapy helps in MAGI. Due to co-existing sexual dysfunction, tadalafil may improve semen parameters.[3,12]

14. What are the antibiotic regimens and their duration for MAGI?

Ans: Infertile men with positive semen culture should be treated with an appropriate course of antibiotics guided by bacterial colonies in the ejaculate and sensitivity testing. Duration depends on the site involved and the pathogen(s) identified, however, it is usually given for 3 to 4 weeks.[2,3]

According to EAU, acute bacterial prostatitis should be considered as complicated UTI; aminoglycoside with second-generation cephalosporin or amoxicillin should be advised. Tetracycline is the gold standard for epididymitis in the absence of STD. If STD is suspected, the administration of cephalosporin is preferred (Tables 7.4 and 7.5).[2,3,13]

TABLE 7.4: Antimicrobial therapy according to pathogen[13]

S.No.	*Pathogen*	*Antimicrobial*	*Dosage and duration of therapy*
1	Gonococcal infection	Ceftriaxone Azithromycin	1 g IM or IV sd 1 g po, sd
2	Non-gonococcal infection (non-identified pathogen)	Doxycycline	100 mg b.i.d, p.o., 7 days
3	*Chlamydia trachomatis*	Azithromycin Or Doxycycline	1.0–1.5 g po, sd 100 mg b.i.d, po., for 7 days
4	*Mycoplasma genitalium*	Azithromycin	500 mg p.o., day 1, 250 mg p.o., 4 days
5	*Ureaplasma urealyticum*	Doxycycline	100 mg b.i.d, p.o., 7 days
6	*Trichomonas vaginalis*	Metronidazole Tinidazole	2 g p.o., sd 2 g p.o., sd

TABLE 7.5: Antimicrobial therapy for chronic bacterial prostatitis[13]

S.No.	Antimicrobial	Daily dose	Duration of therapy
1	Fluoroquinolone	Optimal oral daily dose	4–6 weeks
2	Doxycycline	100 mg b.i.d	10 days (only for *C. trachomatis* or mycoplasma)
3	Azithromycin	500 mg once daily	3 weeks (only for *C. trachomatis*)
4	Metronidazole	500 mg t.i.d.	14 days (only for *T. vaginalis*)

15. What are the outcomes of antibiotic treatment for MAGI?

Ans: Literature regarding anti-bacterial therapy and fertility outcomes has conflicting reports. Bacteriospermia can persist after treatment with antimicrobials. The eradication rate of infection is inversely related to the spectrum of the inflammatory process, being very high (92.5%) in patients with prostatitis alone, intermediate (70.4%) in prostato-vesiculitis, and lowest (52%) in prostato-vesciculo-epididymitis after antibiotic therapy. Patients with eradicated infection had improvement in sperm parameters compared to patients with persistent infection.[2]

Even if infection is eradicated, semen quality may not improve completely due to chronic inflammatory state persisting.[7]

16. What are the reasons for low eradication rate in patients with chronic bacterial prostatitis?

Ans:

- Poor penetration of antibiotics within the prostatic tissue
- Inflammation of glands
- Altered pharmacokinetics
- Antibiotic resistance of microorganisms
- Adverse effects of antibiotics
- Presence of calcifications in prostate
- Micro colony formation and biofilm in the acinar and ductal inflamed walls

17. What are the effect of MAGI on ART outcomes?

Ans: Recent studies have not reported any significant effect of leukocytospermia on ART outcomes.[12] However, MAGI results in a higher percentage of sperms with fragmented DNA and sperm DNA is a prognostic factor for ART outcome. MAGI has been shown to alter sperm parameters leading to poorer reproductive outcomes, lower pregnancy rates and higher miscarriage rates with ART; some studies suggest using testicular sperm ICSI.[2,14]

18. What is the relation of MAGI and oxidative stress/ DNA fragmentation?

Oxidative stress (OS) and consequent damage to DNA integrity is an important modulator of human sperm function and conception outcomes. DNA damage is most commonly measured outcome to examine the balance of antioxidants and ROS. OS is signified by ROS and imbalance in the antioxidant defences. An increase in ROS by 25% can lead to a 10% increase in sperm DNA fragmentation. A positive association is also found between leukocytospermia, ROS, and SDF levels.[6]

Three main mechanisms can lead to DNA damage—abortive apoptosis, abnormal chromatin packaging/maturation, or increased OS.[1] This results in asthenospermia, reduced sperm-oocyte fusion, hyperviscous semen, oocyte penetration and also damages sperm chromatin/DNA integrity (Fig. 7.2).[12]

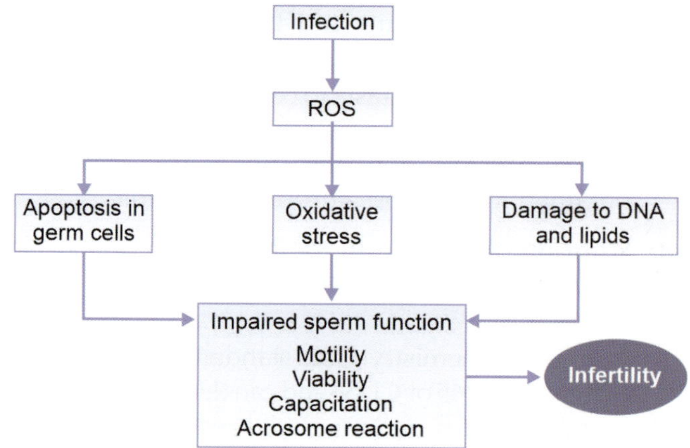

Fig. 7.2: Mechanism of ROS production and infertility in MAGI[12]

19. How will you counsel an anxious patient with MAGI?

Ans: The patient needs to be reassured that MAGI is a possibly curable cause with good resolution rates in infertile men. Patient should also be made aware of the low diagnostic value of leukocytospermia alone for bacteriospermia and altered semen quality. Furthermore, it is not a predictive determinant of positive semen culture.[6,16]

20. What are the effect of MAGI on female fertility/ female genital tract infection?

Ans: Nearly 60% of acute salpingitis in young women are caused by Chlamydia. There is an increased risk of tubal–peritoneal damage leading to pelvic inflammation and subsequent pelvic adhesions. Thus, chances of tubal infertility and ectopic pregnancy are considerably increased with each infectious episode.[5] MAGI can potentially result in the male accessory sex glands functioning as reservoirs for the infective organism, thus women have a higher chance of infection.[15] Also, DNA fragmentation, a possible outcome of MAGI, negatively affects fertility rates, embryo quality and implantation. It also has a positive correlation with miscarriage and neonatal diseases.[3]

21. What is the role of uroflowmetry, alpha blockers and NSAIDs in the treatment of prostatitis?

Ans: Obstruction due to enlarged prostate is a predisposing factor for prostatitis, uroflowmetry will objectively document the flow rate and guide further treatment. Alpha blockers are the mainstay of therapy for outlet obstruction due to prostate. NSAIDs alleviates the inflammation associated with chronic prostatitis and contributed to positive clinical outcomes.[3]

KEY POINTS

- Male accessory gland infection (MAGI) is an often overlooked but important and modifiable risk factor for male infertility
- It is a clinical and laboratory based diagnosis.
- Infection and inflammation can lead to direct reduction in sperm parameters or indirectly can lead to elevated oxidative stress and sperm DNA fragmentation.
- Treatment is based on cause; includes diet, lifestyle changes, specifically treating prostate-seminal vesiculitis, and antioxidants.

REFERENCES

1. Weidner W, Krause W, Ludwig M. Relevance of male accessory gland infection for subsequent fertility with special focus on prostatitis. Hum Reprod Update. 1999;5:421–432.
2. Noweir HA, Modgil V, Pearce I. Male accessory gland inflammation (MAGI): an evolving entity. *Journal of Clinical Urology*. 2022;15(5):414–423.
3. Calogero AE, Duca Y, Condorelli RA, La Vignera S. Male accessory gland inflammation, infertility, and sexual dysfunctions: a practical approach to diagnosis and therapy. Andrology. 2017 Nov;5(6):1064–1072.
4. Walter K.H. Krause (April 2008). "Male accessory gland infection". *Andrologia*. 40 (2): 113–116.
5. Henkel R. Infection in Infertility. In: Parekattil SJ, Esteves SC, Agarwal A, editors. Male Infertility: Contemporary Clinical Approaches, Andrology, ART and Antioxidants. 2nd ed. Cham: Springer; 2020:409–24.
6. Calogero AE, La Vignera S, Condorelli RA, Agata RD, Vicari E. Effects of male accessory gland infection on sperm parameters. In: Zini A, Agarwal A, eds. Sperm chromatin, biological and clinical applications in male infertility and assisted reproduction. New York: Springer; 2011; 375–394.
7. La Vignera S, Vicari E, Condorelli RA, D'Agata R, Calogero AE. Male accessory gland infection and sperm parameters (review). Int J Androl. 2011;34:e330–47.
8. Robbins SL, Cotran RS, Kumar V, Collins T (1998). *Robbins Pathologic Basis of Disease*. Philadelphia: W.B Saunders Company. ISBN 978-0-7216-7335-6.
9. Comhaire F, Verschraegen G and Vermeulen L. Diagnosis of accessory gland infection and its possible role in male infertility. Int J Androl 1980; 3: 32–45.
10. La Vignera S, Crafa A, Condorelli RA, Barbagallo F, Mongioì LM, Cannarella R, Compagnone M, Aversa A, Calogero AE. Ultrasound evaluation of patients with male accessory gland inflammation: a pictorial review. Andrology. 2021 Sep;9(5):1298–1305.
11. Krieger JN, Nyberg LJ, Nickel JC. NIH consensus definition and classification of prostatitis. JAMA. 1999;282:236–7.
12. Sharma R, Gupta S, Agarwal A, *et al*. Relevance of leukocytospermia and semen culture and its true place in diagnosing and treating male infertility. World J Mens Health. 2021;40:191–207.
13. EAU Guidelines: Urological Infections I Uroweb. [online] Uroweb. Available at: https://uroweb.org/guideline/urological-infections/(2023).
14. Agarwal A, Farkouh A, Parekh N, Zini A, Arafa M, Kandil H, *et al*. Sperm DNA fragmentation: A critical assessment of clinical practice guidelines. World J Mens Health. 2022; 40:30–7.
15. Purvis K, Christiansen E. Infection in the male reproductive tract. Impact, diagnosis and treatment in relation to male infertility. International Journal of Andrology. 1993;16(1):1–3.
16. Depuydt, C., Mahmoud, A., Everaert, K. (2006). Infection/Inflammation of the Male Genital Tract as Cause of Abnormal Spermatozoa. In: Schill, WB., Comhaire, F., Hargreave, T.B. (eds) Andrology for the Clinician. Springer, Berlin, Heidelberg. https://doi.org/10.1007/3-540-33713-X_65.

Chapter

8

Obstructive Azoospermia

• Karthikeyan VS • Datteswar Hota

LEARNING OBJECTIVES

- To make a confident diagnosis of obstructive azoospermia.
- To identify the etiology of obstructive azoospermia and perform appropriate evaluation.
- To be able to counsel couple regarding assisted reproduction and appropriate surgical sperm retrieval technique.

INTRODUCTION

CBAVD is a relatively rare condition (1–2% of male infertility and 1:1000 men) and causes obstructive azoospermia. Normal testicular volume and FSH suggest an intact spermatogenesis. Genetic evaluation especially for CBAVD with unilateral renal agenesis can identify mutations in the cystic fibrosis transmembrane conductance regulator (CFTR) gene. Wife evaluation, genetic evaluation and counselling and counselling about assisted reproduction go hand-in-hand. Surgical sperm retrieval in the form of testicular sperm aspiration (TESA) and percutaneous epididiymal sperm aspiration (PESA) are the options, in this patient. These sperms would be used for IVF-ICSI.

Case Scenario

A 29-year-old male, 28-year-old lady, married for 8 years; husband has azoospermia, 0.5 ml; FSH 4.5; wife AMH is 3.3; On male examination, bilateral vas absent—how to proceed?

1. **What is the diagnosis?**

   Ans: In view of absent vas on bilateral clinical examination and azoospermia with low volime ejaculate on semen analysis (Fig. 8.1), the most likely diagnosis is congenital bilateral absence of vas deferens (CBAVD) leading to obstructive azoospermia.[1,2]

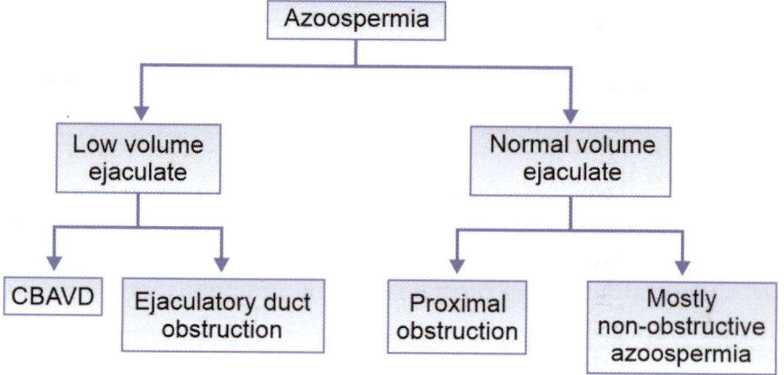

Fig. 8.1: Workup of azoospermia

2. **Is this information enough on clinical examination?**

   Ans: The next step is to perform a thorough clinical examination to assess the androgenization, bilateral testis volume and epididymal fullness. Also, confirm absence of vas deferens on both sides.

3. **What is the next step in the management of this patient?**

   Ans: Hormonal evaluation is the next logical step in the management of this patient. It has been mentioned that the follicle stimulating hormone (FSH) is 4.5 IU/L and this falls in the normal range.

4. **What are the other hormone tests you would like to do?**

   Ans: In this patient, since his testicular volume is normal, both vasa are absent and FSH is within the normal range, it is sufficient to proceed to the next treatment step and no other hormone evaluation are routinely required. It is presumed that this patient has a normal functioning testis and because of the obstruction due to CBAVD these sperms have not been able to reach the semen.

Patients do come with other reports such as luteinizing hormone (LH), total testosterone and estradiol (E2). These hormones could be considered in case of additional factors like smaller testes, erectile dysfunction or obesity. Here, there can be a rare coexistence of both components of hormonal dysfunction and obstruction.[2]

5. **Why is it important to identify obstruction?**

Ans: It is essential to identify obstruction for two reasons. It is deemed that in case obstruction is proven, then the spermatogenesis is usually intact and it has better assisted reproduction (ART) outcomes. This particular patient has CBAVD and hence the only option which remains in surgical sperm retrieval. However, in case of an otherwise palpable bilateral vasa and suspected obstructive cause, or a proven vasal or epididymal obstruction amenable to surgical correction, the couple stand a chance for natural conception. These are two reasons why identifying an obstruction is beneficial for the patient.[2]

6. **How to suspect obstructive cause for azoospermia?**

Ans: The parameters to consider for deciding the probable etiology for azoospermia are listed in Table 8.1.[2,3]

In men with vasal block, epididymis is usually full; In CBAVD the epididymis may be empty or full based on the involvement.

7. **What are the other important examination findings which can suggest obstruction?**

Ans: The other findings which guide towards a diagnosis of obstruction especially when the vasa are palpable is the epididymal fullness. A flaccid epididymis usually points towards a non-obstructive etiology. A turgid epididymis may point towards an obstructive pathology.

8. **What is the role for imaging in obstructive azoospermia?**

Ans: CBAVD is a clinical diagnosis. There is no recommendation for imaging studies to diagnose CBAVD. However, transrectal ultrasound can confirm the physical findings and give more clarity to the clinical picture. Bilateral absent vas on TRUS, along with hypoplastic or absent seminal vesicles would clearly show that this patient would have surgical sperm retrieval and intracytoplasmic sperm injection (ICSI) as the only therapeutic option.

There is no role to routinely perform ultrasound scrotum in men with CBAVD. Some patients do come with scan reports showing varicocele or epididymal cysts. Varicocele is a clinical diagnosis in these men because only a significant palpable varicocele may change the overall treatment plan in obstructive azoospermia. Subclinical varicoceles detected on ultrasound usually do not warrant surgical treatment. Epididymal cysts detected on ultrasound again may not add significantly to treatment. A dilated rete testis on ultrasound scrotum may suggest obstruction.

9. **Discuss the role of TRUS in obstructive azoospermia (EDO)?**

Ans: TRUS is the most useful imaging modality for ejaculatory duct obstruction, with a midline ejaculatory duct cyst with dilated seminal vesicles suggesting a possibility of correction via a TURED (transurethral resection of the ejaculatory duct). Calcification along the vas, in absence of a sizable midline cyst could represent a high intraprostatic block, which is usually not accessible by TURED.

TABLE 8.1: Differentiating various causes of azoospermia

Parameter	*Obstructive azoospermia (Epididymal)*	*CBAVD or EDO*	*Non-obstructive azoospermia*
Androgenisation and general body habitus	Usually normal	Usually normal	May be normal or reduced; Patient may be obese
Testicular volume	Usually normal	Usually normal	May be normal or reduced
Presence or absence of vas	Present	CBAVD—absent EDO—present	Usually present
Semen volume	Usually normal	Usually reduced	Usually normal
Semen pH	Alkaline	Acidic	Usually alkaline
Semen fructose	Usually positive	Negative (low volume ejaculate insufficient for analysis)	Usually positive
FSH	Usually normal		Normal or elevated

10. What is the next step in the management of this couple (CBAVD)?

Ans: Before proceeding to evaluate the male, it is wise to have a clear picture of the female partner's reproductive potential. In this case, the wife's age is 28 years and her anti-mullerian hormone (AMH) is 3.3 U/L, which is normal. Wife's evaluation is typically performed by a reproductive medicine expert or a gynecologist. The most important tests are ovarian reserve (as assessed by AMH and antral follicle count-AFC), tubal patency and uterine cavity assessment. In this couple, in view of CBAVD, the only treatment possible is ICSI and hence she should be evaluated for the same. The gynecologist would also assess the regularity of menstrual cycles, other comorbid conditions such as diabetes mellitus, thyroid dysfunction and counsel her for stimulation for oocyte aspiration and ICSI.

11. Is there a role for genetic evaluation in this couple?

Ans: CBAVD may be part of the spectrum of cystic fibrosis. Cystic fibrosis transmembrane conductance regulator (CFTR) gene mutations are observed in men with CBAVD. Though this represents a milder variant of cystic fibrosis, it is essential to understand the cystic fibrosis is a genetic disorder which is transmitted by autosomal recessive inheritance. So the child is at risk for a severe form of cystic fibrosis if alleles from both partners are inherited. If the wife is a carrier for the mutation, then it is possible for this situation to arise. A genetic counselling should be done for the couple.

Genetic evaluation starts from the husband because he has the phenotype of a possible CFTR gene mutation. In men with CBAVD, an ultrasound of both kidneys should be done to look for unilateral renal agenesis. In case of unilateral renal agenesis with vasal aplasia, CFTR testing is not required as it suggests a mesonephric duct development anomaly. The best genetic test in the setting of CBAVD would be to do the complete gene sequencing for cystic fibrosis (NGS: Next generation sequencing). The rationale behind this is that the genetic variations in Indian population are different from Caucasian patients and it is not sufficient to test only for the common variants observed in western population (standard testing done at most centers) as our population might harbour selective variants which are common in our patients. If CFTR testing shows no mutation in the CFTR gene, then there is no significant risk of the child being affected by cystic fibrosis. If the CFTR gene mutation in the husband is positive, then those corresponding mutations can be checked in the wife and if negative, can safely undergo ICSI after surgical sperm retrieval. It is important to be sure of the genetic pattern in both partners, minor and major mutations and decide the risk of transmission to the fetus before performing ICSI.[3–5]

12. In case the wife tests positive for the corresponding mutations, what are the options?

Ans: In case both partners have similar positive mutations (major), the couple should undergo thorough genetic counselling to understand the pattern of inheritance and the risk of transmission should be clearly explained. It would probably be wise to advise against ICSI with gametes from the male partner.

There is a newer option of preimplantation genetic testing where an embryo biopsy can be done to identify if that particular embryo that would be transferred has CFTR gene mutations. This is because the disease is transmitted by autosomal recessive mode of inheritance, not all embryos would be affected.[3–5]

13. What are the options for surgical sperm retrieval?

Ans: In case of CBAVD, both options of testicular (TESA) and percutaneous epididiymal (PESA) sperm aspiration are available. If the epididymis is developed and turgid, PESA offers motile mature sperms and can be used for IVF (*in vitro* fertilization) or ICSI. If the epididymis is not well developed or is flaccid, then TESA-ICSI is the only option. An option of microdissection testicular sperm extraction is very rarely required in men with CBAVD with normal FSH levels and no suspicion of non-obstructive component.

14. What are the surgical options for a patient with suspected obstructive etiology with palpable bilateral vasa? (Epididymal Obstruction)

Ans: The ideal method to prove obstruction is testicular biopsy and to prove normal spermatogenesis. This is one of the very few indications for testicular biopsy in modern urological practice. It is best to perform it in a centre with facilities for testicular sperm cryopreservation. This can be combined with a surgical corrective procedure at the same time based on availability of the operating microscope and after adequate patient counselling.

Once obstruction with normal spermatogenesis is proven, microsurgical vasoepididymal anastomosis is a possibility depending on the etiology of obstruction (filarial infection has worst prognosis) and nature of epididymis (turgi, beaded, firm). Intraoperative vasal fluid analysis guides the ideal level at which the anastomosis should be done. Semen analysis should be repeated after 3–6 months.

In men with previous vasectomy, microsurgical vasectomy reversal (vaso-vasostomy) can yield good results based on the duration after vasectomy, nature of spermatogenesis on preoperative testicular biopsy and length of defect which has to be bridged during the vasectomy reversal. Conversion to vasopeididymal anastomosis is often required.

15. What is the postoperative management for TESA/PESA?

Ans: These procedures are usually done as day-care surgeries. Scrotal support, ice packs and analgesics are sufficient. The patient should be explained about scrotal swelling (due to hematoma) and rare instances of bleeding.

KEY POINTS

- Obstructive azoospermia is mainly a clinical suspicion.
- Factors favoring a diagnosis of OA include normal sized testes, turgid epididymis and normal FSH values.
- In case of low semen volume, absent fructose and acidic pH, it suggests an obstruction.
- Congenital bilateral absent vas deferens is a clinical diagnosis where both vasa are not palpable. The head of the epididymis may be turgid.
- Surgical sperm retrieval in OA may be with percutaneous epididymal sperm aspiration (PESA) or testicular sperm aspiration (TESA).
- A strong genetic background is essential for the urologist to workup these men:

SUMMARY

- CBAVD is a relatively rare condition (1–2% of male infertility and 1:1000 men) and causes obstructive azoospermia. Normal testicular volume and FSH suggest an intact spermatogenesis. Genetic evaluation especially for CBAVD with unilateral agenesis can identify mutations in the cystic fibrosis transmembrane conductance regulator (CFTR) gene. Wife evaluation, genetic evaluation and counselling and counselling about assisted reproduction go hand-in-hand. Surgical sperm retrieval in the form of testicular (TESA) and percutaneous epididiymal (PESA) sperm aspiration are the options, in this patient. These sperms would be used for IVF-ICSI.

REFERENCES

1. Baker K, Sabanegh E Jr. Obstructive azoospermia: reconstructive techniques and results. Clinics (Sao Paulo). 2013;68 Suppl 1(Suppl 1):61–73.
2. Practice Committee of the American Society for Reproductive Medicine in collaboration with the Society for Male Reproduction and Urology. Electronic address: asrm@asrm.org. The management of obstructive azoospermia: a committee opinion. Fertil Steril 2019;111(5):873–880.
3. Cioppi F, Rosta V, Krausz C. Genetics of Azoospermia. Int J Mol Sci 2021;22(6):3264.
4. de Souza DAS, Faucz FR, Pereira-Ferrari L, Sotomaior VS, Raskin S. Congenital bilateral absence of the vas deferens as an atypical form of cystic fibrosis: reproductive implications and genetic counseling. Andrology 2018;6(1):127–135.
5. Gaikwad A, Khan S, Kadam S, *et al*. Cystic fibrosis transmembrane conductance regulator-related male infertility: Relevance of genetic testing and counselling in Indian population. Indian J Med Res 2020;152(6):575–583.

Chapter

9

Hypogonadotropic Hypogonadism and Infertility

• *Pramod Krishnappa*

LEARNING OBJECTIVES

- Diagnose, classify and identify the etiology of hypogonadotropic hypogonadism (HH).
- To understand sperm induction protocol and follow-up.
- To fix appropriate deadlines to proceed to ART.

INTRODUCTION

There are both congenital and acquired causes of which congenital appears to be the common cause of HH. HH is a combination of low FSH and LH with low testosterone levels. Gonadotropin therapy is the treatment of choice. Inj hCG is started first to normalize testosterone levels and then inj HMG is added to induce spermatogenesis. High cost and long duration of treatment must be clearly explained and counselled. A sperm retrieval procedure is to be considered after a reasonable period of gonadotropin therapy.

Case Scenario

A 28-year-old male, married to a 24-year-old lady for 2 years has primary infertility. his semen analysis has low volume with occasional sperm per HPF. His primary infertility; semen analysis (vol 0.7 ml) shows occasional sperms per HPF; Testosterone is 110 ng/dl and FSH 0.4; how to proceed?

Here is a young couple in their 20s who are married since 2 years and unable to conceive. The man has low volume ejaculate (<1.5 ml), severe oligospermia (< 1 million/ml), low total testosterone (< 300 ng/dl) and low FSH (< 1.5 mIU/ml). From the above clinical information, it appears to be a case of ***hypogonadotropic hypogonadism (HH).*** Hypogonadism (low testosterone) can be due to problem in the testis (hypergonadotropic) or disorder of the hypothalamic-pituitary axis (hypogonadotropic). "Hypogonadotropic" means low gonadotropins (FSH, LH) and "hypogonadism" means low testosterone.

1. **What are the various causes of hypogonadotropic hypogonadism (HH) ?**

   Ans: The various causes are mentioned in Table 9.1.

Table 9.1: Hypogonadotropic hypogonadism: Etiology[1–2]

Congenital causes	
• Kallmann syndrome • Idiopathic secondary hypogonadism • Prader-Willi syndrome • Laurence-Moon syndrome • Moebius syndrome	• Hyperprolactinaemia • Pituitary dysfunction (e.g., tumour, surgery, trauma, infections or infiltrative diseases) • Hypothalamic dysfunction (e.g., tumours or intracranial masses) • Chronic conditions (e.g., type 2 diabetes mellitus, haemochromatosis, hepatic steatosis and cirrhosis or coronary artery disease) • Drug use (i.e., glucocorticoid, opioids, androgen, progestins, oestrogens or gonadotropin-releasing hormone analogs) • Obesity • Older age (with associated co-morbidities)

Though Kallmann syndrome is the commonest cause of congenital HH, idiopathic secondary hypogonadism is proposed to be a commoner etiology by some authors.[3–5] Kallmann syndrome should be considered in HH men with anosmia or hyposmia.

2. What are the clinical characteristics of hypogonadotropic hypogonadism?

Ans: The clinical features of HH are androgen deficiency and interruption in sexual maturation around puberty. HH is idiopathic when there is deficiency of gonadotropin releasing hormone (GnRH) beyond 18 years of age. HH is properly defined as pubertal delay in boys <18 years of age. ***HH must be confirmed only after the patient has crossed 18 years.***[6]

3. What are the clinical features of HH?

Ans:

- Normal stature and normal voice
- Gynecomastia
- Thin facial, pubic and axillary hair
- Small/normal size testes
- Infertility
- Reduced libido
- Reduced bone mineral density
- Reduced muscle mass, elevated body fat percentage
- Mild anemia
- Hot flashes

4. How do you proceed with evaluation?

Ans: Lab investigations include:

- Two reports of total testosterone for confirmation of hypogonadism
- FSH, LH, prolactin

Testosterone estimation is best done before 10 am because of diurnal variation. Free testosterone, sex hormone binding globulin (SHBG) and albumin may not be of much clinical significance in HH. ***Low FSH, low LH and low total testosterone confirms the diagnosis of HH*** (Table 9.2). A cut-off of early morning ***total testosterone of 300 ng/dl in adults is considered as reasonable lower limit [Expert opinion].***[7]

In Kallmann syndrome, MRI of brain can show anomalous morphology or the absence of the olfactory bulb. A normal MRI scan does not rule out a diagnosis of Kallmann syndrome, as normal olfactory bulbs can still be visualized in 20% of cases.[8]

5. Is MRI brain compulsory in all patients with HH?

Ans: MRI is recommended by The Endocrine Society in secondary hypogonadism where total testosterone levels are <150 ng/dL with ***persistent hyperprolactinemia***, panhypopituitarism or with symptoms of tumour mass effect (headache, visual impairment or visual field defect) and MRI has a better yield.[9] Anatomic lesions are likely to be present when men have low testosterone and concomitant ***hyperprolactinemia***. A study reported that 18.8% had abnormal MRI, with microadenoma or empty sella and no meaningful surgical treatments are offered.[10]

6. Is there a genetic basis for HH?

Ans: Congenital HH has significant phenotypic and genotypic heterogeneity, with over 30 genes implicated. Genetic etiology is obscure in at least 50%; ***congenital HH is a diagnosis of exclusion.*** Congenital HH can be autosomal dominant, autosomal recessive, X-linked, and oligogenic inheritance, with variable penetrance. Pituitary tumours, genetic causes, infiltrative diseases like hemochromatosis, functional hypogonadism (drugs/medical conditions) should be ruled out before labelling as congenital HH.

7. What is the genetic testing done for HH?

Ans: Next-generation sequencing is recommended unless there is a known familial mutation or a clear pattern of familial inheritance and includes at least genes for Kallmann and normosmic HH (ANOS1, CHD7, FGFR1, GNRHR, IL17RD, PROKR2, SOX10 and TACR3). Genetic testing may aid in prognostication and for personalized management of patients, but at this time increased likelihood of detecting insignificant variants.[11]

8. What are the goals of treatment in this case?

Ans:

- Improve testosterone levels
- Fertility preservation and conception

9. Is testosterone therapy indicated in this patient?

Ans: Gonadotropin therapy will be the mainstay of treatment in HH to improve testosterone levels when the goal of treatment is fertility enhancement.

TABLE 9.2: Hormone levels in severe oligospermia due to spermatogenic defect, obstructive azoospermia and hypogonadotropic hypogonadism

	Severely impaired spermatogenesis	*Obstructive azoospermia*	*Hypogonadotropic hypogonadism*
LH	High/normal	Normal	Low
FSH	High/normal	Normal	Low
Testosterone	Low/normal	Normal	Low

Exogenous testosterone is contraindicated in men desiring fertility as it suppresses intratesticular testosterone production which is essential for spermatogenesis. The contraceptive effect of exogenous testosterone is well known. Exogenous testosterone inhibits spermatogenesis due to reduction in intratesticular testosterone, feedback inhibition of GnRH and inhibition of LH synthesis. Inhibiting GnRH production also inhibits FSH release and impairs spermatogenesis in Sertoli cells. ***Hence testosterone therapy should never be prescribed in men seeking fertility care.***[12]

10. What is the treatment for hyperprolactinemia?

Ans: ***In men with hyperprolactinemia, medical therapy should initially be provided with dopamine receptor agonists before starting gonadotropin therapy.***[13] Hyperprolactinemia suppresses GnRH release from hypothalamus. Cabergoline (0.5–1.0 mg orally twice weekly) is the most commonly used drug. It has been specifically demonstrated to improve fertility by normalizing sperm quality in men with hyperprolactinemia.

11. How is gonadotropin replacement therapy started?

Ans: Human chorionic gonadotropin (hCG), an LH analog, is typically the first drug prescribed for HH, intramuscularly or subcutaneously at doses from 2000 to 3000 IU 2 to 3 times weekly, to first correct the LH deficiency.[13] HCG dosing is adjusted to achieve serum total testosterone levels in the mid-normal range (350–400 ng/dL).

Once testosterone levels have normalized or spermatogenesis is initiated, FSH is added in the form of:

- Human menopausal gonadotropin (HMG), containing both LH and FSH activity, in doses of 75–150 IU subcutaneously 2 to 3 times per week.[14] Therapy with both hCG and HMG (combined therapy) is required for optimal spermatogenesis in men with the onset of **prepubertal** HH, where testis volumes are typically <4 ml. In special circumstances, recombinant human FSH (rFSH) in doses of 75 to 150 IU can be used subcutaneously 2–5 times weekly.[14]
- Men with baseline severe testicular atrophy (volume <4 ml) or cryptorchidism should be counselled that monotherapy with hCG alone yields poor success and hCG + HMG/rFSH from the beginning.[3]
- Portable GnRH-infusion pumps can be used which administer pulses of GnRH into the subcutaneous tissue of the abdominal wall every 2 hours, with doses ranging from 100 to 400 ng/kg. The duration of therapy is only for 4 months and is shorter than that of gonadotropin therapy. It is difficult to practice due to high costs and availability only in specialized tertiary hospitals.[6]

12. What are the favourable factors for success of gonadotropin therapy ?

Ans:

- Larger testis volume> 4 ml
- Pre-pubertal onset of HH
- Prior gonadotropin use

Testis volume is determined by the number of functional seminiferous tubules inside the testis. This is decided by prior exposure to gonadotropins and can predict spermatogenesis. Gonadotropins at the time of puberty "prime" the testis for spermatogenesis. Cryptorchidism indicates poor prognosis for fertility enhancement. Men with congenital HH and cryptorchidism require extended courses of gonadotropin treatment (18–24 months).[15]

13. Is prior testosterone therapy a negative predictor for gonadotropin therapy?

Ans: Conflicting data is available.[16,17] ***It is a common practice to keep young men proven to have HH, on testosterone replacement therapy and switch over to hCG therapy when they seek fertility.***

14. How long does it take to normalise testosterone levels after starting gonadotropin therapy ?

Ans: Time taken to reach normal serum testosterone level depends on testis volume and testosterone levels at the beginning. It can range from 1 week to 6 months or even more.[18–19]

15. What are the spermatogenesis outcomes of gonadotropin therapy in HH?

Ans: Many men may not reach normal sperm counts but this does not preclude fertility (median: 5–8 million/ml). Smaller the testes size, longer is the duration of therapy typically required, ranging even up to 24 months for spermatogenesis. hCG + HMG therapy has been shown to induce spermatogenesis in up to 84% of patients; 69% of these men had sperm concentrations >1.5 million/ml.[20]

16. When should a couple seek assisted reproductive techniques (ART) in HH?

Ans: ART may be considered if spontaneous conception is not occurring:[21]

- Even after 20 months of starting gonadotropin therapy or
- Even after 6–8 months of achieving a sperm concentration of >5 million/ml or

- if there is associated significant female factor infertility (poor ovarian reserve, tubal blockage)

The time durations mentioned above can vary based on the personal needs/priority of the couple to seek early or delayed fertility treatment. Not only male factor evaluation is enough; reproductive potential of the female partner should also be simultaneously tested.

Assisted reproductive techniques (ART) have changed the landscape of treatment in couples with male HH. Intrauterine insemination (IUI) is good if the patient has a total motile sperm concentration higher than 5 million/ml with gonadotropin therapy but couple did not have spontaneous conception despite the female partner having patent fallopian tube and good ovarian reserve. Intracytoplasmic sperm injection (ICSI) is the treatment of choice for patients who have completed at least one year of gonadotropin therapy and exhibit sperm concentrations of <1 million/ml or failed to conceive. Pregnancy rates of 30–55% per cycle have been reported with ICSI.[21–22]

17. When do you plan surgical sperm retrieval if this HH patient presented with azoospermia and remains azoospermic during gonadotropin therapy? How long do you wait after gonadotropin therapy to perform surgical sperm retrieval?

Ans: Yilmazel *et al* reported that 5/65 (7.7%) patients with HH with azoospermia continued to be azoospermic despite the long-term gonadotropin treatment (>2 years).[23] Microdissection TEsticular Sperm Extraction (MicroTESE) was successful in retrieving sperms in 3 out of these 5 patients. Fahmy *et al* reported that testicular sperm extraction (TESE) was successful in retrieving sperms in 11 out of 15 (73%) HH patients (73%) with azoospermia after 6 months of combined gonadotropin therapy (hCG + HMG). [24]

18. When do you stop the gonadotropin therapy?

Ans:

- hCG + HMG for fertility restoration should be continued till pregnancy is achieved.
- Medications should be continued until the beginning of the second trimester, beyond which the risk of miscarriage is negligible.
- If the couple plans to have another child soon, then hCG monotherapy may be continued. This is not very expensive. However, if the expected interval is anticipated to be long, the patient can switch to testosterone replacement therapy.
- Sperm cryopreservation is an option for fertility preservation.

19. How is the compliance of patients for gonadotropin therapy?

Ans:

- As for chronic conditions, adherence to long-term therapy is difficult.
- Mild, moderate or severe depressive symptoms along with low adherence to injections has been reported.[25]
- It is essential to spend adequate time with the couple and motivate the male partner to continue injections.
- Gynecomastia is the most common side effect of gonadotropin therapy and is due to hCG stimulation of aromatase causing increased secretion of estradiol. This undesirable side effect can be prevented by using the lowest dose of hCG capable of maintaining serum testosterone levels towards the lower end of the normal range.[1]

20. Is there a role of less expensive oral medications like clomiphene in HH?

Ans: Very few studies[26] with small numbers have used clomiphene in adult-onset HH, but no good quality study have established the role of clomiphene in congenital causes of HH.

21. When do you start testosterone replacement therapy (TRT) in HH?

Ans: TRT is initiated when

- Not concerned about fertility
- The couple have not benefitted in terms of fertility outcomes with gonadotropin therapy and have decided to proceed with donor sperms for conception, or
- After the childbirth

SUMMARY

- Repeat blood test to confirm low total testosterone and rule out hyperprolactinaemia
- ***Clearly explain about the high costs of treatment before starting on gonadotropin therapy.***
- Initiate on sperm induction protocol. Add HMG after adequate improvement in testosterone levels and after an adequate period of hCG.
- If unable to conceive during the gonadotropin therapy of 12–18 months, then offer the options of assisted reproductive techniques (IUI and IVF/ICSI) depending on female factor.
- Genetic testing in HH is not mandatory as it will not change the treatment plan.
- After conception or if he is not affordable, he can stop the hormonal therapy, cryopreserve sperms and switch over to lifelong testosterone replacement therapy.

REFERENCES

1. Boeri L, Capogrosso P, Salonia A. Gonadotropin Treatment for the Male Hypogonadotropic Hypogonadism. Curr Pharm Des. 2021;27(24):2775–2783.
2. Berookhim BM, Schlegel PN. Azoospermia due to spermatogenic failure. Urol Clin North Am. 2014 Feb;41(1):97–113.
3. Boehm U, Bouloux PM, Dattani MT, *et al*. European consensus statement on congenital hypogonadotropic hypogonadism—pathogenesis, diagnosis and treatment. *Nat Rev Endocrinol* 2015;11:547–64.
4. Yılmazel FK, Karabulut i, Yılmaz AH, Keskin E, Bedir F, Özbey i. A review of hypogonadotropic hypogonadism cases followed up in our clinic in the last decade. Urologia 2021 Feb;88(1):50–55.
5. Whitten SJ, Nangia AK, Kolettis PN. Select patients with hypogonadotropic hypogonadism may respond to treatment with clomiphene citrate. Fertil Steril. 2006 Dec;86(6):1664–8.
6. Fraietta R, Zylberstejn DS, Esteves SC. Hypogonadotropic hypogonadism revisited. Clinics (Sao Paulo). 2013;68 Suppl 1(Suppl 1):81–8.
7. Trost LW, Mulhall JP. Challenges in Testosterone Measurement, Data Interpretation, and Methodological Appraisal of Interventional Trials. J Sex Med. 2016 Jul;13(7):1029–46.
8. Silveira LF, MacColl GS, Bouloux PM. Hypogonadotropic hypogonadism. *Semin Reprod Med* 2002;20:327–38.
9. Bhasin S, Brito JP, Cunningham GR, *et al*. Testosterone therapy in men with Hypogonadism: An Endocrine society clinical practice guideline. *J Clin Endocrinol Metab*. 2018; 103: 1715–1744
10. Das G, Surya A, Okosieme O, Vali A, Tennant BP, Geen J, Abusahmin H. Pituitary imaging by MRI and its correlation with biochemical parameters in the evaluation of men with hypogonadotropic hypogonadism. EndocrPract. 2019 Sep;25(9):926–934.
11. Millar AC, Faghfoury H, Bieniek JM. Genetics of hypogonadotropic hypogonadism. TranslAndrol Urol. 2021 Mar;10(3):1401–1409.
12. Patel AS, Leong JY, Ramos L, Ramasamy R. Testosterone Is a Contraceptive and Should Not Be Used in Men Who Desire Fertility. World J Mens Health. 2019 Jan;37(1):45–54.
13. Berookhim BM, Schlegel PN. Azoospermia due to spermatogenic failure. Urol Clin North Am. 2014 Feb;41(1):97–113.
14. Dabaja AA, Schlegel PN. Medical treatment of male infertility. Transl Androl Urol. 2014 Mar;3(1):9–16.
15. Liu Z, Mao J, Xu H, Wang X, Huang B, Zheng J, Nie M, Zhang H, Wu X. Gonadotropin-Induced Spermatogenesis in CHH Patients with Cryptorchidism. Int J Endocrinol 2019 Dec 18;2019:6743489.
16. Liu PY, Baker HW, Jayadev V, Zacharin M, Conway AJ, Handelsman DJ. Induction of spermatogenesis and fertility during gonadotropin treatment of gonadotropin-deficient infertile men: predictors of fertility outcome. J Clin Endocrinol Metab. 2009 Mar;94(3):801–8.
17. Rastrelli G, Corona G, Mannucci E, Maggi M. Factors affecting spermatogenesis upon gonadotropin-replacement therapy: a meta-analytic study. Andrology. 2014 Nov;2(6):794–808. doi: 10.1111/andr.262. Epub 2014 Oct 1. PMID: 25271205.
18. Delemarre-Van De Waal HA. Induction of testicular growth and spermatogenesis by pulsatile, intravenous administration of gonadotrophin-releasing hormone in patients with hypogonadotrophic hypogonadism. Clin Endocrinol (Oxf) 1993;38(5):473–480.
19. Spratt D, Finkelstein J, O'Dea L. Long-term administration of gonadotropin-releasing hormone in men with idiopathic hypogonadotropic hypogonadism: a model for studies of the hormone's physiologic effects. Ann Intern Med. 1986;105(6):848–855.
20. Prior M, Stewart J, McEleny K, Dwyer AA, Quinton R. Fertility induction in hypogonadotropic hypogonadal men. Clin Endocrinol (Oxf). 2018 Dec;89(6):712–718.
21. Bakircioglu ME, Erden HF, Ciray HN, Bayazit N, Bahçeci M. Gonadotrophin therapy in combination with ICSI in men with hypogonadotrophic hypogonadism. Reprod Biomed Online. 2007 Aug;15(2):156–60.
22. Zorn B, Pfeifer M, Virant-Klun I, Meden-Vrtovec H. Intracytoplasmicsperm injection as a complement to gonadotrophin treatment in infertile men with hypogonadotrophic hypogonadism. Int J Androl. 2005;28(4):202–7.
23. Yılmazel FK, Karabulut, Yılmaz AH, Keskin E, Bedir F, Özbey. A review of hypogonadotropic hypogonadism cases followed up in our clinic in the last decade. Urologia. 2021 Feb;88(1):50–55.
24. Fahmy I, Kamal A, Shamloul R, Mansour R, Serour G, Aboulghar M. ICSI using testicular sperm in male hypogonadotrophic hypogonadism unresponsive to gonadotrophin therapy. Hum Reprod. 2004 Jul;19(7):1558–61
25. Dwyer AA, Tiemensma J, Quinton R, Pitteloud N, Morin D. Adherence to treatment in men with hypogonadotrophic hypogonadism. Clin Endocrinol (Oxf). 2017 Mar;86(3): 377–383.
26. Liel Y. Clomiphene citrate in the treatment of idiopathic or functional hypogonadotropic hypogonadism in men: a case series and review of the literature. EndocrPract. 2017 Mar;23(3):279–287.

Chapter

10

Klinefelter's Syndrome

• *Chirag Gupta* • *Priyank Kothari*

LEARNING OBJECTIVES

- Diagnosis of Klinefelter's syndrome in infertile men.
- Phenotype and genotype of Klinefelter's syndrome.
- Fertility considerations in Klinefelter men.
- Sperm retrieval for Klinefelter's men.
- Genetic considerations in offsprings.

INTRODUCTION

Klinefelter syndrome is the most prevalent chromosomal disorder in humans, with an estimated frequency of 1:500 to 1:1,000 men.[1] It is also the most frequent genetic cause of azoospermia.[2,3] Most men with Klinefelter syndrome are diagnosed when they have failed to achieve a pregnancy and are diagnosed with azoospermia. The cardinal stigmata include small testes in virtually all KS, hypergonadotropic hypogonadism, gynecomastia, learning difficulties, and infertility.

The phenotype of"Klinefelter syndrome" was first described in 1942 by Harry Klinefelter.[4] He reported nine men with gynecomastia, small testes, and azoospermia. Men with Klinefelter syndrome have an additional X chromosome, resulting in a 47,XXY karyotype.[5] It is known that a 47,XXY karyotype is found in 80–90% of men with Klinefelter syndrome, whereas the remaining cases show a mosaic karyotype (46,XY/47,XXY), additional X chromosomes (e.g., 48,XXXY or 48,XXYY), or structurally abnormal X chromosomes (e.g., 47,X,iXq,Y).[1,6]

Case Scenario

A 22-year-old male, 20-year-old lady; Married for 3 years; Fructose positive Azoospermia; couple is keen on own sperm.

FSH 21; Karyotyping 47 XXY

What is the best way to proceed?

1. How will one diagnose a case of Klinefelter's syndrome? Which are the modifiable and non modifiable features?

Ans: Modifiable, partially modifiable and unmodifiable features, are discussed in Table 10.1.

2. What are the relevant genetics of Klinefelter's syndrome?

Ans: Prior to the first meiotic division, the amount of DNA is doubled (replication), resulting in 46 chromosomes, each consisting of two chromatids (2n, 4c). The first meiotic division (reduction division) involves segregation of homologous chromosomes (2n, 4c) and gives rise to haploid (23 chromosomes; 1n, 2c) germ cells: two secondary spermatocytes (male meiosis) or one secondary oocyte and one polar body (female meiosis).

In cases of Klinefelter syndrome with an additional maternal X, nondisjunction in either the first or second meiotic division occurs. In paternal cases, the additional X chromosome is usually the result of nondisjunction in the first meiotic division, because a meiosis II error will result in either XX or YY gametes (and therefore XXX or XYY zygotes).[7]

3. Discuss fertility potential of Klinefelter's patients?

Ans: Very few Klinefelter's males have enough spermatogenic capability to father a child naturally. A few have either very scare sperm in the ejaculate good enough for ICSI while majority are azoospermic

TABLE 10.1: Klinefelter syndrome—factors

	Modifiable features	*Partially modifiable features*	*Unmodifiable features*
Signs	Sparse body and facial hair Female pubic escutcheon Weight, BMI, WC, WHR Reduced muscle mass Bilateral gynecomastia Impaired estradiol/testosterone ratio		Longer legs Small testes Eunchoid habitus Tall stature Elevated gonadotropins
Symptoms	Impaired sexual desire Erectile dyfunction Weakness and loss of vigor Impaired well-being Impaired QoL		Azoospermia/infertility
Comorbidities	Metabolic abnormalities (overweight, obesity) Mood disturbances	Reduced bone mineral density	

and may have spermatozoa located in a few individuals and randomly spaced seminiferous tubules discovered and harvested during microsurgical testicular sperm extraction (mTESE).

In men with non-obstructive azoospermia (NOA), *in vitro* fertilization with intracytoplasmic sperm injection (ICSI) is the most promising method of conception. As a single sperm is required for the procedure, a low sperm yield in the ejaculate may preclude invasive sperm retrieval techniques. With no sperm in the ejaculate, sperm retrieval with mTESE is the last resort.

4. **Where do the spermatozoa actually come from?**

Ans: Sciurano *et al.*[8] demonstrated that only a small proportion (< 25%) of all tubules contained germ cells. They analyzed multiple meiotic spermatocytes using fluorescence *in situ* hybridization (FISH) with X-centromeric probes and with immunolocalization of meiotic proteins, and all were euploid, 46,XY and thus capable of producing haploid spermatozoa. All Sertoli cells analyzed were 47,XXY. Thus, the spermatogenic foci probably originate from clones of spermatogonia which have randomly lost one of the X chromosomes during periods of life when high spermatogonial mitotic activity occurs.[8] Random loss of the extra X chromosome gives rise to a small number of 46,XY spermatogonial clones that may indeed undergo meiosis and spermiogenesis, even within the dysfunctional environment provided by 47,XXY Sertoli cells.

5. **Can sperm retrieval be done in men with Klinefelter's syndrome?**

Ans: Microdissection testicular sperm extraction (mTESE) with intracytoplasmic sperm injection has become the first-line treatment for patients with nonobstructive azoospermia (NOA). The small testis (usually 2–6 cc) is bivalved under optical magnification (×10 to 15 power) to visualize the vascular anatomy. Direct examination of the testicular parenchyma is performed via magnification under the operating microscope to identify individual seminiferous tubules that are larger than other tubules in the testicular parenchyma. Small (2 to 10 mg) samples are removed containing tubules that were larger and typically more opaque Each excised testicular tissue specimen is processed by an embryologist and further cut or teased into smaller pieces to allow spermatozoa to be released from the inside of the seminiferous tubules. A few protocols use enzymatic lysing agents to break the tissue for release of sperms. The resulting suspension is examined for spermatozoa. The procedure is terminated when spermatozoa were retrieved or all areas of testicular tissue had been examined and representative samples taken. Rarest of foci of spermatozoa production can thus be harvested with microdissection TESE. Dissection under the microscope parallel to the vascular anatomy avoids injury to the vessels. Individual tubules can be picked up which provides precision.

6. **What are the sperm retrieval rates in Klinefelter's males?**

Ans: The 2020 AUA/ASRM guidelines reports that the rate of spermatozoa found upon microdissection-testicular sperm extraction (micro-TESE) is up to 50–60% of 47, XXY men (2020 by the American Urological Association and American Society for Reproductive Medicine) while other studies have reported SRR in 20–60% of men with Klinefelter.[9] A study comparing rates of sperm retrieval between Klinefelter's syndrome (KS) patients and other NOA patients with normal karyotype using skewed regression analysis showed a success rate of 28.4% for the KS group compared to 22% for the NOA with normal karyotype group. Statistically significant difference existed, with higher testosterone levels in the successful SSR group.[10] The retrieval rates in KS patients are variable and testosterone levels could be an indicator for predicting success. Further studies and analysis for the same will provide further evidence for the same.

In summary currently, the SSR rates using m-TESE in patients with Klinefelter syndrome are very variable and low (success rates are lower than non-KS men). Therefore, m-TESE for Klinefelter syndrome can be performed after explaining realistic success rates to patients. Future research is warranted to enhance SSR in this selected category of patients. High volume mTESE centers may have better success in SSR in Klinefelter patients.

7. **Should the retrieval be performed in conjunction with ovum pick up or trial mTESE to confirm spermatogenesis also gives realistic chance of success?**

Ans: The sperm retrieval procedures can be performed in conjunction with programmed *in vitro* fertilization cycles. Sperm retrieval is usually done on the day before or on the day of oocyte retrieval. As the number of sperm retrieved in these patients is usually less in number, we usually prefer simultaneous partner preparation. In a few cases where finances are an issue or the couple so chooses trial mTESE with cryopreservation followed by partner preparation is a valid option. Although literature suggests that rates for fertilization are equal in both cases,[11] we would prefer fresh sperms due to the very small number of sperms usually retrieved.

8. **What is the genetic risk to offspring born via ICSI in these couples? What is the role of PGT?**

Ans: The safety concerns identified among couples using TESE-ICSI, are in terms of chromosomal, congenital, or developmental abnormalities in their offspring.[12] The majority of offspring born to men with KS have been healthy, with a normal 46,XX or 46,XY chromosomal complement.[13] However, the conception of 47,XXY pregnancies has certainly been reported, resulting in spontaneous early abortion or elective termination.[14,15]

An increased rate of sex and autosomal chromosomal aneuploidy has been reported in sperm from men with KS.[16–20] Whether this increased rate is specific to KS offspring, or reflective of the rate seen in ICSI offspring in general, is unknown. The largest series on this topic was published by Levron, *et al.*[20] who showed chromosomal abnormalities in 7 of 112 (6.3%) patients, of which five were related to sex chromosomes and two to chromosome.[18]

Given the potential for increased chromosomal abnormalities in the offspring of men with KS, preimplantation genetic diagnosis of embryos obtained using TESE-ICSI has been recommended. Staessen *et al.*[19] showed the rate of normal embryos for KS couples was significantly lower than that for normal controls (54% vs. 77.2%).[19] However, preimplantation genetic diagnosis is not routinely used by many centers, either due to lack of availability, or because the majority of offspring of KS couples are normal.[21] A recent study with cryopreserved sperms from microTESE resulted in Euploidy in 29 of 45 (64.4%) embryos. Thus, the paternal genetic risk of sex chromosome abnormalities in their offspring is extremely low in men with KS.

Direct intracytoplasmic sperm injection (ICSI) is comparably effective and more economical for young nonmosaic KS couples.[22] ICSI should be offered as an option for such couples, but monitoring by prenatal genetic diagnosis is recommended in couples wanting but be sure. In summary, the use of preimplantation genetic diagnosis in KS couples undergoing ICSI should, therefore, be considered and decision should be taken in consultation with the couple. The cost of PGT and the newer PGT-NGS (next generation sequencing) techniques is also a hinderance in the Indian situation.

9. **Which are the newer non-invasive prenatal diagnosis test (recent advance)?**

Ans: The traditional PGD depending on segmentation-sphere biopsy can identify the extra chromosome in the KS fetus. Blastomere biopsy does directly assess the genomic DNA of *in vitro* fertilized embryos, but this invasive procedure is likely to result in reducing the developmental potential of embryos and may increase the risk of abortion.[23]

The critical diversity of the offspring lies in maternal chromosomes. In 1997, Y M Dennis Lo *et al.* pioneered a non-invasive prenatal diagnosis by detecting fetal DNA in maternal plasma and serum.[24] Subsequently, this method was extended to detect a single copy fetal DNA sequence, RhD status, beta-thalassemia gene, and so on.[25–27] On the basis of this a new concept was developed, namely, non-invasive PGD during the KS patients' ICSI cycle. The a new non-invasive chromosome screening (NICS) method was based on sequencing the genomic DNA secreted into the culture medium from the human blastocyst was developed. A positive genetic link between the embryo and the spent culture medium was established. Currently, it has been widely used to screen aneuploid diseases, including Down's syndrome, Turner syndrome, XYY syndrome, and KS.[28–30] The genetic diagnosis in this stage is not as reliable, especially in embryos with mosaicism.[31] Further study revealed that genomic DNA was present in approximately 90% of blastocyst fluid samples harvested during the vitrification procedure.[32] Therefore, noninvasive PGD by determining the spent culture medium could provide an optimal approach to avoiding the birth of KS infants to the KS couples who are seeking ART medical therapy.

10. Discuss the role of TRT in Klinefelter's syndrome.

Ans: These patients usually need testosterone replacement therapy for their hypergonadotropic hypogonadism. Three monthly depot preparations can be used, or monthly injections can be used with the aim of maintaining the total testosterone levels in the therapeutic range (full details in Hypogonadism chapter).

11. Discuss management of the index case.

Ans: As is often the case, this couple presented with primary infertility and subsequently the husband was evaluated for male factor, and found to be azoopsermic with karyotpe suggestive of Klinefelter's syndrome. Among the phenotypical abnormalities he has taller with non-muscular body and small testicles. Both the testis are 3 cc in volume.

Evaluation

- Hormones: FSH–21 (is usually raised)—suggesting testicular failure
  Testsoterone: 220 ng/dl (lower than normal)
- Karyotype: 47 XXY (can be mosaics, mosaics with partial 46XY have better outcomes)
- Female evaluation assessment is mandatory—was normal in this case

As the male is 25 years old, one should bear in mind that the chances of successful sperm retrieval is better than with older males in their 30s and 40s.

Testosterone levels are usually lower than normal, and there is general consensus that higher testosterone levels have a better prognosis although this has not been proven by robust evidence.

Options for Fertility in Indian Setting

1. If the couple is not affording and okay with donor sperm–donor IUI

   The man requires hormonal supplementation probably lifelong (not to be forgotten).

   Usually depot preparations would be required for long-term supplementation, although initial supplementation with shorter acting injectables followed by depot might be preferred (details in hypogonadism chapter).
2. Couple wants self-sperms but wants to ensure the presence of sperms before wife stimulation: Trail microdissection TESE with cryopreservation (vitrification—best chances of sperm survival).

   Counselling about realistic chances with the possibility of loss during cryopreservation especially if it is not a high volume center or conventional methods of tissue preservation are used (not vitrification).

   Thawed sperm can be used for ICSI and successful outcomes can be achieved.
3. Financially stable couple wants the best chances for offspring.

   Wife stimulation with sperm retrieval on the day of ovum pick up, enabling use of fresh sperm and fresh oocytes, which as a general consensus has the best outcomes for embryo formation and later pregnancy. (Entire process is labour and cost intensive.)

Counselling for Offspring

There is enough data to suggest that aneuploidy in the offspring is only marginally more than the risk in general population and even risk of child with Klinefelter's is similar to that in general population. Many studies have reported normal healthy offsprings in these couples. If a couple wants to guarantee that the child does not have any chromosomal aberrations or abnormalities, then PGT or non-invasive PGT can be offered. A consult with a genetic counselling can be useful and reassuring and can help the couple take an informed decision for PGT or need for advanced PGT-NGS depending on their affordability and risk to the the embryo.

KEY POINTS

- Klinefelter syndrome is characterised by 47XXY on karyotyping.
- The usual presentation is non-obstructive azoospermia.
- Clinical features suggestive of Klinefelter syndrome include small testis, gynecomastia and classic body habitus.
- Genetic diagnosis and counselling are mandatory.
- MicroTESE is the only option for sperm retrieval in these men.

SUMMARY

- Klinefleter syndrome is one of the commonest chromosomal abnormalities causing non-obstructive azoospermia. The patients present with elevated LH and FSH values with variable but usually low testosterone. Urologists should identify these men and counsel about their genetic problem after performing karyotyping. The window for successful sperm retrieval reduces with advancing paternal age. MicroTESE is successful in a few men with Klinefelter syndrome.

REFRENCES

1. Bojesen A, Juul S, Gravholt CH. Prenatal and postnatal prevalence of Klinefelter syndrome: a national registry study. J Clin Endocrinol Metab 2003;88:622–6.
2. Tuttelmann F, Werny F, Cooper TG, Kliesch S, Simoni M, Nieschlag E. Clinical experience with azoospermia: aetiology and chances for spermatozoa detection upon biopsy. Int J Androl 2011;34:291–8.
3. Vincent MC, Daudin M, De MP, Massat G, Mieusset R, Pontonnier F, *et al.* Cytogenetic investigations of infertile men with low sperm counts: a 25-year experience. J Androl 2002;23:18–22; discussion 44–5.
4. Klinefelter HF, Reifenstein EC, Albright F. Syndrome characterised by gynecomastia, aspermatogenesis without a-leydigism, and increased excretion of follicle-stimulating hormone. J Clin Endocrinol 1942;2:615–27.
5. Jacobs PA, Strong JA. A case of human intersexuality having a possible XXY sex-determining mechanism. Nature 1959;183:302–3.
6. Lanfranco F, Kamischke A, Zitzmann M, Nieschlag E. Klinefelter's syndrome. Lancet 2004;364:273–83.
7. Sciurano RB, Luna Hisano CV, Rahn MI, Brugo Olmedo S, Rey Valzacchi G, Coco R, *et al.* Focal spermatogenesis originates in euploid germ cells in classical Klinefelter patients. Hum Reprod 2009;24:2353–60.
8. Siffroi JP, Chantot-Bastaraud S, Ravel C. Genetic origin of spermatogenesis impairments: clinical aspects and relationships with mouse models of infertility [in French]. Gynecol Obstet Fertil 2003;31:504–15.
9. Caroppo E, Colpi GM. Update on the Management of Non-Obstructive Azoospermia; Current Evidence andUnmet Needs. J Clin Med. 2021 Dec 23 11(1):62.
10. Chehrazi M, Rahimiforoushani A, Sabbaghian M, *et al.* Sperm Retrieval in Patients with Klinefelter Syndrome: A Skewed Regression Model Analysis. *Int J Fertil Steril*. 2017;11(2):117–122. doi:10.22074/ijfs.2017.4702.
11. Wu S, Zhao J, Wu Y, Hu Y, Fang L, Chen W. Comparison of pregnancy and neonatal outcomes of intracytoplasmic sperm injection performed with frozen versus fresh testicular sperm. *Transl Androl Urol*. 2022;11(4):472–479. doi:10.21037/tau-22-125.
12. Maiburg MC, Hoppenbrouwers AC, van Stel HF, Giltay JC. Attitudes of Klinefelter men and their relatives towards TESE-ICSI. J Assist Reprod Genet 2011;28:809–14.
13. Schlegel PN. Nonobstructive azoospermia: a revolutionary surgical approach and results. Semin Reprod Med 2009;27: 165–70.
14. Ron-El R, Strassburger D, Gelman-Kohan S, Friedler S, Raziel A, Appelman Z. A 47,XXY fetus conceived after ICSI of spermatozoa from a patient with nonmosaic Klinefelter's syndrome: case report. Hum Reprod 2000;15:1804–6.
15. Hinney B, Guttenbach M, Schmid M, Engel W, Michelmann HW. Pregnancy after intracytoplasmic sperm injection with sperm from a man with a 47,XXY Klinefelter's karyotype. Fertil Steril 1997;68:718–20.
16. Foresta C, Galeazzi C, Bettella A, Stella M, Scandellari C. High incidence of sperm sex chromosomes aneuploidies in two patients with Klinefelter's syndrome. J Clin Endocrinol Metab 1998;83:203–5.
17. Hennebicq S, Pelletier R, Bergues U, Rousseaux S. Risk of trisomy 21 in offspring of patients with Klinefelter's syndrome. Lancet 2001;357:2104–5.
18. Rives N, Joly G, Machy A, Simeon N, Leclerc P, Mace B. Assessment of sex chromosome aneuploidy in sperm nuclei from 47,XXY and 46, XY/47,XXY males: comparison with fertile and infertile males with normal karyotype. Mol Hum Reprod 2000;6:107–12.
19. Staessen C, Tournaye H, Van Assche E, Michiels A, Van Landuyt L, Devroey P, *et al.* PGD in 47,XXY Klinefelter's syndrome patients. Hum Reprod Update 2003;9:319–30.
20. Levron J, Aviram-Goldring A, Madgar I, Raviv G, Barkai G, Dor J. Sperm chromosome analysis and outcome of IVF in patients with non-mosaic Klinefelter's syndrome. Fertil Steril 2000;74:925–9.
21. Vernaeve V, Staessen C, Verheyen G, Van Steirteghem A, Devroey P, Tournaye H. Can biological or clinical parameters predict testicular sperm recovery in 47,XXY Klinefelter's syndrome patients? Hum Reprod 2004;19: 1135–9.
22. Tong J, Zhao XM, Wan AR, Zhang T. PGT or ICSI? The impression of NGS-based PGT outcomes in nonmosaic Klinefelter syndrome. *Asian J Androl*. 2021;23(6):621–626. doi:10.4103/aja.aja_30_21.
23. De Vos A, Staessen C, De Rycke M, Verpoest W, Haentjens P, Devroey P, *et al.* Impact of cleavage-stage embryo biopsy in view of PGD on human blastocyst implantation: a prospective cohort of single embryo transfers. Hum Reprod. 2009;24(12):2988–96. https://doi.org/10.1093/humrep/dep251. J Assist Reprod Genet.
24. Lo YM, Corbetta N, Chamberlain PF, *et al.* Presence of fetal DNA in maternal plasma and serum. *Lancet*. 1997;350(9076):485–487. doi:10.1016/S0140–6736(97)02174–0.
25. Bischoff FZ, Hahn S, Johnson KL, Simpson JL, Bianchi DW, Lewis DE, *et al.* Intact fetal cells in maternal plasma: are they really there? Lancet. 2003;361(9352):139–40. https://doi.org/10. 1016/S0140–6736(03)12191–5.
26. Lo YM, Hjelm NM, Fidler C, Sargent IL, Murphy MF, Chamberlain PF, *et al.* Prenatal diagnosis of fetal RhD status by molecular analysis of maternal plasma. N Engl J Med. 1998;339(24):1734–8.
27. Lo YM, Patel P, Sampietro M, Gillmer MD, Fleming KA, Wainscoat JS. Detection of single-copy fetal DNA sequence from maternal blood. Lancet. 1990;335(8703):1463–4.
28. Lo YD, Chiu RW. Non-invasive prenatal diagnosis of Down's syndrome. Lancet. 2007;369(9578):1997. https://doi.org/10. 1016/S0140–6736(07)60935–0.
29. Hulten M. Non-invasive prenatal diagnosis of Down's syndrome. Lancet. 2001;357(9260):963–4. https://doi. org/10.1016/S0140–6736(05)71670–6.
30. Kou KO, Poon CF, Kwok SL, Chan KY, Tang MH, Kan AS, *et al.* Effect of non-invasive prenatal testing as a contingent approach on the indications for invasive prenatal diagnosis and prenatal detection rate of Down's syndrome. Hong Kong Med J. 2016;22(3): 223–30. https://doi.org/10.12809/hkmj154730.
31. Gleicher N, Vidali A, Braverman J, Kushnir VA, Barad DH, Hudson C, *et al.* Accuracy of preimplantation genetic screening (PGS) is compromised by degree of mosaicism of human embryos. Reprod Biol Endocrinol. 2016;14(1):54. https://doi.org/10. 1186/s12958–016–0193–6.
32. Palini S, Galluzzi L, De Stefani S, Bianchi M, Wells D, Magnani M, *et al.* Genomic DNA in human blastocoele fluid. Reprod BioMed Online. 2013;26(6):603–10. https://doi.org/10.1016/j. rbmo.2013.02.012.

Section

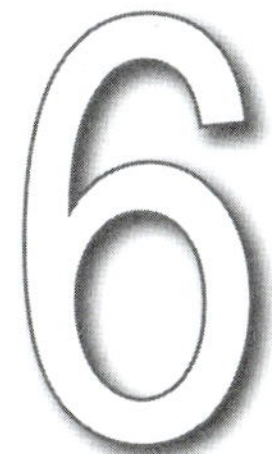

Renal Transplant

Chapter

1

Recipient for Kidney Transplant: Pre-transplant Evaluation

• Amit K Devra • LP Choudhary

LEARNING OBJECTIVES

- To understand the management options for chronic kidney disease (CKD).
- To understand the indications and contraindications for kidney transplantation.
- To understand the recipients evaluation before transplant.

INTRODUCTION

Patients suffering from chronic kidney disease (CKD) that has progressed to end stage renal disease (ESRD) require some form of renal replacement therapy (RRT) for survival. Currently there are two forms of RRT: Dialysis and kidney transplantation. Kidney transplantation is preferred over dialysis as it provides better quality of life, improved recipient survival and is cost effective over a long-term basis. However, unlike dialysis, kidney transplantation is not 'by default' form of RRT. Careful patient selection and evaluation is required to maximise transplant outcome.

Case Scenario 1

A 56-year-old male with stage 5 CKD, diabetes and hypertension has presented with breathlessness and fatigue. He has been started on haemodialysis by his nephrologist. Discuss about the further plan of action.

1. **Enumerate the RRT options available to him.**

   Ans: Dialysis and renal transplantation. There are two types of dialysis—peritoneal and hemodialysis. Peritoneal dialysis involves exchange of fluid and electrolytes through peritoneal membrane, while in hemodialysis, it is achieved through blood catheter and hemodialysis machine.

2. **What are the types of renal transplantation based upon the types of donor?**

   Ans: Renal transplantation can be categorized based on the types of donors, each presenting unique considerations and implications. Here is an overview of renal transplantation based on donor types:

   - Deceased donor transplantation involves procuring kidneys from individuals who have been declared brain dead or have died due to circulatory arrest.
   - Living donor transplantation involves the voluntary donation of a kidney from a healthy individual, often a family member or close friend, to the recipient. In India, living donor transplant is governed by Transplant of Human Organ Act, 1994.

3. **What is pre-emptive renal transplantation?**

   Ans: Transplantation done before initiation of dialysis is called pre-emptive transplantation. It is associated with better patient and graft outcome. Long-term graft survival is higher in patients who were < 6 months on dialysis or who never had dialysis in comparison to those on dialysis for more than 2 years.[1] Pre-emptive transplantation should be considered when eGFR is <20 ml/min/1.75 m^2 or earlier if symptomatic.

4. **Who are eligible candidates for kidney transplant and what are the conditions where transplant is not recommended?**

   Ans: Any patient with ESRD can be a candidate for kidney transplant. ESRD patients having the following conditions are not suitable for undergoing kidney transplantation.

Absolute contraindications for renal transplantation:

- Active or metastatic cancer disease
- Severe chronic illness with expected survival <2 years
- Active untreated infection
- Uncontrolled psychiatric illness impairing compliance or consent
- Non-compliance to treatment
- Active substance or alcohol abuse
- Severe irreversible obstructive or restrictive lung disease

5. **What is the aim of pretransplant recipient evaluation?**

Ans: The successful long-term outcome of transplant is dependent on careful case selection. Pretransplant recipient evaluation is directed towards specific goals.

- To assess fitness to undergo major surgery.
- To rule out comorbidities which decrease survival of patient.
- To rule out disease which may flare up or have high recurrence after transplant
- To assess emotional and psychological well-being needed for lifelong adherence to treatment and follow-up
- To know technical feasibility of transplant surgery (vascular and lower tract evaluation).

The kidney recipient should be evaluated systematically by detailed history taking and physical examination to cover all the important domains of evaluation.

Proforma should cover following domains of recipient evaluation	
a.	Understanding basic kidney disease
b.	Duration and status of dialysis mode
c.	Vaccination prophylaxis
d.	Identifying the existing chronic infection
e.	History of any pre-existing malignancy along with treatment received.
f.	Cardio-pulmonary evaluation
g.	Evaluation of peripheral vascular disease including recipient's pelvic vessels
h.	Lower tract (bladder) evaluation
i.	Psychiatric evaluation
j.	Assessment general fitness and PAC workup
k.	Immunological workup

6. **Why is it important to identify the etiopathogenesis of ESRD?**

Ans: Native kidney disease causing ESRD is not always known because kidney biopsy is not routinely done. However, the cause of ESRD in candidates for transplant should be determined whenever possible, to counsel the patients for risks of recurrence of disease in transplanted kidney and sometimes different management guidelines after kidney transplantation. Sometimes patients with specific pathology may need pretransplant removal of affected renal unit.

7. **What are the common kidney disease with high risk of recurrence?**

Ans: Recurrence of disease accounts for < 2% of all graft failure.[2] On long-term follow-up recurrent glomerular disease is third most common cause of graft loss.[3] The common kidney diseases with high risk of recurrence are focal segmental glomerulosclerosis, MPGN type I and II, IgA nephropathy, membranous glomerulonephritis, anti-glomerular basement membrane (GBM) disease, antibody glomerulonephritis (Table 1.1). These patients can be appropriately counselled regarding risk of recurrence and potential graft loss.

TABLE 1.1. Risk of kidney disease recurrence post-transplant and risk of graft loss

Primary disease	*Risk of recurrence*	*Risk of graft loss due to recurrence*
IgA nephropathy	50%	15%
FSGS	20–50% (80% if prior graft loss)	50%
MPGN type I	20–50%	15%
MPGN type II	80–100%	15–30%
Membranous GN	10–30%	20–50%
Anti-GBM disease	Rare (if quiescent at time of transplant)	Rare
ANCA vasculitis	15–20%	6–8%
SLE	2–9%	2–4%
HUS/TTP	15–25%	50%
Diabetic nephropathy	100%	Rare
Immunoglobulin deposition diseases	50%	30%
Amyloidosis	40%	20%
Fabry disease	100%	Rare
Scleroderma	20%	50%
Oxalosis	100%	50%
Cystinosis	0%	0%

Source: Melissa Yeung MD, FRCPC (auth.), Anil Chandraker, Mohamed H. Sayegh, Ajay K. Singh (eds.)-Core Concepts in Renal Transplantation: Springer US (2012).

8. **What are the indications of pre-transplant nephrectomy?**

Ans:

- ADPKD kidneys—symptomatic, large extending below iliac crest, infected or containing solid tumor
- Persistent anti-GBM antibody levels
- Recurrent pyelonephritis
- Grossly hydronephrotic kidneys
- Solid renal tumors with or without acquired renal cystic disease
- Significant proteinuria persisting after medical therapy.

9. **Why is important to screen immunity against potential viral infection in a kidney recipient and what are the common infection for which screening is recommended?**

Ans: Renal transplant recipients have increased risk of infection because of immunosuppressants. Infections are the second most common cause of death after cardiovascular diseases. Hence, it is imperative to vaccinate them against preventable diseases. The antibody response to vaccination decreases with progression of CKD and is even less in patients on dialysis. So, vaccination should be completed as early as possible in the course of CKD.

Screening for CMV with CMV IgG, and Varicella-zoster virus (VZV) with VZV IgG is recommended (Table 1.2). Anti-HBS titre is also recommended if patient has already received hepatitis vaccination in the past.

10. **How do you plan vaccine prophylaxis in a kidney transplant patient?**

Ans: Kidney transplant patients should receive ancillary inactivated vaccine based on the risk factors for the respective disease (Table 1.3). Any live attenuated vaccine should only be administered prior to kidney transplantation. Live vaccines carry risk of shedding of organism and potential cross infection in transplant recipients.[4,5]

TABLE 1.2: Screening for viral and non-viral infection in kidney recipient evaluation

Recommendations for initial and follow-up screening of viral and non-viral pathogens in kidney transplant candidates

Pathogen	*Test*	*Repeating*
Viral infections		
HIV	IgG	If negative, repeat annually and at time of transplant
HCV	IgG	If negative, repeat annually and at time of transplant
HBV	Anti-HBs, Anti-HBc, HBsAg	If negative, repeat annually and at time of transplant
CMV	IgG	If negative, repeat at time of transplant
EBV	VCA IgG or EBNA IgG	If negative, repeat at time of transplant
HSV	IgG	If negative, repeat at time of transplant
VZV	IgG	If negative, repeat at time of transplant and 4 weeks post-vaccination
Measles, mumps, rubella	IgG	If negative, repeat at time of transplant and 4 weeks post-vaccination
HTLV	IgG	None unless ongoing risk of exposure
Non-viral infections		
Syphilis	IgG with confirmatory testing if IgG positive	None
Strongyloides	IgG	None
Chagas disease	IgG	None
Tuberculosis (in low prevalence areas)	Tuberculin skin test or interferon-gamma release assay (IGRA)	Annually if ongoing risk of exposure
Malaria	Blood smear if clinically indicated	None

Anti-HBc, hepatitis B core antibody: Anti-HBs, hepatitis B surface antibody; CMV, cytomegalovirus; EBNA, EBV, Epstein-Barr virus; HBV, hepatitis B virus; HBsAg, hepatitis B surface antigen; HCV, hepatitis C virus; HIV, human immunode3ficiency virus; HSV, herpes simplex virus; HTLV, human T-lymphotropic virus; IgG, immunoglobulin G; VCA, viral capsid antigen; VZV, varicella zoster virus.

Source: Kidney disease: Improving global outcomes (KDIGO) Kidney Transplant Candidate Work Group. KDIGO Clinical Practice Guideline on the Evaluation and Management of Candidates for Kidney Transplantation. Transplantation.2020;104: S1–S103.

TABLE 1.3: Vaccine prophylaxis for kidney transplant recipients

Summary of routine vaccinations for kidney transplant candidates

Routine vaccines	Dosing guidelines*	Comment
Inactive vaccines		
Diphtheria, pertussis, polio, tetanus, HiB	Generally given in childhood; Ensure these are up-to-date	
Pneumococcal vaccination: PCV13, PPV23	One dose of PCV13 following by one dose of PPV23 with a minimum of 8-week interval in between	One booster of PPV23 five years from previous PPV23
Influenza	One dose annually	
Hepatitis B	Three doses at 0, 1, 6 months	Check anti-HBs titer Monitor annually and give booster dose if titers decline < 10 IU/ml
Hepatitis A	Two doses at 0, 2 months	Check titers; If not immune, give vaccination again (i.e. repeat of no response to first series)
Human papillomavirus	Three doses in both males and females if not previously given (ages 9 to 45)	No boosters
Meningococcal quadrivalent conjugate (serogroups A, C, Y, W-135)	Two doses given 8 weeks apart; Indicated for travel to endemic areas, prior or planned splenectomy or planned use of eculizumab	Repeat one dose every five years in patients at risk
Meningococcal B vaccine	One dose if planned use of eculizumab	
Shingles (herpes zoster subunit)	Two doses at 0, 2–6 months for those age ≥ 50 years and VZV IgG positive	Unknown if benefit in less than 50 years of age. No boosters
Measles, mumps, rubella	Two doses given 4 weeks apart. Considered immune after two doses regardless of seroconversion	Check serology and provide vaccination if negative
Varicella	Two doses given 4 weeks apart. Considered immune after two doses regardless of seroconversion	Check serology and provide vaccination if negative
Shingles (herpes zoster Live)**	One dose in those > age 50 years and VZV IgG positive	Unknown if benefit in less than 50 years of age. No boosters

*Duration and doses are suggestive only as they may be variable in different regions. Please check your local guidelines.

**The herpes zoster subunit inactivated vaccine is preferred over the herpes zoster live vaccine. If the herpes zoster live vaccine has already been administered, the transplant candidate can be reimmunized with the inactivated vaccine a minimum of one year after the live vaccine.

Anti-HBs, hepatitis B surface antibodies; HiB, *hemophilus influenzae* type b; IgG, immunoglobulin g; IU, internationl unit; PCV13 pneumococcal conjugate vaccine-13 valent; PPV23, pneumococcal polysaccharide vaccine-23 valent; VZV, varicella zoster virus.

Source: Kidney Disease: Improving Global Outcomes (KDIGO), Kidney Transplant Candidate Work Group. KDIGO Clinical Practice Guideline on the Evaluation and Management of Candidates for Kidney Transplantation. Transplantation. 2020;104: S1–S103.

It is recommended to delay kidney transplantation by 4 weeks if a live vaccine like MMR, VZV, shingles, yellow fever, oral typhoid, oral polio vaccine is administered.

Hepatitis B vaccination should be administered to kidney transplant recipients who do not have protective antibody titres (>10 IU/ml). Pneumococcal vaccination with both 23 valent polysaccharide vaccine (PPSV23) and 13 valent conjugate vaccine (PCV13) is recommended for general adults. The first dose of PCV13 should be followed by PPSV23 8 weeks later. A PCV13 dose should be repeated after a year only, if he had received PPSV23 in the past.

Ideally household contacts and pets should also be vaccinated with inactivated vaccines.

Case Scenario 2

A 45-year-old male, on maintenance hemodialysis for 2 years, has history of incomplete vaccination. During pre-transplant work up he is found to be hepatitis B antigen positive (HBsAg positive).

1. **Should you offer renal transplant to this patient with hepatitis B infection?**

   Ans: Although kidney transplantation is not contraindicated in hepatitis B positive ESRD patients, they have significant risk of reactivation of viral replication and progression of liver disease due to post-transplant immunosuppression.[6,7] Patients should be fully informed that both long-term patient and graft survival are less in these patients in comparison to hepatitis B negative transplant recipients.

2. What is the next line of management in this patient?

Ans: All hepatitis B positive transplant candidates (HBsAg positive) should undergo further testing with liver enzymes (AST/ALT), HBV DNA and HBeAg to know status of viral replication. They should also undergo ultrasound elastography (fibro scan) and if indicated liver biopsy. Those who have cirrhosis on biopsy are not a candidate for renal transplantation alone. They may be considered for combined liver and kidney transplantation.

Patients without cirrhosis who have evidence of active viral replication should receive antiviral therapy before transplant. Tenofovir or Entecavir are antiviral drugs of choice because of low risk of development of viral resistance and less nephrotoxicity.[4,8] However, even in patients without active replication there is risk of reactivation of viral replication and progression of liver disease in the post-transplant period.

3. How will you counsel HCV positive ESRD patient on dialysis for renal transplant?

Ans: Presence of hepatitis C infection in a dialysis patient is not a contraindication for renal transplant. Allograft and patient survival is less in these patients but transplant is still considered better option as HCV infected patients on dialysis have comparatively worse outcome than HCV positive kidney transplant recipients.

Patients with no cirrhosis or compensated cirrhosis without portal hypertension can proceed with renal transplant. They should receive 24 weeks of direct acting antiviral (DAA) therapy pre- or post-transplant depending upon anticipated waiting time for transplant surgery.[9]

4. How will you evaluate for viral infection before transplant?

Ans: The importance of assessment for infection cannot be overemphasized. Presence of active infection of any kind, bacterial, viral or fungal is a contraindication to transplant. Therefore, transplant must be delayed until infection is completely treated.[10]

Careful evaluation involves history, physical examination and relevant lab investigations. Patient should be enquired about symptoms suggestive of infection, e.g. fever, cough, dysuria, loose motion, etc., presence of any wound, past history of TB, syphilis, any history of contact, endemic disease, recurrent UTI, pyelonephritis, peritonitis in patients on peritoneal dialysis, etc. Physical examination to rule out dialysis access site infection, dental examination or focused examination for symptoms must be done.

Routine laboratory investigations consist of complete blood count (CBC), urine c/s, chest X-ray, serology for HIV I/II, hepatitis B, C, CMV, varicella zoster, Epstein-Barr virus, VDRL/RPR for syphilis, interferon-gamma release assay- (QuantiFERON® TB Gold test) or Mantoux test for TB. Active TB must be treated before transplant. For latent TB prophylaxis should be started before or soon after transplant.[11,12]

Case Scenario 3

A 50-year-old female with ESRD on dialysis is a prospective renal transplant recipient. She is incidentally detected with a solitary 1.5 cm bladder tumor on USG KUB. She undergoes cystoscopy and TURBT. HPE is suggestive of low grade NMIBC.

1. Why is it important to evaluate recipients for pre-existing malignancy and what are the common screening tests?

Ans: Pre-kidney transplant malignancy was considered a relative contraindication for transplant due to four major concerns: (a) Recurrence of primary tumours (b) progression of *de novo* malignancy (c) adverse effects on patient survival (d) graft-specific outcomes such as rejection.[13,14]

Screening for cancers in potential kidney transplant recipients is similar to those for general population.[15,8] It includes chest X-ray, USG abdomen and pelvis, serum PSA in males and mammography and Pap smear in females. Further, screening depends on presence of risk factors such as family history, history of smoking, presence of inflammatory bowel disease, etc.

2. What is the recommended waiting period for patients undergoing treatment for malignant neoplasm before transplant?

Ans: Historically, a recurrence free waiting period of 2–5 years depending upon type of neoplasm was required before patient was considered fit for transplant (Table 1.4). More recently, with considerable progress in staging and treatment of various cancers, a personalised approach for risk of relapse is advised.

Recent studies have highlighted that successfully treated cancers like superficial non-melanoma skin cancer, carcinoma *in situ* of cervix, ductal carcinoma *in situ* of breast, solitary low grade bladder tumor

TABLE 1.4: Recommended waiting time for cancer remission and kidney transplantation

Cancer type	*Stage*	*Waiting time*
Breast	Early	At least 2 years
	Advanced	At least 5 years
Colorectal	Dukes A/B	At least 2 years
	Dukes C	2–5 years
	Dukes D	At least 5 years
Bladder	Invasive	At least 2 years
Kidney	Incidentaloma (<3 cm)	No waiting time
	Early	At least 2 years
	Large and invasive	At least 5 years
Uterine	Localized	At least 2 years
	Invasive	At least 5 years
Cervical	Localized	At least 2 years
	Invasive	At least 5 years
Lung	Localized	2–5 years
Testicular	Localized	At least 2 years
	Invasive	2–5 years
Melanoma	Localized	At least 5 years
	Invasive	Contraindicated
Prostate	Gleason ≤6	No waiting time
	Gleason 7	At least 2 years
	Gleason 8–10	At least 5 years
Thyroid (papillary/ follicular/ medullary)	Stage 1	No waiting time
	State 2	At least 2 years
	Stage 3	At least 5 years
	Stage 4	Contraindicated
	Anaplastic	Contraindicated
Hodgkin lymphoma	Localized	At least 2 years
	Regional	3–5 years
	Distant	At least 5 years
Non-Hodgkin lymphoma	Localized	At least 2 years
	Regional	3–5 years
	Distant	At least 5 years
Post-transplant lymphoproliferative disease	Nodal	At least 2 years
	Extra-nodal and cerebral	At least 5 years

Adapted from the KDIGO Clinical Practice Guideline on the Evaluation and Management of Candidates for Kidney Transplanation

(pTa), incidentally detected small renal tumor (< 3 cm), low grade follicular/papillary carcinoma of thyroid <2 cm in size, low risk prostate cancer (T1c-T2a, Gleason score <6 Grade group 1, PSA <10) do not require any waiting period for kidney transplantation. But kidney transplant should be avoided in some invasive tumors because of a high risk of recurrence or metastasis after transplantation.[15]

For hematologic malignancy, decision regarding eligibility for transplant candidacy should be made in consultation with hematologist. Factors to be considered are completion of therapy, duration of remission and risk of progression after transplant.

3. What are the measures one should take before transplant in presence of coexisting gastrointestinal diseases?

Ans: Although screening for peptic ulcer disease, gall stone disease or diverticulosis is not recommended, evaluation in symptomatic patient is important. Although ADPKD patients have high prevalence of diverticulosis, screening recommendation is no different than general population.[16]

Active peptic ulcer disease should be treated before transplant. Elective cholecystectomy should be done for symptomatic gall stone disease or recurrent acute cholecystitis. However, need for prophylactic cholecystectomy is controversial for incidentally detected asymptomatic gall stones.

Acute diverticulitis, pancreatitis and active inflammatory bowel disease should be treated first. Transplant should be delayed until after resolution of symptoms. Prophylactic colectomy is not recommended for asymptomatic colonic diverticulosis, however, it may be considered in select patients with history of severe acute diverticulitis. Transplant should be deferred by at least 6 months after an episode of acute pancreatitis. Chronic pancreatitis should be inactive for 1 year before proceeding with transplant.[8]

4. Why do you need cardiopulmonary evaluation before kidney transplant surgery?

Ans: CKD is an independent risk factor for cardiovascular disease. Thorough cardiac evaluation is important because it is the most common cause of mortality after kidney transplantation.[17,18] The focus of evaluation is coronary artery disease, left ventricular dysfunction and peripheral arterial disease. Extent of evaluation depends on presence or absence of symptoms and risk factors.

5. How do you evaluate to define cardiac risk in kidney recipients?

In general, basic evaluation consists of history, physical examination, chest X-ray and 12 lead ECG. Low-risk patients who are asymptomatic, less than 40 years of age, non-smoker with no other risk factors, no further evaluation is required.

High risk patients who are symptomatic, abnormal finding on basic evaluation, diabetic, hypertensive, smoker, family history of ischemic heart disease, >50 years of age, more than 2 years on dialysis, dyslipidaemia, further testing with stress echocardiography, nuclear myocardial perfusion scan or Holter is done.

Very high risk patients having multiple risk factors or positive stress ECHO test/myocardial perfusion study should undergo angiography.

Ongoing symptoms of angina or myocardial infarction within 6 months are contraindications to transplant surgery.[19] Left ventricular dysfunction(LVD) is also quite prevalent in CKD patients.[20] Left ventricular dysfunction is not necessarily a contraindication for transplant because it may improve after transplant.

6. What kind of lung diseases are contraindication to kidney transplant surgery?

Ans: Kidney transplant surgery, like any major surgery, is performed under general anesthesia and requires pulmonary evaluation. In transplant candidates, chronic or latent lung infections are another major concern.

Patients with following lung conditions are not suitable transplant candidates given the very poor prognosis associated with them.[8]

- Uncontrolled asthma
- Irreversible severe pulmonary hypertension
- Severe cor pulmonale
- On home oxygen therapy
- Severe pulmonary fibrosis or restrictive lung disease
- Severe COPD

7. Why is it important to do evaluation for peripheral vascular disease (PAD) and what tests will you do for arterial and venous evaluation?

Ans: PAD is associated with increased mortality both in general population and in patients on dialysis.[21] Patients with symptomatic recurrent PAD have low post-transplant survival.[20] CKD patients have high prevalence of diabetes, hypertension, dyslipidemia and history of smoking. These are also risk factors for peripheral arterial disease. CKD is itself a risk factor and degree of iliac artery calcification increases with increasing duration on dialysis.[22]

Evaluation includes history for symptoms like intermittent claudication, rest pain, lower limb swelling, femoral vein canulation for hemodialysis and physical examination. Non-invasive test like Doppler USG study should be done in high risk patients. In patients with significant findings on non-invasive tests or clinical evidence of PAD, non-contrast CT imaging to assess degree on vascular calcification's and pelvic with lower limb angiography or venography is advised.

8. What kind of risk is anticipated with suboptimal recipient vessels?

Ans: Heavily calcified or atherosclerotic recipient iliac arteries may cause reduced graft perfusion or pose technical challenge during anastomosis, may cause intimal dissection, arterial thrombosis or pseudoaneurysm formation postoperatively.[23] Similarly, fibrosed, thick walled iliac veins or atretic lumen may cause venous thrombosis, poor distal venous run off and graft turgidity with risk of hematuria, anastomotic site bleeding or even graft rupture.

Patients with large uncorrectable abdominal aneurysm, severe occlusive common iliac disease, active gangrene or history of recent atheroemboli should be excluded from transplant.[8]

9. What is disuse bladder and how do you evaluate lower tract in kidney recipient?

Ans: Defunctionalized or disuse bladder has been defined one with urinary output < 300 ml/24 hours[24] or a bladder that has not been used for several years.[25] An unfavourable lower urinary tract may jeopardize graft function after transplant. Normal urinary bladder that stores urine at low pressure, does not leak and completely empties by natural voiding is essential for stable graft function. However, there is a little evidence to suggest that initial evaluation beyond history, urine R/E, culture and sensitivity, uroflowmetry and ultrasound KUB with postvoid residual urine is necessary in patients without significant urinary complaints.[26,27]

Further evaluation with retrograde urethrography, MCU, urodynamic study or cystoscopy should be done in those with history of genitourinary abnormalities or in children with dysfunctional voiding.[28]

Most of the voiding dysfunction can be managed with self-intermittent catheterization.[29] The need for urinary diversion or bladder augmentation should be decided on case to case basis.

10. Why is important to do psychosocial evaluation in kidney recipient?

Ans: Psychosocial evaluation of transplant candidates is of utmost importance. Successful long-term graft outcome requires lifelong adherence to medications, regular follow-up visit to transplant clinic, discipline to follow safe practices to prevent infection and financial stability to bear the cost of medicines, lab investigations and treatment of any complications. Non-compliance with medication intake is one of the most important causes of graft rejection and graft loss.[30–32]

So, the crux of psychosocial evaluation is to ensure compliance. Any condition which is deemed to interfere with compliance such as drug or substance abuse, cognitive impairment or psychiatric illness has to be addressed.

Psychiatric illness in itself is not a contraindication to transplant, provided patient symptoms are well under control. Similarly, recipient with cognitive impairment can also be offered kidney transplant provided a responsible caretaker is available to assist them. They should have a legal guardian or family member to give consent for surgery.[33]

KEY POINTS

- It is important to know the etiology of ESRD.
- Some native kidney diseases have high risk of recurrence in renal allograft.
- High risk of recurrence is not a contraindication for renal transplant but patient should be counselled.
- Infection is common in renal transplant recipients because of immunosuppression.
- It is an important cause of both graft and patient loss.
- Active infection is a contraindication for transplantation.
- Patients must be screened for common viral and bacterial infections.
- They should be immunized against preventable disease as early as possible.
- Live attenuated vaccines are contraindicated in post-transplant setting.
- Hepatitis B or Hepatitis C positive status in recipient is not a contraindication for kidney transplant.
- There is a risk of flare up of infection and rapid progression of liver disease after transplant.
- Long-term graft and patient survival is less in these patients.
- They must receive anti-viral therapy after transplant.
- In general, a waiting period of 2–5 years is recommended after treatment completion of malignancy before listing patient for renal transplant.
- In case of low risk and low grade malignancy, transplant can proceed without any waiting period.
- Ideally, risk of recurrence of malignancy and life expectancy of patient should be assessed on a case to case basis.
- Screening for asymptomatic gall stone disease, diverticulosis or peptic ulcer disease is not recommended.
- Role of prophylactic cholecystectomy for asymptomatic gall stone is controversial.
- Active peptic ulcer, acute diverticulitis, acute cholecystitis or acute pancreatitis should be treated first.
- There is high prevalence of cardiovascular disease in CKD patients.
- Cardiovascular disease is the leading cause of mortality in transplant recipients.
- Basic cardiology work up in asymptomatic low risk patients consists of history, physical examination, chest X-ray and 12 lead ECG.
- High risk patients require further evaluation with 2D ECHO, myocardial perfusion scan or Holter.
- Coronary angiography should be advised for symptomatic patients or those with positive findings on evaluation.
- Symptomatic angina or myocardial infarction within 6 months are contraindications for renal transplant
- Pulmonary assessment consists of evaluation of fitness for major surgery under general anesthesia and screening for chronic or latent lung infections.
- CKD in itself as well as frequently co-existing co-morbidities are risk factors for vascular disease.
- Significant vascular disease is associated with poor patient survival.
- Goal of vascular evaluation is to ensure suitable recipients vessels for graft anastomosis and long-term survival of patients.
- Lower urinary tract evaluation is important to ensure stable graft function.
- In patients without history of lower urinary tract symptoms, evaluation should be limited to urine examination, uroflowmetry and USG KUB.
- Children with dysfunctional voiding or patients with genitourinary abnormalities or significant LUTS need further work up with RGU, MCU, urodynamic study or cystoscopy.
- Urinary diversion or bladder augmentation is required in select cases as self-intermittent catheterisation is sufficient to manage most of voiding dysfunctions.
- Psychosocial evaluation should be directed towards assessment of compliance and cognitive function.

SUMMARY

- This chapter will provide a comprehensive overview of the treatment options for ESRD, criteria for kidney transplantation, and the meticulous evaluation process for potential transplant recipients. By understanding these aspects, urologist can better manage and support patients with ESRD in their journey towards optimal renal replacement therapy.

REFERENCES

1. Goldfarb-Rumyantzev A, Hurdle JF, Scandling J, *et al.* Duration of end-stage renal disease and kidney transplant outcome. Nephrol Dial Transplant. 2005;20:167–75.
2. Timothy Hamish Mathew, Recurrence of Disease Following Renal Transplantation, American Journal of Kidney Diseases, Volume 12, Issue 2, 1988, Pages 85–96, ISSN 0272–6386.
3. Briganti EM, Russ GR, McNeil JJ, *et al.* Risk of renal allograft loss from recurrent glomerulonephritis. N Engl J Med 2002;347(2):103–9.
4. ISSN 0272–6386, Kidney Disease: Improving Global Outcomes (KDIGO) Kidney Transplant Candidate Work Group. KDIGO Clinical Practice Guideline on the Evaluation and Management of Candidates for Kidney Transplantation. *Transplantation*. 2020;104: S1–S103.

5. Indian Society of Nephrology Guidelines for Vaccination in Chronic Kidney Disease. Indian Journal of Nephrology. Supplement 1–2016–Volume 26.
6. Fornairon S, Pol S, Legendre C, *et al.* The long-term virologic and pathologic impact of renal transplantation on chronic hepatitis B virus infection. Transplantation 1996;62(2):297–9
7. Fabrizi F, Martin P, Dixit V, Kanwal F, Dulai G. HBsAg seropositive status and survival after renal transplantation: meta-analysis of observational studies. Am J Transplant 2005;5(12):2913–21.
8. Knoll G, Cockfield S, Blydt-Hansen T, *et al.* Canadian Society of Transplantation consensus guidelines on eligibility for kidney transplantation. *CMAJ*. 2005; 173: 1181–1184.
9. KDIGO 2022 Clinical Practice Guideline for the Prevention, Diagnosis, Evaluation, and Treatment of Hepatitis C in Chronic Kidney Disease. Kidney International (2022) 102 (Suppl 6S), S129–S205.
10. Malinis M, Boucher HW. Screening of donor and candidate prior to solid organ transplantation-Guidelines from the American Society of Transplantation Infectious Diseases Community of Practice. Clin Transplant. 2019: e13548.
11. Rogerson TE, Chen S, Kok J, *et al.* Tests for latent tuberculosis in people with ESRD: a systematic review. Am J Kidney Dis. 2013; 61:33–43.
12. Krishnamoorthy S, Kumaresan N, Zumla A. Latent tuberculosis infection and renal transplantation-Diagnosis and management. Int J Infect Dis. 2019 Mar; 80S:S73–S76.
13. Gutierrez-Dalmau A, Campistol JM. Immunosuppressive therapy and malignancy in organ transplant recipients: a systematic review. Drugs. 2007;67(8):1167–98.
14. Acuna SA, Huang JW, Daly C, Shah PS, Kim SJ, Baxter NN. Outcomes of Solid Organ Transplant Recipients With Preexisting Malignancies in Remission: A Systematic Review and Meta-Analysis. Transplantation. 2017 Mar;101(3):471–481.
15. Wong G, Chapman JR, Craig JC. Cancer screening in renal transplant recipients: what is the evidence? *Clin J Am Soc Nephrol*. 2008;3 Suppl 2: S87–S100
16. Kasiske BL, Cangro CB, Hariharan S, *et al.* The evaluation of renal transplant candidates: clinical practice guidelines. Am J Transplant 2001;1 suppl 2:3–95.
17. Lentine KL, Brennan DC, Schnitzler MA. Incidence and predictors of myocardial infarction after kidney transplantation. J Am Soc Nephrol. 2005;16:496–506.
18. Kasiske BL, Maclean JR, Snyder JJ. Acute myocardial infarction and kidney transplantation.J Am Soc Nephrol. 2006;17:900–7.
19. American College of Physicians. Guidelines for assessing and managing the perioperative risk from coronary artery disease associated with major noncardiac surgery. Ann Intern Med 1997;127(4):309–12.
20. Parfrey PS, Foley RN, Harnett JD, *et al.* Outcome and risk factors for left ventricular disorders in chronic uremia. Nephrol Dial Transplant 1996;11(7):1277–85.
21. Criqui MH, Langer RD, Fronek A, *et al.* Mortality over a period of 10 years in patients with peripheral arterial disease. N Engl J Med 1992;326(6):381–6
22. Sung RS, Althoen M, Howell TA, *et al.* Peripheral vascular occlusive disease in renal transplant recipients: risk factors and impact on kidney allograft survival. *Transplantation*. 2000; 70: 1049–1054
23. Kahn J, Ram LM, Eberhard K, *et al.* Calcification score evaluation in patients listed for renal transplantation. *Clin Transplant*. 2017; 31.
24. Errando C, Batista JE, Caparros J, Vicente J, Arano P. Urodynamic evaluation and management prior to renal transplantation. Eur Urol. 2000;38:415–8.
25. Kogan SJ, Levitt SB. Bladder evaluation in paediatric patients before undiversion in previously diverted urinary tracts. J Urol. 1976;118:443–6.
26. Shandera KC, Rozanski TA, Jaffers G. The necessity of voiding cystourethrogram in the pre transplant urologic evaluation. Urology 1996;47(2):198–200.
27. Glazier DB, Whang MI, Geffner SR, *et al.* Evaluation of voiding cystourethrography prior to renal transplantation. Transplantation 1996;62(12):1762–5.
28. Crowe A, Cairns HS, Wood S, *et al.* Renal transplantation following renal failure due to urological disorders. Nephrol Dial Transplant 1998;13(8):2065–9.
29. Gill IS, Hayes JM, Hodge EE, *et al.* Clean intermittent catheterization and urinary diversion in the management of renal transplant recipients with lower urinary tract dysfunction. J Urol 1992;148(5):1397–400.
30. Greenstein S, Siegal B. Compliance and noncompliance in patients with a functioning renal transplant: a multicenter study. Transplantation 1998;66(12):1718–26.
31. De Geest S, Borgermans L, Gemoets H, *et al.* Incidence, determinants, and consequences of subclinical noncompliance with immunosuppressive therapy in renal transplant recipients. Transplantation 1995;59(3):340–7.
32. Hilbrands LB, Hoitsma AJ, Koene RA. Medication compliance after renal transplantation. Transplantation 1995; 60(9):914–20.
33. Benedetti E, Asolati M, Dunn T, *et al.* Kidney transplantation in recipients with mental retardation: clinical results in a single-center experience. Am J Kidney Dis 1998;31(3): 509–12.

Chapter 2

Histocompatibility Testing in Renal Transplant

• Renuka Soni • Priyadarshi Ranjan

LEARNING OBJECTIVES

- To understand the role of immunology in the success of transplant.
- To understand the immuno-compatibility testing for detection of antibodies and how to address them.
- To understand the role of HLA and anti-HLA antibodies
- To understand the ABO incompatible transplant.
- To understand the kidney graft failure due to rejection.
- To understand the existing and newer evolving laboratory assays for antibody detection.

Human Leukocyte Antigen and its Role in Kidney Transplant

In humans, the major histocompatibility complex (MHC) encodes several cell surface proteins called human leukocyte antigens (HLA) that play an essential role as immunological barriers in kidney transplantation. HLA antigen genes are co-dominantly expressed on the short arm of chromosome 6. In the human genome, the HLA region spans 3.6 million base pairs and is the most gene-dense region with about 224 gene loci.[1] The HLA genes are classified into three classes, Class I, II genes encode for HLA molecules that are important in kidney transplantation, whereas class III genes encode proteins (cytokines, complement factors, heat shock proteins) involved in other immune system pathways. HLA genes are highly polymorphic, with more than 36,061 allelic variations, thus contributing to 10% of human genetic diversity.[1,2]

Histocompatibility antigens HLA Class I includes HLA-A, B, and C genes, and HLA Class II includes HLA-D (DP, DQ, DZ/DO and DR) genes. Class I HLA genes are expressed on all cells and class II HLA genes are expressed on antigen-presenting cells (dendritic cells, Langerhans cells, macrophages, B-cells, and capillary endothelium).[3,4] One set of HLA genes is called a haplotype, and an individual has two sets of haplotypes that are inherited from four different combinations of haplotypes from their parents.[5] The human immune system uses HLA molecules as protective mechanisms for the processing and presentation of peptide antigen as fragments to T lymphocytes. Class I HLA genes expressed on human nucleated cells are presented as non-self-antigen to cytolytic CD8 T cells, and class II HLA genes expressed on APCs present the antigen to CD4 T helper cells. HLA has a huge diversity as it involves numerous alleles for any antigen. HLA molecules are surface glycoproteins with peptide-binding affinity and associated peptide-binding regions and mismatch may occur at antigenic or allelic levels.[5,6] The antigenic ones have amino acid substitutions in both the T-cell recognition and peptide-binding regions, whereas the allelic ones have amino acid substitutions in the peptide-binding region only.

Kidney failure due to rejection occurs when the immune system of the recipient produces *de novo* or has pre-preformed anti-HLA antibodies against the donor organ and recognises the organ as foreign.[6] HLA matching reflects the immune reactivity of a host, is considered more important in the case of renal transplantation than other organs. It has been proven that better survival of a grafted kidney is achieved with HLA matching. Thus, before any kidney transplant, it is mandated to determine donor-recipient compatibility via HLA antibody testing to assess the potential risk for graft loss. The results from HLA typing decides the physician's decisions regarding donor selection, immunosuppressive regimens, and post-kidney transplant patient care.[7]

Case Scenario

A 32-year-old young woman has developed end stage renal disease due to pregnancy-induced complications and is interested for a renal transplant and her husband and mother have offered to be her donor. Her blood group is O+ and her husband is also O+ but is unmatched on tissue typing (0/6 HLA match), the mother is 60 years healthy but has B+ blood group. She received multiple transfusions due to her pregnancy related complications. How would you proceed for immunological workup?

A complement dependent crossmatch, flow crossmatch and Luminex bead single antigen assay should be performed along with anti-B titres in the recipient.

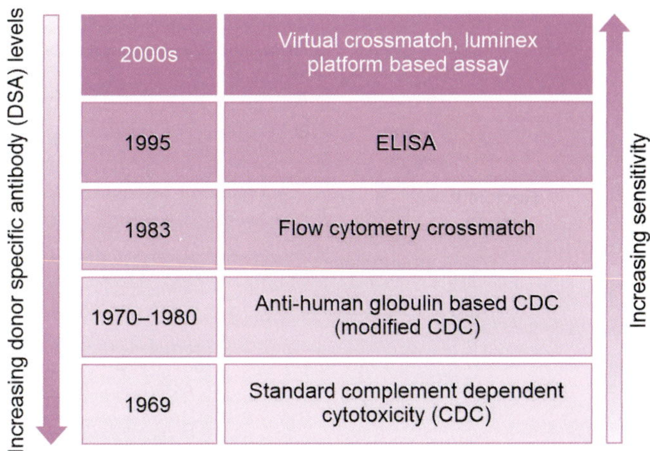

Fig. 2.1: Development of sensitive HLA antibody detection tests for assessing the percentage of donor specific antibody in recipient sera

HLA Antibody Detection Assays

For a kidney transplant to be successful, HLA detection assays are done prior to the transplant to ensure that the recipient is devoid of any antibodies against the donor tissue and to determine the degree of sensitization of the recipient towards the donor. For HLA detection, crossmatch is considered an important test. Several crossmatch detection assays have evolved over the years with an increased level of specificity and sensitivity (Fig. 2.1).

Standard Cell-Based Assays: CDC

The complement dependent cytotoxicity (CDC) is a (lymphocyte-based) standard cell-based biological assay developed by Terasaki and McClelland in 1964.[8] CDC assay requires antibody binding, complement activation, and cellular damage for a positive reaction (Figs 2.2A and 2.2B). The CDC crossmatch test detects the functional potential of anti-HLA antibodies in the recipient's circulation which can immediately bind to complement and cause cell lysis, providing direct evidence for the presence of likely pathogenic (i.e. cytotoxic) antibodies resulting in hyperacute rejection. It is an *in vitro* test in which recipient serum is mixed with donor lymphocytes (T or B cells). Complement (usually from rabbit serum) is added to the mixture. The readout of this test is the detection of percentage of donor cell death. The results are scored using a standardized ranking system by the National Institutes of Health (NIH). However, different scoring systems are also used. CDC crossmatch (CDCXM) test is a working paradigm before any renal transplant and a positive T cell CDCXM has traditionally been considered an absolute contraindication to perform a kidney transplant.[9]

Scoring and Interpretation of Results in Both Standard CDC and AHG-CDC

Score in each well is determined by the percentage of nonviable cells. Viable cells retain the carboxyfluorescein diacetate (CFDA) and appear green. Dead cells take up Ethidium bromide (EB) and appear red.

For appropriate results, positive and negative control should also be assessed simultaneously to rule out non-complement fixing antibodies or autoantibodies. Positive control should show 80% cell death, whereas negative control should have 80% of cell viability. Cytotoxicity scoring system and its interpretation are shown in Tables 2.1 and 2.2 respectively.[10]

TABLE 2.1: CDC crossmatch scoring system

Score	*% Dead cells*	*Interpretation*
0	Not readable	Invalid (technical issue)
1	0–10	Negative
2	11–20	Doubtful negative
4	21–50	Weak positive
6	51–80	Positive
8	>80	Strong positive

CDC crossmatch scoring system

TABLE 2.2: How to interpret the results of a CDC crossmatch assay?

B-cell Crossmatch	*T-cell Crossmatch*	*Interpretation*
Negative	Negative	No or very low titre levels of donor specific antibodies to cause a positive reaction
Negative	Positive	Result invalid. Test needs to be repeated. Technical error as B-cell crossmatch should be positive for a T-cell crossmatch to be positive
Positive	Negative	One or more HLA Class II donor-specific antibody. No or low levels of Class I donor-specific antibody with higher lysis of B-cells, rituximab administration
Positive	Positive	Multiple donor-specific antibodies to both the HLA Class I and Class II donor specific antibody

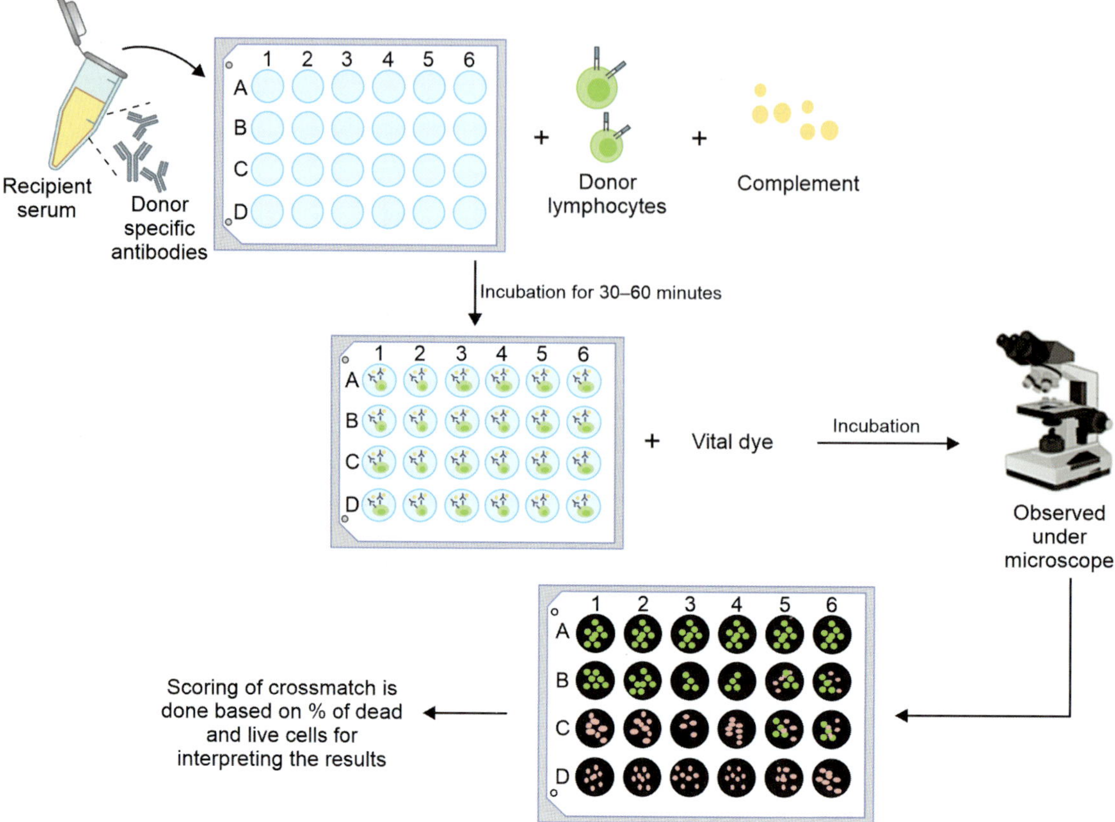

Fig. 2.2A: Brief description of steps involved in the CDC crossmatch assay

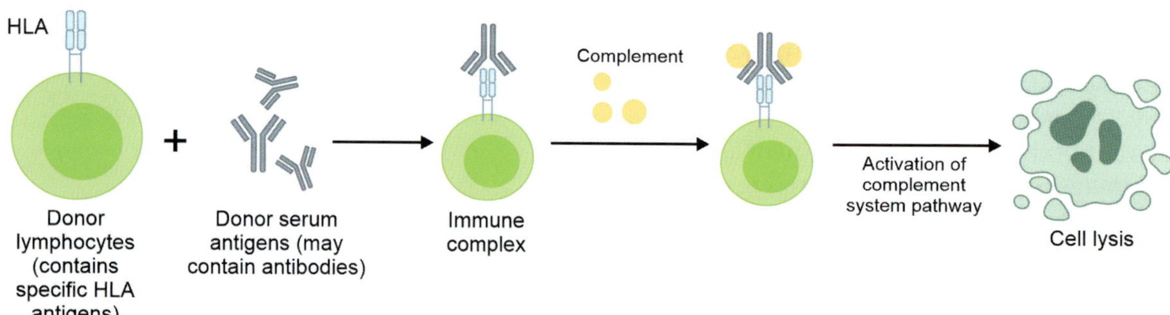

Fig. 2.2B: Immunopathological pathway involved in the CDC crossmatch assay

1. **How can we improve the sensitivity and specificity of standard CDC assay?**

   Ans: Modified lymphocytotoxicity assays are advanced version of standard CDC method with increased specificity and sensitivity. Several modifications or steps are added to improve the overall yield of CDC crossmatch. A brief overview is outlined in Table 2.3.

2. **What is PRA and what is its clinical importance?**

   Ans: Panel reactive antibody (PRA) is an assay that identifies sensitized patients who have pre-existing antibodies and estimates their likelihood of finding a crossmatch-compatible donor.[12] PRA is primarily indicated when a living donor is unavailable and a potential recipient is being waitlisted to receive a kidney from a deceased donor. The assay assesses the antibodies to a prevailing HLA antigen pattern of a specific geographic location. These antigens form the testing panel against which the strength of antibodies is determined. Percentage of cells in a panel with a positive cytotoxic reaction (%PRA) indicates their sensitization against the panel. Percent PRA depends on serum sample and antigenic composition of test cell panel which may differ from kit to kit and region to region. Though commercial based cell panels are available, CDC-based PRA testing has a limited degree of consistency and possess drawbacks such as non-specificity of the antibody and positive result from non-HLA antibodies.[12]

TABLE 2.3: Steps to improve the sensitivity and specificity of standard CDC assay

Procedure step	*Modification*	*Remarks*
Before complement: Addition	Addition of washing steps	Effective removal of anti-complementary factors
	Addition of antihuman globulin (AHG)	AHG binds to all the available donor specific anti-HLA antibodies on donor cells leading to the amplification of F_c receptor for complement binding, activation for cell lysis.[2,11] Thus, increasing the sensitivity to detect low titer non-complement antibodies
Incubation time	60 minutes serum and cells; 120 minutes complement	Effective binding of low avidity antibodies
Dithiothreitol (DTT) treatment	Recipient serum treatment with DTT	DTT reduce the pentameric form of immunoglobulin M (IgM) to monomers making them capable of binding to complement components
Cell panels	Use of randomly selected donor HLA-typed cell panels	Reciprocate the natural distribution of HLA antigens.

Calculated PRA

The dynamic evolution of PRA is Calculated Panel Reactive Antibody (cPRA) that uses a computer software based on the HLA frequencies derived from HLA types of different ethnic population. In 2007, the use of cPRA was approved by the United Network of Organ Sharing. cPRA provides the percentage of deceased organ donor antigens that will be crossmatch incompatible for a candidate. It is highly sensitive as it provides the accurate HLA frequencies of both Class I and Class II antigens together including the donor's unacceptable HLA.[12]

3. **What is flow cytometry crossmatch? What are its advantages and limitations?**

   Ans: Flow cytometry is the next evolution to measure/titrate the strength of pre-existing anti-HLA antibodies in the recipient. The flow cytometric crossmatch is now becoming an emerging standard technique for evaluating the immunological compatibility between the donor–recipient pair. The flow cytometry assay involves the detection of cell-bound anti-HLA antibodies in the recipient serum treated with the donor's mononuclear cells, followed by the addition of fluorescently conjugated, secondary antihuman IgG and analysis by flow cytometry.

Advantages

1. It is more sensitive as compared to CDC crossmatch.
2. Evaluation of both the T-cell and B-cell reactivities simultaneously. An additional incubation step is involved with anti-CD3 for the identification of both T- and B-cell populations, respectively.[13,14]
3. This test can be performed with the use of damaged cells also.
4. Testing of different isotypes of IgG, IgM, or IgA immunoglobulin by using secondary detection antibody.[10]

Limitations

1. Nonspecific binding of Ig to Fc receptors can be mistaken as positive result.
2. Non-HLA antibodies as well as monoclonal antilymphocyte antibodies such as thymoglobulin, rituximab, and alemtuzumab used for immunosuppression can also interfere with the assay giving a false-positive result.[15,2]
3. Can even be positive by non-complement fixing antibodies which may not be important in kidney transplant.

4. **How do we analyse the test results of flow crossmatch?**

   Ans: In flow cytometry crossmatch, the strength of antibodies is calculated based on channel shift phenomenon. Channel shift refers to the fluorescence intensity above control. It is used for assessing positive and negative matches in flow cytometry crossmatch.[10] It is expressed as the degree of positivity and the fluorescent intensity. A 40-channel shift for T cells and an 80-channel shift for B cells are generally considered a positive test.[16]

5. **What would be the crossmatch result interpretation in the following cases?**

   Ans:
   1. **CDC (B and T-cells) negative and flow crossmatch is positive:** Hyperacute rejection may occur and further testing is required due to the low-titer of anti-class I antibodies, these patients might need desensitization measures.
   2. **CDC (T-cell negative, B-cell positive) and flow crossmatch is negative:** Low risk of rejection as autoantibody IgM is likely to be present. Treatment with DTT is required to eradicate IgM antibody.[15]

ELISA

Kao *et al* developed an ELISA-based HLA antibody detection method using affinity-purified HLA class I from platelets as the target antigens for the detection of HLA antibodies in patient sera.[17] Several rapid and sensitive ELISA-based assays to detect HLA antibodies were developed in the 1990s.[14] ELISA is used as a routine procedure in laboratories for detecting PRA. However, it is now replaced by bead-based assays due to tedious procedure and higher chances of cross-contamination.

6. **What is Luminex platform for testing antibodies?**

   Ans: Luminex platform is the most modern and a highly sensitive (solid phase) assay for assessing the pre-formed antibodies in the recipient. Luminex crossmatch detects donor-specific anti-HLA IgG antibodies against donor's class I and/or class II antigens in a single well. In this assay, synthetic beads coated with single or multiple HLA class I and II antigens are treated with the recipient's sera, and a fluorescently labelled secondary antibody detects and binds the bead-bound recipient antibody. A beam laser is used for the detection of bound secondary antibodies and specific beads (Fig. 2.3). It is an ideal technique for both pre- and post-transplant testing as frozen donor lysate can be used, avoiding cell viability issues. However, it is always used in combination with other testing assays due to its inability to detect class II antibodies, especially against DQ and DP antigens.[18,19]

7. **What is virtual crossmatch?**

   Ans: Virtual crossmatch is a risk assessment tool used to ascertain the presence of HLA antibodies in the recipient's serum and to determine the potential crossmatch results with an available donor virtually. Recipient sensitization towards different HLA can be predicted before performing actual CDC and flow cytometry crossmatch. For a virtual crossmatch, we first analyse and titrate the levels of anti-HLA antibody in the recipient's serum by means of Luminex platform. The level of these antibody is measured in terms of Mean Fluorescence Intensity (MFI). MFI >1000–2000 is considered highly significant which has the potential to convert a CDC/flow cytometry crossmatch positive. These antibody levels are then directly corelated to donor's HLA antigen profile and a virtual crossmatch is established.[20–22]

Applications

1. Used in case of both the sensitized and non-sensitized patients.
2. Predicts actual flow cytometry crossmatch results, facilitating rapid allocation of organs in highly sensitized recipients.
3. Some studies have shown the statistically significant reduction in cold ischemia time with the use of virtual crossmatch.
4. Virtual crossmatch is possible both at the time of organ allocation and after organ allocation (Table 2.4).

8. **What is ABO incompatible (ABO-I) transplantation?**

   Ans: ABO-I refers to the transplantation from the individuals having different blood group. It has been considered as a significant barrier to a successful kidney transplantation due to anti-blood group antibody-mediated rejection of the graft. However, the successful breakthrough of ABO-incompatible kidney transplantation in Boston, US in 1954 has opened the doors of hope for patients waiting for a transplant. In ABO-I transplant, patients are pre-operatively treated with immunosuppressive drugs to remove or reduce antibody levels in recipient's blood. ABO-I transplantation of kidney is performed when recipient is highly in need of a transplant and a blood group compatible kidney is not available.[23]

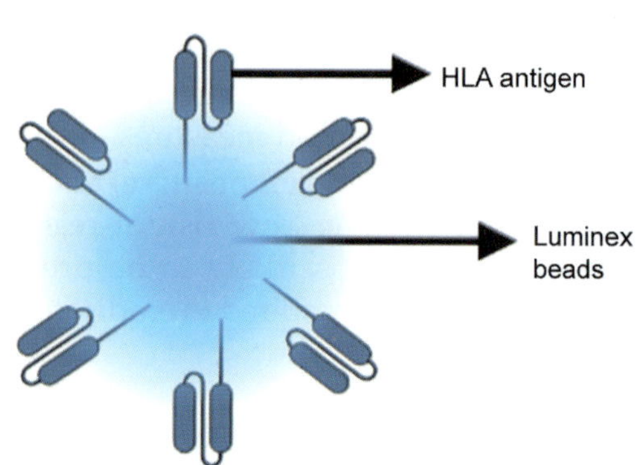

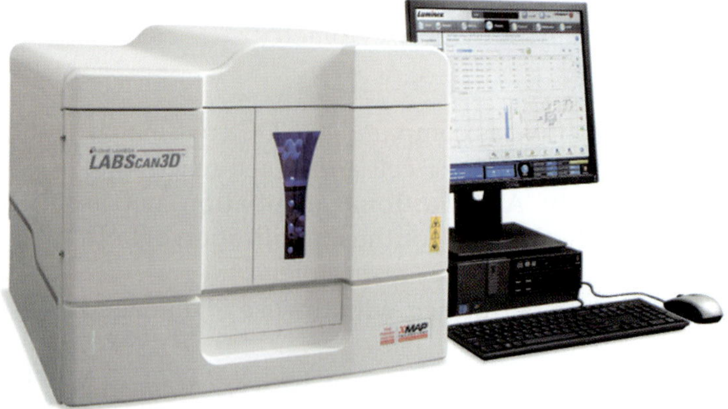

Fig. 2.3: Luminex antigen bead and LABScan3D™
(*Source:* One Lambda Thermo Fisher Scientific Inc.)

TABLE 2.4: How to interpret contradictory results of flow cytometry crossmatch and virtual crossmatch?

Scenarios	*Flow cytometry crossmatch*	*Virtual Crossmatch*	*Factor responsible*
1	Positive	Negative	Presence of autoantibodies Incomplete/incorrect HLA typing Non-specific binding Antibodies may be under presented due to the dispersion of the antibody across many beads
2	Negative	Positive	Low HLA expression Presence of low affinity/avidity donor specific antibody Antibody reactivity towards denatured HLA

The evolution of HLA antibody detection assays has been summarized in Fig. 2.4.

HLA antibody detection assays		Remarks
Cell-based crossmatch	Complement dependent cytotoxicity	• Time consuming and tedious to perform • No difference between IgG and IgM antibodies • Low sensitivity and specificity • High background reading of non-HLA antibodies due to spontaneous cell death leading to false positive • Dependent on cell surface expression of HLA antigen • Detection of complement-fixing antibodies only
	Anti-human globulin CDC	• High background reading of non-HLA antibodies due to spontaneous cell death leading to false positive • Dependent on cell surface expression of HLA antigen • Detection of complement-fixing antibodies only
Flow cytometry	Flow cytometry crossmatch	• More sensitive than CDC • This test can be performed with the use of damage cells also • Detection of T and B-cells reactivities together • Optimal channel shift an issue • Nonspecific binding of Ig to Fc receptors can be mistaken as positive result • Difficult to standardize due to variability among cytometers, fluorochromes, antiglobulin reagents and variation in cell to serum ratio

(Contd.)

(Contd.)

HLA antibody detection assays		Remarks
Solid based assay	Luminex bead crossmatch	• Highly sensitive, semi-quantitative and enables precise definition of anti-HLA antibodies • Dectection and characterization of anti-MICA antibodies • Problems of false positivity and false negativity • Do not cover the whole diversity of HLA alleles

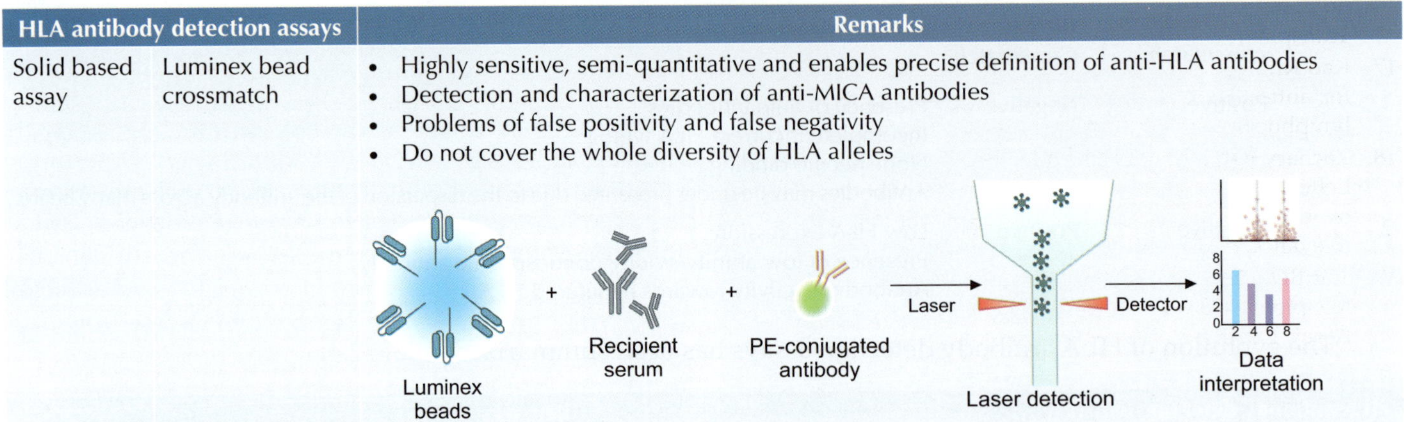

Fig. 2.4: Evolution of HLA antibody typing assay[2]

In these recipients, the titer levels of respective anti-A or anti-B blood group antibodies is measured/titrated by means of gel/card method. There are several techniques based on double dilution of serum for detection of the level of antibodies. The titre is marked as 1:1, 1:2, 1:4, 1:8, 1:16, 1:32 and so on. These antibodies are subsequently removed/suppressed prior to ABO incompatible transplant.

Future Directions

Cell surface is a jungle which has numerous antigens that includes both HLA and non-HLA antigens. Although HLA comprises immunologically the most important antigen, triggering a rejection, however, non-HLA antigens such as MICA, endothelin, etc are recently discovered and antibodies against them may also play a significant role in the rejection process. The antigen profiling and characterization of these newer antibodies is the newer direction to standardize the antibody profiling in the recipient. In the existing anti-HLA antibody titration, there are several limitations present mainly due to the genetic and geographical variations of antigens. The antibody profiling is gaining a widespread application for monitoring the rejection post-transplant. Additionally, there are several triggers which might lead to production of newer *de novo* antibodies making the entire assessment unpredictable. Hence, attention is being directed towards them as well.

REFERENCES

1. Horton R, Wilming L, Rand V, *et al.* Gene map of the extended human MHC. Nature Reviews Genetics. 2004;5(12):889–899.
2. Bhargava V, Sahay M, Meena P, Sakhuja V, Gupta A. Textbook of Kidney Transplantation. 2022.
3. Mongkolsuk T., Tammakorn C., Kitpoka P. A rare HLA-DRB1*14:22–DQB1*04:01 haplotype in a kidney donor: implication in the interpretation of donor-specific antibody in kidney transplantation—a case report. Transplantation Proceedings. 2016;48(3):943–945.
4. Schreuder GM, Hurley CK, Marsh SG, Lau M, Fernandez-Vina M, Noreen HJ, *et al.* The HLA Dictionary 2004: a summary of HLA-A,-B,-C,-DRB1/3/4/5 and-DQB1 alleles and their association with serologically defined HLA-A,-B,-C,-DR and-DQ antigens. Tissue Antigens. 2005;65(1):1–55.
5. Trivedi VB, Dave AP, Dave JM, Patel BC. Human leukocyte antigen and its role in transplantation biology. Transplant Proc. 2007;39(3):688–93.
6. Alelign T, Ahmed MM, Bobosha K, Tadesse Y, Howe R, Petros B. Kidney Transplantation: The Challenge of Human Leukocyte Antigen and Its Therapeutic Strategies. J Immunol Res. 2018:5986740.
7. Barlow AD. Kidney transplantation. Surgery. 2017;35(7):378–384.
8. Terasaki PI, McClelland JD. Microdroplet Assay of Human Serum Cytotoxins. Nature. 1964:998–1000.
9. Bhaskaran MC, Heidt S, Muthukumar T. Principles of Virtual Crossmatch Testing for Kidney Transplantation. Kidney Int Rep. 2022;7(6):1179–1188.
10. Peña JR, Fitzpatrick D, Saidman SL. Complement-dependent cytotoxicity crossmatch. Methods Mol Biol. 2013;1034: 257–83.
11. Mulley WR, Kanellis J. Understanding crossmatch testing in organ transplantation: A case-based guide for the general nephrologist. Nephrology (Carlton). 2011 Feb;16(2):125–33.
12. Santos RD, Langewisch ED, Norman DJ. Immunological assessment of the Transplanted Patient. In: Weir MR, Lerma EV, eds. Kidney Transplantation. New York, NY: Springer New York; 2014:23–34.
13. Cecka J.M. Calculated PRA (CPRA): the new measure of sensitization for transplant candidates. Am J Transplant. 2010;10:26–29.
14. Bray RA, Nickerson PW, Kerman RH, Gebel HM. Evolution of HLA antibody detection: technology emulating biology. Immunol Res. 2004;29(1–3):41–54.
15. Bray RA, Lebeck LK, Gebel HM. The flow cytometric crossmatch. Dual-color analysis of T cell and B cell reactivities. Transplantation. 1989;48(5):834–40.

16. Ettenger RB, Jordan SC, Fine RN. Cadaver renal transplant outcome in recipients with autolymphocytotoxic antibodies. Transplantation. 1983;35(5):429–31.
17. Kao KJ, Scornik JC, Small SJ. Enzyme-linked immunoassay for anti-HLA antibodies-an alternative to panel studies by lymphocytotoxicity. Transplantation. 1993;55(1):192–6.
18. Zachary AA, Ratner LE, Graziani JA, Lucas DP, Delaney NL, Leffell MS. Characterization of HLA class I specific antibodies by ELISA using solubilized antigen targets: II. Clinical relevance. Hum Immunol. 200;62(3):236–46.
19. Tait BD. Detection of HLA Antibodies in Organ Transplant Recipients-Triumphs and Challenges of the Solid Phase Bead Assay. Front Immunol. 2016;7:570.
20. Pinelli DF, Tambur AR. Virtual crossmatching for deceased donor transplantation: one size does not fit all. Kidney Int. 2020;97:659–662.
21. Clifford Sullivan H, Krummey SM, Gebel HM, *et al.* Physical crossmatching vs virtual crossmatching: the end of an era? or why give up a good thing?. Hum Immunol. 2020;81: 401–406.
22. Rao, Prakash; Deo, Dayanand; Marchioni, Misty; Harris, Patricia. 117.4: The virtual crossmatch: A useful tool to improve organ allocation. Transplantation 103(11S):pS12. 2019.
23. Wang Yi. ABO-incompatible Organ Transplantation. Springer Singapore. 2019.

Chapter

3

Immunosuppression in Renal Transplant

• *Sanjay P Kolte*[1] • *Kapil Sejpal*[2]

LEARNING OBJECTIVES

- To understand the various immunosuppressive agents used in clinical practice for kidney transplantation.
- To understand their mechanisms of action, indications, contraindications, side-effects and various therapeutic regimens.

Case Scenario 1

A 44-year-old male, known case of CKD, ESRD on maintenance haemodialysis who is registered for deceased donor transplant, gets a call for kidney transplant. He is found to have DSA titre of HLA II of 1100 MFI. His CDC crossmatch is negative. It is decided to give him ATG (anti-thymocyte globulin) induction.

1. What are different types of immunosuppressive medications used in renal transplant?

Ans: There are three types of immunosuppressive medications used in renal transplant. They are as follows:

1. Induction agents
2. Maintenance agents
3. Anti-rejection drugs

2. What is the purpose of induction agents? How are they classified?

Ans: Immediately after transplantation, when the blood flow to the graft is restored, recognition of donor antigens by T cells of the host initiates an adaptive immunogenic response which leads to rejection of allograft. Induction agents are highly potent and cause intense immunosuppression. In a nutshell, the purpose of their use is to:

a. Deplete or modulate T-cell responses at the time of antigen presentation,
b. Reduce the risk of acute rejection and
c. Allow reduction in maintenance immunosuppression.

They are classified into:

a. Depleting agents—act by causing T cell lysis. They also interfere with T cell dependent activation of B cells and affect antibody formation too.[1]
b. Non-depleting agents—bind to receptors which prevent T cell stimulation during antigen recognition.

Table 3.1 shows the classification of induction agents. ATG (anti-thymocyte globulin) and Basiliximab are the most common induction agents used in renal transplant in India and worldwide.

TABLE 3.1: Classification of induction agents
Depleting agents
• ATG (thymoglobulin)
• Alemtuzumab (monoclonal anti-CD52 antibody)
• OKT3 (monoclonal anti-CD3 antibody)
Non-depleting agents
• Basiliximab (chimeric monoclonal anti-CD25 antibody)
• Daclizumab (humanized monoclonal anti-CD25 antibody)

3. Is it necessary to use induction agents in all patients before transplant?

Ans: It is not mandatory to use induction agents in all patients before transplant. However, it can be considered in situations like:

1. In sensitized individuals (patients with prior history of transplant, transfusions, or multiple pregnancies),

2. Patients in whom late introduction of calcineurin inhibitors (CNI) is desirable such as recipients of extended criteria donor organs,
3. As a part of steroid-minimization or withdrawal regimens,
4. Patients with positive DSA

4. How do we decide on the choice of induction agent?

Ans: ATG is usually preferred for transplants with high risk, and Basiliximab is used for low or intermediate risk transplant. High risk transplant implies a transplant with a high risk of rejection. Risk factors for rejection are given in Table 3.2. Meta-analysis of 9 RCTs found no difference between the two agents with respect to patient and graft survival.[2] However, a landmark RCT comparing ATG with Basiliximab in high-risk transplant recipients showed reduction in acute rejection episodes with ATG. But there was no difference in graft survival in both these groups.[3]

TABLE 3.2: Risk factors for acute rejection[4]

- Number of human leukocyte antigen (HLA) mismatches
- Younger recipient age
- Older donor age
- Positive PRA
- Presence of DSA (donor-specific antibody)
- Blood group incompatibility (ABOi)
- Delayed onset of graft function
- Cold ischemia time >24 hours

5. How do we stratify the immunological risk based on recipient sensitization in a transplant patient?

Ans: The risk can be classified as low, intermediate, or high as follows (Table 3.3):

TABLE 3.3: Immunological risk stratification

Low risk	No donor directed sensitisation of HLA.
Intermediate risk	Absence of history of DSA or presence of low levels of DSA at the time of transplantation.
High risk	Presence of high levels of circulating antibodies specific to the donor HLA at the time of transplantation.

6. What is the recommended dose for ATG?

Ans: ATG is extracted and purified from serum of thymic tissue-immunised rabbits. In India it is available as a 25 mg vial, labelled as thymoglobulin (rATG, Genzyme-Sanofi).

Usual dose of ATG varies from 1 to 1.5 mg/kg for 4–10 days and it differs according to centre specific practices. It should be administered in the immediate perioperative period over 4–6 hours, preferably infused via central line. Peripheral line must not be used due to increased chances of thrombophlebitis. Allergic reactions are common with ATG and hence a pre-medication with hydrocortisone, anti-histaminic and paracetamol is usually warranted 30 minutes before ATG infusion.

7. What are the side effects expected with ATG?

Ans: Being polyclonal, ATG acts on multiple targets, both lymphocyte and non-lymphocyte cell types. Though, their main function is lymphocyte depletion but cross reactivity with other hematopoietic cell types results in anaemia, thrombocytopenia and leukopenia. These side-effects frequently become reasons for their dose limitations and, at times even their discontinuation. Allergic infusion reactions should always be watched for. Subsequent doses of ATG should be halved if platelet count is low, i.e. between 50000 and 100000/ml and withheld if platelet count <50000/ml or WBC count <3000/ml. CMV infection is an important consequence of ATG administration and thus CMV prophylaxis with Valgancyclovir for 3 months following ATG administration may be advisable.[5]

8. What is the mechanism of action of basiliximab?

Ans: Basiliximab is a monoclonal antibody; an IL-2 (interleukin-2) receptor antagonist. It does not deplete T cells, only causes their dysfunction. On recognition of antigen by the recipient T cells (Fig. 3.1), there is release of IL-2 by T cells which leads to their proliferation and differentiation. This process proliferation is prevented by basiliximab.

9. What is the recommended dose for basiliximab?

Ans: Basiliximab (Simulect) is available in the form of 10 or 20 mg powders for injection. Usual dose is 20 mg IV 2 hours prior to surgery and at day 4 of transplantation. First dose reactions and anaphylaxis are occasionally described, otherwise basiliximab is notably free of any major side effects (Table 3.4).

TABLE 3.4: Comparative analysis of side-effects of ATG and basiliximab[5]

SN	*Parameter*	*rATG*	*Basiliximab*
1	Biopsy proven acute rejection	15.6%	25.5%
2	Infection rate	85.8%	75.2%
3	Myelosuppression	More	Less
4	CMV infection	7.8%	17.5%
5	Malignancy	5/141 (3.54%)	1/137 (0.73%)

10. What is the role of rituximab in induction regimens?

Ans: Rituximab is not used alone as an induction agent. It is mainly used as part of induction therapy in ABOi kidney transplant and as part of de-sensitization protocol prior to renal transplant in highly sensitized patients. It is an anti-CD20 monoclonal antibody directed against the CD20 antigen present on naive B-cell lymphocytes. It creates a rapid and sustained depletion of circulating naive B cells which lasts for approximately 6 months. Because of its specific activity against B-cells, it is used to target the humoral arm of the immune response which limits B-cell activity and antibody production (Fig. 3.1).

Case Scenario 2

A 38 years old male receives a kidney from his father and is shifted to renal transplant ICU. His post-op prescription includes Cap Tacrolimus 2 mg BD, Tab MMF 1g BD and Inj Methyl prednisolone 500 mg OD.

1. What is the purpose of maintenance immunosuppression? Which are the commonly used drugs for this purpose?

Ans: Maintenance immunosuppression is given with the purpose of maintaining tolerance to the renal allograft (prevent further episodes of acute rejection) and to prevent formation of anti-HLA antibodies against the donor kidney, with passage of time. They are usually supposed to be taken lifelong. Drugs used for this type of immunosuppression are classified based on their mechanism of action (Table 3.5).

TABLE 3.5: Classification of maintenance immunosuppression
Calcineurin inhibitors
• Cyclosporine
• Tacrolimus
Antimetabolites
• Mycophenolic acid
• Azathioprine

(Contd.)

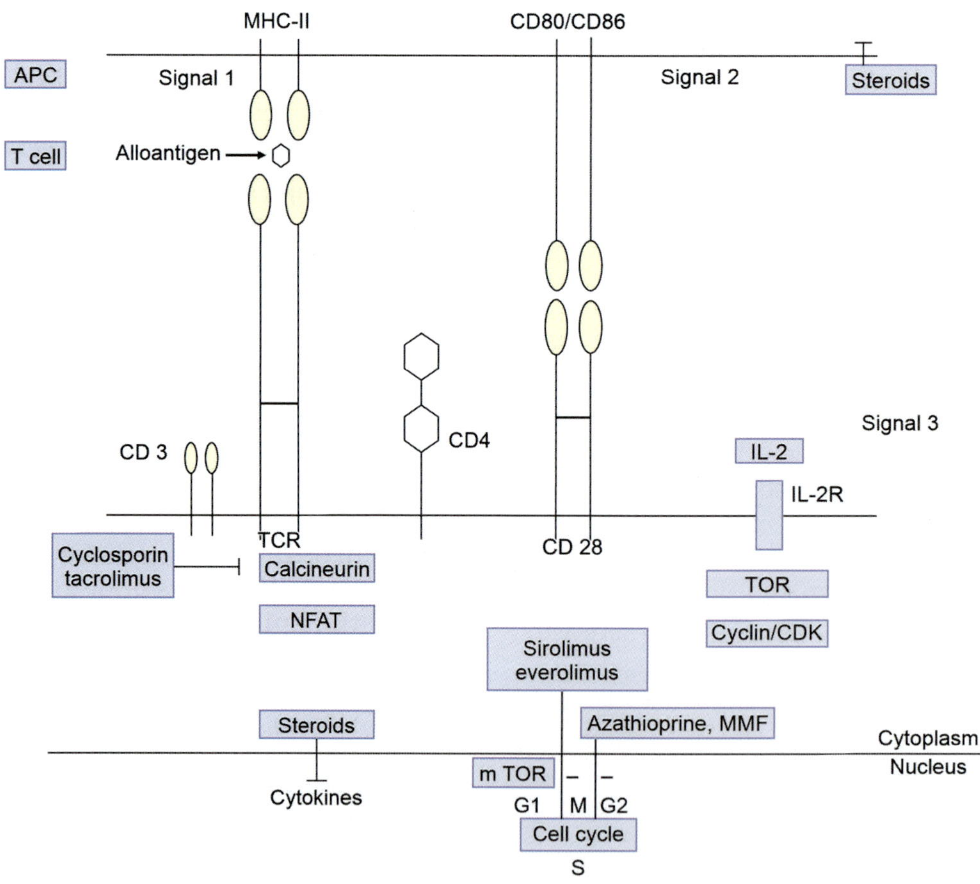

Fig. 3.1: Mechanism of immunosuppression: Target signalling pathways for the T cell activation, proliferation, and polarization. Activation of T cells results from alloantigen recognition via the T cell receptor (TCR)—CD3 complex with the MHC-II on the APC (signal 1) and a co-stimulatory signal (Signal 2) from CD28-CD80/CD86 on the APC. Stimulation by IL-2 (signal 3) results in cell proliferation and polarization. Immunosuppressive agents (shown in red boxes) act by inhibiting different targets. G1 (first growth phase), S (synthesis of DNA), G2 (second growth phase), and M (cell division) represent the different phases of the cell cycle.

APC, antigen-presenting cell; CD, cluster of differentiation; CDK, cyclin-dependent kinase; IL-2, interleukin-2; IL-2R, interleukin-2 receptor; MHC, major histocompatibility complex; MMF, mycophenolate mofetil; NFAT, nuclear factor of activated T cells; TCR, T cell receptor; TOR, target of rapamycin protein.

TABLE 3.5: Classification of maintenance immunosuppression *(Contd.)*
Mammalian target of Rapamycin (m-TOR) inhibitors
• Sirolimus
• Everolimus
Steroids
• Prednisolone

2. **What is the mechanism of action of calcineurin inhibitors (CNI)?**

   Ans: Tacrolimus and cyclosporine are both calcineurin inhibitors (CNI) which are the back bone for renal transplant medication for the past 30 years. These drugs enter the T cells and bind to their cytoplasmic receptor (Fig. 3.2). This complex then enters the nucleus and inhibits calcineurin which leads to inhibition of cytokine production causing inhibition of T cell activation and proliferation. Mechanism of action of both these drugs is similar and is mentioned in Fig. 3.2. The only difference is the cytoplasmic receptor to which they bind inside the cell cytoplasm. It is FKBP for tacrolimus and cyclophilin for Cyclosporine. The adverse effect profile of these two drugs is also similar.

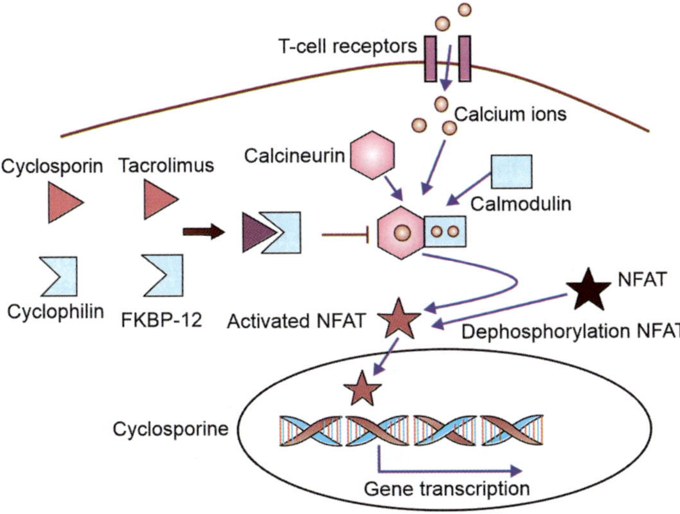

Fig. 3.2: Tacrolimus binds to the immunophilin FKBP-12, inhibiting the phosphorylation activity of calcineurin and preventing the translocation of nuclear factor of activated T cells (NFAT) into the nucleus and transcription of NFAT dependent genes. Inhibition of NFAT suppresses T-cell activation

3. **What is the usual recommended dose for CNIs?**

   Ans: Tacrolimus is universally available in an immediate release capsule form. The bioavailability of oral tacrolimus is about 25%. Maximum blood concentration is reached in one to three hours of consumption of the drug. The usual dose of tacrolimus is 0.1 mg/kg/day, in two divided doses. Cyclosporin has a bioavailability of around 30% and reaches peak blood concentration in two hours. Its dose is 3–5 mg/kg/day given in two divided doses.

4. **What are the adverse effects of CNI?**

   Ans: Calcineurin inhibitors are the most frequently used drugs in renal transplant and hence knowledge about their adverse effects is crucial. They cause reversible, dose dependant vasoconstriction of the afferent arteriole in the glomerulus. This may manifest as a transient and reversible rise in serum creatinine levels. Long-term use at high dose may lead to chronic damage to allograft in the form of interstitial fibrosis. Adverse effects are mentioned in Table 3.6.

TABLE 3.6: Adverse effects of CNI[6]
• Nephrotoxicity
– Acute reversible reduction in GFR
– Chronic interstitial fibrosis (with long-term use of CNIs)
• Hypertension
• Volume overload
• Hypomagnesemia
• Post-transplant diabetes mellitus
• Type IV renal tubular acidosis
• Hyperlipidemia
• Neurotoxicity (peripheral neuropathy)
• Hyperuricimia (gout)

Cyclosporine and tacrolimus have the similar side effect profile, however, the extent to which they affect the different parameters varies between the two. Comparative analysis of their side effects is given in Table 3.7:

TABLE 3.7: Comparison between the adverse effects of cyclosporine and tacrolimus

Feature	*Cyclosporine*	*Tacrolimus*
Hypertension	++	+
Nephrotoxicity	+	+
Pancreatic Islet toxicity	+	++
Neurotoxicity	+	++
Hirsutism	+	-
Hair loss	-	+
Gum hypertrophy	+	-
Hyperuricimia (gout)	++	+
Hypercholesterolemia	+	-

5. **What are the drug interactions of CNI?**

Ans: Both cyclosporine and tacrolimus are metabolised by cytochrome P450 enzymes especially 3A4 and 3A5.[7] Cytochrome 450 also metabolizes a host of other drugs. Thus, co-administration of such drugs would lead to changes in the blood levels of CNI. Table 3.8 shows drugs that affect the blood levels of CNIs.

TABLE 3.8: Drug interactions of CNIs

Drugs causing reduction in CNI levels (CYP3A inducers)

- Carbamazepine
- Phenytoin
- Rifampicin
- Bosentan
- Efavirenz

Drugs causing increase in CNI levels (CYP3A inhibitors)

- Ketoconazole
- Voriconazole
- Lopinavir/Ritonavir
- Fluconazole
- Imatinib
- Verapamil

6. **What are the target blood levels of CNI post-transplant?**

Ans: Monitoring and titration of CNI drug levels is an integral part of transplant immunosuppression as both these drugs have large inter-individual variability. There are many methods to determine the blood levels of these drugs. However, LCMS (liquid chromatography mass spectroscopy) is the most widely used method. Drug levels are usually measured on post-operative day two or three or whenever there is unexplained rise in serum creatinine. Drug levels can be measured just before the next dose (C_0) or 2 hours after consuming the drug (C_2). Tables 3.9 and 3.10 show the target blood level of CNI which should be maintained in the post-transplant period.

TABLE 3.9: Target levels of tacrolimus in post-transplant period

Period post-transplant	*Tac C0 level (ng/ml)*
0–3 months	8–10
3–12 months	6–8
>12 months	4–6
>5 years	3–5

TABLE 3.10: Target levels of cyclosporine post-transplant

Period post-transplant	*Cyclosporine C2 levels (ng/ml)*
0–3 months	1200–1500
4–6 months	1000–1200
>6 months	800–1000

7. **Which CNI is superior? Tacrolimus or cyclosporine?**

Ans: In clinical transplant, cyclosporine was used initially in the late 1970s, whereas tacrolimus was introduced in renal transplant in 1997. Over the last 20 years, tacrolimus has largely replaced cyclosporine. Meta-analysis have shown tacrolimus to be superior to cyclosporine in terms of graft loss and acute rejection rates.[8]

Case Scenario 3

A 42 years old patient who had a renal transplant 1 month ago, is readmitted with pneumonia. His MMF (mycophenolate mofetil) is stopped and dose of Tacrolimus reduced to half. Why was MMF stopped?

1. **What is the mechanism of action and dose of MMF?**

Ans: MMF is a reversible inhibitor of the enzyme inosine monophosphate dehydrogenase (IMPDH).[9] It leads to anti-proliferative effect on lymphocytes. This causes inhibition of proliferation of T cells and B cells and also inhibits antibody formation.

2. **What is the dose of MMF?**

Ans: MMF is available in two formulations. One is immediate release ester formulation that comes as 500 mg immediate release tablets. The usual dose of this formulation is 1gm twice a day. The other formulation is an enteric coated formulation, available as 360 mg tablets. Usual dose of these enteric coated tablets is 720 mg twice a day.

3. **What are the adverse effects of MMF?**

Ans: The most common side effects of this drug are related to GI tract and commonly include diarrhoea (occurring in 1/3 of the patients) and vomiting (20%).[10]

Because MMF cause bone marrow suppression, it renders all patients more prone to infections compared to CNIs. Hence, the usual practice in the event of any infection occurring after transplant depends on the severity of the infection. In severe infections MMF is stopped and dose of tacrolimus is reduced to half with frequent trough level monitoring, whereas in milder infections it may suffice to halve the dose of MMF. When GI side effects occur, change of formulation of MMF/ reducing the dose is usually enough.

Mycophenolates are known to produce congenital malformations and thus are unsafe for use in pregnancy. It is advisable to discontinue them one month before a planned pregnancy both in the male and female.

4. **What is the role of azathioprine in renal transplant?**

Ans: Azathioprine has largely been replaced by MMF in most transplantation programmes. It still has roles in place of MMF in patients with recurrent severe infections, refractory GI side effects of MMF and low-cost immunosuppressive regimen. A systematic review comparing MMF with azathioprine showed that MMF significantly reduced the risk of acute rejections and graft loss.[11]

Case Scenario 4

A 42-year-old male patient undergoes a live related renal transplant. He received IV methyl prednisolone 500 mg intraoperatively and on POD 1 and 2. Oral prednisolone 30 mg daily was started from POD3. The dose was tapered at the rate of 5 mg/week to reach a dose of 5 mg daily from 3rd month post-transplant.

1. **What is the usual dose of steroids in kidney transplant?**

Ans: Steroids were initially used in kidney transplantations to reverse acute rejection. Just a single dose administration of steroids would lead to the improvement in kidney function.[12] However, soon steroids became an integral part of transplant immunosuppression and are used regularly in most protocols. Their doses are progressively minimised in most protocols. Steroids have anti-inflammatory and immunosuppressive properties.

Most of the transplant centres have a practice of administering methyl prednisolone 500 mg intra-operatively which is continued till post-operative day two, as a single dose daily. Oral prednisolone is tapered to the physiological dose of 5 mg/day over a few weeks following transplant.[13]

2. **What are the side effects associated with steroid therapy?**

Ans: Steroids are given lifelong post renal transplant. Knowledge about their side effects becomes important as they may lead to significant morbidity. Adverse effects associated with steroid therapy are given in Table 3.11.

TABLE 3.11: Adverse effects of steroids in kidney transplant patients
Hypertension
Dyslipidemia
Osteoporosis
Post-transplant diabetes mellitus (PTDM)
Cataract
Growth retardation

3. **Can we avoid giving steroids in kidney transplant?**

Ans: Introduction of CNI and anti-proliferative drugs facilitated steroid withdrawal immunosuppressive regimen. As per USRDS data, around 23% of the patients were discharged after transplant without steroids. Also, KDIGO in its 2009 guideline recommends steroid withdrawal in the first week post-transplant in low-risk patients.[4] RCTs comparing early steroid withdrawal (at 7 days) with steroid maintenance have shown comparable graft function at 1 year but increased incidence of biopsy proven acute rejection in early steroid withdrawal group.[14] Steroid withdrawal may be considered in low-risk transplant recipients but such patients should be on regular follow-up as these patients are at increased risk for rejections.

Case Scenario 5

A 45-year-old male, 5 years post-transplant, comes for follow-up with a marginal rise in creatinine to 1.8 mg/dl from an earlier nadir of 1.1 mg/dl. He undergoes a graft kidney biopsy. After seeing the report, the nephrologist changes his prescription from tacrolimus to sirolimus.

1. **Why was this done? What is the role of mTOR inhibitors in renal transplant?**

Ans: Long-term use of CNIs leads to interstitial fibrosis and tubular atrophy. Thus, CNI minimization, CNI avoidance and CNI conversion to safer alternative regimens have been tried. Mammalian target of Rapamycin inhibitors (mTOR inhibitors—sirolimus and everolimus) have been successfully used for this purpose. The shift over to sirolimus was done after the biopsy report showed evidence of interstitial fibrosis (CNI induced). Like CNIs, mTOR inhibitors act through a cytoplasm binding protein. This protein inhibits the action of another protein called target of rapamycin. This inhibition reduces cellular proliferation at G1 to S phase of cell division (Fig. 3.1). Sirolimus has unique antiatherogenic and antineoplastic properties. It has been shown to promote immunological tolerance and reduce the incidence of chronic allograft nephropathy.

2. **What is the usual recommended dose for sirolimus?**

Ans: There are 2 ways in which Sirolimus is administered post-transplant. One is CNI minimization in which it is given with low dose CNI and other is CNI avoidance in which it is given without CNI.

Calcineurin inhibitor minimization:[15]

Oral 6 mg loading dose on day 1, followed by 2 mg once daily in combination with calcineurin inhibitor (CNI) and corticosteroids. The target trough concentration to maintain is between 3 and 8 ng/ml.[16]

Calcineurin inhibitor avoidance:[17]

Oral 12 to 15 mg loading dose between 4 and 24 hours after last CNI dose, followed by 4 to 8 mg once daily thereafter (in combination with adjunctive agents and corticosteroids). The target trough concentration to maintain is between 8 and 12 ng/ml.

Steady-state concentrations of sirolimus occur five to seven days after initiation of therapy or a change in dose. Its whole-blood concentrations can be measured by both chromatographic and immunoassay methods. The recommended time for collection is one hour prior to the next oral dose.

3. **What are the adverse effects of sirolimus?**

Ans: mTOR inhibitors affect cell division of both haemopoietic and non-haemopoietic cells. Thus, with myelosuppression, wound healing is also affected. Other adverse effects seen are hyperlipidaemia, proteinuria, oedema, pneumonitis and thrombotic microangiopathy. Sirolimus may impair fertility. Ovarian cysts, amenorrhea, menorrhagia, azoospermia, or oligospermia have been observed following use of oral sirolimus. Sperm banking prior to sirolimus treatment may be considered. Use of sirolimus in early postoperative period involves risk of delayed wound healing and lymphocele formation.

Case Scenario 6

A 30 years old male, underwent renal transplant with mother as the donor. One month ago, he skipped his immunosuppressive medications for 2 weeks and came for follow-up with a serum creatinine of 4.1 mg/dl. He was managed with Inj methyl prednisolone 500 mg IV for 3 days and underwent graft kidney biopsy which revealed acute T cell mediated rejection.

1. **When should we suspect acute rejection?**

Ans: Rejection should always be suspected when there is an unexplained rise in serum creatinine.

2. **What is the treatment for acute T cell mediated rejection?**

Ans: Historical symptoms of rejection including fever and graft tenderness are rare with the advanced immunosuppressive regimen, hence a high index of suspicion is needed to diagnose it in early phase. Graft biopsy is essential to diagnose rejection (B or T cell mediated or mixed). The treatment depends on the type of rejection. The goal of therapy is to reverse the rejection and return kidney allograft function as close to baseline as possible. Acute T cell mediated rejection is treated with pulse methyl prednisolone with or without ATG depending on the histologic grade of rejection. Usual initial treatment is pulse methyl prednisolone 250–500 mg daily for 3–5 days.[1] For severe acute T cell mediated rejections (grade IB and above), ATG at a dose of 1–1.5 mg/kg/day is added for 5–7 days. Treatment with ATG leads to reversal of acute rejection in 70–80% of the patients.[18]

Banff grading system: The severity of acute TCMR is graded using the Banff classification:[19]

- Borderline: 25 percent interstitial inflammation (i1) with any tubulitis (t1, t2, or t3) or >25 percent interstitial inflammation (i2 or i3) with mild tubulitis (t1)
- Type IA: 25 percent interstitial inflammation (i2 or i3) with moderate tubulitis (t2)
- Type IB: 25 percent interstitial inflammation (i2 or i3) with severe tubulitis (t3)
- Type IIA: Mild to moderate intimal arteritis (v1) with or without interstitial inflammation and tubulitis
- Type IIB: Severe intimal arteritis (v2) with or without interstitial inflammation and tubulitis
- Type III: Transmural arteritis and/or arterial fibrinoid change and necrosis of medial smooth muscle cells with accompanying lymphocytic inflammation (v3)

3. **What is the treatment of antibody mediated rejection (ABMR)?**

Ans: ABMR is considered to occur early when it occurs within first 6 months of transplant and late when it occurs after that.[20] Principles of treatment of ABMR include:

- Depletion of B cells which produce donor specific antibodies (DSA),
- Removal of the existing antibodies (DSA).
- Prevention of complement activation
- Reduce resultant endothelial injury and preserve graft function

Treatment involves a combination of glucocorticoids and IVIG along with the addition of plasmapheresis and/or rituximab in selected patients. Plasma exchange (PLEX) and IVIG has remained the standard of care for treatment of ABMR.[21] Most commonly used regimen for treatment of ABMR is PLEX alternate day followed by IVIG at 100–200 mg/kg with or without a single dose of Rituximab after the last session of PLEX.[22] Some centres prefer PLEX alone and some centres prefer IVIG to be added after PLEX. An observational study found superior results with PLEX and IVIG compared to PLEX alone.[23]

Early ABMR

Initial therapy is combination of glucocorticoids, plasmapheresis, and IVIG. Rituximab is considered when biopsy shows less chronicity, in younger subset population and those who has better allograft function.

Dosing of glucocorticoids: Intravenous (IV) methylprednisolone at a dose of 300 to 500 mg daily for three to five days, followed by a rapid oral prednisone taper to the maintenance dose.

Plasmapheresis regimen: Plasmapheresis is performed daily or every alternate day for a maximum of 6 to 8 sessions or until the serum creatinine is within 20 to 30 percent of the baseline. The initial exchange is typically a one or one-and-one-half-volume exchange with albumin. Alternate day exchange allows interval time for recovery of the prothrombin time, partial thromboplastin time, and fibrinogen to acceptable levels without the need to administer fresh frozen plasma. This avoids the risk of antigen sensitization; however, one to two units of fresh frozen plasma may be used for replacement at the end of a plasmapheresis treatment to reduce bleeding risk in the appropriate clinical setting, such as a same-day kidney allograft biopsy or in immediate post-transplant cases.

Dosing of IVIG: Administer IVIG at a dose of 100 mg/kg after each session of plasmapheresis.

Dosing of rituximab: Administer a single dose of either 200 mg or 375 mg/m^2 after completion of plasmapheresis and IVIG.

Late ABMR

Initial therapy comprises pulse steroids and IVIG.

Use of plasmapheresis is controversial in such patients because of the lack of evidence supporting the safety and efficacy of plasmapheresis in later-onset ABMR. Rituximab can be used if the patient is young, has better allograft function (e.g., eGFR 20 ml/min/1.73 m^2) and lower chronicity scores on biopsy and has evidence of severe disease on biopsy.

Prophylactic measures for all patients: In all patients who are treated for active ABMR, it is prudent to give prophylaxis against PCP pneumonia and CMV infection.

Most patients with ABMR who have a successful response to antirejection therapy will demonstrate an improvement in serum creatinine within seven days of treatment.

Modification of therapy is based upon the response to initial therapy.

In patients who respond to therapy with a decrease in serum creatinine, it is advisable to increase the maintenance tacrolimus dose so as to achieve a trough level that is 20 to 25 percent above the level at the time of rejection and resume routine monitoring of allograft function.

Typically, maintenance immunosuppression is also augmented by increasing the daily dose of oral prednisone and maximizing the dose of the antiproliferative agent (mycophenolate).

Patients without any decrease in serum creatinine after seven days of rejection treatment are considered to be unresponsive to initial treatment. In such patients, ongoing rejection and/or another cause of kidney allograft dysfunction should be suspected, and a repeat kidney allograft biopsy should be performed.

Second-line agents for the treatment of ABMR can be used **as rescue therapy** if repeat biopsy shows ongoing active ABMR.

Proteasome inhibitors: Bortezomib is a proteasome inhibitor is particularly effective against differentiated plasma cells.

Complement inhibitors: Eculizumab is a fully humanized, monoclonal antibody directed against the C5 fragment of the complement cascade and inhibits the generation of the membrane attack complex. Eculizumab has not been shown to be effective for the treatment of C4d-negative active and chronic ABMR, suggesting that its efficacy may be limited to acute, complement-mediated processes.

KEY POINTS

- A sound knowledge of immunosuppression (various agents, their indications, drug-interactions, side-effects, etc.) is a must for a transplant surgeon.
- Immunosuppression agents are classified into induction agents, maintenance agents and anti-rejection therapies.
- Induction agents are highly potent agents, used prophylactically at the time of transplantation to ensure maximum immune suppression immediately post-transplant when the risk of acute 'allograft-decimating' immunological events is at its highest.

(Contd.)

KEY POINTS *(Contd.)*

- The agents used for maintenance therapy are less potent and also less toxic than induction agents. They are given for long period (life-long). Triple drug maintenance therapy comprising of steroids, calcineurin inhibitors (tacrolimus) and anti-proliferative agent (mycophenolate) is standard of care for maintenance immunosuppression worldwide.
- CNIs have narrow therapeutic index and drug needs regular monitoring of blood levels and frequent dose modifications to maintain desirable levels. High levels lead to toxicity and graft damage and low levels may result in rejection.
- Any amount of graft dysfunction (evident by a rise in serum creatinine) needs proper investigation like CNI drug levels and even graft biopsy.
- Anti-rejection rescue therapies are instituted for biopsy-proven rejection episodes and are guided by biopsy findings.

REFERENCES

1. Abecassis M, Bartlett ST, Collins AJ, Davis CL, Delmonico FL, Friedewald JJ, *et al.* Kidney Transplantation as Primary Therapy for End-Stage Renal Disease: A National Kidney Foundation/Kidney Disease Outcomes Quality Initiative (NKF/KDOQI^{TM}) Conference. Clin J Am Soc Nephrol CJASN. 2008 Mar;3(2):471–80.
2. Ghelichi-Ghojogh M, Ghaem H, Mohammadizadeh F, Vali M, Ahmed F, Hassanipour S, *et al.* Graft and Patient Survival Rates in Kidney Transplantation, and Their Associated Factors: A Systematic Review and Meta-Analysis. Iran J Public Health. 2021 Aug;50(8):1555–63.
3. Bamoulid J, Staeck O, Crépin T, Halleck F, Saas P, Brakemeier S, *et al.* Anti-thymocyte globulins in kidney transplantation: focus on current indications and long-term immunological side effects. Nephrol Dial Transplant Off Publ Eur Dial Transpl Assoc-Eur Ren Assoc. 2017 Oct 1;32(10):1601–8.
4. Wang K, Xu X, Fan M. Induction therapy of basiliximab versus antithymocyte globulin in renal allograft: a systematic review and meta-analysis. Clin Exp Nephrol. 2018 Jun;22(3):684–93.
5. Brennan DC, Daller JA, Lake KD, Cibrik D, Del Castillo D. Rabbit Antithymocyte Globulin versus Basiliximab in Renal Transplantation. N Engl J Med. 2006 Nov 9;355(19):1967–77.
6. Kasiske BL, Zeier MG, Chapman JR, Craig JC, Ekberg H, Garvey CA, *et al.* KDIGO clinical practice guideline for the care of kidney transplant recipients: a summary. Kidney Int. 2010 Feb;77(4):299–311.
7. Razonable RR, Humar A. Cytomegalovirus in solid organ transplant recipients-Guidelines of the American Society of Transplantation Infectious Diseases Community of Practice. Clin Transplant. 2019 Sep;33(9):e13512.
8. Matas AJ. Calcineurin inhibitors: short-term friend, long-term foe? Clin Pharmacol Ther. 2011 Aug;90(2):209-11. doi: 10.1038/clpt.2011.77. PMID: 21772297; PMCID: PMC3627685.
9. Fernando ME, Sellappan M, Srinivasa Prasad ND, Suren S, Thirumalvalavan K. Influence of CYP3A5 and ABCB1 Polymorphism on Tacrolimus Drug Dosing in South Indian Renal Allograft Recipients. Indian J Nephrol. 2019 Aug;29(4):261.
10. Azarfar A, Ravanshad Y, Mehrad-Majd H, Esmaeeli M, Aval SB, Emadzadeh M, *et al.* Comparison of tacrolimus and cyclosporine for immunosuppression after renal transplantation: An updated systematic review and meta-analysis. Saudi J Kidney Dis Transplant Off Publ Saudi Cent Organ Transplant Saudi Arab. 2018;29(6):1376–85.
11. Allison AC, Eugui EM. Mycophenolate mofetil and its mechanisms of action. Immunopharmacology. 2000 May 1;47(2):85–118.
12. Halloran P, Mathew T, Tomlanovich S, Groth C, Hooftman L, Barker C. Mycophenolate mofetil in renal allograft recipients: a pooled efficacy analysis of three randomized, double-blind, clinical studies in prevention of rejection. The International Mycophenolate Mofetil Renal Transplant Study Groups. Transplantation. 1997 Jan 15;63(1):39–47.
13. Knight SR, Russell NK, Barcena L, Morris PJ. Mycophenolate mofetil decreases acute rejection and may improve graft survival in renal transplant recipients when compared with azathioprine: a systematic review. Transplantation. 2009 Mar 27;87(6):785–94.
14. Starzl Te, Marchioro Tl, Waddell Wr. The Reversal Of Rejection In Human Renal Homografts With Subsequent Development Of Homograft Tolerance. Surg Gynecol Obstet. 1963 Oct;117:385–95. Pmid: 14065716; Pmcid: Pmc2581919.
15. Steiner RW, Awdishu L. Steroids in kidney transplant patients. Semin Immunopathol. 2011 Mar;33(2):157–67. doi: 10.1007/s00281–011–0259–7. Epub 2011 Feb 18. PMID: 21331501; PMCID: PMC3082701.
16. Vincenti F, Schena FP, Paraskevas S, Hauser IA, Walker RG, Grinyo J. A Randomized, Multicenter Study of Steroid Avoidance, Early Steroid Withdrawal or Standard Steroid Therapy in Kidney Transplant Recipients. Am J Transplant. 2008 Feb 1;8(2):307–16.
17. Chinnock TJ, Shankel T, Deming D, Cutler D, Sahney S, Fitts J, *et al.* Calcineurin inhibitor minimization using sirolimus leads to improved renal function in pediatric heart transplant recipients. Pediatr Transplant. 2011 Nov;15(7):746–9.
18. Cucchiari D, Molina-Andujar A, Montagud-Marrahi E, Revuelta I, Rovira J, Ventura-Aguiar P, *et al.* Use of De Novo mTOR Inhibitors in Hypersensitized Kidney Transplant Recipients: Exerience From Clinical Practice. Transplantation. 2020 Aug;104(8):1686–94.
19. Haller M, Oberbauer R. Calcineurin inhibitor minimization, withdrawal and avoidance protocols after kidney transplantation. Transpl Int Off J Eur Soc Organ Transplant. 2009 Jan;22(1):69–77.
20. Cooper JE. Evaluation and Treatment of Acute Rejection in Kidney Allografts. Clin J Am Soc Nephrol. 2020 Mar;15(3):430.
21. Loupy A, Haas M, Roufosse C, Naesens M, Adam B, Afrouzian M, *et al.* The Banff 2019 Kidney Meeting Report (I): Updates on and clarification of criteria for T cell-and antibody-mediated rejection. Am J Transplant Off J Am Soc Transplant Am Soc Transpl Surg. 2020 Sep;20(9):2318–31.
22. Budde K, Dürr M. Any Progress in the Treatment of Antibody-Mediated Rejection? J Am Soc Nephrol JASN. 2018 Feb;29(2):350–2.
23. Wan SS, Ying TD, Wyburn K, Roberts DM, Wyld M, Chadban SJ. The Treatment of Antibody-Mediated Rejection in Kidney Transplantation: An Updated Systematic Review and Meta-Analysis. Transplantation. 2018 Apr;102(4):557–68.

Chapter

4

Recipient with Peripheral Vascular Disease (Atherosclerotic Vessels, Orthotopic Transplant)

• Ravindra B Sabnis • Abhijit Patil

LEARNING OBJECTIVES

- To understand the evaluation and technical challenges in recipient with peripheral vascular disease or calcified vasculature.
- To understand the indications and technique of orthotopic kidney transplant (OKT).
- To understand the evaluation and management of kidney donors with plaque at the origin of renal arteries.
- To understand the evaluation and selection of kidney donors with fibromuscular dysplasia.

Recipient with atherosclerotic vascular disease

Case Scenario 1

A 53 years old, diabetic and hypertensive male with ADPKD and ESRD came for second renal transplant with wife as a prospective donor. He was asymptomatic with all peripheral pulses well felt. He received first kidney from sister-in-law in 2017; but eventually he had graft failure due to interstitial fibrosis and tubular atrophy (IFTA). On evaluation, there was extensive calcification of abdomen and pelvic vessels (Figs 4.1 and 4.2).

1. **How to investigate this patient for renal transplant?**

Ans: A detailed history needs to be elicited, which should include history of intermittent claudication or rest pain. Details should be obtained for cardio-vascular risk factors like smoking, tobacco consumption, co-morbidities like diabetes and hypertension, which are also the risk factors for PVD.

Examination should include palpation of femoral and lower limb vessels up to dorsalis pedis. Ankle brachial pressure index (ABPI) is an

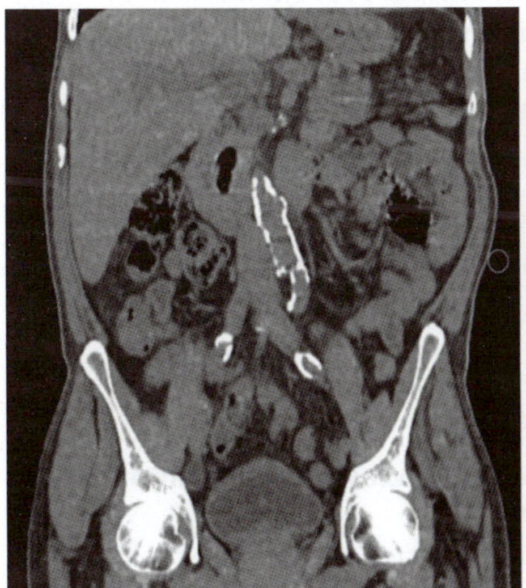
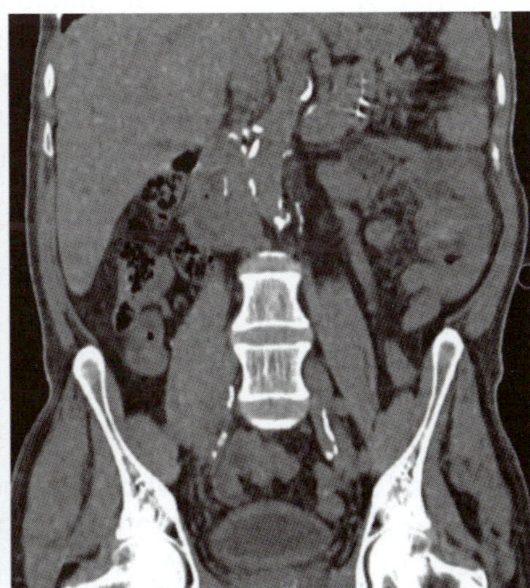
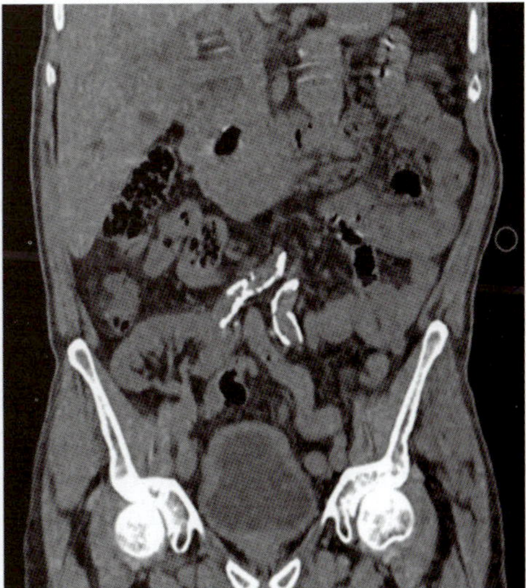

Fig. 4.1: NCCT of abdomen of recipient with calcifications in aorta, common iliac artery and bilateral external iliac artery

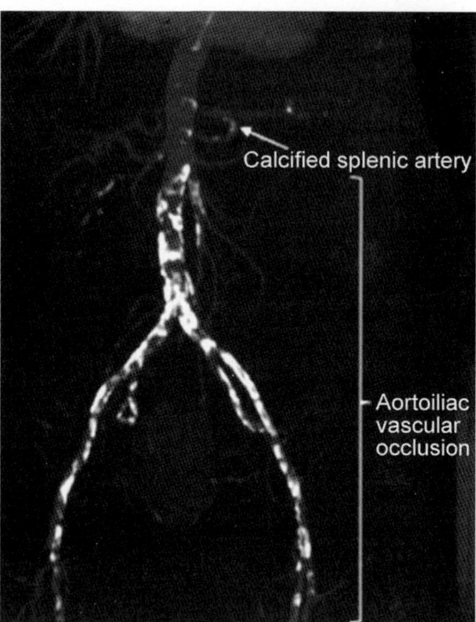

Fig. 4.2: NCCT abdomen showing marked calcifications in aorta, common iliac artery bilateral internal and external iliac arteries

important test, which tells about the quality and patency of peripheral lower limb vessels.

2. **What is the investigation of choice in this case: Iliofemoral Doppler or angiography?**

   Ans: Bilateral iliofemoral Doppler is routinely done in evaluation of all recipients. This patient's iliofemoral Doppler was suggestive of marked wall calcification seen in bilateral common iliac and internal iliac arteries. Mild wall calcification was seen in bilateral external iliac arteries. No dampening of flow was seen. The role of CT angiography is limited to selected cases.[1]

   One can have rough idea about the amount of vascular calcification especially in the internal iliac artery from the X-ray KUB. If the recipient is undergoing conventional cardiac angiography, then we can ask for iliofemoral shoots to look for the vascular luminal status.

   The gold standard test to understand the quality of iliofemoral vasculature would be CT angiography. The NCCT scan would help us assess the location and amount of calcification.

   The location of calcification would help us locate the probable site of vascular clamping and arterial anastomosis.

   The arterial phase would help us understand the lumen of the iliofemoral vessels.

   This patients NCCT (Fig. 4.1) was suggestive of marked calcification seen in abdominal aorta, bilateral common iliac arteries and internal iliac arteries. Minimal calcification was seen in right external iliac artery and in distal left external iliac artery.

3. **Whether to proceed with transplant or not?**

   Ans: In this case, the patient did not have any lower limb claudication. His peripheral pulses including bilateral dorsalis pedis were palpable. His ileo-femoral Doppler showed no dampening of blood flow. We could find an area without calcification in proximal external iliac artery. So, we proceeded in this case.

   On the contrary, if the patient had lower limb claudication with non-palpable peripheral pulses and severe complete calcification of aorta, common iliac and external iliac vessels (Fig. 4.2), then we would not proceed. The outcomes of grafts in patients with peripheral vascular disease is inferior to that with normal arterial vasculature.[2]

4. **Explain the salient surgical tips and tricks on anastomosis in atherosclerotic vessels.**

   The most important problem for anastomosis in severe atherosclerotic vessels is inability to clamp the vessels with bull dog clamps and sub-intimal dissection of external iliac artery. We should choose the relatively less atherosclerotic and calcified area of vessels for clamping.

   Regarding the suturing technique, the following points are to be kept in mind:
   - The lightest and smallest but adequate clamps are useful for these arteries.
   - Choose proper site for suturing based on amount of calcification (preoperative imaging and intraoperative assessment with inspection and palpation)
   - Gentleness in suturing
   - Minimal traction of suture by the assistant to prevent cut-through of vessel wall.
   - The recipient vessel sutures should always be sutured inside to outside in order to fix the intima to media and prevent dissection.
   - If there is intimal flap, then it can be fixed with the media with fixing sutures at 6 points with prolene suture (quilting sutures)
   - Ensure that the needle passes as atraumatic as possible from the adventitia of the artery through to the lining of the artery.
   - Force should be applied so that the needle advances according to the curvature of the needle.
   - When tying the thread, ensure that sufficient tension is applied.

5. **What are the intricacies in transplantation in a synthetic graft?**

   Ans: In prior iliac artery prosthetic replacement, intravenous heparin (1250 IU) should be given prior to prosthesis clamping and the renal artery should be anastomosed with the iliac prosthesis. All patients should receive short-term prophylactic antibiotic therapy (generally, vancomycin 2 g) and heparinization intraoperatively. Twelve hours after vascular procedure, sodium enoxaparin and clopidogrel 75 mg should be given to all patients. Enoxaparin can be given to all patients for 1 month postoperatively and the dose must be adjusted based on glomerular filtration rate (GFR) estimated with the Cockroft–Gault formula (2000 IU with GFR <30 ml/min, 4,000 IU with GFR 30 ml/min) and substituted with aspirin 75 mg in association with clopidogrel thereafter. A study revealed 1-year post-operative, graft survival rate was 100%.[3]

6. What is the role of orthotopic transplant in severe pelvic vascular atherosclerosis?

Ans: Indications for orthotopic kidney transplant:[4]

- Unsuitable candidates for heterotopic kidney transplant
- Severe vascular pathology
- IVC thrombosis/agenesis
- Severe atheromatosis
- Iliac fossa occupied by previous grafts (especially 3rd or 4th grafts) or previous pelvic surgery
- Patients with urinary diversion

The graft survival after orthotopic kidney transplant at 1 year is more than 80% (Table 4.1).

7. Explain the technique of orthotopic kidney transplant (OKT).

The workup starts with recipient CT angiography—for vascular evaluation. Abdominal vascular branches to be evaluated are mainly aorto-iliac segment, native renal vessels, IVC and splenic artery.[5]

The surgical technique of OKT was first described by Gil-Vernet *et al* in 1978. It was a retroperitoneal approach to the splenic hilum via lumbotomy. It was meant to treat hypertension due to left renal artery stenosis. The steps of OKT are as follows:

1. Nephrectomy is performed via a left lumbotomy
2. Native renal vein is ligated near the renal parenchyma including its bifurcation.
3. Artery revascularization: End-to-end anastomosis between the graft renal artery and the native splenic artery (or renal artery or inferior mesenteric artery). The native renal artery may often be narrow and unfit for anastomosis.
4. Vein revascularization: End-to-end anastomosis between the graft renal vein and the native renal vein or splenic vein.
5. Urinary reconstruction: Pyelo-pyelic anastomosis with ureteral stent.[6]

TABLE 4.1: Outcomes of orthoptic kidney transplants.[4]

Author	*Year*	*Sample*	*Indications*	*Complication rate*	*Graft survival*
Gil-Vernet *et al*	1989	139	Alternative to elective surgery	Vascular: 2.8% Urinary: 2.8%	Graft loss rate: 5%
Paduch *et al*	2001	5	Severe iliac atherosclerosis: 3 Retained bilateral iliac fossa kidney transplant: 2	NA	Graft survival: 100% during follow-up (from 6 months to 5 years)
Rodrigues *et al*	2004	4	Bilateral occlusion of common iliac arteries: 4	NA	Graft survival: 100% (9 days–14 months)
Musquera *et al*	2010	223	Severe iliac atherosclerosis: 41.7% Bilaterally retained iliac fossae from a previous kidney transplant: 28.9% Elective: 4.5%	Vascular: 13/84 (9.6%) Urinary: 16/84 (19.1%)	Graft survival at 1 year: 86.4%
Hevia *et al*	2014	9	Unsuitable iliac region: 67% LUT abnormalities/urinary diversion: 33%	Early: 33.3% (3/9) Late: 22.2% (2/9)	Graft survival at 1 year: 88.9%
Chan *et al*	2019	3	IVC thrombosis or stenosis	Early: 100% (2 Clavien grade 2 and 1 Clavien grade 3a)	NA
Medina *et al*	2022	21	Mentioned above	Early: 66.67% (23.81% of Clavien grade 3b) 2 arterial thrombosis and one hypoperfusion requiring graft nephrectomy	At 12 months, the survival rate was 84.9%.

Donor with Vascular Anomalies

Atherosclerosis

Case Scenario 2

A 59-year-old female, with no comorbidity, was mother to the recipient. Her serum creatinine was 0.67 mg/dl (eGFR:101 ml/min/1.73 m^2). Her right kidney size was 10.3 x 3.3 cm while the left kidney size was 10.9 x 4.9 cm. On CT angiography, she had bilateral single renal artery and single renal vein. Her both renal arteries had atherosclerotic plaques at their origin with no evidence of stenosis on either side. Her CT images are given in Fig. 4.3.

1. **Will you accept this donor?**

   Ans: This donor does not have any comorbidity. Her eGFR is 101 ml/min/1.73 m^2. Her CT angiography shows calcification at origin of both the renal arteries, but without causing any stenosis.

   This donor should be counseled about the stringent follow-up to evaluate the remaining kidney. This donor should also be counseled to strictly maintain her blood pressure on follow-up.

2. **What precaution should be taken when there are plaques at origins of donor renal arteries?**

   Ans: The donor artery should be cautiously clipped and the clip application over the plaque should be avoided. The donor artery should be clipped above the level of the plaque. 1 mm of donor artery cuff should be left above the second clip before transecting the artery. The remaining donor artery should be inspected for atherosclerotic plaque.

   While performing arterial anastomosis, the sutures should pass inside out of donor artery, so as to fix the atherosclerotic plaque.

3. **When should such donor be rejected?**

   Ans: Donor with the following features should be rejected:
   - Significant atheromatous plaques at both renal artery ostia
   - Renovascular hypertension
   - Size discrepancy on imaging
   - DTPA suggestive of significant difference in function of both kidneys
   - Low or borderline global eGFR
   - Cardiovascular co-morbidity

Donor with Fibromuscular Dysplasia (FMD)

Introduction

FMD is a fibrous non-atherosclerotic and non-inflammatory disease of medium and small caliber arteries.[7] This disease with unknown etiology, is reported in 2–6% potential living renal donors.[8–11] If not treated, it may be asymptomatic or lead to arterial hypertension, thrombosis or aneurysms due to vascular stenosis and dilatation.[12,13] It is more common in females and hypertension is the most common clinical manifestation. Three subtypes of FMD are described: Intimal, medial (most common) and adventitial.

Severity of FMD (assessed on the basis of the degree of arterial stenosis) is as follows:
- Mild FMD: Mild irregularity of the artery without significant stenosis
- Moderate FMD: arterial irregularity and stenosis < 50% of the arterial caliber.[14]

Case Scenario 3

A40-year-old female donor for her husband without any comorbidities was evaluated and her CT angiography revealed beaded appearance of right renal artery (Fig. 4.4). Her serum creatinine is 1.1 mg/dl.

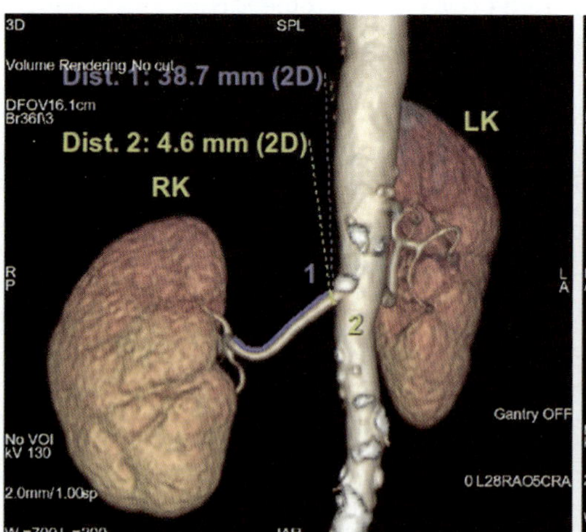

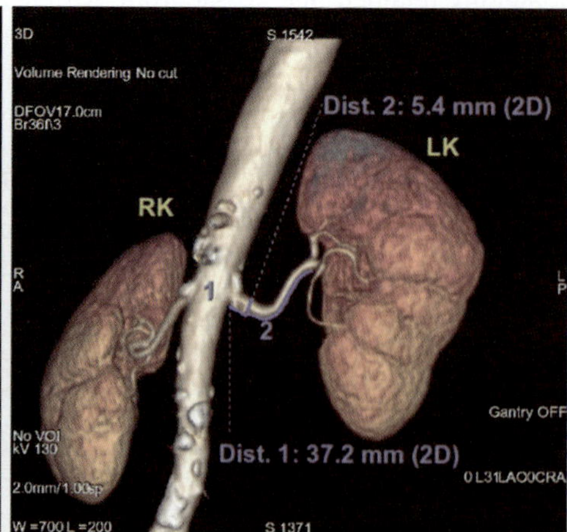

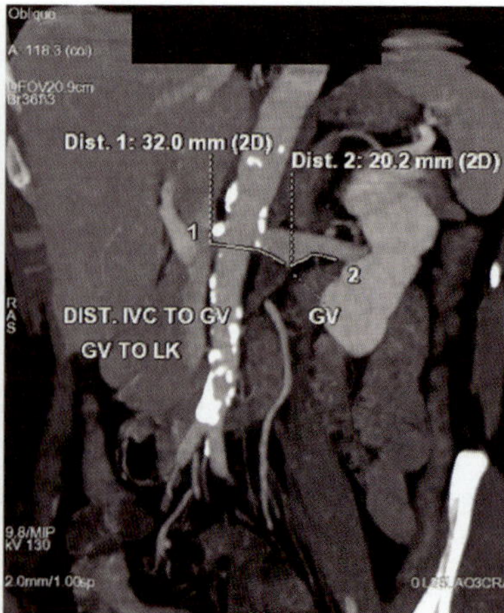

Fig. 4.3: CT angiography showing calcified plaque at the origin of bilateral renal arteries

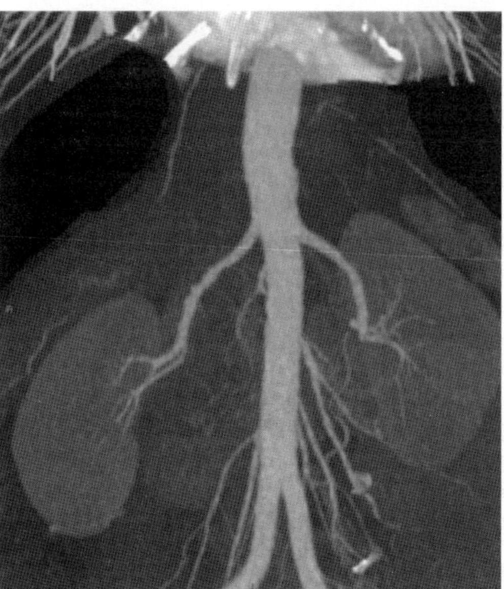

Fig. 4.4: CT angiography showing beaded appearance of right artery

1. **Would you accept or reject this donor?**

   Ans: This donor can be accepted as she has unilateral FMD (right side). The involved right kidney should be accepted, leaving behind the better left kidney with the donor. If need be, the affected donor artery can be resected and an internal iliac artery graft can be used for anastomosis.

2. **How frequent is this disease unilateral or bilateral?**

   Ans: FMD presents as bilateral disease in 32–40% of FMD cases published in the literature. The left kidney is generally less affected.[15]

3. **What are the criteria for accepting such donor?**

   Ans: The criteria for accepting a donor with FMD would be as follows:[16]

   The important aspect for selecting FMD kidney donor is to have a written consent from both donor and recipient, preferably avoid pregnancy after kidney donation and there should be no other living potential donor.

   - Mild FMD disease.
   - No or mild FMD lesions in other arterial beds
   - No or mild hypertension.
   - A few or no cardiovascular risk factors (smoking, obesity, dyslipidemia, etc.).
   - Unilateral or predominantly unilateral renal FMD lesions (in this case, the unaffected or less affected artery/kidney should be left with the donor).
   - No dissection or aneurysm of renal or extra-renal arterial beds (head-to-pelvis CT or MR-angiography required).

4. **What would be the long-term outcome of this donor?**

   Ans: The renal and lung living donor evaluation (RELIVE) study[17] evaluated long-term outcomes of 8922 kidney donors (1963–2007) from the University of Minnesota, University of Alabama–Birmingham and Mayo Clinic–Rochester. Donors with FMD were older and females. Baseline eGFR was also lower in donors with FMD (79 versus 88 ml/min/1.73 m^2, $P < 0.001$).

   After a mean follow-up of 15.5 +/–8.9 years, comparable donors with FMD were alive. There were comparable donors who developed hypertension (22.2% versus 19.8%), proteinuria (20.6% versus 13.7%) and CVD (13.3% versus 13.5%). There was no donor with FMD who developed an eGFR <30 ml/min/1.73 m^2 or ESRD.

   A study from Mayo clinic with evaluation of 2250 donors, 38 donors had FMD with 14 of them having bilateral FMD. There was comparable blood pressure and protein excretion in donor with or without FMD, after a follow-up of 16.6 years. Also, the long-term recipient outcomes were comparable with or without FMD donors.[18]

   So, to conclude

   - Kidney donors with FMD do not appear to have increased risks of hypertension, proteinuria, CVD or reduced eGFR.
   - They can safely donate kidney in carefully selected candidates with no involvement of other vascular beds.

SUMMARY

- Atherosclerotic disease is the most common cause of renal artery stenosis, with a prevalence of 27% at autopsy.
- Recipients with atherosclerotic pelvic vascular disease need detailed evaluation of their disease status and extent of involvement.
- Kidney transplant still remains the best treatment option for these patients, it however requires meticulous surgical planning.
- Orthotopic renal transplant remains a viable option in case of severe atherosclerosis of pelvic vessels; not suitable for anastomosis.
- Donors with atherosclerotic plaque and calcification located at the renal arterial ostium can still donate with good outcome.
- Fibromuscular disease is the second most frequent cause of renal artery stenosis and is more common in females aged less than 40 years, being usually localized to the middle and distal parts of the main renal artery.
- KDIGO Clinical Practice Guideline on the Evaluation and Care of Living Kidney Donors (2017) suggests that a donor candidate with atherosclerotic renal artery disease or fibromuscular dysplasia involving the orifices of both renal arteries should not donate.

- The decision to accept donors with atheromatous plaque should be based on hypertension, global eGFR, presence of comorbidities, differential size and function of the kidney.
- The long-term follow-up of a large number of donors in RELIVE study had demonstrated that kidney donors with FMD appear to do well, do not appear to incur increased risks of hypertension, proteinuria, CVD or reduced eGFR, and perhaps carefully selected candidates with FMD can safely donate as long as involvement of other vascular beds is ruled out.

REFERENCES

1. Smith D, Chudgar A, Daly B, Cooper M. Evaluation of potential renal transplant recipients with computed tomography angiography. Archives of Surgery. 2012 Dec 1;147(12):1114–22.
2. Brar A, Jindal RM, Elster EA, Tedla F, John D, Sumrani N, Salifu MO. Effect of peripheral vascular disease on kidney allograft outcomes: a study of U.S. Renal data system. Transplantation. 2013 Mar 27;95(6):810–5.
3. Tozzi M, Franchin M, Soldini G, Ietto G, Chiappa C, Molteni B, Amico F, Carcano G, Dionigi R. Treatment of aortoiliac occlusive or dilatative disease concomitant with kidney transplantation: how and when? International Journal of Surgery. 2013 Dec 1;11:S115–9.
4. Artiles Medina A, Gómez Dos Santos V, Díez Nicolás V, Hevia Palacios V, Ruiz Hernández M, Laso García I, Mata Alcaraz M, Galeano Álvarez C, Jiménez Cidre MÁ, Arias Fúnez F, Fernández Lucas M. Kidney autotransplantation and orthotopic kidney transplantation: two different approaches for complex cases. Advances in Urology. 2022 Aug 3;2022.
5. Hevia V, Gómez V, Hevia M, Lorca J, Santiago M, Dominguez A, Álvarez S, Díez V, Gordaliza C, Burgos FJ. Troubleshooting complex vascular cases in the kidney transplant recipient: vascular anomalies, challenging vessel diseases, and procedural disasters. Current Urology Reports. 2020 Jan;21:1–6.
6. Musquera M, Peri LL, Alvarez-Vijande R, Oppenheimer F, Gil-Vernet JM, Alcaraz A. Orthotopic kidney transplantation: an alternative surgical technique in selected patients. European urology. 2010 Dec 1;58(6):927–33.
7. Wright C, Corbally MT, Hayes R, McDermott MB. Multifocal infantile myofibromatosis and generalized fibromuscular dysplasia in a child: evidence for a common pathologic process?. Pediatric and Developmental Pathology. 2004 Apr;7:385–90.
8. Cragg AH, Smith TP, Thompson BH, Maroney TP, Stanson AW, Shaw GT, Hunter DW, Cochran ST. Incidental fibromuscular dysplasia in potential renal donors: long-term clinical follow-up. Radiology. 1989 Jul;172(1):145–7.
9. Blondin D, Lanzman R, Schellhammer F, Oels M, Grotemeyer D, Baldus SE, Rump LC, Sandmann W, Voiculescu A. Fibromuscular dysplasia in living renal donors: still a challenge to computed tomographic angiography. European Journal of Radiology. 2010 Jul 1;75(1):67–71.
10. Andreoni KA, Weeks SM, Gerber DA, Fair JH, Mauro MA, McCoy L, Scott L, Johnson MW. Incidence of donor renal fibromuscular dysplasia: does it justify routine angiography? Transplantation. 2002 Apr 15;73(7):1112–6.
11. McKenzie GA, Oderich GS, Kawashima A, Misra S. Renal artery fibromuscular dysplasia in 2,640 renal donor subjects: a CT angiography analysis. Journal of Vascular and Interventional Radiology. 2013 Oct 1;24(10):1477–80.
12. Olin JW, Sealove BA. Diagnosis, management, and future developments of fibromuscular dysplasia. Journal of vascular surgery. 2011 Mar 1;53(3):826–36.
13. Plouin PF, Perdu J, La Batide-Alanore A, Boutouyrie P, Gimenez-Roqueplo AP, Jeunemaitre X. Fibromuscular dysplasia. Orphanet Journal of Rare Diseases. 2007 Dec;2:1–8.
14. Sun IO, Hong YA, Kim HG, Park HS, Choi SR, Chung BH, Park CW, Yang CW, Kim YS, Choi BS. Successful transplant of a kidney with fibromuscular dysplasia having higher glomerular filtration rate than the contralateral kidney. Exp Clinical Transpl. 2012 Jun 1;3:290–2.
15. McKenzie GA, Oderich GS, Kawashima A, Misra S. Renal artery fibromuscular dysplasia in 2,640 renal donor subjects: a CT angiography analysis. Journal of Vascular and Interventional Radiology. 2013 Oct 1;24(10):1477–80.
16. Chrysochou C, Devresse A, Kanaan N, Persu A. Kidney donors with fibromuscular dysplasia, is it time to open the doors?. Nephrology Dialysis Transplantation. 2021 Aug;36(8):1365–8.
17. Adrogue HE, Evans A, Murad DN, Nguyen H, Hebert SA, Nguyen DT, Graviss EA, Ibrahim HN. Long-term outcomes of kidney donors with fibromuscular dysplasia. Nephrology Dialysis Transplantation. 2021 Aug;36(8):1538–45.
18. Gonzalez SM, Amer H, Jaffer I *et al.* Fibromuscular Dysplasia in Living Kidney Donors: Characteristics and Recipient Outcomes. American Transplant Congress, 29 April to 3 May 2017, Chicago, IL.

Chapter

5

Recipient with Adult Polycystic Kidney Disease (ADPKD)

• *Umesh Oza* • *Akshay Deshpande*

LEARNING OBJECTIVES

- To understand the problems of recipient with ADPKD.
- To understand the complications of ADPKD recipient and their outcomes.
- To understand the appropriate donor selection for ADPKD.
- To understand the indications of pretransplant nephrectomy in ADPKD.

INTRODUCTION

Autosomal dominant polycystic kidney disease (ADPKD) is the most common hereditary kidney disease in all ethnicities. ADPKD is the cause of 10% end stage kidney diseases (ESRD) and a cause of major health burden.[1] It is a systemic disease and can involve kidneys, liver, pancreas, spleen, epididymis, seminal vesicles, etc. More than 70% of patients with ADPKD will develop ESRD with total volume of the functioning kidney being the strongest predictor.[2]

Renal transplantation is the most appropriate renal replacement therapy for patients with APDKD.[3–8] With the known diagnosis, family history and slow progress of the renal failure, pre-emptive transplant is the ideal choice of management. Pre-transplant evaluation and counselling of the recipient and the related donor is important for the optimum outcome for these patients.

Case Scenario

A 45-year-old man with a known case of autosomal dominant polycystic kidney disease (ADPKD) and chronic kidney disease (CKD) was being evaluated for a renal transplant. The patient was not on dialysis, but his renal function was gradually deteriorating. Therefore, a decision was made to proceed with a pre-emptive transplant.

The patient presented with fever and right flank pain with mild hematuria. Ultrasonography and MRI were not conclusive of the diagnosis; however, positron emission tomography (PET) clinched the diagnosis of cyst infection (Figs 5.1 and 5.2). He was treated conservatively with appropriate antibiotics but his fever and right flank pain continued. It was decided to proceed with pre-transplant right nephrectomy (Fig. 5.3).

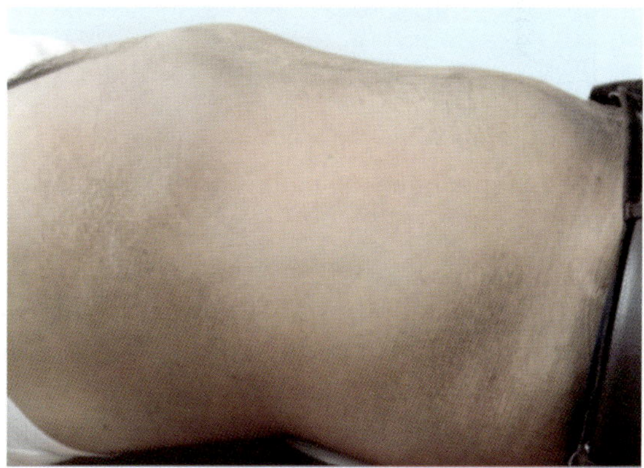

Fig. 5.1: Clinical image of ADPKD showing flank fullness in lying down position

1. **What are the problems expected in this recipient?**

   Ans: This patient had infection in polycystic kidney which was symptomatic. Initially treatment with appropriate antibiotics was tried, but he required pre-transplant nephrectomy. Presence of infection in immunocompromised patients, if not treated adequately, may remain source of infection post-transplant.

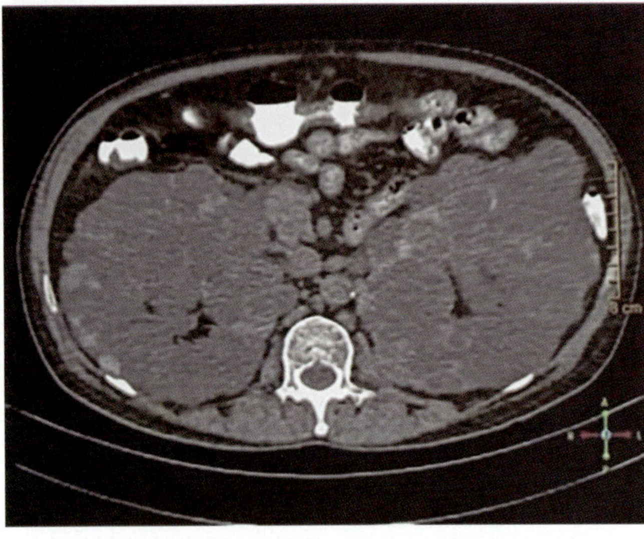

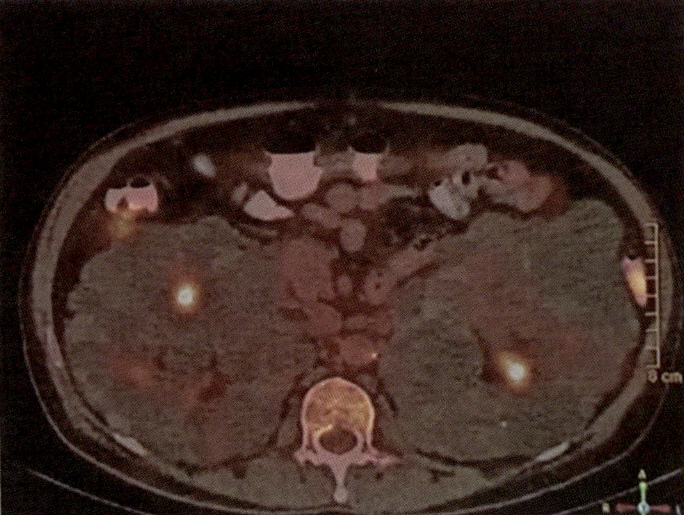

Fig. 5.2: PET CT scan showing infected cyst

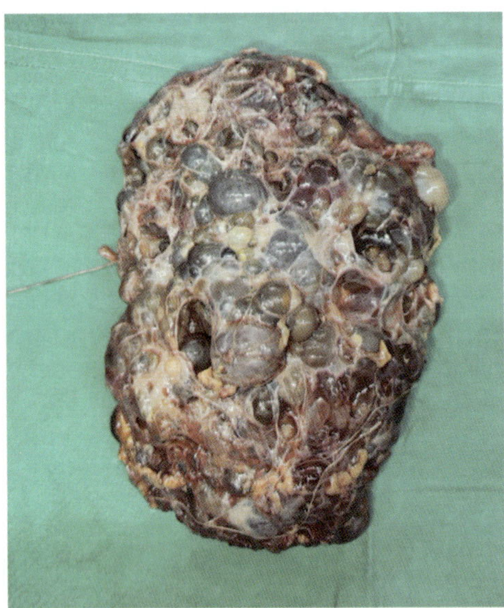

Fig. 5.3: Gross specimen of native pre-transplant ADPKD nephrectomy

Timely decision in patients who are on dialysis and who are immunocompromised can avoid life-threatening septicaemia.

Ronsin *et al*[9] concluded that cyst infection rate post-transplant was found to be 1.6 events per 100 years.

There is no role for routine/elective pretransplant nephrectomy. Pretransplant nephrectomy is indicated only in patient with recurrent infections not responding to medical management or life-threatening infections. It has been observed by Ronsin and Charles *et al* that incidence of cyst infection post-transplant is not common in those who have been treated successfully for cyst infection pre-transplant. It is challenging to diagnose the cyst infection due to non-specific symptoms, however, diagnostic tools like PET-CT helps in the diagnosis.[9]

2. **How will you evaluate this recipient?**

Ans: In addition to routine evaluation as carried out in other recipients, following points should be considered.

History

- History of past episodes of urinary tract infection or cyst infection
- History of stone disease or any surgical intervention for the same.
- History of intracerebral bleed due to aneurysm in the relatives or patient.

Physical Examination

- Size of the kidneys to assess availability of space to transplant kidney in the iliac fossa.
- Any clinical evidence of infection or scar of previous surgery
- Examinations of genitals in males for presence of cysts in epididymis and to make a note of the same, however, its presence does not come in the way of renal transplantation.

Imaging

In a polycystic kidney disease, imaging plays an important role.

Ultrasonography reveals renal as well as extrarenal cysts. It formulates diagnostic criteria for individuals with 50% risk of developing disease as:

1. At least 3 unilateral or bilateral cysts before age of 40 years
2. 2 cysts in each kidney in individuals between 40 and 59 years
3. 4 cysts in each kidney above 60 years

For PKD1 patients aged 30 years or older, the criteria exhibits a sensitivity of 100%, ensuring reliable detection in this age group. However, in younger patients, the false-negative rates are higher, with PKD2 showing a 23% false-negative rate and PKD1 showing a 5% false-negative rate. In cases where the family history is unknown or negative, these criteria may not be fully applicable. In such situations, it is advisable to consider mutation analysis for both disease exclusion and diagnostic purposes to ensure accurate and effective assessment.[10]

Advanced imaging like CT scan and MRI are superior to ultrasonography for diagnosing extrarenal cysts and complications in ADPKD. They help identify nephrolithiasis, hemorrhage, infection, and malignancy in native kidneys.[17] F-18 FDG PET CT scan is useful for localizing cyst infections and malignancy through metabolic activity assessment.[18]

Evaluation for Intracranial Aneurysm (ICA)

Intracranial aneurysm rupture is one of the most serious complications of ADPKD with increased morbidity and mortality.[19]

Very little is known about the natural history of ICA in ADPKD. Screening for asymptomatic ICA in ADPKD patients should be performed in those with personal or family history of ICA. Patients with unknown history should be counselled about the risks and if anxious, screening should be done. CT angiography or MR angiography can be done but MR angiography is the screening of choice.[19]

3. **How will you evaluate a live related donor for this recipient?**

Ans: APDKD is hereditary disease. it is found equally in male and female offspring and each offspring has 50% chance of inheriting the disease. This makes it difficult to find a related healthy donor.

Selecting donor from the relative needs proper imaging and molecular genetic testing in selected donors (Fig. 5.4).

For donor evaluation, ultrasonography is a baseline investigation and has an excellent negative predictive value for the donors above age of 40 years.[11] However, with age between 30 and 39 years ultrasonography has false negative value of 0.7%. MRI becomes a preferred mode of imaging in this group of patients for the diagnosis of presence of cysts. Even if USG and MRI is normal, molecular genetic testing by linkage analysis using polymorphic PKD1 and PKD2 markers or mutational screening of PKD1 and PKD2 should be done if family members are available, in young less than 30 years old donor. Donation is contraindicated in confirmed case of ADPKD in a living donor kidney transplantation.[12–15]

The kidney donation, after considering clinical scenario, may be deferred, if the mutation analysis is inconclusive.[16] This approach ensures that donors are thoroughly evaluated, and their safety is prioritised.

MRI

MRI is useful for obtaining the diagnosis and exclude the possibility of ADPKD in the donors. Among subjects who are at risk of ADPKD at the ages of 16 to 40 years, presence of more than 10 cysts can be diagnostic. And the finding of less than 5 cysts can be considered as a disease exclusion.[17]

4. **What are the indications of pre-transplant nephrectomy in ADPDKD recipient?**

Ans: Pre-transplant nephrectomy of native kidneys is generally not recommended in all the patients of

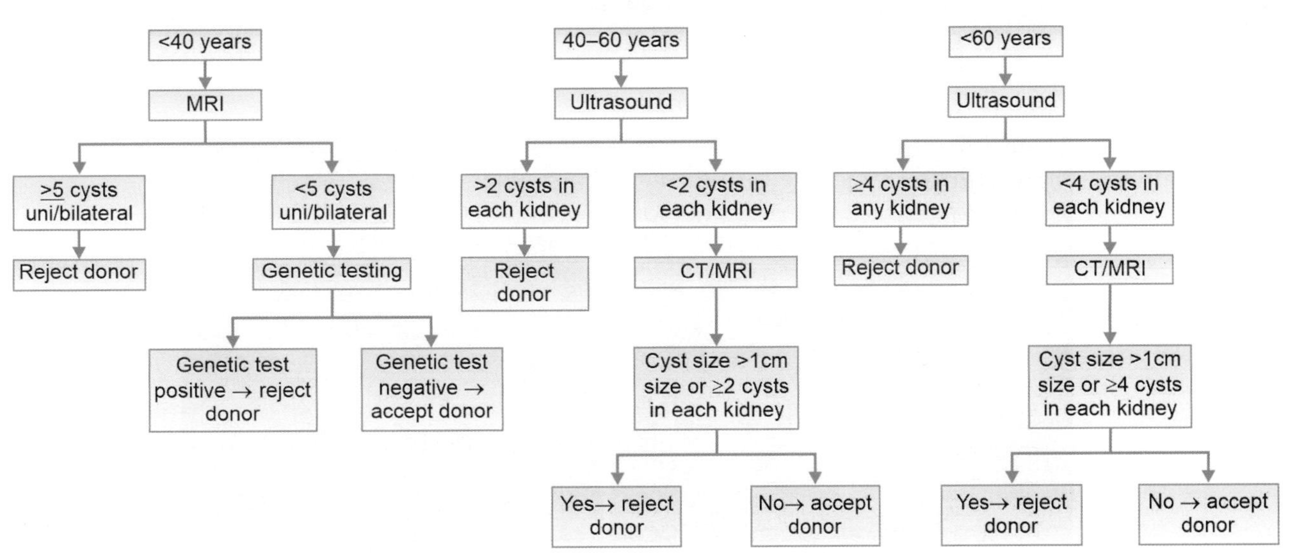

Fig. 5.4: Role of imaging and genetic testing in donor evaluation

ADPKD undergoing kidney transplantation except following conditions:[20]

- Insufficient space for the kidney graft
- Recurrent cyst infection
- Recurrent or obstructive stone disease
- Possibility of malignancy (Figs 5.5 and 5.6)
- Large size responsible for symptoms of pain, heaviness or gastrointestinal symptoms

It is also known that native kidneys shrink after kidney transplantation. In a study of 28 ADPKD recipients, it was found that, size of ADPKD kidneys reduced significantly (40%) after renal transplant. So pre-transplant nephrectomy

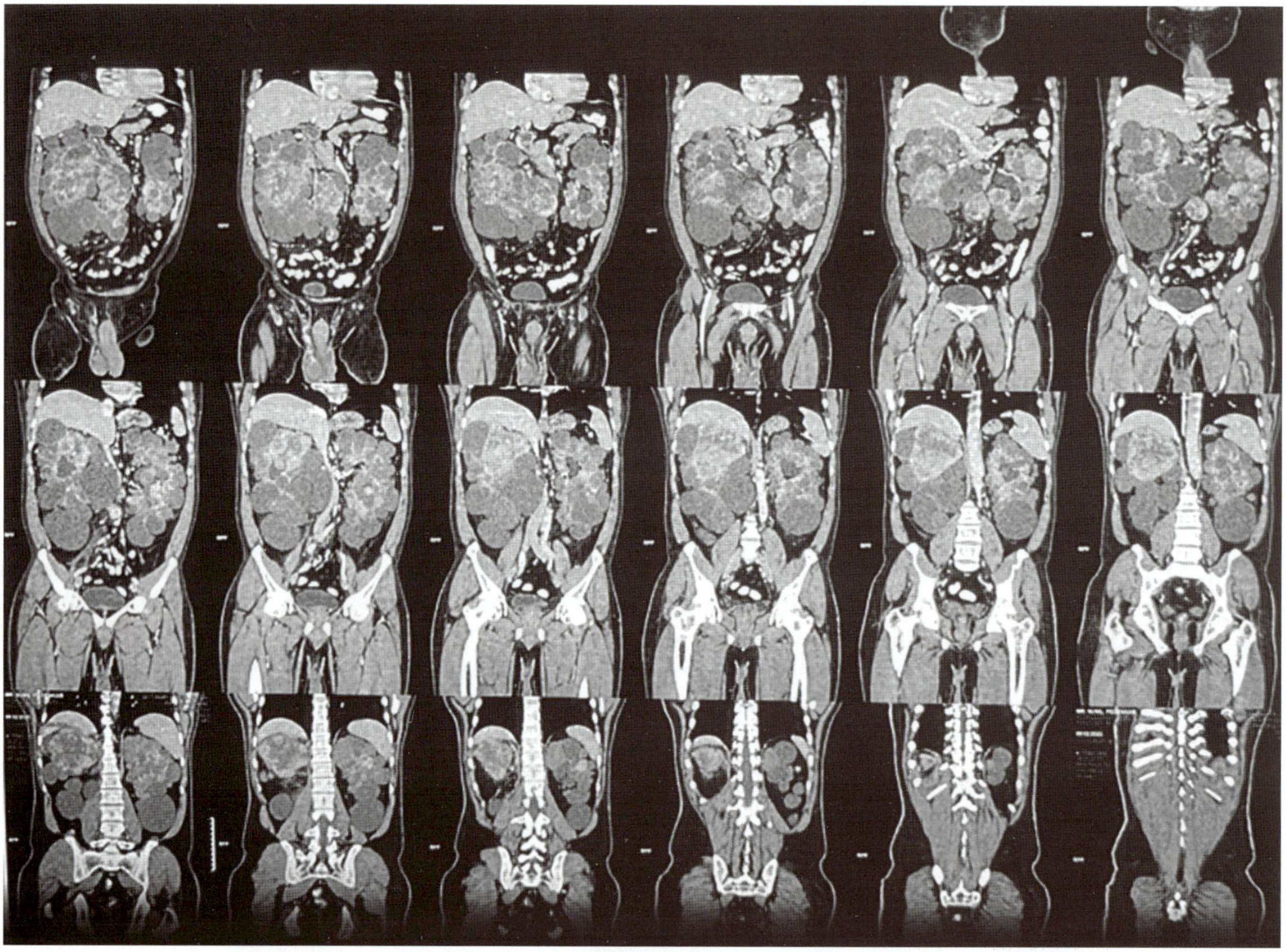

Fig. 5.5: CECT abdomen showing solid components in cysts symptoms of renal mass in both kidneys

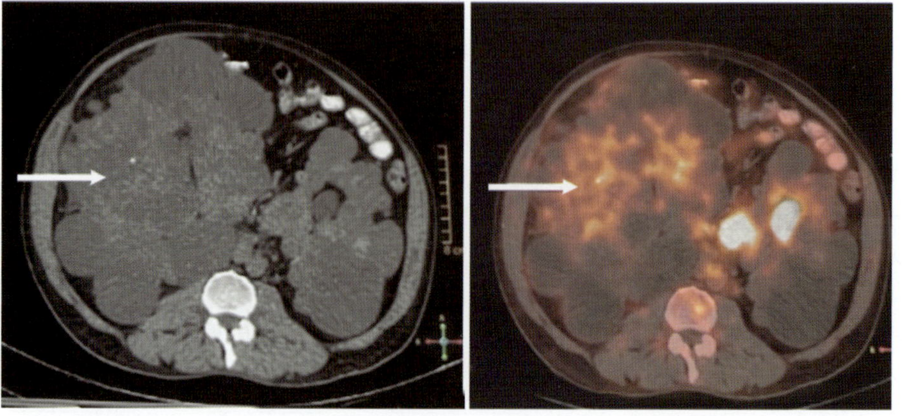

Fig. 5.6: ADPKD kidney showing renal malignancy in FDG PET scan

in asymptomatic patients with space available for transplant is not recommended.[21]

It is important to understand, nephrectomy of polycystic kidney in a patient of chronic kidney disease is not an easy operation. It has its own morbidity and complications. Requirement of blood transfusions, proximity of vena cava with short renal vein and duodenum on the right side, large size of the cysts covering the hilum and the bulk of the kidney makes this surgery more challenging. On left side, injury to spleen, pancreas (more so if it has large cysts) is also significant. High level of expertise, support and infrastructure for the perioperative care is recommended. Complications can jeopardise the subsequent renal transplantation.

5. **Which approach would you opt and the timing of pretransplant nephrectomy?**

Ans: Despite different views on timing, approach, indications, for native kidney nephrectomy, following are the valuable points.

Timing of native nephrectomy

- Pre-transplant nephrectomy a few weeks before transplant surgery
- Concomitant with transplant surgery
- Post-transplant nephrectomy

Generally, unilateral nephrectomy is required in indicated patients for the reasons described earlier. Some patients do require bilateral nephrectomy for native kidneys.

Recent published data do not find significant difference in the complications and outcome of results when nephrectomy was done before transplantation or during kidney transplantation.[22] Proponents of simultaneous transplantation believe that this approach offers a single operation and avoidance of dialysis pre-transplant if it is a pre-emptive transplantation.

However as mentioned earlier, it is a challenging surgery and it may be safer to stage the procedure to assure smooth outcome of the transplant surgery. It has to be a collective decision of surgeons, nephrologists and the anaesthesiologist to decide about the timing of the nephrectomy. The final decision will depend on the clinical condition of the patient and the confidence of the medical team to give best results. In case of bilateral nephrectomy, it may be better to adopt staged approach.[23]

Bilateral nephrectomy is more difficult and has increased morbidity. Maintaining anephric patient on dialysis is very challenging for nephrologists. It is equally important for transplant surgeon to look after vascular access in these patients. Significant drop in blood pressure or pressure on the extremity due to the positioning of the patient during the surgery may close down arterio-venous fistula. This may become a bigger challenge for the patient undergoing dialysis.

Approaches for native nephrectomy

Traditionally open surgical approach has been followed in most of the centres. Recently there are reports of laparoscopic and robotic approach for ADPKD native nephrectomy. They have shown excellent results with better post-operative outcome and less morbidity. However, it requires high degree of expertise and centre of excellence to give desired results.[24]

6. **Are there any alternatives to pre-transplant nephrectomy in ADPKD?**

Ans: Transcatheter unilateral arterial embolization is an emerging alternative to pretransplant nephrectomy. It has shown significant promise in reducing the size of native kidney.

Meta-analysis shows renal transcatheter arterial embolization reduces kidney volume by 46% to 54% on average in 12 months in patients with enlarged kidneys due to autosomal dominant polycystic kidney disease.[25]

SUMMARY

- Patients with ADPKD have excellent patient and graft survival rates following kidney transplantation. Pre-emptive transplantation should be planned, if possible.
- Prophylactic native kidney nephrectomy is typically reserved for ADPKD patients who experience severe pain, early satiety or disturbing gastrointestinal symptoms, recurrent bleeding, infection, recurrent stones, or require additional space to implant the graft. This approach should be tailored to the individual patient's needs and may not be necessary for all transplant recipients. Pre-transplant nephrectomy of ADPKD kidney can be a challenging surgery.
- Timing of native nephrectomy whether staged, simultaneous with transplant or post-transplant, should be a joint decision of surgeon, nephrologist and anaesthesiologist tailored for each patient.
- Laparoscopic or robotic native ADPKD kidney nephrectomy is possible but should be done only by surgeons with adequate experience and reasonable expertise.
- General recommendations for screening intracranial aneurysms in ADPKD patients should be followed to identify individuals who may benefit from pretransplant screening.
- In young < 30 years live related donors, when imaging is normal or equivocal, genetic testing should be performed. This highlights the importance of genetic screening in identifying potential donors who may carry the ADPKD gene mutation, even if they do not display symptoms of the disease.

REFERENCES

1. Singh, Shivendra; Sreenidhi, HC; Das, Parimal1; Devi, Chandra1. Predicting the Risk of Progression in Indian ADPKD Cohort using PROPKD Score –A Single-Center

Retrospective Study. Indian Journal of Nephrology ():10.4103/ijn.ijn_69_22, March 07, 2023. | DOI: 10.4103/ijn.ijn_69_22.

2. Harris, P. C. *et al.* Cyst number but not the rate of cystic growth is associated with the mutated gene in autosomal dominant polycystic kidney disease. J. Am. Soc. Nephrol. 17, 3013–3019 (2006).
3. Alam, A. and Perrone, RD. Management of ESRD in patients with autosomal dominant polycystic kidney disease. Adv. Chronic. Kidney Dis. 17, 164–172 (2010).
4. Haynes, R., Kheradmand, F. & Winearls, C. G. Survival after starting renal replacement treatment in patients with autosomal dominant polycystic kidney disease: a single-centre 40-year study. Nephron Clin. Pract. 120, c42–c47 (2012).
5. Mosconi, G. *et al.* Renal transplant in patients with polycystic disease: the Italian experience. Transplant. Proc. 45, 2635–2640 (2013).
6. Jacquet, A. *et al.* Outcomes of renal transplantation in patients with autosomal dominant polycystic kidney disease: a nationwide longitudinal study. Transpl. Int. 24, 582–587 (2011).
7. Orskov, B., Romming Sorensen, V., Feldt Rasmussen, B. and Strandgaard, S. Improved prognosis in patients with autosomal dominant polycystic kidney disease in Denmark. Clin. J. Am. Soc. Nephrol. 5, 2034–2039 (2010).
8. Perrone, R. D., Ruthazer, R. and Terrin, N. C. Survival after end-stage renal disease in autosomal dominant polycystic kidney disease: contribution of extrarenal complications to mortality. Am. J. Kidney Dis. 38, 777–784 (2001).
9. Ronsin C, Chaba A, Suchanek O, Coindre JP, Kerleau C, Garandeau C, Houzet A, Cantarovich D, Dantal J, Blancho G, Giral M. Incidence, risk factors and outcomes of kidney and liver cyst infection in kidney transplant recipient with ADPKD. Kidney International Reports. 2022 Apr 1;7(4): 867–75.
10. Pei, Y. *et al.* Unified criteria for ultrasonographic diagnosis of ADPKD. J. Am. Soc. Nephrol. 20, 205–212 (2009).
11. Peral, B. *et al.* Evidence of linkage disequilibrium in the Spanish polycystic kidney disease I population. Am. J. Hum. Genet. 54, 899–908 (1994).
12. Zhao, X. *et al.* Molecular diagnostics in autosomal dominant polycystic kidney disease: utility and limitations. Clin. J. Am. Soc. Nephrol. 3, 146–152 (2008).
13. Rossetti, S. *et al.* Comprehensive molecular diagnostics in autosomal dominant polycystic kidney disease. J. Am. Soc. Nephrol. 18, 2143–2160 (2007).
14. Garcia-Gonzalez, M. A. *et al.* Evaluating the clinical utility of a molecular genetic test for polycystic kidney disease. Mol. Genet. Metab. 92, 160–167 (2007).
15. Huang, E., Samaniego-Picota, M., McCune, T., Melancon, J. K., Montgomery, R. A., Ugarte, R., Kraus, E., Womer, K., Rabb, H., and Watnick, T. (2009). DNA Testing For Live Kidney Donors At Risk For Autosomal Dominant Polycystic Kidney Disease. Transplantation, 87(1), 133. https://doi.org/10.1097/TP.0b013e318191e729.
16. Pei Y, Hwang YH, Conklin J, Sundsbak JL, Heyer CM, Chan W, Wang K, He N, Rattansingh A, Atri M, Harris PC, Haider MA. Imaging-based diagnosis of autosomal dominant polycystic kidney disease. J Am Soc Nephrol. 2015 Mar;26(3):746–53. doi: 10.1681/ASN.2014030297. Epub 2014 Jul 29. PMID: 25074509; PMCID: PMC4341484.
17. Zhang W, Blumenfeld JD, Prince MR. MRI in autosomal dominant polycystic kidney disease. J Magn Reson Imaging. 2019 Jul;50(1):41–51. doi: 10.1002/jmri.26627. Epub 2019 Jan 13. PMID: 30637853.
18. Jouret, F. *et al.* Positron-emission computed tomography in cyst infection diagnosis in patients with autosomal dominant polycystic kidney disease. Clin. J. Am. Soc. Nephrol. 6, 1644–1650 (2011).
19. Rozenfeld MN, AnsariSA, Shaibinia *et al.* Should patients with ADPKD be screened for Cerebral Aneurysm? Am J of Neuroradiology 2014, 35, 3–9.
20. Patel, P. *et al.* Native nephrectomy in transplant patients with autosomal dominant polycystic kidney disease. Ann. R. Coll. Surg. Engl. 93, 391–395 (2011).
21. Yamamoto, T. *et al.* Kidney volume changes in patients with autosomal dominant polycystic kidney disease after renal transplantation. Transplantation 93, 794–798 (2012).
22. Fuller, T.F.; Brennan, T.V.; Feng, S.; Kang, S.M.; Stock, P.G.; Freise, C.E. End stage polycystic kidney disease: Indications and timing of native nephrectomy relative to kidney transplantation. J. Urol. 2005, 174, 2284–228.
23. Kirkman MA, van Dellen D, Mehra S, Campbell BA, Tavakoli A, Pararajasingam R, Parrott NR, Riad HN, McWilliam L, Augustine T. Native nephrectomy for autosomal dominant polycystic kidney disease: before or after kidney transplantation? BJU Int. 2011 Aug;108(4):590–4. doi: 10.1111/j.1464–410X.2010.09938.x. Epub 2010 Dec 16. PMID: 21166760.
24. John M. Masterson, Hanson Zhao, Lior Taich *et al.* Robotic Bilateral Nephrectomy for Large Polycystic Kidney Disease, 13 September 2022, PREPRINT (Version 1) available at Research Square [https://doi.org/10.21203/rs.3.rs–2043107/v1].
25. Oda Y, Sawa N, Suwabe T, Hoshino J, Ubara Y. Renal Transcatheter Arterial Embolization for ADPKD. Kidney Int Rep. 2020 Mar 3;5(4):546–549. doi: 10.1016/j.ekir.2020.01.014. PMID: 32274461; PMCID: PMC7136319.

Chapter

6

Transplantation in Abnormal Urinary Tract

• *Ruchir Maheshwari* • *Anant Kumar*

LEARNING OBJECTIVES

- To understand the different possible scenarios of difficult bladder encountered during evaluation of prospective kidney transplant recipient.
- To understand the evaluation of each of these possible conditions.
- To understand the available treatment options.
- To understand the follow-up care in case of transplant in abnormal urinary tract.

INTRODUCTION

A functional lower urinary tract, normally compliant urinary bladder having age appropriate capacity and ability to empty at volition within physiological pressures, is of paramount importance for upper urinary tract. Any dysfunction here may lead to damage to upper tracts—native or transplanted.

The aetiology of renal failure secondary to lower urinary tract dysfunction usually varies between different age groups (Table 6.1). Posterior urethral valves (PUV) and prune belly syndrome (PBS) usually lead to end stage renal disease (ESRD) in childhood/adolescence. Vesico-ureteric reflux (VUR) and neurogenic bladder dysfunction secondary to congenital spinal dysraphism, though paediatric issues, lead to ESRD in early adulthood. Genitourinary tuberculosis (GUTB) associated thimble bladder is not common in paediatric age-group. Conditions like stricture urethra, overactive bladder (OAB), underactive detrusor and benign prostatic hyperplasia (BPH) associated bladder outlet obstruction (BOO) are encountered in adult population.

TABLE 6.1: Etiologies of renal failure secondary to lower urinary tract dysfunction in paediatric and adult population

Paediatric population	*Adult population*
Posterior urethral valves (PUV)	Genito-urinary tuberculosis (GUTB)/thimble bladder
Prune belly syndrome	Benign prostatic hyperplasia (BPH)
Neurogenic bladder dysfunction secondary to spinal dysraphism	Stricture urethra
Vesico-ureteric reflux	Overactive bladder (OAB)
	Underactive detrusor
	Stress urinary incontinence (SUI)
	Vesico-ureteric reflux

During initial years of renal transplantation, surgeons were wary of transplanting a patient with abnormal bladder. If a lower tract can damage native kidneys, transplanted kidney will be at equal, if not greater, risk—was the logical explanation. It was not until 12 years after first successful kidney transplant, when Kelly reported first transplant in a patient with abnormal urinary bladder.[4]

A thorough assessment of lower urinary tract is a cornerstone of pre-transplant evaluation. All unstable/high pressure lower tracts should be converted to low pressure good compliance bladders before embarking upon kidney transplantation.[2–4] In this chapter, we will be discussing about various situations encountered in both paediatric as well as adult population, the evaluation methodology and management protocols.

PUV

Case Scenario 1

A 16-year-old boy with history of PUV diagnosed at 1 month of age was managed immediately with per-urethral catheterisation followed by transurethral fulguration of valve. His creatinine stabilised to 0.8 mg/dL. He was under regular follow-up with a paediatrician. Recently, he had history of recurrent febrile UTI that were managed conservatively. On evaluation, he had high PVR and was advised regular CIC, but compliance was poor. Gradually his serum creatinine deteriorated and now has reached a level of 5 mg/dl.

The PUV, with an incidence of 1.2 to 2.1 per 10,000 live male births, is a unique congenital anomaly of lower urinary tract. In contemporary times, it is usually diagnosed early and managed via minimally invasive method in a seemingly straightforward method (Fig. 6.1). Yet, the insult suffered during developmental phase in *utero*, effects both the lower tract as well as upper tract and leads to end stage renal disease in almost 20–50% of these boys.[5,6] Renal transplant, the best treatment for ESRD has mixed result in cases of PUV. It has been observed that 13–38% of these patients develop valve bladder syndrome, which can negatively affect the transplant outcomes.[7]

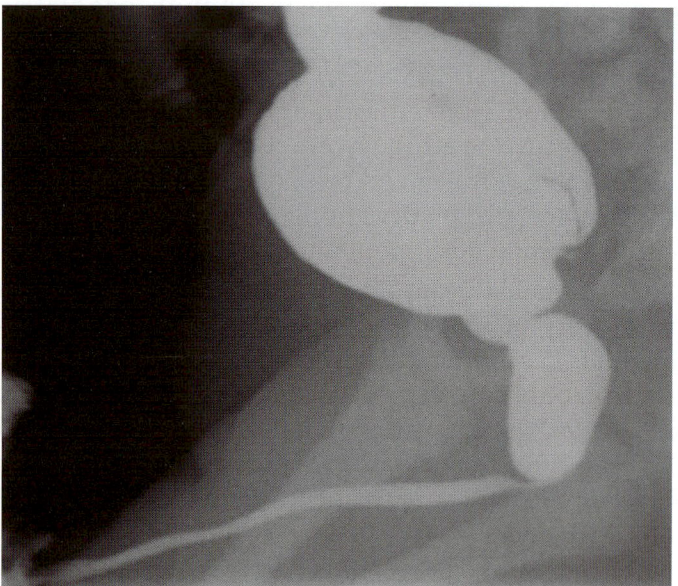

Fig. 6.1: MCU of posterior urethral valve

1. **What is the pathophysiology of valve bladder?**

   Ans: *In utero* phase, the developing urinary bladder has to generate high pressures leading to compensatory hypertrophy of detrusor muscles. These high pressures also affect developing glomeruli leading to dysplasia. The combination of polyuria by dysplastic kidneys, bladder insensitivity and incomplete emptying by high pressure urinary bladder leads to bladder decompensation (high capacity atonic bladder or hypercontractile bladder), also known as valve bladder syndrome. The valve bladder along with high grade vesico-ureteric reflux in these patients causes further injury to already dysplastic kidneys.[7]

2. **How will you evaluate an ESRD patient with h/o PUV for renal transplant?**

   Ans: Before proceeding for transplantation, it is of paramount importance to thoroughly evaluate urinary bladder or the lower tract.
   1. *Bladder diary*: It gives objective assessment of urine output, assesses polyuria, urinary frequency and gives baseline parameters for urodynamic study.
   2. *Uroflowmetry + post-void residual urine*: Non-invasive modality for evaluating functional status of lower urinary tract
   3. *Video-urodynamic study*: It provides both anatomical and functional assessment of lower urinary tract and provides targets for stabilising lower urinary tract before proceeding for renal transplant. In the absence of facility for video-urodynamic study, urodynamic assessment along with micturating cysto-urethrogram can be done for the assessment.
   4. *Ultrasound (USG)*: It provides anatomical assessment of the urinary tract.
   5. *Urine culture/sensitivity:* A sterile urine culture is *sine qua non* before proceeding for renal transplantation. Bacterial colonisation is very common in abnormal/augmented urinary bladders.
   6. *Cystoscopy:* If there is any history of sterile pyuria, hematuria or history of bladder augmentation.

3. **How will you optimise the valve bladder before proceeding for renal transplantation?**

   Ans: Before going for renal transplantation, lower urinary tract should be able to hold physiological amount of urine at low pressure (less than 30 cm H_2O) and be able to empty it to completion.[8] Depending upon urodynamic study findings, treatment can be tailored for optimising bladder function. Multiple treatment modalities can be combined as per need:
   1. *Anti-cholinergic medicines*: For poor compliance/overactive bladders
   2. *Clean intermittent self catheterisation (CIC)*: In case of myogenic failure/high capacity bladder/

polyuria with high PVR/dilated upper tracts. Multiple studies have favoured continuous night-time drainage using indwelling catheter to ensure completely empty bladder during average of 8 hours of sleep in these boys. It ensures optimal drainage of upper tract and has been proved to delay onset of ESRD.[7,9]

3. *Mitrofanoff catheterisable stoma*: Many patients have demonstrated poor compliance to the strict CIC regimen advised. A major reason being discomfort/pain during catheterisation of sensitive urethra. A catheterisable stoma using Mitrofanoff principle (Fig. 6.2) significantly improves the compliance in these patients. This procedure can be done using laparoscopy or surgical robot, thereby decreasing surgical morbidity.[6]

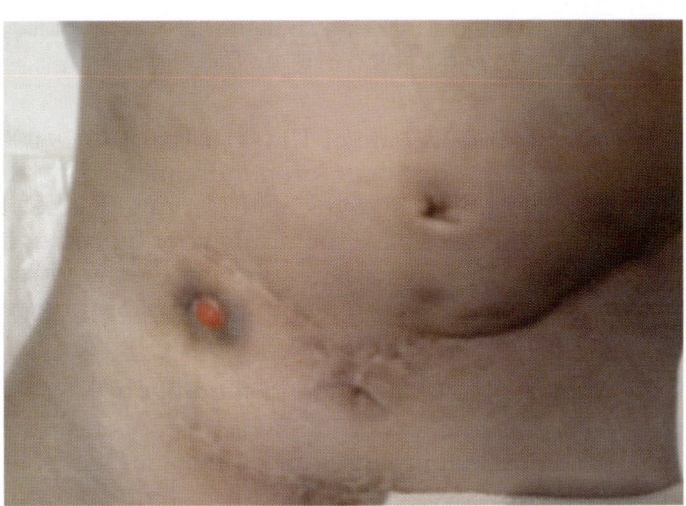

Fig. 6.2: Mitrofanoff stoma *in situ*

4. *Bladder augmentation*: In patients with high pressure poor compliance small capacity bladder, augmentation gives a high capacity low pressure reservoir. It can be done using ileum, sigmoid or the dilated ureter (Fig. 6.3), if available. Augmentation with urothelium lining has obvious advantages.

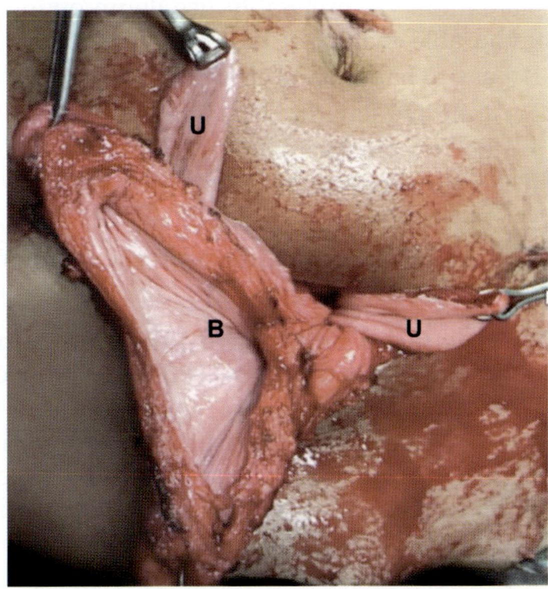

Fig. 6.3: Ureterocystoplasty using dialated native ureters (U) to augment urinary bladder (B)

Gastrocystoplasty (Fig. 6.4), a common procedure in the past, has fallen out of favour owing to complications associated with acid secreting gastric mucosa. It is especially difficult to manage in anuric patients.

There is enough evidence in literature regarding usefulness of bladder augmentation as well as

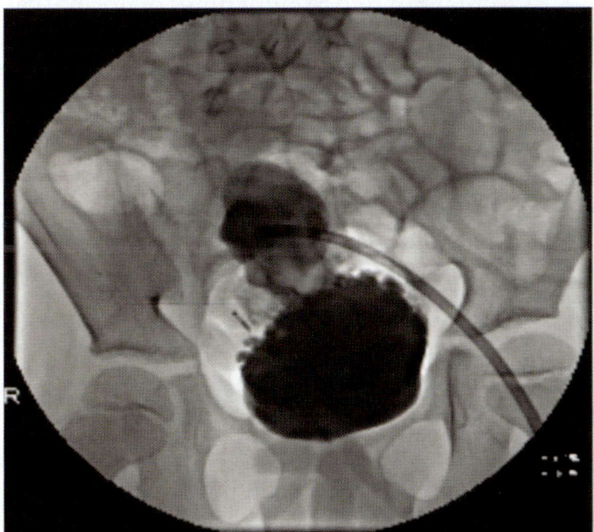

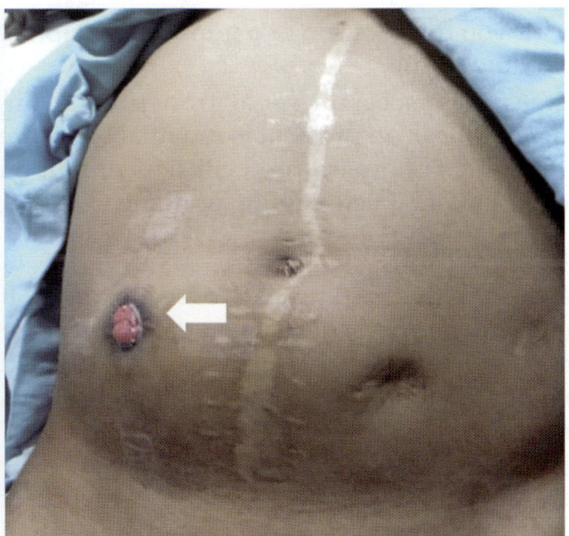

Fig. 6.4: Gastrocystoplasty with Mitrofanoff appendicovesicostoma (white arrow)

comparable renal transplant outcomes of patients with normal urinary bladder. The debate is still on regarding timing of surgery with respect to renal transplantation surgery. Majority of authors prefer pre-transplant augmentation.[10–14]

The authors prefer to do augmentation enterocystoplasty four weeks prior to renal transplantation. We preferably use ileum owing to its favourable characteristics

1. Easy to handle and configure
2. Abundant length
3. Robust vascularity
4. Good compliance
5. Moderate mucous production
6. Favourable complication profile compared to stomach or colon

4. What is the place of pre-transplant bladder augmentation in a case of ESRD with valve bladder syndrome?

Ans: A number of authors have questioned regarding bladder augmentation procedure prior to renal transplantation in valve bladder patients. It is said that instead of the bladder, it is nephrogenic diabetes insipidus induced polyuria which has led to abnormal urodynamic findings in this subset of patients. Once renal transplant is done, functioning graft kidney controls polyuria. With more physiological urine output, bladder dynamics return to normal; thus, obviating the need for bladder augmentation. A bladder diary is invaluable in this decision making.[15]

5. What are the indications of pre-transplant nephrectomy in a case of ESRD with PUV?

Ans: Pre-transplant nephrectomy is required only in some very specific indications—polyuria causing hemodynamic instability or gross proteinuria.[16]

6. How will you do follow-up of a transplant recipient with history of PUV?

Ans: After successful renal transplantation, stringent follow-up protocol is essential to ensure graft safety. Follow-up protocol depends upon whether patient is self-voiding or doing CIC.[17]

Self-Voiding Patients

These patients are followed up like routine patients. If there is any evidence of renal function deterioration or urinary tract infection, the patients must be evaluated with urine cultures, uroflowmetry + PVRU and imaging. In case of deterioration of uroflowmetry parameters/increasing PVRU, CIC should be instituted. Urodynamic studies are to be undertaken if there is evidence of bladder outflow obstruction/decreased functional bladder capacity or upper tract dilation.

Patients on CIC

It is important to ensure compliance with CIC. In case the child is non-compliant due to sensate urethra, Mitrofanoff procedure should be undertaken. Asymptomatic bacteriuria is common and treatment with antibiotics is instituted in only certain conditions:

1. Patient develops fever
2. Suprapubic discomfort/urine leak between CIC intervals
3. Colonisation with urea splitting bacteria like Proteus

Prune Belly Syndrome (PBS)

Case Scenario 2

A 20-year-old male with history of unilateral nephroureterectomy in childhood for some congenital anomaly and recurrent UTI has now presented with symptoms and signs of uraemia. On examination, he is pale, with pot belly. His serum creatinine is 6 mg/dl and USG revealed right kidney with raised echogenicity and loss of CMD and high PVRU 500/800 ml.

PBS has an incidence rate of 1 in 40,000 to 1 in 29,000 live births with high male preponderance (95%). It affects a multitude of systems, with varying degree of severity. Type I cases have uniformly poor outcomes if not stillborn. Type III cases require intervention only if there is evidence of upper tract deterioration or recurrent urinary tract infection.[18–21]

1. What are the features found in category II PBS?

Ans: It is category II PBS which is of concern to paediatric nephrologist and transplant surgeons as it may progress to ESRD in childhood or early adolescent. The ureters are usually dilated, tortuous and redundant; up to 75% have vesicoureteric reflux. The unobstructed urinary bladder is enlarged two to eight times of normal capacity with urachal pseudodiverticulum. Twenty-five to 30% of children have patent urachus at birth. The bladder wall is smooth, thick with abnormal muscle to collagen ratio. Under electron microscopy, disorganisation of smooth muscle cells is well appreciated. The ability to empty urinary bladder is variable in these patients. On urodynamic assessment, the bladder is high capacity, normal to high compliance with delayed first sensation and poor contractility.[20]

2. What are the factors leading to progression to ESRD?

Ans: The causative factors considered for progression to ESRD can be

1. Congenital dysplasia of kidney with polyuria
2. High grade VUR with reflux nephropathy

3. Persistent high PVR with resultant back pressure changes
4. Recurrent urinary tract infections

It goes without saying that stabilisation of bladder dynamics is to be ensured before proceeding for renal transplantation; and regular monitoring post-transplant is important.

3. **What is the indication for nephro-ureterectomy?**

Ans: Dysplastic kidney with high grade VUR can be a source of recurrent infection and needs to be removed (nephroureterectomy) prior to transplantation.

4. **What are the steps needed for stabilisation of lower urinary tract prior to transplantation?**

Ans: Lower tract dysfunction is a combination of deficient abdominal wall, high capacity urinary bladder and bladder outlet obstruction. Each patient needs individualised assessment to look at the key components and treatment is tailored accordingly. Reconstruction of abdominal wall can improve intra-abdominal dynamics and improve bladder emptying.[22] In some patients, reduction cystoplasty of urachal diverticulum can improve bladder pressure characteristics and reduce postvoid residue. Similarly, evaluation of urethra for any obstruction and appropriate management will help in reducing leak point pressure into physiological range.[20]

Polyuria-induced high PVR can be expected to get resolved after transplantation. Behavioural reinforcement for double voiding is attempted. CIC, if required, is better done through Mitrofanoff appendico-vesicostomy.

5. **What is the key point for evaluation in post-transplant period?**

Ans: In post-transplant follow-up, for volitionally voiding patients, PVRU is the most important parameter to be monitored and, if required, corrective methods applied as discussed above.

Neurogenic Bladder Dysfunction

Case Scenario 3

A normally born female child with normal milestones, developed urinary incontinence at 8 years of age. Coming from a poor family from remote village, she was evaluated and managed with alternative medicines. Over years, her condition worsened and now she has presented at 16 years of age with uremic symptoms. On evaluation, bladder is grossly distended (reaching up to umbilicus), serum creatinine is 8 mg/dl, and USG shows grossly overdistended urinary bladder with B/L hydro-ureteronephrosis with thinned out cortex.

Unlike the previous two conditions, upper tract damage leading to ESRD is a preventable condition. However, in poorly managed neuropathic voiding disease (NVD), patients do land up in ESRD. Prior to renal transplant, it is of paramount importance to assess urinary bladder dynamics and stabilize it, well in advance.

1. **How will you evaluate an ESRD patient with neurogenic bladder for renal transplantation?**

Ans: Evaluation starts with a careful history about onset, progression, interventions and surgical procedures done. In patients with sufficient volume of voided urine, a carefully maintained bladder diary provides invaluable information about the bladder. It forms a baseline for urodynamic assessment. In anuric patients, history of voiding pattern can provide some hint regarding possible bladder dynamics. A careful physical examination gives details about previous surgical scars and stomas. If available, previous surgical details prepare the surgeon to avoid any unpleasant surprises.[23]

Uroflowmetry with PVRU is the non-invasive way for preliminary assessment of bladder function.[24] Careful analysis of tracing can give hint regarding possible underactive detrusor or outlet obstruction. Urine culture is to be done prior to any invasive investigation and before scheduling transplant surgery.

If history is suggestive of urethral trauma/traumatic catheterisation, RGU + MCU can provide information regarding possible urethral stricture, status of bladder neck and posterior urethra, bladder capacity, diverticula, postvoid residue and vesicoureteric reflux.

Video-urodynamic study is the ideal test to study lower urinary tract. However, this facility is very rare, at least in Indian subcontinent. Urodynamic study along with MCU is an acceptable alternative.[8]

2. **How will you stabilise lower tract in a case of neuropathic voiding disorder?**

Based on urodynamic study findings, management can be planned:

1. *High capacity normal compliance urinary bladder with underactive detrusor*: Patient will require CIC to maintain upper tract. A Mitrofanoff appendico-vesicostomy is a useful adjunct to ensure good compliance and has been proven in various series. If appendix is not available, catheterisable stoma can be configured from ileum (Yang-Monti's catheterisable stoma).[8,25]

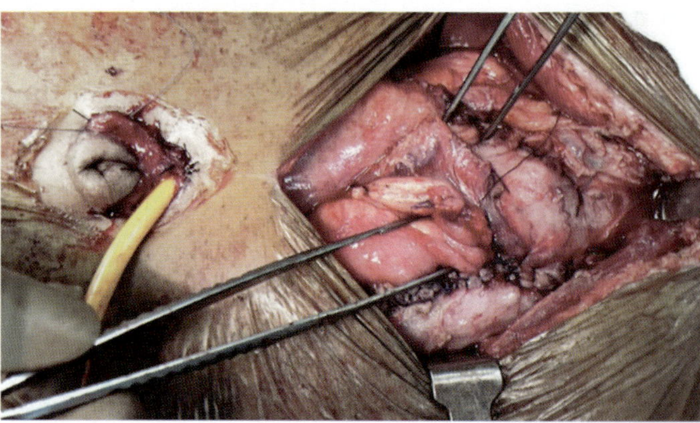

Fig. 6.5: Augmentation enterocystoplasty with catheterisable Yang-Monti's catheterisable stoma in periumbilical region

2. *Normal or high capacity bladder with poor compliance*: Anticholinergic medications should be tried.

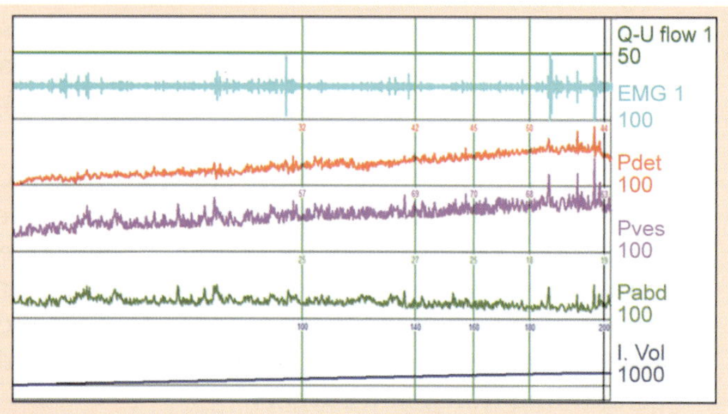

Fig. 6.6: Urodynamic tracing showing poor compliance

3. *Overactive detrusor*: Anticholinergic medications are the first line therapy. Various pharmacological options are commercially available and can be tailored according to each patient's tolerability. A combination of antimuscarinic drugs and β adrenoreceptor agonists can be used with advantage of reduced adverse effects. In recalcitrant cases, intravesical Botox® injection can be used. Botox® had disadvantages of possibility of detrusor paralysis, requiring CIC. Also, Botox® needs to be re-injected every 6–8 months.
4. *Low capacity poor compliance urinary bladder*. A bladder capacity of less than 100 ml or voiding pressure of more than 100 cm H_2O is hazardous for upper tract safety. Transplanting kidney into such bladder is doomed to fail. Pharmacological management is unlikely to succeed. The best management option is bladder augmentation.[12]
5. *Low detrusor leak point pressure–urinary incontinence*. This is the other end of the spectrum. Post-transplant, urinary incontinence presents as a major quality of life issue. Artificial urinary sphincter is considered to be the treatment of choice and should be placed prior to transplantation.[26–28] However, affordability is a major issue in our part of the world. In such case, bladder neck closure with Mitrofanoff appendicovesicostomy is a reasonable alternative.

3. What is the optimal time for bladder augmentation?

Ans: Regarding timing of bladder augmentation with respect to kidney transplantation, there are two schools of thoughts:

a. Before renal transplantation:
   i. *Advantages:* Patient not on immunosuppressants, less risk of infection, better wound healing.
   ii. *Disadvantages:* In anuric patients, dry cystoplasty—accumulation of mucous plugs which is a nidus for infection.[29]

b. After renal transplantation:
   i. *Advantages:* No dry cystoplasty
   ii. *Disadvantages:* Risk of graft dysfunction till augmentation is done, higher rate of wound infection and delayed wound healing.[11–14]

4. How will you manage dry enterocystoplasty?

Ans: Most centres who are doing pre-transplant enterocystoplasty in anuric patients start with "recycling regimen". The augmented bladder is filled with 300 ml of normal saline solution twice daily to maintain adequate bladder volume. This also aids to remove enteric secretions, that can accumulate and become a source of infection or obstruction.[30]

In contemporary times, distal ileum or sigmoid colon are the most favoured intestinal segments to be used for augmentation. Gastrocystoplasty has advantages of being less permeable to urinary solutes, less secretion of chloride and less mucous secretion; however, is not favoured by many surgeons now.[29]

Most of the surgeons prefer doing modified Lich-Gregoir ureteroneocystostomy with native-bladder wall in cases of augmented bladder. In cases of having too small native bladder wall, graft ureter can be anastomosed with enteric wall of augmented bladder also. With careful dissection, mucosal tunnel can be made here.

5. How will you manage a case of renal transplant with augmented enterocystoplasty (augmented bladder)?

Ans: Any patient with augmented enterocystoplasty is predisposed to higher rate of UTI and pyelonephritis. Kidney transplant recipients are no different. Multiple series have confirmed higher rate of asymptomatic bacteriuria, symptomatic UTI as well as graft pyelonephritis in patients with augmented urinary bladder as compared with normal urinary tracts. However, no significant differences between graft outcomes have been found between the two cohorts.

These patients require rigorous follow-up with close watch on renal profile. Patients on CIC are constantly motivated for compliance as well as proper technique. Any deterioration in renal profile warrants detailed work up, including urine culture, upper tract (graft kidney) imaging and uroflowmetry + PVRU (in self-voiding patients). In series from Indian subcontinent, incidence of UTI in patients doing CIC is much higher than compared to publications from developed world. The reason ascribed was less than optimum level of hygiene in these countries. The authors have emphasised on rigorous follow-up and timely treatment for optimal graft survival.[31,11]

Vesico-Ureteric Reflux (VUR)

Case Scenario 4

During evaluation of 2-year-old male child for single episode of febrile UTI, B/L grade III VUR was diagnosed. After detailed discussion, he was started on low dose suppressive antibiotic prophylaxis, and did not suffer from any other febrile UTI episode. He was kept on regular follow-up for next 5 years, thereafter, he was lost to follow-up. Now, at 24 years of age, he has presented with incidentally detected high creatinine levels.

VUR can be primary or secondary. Secondary VUR is managed by treating the primary cause (e.g. PUV, neuropathic voiding disorders) and in these cases, peri-transplant management is done for primary disorder.[32]

In primary VUR, low grades are usually followed expectantly. If there is no evidence of UTI, no active urological intervention is advocated. It is the high grade VURs which are of concern. Recent literature suggests that high grade VURs are associated with renal hypoplasia or dysplasia. Cochrane review has questioned the benefit of antibiotic prophylaxis for VUR associated recurrent UTI.[33] Another study did not find any benefit of surgical correction over antibiotic prophylaxis.[34]

1. **What is the role of native nephrectomy in a case of primary VUR prior to renal transplantation?**

   Ans: During evaluation of patients with primary VUR for transplant, it is important to decide regarding need for native nephrectomy. In absence of recurrent culture proven UTI, native nephrectomy

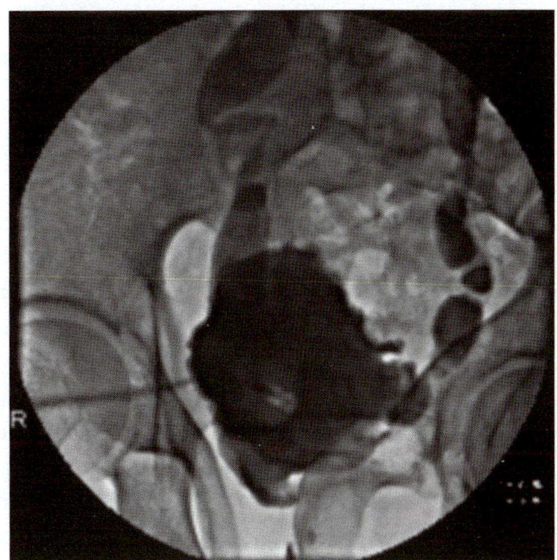

Fig. 6.7: MCU in a case of neurogenic bladder showing B/L VUR grade 5 (secondary VUR)

does not add any advantage. The indications for pre-transplant native nephrectomy are:
1. Recurrent upper tract infections
2. Uncontrolled hypertension
3. Nephrotic syndrome with massive protein loss

In post-operative period, native nephrectomy should be considered only if the patient is suffering from recurrent UTI and no other source is identified.[16]

Genitourinary Tuberculosis with Thimble Bladder

Case Scenario 5

A 43-year-old female presented with extreme urinary frequency, dysuria, intermittent haematuria with clots, loss of weight and appetite and low-grade fever. On evaluation, she was anaemic, with deranged renal functions, and sterile pyuria. USG revealed left-sided pyonephrosis and right-sided hydroureteronephrosis. She could not hold urine, bladder could not be properly assessed.

India holds the dubious distinction of having the largest number of tuberculosis cases in the world. Extrapulmonary tuberculosis accounts for 20–25% of total disease burden; out of which, genitourinary tuberculosis accounts for four percent. Signs and symptoms of GUTB are often masked, usually like UTI, leading to delayed diagnosis. Kidney is the primary organ affected and other organs are involved by direct extension. Neglect casts a huge toll on genitourinary system with destruction of kidneys, extensive scarring/stricture formation of ureters leading to CKD. *Mycobacterium spp* causes patchy cystitis, ultimately leading to healing by fibrosis, leading to bladder contracture.

1. **What is tubercular urinary bladder?**

   Ans: Tubercular bladder is characterised by two types of lesions

   1. Active infection causes reduction in capacity of bladder to 150–200 ml. Timely anti-tubercular therapy (ATT) is often successful in preventing disease progression and restoring bladder capacity to a large extent.
   2. Structural bladder contracture—cicatrisation happens, leading to bladder permanently losing its capacity and reservoir function. ATT is not helpful in restoration; patient will need surgical intervention to restore low pressure normal capacity reservoir.
      a. Small capacity poor compliance bladder wherein dome has contracted, but trigone and bladder neck are relatively spared—augmentation cystoplasty
      b. Tubercular thimble bladder, wherein bladder has shrunken to very small size (reduced elasticity and compliance)—consider for orthotopic neobladder or ileal conduit.

2. **What is the optimal time for lower tract reconstruction in a case of GUTB?**

   Ans: In all cases of GUTB, at least four weeks of ATT is required to take care of active infection, reduce infective potential and stabilise patients.[35]

   The bladder should be reconstructed before transplant surgery. In case of anuric patients, bladder recycling should be instituted with normal saline solution, twice daily (as discussed above)

   In case of very small, scarred, friable urinary bladder, it may be difficult to augment urinary bladder. Another option is ileal conduit, into which transplant kidney ureter can be implanted.[36]

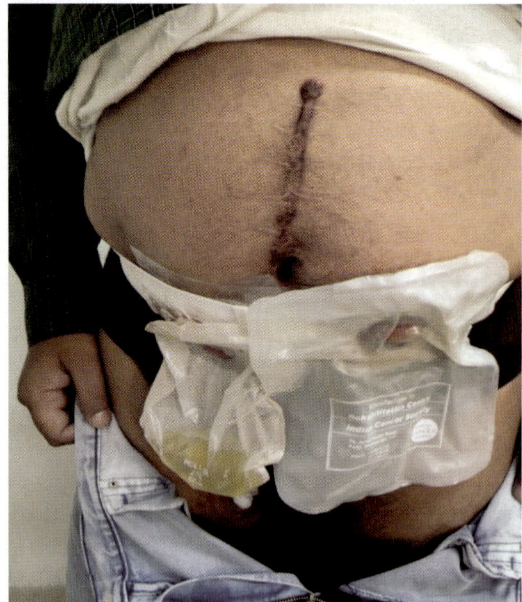

Fig. 6.8: Transplant in a case of ileal conduit

Benign Prostatic Hyperplasia (BPH)

Case Scenario 6

A 63-year-old diabetic male has come for evaluation for renal transplantation. Currently he is dialysis dependent and is anuric. Prior to dialysis, he had moderate severity LUTS and was not very satisfied with medical management. On evaluation, USG revealed estimated prostatic weight of 76 gm. What will be your plan for management of LUTS?

1. **Is there any association between BPH and CKD?**

   Ans: Incidence of both BPH and CKD increases with age. In some cases, bladder outlet obstruction (BOO) can lead to obstructive nephropathy.[37] The size of prostate gland has got no correlation with severity of symptoms or urodynamic study proven BOO.

2. **How to evaluate ESRD patient for BPH?**

   Ans: In non-oliguric patients, LUTS can be evaluated as in other patients. However, high index of suspicion should be there in oliguric patients, when LUTS can be masked. This subset of patients is gradually increasing in number as more and more elderly patients are being accepted for renal transplant. Patients should be carefully interrogated for any evidence of LUTS prior to progressing to oliguric/anuric stage. A careful clinical examination, and relevant investigations like USG, cystoscopy, etc. should be done for proper assessment.[38,39]

3. **In ESRD patient, what are the deciding factors for management of BPH?**

   In a diagnosed ESRD patient, management of BPH is dependent upon the following factors:

   1. Severity or bothersome of LUTS (in non-anuric patients)
   2. Size of the gland
   3. UTI—active or recurrent
   4. BPH-induced complications
   5. Tolerability to pharmacotherapy

   There have been concerns regarding higher complication rates in CKD/ESRD patients. At the same time, the lower tract should be stable enough before transplantation to manage post-transplant diuresis. Post-transplant surgery also carries risk of infection in immunocompromised patients, justifying pre-transplant procedure.[38–40]

In non-oliguric patients, surgical intervention can be planned as per standard treatment guidelines.

1. Size of the gland to decide appropriate surgical modality—TURP (monopolar/bipolar) vs HoLEP (or any other LASER) vs open/robot assisted simple prostatectomy
2. Recurrent UTI
3. Recurrent haematuria
4. Vesical calculi
5. LUTS refractory to pharmacotherapy

The patients should be optimized prior to surgery with pre-procedure dialysis.

In oliguric patients, there have been concerns regarding formation of post-operative bladder neck contracture. This can be mitigated by planning the surgery approximately 6 weeks prior to kidney transplantation.[38,39]

Stricture Urethra

Case Scenario 7

A 56-year-old male ESRD patient presented for evaluation for transplantation. He had history of RTA with prolonged catheterisation, and history of analgesic abuse. Currently he is anuric, and does not give any specific history for bothersome LUTS.

1. **How will you evaluate ESRD patient with suspicion of urethral stricture?**

   Ans: Stricture urethra can be diagnosed during workup for renal transplantation. In non-anuric patients, careful history regarding LUTS can indicate presence of outflow obstruction. Standard workup includes uroflowmetry and RGU + MCU under antibiotic cover. In anuric patients, history about LUTS should be elicited for pre-anuric phase and in case of suspicion, RGU + MCU should be performed.[38,39]

   Rarely, in patients with neglected stricture, obstructive uropathy can develop and proceed to ESRD. These patients are usually non-oliguric and standard workup should be done to characterise stricture.

2. **How will you manage stricture urethra in a case of ESRD patient scheduled for transplantation?**

   Ans: Urethroplasty should be preferred over optical internal urethrotomy (except in case of flimsy short segment stricture) for

   1. Higher success rates
   2. No need for regular self-calibration and thus, reduced risk of UTI.

   Appropriate urethroplasty technique should be utilized to manage stricture prior to proceeding for renal transplantation, thereby stabilising lower urinary tract.

3. **What is the optimal time for urethroplasty in a case of ESRD patient?**

   Ans: Preferably, urethroplasty should be done 6 weeks prior to transplantation.[38,39]

Overactive Bladder (OAB)

Case Scenario 8

A 38-year-old female ESRD patient presented for evaluation for pre-emptive renal transplant. She has history of bothersome urinary frequency with urgency. Physical examination was normal and urinalysis/urine culture were normal. Uroflowmetry was normal.

1. **What is the differential diagnosis for high urinary frequency in a young, neurologically intact patient?**

   Ans: Detailed history should be taken to evaluate OAB, any possible treatable factors and its overall impact on quality of life of the patient. In anuric patients, history of pre-anuric phase is to be elicited.[40]

   It is important to rule out the following conditions

   1. Urinary tract infection
   2. Contracted small capacity bladder
   3. High postvoid residue
   4. Bladder pain syndrome or interstitial cystitis
   5. Carcinoma *in situ*

   Complete urinalysis and culture, ultrasound of kidney–ureter–bladder (USG–KUB) region, diagnostic cystoscopy and urodynamic studies should be conducted for proper evaluation prior to transplant. If required, urine for cytology and bladder biopsy should be ordered.

   If the patient is polyuric, symptoms can get relieved post-successful transplant surgery. In other cases, standard line of management is followed as discussed previously in neurogenic bladder condition.

   1. Antimuscarinics and beta-adrenergic agonists
   2. Botulinum toxin
   3. Neuromodulation
   4. Bladder augmentation[41]

Detrusor Underactivity (DUA)

Case Scenario 9

A 53-year-old diabetic female presented for evaluation for pre-emptive renal transplantation. She has history of rectosigmoid carcinoma 10 years back, for which she had undergone low anterior resection and chemoradiation. Her malignancy is under control. During evaluation, she was found to have chronic urinary retention.

1. **What are the possible etiological factors for DUA?**
   Ans: Like OAB, detailed history is to be taken to rule out the following conditions
   1. Neurological conditions
   2. Diabetes mellitus—diabetic cystopathy
   3. Bladder outlet obstruction–BPH associated BOO can lead to chronic urinary retention and DUA.
   4. H/o pelvic surgery–during radical surgeries, iatrogenic denervation can lead to DUA
   5. Drug history

   Unlike other lower urinary tract conditions, DUA has got no universally accepted criteria. Urodynamic study is the only acceptable modality for diagnostic evaluation.[42]

2. **How will you manage DUA prior to renal transplantation?**
   Ans: In non-oliguric patients with evidence of prostagomegaly or BOO can be offered transurethral resection of prostate to reduce detrusor leak point pressure and improve voiding. The other defined modalities of treatment are:
   1. Timed voiding
   2. CIC
   3. Neuromodulation[42]

Stress Urinary Incontinence

Case Scenario 10

A 58-year-old diabetic CKD patient underwent HoLEP for bothersome LUTS with high PVRU refractory to medical management. One-year post surgery, he is still totally incontinent. With rising creatinine, he wants to go for pre-emptive renal transplantation.

1. **How will you evaluate SUI in a case of CKD patient?**
   Ans: This is an overt problem in non-oliguric patients; can remain masked in anuric, dialysis dependent patients. It is important to take detailed history in all patients for any previous trauma/surgical intervention which might have damaged external urethral sphincter. A diagnostic cystoscopy is warranted to assess volitional control of sphincter complex.

2. **What is the optimal time for AUS surgery in an ESRD patient?**
   Ans: Artificial urethral sphincter (AUS) can be placed prior to transplant surgery. However, the patient must be counselled regarding higher risk of re-operation in view of CKD. Once the wounds have settled down, patient can proceed for renal transplantation. During peri-operative period, it is important to keep AUS cuff deflated to avoid erosion of urethra due to per-urethral catheter *in situ*.[27,28]

SUMMARY

- Transplant in abnormal bladder can have sub-optimal outcomes, but is not a contraindication anymore.[43]
- Thorough pre-operative assessment and stabilization is of paramount importance for optimal outcomes.
- Pre-operative management involves both medical and surgical options.
- Any surgical intervention should be optimally timed for best outcomes.

REFERENCES

1. Kelly WD, Merkel FK, Markland C. Ileal urinary diversion in conjunction with renal homotransplantation. Lancet 1966;1:222–6.
2. Peters CA, Lorenzo AJ. Urologic considerations in paediatric renal transplantation in Partin AW, Dmochowski RR, Kavoussi LR, Peters CA (ed.) Campbell-Walsh-Wein Urology, 12th ed. 2022, Elsevier Inc. ISBN 9780323546423.
3. Kahokehr AA, Peterson AC. Transplantation and the abnormal bladder in Knechtle SJ, Marson LP, Morris PJ (ed.) Kidney transplantation: Principles and practice, 8th ed. 2020.. Elsevier Inc. ISBN 978-0-323-53186-3.
4. Sullivan ME, Reynard JM, Cranston DW. Renal transplant into the abnormal lower urinary tract. BJU Int. 2003; 92: 510–515.
5. Shukla AR, Srinivasan AK. Posterior Urethral Valve. in Partin AW, Dmochowski RR, Kavoussi LR, Peters CA (ed.) Campbell-Walsh-Wein Urology, 12th ed. 2022, Elsevier Inc. ISBN 9780323546423.
6. Rickard M, Chua ME, Zu'bi F, Dos Santos J, Koyle MA, Lorenzo AJ, Farhat WA. Comparative outcome analysis of pediatric kidney transplant in posterior urethral valves children with or without pretransplant Mitrofanoff procedure. Pediatr Transplant. 2020;00:e13798.
7. Koff SA, Mutabagani KH, Jayanthi VR. The valve bladder syndrome: pathophysiology and treatment with nocturnal bladder emptying. J Urol 2002;167:291e7.
8. Mishra SK, Muthu V, Rajapurkar MM, Desai MR. Kidney transplantation in abnormal bladder. Indian J Urol 2007;23:299–304

9. Kogan SJ, Weiss R, Hanna M, Levitt SB. Successful renal transplantation in a patient with a neurogenic bladder managed by clean intermittent catheterization. J Urol. 1986; 135: 563–565.
10. Gueguen J, Timisit MO, Scemla A, Boutin J-M, Bruyere F, Longuet H, Sberro-Soussan R, Legendre C, Anglicheau D, Büchler M. Outcomes of kidney-transplanted patients with history of intestinal reconstruction of the urinary tract. Outcomes of kidney-transplanted patients with history of intestinal reconstruction of the urinary tract. BJUI Compass. 2022;3(1):75–85.
11. Mohsin R, Hashmi A, Mubarak M, Shehzad A, Sultan G, et al. Renal Transplantation in Patients with Lower Urinary Tract Dysfunction: A Single Centre Experience from a Developing Country. J Transplant Technol Res. 2012; 2:115. doi:10.4172/2161–0991.1000115.
12. Capizzi A, Zanon GF, Zacchello G, Rigamonti W. Kidney transplantation in children with reconstructed bladder. Transplantation 2004; 77: 1113–1116.
13. Franc-Guimond J, González R. Kidney transplantation in children with reconstructed bladder. Transplantation 2004; 77: 1116–1120.
14. Theodorou CH, Kostakis A, Bokos J, Plastiras D, Vosnides G. Lower urinary tract reconstruction in association with renal transplantation. Int Urol Nephrol. 1997; 29: 695–699.
15. Lo'pez Pereira P, Ortiz R, Espinosa L, Martínez Urrutia MJ, Lobato R, Alonzo A, Jaureguíjar E. Does bladder augmentation negatively affect renal transplant outcome in posterior urethral valve patients?, Journal of Pediatric Urology (2014), http://dx.doi.org/10.1016/j.jpurol.2014.01.011.
16. Sharbaf FG, Bitzan M, Szymanski KM, Bell LE, Gupta I, Tchervenkov J, Capolicchio J-P. Native nephrectomy prior to paediatric kidney transplantation: biological and clinical aspects. Pediatr Nephrol. 2012; 27: 1179–1188.
17. Amesty MV, García-Vaz C, Espinosa L, Martínez-Urrutia MJ and López-Pereira P. Long-Term Renal Transplant Outcome in Patients With Posterior Urethral Valves. Prognostic Factors Related to Bladder Dysfunction Management. Front. Pediatr. 2021; 9:646923. doi: 10.3389/fped.2021.646923
18. Yalcinkaya F, Bonthuis M, Erdogan B. D., van Stralen K. J., Baiko S., et al.. Outcomes of renal re-placement therapy in boys with prune belly syndrome: findings from the ESPN/ ERA-EDTA Registry. Pediatric Nephrology, In press, 33 (1), pp.117–124. 10.1007/s00467–017–3770–9 . hal–03101597.
19. Dénes FT, Lopes RI. Prune Belly Syndrome in Partin AW, Dmochowski RR, Kavoussi LR, Peters CA (ed.) Campbell-Walsh-Wein Urology, 12th ed. 2022, Elsevier Inc. ISBN 9780323546423.
20. Lopes RI, Baker LA, Dénes FT. Modern management of and update on prune belly syndrome, J Pediatr Urol. 2021 August; 17(4): 548–554. doi:10.1016/j.jpurol.2021.04.010.
21. Fusaro F, Zanon GF, Ferreli AM, Giuliani S, Zacchello G, Passerini-Glazel G, Rigamonti W. Renal Transplantation in Prune Belly Syndrome. Transpl Int (2004) 17: 549–552.
22. Smith CA, Smith EA, Parrott TS, Broecker BH, Woodard JR. Voiding function in patients with the prune-belly syndrome after Monfort abdominoplasty. J Urol 1998; 159:1675.
23. Barry JM. Kidney transplantation into patients with abnormal bladder. Transplantation 2004; 77: 1120–1123.
24. Cairns HS, Leaker B, Woodhouse CRJ, Rudge CJ, Neild GH. Renal transplantation into abnormal lower urinary tract. The Lancet. 1991; 338: 1376–1379.
25. Neild GH, Dakmish A, Wood S, Nauth-Misir R, Woodhouse CRJ. Renal transplantation in adults with abnormal bladder. Transplantation 2004; 77: 1123–1127.
26. Carlos DM, Antonio MS, Virginia A, Susana R, María JM, Pedro P. Artificial urinary sphincter in congenital neuropathic bladder: Very long-term outcomes. Int J Urol. 2022; 29: 692–697.
27. O'Malley KJ, Hickey DP, Kapoor A, Goldfarb DA, Murphy DM, Flechner SM. Artificial urinary sphincter insertion in renal transplant recipients. Urology. 1999; 54: 923.
28. Thomalla JV, Mitchel ME, Leapman SB, Filo RS. Renal transplantation in a patient with an artificial urinary sphincter device. J Urol. 1988; 139: 573–574.
29. Ashraf Abou-Elela. Augmentation Cystoplasty: in Pretransplant Recipients, Understanding the Complexities of Kidney Transplantation, Prof. Jorge Ortiz (Ed.), 2011; ISBN: 978-953-307-819-9, InTech, Available from: http://www.intechopen.com/books/understanding-the-complexities-of-kidney-transplantation/augmentation-cystoplasty-in-pretransplant-recepients
30. Pozza G, Iafrate M, Mancini M, Silvestre C, Neri F, Furian L, Rigotti P, Geletti TP. Outcome and quality of life of patients with augmented bladder or urinary diversion after kidney transplantation. Archivio Italiano di Urologia e Andrologia. 2020; 92: 286–290
31. Desai P, Yadav R, Chaturvedi S, Maheshwari R, Gulia A, Kumar A. Kidney transplant in patients with abnormal bladder: Experience of tertiary care centre in developing country-Is the outcome same?. Indian J Transplant 2018;12:136–42.
32. Koury AE, Wehbi E. Management strategies for vesicoureteric reflux in Partin AW, Dmochowski RR, Kavoussi LR, Peters CA (ed.) Campbell-Walsh-Wein Urology, 12th ed. 2022, Elsevier Inc. ISBN 9780323546423.
33. Williams G, Hodson EM, Craig JC. Interventions for primary vesicoureteric reflux. Cochrane Database of Systematic Reviews 2019, Issue 2. Art. No.: CD001532. DOI: 10.1002/14651858.CD001532.pub5.
34. Veridiana A, Rodrigo R, Wilson A. Primary Vesicoureteral reflux and chronic kidney disease in pediatric population. What we have learnt? Int Braz J Urol. 2020; 46: 262–8.
35. Gupta NP, Kumar A, Sharma S. Reconstructive bladder surgery in genitourinary tuberculosis. Indian J Urol 2008;24:382–387.
36. Gupta NP, Kumar A, Sharma S. Reconstructive bladder surgery in genitourinary tuberculosis. Indian J Urol 2008;24:382–387.
37. Ricardo Leão, Bruno Jorge Pereira and Hugo Coelho (2012). Benign Prostate Hyperplasia and Chronic Kidney Disease, Chronic Kidney Disease, Prof. Monika Gö z (Ed.), ISBN: 978-953-51-0171-0, InTech, Available from: http://www.intechopen.com/books/chronic-kidney-disease/benign-prostate-hyperplasia-and-chronic-kidney-disease.
38. Kabler RL, Cerny JC. Pre-transplant urologic investigation and treatment of end stage renal disease. J Urol 1983; 129: 475–478.

39. Shenasky-II, JH, Renal transplantation in patients with urologic abnormalities. J Urol 1976; 115: 490–493.
40. Marialaura R, Mariangela M, Daniele M, Arturo C, Paolo B, Fabrizio DM. Patients with renal transplant and moderate-to-severe LUTS benefit from urodynamic evaluation and early transurethral resection of the prostate. World J Urol. 2021; 39: 4397–4044.
41. Reynolds WS. Overactive Bladder in Partin AW, Dmochowski RR, Kavoussi LR, Peters CA (ed.) Campbell-Walsh-Wein Urology, 12th ed. 2022, Elsevier Inc. ISBN 9780323-546423.
42. Chapple CR, Osman NI. The underactive detrusor in Partin AW, Dmochowski RR, Kavoussi LR, Peters CA (ed.) Campbell-Walsh-Wein Urology, 12th ed. 2022, Elsevier Inc. ISBN 9780323546423.
43. Salman B, Hassan A, Sultan S, Tophill P, Halawa A. Renal transplant in abnormal bladder: Long term follow up. Exp and Clin Transplant. 2018; 1: 10–15.

Chapter 7

Liver Disease in Kidney Transplant Recipient

• *Aditya Pradhan*

LEARNING OBJECTIVES

- To have a working knowledge of the assessment and management of both Hepatitis B and C, which are commonly encountered in patients on dialysis.
- To outline prevention, diagnosis and management of liver diseases in a transplant recipient.

1. What is the extent of Hepatitis B and C?

Ans: Hepatitis B virus (HBV) is a hepatotropic DNA virus of which about eight genotypes exist. Hepatitis C virus (HCV) is a single-stranded RNA virus of the Flavivirus family, and six genotypes exist. In India, types 1 and 3 genotypes of HCV are the most prevalent.

About 269 million persons are infected with chronic hepatitis B (CHB) globally, resulting in 820,000 deaths annually. More than 90% of the deaths and disability due to viral hepatitis can be attributed to CHB and chronic hepatitis C (CHC) infections.[1] India falls in the intermediate HBV endemicity group, with a prevalence rate of 2% to 4% in the general population. India harbors 10% to 15% of the global pool of HBV and has 40 million HBV carriers, of whom 15% to 25% develop cirrhosis and complications.[2] The prevalence of HBV seropositivity in dialysis patients is 5% to 13%; the leading causes being the reuse of dialyzers and multidose vials of heparin or injectable iron.[3] Another study quoted the prevalence of HCV among dialysis patients to be very high, 20-80%, and for HBV, between 3.4 and 4.3%.[4]

> In dialysis patients in India, HBV seropositivity is about 5–13%, and HCV positivity is 20–80%.

2. What is the course of HBV and HCV infections?

Ans: HBV infection can result in acute hepatitis, which is often resolved. It is considered chronic when there is evidence of viral positivity and elevated liver transaminase levels after six months. In HCV infection, there is an onset of mild acute disease progressing to chronicity in 85% of the cases.

Chronicity with both HBV and HCV can progress to hepatic cirrhosis and hepatocellular carcinoma.[5] An added risk in dialysis-acquired infections is poor viral clearance due to suppressed cellular and humoral immune status.

> Most hepatitis B infections will resolve without progressing to chronicity. HCV infections present with a mild infection and most progress to chronicity.

3. What is the immunization schedule for preventing HBV and HCV infections?

Ans: One of the most critical aspects in preventing hepatitis B disease in patients on dialysis is immunization and monitoring of anti-HBs antibody levels. Ideally, immunization has to be initiated early and 3–4 doses of vaccination are given for good efficiency. The recommended doses are 40 µg IM at 0, 1, 2, and 6 months with booster doses whenever the anti-HBs antibody falls below 10 IU/ml[6] with a protection rate of 73-92%. HCV has a high mutagenic potential, and hence to date, no effective vaccine is available.

> While effective vaccination is available for HBC, no vaccine is available for HCV

4. What are the serological tests for HBV virus?

Ans: The aims of screening tests are to screen potential donors and recipients for the presence of acute or chronic disease, level of viremia, and risk of transmission and monitor the effects of therapy The commonly used serological tests for HBV and their interpretations are given in Table 7.1.

Measurement of HBV DNA (NAT)

Plasma HBV DNA concentrations are quantified by real-time polymerase chain reaction (PCR) test. This is used for the following information:

a. To correlate with disease progression
b. To differentiate chronic active (HBeAg negative) disease from chronic inactive infection.
c. For decisions to treat and for optimal monitoring of response to antiviral therapy, a rise may indicate the emergence of resistant variants.

For HBV—a combination of serological tests, NAT, and ALT levels are needed for assessing disease activity.

5. What are the tests used for hepatitis C?

Ans: The anti-HCV antibody test is used in conjunction with the HCV NAT test to determine the chronicity of the disease. The anti-HCV test is positive for life. Hence anti-HCV positive, and HCV-NAT test negative indicates past infection. However, if the anti-HCV and HCV-NAT test are positive, this indicates current HCV infection.

HCV quantitative assessments are used for assessing the therapy responses.

6. How the impact of chronicity of HBV and HCV on the liver is assessed?

Ans: There are two types of tests to assess the liver damage:

- Invasive test like liver biopsy
- Non-invasive tests

7. Explain the role of liver biopsy in assessment of liver injury.

Ans: In HBV and HCV infections, liver biopsy is the gold standard for assessing the degree of liver injury, including both inflammatory activity and fibrosis stage. It is also used to confirm hepatocellular carcinoma. In HBV, there is a varying degree of predominantly lymphocytic portal inflammation with interface hepatitis and spotty lobular inflammation. Bridging necrosis and confluent necrosis can be seen. Knodell, Ishak, and METAVIR systems are the histological scoring systems more routinely used to assess the disease activity and treatment response. The METAVIR system, the scores range from F0 (no fibrosis) to F4 (cirrhosis).

There are several disadvantages of liver biopsy: Risk of complications, observer variability in reading the biopsy, and cost. So a biopsy is not used unless the non-invasive tests are inconclusive.

8. What are the non-invasive tests to assess the degree of liver damage?

Ans: Non-invasive tests for the assessment of liver parenchyma:

1. **APRI (AST-to-platelet ratio index) and FIB 4** are recommended as preferred non-invasive tests to evaluate for the presence of cirrhosis (APRI score >2: FIB 4 >3.25 in adults). The variables entered in the FIB-4 are aspartate aminotransferase (AST), alanine aminotransferase (ALT), and platelet (PLT) count.
2. **USG:** This inexpensive bedside assessment can diagnose steatosis (fatty liver), fibrosis parenchymal nodularity, and coexisting hepatocellular Ca. The additional information available includes evidence of portal hypertension, ascites, and the size of the liver. Abdominal ultrasound had a sensitivity of 81% and a specificity of 79% to detect cirrhosis.[8]
3. **Fibroscan (transient elastography):** With this device, a rapid assessment of the degree of fibrosis and amount of fat in the liver parenchyma is assessed non-invasively.[9] Values of shear in the liver are measured as Pascal and range from 2 to 75 kPa. Values of 2 to 7 are normal. With a cut-off value of 17.6 kPa, negative

TABLE 7.1. Screening tests for hepatitis B[7]

Screening test results				
HBsAg	***Anti-HBc***	***Anti-HBs***	***Interpretation***	***Management***
+	+	–	Chronic hepatitis B	Additional testing and management needed
–	+	+	Post-HBV infection, resolved	No further management unless immunocompromised or undergoing chemotherapy or immunosuppressive therapy
–	+	–	Post-HBV infection, resolved or false-positive	HBV DNA testing if immunocompromised patient
–	–	+	Immune	No further testing
–	–	–	Uninfected and not immune	No further testing

and positive predictive values for the diagnosis of cirrhosis were 92% and 91%, respectively.[10]

The corresponding degree of fibrosis is as follows:

a. A fibrosis score of F0 to F1 (2 to 7 kPa) means there is a little or no scarring on the liver.
b. A fibrosis score of F2 (7.5 to 10 kPa) indicates moderate scarring.
c. A fibrosis score of F3 (10 to 14 kPa) indicates severe scarring, which has spread and disrupts normal blood flow.
d. A fibrosis score of F4 (14 kPa or higher) means late-stage scarring or cirrhosis, where the scarring is permanent, and the damage is irreversible.

The fibroscan also measures the degree of steatosis in the liver by the CAP (combined attenuation parameter) score

4. The **upper GI endoscopy** is used to assess the severity of varices and also treat active bleeding varices.
5. **MELD score:** This is a quantitative assessment based on four laboratory parameters to assess the severity of liver failure. Serum creatinine, serum bilirubin, serum sodium and INR value. The score is often used to assess the severity of hepatic failure to allocate deceased donor organs.

> Liver biopsy is uncommonly used in these high-risk patients. Most often, noninvasive tests permit adequate patient assessment of the status of the liver in chronic HBV and HCV infections.

9. What are the risks and benefits of kidney transplant with HBV and HCV infection?

Ans: In both HBV and HCV infections, outcomes of kidney transplantation, both in terms of graft survival and liver disease, are worse compared to non-infected patients.[7] In an immunosuppressed environment, there is increased viral replication and liver damage. The extreme manifestation of this is direct fulminant hepatic toxicity causing fibrosing cholestatic hepatitis which is rarely salvageable.

The post-transplant course in HCV-positive recipients is also complicated by a higher incidence of post-transplant diabetes mellitus (PTDM), *de novo* onset of glomerulopathy, and rejection. Given that in HCV-positive patients, there is a higher incidence of PTDM, there is a need to maintain immunosuppression at the minimum doses needed to prevent rejection. Yet the overall mortality in the transplanted patient is less than maintaining dialysis, and hence transplant is recommended in HCV and HBV-positive patients.

In those patients of ESRD where there is cirrhosis, the patient should be considered for a combined liver–kidney transplant.

10. What is the current status of kidney transplantation from HBV-positive donors?

Ans: Traditionally, transplantation of kidneys from HBsAg+ donors is contraindicated for HBV-recipients. However, it has been found that the risk of donor-derived infection is low in kidney transplantation. If a donor is positive for HBsAg but has anti-HBc antibody and negative NAT for HBV, there is minimal risk of HBV transmission. At the same time, the levels of anti-HBs antibody should be maintained greater than 10 IU/ml in the recipient. These recipients need monitoring and possible lifelong treatment. Still, the recipient should be informed of the potential risk of disease transmission and need for lifelong monitoring.[11] Many reports of successful renal transplants with HBsAg-positive donors to HBsAg–ve recipients with promising outcomes[12] are available. In a known case of HBsAg positive recipient undergoing transplant, treatment is started preoperatively in most and post-transplant continued indefinitely. Pegylated interferon is not used.

> While traditionally, HBsAg positive donors were contra-indicated for renal transplantation to a HBsAg negative recipient; there is now evidence of good outcomes with low-risk donors.

11. What is the current status of kidney transplantation from HCV-positive donors?

Ans: The availability of DAAs active against all genotypes has opened the possibilities of utilizing donors who are known HCV positive status to HCV negative recipients.

The 2013 US PHS guideline recommends that all living donor candidates should be tested for both anti-HCV antibodies and for HCV RNA by NAT, and most centers follow this practice. In those donors who are considered suitable for organ donation, a 12-week duration of DAAs (Directly Acting Antivirals) is used to achieve good reductions in viral load. Major clinical trials have demonstrated the safety, efficacy, and feasibility of using DAAs in treating HCV-uninfected kidney transplant recipients of HCV-infected donors.

All kidney donors should be screened with anti-HCV antibodies and NAT.

The use of HCV-positive donors to negative recipients is increasingly being suggested as a safe procedure with the availability of highly efficient DAAs.

In those recipients with known hepatitis C positive status, DAA therapy is started preoperatively if there is evidence of advanced liver disease or extrahepatic manifestations. In other circumstances, DAA therapy can be started after renal transplantation.[13]

Pathway of management of recipient with HBV or HCV positive status—refer to Appendices B and C.

12. How dual organ failure (simultaneous liver and kidney failure) is dealt?

Ans: Dual organ failure is an uncommon entity. In 2020, 777 combined liver–kidney transplants were performed (OPTN database). Management of these patients is a challenge. There is increased mortality in patients with liver failure with renal failure while waiting on a liver transplant waitlist. Poor results have been noted for liver transplants if the kidney function does not improve after the liver transplant. Simultaneous liver–kidney transplant (SLKT) is presented as a strategy to improve survival. The first successful SLKT was performed by Margreiter *et al* in 1983. SLKT transplants have the advantage of a single surgery for the recipient. The liver also exerts a protective immunological effect on kidneys due to the secretion of soluble HLA antibodies and phagocytosis of reactive antibodies by Kupffer cells.

A clinical dilemma exists when deranged renal function is present in a patient with chronic liver disease (CLD). The concept of hepatorenal syndrome in patients of CLD is well established. Therein, vasoconstriction in the renal vasculature leads to renal impairment in the absence of pathological changes of glomerulopathy. These changes reverse on recovery of hepatic function. However, once chronicity of glomerulopathy is established, then renal dysfunction is irreversible, needing consideration of kidney transplant also. So the main concern remains to determine the reversibility of deranged renal function. The major criteria described for determining irreversibility is the duration of CKD 3 more than three months and pathological changes on renal biopsy (glomerulosclerosis more than 40%, and tubule interstitial fibrosis more than 30% with arteriosclerosis.[14] Often, it is difficult to perform a renal biopsy in liver failure patients due to risks of bleeding. Hence in those situations where a renal biopsy is needed, a transjugular route is used to perform the renal biopsy.

13. What are the indications for considering Simultaneous liver kidney transplant (SLKT)?

Ans: These are broadly considered kidney-pulling liver or liver-pulling kidney.[15]

ESRD: End-stage renal disease; ESLD: End-stage liver disease

A. Patients with ESRD listed for a kidney transplant and have liver disease (kidney-pulling liver)
   1. ESRD patients with liver cirrhosis
   2. ESRD because of hyperoxaluria
   3. Polycystic kidney and liver disease with ESRD
B. Patients with ESLD (cirrhosis and liver failure) listed for a liver transplant, who have the renal disease (liver pulling kidney) [defined by the OPTN criteria[#]]
   1. ESLD with chronic kidney disease
   2. ESLD with acute kidney injury

#The OPTN 2017 criteria[16]

CKD patient criteria GFR 60 ml/min for 3 months with recent GFR 30 ml/min or on hemodialysis

AKI criteria dialysis for >6 weeks GFR ≤ 25 for > six weeks documented every seven days. Combination of the above two criteria and meeting six weeks duration.

14. What is primary hyperoxaluria (PH) and how is it managed?

Most often, the disease presents with a history of multiple stone episodes or early failure of the graft kidney. It results from autosomal recessive genetic alterations in 3 pathways of oxalate synthesis. SLKT provides enzymatic synthesis from the grafted liver to correct the underlying metabolic defect.

The most familiar type is **Type 1**, caused by alanine-glyoxalate aminotransferase deficiency leading to the overproduction of oxalate by LDH acting on glycoxalate. It accounts for ~80% of all PHs, with a prevalence of 1–3 cases per million people. It is the most severe form of the disease, with nearly all patients with PH1 progressing to ESRD.

Type 2 disease is caused by functional loss of GRHPR, encoded by GRHPR gene, which decreases the metabolism of glyoxylate and leads to increased LDH-mediated oxalate synthesis. It causes about 10% of cases which are usually less severe, and ESRD is caused in 20–30% of patients.

PH **type 3** involves functional loss of HOGA1. It is less severe than PH1 and PH2 and tends to present with early symptomatic nephrolithiasis in the first months to years of life. For more details on the evaluation and management of primary hyperoxaluria, the reader is referred to an excellent review on the subject.[17]

In the case of liver failure with end stage renal disease, the transplant strategy is defined strongly by the environment of organ donation. In major parts of America and Europe, dual transplants have been done using cadaver donation. The practice has evolved from sequential transplant (liver transplant followed by kidney transplant) to simultaneous liver–kidney transplant. In many parts of Asia and particularly in India, cadaver donations are not common. In this scenario dealing with dual organ failure with a living donor has to be optimized to accommodate the safety of both donors and recipients.

Most literature on simultaneous liver and kidney transplants arises from cadaver transplant programs. Most of the available data is from large patient databases. Fong Tse Ling *et al* analysed outcomes in cirrhotic patients in renal failure from the OPTN/UNOS database from 2002 to 2008. In the 4275 cases, 2774 were liver transplants alone, and 1501 were SLKT. The SLKT outcomes were superior in graft and patient survival at 5-year follow-up.[18]

A subsequent assessment of the same database presented at the 2017 American Transplant Congress showed the equivalence of Sequential liver–kidney transplantation compared to SLKT.

Another study on SLKT over ten years, from 2004 to 2014, was reported by Lunsford *et al*, from a single center. One hundred forty-five underwent SKLT, and 15 underwent liver transplants alone. They experienced a high graft loss of 20% in the short term, probably a reflection of the poor quality of allocated renal grafts and poor-risk patients.[19]

There is very scarce data on SLKT using living donors in the literature. This data originates from those areas where the cadaver organ donation program is not active, and most transplants are from living donors.

The first approach is using a single living donor for both the liver and kidney grafts, Unek *et al* reported their experience in Turkey with to six patients treated from 2001–2009. Of the recipients, five were of primary hyperoxaluria type 1, and 1 patient had CHB. All the donors were young females (median age 27.5 years). After the hepatectomy and engraftment of the liver graft, the right kidney was harvested and transplanted in the recipient. In one case, a sequential transplant was done kidney first; followed by liver after 11 days later. The mean operative time was 591 min. Three donors needed a blood transfusion, and one patient had prolonged ileus. The mean duration of hospital stay was 11.4. All donors were well on follow-up. The authors concluded that meticulous technique and patient evaluation allowed the procedure to be done safely.[20]

In a study from Taiwan, the authors mention that the rates of cadaver donation are low and allocation of 2 organs to a single recipient rare. So they, too, adopted SLKT from different living donors. 5 SLKT were done with a different living donor. In these 5 cases, two recipients had an average recovery, one patient had hyperacute rejection of renal allograft from presensitisation. 1 case was reexplored for persistent bleeding, and 1 case had biliary stenosis.[21]

A recent retrospective analysis of 2742 patients with living donors was reported. In this cohort, 47 patients of CKD 3 to 5 were assessed, wherein 1 group of 25 underwent liver transplant alone (LTA), and the other group of 22 underwent SLKT. Survival was similar at 1, 3, and 12 months, respectively. At the end of the study period, 57% of patients who survived in LTA groups had stabilized renal function (creatinine = 1.8 ± 0.6 mg/d). The authors concluded that LTA alone was not inferior to SLKT in cirrhotic patients.[22]

Based on our experience in the field of SLKT with two different living donors, herein are presented some of the steps followed in our center.

Donor Evaluation and Counselling

The counselling of these patients includes a discussion of deferring the kidney transplant in case of unforeseen situations intraoperatively, like excessive bleeding causing hemodynamic instability during the native liver hepatectomy and engraftment stage. In such situations, it may be prudent to defer donor nephrectomy and kidney transplant till the patient is stabilized. There may be a need for CRRT in the interim period.

All liver donors were blood group compatible with a Graft Recipient Weight Ratio (GRWR) of at least 0.8. As a part of work up donors underwent CT angiography (triple phase) with volumetry, MRCP, and MR fat fraction. The minimally accepted remnant in the donor was 30%. Donors were accepted for hepatectomy if the total liver fat fraction was less than 10%. The decision to implant the right or left lobe was made on GRWR, hepatic venous anatomy, and remnant liver.

All kidney donors were blood group and crossmatch compatible.

In patients of primary hyperoxaluria awaiting transplant, the oxalate levels are monitored, and patients were managed with high flux dialysis daily in the 7 days pre-transplant (until oxalate levels were less than 20 µmol/L).

Two days before surgery, all the patients are started on Tacrolimus 1 mg twice a day and Mycophenolate Mofetil 360 mg twice daily. Postoperatively, Tacrolimus level was maintained around 8–10 ng/ml in the initial 4–5 months and then maintained at 6–8 ng/ml (lower levels than for conventional kidney transplant surgery). Steroids are tapered gradually and eventually stop over one year.

Surgery

The liver transplant was started traditionally. After confirming hepatic artery anastomosis patency with a Doppler study, in the adjacent theatre, donor nephrectomy was started. The kidney graft was implanted in the right or left iliac fossa in the standard fashion.

The abdominal incision was closed routinely. We, however, avoided using right-sided drains in recipients, and both subhepatic and left paracaval drains were inserted from the left side (Figs 7.1 to 7.6).

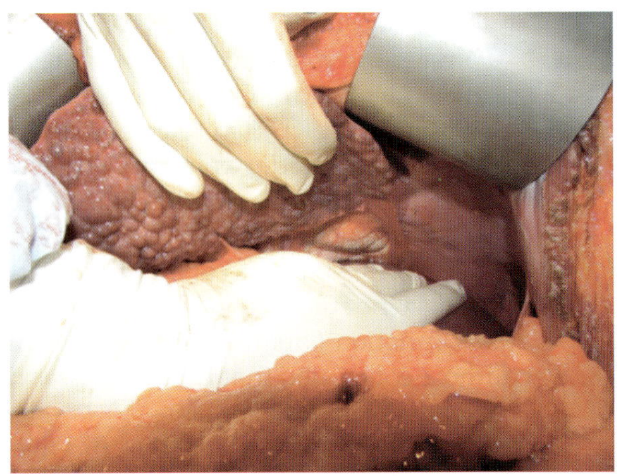

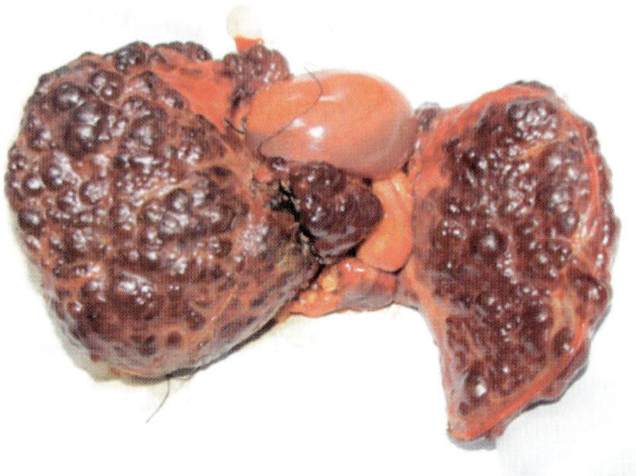

Fig. 7.1: Recipient hepatectomy

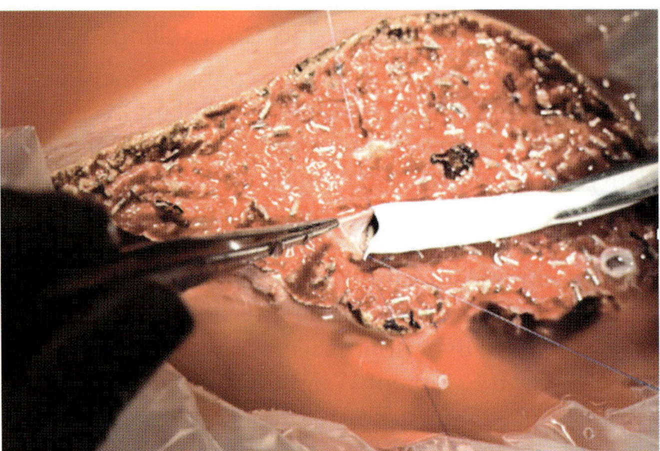

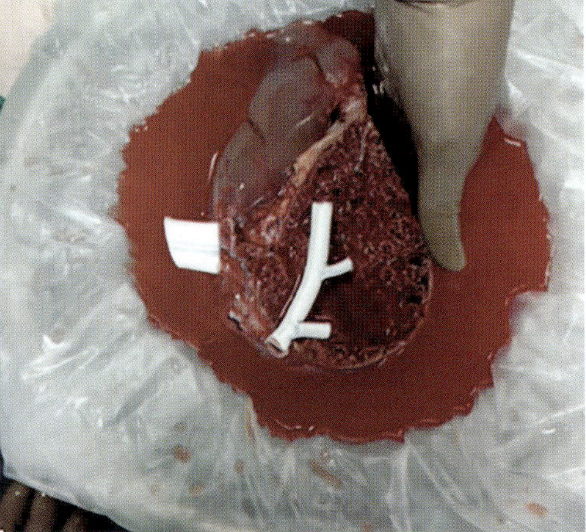

Fig. 7.2: Bench reconstruction of portal vein

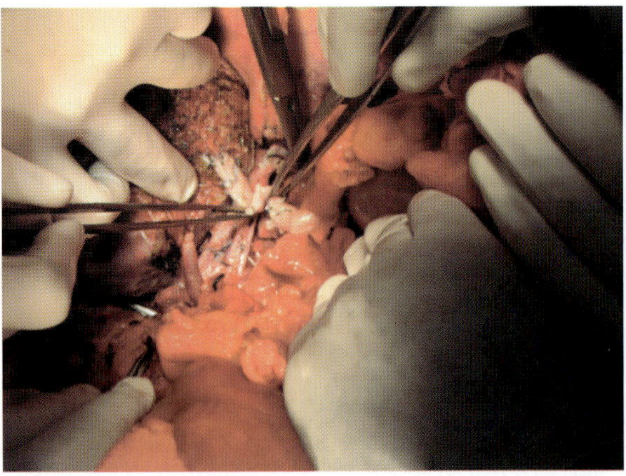

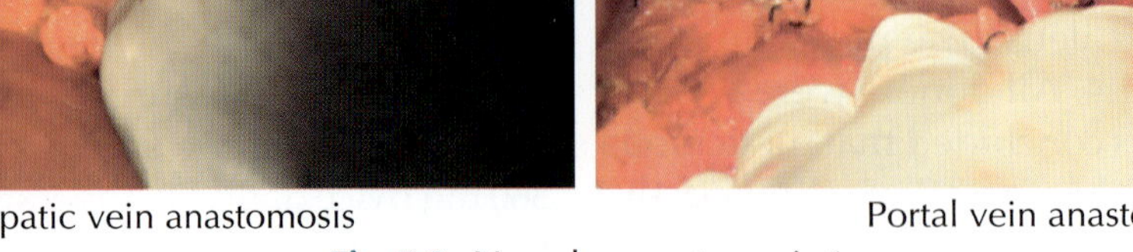

Hepatic vein anastomosis

Portal vein anastomosis

Fig. 7.3: Vascular anastomosis 1

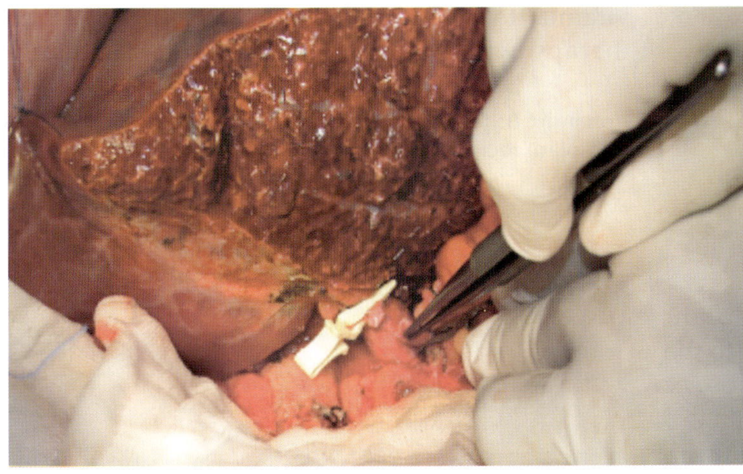

Hepatic artery anastomosis

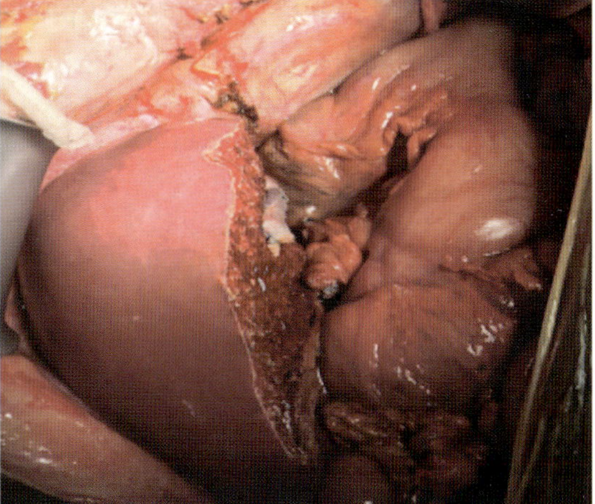

Bile duct anastomosis

Fig. 7.4: Completion of anastomosis

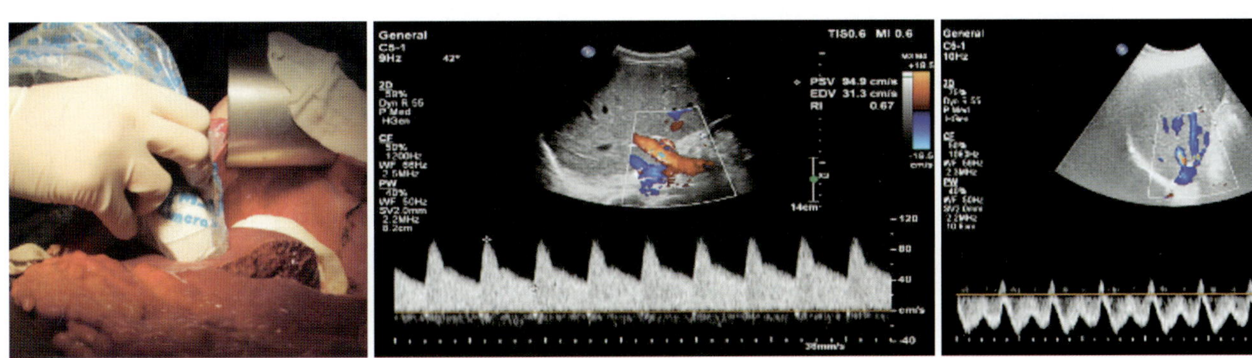

Fig. 7.5: Doppler confirmation of anastomotic patency

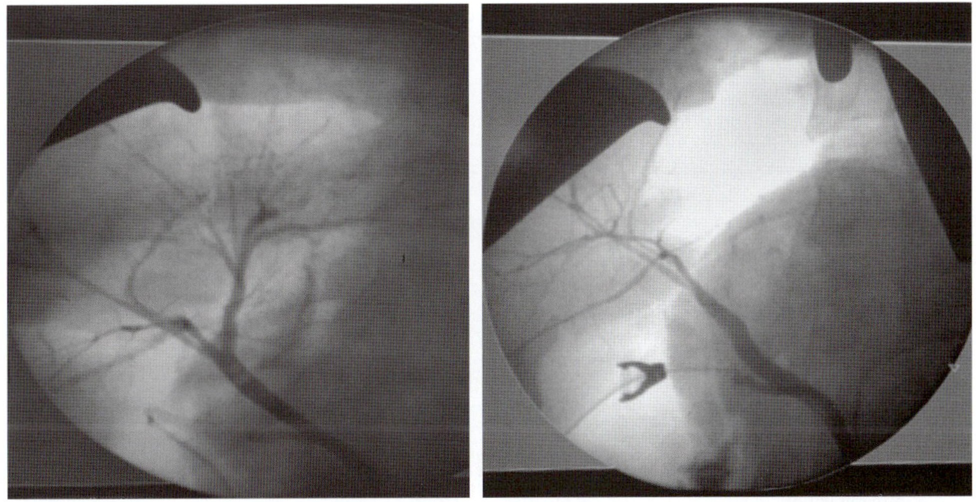

Fig. 7.6: Completion cholangiogram

(*Operative images courtesy:* Dr Abhideep Chowdhary, BLK-Max Superspeciality Hospital, New Delhi)

Appendix A: Drug Therapy for Hepatitis B [Nucleotide/Nucleoside analogues (NAs)]

Though eight genotypes exist of the hepatitis B virus, treatment is not genotype-specific. The earlier agents, Lamivudine and Adefovir, are less commonly used now due to the common occurrence of resistance. The main agents used today are the NAs: Entecavir and Tenofovir.[23]

	Drug	Dose
1	Tenofovir disoproxil fumarate (TDF)	300 mg once daily
2	Entecavir (adult with compensated liver disease and lamivaudine naive)	0.5 mg once daily
3	Entecavir (adult with decompensated liver disease)	1 mg once daily
4	Tenofavir alafenamide fumarate (TAF)	25 mg once daily

TAF is preferred to TDF in renal transplant recipients due to lower nephrotoxicity. Due to the success of NA therapy in these patients, the use of HBIg has almost entirely been abandoned.[24]

Treatment is continued indefinitely, especially in cirrhosis. Cessation can result in decompensation of the liver with virus reactivation.

Drug Therapy for Hepatitis C: Directly Acting Antiviral (DAA) Therapy

Therapy of hepatitis C has evolved today from interferon therapy (which boosts the immune system response to viremia) to DAA drug combination therapy. Interferon therapy was of extended duration (48 weeks), with

Appendix B: Flowchart of management of HBsAg positive kidney transplant recipient

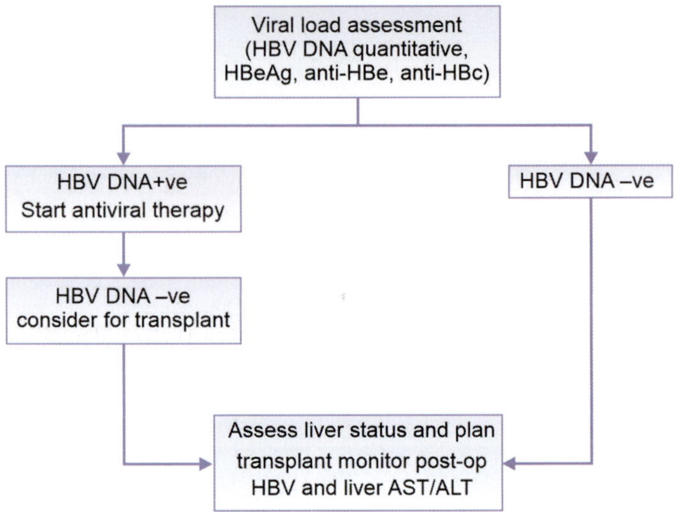

Appendix C: Flowchart for the recipient with HCV

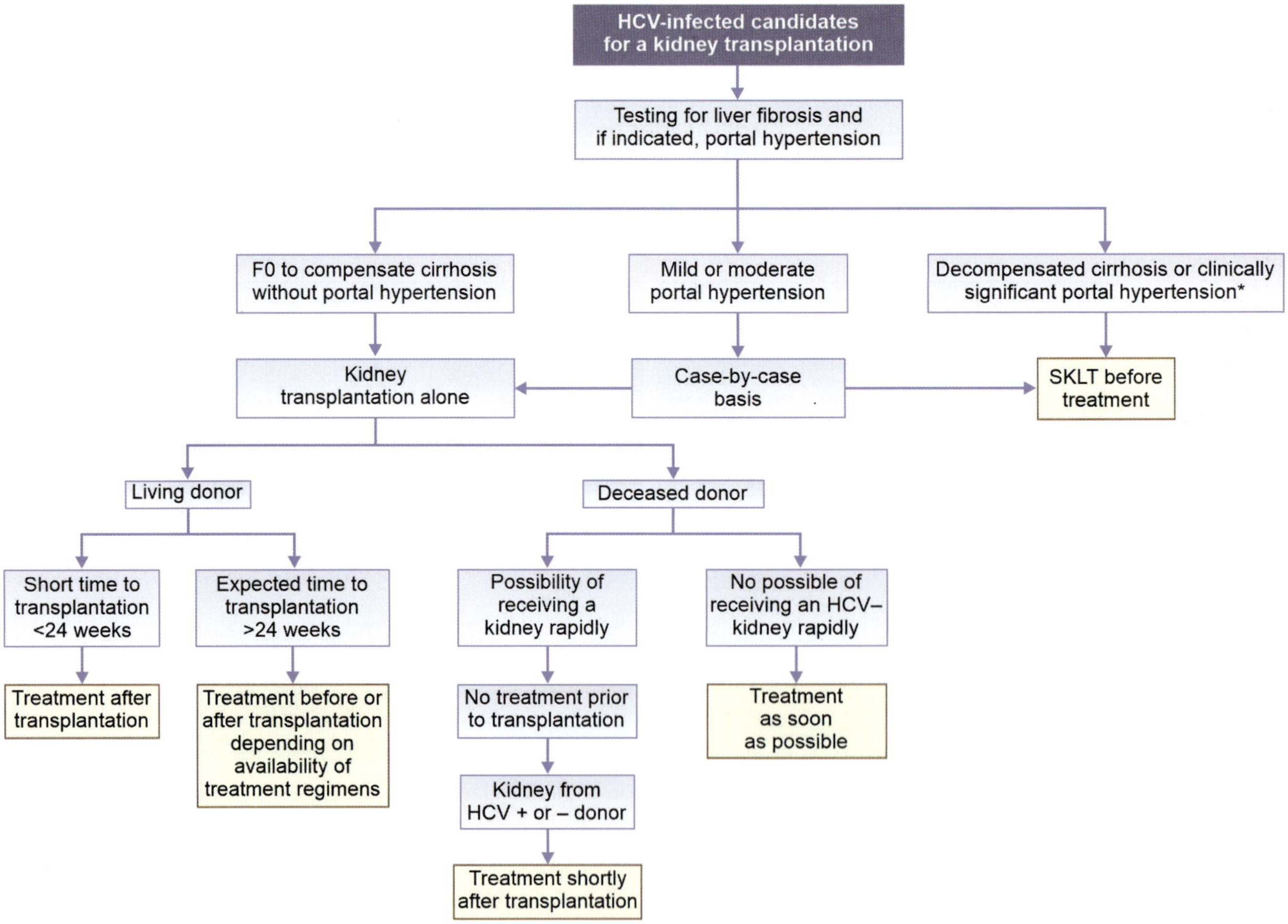

HCV-infected candidates for a kidney transplantation

Testing for liver fibrosis and if indicated, portal hypertension

F0 to compensate cirrhosis without portal hypertension

Mild or moderate portal hypertension

Decompensated cirrhosis or clinically significant portal hypertension*

Kidney transplantation alone

Case-by-case basis

SKLT before treatment

Living donor

Deceased donor

Short time to transplantation <24 weeks

Expected time to transplantation >24 weeks

Possibility of receiving a kidney rapidly

No possible of receiving an HCV– kidney rapidly

Treatment after transplantation

Treatment before or after transplantation depending on availability of treatment regimens

No treatment prior to transplantation

Treatment as soon as possible

Kidney from HCV + or – donor

Treatment shortly after transplantation

Proposed management strategy in a hepatitis C virus (HCV)—infected kidney transplant candidate. *Clinically significant portal hypertension is defined as hepatic venous pressure gradient >or =10 mm Hg or evidence of portal hypertension on imaging or exam, e.g. ascites, esophageal varices, collaterals on imaging. F0, no scarring or fibrosis; SKLT, simultaneous kidney–liver transplantation.

multiple side effects and high costs, and so fell into disrepute. In comparison, DAA therapy is highly effective, 95–98%, in oral therapy of shorter duration (12 weeks). The outcomes are measured in terms of sustained viral response (SVR 12—undetectable virus at 12 weeks).

There are three classes of DAAs presently.

a. NS3/4A protease inhibitors: Voxilaprevir, Glecaprevir, Simrpervir, Ombitasvir, Telapravir
   Due to the common occurrence of viral resistance, these agents are used only as part of combination therapy.
b. NS5A polymerase inhibitors: Ledipasvir, Velpatasvir, Pibrentasvir, Daclatasvir, Pibrentasvir.
c. NS5B polymerase inhibitors: Sofosbuvir, Dasabuvir.
   Commonly used pan-genotypic therapy, combination therapy available in India is as follows:
   i. Sofosbuvir 400 mg + Velapatasvir 100 mg
   ii. Sofosbuvir 400 mg + Daclatasvir 60 mg

The reader is referred to the recent update on HCV management in kidney transplant patients.[25]

SUMMARY

- In dialysis patients in India, HBV seropositivity is about 5–13%, and HCV positivity is 20–80%.
- Most hepatitis B infections will resolve without progressing to chronicity. HCV infections present with a mild infection and most progress to chronicity
- While effective vaccination is available for HBC, no vaccine is available for HCV
- For HBV—a combination of serological tests, NAT, and ALT levels are needed for assessing disease activity.
- For HCV—a combination of anti-HCV antibody, HCV–NAT and quantitative assessment is used for screening, diagnosis and response to therapy respectively.
- Non-invasive tests permit adequate patient assessment of the status of the liver in chronic HBV and HCV. Liver biopsy, though gold standard, is not routinely required. It is reserved for patients in whom the non-invasive tests are inconclusive.
- While traditionally, HBsAg positive donors were contraindicated for renal transplantation to a HBsAg negative recipient; there is now evidence of good outcomes with low-risk donors.
- The use of HCV-positive donors to negative recipients is increasingly being suggested as a safe procedure with the availability of highly efficient DAAs.
- Determination of reversibility of deranged renal function in a case of CLD poses a clinical dilemma; SLK is the option if CKD3 persists for more than 3 months and/or evidence of chronic changes on renal biopsy (preferably done through transjugular route).
- Primary hyperoxaluria (PH) is a disease of liver, wherein there is deficiency of enzymes involved on oxalate synthesis. Kidney failure occurs in childhood especially in type 1. These patients are candidate for SLK. SLK provides enzymatic synthesis from the grafted liver to correct the underlying metabolic defect.
- SLK is a practical challenge in a country like India, where still more than 90% of transplants are living-related. In this scenario dealing with dual organ failure with living donors has to be optimized to accommodate the safety of both donors and recipients.

REFERENCES

1. WHO... H. B. factsheet, "https://www.who.int/news-room/fact-sheets/detail/hepatitis-b.," 25 Mar 2023.
2. Tandon BN, Acharya SK, Tandon A "Epidemiology of hepatitis B virus infection in India.," Gut, vol. 38 (Suppl 2), pp. 56–59, 1996.
3. Premkumar M, Chawla Y "Chronic Hepatitis B: Challenges and Successes in India," Clin Liver Dis (Hoboken), vol. 18, pp. 111–116, 2021.
4. Perumal A, P. Ratnam, S. Nair, P. Anitha and V. Illangovan, "Seroprevalence of hepatitis B and C in patients on hemodialysis and their antibody response to hepatitis B vaccination," J Curr Res Sci Med, vol. 2, pp. 20–23, 2016.
5. Ringehan M, Mckeating JA, Protzer U, "Viral hepatitis and liver cancer," Philos Trans R Soc Lond B Biol Sci, vol. 1372, p. 20160274, 2017.
6. Prasasd N, Chaudhuri et. al, "Indian Society of Nephrology Guidelines for Vaccination in Chronic Kidney Disease, " Ind J Nephr, Vols. Vol 26, Supplement 1, p. s15, 2016.
7. Varughese S. Kidney transplantation–Principles and practice. Indian J Med Res. 2020 Dec;152(6):668–9. doi: 10.4103/ijmr.IJMR_2854_20. PMCID: PMC8224148.Page Number: 511–536.
8. Richard P, Bonniaud P, Barthélémy C, Etaix JP, Veyret C, Audigier JC, Fraisse H. Valeur de l'ultrasonographie dans le diagnostic des cirrhoses. Etude prospective de 128 patients [Value of ultrasonography in the diagnosis of cirrhoses. Prospective study of 128 patients]. J Radiol. 1985 Aug-Sep;66(8–9):503–6. French. PMID: 3912496.
9. Wilder J, Patel K. The clinical utility of FibroScan(®) as a noninvasive diagnostic test for liver disease. Med Devices (Auckl). 2014 May 3;7:107–14. doi: 10.2147/MDER.S46943. PMID: 24833926; PMCID: PMC4014361.
10. Foucher J, Chanteloup E, Vergniol J, Castéra L, Le Bail B, Adhoute X, Bertet J, Couzigou P, de Lédinghen V. Diagnosis of cirrhosis by transient elastography (FibroScan): a prospective study. Gut. 2006 Mar;55(3):403–8. doi: 10.1136/gut.2005.069153. Epub 2005 Jul 14. PMID: 16020491; PMCID: PMC1856085.
11. Kidney disease: improving global outcomes (KDIGO) Living kidney Donor World Group. KDIGO Clinical Practice Guidelines on the Evaluation and Care of Living Kidney Donors. Transplantation; 2017.vol.101, suppl. 8S; Pages S1–S109.
12. Srisuwarn P, Sumethkul V. Kidney transplant from donors with hepatitis B: A challenging treatment option. World J Hepatol. 2021 Aug 27;13(8):853–867. doi: 10.4254/wjh.v13.i8.853. PMID: 34552692; PMCID: PMC8422915.
13. Te H, Doucette K. Viral hepatitis: Guidelines by the American Society of Transplantation Infectious Disease Community of Practice. Clin Transplant. 2019 Sep;33(9):e13514. doi: 10.1111/ctr.13514. Epub 2019 Apr 14. PMID: 30817047.
14. Tanriover B, Mejia A, Weinstein J, Foster SV, Ghalib R, Mubarak A, Cheng SS. Analysis of kidney function and biopsy results in liver failure patients with renal dysfunction: a new look to combined liver kidney allocation in the post-MELD era. Transplantation. 2008 Dec 15;86(11):1548–53. doi: 10.1097/TP.0b013e31818b22cc. PMID: 19077888.

15. Singal AK, Ong S, Satapathy SK, Kamath PS, Wiesner RH. Simultaneous liver kidney transplantation. Transpl Int. 2019 Apr;32(4):343–352. doi: 10.1111/tri.13388. Epub 2019 Feb 21. PMID: 30548094.
16. Boyle G, Simultaneous Liver Kidney (SLK) Allocation Policy.2020. https://optn.transplant.hrsa.gov/media/1192/0815–12_SLK_Allocation.pdf.
17. Shee K, Stoller ML. Perspectives in primary hyperoxaluria-historical, current and future clinical interventions. Nat Rev Urol. 2022 Mar;19(3):137–146. doi: 10.1038/s41585–021–00543–4. Epub 2021 Dec 8. PMID: 34880452; PMCID: PMC8652378.
18. Fong TL, Khemichian S, Shah T, Hutchinson IV, Cho YW. Combined liver-kidney transplantation is preferable to liver transplant alone for cirrhotic patients with renal failure. Transplantation. 2012 Aug 27;94(4):411–6. doi: 10.1097/TP.0b013e3182590d6b. PMID: 22805440.
19. Lunsford KE, Bodzin AS, Markovic D, Zarrinpar A, Kaldas FM, Gritsch HA, Xia V, Farmer DG, Danovitch GM, Hiatt JR, Busuttil RW, Agopian VG. Avoiding Futility in Simultaneous Liver-kidney Transplantation: Analysis of 331 Consecutive Patients Listed for Dual Organ Replacement. Ann Surg. 2017 May;265(5):1016–1024. doi: 10.1097/SLA.0000000000001801. PMID: 27232249.
20. Unek T, Egeli T, Özbilgin M, Çelik A, Atilla K, A alar C, Arslan NÇ, Karademir S, Bora S, Gülay H, Derici ZS, Astarcıo lu I. Long-term Results of Living Donors in Simultaneous Kidney and Liver Transplantations. Transplant Proc. 2017 Apr;49(3):403–406. doi: 10.1016/j.transproceed.2017.01.020. PMID: 28340800.
21. Soh KS, Jeng LB, Yang HR, Li PC, Lee CC, Poon KS, Chen TH, Yeh CC, Lai HC, Su WP, Peng CY, Chen YF, Ho YJ. Simultaneous liver and kidney transplantation from different living donors. Transplant Proc. 2012 Mar;44(2):509–11. doi: 10.1016/j.transproceed.2012.01.061. PMID: 22410057.
22. Verma S, Naganathan SK, Das LK, Agarwal S, Gupta S. Living Donor Liver Transplantation Alone Is Not Inferior to Combined Kidney Liver Transplant for Cirrhotic Patients With Chronic Kidney Disease. Transplant Proc. 2023 Mar 5:S0041–1345(23)00031–3. doi: 10.1016/j.transproceed.2023.02.004. Epub ahead of print. PMID: 36882356.
23. G. O. I. Min of Health and Family Welfare, "https://main.mohfw.gov.in/sites/default/files/Diagnosis%20and%20management%20of%20viral%20Hepatitis%20Final_Reference%20File_0.pdf," 2018. [Online].
24. Park KS, Han DJ, Park JB, Park JS, Park S. Long-term outcome of Hepatitis B-positive renal allograft recipients after development of antiviral treatment. Clin Nephrol. 2012 Nov;78(5):391–8. doi: 10.5414/CN107565. PMID: 22541689.
25. Martin P, Awan AA, Berenguer MC, Bruchfeld A, Fabrizi F, Goldberg DS, *et al.* Executive Summary of the KDIGO 2022 Clinical Practice Guideline for the Prevention, Diagnosis, Evaluation, and Treatment of Hepatitis C in Chronic Kidney Disease. Kidney Int. 2022 Dec;102(6):1228–37.

Chapter 8

Vascular and Lymphatic Complications of Kidney Transplant

• Ajay Oswal • Akshay Mahesh Kriplani

LEARNING OBJECTIVES

- To understand the pathophysiology of the various vascular and lymphatic complications.
- To understand the diagnosis, evaluation, and management of these complications.
- To understand the tips to prevent these complications.

INTRODUCTION

Surgical complications after renal transplantation have a current incidence of 2.9–12.5%[1,2] and can be classified into urological, vascular and lymphatic complications.[3,4] Vascular complications can be further classified into intraoperative (external iliac artery dissection, renal artery kink, venous outflow obstruction), early postoperative (renal artery or vein thrombosis) and late postoperative (renal artery stenosis). Lymphatic complications can have a wide spectrum of presentation ranging from persistent lymphorrhea to lymphocele or lymphocutaneous fistula formation.

Renal Artery Stenosis

Case Scenario 1

A 37-year-old male underwent a live related ABO compatible renal transplant with spatulated end to end anastomosis of donor renal artery to internal iliac artery and end to side anastomosis of donor renal vein to external iliac vein. After the uneventful surgery recipient was discharged with a creatine of 1 mg/dl and had a stable early postoperative course. Six months post-transplant recipient developed hypertension with increasing need of anti-hypertensives and gradual rise of creatinine (up to 2.3 mg/dl). On examination, machinery murmur was audible at the graft site. There were no other clinical or biochemical abnormalities detected. Graft biopsy showed no evidence of rejection.

1. **What is the probable diagnosis?**
   Ans: The probable diagnosis is a graft renal artery stenosis (RAS).

   Transplant renal artery stenosis is a late postoperative complication commonly presenting between 2 months and 2 years post-transplant.[5] It is also the most common transplant vascular complication (1–23%).[6] Stenosis can be silent and incidentally detected during routine Doppler ultrasound or be significant (>50% occlusion) causing symptoms.[7] Activation of renin-angiotensin-aldosterone system (RAAS) leads to sodium and fluid retention causing worsening or refractory hypertension, flash pulmonary edema or congestive cardiac failure with graft dysfunction (Pickering syndrome).[8]

2. **What causes renal artery stenosis?**
   Ans: Arterial injury during retrieval or anastomosis like clamping, suturing, intimal injury, kinking or torsion of the artery or narrow anastomosis can cause early stenosis. Atherosclerosis of renal or iliac artery, cytomegalovirus infection, immunological injury or drug toxicity can cause late stenosis.[9] Predisposition with type of anastomosis (end to end or end to side), choice of artery (external or internal iliac) have been debated but yet not proven.[10]

3. **What is the next step in the management?**
   Ans: Graft Doppler ultrasound is the first screening test with a sensitivity of 60–100% to detect RAS.[11] Peak systolic velocity (PSV) >2.5 m/s at the renal artery (sensitivity 70–80%, specificity 67–100%) implies stenosis. Intrarenal parvus et tardus pattern, ratio of PSV at the renal artery (stenotic segment) and the iliac artery (pre-stenotic segment)

>1.8, high acceleration time at renal and intrarenal artery ≥0.1 seconds, inter-segmental artery RI <0.5 has a sensitivity of 90–100% and a specificity of 87–100%.[11–14]

CT (Fig. 8.1) or MR angiography can confirm the diagnosis but carry a risk of contrast-induced nephropathy.

4. What is the 'gold standard' management?

Ans: Percutaneous transluminal angioplasty (PTA) (Fig. 8.2) (Video 17) with or without stenting is safe and effective and considered as the current standard of management with a technical success rate of 85–93% and clinical success rate of 75–86% (Video 18).[15,16] Prerequisite for a successful PTA is maintained flow distal to the stenotic segment for a successful cannulation and dilatation. Best results are for a short segment, linear, and non-ostial stenosis.[12] Results of allograft survival are comparable for PTA only versus PTA with stenting groups but restenosis is lesser in the stenting group.[17,18] Therefore, reintervention rate in PTA only versus PTA with stenting is 16–62% versus <10%.[16] Potential complications include bleeding, hematoma formation, arterial dissection (Fig. 8.3) (Video 19), aneurysm formation or restenosis.

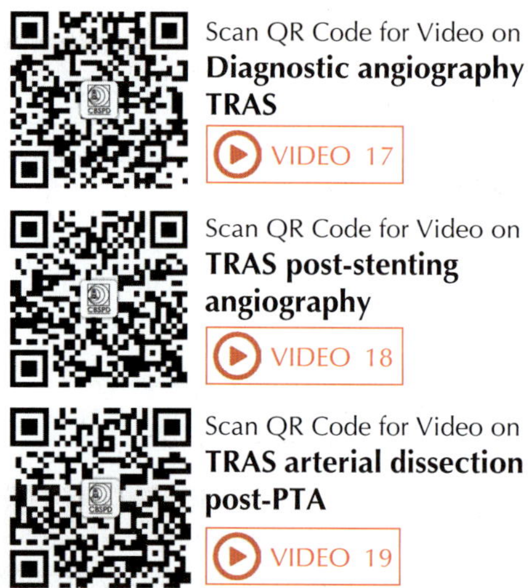

5. What are the options after a failed PTA?

Ans: Complex, long segment, non-ostial or multiple segment stenosis have a high failure rate for PTA. Technical difficulties in cannulation in nonlinear segments or arterial kink or torsion is unfavorable for PTA (Fig. 8.4) (Videos 20, 21, 22). Open surgical re-exploration with revision of anastomosis can be attempted. Vascular grafts can be used in select complex cases or failed angioplasty to bypass circulation from common or external iliac artery to distal renal artery (Fig. 8.5).[19]

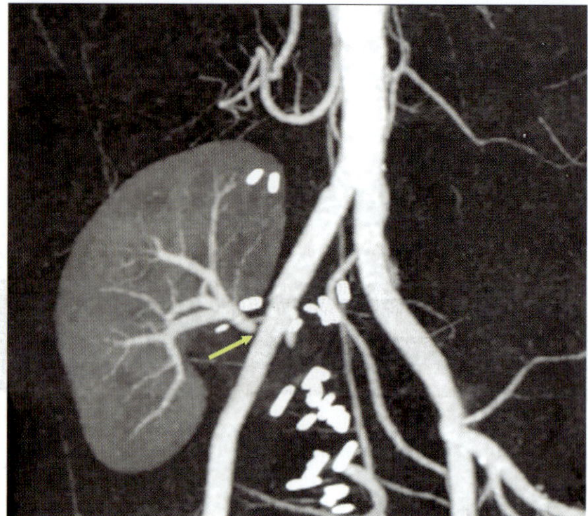

Fig. 8.1: CT angiography showing anastomotic stenosis (yellow arrow) in a case of end to side anastomosis of renal artery and external iliac artery

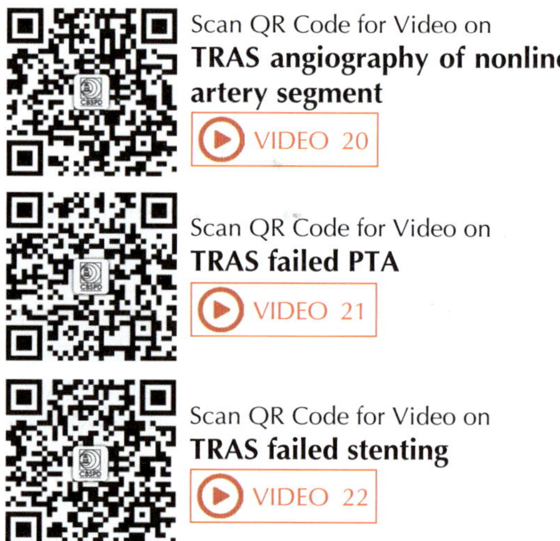

6. What is the role of CO_2 angiography?

Ans: In an attempt to avoid contrast-induced nephrotoxicity in post-transplant patients, CO_2 angiography is a potential tool replacing contrast angiography.[20] Small volume (15–20 ml) CO_2 infusion can produce a negative contrast as compared to the surrounding tissues and guide intervention.[21] Use of capnography during the procedure allows patient monitoring of ventilatory and hemodynamic function.[22] Risk of transient mesenteric ischemia or limb pain is described but is self-limiting.[21]

In this case graft Doppler showed a PSV in renal artery 240 m/s, PSV at stenotic to PSV at pre-stenotic segment ratio 2:1, Parvus et tardus flow in interlobar arteries, increased acceleration time more than 0.1 s.

Patient was taken up for a PTA with a stent placed across the renal artery to internal iliac artery anastomosis.

Fig. 8.2A to D: (A) Graft angiography showing anastomotic stenosis (yellow arrow) between renal artery and internal iliac artery, (B) Stent placed after balloon dilatation, (C) Post-stenting angiography; (D) DSA

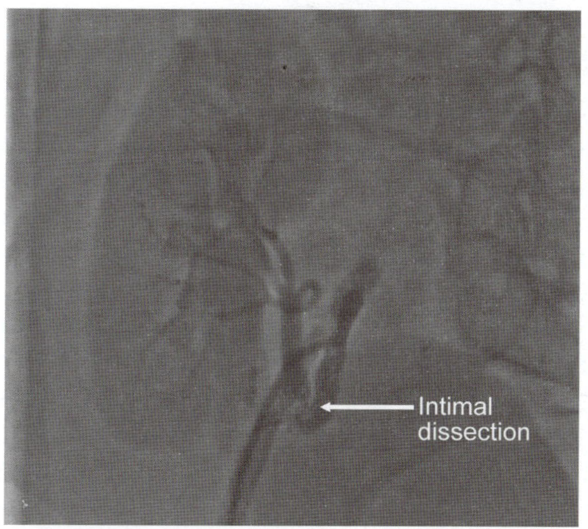

Fig. 8.3: Post-PTA intimal dissection

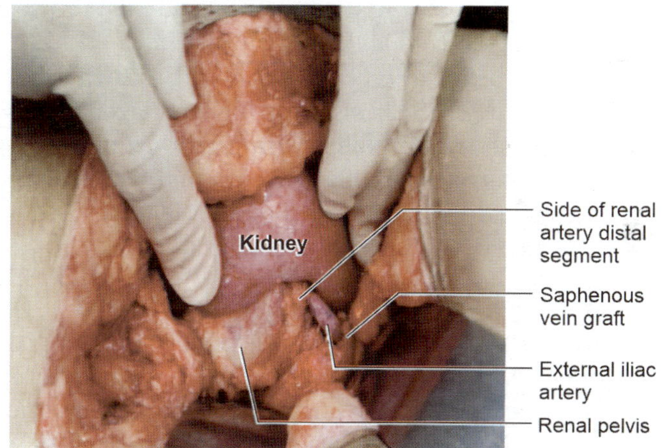

Fig. 8.5: Vascular bypass graft between external iliac artery and distal renal artery in a case of failed PTA for an anastomotic stenosis between renal artery and internal iliac artery

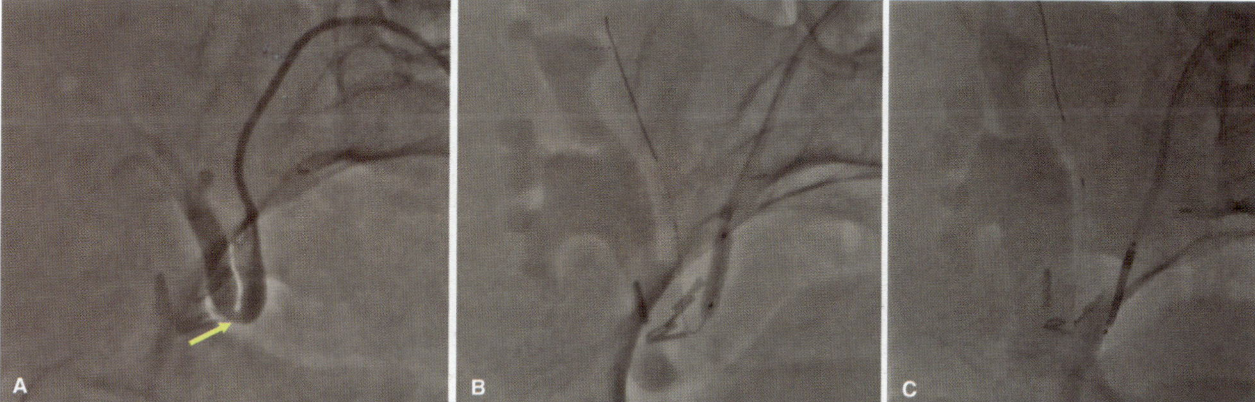

Fig. 8.4A to C: (A) Graft angiography showing an anastomotic stenosis (yellow arrow) and a kinked configuration of renal artery and internal iliac artery complex; (B) Inability to balloon dilate the non-linear stenotic segment; (C) Inability to pass a stent across the kink

Post-procedure requirement for anti-hypertensive medications reduced drastically with improvement in renal function (nadir creatinine 1.2 mg/dl).

Renal Artery Thrombosis

Case Scenario 2

A 49-year-old male underwent a second deceased donor transplant in left iliac fossa with end to side anastomosis of renal artery to common iliac artery and renal vein to external iliac vein. The previous transplant was also a deceased donor transplant but graft nephrectomy was resorted for a nonviable graft. Two years after the second transplant patient turned COVID positive and developed antibody mediated rejection. Serum creatinine rose to 2.5 mg/dl from 1.7 mg/dl but remained stable for next five years. Seven years post-transplant patient suddenly noticed fall in urine output. By the time patient presented to the hospital patient was anuric, had fever, chills, and a palpable left iliac fossa mass. Patient had hypertension and a serum creatinine of 7 mg/dl. Graft Doppler showed no graft perfusion (Fig. 8.6).

1. **What is the probable diagnosis?**
   Ans: The probable diagnosis is graft renal artery thrombosis (RAT).
   Renal artery thrombosis is rare with a prevalence of 0.5–3.5%.[23] Thrombosis in case of a single renal artery can cause sudden fall in urine output, worsening hypertension in an otherwise normal recipient and sudden rise in serum creatinine. It is therefore also considered as a 'silent' cause of graft loss.
2. **What are the common etiological factors?**
   Ans: Graft artery thrombosis is usually an early post-operative complication and can be multifactorial. Acute arterial kink or torsion, external compression or renal artery stenosis are common anatomical causes.[24] Intraoperative intimal injury, arterial dissection or narrow constricting anastomosis are predisposing technical factors. Rarely hyperacute rejection, hypercoagulopathies, decreased cardiac output, severe hypotension, infection like mucor mycosis can also predispose to arterial thrombosis and rupture.[25,26] Theories stating more prevalence in deceased donor kidneys or multiple renal arteries have been debated.[27,28] Certain immunosuppressive agent toxicity like cyclosporine, sirolimus, OKT3 and atherosclerosis of the donor or recipient vessels have been reported to be responsible.[29,30] RAT is more common in children compared to adults.
3. **How do you evaluate this patient?**
   High degree of clinical suspicion is required in the early postoperative period for early diagnosis to prevent graft loss. Ultrasound Doppler is usually the first investigation showing the graft perfusion and flow in the arteries. CT or MR angiography can be diagnostic. Conventional angiography can be both diagnostic and therapeutic. Radionuclide imaging can also show reduction or absence of graft perfusion.[31]
   In this case CT angiogram showed an engorged non-enhancing graft with multiple hypodense areas and a thrombosed graft renal artery with no flow across the thrombosed segment (Fig. 8.7).
4. **What is the possibility of salvaging this graft?**
   Ans: Graft with a thrombosed single supplying artery is a surgical emergency. Immediate exploration with thrombectomy, graft reperfusion and anastomosis for salvage can be attempted but mostly graft nephrectomy is inevitable.
   Endovascular techniques include percutaneous transluminal angiography, thrombectomy, and intra-arterial thrombolysis with TPA or urokinase with or without stent placement.
   In cases with segmental artery thrombosis or thrombosis in one artery of a graft with multiple

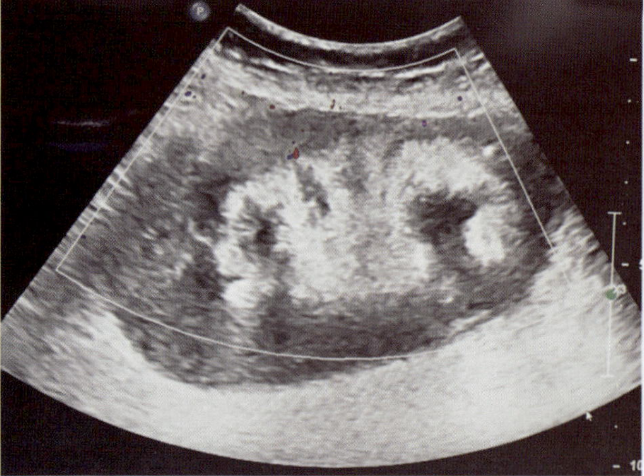

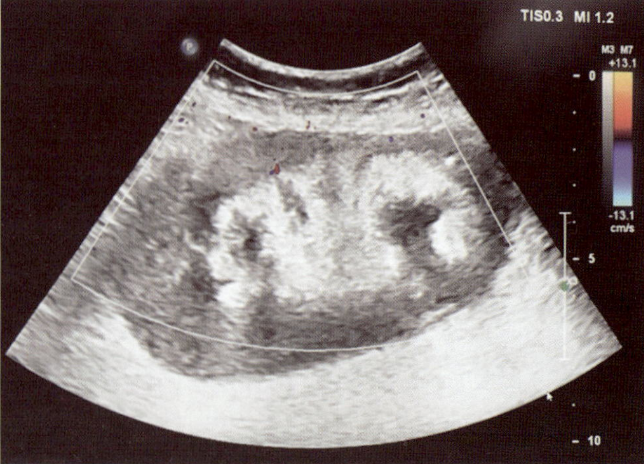

Fig. 8.6: Graft Doppler showing a non-perfused graft

Fig. 8.7: CT angiography showing thrombosed renal artery

arteries, the clinical course is less alarming and catastrophic (Fig. 8.8).

In this case immediate exploration revealed a completely necrotic graft with extensive adhesions and fibrosis around it. Renal artery and vein were ligated and divided. External iliac vein was avulsed during dissection and was reconstructed by a long saphenous vein patch. Graft contained multiple abscess cavities.

On histopathology, renal parenchyma showed diffuse necrosis and patchy neutrophilic infiltration with complete loss of architecture. Renal artery showed a thrombus within.

Transplant Renal Vein Thrombosis

Case Scenario 3

A 52-year-old female underwent a deceased donor renal transplant with end to side anastomosis of left

(Contd.)

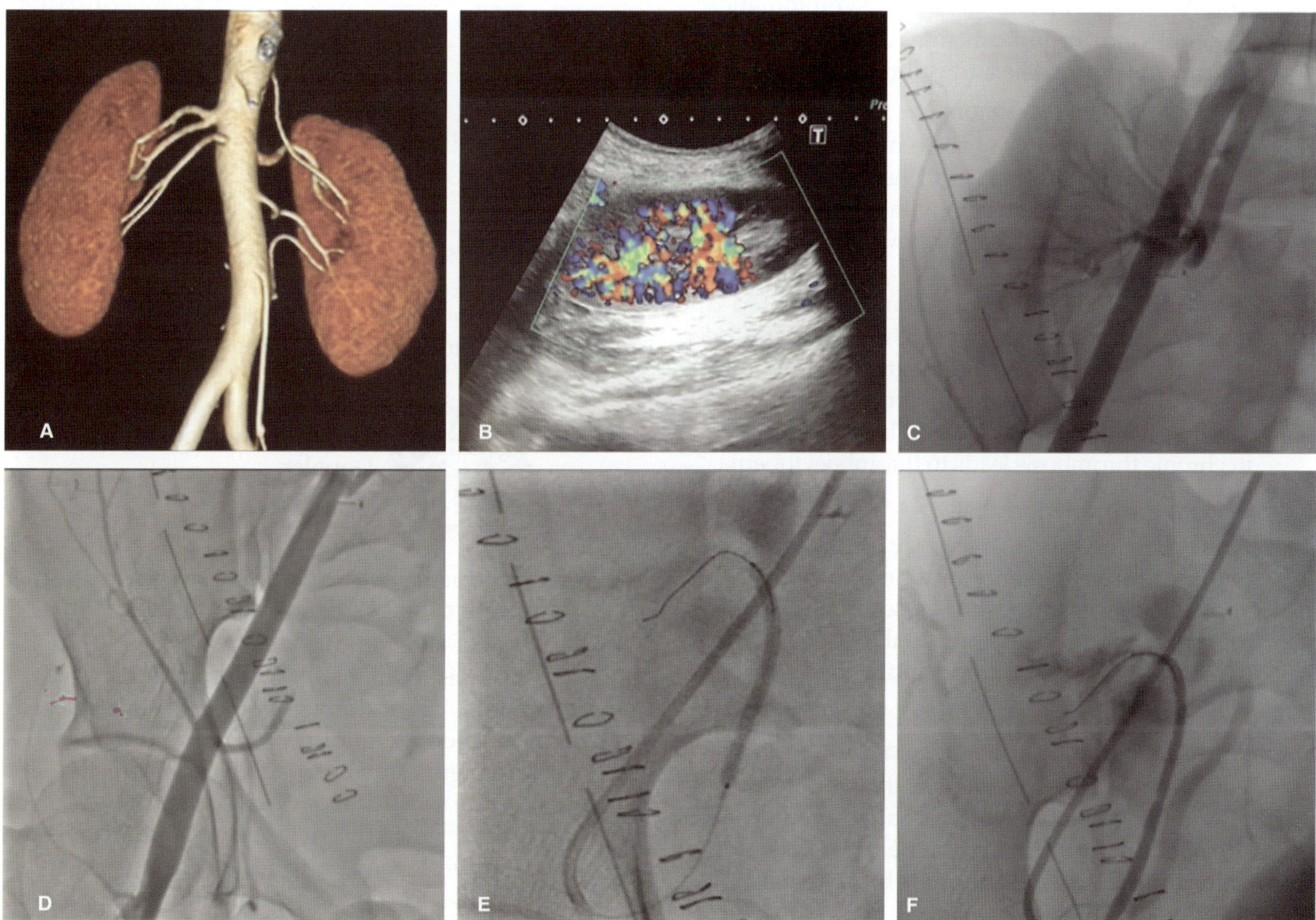

Fig. 8.8A to F: Case of third renal artery thrombosis of right donor kidney after end-to-end anastomosis with inferior epigastric artery: (A) Donor CT angiogram showing 4 left renal arteries and 2 right renal arteries with early branching of upper artery; (B) Graft Doppler showing non-perfused lower pole; (C) Graft angiography showing a nonperfused lower pole; (D) Thrombosed lower polar renal artery with no flow across the inferior epigastric artery; (E) Thrombectomy, balloon angioplasty and stenting; (F) Revascularized lower pole after stent placement.

(Contd.)

renal artery and vein to external iliac artery and external iliac vein respectively. On second postoperative day, patient developed sudden decrease in urine output with hematuria and severe graft site pain. Ultrasound showed an enlarged graft with reversed diastolic flow in renal artery on Doppler. Renal vein was dilated but did not show any flow. Patient had previous history of failure of both radio-cephalic fistulas.

1. **What is the clinical diagnosis?**

   Ans: Diagnosis is renal vein thrombosis (RVT)

   Renal vein thrombosis can be one of the most dreaded and dramatic vascular complication with a prevalence of 0.1–4.2%.[4,32] Classical clinical presentation is graft site pain and tenderness, rapid onset fall in urine output, hematuria with graft dysfunction. Severe venous congestion may also lead to graft rupture, hemorrhage and shock.[33] High index of clinical suspicion is crucial as early diagnosis and timely intervention can help in salvaging the graft. Chronic venous thrombus can be asymptomatic.[34]

   Renal vein thrombosis may be associated with deep vein thrombosis and pulmonary embolism.

2. **What are the investigations?**

   Ans: Conventional gray scale ultrasound showed enlarged graft with peri-graft hematoma. Doppler showed enlarged renal vein with absence of venous flow and reversed diastolic flow in renal artery.[35] High resistive index indicates graft dysfunction. Thrombus in the vein is seldom appreciated due to the large edematous hyperechoic graft and deep anastomosis in pelvis.[36] MR venography can accurately demonstrate the thrombus but time constraints make this investigation uncommon.[7] Platelet sequestration in chronic thrombosis leads to thrombocytopenia.[34]

3. **Discuss graft salvageability.**

   Ans: Thrombolytic therapy and immediate exploration with venotomy and thrombectomy should be attempted but is seldom successful. Severe venous congestion usually makes the graft salvageability difficult and graft nephrectomy is usually resorted.[37]

4. **What is the role of endovascular procedures?**

   Ans: Percutaneous mechanical thrombectomy with or without thrombolysis can be attempted in partial thrombosis and if intervened early. Dissection or vein rupture and thrombolytic therapy may cause life-threatening hemorrhage.[38]

5. **What are the ways to prevent RVT?**

   Ans:

   - Avoid technical errors during retrieval, bench preparation and anastomosis.
   - Adequate length of renal vein should be ensured. Long veins can cause kink and stasis and short veins can cause apposition of vein walls.
   - Monitoring intravascular volume status and ensuring adequate fluid balance especially in children.
   - Large peri-graft collections in high-risk patients should be addressed to avoid external compression on the vein.

   Low molecular weight heparin or low dose aspirin in patients with multiple vessels, hypercoagulable state or multiple failed AV fistulas.[39]

   In this case patient was immediately reexplored to find a severely congested non-viable graft with peri-graft hematomas necessitating graft nephrectomy.

Transplant Artery Pseudoaneurysm

Case Scenario 4

A 37-year-old male underwent a live related renal transplant with end-to-end anastomosis of renal artery with internal iliac artery and end to side anastomosis of renal vein to external iliac vein. Apart from a single febrile episode on POD 5 (managed conservatively) recipient had an uneventful early post-operative course with good urine output, normal serum creatinine and normal routine graft Doppler on POD 14. On POD 36 recipient was incidentally detected to be COVID-19 positive and on POD 38 IgM Dengue positive. Patient developed sudden onset anuria on POD 38. Graft Doppler showed normal kidney size but no graft perfusion with a 5 x 4.5 cm pulsatile aneurysm of renal artery with hyperdynamic circulation (Fig. 8.9) (Video 23).

Scan QR Code for Video on **TRA pseudoaneurysm Doppler**

VIDEO 23

1. **What causes pseudoaneurysm formation in transplant arteries?**

   Ans: Juxta-anastomotic transplant artery pseudoaneurysm is a rare complication occurring in <1% recipients.[40] Pseudoaneurysm can have infective or non-infective etiology.[41] Early post-operative pseudoaneurysms are usually non-infective and occur due to intimal injury or faulty suturing techniques.[42] Infective or mycotic pseudoaneurysms occur in the second or third week post-transplant usually due to fungal (Candida and Aspergillus) or bacterial (Staphylococcus, Pseudomonas, and Klebsiella) infection.[40] The source of infection can be donor derived, infected irrigation fluid, operation theatre contamination or any distant septic foci in an immunocompromised recipient.[43] Immunological

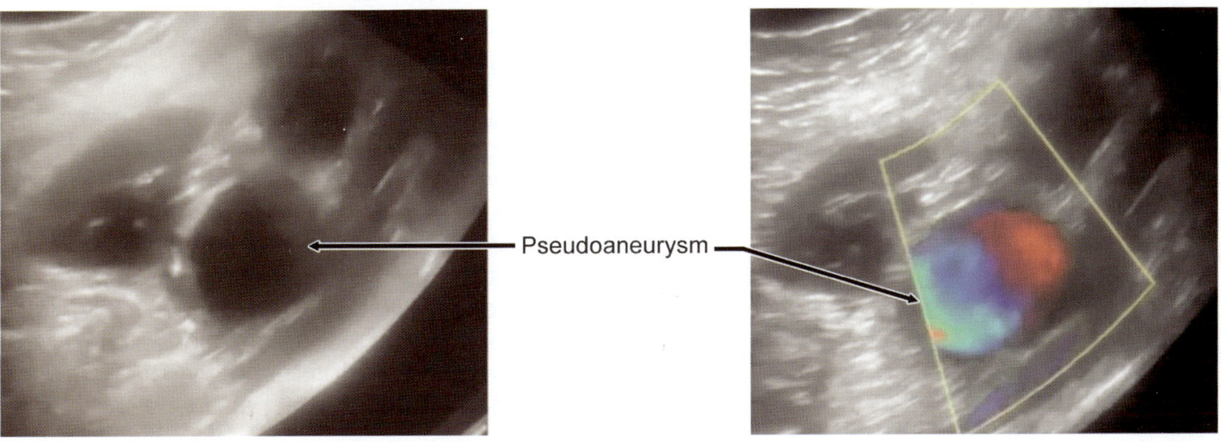

Fig. 8.9: Graft Doppler showing no graft perfusion with a pseudoaneurysm of renal artery

injury due to vascular rejection can cause endothelial damage and pseudoaneurysm formation.[42]

2. **What are the clinical indicators to suspect a pseudoaneurysm?**

   Ans:
   - Small pseudoaneurysms or those in case of multiple supplying renal arteries can be 'silent' or cause asymptomatic graft dysfunction. Routine Doppler followed by contrast CT or MRI usually identifies the condition.
   - Large pseudoaneurysms can compress the graft or iliac vessels causing graft dysfunction or lower limb swelling or ischemia.
   - Infected pseudoaneurysm can cause fever with graft site pain and tenderness.
   - Occasionally in thin patients a pulsatile lump is palpable at the graft site.
   - Ruptured pseudoaneurysms cause hemorrhagic shock and are usually catastrophic.

   In this case a CT angiogram suggested a 5 × 5 × 4 cm narrow neck juxta-anastomotic hyperdense outpouching from the graft renal artery suggesting a pseudoaneurysm, with no distal flow in the renal artery and no contrast uptake of the graft (Fig. 8.10).

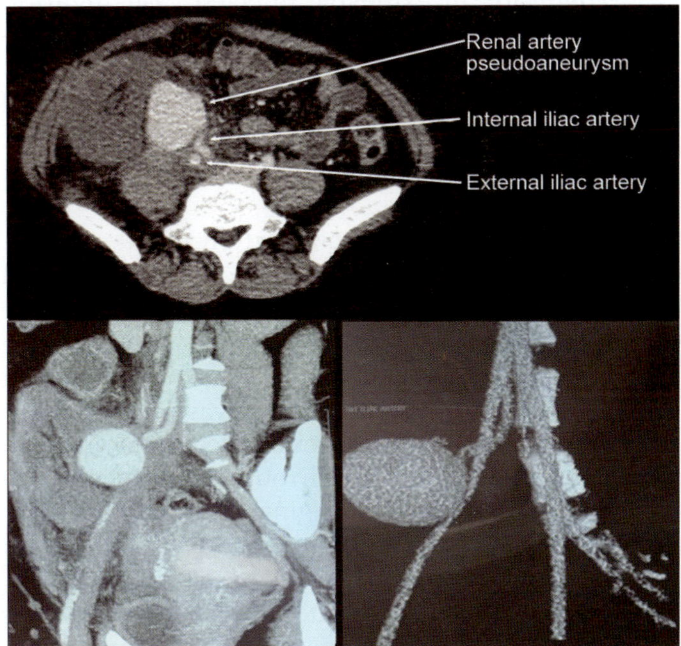

Fig. 8.10: CT angiography and reconstruction showing pseudoaneurysm of renal artery with no graft uptake

3. **Do all pseudoaneurysms need intervention?**

   Ans: Small pseudoaneurysms or those with chronic calcified walls and not compromising the graft function can be managed conservatively.[44] Intervention is indicated in patients with symptoms, size >2.5 cm, rapidly increasing in size, impending rupture, compressive features, or graft dysfunction.[42, 44]

4. **Do endovascular techniques have a role in management?**

   Ans: Endovascular stenting across the artery with exclusion of the pseudoaneurysm can be attempted for small noninfected aneurysms. This less invasive approach has comparatively less risk of compromise to graft vascularity.[45] Maintained circulation across the affected arterial segment, confirmed during angiography is a prerequisite to allow stenting.

   Endovascular coil embolization or ultrasound guided thrombin/glue injection has also been described for small narrow-necked pseudoaneurysms.[46, 47]

5. **What is 'gold standard' management?**

   Open surgery is considered 'gold standard' for large, wide neck, impending rupture pseudoaneurysms where excision with vascular reconstruction is necessary.[41] Open surgical repair is a morbid procedure due to complexity of impending rupture of the pseudoaneurysm in the setting of difficult dissection due to adhesions secondary to previous surgery. Another challenge in this vascular dissection and reconstruction is to salvage the graft and the ipsilateral limb.[42,48] Graft salvage by repairing the artery at the neck of the pseudoaneurysm sac or by patch angioplasty can be attempted in non-infected cases. Bypass vascular grafts can be used to maintain circulation to the allograft and the limb.[41]

For infected cases excision of pseudoaneurysm, graft nephrectomy and vascular reconstruction is the usual course.[49] Vascular stump blowout is a notorious life-threatening complication.[50] Therefore, in extensive infected cases ligation of common or external iliac artery with femoro-femoral bypass may be the only option.[51]

Hybrid approach to re-anastomose the renal artery to common or external iliac artery and exclude the pseudoaneurysm with a stent has been described.[52]

Microbiological examination of the excised specimens with long-term antibiotics and antifungal coverage as per culture sensitivity is important.

In this case due to absence of distal flow in the renal artery success of endovascular intervention was questionable and so patient was explored. Graft kidney had necrotic cortex and seemed nonviable. Large aneurysm with surrounding friable tissues made dissection challenging. Graft nephrectomy was done with excision of pseudoaneurysm and ligation of sac neck.

On histopathology acute tubular injury of the graft with foci of papillary necrosis and inflammatory cells with interstitial oedema and subepithelial myxoid changes were seen. Aneurysmal wall showed inflammation with culture negative for aerobes, anaerobes, and fungal elements.

Bleeding

Case Scenario 5

A 35-year-old male underwent an uneventful renal transplant with end-to-end anastomosis of renal artery to internal iliac artery and renal vein to external iliac vein. Ten hours post-operatively there was a sudden gush of hemorrhagic output (800 ml) in the drain which stopped gradually. Patient had developed hypotension, tachycardia and fall in output. Ultrasound Doppler showed a large peri-graft collection with poor graft perfusion. CT showed a peri-graft hematoma with areas of poorly perfused hypodense patches on the graft (Fig. 8.11).

1. **What can be the cause of bleeding?**

   Post-transplant bleeding is common (0.2–14%) and can be multifactorial.[53] Common causes are anastomotic leak, missed graft perihilar or retroperitoneal vessels, ureteric artery bleed, small bleeder at drain insertion site or abdominal wall. Slipped ligatures of the branches of iliac vessels can cause torrential bleeding. Small arteries spasm during dissection but can bleed postoperatively after relieve of spasm.

2. **Do all hematomas require intervention?**

   Ongoing bleeding can cause hemodynamic instability. Persistent tachycardia, hypotension requiring ionotropic support, peri-graft pain in the background of a serial drop in hemoglobin level with or without high drain output signify ongoing bleeding.

   Graft compression by hematoma or hemodynamic instability can cause graft dysfunction. Expanding hematoma can also cause compartment syndrome. Doppler ultrasound and CT can characterize the hematoma but these clinical indicators necessitate surgical re-exploration.

   In this case, angiography showed a massive leak from renal artery (Fig. 8.12) (Video 9). Immediate re-exploration showed a cyanotic soft kidney with

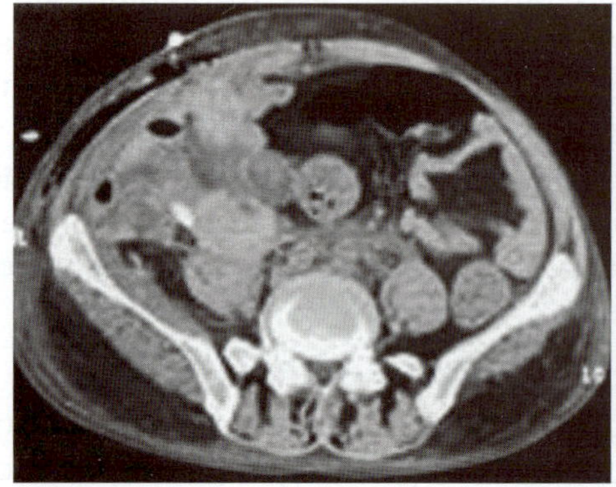
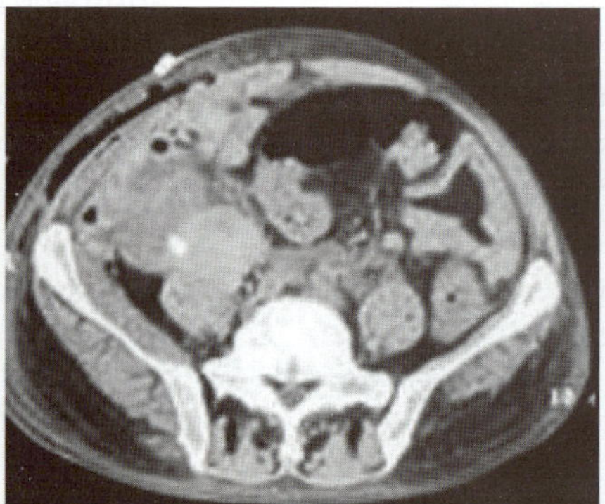
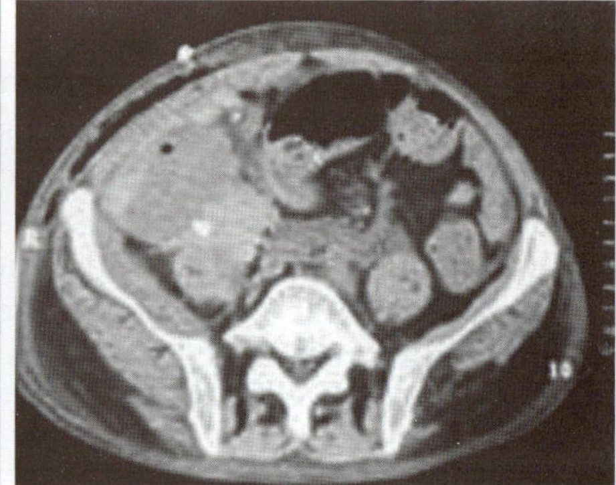

Fig. 8.11: Peri-graft hematoma with poorly perfused graft

a large peri-graft hematoma. A rent on the posterior aspect of renal artery was identified. The injury was retrospectively identified as a cautery hook injury during laparoscopic donor nephrectomy (Fig. 8.13). The weak area of injury was inapparent during bench preparation and anastomosis with no intraoperative leak. Blood pressure fluctuations and relieve of arterial spasm post-operatively might have revealed the rent.

After vascular control, renal artery was cut, refashioned and graft reperfused. Renal artery was re-anastomosed after lengthening with a long saphenous vein graft. Post-operatively patient remained anuric and on dialysis. Eventually graft nephrectomy was done.

Acute Page Kidney

Case Scenario 6

A 55-year-old male underwent a live related kidney transplant following a laparoscopic donor nephrectomy. During bench preparation a small 1cm subcapsular hematoma was observed on the anterolateral aspect. After declamping the graft was well perfused with immediate diuresis. The subcapsular hematoma was not expanding and capsulotomy was differed. Immediate post-operatively patient was hemodynamically stable but urine output dropped gradually and within 4 hours patient went anuric. Graft ultrasound Doppler showed a subcapsular collection, PSV of 240 ml/s, intrarenal RI > 8, reduced cortical perfusion and reversal of diastolic flow (Fig. 8.14).

1. **What is the diagnosis?**

   Ans: Diagnosis is acute graft page kidney.

   Page kidney refers to external compression of the graft by a hematoma, urinoma, lymphocele, or a mass causing parenchymal hypoperfusion and graft dysfunction. Ultrasound confirms the collection with increased intrarenal resistive index, normal peak systolic velocity and absent diastolic flow.[54]

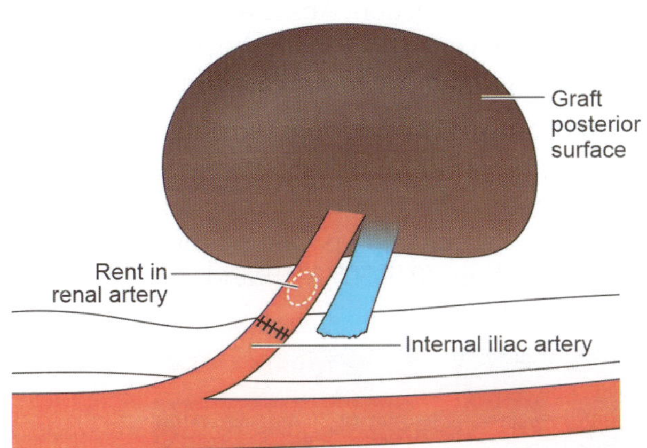

Fig. 8.12: Intraoperative finding of rent on the posterior aspect of renal artery

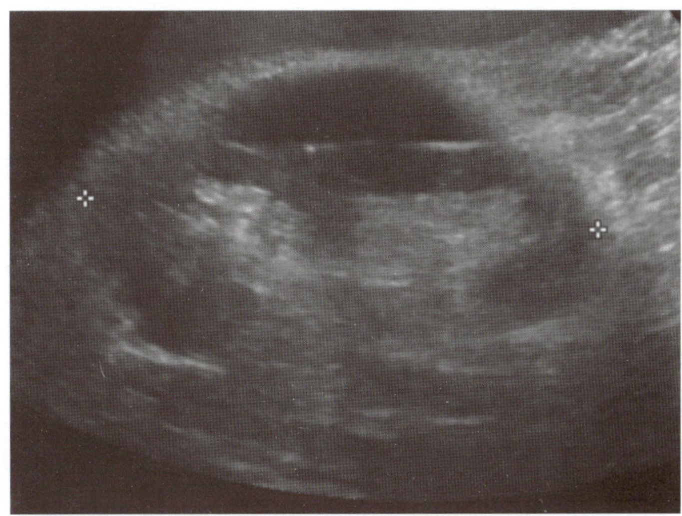

Fig. 8.14: Graft Doppler showing a large subcapsular hematoma with no graft perfusion

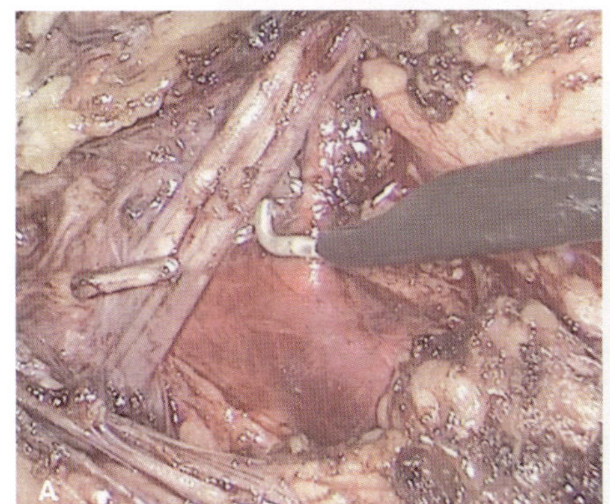

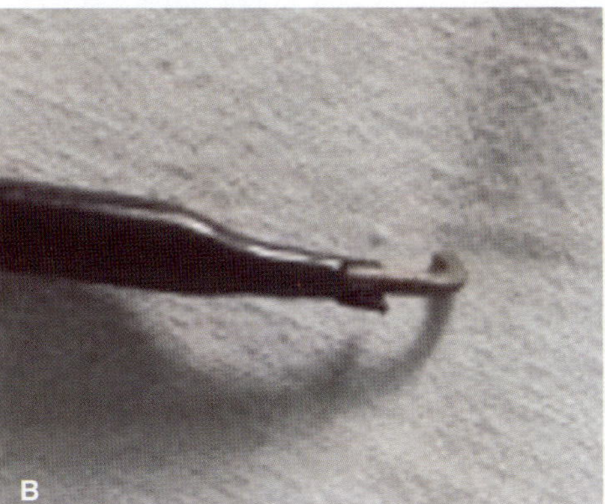

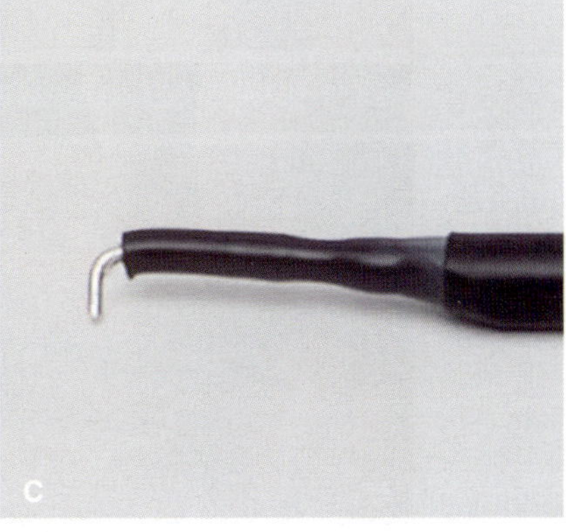

Fig. 8.13A to C: (A) Unidentified cautery hook injury to renal artery during donor nephrectomy; (B) Defective insulation of cautery hook which caused the injury; (C) Ideal cautery hook insulation

2. **How do you manage this patient?**

High index of suspicion in a patient of graft site pain, falling output, rising blood pressure with a peri-graft collection permits early diagnosis.[55] Immediate intervention and decompression can prevent graft dysfunction. In case of subcapsular hematomas wide capsulotomy is necessary to prevent further collections.[56]

In this case, patient was immediately re-explored to find a tense, turgid graft with a large subcapsular hematoma (Fig. 8.15). Capsulotomy done over lateral aspect of the kidney from upper pole to lower pole on the bench to drain the hematoma (100 ml blood clots). No definitive bleeder was identified. Absorbable hemostatic sheet (Surgicel™) was wrapped around the kidney. Immediate diuresis resumed on-table and normal post-operative recovery of graft parameters observed.

Lymphocele

Case Scenario 7

A 55-year-old male underwent an uneventful live related renal transplant with two renal arteries anastomosed with external and internal iliac artery and renal vein anastomosed to external iliac vein. Foley catheter was removed on POD4 and drain was removed on POD5 and patient was discharged with a normal creatinine. Six weeks post-transplant patient developed suprapubic fullness with right lower limb edema extending up to groin. Urine output was maintained with no lower urinary tract symptoms. Creatinine raised to 2.3 mg%. Ultrasound showed moderate graft hydroureteronephrosis with well perfused graft and large peri-graft fluid collection (Fig. 8.16). CT cystogram showed the bladder being pushed to the opposite side of the collection (Fig. 8.17).

1. **What is the differential diagnosis of a peri-graft fluid collection?**

Ans: A peri-graft fluid collection on ultrasound and CT can be a hematoma, urinoma, lymphocele, or abscess. These can be differentiated with a combined clinical, radiological, and biochemical assessment. Hematoma would be a heterogenous density collection on CT with acute bleeding being more hyperdense. Large hematomas would have associated hemodynamic alterations and a drop in hemoglobin. Urinoma and lymphocele would both be hypodense on CT and can only be differentiated by biochemical analysis (creatinine) of aspirated fluid.[57] Urinoma would be associated with fall in urine output with or without graft dysfunction. Microbiological evaluation of the aspirated fluid can rule out infection. Abscess would have a clinical profile of fever, toxicity, graft site pain and tenderness with mixed density on CT and purulent aspirate.

2. **What causes lymphocele formation?**

Ans: Lymphocele is a pseudocyst where peri-graft lymphatic collection is lined by a non-epithelized fibrous capsule.[58] It is one of the most common complications (0.5–50%)[59,60] and can occur between

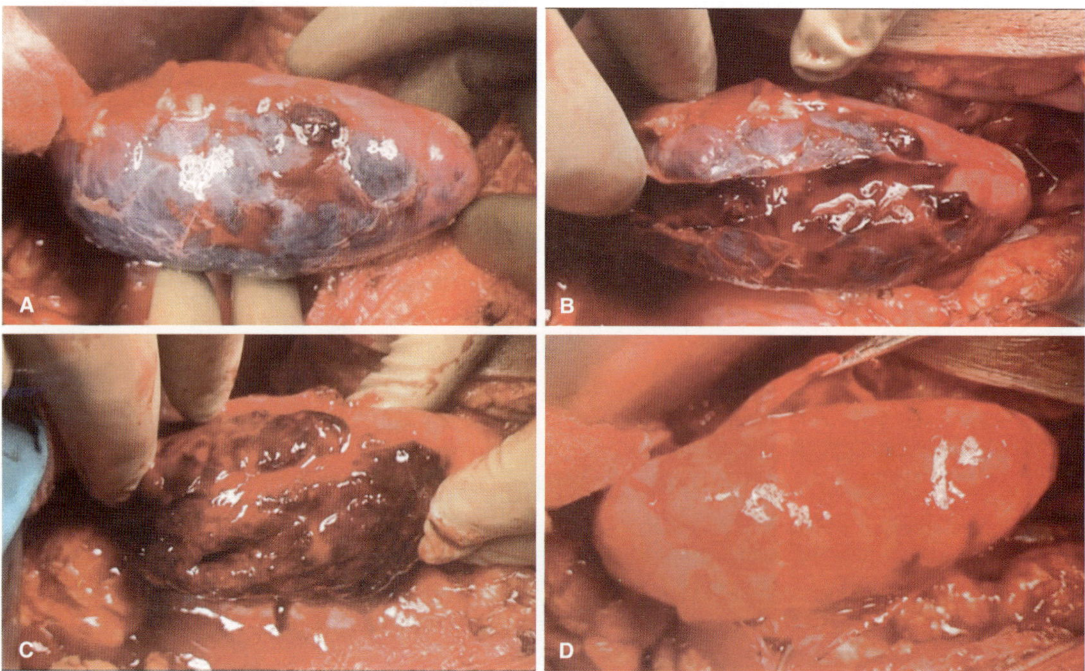

Fig. 8.15A to D: Intraoperative pictures of re-exploration of page kidney: (A) Large subcapsular hematoma; (B) Lateral capsulotomy; (C) Evacuation of hematoma; (D) Well-perfused graft

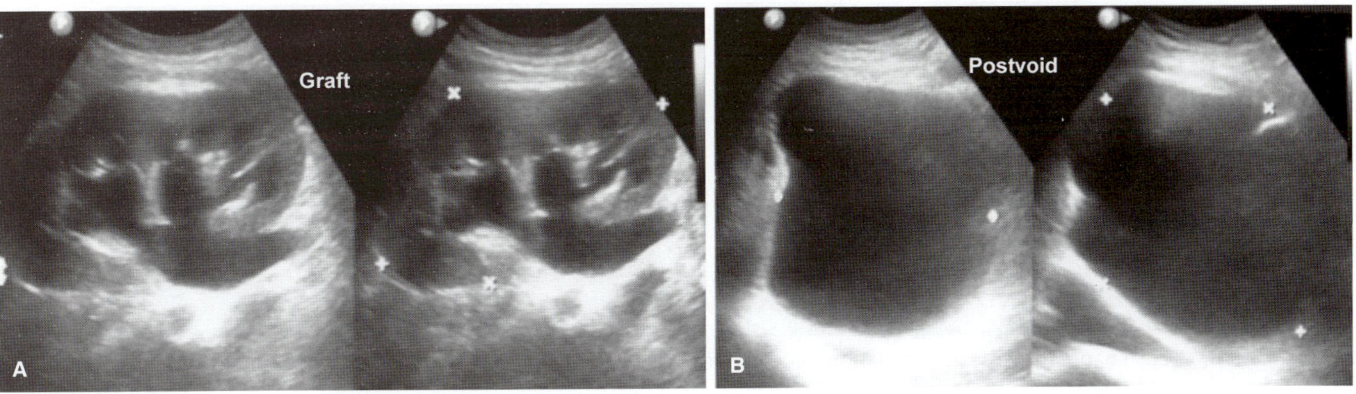

Fig. 8.16A and B: Graft hydroureteronephrosis (A) with peri-graft hypoechoic collection (B) seen on a postvoid ultrasound with empty bladder

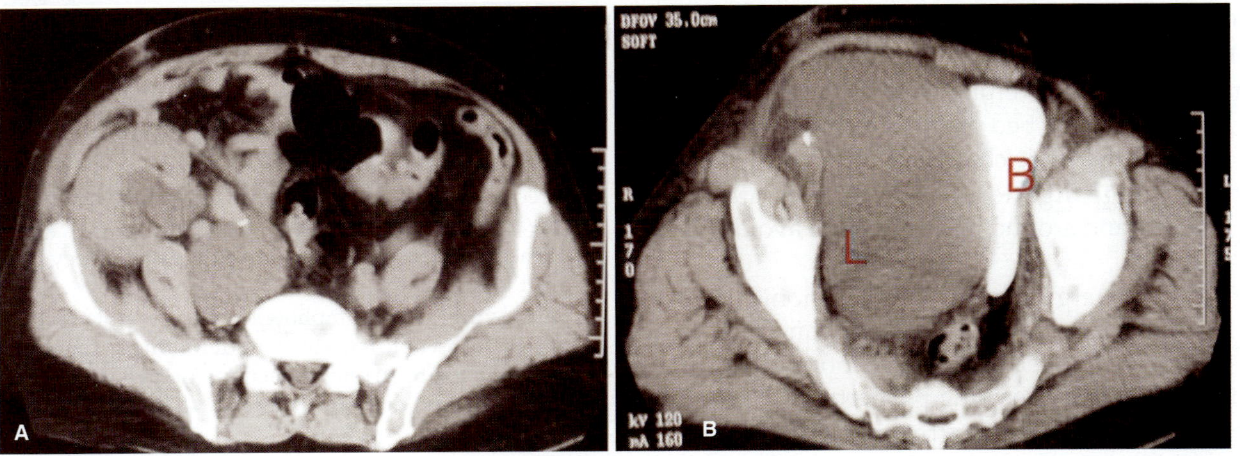

Fig. 8.17A and B: Non-contract CT showing the peri-graft collection; (A) CT cystogram showing the collection compressing the bladder; (B) (L: Lymphocele, B: Bladder)

2 weeks and 6 months post-transplant.[61, 62] The source of lymph leak can be donor lymphatics around the graft hilum or recipient lymphatics along the iliac vessels. Both surgical or medial risk factors contribute to increase lymph ooze. Incomplete ligation of lymphatics along the recipient iliac vessels and donor renal hilum or perinephric fat is the most common etiology.[60] Use of mTOR inhibitors, anticoagulants, high dose steroids or diuretics have also been correlated with lymphocele formation.[63] ABOi transplants, immunocompromised state, hypoalbuminemia, obesity, or delayed graft function/acute rejection have also been implicated as potential risk factors.[64,63]

3. **When can lymphoceles be a matter of concern?**

Ans: Majority of lymphoceles are asymptomatic and are incidentally detected on routine ultrasound. Large lymphoceles can cause pain, swelling at the graft site and fever if infected.[65] Occasionally large lymphoceles especially anteromedial collections can compress on the graft ureter to cause hydroureteronephrosis and graft dysfunction. Compression of iliac vessels can cause ipsilateral limb or genital edema. Bladder compression can cause increased frequency or rarely bladder outlet obstruction.[61] Lymph can tract along the iliac and femoral vessels to cause groin swellings or through the musculofascial plane to cause subcutaneous collections or lymphocutaneous fistula. These can impair wound healing or can even cause wound dehiscence in immunocompromised recipients.[66]

4. **Do all lymphoceles need to be addressed?**

Ans: Small (<100 ml) asymptomatic lymphoceles can be observed. In large symptomatic lymphoceles decompression of the collection by ultrasound guided percutaneous drain placement relieves symptoms.[60] Usually, lymphorrhea resolves with time. In persistent cases sclerosant (povidone-iodine) infiltration has a failure rate of <11%.[62] Lack of aseptic technique during sclerosant instillation can lead to infected lymphocele/abscess formation (Fig. 8.18). In recurrent collections or persistent high output (>300 ml/day) drainage laparoscopic or open fenestration/deroofing or marsupialization into peritoneal cavity can be done.[67]

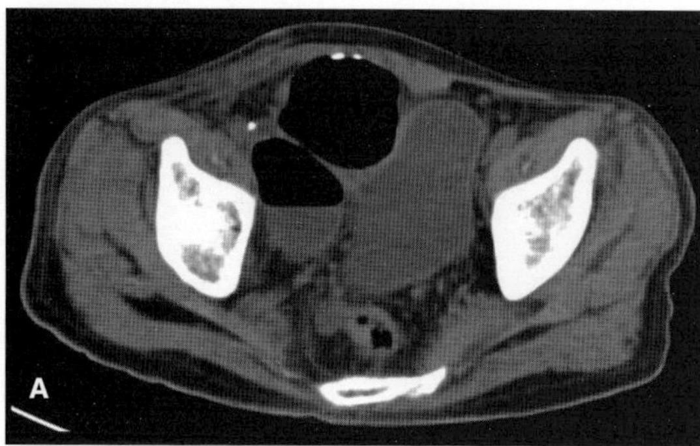

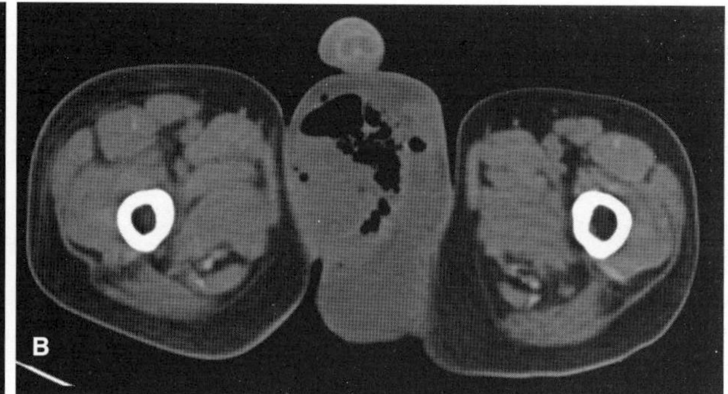

Fig. 8.18A and B: A case of post-sclerosant instillation infected lymphocele by *E.coli* (gas producing organism) tracking up to the scrotum

5. What are the ways to prevent lymphocele in transplant setting?

Ans:

- Limited and careful dissection around the iliac vessels during bed preparation can avoid injury to the lymphatic channels.[68]
- Thorough ligation of lymphatics along the vessels and around the graft hilum avoids lymph leak.[57]
- Use of energy devices like Harmonic scalpel[69] and LigaSure™[58] for dissection have been reported to reduce lymph ooze due to the superior vessel sealing property.
- Maintaining peri-graft drain *in-situ* till drain output reduces <100 ml can avoid peri-graft collections.[70]
- Prophylactic peritoneal fenestration is not popular but has been reported to prevent peri-graft accumulation of lymph.[62]

In this case ultrasound guided drain insertion drained 700 ml clear fluid. Fluid creatine was comparable to serum creatinine and urine leak was ruled out. Graft function improved and lower limb edema subsided within 24 hours. Drain output gradually subsided over 3 weeks and drain was removed. No recurrent collection on long-term follow-up.

SUMMARY

- Post-transplant bleeding is common and serial drop in hemoglobin level with persistent tachycardia, hypotension requiring ionotropic support, peri-graft pain with or without high drain output signify ongoing bleeding requiring intervention.
- Graft renal artery stenosis is the most common post-transplant vascular complication and clinical judgement and specific Doppler findings can guide in early diagnosis.
- Conventional angiography and PTA are the current standard of management with open repair reserved for complex, long segment, non-ostial or multiple segment stenosis.
- Graft renal artery thrombosis is a rare but 'silent' cause of graft failure necessitating immediate re-exploration.
- Graft renal vein thrombosis has a classical clinical presentation but graft salvageability is difficult and graft nephrectomy is usually resorted.
- Small non-infective renal artery pseudoaneurysms <2.5 cm, not increasing in size, without compressive features, graft dysfunction or signs of impending rupture can be managed conservatively.
- Infected pseudoaneurysms are surgically challenging with threat to graft and ipsilateral limb.
- Immediate decompression in acute page kidney can prevent graft loss.
- Large symptomatic lymphoceles can be percutaneously drained with laparoscopic fenestration/deroofing or marsupialization reserved for recurrent collections or persistent high output (>300 ml/day) drainage.

REFERENCES

1. Deininger S, Nadalin S, Amend B, Guthoff M, Heyne N, Königsrainer A, *et al.* Minimal-invasive management of urological complications after kidney transplantation. Int Urol Nephrol. 2021 Jul;53(7):1267–77.
2. Inci MF, Ozkan F, See TC, Tatli S. Renal transplant complications: diagnostic and therapeutic role of radiology. Can Assoc Radiol J J Assoc Can Radiol. 2014 Aug;65(3):242–52.
3. Lempinen M, Stenman J, Kyllönen L, Salmela K. Surgical complications following 1670 consecutive adult renal transplantations: A single center study. Scand J Surg SJS Off Organ Finn Surg Soc Scand Surg Soc. 2015 Dec;104(4):254–9.
4. Pillot P, Bardonnaud N, Lillaz J, Delorme G, Chabannes E, Bernardini S, *et al.* Risk factors for surgical complications after renal transplantation and impact on patient and graft survival. Transplant Proc. 2012 Nov;44(9):2803–8.
5. Baird DP, Williams J, Petrie MC, Smith JR. Transplant Renal Artery Stenosis. Kidney Int Rep. 2020 Dec;5(12):2399–402.
6. Li X, Zhang J, Meng Y, Yang L, Wang F, Li B, *et al.* Transplant renal artery stenosis caused by the stretch of an artey branch: a case report and literature review. BMC Nephrol. 2018 Mar 9;19(1):56.
7. Dimitroulis D, Bokos J, Zavos G, Nikiteas N, Karidis NP, Katsaronis P, *et al.* Vascular complications in renal transplantation: a single-center experience in 1367 renal transplantations and review of the literature. Transplant Proc. 2009 Jun;41(5):1609–14.
8. Pini A, Faggioli G, Pini R, Mauro R, Gallitto E, Mascoli C, *et al.* Assessment and Management of Transplant Renal Artery Stenosis. A Literature Review. Ann Vasc Surg. 2022 May;82:13–29.

9. Nasserala JCL, Oliveira CMC, Cerqueira JBG, Souza S, Silva SL, Santos LC d. O, *et al.* Artery Stenosis of the Renal Graft: Experience of a Center of Northeastern Brazil. Transplant Proc. 2016 Jan 1;48(1):74–80.
10. Szabo-Pap M, Zadori G, Fedor R, Illesy L, Toth F, Kanyari Z, *et al.* Surgical Complications Following Kidney Transplantations: A Single-Center Study in Hungary. Transplant Proc. 2016 Sep;48(7):2548–51.
11. Ardalan MR, Tarzamani MK, Shoja MM. A correlation between direct and indirect Doppler ultrasonographic measures in transplant renal artery stenosis. Transplant Proc. 2007 Jun;39(5):1436–8.
12. Chen W, Kayler LK, Zand MS, Muttana R, Chernyak V, DeBoccardo GO. Transplant renal artery stenosis: clinical manifestations, diagnosis and therapy. Clin Kidney J. 2015 Feb;8(1):71–8.
13. Bruno S, Ferrari S, Remuzzi G, Ruggenenti P. Doppler ultrasonography in posttransplant renal artery stenosis: a reliable tool for assessing effectiveness of revascularization? Transplantation. 2003 Jul 15;76(1):147–53.
14. Qi R, Qi G, Zhu D, Wang J. Diagnosis and Treatment of Early Transplant Renal Artery Stenosis: Experience From a Center in Eastern China. Transplant Proc. 2020;52(1):179–85.
15. Ghazanfar A, Tavakoli A, Augustine T, Pararajasingam R, Riad H, Chalmers N. Management of transplant renal artery stenosis and its impact on long-term allograft survival: a single-centre experience. Nephrol Dial Transplant Off Publ Eur Dial Transpl Assoc-Eur Ren Assoc. 2011 Jan;26(1):336–43.
16. Ngo AT, Markar SR, De Lijster MS, Duncan N, Taube D, Hamady MS. A Systematic Review of Outcomes Following Percutaneous Transluminal Angioplasty and Stenting in the Treatment of Transplant Renal Artery Stenosis. Cardiovasc Intervent Radiol. 2015 Dec;38(6):1573–88.
17. Chen LX, De Mattos A, Bang H, Vu CT, Gandhi M, Alnimri M, *et al.* Angioplasty vs stent in the treatment of transplant renal artery stenosis. Clin Transplant. 2018 Apr;32(4):e13217.
18. Biederman DM, Fischman AM, Titano JJ, Kim E, Patel RS, Nowakowski FS, *et al.* Tailoring the endovascular management of transplant renal artery stenosis. Am J Transplant Off J Am Soc Transplant Am Soc Transpl Surg. 2015 Apr;15(4):1039–49.
19. Shames BD, Odorico JS, D'Alessandro AM, Pirsch JD, Sollinger HW. Surgical repair of transplant renal artery stenosis with preserved cadaveric iliac artery grafts. Ann Surg. 2003 Jan;237(1):116–22.
20. Fujihara M, Kawasaki D, Shintani Y, Fukunaga M, Nakama T, Koshida R, *et al.* Endovascular therapy by CO_2 angiography to prevent contrast-induced nephropathy in patients with chronic kidney disease: a prospective multicenter trial of CO_2 angiography registry. Catheter Cardiovasc Interv Off J Soc Card Angiogr Interv. 2015 Apr;85(5):870–7.
21. Sharafuddin MJ, Marjan AE. Current status of carbon dioxide angiography. J Vasc Surg. 2017 Aug;66(2):618–37.
22. Elmously A, Stern JR, Greenberg J, Agrusa CJ, Schneider DB, Ellozy SH, *et al.* Carbon Dioxide Angiography in the Treatment of Transplant Renal Artery Stenosis. Ann Vasc Surg. 2020 Feb 1;63:198–203.
23. Cavenaghi AS, Cappiello A, Pini R, Faggioli G, La Manna G, Gargiulo M. Urgent endovascular maneuvers to rescue a failing transplant kidney with a T-stent approach. J Vasc Surg Cases Innov Tech. 2023 Mar 29;9(2):101168.
24. Sugi MD, Albadawi H, Knuttinen G, Naidu SG, Mathur AK, Moss AA, *et al.* Transplant artery thrombosis and outcomes. Cardiovasc Diagn Ther. 2017 Dec;7(Suppl 3):S219–27.
25. Zhu X, Liu H, Wang W, Song S, Jin M, Hu X, *et al.* Two cases of transplant renal artery thrombosis and spontaneous rupture caused by mucormycosis. Transpl Infect Dis Off J Transplant Soc. 2015 Jun;17(3):442–8.
26. Srivastava A, Kumar J, Sharma S, Abhishek null, Ansari MS, Kapoor R. Vascular complication in live related renal transplant: An experience of 1945 cases. Indian J Urol IJU J Urol Soc India. 2013 Jan;29(1):42–7.
27. Osman Y, Shokeir A, Ali-el-Dein B, Tantawy M, Wafa EW, el-Dein ABS, *et al.* Vascular complications after live donor renal transplantation: study of risk factors and effects on graft and patient survival. J Urol. 2003 Mar;169(3):859–62.
28. Salehipour M, Salahi H, Jalaeian H, Bahador A, Nikeghbalian S, Barzideh E, *et al.* Vascular complications following 1500 consecutive living and cadaveric donor renal transplantations: a single center study. Saudi J Kidney Dis Transplant Off Publ Saudi Cent Organ Transplant Saudi Arab. 2009 Jul;20(4):570–2.
29. Irish A. Hypercoagulability in renal transplant recipients. Identifying patients at risk of renal allograft thrombosis and evaluating strategies for prevention. Am J Cardiovasc Drugs Drugs Devices Interv. 2004;4(3):139–49.
30. Shankar R, Bastani B, Salinas-Madrigal L, Sudarshan B. Acute thrombosis of the renal transplant artery after a single dose of OKT3. Am J Nephrol. 2001;21(2):141–4.
31. Tavakkoli M, Zafarghandi RM, Taghavi R, Ghoreifi A, Zafarghandi MM. Immediate Vascular Complications After Kidney Transplant: Experience from 2100 Recipients. Exp Clin Transplant Off J Middle East Soc Organ Transplant. 2017 Oct;15(5):504–8.
32. Poli D, Antonucci E, Zanazzi M. Hemostatic Complications in Renal Transplantation. Semin Thromb Hemost. 2017 Oct;43(7):742–9.
33. Sanni A, Wilson CH, Wyrley-Birch H, Vijayanand D, Navarro A, Sohrabi S, *et al.* Donor risk factors for renal graft thrombosis. Transplant Proc. 2007;39(1):138–9.
34. Ponticelli C, Moia M, Montagnino G. Renal allograft thrombosis. Nephrol Dial Transplant Off Publ Eur Dial Transpl Assoc-Eur Ren Assoc. 2009 May;24(5):1388–93.
35. El Zorkany K, Bridson JM, Sharma A, Halawa A. Transplant Renal Vein Thrombosis. Exp Clin Transplant Off J Middle East Soc Organ Transplant. 2017 Apr;15(2):123–9.
36. Santos JE, Gaspar A, Querido S, Jorge C, Weigert A, Gabriel HM, *et al.* Unexpected success in early post-transplantation renal vein thrombosis: A case report and literature review. Clin Nephrol Case Stud. 2021;9:19–25.
37. Khan SA, Al-Huneini MN, Al-Mula Abed YWA, Mohammed SM, Al-Riyami DA. Acute Allograft Renal Vein Thrombosis: A Case Report. Oman Med J. 2014 Sep;29(5):e079.
38. Melamed ML, Kim HS, Jaar BG, Molmenti E, Atta MG, Samaniego MD. Combined percutaneous mechanical and chemical thrombectomy for renal vein thrombosis in kidney transplant recipients. Am J Transplant Off J Am Soc Transplant Am Soc Transpl Surg. 2005 Mar;5(3):621–6.
39. Alkhunaizi AM, Olyaei AJ, Barry JM, deMattos AM, Conlin MJ, Lemmers MJ, *et al.* Efficacy and safety of low molecular weight heparin in renal transplantation. Transplantation. 1998 Aug 27;66(4):533–4.
40. Chung MM, Chan YC, Law Y, Cheng SW. Infectious anastomotic pseudoaneurysm complicating renal allograft: case report and review of literature. Int J Nephrol Renov Dis. 2017;10:55–60.

41. Sharma N, Bidnur S, Caldas M, McNally D, Murray A, Turnbull R, *et al.* Renal transplant anastomotic pseudoaneurysms: Case report of open repair and endovascular management. IJU Case Rep. 2019 Mar;2(2):86–9.
42. Bracale UM, Santangelo M, Carbone F, Del Guercio L, Maurea S, Porcellini M, *et al.* Anastomotic pseudoaneurysm complicating renal transplantation: treatment options. Eur J Vasc Endovasc Surg Off J Eur Soc Vasc Surg. 2010 May;39(5):565–8.
43. Kountidou CS, Stier K, Niehues SM, Lingnau A, Schostak M, Fuller TF, *et al.* Successful repair of post-transplant mycotic aneurysm of iliac artery with renal graft preservation: a case report. Urology. 2012 Nov;80(5):1151–3.
44. Marcu CB, Nijveldt R, Van Rossum AC. Unsuspected chronic traumatic aortic pseudoaneurysm-what to do about it. Late post-traumatic aortic pseudoaneurysm. Can J Cardiol. 2008 Feb;24(2):143–4.
45. Kubal C, Cacciola R, Riley P, Ready A. Internal iliac artery pseudoaneurysm following renal transplant biopsy successfully treated with endovascular stenting and thrombosis: a case report. Transplant Proc. 2007 Jun;39(5):1676–8.
46. Asztalos L, Olvasztó S, Fedor R, Szabó L, Balázs G, Lukács G. Renal artery aneurysm at the anastomosis after kidney transplantation. Transplant Proc. 2006 Nov;38(9):2915–8.
47. Fananapazir G, Hannsun G, Wright LA, Corwin MT, Troppmann C. Diagnosis and Management of Transplanted Kidney Extrarenal Pseudoaneurysms: A Series of Four Cases and a Review of the Literature. Cardiovasc Intervent Radiol. 2016 Nov;39(11):1649–53.
48. Vijayvergiya R, Kasinadhuni G, Sharma A, Lal A. Endovascular Repair of a Post-Renal Transplant Internal Iliac Artery Pseudoaneurysm. Vasc Endovascular Surg. 2021 Aug;55(6):651–3.
49. Leonardou P, Gioldasi S, Zavos G, Pappas P. Mycotic pseudoaneurysms complicating renal transplantation: a case series and review of literature. J Med Case Reports. 2012 Feb 14;6:59.
50. Eng MMP, Power RE, Hickey DP, Little DM. Vascular complications of allograft nephrectomy. Eur J Vasc Endovasc Surg Off J Eur Soc Vasc Surg. 2006 Aug;32(2):212–6.
51. Osmán I, Barrero R, León E, Medina R, Torrubia F. Mycotic pseudoaneurysm following a kidney transplant: a case report and review of the literature. Pediatr Transplant. 2009 Aug;13(5):615–9.
52. Buimer MG, van Hamersvelt HW, Adam van der Vliet J. Anastomotic pseudoaneurysm after renal transplantation; a new hybrid approach with graft salvage. Transpl Int Off J Eur Soc Organ Transplant. 2012 Jul;25(7):e86–88.
53. Hachem LD, Ghanekar A, Selzner M, Famure O, Li Y, Kim SJ. Postoperative surgical-site hemorrhage after kidney transplantation: incidence, risk factors, and outcomes. Transpl Int Off J Eur Soc Organ Transplant. 2017 May;30(5):474–83.
54. Singh Rana AK, Agarwal N, Kumar P. Recognition of Acute Page Kidney following Renal Transplant: Varied Etiologies Requiring High Clinical Suspicion. Saudi J Kidney Dis Transplant Off Publ Saudi Cent Organ Transplant Saudi Arab. 2021;32(4):1134–40.
55. Hori S, Tomizawa M, Maesaka F, Owari T, Morizawa Y, Nakai Y, *et al.* Unexpected presentation of allograft dysfunction triggered by page kidney phenomenon immediately after kidney transplantation: a case report. BMC Nephrol. 2018 Mar 13;19(1):59.
56. Lee TW, Bae W, Choi J, Bae E, Jang HN, Chang SH, *et al.* Page kidney following spontaneous subcapsular hematoma immediately after kidney transplantation: a case report. BMC Nephrol. 2022 Jul 7;23(1):239.
57. Inoue T, Saito M, Narita S, Numakura K, Tsuruta H, Maeno A, *et al.* Evaluation of Persistent Lymphatic Fluid Leakage Using a Strategy of Placing a Drain After Kidney Transplantation: A Statistical Analysis to Assess Its Origin. Transplant Proc. 2017 Oct;49(8):1786–90.
58. Lucan CV, Jurchis I, Suciu M, Selicean SE, Buttice S. Modern lymphatic dissection techniques for preventing post renal transplant lymphocele. Clujul Med 1957. 2017;90(4):416–9.
59. Mehrabi A, Golriz M, Khajeh E, Ghamarnejad O, Kulu Y, Wiesel M, *et al.* Surgical outcomes after pediatric kidney transplantation at the University of Heidelberg. J Pediatr Urol. 2019 May;15(3):221.e1–221.e8.
60. Heer MK, Clark D, Trevillian PR, Sprott P, Palazzi K, Hibberd AD. Functional significance and risk factors for lymphocele formation after renal transplantation. ANZ J Surg. 2018 Jun;88(6):597–602.
61. Singh AG, Jai SJ, Ganpule AP, VijayKumar M, Sabnis RB, Desai MR. Critical appraisal of consecutive 36 cases of post-renal transplant lymphocele: a proposed algorithm. World J Urol. 2017 Sep;35(9):1443–50.
62. Golriz M, Klauss M, Zeier M, Mehrabi A. Prevention and management of lymphocele formation following kidney transplantation. Transplant Rev Orlando Fla. 2017 Apr;31(2):100–5.
63. Isiktas Sayilar E, Ersoy A, Ayar Y, Aydin MF, Sahin AB, Coskun B, *et al.* Factors Influencing Lymphocele Development After Kidney Transplant: Single Center Experience. Exp Clin Transplant Off J Middle East Soc Organ Transplant. 2022 Feb;21(2):116–22.
64. Jänigen BM, Salabè C, Glatz T, Thomusch O, Lässle C, Fichtner-Feigl S, *et al.* Single cohort study: ABO-incompatible kidney transplant recipients have a higher risk of lymphocele formation. Langenbecks Arch Surg. 2019 Dec;404(8):999–1007.
65. Bzoma B, Kostro J, D bska- lizie A, Hellmann AR, Zadro ny D, ledzi ski Z, *et al.* Treatment of the Lymphocele After Kidney Transplantation: A Single-center Experience. Transplant Proc. 2016 Jun;48(5):1637–40.
66. Koch M, Kantas A, Ramcke K, Drabik AI, Nashan B. Surgical complications after kidney transplantation: different impacts of immunosuppression, graft function, patient variables, and surgical performance. Clin Transplant. 2015 Mar;29(3):252–60.
67. Sim A, Ng LG, Cheng C. Occurrence of a lymphocele following renal transplantation. Singapore Med J. 2013 May;54(5):259–62.
68. Burleson RL, Marbarger PD. Prevention of lymphocele formation following renal allotransplantation. J Urol. 1982 Jan;127(1):18–9.
69. Nelson EW, Gross ME, Mone MC, Hansen HJ, Sheng X, Cannon KM, *et al.* Does ultrasonic energy for surgical dissection reduce the incidence of renal transplant lymphocele? Transplant Proc. 2011 Dec;43(10):3755–9.
70. Derweesh IH, Ismail HR, Goldfarb DA, Araki M, Zhou L, Modlin C, *et al.* Intraoperative placing of drains decreases the incidence of lymphocele and deep vein thrombosis after renal transplantation. BJU Int. 2008 Jun;101(11):1415–9.

Chapter

9A

Urological Complications of Kidney Transplant: Urine Leak

• *Arun Chawla*

LEARNING OBJECTIVES

- To understand the causes, diagnosis and management of post-transplant urine leak.

Case Scenario

A 24-year-old male with CKD 5D (medical renal disease: HTN nephropathy) underwent live renal related transplant, ABO compatible with 3/6 HLA mismatch. Immediate graft function was good and discharged after a few days with serum creatinine of 0.8 mg/dl. Catheter and drain removed after 7 days. Stent removal was advised after 3 weeks. Patient was on triple immunosuppression.

Patient presented after 2 weeks after discharge with vague abdomen discomfort and fever of one day and decreased urine output. Ultrasound showed fluid collection in perirenal and perivesical area (Fig. 9A.1). Serum creatinine increased from 0.8 to 1.4 mg/dl.

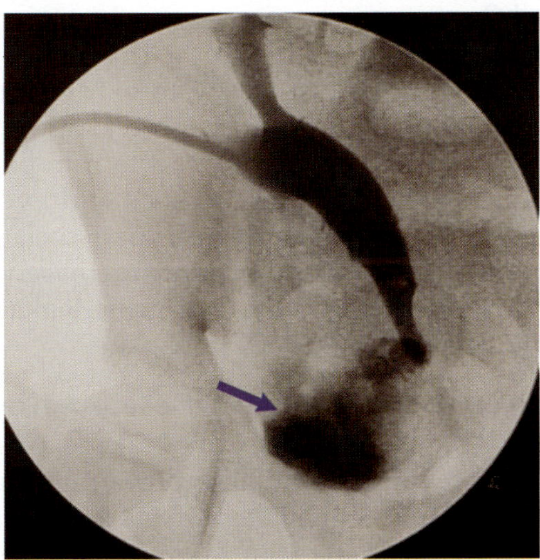

Fig. 9A.1: Antegrade nephrostogram showing contrast extravasation (blue arrow)

1. **What is the probable diagnosis?**

   Ans: Decreased urine output with fluid collection with increase in creatinine points to urine leakage.

2. **How can urine collection be differentiated from lymph or serous collection?**

   Ans: Fluid creatinine is 5–10 times higher than serum creatinine in urinomas and urine leakage.

3. **How will you manage this patient?**

   Ans: Patient will need further imaging. CECT was done that showed significant contrast extravasation that is diagnostic of urinary leak (Fig. 9A.2). Patient was immediately re-catheterised and managed conservatively. Patient was monitored for improvement by ultrasound and serum creatinine. Patient improved with restoration of serum creatinine to normal and ultrasound showing minimal fluid. Patient was discharged on day 8 and underwent stent removal 2 weeks post-discharge.

4. **How does urine leak commonly present in post-renal transplant?**

   Ans: A key clinical finding of urine leak is excessive liquid drain output during the early postoperative period. Drain fluid can be checked to confirm as urine based on fluid creatinine. Other leading clinical findings suggestive of urine leakage decreased urine output, wound fluid drainage, delayed graft function, and swelling and tenderness over the graft, ipsilateral lower limb edema and systemic infection. The clinical presentation can have a more insidious onset

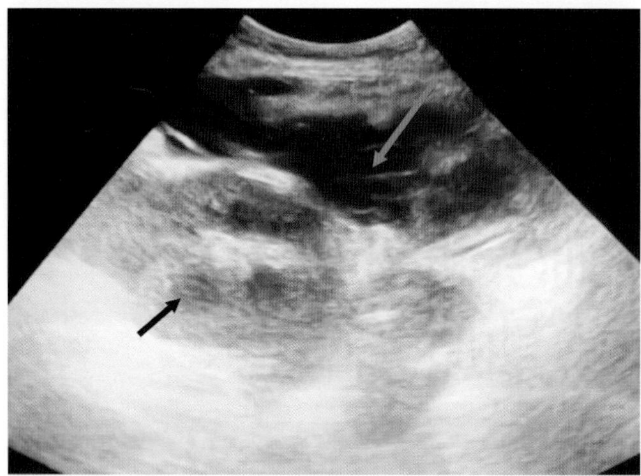

Fig. 9A.2: Peri-graft collection on ultrasound (urinary leak). (Black arrow: Renal graft, Green arrow: Perinephric collection)

because of confounding factors (pre-existing seroma, limited drainage fluid related to delayed graft function). Severe urine leaks can also track along the retroperitoneal space, pelvis, pre-sacral, incision site and scrotal area.[1]

5. How do we decide which patient to explore and which to conserve?

Ans: Indications for exploration include:

1. Large urinoma,
2. Persistent urine leak in patients on conservative management
3. Copius urine collection in the retroperitoneum or urine leaking through the abdominal incision/ wound.

6. What are the common sites of urine leakage post-renal transplant?

Ans: The most common location of urine leak is at site of the ureteroneocystostomy and lower ureter.[2] Urine leakage can occur from other sites like bladder, calyx, pelvi–native ureteric anastomosis.

7. What factors predisposes to urine leakage in a post-transplant patient?

Ans: Cause of urine leakage is multifactorial. The two most common causes are surgical/technical error and ureteric ischaemia with necrosis. Technical errors include misplacement of ureteral sutures and insufficient ureteral length with tension on the anastomosis. Technical errors during retrieval, bench dissection with unrecognised injury to the ureter or implantation contributes to urine leakage. Other causes of urinary leak include outflow obstruction (blocked Foley catheter or urinary retention) with partial disruption of an otherwise technically perfect anastomosis, unrecognized surgical laceration or electrocautery injury of the ureter or renal pelvis, acute ureteral obstruction with perforation of renal calyx, and protrusion of a ureteral stent. Early leaks often occur at the heel of the ureterocystostomy.[3]

Ureteral ischemia secondary to compromised blood supply to distal ureter leading to necrosis can result from loss of a lower pole artery or devascularization of the distal tip of the ureter due to the lack of preservation of the blood supply from mesoureter.

In this patient urine leak could be attributed to full bladder resulting in leak from ureteroneocystostomy.

8. How do we evaluate a patient with post-renal transplant urine leakage?

Ans: Once clinical suspicion of urine leakage is there, initial ultrasonography can be helpful for establishing diagnosis of urinoma secondary to urine leakage. In normal bladder, urinomas appear as well-defined anechoic collections without septations. It would appear echoic collection with septations if infected or mixed with blood. The leak may be extraperitoneal or intraperitoneal.[3,4] Ultrasonography can determine size and site of urine collection and associated hydronephrosis. The obstruction can be associated with urine extravasation.

Computed tomography and MRI can be helpful in diagnosing urine collection area but may not precisely show the source of the urine leak. Renal scintigraphy can be used to contribute to the diagnosis if the patient has good renal function. It is useful for detection of urine leaks after renal transplant.[5]

Cystography imaging with a retrograde opacification can also be used to show bladder leaks.

9. What if urine leakage is left untreated or not treated early?

Ans: Urinomas due to urine leakage can cause hydronephrosis due to extrinsic ureteral obstruction. Persistent urine leakage can lead to infection which can spread to retroperitoneal planes and perinephric tissues and eventually causing perinephric abscess.[6] It is associated with delayed wound healing and increased risk of wound infection, if there is urine leakage from wound site, post-kidney transplant.

10. How can complication of urine leakage avoided?

Ans: As risk factors of urine leakage are known, incidence can be avoided by preventive measures. Meticulous precise tension free watertight ureterovesical anastomosis with vascular distal ureter should be performed with uninterrupted drainage of urinary bladder in early postoperative period. Ureteric ischemia leading to leakage can be prevented by avoiding excessively dissected tissue around the donor ureter during laparoscopic or open kidney harvesting and bench preparation. The preservation of peri-ureteric tissue that contains fine branches of renal artery is crucial to minimizing the risk of devascularization of the ureter. This peri-ureteric tissue should be handled with care and should not be stripped off. Also, preservation of the "golden triangle area" which has lower polar artery, which supplies the distal ureter is of utmost importance. Length of the ureter should also be kept as short as possible, and anastomosis done without any tension to prevent urine leak. A compromised ureter at the time of surgery could be due to failure to bleed after reperfusion, transected lower polar artery, over stripping of ureter should be cut as proximally as necessary to reach well-perfused tissue. If this is not possible, then it may either necessitate anastomosis to the ipsilateral native ureter or by an extension technique of the bladder (psoas hitch, Boari flap). A stent is also advisable in these situations. Regarding techniques of ureteroneocystostomy, Lich-Gregoir technique is associated with lesser incidence of ureteral leaks when compared to the Leadbetter-Politano technique.[7]

11. What is management urine leakage?

Ans: Management depends upon timing of presentation, site and severity of leakage, associated hydronephrosis. It can be conservative, percutaneous or exploration. Indications for exploration include:

1. Large urinoma,
2. Persistent urine leak in patients on conservative management
3. Copius urine collection in the retroperitoneum or urine leaking through the abdominal incision/ wound.

Conservative treatment

In patients with milder urine leakage with no hydronephrosis, conservative management with indwelling catheter can be done. If the patient already had the ureteral stent removed, replacing this stent can be effective. If prior double J stent was not done, retrograde placement is technically a difficult task and should not be attempted in the early postoperative period.

Percutaneous treatment

The objective of this management is to divert urine from the urinary leakage site. If there is a delay in operative intervention, larger urine collection needs drainage to reduce risk of infection.[8–11] It is possible to manage urine leak associated with hydronephrosis by external drainage (percutaneous nephrostomy) or internal drainage (DJ stenting). It is often difficult to place DJ stent via retrograde approach since the neoureteric orifice is located more anterolaterally and lack of periureteral supports. Hence placement of percutaneous nephrostomy (PCN) is done. Antegrade nephrostogram during PCN placement can evaluate the site of extravasation and helps to guide therapeutic management, as illustrated in Fig. 9A.3.An antegrade stent placement at time of PCN placement if possible for 6–12 weeks along with a Foley catheter replacement remains a practical approach.[12,13] This will divert the flow of urine away from the leak site allowing the healing to take place along with decompression of the collecting system. Alcaraz and associates[14] assessed that among those developing urine leak 3 days after

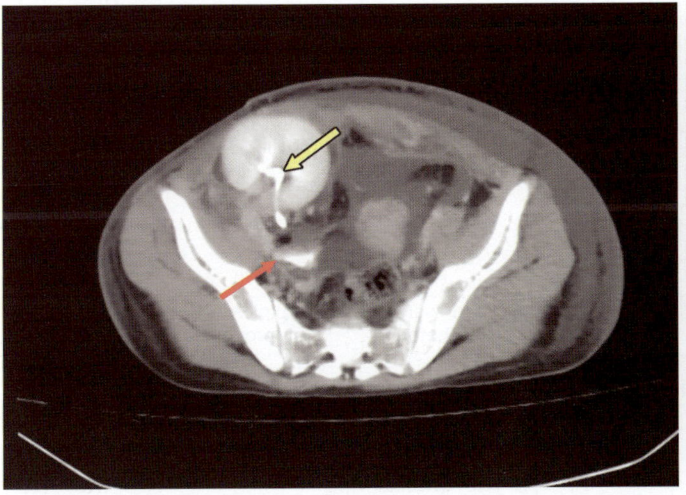

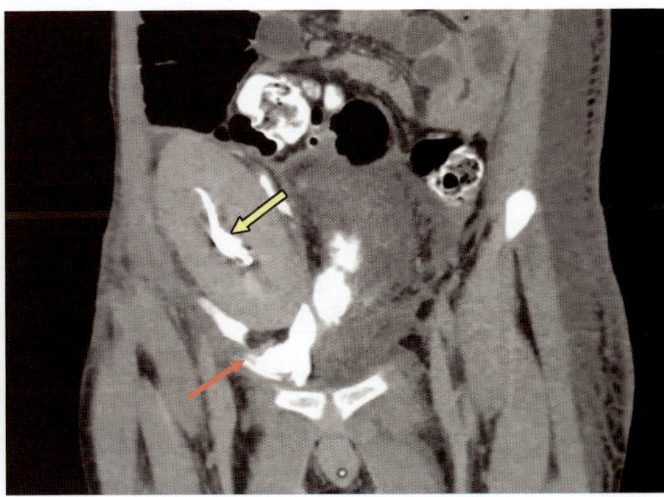

Fig 9A.3: Coronal and axial sections of CECT denoting urinary leak (Yellow arrow: Contrast draining the pelvicalyceal system of graft, Red arrow: Contrast extravasation/leak)

kidney transplant, PCN can result in successful treatment for 60% of recipients. If the conservative treatment fails, surgical exploration is indicated.

Open Exploration

Open exploration should be considered for patients with extensive urine leakage, with proximal fistula, or those not responding despite PCN placement. Large ureteric leaks as a result of anastomotic failure would require reimplantation to the urinary bladder. Urine leak due to ureteral necrosis would need resection of necrosed segment and reimplantation. The reimplantation depends on the ureteric perfusion and length.[15]

If the ureter length and perfusion are adequate, a reimplantation of the preserved transplant ureter is performed. If there is not enough length of well-perfused transplanted ureter, then anastomosis with the native ureter needs to be performed. Native nephrectomy is not required, even if it is side-to-side anastomosis or to the end of native ipsilateral native ureter.[16] Boari flap and psoas hitch are other options. Rarely, other techniques like use of ileum as a neoureter is indicated if there is no native ureter available (for previous bilateral nephrectomy.[17,18]

Although urine leak is associated with significant morbidity, the prognosis is generally excellent if recognized and managed early.

12. What is the management of leakage from other sites?

- Blocked per urethral catheter, replace the catheter.
- If still significant leak → bladder repair indicated (keep per urethral catheter for at least 2 weeks).[19]
- Calyceal leak due to obstruction → remove the obstruction.[20]
- If this leak is attributed to segmentary renal infarction by ligation of a polar artery, conservative treatment is the first choice. Partial nephrectomy (in rare instance).[21]

KEY POINTS

- Most common cause of urine leakage are surgical technical error and ureteral ischemia with necrosis. Rarely urinary retention and blocked Foley's catheter can lead to leakage.
- Later leaks due to ureteral ischemia and necrosis can be due to vascular infringement of ureter during donor kidney harvesting, bench dissection and poor anastomotic technique. Delayed graft function and old donor age are risk factors of ureteral necrosis.
- Urine leakage should be suspected in early postoperative period in case of poor urinary output, new fluid collection, delayed graft function. Fluid creatinine estimation always show raised creatinine values.
- Surgical reconstruction involves transplant ureteroneocystostomy and use of native ureter for anastomosis.
- Prognosis in terms of graft function after effective management of urine leakage is excellent.

SUMMARY

- Urine leakage should be suspected when fluid drain output is excessive and has high creatinine. Decreased urine output, delayed graft function with swelling of ipsilateral lower limb, and tenderness over the graft adds to the suspicion.
- Though urine leak can happen from any part of collecting system, most commonly it is from the site of uretero-neocystostomy site and lower ureter when necrosis and later fistula forms.
- Most common cause leading to urine leakage in early postoperative period is surgical, technical and later due to ureteric ischaemia with necrosis and fistula.
- Poor reconstruction of uretero-vesical anastomosis with misplaced sutures and anastomosis of poor vascularised lower end of ureter with tension are causative factors.
- Technical errors in retrieval and poor bench dissection lead to ischemia, contributing to urine leak. Poor vascularity of terminal ureter due to loss of lower pole renal artery can lead to ureteral necrosis and fistula.
- Post-renal transplant leakage can be diagnosed by presence of urine collection on ultrasound, CT, MRI, renal scintigraphy and cystography.
- Early urine leaks can be prevented. Tension-free watertight uretero-vesical anastomosis with vascular distal ureter should be performed with uninterrupted bladder drainage in the post-operative period.

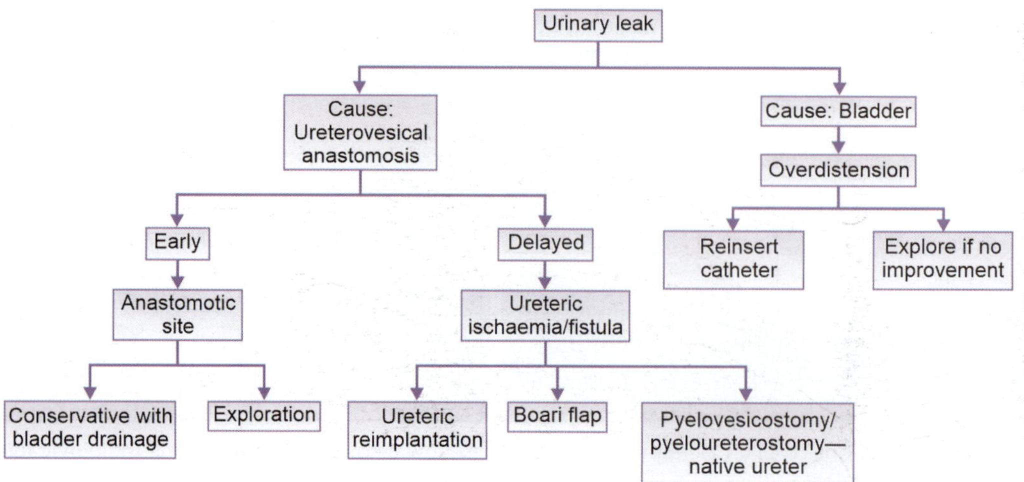

Section 6

- Delayed leaks from ureteral necrosis and fistula can be avoided by careful preservation of vascularity of ureter during harvesting and bench dissection. After renal perfusion during transplant procedure, note should be made of pink ureter with bleeding edges before anastomosis.
- Conservative treatment involves stenting and bladder drainage. In presence of urine leak and associated hydronephrosis, Percutaneous drainage of kidney provides decompression, allows to have an antegrade contrast study to see the site of leakage and antegrade stenting if needed.
- Retrograde stenting is difficult because of ectopic location of uretero-neocystostomy and poorly supported transplant ureter, and it should not be attempted in the early post-operative period.
- Larger urine leaks need reconstruction, transplant uretero-neocystostomy, Boari flap, pyelovesicostomy, pyeloureterostomy with native ureter.
- Though the urine leak from post-transplant ureter is associated with significant morbidity, prognosis is generally excellent if managed early.

REFERENCES

1. Son H, Heiba S, Kostakoglu L, Machac J. Extraperitoneal urine leak after renal transplantation: the role of radionuclide imaging and the value of accompanying SPECT/CT-a case report. BMC Med Imaging [Internet]. 2010 Oct 20 [cited 2023 Aug 1];10. Available from: https://pubmed.ncbi.nlm.nih.gov/20961409/.
2. Obert R, Olfe AW, Alarie V, Shby BA, Dgar E, Ilford LM, *et al.* Number 23 1725 Mortality in Patients on Dialysis and Transplant Recipients. 1999;341.
3. Dinckan A, Tekin A, Turkyilmaz S, Kocak H, Gurkan A, Erdogan O, *et al.* Early and late urological complications corrected surgically following renal transplantation. Transpl Int [Internet]. 2007 Aug [cited 2023 Aug 1];20(8):702–7. Available from: https://pubmed.ncbi.nlm.nih.gov/17511829/.
4. Wilson CH, Bhatti AB, Rix DA, Manas DM. Routine intraoperative ureteric stenting for kidney transplant recipients. Cochrane Database Syst Rev [Internet]. 2005 Oct 19 [cited 2023 Aug 1];(4). Available from: https://pubmed.ncbi.nlm.nih.gov/16235385/.
5. Gunatunga I, Facey P, Bartley L, Rees J, Singh S, Fielding P. Perinephric urinoma secondary to perforated UPJ obstruction diagnosed using Tc-99m mercaptoacetyltriglycine (MAG3) SPECT/CT. Clin Nucl Med [Internet]. 2007 Apr [cited 2023 Aug 1];32(4):317–9. Available from: https://pubmed.ncbi.nlm.nih.gov/17413586/.
6. Arpali E, Al-Qaoud T, Martinez E, Redfield RR, Leverson GE, Kaufman DB, *et al.* Impact of ureteral stricture and treatment choice on long-term graft survival in kidney transplantation. Am J Transplant [Internet]. 2018 Aug 1 [cited 2023 Aug 1];18(8):1977–85. Available from: https://pubmed.ncbi.nlm.nih.gov/29446225/.
7. Dalgic A, Boyvat F, Karakayali H, Moray G, Emiroglu R, Haberal M. Surgical Urologic Complications in 1523 Renal Transplantations: The Baskent University Experience. Transplant Proc. 2006;38:543.
8. Emiro-lu R, Karakayall H, Sevmi S, Akkoç H, Bilgin N, Haberal M. Urologic complications in 1275 consecutive renal transplantations. Transplant Proc [Internet]. 2001 [cited 2023 Aug 1];33(1–2):2016–7. Available from: https://pubmed.ncbi.nlm.nih.gov/11267607/.
9. Campbell SC, Streem SB, Zelch M, Hodge E, Novick AC. Percutaneous management of transplant ureteral fistulas: patient selection and long-term results. J Urol [Internet]. 1993 [cited 2023 Aug 1];150(4):1115–7. Available from: https://pubmed.ncbi.nlm.nih.gov/8371367/.
10. Duty BD, Conlin MJ, Fuchs EF, Barry JM. The current role of endourologic management of renal transplantation complications. Adv Urol [Internet]. 2013 [cited 2023 Aug 1];2013. Available from: https://pubmed.ncbi.nlm.nih.gov/24023541/.
11. Duty BD, Barry JM. Diagnosis and management of ureteral complications following renal transplantation. Asian J Urol [Internet]. 2015 [cited 2023 Aug 1];2(4):202–7. Available from: https://pubmed.ncbi.nlm.nih.gov/29264146/.
12. Dominguez J, Clase CM, Mahalati K, MacDonald AS, McAlister VC, Belitsky P, *et al.* Is routine ureteric stenting needed in kidney transplantation? A randomized trial. Transplantation [Internet]. 2000 Aug 27 [cited 2023 Aug 1];70(4):597–601. Available from: https://pubmed.ncbi.nlm.nih.gov/10972216/.
13. Parapiboon W, Ingsathit A, Disthabanchong S, Nongnuch A, Jearanaipreprem A, Charoenthanakit C, *et al.* Impact of early ureteric stent removal and cost-benefit analysis in kidney transplant recipients: results of a randomized controlled study. Transplant Proc [Internet]. 2012 Apr [cited 2023 Aug 1];44(3):737–9. Available from: https://pubmed.ncbi.nlm.nih.gov/22483481/.
14. Alcaraz A, Bujons A, Pascual X, Juaneda B, Martí J, De La Torre P, *et al.* Percutaneous Management of Transplant Ureteral Fistulae Is Feasible in Selected Cases. Transplant Proc.2005 Jun 1;37(5):2111–4.
15. Haberal M, Boyvat F, Akdur A, K rnap M, Özçelik Ü, Yarbuð Karakayal F. Surgical Complications after kidney transplantation. Exp Clin Transplant. 2016;14(6):587–595.
16. Khoubehi B, Williams G. Re: Ligation of the native ureter in renal transplantation [1]. Journal of Urology. 2003 Jan 1;169(1):292.
17. Shokeir AA, Shamaa MA, Bakr MA, El-Diasty TA, Ghoneim MA. Salvage of difficult transplant urinary fistulae by ileal substitution of the ureter. Scand J Urol Nephrol [Internet]. 1993 [cited 2023 Aug 1];27(4):537–40. Available from: https://pubmed.ncbi.nlm.nih.gov/8159928/.
18. French CG, Acott PD, Crocker JFS, Bitter-Suermann H, Lawen JG. Extravesical ureteroneocystostomy with and without internalized ureteric stents in pediatric renal transplantation. Pediatr Transplant [Internet]. 2001 [cited 2023 Aug 1];5(1):21–6. Available from: https://pubmed.ncbi.nlm.nih.gov/11260484/.
19. Singer J,Gritsch HA, Rosenthal JT. The transplant operation and its surgical complications. In: Danovitch GM, ed. Handbook of Kidney Transplantation. 5th ed. Philadelphia, PA, Lippincott Williams & Wilkins; 2005:193–212.
20. Shoskes D, Jiménez JA. Urological complications after kidney transplantation. In: Morris PJ, Knechtle SJ, eds. Kidney Transplantation: Principles and Practice. 7th ed. Oxford, UK: Saunders; 2013:464–471.
21. Gutierrez-Calzada JL, Ramos-Titos J, Gonzalez-Bonilla JA, Garcia-Vaquero AS, Martin-Morales A, Burgos-Rodriguez R. Caliceal fistula formation following renal transplantation: management with partial nephrectomy and ureteral replacement. J Urol [Internet]. 1995 Mar [cited 2023 Aug 1];153(3 Pt 1):612–4. Available from: https://pubmed.ncbi.nlm.nih.gov/7861495/.

Chapter

9B

Post-transplant Ureteric Stricture

• *Arun Chawla*

LEARNING OBJECTIVES

- To understand the causes, diagnosis and management of post-transplant ureteric stricture.

Case Scenario

Male patient, aged 54 years, CKD with chronic glomerulonephritis on thrice weekly HD since 5 years underwent deceased donor renal transplant (19-year-old brain-dead donor with cold ischemia time of 6 hours). Patient was on triple immunosuppression. Post-transplant serum creatinine was 1.2 mg/dl at one month. DJ stent removed after 4 weeks post-transplant. Four months post-transplant patient presented with vague abdominal pain with ultrasound showing graft hydroureteronephrosis. Serum creatinine increased from 1.2 to 2.1 mg/dl in a week's duration. MRI revealed short segment distal ureteric stricture with hydroureteronephrosis.

1. **What is the probable diagnosis?**

   Ans: Based on increasing creatinine and USG evidence of HUN, the diagnosis would be ureteric obstruction probably due to stricture.

2. **What is the next line of management?**

   Ans: Further evaluation with NCCT/CECT or MRI is needed to document site of obstruction. MRI was done and T2 WI showed lower ureteric stricture. In view HUN and rising creatinine, patient underwent graft PCN insertion. Patient had improvement in serum creatinine and resolution of HUN. Antegrade nephrostogram was done and confirmed obstruction at distal ureter a few centimeters away from bladder, with mild trickle of contrast into the bladder (Fig. 9B.1). Antegrade stenting was unsuccessful.

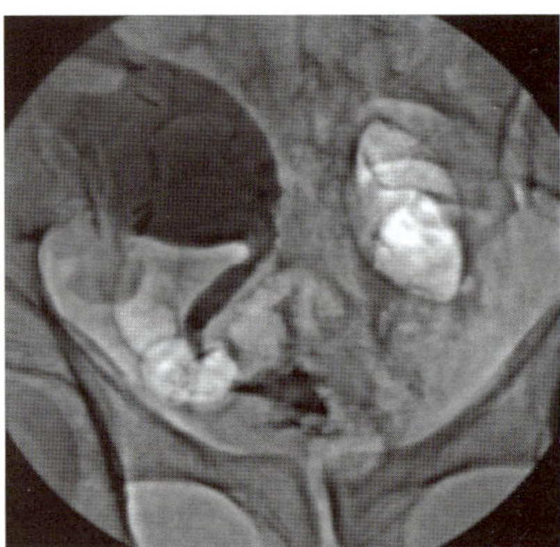

Fig 9B.1: Nephrostogram confirming presence and location of stricture (red arrow depicting site of narrowing)

3. **What are the common causes of ureteric obstruction post-renal transplant?**

   Ans: Ureteral obstruction due to stricture is seen in 1–4.5% of transplant recipients and is most common cause of ureteric obstruction.[1,2] The most common location of stricture is distal ureter (Table 9B.1).

TABLE 9B.1: Causes of ureteric obstruction	
Extra-luminal	Compression from lymphocele, hematoma, and spermatic cord
Ureteric	Poor anastomotic technique, ischemia
Intra-luminal	Stone, sloughed renal papilla, foreign body, fungal ball

4. **What is common presentation of ureteric stricture with obstruction?**

   Ans: These patients rarely develops symptoms of pain due to ureteral obstruction since transplant kidney is denervated. The clinical presentation of ureteral stricture can vary according to its location, degree, and speed of onset. Most commonly, ureteral stricture is gradual and patients are asymptomatic, and are diagnosed with an unexplained increase in serum creatinine and presence of hydronephrosis on Ultrasound or computed tomography.

5. **Which are predisposing conditions for stricture leading to ureteric obstruction?**

Ans: It occurs mainly due to devascularization of ureter with compromised blood supply. It can present early (< 3 months) or a late (>3 months). Early causes include technical errors during the ureteroneocystostomy, extrinsic compression (due to hematoma, lymphocele, and abscess), ureteral kink and edema at anastomosis site. Surgical technique-related factors such as length of ureter used, tissue handling technique too play important role in preventing post-renal transplant ureteric stricture.

Late post-operative causes include ureteral ischemia, vasculitis due to acute rejection, lymphocele and fibrosis due to immunosuppressants usage. Longer duration of ischemia time during ureteroneocystostomy has been reported to be cause of ureteral strictures.[3] Donor age, multiple donor renal arteries and delayed graft function (DGF) are associated with a higher rate of ureteral complications leading to stricture.

6. **How do you evaluate post-transplant ureteric stricture?**

Ultrasound is the first line of investigation in these patients to look for presence and severity of hydroureteronephrosis (Fig. 9B.2). Computed tomography (with or without contrast) should be the next line of imaging if hydroureteronephrosis is present, especially in the early postoperative period, to identify both intrinsic (ureteral calculus, clots) and extrinsic (lymphocele, hematoma) causes of obstruction. Diuretic renogram with Tc 99m MAG-3/EC can be done to confirm obstruction. A diuretic renogram suggests obstruction if the urinary transit time is prolonged, or if the clearance curve shows pelvicalyceal holdup, especially after the diuretic. False-negative results can occur in patients with poor renal function, and false positive results can occur with bladder outflow obstruction or reflux. Voiding cystourethrogram should be considered if there is hydroureteronephrosis without obstruction to rule out VUR. Site and severity of obstruction can be estimated by CECT if renal function is normal, MRI (T2 weighted images), antegrade nephrostogram and combined antegrade and retrograde contrast studies if possible (Fig. 9B.3).

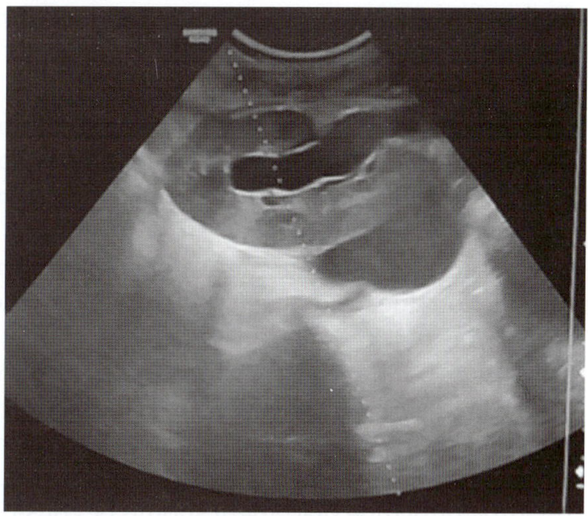

Fig 9B.2: Ultrasound depicting hydronephrosis in transplanted kidney due to ureteric obstruction

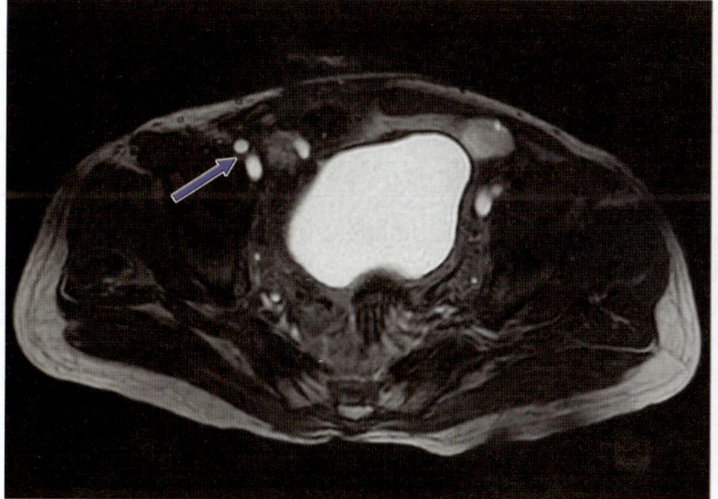

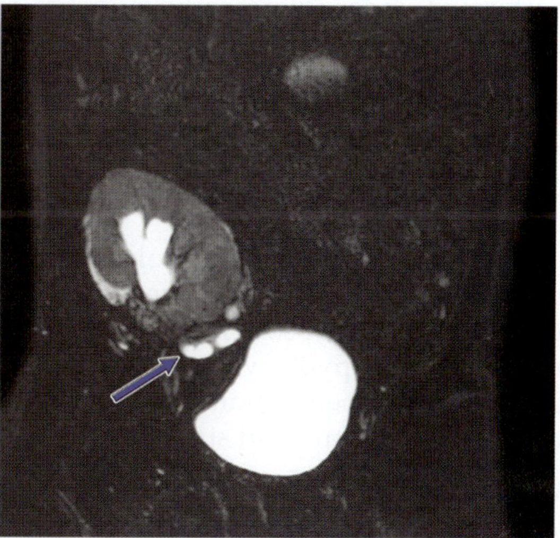

Fig. 9B.3: Blue arrow depicting site of stricture as noted on MR urogram (T2W with reconstructed sequence)

7. **What are management options for ureteric obstruction due to stricture?**

Ans: Management depends upon severity of obstruction, effect on renal function and timing of presentation. Different arms of management include conservative, minimal invasive treatment and surgical reconstruction.

Conservative management alone is sufficient in obstruction due to edema at ureteroneocystostomy site.

Active management in hydronephrosis with effect on graft function includes early decompression of the collecting system to protect renal function of transplant kidney. Percutaneous nephrostomy tube placement should be considered first-line treatment in most patients since DJ stent placement is often difficult due to the anterolateral location of the ureteroneocystostomy, edema at anastomosis site and the lack of strong tissue supports of the transplant ureter. Extrinsic obstruction by urinoma and lymphocele which are smaller should be managed with ultrasound guided percutaneous drainage, percutaneous lap or open drainage based on case scenario.

Length of ureteric stricture is assessed by combination of different imaging means. CECT, MRI, antegrade nephrostogram with or without combined cystogram. Strictures < 1 cm can be managed by endoscopic intervention. More complex and longer strictures need open reconstruction. Strictures > 2 cm require excision and reimplantation of the remaining healthy ureter into the bladder or native ureter. Endoscopic intervention includes ureteral balloon dilation and endoureterotomy. Endoureterotomy can be performed with a cold knife, Acucise balloon-cutting catheter or holmium laser. Ureteral balloon dilation and Acucise endoureterotomy are performed under fluoroscopic guidance making them ideal for both antegrade and retrograde treatment. As a result, treatment of distal strictures frequently requires an antegrade approach. The overall success rate is 51%, 78%, and 79% for balloon dilatation, Acucise balloon–cutting and endoureterotomy respectively.[3–6]

Open reconstruction involves any of the operative approaches discussed previously for ureteral leak (e.g., psoas hitch, Boari flap, ureteropyelostomy, pyelocystostomy, ileal ureter). Successful treatment of transplant ureteral stenosis results in long-term graft survival.[7]

8. **What was done for this patient?**

Ans: Boari flap with DJ stent was performed. PCN tube was retained. Patient underwent anastomosis of the dilated proximal ureter to the bladder after creating a Boari flap. The distal ureter with the strictured segment was unexplored in view of dense adhesions. Nephrostogram on POD 15 showed good contrast drainage into bladder. PCN was clamped and removed after 48–72 hours and stent removal after 6 weeks. Postoperative period was uneventful.

9. **How can post-transplant ureteric strictures be managed with surgical reconstruction?**

Ans: Good preoperative preparation is crucial for success of surgical reconstruction. It is important to understand the site of the leak or stricture prior to repair with antegrade or retrograde imaging. A voiding cystourethrogram (VCUG), urodynamics and cystoscopy for bladder capacity compliance and function compliments the above imaging techniques is important to confirm a competent native ureter and adequate bladder and capacity. Principles of reconstruction involves bypassing obstruction or using the same ureter especially in distal ureteric strictures. A side-to-side or end-to-side anastomosis between the transplant and native ureter is preferred as this preserves both the renal and iliac arterial supply to the native ureter. However, sometimes the proximal native ureter must be ligated in order for it to reach the ureterostomy or pyelostomy. This may decrease the blood supply to the remaining ureter. There are concern of hydronephrosis or pyelonephritis due to native ureter ligation, however, this has not had clinical consequences. There are concerns of hydronephrosis or pyelonephritis due to native ureter ligation.

Distal ureteric strictures can be managed by transplant ureteroneocystostomy, if reasonable length of ureter with good vascularity is available. In cases where there is no native ureter or functional bladder an ileal conduit can be used for the reconstruction. In poor operative risk recipients other techniques such as an extra-ureteric bypass,[8] ante-or retrograde endoureteric surgery or the nitinol stent have been described Burgos *et al*[9] may be performed, with no proven results. The gold standard, however, remains re-anastomosis of the graft to available recipient urologic structures. The post-transplant ureteric strictures are better prevented by taking care of the factors mentioned in Table 9B.2.

TABLE 9B.2: Prevention of transplant ureteric strictures	
During donor nephrectomy	1. Preserve vascularity of the ureter 2. Preserve the fat pad of the golden triangle 3. Preserve the lower polar artery, if any 4. Lower ureter to be brought out safely during retrieval by endo-bag

(Contd.)

TABLE 9B.2: Prevention of transplant ureteric strictures *(Contd.)*

During bench preparation	1. Do not sacrifice the fat between the ureter and lower pole of the kidney while excising the excess perinephric fat
During transplant procedure	1. After clamp removal post-vascular anastomosis, make sure that the lower ureter has bleeding vascular margins 2. Do not strip the lower ureter excessively 3. Use adequate length of the ureter–neither too long nor too short 4. Meticulous and precise mucosa to mucosa anastomosis with adequate cover of the detrusor

KEY POINTS

- Ureteric obstruction can be extraluminal, luminal or intraluminal.
- Common presentation is asymptomatic with unexplained increase in creatinine and presence of hydronephrosis.
- Ureteral ischemia is the commonest cause leading to ureteral stricture.
- Complete evaluation for length of stricture, severity of obstruction, bladder assessment for adequate function and capacity.
- Commonly used investigations after initial USG involves CT, MRI, diuretic renogram, antegrade studies by PCN, MCU.
- Endoscopic management includes balloon dilatation and endoureterotomy with stenting for strictures < 1 cm.
- Surgical reconstruction for longer strictures includes transplant ureteroneocystostomy with or without psoas hitch or techniques bypassing strictures like Boari flap, pyeloureterostomy or ureteroureterostomy with ipsilateral native ureters (very rarely contralateral).
- The transplant can be salvaged with graft survival rates equivalent to a matched control group without ureteral complications and excellent functional outcomes.

SUMMARY

- Ureteric obstruction due to strictures is seen in 1–4.5% of transplant recipients. Ureteric obstruction can be extraluminal, ureteric and intraluminal.
- Clinical presentation of ureteric obstruction by stricture depends upon location, severity of obstruction and speed of onset. Most commonly it is asymptomatic with unexplained increase in creatinine levels and presence of hydronephrosis.
- Strictures in transplanted ureter develop due to devascularisation and ischemia.
- Early causes of ureteric obstruction includes technical errors in ureterovesical anastomosis, edema/hematoma/clots at anastomosis, extrinsic compression by fluid collections and ureter kinking.
- Precise and meticulous surgical technique for tension free anastomosis of a good length of vascular ureter to bladder is important in preventing ureteric strictures.
- Majority of ureteric strictures arising during first year of transplant are ischemic and later causes include rejection, BK virus and recurrent infections.
- Evaluation of ureteric stricture includes Imaging by ultrasound, CT, MRI, diuretic renogram, antegrade and retrograde contrast studies, VCUG, and UDS. Evaluation is directed to confirm obstruction, length and severity of obstruction along with bladder function and capacity.
- Management depends on the cause of obstruction. Percutaneous techniques are used to drain urinoma and lymphocele causing extrinsic ureteric obstruction.
- Endourological management of short ureteral strictures include antegrade and retrograde dilatation of stricture, followed by stenting.
- Surgical reconstruction comprises bypassing transplanted ureter stricture by Boari flap, pyelovesicostomy, pyeloureterostomy with ipsilateral native ureter and transplant ureter-neocystostomy with or without psoas hitch.

Management of Ureteric Obstruction

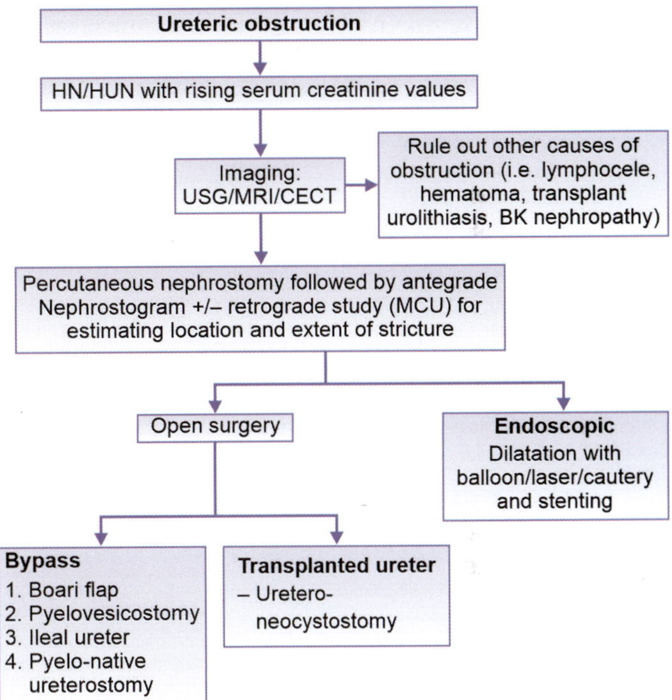

REFERENCES

1. Mano R, Golan S, Holland R, Livne PM, Lifshitz DA. Retrograde endoureterotomy for persistent ureterovesical anastomotic strictures in renal transplant kidneys after failed antegrade balloon dilation. Urology [Internet]. 2012 Aug [cited 2023 Apr 18];80(2):255–9. Available from: https://pubmed.ncbi.nlm.nih.gov/22497983/.
2. Lempinen M, Stenman J, Kyllönen L, Salmela K. Surgical complications following 1670 consecutive adult renal transplantations: A single center study. Scand J Surg [Internet]. 2015 Dec 1 [cited 2023 Apr 18];104 (4):254–9. Available from: https://pubmed.ncbi.nlm.nih.gov/25567856/.
3. Rahnemai-Azar AA, Gilchrist BF, Kayler LK. Independent risk factors for early urologic complications after kidney transplantation. 2015 [cited 2023 Aug 1]; Available from: https://onlinelibrary.wiley.com/doi/10.1111/ctr.12530.

4. Arpali E, Al-Qaoud T, Martinez E, Redfield RR, Leverson GE, Kaufman DB, *et al* Impact of ureteral stricture and treatment choice on long-term graft survival in kidney transplantation. Am J Transplant [Internet]. 2018 Aug 1 [cited 2023 Aug 1];18(8):1977–85. Available from: https://pubmed.ncbi.nlm.nih.gov/29446225/.
5. Dalgic A, Boyvat F, Karakayali H, Moray G, Emiroglu R, Haberal M. Surgical Urologic Complications in 1523 Renal Transplantations: The Baskent University Experience. Transplant Proc. 2006;38:543.
6. Kumar A, Verma Bs, Srivastava A, Bhandari M, Gupta A, Sharma R. Evaluation of the urological complications of living related renal transplantation at a single center during the last 10 years: impact of the Double-J* stent. J Urol [Internet]. 2000 Sep [cited 2023 Aug 1];164(3 Pt 1):657–60. Available from: https://pubmed.ncbi.nlm.nih.gov/10953120/.
7. Aytekin C, Boyvat F, Harman A, Özyer U, Colak T, Haberal M. Percutaneous therapy of ureteral obstructions and leak after renal transplantation: long-term results. Cardiovasc Intervent Radiol [Internet]. 2007 Nov [cited 2023 Aug 1];30(6):1178–84. Available from: https://pubmed.ncbi.nlm.nih.gov/17508243/.
8. Iwaszko MR, Krambeck AE, Chow GK, Gettman MT. Transureteroureterostomy revisited: long-term surgical outcomes. J Urol [Internet]. 2010 Mar [cited 2023 Aug 1];183(3):1055–9. Available from: https://pubmed.ncbi.nlm.nih.gov/20092851/.
9. Burgos FJ, Bueno G, Gonzalez R, Vazquez JJ, Diez-Nicolás V, Marcen R, *et al* Endourologic implants to treat complex ureteral stenosis after kidney transplantation. Transplant Proc [Internet]. 2009 Jul [cited 2023 Aug 1];41(6):2427–9. Available from: https://pubmed.ncbi.nlm.nih.gov/19715941/.

Chapter

9C

Post-transplant Ureteric Stones

• *Arun Chawla*

LEARNING OBJECTIVES

- To understand the causes, diagnosis and management of post-transplant ureteric stones.

Case Scenario

A 55-year-old male, voluntary renal donor, for ABO compatible: Live related transplant, on evaluation was found to have a 6 mm left lower pole calculus (Fig. 9C.1). He had history of right PCNL 2 years back. Left donor nephrectomy was planned.

During donor nephrectomy, after kidney was prepared on bench pyelolithotomy was done to successfully retrieve this stone. Pelvis was closed with Vicryl 4.0 sutures.

Post-transplant graft function was good and patient discharged after a week with serum creatinine of 0.8 mg/dl. Eight months later, patient (recipient) presented with decreasing urine output and rising serum creatinine levels of 2.0 mg/dl. On ultrasound, graft hydroureteronephrosis was noted and NCCT done (Fig. 9C.2).

1. **What is common presentation of transplant ureterolithiasis**

   Ans: Ureteric stones occurs in less than 1% in the transplant kidney recipients.[2] These patients rarely develop ureteric colic since the transplant kidney is denervated and can lead to delay in diagnosis. However, they might present with vague abdominal pain, hematuria, reduced or absent urine output, impaired renal function, urinary infection or hydronephrosis.[3] Routine

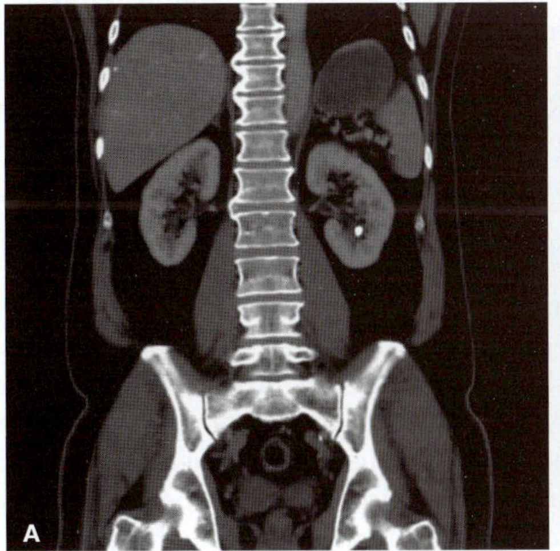

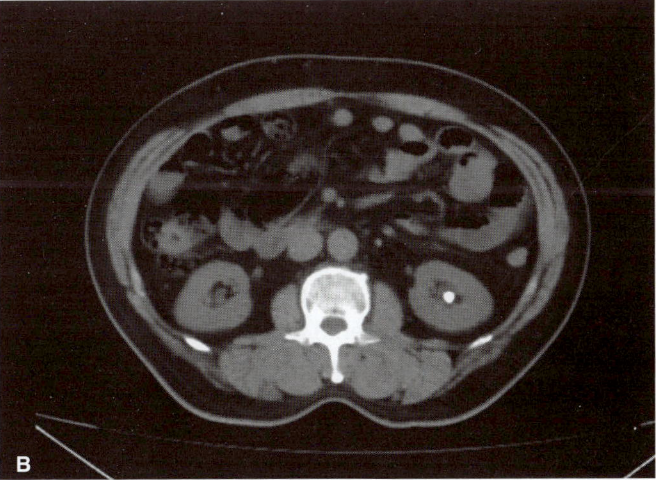

Fig. 9C.1A and B: Donor lower pole renal calculi on CT

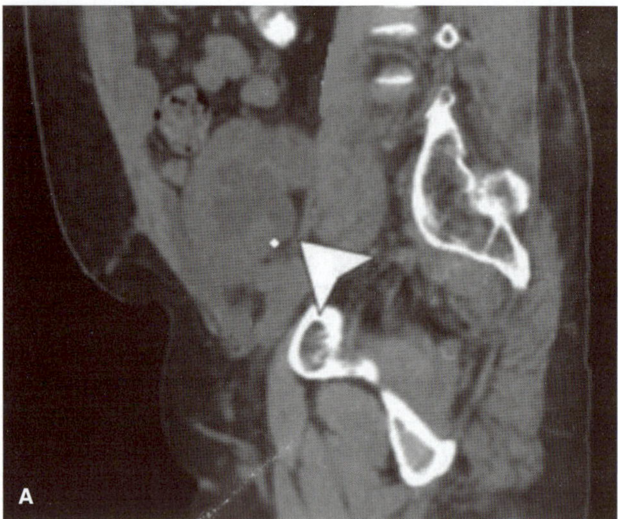

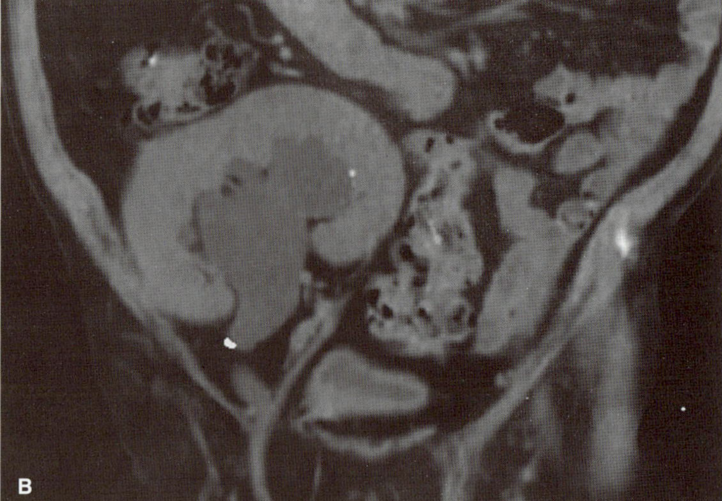

Fig. 9C.2A ann B: Graft hydronephrosis post-ureteric calculi

imaging or evaluation of graft dysfunction may discover asymptomatic stones.

2. **What conditions predispose to transplant urolithiasis?**

   Ans: Pathogenesis of transplant urolithiasis is multifactorial. Most commonly it is due to asymptomatic renal stones from the renal donor. Other causes can be due to urinary stasis due to ureteral obstruction, foreign bodies like retained suture, immunosuppressants (cyclosporine)–induced hyperuricemia, or calcineurin-induced hyperoxaluria or hypocitraturia, secondary hyperparathyroidism and recurrent urinary infections.[4]

3. **What are common underlying metabolic abnormalities in these patients?**

   Ans: Metabolic evaluation of transplant recipients who form stones most commonly reveals hypocitraturia, hyperparathyroidism, hypophosphatemia, and hypercalcemia.[5] Hypocitraturia has been linked with the use of calcineurin inhibitors.[6]

4. **How can donor kidney with stones be treated to reduce post-transplant complications?**

   Ans: When a stone is identified in a living donor, stone bearing kidney is always selected for transplantation. Donor kidney with stones can be treated for stones by ESWL, RIRS or mini PNL based on stone factors and renal anatomy. Donor nephrectomy can be planned a month after kidney has fully recovered from the surgical insult.

   Successful stone retrieval has been reported using ureteroscopy or nephrolithotomy, pyelolithotomy on the back table. Caution and care in avoiding severe injuries to collecting system by instruments or energy to pulverise the stones. Restoration of parenchymal integrity is advised in case of nephrotomy done to remove stones to prevent post- transplant bleeding.

5. **How are you going to manage this case?**

   Ans: For this clinical scenario, various options are conservative, ESWL, PCN followed by antegrade stone removal. This patient underwent PCN because of oliguria and rising serum creatinine. Patient had good output from PCN and drop in serum creatinine to 1.2 mg/dl. Mini PCNL with stenting was done after 10 days.

6. **What is the management options in transplant ureterolithiasis?**

   Ans: Treatment is similar to that of native kidney stone disease. Stone numbers, location, size, Hounsfield units are best delineated by CT scan. Many small stones pass spontaneously. Anuria requires emergent intervention, usually first with a percutaneous nephrostomy followed by antegrade RIRS, or ESWL later, depending upon stone factors.

   Larger stones and stones causing obstruction or symptoms need to be managed actively.

   It includes ESWL, RIRS, percutaneous ureteroscopy via antegrade approach and open surgical approach.[7] Since the transplant kidney is located ectopically in the pelvis, special consideration should be taken regarding ESWL to avoid pelvic bones during stone lithotripsy.[8] Antegrade access is easier because of the easier accessibility of the transplant kidney in the pelvis, and retrograde techniques are more difficult because of the ectopic position and course of the ureter.

7. **How was this patient followed up?**

Ans: Patient had PCN removal 48 hours after mini PNL followed by stent removal after one month. Metabolic evaluation revealed hypocitraturia and hypovolemia. Patient was advised for increased fluids and evaluation by ultrasonography every 6 months.

KEY POINTS

- As more transplant kidneys from living donors with known asymptomatic renal stones are used, the incidence of transplant ureterolithiasis may increase.[9]
- Transplant ureterolithiasis is multifactorial.
- Donor kidney bearing stones can be treated by ESWL, RIRS or mini PNL depending upon stone factors. Bench removal of stones from donor kidney by URS, nephrolithotomy, pyelolithotomy have been reported.
- Post-transplant ureterolithiasis is managed in the same way as stones in native kidneys. ESWL is one of the options but consideration to be given in view of graft being in pelvic position.
- Antegrade techniques are easier as the graft kidney in pelvis is readily accessible. At the same time, ectopic position of ureter and the tortuous course of ureter leads to difficult retrograde techniques.

SUMMARY

- Urolithiasis in renal transplant recipients is uncommon with incidence ranging from about 1% to 5% of transplants performed.[1] Strong risk factors are female sex and prior history of stone disease.
- Due to shortage of living donors, more centers are accepting transplant kidneys from living donors with known asymptomatic renal stones, which may lead to increased incidence of transplant urolithiasis.
- The clinical presentation of transplant urolithiasis varies as transplant kidney is denervated. Patients may have graft pain, oligo or anuria or hematuria. Routine imaging or evaluation of graft dysfunction may discover asymptomatic stones.
- Metabolic evaluation of transplant recipients who form stones most commonly reveals hypocitraturia, hyperparathyroidism, hypophosphatemia, and hypercalcemia.
- Before transplant surgery, stones in donor kidneys can be treated by EWSL, RIRS or mini PNL followed by donor nephrectomy a month later. Successful stone retrieval from donor kidneys have been reported after transplant nephrectomy using ureteroscopy on the back table or pyelolithotomy/pyelo-nephrolithotomy depending upon the location, size and number of stones. Care and caution need to be exercised to avoid injury to kidney and its collecting system due to instruments and energy used for pulverisation.
- Post-transplant ureterolithiasis can be treated by ESWL or antegrade procedures. Retrograde procedures are difficult because of ectopic position and course of ureter. Anuria requires emergent intervention, usually with a percutaneous nephrostomy.

REFERENCES

1. Khositseth S, Gillingham KJ, Cook ME, Chavers BM. Urolithiasis after kidney transplantation in pediatric recipients: a single center report. Transplantation [Internet]. 2004 Nov 15 [cited 2023 Aug 1];78(9):1319–23. Available from: https://pubmed.ncbi.nlm.nih.gov/15548970/.
2. Obert R, Olfe AW, Alarie V, Shby BA, Dgar E, Ilford LM, *et al.* Number 23 · 1725 Mortality in Patients on Dialysis and Transplant Recipients. 1999;341.
3. Opelz G, Döhler B. Association of HLA mismatch with death with a functioning graft after kidney transplantation: a collaborative transplant study report. Am J Transplant [Internet]. 2012 Nov [cited 2023 Aug 1];12(11):3031–8. Available from: https://pubmed.ncbi.nlm.nih.gov/22900931/.
4. Sellarés J, De Freitas DG, Mengel M, Reeve J, Einecke G, Sis B, *et al.* Understanding the causes of kidney transplant failure: the dominant role of antibody-mediated rejection and nonadherence. Am J Transplant [Internet]. 2012 Feb [cited 2023 Aug 1];12(2):388–99. Available from: https://pubmed.ncbi.nlm.nih.gov/22081892/.
5. Harper JM, Samuell CT, Hallson PC, Wood SM, Mansell MA. Risk factors for calculus formation in patients with renal transplants. Br J Urol [Internet]. 1994 [cited 2023 Aug 1];74(2):147–50. Available from: https://pubmed.ncbi.nlm.nih.gov/7921929/.
6. Stapenhorst L, Sassen R, Beck B, Laube N, Hesse A, Hoppe B. Hypocitraturia as a risk factor for nephrocalcinosis after kidney transplantation. Pediatr Nephrol [Internet]. 2005 May [cited 2023 Aug 1];20(5):652–6. Available from: https://pubmed.ncbi.nlm.nih.gov/15782300/.
7. Dalgic A, Boyvat F, Karakayali H, Moray G, Emiroglu R, Haberal M. Surgical Urologic Complications in 1523 Renal Transplantations: The Baskent University Experience. Transplant Proc. 2006;38:543.
8. Kumar A, Verma BS, Srivastava A, Bhandari M, Gupta A, Sharma R. Evaluation of the urological complications of living related renal transplantation at a single center during the last 10 years: impact of the Double-J* stent. J Urol [Internet]. 2000 Sep [cited 2023 Aug 1];164(3 Pt 1):657–60. Available from: https://pubmed.ncbi.nlm.nih.gov/10953120/.
9. Devasia A, Chacko N, Gnanaraj L, Cherian R, Gopalakrishnan G. Stone-bearing live-donor kidneys for transplantation. BJU Int [Internet]. 2005 Feb [cited 2023 Aug 1];95(3):394–7. Available from: https://pubmed.ncbi.nlm.nih.gov/15679801/.

Chapter

10

Pediatric Renal Transplantation

• Abhinav Jain • Sumit Bansal

LEARNING OBJECTIVES

- To understand the difference between adult and pediatric transplant.
- To understand the difficulties that may be encountered in the immediate intra- and post-operative period.

INTRODUCTION

The incidence of chronic kidney disease (CKD) requiring renal replacement therapy is on a rise and even children are not spared from this menace. CKD may hinder growth and neurocognitive development of the children, so the management requires a special focus on this aspect. Children have a longer lifespan ahead compared to adults and so every effort should be made to maximize graft function. As with adults, organ transplantation remains the treatment of choice in pediatric population too providing better quality of life, lesser morbidity and mortality compared to any other form of renal replacement therapy. Historically, the outcomes of renal transplant in children were inferior to those in adults[1] but, in recent years, owing to better understanding of immunosuppression, pediatric anatomy and physiology, the results are comparable to adult population.[2] The 5-year patient and graft survival in children in many series has been reported up to 94%.[3]

Case Scenario

A 10 years old male child presents with left mid-ureteric 8 mm obstructing calculus and right pelvi-ureteric junction calculus measuring 15 mm. There is bilateral marked thinning of parenchyma with a serum creatinine of 6.1. He has history of multiple interventions for stones since he was 5 years of age. Stones were cleared and a nadir serum creatinine of 5.4 obtained. Parents were counselled regarding the need for renal replacement therapy and genetic testing for primary hyperoxaluria.

1. **What are the causes of ESRD (end stage renal disease) in pediatric population?**

   Ans: The causes of end stage renal disease (ESRD) in children are markedly different than those in adults (Table 10.1). Congenital anomalies are responsible in over 1/3rd cases followed by chronic glomerulonephritis and focal segmental glomerulosclerosis. Other important causes are renal dysplasia, obstructive uropathy, neurogenic bladder, primary hyperoxaluria, secondary glomerulonephritis and reflux nephropathy.[1, 3]

TABLE 10.1: Percentage wise causes of renal failure in children

Etiology of ESRD in children[4,5]	*Percentage*
Focal segmental glomerulosclerosis	7.4
Glomerulonephritis	5.1
Congenital anomalies	38.3
Other or unknown	49.2

2. **What are the indications of pediatric kidney transplant?**

   Ans: Any patient who is CKD stage 5 needing renal replacement therapy is a candidate for renal transplantation.

3. **What are the contraindications of transplant in children?**

   Ans: The contraindications may be divided into absolute and relative (Table 10.2).

TABLE 10.2: Contraindications of pediatric renal transplant

Absolute contraindications	*Relative contraindications*
• Active infection in body	• Active anti-glomerular basement membrane (GBM) disease
• Active malignancy	• Active hemolytic-uremic syndrome
• Treated malignancy but not having waited for appropriate time[17]	• Active lupus and active anti-neutrophil cytoplasmic antibody (ANCA) vasculitis
• Untreated lower tract pathologies	• Focal segmental glomerulosclerosis (FSGS) or membranoproliferative glomerulonephritis
	• Progressive neurodegenerative disorders

The weight and height of the child is a very subjective criteria on which the decision to transplant a kidney should be based as it may pose a risk of vascular thrombosis owing to graft and patient size mismatch.[18]

4. Who is the ideal kidney donor for children: Deceased vs living donor?

Ans: Recipient outcomes are better with living kidney donors compared to deceased donor kidney.[24] This is most likely due to reduced ischemia time, better preoperative recipient preparation and HLA crossmatching. Much of the research has gone into studying the various aspects and suitability of deceased kidney donation in pediatric population and the following are some of the conclusions:

1. Small sized vessels in young donors may come with the inherent risk of vascular thrombosis. In various analyses best outcomes were seen with donor age of more than 6 years and lesser than 45 years.
2. Suitability of marginal donors and cardiac death donors is questionable owing to the possibility of delayed graft function and decreased graft survival.
3. A practical approach may be "Share 35," which involves allocating kidneys from deceased donors aged <35 years to pediatric recipients aged <18 years.[7]

5. How is the transplant immunology and immunosuppression protocol different in children?

Ans: In children, reduced T-cell effector function, lower titers of anti-HLA antibodies, lower expression of CD40 co-stimulatory ligands, and fewer T-lymphocytes with specific antigen affiliation make the allograft more tolerable, with better post-transplant outcomes.[15]

Several transplant centers may utilize similar protocols for children as adults. However, a trend has been towards shifting away from excessive steroid dependence. The usage of steroids causes various adversities including metabolic bone deformities, hypertension, glucose intolerance, hyperlipidemia, cataract formation and diabetes. Hence a practical approach is early or late steroid withdrawal or complete steroid avoidance, among others.[16]

6. What work up is needed in a recipient before surgery?

1. The work up includes all the basic and routine investigations as done for an adult transplant recipient. Apart from these, a detailed and thorough history and examination is must and the child may need further evaluation of the lower tracts if the history shows presence of lower urinary tract dysfunction or congenital urologic anomaly/voiding abnormalities like urgency, increased urinary frequency, urinary incontinence or bladder and bowel dysfunction that might be attributable to kidney failure. Of importance is to rule out posterior urethral valves, valve bladder, and neurogenic bladder or reflux nephropathy.
2. MCUG must be done in children where reflux nephropathy is strongly suspected or the child has recurrent culture positive urinary tract infection episodes in the past.
3. Detailed metabolic evaluation is recommended in cases of urological stone disease. Genetic testing should be done if primary hyperoxaluria is suspected (*as with the reference case*). If confirmed, ESRD due to primary hyperoxaluria, it requires simultaneous liver and kidney transplant.
4. Urodynamic evaluation is a must for children with voiding dysfunction or those who have undergone some form of urinary tract surgeries in the past. Warning signs may include low capacity bladder, poorly compliant detrusor or high storage or voiding pressures. These may need optimization with appropriate medical or surgical therapy prior to subjecting the patient to renal transplantation.

7. What are the non-surgical complications post-renal transplant in children?

A. Cardiovascular complications

The overall picture following pediatric transplantation is grim as far as the cardiovascular risks are concerned and the same continues to be one of the most feared complications following transplantation.[6] This can be explained partly because of the greater propensity of the development of persistent metabolic derangements during dialysis in children including hypertension. Owing to the significant differences in the body size of recipient and donor, the heart remains in an additional strain with the risks decreasing but not diminishing after the surgery. This is because kidney transplantation in them usually involves adult donors due to the scarcity of pediatric donors and even if pediatric donors do become available, they pose a technical challenge during surgery due to risks of thrombosis owing to anastomosis between small vessels. The chances of future development of left ventricular hypertrophy are real and existent.

B. **Graft dysfunction**

The small size of the patient as compared to the large size of the transplanted kidney usually causes graft hypoperfusion which is accentuated by the lower resting blood pressure of the small recipients. Hence delayed graft function is a practical problem encountered in these settings and is not so rare.[7] The practical problem lays in the fact that usage of inotropes and crystalloids to improve the renal perfusion may exacerbate the cardiovascular strain and compromise.

C. **Post-transplant lymphoproliferative disorder (PTLD) and malignancy**

This is also a troublesome issue and the chances of pediatric patients developing PTLD is more as compared to their adult counterparts probably owing to the higher probability of them being EBV negative (49% vs. 8%).[8] Occurrence of non-PTLD malignancies is also higher in children with renal cell carcinoma being the most common of all.[9]

D. **Retarded growth and bone complications**

These set of complications cannot be ignored and can lead to severe loss of bony function and morbidities as the child grows. To name a few, these may include skeletal deformities, bone pain, fracture, osteonecrosis, growth failure, and ectopic calcification.[10,11] Some of the prudent strategies to reduce this include transplantation at a younger age, obtaining the graft from living donors, improving and maintaining adequate function of the graft kidney and restricting the usage of steroids.[12]

E. **Nonadherence to protocol**

A pediatric individual may be non-compliant and non-adherent to the transplant physician's advice and is seen in up to 75% of the people as they advance into adolescence[13,14] and this is considered to be a major issue that leads to decrease in renal graft function.

8. What is the prognosis after pediatric renal transplant?

Ans: Table 10.3 outlines the graft failure as a function of time after deceased and living donor kidney transplantation:[19]

TABLE 10.3: Percentage of graft failure as a function of time

	Percentage graft failure	*Percentage graft failure*
	After deceased donor transplant	*After living donor transplant*
6 months	1.9	0.8
1 year	2.8	1.6
3 years	6.4	2.7
5 years	15.2	8.2
10 years	32.1	21.7

9. Are surgical steps in child different from an adult?

Ans:

1. *Larger children:* The surgical steps in them are essentially the same as those in an adult kidney transplant. The abdomen is opened with Gibson incision and the renal graft is placed extraperitoneally. The choice of anastomosis in internal or external iliac artery rests with the transplant surgeon and there are no particular advantages or disadvantages of using a particular artery for anastomosis.
2. *Smaller children:* The surgical steps need modification for infants and smaller children. However, the same surgical steps may also be followed in them, they usually receive kidney from an adult donor, hence, some surgeons prefer to enter into the peritoneal cavity using a midline abdominal incision. The vessels used for the anastomosis are aorta and inferior vena cava although common iliac arteries/veins may also be utilized (Figs 10.1 and 10.2).
3. Various studies have been done comparing extraperitoneal and intraperitoneal approaches. They have found out a similar rate of complications, hospital stay and early/late graft function.[20]

10. What are the surgical complications after renal transplant surgery?

Ans: The most worrisome surgical complication in pediatric transplantation is higher propensity of vascular thrombosis (both artery and vein). This is because of small caliber vessels available for anastomosis; more so in younger children. Robust

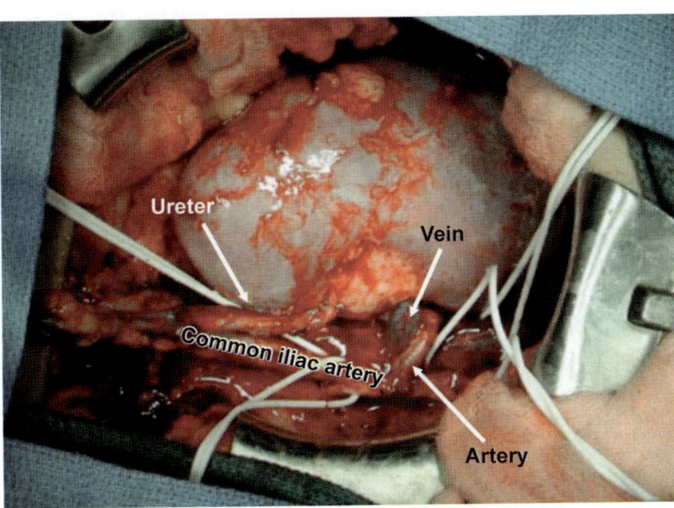

Fig. 10.1: Anastomosis done with common iliac artery

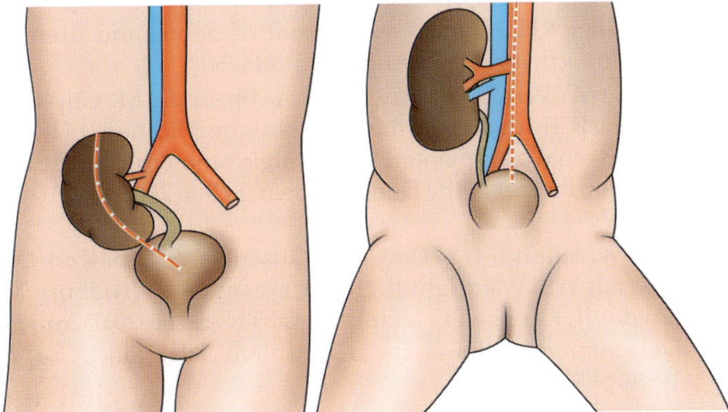

Fig. 10.2: Different operative approaches (extraperitoneal and intraperitoneal)

surgical expertise in handling small vessels and sticking to the principles of vascular anastomosis are best possible ways to avoid them. Routine anti-coagulation is not recommended but the choice is entirely individual. Below are some of the complications:

1. **Lymphocele:** This may occur in 1 to 10 percent of pediatric patients and may manifest as swelling at the site of renal transplant, fullness, pain or worsening renal functions. It is usually attributable to the lymphatics of the donor kidney and may be managed either conservatively or surgically by creating a window between the collection and the peritoneal cavity.
2. **Renal venous thrombosis (RVT):** Pediatric recipients are at higher risk of vascular thrombosis owing to small-caliber vessels. RVT is an emergency and manifest usually 7 to 10 days after transplant. The presentation may be graft pain, hematuria or worsening graft functions. This entity needs **emergency** exploration and thrombectomy.
3. **Renal artery stenosis:**[21] This may also manifest as decreasing urine output and worsening creatinine. Digital subtraction angiography is the most sensitive modality for its diagnosis and may be managed by percutaneous interventions.
4. **Urinary obstruction:**[22] This occurs because of stenosis of ureteric anastomosis and may be managed by per cutaneous nephrostomy and antegrade DJ stenting.
5. **Urinary leakage:**[23] This may manifest as increasing drain output and is diagnosed with a high drain fluid creatinine. Management may be conservative if the leak is small and if the drain output is reducing or may need open intervention and re-exploration.

SUMMARY

- Like adults, kidney transplant remains the best treatment option for ESRD even in pediatric population.
- Results are similar to adult population and 5-years graft survival has been reported to be more than 95%.
- The causes of renal failure in children are different from adult and include congenital anomalies and glomerulopathies.
- Various immunological factors in children make the allograft more tolerable, with better post-transplant outcomes.
- Most centers prefer early or late steroid withdrawal or complete steroid avoidance in children.
- Pediatric recipients require a rather detailed work-up to identify and address underlying etiologic factors and corrective measures need to be taken before hand only.
- The important non-surgical complications include cardiovascular issues, graft dysfunction, higher risk of PTLD and other malignancies and bone complications owing to steroid-based immunosuppression regimens.
- Non-compliance to drugs especially as they advance into adolescence is a major issue and cause of graft dysfunction.
- Surgical approach in older children is no different from adult population; however, in younger children, an intraperitoneal approach may be required, with anastomosis in common iliacs or aorta/IVC.
- Pediatric recipients are at higher risk of vascular thrombosis because of small-caliber vessels; which may require urgent interventions to save the graft.
- Children have a longer lifespan ahead compared to adults and so every effort should be made to maximize graft function.

REFERENCES

1. Dharnidharka VR, Fiorina P, Harmon WE. Kidney transplantation in children. *N Engl J Med.* 2014; 371:549–58.
2. Peruzzi L, Amore A, Coppo R. Challenges in pediatric renal transplantation. *World J Transplant.* 2014;4:222–8
3. Shapiro R, Sarwal MM. Pediatric kidney transplantation. *Pediatr Clin North Am.* 2010;57:393–400.
4. Lentine KL, Smith JM, Hart A, Miller J, Skeans MA, Larkin L, *et al.* OPTN/SRTR 2020 Annual Data Report: Kidney. *Am J Transplant.* 2022 Mar. 22 Suppl 2:21–136

5. Ullman E. [Experimental kidney transplantation. 1902]. *Wien Klin Wochenschr*. 2002 Feb 28. 114 (4):126–7.
6. Kaidar M, Berant M, Krauze I, Cleper R, Mor E, Bar-Nathan N, *et al.* Cardiovascular risk factors in children after kidney transplantation: from short-term to long-term follow-up. *Pediatr Transplant*. 2014;18:23–8.
7. Donati-Bourne J, Roberts HW, Coleman RA. Donor-recipient size mismatch in paediatric renal transplantation. *J Transplant*. 2014;2014:317574.
8. Srivastava T, Zwick DL, Rothberg PG, Warady BA. Posttransplant lymphoproliferative disorder in pediatric renal transplantation. *Pediatr Nephrol*. 1999;13:748–54.
9. Smith JM, Martz K, McDonald RA, Harmon WE. Solid tumors following kidney transplantation in children. *Pediatr Transplant*. 2013;17:726–30.
10. Harambat J, Cochat P. Growth after renal transplantation. *Pediatr Nephrol*. 2009; 24:1297–306.
11. Haffner D, Schüler U. Metabolic bone disease after renal transplantation. *Curr Opin Pediatr*. 2014; 26:198–206.
12. Laster ML, Fine RN. Growth following solid organ transplantation in childhood. *Pediatr Transplant*. 2014; 18:134–41.
13. Pai AL, Ingerski LM, Perazzo L, Ramey C, Bonner M, Goebel J. Preparing for transition? The allocation of oral medication regimen tasks in adolescents with renal transplants. *Pediatr Transplant*. 2011; 15:9–16.
14. Dharnidharka VR, Fiorina P, Harmon WE. Kidney transplatation in children. *N Engl J Med*. 2014 Aug 7. 371 (6):549–58.
15. Shemesh E, Annunziato RA, Arnon R, Miloh T, Kerkar N. Adherence to medical recommendations and transition to adult services in pediatric transplant recipients. *Curr Opin Organ Transplant*. 2010; 15:288–92.
16. Grenda R, Webb NJ. Steroid minimization in pediatric renal transplantation: Early withdrawal or avoidance? *Pediatr Transplant*. 2010;14:961–7.
17. Knoll G, Cockfield S, Blydt-Hansen T, Baran D, Kiberd B, Landsberg D, *et al.* Canadian Society of Transplantation consensus guidelines on eligibility for kidney transplantation. *CMAJ*. 2005 Nov 8. 173 (10):1181–4.
18. Jalanko H, Mattila I, Holmberg C. Renal transplantation in infants. *Pediatr Nephrol*. 2016 May. 31 (5):725–35.
19. Lentine KL, Smith JM, Hart A, Miller J, Skeans MA, Larkin L, *et al.* OPTN/SRTR 2020 Annual Data Report: Kidney. *Am J Transplant*. 2022 Mar. 22 Suppl 2:21–136.
20. Heap SL, Webb NJ, Kirkman MA, Roberts D, Riad H. Extraperitoneal renal transplantation in small children results in a transient improvement in early graft function. *Pediatr Transplant*. 2011 Jun. 15 (4):362–6.
21. McDonald RA, Smith JM, Stablein D, Harmon WE. Pretransplant peritoneal dialysis and graft thrombosis following pediatric kidney transplantation: a NAPRTCS report. *Pediatr Transplant*. 2003 Jun. 7 (3):204–8.
22. Whitaker RH. Clinical assessment of pelvic and ureteral function. *Urology*. 1978 Aug. 12 (2):146–50.
23. Kumar A, Verma BS, Srivastava A, Bhandari M, Gupta A, Sharma R. Evaluation of the urological complications of living related renal transplantation at a single center during the last 10 years: impact of the Double-J stent. *J Urol*. 2000 Sep. 164 (3 Pt 1):657–60.
24. Hart A, Smith JM, Skeans MA, Gustafson SK, Stewart DE, Cherikh WS, Wainright JL, Kucheryavaya A, Woodbury M, Snyder JJ, Kasiske BL, Israni AK. OPTN/SRTR 2015 Annual Data Report: Kidney. Am J Transplant. 2017 Jan;17 Suppl 1(Suppl 1):21–116.

Chapter

11

Surgical Technique of Kidney Transplant Including Graft Nephrectomy

• Nitesh Jain

LEARNING OBJECTIVES

- To understand all the operative steps of renal allografting in iliac fossa (recipient surgery).
- To understand the different approaches and steps involved in graft nephrectomy.

INTRODUCTION

Kidney transplantation is the optimal treatment for kidney failure, associated with a lower risk of mortality compared with dialysis[1] and improved quality of life.[2] The incidence of surgical complications after kidney transplant has improved over the last two decades, from as high as 30% to less than 6% currently, which is attributed to the refinement of operative technique in kidney procurement, preparation, and transplantation.[3]

Case Scenario 1

A 36 years old male with ESRD is planned for renal transplant with mother as living donor. Left kidney with single artery and vein procured laparoscopically from donor. Implantation is planned in right iliac fossa.

1. **How the patient is prepared for the surgery?**

   Ans: Surgery is done under general anaesthesia (GA), with patient lying supine on operating table. Sometimes, in view of high cardio-pulmonary risk involved, surgery may also be contemplated under combined spinal-epidural anaesthesia. Following this, with all aseptic precautions, catheterisation with a 3-way Foley catheter is done. One channel of this 3-way catheter is connected to 500 ml saline as the bladder filling will be required at the time of bladder dissection. A hockey stick incision (Fig. 11.1) is made in the right iliac fossa and deepened to enter the retroperitoneum to access to the iliac vessels. Attempt should be made to split, rather than cut the muscles of anterior abdominal wall. Bed preparation is done by ligating the multiple small tributaries of the external iliac vein. The external iliac artery is dissected off its lymphatics (Fig. 11.2). Clamps and bull dogs are checked prior to their application.

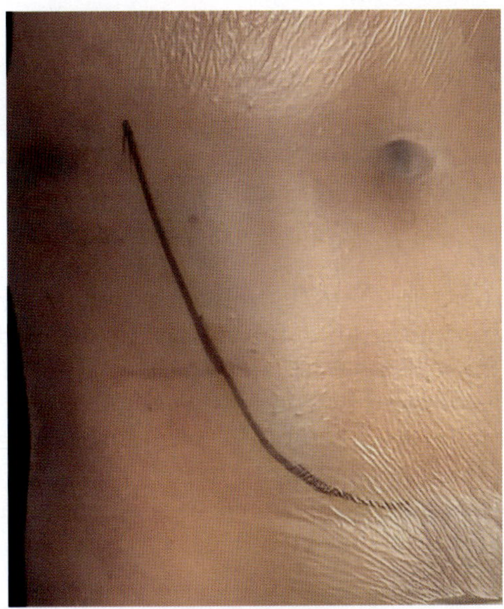

Fig. 11.1: Incision

2. **Describe the steps in renal vein anastomosis.**

   Ans: The renal vein is first anastomosed in an end-to-side fashion to the external iliac vein. Stay sutures are taken at 12 and 6 o' clock position (Fig. 11.3) on the external iliac vein that helps in retraction of the vein with very minimal handling and ensures that intimal layer is included in the anastomosis. The

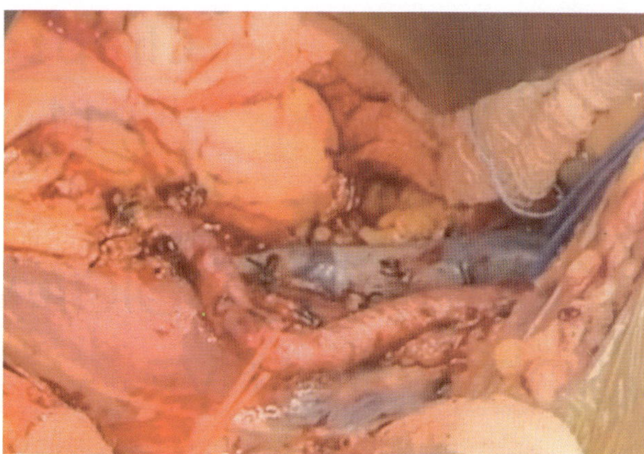

Fig. 11.2: Bed preparation—space adequate enough to apply vascular clamps

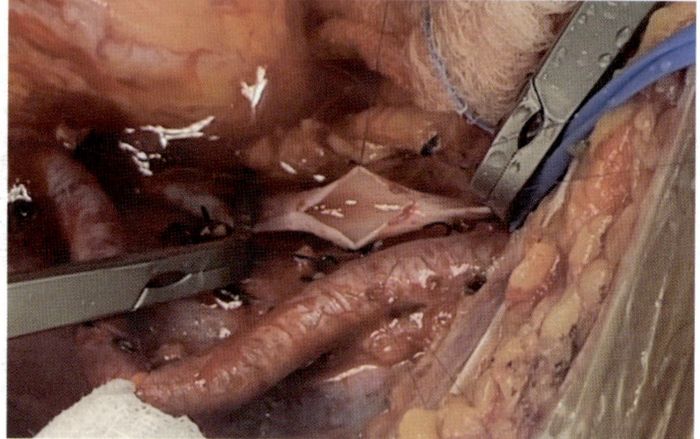

Fig. 11.3: Stay sutures taken at 3 and 6 o'clock position on the external iliac vein

corner sutures (6/0 Prolene) are placed while the kidney allograft is first placed at the medial side of the incision. The lateral side of the renal vein is anastomosed by continuous suture using the 6/0 Prolene (needle length 9.3 mm) suture. The kidney allograft is then flipped to the lateral side and the medial side of the renal vein is anastomosed to the external iliac vein (Fig. 11.4).

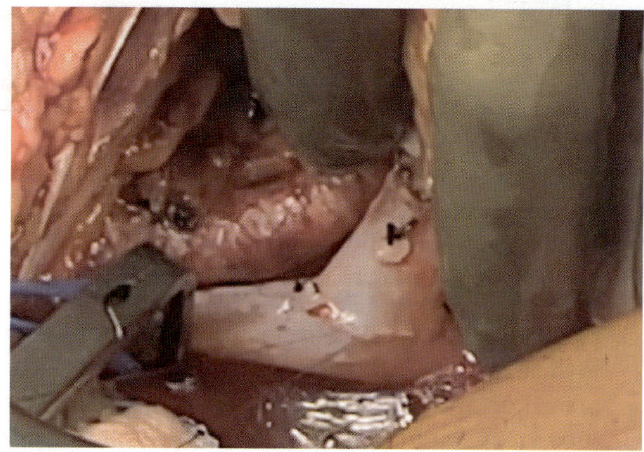

Fig. 11.4: Completed anastomosis of the renal vein to external iliac vein

3. Describe the steps in renal artery anastomosis.

Ans: Arterial anastomosis can either be done with external iliac artery (EIA) in an end-to-side manner or internal iliac artery (IIA) in an end-to-end manner.

External iliac artery anastomosis: An incision is made using no. 11 blade at the desired site on EIA. This is enlarged with Pott's scissors (Fig. 11.5) and an aortic punch is used to make a good size clean button hole on the EIA, the size of which is comparable to the calibre of the donor renal artery. Two corner sutures (6/0 Prolene) are placed first, then the lateral side of renal artery anastomosis is created with continuous sutures from inside the lumen, and then medial side anastomosis is performed by continuous sutures from the outside of the lumen. Integrity of the anastomosis is checked by placing a bull dog clamp over the graft renal artery (Fig. 11.6) and then releasing the vascular clamp on the external iliac artery (Fig. 11.7).

Venous anastomosis integrity is confirmed and the kidney is re-perfused by sequentially releasing

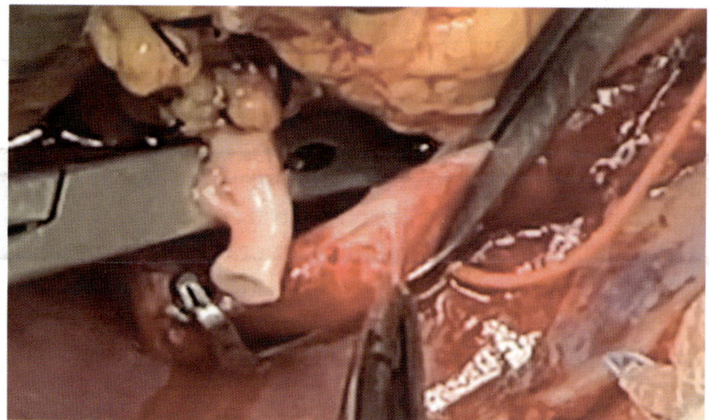

Fig. 11.5: Slit on the external iliac artery

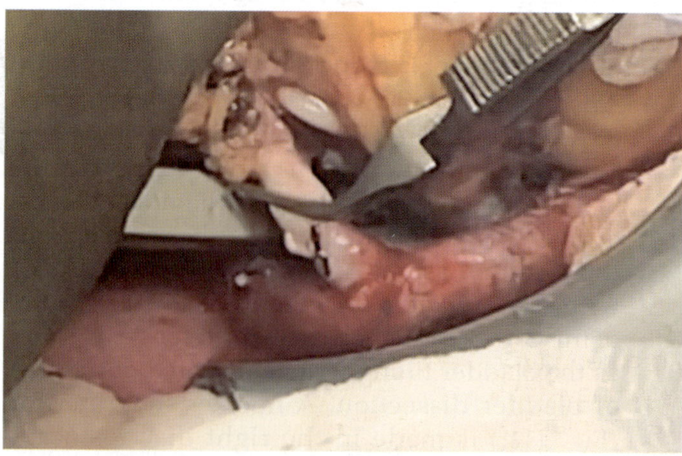

Fig. 11.6: Checking for anastomotic integrity by applying clamp over the graft artery and releasing the clamp off the external iliac artery

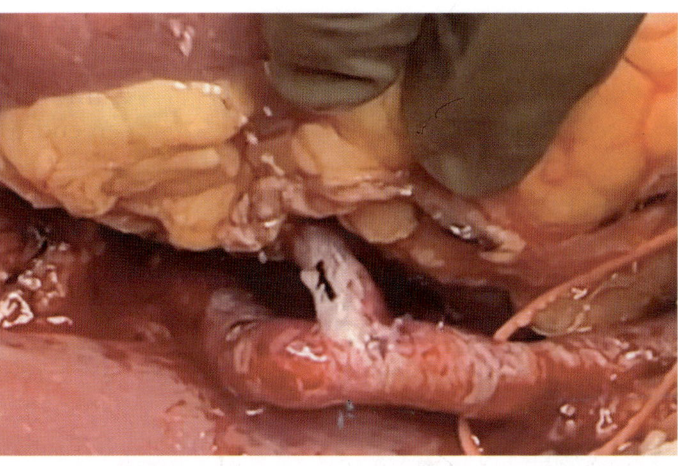

Fig. 11.7: Final appearance of the completed anastomosis of graft renal artery with EIA

the renal artery clamp followed by venous vascular clamp.

Internal iliac artery anastomosis: The bed preparation steps are the same as the preparation for external iliac artery. The internal iliac artery is identified and its branches are ligated as the anastomosis here is going to be end to end. After assessing the luminal diameter of the internal iliac artery it is decided to procced with the anastomosis. In case the lumen diameter is inadequate, the surgeon can get back to the external iliac artery for anastomosis.

4. **Describe the steps in uretero-vesical anastomosis.**
Ans: Ureteroneocystostomy is performed by using modified Lich-Gregoir technique with a 5/0 polydioxanone suture. The bladder is inflated with betadine saline irrigation as there is a 3-way Foley already in place. Lifting the ends of the anastomotic site of the bladder mucosa with vicryl sutures again helps in ensuring that mucosa is included in the repair. A ureteric stent (5 Fr × 16 cm) is routinely placed *in-situ*.

After completion of all the anastomosis and ensuring good diuresis, adequate haemostasis is achieved. A 20 size drain tube is placed at the surgical bed and the wound is closed in layers.

Graft Nephrectomy

Case Scenario 2

A 42 years old female received a live-related graft from her mother 1-month back. Peri-operative period was uneventful and she had a good graft function (serum creatinine 1.3 mg/dl) till last week. Yesterday, she presented in emergency room with acute onset severe pain at graft site and marked drop in urine output. She had profound hypotension (BP 80/40) in ER. After initial resuscitation, the graft Doppler revealed an aneurysm of size 3.3 × 2.9 cm at the anastomotic site, with large expanding peri-graft hematoma. There was hardly any blood flow noticed in the graft. She was immediately rushed to operating room for a life-saving graft nephrectomy.

The removal of the transplant kidney is known as graft nephrectomy (GN) and it becomes imperative sometimes to save the life of the patient like in the present case scenario. It is considered to be a procedure with high morbidity (17–60%) and mortality (1.5–14%) rates due to immunosuppression, co-morbid conditions of patients and the technical difficulty of the procedure.

1. **What are the indications of graft nephrectomy?**
Ans: Various situations might arise in a post-transplant patient that warrant the removal of the graft kidney, viz. renal artery or vein thrombosis, transplant pyonephrosis not responding to medical management, pain due to uncontrolled rejection or malignancy in the transplant kidney.[4]

2. **Describe the surgical approach to graft for removal.**
Ans:
   - GN is performed using the same oblique incision in the iliac fossa as the original transplantation.[5]
   - There are three recognised surgical techniques for GN: Intraperitoneal; extraperitoneal with an intra-capsular (IC) approach; or extraperitoneal with an extra-capsular (EC) approach.[6]
   - The favoured technique is determined by multiple factors, including the original method of graft implantation, the timing of GN after transplantation, the possible presence of intraperitoneal disease, and the surgeon's preference.
   - Early graft nephrectomy done within 3 weeks of transplant can be done by EC technique. Usually after this time frame intra IC approach is usually preferred by many surgeons. Whenever previous vascular anastomosis details are not available, it is relatively safer to go ahead with IC approach.

3. **Describe the surgical steps in intracapsular (IC) approach.**
Ans: The same incision of the transplant is utilised and layers are opened and one can expect adhesions due to previous surgery. Good hemostasis as the layers are being opened is essential. If there are a lot of adhesions around the kidney, then it is ideal to go ahead with IC technique. The peritoneum over the graft kidney is incised. Then the capsule of the kidney is opened and with finger dissection

(Fig. 11.8) *get* all around and keep the kidney hanging on its hilum. Once this stage is reached, apply clamp to entry of renal vessels and then feel the clamp on opposite side of hilum. Once double clamps are safely applied across the hilum, transect the remaining portion of the kidney. With 2–0 prolene sutures run over and suture the hilum.[7] During all the steps keep feeling the femoral pulse; right from application of clamp to completion of sutures. Remove clamps gently after tying the sutures. Achieve good hemostasis and any extra capsule can be dissected at this point. Saline check for hemostasis and betadine check for lymphatics can be done at this stage. Make sure no expanding hematoma along the iliac vessels prior to closure.

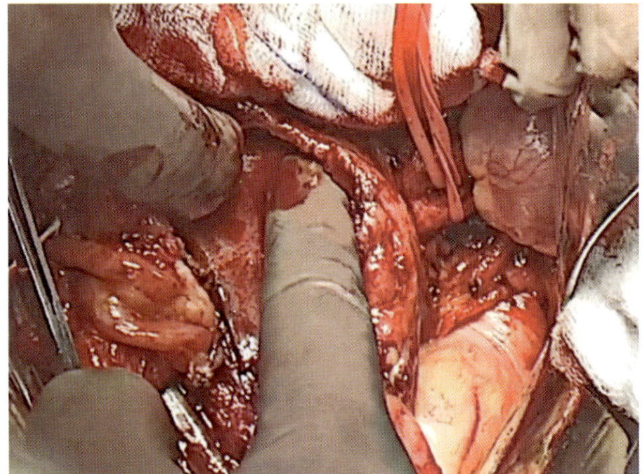

Fig. 11.8: Intracapsular graft nephrectomy (the surgeon's finger dissection is being shown)

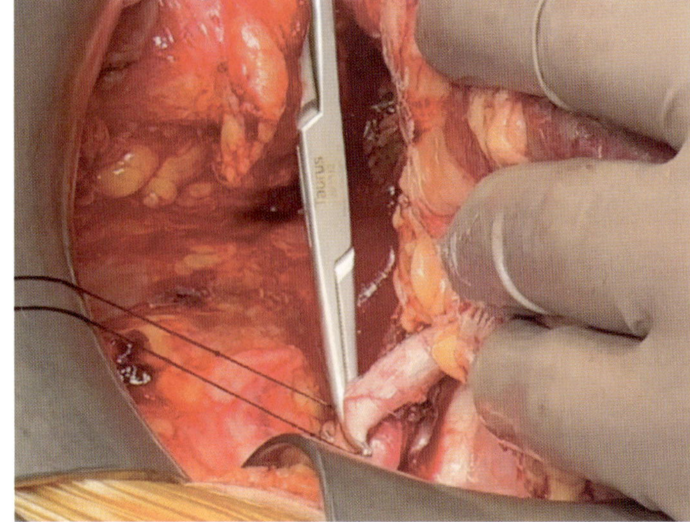

Fig. 11.9: Clamp applied over the graft renal artery and the vessel tie is being applied

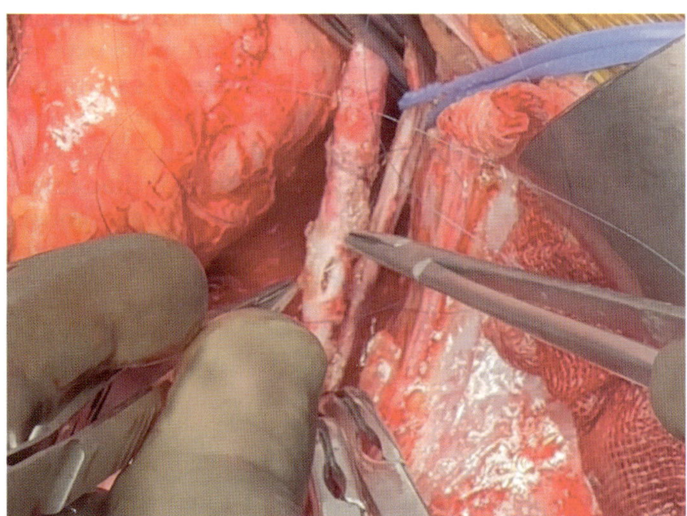

Fig. 11.10: Closure of the anastomotic site on the external iliac artery in graft nephrectomy

4. **Describe the surgical steps in extra-capsular (EC) approach.**

   Ans: With the same incision and by retroperitoneal or extra peritoneal approach, the graft kidney is mobilised all around. Dissection planes is relatively easy as procedure is done within 3 weeks of transplant. The vessels are dissected (Fig. 11.9) and the disconnection of vessels is based on whether slit or aortic punch was used for vascular anastomosis (Fig. 11.10). If punch was used, vessels are clipped or tied a few millimeters away from the anastamotic site. Sometimes a Dacron patch might be needed in these cases. If slit was used, a primary closure or ties a few mm away from the anastomosis is sufficient. Ureter is disconnected at the site of previous anastomosis and kidney is mobilised all around and delivered out.

5. **What are the different incisions to reach the retroperitoneum for a transplant?**

   Ans: The oblique incision, the hockey stick incision, and the pelvic Gibson incision are three conventional incisions that have traditionally been recommended for renal transplant. Because it offers relatively painless and convenient access to the iliac fossa and bladder, the "pelvic Gibson incision," a curvilinear incision in the lower quadrant of the abdomen, is frequently used for kidney transplantation. The oblique incision and the inverted J-shaped incision, also known as the "hockey stick incision," are the other two incisions that are frequently used in some locations. The oblique surgical incision was superior to the hockey-stick incision when Nanni and colleagues compared the two incisions for the likelihood of long-term complications because it resulted in a lower risk of hernia, abdominal wall relaxation, and better cosmetic outcomes.[8] Recently, paramedian, midline, and even transverse incisions have been used in living kidney transplantation for better cosmetic appearance. However, these incisions all have the same inherent disadvantage of making it difficult to expose the operating table, which may be a potential option for special candidates.[9]

6. What are techniques in bed preparation to minimize postoperative lymphocele?

Ans: Although lymphoceles are prevalent after every kidney transplant, their exact cause is still unknown. The best way to manage perivascular lymphatic leakage is either by dividing them between ligatures or sealing them ultrasonic device. When groups were compared based on patient's age, gender, graft source, or repeat transplant, a research contrasting surgical ties to ultrasonic devices in the surgical dissection method for control of lymphatics failed to demonstrate a statistical benefit to either technique.[11]

7. What are the types of retractors used?

Ans:

1. Bookwalter retractor: A self-retaining retractor with movable limbs and blades and a metal frame. It frequently serves for larger incisions and offers a great surgical site exposure (Fig. 11.11).

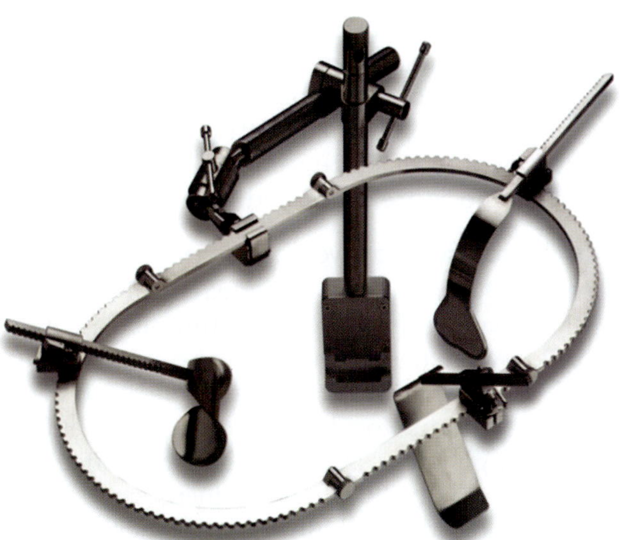

Fig. 11.11: Bookwalter retractor

2. Balfour retractor: This self-retaining retractor has three or four blades on a wide, curved frame. It creates a spacious working area and serves to keep the abdominal wall away from the kidney (Fig. 11.12).
3. Thompson retractor: This device has a flat, curved blade that is connected to a handle by a ratchet mechanism and can be secured into place once it has been properly positioned. Even though it takes time, it is recommended to only use it on recipients who are extremely obese (Fig. 11.13).

With central blade

Fig. 11.12: Balfour retractor

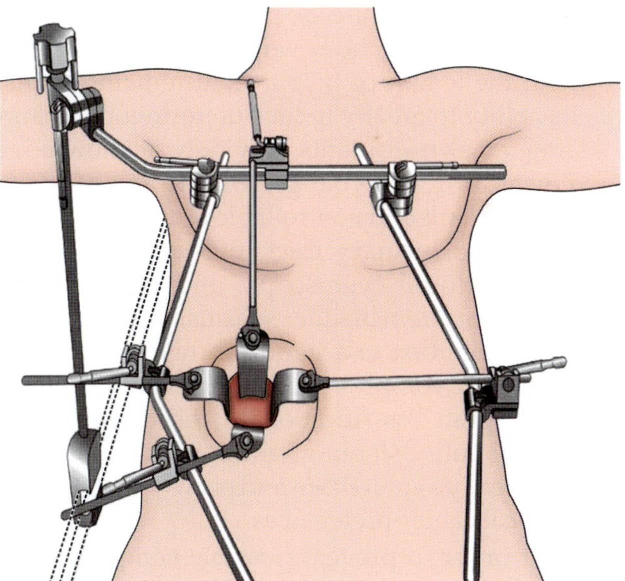

Fig. 11.13: Thompson retractor

4. Denis Browne retractor: Denis Browne ring retractor comes with four fixed blades (two curved and two toothed) and adjustable ratchet with locking (Fig. 11.14).

8. What are the precautions to be taken while applying retractors?

Ans: To achieve optimum exposure, a self-retaining retractor is typically inserted, freeing the assistant's

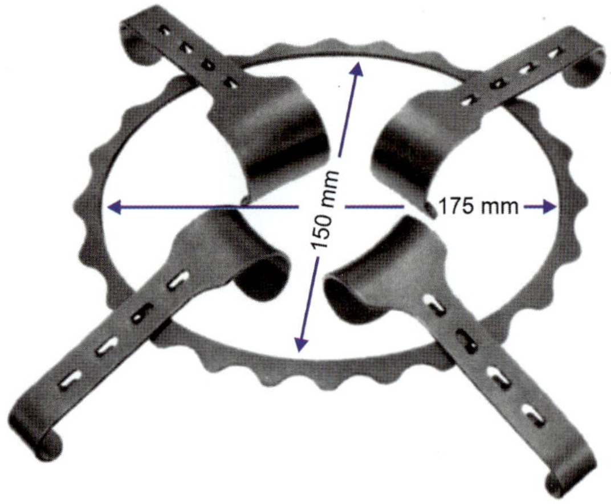

Fig. 11.14: Denis Browne retractor

hands so they can help with the anastomoses. The retractor's position should be carefully examined before being fixed, as the unintentional injury by the retractor was one of the causes of femoral neuropathy, an uncommon complication following kidney transplantation with the main clinical features of reversible muscle weakness or paralysis of hip flexion.[12]

9. What is the role of stents in transplant?

Ans: Major urological complications in kidney transplantation are decreased by prophylactic ureteric stenting; however, morbidity is correlated with the length of time a stent remains in place. Its ability to greatly reduce ureteric complications after renal transplants is widely acknowledged. The minor drawbacks, which are relatively unimportant and controllable are that it increases the risk of urinary tract infection, necessitates an additional cystoscopy, and causes patient discomfort from bladder spasms, cannot outweigh its contribution to a significantly lower incidence of ureteric complications, which can occasionally lead to graft loss. Additionally, the ideal time frame for preventive stenting has not been established. It is typically kept for two and six weeks, depending on local center preferences.

In order to prevent possible complications of bleeding and clot obstruction, it is wise to postpone stent removal in anuric patients with delayed graft function (DGF) and where a transplant biopsy was required.[13]

10. Which is better anastomosis: Renal artery to internal iliac or to external iliac artery?

Ans: It is more of an individual choice rather than any scientific pretext. However, there are a few points to ponder:

When the external iliac artery has already been used or when a Doppler examination reveals that the external iliac artery has atherosclerosis, the internal iliac artery is frequently the only option left. Since the internal iliac trunk can be used at various lengths, this approach offers good feasibility in cases where the transplant renal artery is short. However, the anastomosis is frequently a difficult technique due to lumen incongruity. Internal iliac artery carries the danger of kinking, which can result in vascular occlusion.[14] Due to the internal iliac artery's smaller size and comparatively narrower caliber, as well as the requirement to ligate its branches in order to facilitate the end-to-end anastomosis to the donor renal artery, its use for anastomosis to the donor renal artery is generally not preferred. End-to-end anastomosis carries the potential of endangering the distal arterial supply, which could result in problems such saddle anesthesia, erectile dysfunction (ED), and claudication.[15]

In cases where the first kidney graft had been anastomosed to the opposite internal iliac artery during the first transplant, it was hypothesised that arterial anastomosis to the external iliac artery could lessen the incidence of ED in those situations.[16] Although these complications are uncommon, early obstruction, late stenosis, and the steal phenomenon could result in ischemia of the transplanted kidney during ambulation or vigorous physical activity, which is why proponents of end-to-end internal iliac artery anastomosis are concerned.[17]

11. Is it necessary to give heparin prior to transplant?

Ans: Overall, there is a dearth of research in the area of preventing graft thrombosis. It is yet unknown whether any therapy can lower the rate of early graft thrombosis in any kind of solid organ transplant due to a lack of good quality evidence. Although there is insufficient evidence to say with certainty that heparin increases the risk of serious bleeding in kidney transplant recipients. To inform the necessity for anti-thrombotic therapies in solid organ transplants, there is no evidence from RCTs.[18]

12. Why renal vein anastomosis is done first before the renal artery and can it be done vice versa?

Ans: Renal vein anastomosis is done first to decrease the handling of the renal artery as once the artery anastomosis is completed, it becomes difficult to visualise both the walls of the vein to complete the anastomosis especially in situations where the length of the renal vein is small especially when the right kidney is procured.

On the other hand, the "artery first, vein second" technique involves anastomosing the renal artery before the renal vein (AFVS). The functioning of the kidney graft is satisfactory and comparable to that of the traditional vein-first vascular anastomosis.[19] The renal artery can be anastomosed delicately and with improved exposure using the renal artery first technique. In contrast to the renal vein first strategy, which calls for moving the kidney allograft during the vascular anastomoses, this method has the advantage of keeping it in place during the vessel anastomoses. Less handling of the kidney allograft would be ideal and could lessen vascular kink mistake. Where a little manipulation of the kidney allograft is frequently desired, such as in robotic-assisted kidney transplantation and laparoscopic kidney transplantation, the use of this procedure could be taken into consideration.[19]

13. **How to do arterial anastomosis when artery is calcified?**

Ans: Two unique issues arise from calcified arteries: Problematic clamping (amenable to soft clamp/Fogarty catheter use for control) and decreased patency (amenable to re-permeability or replacement procedures). Soft clamps are preferred over Fogarty catheters whenever practical because they offer superior flow control and surgical comfort during the anastomosis. An important point of technique to handle calcified EIA with plaques is to take the suture inside-out manner, thereby fixing or "tucking" the plaque.

Numerous methods, including the insertion of an autologous long saphenous vein graft to avoid an EIA dissection, have been suggested to increase luminal patency.[20] Despite its value, the use of synthetic material in immunocompromised patients needs to be carefully considered due to the higher risk of infection. Another viable alternative is orthotopic kidney transplantation, but since atherosclerosis is a systemic condition and lesions frequently spread to other native arteries, thorough preoperative evaluation is required.[20]

SUMMARY

- Graft kidney is placed extra-peritoneally, preferably in right iliac fossa. Left iliac fossa is used for second graft or when the RIF is not suitable.
- Modified Gibson muscle—splitting incision usually gives a good exposure of iliac vessels and bladder dome.
- Attempt should always be made to either ligate or seal the lymphatics during bed preparation. It decreases the risk of post-transplant lymphocele.
- For venous anastomosis, EIV is utilised and an end-to-side anastomosis is done.
- For artery, there are two options: EIA and IIA. It is more of individual preference and training. Anastomosis with EIA is done in an end-to-side manner and in an end-to-end manner with IIA, after ligating all its branches.
- Artery first or vein first! Again, it is individual choice and one should adopt a comfortable method to safe anastomosis.
- Stented uretero-neocystostomy is preferred by most, as it is known to decrease ureteric complications.
- Graft nephrectomy is often required in conditions like renal artery or vein thrombosis, transplant pyonephrosis not responding to medical management, pain due to uncontrolled rejection or malignancy in the transplant kidney.
- Normally, the graft is approached through the same incision. There are two ways to accomplish this, intracapsular or extra-capsular.
- When required in an early post-operative period (within 3 weeks), when adhesions are not much and it is relatively easier to take control of vessels; an extra-capsular approach is preferred.
- Late graft nephrectomy or whenever there are dense adhesions; it is not possible to take control of vessels. In this scenario, an intra-capsular approach is safe and quick.

REFERENCES

1. Wolfe RA, Ashby VB, Milford EL, Ojo AO, Ettenger RE, Agodoa LY, Held PJ, Port FK: Comparison of mortality in all patients on dialysis, patients on dialysis awaiting transplantation, and recipients of a first cadaveric transplant. N Engl J Med 341: 1725–1730, 1999.
2. Wyld M, Morton RL, Hayen A, Howard K, Webster AC: A systematic review and meta-analysis of utility-based quality of life in chronic kidney disease treatments. PLoS Med 9: e1001307, 2012.
3. Surgical prevention and management of vascular complications of kidney transplantation. Bessede T, Droupy S, Hammoudi Y, Bedretdinova D, Durrbach A, Charpentier B, Benoit G. *Transpl Int.* 2012;25:994–1001.
4. Akoh JA. Transplant nephrectomy. *World J Transplant.* 2011;1(1):4–12.
5. Sutherland DE, Simmons RL, Howard RJ, Najarian JS. Intracapsular technique of transplant nephrectomy. *Surg Gynecol Obstet.* 1978;146:950–952.
6. Phillips BL, Callaghan CJ. Graft nephrectomy in children. *Pediatr Nephrol.* 2018;33(6):947–955.
7. Touma NJ, Sener A, Caumartin Y, Warren J, Nguan CY, Luke PP. Extracapsular versus intracapsular allograft nephrectomy: impact on allosensitization and surgical outcomes. *Can Urol Assoc J.* 2011;5(1):49–52.
8. Nanni G, Tondolo V, Citterio F, *et al* Comparison of oblique versus hockey-stick surgical incision for kidney transplantation. *Transplant Proc.* 2005;37(6):2479–2481.
9. Park SC, Kim SD, Kim JI, Moon IS. Minimal skin incision in living kidney transplantation. *Transplant Proc.* 2008;40(7):2347–2348.
10. Smyth GP, Beitz G, Eng MP, Gibbons N, Hickey DP, Little DM. Long-term outcome of cadaveric renal transplant after treatment of symptomatic lymphocele. *J Urol.* 2006;176(3):1069–1072.
11. Nelson EW, Gross ME, Mone MC, *et al.* Does ultrasonic energy for surgical dissection reduce the incidence of renal transplant lymphocele?. *Transplant Proc.* 2011;43(10):3755–3759.

12. Sharma KR, Cross J, Santiago F, Ayyar DR, Burke G 3rd. Incidence of acute femoral neuropathy following renal transplantation. *Arch Neurol*. 2002;59(4):541–545.
13. Patel P, Rebollo-Mesa I, Ryan E, *et al*. Prophylactic Ureteric Stents in Renal Transplant Recipients: A Multicenter Randomized Controlled Trial of Early Versus Late Removal. *Am J Transplant*.
14. Fechner G, von Pezold C, Hauser S, Gerhardt T, Klehr HU, Müller SC. Impairment of long-term graft function after kidney transplantation by intraoperative vascular complications. *Int Urol Nephrol*. 2008;40:869–73.
15. Rayt HS, Bown MJ, Lambert KV, Fishwick NG, McCarthy MJ, London NJ, *et al*. Buttock claudication and erectile dysfunction after internal iliac artery embolization in patients prior to endovascular aortic aneurysm repair. *Cardiovasc Intervent Radiol*. 2008;31:728–34.
16. Bitker MO, Benoit g. Surgical aspects of kidney transplantation in France in 1997. Eur Urol. 1998;34:1–5.
17. Humar A, Johnson EM, Payne wD, *et al*. The acutely ischemic extremity after kidney transplant: an approach to management. Surgery. 1998;123:344–50.
18. Surianarayanan V, Hoather TJ, Tingle SJ, Thompson ER, Hanley J, Wilson CH. Interventions for preventing thrombosis in solid organ transplant recipients. *Cochrane Database Syst Rev*. 2021;3(3):CD011557. Published 2021 Mar 15.
19. Ng ZQ, Lim W, He B. Outcomes of Kidney Transplantation by Using the Technique of Renal Artery Anastomosis First. *Cureus*. 2018;10(8):e3223.
20. Garcia LE, González J, Serena G, Ciancio G. Arterial reconstruction with donor iliac vessels during kidney transplantation in a patient with severe atherosclerosis. *J Vasc Surg Cases Innov Tech*. 2019;5(4):443–446. Published 2019 Oct 5.

Access for Renal Replacement Therapy

• Muthu Veeramani

LEARNING OBJECTIVES

- To understand need, pre-requisite, indications and timing for vascular access.
- To understand the various types and techniques of vascular access.
- To understand their complications and management.

Dialysis remained mainstay of the treatment for the patients with ESRD. Worldwide, hemodialysis (HD) is a preferred method (89%) over peritoneal dialysis (11%).[1] In current era, ESRD patients are living longer and may need to be maintained on dialysis for decades. Options of vascular access include central venous catheters (CVCs), arteriovenous grafts (AVGs), and arteriovenous fistulas (AVFs). The AVF is the most durable form of vascular access for HD and is associated with the lowest risks of complications.[2,3] CVCs are primarily intended for acute short-term vascular access. AVG display low primary failure rates but are associated with inferior patency and higher complications (Table 12.1).

The first use of the AV fistula was demonstrated in 1966 by Brescia, Cimino and colleagues, which solved many issues related to previously mentioned external grafts and opened a new era for repeated HD.[4] AVFs should be created pre-emptively whenever possible. As per recent KDIGO guidelines, AV fistula should be offered to each patient with CKD stage 4.

Case Scenario

A 64 years old male presented with anorexia and weight loss. He is known case of rheumatoid arthritis and has been taking NSAIDs for more than 15 years. He is a known diabetic on regular medication. Serum creatinine has gradually risen to 8.5 mg/dl. Ultrasound revealed bilateral echogenic kidney, no stone, no hydronephrosis. Recently he had a history of pulmonary edema, required ICU admission, intubation and 4 cycles of HD via right IJV DLC.

He has lots of reservations regarding dialysis and has many questions regarding best access for dialysis and about the fistula.

1. **What is AV fistula and how one should plan it? What is the patency rate of each of the AVF?**

Ans: AVF is a surgically constructed arterio-venous anastomosis to divert high-pressure arterial blood into the high-capacity venous system leading to "**arterialization**", remodelling and eventual maturation of the veins to carry out effective HD (Figs 12.1 and 12.2). Non-dominant arm should

TABLE 12.1: Different types of vascular access and their complications

Access type	*Patients with complications (%)*	*Distribution of complications (total 100%)*				
		Thrombosis	*Stenosis*	*Infection*	*Bleeding*	*Flow problem*
AV fistula	15.5	36	28	15	15	7
AV graft	37.3	45	26	6	21	2
Chronic CVC	27.5	18	8	47	8	18

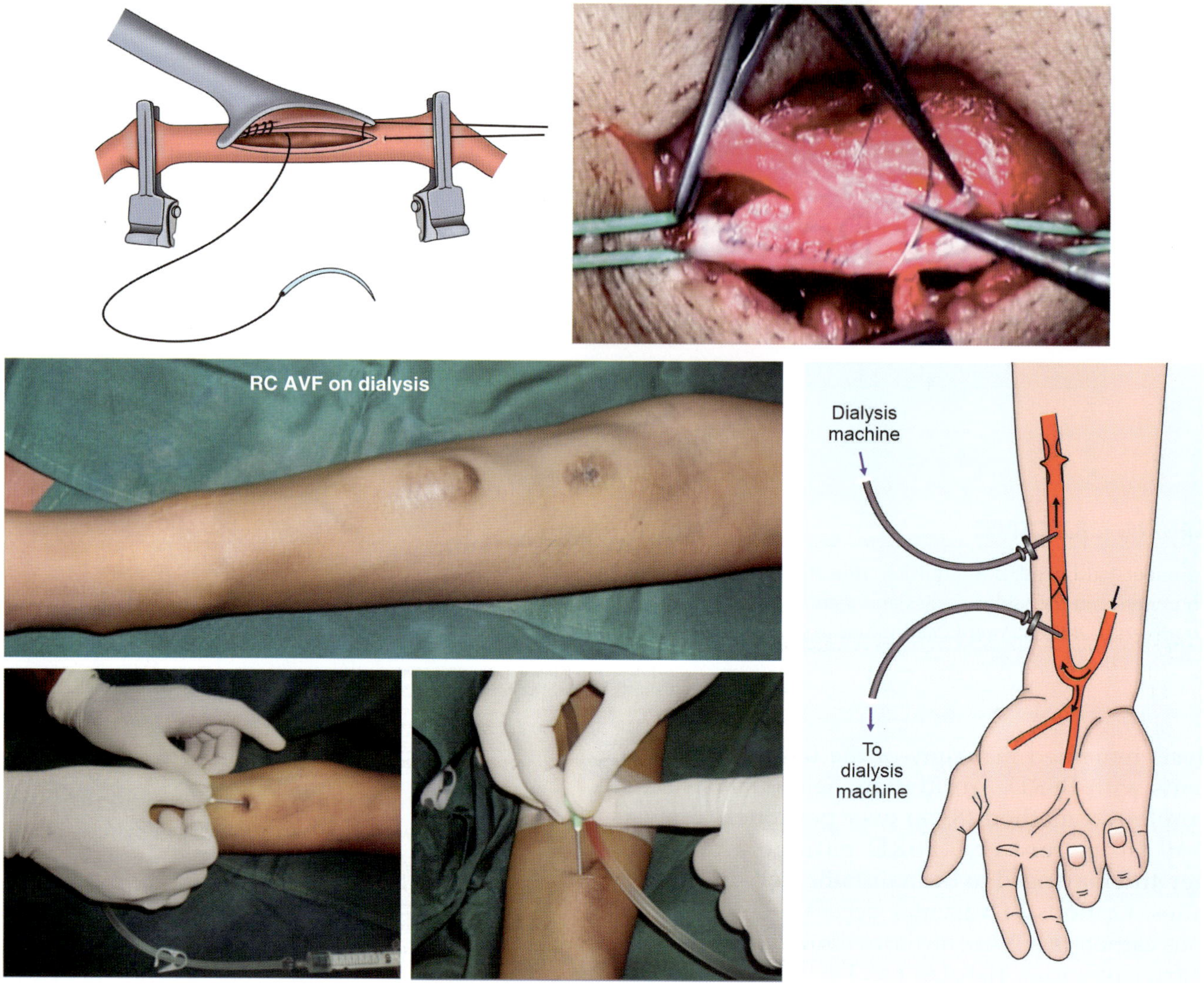

Fig. 12.1: Arteriovenous fistula

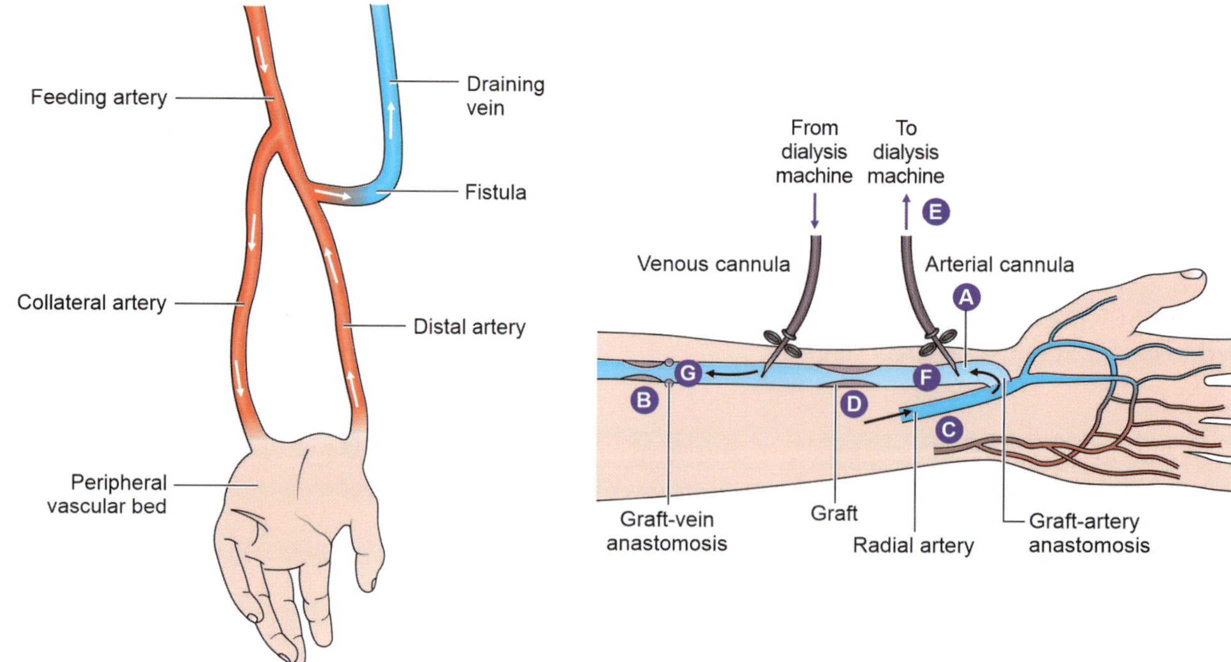

Fig. 12.2: How fistula works

be used. Preference should be for the distal sites as it allows the greatest possible length of vascular conduit and preserves proximal sites for the future. Leg vessels are less preferred and should only be used when other options are exhausted.

Sequence of the fistula sites (Figs 12.3 and 12.4):

1. Anatomical snuff box radio-cephalic (RC AVF).
2. Distal wrist RC AVF (preferred site)
3. Cubital fossa brachiocephalic (BC) AVF
4. Basilic vein transposition
5. When both arms vein get exhausted, consider AV grafts
6. If AVG is not possible, then lower limb AVF (humero-humeral or femoro-femoral AVF with vein superficialization)
7. Long-term tunnelled, cuffed central venous catheter[5]

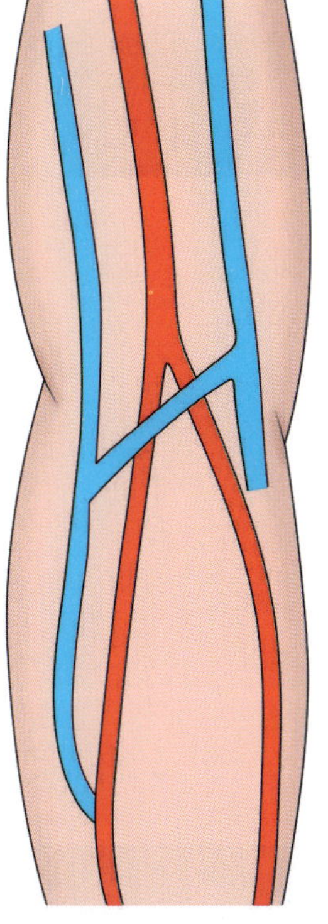

Radio-cephalic (RC AVF)

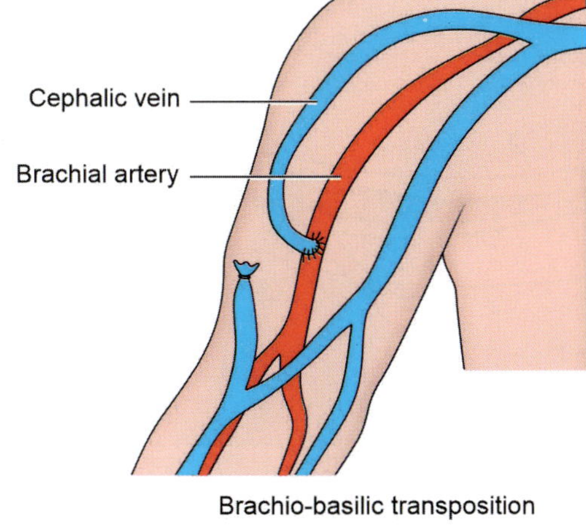

Brachio-basilic transposition

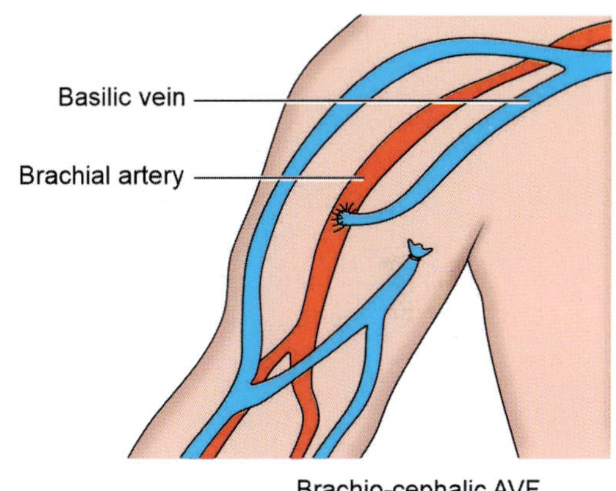

Brachio-cephalic AVF

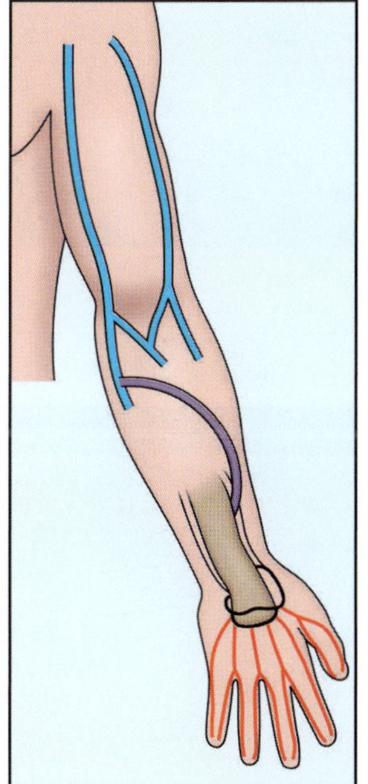

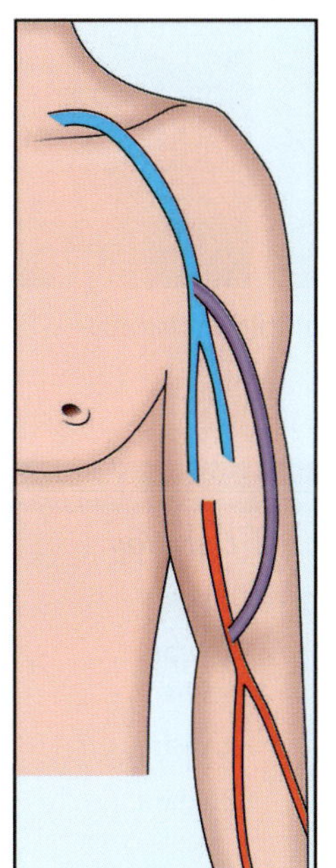

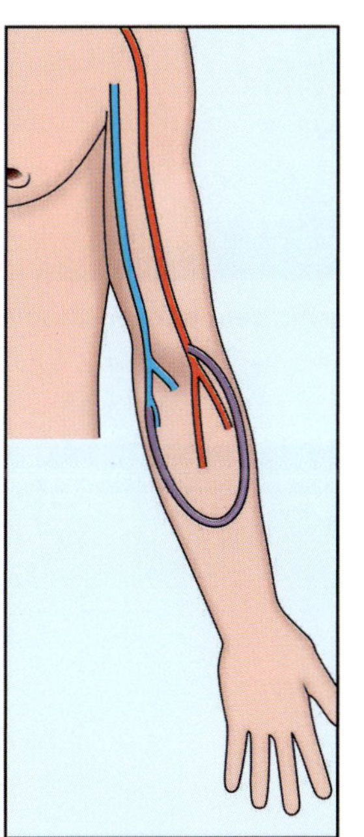

Graft interposition

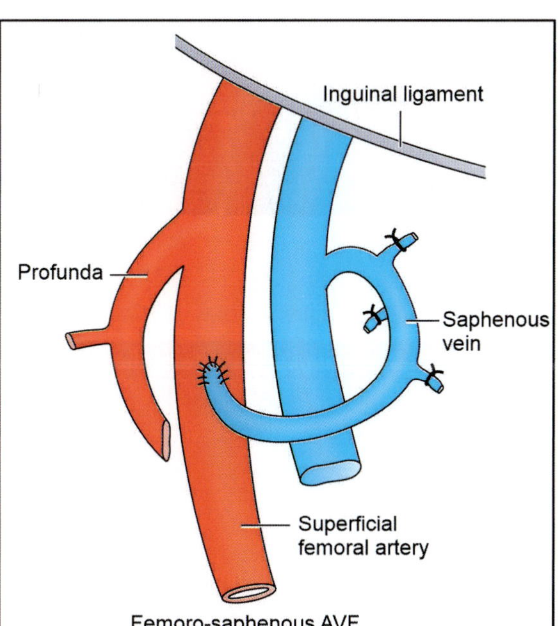

Femoro-saphenous AVF

Fig. 12.3: Different types of AV fistula

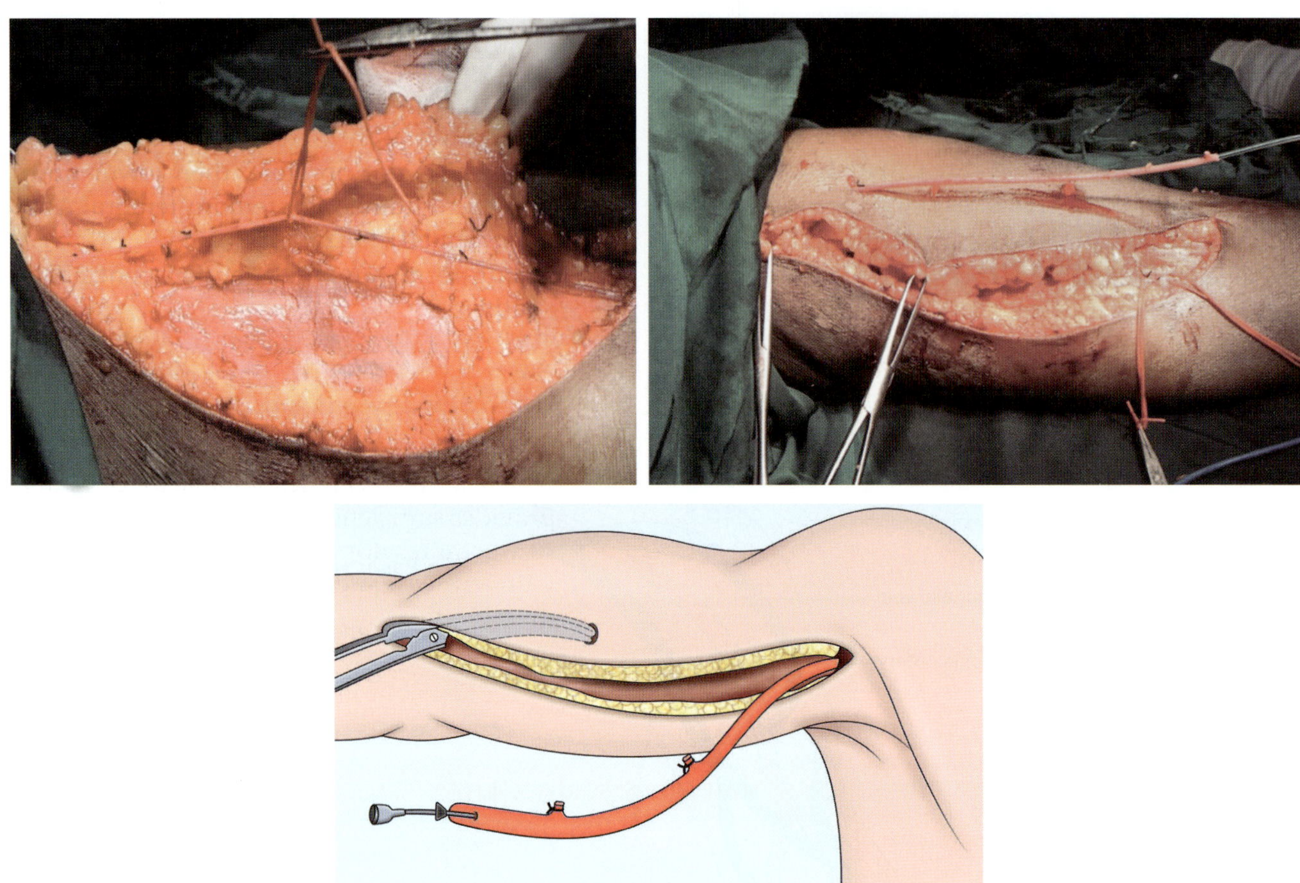

Fig. 12.4(A): Basilic vein transposition (conventional)

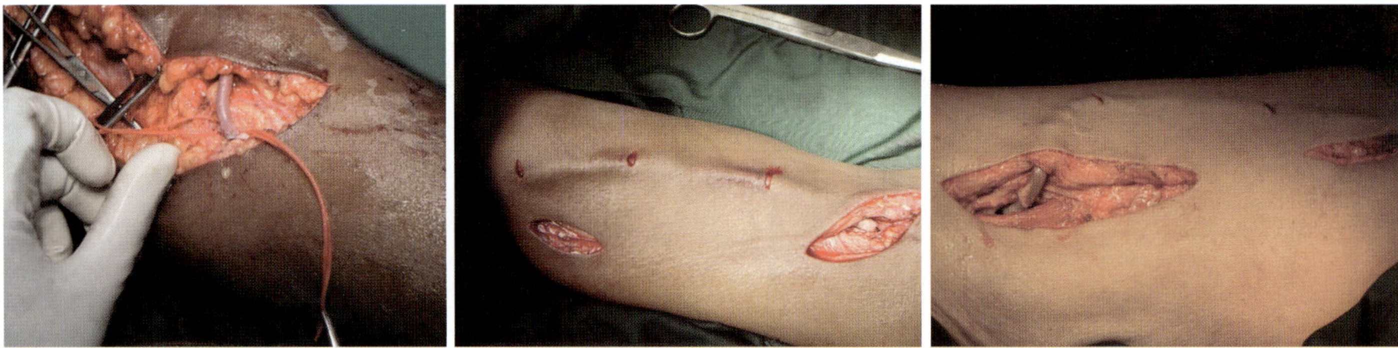

Fig. 12.4(B): Basilic vein transposition (multiple incisions)

TABLE 12.2: Average patency rate of the AVF		
Fistula	***Patency***	***Duration***
RC	80%	2 years
BC	80% 70%	3 years 4 years
Transposed BB	80%	2 years
Autologous saphenous vein interposition	22–60%	2 years
PTFE graft interposition	60%	2 years

Source: Kidney Transplant, Peter Moris

2. **When should dialysis be started?**
   Ans: The ideal trial showed no difference in overall outcomes between early (GFR>10 ml/min per 1.73 m^2) and late HD (GFR<10 ml/min per 1.73 m^2).[10] Other literature also did not find any benefit from the early versus the late start of dialysis in terms of morbidity, mortality and quality of life,[11] especially in the elderly. Thus it is clear that renal replacement therapy (RRT) should not be started until patient becomes symptomatic.

3. **What are the various techniques of making a fistula?**
   Ans:

TABLE 12.3: Different methods of doing fistula

Artery-Vein	*Advantages*	*Disadvantages*
Side–side	Simple, distensibility of prox vein from distal venous limb	Venous hypertension
End–end	Limited flow—prevents hypercirculation	Equal diameters, risk of ischemia, extension of thrombosis, acute angles
Side–end	When A and V are apart, no acute angle, no extension of thrombosis into artery.	-

4. **What are the optimal diameters of artery and vein on Doppler Ultrasound (DUS) before surgery?**
   Ans: Preoperative vein diameter greater than 2.5 mm resulted in a fivefold increase in fistula maturation compared to a vein size less than 2.5 mm.[12, 13] According to guidelines, a minimum internal radial artery diameter of 2 mm is suggested for RC AVF. At the same time, it is possible to successfully create fistulas with diameters of up to 1.5–1.6 mm provided the artery has healthy non-calcified wall.

5. **What is fistula maturation?**
   Ans: Maturation period is defined as time of AVF formation to the first cannulation. Maturation is the high-impact violent remodelling process by which an AVF becomes suitable for canulation and provides sufficient blood flow for adequate HD. An AVF requires approximately 6 weeks to mature,[14] with approximately 25% of AVFs never achieving maturation[15] (Fig. 12.5).

   A. *Positive effect on fistula maturation–"Outward remodelling"*
      Increased blood flow pressure in the vein leads to a violent increase in wall shear stress (WSS) (from 1–6 dyn/cm^2 to 10–70 dyn/cm^2 that of the arterial system).[16] This sets off a cascade of biochemical events to restore the WSS values, which are as follows:
      a. The large amount of nitric oxide (NO), a potent vasorelaxant are produced by the

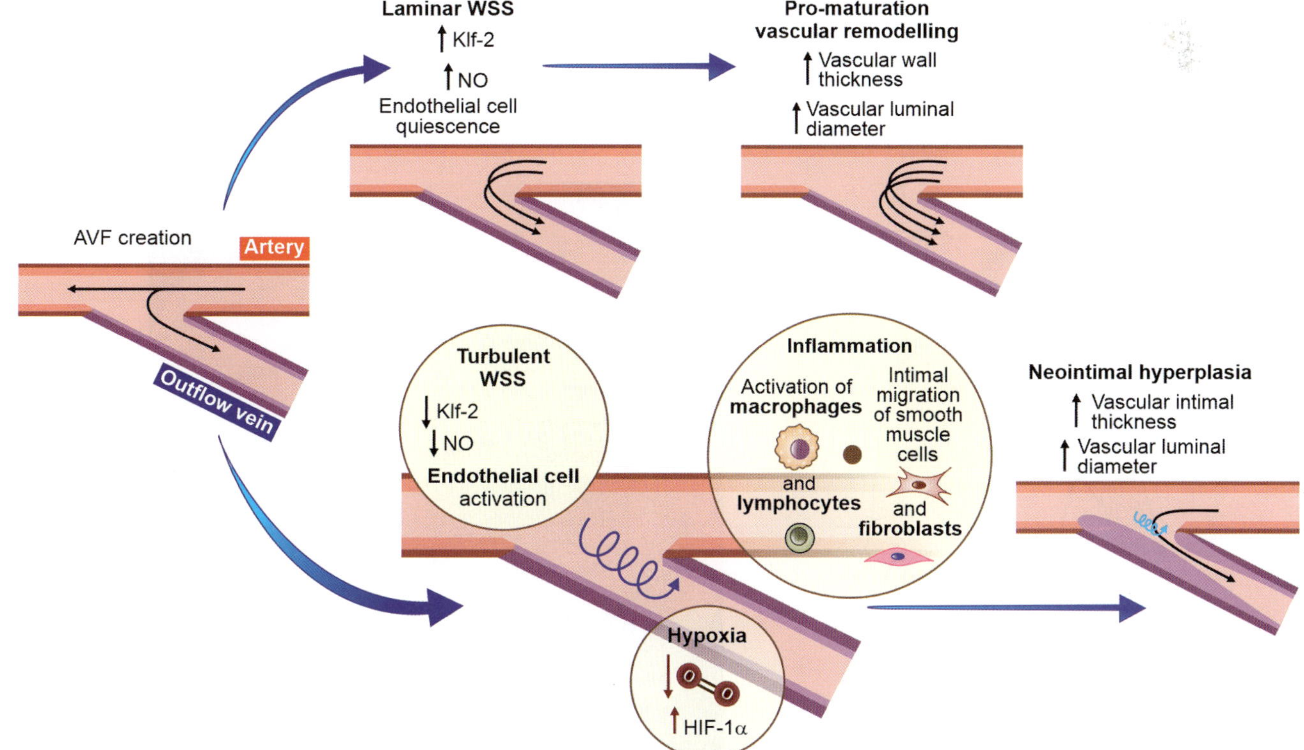

Fig. 12.5: Maturation cycle of AV fistula

endothelial cells NO synthase (eNOS). This expands the inflow artery and outflow vein and inhibits the development of NIH and gradually restores WSS to the baseline level. Overexpression of eNOS results in favourable vascular profiles for AVF maturation.

b. Excessively released NO + free radicals stimulates the matrix metalloproteinases (MMP), triggers extracellular matrix (ECM) degradation and decompose the vascular middle layer elastic fibers resulting in sustained luminal expansion.

c. Eccentric medial hypertrophy resulting from increased circumferential tension due to flow (outward remodelling).

B. *Negative effect on fistula maturation: Venous neointimal hyperplasia (NIH)—inward remodelling*

Synergistic action of turbulent WSS + inflammation +surgical stress + uremia + hypoxia promotes activation of pro-inflammatory macrophages and lymphocyte + intimal migration of smooth muscle cells and myofibroblast leads to NIH and vascular stenosis leading to eventual stasis and thrombosis (inward remodelling).

If prevailing process is outward remodelling, the AVF will successfully mature. But the excessive inward remodelling will lead AVF stenosis and subsequent failure to maturation.[17] The most common site of stenosis is near the anastomotic (juxta-anastomotic) segment (70%) because it is the area most subject to surgical manipulation, flow turbulence and myo-intimal alteration. Other areas are the sites of intravenous puncture and the venous valves.

6. What pre-operative assessment is required? Is pre-operative mapping DUS required in all?

Ans:

Examination: At the wrist the radial and ulnar arteries can be palpated for the adequate pulsations and calcifications. They are usually weak in diabetics and elderly patients. Allen's test confirms the patency of the palmer arch and confirm the dominance of the radial or the ulnar artery (Fig. 12.6).

Veins are best examined with tourniquet in the upper arm and asking the patient to clinch the fist. The patency of the cephalic vein at the wrist as well as in antecubital fossa is checked by tapping the vein and feeling the transmitted wave proximally in the elbow. The patency of the deep veins could only be assessed by imaging (DUS or venography, Fig. 12.6) as central vein stenosis or obstruction is usually asymptomatic.

Preoperative Doppler ultrasound (DUS) mapping is recommended to all patient planned for AVF/AVG[18]

A high bifurcation of brachial artery (20–25% of cases) and modest stenosis of the radial artery (20–30% of cases) could be vital to know before the fistula surgery which may impair the maturation. Table 12.4 shows various venous parameters to be checked on DUS.

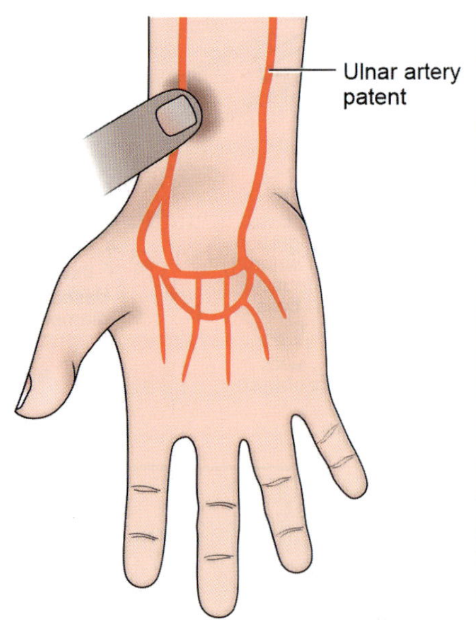

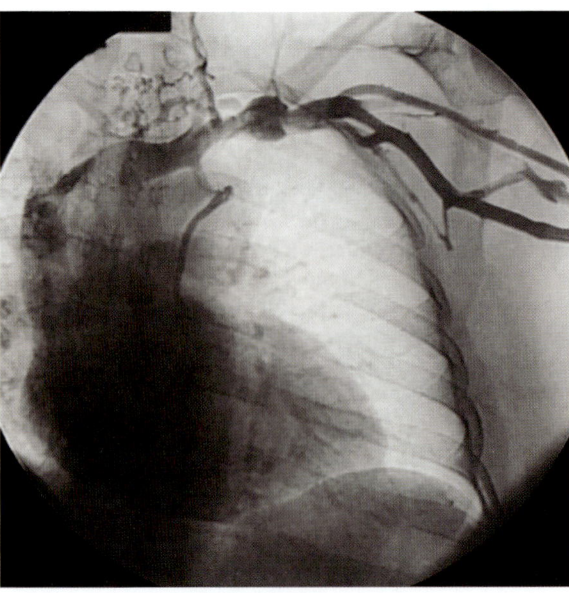

Fig. 12.6: Allen's test and venography demonstrating central vein stenosis

TABLE 12.4: Venous anatomy to be checked on DUS

- Venous diameter > 2.5 mm for AVF > 4 mm for graft.
- Patent venous segments without stenosis or thrombosis.
- Continuity with the deep veins of the upper arm.
- Absence of central venous stenosis.
- Straight segment.
- Vein is within 1cm of surface.
- Compliance—ability to dilate>50% with tourniquet.

Arterial anatomy to be checked on DUS

- Patent palmar arch
- Arterial diameter > 2 mm
- Symmetric UL BP—discrepancy < 20 mmHg
- Reasonable vessel wall

7. **What are the criteria to confirm that fistula has matured?**

   Ans: AVF should be at least 6 mm in diameter, less than 6 mm deep, and with a blood flow of at least 600 ml/min[19] (Table 12.5). Some literature considers minimum flow rates of 300–400 ml/min for mature AVFs.[20,21] The matured vein length should be 6–10 cm to allow for a successful two-needle dialysis.[22] If the segment is tortuous, there should be two straight segments at least 4 cm. Clinical examination is adequate to advice patient when to use the fistula for dialysis.

TABLE 12.5: Fistula maturation parameters

AV fistula

- Minimum flow rate: 350 to 400 ml/min
  < 300 ml/min recirculation problems
  < 200 ml/min clotting problems

PTFE graft

- Minimum flow rate: 800 to 1000 ml/min
  <600 ml/min clotting problems

8. **What is the post-operative follow-up of the patients?**

   Ans: Follow-up at 7–10 days—look for infection or neurological issues

   At 1 month—look for maturation

   At 1 month the fistula can be categorized into[23]

   A. *Mature AVFs:* Qa > 600 ml/min, cannulation segment straight, at least 10 cm long or two straight segments at least 4 cm in length, > 6 mm in diameter, <6 mm deep from skin surface.

   B. *AVFs are maturing well, but not meeting all maturation criteria:* Qa 400 to 600 ml/min, inner diameter of outflow segment 4–6 mm, depth from skin surface 6–8 mm → wait another period of 4 weeks and then a reassess.

   C. *Blood flow is adequate, but AVF cannot be used:* The outflow veins are not fulfilling the above mentioned criteria or situated deep → vein superficialization or USG guided punctures for HD.

9. **Is there a role of anti-platelets or antithrombotic agents for avoiding early thrombosis of the fistula?**

   Ans: There is not enough current evidence to suggest antiplatelet treatment for reducing AVF thrombosis or improve maturation. Double therapy (aspirin plus clopidogrel) and monotherapy with warfarin significantly increased the risk of bleeding without any benefit. Systemic heparinization to avoid early thrombotic events is also debated.[24]

10. **Is there a role of hand exercise after fistula surgery?**

    Ans: Exercise of the AVF hand positively influences the clinical maturation and ultrasound parameters associated with the maturity. So, it is recommended to encourage the patients to perform post-AVF hand-arm exercise program.

11. **Which are the factors associated with AVF maturation?**

    Ans:

    Modifiable: Obesity, peripheral arterial disease, surgeon's experience, previous cannulation, smoking, early cannulation, etc.

    Non-modifiable: Vessels-specific—condition of the vessels—diameter, length, maturation, blood flow

    - Patient-specific—female sex, age, co-morbidities, cardiac output, blood pressure, etc.[27–30]
    - Hypercoagulable states: Factor 5 Leiden, protein C and S, antithrombin III, Cardiolipin IGG AB, factor VIII, homocysteine

12. **What are the complications of the AVF?**

    Ans:

    A. *Early failure/fail to mature/pseudomaturation:* They all are synonymous and are generically defined as the inability of an AVF maturation within 4–6 weeks. Waiting >6 weeks is generally not necessary and does not improve the chances of recovery of access.[31] Pseudomaturation well-matured vein which is in excessive depth due to thick subcutaneous fat. Nearly 80% RC AVF can be recovered by endovascular or surgical correction.[32,33]

    B. *Large hematomas:* Hypertension, inadequate haemostasis at the end of the intervention, excessive use of anticoagulant agents or anti-platelet could be the reasons. To minimize bleeding risk, AVF should be done 24 hours after HD.

    C. *Wound infection:* Must be treated seriously as there are chance of secondary bleeding. Hospitalisation and IV antibiotics may be warranted in certain situations (Fig. 12.7).

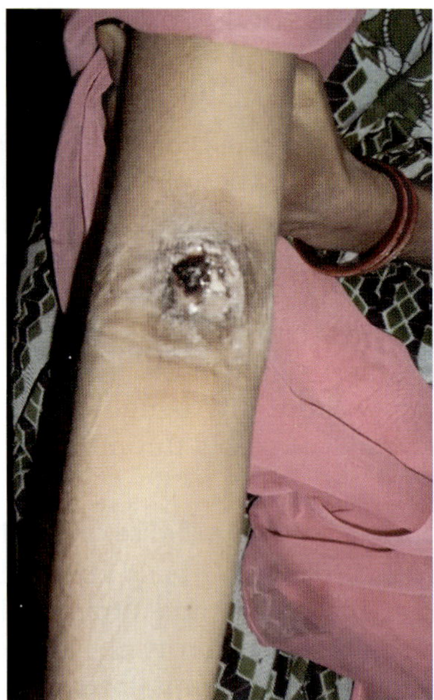

Fig. 12.7: Wound infection at brachio-cephalic fistula site

D. *Venous hypertension:* → Central venous stenosis or occlusion may present clinically with limb edema or ipsilateral neck, face, breast or chest wall edema (Fig. 12.8). Severe cases may also be complicated by venous ulceration. Treatment is endovascular intervention (percutaneous transluminal angioplasty).

E. *Arteriovenous fistula aneurysms:* Generalized outflow vein enlargement is a normal finding. There are two types of aneurysms:

a. True aneurysm—dilatation of all the three layers of the vein → generally related to degenerative changes in the vessel → may be due to venous outflow stenosis. No action is usually required.

b. False aneurysm—which is caused by a small tear in the outflow vein (usually iatrogenic from repeated cannulation), resulting in a persistent defect that allows blood flow into the subcutaneous tissues outside of the wall of the outflow vein (Fig. 12.9).

Indication of the early surgery—rapid enlargement, overlying skin necrosis, or spontaneous bleeding.

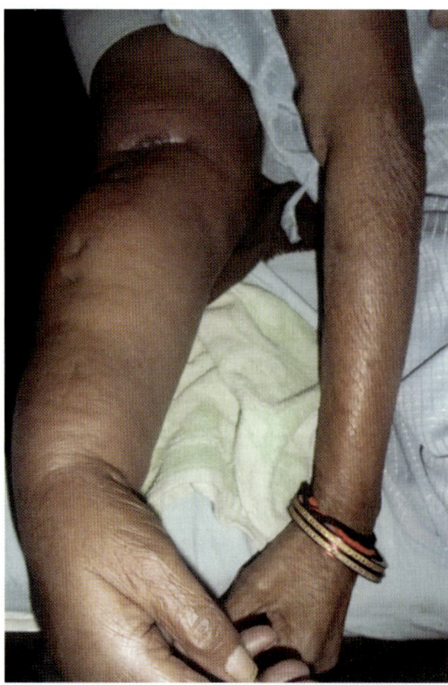

Fig. 12.8: Edematous upper limb secondary to central venous stenosis

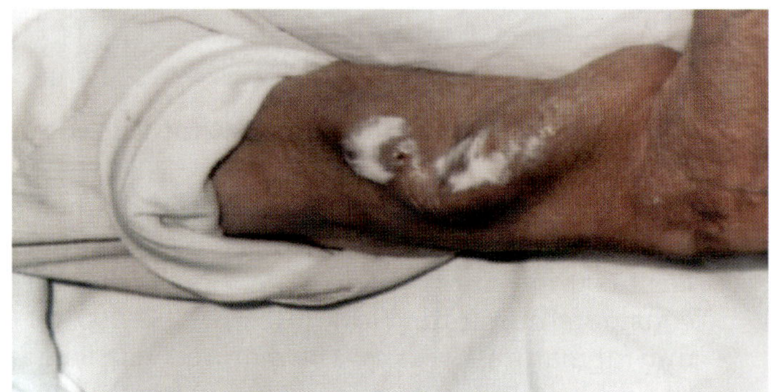

Fig. 12.9: Aneurysmal dilatation at the site of fistula

F. *Steal syndrome and ischemic monomelic neuropathy—also known as hemodialysis access induced distal ischemia (HAIDI)* is caused by inadequate vascularization of the vasa nervorum as arterial inflow is diverted to AVF/AVG which leads to severe sensorimotor dysfunction of the radial, median and ulnar nerves resulting in ischemic symptoms. This usually happens with proximal fistulas in diabetic patients. Preoperative Doppler US may reveal individuals at risk of steal syndrome. Allen's test performed with DUS duplex is more objective in assessing blood flow in palmar arches than physical examination alone.[34]

13. What are the recent advances in AVF?

Ans:

Localized Perivascular Therapeutic Approaches[35]

A. *Mechanical devices:* The use of supportive mechanical devices minimizes NIH by decreasing turbulence through the fistula and modulating pathologic vascular WSS

B. *Targeted drug delivery:* Localized exposure to pharmacologic agents (sirolimus, paclitaxel, simvastatin, 1, 25-dihydroxyvitamin D_3, vonapanitase, bevacizumab) may prevent the anastomotic region from NIH.

C. *Perivascular cell-based therapeutics:* The use of the cells that produce variety of the substances that potentially suppress NIH has been explored in recent studies, mesenchymal stem/stromal cells.

14. What are the indications, advantages and disadvantages of AVG?

Ans: Common graft materials are expanded polytetrafluoroethylene (ePTFE), polycarbonate urethane, polyurethane and multi-material grafts.

- Indications: Patients with limited availability of sites for vascular access.
- Advantages: Early maturation of access.
- Disadvantages: Higher all-cause mortality and fatal infections than AV fistulas.

15. What are the indications, advantages and disadvantages of CVC?

Ans:

Indications: (*Source: Kidney Transplant* by Peter Morris)

- Awaiting maturation of autogenous AVF
- Awaiting maturation of CAPD
- Patients waiting for living related transplantation
- Dialysis bridge after failed previous vascular access/CAPD to allow planning and imaging for long-term access
- Parmanent access—all other sites exhausted, severe cardiac dysfunction, vascular arterial disease

Advantages

- Less demanding technical procedure, universally applicable
- Lower resource usage—easy and low cost for placement and replacement
- Immediate HD provision—maturation time not required
- No need for percutaneous cannulation.
- Preferred as a long-term option in low-resource settings or in patients with multiple comorbidities and limited life expectancy.
- Ease of correcting thrombotic complications.

Complications

- Arterial puncture
- Bleeding
- Pneumothorax
- Hemothorax
- Hemomediastinum
- Atrial perforation
- Air embolus
- Arrhythmias
- Primary failure

16 What are the contraindications, advantages and disadvantages of PD?

Ans:

Absolute contraindications	*Relative contraindications*
• Encapsulating peritoneal sclerosis	• Severe obesity • Severe peritoneal adhesions
• Inflammatory bowel disease • Large irreparable abdominal wall hernias	• Large hernias of anterior abdominal wall • Abdominal wall stomas • Chronic obstructive pulmonary disease • Psychosocial factors likely to result in poor compliance • Physical disability • Learning disability

Advantages

- Better quality of life due to autonomy, flexibility, avoidance of regular hospital visits
- Better cosmesis
- Pain-free repeated cannulation
- Preservation of vascular access sites for further HD and residual renal function
- Literature has shown progressive increase in 5-year survival of patients on PD than those on HD.[6]

Complications

Mechanical complications—leaks, catheter displacement, catheter obstruction, hernias, hydrothorax, peritonitis.

SUMMARY

- AV fistula is the lifeline for patients with ESRD on MHD.
- All patients with CKD stage 4 should be counselled and offered AVF.
- Preservation of veins in the non-dominant hand of a patient with progressive CKD should be the standard of practice.
- Veins can be preserved by avoiding repeated cannulations and blood sampling in non-dominant hand.
- Distal AVF in non-dominant hand is the first choice of majority surgeons.
- A thorough clinical examination of the hand and a pre-op DUS should be done for the assessment of vessels in all patients.
- There are different ways of doing the fistula including end-to-end or end-to-side and it is individual choice of practice and training.
- There is no proven role of peri-opertive heparanization or anti-coagultion to prevent thrombosis.
- Fistula takes 6 weeks to get matured and gentle hand exercises really help in maturation.
- Arterio-venous grafts are reserved for those who do not have good quality suitable veins.
- Lower limb fistulas are done once all the options of upper limb have been exhausted.

REFERENCES

1. Pecoits-Filho R, Okpechi IG, Donner JA, Harris DCH, Aljubori HM. Capturing and monitoring global differences in untreated and treated end-stage kidney disease, kidney replacement therapy modality, and outcomes. *Kidney Int Suppl* (2011) 2020;10(1):e3–9.
2. Zavacka M, Zelko A, Madarasova Geckova A, Majernikova M, Pobehova J. Vascular access as a survival factor for the haemodialysis population: a retrospective study. Int Angiol. 2020;39 (6):525–531.
3. Murad MH, Elamin MB, Sidawy AN, Malaga G, Rizvi AZ, Flynn DN, *et al.* Autogenous versus prosthetic vascular access for hemodialysis: a systematic review and meta-analysis. *J Vasc Surg* 2008;48(5 Suppl):34S–47S.
4. Brescia MJ, Cimino JE, Appel K and Hurwich BJ Chronic hemodialysis using venipuncture and a surgically created arteriovenous fistula. N. Engl. J. Med 275, 1089–1092 (1966).
5. Idrees M, Suthananthan A, Pathmarajah T, Sieunarine K. Snuffbox fistula-a first-line approach to haemodialysis: a review. J Vasc Access. 2020;21 (5):1129729819867817.
6. Bourquelot P, Rawa M, Van Laere O, Franco G. Long-term results of femoral vein transposition for autogenous arterio-venous hemodialysis access. J Vasc Surg. 2012;56(2):440–445.
7. Karam L, Rawa M, Shoenfeld R, Bourquelot P. Brachial vein trans-position is a promising ultimate upper limb autologous arteriovenous angioaccess despite its many pitfalls. J Vasc Surg. 2018;67(1): 236–243.
8. Pham XD, Kim JJ, Ihenachor EJ, *et al.* A comparison of brachial artery-brachial vein arteriovenous fistulas with arteriovenous grafts in patients with poor superficial venous anatomy. J Vasc Surg. 2017;65 (2):444–451.
9. Muthu Veeramani, Jigish Vyas, Ravindra Sabnis, Mahesh Desai, Indian J Urol, Jan-Mar 2010, Vol 26, Issue 1.
10. Rosansky SJ, Clark WF, Eggers P, *et al.* Initiation of dialysis at higher GFRs: is the apparent rising tide of early dialysis harmful or helpful? *Kidney Int* 2009; 76(3): 257–261.
11. Molnar MZ, Ojo AO, Bunnapradist S, *et al.* Timing of dialysis initiation in transplant-naive and failed transplant patients. *Nat Rev Nephrol* 2012; 8(5):284–292.
12. Siddiqui MA, Ashraff S, Santos D, Rush R, Carline T, Raza Z. Predictive parameters of arteriovenous fistula maturation in patients with end-stage renal disease. Kidney Res Clin Pract. 2018;37 (3):277–286.
13. Brimble KS, Rabbat CG, Treleaven DJ, Ingram AJ. Utility of ultra-sonographic venous assessment prior to forearm arterio-venous fistula creation. Clin Nephrol. 2002;58(2):122–127.
14. Robbin ML, Chamberlain NE, Lockhart ME, Gallichio MH, Young CJ, Deierhoi MH, *et al.* Hemodialysis arteriovenous fistula maturity: US evaluation. *Radiology* 2002;225(1):59–64.
15. Kian K, Vassalotti JA. The new arteriovenous fistula: the need for earlier evaluation and intervention. *Semin Dial* 2005;18(1):3–7.
16. Fitts MK, Pike DB, Anderson K, Shiu YT. Hemodynamic shear stress and endothelial dysfunction in hemodialysis access. Open Urol Nephrol J. 2014;7(Suppl1 M5):33–44.
17. Nath KA, Katusic ZS. Predicting the functionality and form of a dialysis fistula. J Am Soc Nephrol. 2016;27(12):3508–3510.
18. Schmidli J, Widmer MK, Basile C, *et al.* Editor's choice-Vascular access: 2018 clinical practice guidelines of the European Society for Vascular Surgery (ESVS). *Eur J Vasc Endovasc Surg* 2018; 55(6): 757–818.
19. Robbin, M.L.; Greene, T.; Allon, M.; Dember, L.M.; Imrey, P.B.; Cheung, A.K.; Himmelfarb, J.; Huber, T.S.; Kaufman, J.S.; Radeva, M.K.; *et al.* Prediction of Arteriovenous Fistula Clinical Maturation from Postoperative Ultrasound Measurements: Findings from the Hemodialysis Fistula Maturation Study. *J. Am. Soc. Nephrol.* 2018, *29*, 2735–2744.
20. Bashar, K.; Conlon, P.J.; Kheirelseid, E.A.H.; Aherne, T.; Walsh, S.R.; Leahy, A. Arteriovenous Fistula in Dialysis Patients: Factors Implicated in Early and Late AVF Maturation Failure. *Surgeon* 2016, *14*, 294–300.
21. Remuzzi, A.; Bozzetto, M. Biological and Physical Factors Involved in the Maturation of Arteriovenous Fistula for Hemodialysis. *Cardiovasc. Eng. Technol.* 2017, *8*, 273–279.
22. Wilson SE. *Vascular Access, principle and practice*. Philadelphia: Lippincott Williams & Wilkins, 2010
23. Mohamed, I.; Kamarizan, M.F.A.; da Silva, A. Medical Adjuvant Treatment to Increase Patency of Arteriovenous Fistulae and Grafts. *Cochrane Database Syst. Rev.* 2021, *7*, CD002786
24. Salimi F, Majd Nassiri G, Moradi M, *et al.* Assessment of effects of upper extremity exercise with arm tourniquet on maturity of arterio-venous fistula in hemodialysis patients. J Vasc Access. 2013;14 (3):239–244.
25. Fontseré N, Mestres G, Yugueros X, *et al.* Effect of a postoperative exercise program on arteriovenous fistula maturation: a randomized controlled trial. Hemodial Int. 2016;20(2):306–314.
26. Monitoring the patients following Radio Cephalic Arteriovenous fistula: a Current prospective, Nicola Pirozzi, Nicoletta Mancianti,Jacopo Scrivano, Loredana Fazzari, Roberto Pirozzi, Matteo Tozzi, Vascular Health and Risk Management 2021:17 111–121.
27. Conte MS, Nugent HM, Gaccione P, Roy-Chaudhury P, Lawson JH. Influence of diabetes and perivascular allogeneic endothelial cell implants on arteriovenous fistula remodeling. J Vasc Surg. 2011;54 (5):1383–1389.
28. Lazarides MK, Georgiadis GS, Antoniou GA, Staramos DN. A meta-analysis of dialysis access outcome in elderly patients. J Vasc Surg. 2007;45(2):420–426. doi:10.1016/j.jvs.2006.10.035.
29. Astor BC, Coresh J, Powe NR, Eustace JA, Klag MJ. Relation between gender and vascular access complications in hemodialysis patients. Am J Kidney Dis. 2000;36(6):1126–1134.
30. Robbin ML, Greene T, Cheung AK, *et al.* Arteriovenous fistula development in the first 6 weeks after creation. Radiology. 2016;279(2):620–629. doi:10.1148/radiol.2015150385
31. Muray Cases S, García Medina J, Pérez Abad JM, *et al.* Importance of monitoring and treatment of failed maturation in radiocephalic arteriovenous fistula in predialysis: role of ultrasound. Nefrologia. 2016;36(4):410–417.
32. Lee T, Ullah A, Allon M, *et al.* Decreased cumulative access survival in arteriovenous fistulas requiring interventions to promote maturation. Clin J Am Soc Nephrol. 2011;6(3):575–581.
33. Habib J, Baetz L and Satiani B. Assessment of collateral circulation to the hand prior to radial artery harvest. *Vasc Med* 2012; 17(5): 352–361.
34. Localized Perivascular Therapeutic Approaches to Inhibit Venous Neointimal Hyperplasia in Arteriovenous Fistula Access for Hemodialysis Use Allan John R. Barcena 1,2, Joy Vanessa D. Perez 1,2, Olivia Liu 1,3, Amy Mu 1,4, Francisco M. Heralde III 2, Steven Y. Huang 1 and Marites P. Melancon 1,5,* *Biomolecules* 2022, *12*, 1367
35. Van de Luijtgaarden MW, Jager KJ, Segelmark M, *et al.* Trends in dialysis modality choice and related patient survival in the ERA-EDTA Registry over a 20-year period. Nephrol Dial Transplant. 2016;31(1):120–8.

Chapter 13

Robotic Kidney Transplant

• *Kishore TA*

LEARNING OBJECTIVES

- To understand the history and current indications for robotic assisted kidney transplant (RAKT).
- To understand the prevalent technique in RAKT.
- To understand the outcomes of RAKT in comparison with open kidney transplantation.
- To understand the technical modifications in RAKT.
- To understand the future status of RAKT.

Case Scenario

A 43-year-old male patient, weight 120 kg and BMI of 37, with end stage renal disease disease is being worked up for transplant. His mother is a donor. She has b/l single renal artery and vein.

1. **What modality would you advise for transplant?**

   Ans: It has also been proven that patients with higher weight are at risk of delayed graft function (DGF) and selected surgical complications, such as infections.[1] Performing kidney transplant is a challenge in obese patient. Vascular anastomosis in obese patients is demanding because of increased abdominal wall thickness, increased intra-abdominal fat and pelvic configuration.[2] Wound complications like infection, dehiscence, seroma are more in obese patients leading to increased hospital stay and secondary procedures.[2] Increased incidence of long-term complications like incision hernia are also prevalent in patients with high BMI.[2] Robotic assisted kidney transplant was introduced in morbidly obese patient who were previous denied kidney transplantation in USA.[3] **Taking into account the high BMI, this patient may benefit from RAKT** (Fig. 13.1).

2. **Where was the first RAKT performed?**

   Ans: This was performed by Giullianotti *et al* at Chicago, USA in a morbidly obese patient.[3]

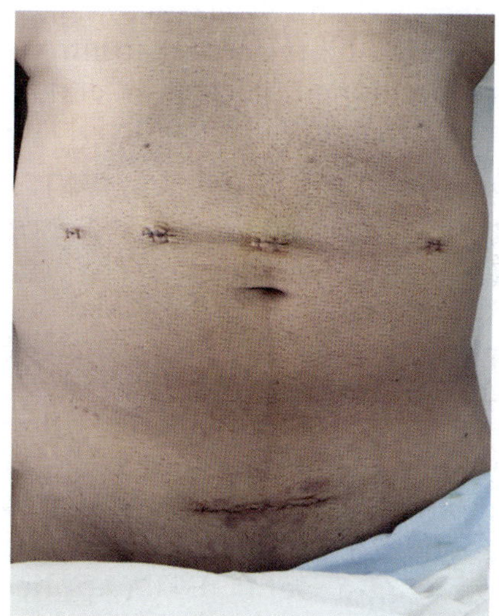

Fig. 13.1: Surgical scar of an obese RAKT recipient

3. **Are there other advantages of RAKT?**

   Ans: Various studies have found out that RAKT is associated with reduced blood loss, decreased pain score and reduced rate of wound complications.[4] RAKT has been implemented in limited centers across the world.[5–8] Early studies primarily focused on evaluating the feasibility and non-inferiority of RAKT when compared to OKT.[9–11] These pioneering studies have addressed the surgical outcomes, short-term graft function and complications.[12] It has been observed in initial series that RAKT is associated with longer rewarming and anastomotic times, yet the graft function remains comparable to that of OKT.[13] To date, there have been two studies that have specifically investigated the long and mid-term outcomes of RAKT. In a study spanning a period of ten years and encompassing 239 patients, Tzveranov and colleagues examined the outcome of RAKT in morbidly obese patients, revealing minimal surgical site infections and excellent graft function.[4] Another study conducted by Ahlawat *et al* compared 126 RAKT patients with 378 patients who underwent open surgery.[14] This study indicated that RAKT was associated with lower blood loss, smaller incisions, reduced postoperative pain, decreased wound complications, and fewer symptomatic lymphoceles.[14]

4. **Is laparoscopic kidney transplant feasible?**

   Ans: Laparoscopic kidney transplant was pioneered by Modi *et al* in 2010 from India.[15] But due to steep learning curve and technical challenges it was not reproduced at other centers.

5. **What is the commonest technique of RAKT performed across the world?**

   Ans: Vattikutti-Medanta technique with regional hypothermia is the widely followed.[5] The technique uses a periumbilical incision to introduce the graft. This is performed utilizing a Gel point. Kidney is covered in a gauze jacket with ice slush.

6. **Is there any risk of performing RAKT?**

   Ans: Most of the studies have determined RAKT to have same graft outcomes. The primary concern surrounding RAKT in the initial era was longer operative time and rewarming time.[16] Significantly longer rewarming times have been reported in previously published literature.[6,13,17] To mitigate longer detrimental effects of warm ischemia time Sood *et al* proposed the regional hypothermia technique.[12] They have adopted a technique by introducing a GeLPOINT (Applied Medicals, CA, USA) through a periumbilical incision.[8] Cold ischemia is achieved by placing ice over the kidney while introducing kidney through GeLPOINT and subsequent reinforcement by placing ice while during anastomosis.

7. **How does RAKT compare with OKT?**

   Ans: RAKT in selected patients from live kidney donors has decreased risk of surgical complications when performed by an experienced surgeon, leading to comparable graft and patient survival, without compromising long-term renal function. RAKT, with minimally invasive benefit, offers an excellent alternative to OKT. RAKT was associated with lower a risk of surgical site infection (Risk ratio (RR) = 0.15, $p < 0.001$), symptomatic lymphocele (RR = 0.20, $p = 0.03$), less postoperative pain (Mean difference (MD) = –1.38 points, $p < 0.001$), smaller incision length (MD = 8.51 cm, $p < 0.001$), and shorter length of hospital stay (MD = 1.69 days, $p = 0.03$) compared with OKT. No difference was found in renal function, graft, and patient survival.[18]

8. **What are the cardinal steps in RAKT?**

   Ans: RAKT is generally performed using da Vinci S/X/Xi system. Five ports are placed and a pfannensteil incision is performed to place the kidney inside. A gel point may be placed to introduce the graft. A peritoneal flap is created before preparing the iliac vessels. The venous anastomoses is performed by applying two Bulldog clamps on EIV and 6/0 Gore-Tex (Gore Medical Inc, AZ, USA) sutures in end to side manner. Similar technique is used for the arterial anastomosis with Gore-Tex 7–0 suture. The ureter is anastomosed to bladder with modified Lich-Gregoir method with 5–0 polydioxanone with 4/16 Fr Double J stent *in situ*.[12]

9. **Why is Goretex the preferred suture in RAKT?**

   Ans: Goretex 6.0 is a preferred suture material due to less memory and better handling.[5]

   For smaller vessels 6.0 and 8.0 Goretex can be used with 9 mm needle. Polypropylene is not favored due to low tensile strength, high memory and tendency to break in minimally invasive surgery.

10. **What is the learning curve for RAKT?**

    Ans: Learning curve of RAKT is to be estimated to be around 35 cases.[9] Various cooling devices have been introduced for maintaining the hypothermia during the learning curve.[19] Robotic simulators have been developed recently to reduce the learning curve.[20]

11. **What are the drawbacks cited for RAKT?**

    Ans: Learning curve, Trendelenburg position, damage to intraperitoneal organ, effect of pneumoperitoneum on graft and recipient are potential concerns for RAKT.[21] Concerns about pneumoperitoneum and its effects on graft kidney were initially raised. Studies have shown that at standard pneumoperitoneal pressures (12–15 mmHg), renal blood flow decreased to 25% of baseline, which becomes more relevant once the graft is reperfused.[21]

12. **Are there any specific complications for RAKT?**

    Ans: Being an intraperitoneal procedure graft is prone for torsion. This can be prevented by hitching the graft to peritoneal flap.[16]

13. **What are contraindications for RAKT?**

Ans: Any contraindication for laparoscopy can considered a contraindication for RAKT. For example, patient with multiple previous abdominal surgery, patients who does not tolerate pneumoperitoneum and steep Trendelenburg position.

14. **Are patients with atherosclerosis and multiple vessels considered a contraindication for RAKT?**

Ans: With increasing experience patient with atherosclerosis can be managed with RAKT. Most of the patients with multiple vessel can be managed extracorporeal bench surgery but with experience multiple robotic vessel anastomosis is also possible in reasonable time (Fig. 13.2).

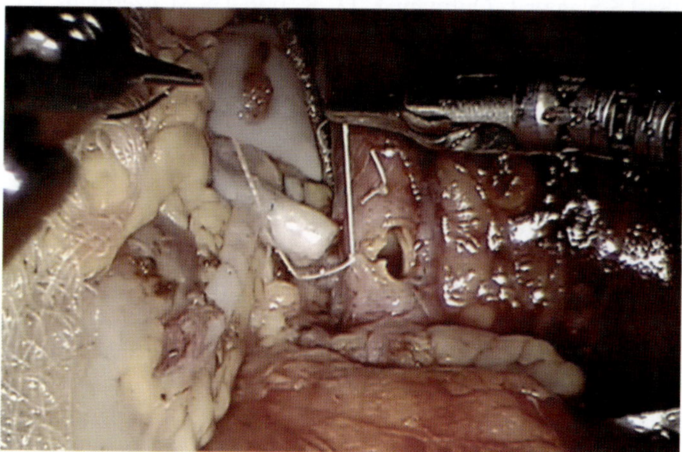

Fig. 13.2: RAKT in atherosclerotic vessel

15. **Can RAKT be performed extraperitoneally?**

Ans: There are a few case reports of total extraperitoneal technique even though it is not standardized.[22] The extraperitonealization of the graft also prevents bowel interference in the operative field if there is an open conversion. Post-operative bleeding is another complication encountered after renal transplantation and requires immediate exploration. When the graft is placed intraperitoneally unimpeded bleeding can occur into peritoneal cavity. Peritoneal cavity can accommodate large quantities of blood before producing any signs and this could lead to delayed detection of hemorrhage. The water tight closure of peritoneum prevents unrestricted catastrophic leakage of blood or urine in the post-operative period into peritoneal cavity. The graft which is placed in the extraperitoneal space allows renal biopsy in the immediate post-operative period without any concern of bowel injury. The extraperitonealization will also prevent bleeding into peritoneal cavity after renal biopsy in the post-operative period.

16. **Can RAKT be performed in pediatric population?**

Ans: RAKT has been performed in children up to 20 kg with good perioperative and cosmetic results (Fig. 13.3).[23]

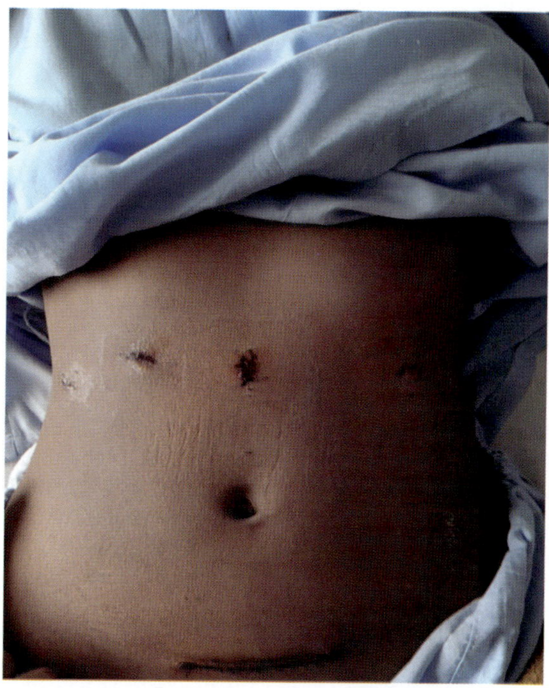

Fig. 13.3: Scars in a pedantic patient

17. **Is natural orifice surgery possible in RAKT?**

Ans: RAKT with transvaginal insertion has been performed to reduce the morbidity.[24]

Transvaginal insertion can obviate the need for incision, thus reducing chances of wound related complications.

18. **Is it possible to perform single port RAKT?**

Ans: Kaouk *et al* reported single port RAKT in a series of 9 patients.[25] This technique was found to be safe and effective, with promising postoperative outcomes and potentially with lesser morbidity.[26]

SUMMARY

- RAKT is useful for obese recipient especially with right renal vein.
- Vattikutti-Medanta technique with regional hypothermia is widely followed.
- RAKT is non-inferior to OKT with regards to long-term graft dysfunction, graft or patient survival.
- Learning curve, Trendelenburg position, damage to intraperitoneal organ, effect of pneumoperitoneum on graft and recipient are potential concerns for RAKT.
- Contraindication to RAKT may include multiple previous abdominal surgery, patients who does not tolerate pneumoperitoneum and steep Trendelenburg position.
- RAKT can also be performed extraperitoneally and single port.

REFERENCES

1. C.J. Hill, A.E. Courtney, C.R. Cardwell, A.P. Maxwell, G. Lucarelli, M. Veroux, F. Furriel, R.M. Cannon, E.K. Hoogeveen, M. Doshi, J.A. McCaughan, Nephrol Dial Transplant 30 (2015) 1403–11.
2. U. Scheuermann, J. Babel, U.-C. Pietsch, A. Weimann, O. Lyros, K. Semmling, H.-M. Hau, D. Seehofer, S. Rademacher, R. Sucher, BMC Nephrol 23 (2022) 37.
3. P. Giulianotti, V. Gorodner, F. Sbrana, I. Tzvetanov, H. Jeon, F. Bianco, K. Kinzer, J. Oberholzer, E. Benedetti, American Journal of Transplantation 10 (2010) 1478–1482.
4. I.G. Tzvetanov, M. Spaggiari, K.A. Tulla, C. Di Bella, O. Okoye, P. Di Cocco, H. Jeon, J. Oberholzer, P. Cristoforo Giulianotti, E. Benedetti, American Journal of Transplantation 20 (2020) 430–440.
5. M. Menon, A. Sood, M. Bhandari, V. Kher, P. Ghosh, R. Abaza, W. Jeong, K.R. Ghani, R.K. Kumar, P. Modi, R. Ahlawat, Eur Urol 65 (2014) 991–1000.
6. A. Breda, A. Territo, L. Gausa, V. Tu cu, A. Alcaraz, M. Musquera, K. Decaestecker, L. Desender, M. Stockle, M. Janssen, P. Fornara, N. Mohammed, G. Siena, S. Serni, L. Guirado, C. Facundo, N. Doumerc, Eur Urol 73 (2018) 273–281.
7. V. Tu cu, N.C. ener, S. ahin, A.H. Yavuzsan, F.G. Akbay, S. Apaydın, Turk Uroloji Dergisi 42 (2016) 295–298.
8. K.T. Adiyat, K.K. Vinod, R. Vishnu, M.K. Ramaprasad, V.N. Unni, R.P. John, J Robot Surg 12 (2018) 535–540.
9. M. Musquera, L. Peri, T. Ajami, R. Campi, V. Tugcu, K. Decaestecker, M. Stockle, P. Fornara, N. Doumerc, F. Vigues, R. Barod, L. Desender, A. Territo, S. Serni, G. Vignolini, S. Sahin, P. Zeuschner, N. Banga, A. Breda, A. Alcaraz, BJU Int 127 (2021) 222–228.
10. G. Vignolini, I. Greco, F. Sessa, L. Gemma, A. Pecoraro, P. Barzaghi, A. Grosso, F. Corti, N. Mormile, M. Martiriggiano, A. Berni, N. Firenzuoli, M. Gacci, S. Giancane, A. Sebastianelli, V. Li Marzi, S. Serni, R. Campi, Front Surg 7 (2020).
11. A. Breda, A. Territo, L. Gausa, V. Tu cu, A. Alcaraz, M. Musquera, K. Decaestecker, L. Desender, M. Stockle, M. Janssen, P. Fornara, N. Mohammed, G. Siena, S. Serni, L. Guirado, C. Facundo, N. Doumerc, Eur Urol 73 (2018) 273–281.
12. A. Sood, P. McCulloch, P. Dahm, R. Ahlawat, W. Jeong, M. Bhandari, M. Menon, International Journal of Surgery 25 (2016) 158–161.
13. R. Maheshwari, S.Y. Qadri, L.R. Rakhul, S. Chaturvedi, P. Desai, R. Grover, G. Chhabra, D. Khullar, A. Kumar, J Endourol 34 (2020) 939–945.
14. R. Ahlawat, A. Sood, W. Jeong, P. Ghosh, J. Keeley, F. Abdollah, V. Kher, P. Olson, G. Farah, H. Wurst, M. Bhandari, M. Menon, J Urol 205 (2021) 595–602.
15. P. Modi, J. Rizvi, B. Pal, R. Bharadwaj, P. Trivedi, A. Trivedi, K. Patel, K. Shah, J. Vyas, S. Sharma, K. Shah, R. Chauhan, H. Trivedi, Am J Transplant 11 (2011) 1320–4.
16. J. Oberholzer, P. Giulianotti, K.K. Danielson, M. Spaggiari, L. Bejarano-Pineda, F. Bianco, I. Tzvetanov, S. Ayloo, H. Jeon, R. Garcia-Roca, J. Thielke, I. Tang, S. Akkina, B. Becker, K. Kinzer, A. Patel, E. Benedetti, American Journal of Transplantation 13 (2013) 721–728.
17. U. Pein, M. Girndt, S. Markau, A. Fritz, A. Breda, M. Stöckle, N. Mohammed, F. Kawan, A. Schumann, P. Fornara, K. Weigand, World J Urol 38 (2020) 795–802.
18. J.S. Slagter, L. Outmani, K.T.C.K. Tran, J.N.M. Ijzermans, R.C. Minnee, International Journal of Surgery 99 (2022).
19. A. Longchamp, R.P.H. Meier, N. Colucci, A. Balaphas, L.A. Orci, A. Nastasi, G. Longchamp, S. Moll, A. Klauser, M. Pascual, F. Lazeyras, J.-M. Corpataux, L. Bühler, Swiss Med Wkly 149 (2019) w20143.
20. R. Uwechue, P. Gogalniceanu, N. Kessaris, N. Byrne, P. Chandak, J. Olsburgh, K. Ahmed, N. Mamode, I. Loukopoulos, J Robot Surg 12 (2018) 541–544.
21. AW. Chiu, KM. Azadzoi, DG. Hatzichristou, MB. Siroky, RJ. Krane, RK. Babyan, J Endourol 8 (1994) 99–103.
22. V. Raveendran, R.M. Koduveli, R. John, D. Varma, K.T. Adiyat, J Robot Surg (2018).
23. A. Bansal, R. Maheshwari, S. Chaturvedi, D. Bansal, A. Kumar, Pediatr Transplant 25 (2021).
24. V. Raveendran, K.T. Adiyat, R.M. Koduveli, R. John, J Robot Surg 11 (2017).
25. J. Kaouk, M. Eltemamy, A. Aminsharifi, Z. Schwen, C. Wilson, M. Abou Zeinab, J. Garisto, L. Lenfant, A. Wee, Eur Urol 80 (2021) 366–373.
26. J.H. Kaouk, A. Khalifeh, H. Laydner, R. Autorino, S.P. Hillyer, K. Panumatrassamee, C. Modlin, H.B. Goldman, Urology 80 (2012) 1171–1175.

Chapter

14

Donor with Medical Conditions

• *Deepak Rathi* • *Varun Mittal*

LEARNING OBJECTIVES

To understand the donor selection dilemmas in situations like:

- Pre-diabetes and diabetes
- Hypertension
- Proteinuria
- Obesity
- Microscopic hematuria
- Elderly donors
- Hepatitis and HIV positive donors

INTRODUCTION

Kidney transplantation is the treatment of choice for most patients with end stage renal disease, offering better quality of life and optimum survival. In a year around 200,000 patients of end stage kidney disease wait for kidney transplant in our country. Less than 10% of these undergo transplant and more than 80% of these are living donor kidney transplants. With this scenario there is a need to expand the kidney donor pool.

While expanding the living donor pool, safety of the donor, recipient's quality of life and survival outcomes remains paramount. If donor's medical condition can affect these parameters, donation need to be discouraged. Overall vigilance in donor and recipient's care and management is essential to ensure that appropriate safeguards are in place to inspire public confidence. This chapter is intended to act as a resource for the transplant community, and to strengthen the best practices in living donor kidney transplantation.

Pre-Diabetes and Diabetes

Case Scenario 1

A 60-year-old male, voluntary kidney donor for his 26-year-old son, found to have fasting blood sugar (FBS) of 120 mg/dl and HBA1c of 6.1. No history of diabetes mellitus (DM). No family history of DM. His routine urine examination did not reveal any abnormality. Urine microalbumin creatinine ratio is 19 mg/g. Split GFR on DTPA renal scan is left kidney 44 ml/min and right kidney 43 ml/min.

1. **What are the concerns for a potential kidney donor with pre-diabetes?**

   Ans: The World Health Organization (WHO) has defined prediabetes as a state of intermediate hyperglycemia using two specific parameters, impaired fasting glucose (IFG) defined as fasting plasma glucose (FPG) 110 to 125 mg/dl and impaired glucose tolerance (IGT) defined as 2 h plasma glucose of 140–200 mg/dl after ingestion of 75 g of oral glucose load or a combination of the two based on a 2 h oral glucose tolerance test (OGTT).[1] The American Diabetes Association (ADA) has additional hemoglobin A1c (HbA1c) based criteria of a level of 5.7% to 6.4%.[2]

   About 5–10% of these may progress over years to become classified as diabetes.[3] This is a matter of great concern as diabetes is now the most common cause of end stage renal disease worldwide as it increases the risk by three times.[4] Risk is even higher in individuals who are overweight and have family history of diabetes. Younger the individual with risk factors, higher is the likelihood of progressing to frank diabetes and subsequent kidney disease.

2. **What will you suggest this donor?**

   Ans: Intervention at an earlier stage with diet and lifestyle changes like exercise and weight loss to normalize glucose metabolism to reduce the risk of progression to diabetes. These changes need to be continued for long term.[5] Repeat FBS, HBA1c are suggested at 12 weeks. In case of no improvement or worsening parameters, he should be excluded from kidney donation.

3. **If his brother who is around 38 years old with similar lab reports come forward for donation, among two of them who would you prefer as donor?**

   Ans: It has been observed that younger the individual with risk factors, higher is the likelihood of having diabetes and subsequent kidney disease. A study of kidney donors with pre-diabetes who proceeded with donation noted higher rates of progression to diabetes (15.6%) compared to donors with normal glucose levels (2.2%), but there is no difference in the remaining kidney function over the first 10 years following donation. I would prefer his father as donor.[6]

4. **Brother is concerned to know his risk of diabetes in near future; can you give rough estimate about this?**

   Ans: I would calculate the risk with available risk calculator to provide accurate, personalized estimates of an individual's risk for diabetes using information based on different parameters.[7]

5. **What are the risk factors associated with prediabetes for progression to diabetes and kidney disease in future?**

   Ans:
   - Increasing age
   - Obesity
   - Ethnicity or race
   - Family history of diabetes in first degree relatives

6. **What are the guidelines recommendations about kidney donation in prediabetes?**

   Ans: Available recommendations regarding eligibility of persons with prediabetes for kidney donation are conflicting.[8,9]
   - The European Best Practice Guideline states that impaired glucose tolerance is not an absolute contraindication to donation.[10]
   - UNOS consider prediabetes a relative contraindication or a condition warranting careful consideration and recommends lifestyle changes including diet change, increased exercise and weight loss to reduce their risk for future diabetes.[11]
   - In view of lack of donor specific data individualized decision to approve donation in persons with prediabetes has been suggested taking long-term risk in consideration.

7. **What if all his sugar readings fall under diabetes range?**

   Ans: Consideration of a diabetic as a potential donor needs a thorough evaluation of the risks and benefits of donation.
   - Careful evaluation for any evidence of target organ damage and assessment of cardiovascular risk factors like obesity, hypertension and hyperlipidemia is paramount.
   - Donor age, GFR and relationship to the potential recipient are important decisive factors.
   - Although uncommon but potential risk of development of diabetic nephropathy should be discussed with the potential donor. A data of 126 cases of ESRD after kidney donation out of 56,458 donors in USA from 1987 and 2003 revealed median time to ESRD after donation was 10.4 years and causes were glomerulonephritis in 33%, hypertension in 25%, and diabetes in 9% only.

   In conclusion, diabetic nephropathy in a kidney donor is not common during the follow-up period but this may not be the case with longer follow-up, particularly in younger donors.[9,12] So as this donor is 60 years old and if no target organ damage is found, can be taken as donor with informed risk.

Hypertension

Case Scenario 2

A 56-year-old female voluntary kidney donor for her daughter found to have to high blood pressure (BP) reading of 156/90 mm of Hg on pre-donation evaluation. There is no past history of hypertension (HTN) and antihypertensive medications. No history of other co-morbidities.

1. **What are the concerns in this donor?**

   Ans: Higher BP readings need further evaluation by confirming measuring BP on a few more occasions or considering ambulatory blood pressure monitoring (ABPM).
   - Hypertension is defined as systolic BP (SBP)/ diastolic BP (DBP) above 140/90 mm Hg in clinic, or at home or mean ABPM measurements of SBP/DBP above 135/85 mm Hg or need medication to control BP.[13]
   - Overall, 20 to 25% of population exhibit white coat hypertension, i.e. at home or ABPM readings are normal.

- Around 10–30% may have a normal blood pressure at clinic but demonstrate hypertension with ABPM or at home readings (masked hypertension).[14]
- Hypertension is one of the causes of chronic kidney disease and/or progression to ESRD in general population.
- Around 30% of patients may develop HTN after unilateral nephrectomy. Reduction in GFR after donor nephrectomy may accelerate progression of HTN due to various physiologic alterations.[3]
- Observational studies of hypertensive donors have documented variable results. Some have found that donors with pre-donation hypertension have a decline in kidney function (evidenced by increasing serum creatinine and decreased estimated GFR), while others found no significant difference in kidney function between normotensive and hypertensive donors.[15–18]

2. How will you proceed further with this donor?

Ans: She needs evaluation for end organ damage including left ventricular hypertrophy, retinopathy, and proteinuria. If at home reading and/or ABPM confirms increased high BP readings, she should be started with antihypertensive medication and target BP should be less than 120/80 (SBP/DBP) mm Hg. In case of no evidence of end organ damage and BP is under control after AHM, then she can be considered for donor nephrectomy.

3. What are the guideline recommendations in donor with high BP readings?

Ans: Younger age of less than 50 years, presence of other cardiovascular risk factors (e.g. obesity, diabetes mellitus, chronic smoking, high salt intake), uncontrolled HTN, need of more than 2 AHMs for adequate control of BP, end organ damage related to HTN including proteinuria, microalbuminuria, left ventricular hypertrophy, and hypertensive retinopathy are contraindications for kidney donation as per most of the guidelines.[8–10]

All potential kidney donors should be evaluated in detail for hypertension which, if present, may exclude donation. However, donation can be considered in the presence of controlled hypertension with no evidence of end organ damage. All donors should be informed that blood pressure may rise after donation, which needs regular follow-up along with lifestyle modifications after donor nephrectomy.[9]

Proteinuria

Case Scenario 3

A 60-year-old female, voluntary kidney donor for her husband, on evaluation was found to have albuminuria. Urine albumin creatinine ratio in random urine sample is 83 mg/g of creatinine. No history of diabetes mellitus, hypertension. Renal functions are within normal limits. Split GFR of each kidney is 45 and 47 ml/min for left and right kidney respectively.

1. What are your concerns regarding this donor?

Ans: Increased urinary protein is one of markers of kidney damage and cardiovascular damage. This can be either increased glomerular permeability (albuminuria) or decreased tubular reabsorption (low molecular weight proteinuria). It predicts progression of CKD in patients with or without diabetics and hypertensive patients.[19,20] Recent meta-analysis suggested 10-fold increase in urinary ACR is associated with three times risk of ESRD over a median follow-up of 4 to 16 years.[4]

2. What are methods of detecting proteinuria?

Ans: Urine protein is composed of small amounts of high molecular weight proteins (principally albumin) that are not normally filtered, low molecular weight serum proteins that are normally filtered by the glomeruli and reabsorbed by the tubules, and proteins secreted by the urinary tract.

- As per KDIGO guidelines gold standard for measurement of protein excretion is a 24-hour urine collection, which is cumbersome and often collected inaccurately.
- A urine albumin /creatinine ratio (ACR) in a spot urine sample is now the preferred methods as it correlates well with 24-hour urinary protein excretion and also minimizes variation due to diurnal variation in albumin excretion and urine concentration.[7] Early morning urine sample is preferred, and 2-stage testing (initial testing followed by confirmatory testing) is recommended.
- Tests for total urine protein as Protein creatinine ratio (PCR) cannot substitute for tests for urine albumin. Urine PCR may reflect only low molecular weight tubular proteinuria or proteinuria due to lymphoproliferative disorder or lower tract disease.
- Albumin excretion rate (mg/day) calculated from ACR is preferred because of variability on ACR. The normal AER is <10 mg per day in healthy young adults and increases with age. Persistent albumin excretion between 30 and 300 mg/day is termed moderately increased albuminuria or microalbuminuria. Albumin excretion >300 mg/day is considered overt proteinuria or severely increased albuminuria or macroalbuminuria.

3. **What are the recommendations, and would you take up this donor?**

Ans: Measurement of albumin rather that total protein is recommended. AER in timed urine collection rather than spot ACR is preferred.

- AER threshold of less than 30 mg/day is acceptable for kidney donation.
- AER between 30 and 300 mg/day meets the criteria of CKD. This is not an absolute contraindication as estimated projected lifetime risk of ESRD in older persons with normal GFR is very low, in the absence of other risk factors including smoking, diabetes, and hypertension.[4,7] So AER of 30 to 300 mg/day or ACR 30 to 300 mg/g is a relative contraindication to donation, although other risk factors for ESRD should be considered.
- AER of > 300 mg/day, ACR of >300 mg/g or PCR of > 500 mg/g is an absolute contraindication for donation.

In view of ACR between 30 and 300 mg/g and no other risk factor for ESRD, she can be taken as donor.

Obesity

Case Scenario 4

A 55-year-old female, voluntary kidney donor for her son, with no history of diabetes and hypertension was evaluated and found to have BMI (Body Mass Index) of 34.

1. **What are the concerns for a potential kidney donor with obesity?**

Ans: Obese individuals in comparison to normal weight people are at increased risk of

- Insulin resistance, diabetes, hypertension, heart diseases, stroke, and sleep apnoea. Obesity is also associated with proteinuria, albuminuria and glomerulopathy.[21]
- The main concern for obese living donors is that it may have an adverse effect on long-term kidney functions and obesity is independently associated with a higher risk of developing end stage kidney disease.[22]

2. **What are the risks of perioperative complications in obese kidney donors in comparison to low BMI donors?**

Ans: Obesity in kidney donors in some studies is associated with an increase in perioperative complications, although these are mostly minor (mostly wound complications), but same low rate of major surgical complications and a similar length of stay as low BMI donors.[23] Overall the data suggest that laparoscopic donor nephrectomy (LDN) is a safe procedure in otherwise healthy obese kidney donors and it does not lead to a higher rate of major perioperative complications.

3. **What should we do in the above case?**

Ans: Being moderately obese (BMI 34) need a thorough pre-donation counselling about the long term risks of including ESRD and cardiovascular morbidity. They should be advised for weight loss before donation and to maintain a healthy body weight after the donation.[8] Dietician advice and exercise to achieve weight loss is imperative. Donation can be considered after documented weight loss.

4. **What are the guidelines recommendations about kidney donation in obesity?**

Ans:

- The data on safety of the very obese (BMI >35 kg/m^2) for kidney donation is very limited and donation should be discouraged.
- Moderately obese donors (BMI 30–35 kg/m^2) should be thoroughly evaluated for cardiovascular, respiratory and kidney diseases. They should be counselled about the increased risk of perioperative complications and also about the long-term increased risk of CKD. They should be advised for weight loss before donation and to achieve ideal body weight after donation.
- Overweight individuals (BMI 25–30 kg/m^2), who are otherwise healthy can safely proceed with kidney donation.[9]

Microscopic Hematuria

Case Scenario 5

A 39-year-old male, voluntary kidney donor for his brother, on pre-donation evaluation was found to have 20 to 30 RBCs per high power field (HPF) on urine microscopy. There is no evidence of protein, casts, or crystals in urine. No history suggestive of lower urinary tract symptoms (LUTS), hematuria, lithuria, recurrent urinary tract infection (UTI). No history of stone disease, urologic intervention. Ultrasonography did not reveal any stone, cyst, or hydronephrosis in kidneys and bladder and prostate were also normal.

1. **What are your concerns in this donor?**

Ans: He is a young male donor with microscopic hematuria. Needs further evaluation to look for cause of hematuria. Nonvisible hematuria has been suggested as term for microscopic hematuria.

- Persistent microscopic hematuria defined as more than 3 to 5 red blood cells per HPF of urinary sediment on 2 to 3 separate occasions, unrelated to exercise, trauma, sexual activity, or menstruation. It is commonly due to urologic abnormalities (e.g. stones, tumors) or glomerular disease. The most common glomerular causes of persistent isolated microscopic hematuria are IgA nephropathy, thin basement membrane nephropathy (TBMN) and Alport syndrome.[8, 24]

- Non-visible hematuria (NVH) is present in 1–21% of the general population with the prevalence increasing with age. Most patients have no urologic symptoms, no proteinuria and normal renal function. Subsequent urine testing is often normal. Such transient hematuria is generally considered insignificant.[9]
- Persistent asymptomatic nonvisible microscopic hematuria (PANVH) is present in about 25% of those with an initial positive test.[9] Its importance has been undermined in a few longitudinal studies. In the Dutch study of 49 patients, those with a normal biopsy developed neither proteinuria nor worsening renal function during 11 years of follow-up. In contrast, proteinuria (10 patients), hypertension (14) and worsening kidney function (4) were found in the 29 patients with an abnormal biopsy.[25] In a Japanese study of 242 living donors, 8.3% had PANVH before donation and 15.3% following donation. None were investigated with a kidney biopsy, but the presence of hematuria predicted the development of proteinuria during a median follow-up of 2.3 years.[25, 26]

This makes further evaluation mandatory of all potential living kidney donors with microscopic hematuria both to exclude urological disease and to identify glomerular pathology that would preclude donation.

2. What urologic work up is needed further in this donor?

Ans: Urologic evaluation includes

- Urine culture
- Urine cytology
- Imaging preferably CECT of urinary system

Look for infection, nephrolithiasis, and urothelial carcinoma. If no cause is found, cystoscopy should be performed to rule out bladder pathology. This is more important if age is more than 40 years.[27]

3. What if a non-obstructing stone is found on CT scan?

Ans: A full metabolic stone workup should be performed and if found normal, then he can be considered for donation. Stone bearing kidney is preferred for donor nephrectomy. Stone removal need to be ensured before transplantation. In case of any significant metabolic stone disease, he should not be considered as donor.[24]

4. What will you do in case all these investigations are non-contributory and microscopic hematuria is persistent?

Ans: Further, evaluation with kidney biopsy is advised to look for glomerular disease. Level of hematuria on urine microscopy or dipstick will determine the further testing.

- A reagent strip 'trace positive' result corresponds to 1–5 red cells/μl, while '1+' corresponds to >10 red cells/μl and is significant in urological practice.
- High degrees of microscopic hematuria (1+ or greater) mandate biopsy inclusive of immunofluorescence before donation.
- Trace hematuria is at present a relative indication.[28]

Incidence of significant disease following the investigation of trace positive hematuria is similar as in normal population and hence considered as a normal variant.

Other than this importance of thin basement membrane nephropathy (TBMN) and IgA nephropathy needs to be highlighted.

5. What should be done if the kidney biopsy shows TBMN?

Ans: TBMN is present in 10–50% of patients biopsied for PANVH. It is an autosomal dominant disorder with mutations in either the COL4A3 or COL4A4 genes (encoding the α_3 and α_4 chains of type 4 collagen). Individuals with mutation in both alleles of either gene may have autosomal recessive Alport syndrome, and TBMN can be regarded as the carrier state for this condition.

Studies have suggested increased risk of proteinuria and hypertension but progression to ESRD is rare.[29] Biopsy should report the presence of any FSGS lesion or IgA nephropathy as this precludes donation. Detailed family history should look at the history of sensory neural deafness, hematuria suggestive of Alport syndrome and if found positive genetic testing is suggested especially when donating to a family member. [29] TBMN must be distinguished from the carrier state of X-linked Alport syndrome (XLAS) caused by mutations in the COL4A5 gene encoding 5 chain of type 4 collagen. It carries 5–20% risk of progressive renal impairment and is excluded from donation especially in female carries of XLAS.[9]

So a donor with TBMN with no hypertension, no proteinuria, normal renal function, no significant family history and no Alport syndrome, can be considered as donor with informed risk.

6. **What if the biopsy shows IgA nephropathy?**

   Ans: Presence of hematuria and glomerular IgA deposits predisposes to progressive kidney disease even in the absence of hypertension and proteinuria. British Transplantation Society guidelines precludes donation in glomerular pathology.[6] Canadian Blood Service's protocol defines IgA nephropathy and Alport syndrome (including carriers) as exclusion from kidney donation.[30]

Age and GFR

Case Scenario 6

A 73-year-old elderly female, with no comorbidity, wants to be a voluntary donor for her granddaughter with ESRD, with DTPA showing GFR of left kidney 41 ml/min and right kidney 42 ml/min.

1. **Will the evaluation be different from a young donor?**

   Ans: Elderly donors need extensive preoperative work up. Firstly, to rule out any cardiovascular and respiratory issues, most centers perform stress echocardiogram and respiratory function tests.[31] Secondly, to rule out malignancy serum PSA is mandatory in elderly males. In females, mammogram, Pap smear and full gynecological evaluation is needed. Bowel function should be assessed in elderly donors and fecal occult blood test should be done. Estimation of GFR by DTPA scan is also an important tool to decide about the donation.

2. **What are the concerns in this donor related to his age?**

   Ans: Following are the concerns:
   1. Increased risk of perioperative complications
   2. Careful assessment of existing comorbidities, if any
   3. Residual function post-donation
   4. Long-term transplant outcome in the recipient associated with reduced donor GFR

3. **Is there any increased risk of perioperative complications?**

   Ans: Due to laparoscopic kidney donation, perioperative outcomes like operative time, blood loss and length of stay in hospital in some recent studies were found to be no different from younger donors in very carefully selected donors >60 years of age.[32]

4. **How are the graft outcomes different in elderly donors as compared to young donors?**

   Ans: In one of the studies, 5-year graft survival after living donor transplantation was 76% for kidneys from donors >60 years and 79% for kidneys from donors aged <60 years. In many studies, serum creatinine levels remained significantly lower in recipients of kidneys from younger donors as compared to donor > 60 years and graft survival was significantly better beyond 5 years after transplantation in younger donors.[33, 34]

5. **What will you do in this case?**

   Ans: In studies, use of older kidney donors appears to be a beneficial alternative to awaiting for deceased donor kidneys.[35] Donor GFR is an important determinant of transplanted kidney function in many studies.[36]

   As in the above case, renal function of the donor is normal, so there is no compelling evidence for excluding kidney donation based only on chronological age.

6. **What are the concerns and guidelines regarding younger donors?**

   Ans: Many transplant centers consider age 18–21 years a relative contraindication for donation. Younger donors usually do not have any risk factor for kidney diseases at the time of evaluation. But they may still develop diabetes, hypertension, obesity or other renal risk factors and have more time for these risk factors to progress to CKD.[37] Careful psychological assessment and pre-donation counseling is recommended before donation. Guidelines do not consider individuals with age less than 18 years fit for kidney donation.

7. **What are the guidelines and recommendations regarding age of the donor?**

   Ans: Old age alone is not a contraindication for kidney donation, but the preoperative workup of the old age donors should be extensive to make sure that they are suitable donors.[9] Both donor and recipient need pre-donation counseling about the facts that old age donors are at increased risk of surgical complications and the long term graft survival can also be compromised in comparison to younger donors.

HBV (hepatitis B virus), HCV (hepatitis C virus) and HIV (human immunodeficiency virus) positive prospective kidney donors

Prospective kidney donors should undergo very careful screening for infectious diseases. This aids in identification of any transmissible infection in the donor and its treatment and subsequent transmission in recipient.

Case Scenario 7

A 58-year-old male, voluntary kidney donor for his son, otherwise healthy with no comorbidities during evaluation was found to be HbsAg positive and recipient is already HbsAg positive.

1. **Does the donor need any further evaluation?**

   Ans: All prospective living donors should be tested for both hepatitis B surface antigen (HBsAg) and hepatitis B core antibody (HBcAb). If the HBcAb is found to be positive, then donor should be tested for HBV DNA and hepatitis B surface antibody (HBsAb).

   i. **Case scenario no 1:**

   Ans: HbsAg+ donor and HbsAg– recipient: As per KDIGO guidelines, transplantation of kidneys from HbsAg positive donors is contraindicated for HBsAg negative recipients.

   ii. **Case scenario no 2:**

   Ans: HbsAg+ donor and HbsAg+ recipient: Kidney donation may be considered for HbsAg positive recipients and recipients with HBV protective immunity, with informed consent of the recipient and antiviral treatment of the recipient and post-operative monitoring.

   iii. **Case scenario no 3:**

   Ans: HbsAg– with anti-HBcAb+ and HBV DNA– donors: The risk of transmission from such donors is very negligible. So, such donors who are HBcAb positive (with negative HBsAg and undetectable HBV DNA) can therefore donate. [38]

   The recipient ideally should be effectively immunized against HBV and if there is suboptimal antibody response, immunization can be repeated post-transplant. Addition of anti-viral drugs may be considered in recipients with a low HBsAb response to vaccination. Advice must always be taken from specialist physicians (hepatologist).[39]

2. **What will you do in this case?**

   Ans: As per KDIGO guidelines, transplantation of kidneys from HbsAg positive donors is contraindicated for HBsAg negative recipients. But, kidney donation may be considered for HbsAg positive recipients or recipients with HBV protective immunity may proceed with transplantation with informed consent of the recipient and antiviral treatment of the recipient and post-operative monitoring.

3. **If the prospective kidney donor is HIV positive, what will you do?**

   Ans: The presence of HIV infection is an absolute contraindication to living kidney donation.

4. **If the prospective donor is HCV antibody positive, how will you proceed?**

   Ans: HCV antibody testing should be done in all potential donors and if HCV antibody is positive, HCV RNA should be checked.

   If donor is HCV RNA negative—transplantation can be considered even into HCV negative recipient, however, the risk should be explained to both the donor and recipient.

   If donor is HCV RNA positive, chances of transmission of HCV infection form such donors to the naïve recipient (HCV negative) is 100 %. [40] So, donor with active hepatitis C infection is a relative contraindication to living kidney donation and also because of the risk of glomerular disease in the donor. [41]

   Nowadays because of very effective anti-viral therapy for HCV infection, there is sustained virological response. If donation from a HCV-infected donor is the only available option, then risks and benefits should be carefully explained to both donor and recipient and advice from a specialist, preferably hepatologist with appropriate expertise should be taken.

5. **What are the guidelines recommendations if the prospective donor is HBsAg, HCV and HIV positive?**

   Ans: As per KDIGO guidelines for HIV, HBV and HCV, screening should be current within 28 days of donation.[8] The presence of HIV infection is an absolute contraindication to living donation. Active HBV and HCV infection in the donor are usually contraindications to living donor kidney donation. Screening for HBV, HCV and HIV infection must be repeated within 30 days of donation.[9]

SUMMARY

- Consideration of a diabetic as a potential donor needs a thorough evaluation of the risks and benefits of donation.
  - Careful evaluation for any evidence of target organ damage and assessment of cardiovascular risk factors like obesity, hypertension and hyperlipidemia is paramount.
  - Donor age, GFR and relationship to the potential recipient are important decisive factors.
- Younger age of less than 50 years, presence of other cardiovascular risk factors (e.g. obesity, diabetes mellitus, chronic smoking, high salt intake), uncontrolled HTN, need of more than 2 AHMs for adequate control of BP, end organ damage related to HTN including proteinuria, microalbuminuria, left ventricular hypertrophy, and hypertensive retinopathy are contraindications for kidney donation as per most of the guidelines.
- Donation can be considered in the presence of controlled hypertension with no evidence of end organ damage. All donors should be informed that blood pressure may rise after donation, which needs regular follow-up along with lifestyle modifications after donor nephrectomy.
- AER of > 300 mg/day, ACR of >300 mg/g or PCR of > 500 mg/g is an absolute contraindication for donation.
- Moderately obese donors (BMI 30–35 kg/m^2) should be thoroughly evaluated for cardiovascular, respiratory and kidney diseases. They should be counselled about the increased

risk of perioperative complications and also about the long-term increased risk of CKD. They should be advised for weight loss before donation and to achieve ideal body weight after donation.

- The most common glomerular causes of persistent isolated microscopic hematuria are IgA nephropathy, thin basement membrane nephropathy (TBMN) and Alport syndrome.
- As per KDIGO guidelines for HIV, HBV and HCV, screening should be current within 28 days of donation.
- The presence of HIV infection is an absolute contraindication to living donation. Active HBV and HCV infection in the donor are usually contraindications to living donor kidney donation. Screening for HBV, HCV and HIV infection must be repeated within 30 days of donation.

REFERENCES

1. World Health Organization. Definition and diagnosis of diabetes mellitus and intermediate hyperglycaemia: report of a WHO/IDF consultation.
2. American Diabetes Association. Diagnosis and classification of diabetes mellitus. Diabetes care. 2014 Jan 1;37 (Supplement_1):S81–90.
3. Tabák AG, Herder C, Rathmann W, Brunner EJ, Kivimäki M. Prediabetes: a high-risk state for diabetes development. The Lancet. 2012 Jun 16;379 (9833):2279–90.
4. Grams ME, Sang Y, Levey AS, Matsushita K, Ballew S, Chang AR, Chow EK, Kasiske BL, Kovesdy CP, Nadkarni GN, Shalev V. Kidney-failure risk projection for the living kidney-donor candidate. New England Journal of Medicine. 2016 Feb 4;374(5):411–21.
5. Ferrannini E. Definition of intervention points in prediabetes. The lancet Diabetes & endocrinology. 2014 Aug 1;2(8):667–75.
6. Chandran S, Masharani U, Webber AB, Wojciechowski DM. Prediabetic living kidney donors have preserved kidney function at 10 years after donation. Transplantation. 2014 Apr 15;97(7):748–54.
7. Heikes KE, Eddy DM, Arondekar B, Schlessinger L. Diabetes Risk Calculator: a simple tool for detecting undiagnosed diabetes and pre-diabetes. Diabetes care. 2008 May 1;31(5):1040–5.
8. Lentine KL, Kasiske BL, Levey AS, Adams PL, Alberú J, Bakr MA, Gallon L, Garvey CA, Guleria S, Li PK, Segev DL. Summary of Kidney Disease: Improving Global Outcomes (KDIGO) clinical practice guideline on the evaluation and care of living kidney donors. Transplantation. 2017 Aug;101(8):1783.
9. Andrews PA, Burnapp L. British Transplantation Society/ Renal Association UK guidelines for living donor kidney transplantation 2018: Summary of updated guidance. Transplantation. 2018 Jul;102(7):e307.
10. Abramowicz D, Cochat P, Claas FH, Heemann U, Pascual J, Dudley C, Harden P, Hourmant M, Maggiore U, Salvadori M, Spasovski G. European Renal Best Practice Guideline on kidney donor and recipient evaluation and perioperative care. Nephrology Dialysis Transplantation. 2015 Nov 1;30 (11):1790–7.
11. AST/ASTS/NATCO/UNOS Joint Societies Work Group. Evaluation of the Living Kidney Donor—a Consensus Document from the AST/ASTS/NATCO/UNOS Joint Societies Work Group.
12. Ibrahim HN, Kukla A, Cordner G, Bailey R, Gillingham K, Matas AJ. Diabetes after kidney donation. Am J Transplant 2010; 10: 331–7.
13. Chobanian AV, Bakris GL, Black HR, Cushman WC, Green LA, Izzo Jr JL, Jones DW, Materson BJ, Oparil S, Wright Jr JT, Roccella EJ. Seventh report of the joint national committee on prevention, detection, evaluation, and treatment of high blood pressure. hypertension. 2003 Dec 1;42(6):1206–52.
14. Stergiou GS, Asayama K, Thijs L, Kollias A, Niiranen TJ, Hozawa A, Boggia J, Johansson JK, Ohkubo T, Tsuji I, Jula AM. Prognosis of white-coat and masked hypertension: International Database of Home Blood Pressure in Relation to Cardiovascular Outcome. Hypertension. 2014 Apr;63 (4):675–82.
15. Ibrahim HN, Foley R, Tan L, Rogers T, Bailey RF, Guo H, Gross CR, Matas AJ. Long-term consequences of kidney donation. New England Journal of Medicine. 2009 Jan 29;360(5):459–69.
16. Srivastava A, Sinha T, Varma PP, Karan SC, Sandhu AS, Sethi GS, Khanna R, Talwar R, Narang V. Experience with marginal living related kidney donors: are they becoming routine or are there still any doubts?. Urology. 2005 Nov 1;66(5):971–5.
17. Kiberd BA. Estimating the long term impact of kidney donation on life expectancy and end stage renal disease. Transplantation research. 2013 Dec;2:1–6.
18. Textor SC, Taler SJ, Driscoll N, Larson TS, Gloor J, Griffin M, Cosio F, Schwab T, Prieto M, Nyberg S, Ishitani M. Blood pressure and renal function after kidney donation from hypertensive living donors. Transplantation. 2004 Jul 27;78(2):276–82.
19. The British Transplantation Society and The Renal Association. The United Kingdom guidelines for living donor kidney transplantation. Third Edition, 2011. Available at: https://bts.org.uk/wp-content/uploads/2016/09/19_BTS RA_Living_Donor_Kidney-1.pdf. (Accessed: September 7, 2016).
20. Chronic Kidney Disease Prognosis Consortium. Association of estimated glomerular filtration rate and albuminuria with all-cause and cardiovascular mortality in general population cohorts: a collaborative meta-analysis. The Lancet. 2010 Jun 12;375(9731):2073–81.
21. Nguyen NT, Magno CP, Lane KT, Hinojosa MW, Lane JS. Association of hypertension, diabetes, dyslipidemia, and metabolic syndrome with obesity: findings from the National Health and Nutrition Examination Survey, 1999 to 2004. Journal of the American College of Surgeons. 2008 Dec 1;207(6):928–34.
22. Hsu CY, McCulloch CE, Iribarren C, Darbinian J, Go AS. Body mass index and risk for end-stage renal disease. Annals of internal medicine. 2006 Jan 3;144 (1):21–8.
23. Heimbach JK, Taler SJ, Prieto M, Cosio FG, Textor SC, Kudva YC, Chow GK, Ishitani MB, Larson TS, Stegall MD. Obesity in living kidney donors: clinical characteristics and outcomes in the era of laparoscopic donor nephrectomy. American Journal of Transplantation. 2005 May 1;5(5):1057–64.
24. Davis R, Jones JS, Barocas DA, Castle EP, Lang EK, Leveillee RJ, Messing EM, Miller SD, Peterson AC, Turk TM, Weitzel W. Diagnosis, evaluation and follow-up of asymptomatic microhematuria (AMH) in adults: AUA guideline. The Journal of urology. 2012 Dec;188(6S):2473–81.

25. Nieuwhof C, Doorenbos C, Grave W, De Heer F, De Leeuw P, Zeppenfeldt E, van Breda Vriesman PJ. A prospective study of the natural history of idiopathic non-proteinuric hematuria. Kidney international. 1996 Jan 1;49(1):222–5..
26. Kido R, Shibagaki Y, Iwadoh K, Nakajima I, Fuchinoue S, Fujita T, Teraoka S. Persistent glomerular hematuria in living kidney donors confers a risk of progressive kidney disease in donors after heminephrectomy. American Journal of Transplantation. 2010 Jul 1;10(7):1597–604.
27. Savige J, Rana K, Tonna S, Buzza M, Dagher H, Wang YY. Thin basement membrane nephropathy. Kidney international. 2003 Oct 1;64(4):1169–78.
28. Savige J, Gregory M, Gross O, Kashtan C, Ding J, Flinter F. Expert guidelines for the management of Alport syndrome and thin basement membrane nephropathy. Journal of the American Society of Nephrology. 2013 Mar 1;24(3):364–75.
29. Jais JP, Knebelmann B, Giatras I, De Marchi M, Rizzoni G, Renieri A, Weber M, Gross O, Netzer KO, Flinter F, Pirson Y. X-linked Alport syndrome: natural history and genotype-phenotype correlations in girls and women belonging to 195 families: a "European Community Alport Syndrome Concerted Action" study. Journal of the American Society of Nephrology. 2003 Oct 1;14(10):2603–10.
30. Ierino F, Kanellis J. Donors at risk: haematuria. Nephrology. 2010 Apr;15: S111–3.
31. Older P, Hall A. Clinical review: how to identify high-risk surgical patients. Critical Care. 2004 Oct;8(5):1–4.
32. Jacobs SC, Ramey JR, Sklar GN, Bartlett ST. Laparoscopic kidney donation from patients older than 60 years. Journal of the American College of Surgeons. 2004 Jun 1;198(6):892–7.
33. Fuggle SV, Allen JE, Johnson RJ, Collett D, Mason PD, Dudley C, Rudge CJ, Bradley JA, Watson CJ, Kidney Advisory Group of NHS Blood and Transplant. Factors affecting graft and patient survival after live donor kidney transplantation in the UK. Transplantation. 2010 Mar 27;89(6):694–701.
34. Øien CM, Reisæter AV, Leivestad T, Dekker FW, Line PD, Os I. Living donor kidney transplantation: the effects of donor age and gender on short- and long-term outcomes. Transplantation. 2007 Mar 15;83(5):600–6.
35. Englum BR, Schechter MA, Irish WD, Ravindra KV, Vikraman DS, Sanoff SL, Ellis MJ, Sudan DL, Patel UD. Outcomes in kidney transplant recipients from older living donors. Transplantation. 2015 Feb 1;99(2):309–15.
36. Hawley CM, Kearsley J, Campbell SB, Mudge DW, Isbel NM, Johnson DW, May K, Preston J, Griffin A, Wall D, Burke J. Estimated donor glomerular filtration rate is the most important donor characteristic predicting graft function in recipients of kidneys from live donors. Transplant International. 2007 Jan;20(1):64–72.
37. Gibney EM, King AL, Maluf DG, Garg AX, Parikh CR. Living kidney donors requiring transplantation: focus on African Americans. Transplantation. 2007 Sep 15;84(5):647–9.
38. Feng S, Buell JF, Cherikh WS, *et al.* Organ donors with positive viral serology or malignancy: risk of disease transmission by transplantation. Transplantation. 2002;74:1657–1663.
39. Ouseph R, Eng M, Ravindra K, *et al.* Review of the use of hepatitis B core antibody-positive kidney donors. Transplant Rev (Orlando). 2010;24: 167–171.
40. Pereira BJ, Milford EL, Kirkman RL, *et al.* Prevalence of hepatitis C virus RNA in organ donors positive for hepatitis C antibody and in the recipients of their organs. N Engl J Med 1992; 327: 910–5.
41. Johnson RJ, Gretch DR, Yamabe H, *et al.* Membranoproliferative glomerulonephritis associated with hepatitis C virus infection. N Engl J Med 1992; 328: 465–70.

Chapter 15

Donor with Kidney Issues (Low GFR, Cysts, AML, Calculus Disease)

• M Ramalingam • V Surya Prakash

'Donor with Low GFR'

LEARNING OBJECTIVES

- To highlight the increasing need of living donors as deceased kidney donation is insufficient.[1]
- To understand that a potential donor with marginally low GFR (less than 80 ml/min/1.72 m^2) needs further evaluation to reduce the risk to the donor's life.[2]
- To understand that counselling the prospective marginal donor regarding the risk of progression of CKD is important, especially to the elderly donors.
- To highlight the importance of GFR when accepting a young donor (18–40 years); a GFR of > 90 ml/min/1.73 m^2 is preferred.[3]
- To understand and counsel the prospective renal donor with low GFR, that renal function (GFR) needs to be monitored life long and there is a remote possibility that the GFR might reduce and lead to early CKD.

Case Scenario 1

A 68 years old female with a BMI of 27.4 with a GFR of 75.2 was willing to donate her right kidney (with 35 GFR) (Figs 15.1 and 15.2) to her matching husband. Laparoscopic right donor nephrectomy was done. (Figs 15.3 and 15.4). One year later GFR of the retained left kidney was 55 from 40 before donation.

INTRODUCTION

The preferred renal replacement therapy is allograft transplant. However, the willing living donors' pool is far below the need necessitating deceased donor kidney transplantation. Hence these ESRD patients must be on haemodialysis or CAPD in the waiting period during which about 7% of them die due to conditions like sepsis or pulmonary oedema. It is also noted that among many communities and cultures, individuals are not forthcoming for organ donation for various reasons, resulting in long waiting lists which increases by 10% annually. Thus, marginal renal donors with low GFR, renal calculi, renal cysts and small angiomyolipoma are being considered.

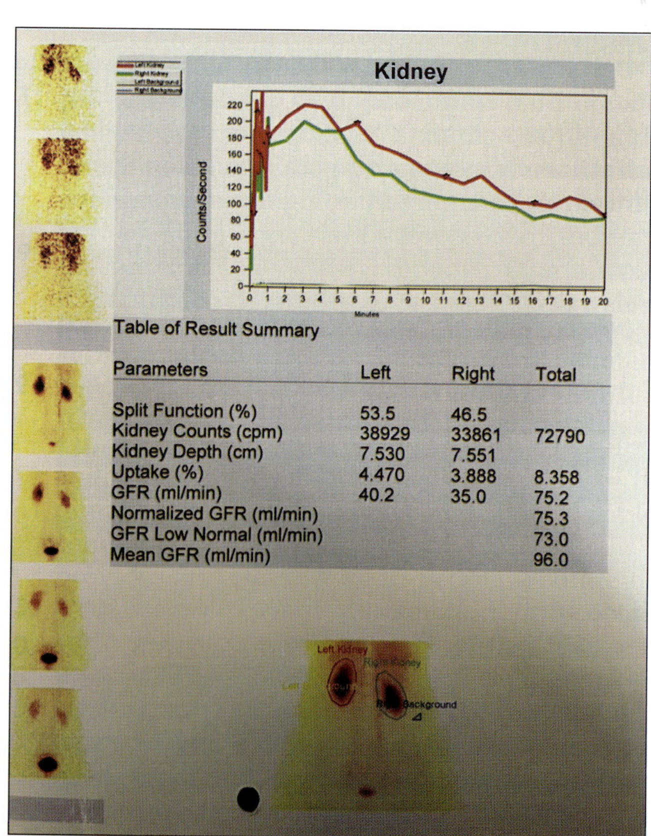

Fig. 15.1: Isotope renal scan (Tc99DTPA) of the index patient

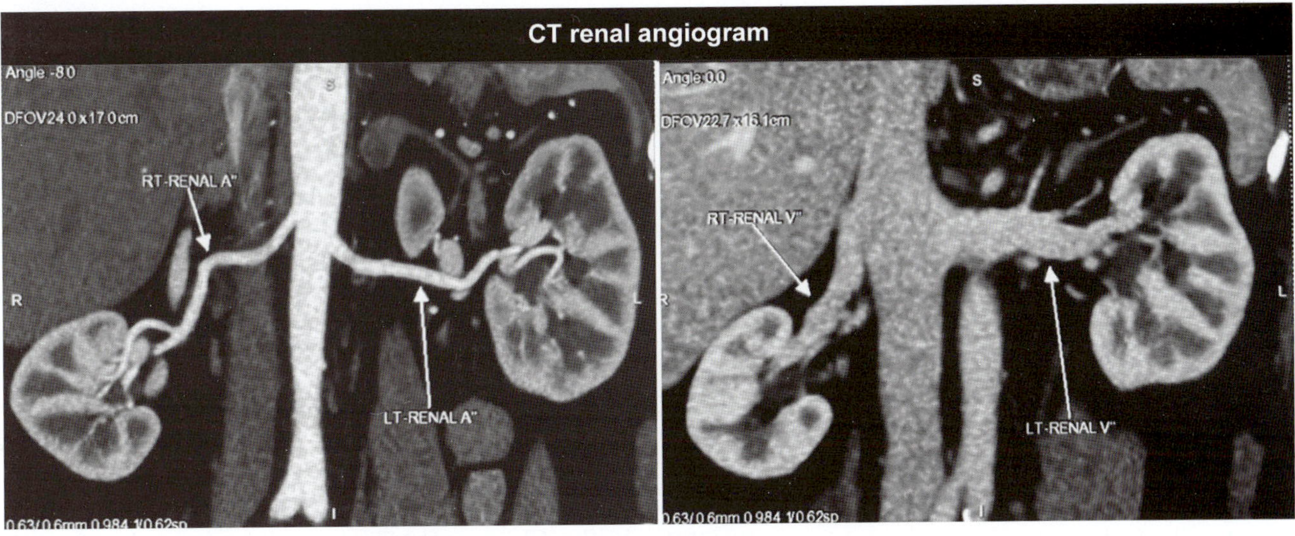

Fig. 15.2: CT renal angiogram of the index patient

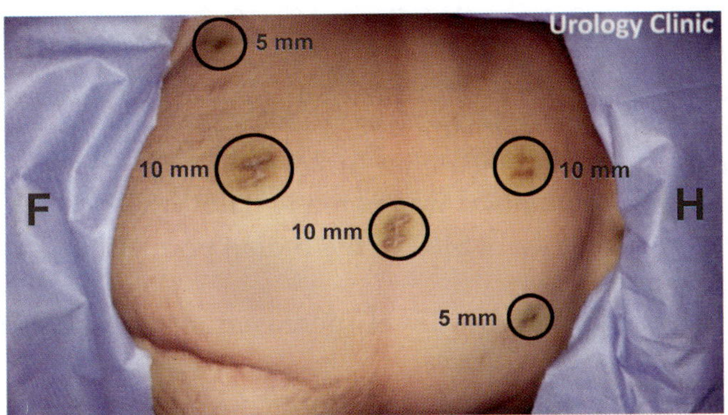

Fig. 15.3: Ports position for right donor nephrectomy

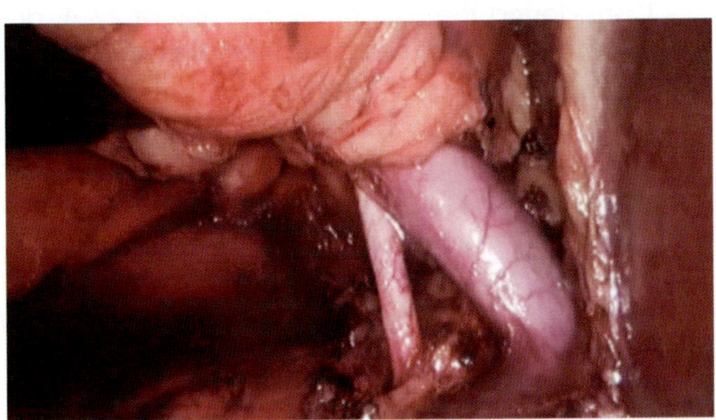

Fig. 15.4: Hilar dissection in right laparoscopic donor nephrectomy

Living Donor with Low GFR

As the age increases, the kidney function decreases. There is higher reduction in individuals with diabetes, hypertension, or dyslipidemia.

Previously living kidney donors with GFR above 80 ml/min/1.73 m^2 was considered as standard, but now lower GFR of even up to 70 ml/min/1.73 m^2 are being accepted provided the BMI is less than 35 and there are no other co-morbidities. In an observational study from JIPMER India, 316 potential young living kidney donors (18–40 years of age) were evaluated over a period of 81 months (July 2011–2018). Among them 22% with GFR less than 70 ml/min/1.73 m^2 were not considered for kidney donation.[3]

One important and reasonable concern for these complex living donors is the marginal increase in the death rate when compared with age matched non-donor population. Hence the donors with low GFR will have to be counselled thoroughly to accept the ground reality even though the individual may be altruistic in attitude.[2] In a large study of 40130 living kidney donors who were followed over 50 years, 39 patients developed ESRD (mean age 62.4 years with mean interval from renal donation to ESRD being 27.1 +/–9.8 years). The majority of renal functional deterioration occurred in smokers. Only two living kidney donors in this robust study had renal cancer in the contralateral kidney.[5]

1. **What is the conventional acceptable age limit for the living donor?**
   Ans: 18 to 65 years.
2. **What is the upper limit of acceptable BMI in a living donor?**
   Ans: BMI less than 35 without any co-morbidity.[6]
3. **What are the other factors that increases the risk to the donor?**
   Ans: Co-morbidities like hypertension, diabetes, obesity, dyslipidaemia and age beyond 65 years increases the risk of renal deterioration in the donor.
4. **What is a minimum GFR that is preferable to accept a renal donor?**
   Ans: 80 ml/min/1.73 m^2 or more is preferable. (KDIGO Guidelines 2017)

5. **What is the standard method to evaluate the GFR in a living donor?**

   Ans: DTPA renogram is the investigation of choice for evaluating donor GFR. It not only tells us the total GFR but also the split GFR. Split GFR guides us in side selection for donor nephrectomy.

6. **What is the acceptable minimum split GFR for kidney donation?**

   Ans: There is no clear-cut answer to this. The important fact to consider here is that, post-donation, the kidney function of the donor should be sufficient enough for him to maintain a normal health without affecting life-span. Therefore, it is mandatory to leave the better kidney with the donor (as done in the present case). Majority of centres in India accept kidneys with a split GFR > 35 ml/min.

7. **Considering the age of 68 and BMI of 27.4, does this index patient need additional investigations?**

   Ans: Perioperative cardiac and long-term risks are increased in patients unable to perform 4 METs of work during daily activities. According to ACC/AHA 2014 guidelines on perioperative cardiovascular evaluation and management of patients going non-cardiac surgery, further cardiac evaluation is required if patients unable to perform 4 METs of work during daily activities.

8. **What is the probability that the index donor may land up in CKD/ESRD?**

   Ans: It takes about 14 years for a patient to progress to CKD as the GFR decreases by 1 ml/min/1.73 m^2 per year.[29]

9. **Does she have a risk to life in undergoing donor nephrectomy?**

   Ans: There is 0.03% (3.1 in 10,000) risk of mortality.[7]

10. **What is the expected decrement in total GFR in this patient 3 months after donation?**

    Ans: Immediately after donor nephrectomy, there is a 25–40% decrease in eGFR associated with hyperfiltration of the remaining kidney.[29]

11. **How much of GFR of the retained kidney will you expect in 1 year (the GFR of left kidney at the time of donation was 40)?**

    Ans: Mean increase in remaining kidney volume was 22.4 ± 23.2% after donor nephrectomy in healthy individuals.[29]

12. **In this index patient in view of age (68 years) which technique will you prefer, laparoscopy or open?**

    Ans: Laparoscopy can be efficacious and as safe as open. The added advantage is shorter hospital stay and early return to work.

Simple Renal Cyst (SRC) in Renal Donor

LEARNING OBJECTIVES

- To learn the incidence of simple renal cysts and their natural history.
- To understand the long-term renal functional loss in recipient and donor.
- To know which patient with simple renal cyst can donate kidney.
- To know if there is an increased risk of complications.
- To know if follow-up of donor or recipient is any different from usual follow-up.

SRC are very common and among 1948 potential donors about 39% of individuals aged 18–49 years and 63% aged 50–75 had cysts.[9]

However, the incidence of SRC was found to be lower in the Chinese (10.7% overall and ranging from 2.38% in the 2nd decade to 35.29% in the 7th decade).[10] Similar incidence was noted in Korean individuals (incidence of 5.43 % of 10261 people followed for 10 years)[11]. Moshrafa *et al* noted an incidence of 4.2% in Middle East (0.6% for patients in their third decade, to 33% in individuals older than 80 years among 8551 people)[12] and Ozveren *et al* reported an incidence of 7.7 % in Turkey.[13] 9.9% of Japanese population was noted to have SRC.[14]

- The incidence of SRC in the Indian population is not known.
- Serum creatinine level increased significantly in individuals with cyst.[12–14]
- Qiu *et al* reported that donor kidney with cysts had more glomerulosclerosis. These kidneys with cysts could affect the long-term renal function in recipients.[15]
- Cysts in younger individuals and multi-loculated cysts grow more rapidly.[11,16]
- Kim *et al* observed that in case of cyst more than 1 cm in size; multiple cysts (more than 2 cysts) and in case of bilateral cyst, there was an increased risk of hypertension.[17]
- Growing SRC are the cysts in which the maximum diameter increased 5% yearly during the follow-up; or when number of cysts increased during follow-up. Renal dysfunction was 10 times higher in patients with growth SRC. Growing SRC had a higher incidence of hypertension and hematuria.[18]
- Among 71468 living kidney donors, 10-unit reduction of 6 months post-donor nephrectomy eGFR was significantly associated with a 28% higher risk of subsequent end-stage renal disease.[19]
- In a retrospective study of 454 living kidney donors, no difference in the eGFR among donors with or without a cyst was noted over a period of 7.8 years median follow-up.[20] There was also no association noted even when the retained cyst was more than 1 cm or multiple.

Case Scenario 2

Mrs M, a 74-year-old female volunteered as a kidney donor for her son. She had 2 normal full-term deliveries and history of hysterectomy for benign disease. Clinical examination revealed midline suprapubic scar and grade 1 cystocele. Height was 150 cm and weight was 62 kg with a BMI of 27.6. Blood pressure was normal. Hemoglobin was 12.1 gm/dl; Serum creatinine was 0.6 mg/dl and blood urea was 23 mg/dl. Urinalysis was normal. 24-hour urine protein was 48.2 mgms. CT scan showed a 3.1 cm cyst in the sinus fat of the left kidney (Fig. 15.5). CT renal angiogram showed bilateral single renal arteries. DTPA isotope renogram showed a GFR of 43 on the left side and 40.2 on the right side.

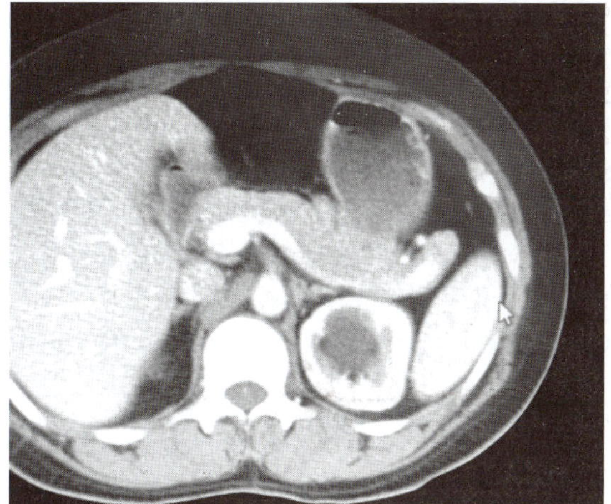

Fig. 15.5: CT scan showing 3.1 cm hilar cyst

1. **Is simple renal cyst a contraindication for being a renal donor?**

   Ans: SRC is not a contraindication. These donors may be accepted for donation if all other factors are favourable.

2. **Are the factors like location, numbers, laterality and size of cysts influence decision-making?**

   Ans: Yes, these factors are important considerations in selecting the donor. Each case has to be individualised.

3. **Is the better functioning kidney selected for donation or the kidney with cyst selected?**

   Ans: When both kidneys have almost comparable function, the kidney with cyst is selected for donation as it is large and hilar in location.

4. **Is surgical treatment of cyst done prior to donor nephrectomy?**

   Ans: Usually the cyst is managed intraoperatively; bench surgery is performed.

5. **Do all cysts need treatment during the surgery?**

   Ans: No. Small cysts which do not pose any risk or challenges in recipient after transplants do not need any intervention. Special circumstances need special treatment, e.g. simple cyst in the hilum may compromise the length of vessels and may cause obstruction. These may need surgical treatment (Fig. 15.6).

6. **Does donor with SRC need any additional follow-up?**

   Ans: Donors with cyst more than 1 cm; more than 2 cysts; and growing SRC are prone to deterioration of renal function and hypertension and hence need close follow-up.

Donor with Kidney Stones

LEARNING OBJECTIVES

- To know the selection criteria for donors with kidney stones during live renal transplantation.
- To know how to manage the stones in a donor eligible for donation.

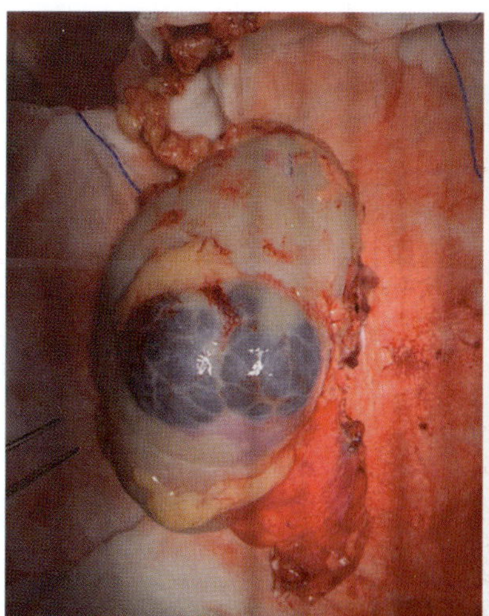

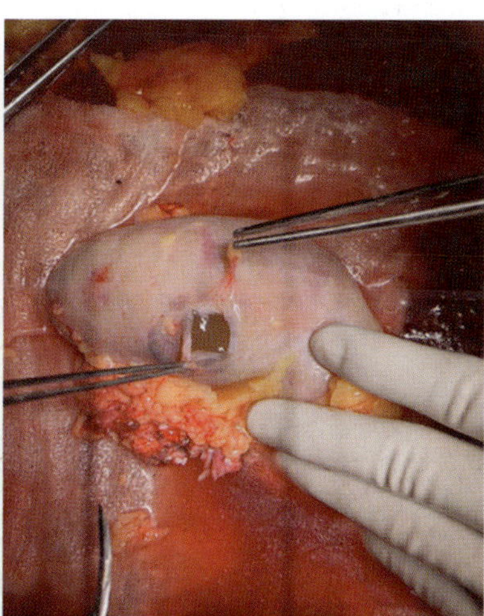

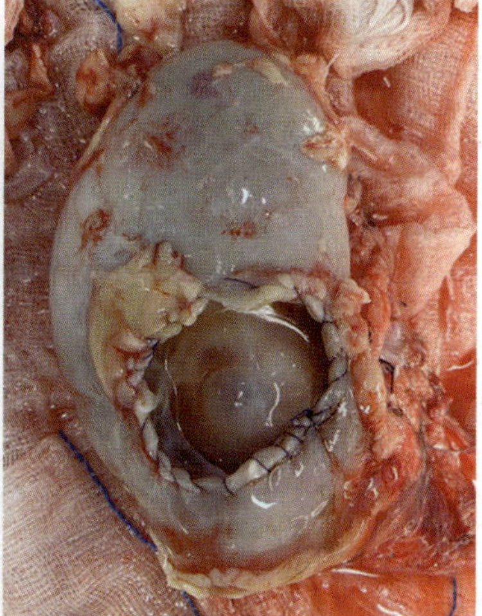

Fig. 15.6: Bench surgery of cyst deroofing

With the use of CT renal angiography (Fig. 15.7) in the evaluation of donors, the diagnosis of small asymptomatic renal calculi in potential living donors has increased. Renal stones in living donors are a concern not only for the donor but also for the recipient. With increasing pool of chronic kidney patients awaiting renal transplant, a select group of donors with kidney stones can be accepted for donation with a calculated risk.

A risk assessment for stone recurrence and understanding of the potential repercussions of kidney stones after donation should be used to determine whether to accept a donor who has a history of kidney stones or who currently has kidney stones.

The Amsterdam forum criteria state that stone formers with the following criteria should not be considered for donation.[21]

1. Recurrent stones
2. Metabolic abnormality
3. Stones associated with urinary infection
4. Multiple calculi.
5. Stone size > 1.5 cm
6. Nephrocalcinosis on CT imaging.

Case Scenario 3

A 45-year-old mother is being worked up as potential donor for her son with chronic kidney disease. The CT renal angio showed left small renal calculi 3 mm in size. There was no other donor in the family.

1. **What history do you elicit in this potential donor with kidney stones?**

   Ans: A thorough history and clinical examination is mandatory in potential donor with nephrolithiasis. Donors are enquired for any symptoms due to kidney stone, history of gravelluria, prior history of any investigations or treatments for kidney stone disease, h/o recurrent urinary infections and h/o inflammatory bowel disease.

2. **How will you evaluate this patient with kidney stones?**

   Ans: Donors with kidney stones need to undergo a complete urine examination, serum chemistries—calcium, uric acid, serum PTH and stone analysis, if stone is available. CT imaging is mandatory to know the stone characteristics (size, number, location and density). Most guidelines recommend 24-hour urine testing on a random diet for calcium, uric acid, oxalate, citrate, sodium, magnesium and creatinine.

3. **Will you accept the donor?**

   Ans: Yes, she can be accepted as donor as she is asymptomatic and the stone is unilateral and small.

4. **Which kidney will be considered for donation?**

   Ans: The kidney with stone is always considered for donation. The dictum of 'primum non nocere' applies best here. Normal better functioning kidney should always be left with the donor.

5. **What is the incidence of asymptomatic kidney stones on imaging in living kidney donors?**

   Ans: Around 5% of donors have asymptomatic stones on CT imaging during the evaluation.

6. **How do you manage the stone detected on CT imaging of the donor?**

   Ans: The decision to remove the stone in the donor prior to the transplant or *ex-vivo* after harvesting or transplanting the stone bearing kidney (donor gifted stone) depends on the size, location and density of the stone.

   ESWL/RIRS can be performed safely in the pre-transplant setting. *Ex-vivo* URS and *ex-vivo* pyelolithotomy are also safe and technically

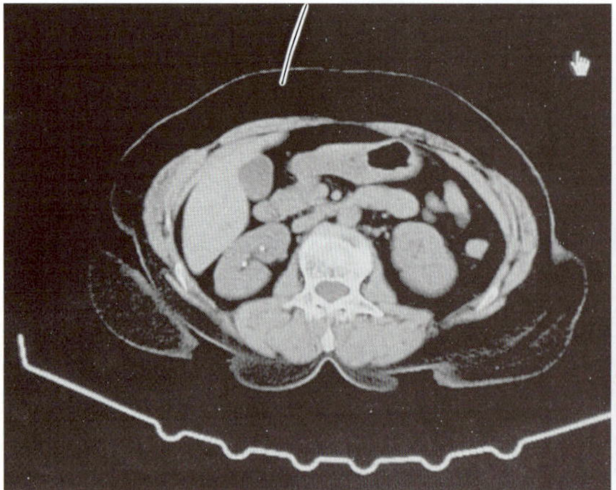

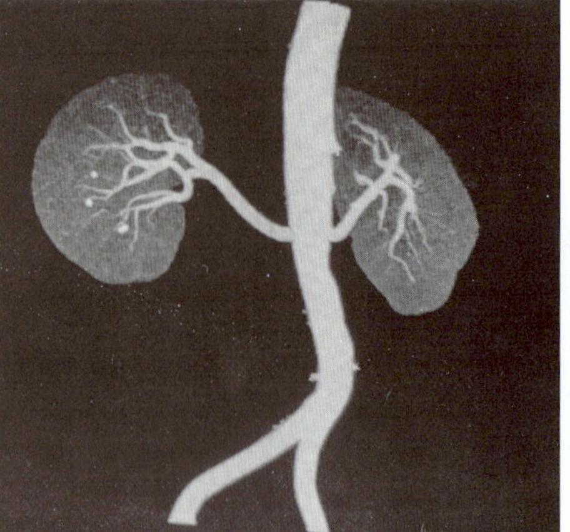

Fig. 15.7: CT images of donor showing small right renal calculi

feasible, to render a stone bearing donor kidney stone free without compromising renal allograft function.

7. **Do all stones warrant removal?**

Ans: Not all stone-bearing kidneys require intervention. There is definite role of expectant management in some patients.

As in the index case; detailed evaluation was done, and all the tests, including a 24-hour urine metabolic test, came out normal. The recipient is doing well at the one-year follow-up after receiving the transplant from the donor who had calculi. Transplantation of kidneys with stones less than 4 mm can be safely accomplished with an expected spontaneous passage rate up to 60%.[22]

In a report by Kim *et al*, eleven recipients were transplanted with allografts containing stones. 10 out of 11 recipients had stable graft function, postoperative ultrasound was negative for nephrolithiasis, and no sequelae from stones. One recipient developed symptomatic nephrolithiasis and was found to have hyperoxaluria, suggesting a recipient-driven propensity for stone formation.[23]

Ganpule *et al* published their experience of managing donors with renal stones. In their study, five patients underwent pretransplant ESWL, one patient pretransplant RIRS with complete stone clearance. *Ex-vivo* URS and *ex-vivo* pyelolithtomy were done in one patient each. In three patients, stone bearing kidney was transplanted with DJ stenting in the recipient and the recipients were followed up for 36 months without any complications. The authors proposed an algorithm for managing stones in donor kidneys (Fig. 15.8).[24]

LIVING DONOR KIDNEYS WITH ANGIOMYOLIPOMA

Introduction

Renal angiomyolipoma is a benign mesenchymal tumour. Small tumours are incidentally detected on imaging. Majority of the lesions are sporadic and are typically solitary, small, unilateral and predominantly seen in middle aged women. Incidentally detected small renal angiomyolipoma on CT renal angiography in the donor poses a dilemma to the transplant surgeon.

The first report of a direct live donor transplant after *ex vivo* excision of the AML was reported in 1993 by Bissada and team.[25]

Case Scenario 4

A healthy male donor on evaluation was found to have a 3 mm exophytic hypodense lesion in the lower pole of left kidney on CT renal angiography suggestive of AML. There is no other eligible donor in the family.

1. **Is this donor eligible for kidney donation?**

Ans: There are reports of donors with small solitary renal AMLs donating AML bearing kidney. In the majority of the reports AML was excised *ex-vivo* and then the kidney was transplanted. Desiree Garcia Anton published a systematic review on the use and outcomes of kidneys from donors with renal angiomyolipoma.[26]

In a retrospective study of 2925 live renal transplants by Zaharan *et al*, 6 donor kidneys with small AMLs were transplanted. The median volume of the AML was 0.96 (range, 0.5–2) cm^2.

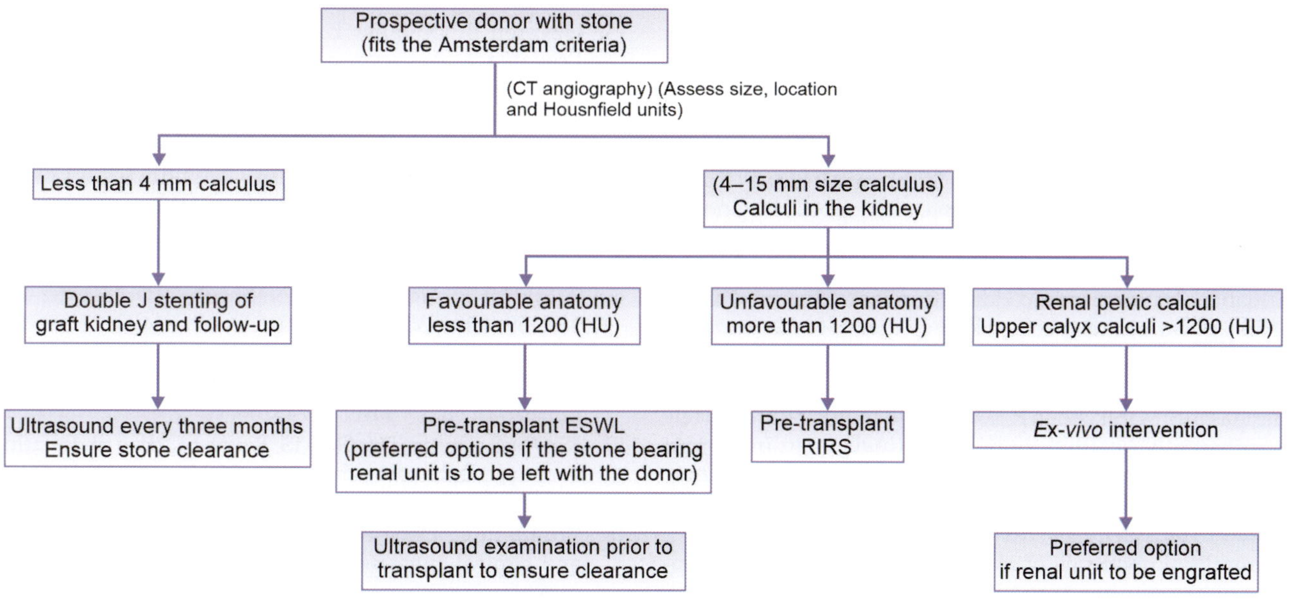

Fig. 15.8: Algorithm for managing stones in living donor kidneys

Two of the six lesions were exophytic and *ex-vivo*-excision was done. Four kidneys with endophytic AMLs were transplanted without excision. After a median follow-up of 82 months, there was no evidence of increase in the AML size or newly developed AML in the grafts. All donors were alive with normal renal function and none developed new AML in the remaining kidney.[27]

The index donor can be accepted as marginal donor. The kidney bearing the AML should be considered for harvesting. As the lesion is superficial and small, *ex-vivo* excision can be considered in this patient.

SUMMARY

- There is a gross disparity between the increasing end stage renal disease patients and suitable living kidney donors or deceased kidney donors. Hence more marginal living kidney donors are explored for a possible donation.
- Although the standard cutoff of GFR for donor is 80 ml/min/1.73 m^2, GFR of up to 70 ml/min/1.73 m^2 is being accepted provided the BMI is less than 35 and there are no other co-morbidities.
- It is the responsibility of the transplant team to apprise marginal kidney donor of the potential risk of deterioration of the renal function in the long term.
- Unilateral, small (<2 cm) simple renal cyst in donor kidney is not a contraindication for donation.
- Potential living donors with unilateral small renal stones are considered as marginal donors and need a detailed assessment before being considered for kidney donation. Amsterdam forum criteria guidelines should be followed to select patients with kidney stones as eligible kidney donors.
- Incidentally discovered small solitary AML during live-donor evaluation is not a contraindication for donation after proper counselling. The AML bearing kidney should be considered for donation leaving the normal kidney to the donor.
- Genetic evaluation should be considered to rule out hereditary conditions like Tuberous sclerosis complex and pulmonary lymphangioleiomyomatosis (LAM).

REFERENCES

1. Gopalakrishnan G, Gourabathini SP. Marginal kidney donor. Indian J Urol 2007;23:286–93. Source of Support: Nil, Conflict of Interest: None declared. CMC Vellore.
2. Okidi, O., Sharma, V., Piscoran, O. *et al.* The altruistic elderly, a valuable but unrecognised kidney donor group. A case report of an 85-year-old unspecified kidney donor. *BMC Geriatr* 22, 826 (2022). https://doi.org/10.1186/s12877–022–03511–8.
3. Parameswaran S, Kulothungan SA, Ponnusamy M, Reddi S, Haridasan S, Manikandan R, *et al.* Low glomerular filtration rate in apparently healthy young individuals is an important factor preventing kidney transplantation from living kidney donors–A single-center observational study from India. Indian J Transplant 2021;15:325–31.
4. Varma PP. Prevalence of chronic kidney disease in India-Where are we heading? Indian J Nephrol. 2015 May-Jun;25(3):133–5. PMID: 26060360; PMCID: PMC4446915.
5. Matas AJ, Payne WD, Sutherland DE, Humar A, Gruessner RW, Kandaswamy R, *et al.* 2,500 living donor kidney transplants: A single-center experience. Ann Surg 2001; 234:149–64.
6. Lin JS, Muhammad H, Lin T, Kamel I, Baghdadi A, Rizkalla N, Ottmann SE, Wesson R, Philosophe B, Gurakar A. Donor BMI and Post-living Donor Liver Transplantation Outcomes: A Preliminary Report. Transplant Direct. 2023 Jan 12;9(2):e1431. doi: 10.1097/TXD.0000000000001431. PMID: 36700065; PMCID: PMC9835892.
7. Department of Medicine, Oslo University Hospital Rikshospitalet, Oslo, Norway. 2 Department of Surgery, Oslo University Hospital Rikshospitalet, Oslo, Norway. 3 Address correspondence to: Geir Mjøen, M.D., Department of Medicine, Oslo University Hospital Rikshospitalet, Sognsvannsveien 20, 0027 Oslo, Norway. E-mail: geir.mjoen@rikshospitalet.no Received 7 May 2009. Revision requested 27 May 2009. Accepted 27 July 2009. Copyright © 2009 by Lippincott Williams & Wilkins ISSN 0041–1337/09/8811–1273 DOI: 10.1097/TP.0b013e3181bb44fd.
8. Tsoulfas G, Agorastou P, Ko DSC, Hertl M, Elias N, Cosimi AB, Kawai T. Laparoscopic vs open donor nephrectomy: Lessons learnt from single academic center experience. World J Nephrol 2017; 6(1): 45–52.
9. Rule AD, Sasiwimonphan K, Lieske JC, Keddis MT, Torres VE, Vrtiska TJ. Characteristics of renal cystic and solid lesions based on contrast-enhanced computed tomography of potential kidney donors. Am J Kidney Dis. 2012 May;59(5):611–8. doi: 10.1053/j.ajkd.2011.12.022. Epub 2012 Mar 6. PMID: 22398108; PMCID: PMC3328591.
10. Chang CC, Kuo JY, Chan WL, Chen KK, Chang LS. Prevalence and clinical characteristics of simple renal cyst. J Chin Med Assoc. 2007 Nov;70(11):486–91. doi: 10.1016/S1726–4901(08)70046–7. PMID: 1806350.
11. Choi JD. Clinical characteristics and long-term observation of simple renal cysts in a healthy Korean population. Int Urol Nephrol. 2016 Mar;48(3):319–24. doi: 10.1007/s11255–015–1186–7. Epub 2015 Dec 19. PMID: 26685889.
12. Mosharafa AA. Prevalence of renal cysts in a Middle-Eastern population: an evaluation of characteristics and risk factors. BJU Int. 2008 Mar;101(6):736–8. doi: 10.1111/j.1464–410X.2007.07234. x. Epub 2007 Oct 8. PMID: 17922869.
13. Ozveren B, Onganer E, Türkeri LN. Simple Renal Cysts: Prevalence, Associated Risk Factors and Follow-Up in a Health Screening Cohort. Urol J. 2016 Mar 5;13(1):2569–75. PMID: 26945663.
14. Terada N, Arai Y, Kinukawa N, Yoshimura K, Terai A. Risk factors for renal cysts. BJU Int. 2004 Jun;93(9):1300–2. doi: 10.1111/j.1464–410X.2004.04844.x. PMID: 15180627.
15. Qiu W, Jiang Y, Wu J, Huang H, Xie W, Xie X, Chen J, Peng W. Simple Cysts in Donor Kidney Contribute to Reduced Allograft Function. Am J Nephrol. 2017;45(1):82–88. doi: 10.1159/000453078. Epub 2016 Dec 2. PMID: 27907917.
16. Terada N, Ichioka K, Matsuta Y, Okubo K, Yoshimura K, Arai Y. The natural history of simple renal cysts. J Urol. 2002 Jan;167(1):21–3. PMID: 11743266.
17. Kim SM, Chung TH, Oh MS, Kwon SG, Bae SJ. Relationship of simple renal cyst to hypertension. Korean J Fam Med. 2014 Sep;35(5):237–42.
18. Wu Q, Ju C, Deng M, Liu X, Jin Z. Prevalence, risk factors and clinical characteristics of renal dysfunction in Chinese outpatients with growth simple renal cysts. Int Urol Nephrol. 2022 Jul;54(7):1733–1740.

19. Massie AB, Holscher CM, Henderson ML, Fahmy LM, Thomas AG, Al Ammary F, Getsin SN, Snyder JJ, Lentine KL, Garg AX, Segev DL. Association of Early Postdonation Renal Function with Subsequent Risk of End-Stage Renal Disease in Living Kidney Donors. JAMA Surg. 2020 Mar 1;155(3):e195472.
20. Waldram MM, Thomas AG, Yu Y, Holscher CM, Nguyen AQ, Halpern SE, Ottman S, Muzaale AD, Henderson ML, Lentine KL, Al Ammary F, Brennan DC, Garonzik-Wang JM, Segev DL, Massie AB. Long-term renal function in living kidney donors with simple renal cysts: A retrospective cohort study. Clin Transplant. 2020 Sep;34(9): e13905.
21. Delmonico F. Council of transplantation society. A report of the Amsterdam forum on the care of the live kidney donor: Data and medical guidelines. Transplantation 2005;79: S53–S66.
22. K.A. Wong, J. Olsburgh Management of stones in renal transplant.Curr. Opin. Urol., 23 (2) (2013), pp. 175–179
23. I.K. Kim, J.C. Tan, J. Lapasia *et al.* Incidental kidney stones: a single center experience with kidney donor selection.Clin. Transpl., 26 (4) (2012), pp. 558–563.
24. A. Ganpule, J.B. Vyas, C. Sheladia, *et al.* Management of urolithiasis in live-related kidney donors J. Endourol., 27 (2) (2013), pp. 245–250.
25. Bissada NK, Bissada SA, Fitts CT, Rajagopalan PR, Nelson R. Renal transplantation from living related donor after excision of angiomyolipoma of the donor kidney. *J Urol.* 1993;150:174–5.
26. Anton DG, Kovvuru K, Kanduri SR, Aeddula NR, *et al.* Use and outcomes of kidneys from donors with renal angiomyolipoma: A systematic review. Urol Ann. 2021 Jan-Mar;13(1):67–72.
27. Zahran MH, Kamal AI, Abdelfattah A,. Outcome of Live-donor Renal Transplants With Incidentally diagnosed Renal Angiomyolipoma in the Donor. Transplant Proc. 2019 Jul-Aug;51(6):1773–1778.
28. British transplantation society living donor kidney transplantation guidelines 2018.
29. Chen KW, Wu MW, Chen Z, Tai BC, Goh YS, Lata R, Vathsala A, Tiong HY. Compensatory Hypertrophy After Living Donor Nephrectomy. Transplant Proc. 2016 Apr;48 (3):716-9.

Chapter

16

Donor with Vascular Anomalies (Multiple Arteries, Venous Anomalies, Aneurysms)

• Mudit Maheshwari • Aneesh Srivastava

LEARNING OBJECTIVES

- To understand how to predict intra-operative difficulty and prevent unforeseen complications based on preoperative assessment of CT angiography of the donor with protocol-based reporting.
- To understand how to decide on a suitable side for donor nephrectomy.
- To understand various techniques of vascular anastomosis for multiple renal arteries both during bench surgery and recipient surgery.
- To understand complications associated with vascular anomalies in donors as well as recipients and their management strategy.
- To understand the long-term outcome of grafts with vascular anomaly.

Case Scenario

A 57-year-old female voluntary kidney donor (VKD) for her 29-year-old son with end stage renal disease secondary to chronic glomerulonephritis was under evaluation. The DTPA scan showed a global GFR of 70 ml/min with a split function of 35 ml/min in each kidney. Figure 16.1 depicts a protocol-based report of the donor's vascular anatomy and Fig. 16.2 shows 3D reconstructed films of MDCT angiography. Which kidney should be preferred for donation?

Ans: In this VKD both the kidneys have complex vascular anatomy with equivalent function on DTPA scan, however, due to the presence of 1 cm simple cortical cyst left-sided kidney should be preferred for donation.

1. What is the preferred vascular anatomy of a donor?

Ans: A donor with a left-sided single renal artery with adequate length before branching and renal vein with early confluence is ideal (Fig. 16.3). The left renal vein is 6–10 cm long and receives several tributaries including the adrenal vein superiorly, gonadal vein inferiorly, and lumbar vein posteriorly.[1] The right renal vein has a short course of 2–4 cm without tributaries with thin walls. Left-sided donor nephrectomy is favored because of the adequate venous pedicle.[2] Certain anatomic conditions including vascular anomalies, the presence of cyst, and considerable reduction in right kidney renal function compared to the left kidney, prevents the harvesting of the left kidney.[3] In these conditions, a right donor nephrectomy can be done. To obtain the additional length of the right renal vein, an inferior vena cava cuff should be included using an open or laparoscopic-assisted technique.[4]

2. What are the common vascular anomalies seen in donors?

Ans: Super-numerary renal artery is the most frequent vascular anomaly, occurring in around 24% of cases.[5] These arteries are classified as either hilar (accessory) or polar (aberrant). While the accessory arteries enter the kidney from the hilum alongside the main renal artery, the aberrant arteries enter the kidney directly from the capsule outside the hilum. These accessory or aberrant renal arteries typically come from the abdominal aorta or iliac arteries, but they can also, very rarely, come from the lower thoracic aorta, the lumbar, or mesenteric arteries.[1]

Early arterial or prehilar branching diagnosed when the first renal branch emerges within 1.5 cm of the renal artery ostium. This is seen in about 12% of donors.[1]

Apart from the number of arteries and branching pattern variations, structural arterial abnormalities

Right kidney measures: 10.3 × 5.5 cm | Left kidney measures: 10.8 × 5.5 cm

Both kidneys are normal in size, shape, position, and outline with normal cortical enhancement. No obvious hydronephrosis on either side. Small midpolar simple cortical cyst 1cm on left side.

Renal Arteries:

Right: No. 02

Superior: Distance before branching from origin: 39.8 mm
Calibre of renal artery just after origin: 3.6 mm

Inferior: Distance before branching from origin: 61.6 mm
Calibre of renal artery just after origin: 2.3 mm

Distance between superior and inferior branches is 2 mm

Left: No. 03

Superior: Distance before branching from origin: 29 mm
Calibre of renal artery just after origin: 1.6 mm

Middle: Distance before branching from origin: 27.8 mm
Calibre of renal artery just after origin: 2.8 mm

Inferior: Distance before branching from origin: 28.1 mm
Calibre of renal artery just after origin: 5.2 mm

Distance between superior and middle branches is 10 mm
Distance between middle and inferior branches is 2.0 mm

Renal Veins:

Right: No. 02

Superior: Distance from confluence to IVC: 16.9 mm
Calibre of renal vein just after confluence: 9.0 mm

Inferior: Distance from confluence to IVC: 27.1 mm
Calibre of renal vein just after confluence: 4.1 mm

Distance between superior and inferior branches is 5 mm

Left: No. 01
Distance from confluence to lateral margin of aorta: 25.9 mm
Calibre of renal vein just after confluence: 9.5 mm
Preaortic

Abdominal aorta and its major branches are normal.
Bilateral single pelvicalyceal system and ureters seen.

Fig. 16.1: Protocol-based report of MDCT angiography

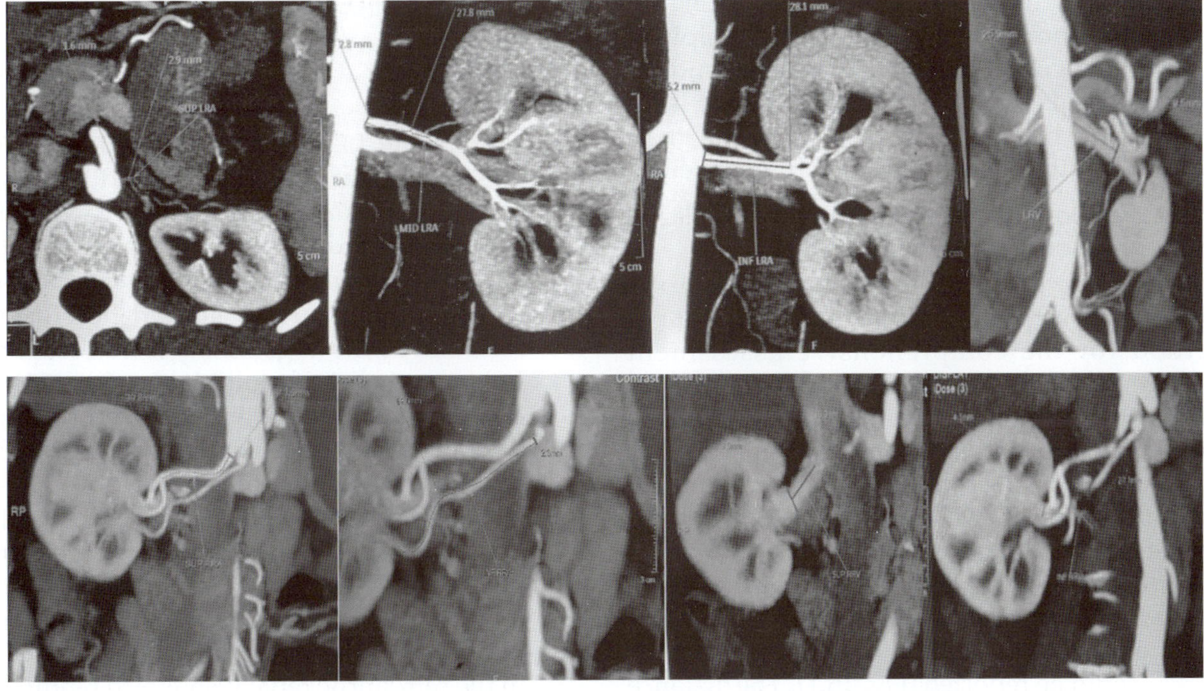

Fig. 16.2: 3D reconstructed films of the left and right kidney of VKD

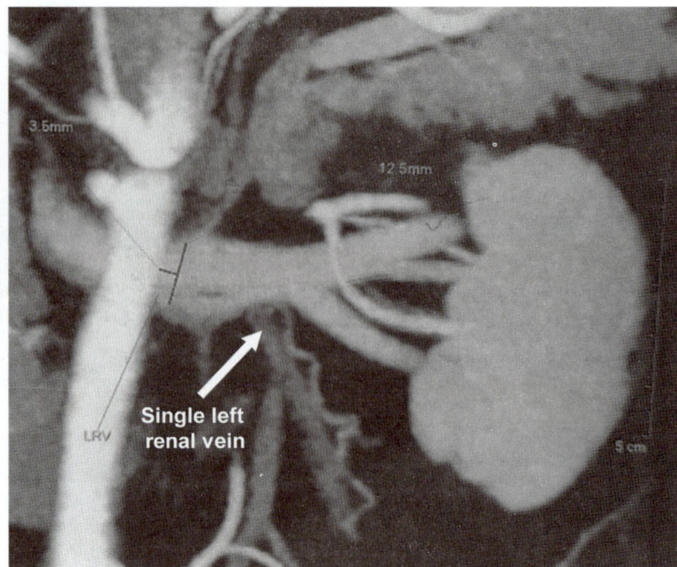

Fig. 16.3: Preferred vascular anatomy of VKD

include renal artery stenosis, aneurysms, arterio-venous malformations, dissection, thrombosis, and fibromuscular dysplasia are also encountered.

Raman *et al.*[7,8] classified renal vein anomalies as major or minor. Major renal vein anomalies are those that necessitate different surgical management, such as vascular anastomoses. It includes supernumerary veins and the presence of a late venous confluence. The major anomalies on the left side also include circumaortic or retroaortic renal veins, as well as a left-sided IVC or a duplicated IVC. Minor venous anomalies are those that impact the planning of donor laparoscopic dissection but do not alter the venous anastomosis procedure in the recipient. These involve lumbar, gonadal, adrenal, and/or retroperitoneal venous anomalies, including large gonadal and lumbar veins (> 5 mm) and their confluence with the main or branch renal veins.

3. **Which preoperative imaging should be utilized for donor vasculature evaluation?**

Ans: Multidetector CT (MDCT) angiography is a quick, dependable, and non-invasive method for the comprehensive assessment of renal vasculature. To create angiographic-quality pictures from axial CT data, various three-dimensional postprocessing approaches are used. Volume rendering and maximum intensity projection (MIP) are the most often used reconstruction algorithms among the numerous available.[9] During evaluation parameters including the calibre of renal artery just after origin and distance before branching from the origin should be reported (Fig. 16.1). The distance from confluence to the lateral margin of the aorta and its trajectory with regard to the aorta is critical for the left renal vein.

4. **Is laparoscopic donor nephrectomy (LDN) a suitable approach?**

Ans: LDN in patients with complex vascular anatomy is safe and efficacious and does not negatively impact the complication rate in donors or recipient outcomes in terms of graft function.[10] Laparoscopy decreases the morbidity of renal donor operation making it attractive to potential donors and leading to an increase in the donor pool which is also true for donors with vascular anomalies.[11]

5. **What additional precautions should be followed during donor nephrectomy with vascular anomalies?**

Ans: In cases of multiple renal arteries while performing LDN traction should be judiciously used, and hilar dissection should be done by an experienced surgeon due to restricted mobility of the kidney. Undue stretching may lead to vascular spasm and injury of smaller renal arteries.

The smaller artery should be clipped first followed by the larger artery to decrease the warm ischemia time-1. If multiple arteries are near each other caution should be exercised during initial artery clipping so as not to jeopardize subsequent arterial and venous clipping.

In the case of multiple renal veins, smaller renal vein with <30% diameter of the larger renal vein can be safely clipped or ligated as they are prone to be injured while traction. While performing left LDN larger calibre tributaries may be encountered in the retroaortic renal vein which require vigilant clipping.

6. **What are the options for arterial reconstruction in multiple renal arteries?**

Ans: Arterial reconstruction is carried out in accordance with transplant surgery expertise and anatomical factors like arterial calibre, site, and orientation utilizing approaches that are most appropriate for the circumstance and the surgeon's comfort level. Anastomotic techniques for multiple renal arteries can be done during bench surgery or intracorporeally by separate anastomosis.

1. *Ex-vivo* bench surgery anastomotic techniques: It enables single anastomosis implantation of the graft and decreases the warm ischemia time-2 of graft kidney. It includes:
   i. Pantaloon or double-barrel anastomosis: In a preferred clinical situation, when 2 renal arteries are comparable in luminal diameter, near to each other with favourable orientation they can be anastomosed side to side after adequate spatulation as shown in Figs 16.4A and 16.4B. The pantaloon technique provides acceptable graft outcomes while utilizing a 30/70 cut-off for the ratio of the diameter of smaller to larger artery.[12] A smaller calibre artery (<2 mm) should not be used for pantalooning as it compromises the calibre of the main renal artery.

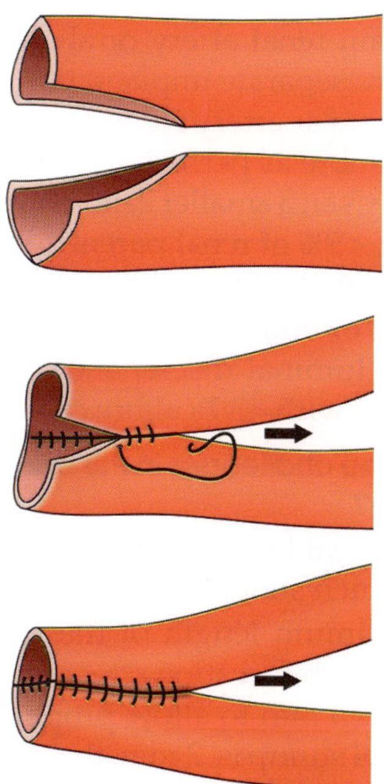

Fig. 16.4A: Steps of pantaloon or double-barrel anastomosis

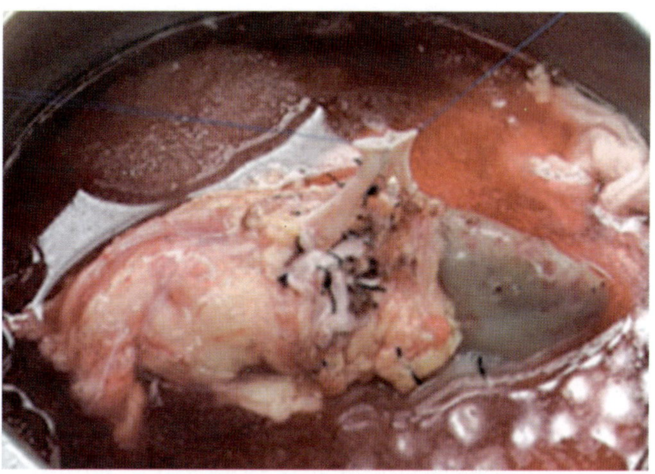

Fig. 16.4B: Bench picture of graft kidney following pantaloon anastomosis

   ii. End-to-side anastomosis: When the arterial anatomy is not suitable for double barrel or the surgeon has more expertise in it, end-to-side anastomosis can be done. It carries the potential risk of compromising the lumen of the larger renal artery.[13] An accessory or aberrant artery with calibre >2 mm should be anastomosed separately in the recipient preferably to the inferior epigastric artery (IEA). The end-to-side procedure, among the anastomosis techniques, theoretically results in the smallest combined diameter of the final artery channel and is thus more prone to stenosis. Thrombus or hyperplasia of the smaller artery in this case could potentially spread to the main artery, leading to chronic ischemia of the entire kidney (Figs 16.5A and 16.5B).[12]

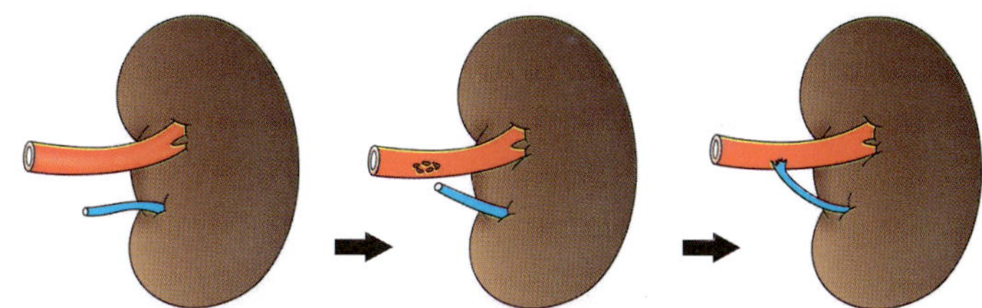

Fig. 16.5A: Steps of end-to-side anastomosis

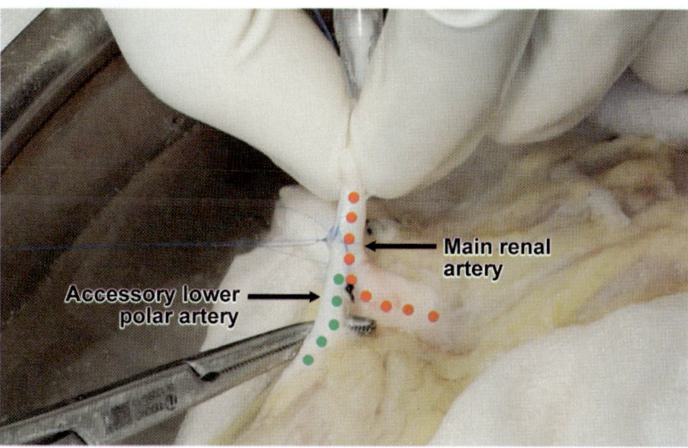

Fig. 16.5B: Bench picture of graft kidney following end-to-side anastomosis

iii. Use of recipient internal iliac artery (IIA): IIA with its branches can be used to anastomose the multiple renal arteries for single implantation.[14]

2. Intracorporeal separate anastomosis: If the aberrant polar artery is present away from the hilum, then bench surgery is not feasible. In the case of similar luminal calibre arteries, separate anastomosis can be done according to the surgeon's preference. External iliac artery (EIA) can be used for end-to-side implantation of both renal arteries as shown in Fig. 16.6. IIA or its branches may be utilized for end-to-end anastomosis of the accessory artery with main renal artery anastomosed to EIA as shown in Figs 16.7A and 16.7B.

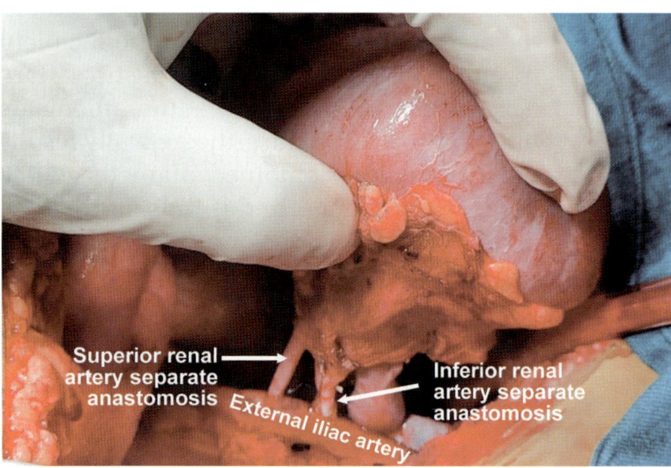

Fig. 16.6: End-to-side anastomosis of both renal arteries to EIA

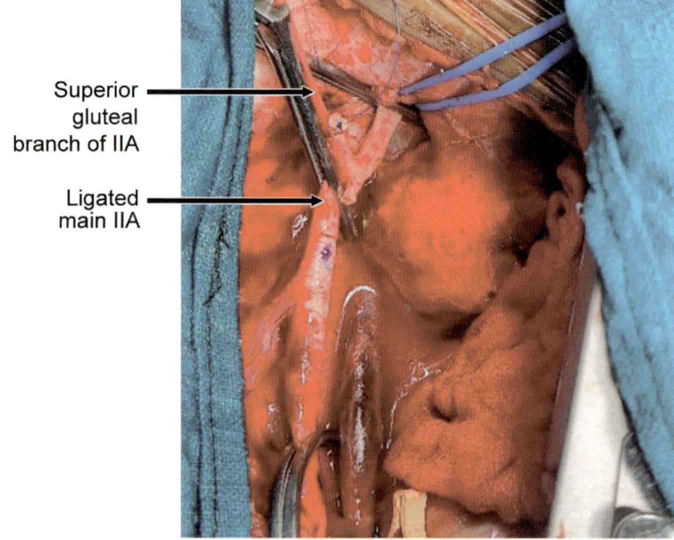

Fig. 16.7A: Dissected superior gluteal branch of IIA

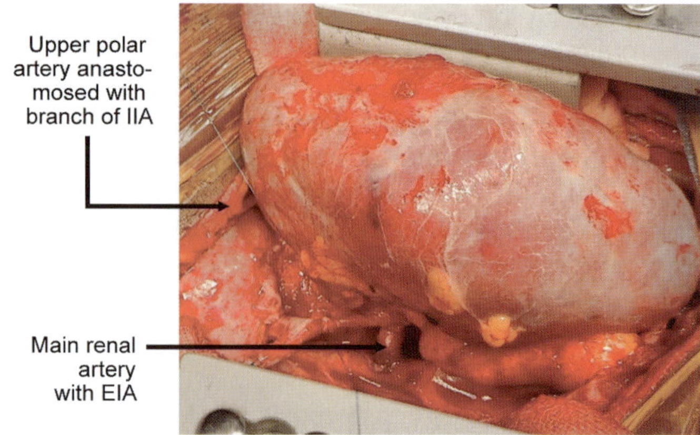

Fig. 16.7B: Separate anastomosis utilizing both EIA and branch of IIA

7. What information on the bench would be useful for deciding technique while dealing with vascular anomalies?

Ans: During bench surgery after perfusion of preservative fluid and dissection of perihilar tissue precise anatomy and orientation of multiple renal vessels can be visualized and reconstruction can be planned. The area of the kidney supplied by the smaller artery can be visualized during perfusion. If the area perfused is < 20% or a polar artery is present, bench surgery can be avoided. Nearby accessory hilar arteries can be anastomosed together with different techniques. An accessory artery away from a main renal artery or aberrant polar artery will require separate implantation in the recipient. The lower polar artery should be preserved even if small in calibre as perfusion of the ureter depends on it. However, a smaller calibre upper polar artery supplying <5% of renal parenchyma as visualized during perfusion can be ligated.[15]

In cases of multiple renal veins or circumaortic veins, the luminal discrepancy is noted. Smaller calibre vein with <3:7 calibre can be safely ligated.

8. What are the challenges in the case of early arterial branching?

Ans: The ideal length of the artery from its origin to first branch should be ≥10 mm.

The optimum length of the residual common stump before bifurcation after donor nephrectomy should be ≥3 mm to allow proper anastomosis. If the residual stump is 2 mm, there may be technical challenges and a risk of injury to the septum or smaller artery (Figs 16.8A and 16.8B).

Technical modifications for arterial anastomosis with small common stump:

1. Parachute technique: By continuously inspecting the vascular lumen, it tries to preserve lumen patency and prevents back wall or septal bites.

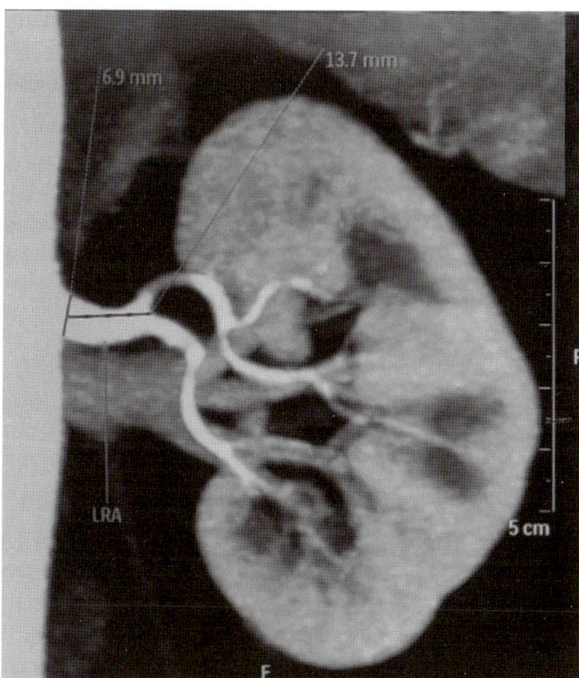

Fig. 16.8A: CT angiography of early branching

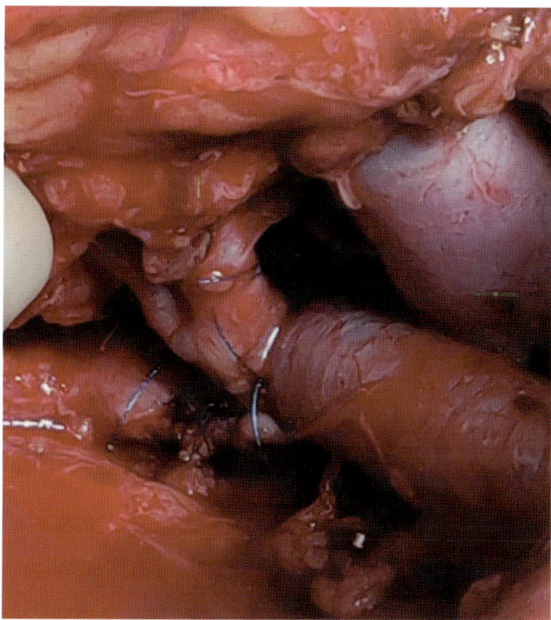
Fig. 16.8B: End-to-side anastomosis to EIA

It also allows for the exact placement of the sutures over the whole width of the vessel, resulting in well-aligned edges while avoiding the crumpling of vessel edges (Fig. 16.9).

2. Multiple interrupted sutures near the septum and smaller vessel.

9. Can smaller branch anastomoses be done off clamp?

Ans: In graft with multiple renal arteries after implantation of the main renal artery, declamping can be done and the smaller accessory or aberrant artery can be sequentially anastomosed off clamp. This reduces the warm ischemia time-2 and the risk of acute tubular necrosis. Sequential anastomosis can be performed utilizing EIA more commonly owing to its superficial location as shown in Fig. 16.10 or a branch of IIA.[16]

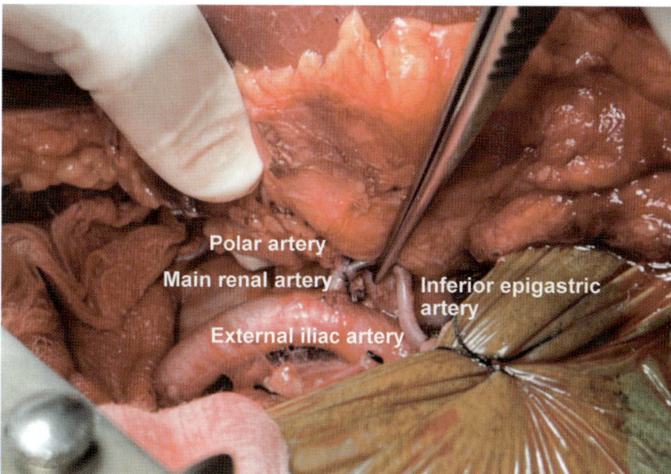

Fig. 16.10: Upper polar artery end-to-end anastomosis to IEA

10. What are the options for multiple renal veins?

Ans: In our experience, if there is a significant luminal discrepancy between the larger vein and smaller vein (ratio>7:3) the smaller vein can be safely ligated, otherwise they require separate anastomosis. Multiple veins with comparable calibre require anastomosis end to side with external iliac vein.

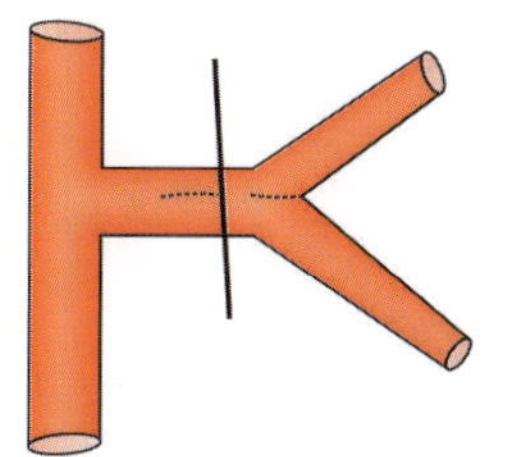
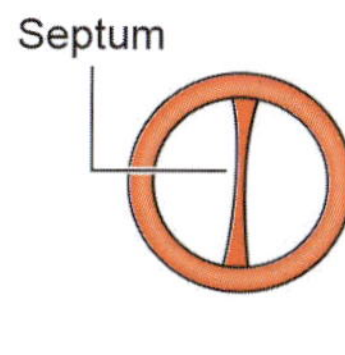

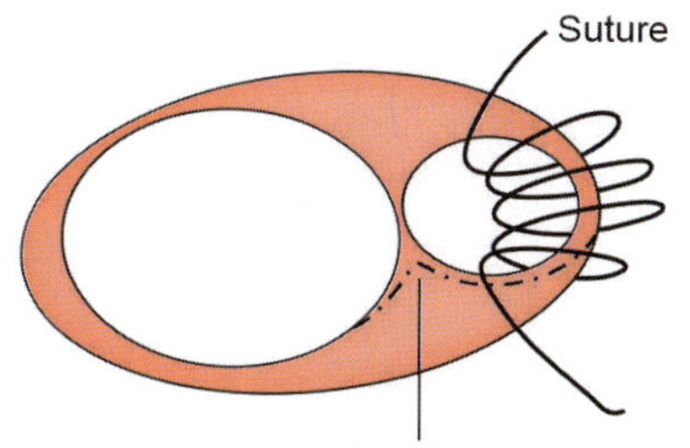

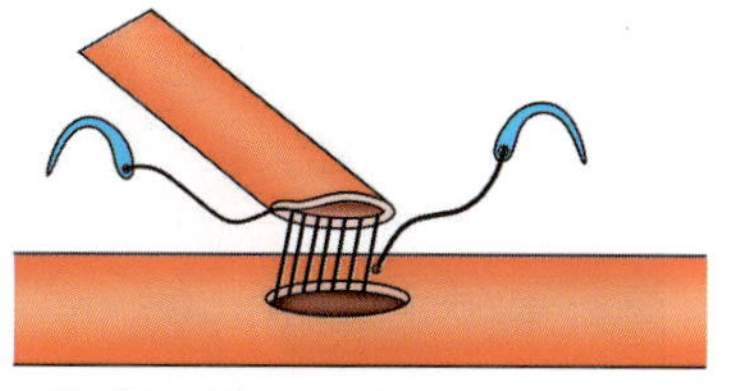

Fig. 16.9: End-on and side view of the parachute technique of anastomosis

11. What are the options for left renal vein anomalies?

Ans: The circumaortic renal vein (Figs 16.11A and 16.11B) is the most common anomaly in the left renal venous system, affecting 4.4–17% of patients.[17] The left renal vein divides into ventral and dorsal limbs that ring the abdominal aorta in this variant. The size of the retroaortic venous component determines the appearance of a circumaortic left renal vein. The retroaortic component frequently joins the IVC at a caudal position. In our experience, the smaller limb of the circumaortic vein usually the retroaortic limb can be safely ligated and a single venous anastomosis is required. However, variations may exist and their discussion is beyond the scope of this book.

A retroaortic left renal vein, a double IVC, and a late confluence of the renal venous trunk are some more major variations of the left renal vein. Less frequently occurring venous anomalies include a solitary retroaortic renal vein, which affects 1.8–3% of patients (Figs 16.12A and 16.12B).[17] Vigilant lower pole dissection is required during laparoscopy as the retroaortic vein runs caudally to insert in IVC and usually has multiple lumbar tributaries, a large adrenal vein, and a large gonadal vein.

Double IVC is a relatively uncommon condition (incidence–0.2–3%).[9,17] The duplicated left IVC usually drains into the left renal vein, and the left renal vein then crosses anterior to the aorta and joins the right IVC in a normal fashion.

12. Do perioperative complications increase in patients with multiple vessels?

Ans: When utilizing allografts with multiple renal vessels comparable outcomes can be achieved in living-donor kidney transplantation with no higher chances of developing delayed graft function (DGF), post-operative (or surgical) complications, lower renal function, or graft loss.[18] However, opinions regarding DGF are variable with certain studies showing increased risk with multiple vessels.[19]

The use of meticulous vascular technique and the surgeon's experience in handling complicated vascular anatomy plays the determining factor.

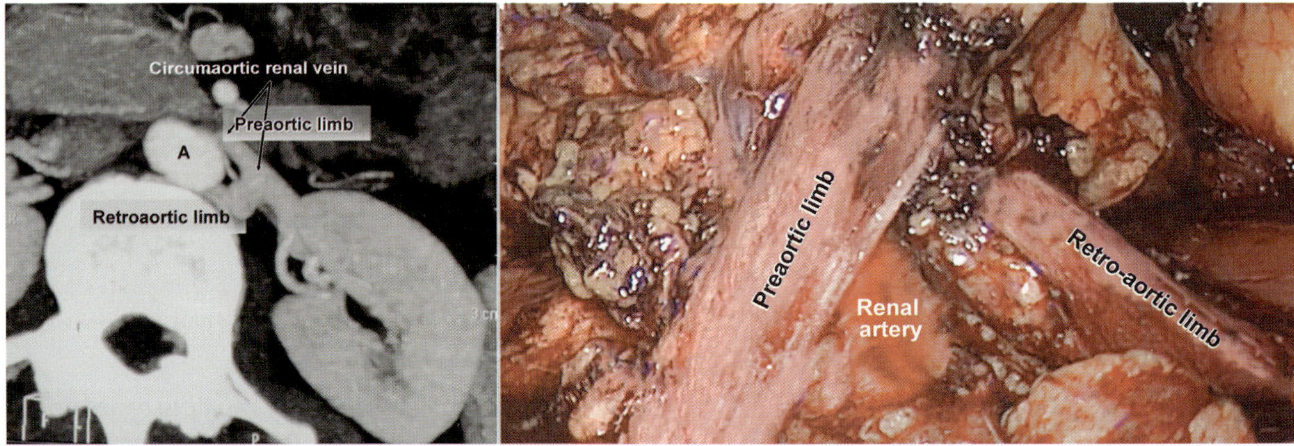

Fig. 16.11A: Circumaortic vein

Fig. 16.11B: Laparoscopic view. Retroaortic component traversing caudally to join IVC

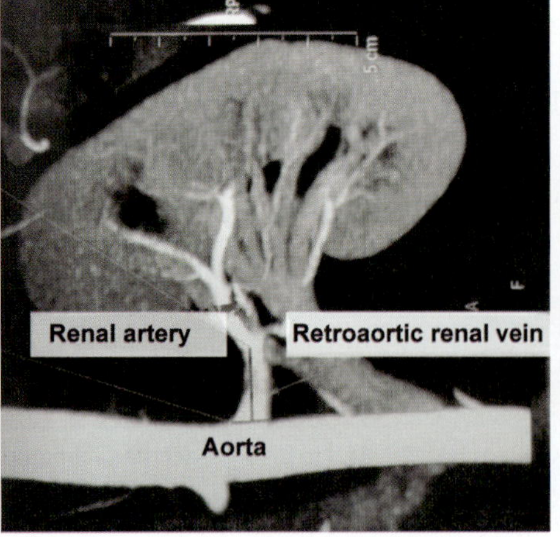

Fig. 16.12A: Retroaortic vein

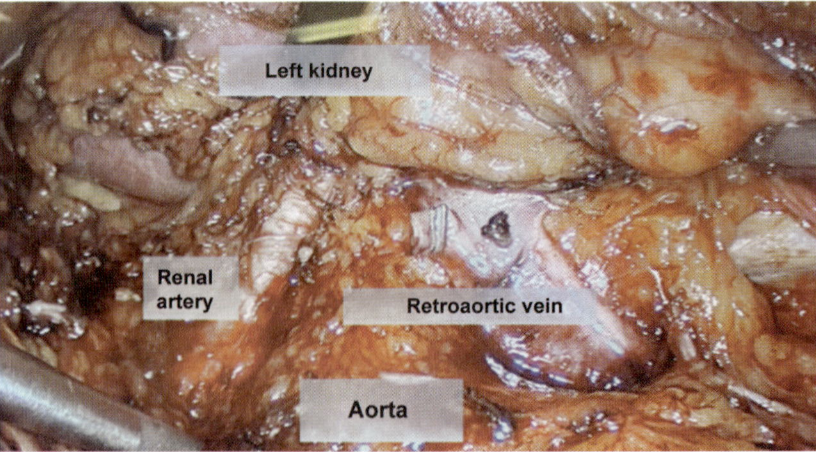

Fig. 16.12B: Laparoscopic view. Retroaortic vein traversing caudally to join IVC

13. What is the long-term outcome of the graft with multiple vessels?

Ans: Similar 5-year graft survival and 5-year patient survival outcomes are seen in comparing the group with multiple renal arteries and another group with a single renal artery in a meta-analysis.[19]

KEY POINTS

- Donors with vascular anomalies can be safely accepted and laparoscopic donor nephrectomy is a suitable procedure with satisfactory outcome.
- MDCT angiography is crucial for assessing renal vasculature and its associated anomalies
- Anastomotic techniques for multiple vessels include separate anastomoses of arteries in the recipient or single anastomosis after bench surgery.
- In donor kidneys with a vascular abnormality and those with straightforward anatomy, the rate of complications and the recipient's short-and long-term results are comparable.

SUMMARY

- Incidence of vascular anomalies in donor kidneys varies from 18% to 30% and presents a challenge for transplant surgeons.
- The presence of multiple renal arteries is the most frequently encountered anatomic variation in kidneys (unilateral 23%; bilateral 10%).
- Multiple renal veins, which are present in 15–30% of patients, are the most frequent venous abnormalities. They are more common on the right side and occur in up to 30% of individuals.
- The primary venous anomalies on the left side also include circumaortic or retroaortic renal veins, as well as a left-sided inferior vena cava (IVC) or a duplicated IVC.
- Multidetector computed tomographic (MDCT) angiography with 3D reconstruction and protocol-based reporting is a reliable, non-invasive investigation for evaluating renal vascular anatomy.
- Laparoscopic surgery is safe in donors with vascular anomalies.
- Donor kidney with multiple vessels is no longer a relative contraindication for renal transplantation. Various vascular techniques like pantaloon, end-to-side anastomosis, or separate implantation can be performed according to the donor's vascular anatomy, the recipient's pelvic anatomy, and the surgeon's expertise.
- Complications rate, short-term, and long-term outcomes in the recipient are comparable in donor kidneys with vascular anomaly and those with uncomplicated anatomy.

REFERENCES

1. Urban BA, Ratner LE, Fishman EK. Three-dimensional volume rendered CT angiography of the renal arteries and veins: normal anatomy, variants, and clinical applications. Radiographics 2001;21:373–386.
2. Jacobs SC, Cho E, Dunkin BJ, Flowers JL, Schweitzer E, Cangro C, *et al.* Laparoscopic live donor nephrectomy: the University of Maryland 3-year experience. J Urol 2000;164:1494–1499.
3. Boorjian S, Munver R, *et al.* Right laparoscopic live donor nephrectomy: a single institution experience. Transplantation 2004;77:437–40.
4. Bollens R, Mikhaski D, Espinoza BP, Rosenblatt A, Hoang AD, Abramowicz D, Donckier V, Schulman CC. Laparoscopic live donor right nephrectomy: a new technique to maximize the length of the renal vein using a modified Endo GIA stapler. Eur Urol. 2007 May;51(5):1326–31.
5. Ozkan U, Og-uzkurt L, Tercan F, Kızılkılıç O, Koç Z, Koca N. Renal artery origins and variations: angiographic evaluation of 855 consecutive patients. Diagn Interv Radiol 2006;12:183–186.
6. Holden A, Smith A, Dukes P, Pilmore H, Yasutomi M. Assessment of 100 live potential renal donors for laparoscopic nephrectomy with multi-detector row helical CT. Radiology 2005;237:973–980.
7. Raman SS, Pojchamarnwiputh S, Muangsomboon K, Schulam PG, Gritsch HA, Lu DS. Utility of 16–MDCT angiography for comprehensive preoperative vascular evaluation of laparoscopic renal donors. AJR Am J Roentgenol 2006;186:1630–1638.
8. Raman SS, Pojchamarnwiputh S, Muangsomboon K, Schulam PG, Gritsch HA, Lu DS. Surgically relevant normal and variant renal parenchymal and vascular anatomy in preoperative 16-MDCT evaluation of potential laparoscopic renal donors. AJR Am J Roentgenol 2007;188:105–114.
9. Chai JW, Lee W, Yin YH, Jae HJ, Chung JW, Kim HH, *et al.* CT angiography for living kidney donors: accuracy, cause of misinterpretation and prevalence of variation. Korean J Radiol 2008;9:333–339.
10. Disick GI, Shapiro ME, Miles RA, Munver R. Critical analysis of laparoscopic donor nephrectomy in the setting of complex renal vasculature: initial experience and intermediate outcomes. J Endourol. 2009 Mar;23(3):451–5.
11. Ratner, L. E., Hiller, J., Sroka, M. *et al.*: Laparoscopic live donor nephrectomy removes disincentives to live donation. Transplant Proc, 29: 3402, 1997.
12. Panwar P, Bansal D, Maheshwari R, Chaturvedi S, Desai P, Kumar A. Management of donor kidneys with double renal arteries with significant luminal discrepancy: A retrospective cohort study. Indian J Urol. 2020 Jul-Sep;36(3):200–204.
13. Popov Z, Stankov O, Stavridis S, Saidi S, Ivanovski O, Spasovski G, Cakalaroski K, Ivanovski N. Management of Multiple Renal Arteries and Unusual Venous Anatomy During Kidney Transplant: From a Simple Technical Problem to a Graft-Saving Procedure. Exp Clin Transplant. 2020 Dec;18(7):763–770.
14. Hiramitsu T, Futamura K, Okada M, *et al.* Impact of arterial reconstruction with recipient's own internal iliac artery for multiple graft arteries on living donor kidney transplantation: strobe study. Medicine (Baltimore) 2015;94(43):e1811.
15. Wijayaratne DR, Sudusinghe DH, Gunawansa N. Multiple renal arteries in live donor renal transplantation; impact on graft function and outcome: A prospective cohort study. Open J Organ Transpl Surg 2018;8:1–11.
16. Kumar, A., Gupta, R.S., Srivastava, A. and Bansal, P. (2001), Sequential anastomosis of accessory renal artery to inferior epigastric artery in the management of multiple arteries in live related renal transplantation: a critical appraisal. Clin Transplantation, 15: 131–135.
17. Reed MD, Friedman AC, Nealey P. Anomalies of the left renal vein: analysis of 433 CT scans. J Comput Assist Tomogr 1982;6:1124–1126.
18. Garcia LE, Parra N, Gaynor JJ, Baker L, Guerra G and Ciancio G (2021) Clinical Outcomes Following Single vs. Multiple Vessel Living-Donor Kidney Transplantation: A Retrospective Comparison of 210 Patients. Front. Surg. 8:693021.
19. Zorgdrager M, Krikke C, Hofker SH, Leuvenink HGD, Pol RA. Multiple Renal Arteries in Kidney Transplantation: A Systematic Review and Meta-Analysis. Annals of transplantation. 2016 Jul 29;21:469–478.

Chapter 17

Laparoscopic Donor Nephrectomy and its Complications

• Jamal Rizvi • Pranjal Modi

LEARNING OBJECTIVES

- To understand the steps of transperitoneal laparoscopic donor nephrectomy.
- To understand the steps of retroperitoneal laparoscopic donor nephrectomy.
- To understand the specific anatomical challenges in donor nephrectomy and how can they be overcome.
- To understand the complications of laparoscopic donor nephrectomy, their prevention and management.

INTRODUCTION

Living donor nephrectomy (LDN) has traditionally been performed by an open approach. While this was an efficacious way to obtain an organ for transplantation, it is associated with significant morbidity of access. Usually, an 11th rib excising incision is made. Long term sequelae include incisional hernias and neuropathic flank pain. In 1995 the first transperitoneal laparoscopic donor nephrectomy was performed.[1] This was a landmark event which has revolutionized the approach to living donor nephrectomy. It has gone a long way in reducing donor morbidity, however, while also increasing certain risks and bringing new surgical challenges.[2] The laparoscopic approach is associated with better pain control, better respiratory function, decreased hospital stays, and earlier return to normal activities and improved cosmetic results, compared to open donor nephrectomy.[3]

LDN by reducing perceived morbidity of living kidney donation[4] has been shown to remove disincentives to kidney donation and thus increase the living kidney donor pool.

Case Scenario

A 55-year-old lady presented herself as a prospective kidney donor for her daughter. She had a history of recent onset hypertension, managed on a single antihypertensive drug. Her BMI was 32.6. On evaluation her blood and urine reports were within normal limits. Ultrasound revealed normal sized kidneys. A DTPA renal scan revealed normally perfused kidneys with a GFR of 53 ml/minute (54%) on the left side and 46 ml/minute on the right side (46%). CT renal angiogram revealed two renal arteries on the left side and a single renal artery on the right side.

1. **Is she acceptable as a renal donor?**

   Ans: Living kidney donors should be rigorously screened for any factor that may contraindicate the removal of a kidney. These are summarised in various guidelines,[5] and have been covered in a preceding chapter. With acceptable renal function, hypertension controlled by a single agent and no morbid obesity, she is acceptable as a kidney donor.

2. **Which modality will you use for kidney retreival?**

   Ans: Laparoscopic donor nephrectomy may be achieved by two approaches: Transperitoneal and retroperitoneal.[6] We hereby discuss the pros and cons of each approach and give a technical description of each operation.

3. **What are the steps of transperitoneal laparoscopic donor nephrectomy?**

   Ans: Transperitoneal laparoscopic donor nephrectomy (TLDN) is by far the most commonly used minimal access approach for donor nephrectomy. Variations include use of hand assistance, either from the outset or at the end. Advantages include wide familiarity with the transperitoneal approach in most urology departments, versatility and ability to create additional ports as per need. The primary disadvantage is that it converts an extra-peritoneal surgery into a transperitoneal one, with the attendant sequelae of peritoneal irritation and post-operative ileus, and the increased potential for injury to intra-peritoneal organs.

Brief description of steps: Exact steps and port placement vary among authors; following is a general description of the operation. For left TLDN, the patient is catheterised and placed in a 60 degree flank up position (Fig. 17.1). Pneumoperitoneum is created by Veress needle. The primary camera port is placed para-rectally slightly cephalic to the umbilicus. Two additional working ports are placed, achieving triangulation with the renal hilum at the apex (Fig. 17.2). Pneumoperitoneum pressure is maintained at 12–15 mm Hg. The descending colon is reflected (Fig. 17.3), taking care to develop the vascular plane between the colon and the Gerota's fascia and avoid creating holes in the mesentery. Some authors advocate mobilizing and dropping down the spleen and tail of pancreas for improved visualization of the kidney and renal hilum. The ureter-gonadal complex is identified caudal to the lower pole and mobilised of the psoas muscle, taking care to preserve maximum peri-ureteric tissue (Fig. 17.4). The kidney is progressively lifted of the psoas muscle in a cephalic direction, until the hilum is reached. Peri-vascular fibro-lymphatic tissue is ablated using a monopolar hook or proprietary bipolar sealing device, taking extreme care to avoid thermal injury to the renal artery and vein (Fig. 17.5). The tributaries of the renal vein are dissected and controlled with energy sealing devices or 5 mm clips. It should be kept in mind that clips can interfere with later application of staples or clips on the main vessel. Dissection of the lumbar vein should be challenging as it is often short and closely applied to the renal artery. Anatomy of the left lumbar vein is variable, anatomy ranges from absence to multiple veins to a complex configuration involving the gonadal vein. It should be carefully dissected with a right-angled forceps, allowing

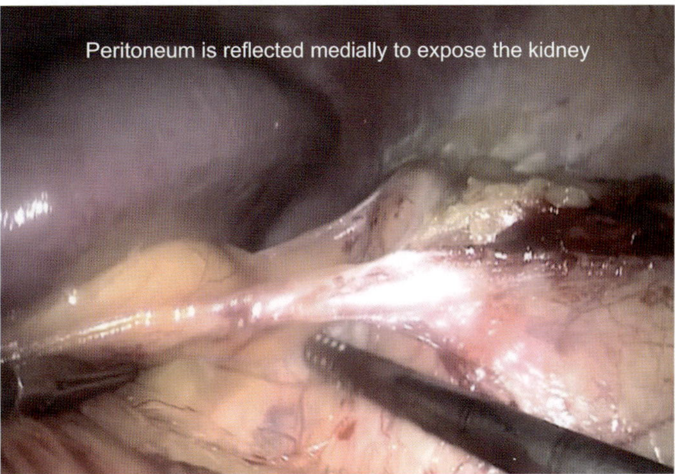

Fig. 17.3: Reflection of the descending colon

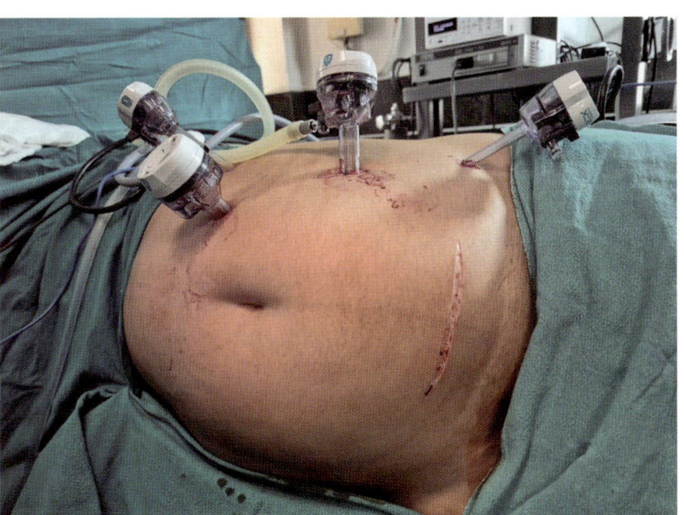
Fig. 17.1: Positioning for left sided TLDN

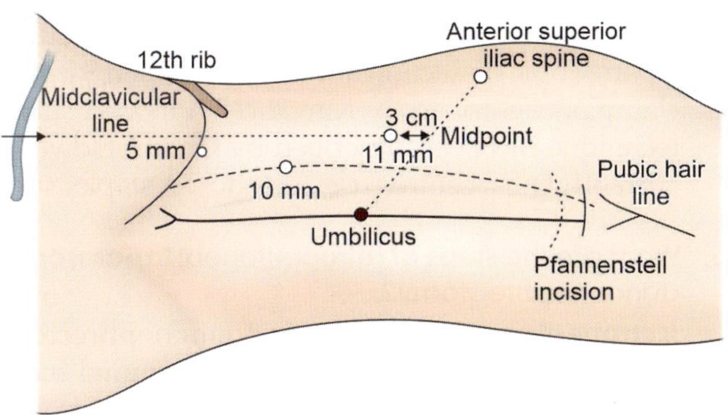

Fig. 17.2: Port placement for TLDN

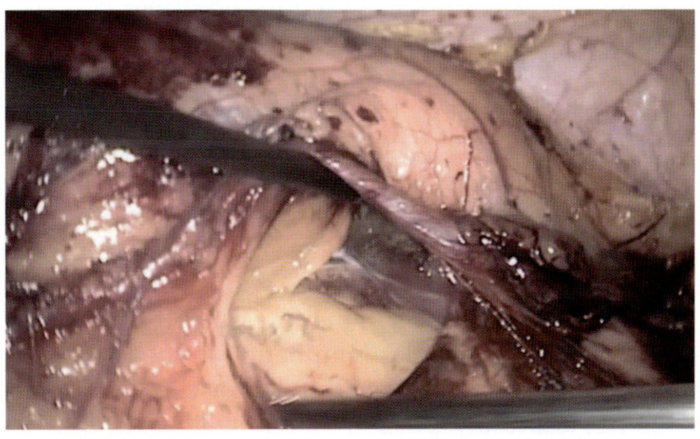
Fig. 17.4: Mobilization of the uretero-gonadal complex

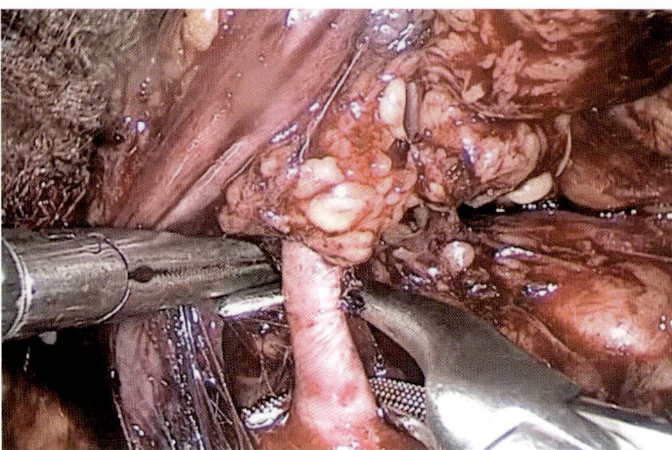

Fig. 17.5: Dissection of the renal hilum

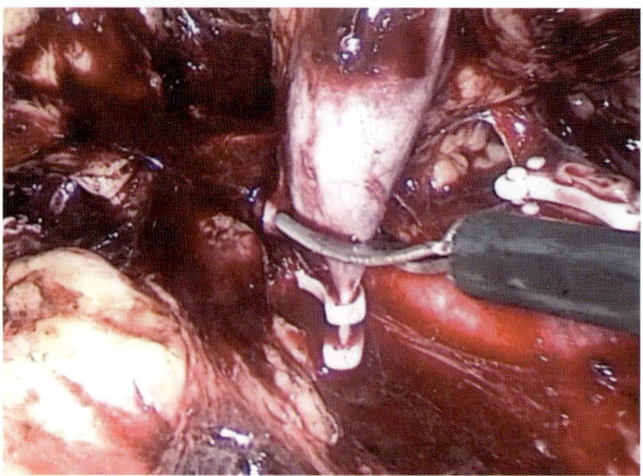

Fig. 17.6: Control of the renal vein

separation from the renal artery, before being securely controlled and divided. If small calibre it may be sealed with energy sources, otherwise 5 mm clips or staples may be used. Division of the lumbar vein allows unimpeded access to the renal artery, which is circumferentially dissected, clearing lymphatic tissue form the aorta for a few millimeters around the origin of the renal artery. The renal vein is dissected as low as possible, to the right of the aorta, where it dips behind the superior mesenteric artery.

The uretero-gonadal complex is dissected distal to the iliac crossing. The kidney is mobilised outside Gerota's fascia, leaving a few lateral attachments to suspend the organ laterally. The retrieval incision is made usually Pfannenstiel or in the ipsilateral groin. Muscle and sheath are incised, leaving the transversalis fascia intact. At this point mannitol may be administered if part of institutional protocol. The ureter is clipped below the iliac crossing and divided. A jet of urine from the cut end confirms a well-perfused kidney. After confirming that arrangements for perfusion are ready, the hilum is controlled. The renal artery is clipped with staplers or clips according to institutional protocol and divided, leaving a 2 mm cuff of tissue distal to the upper clip. The renal vein is similarly controlled and divided (Fig. 17.6). The freed graft may be placed into a retrieval bag, or the surgeon inserts their right hand and extracts the graft, which is placed in ice slush and sent for perfusion. The retrieval incision is closed, and check laparoscopy is performed to look for bleeding. Hemostasis should be assured at low pressures to rule out venous bleeding, that may be masked by higher pressure. It is advisable to clip the perihilar lymphatics on the left side to minimize the chance of chylous ascites. Drains are not routinely placed. Subcuticular skin sutures conclude the operation.

Variations of transperitoneal approach include hand assisted, single port and robot assisted transperitoneal laparoscopic donor nephrectomy.

Right-sided TLDN: Port placement is generally mirror-image of the left side. An additional port may be placed in the epigastrium and used to elevate the liver. A 12 mm port is placed in the right iliac fossa, for placement of an endo-TA stapler. The low position of the port allows the stapler to be passed parallel to the IVC. After the renal artery is divided, the stapler is passed and applied as low as possible at the confluence of the right renal vein with the IVC. Cold shears are used to divide the vein flush with the staple line. In case of early bifurcation of the renal artery, proximal dissection may be achieved by flipping the kidney medially and dissecting behind the IVC. If this gives insufficient access to the renal artery, inter-aortocaval dissection mat be done to control the right renal artery at its origin from the aorta.

4. How do you manage the right renal vein retrieval?

Ans: Various techniques have been described for management of the right renal vein. Hem-o-lok clips are commonly used, in some instances of 15 mm size. Turek described the use of a laparoscopic Satinsky clamp.[7] This is not widely adopted because of the possibility of dislodgement and the need for intracorporeal suturing. A safer option is to open after laparoscopic dissection and use of an open Satinsky clamp, as described by Kim *et al.*[8] A looped silk tie technique has been described by Chon.[9] However, currently most centres use an endo-TA stapler.

5. What are the steps of retroperitoneal laparoscopic donor nephrectomy?

Retroperitoneal laparoscopic donor nephrectomy (RLDN): This operation combines minimal access with the inherent advantages of an extraperitoneal approach. Possibly due to overall unfamiliarity

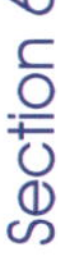

Fig. 17.7: Gaur balloon, made from two fingers of a glove tied on to a K-90 catheter

with the retroperitoneal approach it is less utilized compared to transperitoneal. However, urologists are familiar with retroperitoneal anatomy and this approach replicates open donor nephrectomy, hence it can be easily adopted and taught. Unlike the peritoneal space, the retroperitoneum is a potential space; the space is created by a balloon and then expanded by surgical dissection. No special armamentarium is required besides an indigenously prepared balloon dilator as described by Gaur[10] and small retractors for creation of the first port (Fig. 17.7).

Steps of left RLDN: The donor is catheterised and placed in a left flank up position on the edge of the table (Fig. 17.8). The surgeon and camera person stand at the back of the donor and the scrub nurse stands opposite. Port placement is shown in Fig. 17.9. The first port (camera port) is created one finger-breadth below the junction of the subcostal margin with the mid-axillary line. Port is created by open method, ensuring a limited opening of the muscles and lumbodorsal fascia (Fig. 17.10). This is important to minimize peri-port gas leak and subcutaneous emphysema which can lead to hypercarbia. The balloon is then inserted and

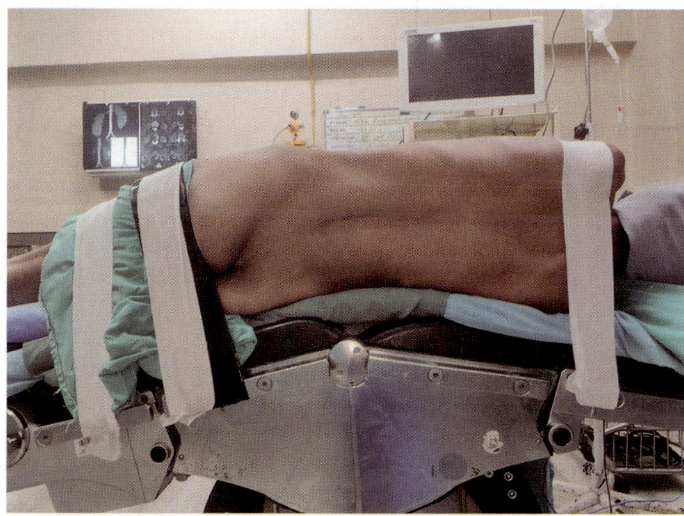

Fig. 17.8: Patient positioning for left RLDN

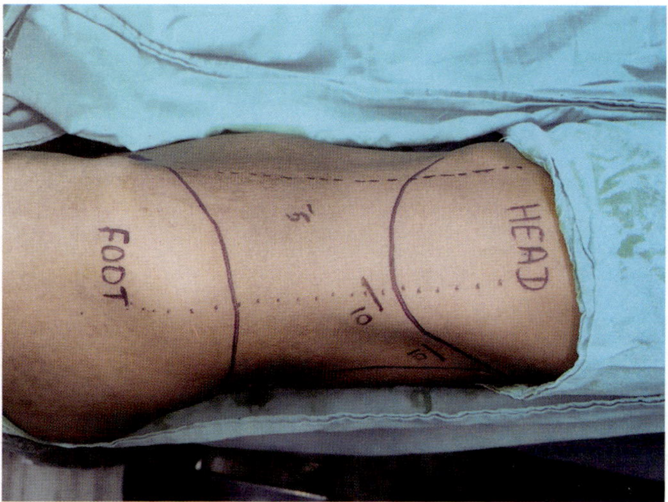

Fig. 17.9: Port placement for RLDN

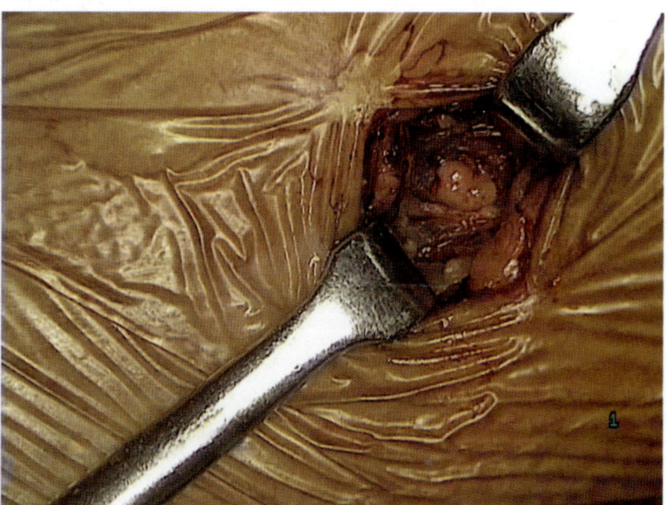

Fig. 17.10: Creation of the first port

inflated to 10–12 ml/kg of patient's body-weight. The anterior port is inserted under vision, ensuring that peritoneum is not transgressed (Fig. 17.11). The posterior port is placed and fixed (Fig. 17.12). Gerota's fascia is opened from upper pole to lower end of the operative field (Fig. 17.13). The uretero-gonadal complex is dissected, preserving the vascularity of the ureter. The gonadal vein is traced up to its confluence with the renal vein (Fig. 17.14). The lumbar vein is identified at this point and dissected free of surrounding fibro-lymphatic tissue (Fig. 17.15). Notably, access to the lumbar vein is superior to that obtained by TLDN, because the posterior approach. The lumbar vein is controlled with energy source or 5 mm Weck clips and then divided. Perihilar lymphatic tissue is controlled with energy sources. The adrenal vein is identified and divided (Fig. 17.16). The kidney is then mobilised, excising the posterior pannus of perinephric fat (Fig. 17.17). The kidney

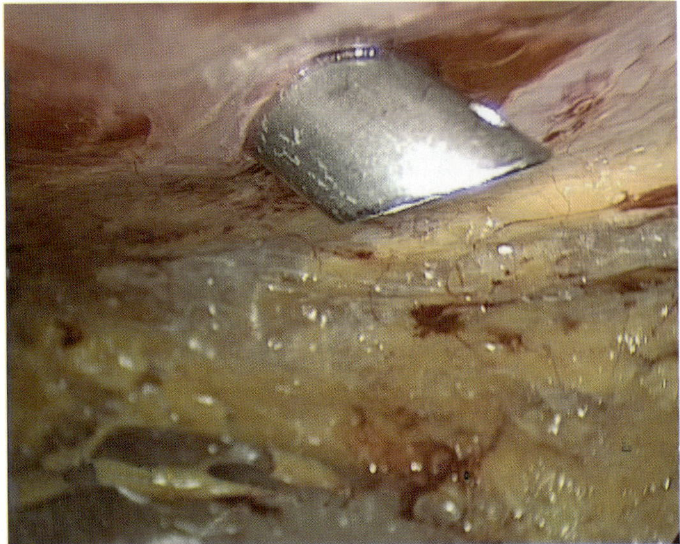

Fig. 17.11: Second (anterior) port

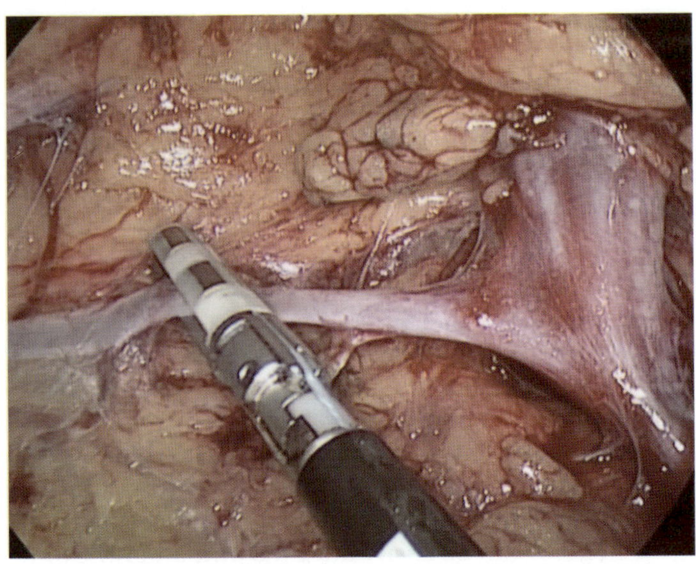

Fig. 17.14: Gonadal vein dissected until confluence with renal vein

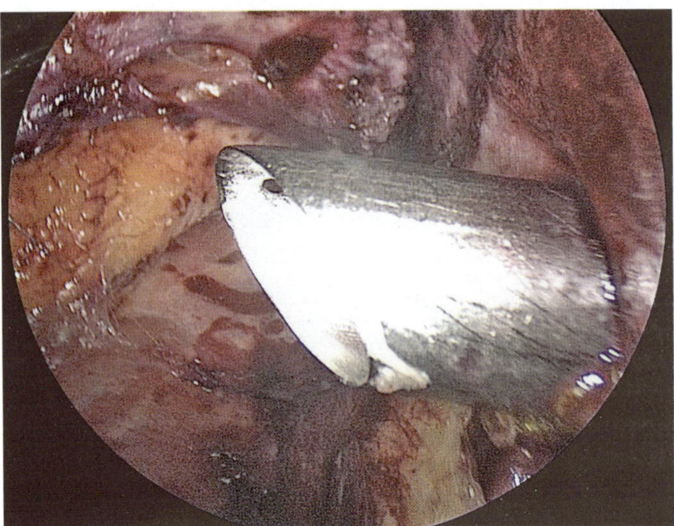

Fig. 17.12: Third (posterior) port

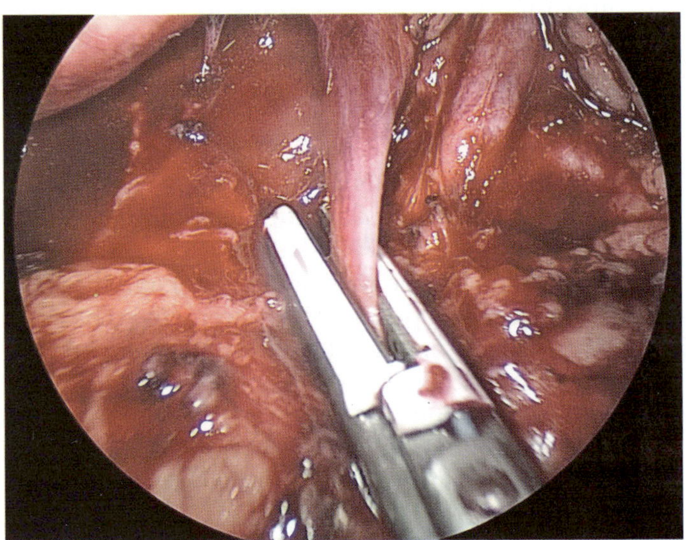

Fig. 17.15: Dissection of the lumbar vein

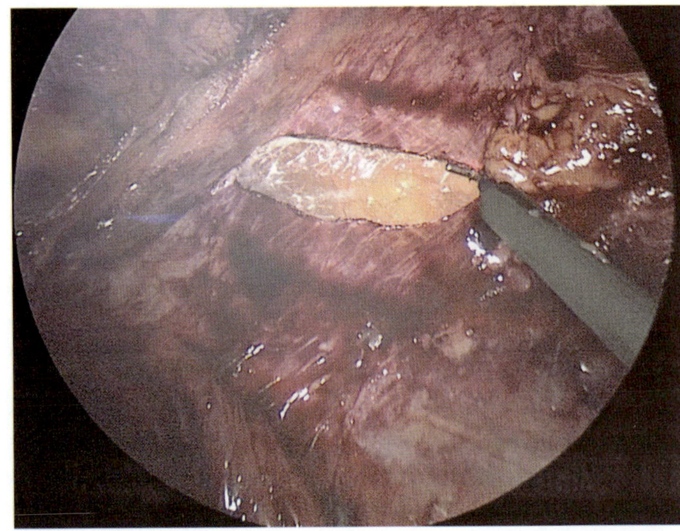

Fig. 17.13: Incision of Gerota's fascia

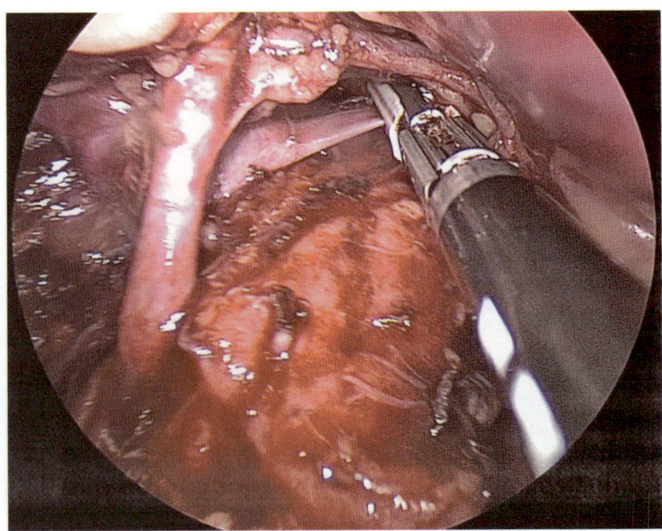

Fig. 17.16: Dissection of adrenal vein

Fig. 17.17: Excision of posterior pannus of perinephric fat

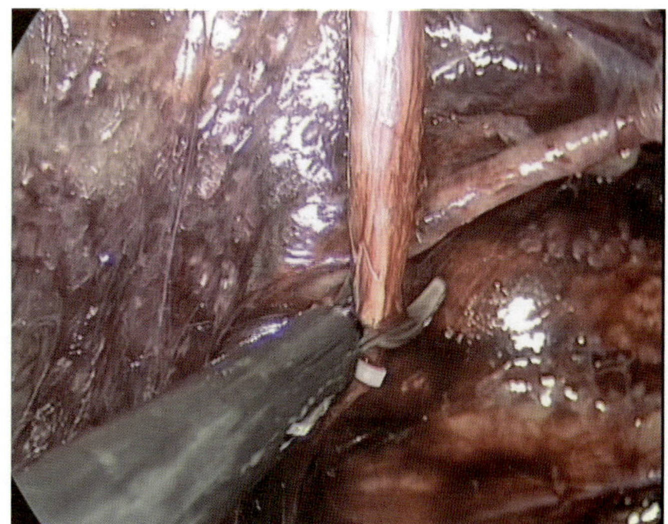

Fig. 17.19: Clipping of the ureter

is flipped laterally, separating the medial avascular attachments with the peritoneum (Fig. 17.18). After the kidney is completely mobilised, the ureter is clipped at the level of the iliac artery bifurcation and divided (Fig. 17.19). A retrieval incision is made in the groin, 1 inch above and parallel to the inguinal ligament (Fig. 17.20). The muscles are divided, preserving the transversalis fascia (Fig. 17.21). The renal artery is controlled either with a stapler or clips as per institutional protocol and divided, leaving a 2 mm cuff of tissue. The renal vein is similarly controlled and divided, freeing the allograft (Fig. 17.22). The left hand of the surgeon is inserted into the abdomen and the graft retrieved and placed in ice slush prior to cold perfusion. The sheath and muscles of the retrieval incision are closed, and check retroperitoneoscopy is performed. Hemostasis is achieved and perihilar lymphatics are clipped

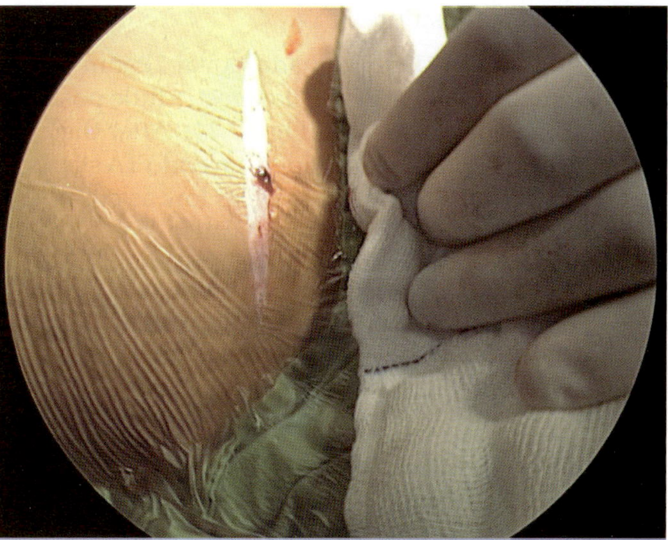

Fig. 17.20: Retrieval incision

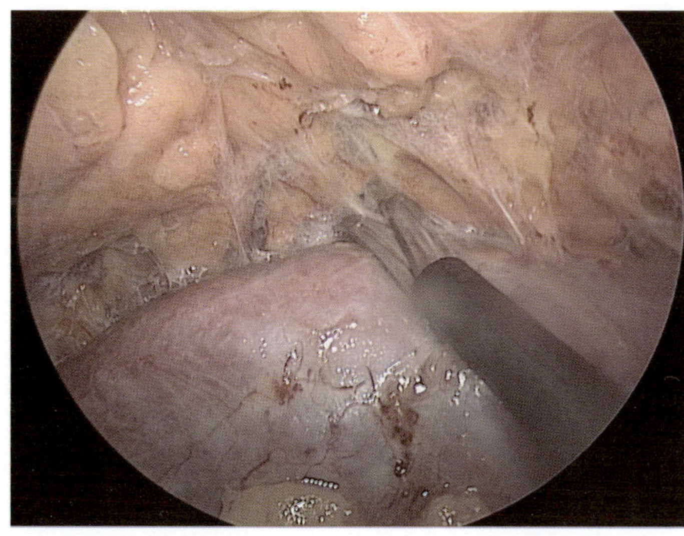

Fig. 17.18: Medial dissection of kidney

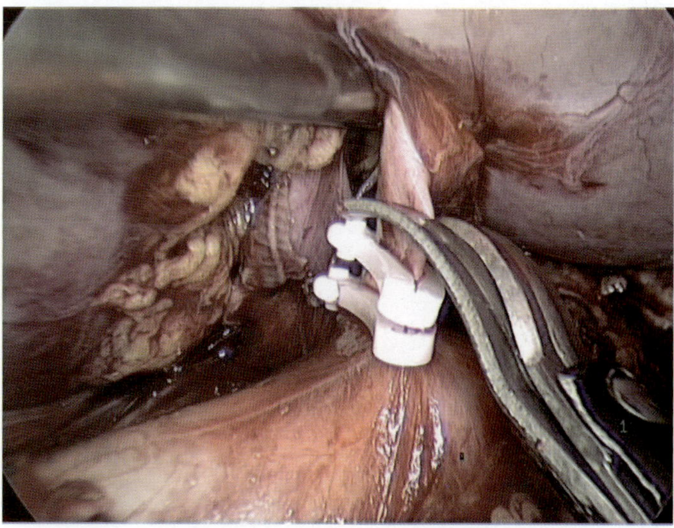

Fig. 17.21: Control of renal artery

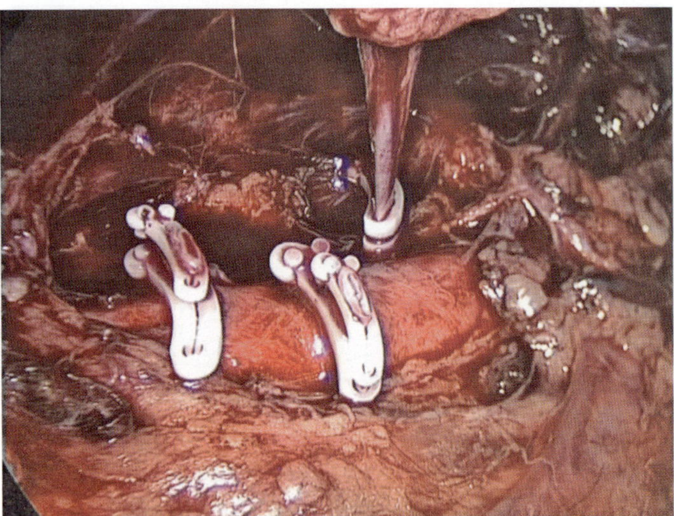

Fig. 17.22: Control of renal vein

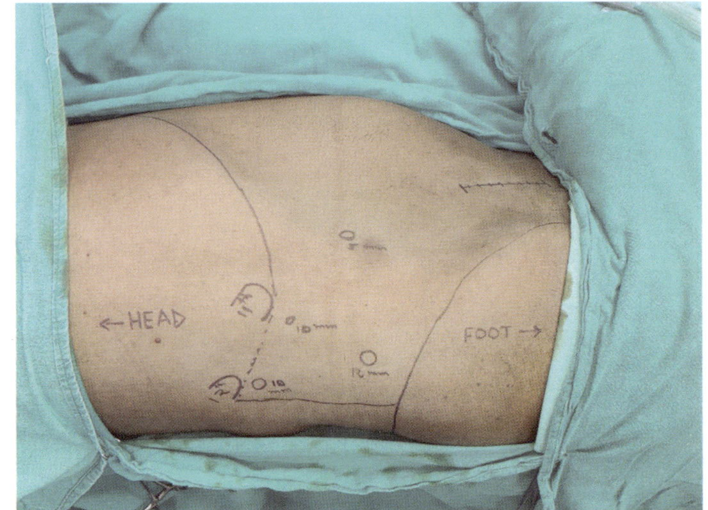

Fig. 17.24: Port placement for right-sided RLDN

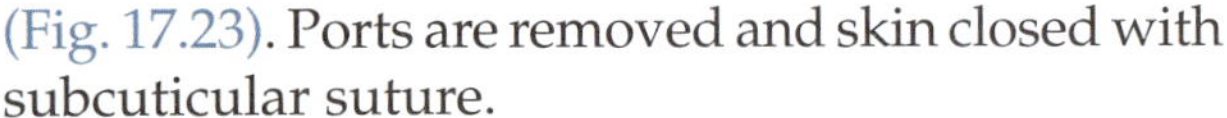

(Fig. 17.23). Ports are removed and skin closed with subcuticular suture.

Right-sided RLDN: An additional 12 mm port is placed at the level of the iliac crest, a little posterior to the mid-axillary line (Fig. 17.24). After the renal artery is clipped and divided, an endo TA stapler is inserted and fired on the IVC as low as possible at the confluence of the right renal vein (Fig. 17.25), as described at our institute.[11] This direction allows the stapler to pass parallel to the IVC, and in most cases it is possible to achieve a cuff of IVC on the renal vein (Fig. 17.26). Presence of a cuff of caval tissue makes anastomosis easier on the recipient side.

Management of peritoneal tears during RLDN: This may hamper surgical progress. A Veress needle should be placed in the peritoneal cavity and the rent close with a row of 5 mm Weck clips (Fig. 17.27).

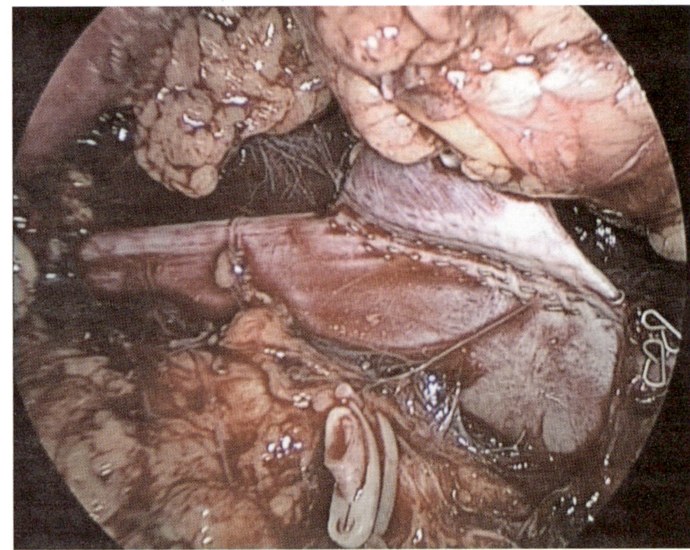

Fig. 17.25: Control of right renal vein using endoscopic stapler

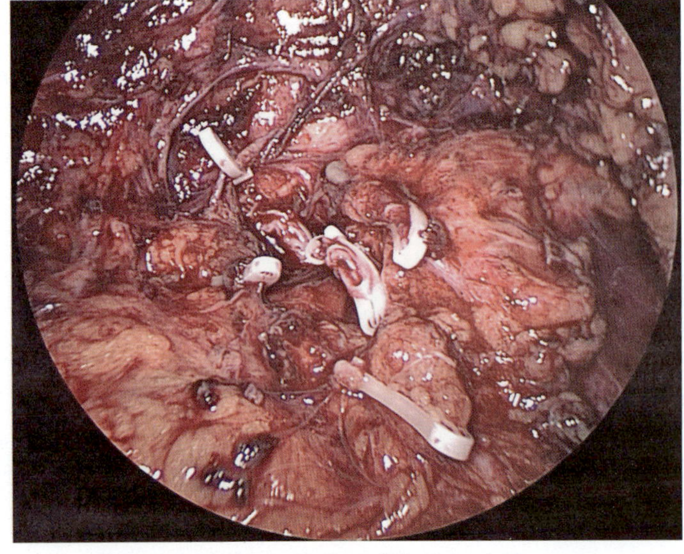

Fig. 17.23: Clipping of perihilar lymphatic tissue

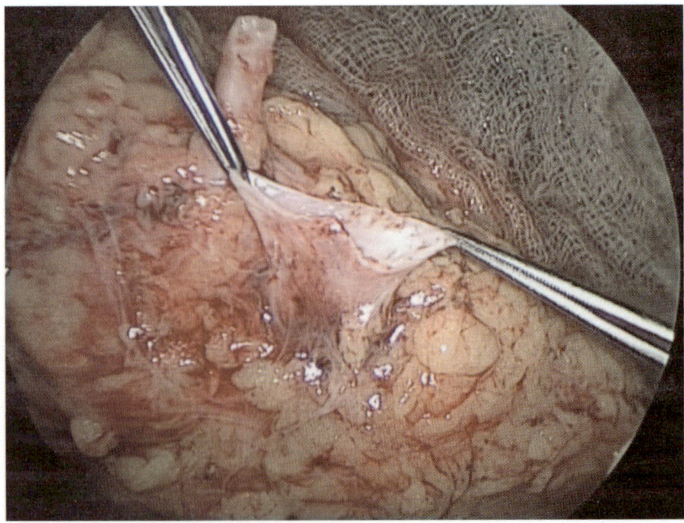

Fig. 17.26: Cuff of IVC on right renal vein

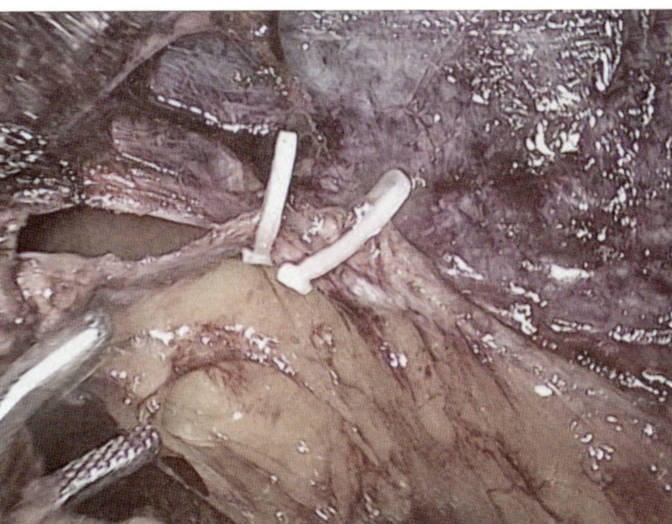

Fig. 17.27: Closure of peritoneal tears using Hem-o-Lok clips

6. What are specific anatomical challenges in donor nephrectomy and how can they be overcome?

Ans:

1. **Multiple renal arteries**: In most cases multiple renal arteries are not a contraindication to laparoscopic donor nephrectomy (Fig. 17.28). The level of complexity that is acceptable is at the discretion of the operating surgeon and team. Renal allografts with two or three renal arteries are commonly utilized in living organ transplantation with results that are similar to allografts with single arteries. Desai *et al* compared the outcomes of TLDN in donors with single versus multiple renal arteries. They reported longer operative time and warm ischaemia times with multiple renal arteries, but similar long-term recipient outcomes.[12] We have reported on our experience with pre- and post-caval renal arteries during right RLDN, and demonstrated its feasibility in this challenging scenario.[13] Small upper polar arteries can be sacrificed. Lower polar accessory arteries must be preserved as they may contribute to ureteric blood supply. During donor nephrectomy it is important to avoid undue traction or kinking of accessory arteries.
2. **Multiple right renal veins**: This presents a challenge because the veins are often short and thin walled. A vein estimated to provide < 30% of venous drainage may be sacrificed. Depending on the anatomy, two renal veins may be taken with a common cuff using a TA stapler, or the stapler may be fired twice. At our institute we have described feasibility of RLDN in right kidneys with two renal veins.[14]
3. **Retro-aortic renal vein**: This anomaly results in a shorter length of left renal vein, as the limit of dissection is the left margin of the aorta, as opposed to the right margin in the usual anatomy. If the vein opens caudally into the IVC as is sometimes the case, available length may be more. RLDN allows excellent dissection of the left renal vein to its passage behind the aorta (Fig. 17.29). TLDN may be challenging in this scenario because of the anterior approach.
4. **Circum-aortic renal vein**: The imaging should be carefully studied to ascertain the relative size of the pre- and retro-aortic components of the vein. In most instances, the retro-aortic component is small and may be sacrificed. RLDN provides unparalleled access to the retrocaval portion of the vein.
5. **Double IVC**: This anomaly creates difficulty on the left side due to the short length of the left renal vein. The renal vein may be divided at its confluence with the left-sided vena cava.

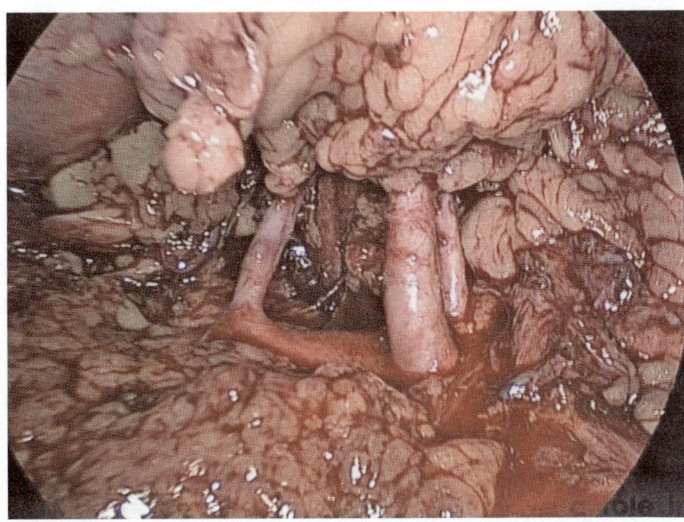

Fig. 17.28: RLDN with 3 renal arteries on the left side

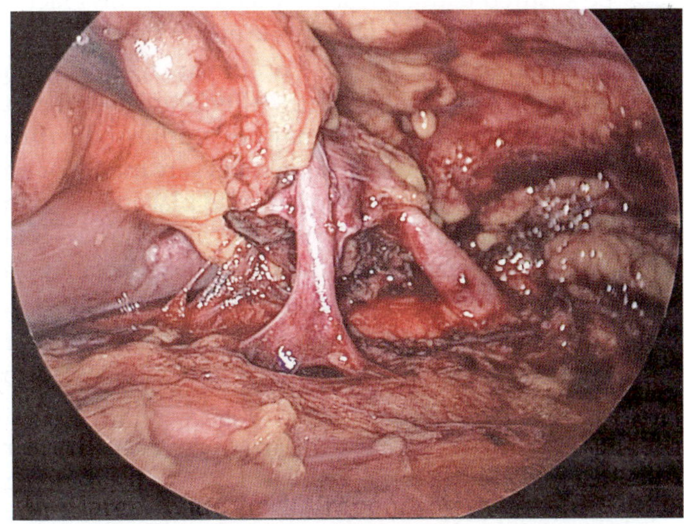

Fig. 17.29: Retro-aortic left renal vein seen at RLDN

Alternatively, TA stapler may be used to divide the left component of the IVC and use it to lengthen the left renal vein.[15] We have described our experience with RLDN in double IVC, where four cases were successfully managed with good donor and recipient outcomes.[16]

6. **Left-sided IVC**: In this situation it may be preferable to perform right DN as a longer length of renal vein will be available. If left DN is done, the cava must be preserved and the vein may be divided at its confluence with the cava using a TA stapler, analogous to a right-sided donor nephrectomy.

7. **What are the complications of laparoscopic donor nephrectomy, their prevention and management?**

Ans: Peri-operative mortality is low, reported as 3.1 per 10,000 living donations over a fifteen year period in the United States.[17] In 2018 in a retrospective review of 1430 TLDN performed over 16 years, Srivastava *et al* reported a 8.6% rate of complications, of which 2.5% were Kocak grade III and IVa.[18]

8. **What are the intraoperative complications?**

Ans: Acute bleeding: Venous causes include injury to the gonadal vein, lumbar vein, adrenal vein or renal vein. Lumbar vein injuries are particularly troublesome because of the location of the lumbar vein posteriorly and often in close approximation to the renal artery. Venous bleeding can often be significantly reduced by increasing pneumoperitoneum to 20 mm Hg. This allows the injury to be identified and dealt with. Partly avulsed tributaries are liable to bleed more because the rent is kept open by traction; clipping and division, or control with a sealing devise will often minimize the bleeding. Rents may occur in the IVC during right-sided DN. Some rents may need to be sutured using a rescue stitch of 5–0 polyglactin with a 5 mm Weck clip at one end.

Arterial bleeding may occur due to laceration of the renal artery or one of its branches. If not threatening, the bleeder may be compressed with a piece of gauze while arrangements are made for an experienced colleague to join, and placement of an additional port, if deemed necessary. Preparation should be made for blood transfusion or open conversion, if the situation warrants.

Liver/spleen injury: Usually involves capsular avulsions or minor lacerations, which respond to compression.

Bowel injury: This may involve laceration or cautery injury to the small or large bowel. Arcing of monopolar current between and active hook and other instrument should be recognized as a potential cause for this injury. If recognized on table, it can usually be repaired laparoscopically. If it goes unrecognized, delayed enteric leak may have more serious consequences.

9. **What are the postoperative complications?**

Ans: Pulmonary atelectasis may be minimised by early ambulation and chest physiotherapy. Deep vein thrombosis is a rare complication, which may be more common on the right side. Use of pneumatic compression stockings and low molecular weight heparin are used for prophylaxis. Elderly male donors may suffer acute urinary retention after catheter removal, and if this is anticipated alpha blocker therapy may be initiated prior to catheter removal.

Paralytic ileus may complicate any abdominal operation. Limited bowel handling and short operative time can reduce the incidence of paralytic ileus. In most cases it is transient and self-limiting, but can delay time to ambulation and discharge. Shoulder-tip pain is unique to TLDN. Paralytic ileus is uncommon after RLDN as small bowel handling is absent.

Post-operative wound collections may occur. Haemorrhagic collections may be managed expectantly, or rarely require exploration if they lead to instability. Chylous collections are a rare occurrence and occur due to disruption of retroperitoneal chyle-bearing lymphatics around the aorta (Fig. 17.30). It is described almost exclusively after left-sided donor nephrectomy, reflecting the preponderance of retroperitoneal lymphatics on the left side. RLDN confines chylous collections to the retroperitoneum, allowing tamponade of the leaking lymphatics. In the setting of TLDN very high volumes of chylous

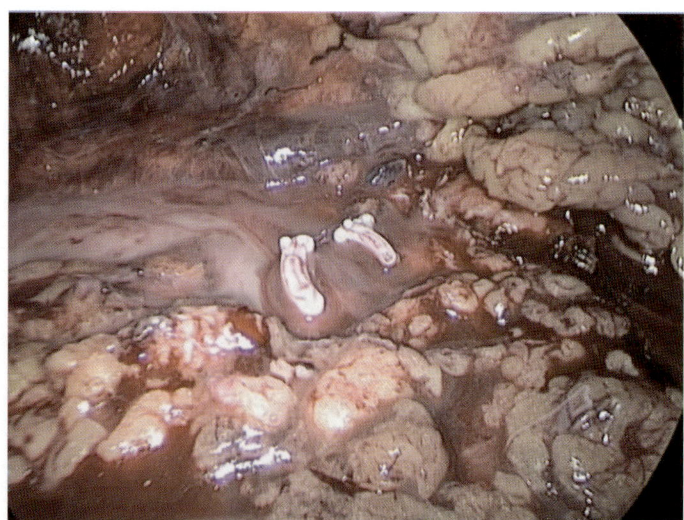

Fig. 17.30: Chylous leakage from disrupted lymphatic during left-sided RLDN

ascites may develop. This complication may be prevented by clipping peri-hilar lymphatics at the end of left laparoscopic donor nephrectomy. Treatment consists of drainage of the collection if necessary, initiation of a low-fat and medium chain triglyceride diet and administration of octreotide.[19]

Incisional hernia has been reported as between 0–4% in several series.[20] Obesity has been reported as a risk factor.[21] Optimum closure techniques should obviate this complication.

10. How should a young transplant surgeon develop a laparoscopic donor nephrectomy program?

Ans: LDN can effectively be taught and replicated. The training should follow a structured program as in any surgical procedure, i.e. theoretical background, observation, assistance, performing steps progressively under guidance of a surgical mentor, and finally performing independently. Takagi *et al* described learning curves in minimal access donor nephrectomy using CUSUM analysis, and found learning curve of 23 cases in LDN, 45 cases in hand-assisted retroperitoneal DN, and 26 cases in robot assisted DN.[22] We have described learning curves for both ablative[23] and living donor retroperitoneal laparoscopic nephrectomy.[24] Learning curve for RLDN at out institute was 35 cases. The learning curve in a high volume institute is expected to be lower than that in a lower volume institute.

Beginner surgeons performing LDN would be well advised to arrange for a senior mentor in the initial cases, and also to be mentally and logistically prepared for open conversion. While preparing for doing LDN for the first time, advantage can be taken of a high number of good quality videos available in the public domain in social media sites such as YouTube. It is also an invaluable practice to record one's own procedure and then review the surgical videos critically.

SUMMARY

- The laparoscopic approach was associated with better pain control, better respiratory function, decreased hospital stay, and earlier return to normal activities and improved cosmetic results, compared to open donor nephrectomy.
- Renal allografts with two or three renal arteries are commonly utilized in living organ transplantation with results that are similar to allografts with single arteries.
- Lower polar accessory artery must be preserved as they contribute to ureteric blood supply. During donor nephrectomy it is important to avoid undue traction or kinking of accessory arteries.
- A vein estimated to provide < 30% of venous drainage may be sacrificed. Depending on the anatomy, two renal veins may be taken with a common cuff using a TA stapler, or the stapler may be fired twice.
- Retro-aortic component of circum-aortic vein is small and may be sacrificed.
- Lumbar vein injuries are particularly troublesome because of the location of the lumbar vein posteriorly and often in close approximation to the renal artery. Venous bleeding can often be significantly reduced by increasing pneumoperitoneum to 20 mm Hg.
- Arcing of monopolar current between and active hook and other instrument should be recognized as a potential cause for bowel injury.
- Peri-operative mortality is low, reported as 3.1 per 10,000 living donations over a fifteen year period in the United States.

REFERENCES

1. Ratner LE, Ciseck LJ, Moore RG, *et al.* Laparoscopic live donor nephrectomy. Transplantation. 1995;60(9):1047-1049.
2. Simforoosh N, Basiri A, Tabibi A, *et al.* Comparison of laparoscopic and open donor nephrectomy: a randomized controlled trial. BJU Int 2005; 95:851–5.
3. Nicholson ML, Kaushik M, Lewis GR *et al.* Randomized clinical trial of laparoscopic versus open donor nephrectomy. Br J Surg. 2010 Jan;97(1):21–8.
4. Chung E, Grant AB, Hibberd AD, Sprott P. Why potential live renal donors prefer laparoscopic nephrectomy: a survey of live donor attitudes. BJU Int. 2007 Dec;100(6):1344–6.
5. Lentine KL, Kasiske BL, Levey AS. KDIGO Clinical Practice Guideline on the Evaluation and Care of Living Kidney Donors. Transplantation 2017:101 (8S–1).
6. Donor Nephrectomy. In Morris PJ, Knechtle SJ. Kidney Transplantation. Edinburgh: Elsevier; 2014.
7. Turk IA, Deger S, Davis JW *et al.* Laparoscopic live donor right nephrectomy: a new technique with preservation of vascular length. J Urol. 2002 Feb;167(2 Pt 1):630–3.
8. Kim BS, Kim KH, Yoo ES, *et al.* Hybrid technique using a Satinsky clamp for right-sided transperitoneal hand-assisted laparoscopic donor nephrectomy: comparison with left-sided standard hand-assisted laparoscopic technique. Urology. 2014 Dec;84(6):1529–34.
9. Chon CH, Chung SY, Ng CS *et al.* Looped silk tie: surgical technique for management of the renal vein during laparoscopic live-donor nephrectomy. J Endourol. 2005 Apr;19(3):401–5.
10. Gaur DD. Retroperitoneoscopy: the balloon technique. Ann R Coll Surg Engl. 1994 Jul;76(4):259–63.
11. Modi P, Kadam G, Devra A. Obtaining cuff of inferior vena cava by use of the Endo-TA stapler in retroperitoneoscopic right-side donor nephrectomy. Urology. 2007 May;69(5):832–4.
12. Desai MR, Ganpule AP, Gupta R, *et al.* Outcome of renal transplantation with multiple versus single renal arteries after laparoscopic live donor nephrectomy: a comparative study. Urology. 2007 May;69(5):824–7.
13. Modi, Pranjal & Rizvi, S.J. & Gupta, Rahul & Patel, Suhag & Trivedi, Amit. (2008). Retroperitoneoscopic Right-Sided Donor Nephrectomy with Pre-and Postcaval Renal Arteries. Urology. 72. 672–4. 10.1016/j.urology.2008.06.006.
14. Modi P and Rizvi SJ. Two Renal Veins Are Not a Contraindication for Retroperitoneoscopic Right-Side Donor Nephrectomy. J Endourol. 2008; 22(07).

15. Rizvi S.J., Prasad T.K., Modi P.R.: Retroperitoneoscopic left donor nephrectomy with duplicated IVC. Indian J Nephrol. 2012; 22: 480–481.
16. Pal, Bipin Chandra; Modi, Pranjal R.; Rizvi, Syed Jamal; *et al.*[3] Pure retroperitoneoscopic donor nephrectomy in duplication of inferior vena cava: A series of four cases. Urology Annals 9(4):p 335–338, Oct–Dec 2017.
17. Segev DL, Muzaale AD, Caffo BS, *et al.* Perioperative Mortality and Long-term Survival Following Live Kidney Donation. *JAMA.* 2010;303(10):959–966.
18. Srivastava A, Bansal A, Sureka S *et al.* A retrospective analysis of complications of laparoscopic left donor nephrectomy using the Kocak's modification of Clavien-Dindo system. IJU 2018; 34(2): 133–139.
19. Sharma S, Rizvi SJ, Modi PR. Medical management of chyloretroperitoneum following retroperitoneoscopic donor nephrectomy. Indian J Nephrol. 2014 Mar;24(2):129–30.
20. Serrano OK, Kirchner V, Bangdiwala A. Evolution of Living Donor Nephrectomy at a Single Center: Long-term Outcomes With 4 Different Techniques in Greater Than 4000 Donors Over 50 Years. Transplantation. 2016 Jun;100(6):1299–305.
21. DuBray BJ, Tompson JJ, Shaffer D. Incisional Hernia Development after Live Donor Nephrectomy: Impact of Surgical Technique. Kidney360. 2023 Jan 1;4(1):78–82.
22. Takagi K, Kimenai HJAN, Terkivatan T *et al.* Learning curves of minimally invasive donor nephrectomy in a high-volume centre: A cohort study of 1895 consecutive living donors. Int J Surg. 2021 Feb;86:7–12.
23. Saifee Y, Nagarajan R, Qadri SJ, *et al.* Retroperitoneoscopic nephrectomy for benign non-functioning kidneys: Training and outcome. Indian J Urol. 2016 Oct-Dec;32(4):301–305.
24. Pal BC, Modi PR, Rizvi SJ *et al.* The Learning Curve of Pure Retroperitoneoscopic Donor Nephrectomy. Int J Organ Transplant Med. 2017;8(4):180–185.

Chapter 18

Deceased Organ Donation (Brain Death Certification, HOTA Rules, DCD, Multi-organ Harvesting)

• *Sunil Shroff*

LEARNING OBJECTIVES

- To understand the concept of deceased organ transplantation.
- To understand the need for deceased organ transplantation and how to improve the deceased organ transplantation rate.
- To understand the Indian Transplant Law.
- To understand the brain stem death criteria.
- To understand the donation after brain death (DBD) and donation after circulatory death (DCD).

INTRODUCTION

Organ transplantation is a lifesaving procedure that has helped millions of people worldwide. Similar to the global scenario, India is also experiencing an increasing need for organ transplantation, but the availability of organs is highly inadequate. India currently performs the highest number of living donor kidney transplants in the world but only a small number of deceased donor transplants. Nonetheless, donation after brain death is gradually getting established, but the rate is still less than one per million population.

The deceased donor transplantation program though complex, is an important initiative to address the issue of organ shortage and increase the availability of organs for transplantation. It is estimated that over 67 per cent of all transplants done worldwide are from deceased donors. So far, only a small number of developing countries have managed to execute this program, and India is among the select few that has achieved some degree of success with it.[1]

Case Scenario 1

A young 28-year-old unmarried male, hypertensive, is ESRD on MHD since 1 year. His parents died of car accident 5 years ago. Currently, he does not have any live related donor.

1. **What are his prospects of receiving deceased donor in India?**

   Ans: In 2022, a total of 904 deceased donations were facilitated in India, contributing to 2765 organs, resulting in an average of 3.05 transplants per donor[2] (Figs 18.1 and 18.2). This amounts to the organ donation rate of 0.7 per million population (pmp) which is significantly lower than many developed countries like Spain, which had a donation rate of 47.02 pmp in 2022.[3]

   According to National Organ and Tissue Transplant Organization (NOTTO), close to 50,000 patients are waiting for an organ transplant,

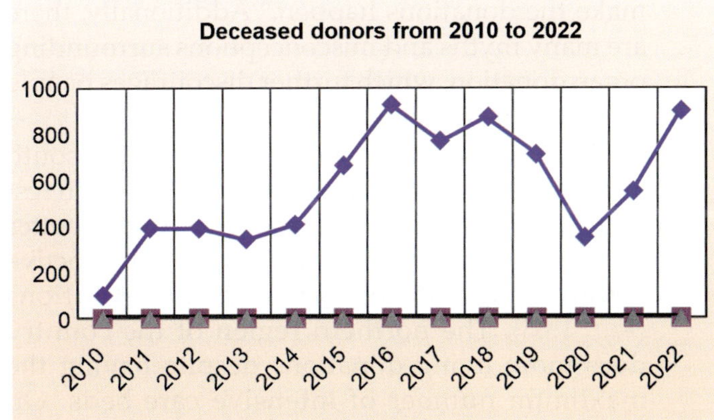

Fig. 18.1: Deceased organ donation in India (*Source*: Union Health Ministry—NOTTO)

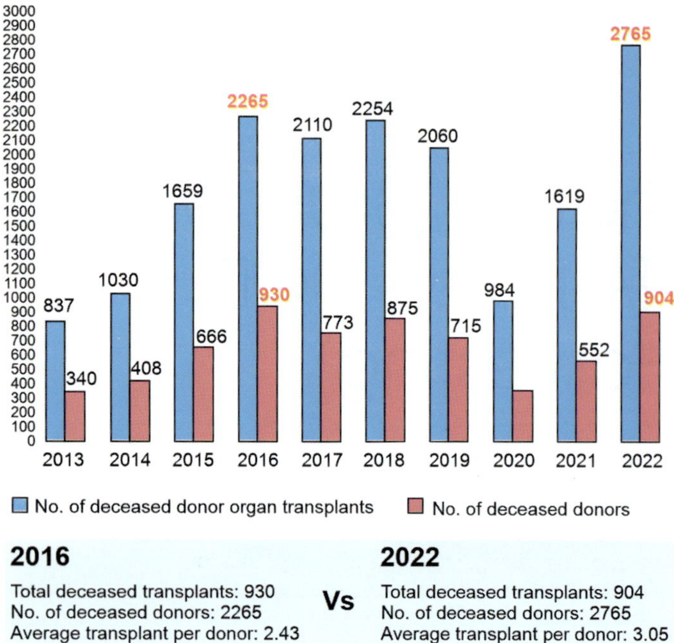

Fig. 18.2: Deceased organ transplants in India (*Source*: Union Health Ministry—NOTTO)

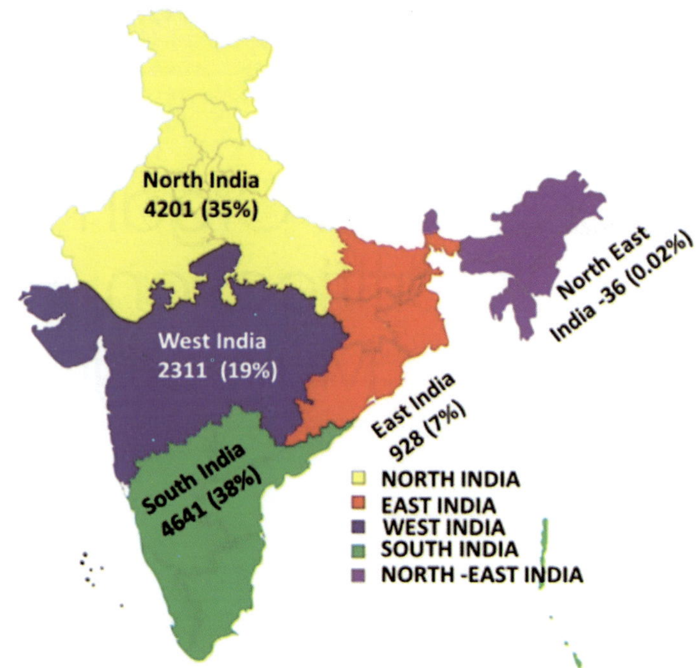

Fig. 18.3: Regional disparity in organ transplantation in India (*Courtesy:* NOTTO)

whereas only 15,561 transplants were performed nationwide in 2022.[4] The incidence of kidney failure is on an increase due to higher incidence of diabetes and hypertension. It is estimated that average crude and age-adjusted incidence rates of end-stage renal disease are estimated to be 151 and 232 per million population, respectively, in India.[5] This huge gap between need and availability of kidneys for transplantation requires multiple strategies including early diagnosis and prevention of kidney failure.

2. **What are the reasons for low donation rate?**

Ans: One of the main reasons for the low rate of donation is the lack of awareness both among the public and medical fraternity and more importantly the lack of processes in tertiary care hospital to make the donations happen.[6] Additionally, there are many myths and misconceptions surrounding organ donation, which further discourages people from donating organs.

There is also regional disparity with the south and west doing more deceased donations than rest of the country and this may partly be due to better healthcare infrastructure, manpower and proactive government and non-government institutions (Fig. 18.3). The northern region of the country does more living donations despite having the maximum number of intensive care beds. On the other hand, the eastern region has only a few transplanting hospitals.

3. **Can you describe the Transplant Law in India ?**

Ans: The organ donation and transplant activities in India are governed by the Transplantation of Human Organs Act (THOA) that was passed in 1994. In 2011 the law was amended and included tissues as well.[7] The law regulates the removal, storage, and transplantation of human organs and tissues. The law also establishes the legal framework for organ donation and transplantation in the country and covers various aspects of organ donation and transplantation, including organ procurement, consent, and registration of transplant centers and tissue banks. The act defines terms such as brain death, organ, and tissue, and establishes guidelines for the harvesting, preservation, and transplantation of organs and tissues. The important provisions of the law are listed in Table 18.1.

4. **What are the penalties under THOA Act?**

Ans: The THOA has had a significant impact on organ donation and transplantation in India. Before the passage of the Act, organ donation and transplantation were largely unregulated, and there were cases of organ trafficking and illegal transplantation. The Act with its legal framework has helped to prevent malpractices and ensure transparency. The penalties for not following the law are severe and can include fine up to Rs. 1 crore and a jail term up to 10 years (Table 18.2).

TABLE 18.1: The important provisions of Transplantation of Human Organs Act (THOA)

Brainstem death	The stage at which all functions of the brain stem have permanently and irreversibly ceased
Appropriate Authority (AA)	One of the key provisions of the law is the requirement for an appropriate authority in every state. The functions of the appropriate authority include: a. Grant / renew registration of hospitals b. Suspend / cancel registration of hospitals c. Enforce standards of care d. Investigate complaints / breach of Act, take appropriate action e. Follow-up and monitoring of hospitals and patients
Authorization committee (AC)	The AC is responsible for approving organ transplantation procedures and ensuring that the transplants are conducted in compliance with the law. The act states that organs and tissues can only be donated with the informed and expressed consent of the donor or their family members in case of deceased donation.
Registration of Hospitals	Doctors to perform donation and transplant procedures only in registered hospitals. The respective hospital is registered with the state authorities a. To undertake organ retrieval, storage and transplantation b. To undertake organ retrieval alone Requirements for hospitals to register as transplant centre / tissue bank / human organ retrieval centre • Specialised services • Skilled manpower • Equipment Registration is valid for 5 years and the renewal of license shall be done after every five years. For each organ, a separate registration is required. There is no separate registration required separately for living and deceased donation.
National Organ and Tissue Transplant Organization (NOTTO)	Another important provision of the THOA is the establishment of a National Organ and Tissue Transplant Organization (NOTTO). NOTTO is responsible for maintaining a registry of donors and recipients, coordinating and facilitating organ donation and transplantation, and ensuring compliance with the provisions of the act.
Transplant Coordinator	The Transplantation of Human Organs (Amendment) Act, 2011, requires hospitals seeking their license as transplant centers to have trained transplant coordinators. Transplant coordinator is defined as a person appointed by the hospital for coordinating all matters related to removal or transplantation of human organs or tissues or both and for assisting the authority for removal of human organs.
Required request	The law has made it mandatory for treating medical doctor in ICU along with transplant coordinator to request relatives of brain-dead patients for organ donation. It also says that recording all brain-dead patients and that of the next of kin who are approached for organ donation should be kept.
Cost for maintenance of cadaver or retrieval or transportation or preservation of organs or tissues	The provisions allow for the cost for maintenance of the cadaver (brain-stem dead declared person), retrieval of organs or tissues, their transportation and preservation, to not be borne by the donor family and may be borne by the recipient or institution or government or non-government organisation or society as decided by the respective state government or union territory administration.

TABLE 18.2: The penalties under THOA Act

Offence	*Imprisonment*	*Fine*
Removal of organs without authority	10 years	Rs. 20 Lakh
Removal of organs without authority by RMP	1st offence: De-registration for 3 years	2nd offence: Permanent de-registration
Commercial dealing in organs falsification of documents	5–10 years	Rs. 20 Lakh–1 crore
Any violation of THOA	5 years	Rs. 20 Lakh

5. **What is the profile of deceased organ donors in India?**

Ans: In contrast to the Western world, where a significant percentage of deceased donors are elderly due to lower rates of road fatalities and increased life expectancy, the donors in India are generally young as the brain deaths are from fatalities due to road traffic accidents. In a report from Tamil Nadu majority of the deceased donations came from this category that were medico-legal in nature and accounted for 76% of the total donations.[8] However, due to late identification of brain death and poor maintenance in busy public care hospitals, the serum creatinine often may go up due to acute insult. Although kidneys from these donors may experience delayed graft function when transplanted, they would generally function eventually. In such a situation, if the donor is not too unstable, the donors can be stabilised and often the creatinine reverses back to normal.

6. **How do you certify brainstem death and donor maintenance?**

Ans: Brainstem death certification criteria and donor maintenance are important aspects of the deceased donor transplantation program. Brainstem death certification is the process of determining brain death due to neurological criteria, which is the legal and medical requirement for organ donation.

Brainstem death certification: To certify brainstem death, a team of four doctors must conduct a series of tests to confirm that all functions of the brain stem have permanently and irreversibly ceased. The concerned doctors are as follows:

1. RMP in charge of hospital
2. Authorized specialist (RMP from Govt. panel approved by appropriate authority)
3. Neurologist/neurosurgeon/surgeon or physician/anaesthetist or intensivist from Govt. panel approved by appropriate authority
4. RMP treating the patient

Establishing loss of 'brainstem reflexes'

Absence of brain stem function is essential for establishing the diagnosis of brain death. In a brain stem dead patient cranial nerve reflexes are tested to observe their motor response to a sensory input. The absence of brainstem function is documented by conducting the following five tests (Table 18.3):

Apnoea test for confirming 'brainstem death'

The aim of apnoea test is to establish death of the respiratory centre in the brainstem. This is the ultimate test to establish brainstem death. It demonstrates that the spontaneous respiratory response fails to occur even in the presence of stimulatory drive from CO_2. The apnoea test may be difficult to perform, in patients with chronic airway disease or severe chest trauma.

- The $PaCO_2$ should be 40 mmHg prior to testing and should rise to at least 60 mmHg during the test.
- The patient should be pre-oxygenated with 100% oxygen for 5–10 minutes prior to testing and baseline arterial blood gases should be taken.
- Disconnect patient from ventilator but oxygen should be administered at 6 L/min via a fine bore catheter down the endotracheal tube.
- Observe patient for 8 to 10 minutes for any respiratory effort
- In the patient who is brain dead the carbon dioxide tension increases at a rate of 2 mmHg/min during apnoea testing. If the initial CO_2 tension before testing is about 40 mmHg, then arterial CO_2 tension after 10 minutes is likely to be 60 mmHg.
- Reconnect patient to the ventilator.
- Discontinue testing if any hypotension, cardiac arrhythmias or hypoxia occurs

Ancillary tests for brain death: These are not required as per the law in India. However, they may be performed to add a layer of comfort for clinicians where there are spontaneous reflexes. They include EEG, four vessel angiography, color Doppler or SPECT isotope.

Donor maintenance: Once a donor is identified, the donor maintenance shifts towards ensuring that the organs are kept well perfused and oxygenated by appropriate medical treatment of the donor, such as maintaining blood pressure, oxygen levels, avoiding hypothermia, hyper-glycemia and hypernatremia. For maintaining the blood pressure infusion of large volume of fluids and vasopressors is required in these ventilated patients.

7. **What are the contraindications to deceased donation?**

Ans: There are very few absolute contraindications to organ donation and include the following:

- Malignancy (except primary brain tumours, low grade skin malignancies and carcinoma *in situ* of the cervix)
- Uncontrolled sepsis
- Active transmissible viral infections such as HIV-AIDS, neurotropic virus—such as rabies and Creutzfeldt-Jakob disease
- Chronic organ failure

TABLE 18.3: Clinical testing for cranial nerves to diagnose absence of brainstem reflexes

S. No	*Brainstem reflexes*	*Brainstem death testing illustrations*	*Sensory and motor cranial nerve (respectively)*	*Region tested*
1.	Absence of pupillary response to light		II, (III)	Upper brainstem
2.	Absence of corneal reflexes	Sclera Cornea	V, (VII)	Mid-upper brainstem
3.	Absence of cranial nerve response to pain	Supraorbital pressure Nailbed pressure	V, (VII)	Brainstem/cerebral hemispheres
4.	Absence of vestibulo-ocular reflex	(Fast phase nystagmus) (Slow phase nystagmus) Brainstem intact (reflex present) Brainstem not intact (reflex absent)	VIII, (III, VI)	Mid-brainstem
5.	Absence of gag and cough reflexes	Palatoglossal arch Uvula	X, (IX)	Lower brainstem

Case Scenario 2

A 30-year-old female is ESRD on MHD since 2 years awaiting deceased donor kidney transplant. She receives a call for a deceased donation from a 70-year-old hypertensive male died of road traffic accident with serum creatinine of 1.2 mg/dl.

1. **What is standard criteria and expanded criteria donor?**

   Ans: A marginal deceased donor is a donor who does not meet the standard criteria for organ donation. Marginal donors may be older, have medical conditions, or have suffered from trauma or disease. While the organs of marginal donors may not be suitable for all recipients, they can be used for certain patients who may benefit from the transplantation.

   Metzger *et al* in 2002 was the first to look at marginal kidneys critically and describe a classification that divided deceased donor kidneys into standard criteria and expanded criteria donor (ECD).[9]

   Standard criteria kidneys were defined when
   - Donor age 10–39 years
   - Death was non-CVA death (stroke)
   - There was no hypertension
   - And the terminal creatinine was below 132 μ mol/L or below 1.5 mg

   Expanded criteria deceased (ECD) donors were defined as where the kidneys were from deceased donors aged 60 years or above or from donors aged 50–59 years with at least two of the following:
   - Cerebrovascular accident (CVA) as cause of death
   - Serum creatinine >1.5 mg/dL or a history of hypertension

   Although in the ECD donor the potential for less than optimum result was present but if used prudently the long-term results from these donor kidneys yielded good results. Keitel E *et al* in 2004 analyzed the outcome of transplants using expanded donor criteria (EDC) which contributed to 25.4% of the total transplants.[10] The study showed that the patient survival at 1 and 5 years was 87% vs 92% and 81% vs 79%, respectively. The graft survival at 1 and 5 years was 74% vs 82% and 57% vs 59%, respectively for EDC and ideal donors (ID).

Case Scenario 3

A 45-year-old male with ESRD on MHD since 3 years awaiting kidney transplant from deceased donor receives a call for deceased donation from a 50-year-old female died of sudden cardiac death. Should he accept this deceased donor offer?

1. **Donation after circulatory death**

   Ans: Donation after circulatory death or donation after cardiac death or non-heart beating donor is a type of deceased donation where the organs are recovered after the heart that has stopped beating. This type of donation is usually done in cases where brain death cannot be certified or in case where the family decides to withdraw life support. The first human heart transplant, performed by Christiaan Barnard in 1967, was made possible by a DCD donor and a recipient who was located in an operating room adjacent to the donor.[11]

   However, this medical achievement was not without ethical controversy, which led to the Harvard criteria for brain death in 1968.[12] As brain death was a more controlled situation, the immediate graft outcomes were superior and organ donation after brain death became a standard practice in many countries.

   DCD organs were considered inferior out of concern for ischemic injury to the organ and hence this type of donations was abandoned. However, with advancement in intensive care techniques and the ongoing shortage of organs for transplantation, coupled with many studies showing that kidneys from DCD donors yielded equivalent long-term outcomes as those from DBD donors led to reconsider about DCD programs. Additionally, while these revitalized DCD initiatives primarily concentrated on kidney procurement initially, they are now increasingly retrieving and successfully transplanting organs with lower warm ischemia tolerance, such as the liver, pancreas, and lungs. Currently in countries such as the UK, 44% of overall deceased donation rate comes from DCD organs in 2021–2022.[13]

   DCD for India: In India, brain death as a concept can be difficult to accept for both the public and professionals and in medico-legal cases the donation pathway is longer and more complex compared to the DCD pathway (Fig. 18.2). DCD provides an opportunity to people who are not comfortable with brain death concept to donate organs of their loved ones. The transplantation law in India does have provision for DCD as the law defines death under Section 2(e) of THOA as follows: Death is 'the permanent disappearance of all evidence of life by reason of brainstem death or in a cardiopulmonary sense at any time after live birth has taken'.[14] However, at present we do not have rules and guidelines for conducting DCD donations.

To push forward DCD in India, an important consensus was reached and a position paper was published in 2022 which was endorsed by eight societies.[15]

- Indian Society of Organ Transplantation
- Indian Society of Critical Care Medicine
- Society of Neuro-Critical Care
- Indian Academy of Neurology
- Indian Association of Palliative Care
- Liver Transplantation Society of India
- Indian Society for Heart and Lung Transplantation
- Indian Academy of Paediatrics

Issues to be considered with DCD donations: In 1995, the Maastricht classification for DCD was published by Koostra *et al* after the 1st **International workshop on NHB (non-heart beating) donors in Maastricht.**[16] It distinguished four categories:

- Category I: Dead on arrival
- Category 2: Death with unsuccessful reanimation
- Category 3: Awaiting cardiac death
- Category 4: Cardiac arrest while brain dead

This underwent further changes and a consensus modified the original Maastricht categories was issued at the 6th International Conference in Organ Donation held in Paris in 2013. This new criterion is based on the location and whether the procedure was controlled or uncontrolled.[17]

Modified Maastricht Classification of DCD

Warm ischemia time: The challenge in DCD donation is the prolonged warm ischemia time that can occur to the organ that can lead to rapid organ deterioration. The functional warm ischemia starts when the systolic blood pressure falls below 50 mm Hg and oxygen saturation is below 70%. The functional warm ischemia for liver and pancreas is 30 minutes, for lungs 60 minutes and for kidneys 120 minutes.

To overcome this issue, *in-situ* perfusion with cold fluid via direct cannulation of the aorta via the femoral is possible and conducting rapid laparotomy and organ retrieval. This may mean anticipating the state of asystole in operation theatre or keeping it ready. External machine perfusion of the organs is another practice to improve the quality of the organs after they have been retrieved.

No touch time in DCD: This is time from asystole to starting organ retrieval to rule out the possibility of self-resuscitation of the heart without any treatment. This time varies from country to country anywhere from 5 to 20 minutes. However, 5 minutes is the consensus that most countries tend to follow. The Academy of Medical Royal Colleges Code of Practice for the diagnosis and confirmation of death says—"the individual should be observed by the person responsible for confirming death for a minimum of five minutes to establish that irreversible cardio-respiratory arrest has occurred".[18]

Multi-Organ Retrieval Protocol (Fig. 18.4) **and Video**

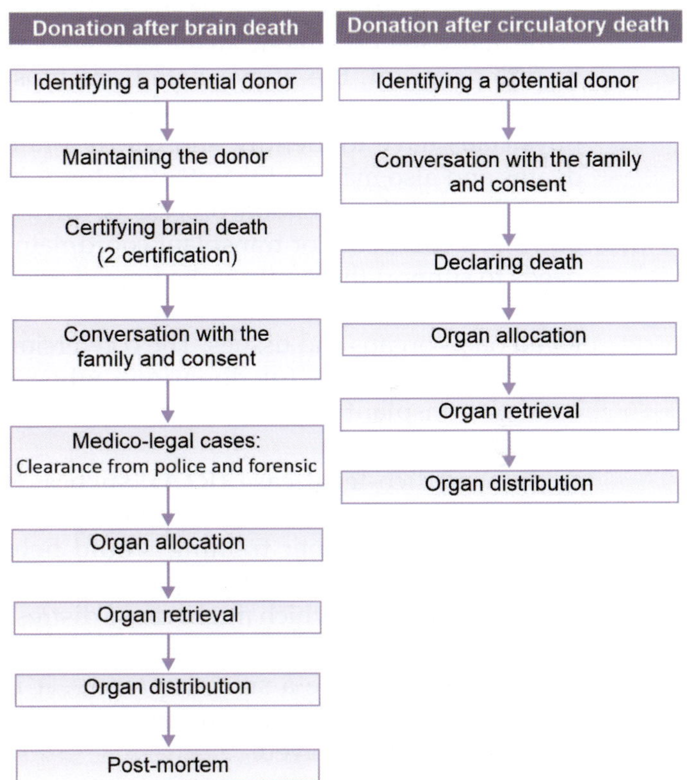

Fig. 18.4: DBD and DCD protocol

TABLE 18.4: Definition of deceased donors

Criteria	*Alternate terms*	*Diagnosis of death*
Determination of death by neurologic criteria (DDNC)	Brain death Whole brain death Brainstem death Donation after brain death (DBD)	Diagnosis and confirmation of death based on the irreversible cessation of functioning in the whole brain, including the brainstem
Determination of death by circulatory criteria (DCD)	Non-heart beating donor Donation after cardiac death	Diagnosis and confirmation of death based on the irreversible cessation of circulation followed by cardiac arrest, cardio-circulatory arrest, and respiratory arrest

This presentation will show you a standard multi-organ retrieval.

2. **What are the solutions to improve the deceased donation rate?**

Ans: To improve the deceased donation rate in India, several measures need to be taken.

a. **Awareness:** Raising awareness is crucial not only among the general public but also among medical and paramedical professionals. Effective use of print and visual media can play an important role along with celebrities and religious leaders endorsing the noble cause. The potential of social media to reach the general public in recent times should be leveraged to promote awareness on a wider scale.

b. **Capacity Building:** Structured training is a fundamental and ongoing requirement for medical professionals, especially those involved in intensive care, neurosurgery, emergency care, counselling or transplant coordination as well as at the police station. Among all the stakeholders in this program, the above listed are most important. The intensivists, neurosurgeons or physicians have to identify and certify brain deaths and also manage the potential donor in the ICU until the donation process is carried out.[19] The counsellor or transplant coordinator needs to support the family at the time of grief, help them in making a decision of donating their loved one's organs and tissues. The conversion rate for getting "yes for donation" when a trained transplant coordinator counsel is as much as 65%.[20]

In a medico-legal case (RTA), such as a road traffic accident (RTA), the police play a significant role. Proper training would help overcome undue delays in the inquest and post-mortem procedures which might cause distress among the grieving family often.[21]

In order to ensure a smooth process, it is essential to provide adequate training to all the key stakeholders involved.

c. **Transparent organ distribution system:** After the retrieval, organs and tissues are distributed as per the waiting list of the state in a very transparent and ethical manner without any ambiguity on predetermined criteria for organ sharing.[22]

d. **Strengthen the functioning of the apex body for organ donation and transplantation:** The apex national body for organ donation and transplantation is called National Organ Transplant and Tissue Organization (NOTTO) and was formed in 2014. Under NOTTO, there are five regional (ROTTO) and about 20 state level bodies (SOTTO) to oversee the coordination and networking for procurement and distribution of organs and tissues.[23] These organisations need to be supported and function with more financial autonomy.

e. **Improve donations in public sector hospitals:** The private hospitals have contributed to the growth and progress of deceased donor transplant program and almost 80 to 85% deceased donations and transplantation happen in private hospitals.

However, the true potential of the deceased donor program lies in public care hospitals. This is because 75% to 80% of all deceased donors are from road traffic accidents and because of the medico-legal nature, they are admitted to the government hospitals. If a step is taken to convert all 540 medical college hospitals or at least the 280 government medical colleges to be made organ retrieval centre in the first phase and then start kidney transplants, it not only helps boost the donation rate but also bring equity and access in this program. Currently due to lack of universal healthcare and due to transplants being expensive surgery, there is lack of access to the less affordable and the equity is tilted towards only the affordable class of citizens.[24]

f. **Enlarge potential donor pool by including donation after circulatory death:** This concept of death maybe more acceptable to the public who are not comfortable with brain death as a concept of death. Some countries have increased their donation rate by 20 to 46% by using this pool of potential donors.

KEY POINTS

- Over the past 28 years, India has made significant strides in deceased organ donation since the transplant law was enacted, resulting in the saving of over 15,000 lives.
- The benefits of this initiative extend beyond kidney failure patients, with individuals requiring heart, lungs, liver, pancreas, small intestine, and hand transplants all benefiting.
- Additionally, there has been an increase in the donation of corneas, skin, and bones.
- However, the progress has been skewed towards the private sector, with affording patients from private sector hospitals being the primary beneficiaries.
- With an increase in government spending on healthcare and the introduction of schemes such as Ayushman Bharat and state-sponsored programs to aid with transplants, we can expect to see a rise in the rate of deceased donations and an increase in such transplants.
- India's robust laws pave the way for the initiation of DCD transplants, providing a new opportunity for the development of transplant sciences, which will ultimately benefit patients and offer a new career pathway for young graduates.

ACKNOWLEDGEMENTS

My heartfelt thanks to MOHAN Foundation for the images and flow diagrams from their resource material and Ms.Sujatha Surtyamoorthi, Associate Course Director from the Foundation for her help with checking facts and stats of the article.

REFERENCES

1. Georgi Abraham, Yuvaram N.V. Reddy, Yogesh N.V. Reddy, Sunil Shroff, Milly Mathew, Sundarajan Saravanan, Evolution of deceased-donor transplantation in India with decline of commercial transplantation: a lesson for developing countries, Kidney International Supplements, Volume 3, Issue 2, 2013, Pages 190–194, ISSN 2157–1716, https://doi.org/10.1038/kisup.2013.12.
2. Shroff S, Sujatha S. Progress with Deceased Donation in India. Indian Transplant Newsletter. Vol.22 Issue No.67, November 2022-February2023. Available at: https://www.itnnews.co.in/indian-transplant-newsletter/issue67/Progress-with-Deceased-Donation-in-India-1199.htm.
3. https://www.transplant-observatory.org/
4. https://www.newindianexpress.com/nation/2023/mar/28/nearly-50000-people-waiting-for-organ-replacement-in-india-says-centre-2560389.html.
5. Modi GK, Jha V. The incidence of end-stage renal disease in India: a population-based study. Kidney Int. 2006 Dec;70(12):2131–3. doi: 10.1038/sj.ki.5001958. Epub 2006 Oct 25. PMID: 17063176.
6. Kute V, Ramesh V, Shroff S, Guleria S, Prakash J. Deceased-Donor Organ Transplantation in India: Current Status, Challenges, and Solutions. Exp Clin Transplant. 2020 Jul;18(Suppl 2):31–42. doi: 10.6002/ect.rlgnsymp2020.L6. PMID: 32758118.
7. https://main.mohfw.gov.in/acts-rules-and-standards-health-sector/acts/transplantation-human-organs-acts-and-rules.
8. Dr. P. Balaji, Dr. S. Shroff, Mr. Karunakaran C.E., Annual Report from Tamil Nadu Organ Sharing Registry for the year April 2016-March 2017.
9. Metzger RA, Delmonico FL, Feng S, Port FK, Wynn JJ, Merion RM. Expanded criteria donors for kidney transplantation. Am J Transplant 2003;3 Suppl 4:114–25.
10. Keitel E, Michelon T, dos Santos AF, Bittar AE, Goldani JC, D'almeida Bianco P, Bruno RM, Losekann A, Messias AA, Bender D, Bianchini JJ, Duro Garcia V. Renal transplants using expanded cadaver donor criteria. Ann Transplant. 2004;9(2) 23–24. PMID: 15478909.
11. Barnard CN. The operation. A human cardiac transplant: an interim report of a successful operation performed at Groote Schuur Hospital, Cape Town. S Afr Med J. 1967 Dec 30;41(48):1271–4. PMID: 4170370.
12. A definition of irreversible coma. Report of the Ad Hoc Committee of the Harvard Medical School to Examine the Definition of Brain Death. JAMA. 1968 Aug 5;205(6):337–40. PMID: 5694976.
13. https://www.odt.nhs.uk/deceased-donation/best-practice-guidance/donation-after-circulatory-death/
14. https://main.mohfw.gov.in/sites/default/files/Act%20 1994.pdf.
15. Seth AK, Mohanka R, Navin S, Gokhale AG, Sharma A, Kumar A, Ramachandran B, Balakrishnan KR, Mirza D, Mehta D, Zirpe KG, Dhital K, Sahay M, Simha S, Sundaram R, Pandit R, Mani RK, Gursahani R, Gupta S, Kute VB, Shroff S. Organ Donation after Circulatory Determination of Death in India: A Joint Position Paper. Indian J Crit Care Med. 2022 Summer;26(4):421–438. doi: 10.5005/jp-journals-10071–24198.
16. Kootstra G, Daemen JH, Oomen AP. Categories of non-heart-beating donors. Transplant Proc. 1995 Oct;27(5):2893–4. PMID: 7482956.
17. Thuong M, Ruiz A, Evrard P, Kuiper M, Boffa C, Akhtar MZ, Neuberger J, Ploeg R. New classification of donation after circulatory death donors definitions and terminology. Transpl Int. 2016 Jul;29(7):749–59. doi: 10.1111/tri.12776. Epub 2016 May 4. PMID: 26991858.
18. https://www.aomrc.org.uk/wp-content/uploads/2016/04/Code_Practice_Confirmation_Diagnosis_Death_1008–4.pdf
19. Palaniswamy V, Sadhasivam S, Selvakumaran C, Jayabal P, Ananth SR. Organ donation after brain death in India: A trained intensivist is the key to success. Indian J Crit Care Med. 2016 Oct;20(10):593–596. doi: 10.4103/0972–5229.192049. PMID: 27829715; PMCID: PMC5073774.
20. Abraham G, Vijayan M, Gopalakrishnan N, Shroff S, Amalorpavanathan J, Yuvaraj A, Nair S, Sundarrajan S. State of deceased donor transplantation in India: A model for developing countries around the world. World J Transplant. 2016 Jun 24;6(2):331–5. doi: 10.5500/wjt.v6.i2.331. PMID: 27358778; PMCID: PMC4919737.
21. Thyagarajan, Ishwarya; Shroff, Sunil, Vincent, Britzer Paul; Rajendran, Juhija; Kanvinde, Hemal; Shankar, Siva; Aneesh, Kavitha. Knowledge and Practice of Organ Donation Among Police Personnel in Tamil Nadu: A Cross-Sectional Study. Indian Journal of Transplantation 14(2):p 141–146, Apr–Jun 2020. | DOI: 10.4103/ijot.ijot_56_19.
22. Shroff, Sunil. "Challenges in setting up of a deceased donor transplant program in South Asia." *Indian Journal of Transplantation*, vol. 12, no. 3, July-Sept. 2018, p. 161.
23. https://notto.gov.in/
24. Shroff, JS Gill. Bold policy changes are needed to meet the need for organ transplantation in India. S American Journal of Transplantation 21 (9), 2933-2936.

Section

7

Endourology

Chapter

1

Renal Colic in Young Lady

• *Mahesh Desai* • *Niramya Pathak*

LEARNING OBJECTIVES

To understand

- The pathophysiology of ureteral colic.
- The important points in history taking in a case of ureteral colic.
- How to approach and investigate a patient with ureteral colic.
- The emergency management options in acute colic.
- The management options depending on host and stone characteristics.
- Recurrence prevention measures and follow-up protocol.
- The recent advances.

Case Scenario

A 30 years old lady presented with left flank radiating colicky pain for 2 days. USG showed left mild to moderate hydronephrosis. NCCT scan was done which was suggestive of left mid-ureter calculus of about 7.8 × 7.4 × 9.9 mm with proximal moderate hydroureteronephrosis with HU of 903 (Fig. 1.1).

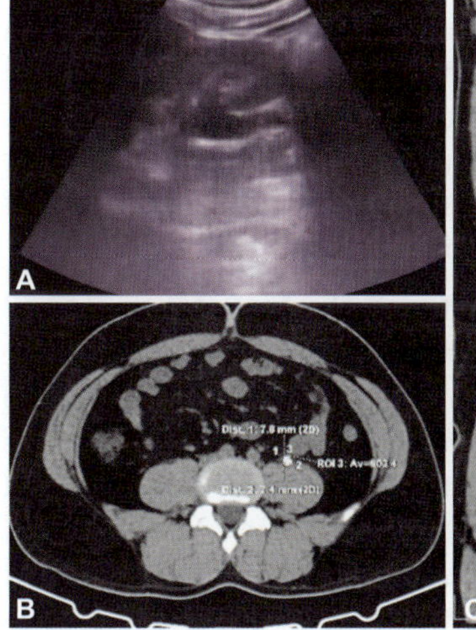

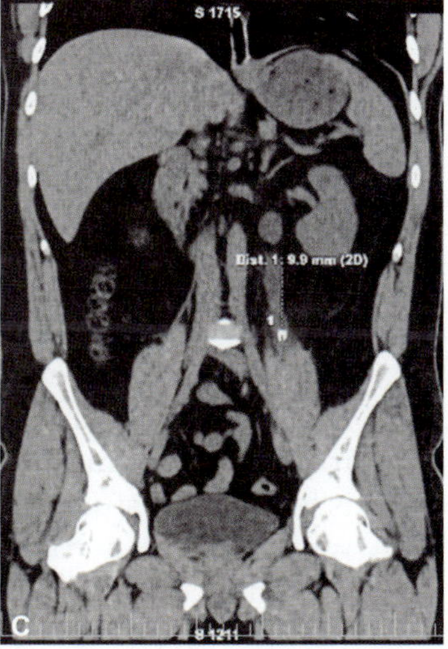

Fig. 1.1A to C: (A) USG KUB (upper left): Image of left kidney showing hydronephrosis with preserved parenchyma; (B) CT scan KUB (lower left): Axial image, through the stone showing cross sectional stone size; (C) Reconstructed CT KUB image (right side): Coronal view showing stone dimensions

1. **What are the important points in history?**

   Ans: The history of present illness is important. The pain needs to be classified as acute or chronic, continuous, or intermittent, localised, or radiating, mild-moderate-severe in intensity, colicky in character, changes on change in position, timing and aggravating and relieving factors for the same. Associated symptoms like nausea, vomiting and its relation with pain episode needs to be looked into. Hydration status of patient, urine output, date of the last menstrual period, family history, medication history, dietary excess, fluid intake, intestinal disease, skeletal fractures, gout, solitary kidney, anatomical abnormalities, renal insufficiency, metabolic stones history are the other additional points to be considered while taking the history of the patient.[1]

2. **What next? What are the baseline investigations?**

   Ans: Since the patient has come to us with ureteral colic, we will subject the patient to baseline investigations in the form of urine routine and microscopy and blood investigations in the form complete blood count, serum creatinine. This is followed by a screening imaging study in the form of ultrasound of KUB region and thereafter a definitive imaging study will be done for further characterization of the stone in the form of non-contrast CT scan of KUB region (NCCT).[1,2]

3. **Can serum creatinine be raised in unilateral ureteral stone? If yes, when?**

   Ans: Yes, serum creatinine and overall kidney function can be affected even in presence of unilateral ureteral stone in following conditions—sepsis, dehydration, solitary functioning kidney with ureteral stone, nephrotoxic drugs, obstruction due to non-stone pathology in contralateral kidney, reflex vascular constriction and ureteral spasm in contralateral kidney.[2]

4. **What is the role of USG KUB?**

   Ans: Ultrasound KUB is the screening or bedside investigation of choice and has a sensitivity of 61% and specificity of 97%. Its advantages include safety, availability, less learning curve, no radiation, kidney architecture can be made out, anatomical abnormalities can be known, parenchymal thickness can be seen and pathology like dilation of PCS/ureter and degree of severity can be known. Disadvantages include low sensitivity, subjective investigation, underestimation of size, mid and lower ureter difficult to visualize due to interposing bowel segments. Ultrasound KUB also helps in getting an idea on the severity and chronicity of the obstruction by focussing on the degree of hydronephrosis and the thickness of parenchyma. There are various classifications for the degree of hydronephrosis. The one that is used most commonly is the SFU classification that grades hydronephrosis into four grades. Grade 1 is mild dilation of the renal pelvis without calyceal dilation, grade 2 is dilation of renal pelvis and major calyces, grade 3 is minor calyceal dilation and grade 4 is parenchymal thinning. The sensitivity of ultrasound can be improved upon by looking for certain things like post-acoustic shadowing and looking for twinkling sign and seeing the ureteral jet on the affected side by focussing on the bladder and by measuring the RI which is elevated on the ipsilateral side during acute colic episode.[1,3,4]

5. **What is the role of X-ray KUB? Is there any role in emergency in acute colic?**

   Ans: It does not have a definitive role in emergency if CT scan is available. With a sensitivity of 57% and specificity of 76%, X-ray KUB is used as a baseline work-up, to identify stone opacity and predict stone type and as part of follow-up regimen. Its drawbacks are that it has low sensitivity and the minimum stone size required to be seen on image is 3 mm.[1]

6. **What is the role of intravenous urography? Should it be done in acute colic?**

   Ans: Intravenous urography should be avoided in acute colic since the kidney function on the side is generally affected due to tubuloglomerular feedback and the contrast would not concentrate or excrete in the pelvicalyceal system. It may not help in most situations and may need prolonged study to identify function. With a sensitivity of 70% and specificity of 95%, intravenous urography is used as a baseline investigation for kidney function, to know opposite kidney function, to delineate pelvicalyceal and ureteral anatomy and visualize lucent stones. Its drawbacks are IV contrast use and its attendant complications of contrast.[1]

7. **What is the role of CT scan?**

   Ans: With a sensitivity of 98% and specificity of 97%, NCCT is the investigation of choice or gold standard for diagnosis. Its advantages include non-subjective investigation, exact size can be estimated, mid and lower ureteral stones can be visualized, kidney pathology, hydronephrosis, anatomical abnormalities can be detected, parenchymal thickness can be known, retrorenal colon can be identified, perinephric collection can be identified, identification of any other organ pathology may be detected, can help detect impaction of the stone by measuring the ureteral wall thickness at the site of impaction, can also help to differentiate infected hydronephrosis vs pyonephrosis in an infected system. The disadvantages include radiation risk, availability, cost.[1,3] Sometimes in non-dilated system, differentiation of lower ureteric stone from phlebolith may be difficult.

8. **Can we reduce the radiation of NCCT by a low dose protocol?**

   Ans: If the radiation dose used is less than 3 mSV, then it is called low dose CT scan. The intention is to preserve the diagnostic accuracy of NCCT and reduce the radiation exposure.[1] Overall utilization has been low. Accuracy is less in patients with a high BMI more than 30. The sensitivity and specificity are more than 90%. If less than 1 mSV is used, then it is called ultra-low dose CT scan, but it is less accurate with specificity and sensitivity of 70–80% and stones 3 mm or less can be missed.[2]

9. **What is the role of CT urography for ureteral stone?**

   Ans: If good parenchymal thickness and stone location is mid and lower ureter, then there is no role of CT urography. But if parenchymal thickness is less, then a study with CT urography is required which gives a rough estimate of function. If proximal ureteral stone and abnormal USG and risk of retropulsion is there, then CT urography is recommended.[5]

10. **What is stone protocol in NCCT?**

    Ans: Thin axial slices of CT scan less than 5 mm from upper pole of kidney to base of urinary bladder.

With 120 kVp with manufacturer recommended settings.[6]

11. **What is dual energy CT (DECT) scan?**

Ans: Simultaneous scanning using two different energies which permits differentiation of stone composition is called dual energy CT scan. It helps to differentiate stone composition such as uric acid, calcium phosphate, cystine, struvite and calcium oxalate. It is not useful during acute episode of colic.[1]

12. **What additional information would you get from CT urography vs NCCT scan?**

Ans: CT urography gives 3D reconstruction of PCS and stone helps in precise knowledge of anatomy of PCS and stone. It is a functional study which helps to visually compare function of both kidneys. Anatomical and functional or physiological obstruction can be differentiated. Postoperative urinoma or collection evaluation can be done.[5]

13. **What is UWT? What is its significance?**

Ans: Ureteral wall thickness is the thickness of ureteral wall as seen on non-contrast CT scan at the site of stone in the ureter. It is useful in predicting the spontaneous passage of ureteral stones less than 10 mm size and success or failure of MET. Cut-off values are variably reported as 2.71/3.49/3.8 mm as per different publications. Higher UWT value correlates positively with presence of ureteral oedema, polyps, stone impaction, longer operating times, lower stone free rates, lower chances of ESWL success and lower risk of spontaneous passage (Fig. 1.2).[7–9]

14. **What is ureteral colic? What is its pathophysiology?**

Ans: Intermittent spasmodic flank pain radiating in nature from flank to groin is a typical ureteral colic. Its pathophysiology is as follows:

When there is ureteral obstruction due to stone, there is spasm due to irritation of ureteral smooth muscle, there is an increase in intra-pelvic pressure, causing stretch on renal pelvis and renal capsule causing flank pain. This will increase hydrostatic pressure and failure of peristalsis. This will reduce the pressure and reduce the pain. Also, stone movement down the ureter also causes intermittent obstruction. When complete obstruction, then again, the above-mentioned cycle repeats. So, pain is intermittent and colicky pain is due to smooth muscle of ureter irritation and spasm. Radiating pain is due to similar dermatomal distribution of parietal and visceral nerves meeting in the spinal cord along the ilio-hypogastric, ilio-inguinal and genito-femoral somatic nerves respectively for upper, mid and lower ureter.[10]

15. **What are the percentage chances of spontaneous evacuation ureteral stone?**

Ans: It depends on stone location and stone size in the form of transverse diameter. For distal ureteral stone spontaneous passage chances are high at 71% and for proximal ureteral stone it is low at 22%. For stones sizes less than or equal to 5 mm in transverse diameter it is 68%, and for 6 to 10 mm it is 47%.[1]

16. **What is MET? What are its indications and contraindications? Medicines used? What is duration of MET? What factors affecting MET?**

MET is medical expulsion therapy, where medicines are administered to relax the ureter

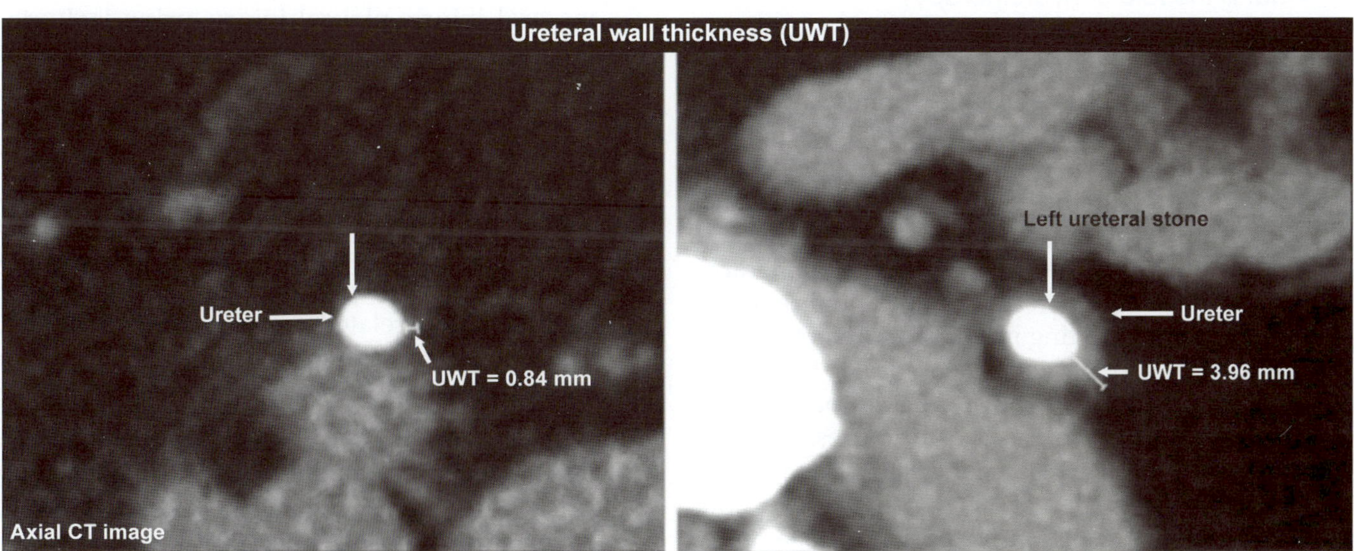

Fig. 1.2: Non-contrast CT scan of UWT. [9] (CT KUB axial images at the level of the stone showing ureteral stone with increased ureteral wall thickness in left image vs right image)

to allow spontaneous passage of ureteral stone. Its advantage is that there is 57% increase in spontaneous passage for distal ureteral stone of more than 5 mm size. The indications of MET are absence of UTI, ureteral stone less than 10 mm in size, compliant and well-informed patient and tolerable symptoms. Its contraindications include active UTI, ureteral stone in solitary functioning kidney, non-tolerable intractable pain, elevated creatinine levels.

Medicines used in MET are the following class of drugs.

a. Alpha blocker: Relaxes lower ureteral smooth muscle alpha-1A receptor, tamsulosin and silodosin. Only drug class which are guideline and FDA approved.
b. Deflazocort: Decreases inflammation and oedema that are associated with stone. Not in guidelines as not supported by high level evidence.
c. PDE5 inhibitors: Tadalafil. It affects cGMP pathway and causes smooth muscle relaxation. Not in guidelines.
d. Calcium channel blockers: Nifedipine—smooth muscle relaxant. Not supported by guidelines.

Duration of MET is up to a period of 4 weeks if no contraindications as mentioned above.

Factors affecting MET include location of stone in ureter, transverse diameter of stone, multiple stones, recurrent stone, degree of dilation proximal to stone.

Combination therapy with alpha blocker has poor evidence for support.[1,3,11] Recent meta-analysis and systematic review suggests better efficacy of silodosin vs tamsulosin.[12]

17. What is the role of hydrotherapy?

Ans: Hydrotherapy is often used for acute colic by family physicians or general practitioners. Sadly, there is no literature data, expert opinion or level 1 evidence for this treatment. In this method, patient is hospitalised and infused with high volume fluids and diuretics with the hope that the fluid pressure builds up in the pelvicalyceal system will force the urine to push the stone distally. This therapy is practically found to reduce the time that the patient spends waiting in MET for ureteral stones less than 10 mm in size.[10] Theoretically, this is not advisable, because if the stone is impacted, the resultant build-up of hydrostatic pressure will cause tubuloglomerular feedback to cause afferent arteriolar constriction at the glomerular level and affect the renal function further and it is akin to 'flogging an already tired horse'.[13] It has also been shown to result in urinoma formation.

18. What is role of analgesics?

Ans: Orally, NSAIDs are better than paracetamol and that is better than opioids. Amongst analgesics, oral ibuprofen is better than ketorolac. Parenterally, intramuscular diclofenac is better than intravenous ibuprofen and IV ketorolac. Antispasmodic addition to analgesic though done routinely does not result in better pain control. For the prevention of recurrent pain, NSAID tablets like diclofenac help reduce inflammation and pain.[3] Although diclofenac can affect renal function specially in patients with already reduced function, it has no functional effect in patients with normal renal function.[14]

19. What is a better technique for deobstruction in a case of obstructive uropathy due to stone–PCN or DJ stenting?

Ans: If analgesia cannot be achieved medically in a patient with acute colic, drainage methods such as stenting, percutaneous nephrostomy or active stone removal are indicated.[3] If there is sepsis with anuria in a patient with ureteral colic, then only decompression via stenting or PCN is to be done and definitive stone treatment is to be done after sepsis resolves.[3] PCN is generally considered to be a better method for decompression if there is an additional component of infection such as pyonephrosis, otherwise DJ stent is better.

Advantages of PCN placement are better drainage, can be flushed if tube gets blocked, can be placed under local anaesthesia, nephrostogram can be done for evaluation of obstruction on follow-up, differential function can be estimated. Disadvantages include maintenance of the tube is difficult, tube dislodgement is possible and complications while PCN placement like bleeding, visceral injury, pleural injury, urine leak, poor quality of life, longer fluoroscopy time, longer hospital stay.

The advantages of DJ stent placement include no tube outside, hence no problem of maintenance. No PCN placement complications with safety, shorter fluoroscopy time, shorter hospital of stay and a better quality of life. Disadvantages are that it cannot be done under local anaesthesia, patient may have stent related symptoms and obviously a nephrostogram, assessment of differential function are not possible. Stents can get blocked since the lumen is very small.[15,16]

20. How to prevent recurrent colic?

Ans: The prevention of recurrent colic essentially is prevention of stone recurrence. This will depend on three factors such as stone composition analysis is available, evaluation of risk factors for recurrence and basic evaluation which includes evaluation of urine and blood such as calcium, phosphorus and uric acid. If the patient is at a low risk for recurrence, then he is advised for general preventive measures which include fluid intake advice, nutritional advice for a balanced diet and lifestyle to normalise general risk factors. If the patient is at a high risk for recurrence, then he is subjected to metabolic evaluation for stone and thereafter he is put on stone specific recurrence preventive measures.[3]

21. **What nutritional advice is to be given during colic episode?**

Ans: The fluid intake advice is as follows: Fluid amount of 2.5–3 litres per day, neutral pH beverages consumption, and urine output target of 2–2.5 litres per day. The nutritional advice is as follows: Consumption of a balanced diet, rich in vegetables and fibre, normal calcium content of 1 gm per day, limited salt content of 4–5 gm per day, limited animal protein content of 1 gm per kg per day.[3]

22. **What is MIMIC calculator?**

Ans: MIMIC is spontaneous stone passage (SSP) prediction calculator that provides an estimated prediction for SSP based on collected multi-centre data. This nomogram is an adjunctive tool developed to guide patient counselling on the predicted probability of SSP. This calculator is based on data from MIMIC which was a multi-centre cohort study assessing the predictors of spontaneous stone passage amongst 4171 patients in 71 sites across 7 different countries.[17,18]

23. **What is the role of antibiotics in ureteral colic? When is it to be given? How is it to be given? Which antibiotics are better?**

Ans: Antibiotics have no role in ureteral colic in absence of any infection. The indication of antibiotics is in the following conditions, ureteral colic with culture proven urinary tract infection and if an intervention is planned and preprocedural culture proven infection is present. If an intervention is planned and there is no infection preoperatively, then the antibiotic should be ideally given as a single preoperative antibiotic dose. The available literature and guidelines do not recommend postoperative antibiotics. Finally, the choice of antibiotic duration dose and should be as per institutional antibiogram.[3,19,20] Fluoroquinolones, second or third generation cephalosporins and carbapenems NFT is not advised for upper tract in fections are the drug classes which have good sensitivity for the common urinary pathogens.[1] Routine total leukocyte count and CRP can be done as part of initial complete blood count to provide information on the severity of inflammation but it should not be the indication for starting antibiotics.[21] In fact, they are used to predict the rates of spontaneous stone passage.[22]

24. **What is role of ureterorenoscopy during acute colic? What are the advantages and disadvantages?**

Ans: Ureterorenoscopy and active removal of stone is indicated in the following situations—stones with a low likelihood of spontaneous passage, persistent pain despite adequate analgesic medication, persistent obstruction, renal insufficiency. The advantages are that it can be done safely in bleeding disorders, lesser need of reinterventions, safe in obese patients, better stone free rate. Disadvantages are greater complication rates, longer hospital stay and more need of adjunctive procedures like stent placement and removal.[23]

25. **What is the role of SWL in acute colic?**

Ans: The indications of SWL are the same as those for URS as mentioned above. The advantages being lower morbidity, shorter hospital stay and lesser need of adjunctive procedures. The disadvantages being need of reinterventions, cannot be done safely in obese patients and stone free rates are less.[23,24]

26. **If the patient is a foreigner who is in India for family function and want to travel back to his native country, is air travel permitted? What are the guidelines?**

Ans: This patient with stone in ureter at present has a high risk of pain without any intervention, hence is currently unfit to work and overseas travel. He requires treatment like stenting or active stone removal to reduce the risk and make him fit for travel.[25]

27. **What are the indications of DJ stenting after URSL?**

Ans: The indications of DJ stenting after URSL are ureteral perforation, ureteral oedema, preoperative significant hydroureteronephrosis, infected system, residual fragments, solitary functioning kidney, prolonged surgery, pregnancy and bleeding. The ideal duration of stent placement is 7 to 14 days.[3]

28. **What if the patient in the question presents with UPT (urine pregnancy test) positivity?**

Ans: Evaluation is done with USG with Doppler to see for urine jet. Can assess the resistive index if stone is impacted. CT scan and X-ray are contraindicated amongst investigations. ESWL is contraindicated amongst treatment options. First trimester or third trimester and symptomatic patient, MET can be done if eligible, since it has a higher success rate in view of physiological dilation. If MET fails or patient is not eligible, then DJ stenting needs to be done but it requires to be changed repeatedly due to early encrustation. In the second trimester, URS with laser or pneumatic lithotripsy is considered safe.[3,1]

29. **How to follow-up after stone clearance?**

Ans: Follow-up of stone disease patients is based on whether the patient is rendered completely stone free and based on whether he is at a high risk for stone recurrence. If patient is completely stone free, then he is subjected to X-ray or ultrasound follow-up based on stone opacity every six months for 1 year and then yearly for a minimum duration of 5 years. If the patient has residual stone fragments which are 4 mm or less, then he is subjected to the same protocol as above but if the residual stone fragments are more than 4 mm, then he is scheduled for a re-intervention and thereafter put on follow-up as above. If there are high risk factors for stone recurrence, then patient is put on the same imaging protocol as above and in addition he is advised for metabolic evaluation and advised medical treatment with follow-up for minimum duration of 4 years and discharge from follow-up only if non-progressive disease. If the patient opts out of medical treatment, then he is advised follow-up as above for a period of 10 years.[3]

SUMMARY

- Screening or primary bedside investigation for suspected ureteral colic is USG KUB.
- Investigation of choice or gold standard for diagnosis in a suspected case of ureteral colic is NCCT KUB.
- Serum creatinine can be elevated even in unilateral colic when associated with sepsis, dehydration or in patients with solitary functioning kidney. Nephrotoxic drugs, obstruction due to non-stone pathology in contralateral kidney, reflex vascular constriction and ureteral spasm in contralateral kidney may also play a role.
- Stone treatment varies as per stone location and transverse diameter of the stone.
- Chances of spontaneous stone passage are as follows:
  - Distal ureteral stone = 71%
  - Proximal ureteral stone = 22%
  - Less than 5 mm size = 68%,
  - 6 to 10 mm = 47%
- MET increases the spontaneous passage for distal ureteral stone more than 5 mm size by 57%.
- Alpha blocker is the only approved therapy as per guidelines for MET.
- Silodosin is better than tamsulosin as MET.
- PCN vs DJ stenting in obstructive uropathy with infection, both have specific advantages and disadvantages, DJ stenting is a better overall option as per recent meta-analysis and systematic review.
- Hydrotherapy is not recommended.
- NSAIDs are better than opioids as painkiller and can be safely used in patients with normal renal function.
- If analgesia cannot be achieved medically in a patient with acute colic, drainage methods such as stenting, percutaneous nephrostomy or active stone removal is indicated. If there is sepsis with anuria in a patient with ureteral colic, then only decompression via stenting or PCN is to be done and definitive stone treatment is to be done after sepsis resolves.
- MIMIC is spontaneous stone passage (SSP) prediction calculator that provides an estimated prediction for SSP.
- Antibiotics have no role in ureteral colic in absence of any infection.
- Ureterorenoscopy and active removal of stone is indicated in the following situations—stones with a low likelihood of spontaneous passage, persistent pain despite adequate analgesic medication, persistent obstruction, renal insufficiency.
- Ureteral wall thickness seen on NCCT scan at stone site helps predict ureteral wall oedema, operating times, stone free rates, ESWL success and risk of spontaneous passage of stones.

REFERENCES

1. Partin AW, Wein AJ, Kavoussi LR, Peters CA, Dmochowski RR. Campbell Walsh Wein Urology, E-Book. Elsevier Health Sciences; 2020. 5215 p.
2. Kazama I, Nakajima T. Postrenal acute kidney injury in a patient with unilateral ureteral obstruction caused by urolithiasis: A case report. Medicine (Baltimore). 2017 Oct;96(43):e8381.
3. EAU Guidelines on Urolithiasis-GUIDELINES-Uroweb [Internet]. Uroweb-European Association of Urology. [cited 2023 Apr 11]. Available from: https://uroweb.org/guidelines/urolithiasis/chapter/guidelines
4. Onen A. Grading of Hydronephrosis: An Ongoing Challenge. Front Pediatr. 2020 Aug 27;8:458.
5. Silverman SG, Leyendecker JR, Amis ES. What Is the Current Role of CT Urography and MR Urography in the Evaluation of the Urinary Tract? Radiology. 2009 Feb;250(2):309–23.
6. Pai R, Modh R, Lamoureux RH, Deitte L, Wymer DC, Mench A, *et al*. Image Quality and Patient-Specific Organ Doses in Stone Protocol CT: A Comparison of Traditional CT to Low Dose CT with Iterative Reconstruction. Biomed Res Int. 2018 Sep 27;2018:5120974.
7. Güler Y. Non-contrast computed tomography-based factors in predicting ESWL success: A systematic review and meta-analysis. Prog Urol. 2023 Jan;33(1):27–47.
8. Yoshida T, Inoue T, Omura N, Okada S, Hamamoto S, Kinoshita H, *et al*. Ureteral Wall Thickness as a Preoperative Indicator of Impacted Stones in Patients With Ureteral Stones Undergoing Ureteroscopic Lithotripsy. Urology. 2017 Aug;106:45–9.
9. Yoshida T, Inoue T, Taguchi M, Omura N, Kinoshita H, Matsuda T. Ureteral wall thickness as a significant factor in predicting spontaneous passage of ureteral stones of 10 mm: a preliminary report. World J Urol. 2019 May;37(5):913–9.
10. Travaglini F, Bartoletti R, Gacci M, Rizzo M. Pathophysiology of reno-ureteral colic. Urol Int. 2004;72 Suppl 1:20–3.

11. Campschroer T, Zhu X, Vernooij RW, Lock MT. Alpha-blockers as medical expulsive therapy for ureteral stones. Cochrane Database Syst Rev. 2018 Apr 5;4(4):CD008509.
12. Özsoy M, Liatsikos E, Scheffbuch N, Kallidonis P. Comparison of silodosin to tamsulosin for medical expulsive treatment of ureteral stones: a systematic review and meta-analysis. Urolithiasis. 2016 Nov;44(6):491–7.
13. Kallidonis P, Liourdi D, Liatsikos E. Medical Treatment for Renal Colic and Stone Expulsion. European Urology Supplements. 2011 Oct 1;10(5):415–22.
14. Lee A, Cooper MG, Craig JC, Knight JF, Keneally JP. Effects of nonsteroidal anti-inflammatory drugs on postoperative renal function in adults with normal renal function. Cochrane Database Syst Rev. 2007 Apr 18;2007(2):CD002765.
15. Zhang KP, Zhang Y, Chao M. Which is the best way for patients with ureteral obstruction? Percutaneous nephrostomy versus double J stenting. Medicine (Baltimore). 2022 Nov 11;101(45):e31194.
16. Goldsmith ZG, Oredein-McCoy O, Gerber L, Bañez LL, Sopko DR, Miller MJ, *et al*. Emergent ureteric stent vs percutaneous nephrostomy for obstructive urolithiasis with sepsis: patterns of use and outcomes from a 15-year experience. BJU International. 2013;112(2):E122–8.
17. Shah TT, Gao C, Peters M, Manning T, Cashman S, Nambiar A, *et al*. Factors associated with spontaneous stone passage in a contemporary cohort of patients presenting with acute ureteric colic: results from the Multi-centre cohort study evaluating the role of Inflammatory Markers In patients presenting with acute ureteric Colic (MIMIC) study. BJU International. 2019;124(3):504–13.
18. BURST Urology [Internet]. [cited 2023 Apr 23]. Available from: https://www.bursturology.com/Studies/Mimic/Overview/
19. Schnabel MJ, Wagenlehner FME, Schneidewind L. Perioperative antibiotic prophylaxis for stone therapy. Curr Opin Urol. 2019 Mar;29(2):89–95.
20. Mariappan P, Smith G, Bariol SV, Moussa SA, Tolley DA. Stone and pelvic urine culture and sensitivity are better than bladder urine as predictors of urosepsis following percutaneous nephrolithotomy: a prospective clinical study. J Urol. 2005 May;173(5):1610–4.
21. Alleemudder A, Tai XY, Goyal A, Pati J. Raised white cell count in renal colic: Is there a role for antibiotics? Urol Ann. 2014 Apr;6(2):127–9.
22. Özcan C, Aydo du O, Senocak C, Damar E, Eraslan A, Oztuna D, *et al*. Predictive Factors for Spontaneous Stone Passage and the Potential Role of Serum C-Reactive Protein in Patients with 4 to 10 mm Distal Ureteral Stones: A Prospective Clinical Study. J Urol. 2015 Oct;194(4):1009–13.
23. Drake T, Grivas N, Dabestani S, Knoll T, Lam T, Maclennan S, *et al*. What are the Benefits and Harms of Ureteroscopy Compared with Shock-wave Lithotripsy in the Treatment of Upper Ureteral Stones? A Systematic Review. Eur Urol. 2017 Nov;72(5):772–86.
24. Tzelves L, Geraghty R, Mourmouris P, Chatzikrachtis N, Karavitakis M, Somani B, *et al*. Shockwave Lithotripsy Complications According to Modified Clavien-Dindo Grading System. A Systematic Review and Meta-regression Analysis in a Sample of 115 Randomized Controlled Trials. Eur Urol Focus. 2022 Sep;8(5):1452–60.
25. Borley NC, Rainford D, Anson KM, Watkin N. What activities are safe with kidney stones? A review of occupational and travel advice in the UK. BJU Int. 2007 Mar;99(3):494–6.

Chapter

2

Incidental Staghorn in Elderly

• *Rahul Yadav* • *Madhu Sudan Agarwal*

LEARNING OBJECTIVES

- To understand the epidemiology, mechanism of lithiasis, and natural history of staghorn stones in the elderly.
- Salient points to note in history taking and physical examination.
- Stratification of surgical risk using the Charlson comorbidity index.
- When to order the metabolic workup in staghorn stones?
- Imaging strategy and renal reserve assessment.
- Options in the management of bilateral staghorn stones in elderly high-risk individuals.
- Treatment options for surgically unfit patients.
- Details of conservative therapy for staghorn stones.
- Step-wise algorithm for management of staghorn stones.

INTRODUCTION

Globally, although the renal stone disease is on the rise, staghorn stones account for a small proportion of the total burden of stone (and stone variety) in the society. Still, they can be a cause of major morbidity, renal functional loss and mortality in people of all ages, including the elderly population.

Percutaneous nephrolithotomy (PCNL), single or multitract, is the most widely accepted surgical treatment for staghorn stones, which can be combined with flexible nephoscopy and flexible ureteroscopy (FURS) to achieve complete stone clearance with minimal morbidity and complications.

Elderly patients with multiple comorbidities are usually poor surgical candidates for major surgeries (like PCNL), and literature evidence is scarce on how to manage, follow-up conservatively and when to intervene during follow-up despite being high-risk surgical candidates.

With advancements in healthcare, improved outcomes have been achieved for treating diseases of the most kind, if not all. Similarly, conservative management in this subset of high surgical-risk elderly with staghorn stones has also improved compared with the past. Conservative practices in managing staghorn stones comprise complete history taking, thorough physical examination, tailored imaging, comprehensive metabolic workup, renal reserve assessment, treating comorbidities, targeted therapy for metabolic abnormality, control of urinary tract infections (UTI), individualised follow-up strategies, timely management of infective complications and thus preventing progressive renal deterioration.

The authors of this chapter attempt to collaborate on current literature evidence to formulate a step-wise algorithm to conservatively follow high-risk surgical staghorn patients, mention trigger points for intervention during follow-up, and an essential pre-requisite of informed consent that explains the pros and cons of conservative management of staghorn calculus disease.

Case Scenario

A 70-year-old lady underwent an ultrasonography (USG) for mild dyspepsia and was incidentally found to have a staghorn renal stone (Fig. 2.1). There was no flank pain and non-bothersome nocturia was the only complain. She has been a well-controlled hypertensive (two antihypertensive medications) for 30 years and a sub-optimally controlled type II diabetic for the last 25 years with a body mass index (BMI) of 29. Her recent HbA1c is 8.5. She was also

(Contd.)

Case Scenario *(Contd.)*

being irregularly treated for bronchial asthma although has no pulmonary complaints at present. She had coronary artery disease (CAD) and underwent percutaneous angioplasty (PTCA) before 20 years with the last documented (3 months prior) ejection fraction (on echocardiography) of 30%. She was operated for mitral valve prolapse and had open mitral valve replacement (MVR) 12 years back and is currently on warfarin.

She had an unremarkable physical examination.

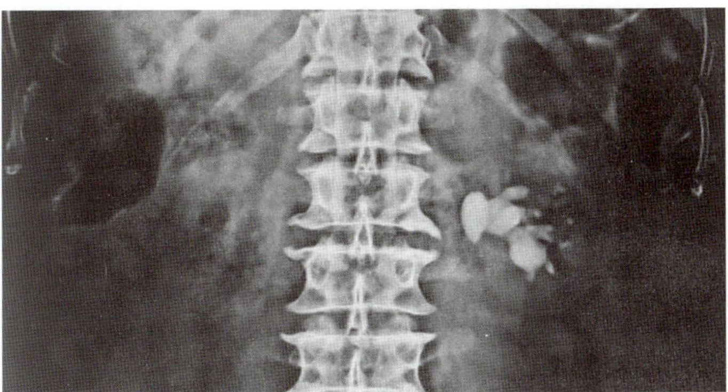

Fig. 2.1: X-ray of the patient showing left-sided staghorn stone

1. **How common are staghorn stones in elderly people?**

   Ans: Globally, nephrolithiasis affects roughly 12% of the population and staghorn stones (SS) account for 10% to 20% of all urinary stones. Women are more likely to have SS and the incidence is rising across all age groups, including the elderly over 60, due to metabolic syndrome and polypharmacy.[1]

2. **How do these stones form? What are the predisposing factors in elderly people?**

   Ans: Physiological factors that predispose geriatric population to kidney stones:
   - Reduced estrogen levels (after menopause in females) and increased sex hormone binding globulin (SHBG) in males during ageing alter calcium regulation, increasing bone resorption and urinary calcium excretion.[2]
   - Increased propensity for urinary tract infection (UTI) due to various age-related changes.[3]
   - Recurrent UTI raises urinary pH, decreases urinary citrate levels and exposes the urinary tract to urea-splitting organisms facilitating infective renal stones.[3]
   - Higher urinary oxalate and lower pH are common in older age.
   - Predisposing factors for stone formation include lifestyle diseases such as obesity, diabetes, metabolic syndrome, and hypertension, which rise with age.

3. **Discuss natural history of staghorn stones in the elderly.**

   Ans: Untreated staghorn stones can cause recurrent UTI, severe urosepsis, progressive renal deteroration leading to end-stage renal disease (ESRD), and even death.[4,5] Previously, a few studies have reported that nearly half of the patients with SS led to renal failure and finally died over a period of 17 years when managed conservatively.[4] However, a recent study suggests better outcomes, with only 14% experiencing progressive renal failure over an eight-year observation.[5] In this study, however, statistically significant differences in disease-specific mortality (0 vs 40%) and morbidity (12 vs 80%) were observed between unilateral and bilateral staghorn stones managed conservatively. With advancements in healthcare and in the absence of life-threatening surgical risks or morbidities, the present data still supports aggressive surgical treatment for staghorn stones.

4. **What is essential to note in the history and physical examination?**

   Ans: With incidentally detected SS, history to be elicited for the presence of fever, hematuria, lower urinary tract symptoms (LUTS), recurrent UTI, features of pyelonephritis, dysfunctional voiding, urinary tract anomalies, and past history of medical or surgical treatment of kidney stones.

5. **What is Charlson Comorbidity Index (CCI) and why is it important?**

   Ans: The Charlson comorbidity index (CCI) predicts 10-year survival in patients with multiple comorbidities. The index consists of 17 items, scored on a scale of 0 to 6 to calculate a cumulative score. For each decade over 50, 1 additional point is added, and a high score predicts a poorer prognosis.[6]

   In the context of the index case, CCI aids in surgical risk stratification and treatment decision-making, whether conservative, active surveillance or surgical.

6. **Is there a role of metabolic workup in staghorn stones?**

   Ans: In contrast to previous data, recent statistics shows that 48–61 percent of SS patients have some type of metabolic abnormality.[7,8] Calcium phosphate is the most predominant stone component, followed by uric acid and calcium oxalate in SS.[8] Most infective staghorn stones are mixed infected stones, meaning they are associated with some metabolic abnormalities and approximately 50% of the cases of pure struvite stones are associated with an underlying metabolic abnormalities.[9]

The most common metabolic abnormality discovered in patients with SS (>40% prevalence) are hypercalciuria, hypocitraturia, and hypernatriuria.[10] Sadly majority of guidelines do not prescribe metabolic evaluation as a part of routine evaluation,[10] but directed therapy can correct metabolic abnormalities, slow progression and reduce recurrence, hence metabolic examination should be individualised in SS and can reasonably be performed in all the patients.

7. **What are the key benefits of urinalysis and urine culture in elderly with SS?**

Ans: Urinalysis detects active infection (white blood cells, red blood cells, nitrite and Leucocyte esterase,[11] proteinuria signalling ongoing kidney damage, and crystals which could identify the type of stone. Urine cultures, in particular, identifies the exact pathogen, which may be a urea-splitting organism indicating struvite stone and help prescribe tailored antibiotics during the peri-operative period and to patients on non-interventional protocols in the case of active UTI or urosepsis. Sensitivity profiles can also assist in advising intermittent or continuous antibiotic prophylaxis in individuals with recurrent UTI or pyelonephritis and increasing renal impairment with stones.[12]

8. **Which is better: Ultrasonography of kidney-ureter-bladder region (USG-KUB)/ intravenous pyelography (IVP)/non-contrast computed tomography of KUB region (NCCT-KUB) / NCCT-KUB with 3D reconstruction/ Contrast-enhanced CT scan of KUB region (CECT-KUB) with urography, in staghorn stones?**

Ans: Detailed imaging of the stone, renal anatomy and function is a must before deciding and planning operative intervention. Various imaging modalities play different roles in the evaluation of renal stones:

- **USG KUB:** Generally an initial investigation due to widespread availability. The disadvantages are low sensitivity (61%), disagreement with the actual size of the stone, misses secondary small stones, and a lack of information on stone hardness.[13]
- **NCCT KUB with or without 3D reconstruction:** Recommended investigation of choice for renal stones by most guidelines. Provides information about the accurate stone burden, hardness [Hounsfield unit (HU)], involved calyces and pelvicalyceal anatomy, renal parenchyma thickness (indirect rough estimate of renal function), and a sensitivity reaching up to 100% with axial cuts spacing less than or equal to 2 mm. Furthermore, it facilitates in the planning of percutaneous nephrolithotomy (PCNL) access with 3D reconstruction.[14–17]
- **IVP:** Low sensitivity (70%), frequently miss small/radiolucent stones, not useful more than a plain X-ray KUB in cases of poorly/non-functioning one-side renal unit with stones and the need for intravenous contrast use and its associated problems. It does have the advantage of delivering anatomical and functional information within a single study, the depiction of images that are close to the intraoperative fluoroscopic images.[13]
- **CECT KUB with urography:** This combines the benefits of an NCCT KUB with functional assessment and more detailed PCS anatomy delineation. Disadvantages are additional cost and radiation exposure.

9. **Renal Scintigraphy studies: Technetium (Tc-99m) labelled diethylenetriamine pentaacetate (DTPA)/ mercaptoacetyltriglycine-3 (MAG-3)/ (Dimercapto succinic acid) DMSA and their role in relation to staghorn stones.**

Ans: Renal scintigraphy is not recommended in the routine evaluation of patients with SS patients, but most accurate in quantifying differential renal function. When imaging modalities indicate reduced function with renal impairment of the affected kidney with stone, a precise function assessment outlines treatment options and aids in prognosis. This could potentially be used to monitor patients on active surveillance or conservative treatment to determine the deterioration of renal function with time. When the obstruction is evident (which is more likely with SS), MAG-3 and DMSA can better assess functioning parenchyma compared to a DTPA scan.[18]

10. **When and how to proceed in case of bilateral SS: Which renal unit first?**

Ans: Bilateral (B/L) staghorn stones threaten the patient's renal reserve. Conservative care is only recommended when surgical treatment is not possible owing to comorbidities, unavailability of such facilities or poses a very high risk. In view of the large stone burden in SS and the age factor in the elderly, kidney stones are better removed in stages rather than simultaneously (consensus statement). The better functioning renal unit must be prioritised based on renal parenchymal thickness or differential GFR on renal scintigraphy. In case of less than a 10% difference in differential function or similar parenchymal thickness on both sides, the symptomatic side, if any to be cleared first (Consensus statement). With similar differential function on both the sides and bilateral asymptomatic staghorn calculi, the easier side which can be surgically cleared may be handled in first stage. In the event of infection in either side, affected renal unit to be drained (via percutaneous nephrostomy or double J stent, depending upon severity of infection) initially.

As such, there are no recommendations regarding a safe interval between two stages when attempting one side after another. However, depending on the patient's condition as well as considering recovery from previous surgery, a gap of one to four weeks may seem reasonable.

11. Is there any choice of pre-operative antibiotic for staghorn stones in the elderly?

Ans: Urea splitting, and other infective pathogens are commonly found in staghorn stones. Preoperative cultures are mandatory and patients should be treated with a culture specific antibiotic for 5 to 7 days pre-operatively. Even if urine culture is sterile, the American Urological Association (AUA) guidelines recommends a single-dose intravenous (IV) antibiotic prophylaxis covering both gram-positive and negative organisms.[19] However, there are studies which categorized patients with staghorn stones into low risk and high risk groups depending upon absence or presence of risk factors like preoperative nephrostomy, diabetes mellitus or previous/ baseline positive urine cultures and advised seven days of prophylactic antibiotics.[20,21]

In practice, the authors of this chapter continue intravenous (IV) antibiotics for a period of stay in hospital and discharge such patients with at least one week of oral antibiotics.

12. What is the role of active surgical management for the staghorn stone in the geriatric population?

Ans: Given the high rates of progressive renal impairment, morbidity, and mortality associated with conservative care, surgery is still the best option for staghorn calculus in any age group. However, surgical clearance of staghorn requires prolonged surgical and anaesthesia time, and often multi-tract or multistage PCNL with additional procedures such as flexible nephroscopy or flexible ureteroscopy (FURS) that may additionally impose risk, especially in geriatric patients.

Stones in solitary kidneys or bilateral (B/L) staghorn has higher risk of progressive renal deterioration and mortality, therefore, conservative therapy may not be appropriate in these patients.

13. Whom to offer active surgical management?

Ans: Any patient who can withstand surgery with acceptable anaesthesia and surgical risk, regardless of age, must be offered surgery. This is a personalised approach that varies with surgeons, anaesthetists, and the facilities available for surgery and involves a multidisciplinary team. Concerning our index case, relevant disciplines (like endocrine, anaesthesiology, cardiology, pulmonology, and cardiovascular surgery) must be consulted to accurately risk stratify before surgery to tackle the correctable components of her comorbidities. Once the patient is optimised by treating comorbidities, the surgical treatment can still be offered with informed consent about the pros and cons of the surgery.

However, in our case, a multidisciplinary team meeting (involving a urologist, anaesthetist, endocrinologist, cardiologist, pulmonologist, cardiothoracic surgeon, intensivist and geriatric physician) was conducted. After comprehensively assessing intraoperative and immediate post-surgical risk, conservative treatment was decided due to the potential risk of morbidity and mortality of surgical intervention and the unacceptability of the same by the patient and attendants.

14. What is the role of conservative or medical management of the staghorn calculi in the geriatric population?

Ans: Recent studies over the last decade have shown that conservative management offers better results than previous conservative trials. There has been a reduction in mortality (3.4–9%), dialysis need (0–9%), and an improved morbidity profile compared to previous results.[5,22–24] In the present era of improved healthcare, conservative management can be offered in carefully selected patients who are either unfit for surgery, refuse surgical intervention, or have limited life expectancy and must be individualised.

15. Which patients to treat conservatively?

Ans: Patients at a high risk of peri-operative death and morbidity should be managed conservatively. Scoring systems such as the Charlson comorbidity index (CCI) are used to assess this risk. Patients with high and very high CCI (6–7 and 8 or more) have a 2-year overall survival rate of 55% and 35%, respectively, making them poor surgical candidates and favoured conservative treatment.

16. Mention protocol to follow-up patients who are on conservative management.

Ans: Different institutions may have different protocols for such patients and no clear-cut guidelines for follow-up in the literature.

The authors prefer 6–12-monthly follow-up.

Each visit includes:

- History and examination
- Renal function test [estimated glomerular filtration rate (eGFR) calculation]
- Urine routine/microscopy (R/M) and culture/sensitivity (C/S)
- Imaging (X-ray/ USG KUB region) to reassess stone load, development, or progression of hydronephrosis, and thickness of renal parenchyma at the upper, mid, and lower poles (as an indirect assessment of deterioration of renal function).
- Renal scintigraphy to assess the renal deterioration of the affected kidney.
- Repeat assessment of metabolic abnormality to ensure adequate correction if found in the first-time evaluation.

Candidates showing progressive renal deterioration, worsening symptoms, recurrent UTI, and pyelonephritis are reconsidered for surgical management subject to their surgical fitness.

17. How to manage complications of staghorn stones during active surveillance?

Ans: The main complications of staghorn stones are urinary tract infections, pyelonephritis, urosepsis, and renal function deterioration.

Infectious complications (UTI/pyelonephritis/urosepsis): Incidences of up to 50% have been recorded in various studies.[17] The mainstay of treatment is broad-spectrum antibiotics, which are either oral or intravenous, depending on the severity of the illness. In severe circumstances, the patient may also require ICU admission.

Patients with recurring infections should be considered for intermittent or continuous antibiotic prophylaxis.

Progressive renal deterioration: This is the most prevalent complication encountered by patients on non-intervention regimens, affecting an average of 27.5 per cent of participants across studies.[24] It is far more common in bilateral (B/L) stone disease, with studies indicating a 44% prevalence compared to 9% in unilateral stone disease.[4] With progressive azotemia in the presence of obstruction, internal or external drainage procedure of the affected renal unit (like double J stenting/percutaneous nephrostomy) will help improving kidney function and may prevent further deterioration. In cases with renal failure, development of uraemia, and/or the requirement for dialysis, nephrology care may be required.[25]

18. What is the role of urease inhibitor?

Ans: Acetohydroxamic acid (AHA) is the only urease inhibitor approved for treating struvite stones. Because of its low efficacy and adverse effect profile, its acceptability as a frontline therapy has been limited. It has been demonstrated in studies to reduce stone growth;[21] therefore, it can be considered in patients who are unfit to undergo surgery, coupled with antibiotics and metabolic abnormality correction.

Dose of AHA: 250 mg, three times a day

Side effects: Tremor, headache, palpitation, gastrointestinal disturbances, alopecia, anaemia, and deep vein thrombosis (DVT).

Contraindications: Pregnancy and renal impairment (creatinine >2.5 mg/dl).

19. Discuss role of antibiotic prophylaxis in conservative management protocols.

Ans: There is no formal recommendation in the literature for the use of antibiotic prophylaxis. Diverse researchers used varied conservative protocols, but most did not use long-term prophylaxis and solely treated clinical infection. It is important to note that the purpose of antibiotic prophylaxis is to suppress infection rather than to eradicate it. Aggressive use of antibiotics for eradication risk the emergence of resistant strains and should be avoided.[12] Therefore, it is at the clinician's discretion whether to adopt this approach or not.

20. Is there a role of chemolysis or stone dissolution therapy?

Ans: Chemolysis for staghorn therapy has limited but of historical significance. In the past, the most widely utilised agents were:

- **Suby solution (Solution G):** Citrate + magnesium oxide + sodium bicarbonate
- **Renacidin:** Malonic acid + gluconic acid + citric acid + magnesium

It acts by reducing the pH to 4, causing the dissolution of calcium carbonate, calcium phosphate, and struvite stone.

Dissolution therapies are not preferred due to the intensive irrigation regimens and extended indwelling nephrostomy, which can last for 1–3 weeks, as well as the high rate of infective complications.

Chemolysis, while nonsurgical, is an invasive method, as explained above, and is thus not suggested for even surgically unfit patients (as our index patient).

21. What are the dietary modifications advised for stones?

Ans: It includes:

- Match water or fluid intake to maintain a 2 to 2.5 L urine output daily.
- Reduced intake of animal proteins.
- Limit sodium intake to less than 2 to 5 gm/day

22. What are the outcomes of conservative management?

Ans: Conservative management has improved outcomes, as reported in the last decade. Mortality (3.4–9%), dialysis dependence (0–9%), and morbidity have decreased with conservative management compared with studies in the past.[5,22–24]

23. What is the algorithm for conservative treatment?

Ans: Due to the scarcity of literature on the conservative management of staghorn calculus, there is no formal recommendation or guidelines on this subject. The authors, on a consensus based on available literature and opinion, formulated a management algorithm in staghorn stones, as highlighted in Flowchart 2.1. The below mentioned recommendations must be individualised based on the urologist's discretion.

KEY POINTS

- Hormonal changes, urinary tract infection (UTI), increased urinary oxalate, diabetes mellitus (DM), and obesity predisposes older people to develop kidney stone(s).
- Bilateral or solitary functioning kidney with staghorn stones in the elderly may jeopardise renal reserve and even progress to end-stage renal disease (ESRD).
- Urinalysis, imaging, surgical risk stratification, and metabolic evaluation should all be performed on patients with SS.
- NCCT KUB region is the imaging modality of choice for diagnosis and evaluation of anatomy.
- The thickness of the renal parenchyma in a USG/ CT scan can roughly predict function. Some patients, however, require renal scintigraphy to measure function accurately.
- Staghorn stones are best treated with percutaneous nephrolithotomy (PCNL) whenever feasible.
- For elderly patients with staghorn stones (SS), multiple comorbidities, and poor performance status, conservative management is a viable option.
- Improved medical management of infective complications has improved the outcomes of conservative management.
- Targeted therapy for metabolic disorders can help reduce stone formation and related complications.

(Contd.)

Flowchart 2.1: Management algorithm for staghorn calculus in the elderly (insights from various papers and author's current practice)

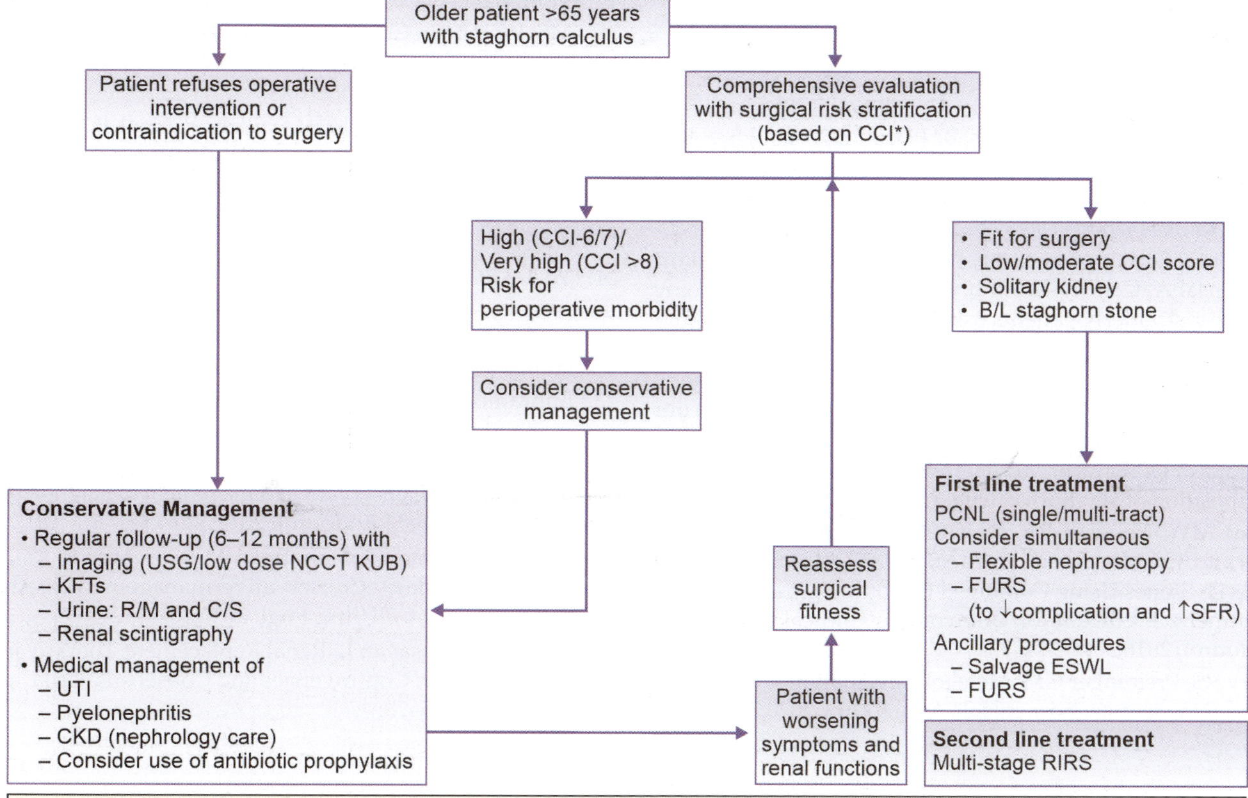

KEY POINTS *(Contd.)*

- Patients under the conservative arm must be closely monitored and treated for any complications during follow-up promptly.
- The role of antibiotic prophylaxis and urease inhibitors is unproven and is left to the clinician's discretion.
- Charlson comorbidity index calculator https://www.mdcalc.com/calc/3917/charlson-comorbidity-index-cci#use-case

ACKNOWLEDGEMENT

The authors gratefully acknowledge the immense contribution of Dr Vishrut Bharti (Consultant, Urologist, Tender Palm Super Specialty Hospital, Lucknow; Email: vishrutbharti07@gmail.com,) for preparing this manuscript.

REFERENCES

1. Alelign T, Petros B. Kidney Stone Disease: An Update on Current Concepts. Adv Urol. 2018;2018:3068365.
2. Usui Y, Matsuzaki S, Matsushita K, Shima M. Urolithiasis in geriatric patients. Tokai J Exp Clin Med. 2003;28(2):81–7.
3. Hedelin H. Uropathogens and urinary tract concretion formation and catheter encrustations. Int J Antimicrob Agents. 2002;19(6):484–7.
4. Singh M, Chapman R, Tresidder GC, Blandy J. The fate of the unoperated staghorn calculus. Br J Urol. 1973;45(6):581–5.
5. Deutsch PG, Subramonian K. Conservative management of staghorn calculi: a single-centre experience. BJU Int. 2016;118(3):444–50.
6. Resorlu B, Diri A, Atmaca AF, Tuygun C, Oztuna D, Bozkurt OF, Unsal A. Can we avoid percutaneous nephrolithotomy in high-risk elderly patients using the Charlson comorbidity index? Urology. 2012;79(5):1042–7.
7. Akagashi K, Tanda H, Kato S, Ohnishi S, Nakajima H, Nanbu A, *et al.* Characteristics of patients with staghorn calculi in our experience. Int J Urol. 2004;11(5):276–81.
8. Viprakasit DP, Sawyer MD, Herrell SD, Miller NL. Changing composition of staghorn calculi. J Urol. 2011;186(6):2285–90.
9. Iqbal MW, Youssef RF, Neisius A, Kuntz N, Hanna J, Ferrandino MN, *et al.* Contemporary Management of Struvite Stones Using Combined Endourologic and Medical Treatment: Predictors of Unfavorable Clinical Outcome. J Endourol. 2016;30(7):771–7.
10. Terry RS, Preminger GM. Metabolic evaluation and medical management of staghorn calculi. Asian J Urol. 2020;7(2):122–9.
11. Bonkat G., *et al.* EAU Guidelines on Urological infections. In: EAU Guidelines, edition presented at the annual EAU Congress Milan 2023. ISBN 978-94-92671-19-6.
12. Wollin DA, Joyce AD, Gupta M, Wong MYC, Laguna P, Gravas S, *et al.* Antibiotic use and the prevention and management of infectious complications in stone disease. World J Urol. 2017;35(9):1369–79.
13. Klein I, Gutiérrez-Aceves J. Preoperative imaging in staghorn calculi, planning and decision making in management of staghorn calculi. Asian J Urol. 2020;7(2):87–93.
14. Sfoungaristos S, Gofrit ON, Pode D, Landau EH, Duvdevani M. Percutaneous nephrolithotomy for staghorn stones: Which nomogram can better predict postoperative outcomes? World J Urol. 2016;34(8):1163–8.
15. Winoker JS, Chandhoke RA, Atallah W, Gupta M. Morphometry scores: Clinical implications in the management of staghorn calculi. Asian J Urol. 2020;7(2):78–86.
16. Yarimoglu S, Bozkurt IH, Aydogdu O, Yonguc T, Sefik E, Topcu YK, Degirmenci T. External validation and comparison of the scoring systems (S.T.O.N.E, GUY, CROES, S-ReSC) for predicting percutaneous nephrolithotomy outcomes for staghorn stones: A single center experience with 160 cases. Kaohsiung J Med Sci. 2017;33(10):516–22.
17. Mishra S, Sabnis RB, Desai M. Staghorn morphometry: a new tool for clinical classification and prediction model for percutaneous nephrolithotomy monotherapy. J Endourol. 2012;26(1):6–14.
18. Keramida G, James JM, Prescott MC, Peters AM. Pitfalls and Limitations of Radionuclide Renal Imaging in Adults. Semin Nucl Med. 2015;45(5):428–39.
19. Preminger GM, Assimos DG, Lingeman JE, Nakada SY, Pearle MS, Wolf JS, Jr. Chapter 1: AUA guideline on management of staghorn calculi: diagnosis and treatment recommendations. J Urol. 2005;173(6):1991–2000.
20. Gravas S, Montanari E, Geavlete P, Onal B, Skolarikos A, Pearle M, *et al.* Postoperative infection rates in low risk patients undergoing percutaneous nephrolithotomy with and without antibiotic prophylaxis: a matched case control study. J Urol. 2012;188(3):843–7.
21. Yu J, Guo B, Yu J, Chen T, Han X, Niu Q, *et al.* Antibiotic prophylaxis in perioperative period of percutaneous nephrolithotomy: a systematic review and meta-analysis of comparative studies. World J Urol. 2020;38(7):1685–700.
22. Subramonian K, Barba HS, Darrad M. Role of conservative management of stones. Turk J Urol. 2020;46(Supp. 1):S64–s9.
23. Morgan TN, Shahait M, Maganty A, Ost M, Jackman S, Averch T, Semins MJ. Conservative Management of Staghorn Calculi: When Is It Safe? J Endourol. 2018;32(6):541–5.
24. Alsawi M, Amer T, Mariappan M, Nalagatla S, Ramsay A, Aboumarzouk O. Conservative management of staghorn stones. Ann R Coll Surg Engl. 2020;102(4):243–7.
25. Heung M, Yessayan L. Renal Replacement Therapy in Acute Kidney Injury: Controversies and Consensus. Crit Care Clin. 2017;33(2):365–78.

Chapter 3

Staghorn Stone in a Diabetic

• *Janak Desai* • *Akshay Nathani*

LEARNING OBJECTIVES

To understand

- The pathophysiology of staghorn calculus.
- How to approach and investigate a patient with staghorn calculus.
- Whether there is any role of medical therapy for staghorn calculus.
- The management options.
- Recurrence prevention measures and follow-up protocol.

INTRODUCTION

It is not uncommon in clinical practice to come across diabetic patient with a staghorn stone. This scenario presents a particularly intricate and challenging manifestation. Diabetes mellitus is notorious for its multifaceted impact on various organ systems, including the urinary tract. Staghorn stones are known to predispose to and are known to be an aftermath of chronic urinary tract infections. This chapter describes the intricate relationship between diabetes and staghorn stones, exploring the pathophysiological underpinnings, clinical presentation, diagnostic modalities, management strategies, and prognostic implications of this challenging clinical entity.

Case Scenario

A 55-year-old lady, diabetic and hypertensive for the past 10 years, presented with complaints of left flank pain for 15 days, associated with occasional fever and burning micturition. There was no history of lithuria, pyuria or hematuria. She had a history of right percutaneous nephrolithotomy (PCNL) 3 years back with an uneventful post-operative course at that time. On examination, she was well nourished, pre-obese, vitally stable with a mild tenderness on the left flank. The rest of the systemic examination was normal. She was not on any blood thinners. She did not have any significant family history of urolithiasis.

1. **What would you like to do next?**

   Ans: I would like to investigate her for the above complaints in the form of laboratory evaluation and radiological imaging.

Laboratory findings

- Hemoglobin 12.3 gm/dl. This helps me to know her baseline hematocrit and if planned for any surgical treatment then to have idea about adequacy of her reserve.
- Random blood sugars:149, HBA1c: 10.9%, which makes me think that I have to spend more time counselling her pre- and post-surgery for importance of her glycemic control.
- Serum creatinine 0.74 mg /dl which is normal so that I can plan for contrast imaging and calculate her e-GFR (estimated glomerular filtration rate).
- Urine analysis pH 6, trace proteins, 2+ sugar, 30–40 RBC and 10–15 white blood cells per high power field.
- Urine culture—sterile to rule out underlying urinary tract infection.
- Imaging: X-ray KUB, USG KUB, CT IVU

2. **How do you define staghorn calculus? What are the common clinical presentations of a patient with staghorn stones?**

   Ans: Staghorn calculi are branched, usually infection stones that occupy a large portion of the collecting system, typically filling the renal pelvis and branching into several or all of the calyces. Staghorn calculi most often present with urinary tract infection hence they are more commonly seen in female patients.[1] Other clinical presentations include haematuria, lower urinary tract symptoms (LUTS), fever, flank pain with or without palpable kidney. They may present with features of acute kidney injury like breathlessness, facial puffiness, pedal oedema or reduced urine output. Advanced cases in individuals with large struvite stones may demonstrate general symptoms such as fatigue, lethargy, malaise, intermittent fever, loss of appetite, and weight loss.

3. Who are high risk patients for struvite /staghorn calculus?

Ans: Predisposing factors[2]

• Neurogenic bladder	• Urethral stricture
• Spinal cord injury/paralysis	• Benign prostatic hyperplasia
• Continent urinary diversion	• Bladder diverticulum
• Ileal conduit	• Cystocele
• Foreign body	• Calyceal diverticulum
• Indwelling urinary catheter	• UPJ obstruction

4. What organisms are associated with struvite stones?

Ans:

- Obligate urease-producing bacteria (> 98%) 1. Proteus spp. 2. *Providencia rettgeri* 3. *Morganella morganii* 4. *Corynebacterium urealyticum* 5. *Ureaplasma urealyticum*.
- Facultative urease-producing bacteria 1. *Enterobacter gergoviae* 2. Klebsiella spp. 3. *Providencia stuartii* 4. *Serratia marcescens* 5. *Staphylococcus* spp.
- 0-5% of *Escherichia coli*, *Enterococcus* spp. and *Pseudomonas aeruginosa* strains may produce urease.[2]

5. This patient is asymptomatic, why do you want to treat her? What will happen if we do not treat the stone?

Ans: Although asymptomatic, she still needs to undergo surgical treatment for stone removal as there is enough evidence to support that untreated staghorn calculi due to their natural history may cause recurrent urinary tract infections, episodes of sepsis and eventually loss of renal function.[3–8] Alsawi et al in a systematic review based on 10 studies involving 304 patients who were managed conservatively, concluded that 50% patients developed recurrent infections, 27.5%, suffered progressive renal deterioration and 9% patients required dialysis.[9]

6. In such a case what would be your investigations?

Ans: As already discussed, investigations will be divided into two categories:

1. Laboratory investigations: Complete blood counts, renal function test, blood sugar levels with HbA1c, coagulation profile, prothrombin time and INR, urine routine and microscopy and urine culture.
2. Imaging: *USG KUB* (ultrasonography kidney ureter bladder) as an extension of clinical examination which is safe without any radiation exposure and is readily available. It can determine number and location of stones, renal parenchymal thickness degree of hydronephrosis and hydroureter. The disadvantage of USG is that it is subjective, can underestimate the size of the stone and lower ureter can be difficult to trace. USG has a sensitivity of 45% and specificity of 88% for renal stones.[10]

   X-ray KUB is a part of baseline work-up and helps to identify radio-opaque or lucent stones for further follow-up. It has a sensitivity and specificity of 57% and 76% respectively.[11]

   X-ray obviously gives a radiation exposure to the patient and needs bowel preparation for proper identification of calculi.

   CT urogram—for surgical planning as shown in Fig. 3.1. (Discussed in the next question.)

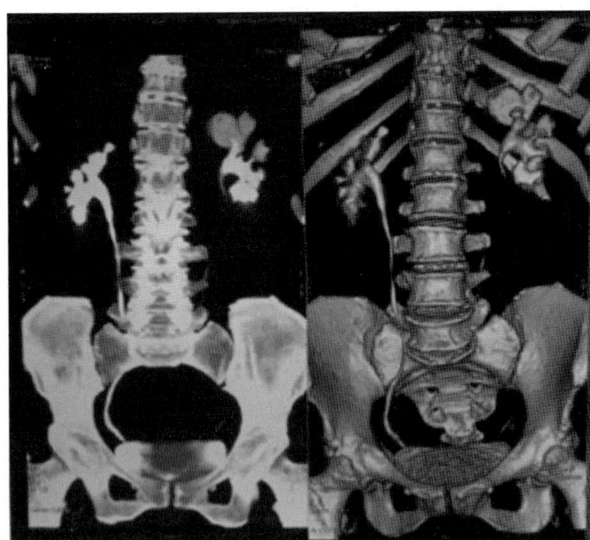

Fig. 3.1: Reconstructed coronal images of CTU with complete staghorn calculus on left side with dilated calyces and left-sided excretion of contrast and right-sided normal system

7. What should we prefer: Conventional intravenous urography (IVU) or CT urography (CTU)?

Ans: CT urography has multiple advantages over IVU:

1. No bowel preparation is required.
2. Number, size and sites of stone can be determined

3. Distance from skin to stone can be assessed (helps in choice of renal access sheath in morbidly obese patients)
4. Stone morphometry and assessment of bulk of stone using 3D reconstruction software.
5. Anatomical abnormalities and aberrations like retrorenal colon can be identified.
6. Perinephric fat stranding or collection/urinoma if any can be detected.
7. Rarely long standing stones may be associated with parenchymal lesion like squamous cell carcinoma. These can be detected on CTU. Their presence can change whole of management.
8. Localizing peripheral stones to anterior or posterior calices is possible.
9. Determining the direction of caliceal extensions of staghorn calculi, visualizing poorly radio-opaque calculi[12] and documenting the parenchymal thickness which is a surrogate marker of the renal function.

The only disadvantages of CTU are the cost and high radiation exposure. Although CTU has proven superiority to IVU, IVU is less expensive and is easily available.

8. Would you ask for a CT IVU or a NCCT and why?

Ans: Investigation of choice will be computed tomography urography (if renal functions are normal) as it provides anatomical as well as functional status of kidney which help to further plan surgical treatment for staghorn calculus and helps counsel the patient regarding number of tracts and number of stages for clearance of stone. In addition, we can calculate stone morphometry and assess infundibulo pelvic angle, length and width which helps to predict the requirement of number of tracts and stages for stone clearance.

If deranged renal functions, CT KUB (computed tomography kidney ureter bladder) without contrast need to be ordered and pelvicalyceal anatomy to assessed at the time of PCNL by retrograde pyelogram.

9. What do you think looking at this CT?

Ans: The CT image as depicted in Fig. 3.2 is a reconstructed film of CTU sequence which depicts normal right-sided kidney with normal contrast excretion. On left side, there is large radiodense complete staghorn calculus with moderate hydronephrosis with faint contrast excretion seen in ureter. Based on these images, a lower posterior tract may give a good access to the major stone bulk. An additional puncture may be required for middle calyceal stone clearance. Before deciding

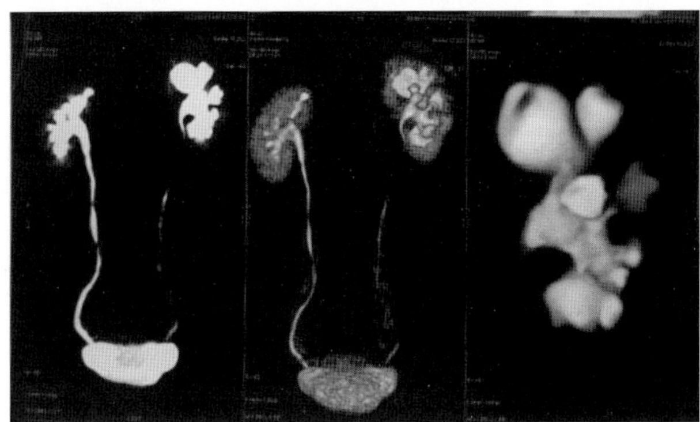

Fig. 3.2: Coronal plate with reconstruction

the site for puncture, it is important to look at axial sections to rule out retrorenal colon and skin to stone distance.

10. What is the role of nuclear scan in patients with staghorn calculi?

Ans: Not done routinely in all patients with staghorn calculi, but if suspicious with poor parenchyma on USG/CT, poor contrast uptake, nuclear scan can be done. Various studies have tried to corelate renal parenchymal thickness on CT scan and differential function on scintigraphy but these are only estimate not accurate.[13,14] In 2019 Sharbaugh et al recommended nuclear renal scan in all patients with staghorn calculi.[15] Common radiotracers such as DTPA (technetium-99m diethylenetriamine pentaacetic acid) or MAG-3 (technetium-99m mercaptoacetyltriglycerine) or EC (ethylene cysteine) are used.

Nephrectomy as treatment should be offered if the involved kidney has negligible function (<10%).[16]

11. What is staghorn morphometry? How does it help you to decide your management?

Ans: Morphometry is a scoring system to objectively determine the complexity of renal stones using various stone factors.[17]

Where morphology and volume calculations done separately are inadequate, morphometry attempts to objectively define the complexity of a staghorn calculus by using both shape and size. It helps for surgical planning, and accurately predicts the rate of both surgical success and complications following PCNL as it is easy to use and reproducible.

12. How would you estimate stone burden? What are the various methods? Which one is reliable?

1. Guy stone scoring for complexity (Fig. 3.3):[18]
   Type I: Solitary stone mid/lower calyx or in pelvis with normal anatomy

Type II: Solitary stone in upper calyx
Multiple stone in mid-calyx, lower calyx
Solitary stone in abnormal anatomy
Type III: Partial staghorn
Diverticular stone
Multiple stone in abnormal anatomy
Type IV: Complex staghorn, stone in spina bifida and spinal injury

2. STONE score: [Stone size (S), Tract length (T), Obstruction (O), Number of involved calyces (N), and Essence or stone density (E)]
   Size Size: 0–399 mm^2: 1 point
   Size: 400–800 mm^2: 2 points
   Size: 800–1600 mm^2: 3 points
   Size: >1600 mm^2: 4 points
   Tract length: < 10 cm: 1 point
   > 10 cm: 2 points
   Obstruction: Yes: 2 points
   No: 1 point
   Number of calyces involved:
   1 point: 1 calyx
   2 points: 2–3 calyx
   3 points: Staghorn
   Essence: HU 1 point < 950 HU
   2 points > 950 HU

Total score between 5 and 13 and the complications, need for blood transfusion and risk of residual calculi increased as the stone score increased. Score also significantly correlated with operation time, estimated blood loss, duration of fluoroscopy, duration of hospital stay, and number of punctures.[19]

3. CROES (Clinical Research Office of the Endourology Society) nomogram
4. Seoul National University Renal Stone Complexity (S-ReSC) score
5. Stone Morphometric Classification:[17]
   Depends upon total stone volume (*TSV*) and unfavourable calyx stone percentile volume (*UCSPV*)
   Type I: < 5000 mm^3 TSV + < 5% UCSPV
   Type II: 5000–20000 mm^3 TSV + < 5% UCSPV
   Type II-b: 5000–20000 mm^3 TSV + > 5% UCSPV
   Type III: > 20000 mm^3 and any unfavourable calyx

Favourable calyx: Defined as calyx having obtuse angle and infundibular width > 8 mm.

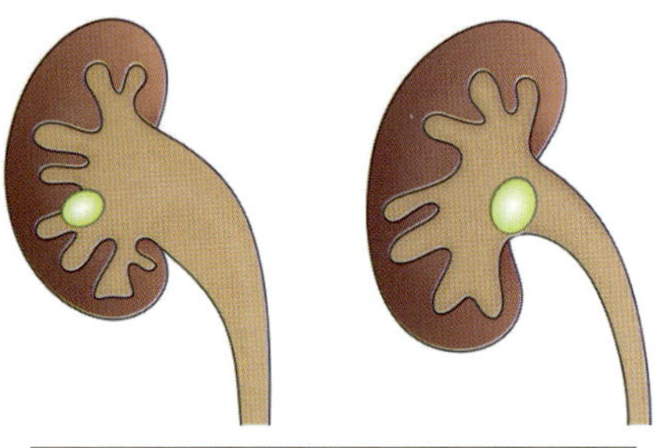

Grade I: A solitary stone in mid/lower pole with simple anatomy or A solitary stone in pelvis with simple anatomy

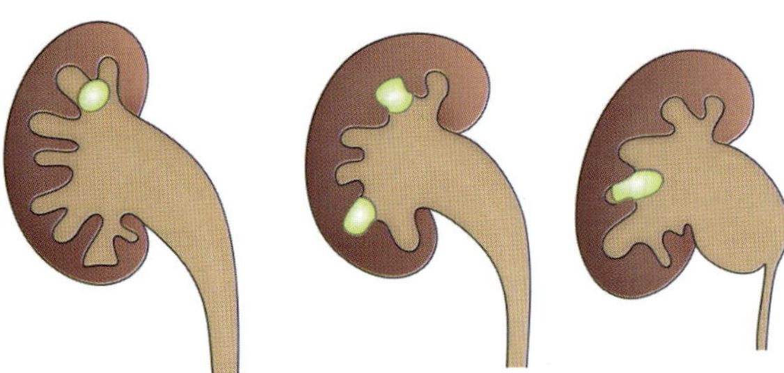

Grade II: Solitary stone in upper pole with simple anatomy Or multiple stones with simple anatomy Or solitary stone with abnormal anatomy

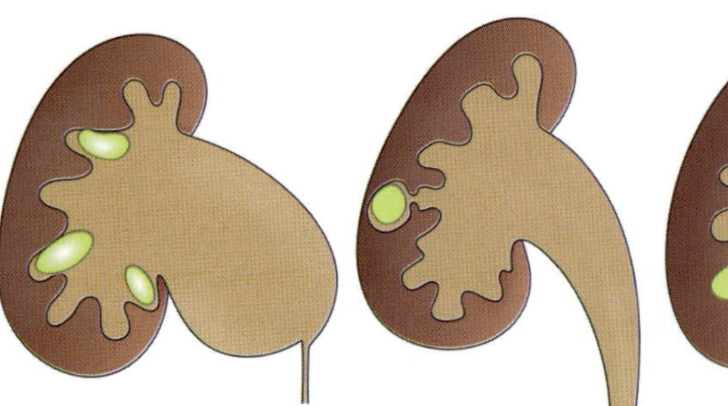

Grade III: Multiple stone with abnormal anatomy Or stones in calyceal diverticulum Or partial staghorn calculus

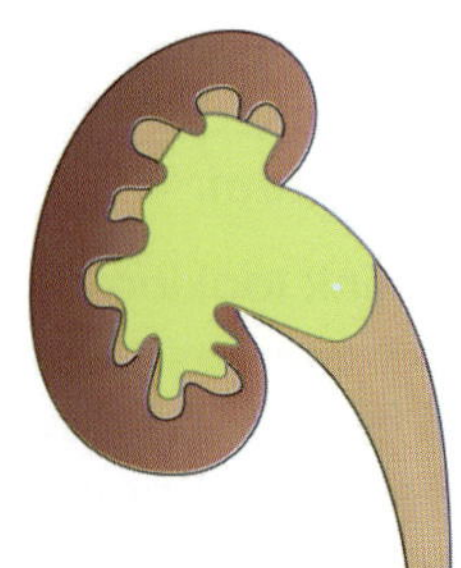

Grade IV: Staghorn calculus Or any stone in patient with spina bifida or spinal injury

Fig. 3.3: (A) Grade I/Type I; (B) Grade II/Type II; (C) Grade III/Type III; (D) Grade IV/Type IV

Fallacies: (A) No consideration for stone size, density, and composition. (B) Same group for abnormal spine patient and staghorn stone patient

An unfavourable calyx, on the contrary, has an acute angle and infundibular width of less than 8 mm.

The number of tracts and stages can be predicted in PCNL with the help of staghorn morphometry. Type 1 (single tract and stage), Type 2 (single tract–single/multiple stage, or multiple tract–single stage), and Type 3 (multiple tract and stage).

Guy stone scoring system and STONE score are doable and can be reproduced while for morphometry there should be a separate software available to measure stone burden.

13. What is the composition of staghorn calculus and are struvite stones same as staghorn? What is pathophysiology of struvite stones?

Ans: Staghorn calculi are most frequently composed of mixtures of magnesium ammonium phosphate (struvite) and/or calcium carbonate apatite. Recently it has been revealed an increasing number of calcium phosphate staghorn stones, supporting the link between staghorn and metabolic stones which leads us for metabolic evaluation of such patients. Cystine and uric acid stones or mixed can also present in staghorn configuration.

Struvite/calcium carbonate apatite stones are also referred to as "infection stones" because they are associated with UTI caused by urease producing organisms[20] Alkaline urinary pH + high ammonia + phosphate + magnesium promotes crystallization of magnesium ammonium phosphate (struvite) calculus formation. Incorporation of mucoproteins and formation of biofilm are other factors that help formation of struvite stones. Culture from both surface and core of the stone have grown urea splitting organisms leading to fact that stone itself is the culprit for these patients for suffering from recurrent UTIs.[21]

14. How will you counsel this patient? What are the treatment options?

Ans: Counselling of this patients must be done.
1. For risk factors: DM control, HTN control and antibiotics for UTI
2. Surgical planning: Procedure, related complications
3. Postoperative course and hospital stay.
4. Need for follow-up imaging after 4 weeks and if required need for auxiliary procedure (PCNL, RIRS, ESWL, etc)
5. Need for stent removal after 3–4 weeks.
6. Stone analysis and prevention strategy (dietary modifications, medications)

Treatment options
1. PCNL: Multiple tracts, multiple stages may be required.
2. Anatrophic nephrolithotomy can be open, laparoscopic or robotic, but PCNL remains the preferred modality (Flowchart 3.1).

Flowchart 3.1: Management algorithm for staghorn calculus

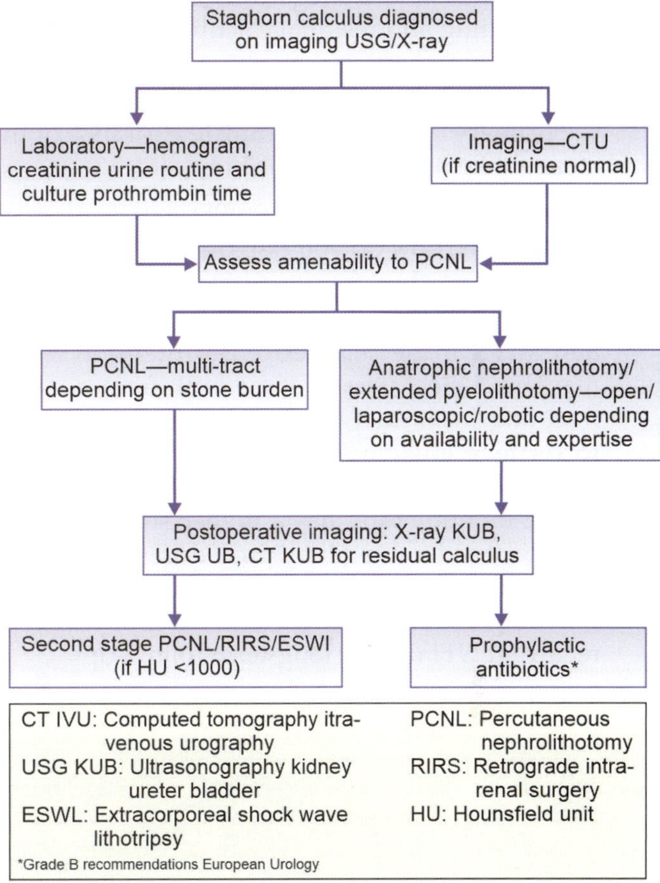

15. How to manage pre-operative positive urine culture?

Ans: Every institute has a different antibiotic policy. Common protocol is to start culture specific oral antibiotics minimum 7-days before surgery and then shift to parenteral antibiotics a day prior surgery. Proper antibiotic cover in these infective stones is important to prevent postoperative sepsis. If the patient presents with sepsis, it is important to hospitalise the patient, get associated diabetes controlled and start parenteral antibiotics. Definitive surgery should be delayed till sepsis is controlled. PCN (percutaneous nephrostomy) placement preoperatively for high risk patients with comorbidities may improve outcomes by drainage of infected and stagnant urine from collecting system additionally to obtain renal pelvis urine for culture for better targeted antibiotic therapy as hypothesized by Benson and colleagues which helps reduce post-PCNL infectious complications and with added advantage of pre-placed access for stone clearance.[22]

16. If you decide to treat her with PCNL, how many tracts will be required?

Ans: Approach to this case will be multiple tracts and if required multistage with thorough counselling of patient regarding the complications like bleeding and residual calculi.

The debate continues over the use of single-tract versus multiple-tract PCNL with either method, the primary objective is complete clearance of the stone while minimizing morbidity (Fig. 3.4).[23]

17. One large tract and other small tracts or multiple small tracts, how do you decide?

Ans: Depending on contrast imaging: Stone volume and dilatation of system, tract numbers and size can be planned with intention being maximum clearance of stone bulk from a single tract and fresh tract (preferably miniperc < 20 fr) to retrieve elusive stones whenever the stones are present in peripheral calyces. A multiple tract PCNL monotherapy has a higher stone free rate and less need for auxiliary procedures. The higher SFR achieved with a multi-tract, could result in a lower stone recurrence rate, and lower incidence of recurrent UTI during long-term follow-up.

18. How to plan multiple tracts?

Ans: After gaining access to target calyx from which maximum stone bulk can be cleared and before dilatation of target calyx another puncture/punctures can be made and guidewire can be pre-placed in unfavourable and peripheral calyx with advantage to gain access, retrograde contrast study to make other puncture will be difficult if attempted after dilatation of primary tract, If guidewire placed in unfavourable tract can be accessed from primary dilated tract and if possible stones can be removed, then another tract dilatation can be avoided disadvantage being that if purchase of pre-placed wire/wires is less, then it can slip off. If pre-placed tract is not done, then stone guided puncture can be obtained.

Ganpule et al reviewed various papers on multitract vs single tract PCNL concluded that various techniques are associated with inherent problems.With a single tract, access to all the calyces will be difficult because of the peculiarities of the renal collecting system, in which case, multiple tract PCNL will be the mainstay of the treatment. The crucial point to understand is that all cases should be individualized.[23]

19. What are the likely complications?

Ans: To enumerate the list of complications:

1. *Position:* Ocular injury, spinal injury, neuropraxia
2. *Puncture:* Surrounding organ injury (colon, spleen, liver, gall bladder). Pneumothorax or

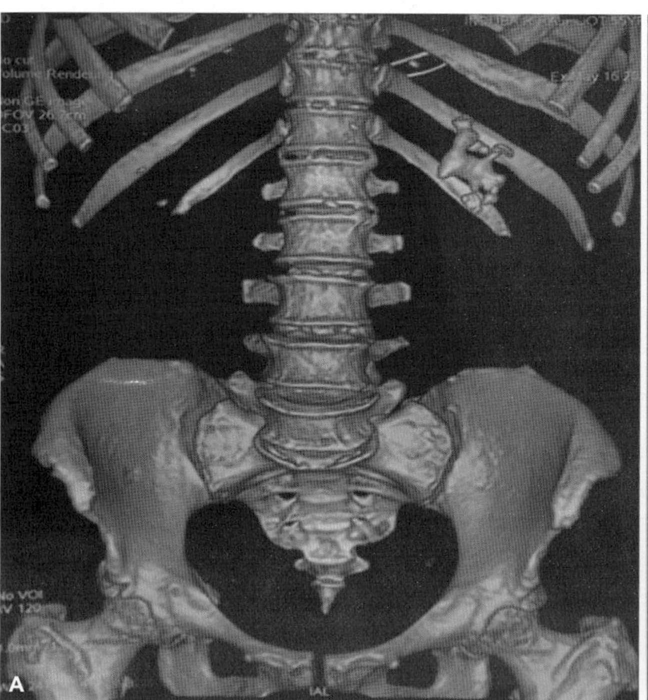

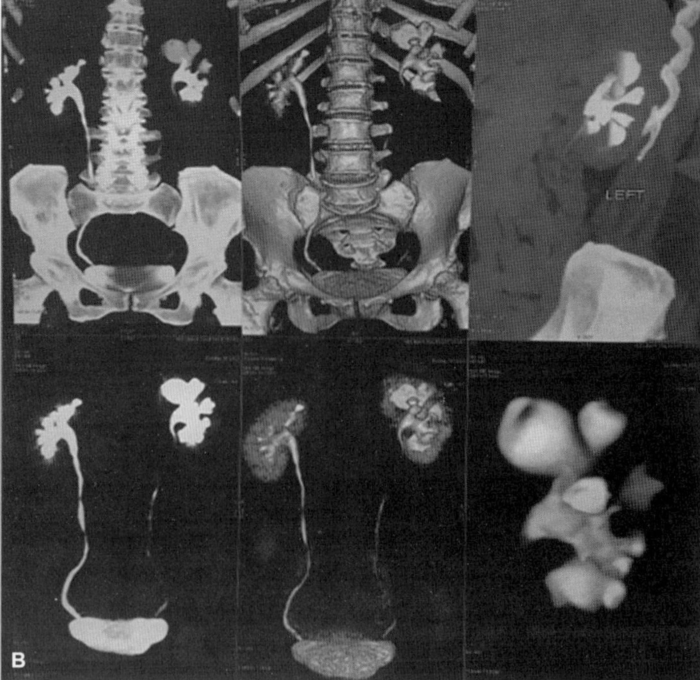

Fig. 3.4A and B: (A) Coronal reconstructed showing stone bulk, complete staghorn; (B) Contrast films showing dilated system

hydrothorax or hemothorax during supracostal access.

3. *PC system:* Under or overdilatation of the tract, infundibular tear or renal pelvis perforation.
4. *Hemorrhage:* Bleeding is the most significant complication of PCNL, with transfusion rates varying between 1% and 10%. Delayed hemorrhage is usually from an arteriovenous fistula or a pseudoaneurysm and this needs an emergency embolization (<0.5% of patients).
5. Air embolism
6. Infection, sepsis
7. Tube dislodgement

20. Is there any role of tranexamic acid for reducing bleeding?

Ans: If there is no contraindication for the drug (renal insufficiency), tranexamic acid can be used prior to PCNL for staghorn stones. A recent RCT showed that tranexamic acid group had a significant reduction in post-op hemoglobin drop (1.39 vs. 2.31 mg/dl) and blood transfusion rate (2% vs. 11%).[24]

21. What are the risk factors affecting bleeding?

Ans: Factors contributing to the bleeding risk during PCNL.[25]

Patient related factors: Older age, uncontrolled hypertension and diabetes, urinary infection, elevated serum creatinine, past ipsilateral interventions like open surgery, PCNL, or SWL, reduced function of affected kidney, mild hydronephrosis, multiple tracts and larger stone surface area.

Procedure related factors: Experienced surgeon. prior-PCN tract, ultrasound guided puncture if available as ultrasonography offers real-time three-dimensional monitoring of the puncture, including the needle and the collecting system, in the same plane, thereby minimizing the chance of segmental vessel injuries, entry of calyx through cup rather than infundibulum associated with lower bleeding risk and factors which increase risk of bleeding urine from puncture needle (clear or hemorrhagic).

Method of tract dilatation preferably single step Amplatz as with its bevelled-edge fascial dilators, spreads the parenchymal tissue rather than lacerating it. Large size of the tract, number of tracts, intraoperative complications like infundibular shear, pelvis perforation, long operating time.

22. On post-operative day 2 she has 500 ml blood in her nephrostomy. What are your thoughts as regards management and prognosis?

Ans: Secondary hemorrhage is mostly due to arteriovenous fistula or malformation. Initial conservative management can be done like close monitoring of vitals, observe haematocrit and replace blood, if necessary, PCN to be clamped. If there is a significant drop in haemoglobin or the patient becomes vitally unstable have a low threshold for endovascular intervention.

Post-PCNL Bleeding

Intraoperative: Small parenchymal bleeding is controlled by renal compression. If surgery is uneventful, then postoperative hematuria will be resolved by 1 or 2 days.

If severe intraoperative bleeding, then put nephrostomy and terminate the procedure. Intensive care monitoring of patient. Give IV fluids. Can give IV 1 gm of tranexamic acid.

Reactionary hemorrhage is mostly due to arteriovenous fistula or malformation, conservative management can be done initially.

If *persistent bleeding* and drop in haematocrit warrants urgent angiography and coiling of fistula. In very rare situations nephrectomy may be needed as a last resort.

Secondary hemorrhage is mostly due to infection. Conservative management along with antibiotics are required for such cases.

23. If she continues to bleed, when would you consider endovascular intervention?

Ans: Persistent bleeding and drop in haematocrit warrant urgent angiography and coiling of fistula.

24. What are your thoughts if a similar presentation happens after 10 days with fever?

Ans: Post-operative fever may be reactionary, systemic inflammatory reaction or due to sepsis. Conservative management with IV fluids, antibiotics and supportive measures are required. Usually, higher antibiotics are needed. Monitor for vitals and leukocytes count.

25. What are the risk factors for colon injury during PNL?

Ans: A retrorenal colon is more frequently noted on the left side.[26]

Risk factors include anterior calyceal puncture, jejunoileal bypass patients resulting in an enlarged colon, previous kidney operations, horseshoe kidney and kyphoscoliosis.

Punctures lateral to the posterior axillary line-risk of colon injury as the position of the retroperitoneal colon is usually anterior or anterolateral. In elderly and thin females, the incidence of posterior colonic displacement is more so the risk of colonic injury.

26. If injury to the colon is diagnosed after PNL, what is the preferred management? Do they present with peritonitis?

Ans: As the injury being retroperitoneal, signs of peritonitis are infrequent and colonic injuries are usually diagnosed postoperatively with visible feculent matter in nephrostomy tube. Further, the aim would be separate renal drainage from colonic one by placement of JJ stent in renal unit and by withdrawing the nephrostomy tube from an intrarenal position to an intracolonic position, thus serving as a colostomy tube.

The colostomy tube is left in place for a minimum of 7 days and is removed, check nephrostogram or a retrograde pyelogram can be done to document no communication between the colon and the kidney.

27. Is there a role of open/laparoscopy or robotic anatrophic nephrolithotomy?

Ans: Limited role as morbidity of PCNL is much lower. Anatrophic nephrolithotomy is performed in select cases with large volume stones with multiple infundibular stenosis that may need multiple tracts, and also in situations where there is lack of expertise or facilities for PCNL or in patients with failed PCNL.

Indications and outcomes for open anatrophic nephrolithotomy in modern era was assessed by Keshavamurthy et al, concluded that it is a valid approach for managing large staghorn calculi, failed minimally invasive approaches, patients with comorbidities like COPD and achieves 80–100% clearance without much secondary interventions, renal function is fairly preserved. With the emergence of laparoscopy and robotic assistance, postoperative stay is minimized with expedited recovery and comparable results with gold standard open surgery.[27] Potential advantages of the anatrophic nephrolithotomy

1. Ability to remove large calculi volume in a single surgery procedure in complex cases.
2. Minimizes the morbidity associated with flank incision—advantage of laparoscopy/robotic
3. Intraoperative direct nephroscopy can inspect for residual fragments.

Literature regarding laparoscopic anatrophic nephrolithotomy suggests that renal function may temporarily decrease after anatrophic nephrolithotomy, but these changes are not clinically significant. In those kidneys that are severely infected or obstructed, the postoperative functional improvement may be important.

Choice of open vs laparoscopy vs robotic depends on availability of expertise and cost constraints.[28–30]

While laparoscopy and robotic techniques for stone removal are feasible with relatively good stone-free rates, they remain second-line therapies when compared with less invasive endourological techniques secondary to cost and lack of outcomes demonstrating superiority.[31,32]

28. If she presented with staghorn calculi in a nonfunctioning kidney, is she a candidate for nephrectomy? If yes, what will be your approach?

Ans: If the contralateral renal unit has satisfactory function, nephrectomy may be considered if the stone-laden kidney has poor function.

Laparoscopic nephrectomy is an option if facilities and expertise are available, but open surgical nephrectomy can be a safer approach if there is intense perirenal inflammation that may occur with xanthogranulomatous pyelonephritis. So accordingly, patient should be counselled and consented.[33–34]

29. How will you counsel and treat residual stones after treatment? What are CIRF?

Ans: CIRFs (clinically insignificant residual fragments) defined as asymptomatic, non-infectious stone fragments less than 4 mm (some consider 2 mm as cut off).

Counselling of patients preoperatively plays an important role for management of residual stone fragments. Residual fragments can be removed by ureteroscopy at the time of stent removal especially if one anticipates complications from residual fragments.

Management CIRFs is to be done when there are possible complications of residual stones related to dislocation of fragments with obstruction and symptoms, persistent urinary tract infection and the risk of developing new stones from the nidus.[35–38]

30. Can we prevent new struvite stone formation? what are preventative measures for other types of stones?

Ans: To prevent recurrence of struvite calculi it is important to eradicate infection after complete clearance of stone. Regarding the duration of postoperative antibiotic administration the evidence remains inconclusive.

General preventive measures are recommended for fluid intake and diet. Specific measures include complete surgical stone removal,[39] short-or long-term antibiotic treatment,[40] maintaining urinary pH below 6.5, avoid crystallization of matrix stones using methionine[41] or ammonium chloride.[42] Acetohydroxamic acid may be an alternative for persistent infections or colonisation.[43,44]

Side-effects such as tremors and embolic events should be kept in mind while prescribing Acetohydroxamic acid. Antibiotics—as mentioned complete clearance of stone is a major determinant specially in struvite. Recurrence can be partly prevented by long-term suppressive antibiotics may be for a period of 3–6 months depending on the merit of the case. However, residual fragments make eradication of infection quite difficult as it being the source of recurrent infection. Complete stone clearance is much more important than antimicrobial therapy.[45]

Also for other types of stones, 24 hours urinary chemistry should be done after 2–3 months of starting therapy, i.e preventative treatment and repeated once after 1 year once therapy is stabilized.

1. For **primary hyperoxaluria:** Alkalinization of urine + Pyridoxine therapy + high fluid intake

   In secondary hyperoxaluria, to decrease calcium absorption, calcium supplements to added in meals.
2. **Calcium stone formers**: Hydrocholorthiazide (thiazide diuretic) + potassium citrate in the case of hypercalciuria.
3. **Hypocitraturia:** Potassium citrate 40–60 mEq per day.
4. In calcium stone former in hyperuricosuric patients, allopurinol when used decreases stone recurrence rates.
5. **Uric acid stone formers**: Maintaining urine pH between 6 and 6.5 will be primary aim in follow-up for which allopurinol can be helpful.

   Just by measuring urinary pH, hyperuricosuric calcium oxalate stone formation can be distinguished from the uric acid stone formation which is less than 5.5 in uric acid stone formation and more than 5.5 in calcium oxalate stone formation.
6. **For cystine stone formers** (cystinuria): Reduce intake of methionine + alkalinization of urine to pH up to 7.5 + fluid intake. For refractory cases, D-penicillamine and tiopronin can be an option.[46]

31. Discuss the role of metabolic evaluation.

Ans: Up to 50% of infectious stones have concomitant metabolic abnormalities and therefore, a comprehensive metabolic evaluation should be pursued.[47] in the form of 24-hour urinary metabolites measurments (for calcium, oxalate, uric acid, citrate, phosphate, uric acid, magnesium, sodium, total volume, and pH) also serum biochemistry for calcium, uric acid, electrolytes, and phosphate are indicated. If the serum calcium level is elevated, serum parathyroid hormone levels should be checked.

If the patient has undergone prior stone removal surgery, information regarding the chemical composition of any previous stones will be helpful.

32. What does the literature say as regards RIRS in such patients?

Ans: RIRS is inferior to PCNL for staghorn calculus in terms of complete stone clearance.

The guidelines recommend PCNL as a primary treatment modality for staghorn calculi by the European and American associations.

For renal calculi more than 2 cm, prospective randomized studies compared efficacy and safety of PCNL and RIRS which concluded PCNL as a upper hand as far as stone free rates were concerned, however, RIRS had less morbidity.[48]

Investigators picked up morbidity as a major factor and proposed RIRS as an alternative option for larger stones with acceptable clinical efficacy with lower morbidity than PCNL when treating renal stones with a diameter >2 cm,[49] >2.5 cm,[50] 1.5 to 3 cm[8] or 2 to 3.5 cm.[51]

33. Disscuss the role of ESWL/sandwich therapy.

Ans: Sandwich therapy typically involves an initial PCNL reducing the stone load, followed by ESWL to stone fragments that are difficult to access endoscopically. ESWL, in turn, precedes a second PCNL to extract residual stone fragments.[52]

SWL was generally thought to be an adjunct treatment to minimize the number of access points required during PCNL but is not recommended as a monotherapy due to lower stone-free rates.[53] In 2005, meta-analysis concluded that PCNL alone has the highest stone-free rate of 78%, while 68% were of PCNL combined with ESWL and 54% stone free rate with SWL alone.[5] Improved PCNL techniques and armamentarium, including the incorporation of flexible nephroscopy, mini PCNL <20 fr tract have provided complete or nearly complete clearance of stone material and reduced tract size reduced risk of bleeding, which decreased the need of SWL treatment as an adjunct.[5] Also, if combination therapy is undertaken, PCNL should be the last procedure to maximize stone fragment removal.[54,55] Flexible ureteroscopy can also be used as a second-stage procedure, if minimal burden remains.

34. Is there any role of non-surgical management for staghorn calculi?

Ans: Conservative management of staghorn calculi is controversial but sometimes necessary in select group of patients with significant comorbidities. Achieving a stone-free state is the aim which often involves multistage or multitract procedures, with procedural risks such as sepsis, bleeding, renal colic, cardiothoracic events, and even death.[47,56,57] These select group of infectious stone patients require close observation as recurrent infections and inflammation act as a precursor for decline in renal function.[58] Three recent studies have concluded that conservative management could be safe in select patients with appropriate monitoring but the mainstay of the treatment of all staghorn stones is surgical.[59–61] Surgical interventions are often long and require multiple procedures, with early complication rates up to 50% in some series, especially in patients with a high Charlson co-morbidtity score.[56,57] Shared decision-making remains mainstay in such clinical situations and as always, the risks and benefits associated with both active and conservative management options must be informed to the patients.

35. How will you follow-up?

Ans: The management of patients with staghorn calculi continues after stone removal as these patients are at risk for stone recurrence.

X-ray KUB and USG KUB (CT KUB in select patients)—1 month

↓

JJ stent removal if imaging is clear. (If residual fragments large enough, then RIRS and stent removal on the merit of the case).

↓

Urine examination after one month (if significant pus cells, then urine culture sensitivity test).

↓

After JJ stent removal and stone clearance to check for any metabolic abnormality and correct if any (comprehensive metabolic work up is indicated).

↓

Some centres prefer suppressive antibiotics for 3 months in matrix stones, anti-hyperuricemic drugs in cases of hyperuricemia, etc. Nephrology consultation in CKD cases.

KEY POINTS

- Staghorn stones are large and branching stones that fill part or all of the pelvicalyceal system. They are usually unilateral and present with UTI with female preponderance. They are linked to urease-producing bacterial infections and, hence, known as struvite infection stones.
- Urinary stasis, urinary tract obstruction, long-term urethral catheter, previous urinary diversion, and neurogenic bladder are well-recognized predisposing factors.
- Untreated staghorn stones are detrimental to the kidney and treatment objectives are complete stone removal, successful treatment of the causative bacteria, preserving renal function and prevention of stone recurrence.
- PCNL should be the recommended first-line treatment for staghorn stones with complete stone clearance as the aim.
- Conservative treatment (in patients with high risk for anaesthesia) can be adopted with suppressive antibiotics.
- Although measures to prevent staghorn stone recurrence are currently available, their clinical utility is still questionable.

REFERENCES

1. Singh P, Enders FT, Vaughan LE, *et al.* Stone Composition Among First-Time Symptomatic Kidney Stone Formers in the Community. *Mayo Clin Proc.* 2015;90(10):1356–1365. doi:10.1016/j.mayocp.2015.07.016.
2. Uroweb-European Association of Urology [Internet]. [cited 2023 Jul 8]. EAU Guidelines on Urolithiasis-Metabolic evaluation and recurrence prevention-Uroweb. Available from: https://uroweb.org/guidelines/urolithiasis/chapter/metabolic-evaluation-and-recurrence-prevention.
3. Blandy JP, Singh M. The case for a more aggressive approach to staghorn stones. *J Urol.* 1976;115(5):505–506. doi:10.1016/s0022-5347(17)59258-7.
4. Koga S, Arakaki Y, Matsuoka M, Ohyama C. Staghorn calculi--long-term results of management. *Br J Urol.* 1991;68(2):122–124. doi:10.1111/j.1464-410x.1991.tb15278.x.
5. Preminger GM, Assimos DG, Lingeman JE, *et al.* Chapter 1: AUA guideline on management of staghorn calculi: diagnosis and treatment recommendations. *J Urol.* 2005;173(6):1991–2000. doi:10.1097/01.ju.0000161171.67806.2a.
6. Rous SN, Turner WR. Retrospective study of 95 patients with staghorn calculus disease. *J Urol.* 1977;118(6):902–904. doi:10.1016/s0022-5347(17)58242-7.
7. Segura JW, Preminger GM, Assimos DG, *et al.* Nephrolithiasis Clinical Guidelines Panel summary report on the management of staghorn calculi. The American Urological Association Nephrolithiasis Clinical Guidelines Panel. *J Urol.* 1994;151(6):1648–1651. doi:10.1016/s0022-5347(17)35330-2.
8. Teichman JM, Long RD, Hulbert JC. Long-term renal fate and prognosis after staghorn calculus management. *J Urol.* 1995;153(5):1403–1407.
9. Alsawi M, Amer T, Mariappan M, Nalagatla S, Ramsay A, Aboumarzouk O. Conservative management of staghorn stones. *Ann R Coll Surg Engl.* 2020;102(4):243–247. doi:10.1308/rcsann.2019.0176.
10. Ray AA, Ghiculete D, Pace KT, Honey RJ. Limitations to ultrasound in the detection and measurement of urinary tract calculi. *Urology.* 2010;76(2):295–300. doi:10.1016/j.urology.2009.12.015.
11. Fulgham PF, Assimos DG, Pearle MS, Preminger GM. Clinical effectiveness protocols for imaging in the management of ureteral calculous disease: AUA technology assessment. *J Urol.* 2013;189(4):1203–1213.
12. Ghani KR, Patel U, Anson K. Computed tomography for percutaneous renal access. *J Endourol.* 2009;23(10):1633–1639. doi:10.1089/end.2009.1529.

13. Feder MT, Blitstein J, Mason B, Hoenig DM. Predicting differential renal function using computerized tomography measurements of renal parenchymal area. *J Urol*. 2008;180(5):2110–2115. doi:10.1016/j.juro.2008.07.057.
14. Morrisroe SN, Su RR, Bae KT, *et al*. Differential renal function estimation using computerized tomography based renal parenchymal volume measurement. *J Urol*. 2010;183(6):2289–2293. doi:10.1016/j.juro.2010.02.024.
15. Sharbaugh A, Morgan Nikonow T, Kunkel G, Semins MJ. Contemporary best practice in the management of staghorn calculi. *Ther Adv Urol*. 2019;11:1756287219847099. Published 2019 May 9. doi:10.1177/1756287219847099.
16. Assimos D, Krambeck A, Miller NL, *et al*. Surgical Management of Stones: American Urological Association/Endourological Society Guideline, PART I. *J Urol*. 2016;196(4):1153–1160. doi:10.1016/j.juro.2016.05.090.
17. Mishra S, Bhattu AS, Sabnis RB, Desai MR. Staghorn classification: Platform for morphometry assessment. *Indian J Urol*. 2014;30(1):80–83. doi:10.4103/0970–1591.124212.
18. Thomas K, Smith NC, Hegarty N, Glass JM. The Guy's stone score-grading the complexity of percutaneous nephrolithotomy procedures. *Urology*. 2011;78(2):277–281. doi:10.1016/j.urology.2010.12.026.
19. Danis E, Polat EC, Bozkurt M, *et al*. Application of S.T.O.N.E. Nephrolithometry Score for Prediction of Stone-Free Status and Complication Rates in Patients Who Underwent Percutaneous Nephrolitotomy for Renal Stone. *J Laparoendosc Adv Surg Tech A*. 2022;32(4):372–377. doi:10.1089/lap.2021.0197
20. Bruce RR, Griffith DP. Retrospective follow-up of patients with struvite calculi. In Urolithiasis: clinical and basic research 1981 (pp. 191–193). Boston, MA: Springer US.
21. Nemoy NJ, Stamey TA. Surgical, Bacteriological, and Biochemical Management of "Infection Stones". *JAMA*. 1971;215(9):1470–1476. doi:10.1001/jama.1971.03180220052010.
22. Benson AD, Juliano TM, Miller NL. Infectious outcomes of nephrostomy drainage before percutaneous nephrolithotomy compared to concurrent access. *J Urol*. 2014;192(3):770–774. doi:10.1016/j.juro.2014.03.004.
23. Ganpule AP, Naveen Kumar Reddy M, Sudharsan SB, Shah SB, Sabnis RB, Desai MR. Multitract percutaneous nephrolithotomy in staghorn calculus. *Asian J Urol*. 2020;7(2):94–101. doi:10.1016/j.ajur.2019.10.001.
24. Kumar S, Randhawa MS, Ganesamoni R, Singh SK. Tranexamic acid reduces blood loss during percutaneous nephrolithotomy: a prospective randomized controlled study. *J Urol*. 2013;189(5):1757–1761. doi:10.1016/j.juro.2012.10.115.
25. Kukreja R, Desai M, Patel S, Bapat S, Desai M. Factors affecting blood loss during percutaneous nephrolithotomy: prospective study. *J Endourol*. 2004;18(8):715–722. doi:10.1089/end.2004.18.715.
26. Atar M, Hatipoglu NK, Soylemez H, *et al*. Relationship between colon and kidney: a critical point for percutaneous procedures. *Scand J Urol*. 2013;47(2):122–125. doi:10.3109/00365599.2012.707685.
27. Keshavamurthy R, Karthikeyan VS, Mallya A, Sreenivas J, Nelivigi GG, Kamath AJ. Anatrophic Nephrolithotomy in the Management of Large Staghorn Calculi-A Single Centre Experience. *J Clin Diagn Res*. 2017;11(5):PC01–PC04. doi:10.7860/JCDR/2017/24723.9837.
28. Thomas R, Lewis RW, Roberts JA. The renal quantitative scintillation camera study for determination of renal function after anatrophic nephrolithotomy. *J Urol*. 1981;125(3):287–288. doi:10.1016/s0022–5347(17)55011–9.
29. Morey AF, Nitahara KS, McAninch JW. Modified anatrophic nephrolithotomy for management of staghorn calculi: is renal function preserved?. *J Urol*. 1999;162(3 Pt 1):670–673. doi:10.1097/00005392–199909010–00007.
30. Kaouk JH, Gill IS, Desai MM, *et al*. Laparoscopic anatrophic nephrolithotomy: feasibility study in a chronic porcine model. *J Urol*. 2003;169(2):691–696. doi:10.1097/01.ju.0000036471.82870.23.
31. Borofsky MS, Lingeman JE. The role of open and laparoscopic stone surgery in the modern era of endourology. *Nat Rev Urol*. 2015;12(7):392–400. doi:10.1038/nrurol.2015.141.
32. King SA, Klaassen Z, Madi R. Robot-assisted anatrophic nephrolithotomy: description of technique and early results. *J Endourol*. 2014;28(3):325–329. doi:10.1089/end.2013.0597.
33. Bercowsky E, Shalhav AL, Portis A, Elbahnasy AM, McDougall EM, Clayman RV. Is the laparoscopic approach justified in patients with xanthogranulomatous pyelonephritis?. *Urology*. 1999;54(3):437–443. doi:10.1016/s0090–4295(99)00261–7.
34. Shekarriz B, Meng MV, Lu HF, Yamada H, Duh QY, Stoller ML. Laparoscopic nephrectomy for inflammatory renal conditions. *J Urol*. 2001;166(6):2091–2094.
35. Altunrende F, Tefekli A, Stein RJ, *et al*. Clinically insignificant residual fragments after percutaneous nephrolithotomy: medium-term follow-up. *J Endourol*. 2011;25(6):941–945. doi:10.1089/end.2010.0491.
36. Osman MM, Alfano Y, Kamp S, *et al*. 5-year-follow-up of patients with clinically insignificant residual fragments after extracorporeal shockwave lithotripsy. *Eur Urol*. 2005;47(6):860–864. doi:10.1016/j.eururo.2005.01.005.
37. Balaji KC, Menon M. Mechanism of stone formation. *Urol Clin North Am*. 1997;24(1):1–11. doi:10.1016/s0094–0143(05)70350–5
38. Shigeta M, Kasaoka Y, Yasumoto H, *et al*. Fate of residual fragments after successful extracorporeal shock wave lithotripsy. *Int J Urol*. 1999;6(4):169–172. doi:10.1046/j.1442–2042.1999.06443.x.
39. Gettman MT, Segura JW. Struvite stones: diagnosis and current treatment concepts. *J Endourol*. 1999;13(9):653–658. doi:10.1089/end.1999.13.653.
40. Wong HY, Riedl CR, Griffith DP. Medical management and prevention of struvite stones. Kidney stones: medical and surgical management. 1996:941–50.
41. Jarrar K, Boedeker RH, Weidner W. Struvite stones: long term follow up under metaphylaxis. *Ann Urol (Paris)*. 1996;30(3):112–117.
42. Wall I, Tiselius HG. Long-term acidification of urine in patients treated for infected renal stones. *Urol Int*. 1990;45(6):336–341. doi:10.1159/000281732.
43. Griffith DP, Gleeson MJ, Lee H, Longuet R, Deman E, Earle N. Randomized, double-blind trial of Lithostat (acetohydroxamic acid) in the palliative treatment of infection-induced urinary calculi. *Eur Urol*. 1991;20(3):243–247. doi:10.1159/000471707.
44. Williams JJ, Rodman JS, Peterson CM. A randomized double-blind study of acetohydroxamic acid in struvite nephrolithiasis. *N Engl J Med*. 1984;311(12):760–764. doi:10.1056/NEJM198409203111203.
45. Diri A, Diri B. Management of staghorn renal stones. *Ren Fail*. 2018;40(1):357–362. doi:10.1080/0886022X.2018.1459306.

46. Abou Chakra M, Dellis AE, Papatsoris AG, Moussa M. Established and recent developments in the pharmacological management of urolithiasis: an overview of the current treatment armamentarium. *Expert Opin Pharmacother*. 2020;21(1):85–96. doi:10.1080/14656566.2019.1685979.
47. Viprakasit DP, Sawyer MD, Herrell SD, Miller NL. Changing composition of staghorn calculi. *J Urol*. 2011;186(6):2285–2290. doi:10.1016/j.juro.2011.07.089.
48. Choi SW, Bae WJ, Ha US, *et al*. Prognostic Impact of Stone-Scoring Systems After Percutaneous Nephrolithotomy for Staghorn Calculi: A Single Center's Experience Over 10 Years. *J Endourol*. 2016;30(9):975–981. doi:10.1089/end.2016.0188.
49. Sfoungaristos S, Gofrit ON, Pode D, Landau EH, Duvdevani M. Percutaneous nephrolithotomy for staghorn stones: Which nomogram can better predict postoperative outcomes?. *World J Urol*. 2016;34(8):1163–1168. doi:10.1007/s00345–015–1743–9.
50. Breda A, Angerri O. Retrograde intrarenal surgery for kidney stones larger than 2.5 cm. *Curr Opin Urol*. 2014;24(2):179–183. doi:10.1097/MOU.0000000000000030.
51. Ghani KR, Sammon JD, Bhojani N, *et al*. Trends in percutaneous nephrolithotomy use and outcomes in the United States. *J Urol*. 2013;190(2):558–564. doi:10.1016/j.juro.2013.02.036.
52. Streem SB, Yost A, Dolmatch B.. Combination "sandwich" therapy for extensive renal calculi in 100 consecutive patients: immediate, long-term and stratified results from a 10-year experience. *J Urol*. 1997;158:342–345.
53. Meretyk S, Gofrit ON, Gafni O, *et al*. Complete staghorn calculi: random prospective comparison between extracorporeal shock wave lithotripsy monotherapy and combined with percutaneous nephrostolithotomy. *J Urol*. 1997;157(3):780–786. doi:10.1016/s0022–5347(01)65039–0.
54. Pearle MS, Watamull LM, Mullican MA. Sensitivity of noncontrast helical computerized tomography and plain film radiography compared to flexible nephroscopy for detecting residual fragments after percutaneous nephrostolithotomy. *J Urol*. 1999;162(1):23–26. doi:10.1097/00005392–199907000–00006.
55. Segura JW, Patterson DE, LeRoy AJ. Combined percutaneous ultrasonic lithotripsy and extracorporeal shock wave lithotripsy for struvite staghorn calculi. World Journal of Urology. 1987 Dec;5:245–7.
56. Osman M, Wendt-Nordahl G, Heger K, Michel MS, Alken P, Knoll T. Percutaneous nephrolithotomy with ultrasonography-guided renal access: experience from over 300 cases. *BJU Int*. 2005;96(6):875–878. doi:10.1111/j.1464–410X.2005.05749.
57. Unsal A, Resorlu B, Atmaca AF, *et al*. Prediction of morbidity and mortality after percutaneous nephrolithotomy by using the Charlson Comorbidity Index. *Urology*. 2012;79(1):55–60. doi:10.1016/j.urology.2011.06.038.
58. Boonla C, Krieglstein K, Bovornpadungkitti S, *et al*. Fibrosis and evidence for epithelial-mesenchymal transition in the kidneys of patients with staghorn calculi. *BJU Int*. 2011;108(8):1336–1345. doi:10.1111/j.1464–410X.2010.10074.x.
59. Charlson M, Szatrowski TP, Peterson J, Gold J. Validation of a combined comorbidity index. *J Clin Epidemiol*. 1994;47(11):1245–1251. doi:10.1016/0895–4356(94)90129–5.
60. Deutsch PG, Subramonian K. Conservative management of staghorn calculi: a single-centre experience. *BJU Int*. 2016;118(3):444–450. doi:10.1111/bju.13393.
61. Flamm J, Forstik F. Zur konservativen Behandlung von Ausgusssteinen [Conservative treatment of staghorn calculi]. *Z Urol Nephrol*. 1987;80(7):395–400.

Chapter

4

Ureteric Calculus during Pregnancy

• Kandarp Parikh • Aditya Parikh

LEARNING OBJECTIVES

- Common presentation
- Investigations
- Treatment options

INTRODUCTION

Urolithiasis during pregnancy is a significant health issue and a frequent cause of non-obstetrical abdominal pain, resulting in hospitalization of pregnant women. The incidence of urinary calculi during pregnancy ranges from 1 in 200 to 1 in 2000, which is comparable to the incidence reported in non-pregnant women.[1] Ureteric stones are a frequent cause of pain during pregnancy. Ureteric stone in pregnancy needs prompt treatment as it can trigger pyelonephritis and premature labour.

Case Scenario

A 25-year-old female who is 20 weeks pregnant has a left upper ureteric 10 mm calculus.

Since this patient was symptomatic with significant hydronephrosis (Fig. 4.1) and had normal blood counts and no fever she was treated with left URS with a 4.5 Fr semirigid ureteroscope. The energy device used was a holmium laser (1 J 10 Hz). Fragments were retrieved with a basket. No DJ stent was kept as the stone was not impacted and the ureter was dilated. Obstetrician under whose care the patient was kept, advised tocolysis to prevent premature contractions. Amoxicillin-Clavulanic acid was used as antibiotic.

1. **What is the incidence of urolithiasis during pregnancy**

   Ans: The incidence of urolithiasis during pregnancy ranges from 1/200 to 1/2000.[1]

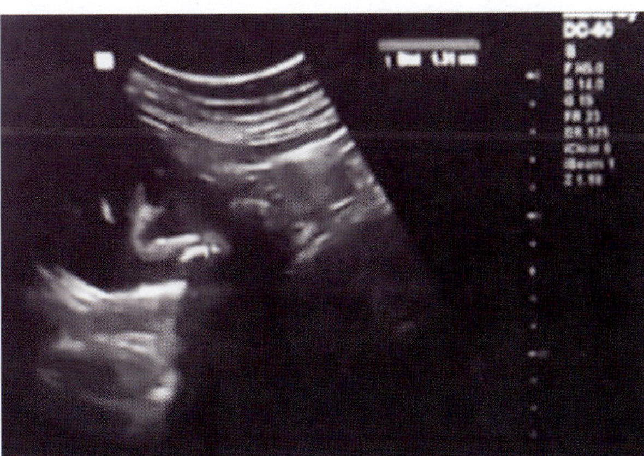

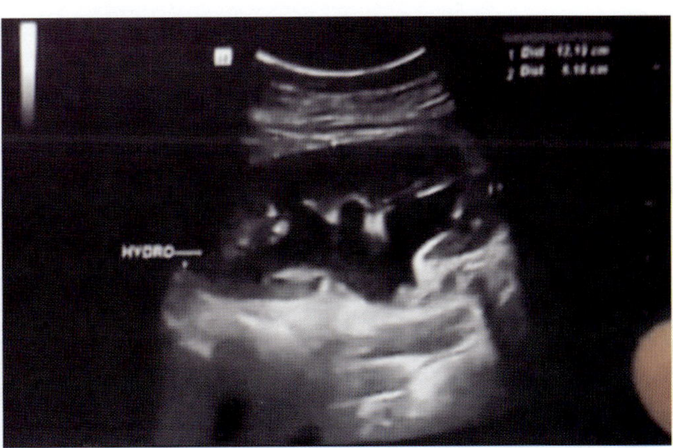

Fig. 4.1: Left hydronephrosis

2. Why is early intervention important?

Ans: Early intervention is important to avoid complications such as renal colic, pyelonephritis, and premature labour. Other pregnancy related complications are obstructive uropathy, hypertension, higher incidence of caesarean section, gestational diabetes mellitus, recurrent abortions and pre-eclampsia.[2]

3. What is the common presentation of ureteric stone in pregnancy?

Ans: Stone can be incidentally diagnosed on routine obstetric sonography. However, the common presentation is ureteric colic. A few patients have urinary tract infection as the antecedent even leading to the diagnosis.

There is often a diagnostic dilemma because there are many overlapping cause of pain.[3]

4. Which diagnostic modalities are used in pregnancy?

Ans:

Laboratory: Urine routine microscopy and a urine culture should be done. Microscopic haematuria is present in 95–100% cases.[4]

Renal function and complete blood count should be checked.

Radiological: USG is the workhorse investigation in pregnancy. However, it has poor sensitivity for ureteric stone. It is difficult to differentiate hydronephrosis due to stone from physiological hydronephrosis.[5]

MR urography is an alternative in patients with stone not detected on USG but with strong clinical suspicion. The use of gadolinium contrast with MRI should be limited; it may be used as a contrast agent in a pregnant woman only if it significantly improves diagnostic performance and is expected to improve foetal or maternal outcome.[6]

There has been concern of the teratogenic and harmful effects of ionizing radiation on the growing foetus and thus the otherwise commonly used modalities of X-ray and CT scan are seldom used in pregnancy. The EAU guidelines state that an X-ray should not be denied to the patient if there is need to confirm diagnosis. Low dose or ultralow dose CT should be used in patients as a last resort.[7]

Tables 4.1 and 4.2 give an idea about the permissible dose of radiation in pregnancy and the dose of radiation in various modalities.[7]

TABLE 4.2: Radiation dose in various imaging modalities

Very low-dose examinations (<0.1 mGy)	
Cervical spine radiography (anteroposterior and lateral views)	<0.001
Head or neck CT	0.001–0.01
Radiography of any extremity	<0.001
Mammography (two views)	0.001–0.01
Chest radiography (two views)	0.0005–0.01
Low-to moderate-dose examinations	(0.1–10 mGy)
Abdominal radiography	0.1–3.0
Lumbar spine radiography	1.0–10
Intravenous pyelography	5–10
Double-contrast barium enema	1.0–20
CT	
Chest CT or CT pulmonary angiography	0.01–0.66
Limited CT pelvimetry (single axial section through the femoral heads)	<1
Nuclear medicine	
Low-dose perfusion scintigraphy	1–5
Technetium-99m bone scintigraphy	4–5
Pulmonary digital subtraction angiography	5
Higher-dose examinations	***(10–50 mGy)***
Abdominal CT	1.3–35
Pelvic CT	10–50
^{18}F PET/CT whole-body scintigraphy	10–50

TABLE 4.1: Effect of gestational age and radiation dose on radiation-induced teratogenesis

Gestational period	***Effects estimated***	***Threshold dose***
Before implantation (0–2 weeks after fertilization) (all or none)	Death of embryo or no consequence	50–100 mGy
Organogenesis (2–8 weeks after fertilization)	2–8 weeks congenital anomalies (skeleton, eyes, genitals) Growth restriction	200 mGy 200–250 mGy
Fetal period	**Effects estimated**	**Threshold dose**
8–15 weeks	Severe intellectual disability (high risk)! Intellectual deficit Microcephaly	60–310 mGy 25 1Q-point loss per 1,000 mGy 200 mGy
16–25 weeks	Severe intellectual disability (low risk)	250–280 mGy

5. **When should intervention be considered for ureteric calculi during pregnancy?**

Ans: The management of ureteric calculi during pregnancy should be individualized based on the size, location, and symptoms of the stone, as well as the gestational age of the patient.

If the stone is <10 mm in size, observation with close follow-up is recommended.

However, if the stone is >10 mm or associated with hydronephrosis or symptoms such as pain or infection, intervention is warranted.

Flowchart 4.1 depicts a good management algorithm for stones in pregnancy.[8]

Flowchart. 4.1: Algorithm for management of stones in pregnanacy (Thakur APS, Sharma V, Ramasamy V, Choudhary A, Patel P, Singh S, *et al*. Management of ureteric stone in pregnancy: a review. Afr J Urol. 2020 Dec;26(1):1–18.)

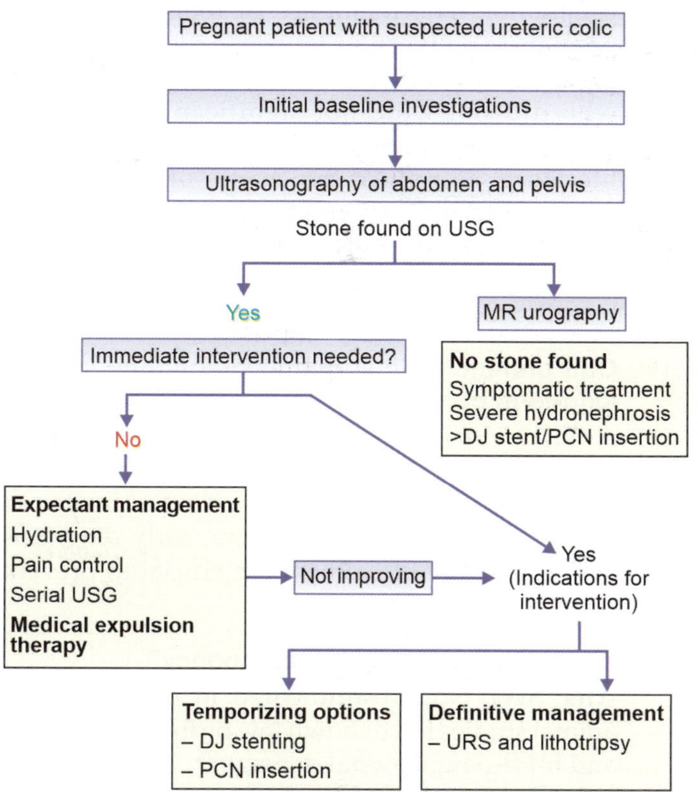

6. **What is the role of expectant management in pregnant patients with urolithiasis?**

Ans: Due to the high incidence of spontaneous passage of stones, the majority of pregnant females with symptomatic ureteric stones can be treated conservatively. With conservative care, 60 to 80 percent of patients naturally pass their stones without any complications. Additionally, the AUA recommendations advised conservative therapy for small non-obstructive calculi (less than 1 cm) in clinically fit patients.[9]

For analgesia	Acetaminophen (paracetamol) 500 mg for mild pain is preferred.
	Morphine in small dose for severe pain can be used.
For antiemetics	Metoclopramide 5–10 mg orally before food is safe in pregnancy,
	Antacids—pantoprazole 20/40 mg.

7. **What is the role of medical management in the treatment of ureteric calculi during pregnancy?**

Ans: Medical management can be considered as an alternative or adjunct to surgical intervention for ureteric calculi during pregnancy. It involves the use of medications such as analgesics, alpha blockers, and antibiotics to manage pain, facilitate stone passage, and prevent infection.

Stone expulsion rate improved by 24% with the use of tamsulosin without any adverse foetal or maternal outcomes.

Calcium channel blocker is a safer drug which is commonly used during pregnancy for the management of preterm labour and gestational hypertension.

The recent AUA guideline supports that if MET is being advised in pregnancy, the patient should be warned that usage of these drugs in pregnancy is not well documented and they are being utilized for an off-label purpose.[10]

8. **What is the role of stenting in managing ureteric calculi during pregnancy?**

Ans: Stenting is one of the options for intervention in patients with ureteric calculi. It can relieve the obstruction and provide drainage of the urine, which can help prevent complications such as infection or sepsis. Additionally, stenting can be performed as a temporary measure to relieve obstruction and allow for the passage of the stone.[11] It is indicated in the following conditions.

- Failure of conservative treatment,
- Complex anatomy,
- Large stone burden,
- Transplanted kidney,
- Presentation very early or very late in the pregnancy,
- Obstetric concerns or complications,
- Active UTI and
- Contraindications to definitive stone management.

9. **Why is frequent stent change required in pregnancy?**

Ans: The physiological hydronephrosis that occurs during pregnancy makes stent migration more common. Due to the high rate of encrustation caused by the metabolic changes in urine chemistry that take place during pregnancy, such as hypercalciuria and hyperuricosuria, it needs to be exchanged every 4–6 weeks. An increased risk of bacteriuria, urinary tract infections, and possible blockage may be linked to extended stenting. Every time an indwelling stent-related UTI is identified, antibiotics should be taken. DJ stenting is preferable to PCN implantation in patients who are at high risk of premature labour.

10. What are the advantages of PCN and when should and should it not be used?

Ans: Main advantages of PCN tube are that it can be performed under local anaesthesia with ultrasound guidance, has high success rate and is safe in pregnancy.

Placement of PCN tube is technically difficult in the third trimester and is preferred as a technique of choice for pregnancies <22 weeks.

PCN affords considerable therapeutic versatility in addressing ureteric stones during pregnancy. It obviates the necessity for extensive surgeries, which pose augmented risks to the pregnant patient and the developing fetus, by effectuating urine diversion and symptom palliation, thereby permitting stone passage via spontaneous means or facilitating safer interventions at subsequent stages.

It has significant benefit in patients with urosepsis.[12]

11. Which is the preferred method for treatment of ureteric stone in pregnancy?

Ans: URS has become a preferred first-line option for the definitive management of ureteric stones in pregnancy, thanks to technological advancements like the development of smaller size, semirigid or flexible ureteroscopes, improved visualisation, improved deflection, better fibre optics, refinement in the design of retrieval baskets, availability of lasers, and advanced obstetrics care with improved monitoring technology.[13]

12. When should ureteroscopy be performed?

Ans: The ACOG guidelines recommend doing any elective procedures, in the second trimester of pregnancy to reduce the risk of premature contractions and spontaneous abortion.[6] If possible one must perform ureteroscopy in the second trimester.

13. What is the intracorporeal lithotripsy device and when is it used?

Ans: Pneumatic lithotripters and holmium YAG lasers are currently advised procedures for intracorporeal stone fragmentation during pregnancy since they are thought to be safe. Holmium: YAG laser does not transmit energy to the foetus and has minimal thermal effects on the periureter. Due to its extremely high peak pressure, electrohydraulic lithotripters may induce uterine contractions during pregnancy by increasing stress throughout the uterine wall. The use of ultrasonic lithotripters should be avoided since they create high-frequency sound (acoustic waves with a frequency of 23–25 kHz) and a high level of noise that is imperceptible to human ears and can exceed 98 dB. These noise levels may negatively impair foetal ear development (theoretically).[14]

14. What is the safety of intracorporeal lithotripsy during pregnancy?

Ans: Intracorporeal lithotripsy is safe and efficient treatment for ureteric calculi during pregnancy. The incidence of foetal deformity, premature delivery, or low birth weight between patients who underwent lithotripsy and those who did not were not significantly different, according to a comprehensive assessment of the literature. To reduce the chance of harm to the foetus, lithotripsy should be carried out by skilled urologists and obstetricians, and safety measures including foetal monitoring and shielding should be followed.[15]

15. Can ureteric calculi during pregnancy lead to long-term complications?

Ans: Ureteric calculi during pregnancy can lead to long-term complications such as chronic kidney disease or hypertension if left untreated or managed improperly. Therefore, early diagnosis and appropriate treatment are crucial to prevent these complications.

16. What is the role of SWL in pregnancy?

Ans: SWL is contraindicated in pregnancy, as animal studies have shown low birth weight babies and intra-parenchymal damage.[16]

KEY POINTS

- Ureteric calculi during pregnancy should be managed based on the size, location, and symptoms of the stone, as well as the gestational age of the patient.
- Stenting can be used to relieve the obstruction and provide drainage of urine in patients with ureteric calculi. Patients treated with stenting require close follow-up and frequent stent change
- Ureteroscopy is safe in pregnancy.
- Intracorporeal lithotripsy using devices such as pneumatic lithotripsy, laser lithotripsy, or electrohydraulic lithotripsy is an effective treatment for ureteric calculi during pregnancy.

REFERENCES

1. Gorton E, Whitfield HN. Renal calculi in pregnancy. Br J Urol. 1997 Jul;80 Suppl 1:4–9.
2. Kroovand RL. Stones in Pregnancy and in Children. J Urol. 1992 Sep;148(3 Part 2):1076–8.
3. Lewis DF, Robichaux AG, Jaekle RK, Marcum NG, Stedman CM. Urolithiasis in pregnancy. Diagnosis, management and pregnancy outcome. J Reprod Med. 2003 Jan;48(1):28–32.
4. Jones WA, Correa RJ, Ansell JS. Urolithiasis associated with pregnancy. J Urol. 1979 Sep;122(3):333–5.
5. Marchant DJ. Effects of pregnancy and progestational agents on the urinary tract. Am J Obstet Gynecol. 1972 Feb 15;112(4):487–501.
6. Nonobstetric Surgery During Pregnancy: Committee Opinion, Number 696. Obstetrics & Gynecology 129(4):p 777–778, April 2017. | DOI: 10.1097/AOG.0000000000002014
7. Fulgham PF, Assimos DG, Pearle MS, Preminger GM. Clinical effectiveness protocols for imaging in the management of ureteral calculous disease: AUA technology assessment. J Urol. 2013 Apr;189(4):1203–13.
8. Thakur APS, Sharma V, Ramasamy V, Choudhary A, Patel P, Singh S, *et al.* Management of ureteric stone in pregnancy: a review. Afr J Urol. 2020 Dec;26(1):1–18.
9. Parulkar BG, Hopkins TB, Wollin MR, Howard PJ, Lal A. Renal colic during pregnancy: a case for conservative treatment. J Urol. 1998 Feb;159(2):365–8.
10. Assimos D, Krambeck A, Miller NL, Monga M, Murad MH, Nelson CP, *et al.* Surgical Management of Stones: American Urological Association/Endourological Society Guideline, PART II. J Urol. 2016 Oct;196(4):1161–9.
11. Jarrard DJ, Gerber GS, Lyon ES. Management of acute ureteral obstruction in pregnancy utilizing ultrasound-guided placement of ureteral stents. Urology. 1993 Sep;42(3):263–7; discussion 267–268.
12. Kavoussi LR, Albala DM, Basler JW, Apte S, Clayman RV. Percutaneous management of urolithiasis during pregnancy. J Urol. 1992 Sep;148(3 Pt 2):1069–71.
13. Lifshitz DA, Lingeman JE. Ureteroscopy as a first-line intervention for ureteral calculi in pregnancy. J Endourol. 2002 Feb;16(1):19–22.
14. Ulvik NM, Bakke A, Høisaeter PA. Ureteroscopy in pregnancy. J Urol. 1995 Nov;154(5):1660–3.
15. Johnson EB, Krambeck AE, White WM, Hyams E, Beddies J, Marien T, *et al.* Obstetric complications of ureteroscopy during pregnancy. J Urol. 2012 Jul;188(1):151–4.
16. Gümü B, Lekili M, Kandilo lu AR, I isa A, Temelta G, Nazli O, *et al.* Effects of extracorporeal shockwave lithotripsy at different stages of pregnancy in the rabbit. J Endourol. 1997 Oct;11(5):323–6.

Chapter

5

Upper Tract Obstruction and Infection in Diabetic Patients

• Kaushikkumar Shah • Parimalsinh Gharia

LEARNING OBJECTIVES

- To elucidate the relationship between urinary tract infection (UTI), diabetes mellitus (DM) and obstruction.
- To allude the readers about potential danger of missing obstruction in case of infection.
- To educate the readers about pathophysiology of obstruction and the importance of de-obstruction in triad of urosepsis, obstruction and DM.
- To educate reader about need and benefits of de-obstruction by DJ stenting or percutaneous nephrostomy (PCN) to relieve obstruction in presence of UTI.
- To educate the reader as regards to role of endourologic procedure like ureteroscopy (URS), retrograde intrarenal surgery (RIRS) or percutaneous nephrolithotomy (PCNL) to treat and prevent recurrent episodes of infection with obstruction

INTRODUCTION

Urinary tract infection (UTI) may have a varied presentation from harmless asymptomatic bacteriuria to complicated UTI to life-threatening urosepsis. It remains a cause of significant morbidity in a community setting, and significant cause of morbidity and mortality in hospital setting especially when associated with obstruction.

Diabetes has reached an epidemic proportion in India. Glycosuria associated with uncontrolled diabetes and augmented by new class of SGLT2 inhibitors (Sodium-Glucose CoTransporter-2) may lead to increased chances of UTI as per USFDA directives.

Management includes good diabetes control with early and prompt diagnosis and treatment of UTI with obstruction. Management, when infection is still organ confined, may prevent progression to complicated UTI with urosepsis and save significant morbidity.

Urgent hospitalization, institution of life support systems, early collection of urine and blood samples before starting broad spectrum antimicrobial therapy, good control of diabetes and early decompression of obstructed systems by DJ stenting or percutaneous nephrostomy (PCN) as an emergency procedure are important steps in management of urosepsis.[1]

A team approach headed by urologist and assisted by intensivist, diabetologist, infectious disease specialist and nephrologist gives better results.

Definitive treatment of stone, papillary necrosis or other causes of obstruction by URS/RIRS/PCNL must be delayed till the patient has been stabilized and infection free.

Case Scenario

A 50-year-old male was referred for ICU care with history of abdominal pain, nausea and occasional vomiting. He had intermittent fever of 3 days duration not responding to conventional treatment. He was a diabetic patient on irregular treatment. He had started deteriorating in last 24 hours. When presented in emergency, he had tachycardia of 120/min, respiration of 22/min, O_2 saturation of 94 percent and temperature of 100 degrees Fahrenheit. He had history of mild LUTS and fever one month back which was treated with antibiotic. His blood pressure was 100/68 on admission.

Prompt basic evaluation and detailed history taking along with resuscitation in a first golden hour set the tone for future treatment and outcome.

1. **What is your first-hand impression from this information?**

   Ans: Looking into his history, it seems that he is in sepsis and likely to have uncontrolled diabetes. He may have urinary tract infection and it has not responded to conventional line of treatment given by his primary physician. He will require intensive care with urgent evaluation and treatment.

2. **What are the principles in managing a case of UTI and associated complications?**

   Ans: There are a few points to consider.
   1. Confirm that there is an infection.
   2. Evaluate that there is unobstructed flow urine from renal papailla to external urethral meatus.
   3. Evaluate the damage done by infection.
   4. Evaluate any alteration in natural body defence mechanism.
   5. Evaluate any abnormal host response to infection.

3. **How will you manage the case?**

   Ans:
   - Primary management involves hemodynamic resuscitation with evaluation of vital parameter and blood sugar levels.
   - After collecting blood and urinary samples for culture and a basic ultrasound, administration of broad-spectrum antimicrobials is the next priority. The choice of antibiotics should be based on local antibiogram.
   - Bedside USG should be able to convey about his bladder, kidneys and other abdominal gross pathology. If a patient is in retention, urethral catheterisation may be done and urine sample collected for urine routine and microscopy, culture and sensitivity.
   - After this treatment in the emergency department, the patient may be shifted to ICU or all can be done in ICU if the patient is highly unstable.
   - With a 2D echo probe, IVC (inferior vena cava) and heart function can be quickly evaluated to know the status of blood volume and cardiac function.
   - **Multidisciplinary team approach** that includes urologist, and intensivist, diabetologist, infectious disease specialist and nephrologist will produce better results.

In emergency, vitals are to be checked and resuscitation measures to be instituted. Quick evaluation and prompt laboratory samples are to be collected and broad-spectrum antibiotics should be started on suspicion of sepsis. Once stabilized hemodynamically, detailed evaluation should be done. Emergency department has to be well equipped with trained manpower and adequate set up to deliver emergency care and investigations for optimal outcome.

4. **What laboratory tests will you send and why?**

   Ans:
   - Complete hemogram with platelet count, serum creatinine with serum electrolyte (renal function test), HbA1c, liver function test including serum bilirubin, serum lactate and arterial blood gas analysis should be performed. They are important for management of patient.
   - C reactive protein (CRP) and procalcitonin (PCT) are important tests to evaluate inflammatory and infective element in the patient. PCT is very specific for bacterial infection and is used in doubtful cases of infection leading to sepsis. CRP is mainly used for follow-up to evaluate the response to treatment so it is recommended as first line investigations.
   - Urine and blood should be collected for culture and sensitivity before the first dose of antibiotics is given.

5. **What is qSOFA?**

   Ans: qSOFA is quick SOFA score[2]
   1. Altered consciousness (GCS score <15)
   2. Systolic blood pressure <100 mmHg
   3. Respiratory rate >22/min

   If 2 of the 3 are positive in a suspected case of sepsis, qSOFA is considered positive and should create a strong suspicion of infection leading to sepsis and organ dysfunction.[2] qSOFA had the specificity of 0.82 (95% CI: 0.76–0.86) and a sensitivity of 0.46 (95% CI: 0.39–0.53) predicting mortality in suspected sepsis patient.[3]

Proper evaluation of severity of patient's condition will help us to prognosticate the treatment outcome based on objective parameters. In a relatively stressful hostile situation, this will help in counselling the relatives about the possible outcome, need for an expensive prolonged critical medical and surgical care and uncertain outcome.

6. **Why are diabetic patients more prone for UTI and have complicated course?**

   Ans: Diabetic patients are more likely to present with UTI and obstruction due to several reasons[4–8]
   - Increased incidence of upper tract stone diseases especially uric acid urolithiasis.[4]
   - Diabetic nephropathy and associated chronic kidney disease with papillary necrosis.[12]
   - Decreased immunity status.[9,10]
   - Diabetic cystopathy with associated high post void residual urine.[11,12]
   - Chronic or recurrent UTI specially in females.[13]
   - Frequent hospital visits and ICU admissions due to other multiple comorbidities and associated catheterisations and catheter associated UTI.

These patients are more susceptible to nosocomial infection, fungal infection, papillary necrosis and emphysematous pyelonephritis.

7. **How will you decide the antibiotics of choice?**

Ans:

- Antimicrobials must be administered no later than one hour after clinical assumption of sepsis.[14] Data suggests that administration of an effective antimicrobial within the first hour of documented hypotension was associated with a survival rate of 80%. Each hour of delay in the subsequent six hours was associated with an average decrease in survival by eight per cent.[15]
- Maximum recommended doses of antibiotics should be administered intravenously with dose-to-dose interval modifications as required for renal and hepatic failure.
- Choice of antibiotics is decided by local susceptibility pattern in a particular set up, prior use of antibiotics in recent past, renal function, liver function, type of pathogen suspected, tissue and urine concentration of antibiotic, side effects of antibiotics, cost and availability.
- In the absence of microbiological report, broad spectrum intravenous antibiotics covering gram negative should be used.[16,17]
- If the patient has not received any antibiotics in previous three months and no hospitalisation or surgical intervention or catheterisation, he is likely to have community acquired infection. *E.coli* and other Enterobacteriaceae are the commonly isolated organisms in such patients. In such cases a third generation cephalosporin, piperacillin in combination with a beta-lactamase inhibitor or a fluoroquinolone with high urinary concentration (ciprofloxacin, levofloxacin) should be used for empirical therapy.[18,19,22]
- If patient is in septic shock or the above criteria are met, patient will be benefitted by combination therapy of antibiotics.[18]
- For hospital-acquired urosepsis especially following urological interventions, an antipseudomonal third-generation cephalosporin or piperacillin plus beta-lactamase inhibitor in combination with an aminoglycoside or a carbapenem should be started as empirical therapy.[16,18]
- In suspected case of fungal infection or recent history of prolonged course of antibiotics, antifungal agents like fluconazole may be started intravenously pending laboratory results.
- Once available, culture report should guide the choice of antibiotics and antibiotic choice can be tailored according to sensitivity report.
- If urine culture report shows resistance to all including carbapenum group, GeneXpert CARBA-R test should be done to know which antibiotic or combination will be lifesaving.
- Help of infectious disease specialist and an expert microbiologist are the keys to success in difficult cases.
- Three culture policy is useful in recurrent UTI as in diabetic patients. First culture will help us to confirm presence of infection and decide which antibiotics can be effective. During the course of antibiotics after a few days, repeat culture will guide us whether given antibiotic is working *in vivo* and giving us microbiological clearance or not by checking for unresolved bacteriuria during therapy. If the culture is positive, it is a case of unresolved bacteriuria during therapy and need to find out cause for the same. If it is positive for the same organism, it means that organism is not responding or there is a presence of continued source like incomplete relief of obstruction. If this second culture grows different bacteria or strain, it means that we were dealing with multiple strains rather than single bacteria. If the second culture is sterile after completing the required course of antibiotics, third urine culture is conducted a few days after antibiotics were stopped. If third culture is also sterile, it means that we have cured the present infection. If this culture is positive, it means that we are dealing with bacterial persistence or reinfection. In bacterial persistence, we have not eradicated the infection and patient may come back with symptomatic infection when enough load of bacteria has grown in side or patient immunity will go down.[20,21]

Identification of microbes causing sepsis, susceptibility to different antimicrobial and selecting the correct one needs good microbiology lab support and expert in infectious disease.

8. **How will you manage diabetes?**

Ans:

- Diabetic ketoacidosis should be ruled out with the help of serum acetone.
- Oral hypoglycemic agents should be stopped as soon as possible to avoid dangerous hypoglycemia and erratic control due to fluctuating blood sugar levels.
- Proper glycemic control with the help of intensivist and diabetologist using insulin according to serial blood glucose monitoring is a must.

9. **What imaging would you do?**

Ans: Bedside ultrasound will guide us about the status of kidney, bladder and prostate and rule out retention.

- USG will show upper tract changes in form of hydronephrosis or hydroureter, renal abscess, papillary necrosis and emphysematous pyelonephritis by presence of air in renal parenchyma
- All the patient with even subtle sign of obstruction or emphysematous pyelonephritis must be evaluated with NCCT scan of the KUB region.
- NCCT KUB may show us the cause of obstruction like stone or papillary necrosis or stricture and associated emphysematous pyelonephritis.

10. What is papillary necrosis?

Ans: As the name suggest, it is a necrosis of renal papilla with or without renal medulla, primary due to ischaemia. Peculiar blood supply from vasa recta predisposes it to necrosis in varied conditions (Fig. 5.1).

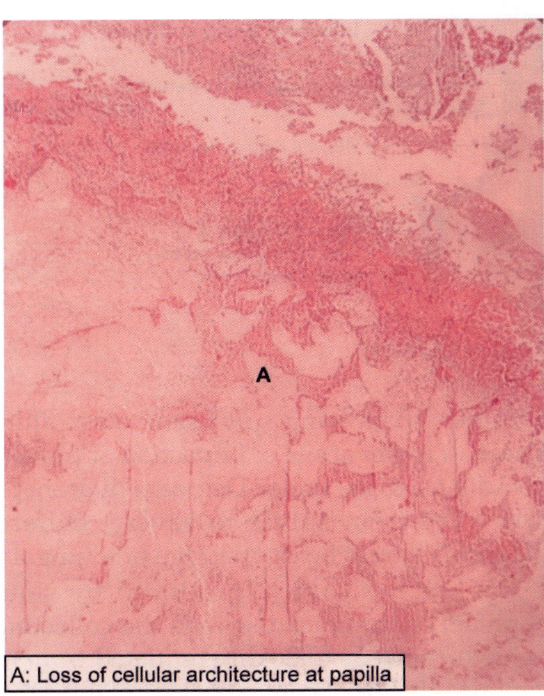

Fig. 5.1: Papillary necrosis

11. What is so peculiar about the blood supply of renal papilla?

Ans: The main renal artery divide into 4–5 segmental arteries which in turn give rise to lobar and interlobar artery. At the base of the renal pyramid, the interlobar arteries give rises to arcuate arteries which runs parallel to renal contour along the corticomedullary junction. Arcuate artery gives rises to multiple radial arterial branches called interlobular arteries which in turn have multiple branches to afferent arterioles and glomeruli. Blood leaves the glomeruli capillary network by efferent arterioles. These arterioles either form secondary capillary network around the urinary tubules in the cortex or descend into the renal medulla as long straight vascular loops called vasa recta. The vasa recta forms wide and plentiful vascular bundles at the base of medullary pyramid but bundle tapers as they continue distally towards apex and papillae. As a result, the papillary tip receives only a marginal blood supply which makes them vulnerable to ischemia and subsequent papillary necrosis. Because of this, the pressure with which blood supply coming from vasa recta is prone to reduce in difficult situations. Hypertonic environment in renal papilla further augments the chances of ischaemia (Figs 5.2 and 5.3).[23]

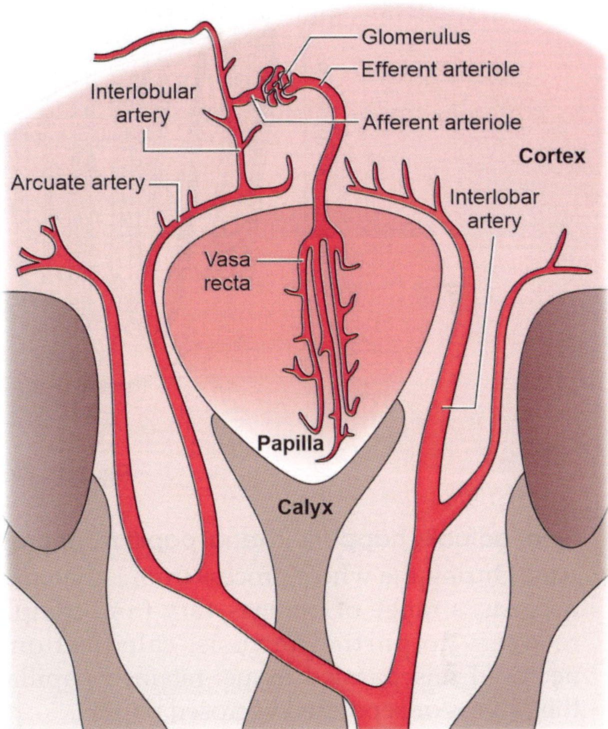

Fig. 5.2: Intrarenal anatomy of renal artery

12. What are those situations in which blood supply from vasa recta may be reduced leading to ischaemia to renal papilla?

Ans: Inflammation of the interstitium by infection causes compression of the vasa recta and produce ischemic change. DM and tuberculosis decrease the perfusion by vasculitis. Hemoglobinopathy, analgesic nephropathy or acute urinary obstruction cause ischemia in medullary pyramids.[23]

13. What causes renal papillary necrosis?

Ans: Renal papillary necrosis is the consequence of an ischemic process in the renal papillae. If normal circulation is not restored within reasonable time or predisposing factors are not corrected, the ischemia leads to irreversible coagulation necrosis, tubular fibrosis and lobar infarcts.[23]

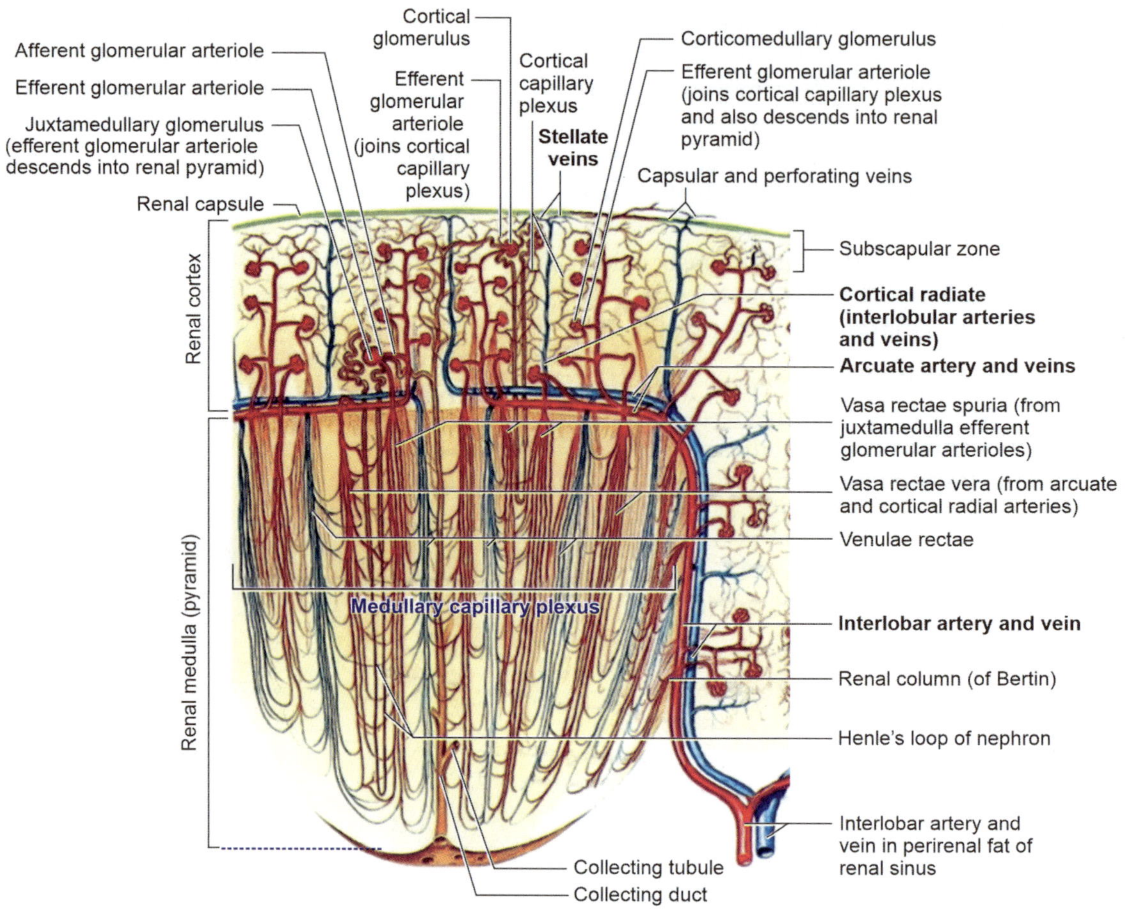

Fig. 5.3: Blood vessels in renal parenchyma

14. What actually happens in renal papillary necrosis?

Ans: During the whole process from ischaemia to necrosis, a range of changes vary from complete recovery to partial necrosis, calcification of necrosed unseparated tissue, retained papilla in the calyces or separated necrosed papilla.

15. What is the significance of renal papillary necrosis?

Ans: Once it gets necrosed, over a period of time the necrosed tissue gets separated from viable tissue and falls into the pelvicalyceal system creating mechanical obstruction to the ureter.[24] Necrosed renal papillae may cause obstruction to the ureter or the renal pelvis just like a stone. If this obstruction is associated with infection, it may lead to serious consequences.

16. What is incidence of development of renal papillary necrosis?

Ans: The incidence of developing RPN in patients with DM is 2.7% to 7.2% and in patients without DM is reported to be less than 0.3 percent.

17. What are the sonographic findings of papillary necrosis?

Ans: Separated sloughed necrosed papilla can be diagnosed by presence of hydronephrosis along with non-shadowing soft tissue mass filling the lumen of ureter at site of impaction or transition to non-dilated distal ureter. Degree of hydronephrosis may vary from subtle to severe. Differential diagnosis would be clot, sludge or a fungal ball

USG shows cavity (produced by sloughed papillae) communicating with the collecting system which needs to be differentiated from hydronephrosis by the irregular contour of the cavity and extension of the cavity up to the arcuate arteries.

Whereas in hydronephrosis, all the calyces are clubbed, whereas in papillary necrosis, one or a few cavities are seen that extend beyond the level of other calyces.

Single calcified necrosed papilla shows the classic ring but if multiple papilla are involved, it will give single garland like calcification of the medulla around the renal sinus echoes.

Isolated distorted calyces should also raise possibility of papillary necrosis.[25–28]

18. What are the CT Imaging findings in cases of renal papillary necrosis?

Ans:

- Poorly perfused papilla area in nephrographic phase

- Signet ring sign, the typical findings in CT scan which is seen due to calyx is filled with contrast material but tip of necrotic papillae is still attached.
- Cavity at calyces due to necrosed sloughed papillae
- Lobster claw appearance due to contrast filling the excavated area at fornix.
- Typical ring-like shadow due to detached necrotic papilla surrounded by contrast material–filled cavity.
- Calcified renal papilla
- Contracted kidney

Secondary changes like filling defect in pelvicalyceal system or ureter and hydronephrosis or hydroureter are typical findings in obstruction caused by sloughed necrosed papilla (Figs 5.4 to 5.7).[29,30]

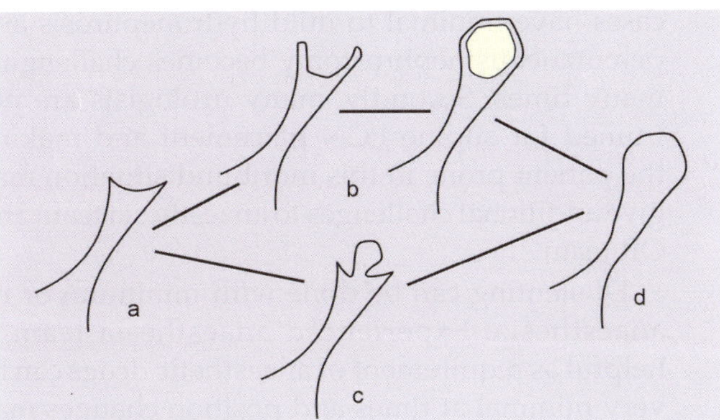

Fig. 5.4: Types of papillary necrosis and end results; (a) Normal papillae; (b) Papillary form of RPN; (c) Medullary form of RPN; (d) Calyceal blunting after sloughing of papillae and epithelialization

19. Why is important to rule out obstruction in cases of patients with urosepsis?

Ans: Ureteric obstruction due to any reasons causes increase in pressure in renal pelvicalyceal system and at certain point of time, this increase may activate the back pressure flow system. There are the backflow system which preserve the renal function when pelvicalyceal system faces high intra-renal pressure.

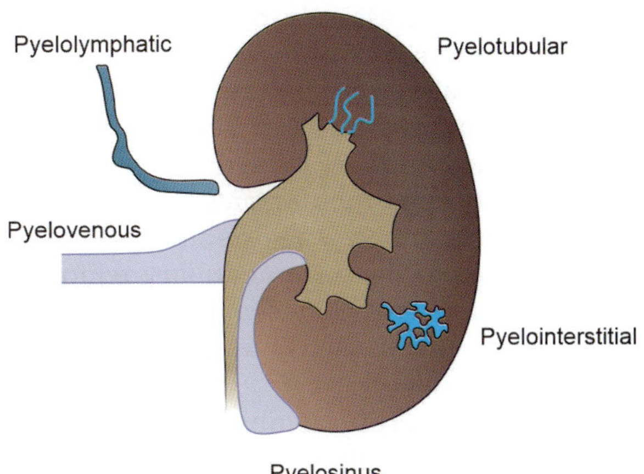

Fig. 5.8: Renal backflow mechanism

When high pressure system is associated with infection, the backflow system will allow bacteria and endotoxins to directly enter the circulatory system and cause septic shock and patient deteriorates very fast.

20. Why only antibiotics does not work in case of obstruction and infection?

Following unilateral ureteric obstruction, renal blood flow (RBF) and ureteral pressure follows triphasic pattern. The first phase lasting 1–2 hours see high ureteral pressure and high RBF. Initial increase in pressure within the renal tubules of

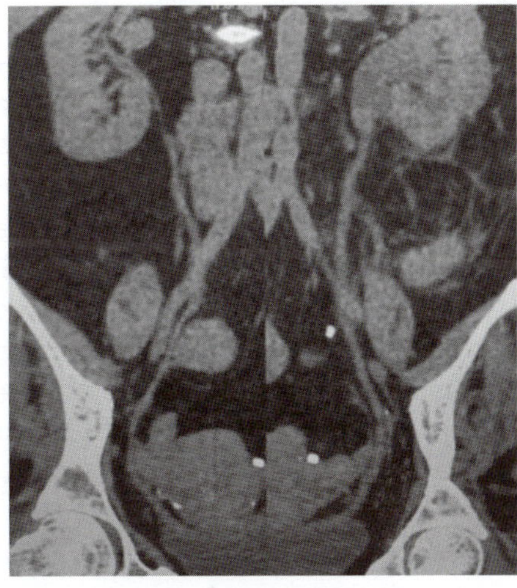

Fig. 5.5: Sloughed papillae at left UPJ causing obstruction

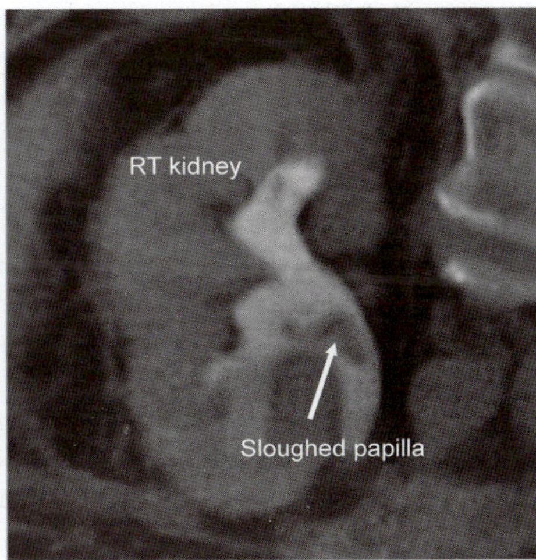

Fig. 5.6: Sloughed papillae as filling defect in CT urography

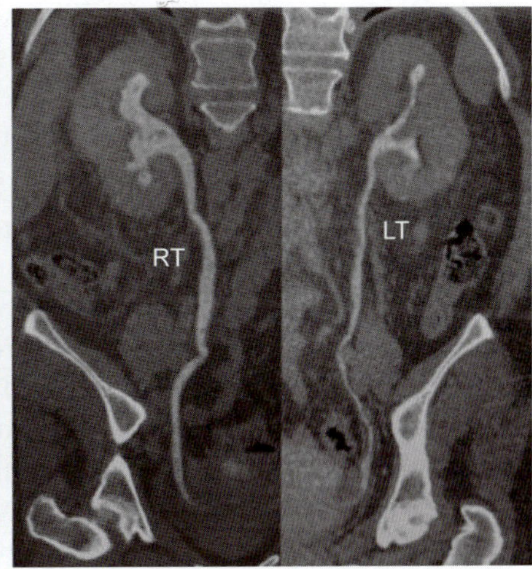

Fig. 5.7: Sloughed papillae as filling defect in CT urography

the affected kidney secondary to obstruction causes decrease in GFR which is compensated by prostaglandin E2 (PGE2) and nitric oxide mediated increase in RBF. During the second phase, lasting 3 to 4 hours, ureteral pressure remains elevated but RBF begins to decline, and, in the final phase, both ureteral pressure and RBF flow progressively decline, resulting in a gradual loss in renal function. This is mediated by an increase in afferent arteriolar resistance which ultimately leads to decrease in effective glomerular capillary pressure and a resulting decrease in renal tubular pressure and decrease GFR. Secondly, there is also a shift in RBF from the outer cortex to the juxtamedullary region of the kidney and large portions of the cortical vascular bed become unperfused or underperfused leading to reduced GFR.

Following ureteral obstruction there is a progressive fall in glomerular filtration rate (GFR) due to a reduction in single nephron glomerular filtration rate (SNGFR) and a reduced number of filtering nephrons.

So antibiotics either stop excretion or antibiotic concentration does not reach to level of minimum inhibitory concentration in pelvicalyceal system and renal parenchyma and hence become ineffective or less effective. In the presence of obstruction, bacterial growth is very fast and they enter into blood circulation causing septicaemia and may not respond at all or have a very poor response. Cases where urinary obstruction is relieved spontaneously, effect of appropriate antibiotics is very good.[31]

21. Why is it imperative to relieve the obstruction in presence of infection?

Ans: As mentioned above, only de-obstruction can relieve the pressure inside pelvicalyceal system and results in decrease the circulatory load of bacteria and endotoxins and only de-obstruction can re-establish the renal blood flow and GFR to become normal and cause good antibiotic concentration inside renal parenchyma as well as PCS.

22. What is the role of source control measure and when should you do?

Ans: It is very important to know the source of infection and it should be controlled at earliest. Source control measures should not be delayed waiting for fever or sepsis to come under control, or waiting for the effect of antibiotics to come. The moment enough blood level of empirical bactericidal antibiotic has reached and some circulatory stability is established; it is better to decompress the system with due precaution not to aggravate the stream of bacterial shower in the blood stream.

Prompt diagnosis and control of source of infection even in difficult situations should be a priority. It is the best, fastest and most effective treatment of sepsis and preservation of kidney function. One should not wait till all parameters improve optimally.

In all cases of suspected or proven cases of obstruction, it is very important to relieve obstruction at an earliest hour. PCN or DJ stenting are the treatment of choice.

23. How would you relieve obstruction?

Ans: Though literature has not proved any difference in the de-obstruction by either percutaneous nephrostomy or DJ stenting,[32] most of the cases have minimal to mild hydronephrosis and percutaneous nephrostomy becomes challenging many times. Secondly, many urologists are not trained for supine PCN placement and making the patient prone in this moribund situation may give additional challenges to anaesthesia team and OR team.

DJ stenting can be done with minimum or no anaesthesia. Experienced anaesthesia team is helpful as requirement of anaesthetic drugs can be very minimal at times and position changes may affect circulatory status in already compromised patients.

24. What precautions will you take during the procedure of de-obstruction?

Ans:

- Adequate dose of appropriate antibiotics should be given intravenously to achieve enough blood level of antibiotics before starting surgical intervention.
- Infected urine sample should be collected from PCS above the obstruction for culture and sensitivity to further guide the choice of antibiotics even if urine culture has been taken on admission.
- Retrograde pyelography (RGP) should be performed with due precautions to prevent reflux of infected urine due to high intrarenal pressure. During RGP, contrast should only be injected after aspiration of fluid from PCS and amount of contrast used should be minimum to avoid intra or extravasation.
- Per urethral catheterisation is a must following the procedure for drainage and monitoring of urine output.

Proper, methodical and gentle operative procedure is the key to success and avoiding complications of the procedure. Do minimum to get maximum result at minimal morbidity of procedure.

25. How do you follow this patient?

Ans: Once out of sepsis and patient should be given adequate antibiotic cover till all inflammatory signs and markers return to normal. Ultimate goal is to achieve nadir serum creatinine and sterile unobstructed system.

26. When do you do reimaging?

Ans: If patient is still febrile or unstable 48–72 hours of de-obstruction and adequate antibiotics, patient requires reimaging to rule out complicating factors like developing renal abscess or perinephric collection, mal-position of DJ stent or PCN and most importantly persistence of obstruction due to any other reason.[33]

27. What would you do if imaging shows persistent obstruction?

Ans: Alternate option of de-obstruction like PCN in case of DJ stenting and additional PCN or DJ stenting in case of PCN should be considered.

28. What do you think why this case deteriorated in spite of hospitalisation?

Ans: This index case patient deteriorated because of inadequate work up and failure to diagnose the obstruction. As discussed above, antibiotics alone may not be adequate in presence of Triad of infection, obstruction and complicating factor like DM or immunocompromised status. Diabetes mellitus, UTI and obstruction aggravate the other two and control of one decrease effect of other two. So, all three should be attacked simultaneously rather than sequentially.

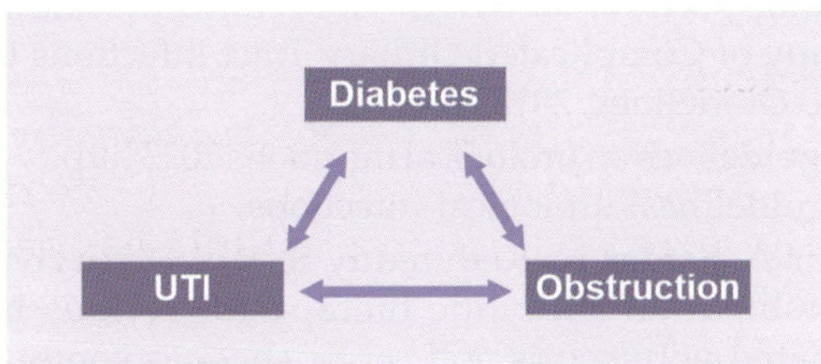

Fig. 5.9: The triad

Adequate resuscitation, prompt work up and localisation of source of sepsis and timely intervention to de-obstruction are key to success in this difficult case.

29. How long will you give parenteral antibiotics?

Ans: It is generally recommended to give antibiotics for 7–14 days. But the duration should be closely related to the treatment of the underlying abnormality. If patient is afebrile and hemodynamically stable for at least 48 hours, duration of antibiotics can be shortened to 7 days.

30. When will you remove DJ stent?

Ans: DJ stent removal can be done after 4 weeks when patient is clinically stable and urine culture with ultrasound are suggestive of complete recovery of infection and obstruction in cases of papillary necrosis.

In cases where stone is the cause of obstruction, stone removal procedure like URS, RIRS or PCNL can be done as early as 2–3 weeks if infection and inflammation have settled clinically and laboratory parameters have improved or came to normal.

31. What are the probable indications of URS or RIRS in cases of papillary necrosis?

Ans: URS/RIRS should be considered in the following conditions at the time of DJ stent removal.

- Those patients who present with recurrent urosepsis associated with papillary necrosis
- Those patients who on imaging show multiple necrosed or sloughed papillae or filling defect in PCS on CT
- Those patients who show filling defect on retrograde pyelography (RGP) either at time of stent placement or DJ stent removal.[34–36]

32. At what time after initial de-obstruction, you consider URS or RIRS in cases of papillary necrosis can be done?

Ans:

- Intervention in form of URS/RIRS should be delayed till patient is free of infection and sterile urine culture can be established.
- It should not be done before 2 weeks to have adequate ureteric dilatation which is imperative to avoid high intrarenal pressure.[37]
- It should not be delayed more than 30 days to decrease stent related sepsis.[38]

33. What precautions are to be taken if patient is planned for URS/RIRS for papillary necrosis?

Ans:

- Patient should be stented and definitive procedure should be delayed for 2 weeks for ureter to dilate and sepsis to settle down as mentioned above.
- It is always safer to do RIRS in a pre-stented patient, major reasons being ease, safety and completeness of intended procedure of removal of necrosed papilla or any obstructive lesion. Chances of access improve, feasibility to keep bigger access sheath is more and possibility of decreased intrarenal pressure are major reasons

to do high risk procedure in cases of infected system 2 to 3 weeks after stenting.

- Urine culture should be sterile or patient should be on culture specific antibiotics for a few days.
- Possibility of fungal infection should be kept in mind and appropriate action should be taken.
- Diabetic control should be optimum.

34. How will you follow-up and what precautions you recommend for these patients?

Ans: The main reasons for RPN is uncontrolled diabetes, UTI and analgesics abuse. Absolute control of DM is prerequisite for prevention of further episodes. Curtailing the use of NSAIDs is recommended. Control of UTI when still it is at level of cystitis will prevent ascending infection.

Upper tract imaging if patient is having persistent or recurrent UTI is must to prevent dangerous urosepsis.

Prophylactic low dose antibiotics has role in preventing ascending infections in cases of persistent UTI without obvious treatable cause even after adequate investigations and imaging.

Any patient with UTI and has undergone surgical procedure like SR/URS/RIRS, they should be followed within next few weeks to have a sterile urine when patient is off the antibiotics for several days to weeks, unobstructed system and control of predisposing factors.

SUMMARY

- UTI is a serious life-threatening infection in presence of obstruction with impaired immune system.
- High index of suspicion with prompt proper work up, resuscitation and management in a well-equipped set up by experienced team gives good result.
- Early institution of proper antimicrobial cover, control of any immunosuppressive condition and early deobstructive measures form the core of management principles guiding treatment decisions.
- UTI in diabetic patient needs special attention to rule out obstruction, papillary necrosis and emphysematous pyelonephritis and if present, consider it as a potentially life-threatening condition.
- PCN and DJ stenting are important to relieve obstruction with minimal risk and should be used at earliest even in suspected cases of urosepsis.
- Stented patients make definitive URS/RIRS a much safer procedure.
- Definitive treatment of obstruction by URS, RIRS or PCNL form the definitive treatment of urinary obstruction.
- Conservative treatment followed by nephrectomy in selected cases have significantly reduced mortality in patients of emphysematous pyelonephritis.

REFERENCES

1. Reyner K., *et al*. Urinary obstruction is an important complicating factor in patients with septic shock due to urinary infection. Am J Emerg Med, 2016. 34: 694.
2. Singer M., *et al*. The Third International Consensus Definitions for Sepsis and Septic Shock (Sepsis-3). JAMA, 2016. 315: 801.
3. Can Wang, A comparison of qSOFA, SIRS and NEWS in predicting the accuracy of mortality in patients with suspected sepsis: A meta-analysis, PLoS One. 2022; 17(4).
4. Michel Daudon et al,Type 2 diabetes increases the risk for uric acid stones, J Am Soc Nephrol 2006 Jul;17(7):2026–33.
5. Patterson JE, Andriole VT. Bacterial urinary tract infections in diabetes. Infect Dis Clin North Am. 1997;11(3):735–750.
6. Joshi N, Infections in patients with diabetes mellitus. N Engl J Med. 1999;341(25):1906–1912.
7. Boyko EJ, Risk of urinary tract infection and asymptomatic bacteriuria among diabetic and nondiabetic postmenopausal women. Am J Epidemiol. 2005;161(6):557–564.
8. Shah BR, Hux JE. Quantifying the risk of infectious diseases for people with diabetes. Diabetes Care. 2003;26(2):510–513.
9. Delamaire M, Maugendre D, Moreno M, Le Goff MC, Allannic H, Genetet B. Impaired leucocyte functions in diabetic patients. Diabet *Med*. 1997;14(1):29–34.
10. Valerius NH, Eff C, Hansen NE, *et al*. Neutrophil and lymphocyte function in patients with diabetes mellitus. *Acta Med Scand*. 1982;211(6): 463–467.
11. Truzzi JC, Almeida FM, Nunes EC, Sadi MV. Residual urinary volume and urinary tract infection–when are they linked? *J Urol*. 2008;180(1): 182–185.
12. Hosking DJ, Bennett T, Hampton JR. Diabetic autonomic neuropathy, Diabetes.1978; 27(10): 1043–1055.
13. Al-Rubeaan KA, Moharram O, Al-Naqeb D, Hassan A, Rafiullah MR. Prevalence of urinary tract infection and risk factors among Saudi patients with diabetes. *World J Urol*. 2013;31(3):573–578.
14. Dellinger, R.P *et al*. Surviving Sepsis Campaign: international guidelines for management of severe sepsis and septic shock, 2012. Intensive Care Med, 2013. 39: 165.
15. Kumar A, Roberts D, Wood KE, Light B, Parrillo JE, Sharma S, *et al*. Duration of hypotension before initiation of effective antimicrobial therapy is the critical determinant of survival in human septic shock. Crit Care Med 2006;34:1589–96.
16. Geerlings, S.E., *et al*. SWAB Guidelines for Antimicrobial Therapy of Complicated Urinary Tract Infections in Adults. SWAB Guidelines, 2013.
17. EAU guidelines on urological infections 2023 https://uroweb.org/guidelines/urological-infections
18. Kumar A, Safdar N, Kethireddy S, *et al*. A survival benefit of combination antibiotic therapy for serious infections associated with sepsis and septic shock is contingent only on the risk of death: a meta-analytic/meta-regression study. Crit Care Med. 2010;38:1651–64.
19. Xu *et al*. Effect of appropriate empirical antimicrobial therapy on mortality of patients with Gram-negative bloodstream infections: a retrospective cohort study, BMC Infectious Diseases (2023) 23:344.
20. Stamey, T. A: Editorial: a clinical classification of urinary tract infection based upon origin. South. Med. J.,68:934, 1975.

21. Campbell's Urology 5th edition, Volume 1,page no 741–743.
22. Gupta, K., *et al.* International clinical practice guidelines for the treatment of acute uncomplicated cystitis and pyelonephritis in women: A 2010 update by the Infectious Diseases Society of America and the European Society for Microbiology and Infectious Diseases. Clin Infect Dis, 2011. 52: e103.
23. Lang EK, Macchia RJ, Thomas R, *et al.* Detection of medullary and papillary necrosis at an early stage by multiphasic helical computerized tomography. J Urol 2003;170(1):94–98.
24. Dae Chul Jung, Renal papillary necrosis: review and comparison of findings at multi-detector row CT and intravenous urography, Review:Radiographics,2006 Nov-Dec;26(6):1827–36.
25. Braden GL, Kozinn DR, Hampf FE Jr, Parker TH, Germain MJ. Ultrasound diagnosis of early renal papillary necrosis. J Ultrasound Med 1991; 10:401–403.
26. Weber M, Brown B, Kohler H. Ultrasound findings in analgesic nephropathy. Nephron 1985; 39:216–222.
27. Boopathy Vijayaraghavan, Sonographic Features of Necrosed Renal Papillae Causing Hydronephrosis, J Ultrasound Med 22:951–956, 2003.
28. Shapeero LG, Vordermark JS. Papillary necrosis causing hydronephrosis in the renal allograft: sonographic findings. J Ultrasound Med 1989; 8:579–581.
29. Lang EK, Macchia RJ, Thomas R, *et al.* Multiphasic helical CT diagnosis of early medullary and papillary necrosis. J Endourol 2004;18(1):49–56.
30. Dyer RB, Chen MY, Zagoria RJ. Classic signs in uroradiology. RadioGraphics 2004;24(Spec Is-sue): S247–S280.
31. S Klahr, K Harris, M L Purkerson, Effects of obstruction on renal functions, Review Pediatr Nephrol 1988 Jan;2(1):34–42.
32. Saskia Weltings, Lessons from Literature: Nephrostomy Versus Double J Ureteral Catheterization in Patients with Obstructive Urolithiasis—Which Method Is Superior? Journal of Endourology, ReviewJ Endourol,2019 Oct;33(10):777–786. doi: 10.1089/end.2019.0309. Vol. 33, No. 10.
33. Om Prakash Kalra, Approach to a Patient with Urosepsis, J Glob Infect Dis. 2009 Jan-Jun; 1(1): 57–63.
34. Rao V C, Bhat SS, Vijayan P, Ramamurthy S. Endoscopic intervention in obstructive renal papillary necrosis. Indian J Urol 2004; 20:29–32.
35. Deepak Ragoori, Role of Retrograde Intrarenal Surgery in the Management of Diabetic Renal Papillary Necrosis, J Endourol 2022 Nov;36(11):1399–1404.
36. Salo JO, Talja M, Lehtonen T. Ureteroscopy in the treatment of ureteral obstruction caused by papillary necrosis. Eur Urol 1987; 13:140–141.
37. Chu L, Sternberg KM, Averch TD. Preoperative stenting decreases operative time and reoperative rates of ureteroscopy. J Endourol 2011;25(5):751e4.
38. Nevo A, Mano R, Baniel J, Lifshitz DA. Ureteric stent dwelling time: A risk factor for post-ureteroscopy sepsis. BJU Int 2017; 120:117–122.

Chapter

6

Ureteric Calculus in Young Man

• *Dilip Kumar Mishra* • *Karthickeyan Naganathan*

LEARNING OBJECTIVES

- How to diagnose obstruction due to upper ureteric stone?
- Emergency management of obstruction and infection due to upper ureteric stone.
- Impacted versus embedded stone.
- Treatment modalities for upper ureteric stone.
- Follow-up of upper ureteric stones and complications.

INTRODUCTION

Upper ureteric stones are almost always formed in the kidneys and migrate to the ureter. Rarely a stone can form *in situ* due to a pre-existing stricture or narrowing in the upper ureter. Studies have shown that the metabolic abnormality in patients harbouring upper ureteric stones is similar to other patients renal.[1]

The presentation is generally of colicky pain in the flank with or without vomiting. Rarely patient may be asymptomatic and in long run may present with infection and loss of renal function.

Diagnosis is primarily by non-contrast computed tomography (CT) of the abdomen and pelvis. Contrast study is needed when there is any suspicion of functional impairment due to obstruction or before any active intervention.

Management revolves around stone clearance and relief of obstruction. The unique position of upper ureteric stones makes them amenable to a myriad of treatment options like shock wave lithotripsy (SWL), semirigid/flexible ureteroscopy (URS), percutaneous nephrolithotomy (PCNL), endoscopic combined intrarenal surgery (ECIRS), laparoscopic ureterolithotomy and open pyelo-ureterolithotomy.[2]

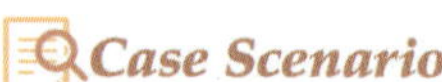

A 28-year-old fit man with a 15 mm upper ureteric calculus presented with discomfort in the right flank for the last one month. He gives history of sharp pain in right flank with vomiting six months back, which subsided after self-medication. There is history of low-grade fever for 3 days. There is no history of haematuria, reduced urine output or swelling on the legs or face. He gives history of stone disease in the family and says his father underwent surgery for stone disease.

He is moderately built and nourished. General physical examination and abdominal examination were normal except for minimal right renal angle tenderness. He has been investigated by local physician and his ultrasonography reveals moderate right hydronephrosis with a suspicious upper ureteric stone.

1. **What is the pathophysiology of loin pain in ureteric colic?**

   Ans: The ureteric stone causes obstruction to the flow of urine and resultant elevated intrarenal pressure with hydronephrosis producing stretching of the renal capsule leading to pain. The ureter undergoes hyperperistalsis with spasms leading to radiating pain to the concerned dermatome. Stone-induced localized inflammatory changes, edema, and irritation also play a role.

   Classically, ureteric stone colic is described as a sudden severe flank pain that originates over the costovertebral angle and extends anteriorly and inferiorly towards the groin or testicle. It is usually waxing and waning type of pain often associated with nausea and vomiting. Loin pain due to renal colic is not related to any physical activity unlike pain due to musculoskeletal pathology. Interestingly, the severity of the pain does not corelate with the stone size or the chance of spontaneous stone expulsion.

2. **What are the other differentials you will consider in this patient with the given history?**

Ans: The other differentials to be kept in mind are right acute pyelonephritis, PUJ obstruction and rarely retrocaval ureter.

3. **Are you happy with the investigation brought by the patient?**

Ans: Ultrasonography (USG) offers a simple non-invasive method for examination of the upper urinary tract. We can easily assess the renal size and location, cortical echogenicity, degree of hydronephrosis, location and size of stones. We can also identify the presence or absence of any echoes within the pelvicalyceal system (suggestive of infection), assess the parenchymal thickness (indirect parameter of renal function) and any perinephric collection (corelates with severity of block). Ultrasound has a sensitivity of 45% in identifying renal and ureteral stones.[3] Easy availability of USG machines, portability, cost-effectiveness, and the ability to identify hydroureteronephrosis makes ultrasound examination the first investigation for renal colic. However, the report brought by the patient seems lacking in many parameters like stone size, echogenicity within the PCS, etc.

4. **What other investigations do you contemplate in this patient?**

Ans: Non-contrast computed tomography (NCCT) is considered the investigation of choice and has significant advantage over USG in the evaluation of loin pain. NCCT provides detailed renal anatomy with its surrounding relations; site, size and density of stone; skin to stone distance, renal parenchymal thickness and perinephric collection if any (Fig. 6.1). The CT can also aid us to predict whether the stone is impacted, embedded.[4]

Apart from CT, other blood and biochemical investigations are needed to look for systemic infection or inflammation and any associated renal failure. A complete hemogram, blood biochemistry, renal function tests, urine routine and urine culture should also be done.

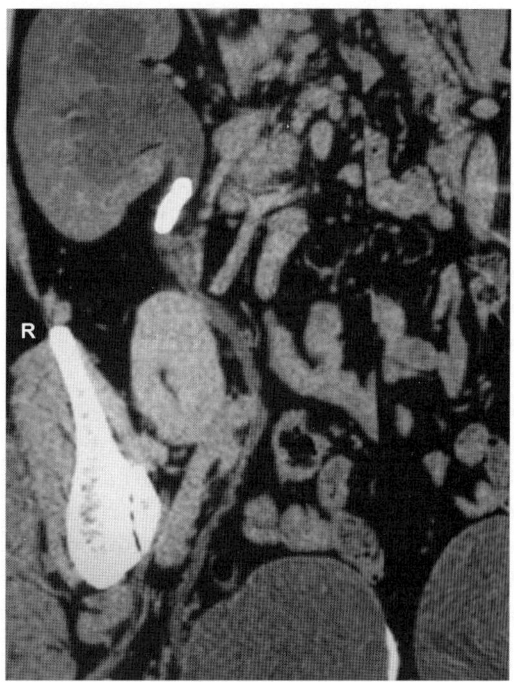

Fig. 6.1: Large upper ureteric stone near PUJ

5. **Is there a need for contrast/functional imaging in this patient? If so, why and which investigation?**

Ans: Functional study enables us not only to assess the function of the individual renal unit, but also to delineate the renal anatomy. Functional imaging is needed before any active intervention for stone disease is planned or when there is a suspicion of renal impairment due to prolonged obstruction. CT-urography, intravenous urogram (IVU) and nuclear scan are the modalities available to assess the same.

Renal and perirenal anatomy, contrast uptake, excretion and drainage all can be assessed with CT urogram apart from stone related parameters. It also helps us to rule out other differential diagnosis. EAU guidelines strongly recommends to perform contrast study when stone removal is planned.[5]

Intravenous urography (IVU) is also a functional imaging which can highlight renal function and anatomical abnormalities; however, it is less informative as compared to CT urography.

In cases of acute colic, the contrast study may give a fallacious report of decreased function and should be interpreted with caution.

Nuclear medicine studies like DTPA scan may be needed in certain cases where we are suspecting loss of renal function due to long standing obstruction and are contemplating a nephrectomy instead of stone removal. However, for anatomical details nuclear scans are inadequate.

6. **Is there a need for urine culture and sensitivity in this patient?**

   Ans: Patient has presented with pain, fever and vomiting pointing towards an infective component. So, urine culture and sensitivity pattern is needed. Bacteriology is also needed before any active intervention like URS/SWL/PNL.

7. **What if this patient also gives history of pedal oedema and reduced output?**

   Ans: These findings are suggestive of renal failure in the setting of ureteric stone. There might be bilateral ureteric stones or stone in a solitary kidney, or the contralateral kidney may have compromised function. In that case, we need to relieve the obstruction at the earliest to prevent irreversible renal injury. Sometimes patients with anuria, severe metabolic acidosis and/or hyperkalaemia might need haemodialysis after consultation with our nephrology colleague for optimization before intervention.

8. **Does this patient need relief of obstruction before definitive management?**

   Ans: No, we can directly plan for definitive stone management procedure in this patient.

   If there are signs of renal failure, sepsis, or impacted stone, it is prudent to relieve the obstruction before definitive stone management. In case of impacted or embedded stone, it is better to leave a double J stent in the ureter to enable drainage of upper urinary tract. This will also allow the mucosal oedema to settle and dilate the ureter so that further intervention can be done at a later time in a hassle-free manner.

9. **What is your choice of diversion: DJ Stent or nephrostomy and why?**

   Ans:

   Double J stent: It is a total internal diversion done in operating room under anaesthesia. Fluoroscopy imaging is needed to confirm its position during the procedure. DJ stent helps to reduce the oedema at the site of obstruction and allows drainage of urine around the stent. Stent inside the ureter acts as a foreign body and initially causes hyperperistalsis of the ureter followed by aperistalsis leading to slow passive dilation of the ureter.[6] In cases of severe obstruction, ureteroscopy may be needed to create a space by the side of the obstructing stone to facilitate passage of a guidewire and DJ stent.

   Patient may experience minor stent related symptoms like dysuria, haematuria and loin pain during voiding.

   Nephrostomy: Nephrostomy can be performed even in unstable patients at bedside under local anaesthesia under USG guidance. In case of suspicious reduced function, the urine output can be analysed for quality and quantity to roughly quantify renal function. Tract for nephrostomy can later be used for a percutaneous nephrolithotomy (PCNL) if desired. Only negative factor for a nephrostomy is the local pain or discomfort to the patient. Some patients might be reluctant to carry the nephrostomy bag due to uneasiness.

   Current available evidence indicates that both nephrostomy and stenting are equally effective in decompressing the system with comparable complication rates.[7] The choice of internal versus external drainage should be based on available resources, local expertise and patient preference.

10. **What are the signs to suggest long standing obstruction?**

    Ans: In case of long-standing obstruction, there will be higher grades of hydronephrosis with thinning of renal parenchyma. Long duration obstruction may also lead to infected hydronephrosis followed by pyonephrosis and loss of renal function. There may be compensatory hypertrophy of the contralateral kidney. At the site of stone impaction, there will be ureteral wall oedema, fat stranding and thickening of ureter.

11. **What do you mean by stone impaction?**

    Ans: Radiologically it is defined as any stone which has remained at the same location for two months or more and failure to visualize contrast in the ureter distal to the stone on IVU films. Surgically, it is a subjective assessment of the endourologist about mobility of stone, ease of dislodging the stone, oedema at the stone site, presence or absence of mucosal polyps and ability to pass a guidewire or stent across the stone in the first instance.[8]

12. **When do you suspect impacted versus embedded stone on CT scan?**

    Ans: Impacted stones may have a greater stone size and volume. Hounsfield unit (HU) value of the ureter distal to the stone, ratio of the HU of the ureteric wall under and above the stone, and degree of hydronephrosis are also elevated. Impacted stones are associated with ureteral wall density value of more than 27 HU below the stone due to oedema and local inflammation.[8,9]

    Embedded ureteral stones may get covered by ureteric mucosa or can become completely submucosal. This can happen in cases of long-standing stones, or post-treatment wherein stone fragments impinge on to the ureteric mucosa.[9]

13. What are the management options in this case?

There are multiple management options available for this type of stone. EAU guidelines (Flowchart 6.1) state that 1st option for stones >10 mm in proximal ureter is URS (antegrade or retrograde) followed by SWL.[10] The other options that can be considered are ECIRS and laparoscopic ureterolithotomy.

Flowchart 6.1: Management options of proximal ureteral stone as per EAU guidelines

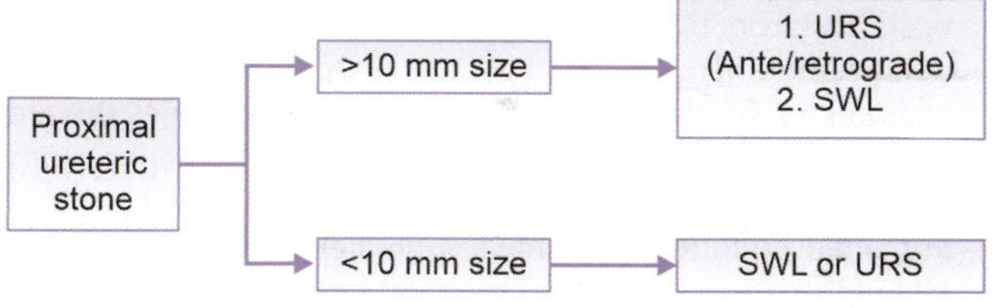

14. Is there a possibility of spontaneous passage of ureteral stones?

Ans: Considering only the stone location, the reported spontaneous stone passage rate of upper, mid and distal ureteric stones was 49%, 58% and 68% respectively. In a meta-analysis conducted by Yallappa et al, almost 75% of stones < 5 mm and 62% of stones > 5 mm passed spontaneously, with an average time to stone expulsion about 17 days (range 6–29 days).[11] Stone diameter rather than length will be a better predictor of spontaneous stone passage. At present with the available evidence, there is no standard recommendation in terms of stone size to predict stone passage spontaneously.[12]

15. What are the factors which will favour use of SWL in these types of cases?

Ans: SWL is one of the preferred modalities of treatment for upper ureteric stones. Stones that are less radiodense (<1000 HU) in a non-obese individual without any distal obstruction are ideally suitable for SWL.[13] Hsiao et al have suggested that SWL is less effective in cases with moderate to severe hydronephrosis.[14]

Double J stenting before SWL can reduce symptomatic steinstrasse formation but does not improve the overall stone free rate. Use of alpha-blockers and diuretics can facilitate spontaneous stone expulsion after SWL, thereby increasing the stone free rates.[13,15]

16. When will you consider ureteroscopy versus PCNL?

Ureteroscopy is the first line of treatment for ureteric stones greater than 10 mm in size.[10] Miniaturisation of scopes, improvements in the optics and image clarity, advancements in the laser technology have made ureteroscopy a safer and more effective method for treatment of ureteric stones. Most upper ureteric stones can be safely accessed with semirigid scopes itself with excellent stone free rates.[16] Flexible ureteroscope is more often required in male patients, in the presence of hydronephrosis or when the stone migrates to regions of pelvicalyceal system that are not accessible with semirigid scope.[17] Sometimes, there is excessive dilation of the upper ureter above the stone due to long standing obstruction which leads to kinks in the ureter and makes ureteroscopy more technically challenging. In such cases, it is better to leave a stent/nephrostomy tube and allow the oedema to settle before proceeding further.

PCNL is an appropriate choice when expertise for flexible ureteroscopy is not available or when the distal ureter is not accessible. In these types of cases, PCNL is generally performed via upper or mid-calyceal access.[18] For an impacted, proximal ureteric stone > 15 mm in diameter, PCNL has better stone-free rates and could simultaneously treat coexisting renal stones.[19] PCNL can be done in both prone as well as supine positions where it can be combined with ureteroscopy for ECIRS. PCNL offers advantage that the stone is approached from the dilated portion of pelvicalyceal system giving wider access, easier manipulations and option to give complete clearance with stone fragments removal.

17. Is there any role of laparoscopic or open surgery in these cases?

Ans: With the advent of improvements in URS/PCNL/SWL techniques, almost all upper urinary tract stones can be safely dealt endoscopically with minimal morbidity. However, on special situations like inaccessible distal ureter, following urinary diversion, multiple upper ureteric stones, impacted upper ureteric stone, failed endoscopic management, obese patients in whom PCNL/SWL have less success rate, open or laparoscopic ureterolithotomy can be offered when the expertise is available.[20]

18. Do you think ECIRS is a good option for this case?

Ans: ECIRS is ideally suitable for patients with large upper tract stone burden where simultaneous antegrade and retrograde access will not only improve stone free rates but also reduce the morbidity by avoiding multiple percutaneous tracts and staged procedure. In large impacted upper ureteric stones, it plays a vital role. Sometimes, the stone is inaccessible by ureteroscopy due to anatomical problems and also there is an ambiguity about the safe feasible access to reach upper ureteric stone. In these cases, the combined technique of ECIRS can be utilized to have an effective solution with good clearance rate in a single sitting.[21]

19. How do you manage an impacted ureteric stone?

Ans: Impacted ureteric stones pose a significant challenge to any endourologist. It is better to disimpact the stone and drain the system with internal stenting or nephrostomy before definitive stone management procedure. Using a semi-rigid ureteroscope and pneumatic lithotripsy probe to disimpact the stone might be safer at times. Due caution should be exercised when we use laser probe for impacted ureteric stone. Laser should be fired at the centre of the stone rather than the periphery to avoid ureteric injury.[8] Laser setting should be adjusted as high frequency has higher chance of ureteric injury than low frequency.[8]

Sometimes, there will be an acute kink just below the site of impaction especially when it is a long-standing stone. The key to negotiate such kinks is to use a new hydrophilic guidewire through the ureteroscope.[22] The ureteroscope should be parked close to the site of kink and good irrigation should be used. Concomitant upward and medial push of the abdomen using the closed fist commonly known as `Mertz manoeuvre' can help to straighten the ureter and aid in passing the guidewire.[23] Flexible ureteroscope might be handy at times in these situations.[8] Antegrade stenting or percutaneous nephrostomy can save the day if nothing works. Definitive stone management in the form of RIRS or PCNL can be done after 10–14 days.

20. How will you follow-up this case?

Ans: Ultrasound, plain X-ray of KUB region, low-dose NCCT can be done before stent removal. If there are any significant residual fragments, it needs to be addressed at the time of stent removal. A long-term follow-up is needed as there is a risk of stone recurrence and of stricture formation at the impacted stone site. A USG should be done at three months and annually thereafter and a CT urography may be needed during the follow-up if stricture development is suspected.

21. What are your options if this patient continues to have hydronephrosis after stent removal?

Ans: Persistent hydronephrosis after stent removal should raise the possibility of ureteric stricture at the site of stone impaction. Ureteric stricture might occur as a sequelae to long standing stone impaction or rarely due to inadvertent ureteric injury during lithotripsy.[24] CT-IVU with delayed films will help us to assess the upper ureteric stricture. Ureteroscopy with retrograde contrast study is another alternative. Subsequent management depends on extent and severity of ureteric stricture and the differential renal function.

KEY POINTS

- Upper ureteric stones generally present as flank pain. Diagnosis rests on ultrasonography and computed tomography (CT) of abdomen.
- Features of sepsis or renal impairment must direct towards acute management in form of double J stent or a nephrostomy tube placement.
- Impacted ureteric stones have a greater stone size, volume, HU of the ureter under the stone, HU under/above ratio, and degree of hydronephrosis and need special attention for management.
- The various treatment options include ureteroscopy, SWL, PCNL, ECIRS, laparoscopic/open ureterolithotomy.
- The treatment should be tailored to the patient requirements, availability and expertise of the treating urologist.
- Follow-up of these patients should be done diligently to recognize formation of stricture at the site of stone impaction.

REFERENCES

1. Husmann DA, Milliner DS, Segura JW. Ureteropelvic junction obstruction with a simultaneous renal calculus: long-term followup. J Urol. 1995 May;153(5):1399–402. PMID: 7714950.
2. Sharma G, Pareek T, Tyagi S, Kaundal P, Yadav AK, Thummala Y, Devana SK. Comparison of efficacy and safety of various management options for large upper ureteric stones a systematic review and network meta-analysis. Sci Rep. 2021 Jun 3;11(1):11811. doi: 10.1038/s41598–021–91364–3. PMID: 34083725; PMCID: PMC8175352.
3. Ray, A.A., *et al.* Limitations to ultrasound in the detection and measurement of urinary tract calculi. Urology, 2010. 76: 295.
4. Tran TY, Bamberger JN, Blum KA, Parkhomenko E, Thai J, Chandhoke RA, Gupta M. Predicting the Impacted Ureteral Stone with Computed Tomography. Urology. 2019 Aug;130:43–47. doi: 10.1016/j.urology.2019.04.020. Epub 2019 Apr 25. PMID: 31029671.
5. A. Skolarikos, H. Jung, A. Neisius, A. Pet ík, B. Somani, T. Tailly, G. Gambaro EAU Guidelines on urolithiasis 2023, *presented at the EAU Annual Congress Milan 2023. ISBN 978-94-92671-19-6.*
6. Venkatesh, Ramakrishna, *et al.* "Impact of a double-pigtail stent on ureteral peristalsis in the porcine model: initial studies using a novel implantable magnetic sensor." Journal of endourology 19.2 (2005): 170–176.
7. Hinojosa-Gonzalez DE, Torres-Martinez M, Villegas-De Leon SU, *et al.* Emergent urinary decompression in acute stone-related urinary obstruction: A systematic review and meta-analysis. Journal of Clinical Urology. 2023;16(1):19–31. doi:10.1177/20514158211017027.
8. Yamashita S, Inoue T, Kohjimoto Y, Hara I. Comprehensive endoscopic management of impacted ureteral stones:

Literature review and expert opinions. Int J Urol. 2022 Aug;29(8):799–806. doi: 10.1111/iju.14908. Epub 2022 Apr 27. PMID: 35475562.

9. Grasso M, Liu JB, Goldberg B, Bagley DH. Submucosal calculi: endoscopic and intraluminal sonographic diagnosis and treatment options. J Urol. 1995 May;153(5):1384–9. doi: 10.1016/s0022–5347(01)67409–3. PMID: 7714947.
10. Geraghty RM, Davis NF, Tzelves L, Lombardo R, Yuan C, Thomas K, Petrik A, Neisius A, Türk C, Gambaro G, Skolarikos A, Somani BK. Best Practice in Interventional Management of Urolithiasis: An Update from the European Association of Urology Guidelines Panel for Urolithiasis 2022. Eur Urol Focus. 2023 Jan;9(1):199–208. doi: 10.1016/j.euf.2022.06.014. Epub 2022 Aug 1. PMID: 35927160.
11. Yallappa S, Amer T, Jones P, Greco F, Tailly T, Somani BK, Umez-Eronini N, Aboumarzouk OM. Natural History of Conservatively Managed Ureteral Stones: Analysis of 6600 Patients. J Endourol. 2018 May;32(5):371–379. doi: 10.1089/end.2017.0848. Epub 2018 Apr 24. PMID: 29482379.
12. Preminger, G.M., *et al.* 2007 Guideline for the management of ureteral calculi. Eur Urol, 2007. 52: 1610.
13. Zhu, Y., *et al.* alpha-Blockers to assist stone clearance after extracorporeal shock wave lithotripsy: a meta-analysis. BJU Int, 2010. 106: 256. https://pubmed.ncbi.nlm.nih.gov/19889063/].
14. Hsiao HL, Huang SP, Wu WJ, Lee YC, Li WM, Chou YH, *et al.* Impact of hydronephrosis on treatment outcome of solitary proximal ureteral stone after extracorporeal shock wave lithotripsy. Kaoh siung J Med Sci. 2008;24(10):507–131.
15. Liu, L.R., *et al.* Percussion, diuresis, and inversion therapy for the passage of lower pole kidney stones following shock wave lithotripsy. Cochrane Database Syst Rev, 2013: Cd008569. https://pubmed.ncbi.nlm.nih.gov/24318643/].
16. Turkan S, Ekmekcioglu O, Irkilata L, Aydin M. Is semirigid ureteroscopy sufficient in the treatment of proximal ureteral stones? When is combined therapy with flexible ureteroscopy needed? Springerplus. 2016 Jan 13;5:30. doi: 10.1186/s40064–016–1677–8. PMID: 26788442; PMCID: PMC4710617.
17. Kartal I, Baylan B, Çakıcı MÇ, Sarı S, Selmi V, Ozdemir H, Yalçınkaya F. Comparison of semirigid ureteroscopy, flexible ureteroscopy, and shock wave lithotripsy for initial treatment of 11–20 mm proximal ureteral stones. Arch Ital Urol Androl. 2020 Apr 6;92(1):39–44. doi: 10.4081/aiua.2020.1.39. PMID: 32255321.
18. Mulawkar PM. Safe PCNL (antegrade URS) in large impacted upper ureteric calculi: A point of technique. Turk J Urol. 2020 Nov;46(6):496. doi: 10.5152/tud.2020.20130. Epub 2020 Aug 20. PMID: 32833617; PMCID: PMC7608543.
19. Bhat A, *et al.* Comparison of antegrade percutaneous versus retrograde ureteroscopic lithotripsy for upper ureteric calculus for stone clearance, morbidity, and complications. Indian J Urol. 2019 Jan–Mar;35(1):48–53. doi: 10.4103/iju.IJU_89_18.
20. Kumar A, Vasudeva P, Nanda B, Kumar N, Jha SK, Singh H. A prospective randomized comparison between laparoscopic ureterolithotomy and semirigid ureteroscopy for upper ureteral stones >2 cm: a single-center experience. J. Endourol. 2015; 29: 1248–52.
21. Mishra DK, Agrawal MS, Shah M, Naganathan K, Hameed Z, Gauhar V. Ambulatory Minimally Invasive Endoscopic Combined Intrarenal Surgery in Management of Large Impacted Proximal Ureteral Calculi: A Feasibility Study at a Tertiary Referral Center. J Endourol. 2023 Mar;37(3):251–256. doi: 10.1089/end.2022.0234. PMID: 36401507.
22. Amasyali AS, Groegler J, Hajiha M *et al.* What guidewire is the best for bypassing an impacted ureteral stone? J. Endourol. 2020; 34: 629–36.
23. JE Lingeman. Mertz maneuver for catheterizing the tortuous ureter. J Endourol. 1987;2:16.
24. May PC, Hsi RS, Tran H *et al.* The morbidity of ureteral strictures in patients with prior ureteroscopic stone surgery: multi-institutional outcomes.J. Endourol. 2018; 32: 309–14.

Chapter

7

Basic evaluation and Lifestyle Modification in Incidentally Detected Stone

• Chandra Mohan Vaddi • Soundarya Ganesan

LEARNING OBJECTIVES

To understand
- The methods of stone analysis.
- The indications for metabolic evaluation.
- How to perform and how to interpret basic metabolic evaluation.
- How to do detailed metabolic evaluation and for which group of patients is it indicated.
- The medical management, individualized treatment for each stone type and disorder.
- The lifestyle changes and dietary modifications to be implemented.
- The common myths in common man's mind and what the actual realities are.

INTRODUCTION

Renal stones have a high recurrence rate of around 50% within the subsequent 10 years.[1] Therefore, prompt evaluation and appropriate medical management matter in a big way to prevent stone recurrence and the associated morbidity.

Case Scenario

A 30-year-old busy executive has bilateral multiple renal stones of size 5–6 mm. He has undergone multiple endourologic interventions in the past. He is asymptomatic now. On follow-up ultrasound, bilateral renal stones are identified. He wants to prevent stone recurrence. He also wants to know the tests to be done, lifestyle modifications, dietary changes and medications to prevent stone formation.

1. **How to do stone analysis? What are the methods available?**

   Ans: Stone analysis can be done by are X-ray powder diffraction crystallography (XRD) or Fourier transform infrared spectroscopy (FTIR). XRD is based on the peculiarity of the crystalline components, while FTIR is based on the energy differences associated with atomic motions.[2–4]

A comprehensive library of standard diffraction or spectroscopic analysis is required for XRD and FTIR respectively. In XRD, the diffraction data is expressed in crystallographic language as interplanar d-spacings in Ångstroms (d[Å]) and as diffraction intensities (I). The interplanar d-spacing indicates the distance between atoms. The diffraction intensity is expressed as either a weak/ strong scale or to a maximum of 100 scale.[5]

The composition is identified by matching the diffraction lines in the sample with the diffraction lines of the standard pattern. The lines that are unmatched are used for identifying other components. In recent times, high resolution XRD cameras and high flux X-ray generators detect the minor stone components also accurately, by making use of monochromators. This is possible because the diffraction lines of the minor components also appear sharper. The limitation of this method is the low sensitivity when the sample is small or when the stone sample is a drug, because the XRD pattern is not established.

In FTIR, the relative percentage of each component of the stone is reported using computer algorithms, based on infrared absorbance of each component. The stone sample is powdered and mixed with powdered potassium bromide. This mixture is compressed into a thin wafer, followed by passage of IR beam. Nowadays, the powdered sample is just grounded and the IR beam is passed to get the attenuated total reflectance. The FTIR spectra of each stone component are represented graphically using the absorption bands at specific wavelengths.

The major advantage of this method is that a small sample is sufficient for analysis and is suitable for drug related stones too. This is because the newly available computer controlled spectrometers mathematically enhance the signals from the sample that make it possible to identify the different components of the stone.

The limitation of FTIR is that the spectral signals from components with similar molecular bonds may overlap and then the differentiation becomes difficult. So both XRD and FTIR can combined to improve the accuracy.

Both XRD and FTIR need standard libraries and their accuracy depends on the same. Many laboratories use patient's sample to generate their standard spectra library, which may be less accurate. Rather, using synthetic stone components for creating standard library would be more accurate. The sensitivity of these methods also depends on the experience of the person who operates the equipment.

Polarising microscopy is a technique in which, the stone is broken, samples are taken from various parts of the stone, and then a polarizing microscope is used to identify the components.[6] The limitation is that small portions of mixed stone cannot be identified and the accuracy is dependent on the experience of the technician.

MicroCT is a newly upcoming non-destructive imaging technique, in which stones are magnified to 1000 times the resolution obtained with clinical CT scanners.[7] This enables to identify the mineral components with nearly the same accuracy as FTIR.

KEY POINTS

- Stone analysis should be done whenever feasible
- Stone analysis should be repeated if there is recurrence even after pharmacological intervention, and even after complete stone clearance[8]
- XRD and FTIR are the most common methods of stone analysis
- MicroCT is an upcoming imaging technique that identifies stone composition

2. What are the indications for metabolic evaluation?

Ans: The indications for metabolic evaluation are listed in Box 7.1.

Box 7.1: Indications for metabolic evaluation

- Pediatric urolithiasis
- Recurrent stone formers
- Strong family history of stones
- Intestinal disease (chronic diarrhoea)
- Pathologic skeletal fractures
- Osteoporosis
- Urinary tract infection with stones
- Personal history of gout
- Solitary kidney
- Anatomical abnormalities
- Renal insufficiency
- Stones composed of cystine, uric acid and struvite
- Patients who cannot tolerate repeat stone procedures

3. How to do basic metabolic evaluation?

Ans: Basic metabolic evaluation for first-time stone formers is depicted in Flowchart 7.1.

Flowchart. 7.1: Evaluation of first time stone formers

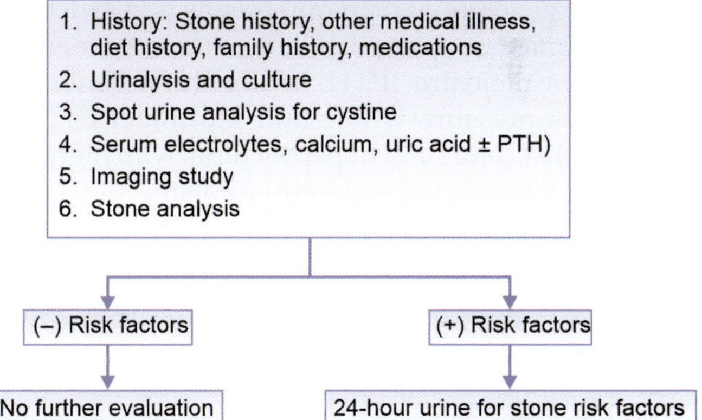

Before embarking upon the initial metabolic work-up, the patient should be preferrably stone free for minimum 3 weeks and they should stick on to their regular diet.[9]

The history should focus on coexisting medical illness (intestinal disease, chronic diarrhoea, gout, osteoporosis, skeletal fractures, renal insufficiency, recurrent urinary infections), dietary history (high salt intake, high animal proteins, weight loss protein diet), occupational history (drivers, primary school teachers, construction workers who are prone to water depletion), family history, drug history (acetazolamide, excess intake of vitamin C, calcium supplements, indinavir, triamterene, and previous episodes of stones.[10–14]

1. Urinalysis is done to assess pH (pH >7.5: Suggestive of infection stones, pH <5.5: Suggestive of uric acid stones) and for crystalluria.
2. Culture is done to rule out infection as the cause of stone.

3. Spot urine analysis for cystinuria
4. Serum electrolytes, calcium, uric acid, intact parathyroid hormone (iPTH) are done to rule out renal tubular acidosis (RTA), primary hyperparathyroidism, and gout.
5. Imaging studies like X-ray KUB, ultrasonogram or CT KUB are done to detect residual stones, anatomy of the pelvicalyceal system and
6. Stone analysis is done to aid in the diagnosis.

4. Would you take any special precautions while sending PTH samples to the laboratory?

Ans: PTH sample is collected in the mid-morning, as it has a circadian rhythm with nadir in mid-morning, but there are no specific recommendations on the timing. The sample can be sent to higher central laboratories in EDTA container (PTH is stable at room temperature in EDTA whole blood for 24 hours, and EDTA plasma for 48 hours. At 4°C, PTH is more stable, hence can be transported in cold packs to the central laboratory at this temperature. Three generations of immune assay (sandwich type immune assay) are available, second-generation assays measure iPTH, while third generation assays measure whole and bio-intact PTH.[15,16] Hypercalcemia and hypercalciuria, with high iPTH point towards hyperparathyroidism.

5. Would the morphology of urine crystals help us in diagnosis? How?

Ans: Urine for crystals aid in the diagnosis as shown in Table 7.1.

TABLE 7.1: Microscopic appearance of urinary stones

Stone type	*Microscopic appearance*
Calcium oxalate monohydrate	Hourglass
Calcium oxalate dihydrate	Envelope
Calcium phosphate—apatite	Amorphous
Brushite	Needle shaped
Struvite	Rectangular, coffin lid shape
Cystine	Hexagonal
Uric acid	Amorphous shards, plates

6. How to diagnose renal tubular acidosis?

Ans: Abnormalities in the serum electrolytes—hypokalemia and low bicarbonates are indicative of RTA. RTA is suspected if 24-hr urine pH is > 6.2 and fasting second morning spot urine pH is > 5.8.[17]

7. Who require detailed metabolic evaluation and how is it done?

Ans: High risk and recurrent stone-formers, patients with multiple stones at initial presentation[18] require more detailed evaluation than single stone-formers.

8. Discuss comprehensive metabolic work-up.

Ans: Comprehensive metabolic work-up includes 24-hour urinary analysis and calcium load test (Box 7.2)

Box 7.2: Comprehensive metabolic work-up

- 24-hour urine analysis
- Fast and Ca load test

24-hour Urinary Analysis: The collecting bottles should be prepared using 1 g thymol per litre in or stored at < 8 °C during collection to reduce bacterial growth.[19] Apart from the basic evaluation, atleast two 24-h urine collections,[20] one on random diet and one after dietary restriction of calcium, sodium and oxalate for seven days.[21] Additional 24-hour urine analysis should be done 8–12 weeks after pharmacologic intervention.[22,23] 24-hour urine sample is collected for the analysis of total volume, pH, calcium, oxalate, uric acid, citrate, sodium, potassium, sulphate, phosphorous, magnesium and creatinine.[18]

9. How do you verify that the patient has collected the sample adequately?

Ans: The average urinary creatinine is 13–21 mg/kg for women and 17–27 mg/kg for men. A lower value indicates under collection and a higher value indicates overcollection.[24]

10. What are the reference values for urinary parameters and what are the red flags?

Ans: The laboratory values for urinary parameters are depicted in Table 7.2.

11. How would you suggest dietary modifications?

Ans: Dietary modifications are advised based on the results of the previous 24-hour urine analyses, before the second round of 24-hour urine analysis, as given in Table 7.3.

Correction of the urinary abnormalities after dietary restrictions, implies **environmental cause**. Persistent abnormalities (espcially urinary calcium, citrate, pH, uric acid, and oxalate) indicate the **need for pharmacologic intervention**.

12. What is the fast and calcium load test?

Ans: Fast and calcium load test: Patient is placed on a diet limited in calcium and sodium for a week. For low calcium diet, one should avoid dairy products like yoghurt, cheese, milk, ice cream, kefir, and greens like spinach, broccoli, food fortified with calcium like instant oatmeal. For low sodium diet, one should avoid smoked fish, salted nuts, pizza, canned food, etc.

TABLE 7.2: Laboratory values for urinary parameters in adults

Urinary parameters	*Reference ranges and limit for medical attention*
pH	Consistently fasting morning spot urine pH > 5.8 and > 6.2 in 24-hour collection (suspicious of renal tubular acidosis)
	Consistently > 7.0 (suspicious of infection)
	Consistently < 5.5 in morning urine and in 24-hour collection (suspicious of acidic arrest)
Specific weight	Specific weight > 1.010
Creatinine	126–234 mg/day (females), 234–324 mg/day (males)
Calcium	90 mg/day
Oxalate	9 mg/day (suspicious of enteric hyperoxaluria) 18 mg/day (suspicious of primary hyperoxaluria)
Uric acid	72 mg/day (females) 90 mg/day (males)
Citrate	Male < 30.6 mg/day, female < 34.2 mg/day
Magnesium	< 54 mg/day
Inorganic phosphate	630 mg/day
Ammonium	900 mg/day
Cysteine	14.4 mg/day

TABLE 7.3: Dietary modifications advised before repeating 24-hour urine analysis

Parameters in 24-hour urine sample	*Modification advised*
Volume < 2 L/day	Increased fluid intake
Sodium >200 mEq/day	Restricted salt intake
Oxalate > 45 mg/day	Restricted intake of oxalate containing food
Calcium >250 mg/day	Restricted calcium intake
Uric acid > 700 mg/day	Restricted animal protein intake
If pH, citrate, potassium is low	Increased intake of citrus fruits

After an overnight fasting, 2-hour urine sample, fasting venous sample are collected. After oral calcium load (1g with a meal), 4-hour urine sample is collected.[24] Parameters analysed in the venous sample include calcium, creatinine, and PTH, and in the urine samples, calcium and creatinine measurement is done.

High fasting urinary calcium **(normal <0.11 mg/dl glomerular filtrate)** implies renal calcium leak or skeletal calcium mobilization, whereas high levels in the 4 hour sample **(>0.2 mg/dl glomerular filtrate or mg/mg creatinine)** with normal serum PTH implies absorptive hypercalciuria.[25]

In most of the patients, the simplified evaluation would suffice. Recurrent and high-risk stone formers warrant a comprehensive evaluation.

KEY POINTS

- First time stone formers should undergo basic evaluation.
- Recurrent and high-risk stone formers should undergo comprehensive evaluation.
- At least two 24-hour urine analyses are done, followed by one more after 8–12 weeks of pharmacologic intervention.

13. How to do pharmacological management for recurrent stone formers?

Ans: Based on the type of the stone detected by stone analysis and the underlying metabolic abnormality detected, pharmacological management is planned. The pharmacological management of calcium oxalate stone (Table 7.5), calcium phosphate stone (Tables 7.6 and 7.7), management of renal tubular acidosis (Table 7.8), management of uric acid stones (Tables 7.9 and 7.10), infection stones (Box 3), cystine stones (Box 4) are described in the following sections.

1. **Calcium oxalate stones**

   The lithogenic risk factors for calcium oxalate stones are hypercalciuria (>250 mg/d), hypocitraturia (<320 mg/d), hyperoxaluria (>40 mg/d), hyperuricosuria(>600 mg/d), hypomagnesuria (<50 mg/d), low urine volume (<2 L/d), or no metabolic abnormality.[23,24] The differential diagnosis of hypercalciuria is detailed in Table 7.4 and the medical management is detailed in Table 7.5.

TABLE 7.4: The differential diagnosis of hypercalciuria

	Absorptive	*Renal*	*Resorptive*
• Serum calcium	Normal	Normal	Elevated
• Parathyroid function	Suppressed (secondarily)	Stimulated (primarily)	Stimulated
• Fasting urinary calcium	Normal	Elevated	Elevated
• Intestinal calcium absorption	Elevated (primarily)	Elevated (secondarily)	Elevated (secondarily)

TABLE 7.5: Medical management of calcium oxalate stones[23]

Biochemical risk factor	Indication for pharmacological therapy	Medication
Hypercalciuria	5–8 mmol/day	Alkaline citrate 9–12 g/day Or sodium bicarbonate 1.5 g TID
	8 mmol/day	Hydrochlorothiazide 25–50 mg/day* Chlorthalidone 25 mg/day
Hypocitraturia	Male < 1.7 mmol/day Female < 1.9 mmol/day	Alkaline citrate 9–12 g/day
Hyperoxaluria	> 0.5 mmol/day (enteric)	Calcium 1000 to 2000 mg/day depending on oxalate excretion **and** magnesium 200–400 mg/day
	> 1 mmol/day (primary)	Pyridoxine 5–20 mg/kg/day Alkaline citrate 9–12 g/day Lumasiran (RNAi agent), subcutaneous [Initial dose once a month for 3 months < 20 kg: 6 mg/kg; > 20 kg: 3 mg/kg Maintenance < 10 kg: 3 mg/kg monthly 10–20 kg: 6 mg/kg every 3 months > 20 kg: 3 mg/kg]
Hyperuricosuria	>4 mmol/day	Alkaline citrate 9–12 g/d **or** sodium bicarbonate 1.5 g tid **plus/or** allopurinol 100 mg/d
	Hyperuricosuria **And** Hyperuricaemia > 380 µmol/L	Alkaline citrate 9–12 g/d **plus** allopurinol 100–300 mg/d **or** Febuxostat 80 mg/day
Hypomagnesiuria	<3 mmol/day	Magnesium 200–400 mg/d (not recommended in renal insufficiency)

*Long-term intake carries risk of skin cancer, non-melanoma skin cancer and some melanomas.[26]

2. Calcium phosphate stones

a. Carbonate apatite

Carbonate apatite crystallisation occurs at a pH > 6.8 and may be associated with infection.[23]

b. Brushite

Crystallises at pH 6.5–6.8 at high urinary concentrations of calcium (> 8 mmol/day) and phosphate (> 35 mmol/day). Its occurrence is not related to UTI.[23]

TABLE 7.6: Medical management of carbonate apatite stones[23]

Hypercalciuria	Hydrochlorothiazide 25–50 mg/day*
Urinary pH > 6.5–6.8 (exclude RTA/ UTI)	Adjust urinary pH between 5.8 and 6.2 (L-methionine 200–500 mg TID)
Elevated serum calcium	Exclude hyperparathyroidism

*Long-term intake carries risk of skin cancer. Non-melanoma skin cancer and some melanomas

TABLE 7.7: Medical management of brushite stones[23]

Hypercalciuria > 8 mmol/d	Hydrochlorothiazide 25–50 mg/day Chlorthalidone 25 mg/day
Urinary pH > 6.5–6.8	Exclude RTA
Elevated serum calcium	Exclude hyperparathyroidism

3. Renal tubular acidosis (RTA) (Table 7.8)

TABLE 7.8: Medical management of renal tubular acidosis[23]

Biochemical risk factor	Indication for pharmacological therapy	Medication
Hypercalciuria	Calcium excretion > 8 mmol/day	Hydrochlorothiazide 25–50 mg/day* Chlorthalidone 25 mg/day
Inadequate urine pH	Hypocitraturia: Male < 1.7 mmol/day Female < 1.9 mmol/day	Alkaline citrate 9–12 g/day Or Sodium bicarbonate 1.5 g TID

*Long-term intake carries risk of skin cancer, non-melanoma skin cancer and some melanomas.

4. **Other disorders associated with calcium stones**
   Granulomatous diseases (may require steroids, hydroxychloroquine or ketoconazole), Nephrocalcinosis (Hyperparathyroidism, primary and enteric hyperoxalurias, RTA, medullary sponge kidney, sarcoidosis, idiopathic hypercalciuria and hypocitraturia, and genetic disorders like Dent's disease, Bartter's syndrome. Management should be based on the underlying metabolic or genetic disease.
5. **Uric acid stones**
   a. Urate acid stones

TABLE 7.9: Medical management of urate acid stones[23]

Biochemical risk factor	*Indication for pharmacological therapy*	*Medication*
Urine pH<5.5	Calcium excretion > 8 mmol/day	Alkaline citrate 9–12 g/day Or Sodium bicarbonate 1.5 g TID [Target pH: prevention: 6.2–6.8, for chemolysis: 6.5–7.2]
Hyperuricosuria	>4.0 mmol/d	Allopurinol 100 mg/d
	> 4.0 mmol/d **and** Hyperuricaemia > 380 µmol	Allopurinol 100–300 mg/d

   b. Ammonium urate stones

TABLE 7.10: Medical management of ammonium urate stones[23]

Urine pH>6.5	Antibiotics for UTI L-methionine 200–500 mg tid [Target urine-pH 5.8–6.2]

6. **Infection stones (struvite/ carbonate apatite/ ammonium urate)**
   Urine pH >6.8: Carbonate apatite; Urine pH> 7.2: Struvite stones.[23]

Box 7.3: Infection stones

- Complete surgical removal, percutaneous chemolysis
- Short or long-term antibiotics
- Urease inhibition (acetohydroxamic acid 15 mg/kg/day)
- Urinary acidification (ammonium chloride 1 g bid or tid or methionine 200–500 mg OD/TID)

7. **Cystine stones**[23]

Box 7.4: Cystine stones

- Appropriate hydration 3.5 L/day (adult), 1.5 L/m^2 (child)
- Adjust urine pH at 7.5–8: Alkaline citrate or sodium bicarbonate
- Recurrence/ cystine excretion >3 mmol/day: Tiopronin** 250–2000 mg/day
  **Side effects can lead to treatment termination (e.g. nephrotic syndrome)

8. **Dihydroxy adenine stones and xanthine stones**
   2, 8 DHA stones: High doses of Allopurinol/ Febuxostat
   Xanthine stones: No medical management available

KEY POINTS

- Defining the underlying abnormality of the particular type of stone is important
- Treatment should aim for correcting the specific abnormality
- Development of side effects, economics of metabolic evaluation and patient compliance are issues in the long-term

14. **What are the general lifestyle and dietary changes to be made to prevent stone recurrence?**
    Ans: The common types of kidney stones and the associated risk factors are given in Table 7.11. Dietary and lifestyle modifications should be done according to the respective risk factors (Table 7.12).
15. **What are the common myths about prevention of stone recurrence?**
    Ans:
    Myth 1: Consuming milk and milk product causes kidney stones.

TABLE 7.11: Dietary modifications for common types of urinary stones

Type of urinary stone	*Risk factors associated*	*Dietary modifications suggested*
Calcium oxalate	Idiopathic hypercalciuria, high-protein diet, high sodium intake, high-oxalate diet, high vitamin C intake, diseases of small bowel, low urine volume	• Decrease meat consumption • Minimize salt intake • Moderate calcium intake (1200 mg/d)
Uric acid	Obesity, acidic urine, high protein/purine intake, low urine volume	• Decrease meat consumption • Encourage citrus juices
Struvite	Recurrent urinary tract infections, alkaline urine	• Encourage fluid intake
Calcium phosphate	Recurrent urinary tract infections, alkaline urine, excessive citrate supplementation, hyperparathyroidism	• Encourage fluid intake

TABLE 7.12: Lifestyle changes for prevention of stone recurrence

Advice on fluid intake	Fluid (water) intake of 2.5–3 L/day **Diuresis: 2–2.5 L/day** Specific weight of urine: < 1,010 g/day
Advice on lifestyle	BMI: Retain a normal BMI level Adequate physical activity Balancing of excessive fluid loss Reduce the intake of alcohol containing fluids Reduce the intake of sodas and calorie-containing fluids
Advice on diet	Balanced diet Rich in vegetables and fibre and fruits Normal calcium content: 1–1.2 g/day Limited NaCl content: 4–5 g/day Limited animal protein content: 0.8–1.0 g/kg/day Limited oxalate intake to 40–50 mg/d Avoid sugar—sweetened soda, dark cola beverages and punch

KEY POINTS

- Increasing water intake reduces the risk of stone recurrence.
- Normal calcium intake, reduced sodium, animal protein and oxalate intake are important to prevent stone recurrence.

Reality: Calcium in milk binds with dietary oxalate and enables its excretion through gut. This actually helps in reducing the risk of stone formation.[27]

Myth 2: Avoid calcium to prevent kidney stone. This can be counter-productive because, restriction of calcium in diet decreases urinary calcium, which in turn leads to secondary hyperparathyroidism and demineralization of bone.[28] One should aim for the dietary reference intake (DRI) of 1000 mg/d. It is better to avoid extremes of calcium intake (>2500 mg/d or < 500 mg/d).[29]

Myth 3: Tomato and other seed containing vegetables cause kidney stones.

Reality: Oxalates in tomatoes is not that high to cause kidney stones because 100 g of tomatoes contain only around 5 mg of oxalates.[30] Stone formers should limit oxalate intake to 40–50 mg/day. One should choose fruits and vegetables with less than 100 mg oxalate per serving.[29] Fruits like watermelon, papaya, apple, plantain are low in oxalate content.[30]

Myth 4: Stone formers should drink 4–5 litres of water a day.

Reality: This would unnecessarily cause increase in the frequency and urgency of micturition. One should drink adequate amount of water sufficient enough to produce atleast 2500 ml of urine per day.[23]

Myth 5: Drinking beer or barley water will flush the kidney stone out.

Reality: Alcohol causes dehydration which may be detrimental, however, as of date, data remain insufficient to claim an association between alcohol intake and renal stone formation.[31] There is no scientific evidence that barley water flushes the stones. As a matter of fact, any stone expulsion can happen with a good urine flow, which happen with any fluid intake (preferably water).

Myth 6: There is a way to dissolve the kidney stones.

Reality: Except small uric acid stones, majority of the stones cannot be dissolved. Medicines can only help in expelling out the stone.

Myth 7: Vitamin supplements are safe if you have kidney stones.

Reality: One should avoid excessive intake of vitamin C, as ascorbic acid is a precursor of oxalate. The DRI for vitamin C is 75 mg/d for women, 90 mg/d for men. Patients who are prone to get oxalate stones should avoid dietary supplements containing more than 1000 mg ascorbic acid per day.[29]

Myth 8: Cranberries can prevent kidney stone formation.

Reality: Cranberries are high in oxalate content and this can increase the risk of stone formation.[32]

Myth 9: Stones form because of poor quality of water.

Reality: Water hardness has no association with the incidence of stones.[33,34] It is beneficial to keep oneself adequately hydrated.

Myth 10: Tea and coffee can increase the risk of stones.

Consumption of tea and coffee does not cause an increase in the risk of stone disease.[35]

Myth 11: Fruits and vegetables cause kidney stones because of their high oxalate content.

Fruit and vegetable intake should be encouraged as they have the beneficial effects of fibre and the high water content.[24,36] The alkaline content of a vegetarian diet increases the urinary pH. However, some dark leafy green vegetables like kale, spinach, and collard greens are extremely high in oxalate (65–750 mg/serving) and must be restricted in patients with hyperoxaluria.[29]

Myth 12: Ramadan fasting can increase the risk of stone formation.

Reality: Fasting and non-fasting conditions do not have a difference in terms of renal stone formation.[37]

Myth 13: Stop non-veg diet completely if you have renal stones.

Reality: 100 g of chicken contains 27 g protein, 100 g mutton contains 25 g protein, 100 g fish contains 22 g protein (*Source*: USDA). Allowable animal protein is around 1 g/kg/day. One need not completely stop non-veg food, instead, they can take in allowable quantities.

KEY POINTS

- Many myths exist about diet and stones
- Thorough knowledge of the realities about the causal relationship is important to break these myths!

REFERENCES

1. Uribarri J, Oh MS, Carroll HJ. The first kidney stone. Annals of internal medicine. 1989 Dec 15;111(12):1006–9.
2. Sutor DJ, Scheidt S. Identification standards for human urinary calculus components, using crystallographic methods. British Journal of Urology. 1968 Feb;40(1):22–8.
3. Berthelot M, Cornu G, Daudon M, Helbert M, Laurence C. Computer-aided infrared analysis of urinary calculi. Clinical chemistry. 1987 Nov 1;33(11):2070–3.
4. Lehmann CA, McClure GL, Smolens I. Identification of renal calculi by computerized infrared spectroscopy. Clinica chimica acta. 1988 Apr 15;173(2):107–16.
5. File PD. International centre for diffraction data. Swarthmore, Pa. 2000;19081.
6. Brien G, Schubert G, Bick C. 10,000 analyses of urinary calculi using X-ray diffraction and polarizing microscopy. European urology. 1982;8:251–6.
7. Borofsky MS, Dauw CA, Cohen A, Williams Jr JC, Evan AP, Lingeman JE. Integration and utilization of modern technologies in nephrolithiasis research. Nature Reviews Urology. 2016 Sep;13(9):549–57.
8. Kourambas J, Aslan P, Teh CL, Mathias BJ, Preminger GM. Role of stone analysis in metabolic evaluation and medical treatment of nephrolithiasis. Journal of endourology. 2001 Mar 1;15(2):181–6.
9. Norman RW, Bath SS, Robertson WG, Peacock M. When should patients with symptomatic urinary stone disease be evaluated metabolically?. The Journal of urology. 1984 Dec 1;132(6):1137–9.
10. Curhan GC, Willett WC, Rimm EB, Stampfer MJ. Family history and risk of kidney stones. Journal of the American Society of Nephrology. 1997 Oct 1;8(10):1568–73.
11. Smith LH, Fromm H, Hofmann AF. Acquired hyperoxaluria, nephrolithiasis, and intestinal disease: description of a syndrome. New England Journal of Medicine. 1972 Jun 29;286(26):1371–5.
12. Griffith DP, Musher DM. Prevention of infected urinary stones by urease inhibition. Investigative urology. 1973 Nov;11(3):228–33.
13. Ettinger B, Oldroyd NO, Sörgel F. Triamterene nephrolithiasis. Jama. 1980 Nov 28;244(21):2443–5.
14. Berns JS, Cohen RM, Silverman M, Turner J. Acute renal failure due to indinavir crystalluria and nephrolithiasis: report of two cases. American journal of kidney diseases. 1997 Oct 1;30(4):558–60.
15. Hanon EA, Sturgeon CM, Lamb EJ. Sampling and storage conditions influencing the measurement of parathyroid hormone in blood samples: a systematic review. Clinical Chemistry and Laboratory Medicine (CCLM). 2013 Oct 1;51(10):1925–41.
16. Smit MA, van Kinschot CM, van der Linden J, van Noord C, Kos S. Clinical guidelines and PTH measurement: does assay generation matter?. Endocrine Reviews. 2019 Dec;40(6):1 468–80.
17. Gambaro G, Croppi E, Coe F, Lingeman J, Moe O, Worcester E, Buchholz N, Bushinsky D, Curhan GC, Ferraro PM, Fuster D. Metabolic diagnosis and medical prevention of calcium nephrolithiasis and its systemic manifestations: a consensus statement. Journal of nephrology. 2016 Dec;29:715–34.
18. Pearle MS, Goldfarb DS, Assimos DG, Curhan G, Denu-Ciocca CJ, Matlaga BR, Monga M, Penniston KL, Preminger GM, Turk TM, White JR. Medical management of kidney stones: AUA guideline. The Journal of urology. 2014 Aug;192(2):316–24.
19. Williams JC, Gambaro G, Rodgers A, Asplin J, Bonny O, Costa-Bauzá A, Ferraro PM, Fogazzi G, Fuster DG, Goldfarb DS, Grases F. Urine and stone analysis for the investigation of the renal stone former: a consensus conference. Urolithiasis. 2021 Feb;49:1–6.
20. Parks JH, Goldfisher E, Asplin JR, Coe FL. A single 24-hour urine collection is inadequate for the medical evaluation of nephrolithiasis. The Journal of urology. 2002 Apr;167(4):1607–12.
21. Rivers K, Shetty S, Menon M. When and how to evaluate a patient with nephrolithiasis. Urologic Clinics of North America. 2000 May 1;27(2):203–13.

22. Assimos DG, Chew B, Hatch MA, Hautmann R, Holmes R, Williams J, Wolf JS. Evaluation of the stone former. Stone Disease 2nd International Consultation on Stone Disease. 2008:33–55.
23. Turk C, Knoll T, Petrik A, Sarica K, Skolarikos A, Straub M, Seitz C. EAU guidelines on urolithiasis 2019. Available from: Uroweb. org. Accessed September. 2020;10.
24. Odvina CV, Pak CY. Medical evaluation of stone disease. Urinary Stone Disease: The Practical Guide to Medical and Surgical Management. 2007:259–68.
25. Menon M, Mahle CJ. Oxalate metabolism and renal calculi. The Journal of urology. 1982 Jan;127(1):148–51.
26. Pedersen SA, Gaist D, Schmidt SA, Hölmich LR, Friis S, Pottegård A. Hydrochlorothiazide use and risk of nonmelanoma skin cancer: a nationwide case-control study from Denmark. Journal of the American Academy of Dermatology. 2018 Apr 1;78(4):673–81.
27. Massey LK, Roman-Smith H, Sutton RA. Effect of dietary oxalate and calcium on urinary oxalate and risk of formation of calcium oxalate kidney stones. Journal of the American Dietetic Association. 1993 Aug 1;93(8):901–6.
28. Byham-Gray L, Burrowes JD, Chertow GM. Nutrition in kidney disease. Humana,; 2014.
29. Massini LA, Han H, Seifter J, Dwyer JT. Diet and kidney stones: myths and realities. Nutrition Today. 2014 Jan 1;49(1):32–8.
30. Ruan QY, Zheng XQ, Chen BL, Xiao Y, Peng XX, Leung DW, Liu EE. Determination of total oxalate contents of a great variety of foods commonly available in Southern China using an oxalate oxidase prepared from wheat bran. Journal of food composition and analysis. 2013 Nov 1;32(1):6–11.
31. Jones P, Karim Sulaiman S, Gamage KN, Tokas T, Jamnadass E, Somani BK. Do lifestyle factors including smoking, alcohol, and exercise impact your risk of developing kidney stone disease? Outcomes of a systematic review. Journal of endourology. 2021 Jan 1;35(1):1–7.
32. Terris MK, Issa MM, Tacker JR. Dietary supplementation with cranberry concentrate tablets may increase the risk of nephrolithiasis. Urology. 2001 Jan 1;57(1):26–9.
33. McDougal WS, Wein AJ, Kavoussi LR, Partin AW, Peters CA. Campbell-Walsh urology 11th Edition review e-book. Elsevier Health Sciences; 2015 Sep 25.
34. Schwartz BF, Schenkman NS, Bruce JE, Leslie SW, Stoller ML. Calcium nephrolithiasis: effect of water hardness on urinary electrolytes. Urology. 2002 Jul 1;60(1):23–7.
35. Barghouthy Y, Corrales M, Doizi S, Somani BK, Traxer O. Tea and coffee consumption and the risk of urinary stones—A systematic review of the epidemiological data. World Journal of Urology. 2021 Aug;39:2895–901.
36. Dussol B, Iovanna C, Rotily M, Morange S, Leonetti F, Dupuy P, Vazi A, Saveanu A, Loundou A, Berland Y. A randomized trial of low-animal-protein or high-fiber diets for secondary prevention of calcium nephrolithiasis. Nephron Clinical Practice. 2008;110(3):c185–94.
37. Amjadi M, Soleimanzadeh F, Ghamatzadeh H, Hajebrahimi S, Hosseinifard H, Pourmehr HS, Tahmasbi F. Ramadan fasting and kidney stones: A systematic review. Urology Journal. 2020 Sep 23;18(04):364–70.

Chapter

8

Renal Stone in Anomalous Kidney

• SK Pal • Harshawardhan Tanwar

LEARNING OBJECTIVES

- To understand the challenges posed in management of stones in pelvic kidney.
- To have a better understanding of evaluation of patients with stones in ectopic pelvic kidney.
- How to choose the best treatment modality for treating patients with stones in ectopic pelvic kidney.
- To know about the challenges in surgical management of these patients.

INTRODUCTION

The development of the definitive kidney occurs as a result of reciprocal inductive effects of ureteric bud and metanephric mesenchyme on each other.[1] This development occurs in sacral region.[2] As the kidneys ascend cranially, they also undergo medial rotation.[1] A complete failure of this ascent results in pelvic ectopic kidney.[3] Failure of ascent also leads to non-rotation of these pelvic kidneys.[1] The estimated incidence of ectopic kidney is 1:2200–3000 patients.[4]

Usually, the patients with ectopic kidneys are asymptomatic and the detection is incidental during radiographic investigations.[5] However, pelvic kidneys have higher incidence of nephrolithiasis and pelviureteric junction obstruction (PUJO) due to associated anatomical and metabolic abnormalities.[5]

In pelvic kidneys due to non-rotation, the pelvis is situated anterior to renal parenchyma and the calyces are directed posteriorly.[6] Sometimes the axis of these kidneys may be tilted laterally, thus making the kidneys lie in horizontal plane.[6] Delayed emptying may occur due to presence of high ureteral insertion in the renal pelvis or due to abnormal crossing vessels obstructing the ureter.[4] The vascular supply is highly variable and frequently anomalous due to persistence of foetal blood supply.[3] Pelvic ectopic kidneys are prone to vesico-ureteral reflux.[3] They may be associated with reproductive structural, cardiac and skeletal anomalies.[6]

Nephrolithiasis is a common complication of pelvic kidneys and treatment may remain challenging due to structural and vascular anomalies.[7] Various radiographic studies including CT scans with angiography phase and functional studies may be needed for understanding detailed anatomy of pelvi-calyceal system and vascular supply.[6,8] Treatment options for pelvic kidney urolithiasis include retrograde intra-renal surgery (RIRS), laparoscopic-assisted percutaneous nephrolithotomy (PCNL), shock-wave lithotripsy (SWL), prone PCNL, laparoscopic or open pyelolithotomy, and robotic pyelolithotomy SWL can be given in prone position, once PUJO has been ruled out, for the stone size less than 15 mm.[9]

- Success rates of RIRS ranges from 75.0% to 84.7% in several studies.[3]
- In stones more than 2 cm in pelvic kidneys confined within true pelvic cavity, laparoscopic assisted PCNL and laparoscopic pyelolithotomy gives excellent stone free rates.[9]

Case Scenario

A 45-year-old man presented with a 6-month history of dull aching left iliac fossa pain. Patient had undergone open pyelolithotomy for stone in ectopic left pelvic kidney 4-years back. On examination patient had a left iliac region scar of previous open surgery and a palpable lump in the same region. Ultrasonography suggested an ectopic left kidney with pelvic calculus of 3 × 2 cm with mild hydronephrosis. A CT scan confirmed the large stone in a malrotated pelvic kidney.

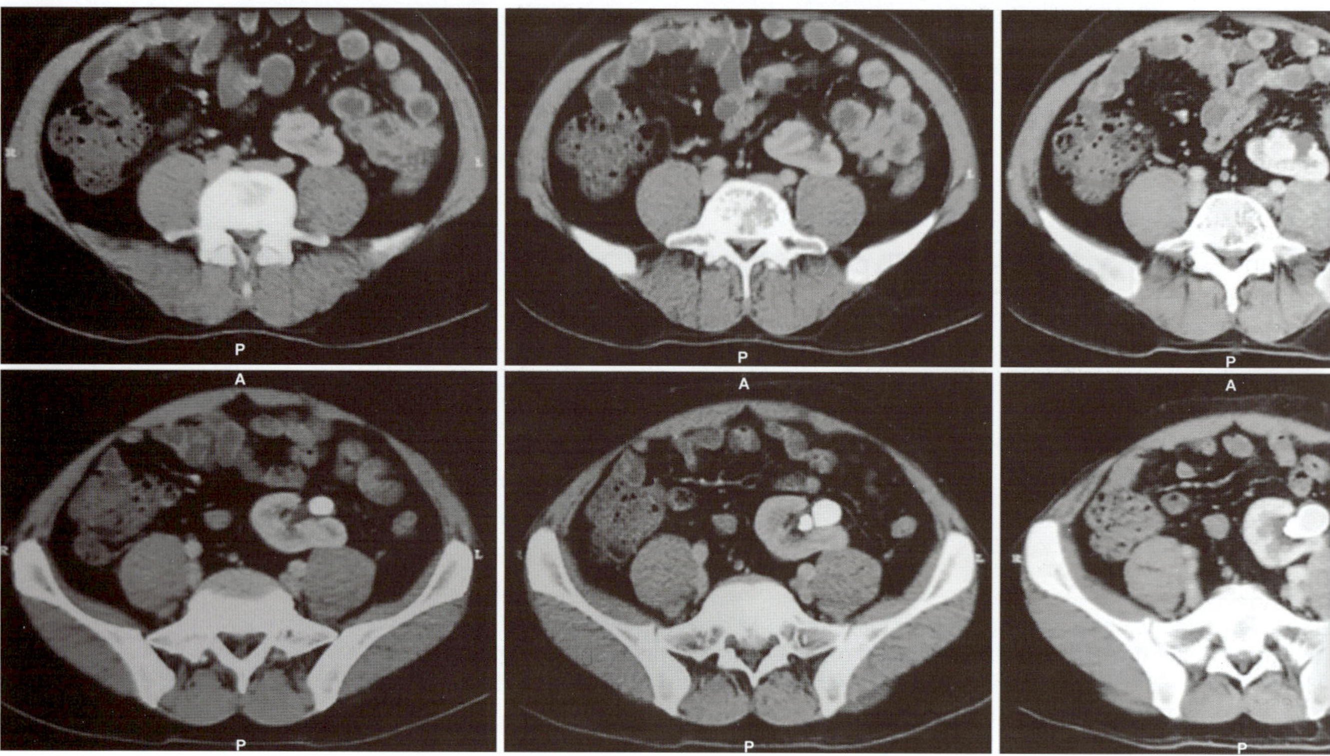

Fig. 8.1: Contrast enhanced computed tomography

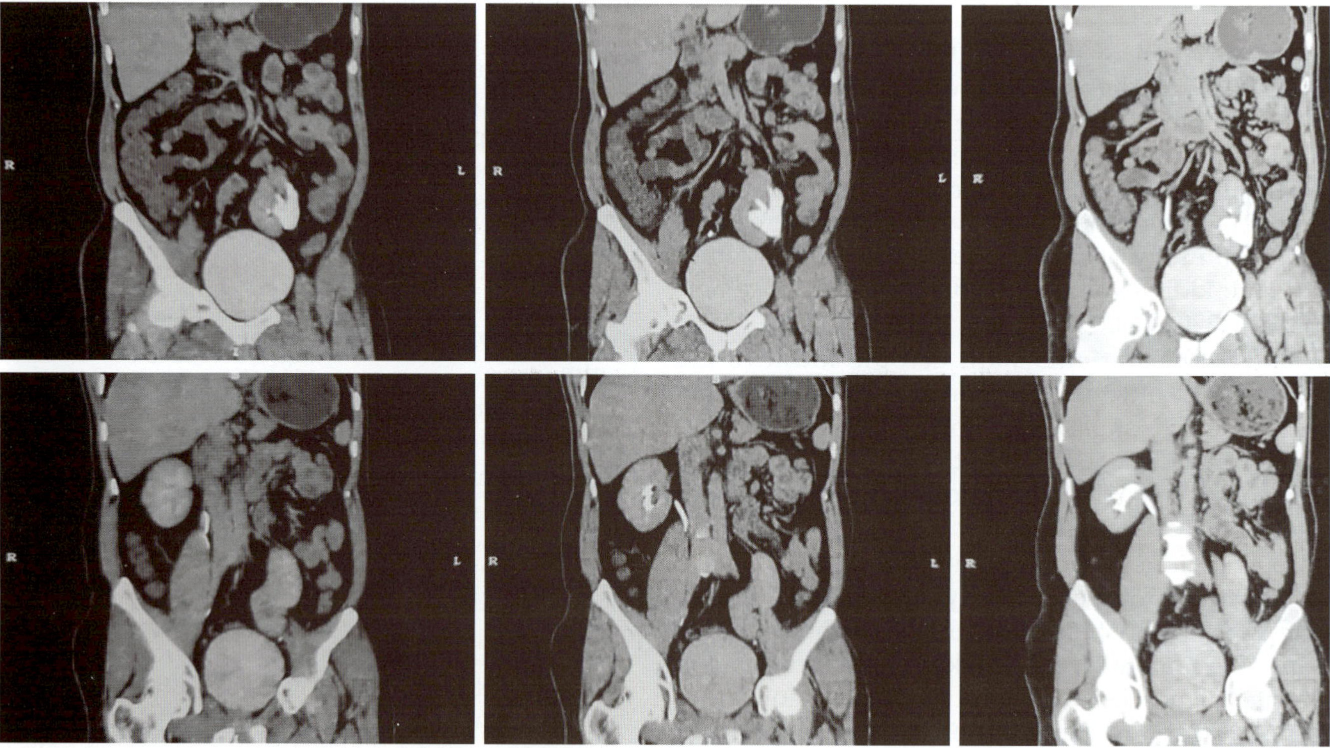

Fig. 8.2: Contrast enhanced computed tomography

1. Which radiological investigations should be done in these cases?

Ans: Ultrasonography: It helps in assessing the orientation of pelvis, as a screening tool to see the anteriorly lying intestine, grade of hydronephrosis, location of major blood vessels. It also helps in stone location and assessing the puncture window in case of USG guided PCNL. The probe of the USG machine can help us to move aside the overlying intestinal loops for ease of puncture.[9] Ultrasound primarily acts as a screening tool. The anatomical details are better delineated by CT scan.

Computed tomography: The most effective imaging for urolithiasis diagnosis is a contrast-enhanced CT scan, which is also the recommended modality for the initial assessment of patients with urinary stones. Its sensitivity can reach 98% and its specificity can reach 96% to 100%.[10] Details of anomalous vasculature of ectopic pelvic kidney are better delineated in the initial arteriographic phase of contrast enhanced CT scan. Exact anatomical location, stone burden, orientation of pelvis, pelvi-ureteric junction obstruction, course of ureter, relationship to visceral organs and functional status of the kidney and other details are noted with CT scan.

In this case CT scan showed an ectopic left kidney measuring 10.8 × 6 cm, in the left iliac fossa with a pelvic calculus of 3.0 × 2.2 cm and a 5 mm calculus in lower pole region. Pelvis was facing anterolateral with anomalous vascularity from left common iliac vessels. Right kidney was found to be in normal location and normal size with no calculus.

2. **What are the challenges in management?**

Ans: The anatomical and structural abnormalities connected to these kidneys make treating ectopic pelvic kidney stones difficult for urologists even today. Following anatomical abnormalities should be anticipated.

- Anomalous vasculature
- Malrotated kidney
- Congenital PUJ obstruction
- High insertion of ureter
- Tortuous ureter
- Narrow ureter
- Crossed ectopia
- Intestinal adhesions
- Proximity to major blood vessels

3. **Which are the factors to be considered for management of ectopic pelvic kidney stones?**

Ans: Multiple factors should be taken in consideration while deciding for treatment in such cases (Table 8.1).

4. **What are the different treatment modalities for management of stones in pelvic kidney?**

Ans:

- SWL: Shock wave lithotripsy
- RIRS: Retrograde intrarenal surgery
- LA-PNL: Laparoscopy assisted percutaneous nephrolithotomy
- L-PL Laparoscopic pyelolithotomy
- Prone PCNL
- Open/robotic pyelolithotomy

SWL is a treatment option for an ectopic kidney with stones in the renal pelvis that are less than 1.5 cm in size or for a patient who declines invasive surgery.[11] LA-"PNL" and RIRS are safe and efficient therapy options for patients with ectopic pelvic kidneys and calyceal calculi. The procedure is best suited for a single big stone situated in the renal pelvis of an ectopic pelvic kidney.[12]

Treatment modalities for management of ectopic pelvic kidney stones

Flowchart 8.1: Algorithm for management of ectopic kidney pelvic stones

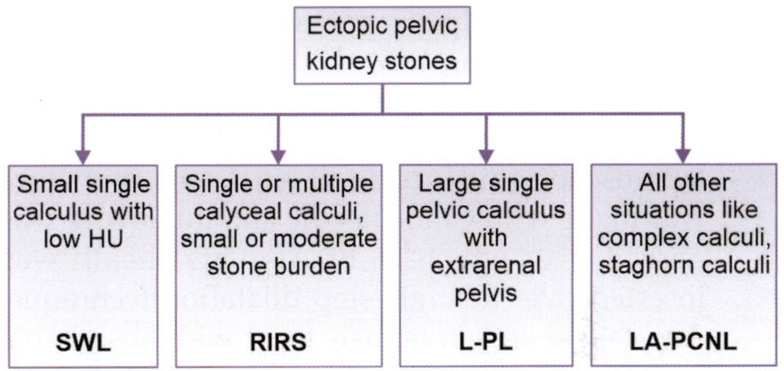

5. **Which is the best treatment option for stone management in a case of ectopic pelvic kidney?**

Ans: The treatment of nephrolithiasis in an ectopic kidney differs from that of an orthotopic kidney with normal anatomy, and the most effective method is still up for debate.[13] Discussion of selecting a treatment option in such cases is multifactorial.

TABLE 8.1: Main factors deciding management

Stone factors	*Anatomical factors*	*Patient factors*
Size of stone	Location of pelvic kidney	Previous surgeries
Location (calyceal/pelvis)	Proximity to major blood vessels	Obesity
Staghorn/single /multiple	Anomalous blood supply	Comorbid conditions
Hounsfield unit	Viscera location	Patients choice
	PUJ obstruction	Sex
	Orientation of pelvis and calyces	Abnormal anatomy

6. Why laparoscopy assisted-PNL was selected in this case?

Ans: Eshghi *et al* in 1985[14] suggested for the first time laparoscopy assisted PNL for ectopic pelvic kidney stones. Holman and Toth (1998) successfully completed 15 transperitoneal laparoscopic aided pelvic kidney laparoscopy procedures for patients with ectopic pelvic kidney stones.[15]

In this case, the kidney was located in pelvis with pelvis facing laterally, with large stone burden of 3 cm in renal pelvis and 5 mm lower pole calculus, with suspected bowel adhesions due to previous surgery. In such scenario laparoscopy-assisted PNL gives the highest stone free rates with minimal complications. Compared to laparoscopic pyelolithotomy, the recurrence rate following laparoscopy assisted PNL is greater, and patients may require postoperative follow-up. Due to its high success rate in treating individuals with ectopic pelvic kidneys that have calyceal calculi, laparoscopy-assisted PNL remains the preferred option for these patients.[16]

7. Describe how you dilate the tract in laparoscopy-assisted PNL.

Ans: With the help of laparoscopy, we first cleared all the overlying bowel loops and identified and delineated the renal pelvis. RGP was done under fluoroscopy. Then under fluoroscopy and laparoscopy guidance direct renal pelvic puncture was made with Chiba needle and guidewire was passed over which 26 Fr Amplatz sheath was inserted over a single step dilatation technique. Amplatz sheath was then fixed with absorbable sutures to avoid slippage. Nephroscope was inserted and complete clearance of the stones was done using pneumatic lithotripsy.

8. What is the role of ultrasonography guidance in planning the initial puncture?

Ans: Using the USG to guide the needle and choose the appropriate calyx is also beneficial. The probe is pressed against the anterior abdominal wall to push the bowel away from the puncture line. When a pelvic stone is present, the target calyx that is selected may be the one that has the stone in it or one that has direct access to the pelvis through the infundibulum.[9] Expert guidance should be used when performing USG guided puncture for an ectopic pelvic kidney.

9. Which is the best exit strategy after completion of laparoscopy-assisted PNL?

Ans: Once stone clearance is achieved and double J stent is placed in antegrade fashion, a thorough inspection of the operative site is done with laparoscopy for any fluid extravasations and organ injuries. Suctioning of the extravasated fluid is done. Drain is placed in the dependent position.

10. Which complications to be anticipated in laparoscopy-assisted PNL?

Ans: Intestinal and major blood vessel injuries are the major and life-threatening complications that can happen. Bladder injury can also happen if the ectopic kidney is posterior to it. Retroperitoneal urinoma, retroperitoneal hematoma and urinary ascites can happen if there is a leak from nephrotomy site or due to extravasated irrigation fluid.

11. What are the specific indications for laparoscopic pyelolithotomy in ectopic pelvic kidney stone?

Ans: Laparoscopic pyelolithotomy is considered as one of the better options for treatment modality for a solitary large pelvic stone in ectopic pelvic kidney.[17] According to Yin *et al*[18] laparoscopy and flexible ureteroscopy work very well together to conduct pyelolithotomy on patients with calculi in inaccessible calcium.

12. Which are the types of approaches for laparoscopic pyelolithotomy?

Ans: With laparoscopic pyelolithotomy, transperitoneal, retroperitoneal, and transmesenteric access are the three most commonly used techniques; each has advantages and disadvantages of its own. The benefit of the transperitoneal approach is that the aberrant arteries and surrounding tissues, including the essential organs, are clearly visible. One benefit of the retroperitoneal laparoscopic method is that it prevents urine from contaminating the peritoneum. The transmesenteric approach offers a quicker way to view the pelvic kidney surface.[4]

13. What is the role of PCNL and SWL in management of kidney stones in ectopic pelvic kidney?

Ans: While some authors recommend using ultrasound or computed tomography guidance to gain percutaneous access for PCNL in patients with ectopic pelvic kidney stones, there is still a significant risk of serious vascular and visceral injuries.[19] Although SWL was thought to be the first-choice non-invasive treatment option for ectopic pelvic kidney stones prior to the widespread use and expertise of RIRS, its success rate was not very high.

For ectopic pelvic kidney with large stone burden and calyceal calculi best and safest treatment modality is laparoscopy-assisted PNL.

14. Why RIRS was not performed in this case?

Ans: RIRS is considered the preferred treatment for small to medium-sized calculi. This case had a 3 cm large pelvic calculus which is a relative contraindication for performing RIRS.

15. What is the success rate of RIRS in ectopic pelvic kidney stone management?

Ans: With improvements in flexible ureteroscope technology, RIRS is becoming a more viable treatment option for small- to medium-sized renal calculi due to its enhanced flexion, deflection, and digital vision. RIRS has a success rate of 75.0% to 84.7% in patients with ectopic pelvic kidney stones, according to studies.[20]

16. Why is RIRS the modality of choice in ectopic pelvic kidney stone management?

Ans: The main advantage of RIRS compared to the other modalities like mini-PCNL and open surgery is the shorter hospital stay, over rate of complications and lesser need for analgesia.[21]

With RIRS we can avoid major vascular, intestinal and other visceral injuries. Nowadays with the availability of newer generation digital flexible scopes with improved vision and easy accessibility, RIRS has emerged as the choice of modality for management of ectopic pelvic kidney stones.

17. What are the challenges in performing RIRS for ectopic pelvic kidney vs orthotopic kidney?

Ans: Performing RIRS in such scenarios is always challenging. Following difficulties can be anticipated in performing RIRS in ectopic pelvic kidneys:

1. Abnormal location of ureteric orifices.
2. Narrow ureters
3. Tortuous ureters
4. Narrow pelvi-ureteric junctions
5. High insertion of PUJ
6. Malrotated kidney and hence poor evacuation of fragments after fragmentation
7. Acute infundibulopelvic angle

18. Is presenting a prerequisite to performing RIRS in pelvic kidneys?

Ans: Many a times the ureters of ectopic pelvic kidneys are not surgeon friendly. By placing a double J stent prior to doing RIRS, we can avoid major ureteric injuries and complications.

Prior double J stenting helps for easy placement of ureteral access sheaths which protects the ureter. The tortuosity of ureter gets straightened up with prior double J stenting to great extent.

The length of DJ stents to be placed in ectopic pelvic kidney should be smaller than that of an orthotopic kidney to avoid stent dysuria.

19. What are the difficulties in performing RIRS in ectopic pelvic kidneys with conventional flexible ureteroscopes?

Ans: The available flexible ureteroscopes made by various companies have working length between 65 and 70 cm.[22]

As the distance from the ureteric orifice of the ectopic pelvic kidney is less than that of an orthotopic kidney, doing RIRS with conventional length flexible scopes is a difficult task.

Due to shorter length of the ureters, the majority of the shaft of the flexible scope remains outside the access sheath or external urethral meatus (when access sheath is not inserted). This leads to difficult manoeuvring and deflection of the scope. Damage to flexible scopes is likely due to excess of bending forces due to long length outside the access sheath. It is highly recommended that specially designed scopes with shorter working length and smaller diameters should be made available for performing RIRS in ectopic pelvic kidneys.

20. What are the Do's and Dont's in performing flexible ureteroscopy in ectopic pelvic kidney?

Ans:

Do's:

1. Presenting helps in placement of access sheath and may also reduce ureteral injuries.
2. Retrograde uretero-pyelography is highly recommended before commencement of flexible ureteroscopy. This helps the surgeon to understand the path of ureter in the ectopic kidney.
3. Use of ureteral access sheath is recommended.
4. Smaller calibre digital flexible ureteroscopes are preferred ones in such scenarios.
5. Use of stone basket to relocate the stone from a difficult calyx to a more favourable calyx should be done.
6. After complete dusting of the stone double J stenting should be done for adequate drainage of the system,

Do you think that this is a situation where a single-use disposable flexible scope would have a advantage?

Dont's:

1. Stone burden of more than 2 cm is a relative contraindication for performing RIRS in pelvic kidney.
2. In case of tight PUJ narrowing on RGP or preoperative imaging studies better to avoid

use of flexible scope to avoid injury/avulsion of pelvi-ureteric junction.

3. Avoid using large calibre flexible ureteroscopes.
4. Avoid using older version scopes with less deflection capabilities. As the kidney is malrotated to reach some stone bearing calyx we might need greater deflection of flexible scopes.
5. Inexperienced RIRS surgeons should avoid performing flexible ureteroscopy in pelvic kidney as it is technically more challenging or should be done under guidance of expert.
6. Sepsis is an absolute contraindication to RIRS.

21. Which complications can happen in performing RIRS in ectopic pelvic kidney?

Ans: RIRS in pelvic kidney is more prone to complications than in normal kidney. Following complications can happen:

1. Ureteric injuries leading to strictures because ureter is usually of smaller calibre in such cases.
2. Ureteric avulsions because of narrow VUJ, narrow PUJ, kinks and narrow calibre ureter.
3. Infundibular stenosis due to injuries while trying to negotiate flexible scopes into calyx in malrotated kidney.
4. Sepsis due to high intrarenal pressures. This happens due to less outflow of irrigation fluid due to tight PUJ, high insertion of PUJ, malrotation of kidney and many a times due to ureters not accommodating ureteral access sheaths.
5. Urinomas due to extravasation of irrigation fluid or calyceal rupture due to high intrarenal pressures.

22. Discuss the role of metabolic evaluation in patients with ectopic pelvic kidney stone disease.

Ans: Patients with ectopic pelvic kidney stones fall under the category of difficult to treat (urinary tract abnormalities/reconstruction). Avoiding recurrence in such cases should be our aim of management. Patients with ectopic pelvic kidney are not at greater risk of any specific metabolic abnormality but to avoid recurrence in this difficult to treat cases, we should do metabolic evaluation. In accordance with the American Urological Association (AUA) policy on medical care of stones, we would urge that patients with recurring stone formers, patients with pelvic kidney stones, or interested first-time stone formers be offered a metabolic examination.[23]

RIRS is the treatment of choice for small to medium sized stones in ectopic pelvic kidney with fair clearance rates and lesser complications but should be done under expert supervision with caution.

23. What was done in this case?

Ans: We did a laparoscopy-assisted percutaneous nephrolithotomy (LA PNL)

LA PNL in this case, as the kidney was located in the true pelvis with large stone burden. Due to previous open surgery, dense adhesions had formed between sigmoid colon and renal pelvis. Laterally facing pelvis was in close proximity to left common iliac vessels.

For detailed surgical steps, see the video by scanning the QR code: https://www.youtube.com/watch?v=Y1heY5fQFAsandt=1s

Scan QR Code for Video on
Laparoscopic assisted PCNL for a left ectopic pelvic kidney stone 3 cm

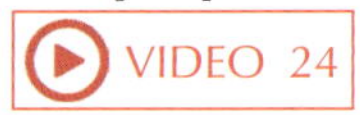

REFERENCES

1. Baskin LS, Cunha G.Embryology of genitourinary tract. In:Partin AW, Dmochowski RR, Kavoussi LR, Peters CA(Eds). Campbell-Walsh-Wein Urology.12th ed.Philadelphia: Elsevier; 2021. p305–340.
2. Eid S, Iwanaga J, Loukas M, Oskouian RJ, Tubbs RS. Pelvic Kidney: A Review of the Literature. Cureus. 2018 Jun 9;10(6):e2775. doi: 10.7759/cureus.2775. PMID: 30109168; PMCID: PMC6084689.
3. Ralitsa Gencheva, Bryce Gibson, ShruthiGarugu, Anthony Forrest, Sumathilatha Sakthi-Velavan, A unilateral pelvic kidney with variant vasculature: clinical significance, Journal of Surgical Case Reports, Volume 2019, Issue 11, November 2019, rjz333.
4. Wang C, Jin L, Zhao X, Li G, Xue B. Minimally invasive treatment of an ectopic kidney stone: a case report and literature review. Journal of International Medical Research. 2019;47(9):4544–4550. doi:10.1177/0300060519865845.
5. Gencheva R, Gibson B, Garugu S, Forrest A, Sakthi-Velavan S. A unilateral pelvic kidney with variant vasculature: clinical significance. J Surg Case Rep. 2019 Nov 29;2019(11):rjz333. doi: 10.1093/jscr/rjz333. PMID: 31803466; PMCID: PMC6883907.
6. Vander Brink BA, Reddy PP. Anomalies of the upper urinary tract. In: Partin AW, Dmochowski RR, Kavoussi LR, Peters CA (Eds). Campbell-Walsh–Wein Urology.12th ed. Philadelphia: Elsevier; 2021.p714–740.
7. Bozkurt IH, Cirakoglu A, Ozer S. Retroperitoneal laparoscopic pyelolithotomy in an ectopic pelvic kidney. JSLS. 2012 Apr-Jun;16(2):325–8. doi:10.4293/108680812x13427982376707. PMID: 23477189; PMCID: PMC3481231.
8. Hermida Pérez JA, del Corral Suárez T, Cerdeiras Martínez G, Agùero Gómez JL, Machado V, PanequeGodefoy P. Riñónderechoectópicohidronefrótico con litiasis de localizaciónpélvica, presentación de un caso [Right ectopic hydronephrotic kidney with pelvic lithiasis. Report of a

case]. Arch Esp Urol. 1998 Apr;51(3):289–93. Spanish. PMID: 9622923.

9. Otaño N, Jairath A, Mishra S, Ganpule A, Sabnis R, Desai M. Percutaneous nephrolithotomy in pelvic kidneys: is the ultrasound-guided puncture safe? Urology. 2015 Jan;85(1):55–8. doi: 10.1016/j.urology.2014.08.015. Epub 2014 Nov 6. PMID: 25440823.
10. Smith RC, Verga M, McCarthy S, Rosenfield AT. Diagnosis of acute flank pain: Value of unenhanced helical CT. AJR Am J Roentgenol. 1996;166:97–101. [PubMed] [Google Scholar].
11. Leavitt DA, Rosette JJMCH, Hoenig DM. Strategies for nonmedical management of upper urinary tract calculi. In: Partin AW, Dmochowski RR, Kavoussi LR, Peters CA (Eds). Campbell-Walsh-Wein Urology.12th ed. Philadelphia: Elsevier; 2021. p2069–2093.
12. Minimally invasive treatment of an ectopic kidney stone: a case report and literature reviewChenglu Wang,* Lu Jin,* Xinyang Zhao, Guobin Li, and BoxinXue.
13. Kamat N, Khandelwal P. Laparoscopic pyelolithotomy–a technique for the management of stones in the ectopic pelvic kidney. Int J Urol 2004; 11: 581–584. DOI: 10.1111/j.1442–2042.2004.00827.x.
14. D'souza N, Verma A, Rai A: Laparoscopic-assisted mini percutaneous nephrolithotomy in the ectopic pelvic kidney: outcomes with the laser dusting technique. Urol Ann. 2016, 8:87–90. 10.4103/0974–7796.171499.
15. Eshghi AM, Roth JS, Smith AD. Percutaneous transperitoneal approach to a pelvic kidney for endourological removal of staghorncalculus.JUrol 1985; 134: 525–527.
16. Holman E, Toth C. Laparoscopically assisted percutaneous transperitonealnephrolithotomy in pelvic dystopic kidneys: experience in 15 successful cases. J LaparoendoscAdvSurg Tech A 1998; 8: 431–435. 10.1089/lap.1998.8.431.
17. Elbahnasy AM, Elbendary MA, Radwan MA, *et al*. Laparoscopic pyelolithotomy in selected patients with ectopic pelvic kidney: a feasible minimally invasive treatment option. J Endourol 2011; 25: 985–989. 10.1089/end.2010.0521.
18. Gupta N, Mandhani A, Sharma D, *et al*. Is laparoscopic approach safe for ectopic pelvic kidneys? UrolInt 2006; 77: 118–121. 10.1159/000093903.
19. Yin Z, Wei YB, Liang BL, *et al*. Initial experiences with laparoscopy and flexible ureteroscopy combination pyeloplasty in management of ectopic pelvic kidney with stone and ureter-pelvic junction obstruction. Urolithiasis 2015; 43: 255–260. 10.1007/s00240–015–0753–9.
20. Desai MR, Jasani A. Percutaneous nephrolithotripsy in ectopic kidneys. J Endourol 2000; 14: 289–292. 10.1089/end.2000.14.289.
21. Demirkesen O, Yaycioglu O, Onal B, *et al*. Extracorporeal shockwave lithotripsy for stones in abnormal urinary tracts: analysis of results and comparison with normal urinary tracts. J Endourol 2001; 15: 681–685. 10.1089/08927790152596235.
22. Wu J, Shen J. The safety and efficacy of mini-percutaneous nephrolithotomy vs. retrograde Intrarenal surgery for treatment of renal lithiasis in pelvic ectopic kidney: an exploratory pilot study. Translational AndrolUrol. 2021;10(4):1734.
23. Paffen ML, Keizer JG, de Winter GV, Arends AJ, Hendrikx AJ. A comparison of the physical properties of four new generation flexible ureteroscopes: (de)flection, flow properties, torsion stiffness, and optical characteristics. J Endourol. 2008 Oct;22(10):2227–34. doi: 10.1089/end.2008.0371. PMID: 18831670.
24. Pearle M.S., Goldfarb D.S., Assimos D.G., Curhan G., Denu-Ciocca C.J., Matlaga B.R. Medical management of kidney stones: AUA guideline. *J Urol.* 2014;192:316–324. [PubMed] [Google Scholar].

Chapter
9

Stone in Calyceal Diverticulum

• *Ramesh Vaman Mahajan*

LEARNING OBJECTIVES

- Calyceal diverticulum (CD) is a known condition. This is compilation of data from literature to plan treatment policies which are practical, workable, and capable of producing good treatment outcomes in the Indian context.

INTRODUCTION

A non-secretary urothelium lined cavity in the renal parenchyma that communicates with the calyx or the renal pelvis that may permit passive urine filling is known as the renal calyceal diverticulum.[1]

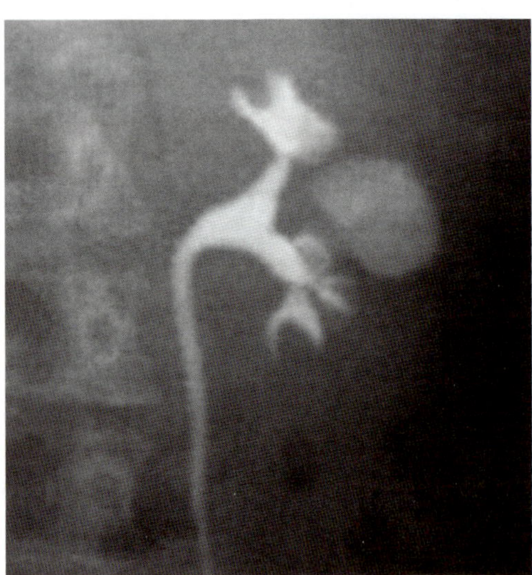

Fig. 9.1: Multiple stones in a calyceal diverticulum

Calyceal diverticula (CD) are found incidentally in no more than 1% of intravenous urograms (IVU) in adults.[2] According to a meta-analysis, 49% of calyceal diverticula are found in upper pole calyces and 21% in lower pole calyces. The anterior and posterior distributions are not investigated.[2,4]

Case Scenario

A 45-year-old male presented with disturbing left flank pain without any comorbidities. Biochemistry was normal. Initial imaging was X-ray KUB and sonography. He underwent SWL initially for 10 mm mid-calyceal calculus and later at 6 months showed failed clearance on imaging and aggravated pain.

1. **How are the CDs formed?**

   The pathogenesis of the CD is thought to be congenital or acquired. The congenital theory is most widely upheld. The "congenital" theory postulates failure of the stimulation of metanephros in terminal fourth and the fifth ureteric bid branching.[3] Proponents of "acquired" pathogenesis theory propose obstructive, traumatic, infective or fibrotic insults at the calyces. However, these theories are not supported by pathology specimens.[4]

2. **How would you classify the CDs?**

   Ans: Wolfsohn's and Dretler's classification systems are commonly used. Wolfsohn's classification:

   - Type I, those communicating with a minor calyx or an infundibulum.
   - Type II, those emanating from the renal pelvis or a major calyx. Type II diverticula are larger, tend to be symptomatic, and are located in the central part of the kidney. (Rare)[5]

Dretler's classification CD (anatomical and therapeutic)[6]:

- Type I has an open mouth and short neck: Suitable for shock-wave lithotripsy (SWL)
- Type II has a closed mouth and short neck: RIRS advisable
- Type III has a closed mouth and long neck: Suitable for percutaneous treatment
- Type IV has an obliterated neck: Percutaneous treatment is the treatment of choice.

3. Why do stones form and are they same as random stone former?

Ans: The basic pathophysiology of stone formation in CD is urinary stasis and supersaturation with calcium oxalate. Control random stone-formers and CD exhibit similar anomalies. For a high remission rate, the anomalies should be rectified with selected medical therapy. It is recommended that individuals with symptomatic calyceal diverticular calculi have a metabolic examination to determine stone formation risk factors and recurrence.[7]

4. Which conditions mimic CD?

Ans:

1. Hydrocalyx: Has a papilla
2. Simple cysts: No communication to PCS, lined with cuboidal epithelium
3. Tubercular cavity and papillary necrosis may mimic CD
4. Rare case of renal tumor is reported[8]

Decisive role of CT urogram is the key.

5. What is a presentation for these patients?

Ans: The vast majority of calyceal diverticula patients are asymptomatic.

Stone formation occurs in around 10–50% of cases with renal calyceal diverticula, although it can result in hematuria, pain, abscess formation, and sepsis.[9]

6. Does this patient need treatment?

Ans: Observation and follow-up is advisable in asymptomatic, uncomplicated and small calyceal diverticulum.[9]

7. How should evaluation be done?

Ans: Routine urine, biochemical investigations and sonography should be done. X-ray KUB will delineate multiple secondary stones (bag of stones). Some stones can be low density detected on sonography or CT. Calyceal diverticula must be identified with a high level of suspicion and contrast-enhanced imaging. The result of evaluation of case showed:

1. Left mid-calyceal calculi
2. Normal urine and biochemical investigations.
3. CT urogram showed left middle posterior calyceal diverticulum with calculi of HU 700.

8. In an era of non-contrast CT, how to derive diagnosis of CD?

Ans: Currently, NCCT is the primary diagnostic modality for kidney and ureteric stones. A contrast study is recommended when kidney stone removal is planned, according to the current EAU guidelines. CTU has limitations due to higher doses of ionizing radiation, in the young cohort of kidney stone patients and cases with comorbidities. CD should be suspected in the following situations, and CTU is advised.[10]

- Prominently symptomatic small renal stone
- Stones refractory to ESWL
- Peripheral or parenchymal location
- Layering of tiny stones
- Grouped secondary stones
- Failed treatment

The success rate and the number of treatments are greatly impacted by the delay in diagnosing CD on contrast CT.[10] Diagnosing CD requires a strong index of suspicion and careful application of contrast imaging.

9. How to plan management?

Ans:

1. Diagnosis and localization
2. Retrograde treatment of CD and stones
3. Percutaneous treatment of CD and stones
4. Marsupialization: Either lap, robotic or open depends on expertise

10. What factors decide 'Preference of Approach'?

Ans: The aim of management is proper identification, approach, and incisions on calyceal opening and stone clearance. Selection of surgery will depend on:

- Polar location of CD[11]
- Anterior or posterior position
- Stone burden
- Number of stones
- Size and protrusion on surface[10]
- Level of sepsis
- Ectopic position of kidney
- Age of patient

Figure 9.2 depicts the preferred choices.

11. Can you elaborate decision making in individual cases in brief?

Ans: Better deflection and optics, slender scope and wider acceptance of pre-stenting procedure, a larger working channel and LASER fibers have improved the efficacy of RIRS. One approach for

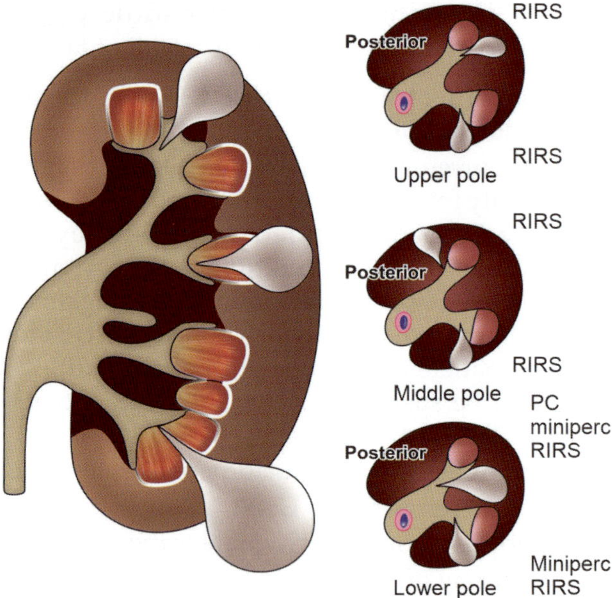

Fig. 9.2: Polar location of CD and choice of approach

treating non-inferior calyx CD calculi is RIRS. Achieving the best postoperative stone-free rate involves taking into account stone sizes less than 1.5 cm. A diverticular neck length under 0.4 cm is more likely to result in a stone-free outcome. Similar results are seen from anterior and posterior calyceal diverticula operations.[12] Selective cases of inferior pole CD, especially anterior, can be managed by RIRS. Limitation can be stone burden in CD, PCNL offers the highest stone-free rates and symptom-free outcomes despite being more invasive. Currently, it is the preferred course of action for bigger stones and diverticula. Multiple studies have shown that PCNL is superior to RIRS but there remains concern for major complications.[13,4]

12. What is the best option in this case?

Ans: RIRS was considered the best option in this case (Fig. 9.3).

Retrograde approach: Most suitable approach for the majority of diverticula (90%) with calculi. Decisive benefit of retrograde approach is precise infundibulotomy.

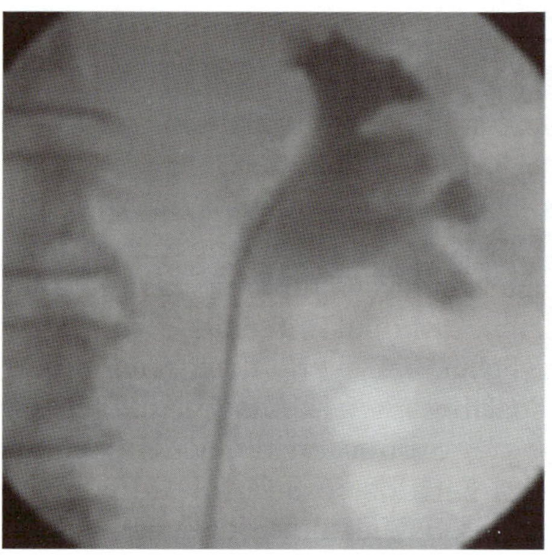

Fig. 9.3: CD with calculi

13. What is the ideal case for RIRS and what would be the standard steps of surgery?

Ans: Ideal CD for RIRS is upper pole locations (Fig. 9.4):

Steps of surgery

- Scout fluoroscopy
- Retrograde pyelography
- RIRS with access sheath

14. How to locate the neck of diverticulum in RIRS?

Ans:

1. **Direct vision:** RIRS is a better modality than PC approach was a choice in this case.

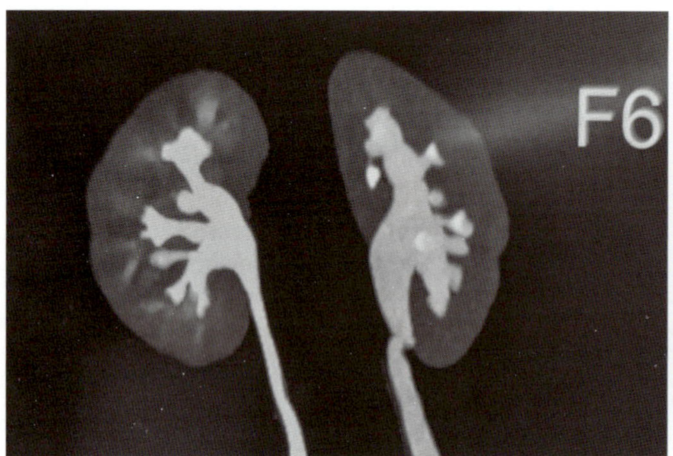

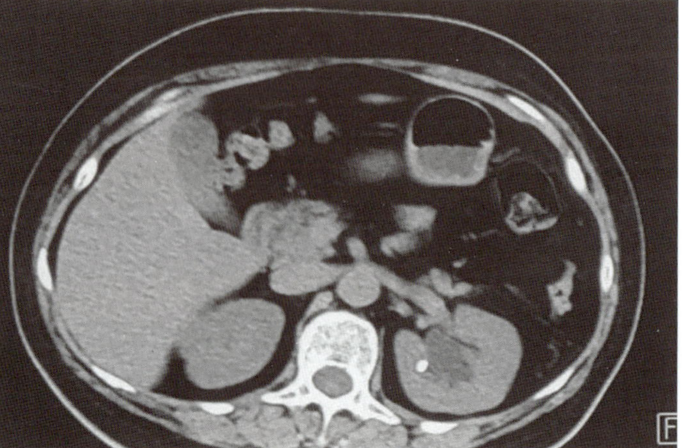

Fig. 9.4: CT urogram

Other options being:

2. **Blue Spritz test:** Blue streak from opening of CD after installation and washing of blue dye (Fig. 9.5).[14]

In this case the opening was identified by direct vision.

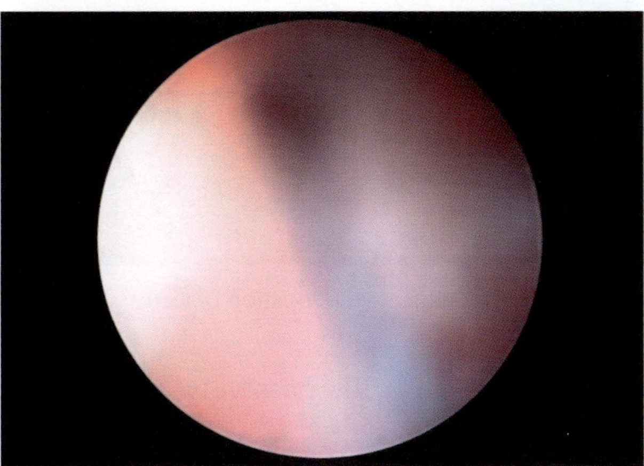

Fig. 9.5: Identification of CD opening

15. How to perform infundibulotomy?

Ans: As the vessel location near papilla (A) and fornix (B) is random, multiple shallow radial laser incisions were made. If the opening is located near infundibulum (C), then lateral 3 and 9 o'clock vessels position should be avoided (Fig. 9.6).

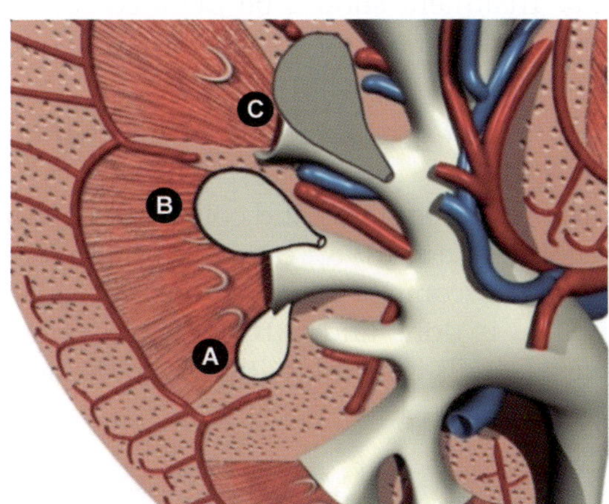

Fig. 9.6: Infundibular vessels

16. Which type of laser can be used?

Ans: The infundibulum of the calyceal diverticulum is usually cut with thin (230 µm) holmium laser optical fiber. This laser also helps in fragmenting the calculi if needed. Usually high energy and low frequency (1.2 J–6 Hz) is used. The aim is to fragment the stone into smaller pieces which can be removed with a small caliber basket. Recently thulium fiber laser also been used with equally good outcome.[15]

17. Does the DJ need to be placed on a CD?

Ans: It depends on operating surgeon's decision. Usually after an adequate infundibulotomy placement of DJ in CD cavity is not needed as the coil will shift to roomy pelvis.[16]

18. Are there any other modalities of treatment?

Ans:

1. **SWL:** SWL surely does not address the underlying anomaly.[8] Diverse case series results have led most authors to conclude that the recurrence and stone-free rates achieved by SWL monotherapy are not optimum.[17] Streem and Yost reported stone-free rates up to 58% but the symptom-free rate was 86%.[18] This strange disparity implies that even if patients still have stones, their symptoms get better.[19] Stones in a CD with short and wide communication with the calyx (Drettler I) can be recommended SWL with poor clearance (20%) but better relief of symptoms.[4]
2. **Marsupialization (open, lap, robotic):** Typically reserved for instances with big stones in anteriorly placed (Fig. 9.5) diverticula with thin overlying parenchyma, as well as those that have failed conventional treatments[18] like recurrence, non-communicating CD and non-accessible CD in ectopic kidney.

   Advantage: CD obliteration with fat or excision is possible (Fig. 9.7).
3. **Percutaneous approach**

19. Which case of CD is ideal for percutaneous approach?

Ans: Percutaneous approach is indicated in large, non-dependent cavity, posterior-calyx location, hard stone.[17] This is ideal case (Fig. 9.8). Advantage: Diverticular cavity can be ablated.

20. How percutaneous approach planned in CD?

Ans: After a detailed review of investigations RGP is done and then proceed for the puncture.

21. What is done on non-visualization of CD on RGP?

Ans: Sonography guided or CT guided direct access can be achieved.

22. What is done if guidewire cannot be coiled in CD?

Ans: Indirect access from remote calyx used to place guidewire in CD is attempted or change to ECIRS.[20]

23. How to identify the neck of a CD in a percutaneous approach?

Ans:

- Direct vision
- Blue Spritz test (Fig. 9.5).

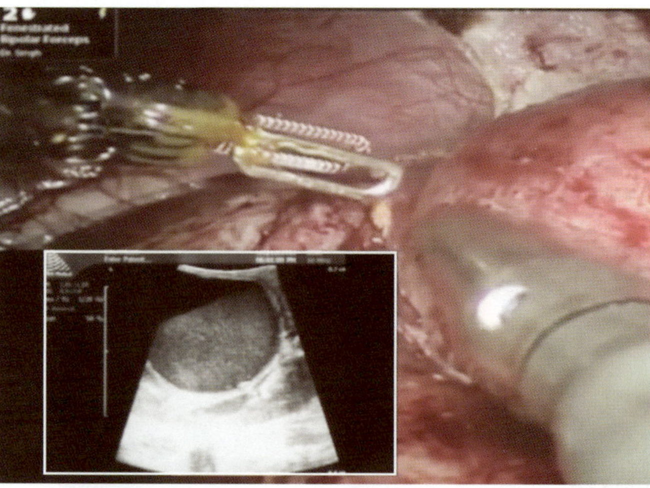

Fig. 9.7: CT anterior location of CD (Intraoperative ultrasound helps to delineate the location of CD)

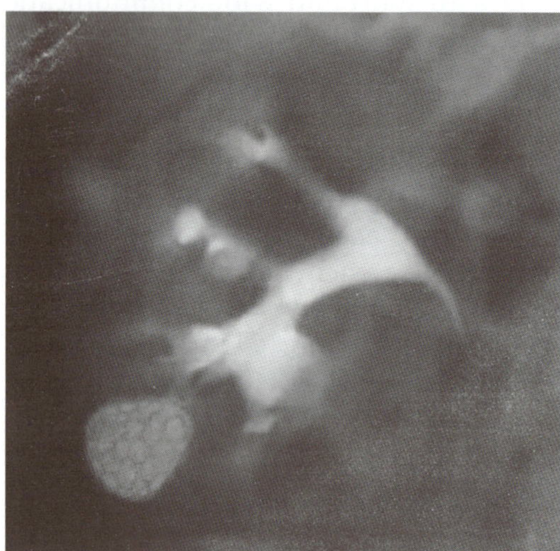

Fig. 9.8: Lower calyceal CD

- Indirect access: PC approach from remote calyx in relatively inaccessible superior calyx
- Air instillation: In PC direct approach[14]

24. How to manage the neck of a CD?

Ans: Before the era of laser, dilatation was the established modality to treat the neck of CD. It is essential to place a GW across the neck and dilate under fluoroscopic control. If the neck is not identified, then neoinfundibulum creation is reported, though not advisable with availability of laser. Laser incisions[21] are under vision precise and bloodless.

25. Should I ablate the CD mucosa? How?

Ans: If a neck of CD is not identified, successful electrocautery ablation of CD mucosa without treatment of neck is reported.[22] If the neck is identified, then laser infundibulotomy is effective to treat CD as CD has non-secretory epithelium and fills passively and ablation is not needed.

26. Should I use a nephrostomy tube across the neck of the CD?

Ans: When a neoinfundibulum is created, placement of a nephrostomy tube across such a neoinfundibulum for a week has been reported.[21] Rest of the cases of dilatation and incision such a nephrostomy is not needed[21] although old literature suggested it.

27. What is the treatment for CD type 2?

Ans: Treatment should be planned on merits of anatomy of renal vessels and structure of CD and complexity of pathology.

28. What about the outcome of intervention and follow-up?

Ans: Stone free status and collapsed diverticulum is achieved in 95 to 98% cases. Symptom relief is the desired outcome of intervention. Interval imaging by USG is done and sufficient in asymptomatic cases. Details imaging with CT can be advised in symptomatic cases (Fig. 9.9).

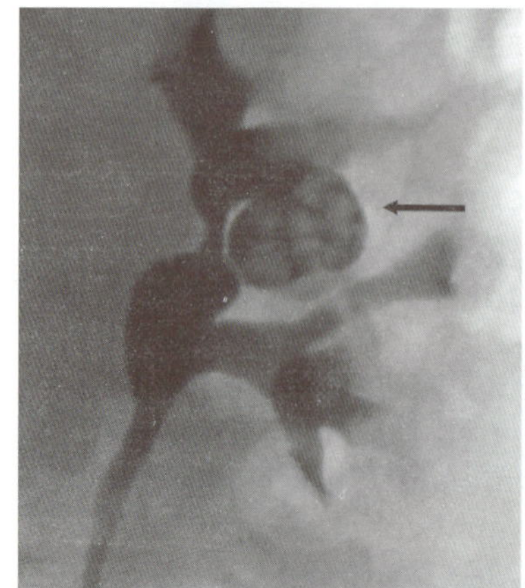

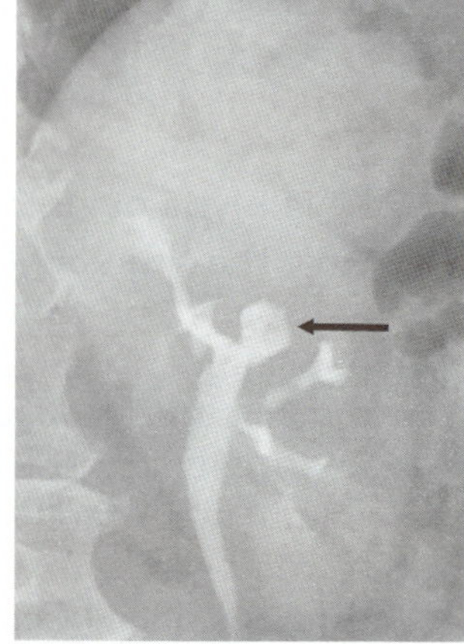

Fig. 9.9: Follow-up Imaging

SUMMARY

- Overall, the most notable development in the treatment of calyceal diverticula and stones appears to be the progressive miniaturization[23] of lasers, Mini-Perc PCNL equipment, and flexible retrograde scopes, which enable efficient CD treatment.
- It seems unlikely that the current methods will be surpassed by the growing accessibility of robotics. Finding a balance between the invasiveness and effectiveness of treatment is crucial for the future of surgical management of this illness.

KEY POINTS

- Calyceal diverticula are of congenital origin.
- Stones can be found in 96% of patients presented with CD.
- Diagnosis is primarily made by computed tomography urogram.
- The vast majority of patients are asymptomatic. Symptomatic CD is an indication for operative intervention.
- Stone-free rates are the lowest with SWL.
- Flexible RIRS is best suited for management of mid-to upper-pole CDs with diverticular stones.
- Percutaneous management is best used in posteriorly located lower-pole CD stones and offers the ability to directly ablate the diverticulum.
- Laparoscopic surgery should be reserved for cases with large stones in anteriorly located diverticula with thin overlying parenchyma, and cases that are refractory to other treatment modalities.

ABBREVIATIONS AND ACRONYMS

CD : Calyceal diverticulum
CT : Computerized tomography
CTU : CT urogram
ESWL : Extracorporeal shock wave lithotripsy
PCNL : Percutaneous nephrolithotomy
RIRS : Retrograde intrarenal surgery

Case Report Video[24,25]

Please Scan

1. Flexible URS Surgery for CD
   https://youtu.be/3NJCMT0ItFw

Scan QR Code for Video on
Calyceal diverticulum RIRS

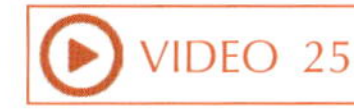

2. PCNL Surgery for CD
   https://www.youtube.com/watch?v=wqq5Y7-L6KA

Scan QR Code for Video on
PCNL for stone in calyceal diverticulum

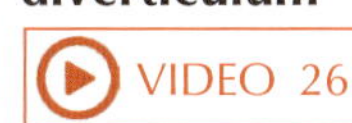

REFERENCES

1. Timmons JW Jr, Malek RS, Hattery RR, Deweerd JH. Calyceal diverticulum. J Urol. 1975;114: 6–9.
2. Pliatsikos EN, Calyceal diverticular calculi: Is there a role for metabolic evaluation? J Urol. 20 00 J ul 1 ;1 64(1):18–20.
3. Wulfsohn MA. Pyelocaliceal diverticula. J Urol. 1980;123:1–8. https://doi.org/10.1016/S0022–5347(17)55748–1.
4. Nikhil Waingankar, MD, Calyceal Diverticula: A Comprehensive Review Rev Urol. 2014;16(1):29–43 doi: 10.3909/riu0581.
5. Yu WW, Zhang DH. Incision and internal drainage treatment of renal cyst and calyceal diverticulum by endoscope. J Clin Urology. 2013;5:337–39+342.
6. Dretler SP. A new useful endourologic classification of calyceal diverticula. *J Endourol.* 1992;6(suppl):81.
7. Brian K Auge Metabolic abnormalities associated with calyceal diverticular stones, Brian K Auge BJU Int 2006 May;97(5):1053–6.
8. Alexandr Kurkov, A Case Report of Calyceal Diverticulum: Differential Diagnosis for Organ-Preserving Operations: Case Report article, Front. Surg., 16 September 2021, Sec. Genitourinary Surgery https://doi.org/10.3389/fsurg.2021.731796.
9. Percutaneous treatment of stone-containing calyceal diverticulum Endourology and ESWL arch. esp. urol. 2009; 62 (1): 42–48.
10. Faris Abushamma, Hiroki Ito, Calyceal Diverticula Disease: Diagnosis and Management Options in the Era of Non-Contrast CT Scan Urol Int 2022;106:688–692.
11. Olivier Traxer https://twitter.com/OTRAXER/status/1051055487502995457/photo/1.
12. Chatporn Chotikawanich: Factors Impacting Stone-Free Rate After Retrograde Intrarenal Surgery for Calyceal Diverticular Calculi Research and Reports in Urology, Volume 12, Issue (2020)Pages 345–350.
13. Tan YK, Cha DY and Gupta M: Management of stones in abnormal situations. Urol Clin North Am 2013; 40: 79.
14. Edward D. Matsumoto, Treatment of Calyceal Diverticula: http://eknygos.lsmuni.lt/springer/508/229–249.
15. Nitin Sharma,Large hydrocalyx mimicking as renal cyst and treated by Thulium fiber,: Urology Case Reports Volume 45, November 2022, 102280.
16. Woei Ming Ng, Retrograde intrarenal surgery in atretic calyceal diverticular stone, a case report: Urology Case Reports Volume 24, May 2019, 100840.
17. S. Hayek. Calyceal diverticula: a comprehensive review: N. Waingankar Reviews in Urology Vol. 16 No. 1•2014.
18. Ricardo Zerati, Marcos Tobias-Machado, Advances in Laparoscopy Minimally Invasive Approach for Treatment of Renal Calyceal Diverticulum, ISSN: 2578-6474 Case Report | Volume 4 | Issue 1 | DOI: 10.36959/367/448.
19. Streem SB and Yost A: Treatment of caliceal diverticular calculi with extracorporeal shock wave lithotripsy: patient selection and extended followup. J Urol 1992; 148: 1043.
20. Cecilia Maria Cracco and Cesare Marco Scoffone: Endoscopic combined intrarenal surgery (ECIRS)-Tips and tricks to improve outcomes: A systematic review: Turk J Urol. 2020 Nov; 46(Suppl 1): S46–S57.

21. Auge BK, Neoinfundibulotomy for the management of symptomatic caliceal diverticula. J Urol 2002; 167: 1616–1620.
22. M Monga Percutaneous ablation of caliceal diverticulum: long-term followup:J Urol 2000 Jan;163(1):28–32.
23. DingX, Xu, Huang-HE,Wei X-D, Zhang-L,WangL-L, *et al.* Management of symptomatic calyceal diverticular calculi: Minimally invasive percutaneous nephrolithotomy versus flexible ureterorenoscopy. Chronic DisTransl Med.2016 Dec;2(4):250–6.DOI:10.1016/j.csmt.2016. 11.016.
24. Case Details Courtesy Dr Pankaj Maheshwari https://www.youtube.com/watch?v=3NJCMT0ItFw
25. Case Details Courtesy Dr Prashant Mulawkar. https://www.youtube.com/watch?v=wqq5Y7-L6KA

Chapter

10

Asymptomatic Lower Calyceal Calculus

• Nanjappa K. Madappa • Abheesh Varma Hegde

LEARNING OBJECTIVES

- Evaluation of aysmptomatic lower pole calculus.
- Indications for intervention.
- Treatment algorithms.
- Follow-up of such calculi.
- Possible long-term outcomes.
- Newer developments.

INTRODUCTION

Urolithiasis is the bulk of urology practice in India. Management of renal calculi has undergone a sea change in recent years with innovations in technology and technique. The prevalence of asymptomatic renal calculus disease today is 8–46%. This figure is even higher in areas with a higher standard of living. The widespread availability and utilization of ultrasound and high-resolution computerized tomography (HRCT) as diagnostic modalities and better access to healthcare facilities are some of the reasons for the higher detection of asymptomatic calculi. Primary asymptomatic renal calculi[3] are detected in patients screened or investigated for other reasons and secondary asymptomatic renal calculi are postoperative residual calculi[3] after primary intervention for renal calculus.[1–3]

A commonly encountered clinical condition for the practising urologist is an asymptomatic lower pole calculus detected on a routine ultrasound scan of the abdomen. This seemingly harmless condition can pose dilemmas for both the anxious patient and the treating urologist. What is watchful waiting? Would the patient be willing for intervention for such calculi when indicated, given the asymptomatic nature of the disease? While guidelines advise watchful waiting for such calculi, there are specific conditions where intervention is required. What would be the ideal procedure and economic implications? The geographical area of practice and the patient would also affect decision-making in such situations. In this chapter, we will deal with the management of such asymptomatic lower pole calculus, when to intervene, follow-up and the latest trends in management.

Case Scenario

Mr X, a 53-year-old software professional presents to the urology OPD with an ultrasound report showing a 6 mm inferior calyceal calculus in the right kidney. He underwent the ultrasound (Fig.10.1) as part of his annual master health check-up. He is asymptomatic for the calculus but anxious to know the further course of action for his condition. His clinical examination is unremarkable and laboratory investigations are normal.

Differential diagnosis of hyperechoic shadow
• Renal sinus fat
• Cyst wall calcification
• Dystrophic calcification
• Renal artery calcification
• Retained DJ stent
• Medullary calcinosis
• Randall's plaque

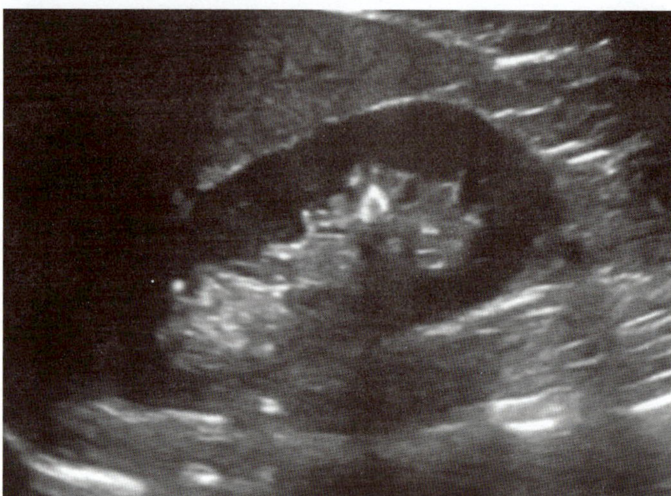

Fig. 10.1. Ultrasound image with a right 6 mm lower calyceal calculus

Management

A NCCT KUB (Fig. 10.2) would be required to confirm the size, location, number and density of the calculi. The dimensional and volumetric assessment of calculus is possible with a CT, while ultrasound can underestimate the actual size of the calculus. This information would help in deciding the further course of action. From his history and based on guidelines, watchful waiting with follow-up annually is the treatment of choice for this patient. If the patient develops symptoms, infection or growth is detected, the follow-up should be more frequent and intervention is advised. Patients who require NCCT for asymptomatic lower calyceal calculus evaluation are those with high risk for stone progression (elaborated later).

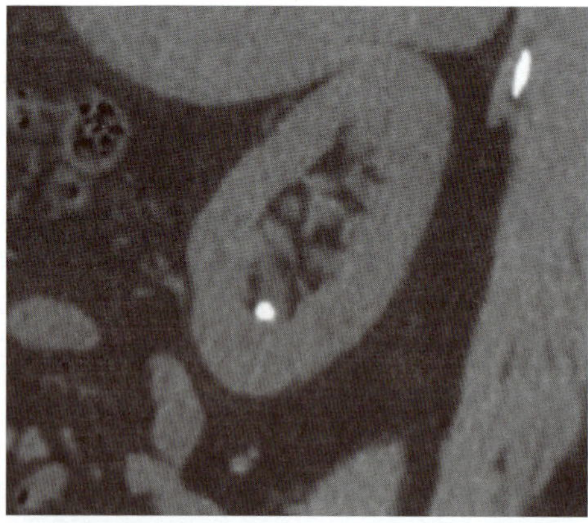

Fig. 10.2. CT image with a 6 mm lower calyceal calculus

1. **What are the EAU and AUA recommendations?**
   Ans: The AUA guidelines recommend no intervention for asymptomatic renal calculi.[1] The EAU guidelines recommend watchful waiting for asymptomatic lower calyceal calculi less than 10 mm with annual re-assessments. If growth is detected, follow-up should be more frequent. Intervention is advised for calculi more than 5 mm showing growth, obstruction, infection, acute or chronic pain.[2]

2. **How do asymptomatic lower pole calculi progress?**
   Ans: The prevalence of such calculi is 8–46%, among various studies in the literature. Natural history is still not precisely known. A recent paper suggested that stone size alone is not a reliable predictor of natural history. For < 1 cm calculi, the percentage of patients becoming symptomatic was 0–59.4%, risk of emergency visit related to the acute episode is 15–20% over 50 months of follow-up. 12–35% of patients required intervention for their calculus over a 36-month follow-up period.[4] The indications for surgery were migration of calculus into the ureter and development of stone-related symptoms.[5]

3. **What are the predictors for stone-related events?**
   Ans: Age ≤ 50 years, a history of prior intervention, annual growth rate, size, location and hyperuricemia are associated with a greater risk of symptom progression and surgical intervention in these patients.[5–8] Spontaneous passage rates for these calculi are 11–20%, with alpha-blockers having no effect on such rates.[9,10] Stone size greater than 5 mm increased the risk for stone-related events and future intervention by over two times compared to smaller stones.[11] Follow-up can be reduced for patients > 50 years old and those with asymptomatic renal calculi less than 5 mm with no history of prior intervention since the need for surgical intervention in such patients was low.[6]

Predictors for progression
• Age ≤ 50 years
• History of prior intervention.
• Stone size > 5 mm.
• Annual stone growth.
• Location.
• Hyperuricemia.

4. **How do you follow-up with these patients?**
   The goals of serial imaging would be to detect:
   - Increase in size of calculus.
   - Change in its location.
   - Hydroureteronephrosis/obstruction.
   - Stone passage.

   Surveillance Protocols (Flowchart 10.1)
   Investigations required and frequency:
   - Abdominal ultrasonography.
   - Serum creatinine.
   - Urine analysis.

All these are done annually. During observation, if symptoms develop or any features as mentioned are seen on sonography, then an NCCT is recommended. The principle remains to keep radiation exposure at a minimum: ALARA—as low as reasonably achievable since such patients would undergo multiple imaging over the years for urolithiasis.[6,7]

Flowchart 10.1: Protocol for evaluation

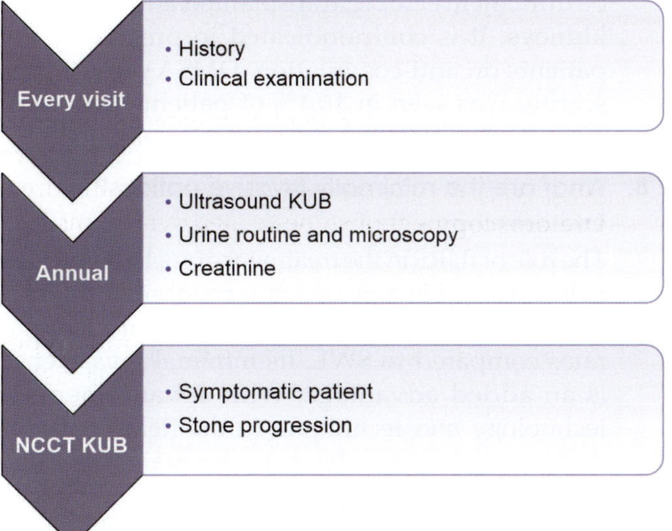

5. What is the role of watchful waiting?

Ans: Ludwig *et al.* reviewed the literature on asymptomatic lower pole calculi and found that about 11–19% of patients required intervention and no intervention was required in the initial two years of diagnosis. They also found the complication rates for SWL and fURS were 20% for immediate intervention at diagnosis for asymptomatic lower pole calculi.[9] Progression (growth, pain or infection) occurs in 33–46% of patients.[10] Another study found that 62% of patients could be safely managed on watchful waiting. However, a growth rate of 1 mm/year could lead to significant adverse events. It was also found that the rate of stone-related adverse events was higher for secondary asymptomatic renal calculi where almost 45% had symptoms or re-intervention post-SWL (average size <4 mm).[12] 43% of patients became symptomatic and 26% required intervention in the post-PCNL group (average size 2 mm). Among post-ureteroscopy residual calculi (average size <4 mm), 20% became symptomatic, 22% passed fragments spontaneously and the remaining were asymptomatic.[3] Hence an initial period of watchful waiting (2–3 years) and intervention after a symptomatic episode is recommended.

6. When to intervene and in which patients?

Ans: Watchful waiting for a silent disease with no threat to life in developing countries is a challenge. There is unequal distribution and access to super specialists, diagnostic modalities and sub-optimal transport facilities for patients living in remote areas. Stone disease is not a priority for many patients and follow-up maybe difficult. As per literature, 2% of asymptomatic lower calyceal calculi on follow-up develop silent hydronephrosis and left unchecked, there may be loss of renal units. Stones >5 mm have a higher progression rate and lesser spontaneous passage rates than those <5 mm. Data is scarce on special groups of patients viz immunocompromised, pregnant ladies, women planning pregnancy, transplanted or reconstructed patients, solitary kidneys, pilots, poorly compliant patients and those living in remote areas.

In summary, follow-up is a reasonable option for motivated patients, those who have access to imaging and laboratory facilities, present for clinical evaluation at least annually and those that do not belong to high-risk or the above categories. For calculi that show progression, intervention is advised.[10] A 10 mm cut-off has been described for lower pole asymptomatic calculi.[3] Prophylactic intervention has been advised for non-inferior calyceal calculi in high-risk patients, poor medical conditions and in certain professions. However, it is not advised for inferior calyceal calculi (Flowchart 10.2).[12]

High risk asymptomatic stones
• Solitary kidney
• Anatomical abnormalities
• Urinary tract reconstruction
• Paediatric patients, familial and recurrent stone formers
• Immunodeficiency
• High risk occupation and environmental factors
• Poor access or compliance
• Hyperuricaemia
• Metabolically active stone formers

Before any intervention, a contrast study (Fig. 10.3) would be recommended to additionally assess the calyceal anatomical factors: Infundibulopelvic angle, length, the width of the infundibulum and the ureter. A CT urogram would be the initial investigation recommended for patients in certain occupations (pilots, seamen, workers on oil rigs), transplanted or reconstructed kidneys, and ectopic kidneys. Metabolic evaluation is to be done for all children and high-risk stone formers.[2]

Flowchart 10.2: Management outline of asymptomatic lower calyceal calculus

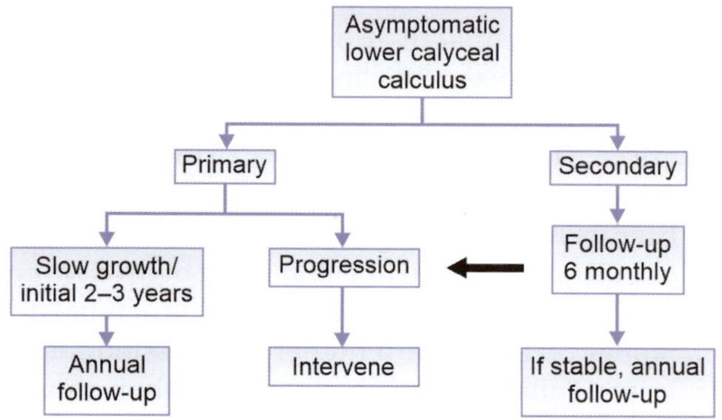

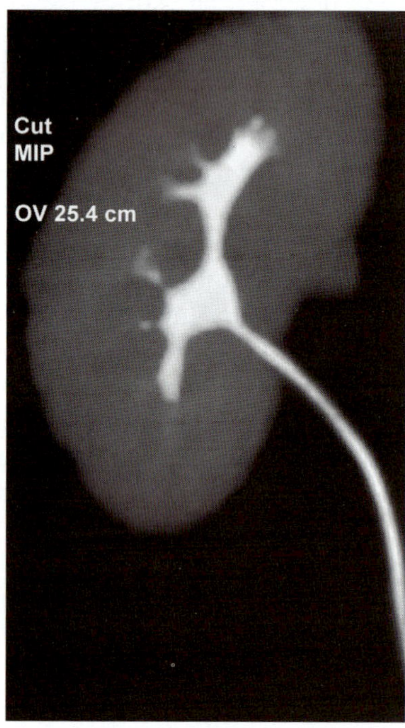

Fig. 10.3: Urogram image of the lower calyceal calculus in Fig. 10.2

7. **What would be the first line of intervention for these patients?**

   SWL would be the first choice for motivated adults with favourable calyceal anatomy. It is also the modality of choice in paediatric patients with asymptomatic lower pole renal calculi after confirming the non-struvite character. Complex lower calyceal drainage, high density of calculi on CT and longer skin-to-stone distance (morbid obesity) lowered SWL success rates. SWL would be difficult in ectopic, transplanted and malrotated kidneys. It is contraindicated in pregnancy and patients on anti-coagulation. DMSA proven renal scaring was seen in 16.1% of patients post-SWL, whereas it was 3.2% in post-PCNL cases.[10–14]

8. **What are the minimally invasive options?**

   Ureteroscopy:

   The role of fURS in the treatment of such calculi is yet to be assessed in a prospective randomized clinical trial setting. However, it has superior clearance rates compared to SWL. Its minimal invasiveness is an added advantage. With advancements in technology and techniques in the field of flexible ureteroscopy, it has become the mainstay in the management of lower calyceal calculi, especially in cases unfavourable for SWL. Challenging lower pole access has become easier with newer digital disposable scopes that are thinner and lighter with better tip deflection. Newer generation of baskets have made it easier to relocate stones from the lower calyx to a favourable position. Advancements in laser technology with thinner fibres and Thulium Fibre Laser (TFL) have made fURS the treatment of choice in many cases. SFR in case of ureteroscopy for lower calyceal calculi has improved in recent years with these advancements (Figs 10.4 and 10.5).[12]

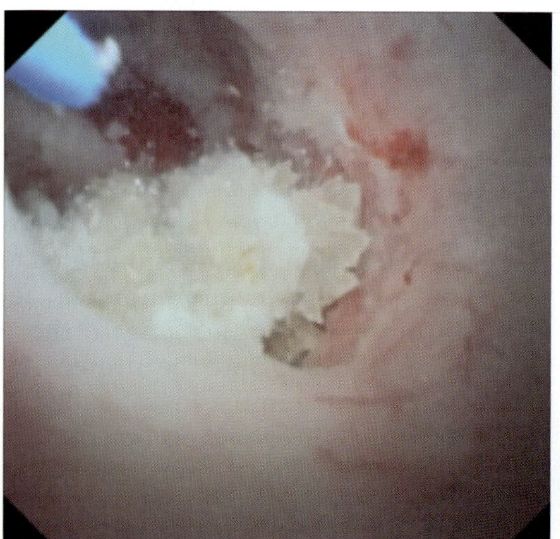

Fig. 10.4: Image of the calculus on fURS

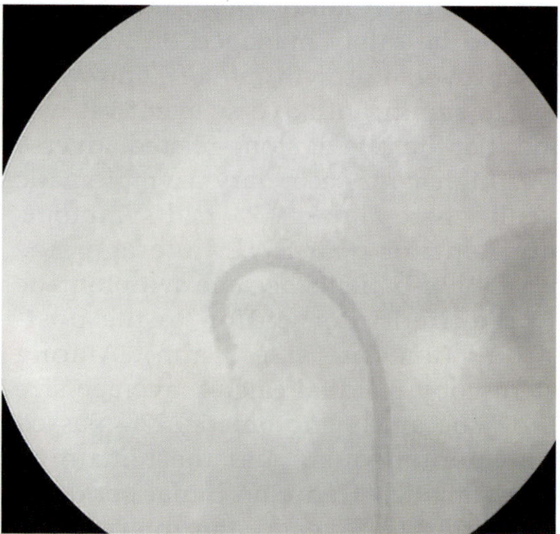

Fig. 10.5: Flouroscopy image of the procedure

Role of PCNL

PCNL offers the highest clearance among interventions for lower pole calculi irrespective of the stone burden.[12] The increased morbidity compared to SWL and ureteroscopy explains its limited role today. With the advancements in miniaturisation–mPCNL, microPCNL can be used in patients who are not suitable for SWL or fURS. It is also recommended in patients with suspected infection, acute IPA and failure to access the lower calyx by the retrograde route due to reconstructive surgeries or in rare cases of transplanted kidneys. Also, the higher cost of treatment for fURS, and the need for pre-stenting, especially in developing countries with low socioeconomic status, might compel patients for PCNL, when SWL is not indicated (Flowchart 10.3).[13]

Flowchart 10.3: Algorithm for intervention in asymptomatic lower calyceal calculus

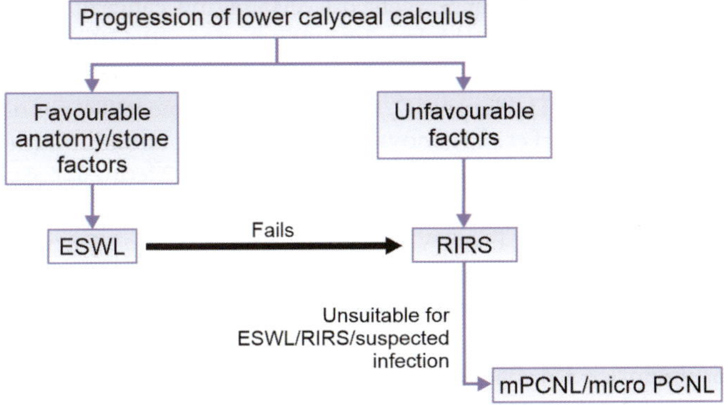

9. Should we treat the asymptomatic lower calyceal calculus when intervening for any other calculi in the PCS—ipsilateral or contralateral?

Ans: Intervention is advised for lower calyceal calculus in all surgeries, even if done on the contralateral side or for distal ureteric calculi. Literature shows that 50% of calculi 5 mm left behind when dealing with calculi at other locations become symptomatic within the first 5 years. Removal of such calculi reduced the relapse rates by 75%. The time to relapse was increased by 75% and the duration of primary surgery increased only by 25.6 minutes. There was also a reduction in the number of visits to the emergency department and surgeries at a later date. The cost benefits of avoiding a second surgery at a later date and potential emergency visits to the hospital, especially for those with difficult access to healthcare are immense.[14]

10. Any recent advances which could change the management of lower calyceal calculus in future?

Ans: One way to reduce radiation exposure to patients on follow-up would be by the use of digital tomosynthesis. It is a low-dose study (effective radiation dose 0.9 mSv) with high resolution, used extensively in dentistry, orthopaedics, breast and chest. It differs from conventional X-ray (ERD 0.59 mSv) in that 74 high-definition images can be obtained from a single scan. Reconstructed images can also be created to show the shape, contour of the kidney and fine details of the renal pelvis. Compared to an X-ray radiograph, it can detect radiolucent calculi too and is less affected by bowel gas. The detection rates for calculi are comparable to that of Unenhanced Multidetector CT (UMDCT) (ERD 2.68 mSv) with a cost advantage.[15] Low-dose CT is another modality that can also provide an alternate diagnosis in suspected cases of urolithiasis with ERD of 1.9±0.6 mSv.[16]

Transcutaneous ultrasonic propulsion as a modality has been proposed to break and expel stones without the need for surgery or anaesthesia. Ultrasonic propulsion to relocate stones to the pelvis or upper ureter can be utilized as an adjunct to surgery and SWL.[17]

Magnetic system for total nephrolith elimination (MagSToNE), a new approach is based on magnetic nanotechnology for efficient stone fragment retrieval. MagSToNE consists of a flexible magnetic wire with a biocompatible plastic sheath and superparamagnetic particles which are functionalized in a gel form to bind to kidney stones. This promising procedure is carried out using flexible ureteroscopy and was found to be better than basketing techniques in an *in vivo* study using porcine tissue (Fig. 10.6).[18]

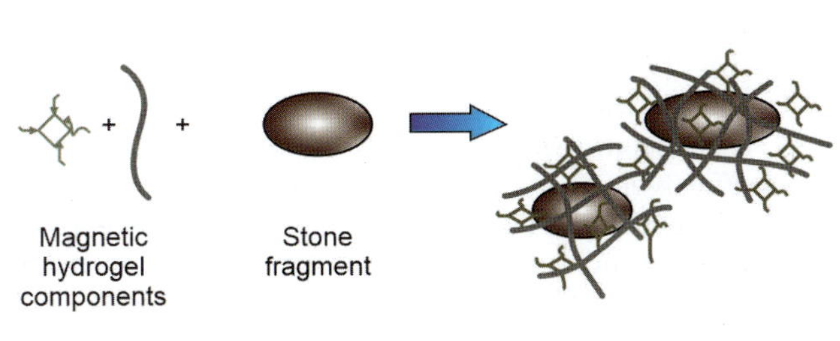

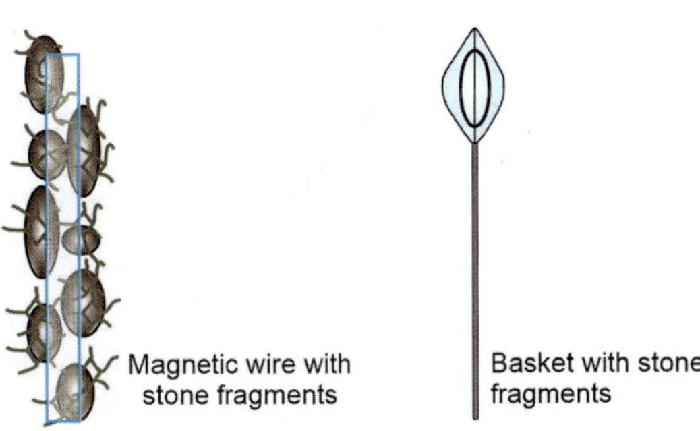

Fig. 10.6: Magnetic system for total nephrolith elimination (MagSToNE)

Newer developments in SWL generators such as twin head, tandem pulse, dual pulse shock wave generators, wide focal zone, low-pressure systems, optimised coupling, automatic location and acoustic tracking systems have shown promise to deal with renal calculi and improve outcomes. Future improvements include burst wave lithotripsy fusion and stone-specific ultrasound imaging algorithms.[19,20]

The ongoing PUrE trial is being carried out to determine the clinical and cost-effectiveness of surgical interventions for lower pole calculi, i.e. fURS vs PCNL and SWL. It looks to provide information on health status, quality of life, clinical outcomes and resource use domains to help make treatment decisions for such patients.[21]

Conclusion

- Asymptomatic lower pole calculi can be a dilemma for the clinician.
- However, most can be followed up.
- Intervention is required in special condition.
- When favourable, ESWL is the first modality of treatment.
- fURS is now becoming the endoscopic intervention of choice due to technologic improvements.

REFERENCES

1. Pearle MS, Goldfarb DS, Assimos DG, Curhan G,Denu-Ciocca CJ, Matlaga BR *et al.* Medical management of kidney stones: AUA Guideline. J Urol 2014; **192:** 316, doi: 10.1016/j.juro.2014.05.006.
2. A. Skolarikos, H. Jung, A. Neisius, A. Pet ík, B. Somani, T. Tailly, G. Gambaro EAU Guidelines on urolithiasis 2023, *presented at the EAU Annual Congress Milan 2023. ISBN 978-94-92671-19-6*
3. Goldsmith, Z. G, Lipkin, M. E. When (and how) to surgically treat asymptomatic renal stones Nat. Rev. Urol. 9, 315–320 (2012) doi: 10.1038/nrurol.2012.43
4. Lovegrove CE, Geraghty RM, Yang B, Brain E, Howles S, Turney B, Somani B. Natural history of small asymptomatic kidney and residual stones over a long-term follow-up: systematic review over 25 years. BJU Int. 2022 Apr;129(4):442–456. doi: 10.1111/bju.15522.
5. Kanno T, Takahashi T, Ito K, Okada T, Higashi Y, Yamada H *et al.* The natural history of asymptomatic renal stones 5 mm: comparison with 5 mm. J Endourol(2020) 34:1188–1194. http://doi.org/10.1089/end.2020.0336.
6. Darrad MP, Yallappa S, Metcalfe J, Subramonian K The natural history of asymptomatic calyceal stones. BJU Int(2018) 122:263–269, doi: 10.1111/bju.14354.
7. Li X, Zhu W, Lam W, Yue Y, Duan H, Zeng G, Outcomes of long-term follow-up of asymptomatic renal stones and prediction of stone-related events. BJU Int (2019) 123:485–492. doi: 10.1111/bju.14565.
8. Ludwig WW, Ziemba JB, Matlaga BR. Difference of opinion-Asymptomatic lower pole stone < 1 cm: to treat or not to treat? Opinion: Do not treat. International Braz j Urol: Official Journal of the Brazilian Society of Urology. 2016 Mar-Apr;42(2):185–187.doi: 10.1590/S1677–5538.IBJU.2016.02.04.
9. Eduardo Mazzuchi, Asymptomatic lower pole stone < 1 cm: to treat or not to treat? Vol. 42 (2): 183–184, March-April, 2016 doi: 10.1590/S1677–5538.IBJU.2016.02.03.
10. Wu T, Liu Z, Ma S, Xue W, Jiang X, Ma J. Should we support prophylactic intervention for asymptomatic kidney stones? A retrospective cohort study with long-term follow-up. Urolithiasis. 2022 Aug;50(4):431–437doi: 10.1007/s00240–022–01331–4.
11. Subramonian K, Sandoval Barba H, Darrad M. Role of conservative management of stones. Turk J Urol 2020; 46(Supp. 1): S64–S69. doi: 10.5152/tud.2020.
12. Mazzucchi E, Berto FCG, Denstedt J, Danilovic A, Batagello CA, Torricelli FCM *et al.* Treatment of renal lower pole stones: an update. Int Braz J Urol. 2022 Jan–Feb;48(1):165–174. doi: 10.1590/S1677–5538.IBJU.2020.1023.
13. Gross AJ, Knipper S, Netsch C. Managing caliceal stones. Indian J Urol. 2014 Jan;30(1):92–8. doi: 10.4103/0970–1591.124214.
14. Sorensen MD, Harper JD, Borofsky MS, Hameed TA, Smoot KJ, Burke BH *et al.* Removal of Small, Asymptomatic Kidney Stones and Incidence of Relapse. N Engl J Med. 2022 Aug 11;387(6):506–513. doi: 10.1056/NEJMoa2204253.
15. Liu S, Wang H, Feng W, Hu X, Guo J, Shang Q *et al.* The value of X-ray digital tomosynthesis in the diagnosis of urinary calculi. Exp Ther Med. 2018 Feb;15(2):1749–1753. doi: 10.3892/etm.2017.5531.
16. Weinrich JM, Bannas P, Regier M, Keller S, Kluth L, Adam *et al.* Low-Dose CT for Evaluation of Suspected Urolithiasis: Diagnostic Yield for Assessment of Alternative Diagnoses. AJR Am J Roentgenol. 2018 Mar;210(3):557–563. doi: 10.2214/AJR.17.18552.
17. Harper JD, Sorensen MD, Cunitz BW, Wang YN, Simon JC, Starr F, *et al.* Focused ultrasound to expel calculi from the kidney: safety and efficacy of a clinical prototype device. J Urol. 2013 Sep;190(3):1090–5. doi: 10.1016/j.juro.2013.03.120.
18. Daniel M R, Jessie T G, Holton G E, Mach K E, Kornberg Z, Sun R *et al.* Efficacy and safety of a magnetic hydrogel for stone fragment removal: an in vitro and in vivo study, J Urol. Apr 2023; 209(4S), e819.
19. Elmansy HE, Lingeman JE. Recent advances in lithotripsy technology and treatment strategies: A systematic review update. Int J Surg. 2016 Dec;36(Pt D):676–680. doi: 10.1016/j.ijsu.2016.11.097.
20. Bach C, Karaolides T, Buchholz N. Extracorporeal shock wave lithotripsy: What is new? Arab J Urol. 2012 Sep;10(3):289–95. doi: 10.1016/j.aju.2012.04.002.
21. McClinton S, Starr K, Thomas R, MacLennan G, Lam T, Hernandez R, Pickard R *et al.* The clinical and cost effectiveness of surgical interventions for stones in the lower pole of the kidney: the percutaneous nephrolithotomy, flexible ureterorenoscopy and extracorporeal shockwave lithotripsy for lower pole kidney stones randomised controlled trial (PUrE RCT) protocol. Trials 21, 479 (2020). https://doi.org/10.1186/s13063–020–04326–x.

ABBREVIATIONS

NCCT : Non-contrast computerised tomography
CT : Computerised tomography
AUA : American Urological Association
EAU : European Association of Urology
KUB : Kidney ureter bladder
fURS : Flexible ureteroscopy
SWL : Shockwave lithotripsy
SFR : Stone free rate
IPA : Infundibular pelvic angle
PCNL : Percutaneous nephrolithotomy
ERD : Effective radiation dose
TFL : Thullium fibre laser

Chapter 11

Moderate Sized Prostate on Blood Thinners

• Mukund G Andankar • Prasad M Brahme

LEARNING OBJECTIVES

- Indications and surgical options for treatment of bladder outlet obstruction (BOO) due to benign prostatic hyperplasia (BPH).
- Surgical management in patients with benign prostatic hyperplasia with large prostatic adenoma on dual antiplatelet agents.
- Efficacy and safety of lasers for benign prostatic hyperplasia in high-risk patients.
- Guidelines for anticoagulant management in urological practice.

INTRODUCTION

Benign prostatic hyperplasia (BPH) is a very common occurrence in elderly men and a significant cause of morbidity and reduced quality of life. The incidence of lower urinary tract symptoms (LUTS) increases with age, affecting approximately 50% of men by 80 years.[1] With increasing life expectancy, men suffering from LUTS due to BPH is also on the rise.[2] Although medical therapy can provide symptomatic relief, it surely does not cure the underlying condition, and often delays intervention.[2] This leads to more older patients, who have associated multiple comorbidities, needing surgical intervention. A lot of these men may have cardiac and neurologic issues necessitating use of anticoagulation (AC) or antiplatelet (AP) therapy.[2] The urologist is faced with surgical challenge of selecting the correct BPH intervention while managing blood thinners in the perioperative period. **In this chapter, we aim to clarify the approach to surgical management of BPH with large prostates in anticoagulated patients.**

Case Scenario

A 65-year-old male, hypertensive diabetic with history of ischemic heart disease (IHD) that needed percutaneous transluminal coronary angioplasty (PTCA) 2-months prior. As a drug eluting stent was placed, he is on dual antiplatelet agents. He has a history of lower urinary tract symptoms since 2-years. Although he was on alpha blockers, he suffered from three episodes of acute painful retention in the last one month. He failed catheter free trial and is on a foley catheter at present. On digital rectal examination, he has a large grade three prostate. USG suggestive of large prostatomegaly-80 gm with thickened irregular bladder wall.

1. What are the indications of surgical intervention in benign prostatic hyperplasia?

Ans: Surgical treatment is indicated for patients with BPH when BPH leads to:

1. Renal insufficiency refractory retention of urine
2. Recurrent urinary tract infections
3. Recurrent bladder stone
4. Gross haematuria
5. Symptoms refractory to medical therapies[3]

2. What are the treatment options for gross prostatomegaly with >= 80 gm prostate?

Ans:

1. Simple prostatectomy (open, laparoscopic, robotic)
2. Anatomic endoscopic enucleation of prostate by holmium, thulium, TFL or bipolar energy.[3]

3. What are the current treatment options for average prostate size (30–80 gm) and small prostate (<30 gm)?

Ans: Average prostate size (30–80 gm):

1. Transurethral resection of prostate (TURP)
2. Holmium laser enucleation of prostate (HoLEP)
3. Thulium laser enucleation of prostate (ThuLEP)

4. Photoselective vaporization of prostate (PVP)
5. Robotic water jet treatment
6. Prostatic urethral lift
7. Transurethral microwave thermotherapy (TUMT)
8. Water vapour thermal therapy

Small prostate (<30 gm)

1. TURP
2. Transurethral incision of prostate (TUIP)
3. HoLEP
4. PVP
5. TUMT

4. What are the surgical intervention options for comorbid patients with BPH at higher risk of bleeding?

Ans: As per the recent *AUA guidelines,* patients who are at higher risk of bleeding, such as those on anticoagulation drugs, can be managed by **HoLEP, PVP, ThuLEP** as the need for blood transfusions in these procedures is very less.[4]

5. Why are laser enucleation procedures considered safe in anticoagulated patients?

Ans: The two major properties that allow holmium laser to be safe and effective when compared with other BPH treatment option are:

1. Low depth of penetration of holmium laser reduces the eschar formation, hence reduces the risk of delayed bleeding.
2. Excellent haemostatic properties of the laser.[5]

6. Can laser enucleation procedures be performed for larger glands >80 gm?

Ans: Most international guidelines including AUA and EAU guidelines, proposes HoLEP or ThuLEP as the treatment of choice for patients with large adenoma as these are **prostate size-independent** options for treatment of LUTS/BPH. The final choice would be based on the surgeon's expertise with these techniques.[4]

7. Can TURP be offered to patients on anticoagulation or with high risk of bleeding?

Monopolar TURP is often not possible in high-risk patients on chronic anticoagulation therapy (i.e. dual antiplatelet therapy after drug eluting stent in coronary artery disease or warfarin in atrial fibrillation) as the risk of bleeding complications is significantly high.[8] If TURP has to be performed, either the anticoagulants should be stopped or bridged with a low molecular weight heparin. Such discontinuation of therapy can potentially increase the risk of cardiovascular complications or thromboembolic events, while continuation would lead to higher bleeding at the surgical site. Bipolar TURP (TURis) can be an alternate option as it is associated with significantly lower risk of clot retention as compared to monopolar TURP, but the transfusion rates are not significantly different.[10]

So if facilities other than monopolar TURP are not available, after initial optimisation in case of gross haematuria or bladder clots, it is advisable to refer the patient to a centre equipped with laser or bipolar equipment.

8. What is the upper limit or cut-off size of prostate while considering TURP?

Ans: Although TURP is an effective treatment option for moderate to severe enlargement of prostate (30–80 gm suitable for M-TURP), there is no data on the optimal cut-off value. It is known that the complications of TURP increase with increasing prostate size,[11] hence **the upper limit for M-TURP is recommended as 80 gm.** The procedure is safest when performed in under 90 minutes.[12] The option of B-TURP should be considered if equipment and expertise is available.[12]

9. What are the recommendations for thulium laser use in BPH for large prostate on anticoagulation?

Ans: The thulium:yttrium-aluminium-garnet laser (Tm:YAG) functions at a wavelength of 2 nm. The depth of penetration is very small and it provides good haemostasis due to high-energy density caused by energy absorption in water.

Two meta-analyses comparing Thu-LEP to M-TURP and B-TURP showed that ThuLEP needed a longer surgical time as compared to M-TURP but a shorter catheterization time. When compared to B-TURP, ThuLEP offered a shorter length of hospitalization.[13,14] The blood transfusion rates were lower when compared to M-TURP, clot retention was less when compared to B-TURP, but overall there were no difference in other.[13,14]

One study[15] comparing ThuLEP to HoLEP reported a significantly shorter enucleation time for ThuLEP, but did not demonstrate much difference in operative, catheterization and hospitalization time, and short-term complication rates. In comparative studies[16] and also in case series of patients with large prostates on anticoagulation or bleeding diathesis, ThuVEP (*Thulium laser Vapoenucleation of prostate*) showed high intra-operative safety.

10. What are the other types of lasers which can be used in vaporization of prostate?

Ans: Laser vaporization of prostate can be performed by Potassium Titanyl-Phosphate (KTP) and the lithium triborate lasers (LBO).[17] KTP laser has a wavelength of 532 nm, a penetration depth is about 0.8 mm and is absorbed by haemoglobin. Non-contact Photoselective vaporization of tissue is achieved with tissue necrosis limited beneath the vaporized area. Along with this, it also ensures an almost bloodless procedure.[17]

The lithium triborate (LBO) laser is a derivative of KTP laser with similar wavelength. LBO-laser has a more efficient and accelerated energy transfer and enhanced working distance (from 0.5 mm for KTP to 3 mm for LBO). A very important disadvantage of this laser is a significant decrease in the haemostatic ability as compared to KTP laser.[17] Currently these lasers are not being used very commonly in treatment of BPH.

11. Can PVP be performed on patients on anticoagulation?

Ans: A study by Knapp, *et al.* compared complications in men undergoing PVP with or without continued anticoagulation. PVP was performed in 59 patients with continued antithrombotic therapy and in 272 patients not on any antithrombotic therapy. There was no difference in total operative or laser time, but patients on antithrombotic treatment needed a longer catheter time (32.4 hr vs 15.6 hr) and hospital stay (46.6 hr vs 23.1 hr). Overall complications were similar in both groups but patients in anti-thrombotic had a higher chance of more severe complications (grade IIIa sepsis 5% vs 0.7%, bladder neck contracture 3.4% vs 0.4% and grade IVb sepsis 1.7% vs 0%). They concluded that continuing anticoagulation at the time of PVP is not associated with an overall increased risk of adverse events; however, it is associated with higher-grade risks.[18] **PVP is safe to be performed in patient on active anticoagulation but should be performed with care.**

12. Can PVP be performed in larger prostate >80 gm?

Ans: A randomized control trial evaluating HoLEP to PVP in men with more than 80 gm prostate showed a comparable symptom improvement but significantly higher flow rates and lower post-void residue after HoLEP at short term follow-up. Also PVP showed 22% conversion to TURP.[19]

EAU guidelines recommend offering laser vaporization of prostate by using 80-W KTP, 120- or 180 W LBO lasers for the treatment of patients receiving antiplatelet or anticoagulant therapy with prostate volume <80 gm.[19]

13. How would you rate the tolerability and safety of bipolar transurethral enucleation in large glands >80 gm?

Ans: One RCT comparing bipolar transurethral enucleation of prostate (B-TUEP) to B-TURP in patients with prostate volume >80 gm with a minimum six month follow-up reported that B-TUEP is superior to B-TURP with respect to operative, catheterization and hospitalization time.[20] The blood transfusion, bladder neck contracture and retrograde ejaculation rates favoured B-TUEP but there was no significant difference in urethral stricture or erectile dysfunction.[20]

Luca Boeri *et al.* compared HoLEP with B-TUEP on patients receiving anticoagulation[21] and concluded that both the procedures are safe in patients with continuous anticoagulation/antiplatelet (AC/AP) medications. Although there was a longer hospital stay and catheter duration in AC/AP therapy patients, it was not clinically significant. Also, patients under AC therapy had an overall higher rate of postoperative complications, but most were of Clavien Dindo grade I and II. Haemoglobin drop, catheterization time and rate of transfusions were not influenced by AC/AP status in B-TUEP patients. There was no difference in post-operative IPSS, haemoglobin drop, and transfusion between the two, both in control group and in AC/AP+ group but the overall complication rates were higher with B-TURP. Overall, these suggest that HoLEP and B-TUEP are equally safe and effective for the treatment of men under continuous AC/AP medications. They can be proposed as minimally invasive treatment option for patients at higher risk of bleeding because of BPH surgery.

Another RCT by Enmar Habib *et al.*[22] compared efficacy and safety of B-TUEP to HoLEP for treatment of large prostate glands >80 gm. They concluded that HoLEP and B-TUEP are comparable in safety and efficacy for treatment of BPH including patients on anticoagulation. However, B-TUEP required a longer catheterization duration and operative time.

14. What is Rezum? What are the recommendations for performing Rezum in large glands >80 gm? Does it have any role in patients on dual antiplatelet therapy?

Ans: Rezum is an emerging minimally invasive surgical treatment which uses convective water vapour thermal therapy for prostatic ablation. Steam is injected within the prostatic transition zone to ablate hyperplastic prostatic tissue. The treatment effect is limited to targeted areas, representing an evolution of thermal ablative techniques like transurethral needle ablation and microwave therapy. Rezum offers effective treatment of BPH with minimum sexual side effects. There is no need for anaesthesia or prolonged hospitalizations.

Even though Rezum is attractive for these reasons, it is only recommended currently for prostate <80 gm. In selected >80 gm prostate patients, it provided short-term symptomatic improvement and improved voiding function. Postoperatively, even though alpha-blocker usage decreased significantly, nearly two-thirds of patients still needed medical management.[23]

There are no bleeding complications usually reported with patients on anticoagulation or platelet aggregation inhibitors. To our knowledge, there is only one study which has stated not to stop anticoagulation prior to Rezum.[27] There are no sufficient published studies or data specifically focusing on safety of Rezum in patients requiring anticoagulants.

15. What are the current recommendations regarding open prostatectomy as a choice of treatment of BPH?

Ans: According to the EAU guidelines, open prostatectomy, although most invasive, is an effective and durable procedure for the treatment of LUTS/BPH. If endourological alternatives like holmium laser or a bipolar system are not available, with appropriate consent and explanation, open prostatectomy can be offered as a reasonable option. There are no studies or case reports in literature evaluating safety of open prostatectomy in patients on continuous anticoagulant medications.

16. What are the current guidelines for patients on anticoagulants in urological practice?

Ans: According to the IUCD-AUA review paper,[24] 'anticoagulation and antiplatelet therapy in urology practice', 2014, it is recommended to

1. Continue aspirin through the perioperative period for patients on clopidogrel or aspirin for secondary stroke prevention, especially after a recent stroke.
2. Obtain a neurological consultation to evaluate competing risks and determine the necessity for bridging therapy.
3. Not to withdraw the dual AP therapy before urological procedures within twelve months of drug eluting stent placement or within three months of bare metal stent placement as there is a high risk of major cardiac and cerebrovascular events. A multidisciplinary approach involving cardiology expertise is essential when urgent urological procedures are required within these time frames. For procedures performed beyond these limits discontinuation of clopidogrel, prasugrel or ticagrelor and continuation of aspirin might be recommended if bleeding risks are acceptable.

Notably intermittent catheterization for treatment of urine retention can reduce the urgency of surgical intervention.

17. Why is it necessary to use dual antiplatelet therapy (DAPT) over aspirin alone in ACS or post-PTCA?

Ans: Studies prove superiority of continuous DAPT over aspirin alone post-PTCA or acute coronary syndrome by reducing the incidence of myocardial infarction, ischemic stroke and other cardiovascular events.[25]

Anti-platelet agents are primarily used to reduce the risk of thrombosis of coronary stents or coronary artery bypass grafts (CABGs). Dual anti-platelets (aspirin with a P2Y12 inhibitor, most commonly, clopidogrel) are indicated both for primary and secondary prevention of ischemic heart disease post-coronary stenting or CABG. According to the updated 2016 American College of Cardiology guidelines, dual AP therapy should be given for at least 12 months in patients with recent acute coronary syndrome treated with either CABG or percutaneous coronary stenting.[25]

SUMMARY

Coming back to our case scenario, how would you manage?

After a thorough review of literature, we conclude

- The patient has history of IHD with PTCA done 2 months back with a drug eluting stent, hence according to IUCD-AUA review paper, the patient has to continue with DAPT at least for 12 months to prevent any adverse cardiac or cerebral thromboembolic event.[24]
- The patient had failed catheter free trial twice being on alpha-blocker with gross prostatomegaly of 80 grams which is an indication for surgical intervention according to AUA and USI guidelines for management of BPH.[3,26]
- Of all the treatment modalities available; HoLEP, ThuLEP, photoselective vaporization of prostate and bipolar TUEP can be safely used in patients with higher risk of bleeding or on anticoagulation with considerably lesser adverse effects.[4,20,22]
- Photoselective vaporization of prostate when used in prostate more than 80 gm have higher grade adverse effects especially sepsis.[18]
- TURP and other minimally invasive surgical techniques like Rezum, Urolift are not very efficacious for gross prostatomegaly and are currently recommended only for moderate prostatomegaly less than 80 gm.[3]

Hence for gross prostatomegaly with 80 gm prostate requiring continuous dual antiplatelet therapy; THULEP, HoLEP and bipolar-TUEP would be an ideal choice with considerably lesser adverse events.

REFERENCES

1. McVary KT. BPH: epidemiology and comorbidities. The American journal of managed care. 2006 Apr 1;12 (5 Suppl):S122–8.
2. Heiman J, Large T, Krambeck A. Best practice in the management of benign prostatic hyperplasia in the patients

requiring anticoagulation. Therapeutic Advances in Urology. 2018 Dec;10(12):431–6.

3. Lerner LB, McVary KT, Barry MJ, Bixler BR, Dahm P, Das AK, Gandhi MC, Kaplan SA, Kohler TS, Martin L, Parsons JK. Management of lower urinary tract symptoms attributed to benign prostatic hyperplasia: AUA guideline part II—surgical evaluation and treatment. The Journal of urology. 2021 Oct;206(4):818–26.
4. Foster HE, Barry MJ, Dahm P, et al. Surgical management of lower urinary tract symptoms attributed to benign prostatic hyperplasia: AUA guideline. J Urol 2018; 11: 43201–43206.
5. Elzayat E, Habib E and Elhilali M. Holmium laser enucleation of the prostate in patients on anticoagulant therapy or with bleeding disorders. J Urol 2006; 175: 1428–1432.
6. El Tayeb MM, Jacob JM, Bhojani N, et al. Holmium laser enucleation of the prostate in patients requiring anticoagulation. J Endourol 2016; 30: 805–809.
7. Bishop CV, Liddell H, Ischia J, et al. Holmium laser enucleation of the prostate: comparison of immediate postoperative outcomes in patients with and without antithrombotic therapy. Curr Urol 2013; 7: 28–33.
8. Descazeaud A, Robert G, Lebdai S, Bougault A, Azzousi AR, Haillot O, Devonec M, Fourmarier M, Saussine C, Barry-Delongchamps N, de la Taille A: Impact of oral anticoagulation on morbidity of transurethral resection of the prostate. World J Urol 2011;29:211–216.
9. Ruhle, A., *et al.* Safety and Effectiveness of Bipolar Transurethral Resection of the Prostate in Patients under Ongoing Oral Anticoagulation with Coumarins or Antiplatelet Drug Therapy Compared to Patients Without Anticoagulation/ Antiplatelet Therapy. J Endourol, 2019. 33: 455.
10. Fagerstrom, T., *et al.* Complications and clinical outcome 18 months after bipolar and monopolar transurethral resection of the prostate. J Endourol, 2011. 25: 1043.
11. Reich, O., *et al.* Morbidity, mortality and early outcome of transurethral resection of the prostate: a prospective multicenter evaluation of 10,654 patients. J Urol, 2008. 180: 246.
12. Riedinger, C.B., *et al.* The impact of surgical duration on complications after transurethral resection of the prostate: an analysis of NSQIP data. Prostate Cancer Prostatic Dis, 2019. 22: 303.
13. Huang, S.-W., *et al.* Comparative efficacy and safety of new surgical treatments for benign prostatic hyperplasia: systematic review and network meta-analysis. BMJ (Clin Res ed.), 2019. 367: l5919.
14. Zhang, Y., *et al.* Efficacy and safety of enucleation vs. resection of prostate for treatment of benign prostatic hyperplasia: a meta-analysis of randomized controlled trials. Prostate Cancer Prostatic Dis, 2019. 22: 493.
15. Xiao, K.W., *et al.* Enucleation of the prostate for benign prostatic hyperplasia thulium laser versus holmium laser: a systematic review and meta-analysis. Lasers Med Sci, 2019.
16. Chang, C.H., *et al.* Vapoenucleation of the prostate using a high-power thulium laser: a one-year follow-up study. BMC Urol, 2015. 15: 40.
17. Dołowy Ł, Krajewski W, Dembowski J, Zdrojowy R, Kołodziej A. The role of lasers in modern urology. Central European journal of urology. 2015;68(2):175.
18. Knapp GL, Chalasani V and Woo HH. Perioperative adverse events in patients on continued anticoagulation undergoing photoselective vaporisation of the prostate with the 180-W Greenlight lithium triborate laser. BJU Int 2017; 5(Suppl. 119): 33–38.
19. Gratzke C, Bachmann A, Descazeaud A, Drake MJ, Madersbacher S, Mamoulakis C, Oelke M, Tikkinen KA, Gravas S. EAU guidelines on the assessment of non-neurogenic male lower urinary tract symptoms including benign prostatic obstruction. European urology. 2015 Jun 1;67(6):1099–109.
20. Tian, J., *et al.* Comparative study of the effectiveness and safety of transurethral bipolar plasmakinetic enucleation of the prostate and transurethral bipolar plasmakinetic resection of the prostate for massive benign prostate hyperplasia (>80 ml). Med Sci Monitor, 2020. 26: e921272.
21. Boeri L, Capogrosso P, Ventimiglia E, Fontana M, Sampogna G, Zanetti SP, Pozzi E, Zuabi R, Schifano N, Chierigo F, Longo F. Clinical comparison of holmium laser enucleation of the prostate and bipolar transurethral enucleation of the prostate in patients under either anticoagulation or antiplatelet therapy. European Urology Focus. 2020 Jul 15;6(4):720–8.
22. Habib E, Ayman LM, ElSheemy MS, et al. Holmium laser enucleation vs bipolar plasmakinetic enucleation of a large volume benign prostatic hyperplasia: a randomized controlled trial. J Endourol. 2020;34(3):330–338.
23. Jenks AM, Damm T, Petrossian R, Delfino K, Dynda D, tadros N. Mp01-10 efficacy of rezūm water vapor thermal therapy for surgical management of benign prostatic hyperplasia in prostates over 80 grams. Journal of Urology. 2022 May 1;207(Supplement 5):e5.
24. Culkin DJ, Exaire EJ, Green D, Soloway MS, Gross AJ, Desai MR, White JR, Lightner DJ. Anticoagulation and antiplatelet therapy in urological practice: ICUD/AUA review paper. The Journal of urology. 2014 Oct 1;192(4):1026–34.
25. Windecker S, Kolh P, Alfonso F *et al* (2014) ESC/EACTS guidelines on myocardial revascularization: the task force on myocardial revascularization of the European Society of Cardiology (ESC) and the European Association for Cardio-Thoracic Surgery (EACTS) developed with the special contribution of the European Association of Percutaneous Cardiovascular Interventions (EAPCI). Eur Heart J 35:2541–2619.
26. Sabnis RB, Mulawkar PM, Joshi RN. The Urological Society of India guidelines on management of benign prostatic hyperplasia/benign prostatic obstruction (Executive summary). Indian Journal of Urology. 2021 Jul 1;37(3):210–3.
27. Ines M, Babar M, Singh S, Iqbal N, Ciatto M. Real-world evidence with the Rezūm system: a retrospective study and comparative analysis on the efficacy and safety of 12 month outcomes across a broad range of prostate volumes. The Prostate. 2021 Sep;81(13):956–70.

Chapter

12A

BPH with Stone

• *Manoj Biswas* • *Apul Goel*

LEARNING OBJECTIVES

- To understand the association between bladder stone and BPH.
- Evaluation of a patient with this association.
- Management of a patient with this association.

INTRODUCTION

Benign prostatic hyperplasia (BPH) affects up to 50% of all men in between 60 and 70 years of age.[1] Urinary tract infections, acute retention of urine, bladder calculi and hematuria, are additional consequences of BPH.[2–4] The association of BPH with bladder calculi has been reported to be up to 10%.[5,6]

Case Scenario

A 68-year-old man presented with voiding and storage lower urinary tract symptoms (LUTS) for the last 2 years. There was history of occasional gross hematuria. There was no history of urinary retention. There was history of regular tobacco intake. DRE showed a grade II prostate with smooth surface and firm consistency. Evaluation revealed normal renal functions, while an ultrasonogram revealed a 4 cm calculus with 50 cc prostate volume and normal upper tracts. There was no history of any surgical intervention in the past. How will you proceed?

1. **What are the predictors of bladder calculi in a patient with BPH?**

   Ans: According to a recent study by Childs, *et al.*[7] the predictors of bladder calculi in BPH patients were advanced age, longer intravesical prostatic protrusion, decreased peak flow on uroflowmetry and higher post-void residual. Bacteria causing cystitis may alter the pH of urine and the urinary citrate concentration that may further contribute to the formation of urinary crystals.

2. **Do these stones form *de novo* or migrate from the upper tracts?**

   Ans: Urinary stasis secondary to bladder outlet obstruction due to BPH, neurogenic bladder, foreign bodies, bladder diverticula or bladder augmentation predisposes to bladder calculi formation, called secondary bladder calculi. However, migratory stones (from upper tracts) are also a possibility.

3. **What investigations are advised for the diagnosis?**

   Ans: Typically, transabdominal ultrasonography is adequate to make a diagnosis. However, for further characterization, either a plain abdominal radiograph (Fig. 12A.1) or non-contrast CT scan (Figs 12A.2 and 12A.3) is needed. Often, bladder

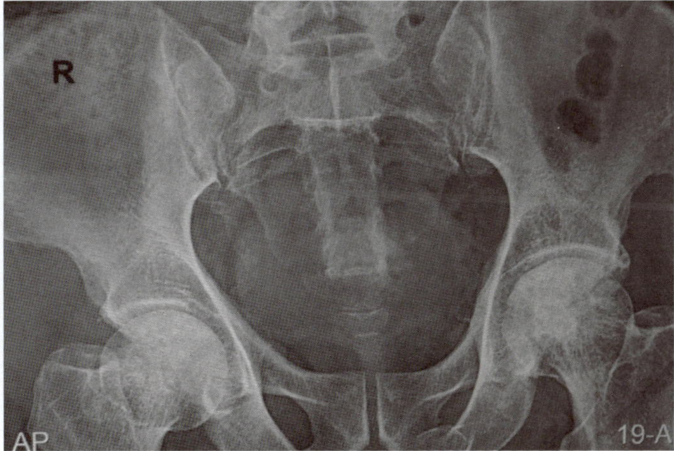

Fig. 12A.1: Plain X-ray does not reveal a large bladder stone

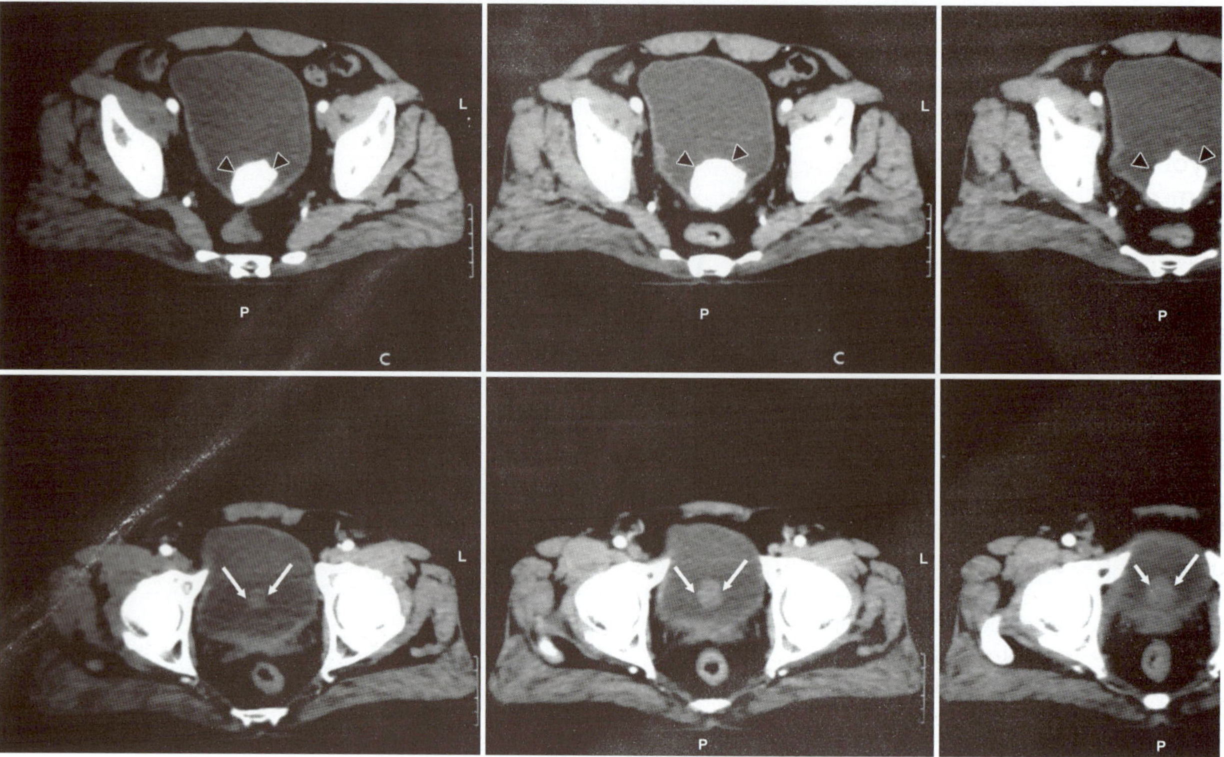

Fig. 12A.2: CT scan (axial cuts) of the same patient shown in Fig. 12A.1 reveals a 6 cm size bladder stone (arrow heads) along with an enlarged prostate gland with a prominent median lobe (arrow)

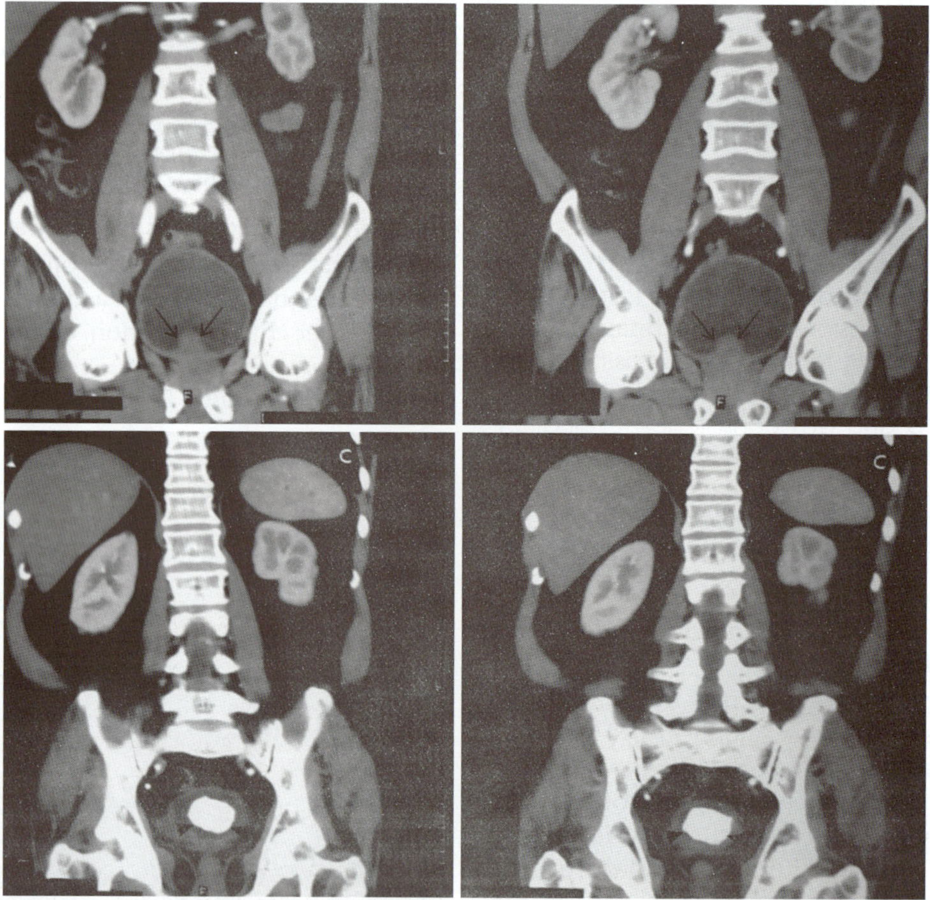

Fig. 12A.3: CT scan (coronal) of the same patient showing bladder stone (arrow head) and enlarge prostate with prominent median lobe (arrow)

stones are not visible on plain abdominal radiographs (Fig. 12A.1). Better characterization of stone is important to plan surgical treatment (Figs 12A.2 and 12A.3).

4. **Do you need other evaluations/investigations, like metabolic evaluation for stone disease or urodynamics in this scenario?**

Ans: Identifying and addressing all potential factors that contribute to the formation of bladder stones can greatly reduce the likelihood of recurrence after successful removal. It is beneficial to conduct a comprehensive assessment to determine the presence of lower urinary tract dysfunction, metabolic predisposition, abnormal materials (such as foreign bodies), and infection when planning treatment of bladder stones.[8] However, the specific metabolic abnormalities responsible for bladder stone formation are not yet well defined.

Assessing the presence of BPH-induced obstruction in presence of bladder stones can be challenging since bladder stones themselves can cause lower urinary tract symptoms.[8] Nonetheless, there were no significant differences observed in both invasive and non-invasive urodynamic findings in men before and after bladder stone removal. Bladder stones are not always associated with bladder outlet obstruction, and the presence of bladder stones does not affect the urodynamic results during testing.[9] Therefore, a urodynamic study is typically unnecessary, and if performed, is done after the removal of the stones.

5. **What is the chemical composition of bladder stones?**

Ans: According to a study involving 86 patients who experienced bladder stones as a result of BPH, the analysis of the stones indicated the following findings: 42% of the patients had stones composed of calcium-based substances such as oxalate and phosphate, 33% had stones made of magnesium ammonium phosphate, 10% had mixed stones consisting of various components, and 14% had stones composed of urate.[10]

6. **Would you do a diagnostic cystoscopy in this patient?**

Ans: A careful cystoscopy is indicated in this patient in view of the symptoms of hematuria and also because of history of tobacco intake. A bladder tumor may be missed in the presence of a bladder stone. Also, if percutaneous cystolithotripsy is performed for bladder stone removal without ruling out bladder tumor, then there is risk of track seeding by tumor.

7. **What are the consequences of bladder calculi when associated with BPH?**

The presence of recurrent bladder stones in men with BPH is a clear indication for surgical intervention.[11–13] These stones not only lead to increased patient discomfort and higher medical expenses but also carry the potential risk of bladder cancer.[14]

While there is a lack of urodynamic evidence to fully support this claim, it has been suggested that BPH is responsible for a significant proportion of bladder stones, ranging from 48% to 80%.[10,15] In line with this, the European Association of Urology (EAU) Guideline on "non-neurogenic male lower urinary tract symptoms (LUTS)" states that bladder stones are considered an "absolute indication for BPH surgery" in men aged 40 years and above.[16]

8. **Can you remove bladder stone alone in this patient or do you need to combine bladder stone removal with prostate removal?**

Ans: The presence of bladder stone in elderly men is considered secondary to outlet obstruction. Accordingly, this scenario was traditionally considered an absolute indication for surgical removal of the prostate gland along with bladder stone removal. However, the newer guidelines by American Urological Association (AUA)[17] suggest that the bladder stone can be removed first followed by a trial of medical therapy. Only if the patient develops recurrent bladder stone, prostate removal is indicated (Box 12A.1).

Box 12A.1

- Bladder stone formation is usually secondary to outlet obstruction caused by enlarged prostate.
- The diagnosis of bladder stone can be made on trans-abdominal ultrasound.
- Bladder stone may be radiolucent.

9. **What are the treatment options in this patient?**

Ans: There is no role of medical therapy in this scenario. There are two options. Removal of bladder stone alone (in view of the fact that this is the first-time bladder stone has formed) and treat BPH medically (combined alpha-blockers and 5-alpha reductase inhibitors) (Box 12A.2).

Box 12A.2

- Recurrent bladder stone is an indication of prostate gland surgery.
- Stone removal should be followed by medical therapy of the prostate (if prostate gland has not been removed).
- There are many surgical methods for bladder stone removal.

The second option is to surgically manage both the bladder stone and BPH. Depending on the size of prostate and bladder stone and the expertise of the surgeon, both the procedures can be combined or done separately (bladder stone removal first followed by prostate gland removal). This patient has a 6 cm bladder stone along with 50 cc prostate. In view of large prostate size, it will be preferable to surgically manage both the conditions. Larger prostates have a higher chance of progression.[18]

10. **How do you remove bladder stone?**

Ans: There are various procedures available for the removal of bladder stones. These procedures encompass cystolithotrity, transurethral cystolithotripsy (TUCL) or percutaneous cystolithotripsy, and open or laparoscopic cystolithotomy. The choice of the specific lithotripsy modality depends on the surgeon's preference and the equipment available. The available modalities include mechanical, laser, pneumatic, or ultrasonic lithotripsy devices.

For stones up to 1.5 cm, cystolithotrity can be performed. Many instruments are available for this procedure and include stone crushing forceps, Hendrickson's Classical Lithotrite, Mauermayer's stone punch. For stones between 1.5 cm and 4–5 cm, transurethral cystolithotripsy can be offered. For stones, larger than these, percutaneous cystolithotripsy or open/laparoscopic cystolithotomy is preferred. Large stones should not be treated transurethrally because of the risk of urethral trauma and subsequent stricture formation.[19]

11. **How would you manage his prostate surgically?**

Ans: The available treatment options consist of either mono-polar or bipolar transurethral resection of the prostate (TURP), holmium LASER enucleation of the prostate (HoLEP), and thulium enucleation. It should be noted that the prostate surgery can be performed either simultaneously with bladder stone removal or as a pre-planned, staged procedure.

In a non-randomized study, 64 men with bladder stones were compared in terms of treatment options: Medical treatment with tamsulosin and finasteride versus TURP.[20] All participants underwent bladder stone removal, followed by either medical therapy or TURP. During a median follow-up period of 39 months, only one patient in the TURP group experienced bladder stone recurrence (3.4% vs. 0%). However, 34% of men in the medication group eventually required TURP. It was found that a higher postvoid residual urine volume before bladder stone removal was predictive of the need for subsequent TURP (odds ratio 1.033, P = 0.014).

12. **Can you do bladder stone and BPH surgery in a same sitting?**

Ans: Three recent retrospective studies have compared the outcomes of different treatment approaches for men with BPH and bladder stones. The studies found that there were no significant differences in complications during surgery or major complications after surgery, and all reported a stone-free rate of 100%.[21–23]

In one retrospective study from China, researchers analyzed 1,078 men who underwent TURP, out of which 297 also had bladder stones. The men with bladder stones underwent simultaneous bladder stone removal (TUCL). The study found that the rate of postoperative urinary tract infections (UTIs) was higher in the group that had simultaneous bladder stone removal (2.0% vs. 0.6%, P = 0.044).[20] However, there was no significant difference in rates of urinary incontinence between the two groups (0.3% vs. 0.3%).

In two studies, men who underwent holmium laser enucleation of the prostate (HoLEP) were compared with or without simultaneous transurethral cystolithotripsy (TUCL). Out of 963 men in one study and 320 men in the other study, 54 and 41 respectively underwent simultaneous TUCL.[19,21] The larger study reported higher rate of urinary tract infection (UTI) (7.4%) and sepsis (1.9%) in patients who had concurrent TUCL compared to those who underwent prostate removal only (3.1% and 0.1%).[21] The smaller study found a higher rate of temporary postoperative urinary incontinence (26.8% vs. 12.5%, P = 0.03), but the long-term continence rates were similar.[19]

These slight increases in minor short-term complications observed in patients undergoing simultaneous TUCL are expected as bladder stones often harbor bacteria,[8] and bladder stones are associated with overactive bladder function.[7]

Based on these findings, it is suggested that simultaneous endoscopic bladder stone removal should be considered along with prostate removal if the stone size is less than 5 cm. For larger stones, it is preferable to stage the procedure due to the longer operating time required (Table 12A.1).

Conclusion

Following the successful removal of bladder stones in men aged 40 years and above, there is a possibility of bladder stone recurrence. In such cases, undergoing surgery for BPH is associated with a lower rate of bladder stone recurrence compared to medical treatment or no treatment for BPH.

TABLE 12A.1: Pros and cons of bladder stone and BPH surgery

Approach	*Pros*	*Cons*
Simultaneous	1. Addresses both conditions at once	1. Longer operating time
	2. Minimizes the need for multiple surgeries	2. Higher risk of complications
	3. Potentially reduces the need for additional hospitalization	3. Increased complexity of the procedure
	4. Single recovery period for both conditions	4. Potential impact on postoperative bladder function 5. Increased risk of postoperative urinary incontinence 6. Higher risk of urinary tract infections
Staged	1. Allows for focused management of each condition separately	1. Requires multiple surgeries
	2. Lower risk of complications for each individual procedure	2. Multiple recovery periods
	3. Better assessment of outcomes for each procedure	3. Potential delay in addressing both conditions
	4. Reduced complexity of each procedure	
	5. Lower risk of postoperative urinary incontinence	
	6. Lower risk of urinary tract infections	

KEY POINTS

- Bladder calculi may be associated with BPH in up to 10% of men.
- Presence of bladder stone is considered an indication for surgical treatment of BPH.
- BPH with bladder stone can be managed simultaneously in a single sitting. In that scenario, the bladder stone should be removed first.
- Bladder stone can be managed by multiple methods as per availability and surgeon preference. The methods include procedures like transurethral cystolithotripsy, percutaneous suprapubic cystolithotripsy or open cystolithotomy.

REFERENCES

1. Yoo TK, Cho HJ. Benign prostatic hyperplasia: from bench to clinic. Korean J Urol 2012;53:139e48.
2. Oelke M, Bachmann A, Descazeaud A, Emberton M, Gravas S, Michel MC, *et al*. EAU guidelines on the treatment and follow-up of non-neurogenic male lower urinary tract symptoms including benign prostatic obstruction. Eur Urol 2013;64: 118e40.
3. Hammad FT, Kaya M, Kazim E. Bladder calculi: did the clinical picture change? Urology 2006;67:1154e8.
4. Douenias R, Rich M, Badlani G, Mazor D, Smith A. Predisposing factors in bladder calculi. Review of 100 cases. Urology 1991; 37:240e3.
5. Papatsoris AG, Varkarakis I, Dellis A, *et al*. Bladder lithiasis: from open surgery to lithotripsy. Urol Res 2006;34:163–7.
6. Huang W, Cao JJ, Cao M, Wu HS, Yang YY, Xu ZM, Jin XD. Risk factors for bladder calculi in patients with benign prostatic hyperplasia. Medicine (Baltimore). 2017 Aug;96(32):e7728. doi: 10.1097/MD.0000000000007728. PMID: 28796057; PMCID: PMC5556223.
7. Childs MA, Mynderse LA, Rangel LJ, Wilson TM, Lingeman JE, Krambeck AE. Pathogenesis of bladder calculi in the presence of urinary stasis. J Urol 2013;189:1347e51.
8. Turk C, Donaldson JF, Neisius A et al. EAU Bladder Stone Guidelines. Presented at the EAU Annual Congress Milan. 978-94-92671-13-4. Arnhem, the Netherlands: EAU Guidelines Office, 2021
9. Millan-Rodrıguez F, Errando-Smet C, Rousaud-Baron F, IzquierdoLatorre F, Rousaud-Baron A, Villavicencio-Mavrich H. Urodynamic findings before and after non-invasive management of bladder calculi. BJU Int 2004; 93: 1267–70.
10. Takasaki E, Suzuki T, Honda M, Imai T, Maeda S, Hosoya Y. Chemical compositions of 300 lower urinary tract calculi and associated disorders in the urinary tract. Urol Int 1995; 54: 89–94. https://pubmed.ncbi.nlm.nih.gov/7538235/
11. Gratzke C, Bachmann A, Descazeaud A, *et al*. EAU Guidelines on the assessment of non-neurogenic male lower urinary tract symptoms including benign prostatic obstruction. Eur Urol 2015; 67:1099–109.
12. McVary KT, Roehrborn CG, Avins AL, *et al*. Update on AUA guideline on the management of benign prostatic hyperplasia. J Urol 2011;185:1793–803.
13. Sabnis RB, Mulawkar PM, Joshi RN. The Urological Society of India guidelines on management of benign prostatic hyperplasia/benign prostatic obstruction (Executive summary). Indian J Urol. 2021 Jul-Sep;37(3):210–213. doi: 10.4103/iju.iju_121_21. PMID: 34465948; PMCID: PMC8388351.
14. Philippou P, Moraitis K, Masood J, *et al*. The management of bladder lithiasis in the modern era of endourology. Urology 2012;79:980–6.
15. Douenias R, Rich M, Badlani G, Mazor D, Smith A. Predisposing factors in bladder calculi: review of 100 cases. Urology 1991; 37: 240–3.
16. Gravas S, Cornus JN, Gacci M, *et al*. EAU guidelines on non-neurogenic male lower urinary tract symptoms. Presented at the EAU annual congress Milan. 978-94-92671-13-4. Arnhem, The Netherlands: EAU Guidelines Office, 2021.
17. Benign Prostatic Hyperplasia (BPH) Guideline-American Urological Association (auanet.org); accessed April 24, 2023.
18. Roehrborn CG, McConnell JD, Lieber M, Kaplan S, Geller J, Malek GH, Castellanos R, Coffield S, Saltzman B, Resnick M, Cook TJ, Waldstreicher J. Serum prostate-specific antigen concentration is a powerful predictor of acute urinary retention and need for surgery in men with clinical benign prostatic hyperplasia. PLESS Study Group. Urology. 1999 Mar;53(3):473–80. doi: 10.1016/s0090–4295(98)00654–2. PMID: 10096369.

19. Torricelli FC, Mazzucchi E, Danilovic A, Coelho RF, Srougi M. Surgical management of bladder stones: literature review. Revista do Colegio Brasileiro de Cirurgioes. 2013;40:227–33.
20. Philippou P, Volanis D, Kariotis I, Serafetinidis E, Delakas D. Prospective comparative study of endoscopic Management of Bladder Lithiasis: Is prostate surgery a necessary adjunct? Urology 2011; 78: 43–7.
21. Shah H, Hegde S, Shah J, Mahajan A, Bansal M. Simultaneous transurethral cystolithotripsy with holmium laser enucleation of the prostate: A prospective feasibility study and review of the literature. BJU Int 2007; 99: 595–600.
22. Guo R, Yu W, Meng Y, *et al*. Correlation of benign prostatic obstruction-related complications with clinical outcomes in patients after transurethral resection of the prostate. Kaohsiung J Med Sci 2017; 33: 144–51.
23. Romero-Otero J, Garcıa Gonzalez L, Garcıa-Gomez B *et al*. Analysis of holmium laser enucleation of the prostate in a high-volume center: The impact of concomitant holmium laser Cystolitholapaxy. J Endourol 2019; 33: 564–9.

Chapter

12B

BPH with Stricture

• Apul Goel • Manoj Biswas

LEARNING OBJECTIVES

- Association of urethral stricture with BPH.
- Criteria for diagnosis of BPH and stricture.
- Plan for endoscopic management of BPH and stricture.
- Intra-operative surprises: What to do?

INTRODUCTION

Urethral stricture disease is typically diagnosed in middle-aged and elderly men[1,2] while benign prostatic hyperplasia (BPH) also commonly presents in men > 50 years of age.[3] Any elderly who consults for lower urinary tract symptoms (LUTS) is often diagnosed to be suffering from BPH, as BPH is more prevalent. Typically, these two conditions are not diagnosed together wilfully. The more common scenario is when transurethral surgery is planned, the urologist incidentally encounters a urethral stricture. Also, when a man being treated with alpha-blocker therapy does not improve, a thorough evaluation for urethral stricture should be performed.

There is a paucity of literature about the simultaneous occurrence of the two conditions and their management. At many places, the authors have used their personal experience in writing this chapter.

Case Scenario

A 70-year-old man goes into acute urinary retention. There is a history of urinary symptoms for last many years. A per-urethral catheterization with 16-Fr Foley was attempted in an emergency ward by a medical officer. The catheter could not be negotiated into the bladder even after repeated attempts. When the medical officer noticed urethral bleed, he abandoned the procedure. A surgeon was called who performed a supra-pubic cystostomy. The patient was then referred to you. The ultrasound shows the prostate size to be 60 ml.

1. **Can BPH and urethral stricture occur together?**

   Ans: Yes. Occasionally, a urologist will incidentally encounter a urethral stricture in a man planned for prostate surgery. The incidence for such a scenario is unknown. Ntia and Dikko evaluated their 10-year experience (between January 1991 and December 2000) in treating BPH and identified 69 patients with this association. They mention that this association tends to occur in 10–12% of BPH patients.[4]

   Another study from Ethiopia involving 65 patients, the authors reported that two (3.0%) cases had urethral stricture with BPH. These patients were treated by DVIU (direct vision internal urethrotomy) and transurethral resection of prostate (TURP).[5]

   However, every attempt should be made to diagnose these conditions pre-operatively and an intra-operative surprise detection should be avoided. A surprise association may lead to medico-legal issues.

   If a man has evident dense stricture with an enlarged prostate, then, this should be diagnosed as stricture only and treated accordingly. Mere enlargement of prostate does not mean that it is a reason for LUTS.[6] BPH is a diagnosis of exclusion.

2. **Can urethral stricture be detected incidentally?**

   Ans: Yes. In a series from Australia the authors shared their 10-year institutional experience in the management of urethral stricture. In a cohort of 360 adult men with median age of 69 years, they reported 122 men (34%) to have incidentally detected urethral stricture.[7] An additional 47 men (13%) presented primarily with urinary retention. Of the 122 men found to have incidental urethral stricture, in 96, it was detected at the time of cystoscopy. In rest 26 men, stricture was identified due to failed urethral catheterization. LUTS as a presentation of urethral stricture is seen in only 54.3% of men.[8]

3. **Can you differentiate clinically between BPH and urethral stricture?**

Ans: The differentiation between urethral stricture and BPH is important. The differences are evident from the symptoms and uroflowmetry patterns. As the urethral stricture is a disease of fibrosis, the urethra lacks elasticity and fails to stretch during micturition. This manifests as a fixed flow rate (box-shaped pattern) (Fig. 12B.1). In men with BPH, on the other hand, the prostatic cavity can distend during different phases of detrusor contraction. This presents as low flow rate (Fig. 12B.2). Also, men with stricture may notice improvement in urinary flow on straining. Investigators have even evaluated the differences in the urodynamic findings between men with BPH and urethral stricture. Bishra and colleagues found that men with urethral stricture disease had lower closure pressures as compared to men with BPH (22.07 vs. 28.4 cm H_2O, $p = 0.0039$, $r = 0.61$). They noted that the slope of passive urethral relation was indistinguishable between the two groups. Of interest was the finding that only 60% of men with symptomatic urethral strictures had unequivocal obstruction based on the Abrams-Griffiths nomogram.[9]

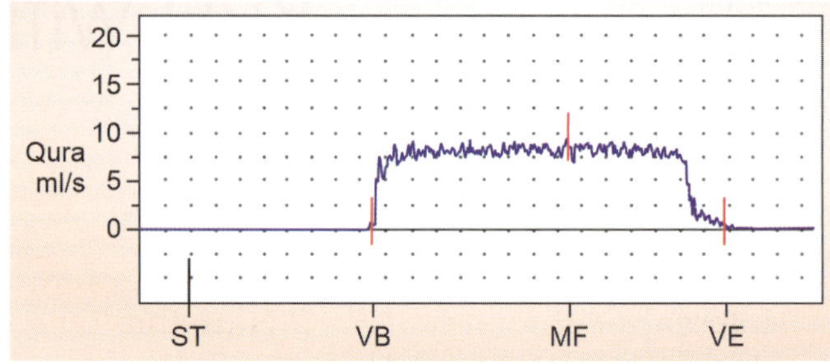

Fig. 12B.1: Fixed flow rate (box-shaped pattern)

4. **Occasionally, in a patient planned for TURP, a urologist encounters a situation where she/he is unable to pass a 26 Fr continuous-flow resectoscope into the urinary bladder. Does this patient have a urethral stricture? What should be done if a 20 Fr cystoscopy can easily be performed while it is difficult to negotiate a 26 Fr continuous-flow resectoscope?**

Ans: The size of urethral lumen is variable and depends on the race. Various authors have used a definition of urethral stricture as lumen size < 10 Fr. The sheath size of a typical continuous flow resectoscope is 26 Fr. In many patients, it is

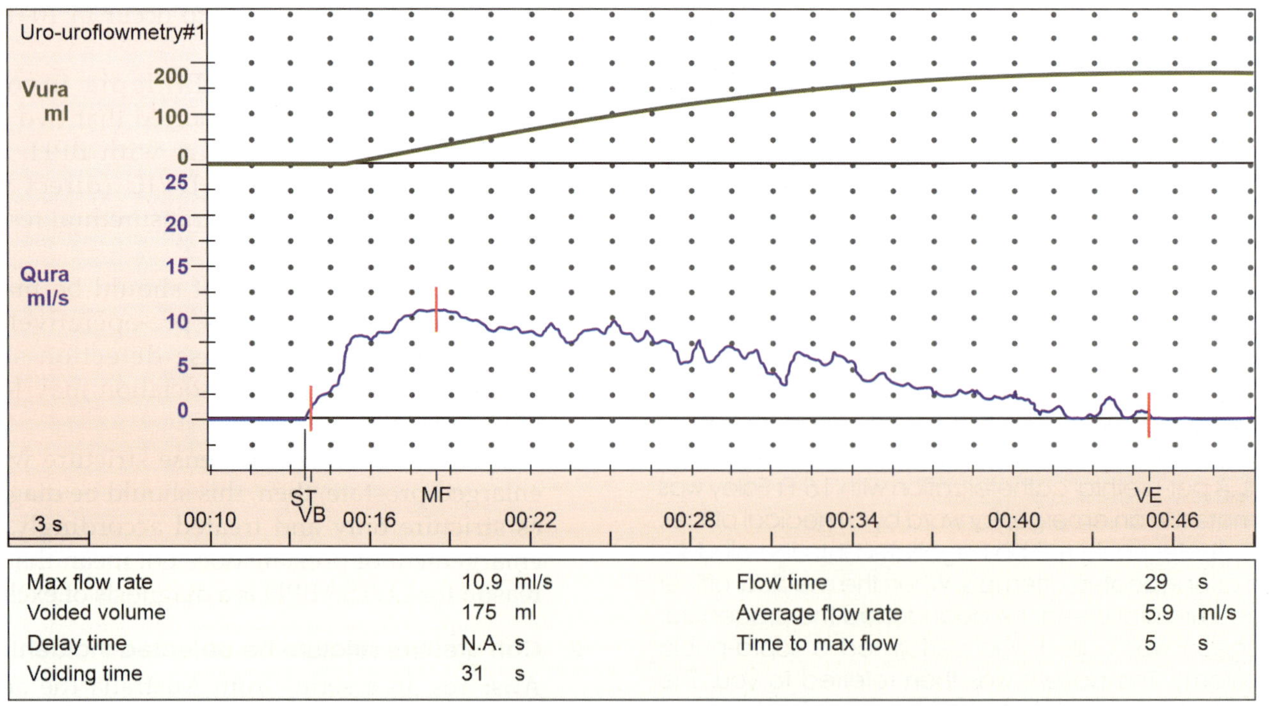

Max flow rate	10.9 ml/s	Flow time	29 s
Voided volume	175 ml	Average flow rate	5.9 ml/s
Delay time	N.A. s	Time to max flow	5 s
Voiding time	31 s		

Fig. 12B.2: Low flow rate in BPH

difficult to safely maneuver the 26 Fr resectoscope sheath into the bladder. In such a scenario, many urologists would either dilate the urethra with metallic bougies or use an Otis urethrotome to increase the size of urethral lumen. Also, some urologists would use a 24 Fr sheath that is not continuous flow (has only inflow). Recently, a smaller size (22 Fr) continuous flow resectoscope has been developed and is available in the market.[10]

5. **Is there evidence that pre-TURP/ holmium laser enucleation of the prostate (HoLEP) urethral dilatation reduce the incidence of post-operative stricture formation?**

Ans: In many centers, urethral dilatation or internal urethrotomy with Otis urethrotome is done routinely before TURP/HoLEP as part of institutional protocol. There is also evidence that pre-prostate surgery urethral dilatation prevents subsequent stricture formation. In a randomized controlled trial involving 72 men, Park and colleagues showed that men who underwent pre-HoLEP urethral dilatation had a lesser chance of developing urethral stricture.[11]

6. **Should all men suspected to have LUTS due to BPH be evaluated for urethral stricture disease?**

Ans: While evaluating a man with LUTS all possible differential diagnosis should be kept in mind, including the possibility of two pathologies simultaneously. The occurrence of two pathologies, stricture urethra with BPH, should be considered in men who fail to improve on medical therapy (alpha-blockers). Also, all men must be examined thoroughly at the time of initial presentation to rule out meatal stenosis or phimosis. Clues that point towards a possibility of urethral stricture include history of previous catheterization and box-shaped pattern on uroflowmetry (Fig. 12B.1).

7. **In the case scenario mentioned in case capsule above, how will you proceed? What are the possible scenarios?**

Ans: This scenario is not uncommon. BPH with a prominent median lobe can be a cause of failed urethral catheterization.[12,13] However, the possible reason for failed catheterization could be either the presence of urethral stricture in man with BPH or it could be normal urethra but failed catheterization due to an enlarged prostate. The traditional understanding that failed catheterization is because of urethral stricture is not absolute. The way forward is to get a micturating cystourethrogram and a retrograde urethrogram after a gap of about 2–3 weeks. It is not uncommon to find a short stricture in the region of proximal bulbar urethra. This stricture has most likely developed due to traumatic catheterization. Also, since the prostate volume is large it is likely that the sequence of events was precipitated due to failed catheterization due to prostate-induced urinary retention and not a pre-existing urethral stricture. However, if the prostate volume was <30 ml, the urologist should also consider the possibility of primary urethral stricture. Currently, there are no guidelines on how to manage these situations. The urologist should take a decision on an individual basis. Simultaneous internal optical urethrotomy and transurethral resection of prostate may be performed in such scenarios with good results. However, the patient needs to be counselled about the possible recurrence of urethral stricture.

8. **If you need to manage only one condition, which one will you manage first surgically?**

Ans: In case the urologist feels that the stricture is dense, or is longer than 1 cm, then, it is likely, that urethral stricture is the primary reason for patient's symptoms (LUTS). The stricture would merit treatment first. The decision algorithm for stricture management must be followed according to the guidelines by various academic societies.

Only, if LUTS persist after correction of urethral stricture, the medical therapy for LUTS should be initiated.

9. **What would be the best management in a man planned for TURP where the urologist encounters a urethral stricture?**

Ans: If the patient has not been counselled before proceeding, it is advisable to talk to the attendants and the patient if he is conscious (mostly the procedure is being done under spinal anesthesia). If the stricture seems soft and short and the patient consents, then simultaneous DVIU and TURP can be performed.[4,5] If the stricture seems firm and long, then, the procedure should be abandoned, and the patient evaluated properly before proceeding further. If needed, a suprapubic cystostomy can be performed.

10. **What is an easy method to rule out urethral stricture in man with BPH?**

Ans: Urethral calibration with a 16 Fr Foley catheter should be done. If calibration happens easily, then the patient is having only BPH. If calibration fails, further evaluation to rule out stricture should be done.

11. **Define urethral stricture. What criteria were used to label a narrowing as stricture? Is it lumen size? Is it inability to negotiate some catheter? Is it some Q_{max} on uroflowmetry?**

Ans: Campbell-Walsh-Wein urology defines urethral stricture as, "The term *urethral stricture* refers to fixed anatomic narrowing of the urethra so that the lumen will not accommodate instrumentation without disruption of the urethral mucosal lining.[14]" The exact lumen size to define stricture is not mentioned in this chapter or in the European Association of Urology guidelines[15] or in the American Association of Urology guidelines.[16] The definition of stricture varies among the authors. It may be based on symptoms, maximum flow rate (Q_{max}) of <10, <12, or <15 ml/s, stricture on retrograde urethrogram or an inability to pass a catheter of size 14 Fr.[17]

SUMMARY

- Association of urethral stricture with BPH is not common but should be kept in mind.
- A diagnosis of simultaneous BPH and urethral stricture should ideally not be made. BPH is a diagnosis of exclusion. Only if the lower urinary tract symptoms cannot be explained by another diagnosis BPH should be diagnosed.
- A man with BPH who goes into urinary retention may sustain urethral trauma at the time of urethral catheterization. Typically, such strictures are short and passable. Such men should be treated for both, stricture and BPH. Often, this can be accomplished endoscopically.
- Sometimes, a man with urethral stricture may be misdiagnosed as BPH. In such a scenario, when medical therapy fails, these patients are planned for endoscopic treatment of BPH (TURP or HoLEP). The surgeon then encounters a urethral stricture. Further treatment should depend on the pre-operative consent taken from the patient and may include surgery for urethral stricture or abandonment of surgery.

REFERENCES

1. Santucci RA, Joyce GF, Wise M. Male urethral stricture disease. *J Urol* 2007;177:1667–74.
2. Palminteri E, Berdondini E, Verze P, *et al*. Contemporary urethral stricture characteristics in the developed world. *Urology* 2013;81:191–6.
3. Berry S.J., Coffey D.S., Walsh P.C., Ewing L.L. The development of human benign prostatic hyperplasia with age. *J Urol.* 1984;132:474–479.
4. Ntia IO, Dikko AA. The Pattern of Association of Urethral Stricture with Benign Prostatic Hyperplasia in Nigerians. Sahel Med. J. 2002; 5(4):190–194.
5. Alemu MH. Transurethral resection of the prostate (TURP)--in the treatment of benign prostatic hypertrophy (BPH) in Mekelle, Ethiopia. Ethiop Med J. 2009 Jan;47(1):65–9. PMID: 19743783.
6. Tanguay S, Awde M, Brock G, Casey R, Kozak J, Lee J, Nickel JC, Saad F. Diagnosis and management of benign prostatic hyperplasia in primary care. Can Urol Assoc J. 2009 Jun;3(3 Suppl 2):S92–S100. doi: 10.5489/cuaj.1116. PMID: 19543429; PMCID: PMC2698785.
7. Hong MKH, Murugappan S, Norton SM, Moore EM, Grills R. Male urethral stricture disease in a regional centre: 10 years of experience. ANZ J Surg. 2019 Jun;89(6):747–751. doi: 10.1111/ans.15244. Epub 2019 May 13. PMID: 31083791.
8. Rourke, K., *et al*. The clinical spectrum of the presenting signs and symptoms of anterior urethral stricture: detailed analysis of a single institutional cohort. Urology, 2012. 79: 1163. https://pubmed.ncbi.nlm.nih.gov/22446349/.
9. Bishara S, Foley C, Peters J, Philp T, Malone-Lee J. Can urodynamics distinguish between urethral strictures and Benign Prostatic Hyperplasia (BPH)? *Journal of Clinical Urology*. 2015;8(4):274–278. doi:10.1177/2051415814565371
10. https://www.karlstorz.com/cps/rde/xbcr/karlstorz_assets/ASSETS/3331222.pdf Accessed June 3, 2023.
11. Park JK, Kim JY, You JH, Choi BR, Kam SC, Kim MK, Jeong YB, Shin YS. Effect of preoperative urethral dilatation on preventing urethral stricture after holmium laser enucleation of the prostate: A randomized controlled study. Can Urol Assoc J. 2019 Nov;13(11):E357–E360. doi: 10.5489/cuaj.5781. PMID: 30817290; PMCID: PMC6877364.
12. Villanueva C, Hemstreet GP 3rd. Difficult male urethral catheterization: a review of different approaches. Int Braz J Urol. 2008 Jul-Aug;34(4):401–11; discussion 412. doi: 10.1590/s1677–55382008000400002. PMID: 18778491.
13. Bianchi A, Leslie SW, Chesnut GT. Difficult Foley Catheterization. [Updated 2022 Nov 28]. In: StatPearls [Internet]. Treasure Island (FL): StatPearls Publishing; 2023 Jan. Available from: https://www.ncbi.nlm.nih.gov/books/NBK564404/
14. Virasoro R, Jordan GH, McCammon KA. Surgery for Benign Disorders of the Penis and Urethra. In: Partin AW, Dmochowski RR, Kavoussi LR, Craig A. Peters CA (editors). Campbell-Walsh-Wein Urology, 12th ed. Philadelphia: Elsevier; 2021. pp. 1814.
15. https://uroweb.org/guidelines/urethral-strictures/chapter/definition-epidemiology-aetiology-and-prevention
16. https://www.auanet.org/guidelines-and-quality/guidelines/urethral-stricture-guideline
17. Pang KH, Chapple CR, Chatters R, Downey AP, Harding CK, Hind D, Watkin N, Osman NI. A Systematic Review and Meta-analysis of Adjuncts to Minimally Invasive Treatment of Urethral Stricture in Men. Eur Urol. 2021 Oct;80(4):467–479. doi: 10.1016/j.eururo.2021.06.022. Epub 2021 Jul 16. PMID: 34275660.

Chapter

12C

BPH with Hernia

• Apul Goel • Manoj Biswas

LEARNING OBJECTIVES

- To explore the relationship between BPH and inguinal hernia.
- To understand if all elderly need evaluation for BPH when being evaluated for hernia surgery.
- Is presence of hernia an indication for surgical removal of prostate?
- Can surgery for prostate and hernia be combined?

INTRODUCTION

Benign prostatic hyperplasia (BPH) and inguinal hernias are two prominent medical diseases that commonly affect older men. While these conditions may appear unrelated, there is evidence suggesting that the elevated abdominal pressure experienced during urination in men with BPH may raise the possibility of getting an inguinal hernia. This chapter focuses on the management of BPH in combination with an inguinal hernia and explores how these conditions can be effectively addressed together. It is reported that among men having prostatectomy, the incidence of inguinal hernia is between 15% and 25%, significantly higher than the approximately 5% prevalence in the general population.[1] Around 30% of patients who are scheduled for inguinal hernia surgery also suffer from lower urinary tract symptoms, which can result in post-operative urinary retention and potentially necessitate urological intervention.[2–4] The abdominal strain exerted during urination, accompanied by a chronically increased intra-abdominal pressure, is the primary factor contributing to the development of inguinal hernias. Hernia formation is further facilitated by the deterioration of the inguinal canal tissues with aging.[5] Urologists often encounter various scenarios involving the simultaneous management of these conditions.

Case Scenario

A 65-year-old male presented with voiding and storage lower urinary tract symptoms (LUTS) of 3 years duration. He also complained of a swelling over the right inguinoscrotal region that he noticed for the last 2 years. His International prostate symptom score (IPSS) was 25. Physical examination revealed a grade-III enlarged prostate on DRE and a right-sided direct inguinal hernia. Investigations revealed a low flow rate on uroflowmetry, serum PSA of 2.6 ng/ml and prostate volume of 54 cc.

1. **Can LUTS due to BPH cause hernia formation?**

   Ans: A study from Taiwan looked at the National Health Insurance Program database (that covered 99% of the population) to identify if LUTS-BPH was a potential danger for inguinal hernia formation. From 1997 to 2013, 22,310 men with LUTS-BPH and 22,310 matched men without LUTS-BPH were included in the data and followed for inguinal hernias. Over a 10-year follow-up period, the authors discovered that 735 (2.53%) of the men without LUTS-BPH and 1,303 (5.84%) of the men with LUTS-BPH had inguinal hernias. It was discovered that LUTS-BPH was linked to a two-fold greater incidence of inguinal hernia after controlling for confounding variables. (HR: 2.25, 95% CI = 2.04–2.49).[6]

   However, the topic remains controversial. A smaller Indian study including only 126 men did not find any correlation between BPH and hernia.[7] In a questionnaire-based study from Finland involving 3143 subjects looked at associated diseases in men suffering from LUTS. These authors found no evidence of an increased risk of inguinal hernias.[8] A small German study involving 105 men also could not show that BPH is associated with an increased chance of developing a hernia.[9]

2. **Can treatment of LUTS-BPH reduce the incidence of inguinal hernia?**

Ans: A study from Taiwan, comprising 3,431,366 men, recruited newly diagnosed men aged 50 years or older with BPH drawn from the 2006–2010 National Health Insurance Research Database. These men were divided into three groups based on the type of treatment they received: Alpha-1 blockers only, transurethral resection of the prostate (TURP), and alpha-reductase inhibitors ± alpha-1 blockers. They followed each patient until the end of 2010 or until the inguinal hernia appeared. The incidence of inguinal hernia in men with BPH was found to be much lower in those undergoing prostate size-reducing therapies, such as TURP and 5ARI, than in those taking alpha-1 blockers.[10]

3. **Does the severity of LUTS correlate with inguinal hernia formation?**

Ans: In a small study involving 52 men, Reis *et al* found that men with inguinal hernia had higher IPSS. However, the authors feel that additional research is necessary to demonstrate the function of IPSS as a marker to predict the development of inguinal hernia.[11] However, another small study involving 100 men could not demonstrate that men suffering from inguinal hernia along with BPH had higher IPSS scores because of voiding dysfunction.[12]

4. **Should uroflowmetry be done in all men > 60 years of age who are planned for hernia repair?**

Ans: There is scant data to answer this question. A small study does recommend uroflowmetry in all elderly men undergoing inguinal hernia repair.[13]

5. **What will be the plan of management?**

Ans: The severity and the clinical picture of both BPH and the inguinal hernia determines how the patient is treated overall.. Depending on the patient's health and the surgeon's decision, both conditions may be managed concurrently or sequentially. The clinical picture of the patient presented above shows that he has an IPSS of 25 with a 54 cc prostate. Naturally, he will need treatment of both the conditions. Simultaneous presence of hernia in a man suffering from LUTS is not considered an indication of operative treatment of BPH. One approach would be to start the patient on combination therapy comprising of an alpha-1 blocker and 5-alpha-reductase inhibitor. The patient can be followed after a gap of about 2 weeks to look for response of these medication on the IPSS. If the symptoms do not improve, then prostate gland removal can be planned. Another approach could be offering upfront surgical treatment of prostate in view of significant symptoms and a large prostate. The reason for recommending upfront surgery is that long-term compliance to medical therapy is about 70% to 80%.[14] Factors that predict failure of medical therapy are poorly understood but include severe symptoms and large prostate at baseline.[14–16]

6. **If there is improvement in LUTS after combination therapy, what advise will you give to the patient?**

Ans: The patient can be advised to undergo hernia surgery alone. In the peri-operative period the patient should continue to consume combination therapy.[17] This could lessen the likelihood of urine retention following surgery.

7. **A 68-year-old man is referred by a surgeon colleague asking for opinion regarding a patient who consulted her for inguinal hernia repair. She was concerned that the hernia might recur because the patient was elderly and might be having prostate enlargement with straining to void. What opinion would you give this patient?**

Ans: This is a common scenario encountered in clinical practice. Standard evaluation of a patient suffering from LUTS is recommended. The symptoms should be quantified using questionnaires, like the IPSS. Further evaluation should include a serum PSA, renal function tests (serum creatinine), uroflowmetry and an abdominal ultrasound to determine the post-void residual urine volume and prostate volume.. Then, first rule out indications for surgery, like, refractory urinary retention, upper tract obstructive changes, azotemia, recurrent hematuria, bladder stone and bladder diverticulum and recurrent urinary tract infection. If the patient does not fall in this group, then a trial of medical therapy is warranted.[18]

If the patient has a similar presentation as in the scenario already discussed above, then you need to proceed accordingly. However, there could be different scenarios. If the evaluation reveals an IPSS of 15 (moderate symptoms), PSA value of 1.1 ng/ml, uroflowmetry result as shown in Fig. 12C.1 and a post-void residual urine volume of 25 ml, and, a prostate volume of 35 ml, then the patient should be kept on alpha-blockers only. This patient can be advised to undergo hernia surgery alone. The patient should be kept on alpha-blockers during the peri-operative period. Alpha-blocker medication may lower the risk of post-operative urine retention, according to evidence.[17]

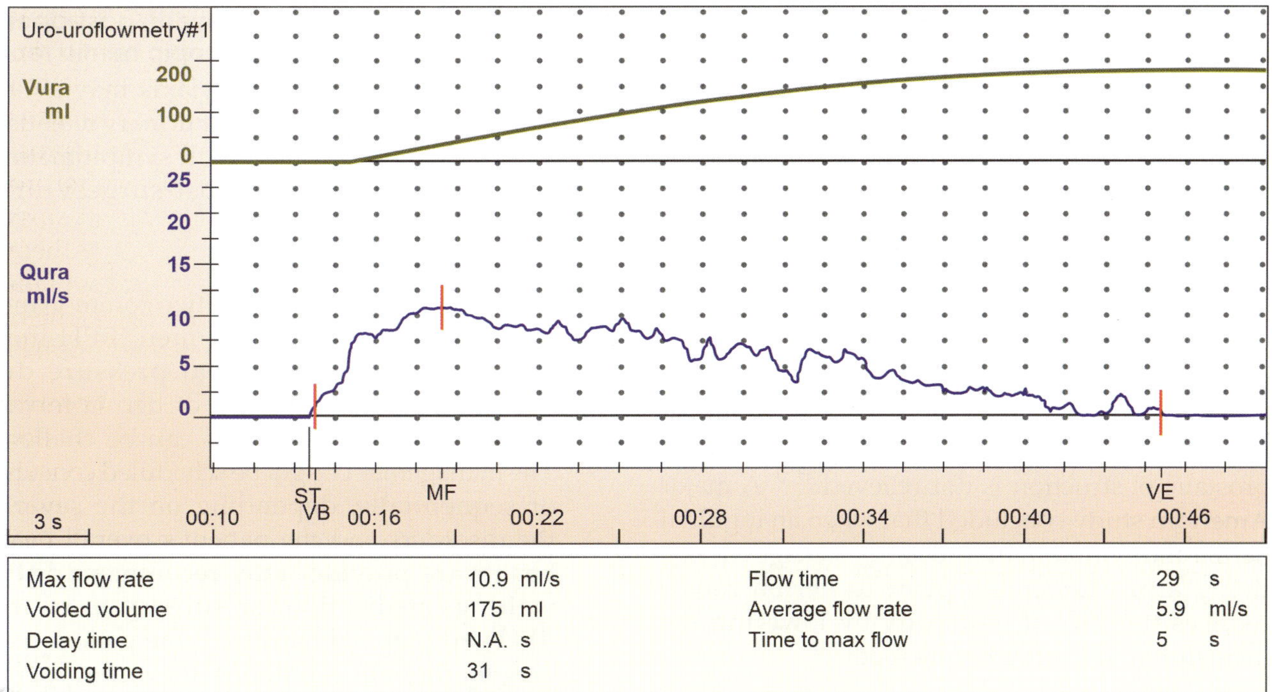

Fig. 12C.1: Uroflowmetry showing low flow rate

Nevertheless, other RCTs have not been able to demonstrate that alpha-blockers have a beneficial effect on post-operative urine retention.[19–22]

For any IPSS, serum PSA < 1.5 ng/ml and prostate volume < 40 ml: Start alpha-blockers alone and look for response. For any IPSS, serum PSA > 1.5 ng/ml and prostate volume > 40 ml: Start combination therapy in the form of alpha-blockers and 5-alpha-reductase inhibitors (finasteride or dutasteride).[23] For mild IPSS a trial of conservative therapy can be offered.[23]

If the patient has concomitant erectile dysfunction, then, consideration for once daily Tadalafil 5 mg can be made.[23] A trial of medical therapy for at least 3–4 weeks can be done. Symptom improvement can be documented objectively using either the IPSS or on uroflowmetry. If the patient does not show improvement with appropriate medical therapy, with persistently raised IPSS, then surgical treatment of prostate can be offered to the patient.

8. Whether one can do TURP and hernia repair in the same sitting?

Ans: Most data regarding combining TURP with hernia surgery is based on small case series[1,24–29] In an earlier era, wound infection was higher when open surgery was performed for both, BPH and for hernia repair.[2,3,30] But in the late 90s, simultaneous TURP with open hernia repair showed promising results. With advancements in laparoscopic technology, laparoscopic hernia repair can now be done simultaneously with TURP.[31]

Combining TURP with inguinal hernioplasty is thought to be a safe and effective surgical technique that lowers hospitalization expenses and permits the treatment of two problems with a single anesthetia and hospital stay.[32] If men with symptomatic BPH undergo hernia repair without treating urinary symptoms, they may develop post-operative urinary retention and are also exposed to an increased risk of urinary tract infection.[31,33]

9. Are there randomized trials (RCT) showing superiority of combined surgery as compared to surgery in two sittings?

Ans: In a small RCT reported from Egypt, 30 men (15 in each group) were randomized to receive either combined surgery (TURP and hernioplasty) while the other group underwent surgery in 2 sittings. When TURP and inguinal hernioplasty procedures were performed concurrently, the authors observed no discernible rise in the complication rate. It was observed that neither group had a hernia recurrence. Doing the two procedures in the same session resulted in a 26% decrease in hospitalization costs.[32] Another non-randomized comparative study evaluated the various outcomes in men undergoing combined TURP and inguinal mesh hernioplasty (n = 44), men undergoing TURP alone (n = 50) and the third group included men undergoing hernia repair only (n = 50). According to the authors, there were no appreciable variations in post-operative problems between the three groups.

There was no mesh infection that they could find. They came to the conclusion that TURP plus inguinal herniorrhaphy is a useful, safe, and efficient treatment.[34] Another small comparative study also showed good results with combined surgery.[35]

10. **If prostate and hernia surgery is done in two different sittings what should be the sequence of surgery? Which surgery should be performed first?**

    Ans: Most authors would prefer to operate the prostate first followed by hernia repair. The rationale is that if hernia surgery is done first then there would be a higher incidence of recurrence if prostatic obstruction is not relieved.[32,36] A major American study concluded that when an inguinal hernia and symptomatic prostatic blockage coexist, doing a prostatectomy prior to hernia repair reduces the risk of morbidity by lowering the incidence of UTI after hernia repair.[37]

11. **Can open prostatectomy be combined with hernia surgery?**

    Ans: There is limited contemporary data that suggests that even open prostatectomy can be combined with simultaneous hernia repair. The authors reported data of 52 men undergoing simultaneous procedure with good results.[38,39]

12. **Which hernia surgery is preferable?**

    Ans: A study on males receiving concurrent transurethral resection of the prostate (TURP) and open hernia repair found no increased infection rate in the group undergoing the combination surgery.[24] This may be attributed to the fact that Lichtenstein's operation, which is an open hernia repair technique, involves placing the mesh anterior to the muscle layer (onlay meshplasty). This is in contrast to the fully extraperitoneal (TEP) technique, in which the mesh is placed in the pre-peritoneal area. TURP can result in micro-injuries and micro-perforations of the prostatic capsule at the bladder neck due to aggressive resection of a large-volume prostate gland, resulting in fluid leakage into the pre-peritoneal area.[40,41]

    Multiple clinical studies and meta-analyses have consistently shown that TEP repair offers advantages over open inguinal hernia repair, including reduced post-operative pain, decreased need for analgesia, earlier return to daily activities, fewer complications, and lower recurrence rates when performed by experienced surgeons. Concurrent TEP and TURP procedures are considered practical, cost-effective, and safe.[31]

13. **What precautions will prevent post-operative urinary retention in laparoscopic hernia repair?**

    Ans: Alpha blocker prophylaxis may avoid the episodes of post-hernia repair urinary retention[42–44] as elderly men and men with symptomatic BPH show high chances of post-surgery urinary retention.

Conclusion

BPH and inguinal hernia are two common medical conditions that can affect men. BPH-induced increased intra-abdominal pressure during voiding may raise the risk of hernia formation. Managing these conditions can be challenging. The management might be scheduled concurrently or sequentially, depending on the severity of the disorders and the patient's overall health. A healthcare provider may recommend watchful waiting, medication, or surgery to treat both BPH and inguinal hernias. If the patient requires surgery for both conditions, they must follow the surgical protocol and make any necessary lifestyle adjustments for a successful long-term outcome. The treatment plan should be individualised.

SUMMARY

- Whether straining for urination, because of BPH, causes inguinal hernia is controversial. Smaller studies have not found an association between the two. However, some large studies have noted an association.
- All elderly (age more than 50 years) with hernia should be asked about urinary symptoms (LUTS). If symptomatic, they should be evaluated for BPH.
- Occurrence of hernia in a man with LUTS is not an absolute indication for prostate surgery (TURP/HoLEP).
- If required, hernia repair and prostate surgery can be combined. However, combined surgery should be undertaken only if facilities are available and the patient is fit.
- If the surgeries are done sequentially, then prostate surgery may be performed first.

REFERENCES

1. Devarajan R, Jaganathan RS, Harriss DR, Chua CB, Bishop MC. Combined transurethral prostatectomy and inguinal hernia repair: a retrospective audit and literature review. BJU Int 1999, 84:637–639.
2. Thompson IM, Wesen CA. Prostatism and inguinal hernia. South Med J 1982, 75: 1342–4.
3. Abramson JH, Gofin J, Makler A, Epstein LM. The epidemiology of inguinal hernia: a survey in western Jerusalem. J Epidemiol Community Health 1978, 32: 59–67.
4. Tundidor-Bermudez AM. Hernia Inguinal y Prostatismo. Arch Esp Urol 1994, 47: 19–21.
5. Gonzalez-Ojeda A, Marquina M, Calva J, Mendoza A, de la Garza L. Combined inguinal herniorrhaphy and transurethral prostatectomy. Br J Surg 1991; 78: 1443–5.
6. Wu Y-H, Juan Y-S, Shen J-T, Wang H-S, Jhan J-H, Lee Y-C, *et al.* (2020) Lower urinary tract symptoms–Benign prostatic

hyperplasia may increase the risk of subsequent inguinal hernia in a Taiwanese population: A nationwide population-Based cohort study. PLoS ONE 15(6): e0234329. https://doi.org/10.1371/journal.pone.0234329.

7. Parthiban SS, Durairaj B. A study on association between inguinal hernia and benign prostatic hyperplasia. Int Surg J, 2019, Vol. 6 No. 6. https://www.ijsurgery.com/index.php/isj/article/view/4176.
8. Koskimäki J, Hakama M, Huhtala H, Tammela TL. Association of non-urological diseases with lower urinary tract symptoms. Scand J Urol Nephrol. 2001 Oct;35(5):377–81. doi: 10.1080/003655901753224431. PMID: 11771864.
9. Jülke M, Schmid R, Thalmann C, Enzler M, Knönagel H, Schwarz H. Leistenhernie als Folge gestörter Blasenentleerung? [Inguinal hernia as a sequela of disordered bladder emptying?]. Helv Chir Acta. 1992 Aug;59(2):331–4. German. PMID: 1385359.
10. Fan YH, Chung HJ, Huang E, Lin A, Chen KK. MP3–10 Reduction of enlarged prostate decreases the incidence of inguinal hernia. https://www.auajournals.org/doi/10.1016/j.juro.2015.02.113.
11. Reis RB, Rodrigues Neto AA, Reis LO, Machado RD, Kaplan S. Correlation between the presence of inguinal hernia and the intensity of lower urinary tract symptoms. Acta Cir Bras. 2011;26 Suppl 2:125–8. doi: 10.1590/s0102–86502011000800023. PMID: 22030828.
12. Sentürk AB, Ekici M, Sahiner IT, Tas T, Cakiroglu B. Relationship between lower urinary tract symptoms and inguinal hernia. Arch Ital Urol Androl. 2016 Dec 30;88(4):262–265. doi: 10.4081/aiua.2016.4.262. PMID: 28073189.
13. Thompson IM, Wesen CA. Prostatism and inguinal hernia. South Med J. 1982 Nov;75(11):1342–4. doi: 10.1097/00007611–198211000–00009. PMID: 6183754.
14. Kaplan SA. Factors in Predicting Failure with Medical Therapy for BPH. Rev Urol. 2005;7 Suppl 7(Suppl 7):S34–9. PMID: 16986060; PMCID: PMC1477626.
15. Hong SJ, Ko WJ, Kim SI, Chung BH. Identification of baseline clinical factors which predict medical treatment failure of benign prostatic hyperplasia: an observational cohort study. Eur Urol. 2003 Jul;44(1):94–9; discussion 99–100. doi: 10.1016/s0302–2838(03)00199–4. PMID: 12814681.
16. Connolly SS, Fitzpatrick JM. Medical treatment of benign prostatic hyperplasia. Postgrad Med J. 2007 Feb;83(976):73–8. doi: 10.1136/pgmj.2006.050724. PMID: 17308208; PMCID: PMC2805943.
17. Shaw MK, Pahari H. The role of peri-operative use of alpha-blocker in preventing lower urinary tract symptoms in high risk patients of urinary retention undergoing inguinal hernia repair in males above 50 years. J Indian Med Assoc. 2014 Jan;112(1):13–4, 16. PMID: 25935942.
18. Helo S, Welliver, RC Jr., McVary KT. Minimally Invasive and Endoscopic Management of Benign Prostatic Hyperplasia. In: Partin AW, Dmochowski RR, Kavoussi LR, Craig A. Peters CA (editors). Campbell-Walsh-Wein Urology, 12th ed. Philadelphia: Elsevier; 2021. pp. 3408–9.
19. Caparelli ML, Shikhman A, Runyan B, Allamaneni S, Hobler S. The use of tamsulosin to prevent postoperative urinary retention in laparoscopic inguinal hernia repair: a randomized double-blind placebo-controlled study. Surg Endosc. 2021 Oct;35(10):5538–5545. doi: 10.1007/s00464–020–08050–0. Epub 2020 Oct 6. PMID: 33025252.
20. Koukoulis GD, Bouliaris K, Perivoliotis K, Tepetes K. Prophylactic Administration of Alpha Blocker for the Prevention of Urinary Retention in Males Undergoing Inguinal Hernia Repair Under Spinal Anesthesia: Interim Analysis of a Randomized Controlled Trial. Cureus. 2021 Nov 17;13(11):e19669. doi: 10.7759/cureus.19669. PMID: 34804757; PMCID: PMC8599459.
21. Drahman A, Ngee-Soon SL, Crawford M. Prophylactic alpha-blockade for prevention of post-operative urinary retention after inguinal hernia repair: a systematic review and meta-analysis. Hernia. 2023 Mar 23. doi: 10.1007/s10029–023–02764–5. Epub ahead of print. PMID: 36952050.
22. Woo HH, Carmalt HL. A placebo-controlled double-blind study using perioperative prazosin in the prevention of urinary retention following inguinal hernia repair. Int Urol Nephrol. 1995;27(5):557–62. doi: 10.1007/BF02564741. PMID: 8775039.
23. https://uroweb.org/guidelines/management-of-non-neurogenic-male-luts/chapter/disease-management.
24. Bawa AS, Batra RK, Singh R. Management of inguinal hernia with benign prostatic hyperplasia: simultaneous inguinal hernioplasty with transurethral resection of prostate. Int Urol Nephrol. 2003;35(4):503–6. doi: 10.1023/b:urol.0000025615.06733.09. PMID: 15198155.
25. Guvel S, Nursal TZ, Kilinc F, Egilmez T, Yaycioglu O, Ozkardes H. Transurethral prostatectomy and inguinal hernia repair in a single session. Urol Int. 2004;73(3):266–9. doi: 10.1159/000080840. PMID: 15539849.
26. González-Ojeda A, Anaya-Prado R, Fuentes-Orozco C, Portilla-de-Buen E, Muciño-Hernández MI, Medina-Meza CO. Combined transurethral prostatectomy and mesh-based tension-free inguinal hernia repair. Hernia. 2003 Sep;7(3):141–5. doi: 10.1007/s10029–003–0127–z. Epub 2003 Apr 24. PMID: 12712366.
27. Dahami Z, Barjani F, Saghir O, Ben Elkhaiat R, Moudouni MS, Sarf I. Cure de hernie inguinale et résection transurétrale de l'adénome de prostate en un seul temps opératoire [Combined inguinal hernia repair and transurethral resection of the prostate (TURP) for benign prostatic hypertrophy]. J Chir (Paris). 2009 Dec;146(6):549–52. French. doi: 10.1016/j.jchir.2009.10.005. Epub 2009 Nov 3. PMID: 19889413.
28. Chong T, Li YQ, Wang ZM, Shi T, Zhang P. [Simultaneous treatment for benign prostate hyperplasia and its concomitant diseases]. Zhonghua Nan Ke Xue. 2006 Jun;12(6):534–6. Chinese. PMID: 16833196.
29. Khiari R, Ghozzi S, Hmidi M, Khouni H, Hammami A, Ktari M, Fkih N, Hellel M, Ben Rais N. Association hypertrophie bénigne de la prostate et hernie inguinale. Cure simultanée à propos de 55 cas [Association of benign prostatic hyperplasia and hernia inguinale. A report of 55 cas]. Tunis Med. 2006 Dec;84(12):790–3. French. PMID: 17288282.
30. McDonald DF, Huggins C. Simultaneous prostatectomy and inguinal herniorrhaphy. Surg Gynecol Obstet 1949; 89: 621–2.
31. Harvitkar RU, Shetty PC, Joshi A. Concurrent laparoscopic totally extraperitoneal inguinal hernia repair and transurethral resection of prostate: Breaking with convention-A retrospective study. J Minim Access Surg. 2022 Jan-Mar;18(1):72–76. doi: 10.4103/jmas.JMAS_260_20. PMID: 35017395; PMCID: PMC8830565.
32. Othman I, Abdel-Maguid AF. Combined transurethral prostatectomy and inguinal hernioplasty. Hernia. 2010

Apr;14(2):149–53. doi: 10.1007/s10029–009–0575–1. Epub 2009 Nov 1. PMID: 19882105.

33. Eubanks S. Hernias. In: Sabiston DC, Lyerly HK, editors. Textbook of Surgery: The Molecular Basis of Modern Surgical Practice. 15th ed. Philadelphia: WB Saunders Company; 1997. pp. 1215–33.
34. Cimentepe E, Inan A, Unsal A, Dener C. Combined transurethral resection of prostate and inguinal mesh hernioplasty. Int J Clin Pract. 2006 Feb;60(2):167–9. doi: 10.1111/j.1742–1241.2005.00630.x. PMID: 16451288.
35. Ather MH, Faruqui N, Abid F, Sulaiman MN. Is there a difference in early perioperative morbidity in transurethral resection of prostate (TURP) versus TURP with cystolitholapaxy and TURP with inguinal herniorrhaphy? Int Urol Nephrol. 2002;33(1):69–72. doi: 10.1023/a:1014457020723. PMID: 12090342.
36. Gueye SM, Fall PA, Ndoye AK, Sylla C, Thiam OB, Ba M, Diagne BA. Cure simultanée de l'hypertrophie bénigne de la prostate et de la hernie inguinale: une vieille procédure revisitée [Simultaneous treatment of benign prostatic hypertrophy and inguinal hernia: an old procedure revisited]. Dakar Med. 1999;44(2):219–21. French. PMID: 11957289.
37. Cramer SO, Malangoni MA, Schulte WJ, Condon RE. Inguinal hernia repair before and after prostatic resection. Surgery. 1983 Oct;94(4):627–30. PMID: 6623362.
38. Granados EA, Villavicencio H, Sole-Balcells F. Se debe practicar la hernioplastia conjuntamente con cirugía de la próstata? [Should hernioplasty be combined with surgery of the prostate?]. Arch Esp Urol. 1998 Oct;51(8):767–70. Spanish. PMID: 9859581.
39. Johnson OK. Simultaneous open preperitoneal repair of inguinal hernia with open prostatectomy for benign prostate hyperplasia. Trop Doct. 2015 Jan;45(1):42–3. doi: 10.1177/00494 75514554640. Epub 2014 Nov 17. PMID: 25406258.
40. Salmela L, Aromaa U, Lehtonen T, Peura P, Olkkola KT. The effect of prostatic capsule perforation on the absorption of irrigating fluid during transurethral resection. British J Urol. 1993 Nov;72(5):599–604.
41. Kenyon HR. Perforations in transurethral operations: Technique for Immediate Diagnosis and Management of Extravasations. JAMA. 1950 Mar 18;142(11):798–802.
42. Mohammadi-Fallah M, Hamedanchi S, Tayyebi-Azar A. Preventive effect of tamsulosin on post-operative urinary retention. Korean J Urol. 2012 Jun 1;53(6):419–23.
43. Li HZ, Cheng YS, Wang XF, Pan W. Caution! The potential overestimated effect of prophylactic alpha-blockade for the prevention of urinary retention following primary inguinal hernia repair in a meta-analysis of randomized controlled trials. American J Surg. 2018 Aug 1;216(2):391–2.
44. Caparelli ML, Shikhman A, Runyan B, Allamaneni S, Hobler S. The use of tamsulosin to prevent post-operative urinary retention in laparoscopic inguinal hernia repair: a randomized double-blind placebo-controlled study. Surgical Endoscopy. 2021 Oct;35:5538-

Chapter

13

Pediatric Vesical Calculi

• Vasudeo Ridhorkar • Siddalingeshwar Neeli

LEARNING OBJECTIVES

- Types of bladder stones in children.
- Clinical features of bladder stones in children.
- Management of bladder stones.
- Technical considerations during surgical interventions for bladder stones in children.
- Prevention of urinary calculi in children and endemic bladder calculi in particular.

INTRODUCTION

Bladder stone disease is rarely seen in the developed western world, however, it is commonly encountered in the Middle East countries, Africa and the Indian subcontinent. They account for 5% of all urinary calculi. In a developing country like India, endemic bladder stones are seen more in the rural areas. In 1999 Bakane *et al.*[1] reported 80% of paediatric urolithiasis in Central India to be bladder stones. Bladder stones are commoner in boys by a factor of 10:1. The incidence of bladder calculi is as old as humanity, as way back in 600 BC, Sushruta, the ancient Indian surgeon, in his book *Sushruta Samhita*, had described various procedures for treating bladder stones.[2]

Bladder stones present as a bimodal peak. One peak occurs in young children where most of the stones are endemic in nature and the other peak in elderly adults where the stones are usually secondary to bladder outlet obstruction.

Traditionally managed by open cystolithotomy, lately more and more of paediatric bladder stones are being managed endoscopically.[3,12] Literature mentions the use of all surgical modalities described for management of urolithiasis for the management of bladder stones. These include SWL (shock wave lithotripsy), endourologic procedures and even robotic surgery. The young male child poses a special challenge since the narrow pediatric urethra can get easily traumatized by instruments and result in stricture.

Education of mothers and healthcare personnel on adequate hydration, dietary modification and weaning practices can reduce the occurrence of vesical calculi in children.[4]

Case Scenario

Three-year-old male child presents with urgency, frequency and dysuria and occasional episodes of hematuria. He typically cries a lot during these episodes of pain and tugs at the penis. His lab reports show very low haemoglobin with significant hematopyuria. Abdominal ultrasound (Fig. 13.1) reveals a 1.2 cm, vesical calculus. X-ray KUB (Fig. 13.2) confirms the bladder stone. He did not have any episode of urinary retention.

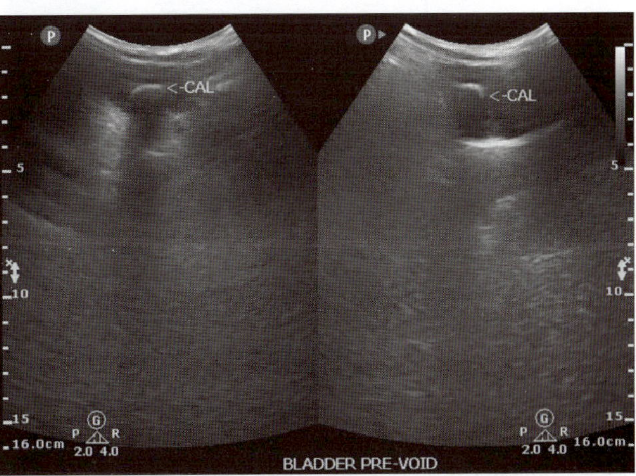

Fig. 13.1: Abdominal ultrasound showing vesical calculus

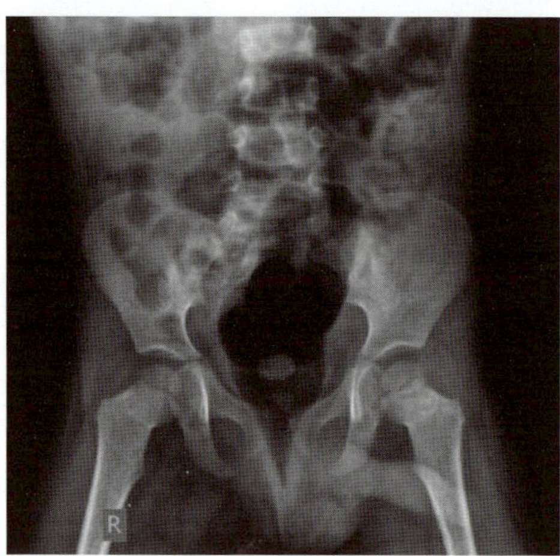

Fig. 13.2: X-ray showing vesical calculus

1. **Why do male children tug at the penis during the episodes of pain?**

   Ans: This is due to trigonal irritation and pain radiating to the penile tip. It is mediated through the sacral-2, 3, 4 reflex arc. Pain may also radiate to the perineum.[5]

2. **How are paediatric bladder stones classified?**

   Ans: In the paediatric population, Soliman and Rizvi[4] have grouped bladder stones as:
   1. Primary—also called endemic or idiopathic.
   2. Secondary—developing due to obstruction, infection, foreign bodies or neurogenic bladder.
   3. Migrant—stones formed in the upper urinary tract, later descending into the bladder.

3. **Are primary or endemic stone commonly seen?**

   Ans: Endemic stone disease is prevalent in the "Afro-Asian stone belt extending from northern Africa, through the Middle East and the Balkans into India, Japan, Thailand and Indonesia. It is uncommon in the southern hemisphere" (Fig. 13.3).[4,6]

   The expansion of industrialization and changes in the western diet has resulted in eradication of endemic calculi in the United States and Europe.[4]

   Primary bladder calculi affect children younger than 10 years of age with a peak incidence at 2 to 4 years. They are usually solitary and recurrence is rare once removed.[6]

4. **What is the composition of endemic bladder stones?**

   Ans: The endemic bladder stones are typically composed of ammonium acid urate (AAU). There might be a subsequent layering of calcium oxalate and uric acid. The nidus of the endemic stones is usually ammonium acid urate.[4]

   The western bladder stones typically resemble adult urolithiasis and can be calcium oxalate, struvite, and uric acid.

5. **What are the three Ds for etiology of endemic bladder stones?**

   Ans:
   1. Dietary deficiency.
   2. Dehydration.
   3. Diarrhoea.

6. **What is the Aetiopathogenesis of endemic bladder stones?**

   Ans: The endemic bladder stones are typically caused by nutritional deficiencies and metabolic problems. Feeding practices which contribute to the problem include prolonged breast feeding and cereal or millet-based diets. Such diet is rich in carbohydrates low in proteins and phosphates and is acidogenic. Low phosphates cannot buffer the increased ammonium production, hence pH is acidic. Due to higher metabolic rate in the growing children, uric acid excretion in urine is more. There

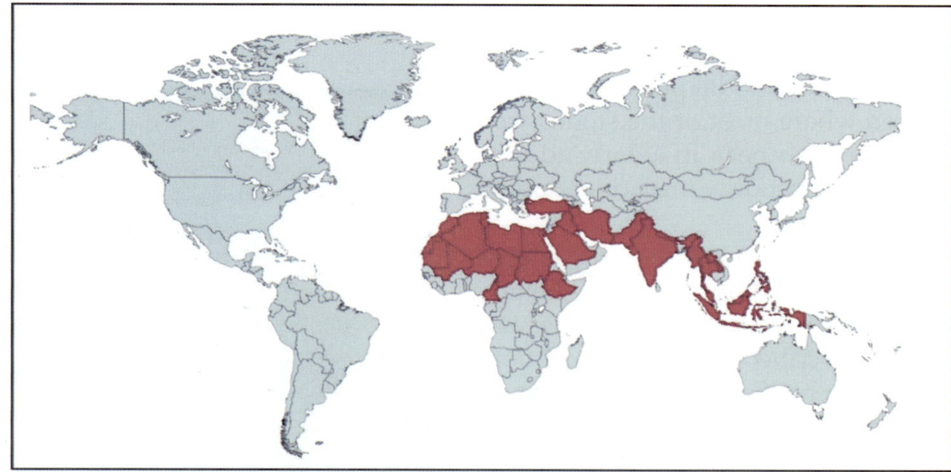

Fig. 13.3: Endemic bladder calculi belt [Drawn using online tools from https://www.mapchart.net/world.html. This work is licensed under a Creative Commons Attribution-Share Alike 4.0 International License (CC BY-SA 4.0). The map data is taken from Soliman NA, Rizvi SA. Endemic bladder calculi in children.)]

is a concomitant deficiency in urinary citrate, potassium and other inhibitors of lithogenesis. Deficiencies of vitamin A, B1, B6, and magnesium also aggravate the issue.

The hot tropical climate increases chances of dehydration and diarrhoea. These again contribute to the endemic bladder stones[6] (Flowchart 13.1).

Flowchart 13.1: Pathogenesis of endemic bladder calculi

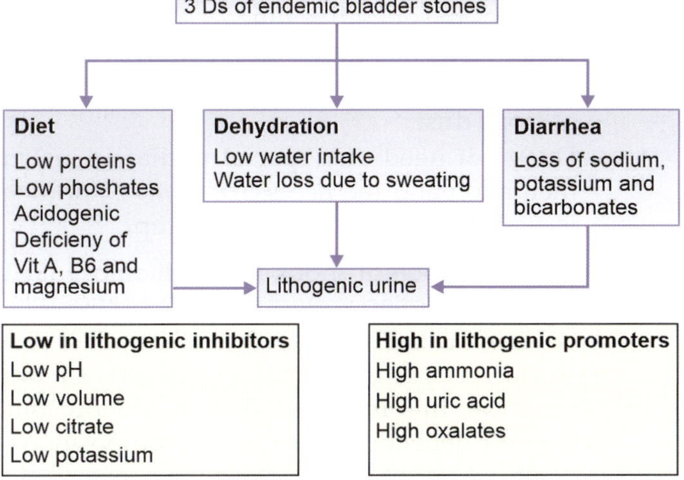

7. **How can we prevent formation of endemic calculi?**

   Ans:
   1. Adequate hydration.
   2. Use of boiled water and improved hygiene to reduce episodes of diarrhoea.
   3. Correction of dehydration by oral rehydration.
   4. Education of mothers on weaning practices.
   5. Use of mixed cereal diet and addition of cow milk and vitamins A and B supplements.[4]

8. **Why are the paediatric bladder stones laminated?**

   Ans: Endemic bladder stones are typically having an ammonium acid urate (AAU) nucleus. Subsequent layers could be due to calcium, oxalate, calcium phosphate or urates, depending on subsequent infections and metabolic changes[7] (Fig. 13.4).

9. **What are the mandatory investigations in case of children with bladder stones?**

   Ans:
   1. Investigations to confirm the bladder stones like ultrasonography of the abdomen and pelvis and X-ray of KUB region
   2. Investigations to rule out other 'secondary causes' contributing to the etiology such as micturating cystourethrogram, MRI spine and cystometry should be done when indicated.
   3. The mandatory cysto-urethroscopy examination can be combined with the definitive management[8]

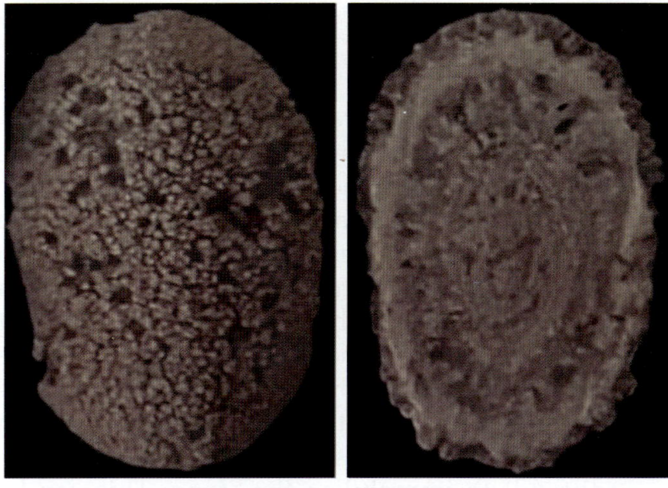

Fig. 13.4: Laminated bladder stone

10. **Enumerate the various management modalities for bladder calculi in children.**

    Ans:
    1. Open cystolithotomy.
    2. Endo-urological management
       a. Transurethral cystolithotripsy (TUCL)
       b. Percutaneous cystolithotripsy (PCCL)
    3. ESWL.
    4. Robot assisted cystolithotomy.[9]

11. **What are the concerns in treating a male child with a large bladder stone?**

    Ans: The size and calibre of the delicate urethra is the main concern. One is worried about urethral trauma and delayed stricture formation. This also limits the size of instruments which is important in removing all stone fragments and stone debris. Adequate sized catheter is important to drain the bladder.

12. **What is the difference between cystolithotrity, cystolitholapaxy and cystolithotripsy?**

    Ans: Cystolithotrity means fragmentation of the stone by mechanical means. The stone dust is cleared by the subsequent acts of voiding. In cystolitholapaxy there is mechanical fragmentation of the stone that is cleared by irrigation and bladder washes using bladder evacuators. Henry Bigelow described a modified lithotrite and bladder evacuator (Bigelow's evacuator) in 1878. Oliver Wendell Holmes coined the term litholapaxy which was *'crushing and flushing'* of the bladder stone fragments.[10] Cystolithotripsy is fragmenting the stone with an energy source like laser or lithoclast.

13. **How would you do a TUCL?**

    Ans: This will depend upon the availability of endoscopes and other armamentarium.

Paediatric cystoscopes are available from various manufacturers from 7.5 to 10 French. However, the limitation is that they have an oblique instrument channel and will only allow the use of laser fibres. The mini PCNL nephroscopes which are available in the size of 7.5 French or optimal for use inside the paediatric urethra. They have the advantage of a straight instrument channel and allowing up to 6 French instrument. The advantage in using a mini nephroscope is that they allow the passage of the probe of a pneumatic lithotripter through the straight instrument channel.[11] Since the available instrumentation is not of the continuous irrigation type, the bladder tends to fill up and it may become difficult to immobilize the stone. This can be overcome by controlling the inflow and keeping the bladder partially distended or else draining the bladder with a suprapubic needle. The other problem is it is not possible to wash the fragments from bladder at the end of the procedure.

14. How would you do a PCCL?

Ans: Suprapubic lithotripsy was first reported by Ganesh Gopalkrishnan *et al*. in 1988.[12] Salah *et al*. published the largest series of PCCL procedure in 117 children with 100% stone free rate. The technique was suitable for low resource setting.[13] This can be done under general anaesthesia using the standard PCNL instruments.

The first step is a preliminary cystoscopy to assess the urethra and bladder and to rule out bladder outlet obstruction.

The patient is placed in a Trendelenburg position and the bladder is distended. One cm incision is made in the suprapubic region 1 to 2 finger breadths above the symphysis pubis. Bladder is punctured using a PCNL initial puncture needle. A guide-wire is inserted and the tract is dilated using the PCNL dilator sets. The dilators could be metallic telescoping dilators, the Amplatz system or the balloon dilator system. This can be done under C-arm fluoroscopy. An adequate sized Amplatz sheath should be put in. One can use Amplatz sheath from 20 to 30 French depending on the size of the stone. A standard adult nephroscope can be inserted and stone fragmented using any of the energy sources used for a PCNL. The fragments can be picked up using forceps and stone dust can be sucked out using a suction cannula. The procedure is terminated by inserting an adequate sized suprapubic catheter and if necessary a urethral Foley's catheter. Dhabaliya *et al*. have published a modification to this technique wherein the trocar is self-retaining. The authors have used this in adults and children too.[14]

The suprapubic catheter can be removed in 24 hours and Foley's catheter in 72 hours.

15. What are the advantages of PCCL over a TUCL?

Ans: Smaller bladder stones may be treated by TUCL, but larger bladder stones are better tackled by PCCL.[15]

Tugcu *et al* have highlighted the following distinct advantages[16]:

1. It spares the urethra.
2. Reduces the operative time.
3. Better stone free rates since it allows for use of forceps for fragment retrieval and suction of stone dust.
4. Does not need any special pediatric instrumentation and the necessary adult equipment is available in a basic urology setup.

16. Can extracorporeal shock wave lithotripsy (SWL) be used for treating vesical calculi?

Ans: Vesical calculi can be pulverized by SWL. The procedure is performed under anaesthesia and placing the child in prone position. The outcome of the SWL depends on the size and composition of the stone. Multiple sittings may be necessary for larger stones and additional procedures such as cystoscopic removal of stone fragments may be required to achieve stone clearance.[5,8]

17. When is open cystolithotomy indicated?

Ans: Open cystolithotomy is employed for removal of large/giant vesical calculus[17] and dealing with associated pathologies such as bladder diverticulum or enterovesical fistula.

However, this procedure is associated with long scars, postoperative pain, prolonged catheterization, extended hospital stay, and risk of wound infection and rarely wound dehiscence and vesicocutaneous fistula.[5]

18. How do you choose among these treatment options?

Ans: The factors that help decide the appropriate surgical intervention for a particular child include the size and composition of the stone, compliance, history of previous lower urinary tract surgery, surgical expertise and equipment available, cost–benefit and risk–benefit of available surgical procedures for each patient (Table 13.1).

19. Should all stones be subjected to analysis?

Ans: Yes. The analysis of the stone by Fourier transform infrared spectroscopy (FTIR) determines the various components of the stone and their relative percentage content.[4] This information helps in modifying the diet to reduce the recurrence of stones.

TABLE 13.1: Factors determining the treatment modality for vesical calculi in children

	Age	Stone bulk	Stone number	HU	Equipment
ESWL	> 5 Years	Small	Solitary	< 900	ESWL access needed
TUCL	> 3 Years (depends on equipment)	Small	Few	Any	Pediatric equipment needed
PCCL	Any age	Large	Multiple	Any	Adult equipment can be used
Open	Any age	Large	Multiple	Any	No access to endourology or associated pathologies needing open surgery.

20. What measures need to be adopted to prevent urinary calculi in children?

Ans:

1. Adequate hydration
2. Restricted salt intake
3. Selective protein intake
4. Increase dietary citrate intake
5. Rational oxalate intake
6. Appropriate calcium intake
7. Adequate physical exercise
8. Avoid excess weight gain[18]

Conclusion: The urologist should be very considerate of the delicate urethra of the male child. Safety of the urethra gets the top priority while choosing the modality for bladder stones in a male child.

PCCL serves the purpose of being both minimally invasive and urethra sparing. It does not need any special instrumentation and uses the readily available standard PCNL instruments. It gives a quick, efficacious, cheap and minimally invasive solution for the patients of the Indian subcontinent.[10]

KEY POINTS

- Primary bladder stones are common in children of Afro-Asian stone belt who are exposed to low-protein, low-phosphate diet.
- Children with bladder stones often present with abdominal pain, dysuria, frequency and hematuria.
- Ultrasound of the abdomen and X-ray KUB can diagnose majority of the bladder stones.
- Appropriate surgical modality should be employed to make the child stone-free
- Male child's urethra needs the greatest respect and care.
- Do not risk the urethra for the sake of a minimally invasive procedure.
- The transurethral procedures should be reserved for small sized stones and in relatively older children.
- PCCL is both cost effective and it safeguards the urethra at the same time. It has all the advantages of a minimally invasive procedure while being maximally effective.
- Open cystolithotomy still is a safe option when facilities are not available.

REFERENCES

1. Bakane BC, Nagtilak SB, Patil B. Urolithiasis: a tribal scenario. *Indian J Pediatr*. 1999;66(6):863–865.
2. Papatsoris AG, Varkarakis I, Dellis A, Deliveliotis C. Bladder lithiasis: from open surgery to lithotripsy. *Urol Res*. 2006;34(3):163–167.
3. Chakraborty RC (1982) Urinary stones their cause and treatment as described in the Sushrutasamhita. Hist Sci Med 17:328–332.
4. Soliman NA, Rizvi SAH. Endemic bladder calculi in children. Pediatr Nephrol. 2017;32(9):1489–1499. doi:10.1007/s00467–016–3492–4.
5. Ho K, Segura J. Lower Urinary Tract Calculi. Wein A, Kavoussi L, Novick A, Partin A, Peters C. *Campbell-Walsh Urology*. 9th. Philadelphia, Pa: Saunders Elsevier; 2007. 3: 2663–73.
6. Gupta NP, Kumar A (2011) Endemic bladder stones. In: Rao PN, Preminger GM, Kavanaugh JP (eds) Urinary tract stone disease. Springer, London, pp 239–243.
7. Teotia, S.P.S., Teotia, M. and Teotia, N.P.S. Primary bladder stone disease in children-crystallisation studies with special reference to urinary excretion of pyrophosphates. *Indian J Pediatr* 1974; **41**, 293–298. https://doi.org/10.1007/BF02829320.
8. Schwartz BF, Stoller ML. The vesical calculus. Urol Clin North Am. 2000 May;27(2):333–46. doi: 10.1016/s0094–0143(05)70262–7. PMID: 10778475.
9. Esposito C, Autorino G, Masieri L, *et al*. Minimally Invasive Management of Bladder Stones in Children. *Front Pediatr*. 2021;8:618756.
10. Haagensen CD, Wyndham EB Lloyd (1999) A hundred years of medicine.
11. Sakly A, Zakhama W, Mahjoubi Z, *et al*. Paediatric cystolitholapaxy using mini PCNL-kit through the Mitrofanoff stoma. *Ann Med Surg (Lond)*. 2021;62:88–91.
12. Gopalakrishnan G, Bhaskar P, Jehangir E. Suprapubic lithotripsy. British Journal of Urology. 1988 Oct 1;62(4):389.
13. Salah MA, Holman E, Tóth C. Percutaneous suprapubic cystolithotripsy for pediatric bladder stones in a developing country. *Eur Urol*. 2001;39(4):466–470.
14. Dhabalia JV, Jain N, Kumar V, Nelivigi GG. Modified technique of percutaneous cystolithotripsy using a new instrument—combined single-step trocar-dilator with self-retaining adjustable access sheath. Urology. 2011 Jun 1;77(6):1304–7.
15. Mishra DK, Bhatt S, Mukhilesh R, Somani BK, Agrawal MS. Mini-percutaneous cystolithotripsy (mPCCL) versus transurethral cystolithotripsy (TUC) in pre-school children:

Prospective comparative non-randomized outcomes over 8 years. *J Pediatr Urol*. 2020;16(6):782.e1–782.e6.

16. Tugcu V, Polat H, Ozbay B, Gurbuz N, Eren GA, Tasci AI. Percutaneous versus transurethral cystolithotripsy. *J Endourol*. 2009;23(2):237–241.
17. Mahran MR, Dawaba MS. Cystolitholapaxy versus cystolithotomy in children. *J Endourol*. 2000;14(5):423–426.
18. Zhong J, Huang Z, Yang T, Wang G, Guo H, Li P, Zhang Y, Zhao Y, Liu J. The current status of preventive measures for urinary calculi in children. Ther Adv Urol. 2021 Aug 14;13:17562872211039581. doi: 10.1177/17562872211039581.

ACKNOWLEDGEMENT

- We sincerely thank Dr Prashant Mulawkar for his critical comments and acquisition of the world map depicting the endemic stone belt.
- Clinical details and images courtesy of Dr Prashant Mulawkar.

Chapter

14

Post-Ureteroscopy Stricture

• Rajeev TP • Abheesh Varma Hegde

LEARNING OBJECTIVES

- Presentation patterns
- Causes
- Pathogenesis
- Preventive strategies
- Management with algorithms

INTRODUCTION

The first rigid ureteroscope was introduced in 1980 when the scope was 50 cm long with dual channel and 12 Fr width.[1] Today's semi-rigid and flexible ureteroscopes have come a long way since then. Improvements in design and functionality, availability of a wide range of accessories, and the addition of laser to the urologist's armamentarium have expanded the use of ureteroscopy (URS) much beyond what it was a few years back. Reduction in complications have made ureteroscopy the most common procedure for urolithiasis today. Ureteric stricture is one such rare complication that can be devastating to patients post-URS due to the risk of renal damage.

The incidence of post-ureteroscopic ureteric stricture is variable in literature, between 0.23% and 3%. Incidence depends on the post-operative imaging being followed and the follow-up. It is a long-term complication and can be difficult to manage. In the Indian scenario, many patients with silent obstruction may not present for evaluation post-stone clearance since their pathology has been treated. The additional cost burden might deter patients from follow-up. Hence, patients suspected to have ureteric stricture post-ureteroscopy need to be counselled well regarding the importance of routine post-operative follow-up and imaging. Ureteric access sheaths (UAS) facilitate repeated access to the collecting system, reduce operative times, protect the scope and provide drainage to the irrigating fluid. Laser lithotripsy has significantly impacted the success rates in ureteroscopy. However, both are also believed to contribute to the rates of stricture post-procedure.[2,3]

Ureteroscopy is safe in children too and is extensively used to treat urolithiasis in these patients today. In this chapter, let us look at the aetiology, pathogenesis, preventive strategies and management of post-ureteroscopy ureteric stricture.

Case Scenario

A 51-year-old male has presented with left flank pain. He has no other urological complaints. His past history is significant for left PCNL (percutaneous nephrolithotomy) 7 years back and left URS done for a proximal ureteric calculus 5 years back. Clinical examination and all laboratory parameters are normal. A kidney, ureter and bladder (KUB) ultrasound reveals left hydro-ureteronephrosis. Rest of the urinary system is normal.

1. **How would you manage this patient?**
   Given the history and imaging findings of this patient, a CT urogram (Fig. 14.1) would be required to identify the cause for the hydronephrosis. With a past history of endoscopic intervention, a diagnosis of post-procedure stricture is a high probability. A CT urogram would help identify the exact site and length of stricture, status of the kidney and ureter, and help plan further management. A diureteric

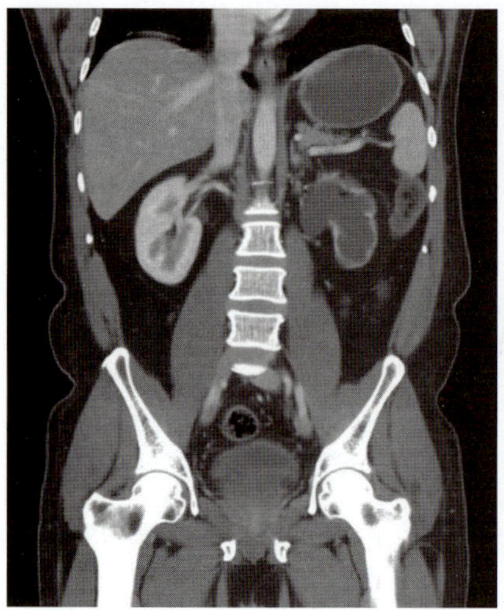
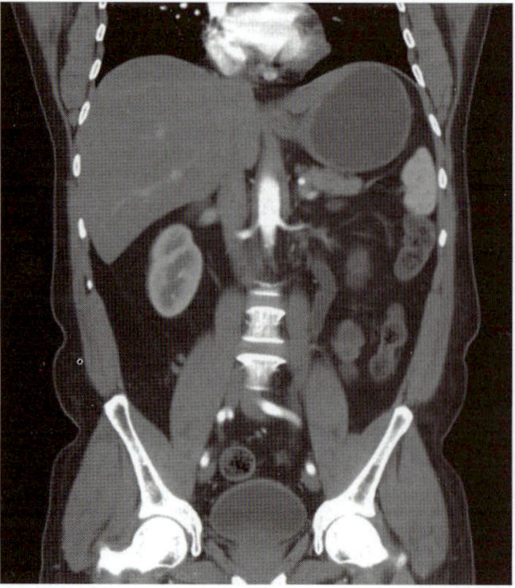
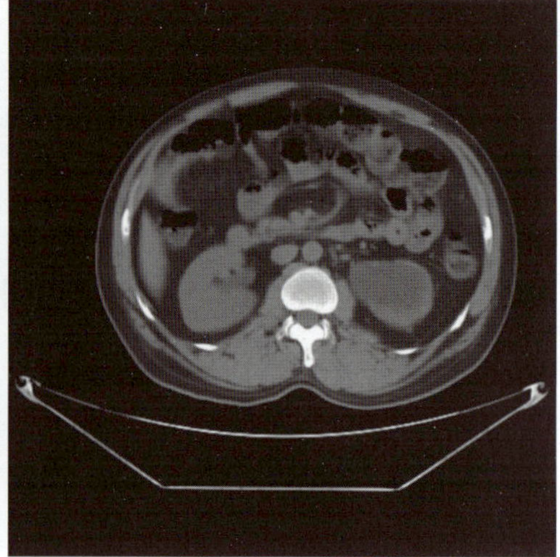

Fig. 14.1: CT urogram showing left proximal ureteric stricture

renogram can be used to confirm the diagnosis. A retrograde ureterography (RGU) would be confirmatory to assess the ureteric mucosa, calibre, length and density of stricture. This could be the only investigation in patients with raised creatinine. Diagnostic ureteroscopy (Fig. 14.2) with a slender ureteroscope (4.5 Fr) practiced by a few centres though has not been advocated in literature. A guidewire can be passed and the ureter stented with or without dilatation after RGU.[4]

2. **What are the causes of post-URS stricture?**

Ans: The most common and significant factor predicting occurrence of post-operative stricture has been stone impaction. 75–100% of post-operative stricture ureter patients had ureteroscopy done for impacted calculi. Larger stones, especially those greater than 2 cm treated by ureteroscopy have a higher chance of post-operative stricture formation. There is an association between double J (DJ) stenting and stricture formation. This could be because of interruption of urine flow through the ureter and patients with impacted calculi or intra-operative trauma undergoing DJ stent placement in most cases.[2,5] With regard to occurrence of post-operative renal pain, intra-operative ureteral dilatation and perforation leading to stricture, data is mixed and no clear consensus exists. Laser lithotripsy was associated with more chances of stricture compared to pneumatic lithotripsy for mid and distal ureteric calculi.[3]

The rates for proximal, mid and distal ureteric stricture were 0.9%, 1,1% and 0.7% respectively. Proximal ureteric calculi had greater chances of ureteric perforation and stricture (Table 14.1).

TABLE 14.1: Etiology of post-ureteroscopy stricture
Patient factors:
• Males
• Older patients

(Contd.)

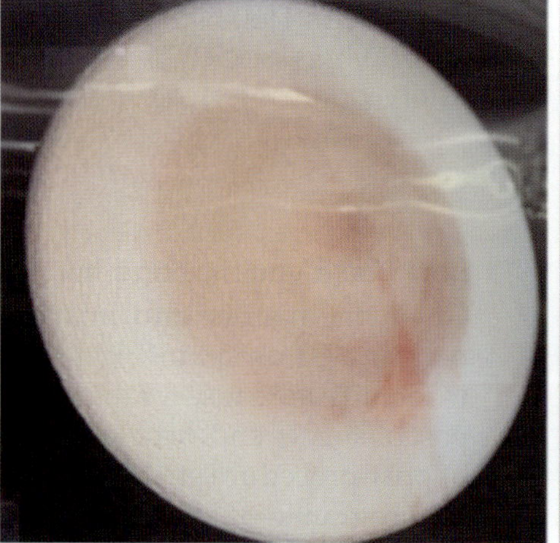
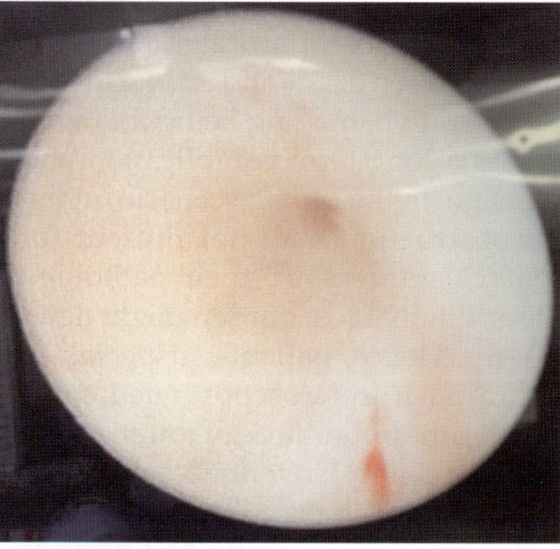

Fig. 14.2: Endoscopic image of the stricture in Fig. 14.1

TABLE 14.1: Etiology of post-ureteroscopy stricture *(Contd.)*
• Stone impaction
• Large stone
Equipment factors
• Laser lithotripsy
• Use of ureteric access sheaths
• Larger scope use
Surgeon factors
• Surgeon experience
• Longer operative time

The use of ureteric access sheaths could cause mucosal ischemia and stricture. But data to establish this fact is lacking and prospective studies with long-term follow-up could help in addressing this knowledge gap.[6] A meta-analysis of 8 studies with 1555 patients comparing stricture rates of HoYAG lasers with pneumatic lithotripters found higher stricture rates in the laser group. However, the results of one study could have significantly affected the overall conclusion. Use of larger scopes and presence of pre-operative hydronephrosis had higher rates of ureteric stricture. Experience of the surgeon also affects rates of ureteric injury and stricture formation[7] Males and older patients were at higher risk of access sheath related injuries. Body mass index, diabetes mellitus, vascular disease, abdominopelvic radiation therapy and operative time were not associated with severe ureteric injury.[8]

3. **What are the preventive strategies for post-URS stricture?**

Ans: Before intervening on such patients, detailed evaluation for previous treatments and imaging must be made to identify high risk factors such as impacted calculi, iatrogenic injuries, infections and multiple lesions. Endoscopic/intraluminal sonography can detect submucosal calculi. Preoperative DJ stenting can significantly reduce ureteric injury rates. Using a smaller ureteroscope produces less mucosal injury. Mucosal injury rates for 8.5–11.5 Fr ureteroscope vs 4.5–6.5 Fr were 13.5% vs 1.9. The use of fluoroscope especially for challenging situations, meticulous technique and patience help reduce the risk of ureteric injury. Choosing the right patient for intervention with respect to stone burden, avoiding prolonged procedures is also important.

Reducing the rates of stone granuloma formation significantly reduces stricture rates. One way of achieving this would be to prevent displacement of stone fragments into the ureteral wall. Keeping the laser tip centrally on the stone and avoiding the urethral mucosa, avoiding lithotripsy use for fragments attached to the ureteric wall, transferring fragments proximally in case of limited working space and avoiding the site of impaction are other methods to reduce post-operative stricture rates.[3] Smaller proximal ureteric diameter on pre-operative CT can predict high grade ureteric injury post-ureteric access sheath insertion. Silodosin 8 mg administered pre-operatively for 3 days reduces the incidence of grade 2 or higher injuries due to ureteric access sheath insertion (Table 14.2).[6]

TABLE 14.2: Preventive strategies
Identify high risk factors: Impacted calculi, previous iatrogenic injuries, infections and multiple lesions
• Preoperative DJ stenting
• Use of smaller ureteroscope
• Endoscopic/intraluminal sonography
• Fluoroscopy for challenging situations
• Meticulous technique
• Proper patient selection
• Avoid prolonged procedures in infection
• Avoid fragment displacement into ureteric wall
• Avoid mucosal injury with laser/lithotripsy
• Avoid working at site of stone impaction
• Careful access sheath insertion
• Silodosin 8 mg pre-operatively for 3 days

4. **What are the various ways such patients present?**

Ans: Ureteric stricture is a late complication which can cause significant morbidity in post-ureteroscopy patients. Most patients are asymptomatic, presenting late with a hydronephrotic kidney on an ultrasound done for other conditions. This can lead to progressive renal loss and non-functional kidney. Others could present with flank pain/features of obstruction, infective complications or secondary calculi.

5. **Explain the pathogenesis.**

Ans: It is multifactorial with ureteric injury and inflammation playing a central role. Ureteric perforation at the site of stone impaction is a significant factor. Impaction causes long-term irritation of ureteric mucosa predisposing to fibrosis and stenosis. There is also epithelial hypertrophy and oedema leading to friable tissue character. Impaction reduces the working space and predisposes to perforation. There is urine infection and extravasation which causes periureteral fibrosis. Ischemia, stone granulomas due to embedded fragments in the mucosa and fibrosis also contribute to stricture. Thermal effects of Ho:YAG laser on ureteric mucosa and in raising the irrigating fluid temperature causes stricture.[6] The ureteric access sheath can cause mucosal ischemia due to overdistention. On removal of the sheath, post-ischemia reperfusion injury with free radicals can cause damage to the ureteric wall.[8]

6. **How do you evaluate such patients?**

Ans: Early diagnosis is critical to preserve renal function in such patients and hence, routine post-operative imaging is advised to detect silent obstruction which occurs in 2.9% of patients. A routine 3 months follow-up is recommended even in the absence of symptoms. In patients with large/impacted proximal ureteric calculi, ureteral injury, pre-existing renal impairment, stricture on endoscopy, post-operative pain or fever, follow-up should extend up to 18 months.[9] For patients who show compromised renal function on laboratory/radiological investigation, a scintigraphy to document the renal function is advised.

Ureteric stricture is ureteric narrowing causing obstruction. Diagnosis necessitates the presence of at least one of the following:

- Luminal narrowing on endoscopy
- Narrowing/obstruction on contrast study: Retrograde/antegrade pyelography or CT urography
- A t ½ > 20 minutes on renal scintigraphy with upper tract dilatation and hydronephrosis[10]

7. **Is there a classification system?**

Ans: Olivier Traxer proposed his classification exclusively for ureteric injury after endoscopic procedures. These injuries were visualised endoscopically while removing the ureteric access sheath at the end of ureteroscopy. Five grades were described (Fig. 14.3). When two or more grades coexist, the highest grade is given.[8] The post-ureteroscopic lesion scale is another classification system for such injuries (Table 14.3).[11]

TABLE 14.3: Endoscopic classification of ureteral wall injury PULS classification[8]

Grade 0	No ureteral lesion/only mucosal petechiae
Grade 1	Mucosal erosion/ flap without smooth muscle injury
Grade 2	Mucosa and smooth muscle injury, adventitia spared (periureteral fat/retroperitoneal tissue not visible)
Grade 3	Full thickness ureteral wall perforation (adventitia included)
Grade 4	Ureteral avulsion with complete rupture of continuity

8. **How do you manage these patients?**

Ans: The general principles for managing ureteric strictures is a prompt diagnosis, relief of obstruction and preservation of renal function. Treatment can be endourological or reconstructive. Endourological procedures are balloon dilatation, laser endoureterotomy and endoscopic dilatation. Reconstructive procedures include pyeloplasty, ureteroureterostomy and ureteroneocystostomy. It is important to follow general principles of reconstruction to perform a tension free, watertight anastomosis with absorbable sutures, preserving the blood supply to the ureter and ensuring drainage. It has been found that reconstructive procedures generally have better outcomes compared to endourological procedures and this was independent of stricture characteristics.

In a population based study looking at data from 3,29,776 patients who underwent ureteroscopy, stricture rate was 3%. Out of these patients, 21% underwent endoscopic management, 5.5% required reconstruction and 2.1% underwent nephrectomy.[12]

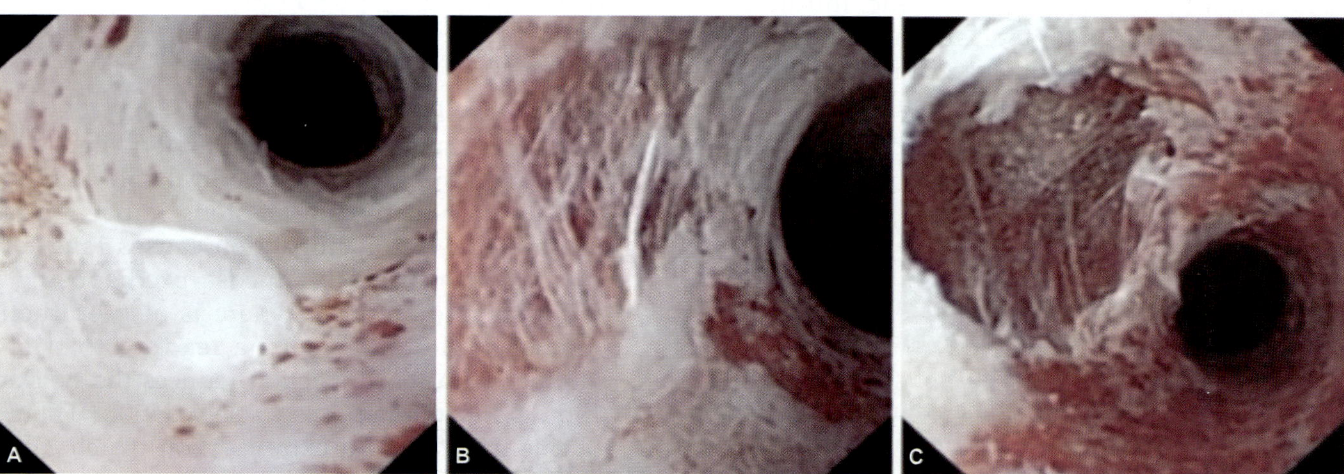

Fig. 14.3: Endoscopic view of ureteric injuries: A. Grade 1, B. Grade 2, C. Grade 3

Success rates for reconstructive procedures are 96–100%, whereas for endourological procedures it is 60.9–71%. However, endourological procedures have shorter operative times, lower intraoperative blood loss, faster post-operative recovery and lower surgical morbidity. These attributes make them the preferred choice for short strictures (less than 1 cm) in the absence of severe hydronephrosis. Longer strictures treated endoscopically have high failure rates. Stricture length more than 2 cm has been associated with recurrence in many studies. Recurrence, almost always occurs in the first year post-operatively. Hence, a follow-up of at least 18 months has been advised in high risk cases (Flowcharts 14.1 and 14.2).[10]

Flowchart 14.1: Follow-up protocol for post-ureteroscopy patients

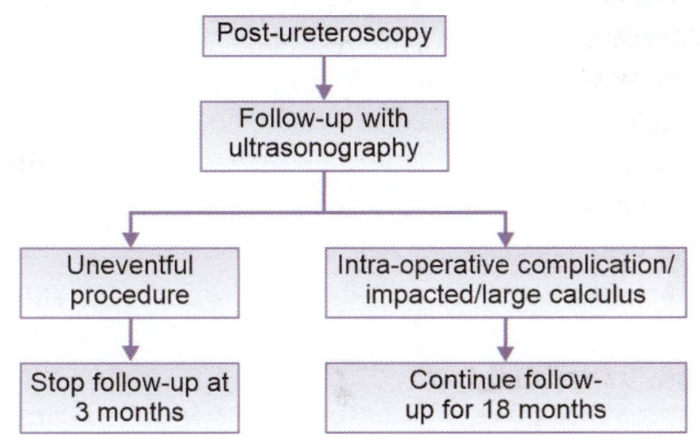

Flowchart 14.2: Intervention for post-ureteroscopy stricture

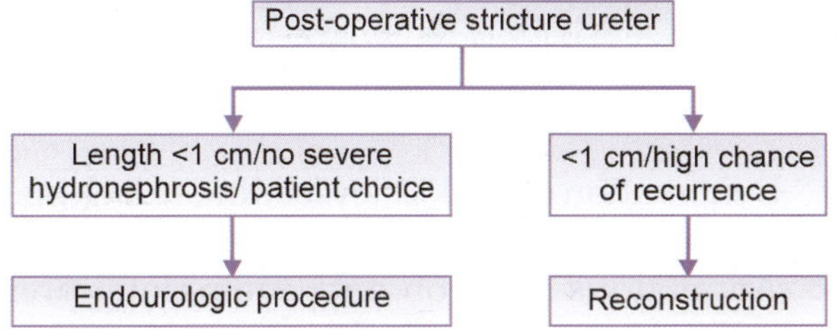

KEY POINTS

- Post-ureteroscopy stricture is a delayed but devastating complication for patients.
- It is adivised to keep post-ureteroscopy patients on follow-up for at least 18 months.
- Diagnosis is made following strict criteria: Radiological/endoscopic/on scintigraphy.
- Endoscopic and reconstructive options exist for management.
- Endoscopic management is appropriate for well-selected patients.
- Reconstructive procedures have higher success rate.

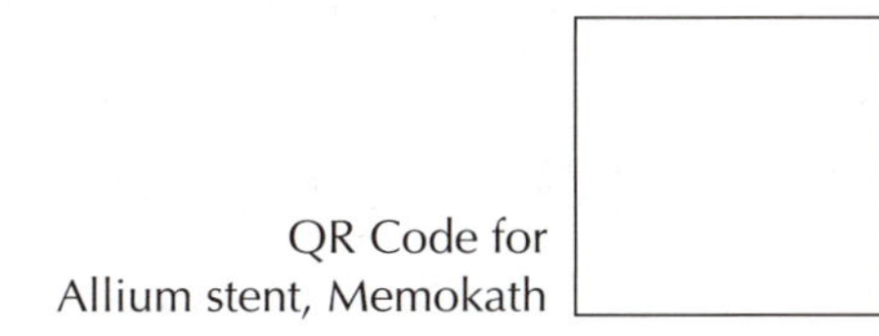

QR Code for Allium stent, Memokath

REFERENCES

1. Wason SE, Monfared S, Ionson A, Klett DE, Leslie SW, Ureteroscopy. [Updated 2022 Nov 28]. In: StatPearls [Internet]. Treasure Island (FL): StatPearls Publishing; 2023 Jan-. Available from: https://www.ncbi.nlm.nih.gov/books/NBK560556.
2. Darwish AE, Gadelmoula MM, Abdelkawi IF, Abdellatif AM, Abdel-Moneim AM, Hammouda HM, Ureteral stricture after ureteroscopy for stones: A prospective study for incidence and risk factors. Urology Annals 11(3) Sep 2019: 276–281.
3. Dong H, Peng Y, Li L, Gao X. Prevention strategies for ureteral stricture following ureteroscopic lithotripsy. Asian J Urol. 2018 Apr;5(2):94–100
4. Fam XI, Singam P, Ho CC, Sridharan R, Hod R, Bahadzor B, Goh EH, Tan GH, Zainuddin Z. Ureteral stricture formation after ureteroscope treatment of impacted calculi: A prospective study. Korean J Urol. 2015 Jan;56(1):63–67.
5. S. Tonyali, A. Pietropaolo, E. Emiliani, M. Ortac, M.F. Von Bargen, S. Turan, M. Glienke, Z. Hamid, T. Tailly, Factors associated with ureteral strictures following ureteroscopy for impacted ureteral stones? A multicenter study by EAU–YAU endourology and urolithiasis working party, Actas Urológicas Españolas (English Edition), 47 (10), 2023, 631–37.
6. Kitrey ND), Juanatey FC, Hallscheidt P, Mayer E, Serafetinidis E, Sharma DM,Waterloos M, EAU Guidelines on Urogenital trauma 2023, *presented at the EAU Annual Congress Milan 2023. ISBN 978-94-92671-19-6*
7. Chen S, Zhou L, Wei T, Luo D, Jin T, Li H, Wang K. Comparison of Holmium: YAG Laser and Pneumatic Lithotripsy in the Treatment of Ureteral Stones: An Update Meta-Analysis. Urol Int. 2017;98(2):125–133.
8. Traxer O, Thomas A. Prospective evaluation and classification of ureteral wall injuries resulting from insertion of a ureteral access sheath during retrograde intrarenal surgery. J Urol. 2013 Feb;189(2):580–4
9. El-Abd AS, Suliman MG, Abo Farha MO, Ramadan AR, El-Tatawy HH, El-Gamal OM, El-Gamal SA, Figenshau R, El Abd SA. The development of ureteric strictures after ureteroscopic treatment for ureteric calculi: A long-term study at two academic centres. Arab J Urol. 2014 Jun;12(2):168–72.
10. Xiong, M., Zhu, X., Chen, D. *et al.* Post ureteroscopic stone surgery ureteral strictures management: a retrospective study. Int Urol Nephrol 52, 841–849 (2020).
11. Schoenthaler M, Wilhelm K, Kuehhas FE, Farin E, Bach C, Buchholz N, Miernik A. Postureteroscopic lesion scale: a new management modified organ injury scale-evaluation in 435 ureteroscopic patients. J Endourol. 2012 Nov;26(11):1425–30.
12. May PC, Hsi RS, Tran H, Stoller ML, Chew BH, Chi T, Usawachintachit M, Duty BD, Gore JL, Harper JD. The Morbidity of Ureteral Strictures in Patients with Prior Ureteroscopic Stone Surgery: Multi-Institutional Outcomes. J Endourol. 2018 Apr;32(4):309–314.

Chapter

15

Miscellaneous Stone Presentations

• Rajesh Kukreja • Mohammed Taif Bendigeri

INTRODUCTION

It is not uncommon in clinical practice to encounter stones with challenging presentations. Often the evaluation and decision making about the treatment plan becomes intriguing. Some of these common situations that one can encounter are:

A. Renal pelvic stone in transplanted kidney
B. Multiple pelvic and lower calyx stones with suspected PUJ obstruction
C. Stone with kyphoscoliosis
D. Stone in morbidly obese patient

A. Renal Pelvic Stone in Post-transplant Kidney

LEARNING OBJECTIVES

- Challenges involved in treating stones in transplanted kidneys.
- Understand the atypical presentation and the reasons for this.
- Anatomical challenges in different treatment modalities and technical considerations to overcome these challenges.

Case Scenario

A 48-year-old lady having undergone renal transplant 3 years back presents with recurrent episodes of urinary infections for last 6 weeks. Ultrasound and a NCCT (Fig. 15.1) revealed a 12.4 mm mobile calculus in the transplanted kidney. She is on regular post-transplant immunosuppressant therapy.

Renal stones in transplanted kidneys are uncommon having an incidence of 0.4 to 4% with calcium oxalate stones being the most common variety.[1–5] Graft stones may occur *de novo* or may be gifted from the donor.

Though not common, treatment of renal stones in transplant kidneys is associated with challenges right from the diagnosis due to the following reasons:

1. Solitary functioning kidney status.
2. Immunocompromised status with increased risk of infection.

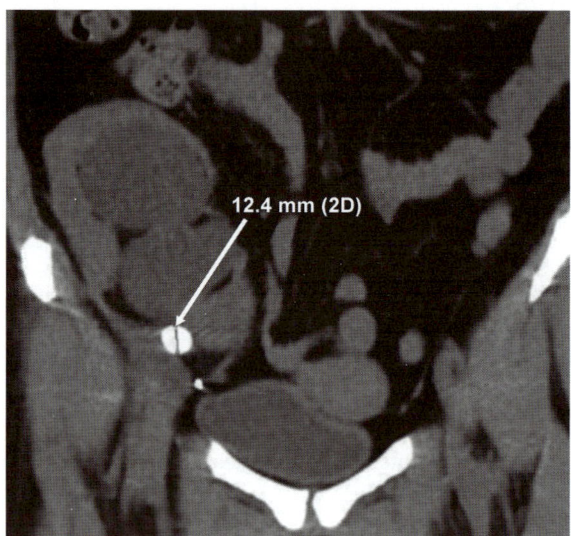

Fig. 15.1: Coronal section CT

3. Denervation of the kidney leading to lack of early symptoms like pain.
4. Anomalous location and anomalous ureteric orifice leading to difficulties in access.

Treatment options are no different from those in managing renal stones in normal kidneys. These include shock wave lithotripsy (SWL), percutaneo-usnephrolithotripsy (PCNL) and retrograde access using flexible ureteroscopy (RIRS). However, the solitary kidney status, presence of immunosuppression and anomalous location make the treatment more challenging.

1. How does the clinical presentation of calculus in transplanted kidney differ from a native renal calculus?

Ans: Clinical presentation is atypical in view of the denervated transplanted kidney with lack of the typical renal colic.[1,2] Rising creatinine, fall in urine output and urinary infection are the most common findings that lead to diagnosis of stones.

In a series of 18 patients by Gerber, Nakada and colleagues, 7 (39%) presented with urinary infection or pyelonephritis, 28% were diagnosed to have stones on routine imaging, 22% presented with haematuria, 5.6% with acute kidney injury and only 5.6% presented with pain.[6] In a multi-centre study by the French Urology Association Transplantation Committee, 55% of the 95 patients were diagnosed incidentally on routine ultrasound examination. Symptomatic stones were diagnosed due to episodes of either urinary tract infection or acute renal failure.[7] The average time to presentation is 1.6–3.5 years post-transplantation.[8]

2. Define risk factors for development of this uncommon condition.

Ans: Surgical risk factors include ureteric obstruction, bladder outlet obstruction and uretero-intestinal anastomosis like augmented bladder.[9] Pathophysiological causes include hyperparathyroidism, hypercalcemia, and hyperuricemia.[1,2,10] There is limited evidence to support role of cyclosporine in development of post-transplant urolithiasis.[11]

3. What are the treatment options?

Ans: Initial management: Initial management depends on the clinical presentation. Patients with significant infection or pyelonephritis or acute renal failure would mandate initial placement of double J stent or percutaneous nephrostomy as an emergency procedure to safeguard the graft function. Definitive treatment in form of SWL or antegrade or retrograde endoscopic access should be offered primarily for silent stones or as a delayed treatment after stabilisation of infection or acute renal failure. Watchful waiting may be considered for small stones (up to 6 mm) with strict and compliant protocol and after explaining risk of acute kidney injury or loss of graft function due to unrecognised obstruction.[3,9] In the French Urology Association Transplantation Committee series, 27% patients underwent initial stenting and 21% underwent percutaneous nephrostomy tube placement.[7]

4. Do you think these procedures would be same as a routine patient or do you expect any anatomical challenges?

Ans: Anatomical considerations with their impact on the treatment method[1,6]

1. Kidneys are transplanted into the right or left iliac fossa. The proximity of the renal graft and the stone to the iliac bones would make fluoroscopic localisation for SWL difficult and also reduce the effectiveness of the therapy.
2. The ureter is typically reimplanted using the Gregor Lich technique near the dome of the bladder. This ectopic location of the orifice along with the unnatural course of the ureter poses challenges in retrograde access.
3. Superficial location of the kidney with surrounding perigraft fibrosis and bowel may pose difficulties in percutaneous access.

5. If you are planning a retrograde access to this kidney, how would you overcome these difficulties?And what about percutaneous access?

Ans:

Modifications while establishing retrograde access.

1. Keeping the bladder partially full along with suprapubic pressure generally helps in identifying and cannulating the ureteric orifice.
2. A 0 or 70 degree telescope could be useful.
3. Flexible cystoscope may be used if above manoeuvres fail.
4. Once the orifice is well visualised, a straight or angle tip glidewire may be used to negotiate the angled orifice and course of ureter and gain access to the kidney.
5. The ectopically located ureteric orifice and angulated course of ureter may make dilatation and placement of access sheath difficult with buckling of the dilators and sheath in the bladder. Proper placement of cystoscope sheath at the orifice with dilation through the sheath would help preventing buckling of the dilators in the bladder.

Modifications while establishing percutaneous access.

- Ultrasound guided access helps in identifying the peripheral desired calyx of access and helps in avoiding bowel injury.
- Use of flexible nephroscope may aid in accessing multiple calyces and upper ureter in an antegrade manner and also help reducing number of tracts and hence the complications.

6. What are the options for definitive treatment of this calculus and what would be the outcomes?

Ans: A meta-analysis of 37 studies with 553 patients of post-transplant urolithiasis was conducted by Boissier and colleagues.[12] The average stone size was 11 mm (2–50 mm). ESWL and retrograde ureteroscopy were the commonly chosen procedures for stones up to 12 mm size, whereas PCNL was the preferred modality for larger stones. The overall stone free rate was 82% (96% with open surgery, 95% with antegrade ureteroscopy, 86% with PCNL, 81% with retrograde ureteroscopy and 75% with SWL.

A. SWL (shock wave lithotripsy)

- The location of the transplanted kidney in the pelvis makes it difficult to locate the stones fluoroscopically. The location also leads to shock wave attenuation and hence reduced efficiency.
- Patients would need to be placed in prone position with a soft water bag placed below the superficial transplanted kidney to prevent compression against the bony pelvis.
- Series by Challacombe and Yuan highlighted the need for multiple sessions (8 out of 13 and 4 out of 5 patients in both the respective series).[3,13]
- 2 out of 13 patients in retrospective analysis by Challacombe and one out of 5 patients in Yuan's series required additional ureteroscopy for removal of stones despite multiple SWL sessions.
- The need for multiple sessions and ancillary procedures along with risk of parenchymal injury and subcapsular haematoma may affect the renal function.[6]

B. PCNL

- Hulber, *et al* first described the use of PCNL for treatment of stones in transplant kidney.[14]
- Krambeck and colleagues published their series of 13 patients with post-transplant nephrolithiasis who underwent PCNL.[15] The average stone size was 1.36 cm. Single tract was made in 12 patients, whereas 1 patient required 2 tracts for a partial staghorn calculus. Ten (77%) patients were stone free after a single procedure while repeat access was required in three patients to make them stone free. With an average follow-up of 5.3 years, only one patient developed recurrence that was treated with ESWL. Mean creatinine stabilised from 2.0 mg% preoperatively to 1.7 mg% at the last follow-up visit.
- Minimally invasive PCNL using a smaller tract size is now the preferred choice for percutaneous access in view of reduced bleeding and reduced trauma to allograft parenchyma. Ji and colleagues presented their data of 11 patients with post-transplant nephrolithiasis treated by MiniPCNL using a 16.5 Fr tract size. All patients were rendered completely stone free with no loss of graft function.[4,16]

C. RIRS

- In a review of 3758 renal transplants at a single centre by Sarier, *et al* 22 patients underwent endoscopic surgery for graft stones.[17] Of the patients who underwent flexible ureteroscopy, 4.5% developed urinary infection and 9% required second look procedure for residual stones. None developed stone recurrence with a mean follow-up of 30.2 months.
- Gerber, Nakada and colleagues recently presented their series of 18 patients who underwent retrograde ureterorenoscopy for post-transplant nephrolithiasis.[6] The mean stone size was 8.6 mm. Flexible ureteroscopy was performed in 16 patients. Retrograde access to the transplanted ureter and kidney was possible in 89% of their patients. Two required antegrade access from previously placed nephrostomy. 61% were stone free after single treatment. Of the 7 patients with residual stones, 4 were managed conservatively, whereas two patients required repeat ureteroscopy within a year.

SUMMARY

- Based on the clinical evidence and the development of thin calibre digital scopes, retrograde flexible ureterorenoscopy or SWL should be the first choice of treatment for post-transplant nephrolithiasis with stones up to 15 mm size. SWL would need prone positioning and may need multiple sessions. Retrograde flexible ureterorenoscopy may not be able to negotiate the ureteric orifice and ureteric angulations in every case but would be associated with better stone clearance rates. Antegrade approach with MiniPCNL may be a better choice for larger stones, in patients with pre-existing nephrostomy and in whom retrograde approach is not possible.[18,19] Definitive treatment should be staged in the presence of pyelonephritis, sepsis, or acute kidney injury.

B. Multiple Pelvic and Lower Calyx Stones with Suspected PUJ Obstruction

LEARNING OBJECTIVES

- Evaluation and diagnosis to plan the line of management.
- Consideration of two stage or single approach.
- Options to clear the PUJO and stones.
- Follow-up and evaluation for metabolic anomalies.

INTRODUCTION

It is not uncommon to come across patients with renal stones with a dilated pelvis creating a suspicion of simultaneous co-existence of pelvi-ureteric junction obstruction (PUJO) and stones. The incidence could be as high as 15–30%.[20] It becomes crucial to evaluate and clarify the suspicion to optimise the outcomes of treatment for the patient.

Case Scenario

A 35-year-old male patient presents with dull aching flank pain for 3 years. The pain was intermittent in nature and not associated with haematuria. He used to take simple over the counter analgesics for achieving pain relief. However, the symptoms have not resolved completely. Clinical examination was unremarkable. Routine evaluation showed normal renal parameters. He was evaluated with ultrasound abdomen and found to have multiple renal stones present in the pelvis and calyces. It was noted that there was significant hydronephrosis as well. Plain CT-KUB (Fig. 15.2) demonstrated that disproportionately severe hydronephrosis along with multiple smooth rounded stones. This created a suspicion of presence of simultaneous PUJO with stones.

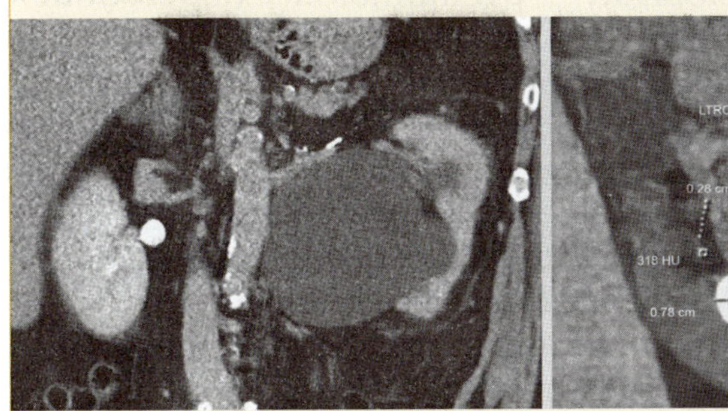

Fig. 15.2: Coronal section CT

1. **What are the diagnostic issues with this case and how do you proceed?**

   Ans: The most important diagnostic dilemma in managing this set of patients is confirmation of the suspicion of PUJO. Confirmation of PUJO and assessment of the degree of impact of the obstruction becomes essential to plan the treatment modality. Confirmation of the PUJO would be on similar lines as any other primary PUJO with renogram being the mainstay of diagnosis. The diagnostic criteria would be like a regular case of PUJO except for extra caution to be given for the presence of stone and its confounding effect. The utility of renogram studies would be meaningful if the location of stone is not at the PUJ area. If the renogram suggests an obstruction, then the plan of management must address both the issues of PUJO and the stone. Intravenous urography (IVU) can also be used if there are constraints of resources for renogram. The major dilemma arises if the location of pelvic stone is close to the PUJ area creating confusion as to whether the stone is the reason for obstructive pattern on imaging. In such scenarios, the confirmation of the PUJO must be done after the clearance of the stone at a later stage. An indirect inference is usually taken from the shape of the stones; if the stone is located at the PUJ and taking the shape of PUJ, then PUJO is unlikely; whereas multiple smooth and rounded stones that are located in dependent calyces and mobile in nature often creates a suspicion that the stones could be secondary in nature with a presence of primary PUJO.[20] Another important aspect to be assessed is the function of the renal moiety especially if there is gross dilatation of the kidney and thinning of the parenchyma. In such scenarios when the function of the kidney is poor, one can consider the option of a nephrectomy.

2. **How would you plan to proceed with treating this case?**

   Ans: Decision about the treatment plan would depend on the reliability of conformation of the suspected PUJO pre-operatively. If the suspected PUJO is confirmed pre-operatively, then the management needs to address both the issues simultaneously. This can often be managed as a single stage approach. However, if the suspicion of PUJO is not confirmed adequately on pre-operative imaging, then a staged approach should be considered and the patient has to be counselled appropriately regarding the dilemma of the situation.

3. **What would be the two staged approach for such case?[20]**

   Ans: Two staged approach: This approach entails a more conservative view towards the suspected PUJO. It might be worthwhile to stage the treatment of PUJO when the diagnosis is uncertain and suspicious. The stones can be cleared in the first stage and followed by interval evaluation of the PUJO during follow-up. The diagnosis of PUJO would be clearer during follow-up after the confounding factor of stone presence is cleared. The confirmatory renogram study has to be done after the stent removal and with an adequate duration of time to allow the effect of stenting to subside. Often a duration of 6 to 12 weeks would suffice to consider for taking up the definitive evaluation. However, borderline indeterminate cases might need longer duration of follow-up prior to second intervention. Options to clear the stones would be percutaneous nephrolithotomy (PCNL) as the first choice depending on the stone burden and the extent of PUJO suspicion. The suspicion of PUJ being not draining adequately would be the major concern for opting of RIRS or SWL.

RIRS would need fragmentation and fragment clearance by basketing and not relying on spontaneous clearance of all the fragments. Suspicious drainage of PUJ might not be able to clear the fragments of SWL similarly. Treating the PUJO as a second stage procedure after a primary endoscopic intervention might be more technically challenging than a primary approach mainly due to the presence of fibrosis from the inflammation and fluid extravasation happening from the endoscopic procedure. Due diligence would be needed to assess the length of obstruction in the presence of peri-pelvic fibrosis during the pyeloplasty (Fig. 15.3).

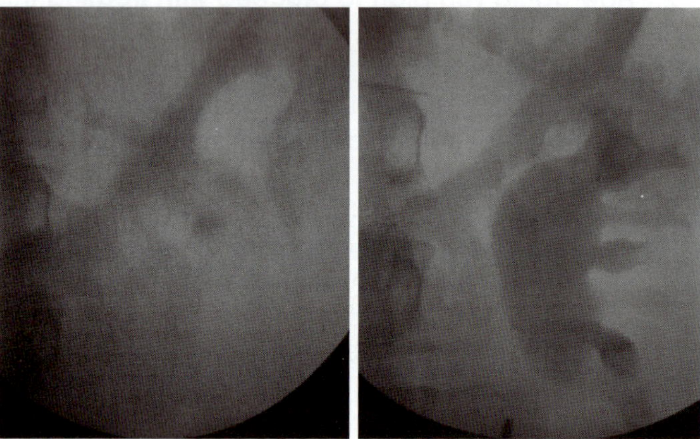

Fig. 15.3: Fluoroscopy images of the stone and the images on retrograde pyelogram showing suspicious delay in drainage of contrast across PUJ.

4. **How would you plan for a single stage approach?**

   Ans: Single stage approach to simultaneously tackle the PUJO and the stones mandate a clear confirmation about the presence and extent of PUJO. It can be treated by three approaches.

   a. Totally endoscopic approach (PCNL + Endopyelotomy)[21,22] considering an endoscopic approach for the PUJO by means of an endopyelotomy or balloon dilatation would give an option to clear both the issues endoscopically. Endopyelotomy can be performed either by antegrade or retrograde approach. Considering the stone burden in mind, antegrade approach with PCNL and endopyelotomy would be a better option rather than a retrograde approach involving RIRS and retrograde endopyelotomy.[23,24] The stone clearance rates is around 80% for the retrograde endopyelotomy and RIRS. The pros of this approach would include single stage addressing both entities in single sitting and the minimal morbidity of the endoscopic approach. The cons of this approach are mainly the lower success rate of endopyelotomy for PUJO and need for re-intervention. The success rate for endopyelotomy has been reported in literature as 70–75%.[25–27] There is mixed opinion about the role of endopyelotomy stents and the impact of stent size to improve the success rate post-endopyelotomy.[28,29] There are post-operative complications of fever and prolonged pain due to extravasation during procedure. Another limitation of this approach is the reduced success rate in the presence of a crossing lower polar vessel.[29–31] As a result of the compromised success rates, limitations of procedure and presence of complications, this approach is usually not the preferred first line of management.

   b. Pyeloplasty + pyelolithotomy (lap/robotic/open)[32–40] in the presence of a confirmed PUJO pre-operatively the preferred line of management would be simultaneous pyeloplasty with pyelolithotomy. The major advantages of this approach are single stage clearance of both issues and high success rate of pyeloplasty for the PUJO as compared to endopyelotomy. The approach for this intervention could preferably be minimally invasive in nature in the form of laparoscopic or robotic approach. The major concern with this minimally invasive pyeloplasty with pyelolithotomy approach is the difficulty in ensuring complete stone clearance intra-operatively. Some of the measures to ensure this are precise enumeration of the number of stones on imaging and patiently ensuring all the stones are retrieved. Often there would be need for nephroscopy to be done through the pyelotomy incision. One can use semi-rigid ureteroscope for this purpose and access through the operating ports. Occasionally there might be need for usage of flexible nephroscope or flexible ureteroscope as well to clear calyceal stones. Care must be taken not to flood the peritoneum with the irrigation fluid during nephroscopic retrieval of stones, else the intra-peritoneal collection of fluid would make the bowel float and hamper the vision and access to complete the further procedure. Frequent washing of the pelvi-calyceal system with the suction-irrigation system often helps in washing out the small calyceal stones. Fluoroscopic guidance if feasible can help in ensuring the clearance. In case of robotic approach, one might need to access through one of the working ports of robotic instruments to have a proper angulation for performing nephroscopy. Occasionally if the calyceal stones cannot be retrieved through a basket, one can use laser for *in-situ* fragmentation and then retrieve the fragments. Usage of ultrasonic energy for lithotripsy and suctioning of fragments is another option for stone clearance with minimal spillage. There are chances of missing out on stone clearance despite performing all the possible maneuvers. Hence, the patient should always be counselled about the probability of an ancillary procedure for clearance of any residual stones.

c. PCNL + minimally invasive pyeloplasty[41] the clearance of stones can be done through PCNL as first part of the procedure and then followed up in the same sitting with minimally invasive pyeloplasty by laparoscopic or robotic approach. The advantage is the ease of clearance of stones by PCNL as compared to the multiple manoeuvres that one might need for stone retrieval during minimally invasive pyelolithotomy. The standard approach for PCNL would ensure the option to utilise all possible accessories including appropriate imaging with fluoroscopy or ultrasound to achieve complete stone clearance. After completion of PCNL, pyeloplasty can be continued in standard manner. There might be increased tissue oedema due to fluid extravasation during the PCNL. The limitation would be the need for the PCNL procedure to be straightforward without any complications. Occurrence of intra-operative bleeding during PCNL or presence of significant level of infection and inflammation of the pelvi-calyceal system would require the pyeloplasty to be staged for a later date. Appropriate counselling has to be done for the possibility of staged clearance.

5. What are the factors to be looked into in post-operative care?

Ans: The main factors to follow-up in patients post-operatively are:

1. Clearance of stone
2. Proper drainage across PUJ
3. Presence of metabolic anomalies for stone formation

Post-operatively patient has to be followed up on these 3 parameters.[42–46] There has been a high incidence of metabolic anomalies in these patients of stones with PUJO. Identification and correction of these anomalies becomes important in order to reduce the risk of future recurrence of stones. There is a synergistic effect of stasis of urine due to PUJO and the metabolic anomaly to form stones. There is high incidence of metabolic anomalies in these patients with hypercalciuria being the most common.[47,48] There can be hyperoxaluria and hypocitraturia as well. Hence clearance of both parameters would be most suitable to reduce risk of stone recurrence.[49,50]

Conclusion

- Clinical decision making and establishing with surety the presence and extent of PUJO remains the crux in managing this clinical scenario.
- Based on the extent of PUJO and stone burden the plan of management can be individualised.
- Single stage minimally invasive pyeloplasty with pyelolithotomy would be the preferred option in cases with confirmed PUJO and multiple stones.
- Total endoscopic approach with PCNL and endopyelotomy is feasible but with reduced success rate for clearing the PUJO.
- In cases of persisting doubt about the presence and extent of PUJO pre-operatively, a staged approach can be adopted.
- Evaluation for metabolic anomalies is worthwhile in order to reduce the risk of recurrence.

C. Renal Stone with Kyphoscoliosis

LEARNING OBJECTIVES

- Understanding anatomic and physiological changes in patients with kyphoscoliosis.
- Treatment options with their limitations.
- Modification in standard treatment approach to suit these patients.

INTRODUCTION

The retroperitoneal and paraspinal position of the kidney makes it well accessible for percutaneous access. The bilateral broad quadrangular posterolateral surface area of the back between the paraspinal muscles, costal margin, iliac crest, and posterior axillary line is ideal for puncturing the calyces and manoeuvring of the nephroscope. Deviation in the alignment of the spinal axis in the coronal or sagittal axis would disturb the renal accessibility with increased surgical risk. Deviation of the spinal curvature by more than 10 degrees as measured by the Cobb angle in the coronal or sagittal axis is termed kyphoscoliosis. This makes the percutaneous renal access difficult and increases the chances of surrounding organ injury (Fig. 15.4).

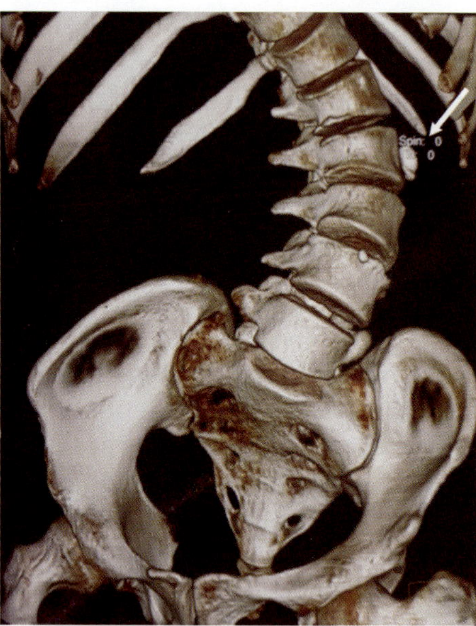

Fig. 15.4: Coronal section CT

Case Scenario

A 40-year-old lady presents with right flank dull ache. She has scoliosis with kyphosis and a surgical history of lumbar spine tuberculosis. Plain CT revealed a large right renal calculus (HU +1200) measuring (2.0 × 1.4 × 2.0 cm) in the right renal pelvis and a spinal Cobb's angle of 60 degrees. Pulmonary function assessment showed a 75% predicted vital capacity. Echocardiography showed 52% left ventricular ejection fraction.

1. What is kyphoscoliosis and what are the common causes?

Ans: Deviation of the spinal curvature by more than 10 degrees as measured by the Cobb angle in the coronal or sagittal axis is termed kyphoscoliosis.[51] Scoliosis specifically refers to lateral deviation in the coronal plane, whereas kyphosis refers to deviation in the sagittal plane. Moderate kyphoscoliosis has a deviation ranging from 25 to 100 degrees, whereas severe kyphoscoliosis has a Cobb angle greater than 100 degrees.

Common causes of kyphoscoliosis include congenital, secondary (related to neuromuscular or skeletal dysfunction or post-traumatic, etc) and idiopathic (unknown etiology).[52]

2. What are the anatomical and physiological changes in patients with kyphoscoliosis?

Ans:

1. These patients are more prone to fall and risk gait changes.
2. Pulmonary function is frequently affected with reduced exercise tolerance and ventilation disorders (both obstructive and restrictive).[53,54] Pulmonary arterial hypertension should be ruled out.
3. The lumbar area on the side of the spinal curvature is stretched and exposes the kidney on that side. Vice versa, the lumbar region on the side opposite to the spinal curvature or convexity is adducted with cramping of abdominal organs. This makes the percutaneous renal access difficult and increases the chances of surrounding organ injury.

3. What investigations are mandatory before planning any treatment?

Ans:

1. Cardiorespiratory assessment is mandatory in view of the frequent associated ventilation disorders.
2. A CT scan should be mandatory to understand the anatomy of the kidney with respect to its drainage system and its relation with the surrounding organs.

4. What are the treatment options? Outline their challenges, success, and modifications.

Ans:

PCNL: PCNL in these patients is challenging. Every case needs to be planned individually depending on the degree of deformity, the cardiorespiratory function, and the stone burden. Most of these patients would be harboring infection stones so antibiotic cover may be needed.

- **Anaesthesia:** General anaesthesia is preferred. Epidural anaesthesia should be avoided due to its cardiopulmonary effects.[53]
- *Position:* Positioning the patient on the operating table is difficult due to the spinal curvature with the associated pelvic tilt and hip ankylosis. Supine position may offer advantages in terms of patient comfort, cardiorespiratory function and ability to do simultaneous combined retrograde access. However, the prone position if possible may offer a wider surface for percutaneous access.[55] Lateral decubitus may be used in specific cases.[56]
- Ultrasound guided puncture would help avoiding surrounding organ injury.[55] CT guided PCNL was performed by Matlaga and colleagues in similar patients.[57] Advantages are precise anatomical details. It, however, is associated with more radiation exposure, requires a two-step procedure and is not easily available at all centres.

- A low-pressure system should be used to reduce fluid absorption and prevent volume overload in these patients with compromised cardiopulmonary function.[58]
- *Success:* In a series of 9 patients with mean stone burden of 372 sq mm, Gourmas, *et al* achieved a complete stone clearance status in 55.5% after single sitting PCNL and 66.6% after two stage PCNL. Using auxiliary procedures (ESWL and RIRS in one case each), the overall stone free rate was 89% at 3 months follow-up.[55] There were no visceral organ injuries while one patient required angiographic embolization. Bleeding incidence may be higher in these scenarios due to difficulty in precise puncture.
- *Impact of Cobb angle:* In a series of 15 patients, Chaudhry and colleagues achieved a stone free rate of 60%. The stone free status correlated with the Cobb angles with a mean Cobb angle of 24 degrees in stone free patients versus a mean Cobb angle of 43 degrees in non-stone free patients.[59]
- *Tract size:* Chen and colleagues compared miniPCNL (18 Fr) and standard PCNL (24 Fr) in patients with renal stones and scoliosis. There was no difference in the stone free rate (55 vs 67%) and the blood loss. The standard PCNL was associated with reduced operative time.[60]

Shock Wave Lithotripsy (SWL)

Stone localisation and patient positioning are the two main challenges in SWL for patients with renal stones and kyphoscoliosis. Patients may be put to a higher risk of vascular and parenchymal injury.[61] Neuwirth and colleagues demonstrated stone free rates of 50% whereas Lazare reported a 73% stone free rate for a mean stone size of 2.9 cm.[62,63]

Retrograde Intrarenal Surgery (RIRS)

Resorlu and colleagues reported the first series of 8 patients with flexible ureteroscopy in patients with renal stones and spinal deformities. They achieved 75% stone clearance rates without any significant complications. Stones on the convex side of scoliosis and narrow lower polar infundibula-pelvic angle were associated with unfavourable outcomes.[64]

SUMMARY

- PCNL is easier when the stone is in the convex side. Flexible retrograde urterorenoscopy may be the better procedure when the stone is in the concave side in patients with kyphoscoliosis. The stone volume and location, pelvicalyceal system anatomy, cardiopulmonary status, other comorbid diseases and urologist experience would determine the ideal treatment choice for each case. SWL is not preferable as the first modality.

D. Stone with Morbid Obesity

LEARNING OBJECTIVES

- Evaluation of patients with morbid obesity and stones.
- Points of concerns while planning the line of management.
- How to choose the treatment options and their limiting factors in obesity

INTRODUCTION

There is an increasing trend in the incidence of obesity and it is not uncommon to come across patients with stones having a morbidly obese body structure.[65] The main concerns with regards to treating these patients is analysing the limiting factors of the treatment options with regards to the obesity and be cautious about the probability of possible complications that might arise.[66] Conventional thumb rules of stone clearance will not be directly applicable due to these two major limitations. One has to be keen to look for the possibility of metabolic anomalies in these patients in view of their high risk for complications during interventions.

Case Scenario

A 40-year-old male presents with complaints of flank pain for past 3 months. It is intermittent in nature and non-radiating. There has been one episode of haematuria. There is no history of fever. He is a known case of renal stone disease with history of spontaneous lithuria in the past. He is on treatment for multiple co-morbid illnesses of diabetes, hypertension, hypercholesterolemia, and obstructive sleep apnoea syndrome. He has undergone treatment for his morbid obesity 4 years back with partial response in terms of weight loss but has regained most of his lost weight. He presently weighs 140 kg with a BMI of 48 kg/m^2. Rest of the physical examination is normal. He was evaluated and found to have a left renal pelvic calculus of 1.5 cm in size with mild hydronephrosis on ultrasound. On further evaluation with plain CT, the findings were reconfirmed, and stone HU was found to be around 800 (Fig. 15.5).

1. **What are the points to keep in mind during evaluation of a morbidly obese patient with stone?**

   Ans: The key points to be kept in mind during evaluation are general assessment and physical fitness for anaesthesia, stone evaluation, and treatment history. The morbidly obese patients typically present with multiple co-morbid issues associated with metabolic syndrome. Proper evaluation of these systemic issues is of paramount importance pre-operatively. Optimisation of co-morbid conditions should be done as much as possible. Respiratory reserves in these patients might be compromised and hence remain a

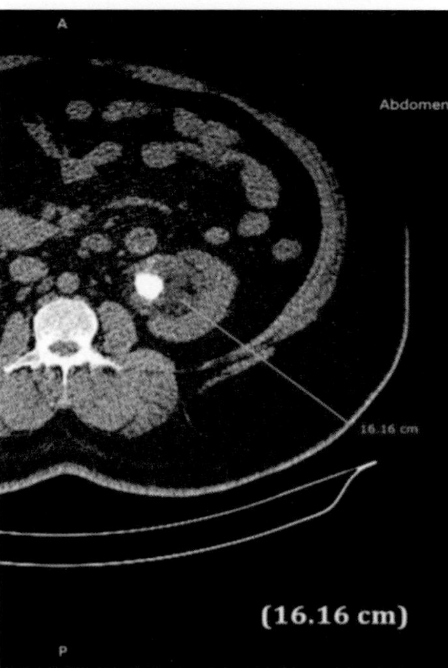

Fig. 15.5: CT scan showing left renal pelvic calculus with skin-stone distance

concern. Often the morbidly obese patients would be on a long list of medications for their metabolic issues. Some of the treatment modalities used for weight reduction might be the risk factor for stone formation and need to be evaluated keenly.

2. **Why obesity increases the risk of stone formation?**

   Ans: Obese patients have multiple risk factors that increase the stone formation tendency. There is increased urinary excretion of calcium, sodium, oxalate, uric acid and low pH. Presence of multiple co-morbid illnesses further can add to their risk of stone formation. Medications being used for obesity treatment can increase the risk of stone formation. Bariatric surgeries can also increase the risk of stone formation due to malabsorption. Evaluation of the risk factors is essential in the management of these patients.

3. **What would be imaging modality of choice for such patients?**

   Ans: The evaluation of these patients with regards to stone remains almost the same as normal non-obese patients. The usual imaging is plain CT-KUB as it would not only give the necessary information about stone in terms of size, location, and density, but also give the crucial information of skin-stone distance (SSD) which is key parameter for SWL and PCNL mode of treatment.

4. **What are the limitations for evaluation with KUB or IVU?**

   Ans: Evaluation with X-ray or IVP would be inadequate to provide the SSD and affected with poor visualisation due to extra fat. Poor visualisation will hamper the decision making in terms of opting the optimal modality of treatment.

5. **What is the technical challenge during CT evaluation for these patients?**

   Ans: The limitation with regards to the acceptable upper limit of weight for the gantry of CT machine has to be kept in mind as it might be inadequate to handle extremely heavy patients. This would be even more difficult if there are any concerns of claustrophobia which is relatively uncommon during CT as compared to MRI.

6. **What are the advantages and limitations of different treatment options?**

   Ans: The treatment options that we can consider are

   1. Shockwave lithotripsy (SWL)
   2. Flexible ureteroscopy and RIRS
   3. Prone PCNL
   4. Supine PCNL

7. **What are the advantages with SWL as the treatment modality?**

   Ans: Shock wave lithotripsy (SWL)[67–73] is one of the options that can be considered for stones in obese patients. However, there are several pros and cons to this treatment modality. The major advantage for this is the chance to avoid anaesthesia and thereby prevent all the possible complications arising out of it. As these patients are more likely to have multiple co-morbidities associated with the metabolic syndrome, possibility of avoidance of anaesthesia could be a major advantage.

8. **What are the disadvantages of SWL in morbidly obese patients?**

   Ans: The basic consideration of stone size and stone density in terms of Hounsfield Units (HU) remain valid even in obese patients. There is higher incidence of calcium oxalate stones in obese patients and hence one has to be careful in selecting the case. The increased skin-stone distance (SSD) is a negative factor that adversely affects the efficiency of SWL. The focussing ability is reduced, and it might have to rely on the principle of blast path effect or extended shock pathway if the stone is beyond the exact zone of focus. One can use abdominal compression to get the stone into the range of focus. The newer devices might be able to mitigate this issue with the ability to adjust the focal length. This has resulted in reduced success rates of around 67% in obese patients for SWL. There is a higher need for multiple sessions for stone clearance as well with retreatment rates of over 30%.[70–72]

9. **What are the concerns about complications of SWL in morbidly obese patients?**

Ans: The incidence for renal hematomas is higher in obese patients, thereby adding another point of concern before opting for SWL as the modality of choice. The reason for increased hematoma formation could be due to the increase in energy used for these patients probably as a compromise for the poorer localisation of stone. Another postulated reason could probably be the increased vascular vulnerability in these patients and the higher incidence of hypertension in this group of patients. [66] However, this can be circumvented with adequate precautions and extra care.

10. **What are the advantages and limitations of flexible ureteroscopy and RIRS in morbidly obese patients?**

Ans: There are major advantages to using retrograde intra-renal surgery (RIRS) as the modality of choice. is that the treatment process *per se* is minimally affected by the body habitus or the BMI of the patient. The success rate with regards to stone clearance is more than 90%.[74–76] The retreatment rates have been less compared to SWL (9% vs 36%).[77–79] When compared to normal non-obese patients, the stone free rates have not been found to be different. Hence, as far as RIRS is considered, the considerations remain exactly the same as those for normal non-obese patients. The size of the stone, location and stone density would be the main factors determining the stone free rates. The main disadvantage would be mainly in terms of need for anaesthesia in the high risk setting of morbid obesity with multiple co-morbidities. One option is to consider pre-stenting electively for these patients under local anaesthesia which might circumvent the inability to access the stone due to narrow ureter after induction of high-risk anaesthesia.

11. **What are the points of concern for opting prone PCNL as the treatment option in morbidly obese patients?**

Ans: Conventional prone PCNL as a modality of treatment is associated with major technical challenges arising from the morbid obesity.[80–86] Positioning the patient in prone position is a major challenge in morbidly obese patients with high risk of injuries. The process has to be extremely cautious and co-ordinated one. Due care must be given to adequately pad and protect all the pressure points to prevent injury. The respiratory distress created might be a major concern from the anaesthesia point of view because of limited ability to achieve free respiratory excursions due to the abdominal compression. There could also be a concern about inferior vena cava compression leading to reduced preload. These parameters have to be kept in mind during the procedure. The skin-stone distance (SSD) is equally relevant in PCNL as it is in SWL mainly because of the length of instruments that are used. One might need to improvise the procedure with the help of extra-long instruments that are now available mainly for usage in morbidly obese patients. Often the Amplatz sheath used for the access might get buried inside the subcutaneous fat in these patients and using a tie to the edge of the sheath might help its retrieval. There could be a need for usage of flexible nephroscope more often if the length of nephroscope remains a concern. These limitations and need for extra precautions translate into longer operative time. However, the most important parameter of stone free rates has been unaffected significantly in obese patients. The success rates and complications have been found to be similar in obese and non-obese patients. There might be a higher radiation exposure and a longer hospital stay. Hence, one can safely consider the option of conventional prone PCNL as an effective treatment modality based on the other stone parameters (Fig. 15.6).

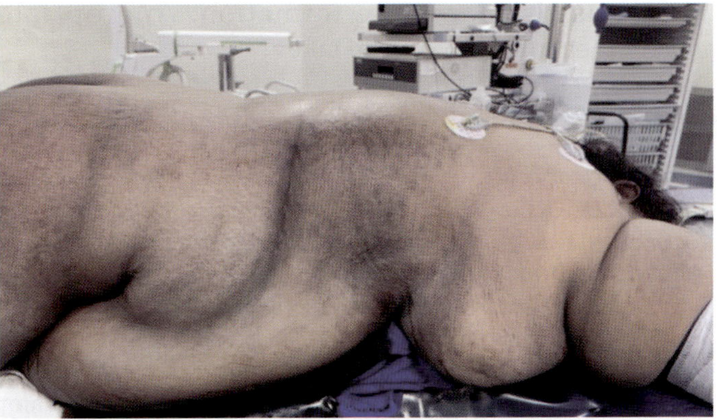

Fig. 15.6: Image showing prone positioned morbidly obese patient for PCNL. Care has to be taken for adequate padding of pressure points and avoiding excessive abdominal compression

12. **What are the advantages and limitations of supine PCNL in morbidly obese patients?**

Ans: The renewed interest in supine PCNL is an important option in morbidly obese patients mainly due to the increased risk of anaesthetic complications from respiratory distress from abdominal compression. The risk factors of prone position can be theoretically mitigated in supine PCNL. However, studies have not found a major difference in the complications rates between supine and prone PCNL in obese patients.[87-90] Along with the limitations of prone PCNL with regards to need for extra-long instruments and accessories, supine position adds to the issue with longer access tracts. Though technically the stone free rates and complications might not be different between the two positions for PCNL, the subjective ease and comfort factor from the anaesthetist point of view remain an advantage for supine over prone PCNL.

13. What are the follow-up points of concern?

Ans: The main concern with regards to the follow-up of these patients is from the point of view of metabolic anomalies found in them. [91–104]

- The incidence and recurrence risk for stones in obese patients is higher.
- There is higher incidence of multiple metabolic anomalies such as increased excretion of calcium, sodium, oxalate, and urate along with reduced pH of urine.
- Metabolic evaluation is necessary to address these risk factors.
- Dosing of medications for stone prophylaxis has to be more frequent in view with higher requirements.
- Treatment modalities for weight reduction such as orlistat, topiramate or bariatric surgeries inducing malabsorption are known to increase the risk for stone formation. Appropriate measures have to be taken.

SUMMARY

- Incidence of obesity and stones is increasing in recent years.
- Evaluation of the general health condition, physical fitness, and treatment history important. Optimisation of general condition important prior to intervention
- Evaluation of the stone needs assessment of SSD along with other parameters of stone.
- ESWL is associated with lower stone free rates, higher retreatment, and complication rates. SSD remains major concern for proper focussing of energy.
- RIRS is preferred modality of treatment for feasible stones as the success rate is comparable to normal non-obese patients.
- Prone PCNL is safe and effective with stone free rates and complication rates being comparable to normal non-obese individuals. Risks associated with anaesthesia and prone positioning remain and adequate precautions have to be taken for the same. Operative time and radiation doses tend to be higher. Extra-long equipment and accessories would be needed in view of longer SSD.
- Supine PCNL mitigates the concerns associated with prone positioning. The success rates and complications have been comparable between supine and prone PCNL in obese patients. The ease and comfort of anaesthetist would be better with supine.
- Metabolic anomalies are common in these patients with wide array of anomalies. Evaluation of these issues and addressing them adequately remain of paramount importance in order to reduce the risk of recurrence.
- Treatment options for weight reduction like itself might be predisposing factors for the patients to develop increased stone formation risk.

REFERENCES

A. Renal Pelvic Stone in Post-transplant Kidney

1. Harraz AM, Kamal AI, Shocker AA. Urolithiasis in renal transplant donors and recipients: An update. International Journal of Surgery 2016;36:693–697.
2. Sabnis RB, Singh AG, *et al*. The development and current status of minimally invasive surgery to manage urological complications after renal transplantation. Indian J Urol 2016;32(3):186–191.
3. Yuan HJ, Yang DD, *et al*. Minimally invasive treatment of renal transplant nephrolithiasis. World J Urol 2015;33(12):2079–2085.
4. Ji ZG, Tian Y, Chen Q, Liu Z, Lin J, Wang JM, Ma LL, Guo HB, Tang YW, Xie ZL, Sun W, Zhang L: A retrospective study of minipercutaneous laser lithotripsy for treatment of allograft kidney lithiasis obstruction. Transplant Proc 2013;45:3298–3301.
5. Hyams E, Marien T, Bruhn A, Quirouet A, Andonian S, Shah O, *et al*. Ureteroscopy for transplant lithiasis. J Endourol. 2012;26:819–22.
6. Gerber RC, Best SL, Hedican SP, and Nakada SY. Flexible Ureteroscopy as the New Standard for the Management of Renal Transplant Urolithiasis <15 mm: A Single-Center Experience. J Endourol2021;35:10,1443–1447.
7. Branchereau J, Timsit MO, Neuzillet Y, *et al*. Management of renal transplant urolithiasis: A multicentre study by the French Urology Association Transplantation Committee. World J Urol2018;36:105–109.
8. Stravodimos KG, Adamis S, Tyritzis S, Georgios Z, Constantinides CA. Renal transplant lithiasis: Analysis of our series and review of the literature. J Endourol. 2012;26:38–44.
9. Verrier C, Bessede T, *et al*. Decrease in and management of urolithiasis after kidney transplantation. J. Urol 2012;187(5):1651–1655.
10. Bolen E, Stern K, Humphreys M, Brady A, Leavitt T, Zhang N, Keddis M. Urine metabolic risk factors and outcomes of patients with kidney transplant nephrolithiasis. Clin Kidney J. 2021 Oct 20;15(3):500–506.
11. Wong KA and Olsburgh J. Management of stones in renal transplant. Curr.Opin.Urol 2013;23(2):175–179.
12. Boissier R, Breda A *et al*. Evaluation of the Effectiveness of Interventions on Nephrolithiasis inTransplanted Kidney. EurUrol Focus 2022 Dec 23:S2405–4569(22)00278–4.
13. Challacombe B, Dasgupta P, Tiptaft R, Glass J, Koffman G, Goldsmith D, *et al*. Multimodal management of urolithiasis in renal transplantation. BJU Int. 2005; 96:385–9.
14. Hulbert JC, Reddy P, Young AT, *et al*. The percutaneous removal of calculi from transplanted kidneys. J Urol1985;134:324–326.
15. Krambeck AE, Leroy AJ, Patterson DE, *et al*. Percutaneous nephrolithotomy success in the transplant kidney. J Urol2008;180:2545–2549.
16. He Z, Li X, Chen L, *et al*. Minimally invasive percutaneous nephrolithotomy for upper urinary tract calculi in transplanted kidneys. BJU Int 2007;99:1467–1471.

17. Sarier M, Duman I, Yuksel Y, Tekin S, Demir M, Arslan F, Ergun O, Kosar A, Yavuz AH. Results of minimally invasive surgical treatment of allograft lithiasis in live-donor renal transplant recipients: a single-center experience of 3758 renal transplantations. Urolithiasis. 2019;47(3):273–278.
18. Ferreira M, *et al*. Lithiasis in 1,313 kidney transplants: incidence, diagnosis, and management. Transpl. Proc., 44 (8) (2012), pp. 2373–2375.
19. Esteban Emiliani, Jose Daniel Subiela, Federica Regis, Oriol Angerri, Joan Palou. Over 30-yr Experience on the Management of Graft Stones After Renal Transplantation. European Urology Focus, Volume 4, Issue 2, 2018, Pages 169–174.

B. Multiple Pelvic and Lower Calyx Stones with Suspected PUJ Obstruction

20. Pearle MS, Lotan Y. Urinary Lithiasis: Etiology, Epidemiology, and Pathogenesis. In: Campbell-Walsh Urology Philadelphia: Saunders Elsevier, 2007, p. 1389.
21. Motola JA, Badlani GH, Smith AD (1993) Results of 212 consecutive endopyelotomies: an 8-year followup. J Urol 149:453–456.
22. Shalhav AL, Guisti G, Elbahnasy AM *et al* (1998) Adult endopyelotomy: impact of etiology and antegrade versus retrograde approach on outcome. J Urol 160:685–689.
23. Meretyk I, Meretyk S, Clayman RV: Endopyelotomy: comparison of ureteroscopic retrograde and antegrade percutaneous techniques. J Urol1992;148:775–782.
24. Knudsen BE, Cook AJ, Watterson JD, Beiko DT, Nott L, Razvi H, Denstedt JD: Percutaneous antegrade endopyelotomy: long-term results from one institution. Urology 2004;63: 230–234.
25. Minervini A, Davenport K, Keeley FX Jr, Timoney AG: Antegrade versus retrograde endopyelotomy for pelvi-ureteric junction (PUJ) obstruction. EurUrol2006;49:536–542.
26. Samarasekera D, Chew BH: Endopyelotomy still has an important role in the management of ureteropelvic junction obstruction. Can Urol Assoc J 2011;5:134–136.
27. Dimarco DS, Gettman MT, McGee SM, Chow GK, Leroy AJ, Slezak J, Patterson DE, Segura JW: Long-term success of antegrade endopyelotomy compared with pyeloplasty at a single institution. J Endourol2006;20:707–712.
28. Anidjar M, Meria P, Cochand-Priollet B, Cussenot O, Desgrandchamps F, Cortesse A, Teillac P, Le Duc A. Evaluation of optimal stent size after antegrade endopyelotomy: an experimental study in the porcine model. Eur Urol. 1997;32(2):245–52. PMID: 9286661.
29. Danuser H, Hochreiter WW, Ackermann DK, Studer UE. Influence of stent size on the success of antegrade endopyelotomy for primary ureteropelvic junction obstruction: results of 2 consecutive series. J Urol. 2001 Sep;166(3):902–9. PMID: 11490243.
30. Knudson BE, Cook AJ, Watherson JD, Beiko DT, Nott L, Razvi, H, Denstedt JD. Percutaneous antegrade endopyelotomy: Long term results from one institution. Urology 2004;63:230–234.
31. Lam JS, Cooper KL, Greene TD, Gupta M. Impact of hydronephrosis and renal function on treatment outcome: antegrade versus retrograde endopyelotomy. Urology 2003;61:1107–1111.
32. Stein RJ, Turna B, Nguyen MM, Aron M, Hafron JM, Gill IS, Kaouk J, Desai M: Laparoscopic pyeloplasty with concomitant pyelolithotomy: technique and outcomes. J Endourol2008;22:1251–1255.
33. Ramakumar S, Lancini V, Chan DY, Parsons JK, Kavoussi LR, Jarrett TW: Laparoscopic pyeloplasty with concomitant pyelolithotomy. J Urol2002;167:1378–1380.
34. Atug F, Castle EP, Burgess SV, Thomas R: Concomitant management of renal calculi and pelvi-ureteric junction obstruction with robotic laparoscopic surgery. BJU Int 2005; 96:1365–1368.
35. Yang C, Zhou J, Lu ZX, Hao Z, Wang J, Zhang L, Liang C. Simultaneous treatment of ureteropelvic junction obstruction complicated by renal calculi with robotic laparoscopic surgery and flexible cystoscope. World J Urol. 2019 Oct;37(10):2217–2223. doi: 10.1007/s00345–018–2608–9. Epub 2019 Jan 19. PMID: 30661106.
36. An LZ, Xiong LL, Chen L, Wang HR, Chen WN, Huang XB. [Laparoscopic pyeloplasty combined with ultrasonic lithotripsy via nephroscope for treatment of ureteropelvic junction obstruction with renal calculi]. Beijing Da XueXue Bao Yi Xue Ban. 2022 Aug 18;54(4):746–750. Chinese. doi: 10.19723/j.issn.1671–167X.2022.04.026. PMID: 35950402; PMCID: PMC9385502.
37. Hong P, Li Z, Zhu D, Zhuang L, Yang K, Hao H, Li X, Zhou L. A Simple Modification for the Usage of Flexible Cystoscope in Modified Laparoscopic Pyeloplasty for Ureteropelvic Junction Obstruction with Renal Calculi: A Flexible Guiding Tube. Urol Int. 2019;102(3):262–268. doi: 10.1159/000495569. Epub 2019 Jan 10. PMID: 30630187.
38. Eden CG, Moon DA, Gianduzzo T: Concomitant management of renal calculi and pelviureteric junction obstruction with robotic laparoscopic surgery. BJU Int 2006;97:653–654.
39. Jensen PH, Berg KD, Azawi NH: Robot-assisted pyeloplasty and pyelolithotomy in patients with ureteropelvic junction stenosis. Scand J Urol2017;51:323–328.
40. Hüttenbrink C, Kelm P, Klein T, Distler F, Pandey A, Pahernik S. Combination of Robotic Pyeloplasty and Percutaneous Renal Surgery for Simultaneous Treatment of Ureteropelvic Junction Obstruction and Calyx Stones. Urol Int. 2021;105(7–8):637–641. doi: 10.1159/000513457. Epub 2021 Mar 10. PMID: 33691328.
41. Agarwal A, Varshney A, Bansal BS. Concomitant percutaneous nephrolithotomy and transperitoneal laparoscopic pyeloplasty for ureteropelvic junction obstruction complicated by stones. J Endourol. 2008 Oct;22(10):2251–5. doi: 10.1089/end.2008.9726. PMID: 18831672.
42. Saussine C, Lechevallier E, Traxer O. Calculs et syndrome de la jonctionpyélo-urétérale [Urolithiasis and ureteropelvic junction obstruction]. Prog Urol. 2008 Dec;18(12):986–8. French. doi: 10.1016/j.purol.2008.09.002. Epub 2008 Oct 31. PMID: 19033067.
43. Rutschik SD, Resnick MI. Ureteropelvic junction obstruction and renal calculi. Pathophysiology and implications for management. Urol Clin North Am 1998;25:317–21.
44. Husman DA, Milliner DS, Segura JW. Ureteropelvic junstion obstruction with a simultaneous renal calculus: long-term followup. J Urol1995;153:1399–402.

45. Husmann DA, Milliner DS, Segura JW. Ureteropelvic junction obstruction with concurrent renal pelvic calculi in the pediatric patient: a long-term followup. J Urol1996;156:741—3.
46. Bernardo NO, Liatsikos EN, Dinlenc CZ, Kapoor R, Fogarty JD, Smith AD. Stone recurrence after endopyelotomy. Urology 2000;56:378—81.
47. Matin SF, Streem SB. Metabolic risk factors in patients with ureteropelvic junction obstruction and renal calculi. J Urol2000;163:1676—8.
48. Tekin A, Tekgul S, Atsu N, Ergen A, Kendi S. Ureteropelvic junction obstruction and coexisting renal calculi in children: role of metabolic abnormalities. Urology 2001;57:542—5.
49. Garcia-Nieto V, Navarro JF, Luis-Yanes MI, Lopez-Mendez M, Garcia-Rodriguez V. Hypercalciuria in pediatric patients with ureteropelvic junction obstruction is of genetic origin. Scand J Urol Nephrol 2007;41:144—8.
50. Skolarikos A, Dellis A, Knoll T. Ureteropelvic obstruction and renal stones: etiology and treatment. Urolithiasis. 2015 Feb;43(1):5–12. doi: 10.1007/s00240-014-0736-2. Epub 2014 Nov 2. PMID: 25362543.

C. Renal Stone with Kyphoscoliosis

51. Papaliodis DN, Bonanni PG, Roberts TT, Hesham K, Richardson N, Cheney RA, Lawrence JP, Carl AL, Lavelle WF. Computer Assisted Cobb Angle Measurements: A novel algorithm. Int J Spine Surg. 2017;11(3):21.
52. Issac S, M Das J. Kyphoscoliosis. [Updated 2022 Aug 30]. In: StatPearls [Internet]. Treasure Island (FL): StatPearls Publishing; 2023 Jan.
53. McPhail GL, Ehsan Z, Howells SA, *et al.* Obstructive lung disease in children with idiopathic scoliosis. J Pediatr 2015; 166: 1018–1021.
54. Tan HT, Yi WT, Shi L, Wang WT, Lin CH. Clinical application of percutaneous nephrolithotomy in a patient with kyphoscoliosis. J Int Med Res. 2021 Jan;49(1):300060520987937.
55. Goumas-Kartalas I, Montanari E. Percutaneous nephrolithotomy in patients with spinal deformities. J Endourol. 2010 Jul;24(7):1081–9.
56. Gofrit ON, Shapiro A, Donchin Y, *et al.* Lateral decubitus position for percutaneous nephrolithotripsy in the morbidly obese or kyphotic patient. J Endourol2002;16:383–386.
57. Matlaga BR, Shah OD, Zagoria RJ, *et al.* Computerized tomography guided access for percutaneous nephrostolithotomy. J Urol2003;170:45–47.
58. Kukreja RA, Desai MR, Sabnis RB, Patel SH: Fluid absorption during percutaneous nephrolithotomy: does it matter?. J Endourol. 2002, 16:221–4.
59. Chaudhry R, *et al.* Percutaneous Stone Surgery in Spina Bifida Patients—Are Stone-Free Rates Worth the Risk? J. Endourol. 2017;S-81-S-86.http://doi.org/10.1089/end.2016.0769.
60. Chen HQ, Zeng F, Qi L, Li Y. Percutaneous nephrolithotomy in patients with scoliosis: our institutional experience. Urolithiasis. 2013 Feb;41(1):59–64.
61. Vaidyanathan S, Johnson H, Singh G, *et al.* Atrophy of kidney following extra corporeal shock wave lithotripsy of renal calculus in a paraplegic patient with marked spinal curvature. Spinal Cord 2002;40:609–614.
62. Neuwirth H, Royce PL, Chaussy C. Use of extracorporeal shock-wave lithotripsy in quadriplegic patients. JAMA 1986;256:1295.
63. Lazare JN, Saltzman B, Sotolongo J. Extracorporeal shock wave lithotripsy treatment of spinal cord injury patients. J Urol1988;140:266–269.
64. BerkanResorlu, EkremOzyuvali, Ural Oguz, Omer Faruk Bozkurt, and Ali Unsal. Retrograde Intrarenal Surgery in Patients with Spinal Deformities. J. Endourol. 2012:1131–1135.

D. Stone with Morbid Obesity

65. Poore W, Boyd CJ, Singh NP, Wood K, Gower B, Assimos DG. Obesity and Its Impact on Kidney Stone Formation. Rev Urol. 2020;22(1):17–23.
66. Kelly, C., Geraghty, R.M. andSomani, B.K. Nephrolithiasis in the Obese Patient. *CurrUrol Rep* 20, 36 (2019).
67. Nussberger F, Roth B, Metzger T, *et al.* A low or high BMI is a risk factor for renal hematoma after extracorporeal shock wave lithotripsy for kidney stones. Urolithiasis. 2017;45:317–21.
68. Dede O, ener NC, Ba O, *et al.* Does morbid obesity influence the success and complication rates of extracorporeal shockwave lithotripsy for upper ureteral stones? Turk UrolojiDergisi. 2015;41(1):20–3.
69. Pareek G, Armenakas NA, Panagopoulos G, *et al.* Extracorporeal shock wave lithotripsy success based on body mass index and hounsfield units. Urology. 2005;65:33–6.
70. Thomas R, Cass AS. Extracorporeal shock wave lithotripsy in morbidly obese patients. J Urol. 1993;150(1):30–2.
71. H-y L, Yang Y-H, Shen J-T, *et al.* Risk factors survey for extracorporeal shockwave lithotripsy-induced renal hematoma. J Endourol. 2013;27:763–7.
72. Raju Thomas, Alexander S. Cass; Extracorporeal Shock Wave Lithotripsy in Morbidly Obese Patients; The Journal of Urology; Volume 150, Issue 1; 1993; Pages 30–32.
73. Pricop C, Radavoi GD, Puia D, Vechiu C, Jinga V. Obesity: a delicate issue choosing the eswl treatment for patients with kidney and ureteral stones? Acta Endocrinol (Buchar). 2019 Jan–Mar;-5(1):133–138.
74. Javanmard B, Razaghi MR, Jafari AA, *et al.* Flexible ureterorenoscopy versus extracorporeal shock wave lithotripsy for the treatment of renal pelvis stones of 10–20 mm in obese patients. J Lasers Med Sci. 2015;6(4):162–6.
75. Doizi S, Letendre J, Bonneau C, *et al.* Comparative study of the treatment of renal stones with flexible ureterorenoscopy in normal weight, obese, and morbidly obese patients. Urology. 2015;85:38–44.
76. Sari E, Tepeler A, Yuruk E, *et al.* Effect of the body mass index on outcomes of flexible ureterorenoscopy. Urolithiasis. 2013;41:499–504.
77. Caskurlu T, Atis G, Arikan O, Pelit ES, Kilic M, Gurbuz C. The impact of body mass index on the outcomes of retrograde intrarenal stone surgery. Urology. 2013;81(3):517–21.
78. Delorme G, Huu YN, Lillaz J, Bernardini S, Chabannes E, Guichard G, *et al.* Ureterorenoscopy with holmium-yttrium aluminum-garnet fragmentation is a safe and efficient technique for stone treatment in patients with

a body mass index superior to 30 kg/m^2. J Endourol. 2012;26(3):239–43.

79. Wang W, Gao X, Peng L and Jin T (2022) Ureteroscopy Is Equally Efficient and Safe in Obese and Morbidly Obese Patients: A Systematic Review and Meta-Analysis. *Front. Surg.* 9:736641.

80. Fuller A, Razvi H, Denstedt JD, *et al*. The Clinical Research Office of the Endourological Society percutaneous nephrolithotomy global study: outcomes in the morbidly obese patient-a case control analysis. Can Urol Assoc J. 2014;8(5–6 JUNE):E393–E97.

81. Alyami FA, Skinner TAA, Norman RW. Impact of body mass index on clinical outcomes associated with percutaneous nephrolithotomy. Can Urol Assoc J. 2013;7:E197–201.

82. TorrecillaOrtiz C, Meza Martinez AI, Vicens Morton AJ, *et al*. Obesity in percutaneous nephrolithotomy. Is body mass index really important? Urology. 2014;84:538–42.

83. Xu Y, Huang X. Effect of Body Mass Index on Outcomes of Percutaneous Nephrolithotomy: A Systematic Review and Meta-Analysis. Front Surg. 2022 Jun 14;9:922451.

84. Kuntz NJ, Neisius A, Astroza GM, Tsivian M, Iqbal MW, Youssef R, *et al*. Does body mass index impact the outcomes of tubeless percutaneous nephrolithotomy? *BJU Int*. (2014) 114:404–11.

85. im ek A, Özgör F, Akbulut MF, Küçüktopçu O, Berberoğlu AY, SarilarÖ, *et al*. Does body mass index effect the success of percutaneous nephrolithotomy? *Turkish J Urol*. (2014) 40:104–9.

86. Keheila M, Leavitt D, Galli R, Motamedinia P, Theckumparampil N, Siev M, Hoenig D, Smith A, Okeke Z. Percutaneous nephrolithotomy in super obese patients (body mass index 50 kg/m): overcoming the challenges. BJU Int. 2016 Feb;117(2):300–6.

87. Mourmouris P, Berdempes M, Markopoulos T, Lazarou L, Tzelves L, Skolarikos A. Patient positioning during percutaneous nephrolithotomy: what is the current best practice? *Res reports Urol*. (2018) 10:189–93.

88. Mazzucchi E, Vicentini FC, Marchini GS, Danilovic A, Brito AH, Srougi M. Percutaneous nephrolithotomy in obese patients: comparison between the prone and total supine position. *J Endourol*. (2012) 26:1437–42.

89. Abouelleil M, Chelluri R, Daugherty M, Bratslavsky G, Shapiro O. In obese patients, the distance between skin and renal collecting system changes with the position of the patient from supine to prone. *J Endourol*. (2015) 29:760–3.

90. Manohar T, Jain P, Desai M. Supine percutaneous nephrolithotomy: effective approach to high-risk and morbidly obese patients. *J Endourol*. 2007;21:44–49.

91. Espino-Grosso PM, Canales BK. Kidney stones after bariatric surgery: risk assessment and mitigation. *BariatrSurgPract Patient Care*. 2017;12:3–9.

92. Park AM, Storm DW, Fulmer BR, *et al*. A prospective study of risk factors for nephrolithiasis after Roux-en-Y gastric bypass surgery. *J Urol*. 2009;182:2334–2339.

93. Salek T, Andel I, Kurfurstova I. Topiramate induced metabolic acidosis and kidney stones—a case study. *Biochem Med (Zagreb)*. 2017;27:404–410.

94. Maalouf NM, Langston JP, Van Ness PC, *et al*. Nephrolithiasis in topiramate users. *Urol Res*. 2011;39:303–307.

95. Astroza GM, Neisius A, Tsivian M, *et al*. Treatment response in patients with stones, and low urinary pH and hypocitraturia stratified by body mass index. *J Urol*. 2016;195:653–657.

96. Heck AM, Yanovski JA, Calis KA. Orlistat, a new lipase inhibitor for the management of obesity. *Pharmacotherapy*. 2000;20:270–279.

97. Davidson MH, Hauptman J, DiGirolamo M, *et al*. Weight control and risk factor reduction in obese subjects treated for 2 years with orlistat: a randomized controlled trial. *JAMA*. 1999;281:235–242.

98. Sjöström L, Rissanen A, Andersen T, *et al*. Randomised placebo-controlled trial of orlistat for weight loss and prevention of weight regain in obese patients. European Multicentre Orlistat Study Group. *Lancet*. 1998;352:167–172.

99. Maalouf NM, Sakhaee K, Parks JH, *et al*. Association of urinary pH with body weight in nephrolithiasis. *Kidney Int*. 2004;65:1422–1425.

100. Taylor EN, Curhan GC. Body size and 24-hour urine composition. *Am J Kidney Dis*. 2006;48:904–915.

101. Pigna F, Sakhaee K, Adams-Huet B, *et al*. Body fat content and distribution and urinary risk factors for nephrolithiasis. *Clin J Am Soc Nephrol*. 2014;9 .

102. Ekeruo WO, Tan YH, Young MD, *et al*. Metabolic risk factors and the impact of medical therapy on the management of nephrolithiasis in obese patients. *J Urol*. 2004;172:159–163.

103. Trinchieri A, Croppi E, Montanari E. Obesity and urolithiasis: evidence of regional influences. *Urolithiasis*. 2017; 45:271–278.

104. Eisner BH, Eisenberg ML, Stoller ML. Relationship between body mass index and quantitative 24-hour urine chemistries in patients with nephrolithiasis. *Urology*. 2010;75:1289–1293.

Chapter 16

Chronic Retention

• Prashant Motiram Mulawkar • Sumeet Gopal Agrawal

LEARNING OBJECTIVES

- Diagnosis of chronic retention.
- Identifying high risk and low risk chronic retention.
- Effective management of chronic retention and its aftermaths.
- Further evaluation of chronic retention of urine.
- Future directives.

INTRODUCTION

Chronic urinary retention (CUR) is defined as a non-painful bladder, which remains palpable or percussible after the patient has passed urine. Such patients may or may not be incontinent.[1] The AUA CUR workgroup defines non-neurogenic CUR as an elevated postvoid residual (PVR) of >300 ml that has persisted for at least six months and is documented on two or more separate occasions.[2] The 300 ml value is widely accepted as at this volume the bladder usually becomes palpable suprapubically.[3] This definition differentiates CUR from either acute/transient urinary retention or urinary retention caused by a temporally related neurologic, oncologic, or situational (iatrogenic or post-procedural) aetiology. These conditions require specific individualised treatment to address the underlying cause of urinary retention, hence are excluded from the definition of CUR. CUR can be secondary to number of factors which either affect bladder outlet resistance (enlarged prostate, stricture urethra) or reduced detrusor contractility (diabetes mellitus, medications). In addition, some medications like antihistamines, alpha adrenergic agonists and antipsychotics increase outlet resistance, whereas anticholinergics, antispasmodics, tricyclic antidepressants, calcium channel blockers, non-steroidal anti-inflammatory agents, opioids, beta-adrenergic agonists, and antipsychotics reduce the bladder contractility. What differentiates acute urinary retention (AUR) from CUR is the suddenness of the event and preserved detrusor function in AUR. Some individuals with CUR do have preserved contractility and typically poor compliance and upper renal tract changes (high-pressure chronic retention).[4,5]

Case Scenario

A sixty-year-old diabetic and hypertensive male patient attended urology outpatient department with history of weak urinary stream, intermittency and straining for urination. He has had long standing lower urinary symptoms (LUTS) and over last few months he was passing small amount of urine at frequent intervals with occasional nighttime bedwetting. Last few days he was having daytime incontinence also. On examination he was afebrile, well oriented, pulse 60/min, blood pressure 140/90 mmHg, SpO_2 94% and bilateral mild oedema feet. Abdominal examination revealed palpable non-tender bladder up to umbilicus. External genitalia was normal but genital and scrotal skin was soiled with urine.

1. **What are the different types of CUR?**

   Ans: CUR is usually classified as low-pressure and high-pressure CUR. In low-pressure CUR there is no hydronephrosis, and renal function is preserved. High-pressure CUR will have hydronephrosis and deranged renal function.

2. **What is a high-risk CUR?**

   Ans: CUR patients who have a high potential for upper tract damage are high-risk CUR. These patients have high-pressure CUR.

Factors important for high-risk CUR:

- Presence of bilateral hydronephrosis and hydroureter
- May have bladder stones
- Elevated creatinine with reduced eGFR (45–59 ml/min/1.73 m^2 or lower.)
- Recurrent symptomatic UTIs

3. **How would these patients present clinically?**

Ans: Clinically CUR may present as lower urinary tract symptoms (LUTS) in the form of poor flow, intermittency, straining, dribbling (overflow Incontinence), urgency, urge incontinence, nocturia, and bed wetting. In patients who have developed renal insufficiency and electrolyte imbalance due to backpressure hydronephrosis and hydroureter can also present with altered sensorium or irritability. Physical examination would reveal palpable bladder. The external genitalia may show phimosis or meatal stenosis. There might be some stigmata of urethral stricture. Digital rectal examination (DRE) may reveal enlarged prostate and in some patients with neurological cause the anal tone and perianal sensations may be impaired. DRE may also reveal faecoliths in some cases as constipation can be a precipitating factor for CUR.

4. **What Investigations would you offer?**

Ans:

- Routine blood investigation: Complete blood count, serum creatinine, electrolytes (sodium, potassium), blood urea, urine routine and microscopy and urine culture.
- Ultrasound to see for upper tract hydronephrosis, bladder assessment, measure pre-void and post-void residue, prostate size any debris or stones in bladder.
- In this index patient initial evaluation revealed: Haemoglobin: 11.02 gm%; TLC: 10,100; polymorph: 79%; Lymphocytes: 18%; Platelets: 2,42,000, Creatinine: 2.7 mg/dl; Blood urea: 69; Na: 137 mEq/L; K: 3.7 mEq/L; Urine routine pus cell: 6–8/hpf
- Abdominal ultrasound: Severe enlargement of prostate with enlarged median lobe with intravesical protrusion: Prostate volume 92 ml; Pre-void volume: 1032; and Postvoid 642 cc, moderate bilateral hydronephrosis and hydroureter (Fig. 16.1).

5. **Why should we check blood urea levels?**

Ans: It helps in management of dehydration and post-obstructive diuresis (details below)

6. **How will you manage this case?**

Ans: The immediate goals are initial assessment, bladder drainage, management of electrolyte disturbance (if present) and management of urinary tract infection.

This patient was catheterized with 16 Fr Foley. Slow decompression of urine was done by hanging the urine bag at higher level and gradually lowering it down. Slowly two-litre urine was drained. He had mild haematuria. Volume correction was done with 0.9% NaCl.

7. **Why do you do slow decompression? What is the logic behind this?**

Ans: Traditionally CUR is being drained gradually with the worry that fast decompression of overfilled bladder may lead to haematuria. Sudden filling of the compressed vessels leading to renal and bladder bleeding is the presumed mechanism. After rapid decompression of the bladder haematuria occurs in 2–16% of patients.[6] It is not clinically significant and not life threatening. But it is still haematuria and would add to the anxiety of the patient. Anecdotal case report of significant bilateral upper tract haematuria following drainage high pressure chronic retention and patient landing in oliguria is reported in literature.[7] However, the methods to decompress bladder gradually are labour intensive and of unproven benefit. Published methods of slow decompression are quite variable from initial release of 500 ml followed by clamping and hourly release of 100–150 ml to clamping after 750 ml or so.[8] In a randomized trial of rapid vs gradual decompression of bladder[8] no statistically significant differences were found with regard to haematuria and circulatory collapse. The process of slow decompression of CRU is of unproven benefit.

8. **What will you prefer perurethral catheterization or suprapubic catheterization?**

Ans: The outcomes with both the catheter is same except that if catheter is expected for longer term, suprapubic could be preferred although the literature does not confirm reduced morbidity with suprapubic catheter.[9]

9. **What is post-obstructive diuresis (POD)?**

Ans: Post-obstructive diuresis (POD) is a polyuric response by the kidneys after relief of urinary retention or similar obstructive uropathy.[10] Copious amounts of salt and water are excreted by the kidneys after relief of obstruction as a normal response. The reported incidence varies from 0.5% to 52%.[11] In POD excess volume and solutes are excreted. Urine output (UOP) after decompression >200 ml/hr for two consecutive hours or >3000 ml in 24 hours is diagnostic of POD.[11]

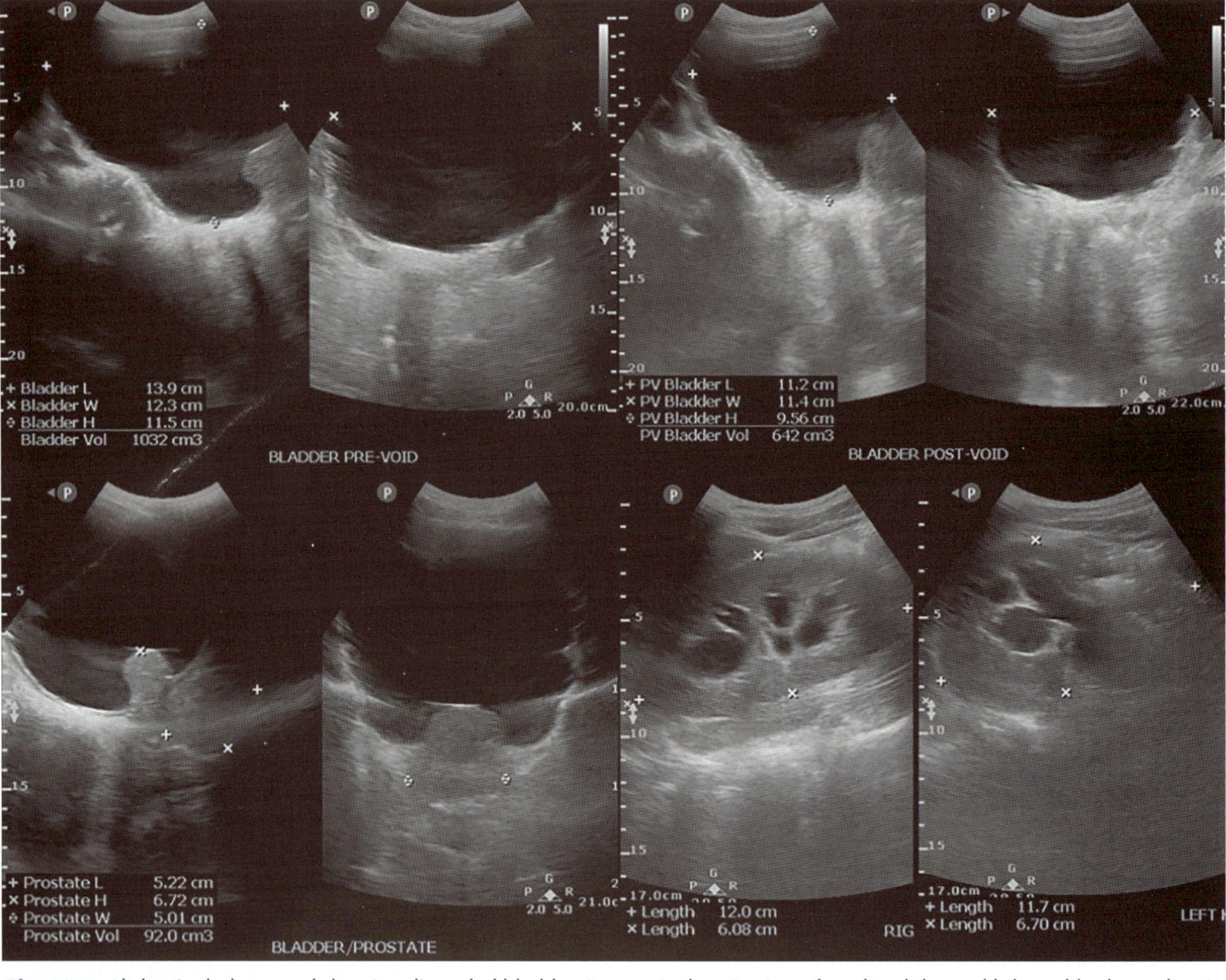

Fig. 16.1: Abdominal ultrasound showing distended bladder, intravesical projection of median lobe and bilateral hydronephrosis

10. What is physiological POD and pathological POD?

Ans: Mostly POD is self-limiting and physiological and goes away once the volume and solute status is restored. It usually resolves in 24 hours. However, in some patients, the salt and water loss continues and then it is called pathological POD. The complications of pathological POD are severe dehydration, electrolyte imbalance, hypovolemic shock and even death. Pathologic POD lasts for >48 hours. It can be exacerbated by excessive IV fluids.[11]

11. How would you manage volume correction in POD?

Ans: Harrrison *et al.* have given detailed outline for management of POD.[10]

In patients with altered sensorium, saline is perfused as per daily requirement and diuresis is to be compensated only in case of hypovolemia and dehydration. One should avoid aggravating the dehydration. Whereas a conscious patient who can drink, oral fluids should be encouraged as per thirst and if required, intravenous fluids may be supplemented. If the patients drink according to thirst, they themselves adjust their fluid balance and natremia. Blood urea levels and urine specific gravity aid in monitoring the adequacy of hydration. If the patients has sodium overload, the fluids need to be curtailed to 75% on second day and still further on the third day. The polyuria takes care of sodium overload by excreting excess sodium.

12. What are the risks in management of POD?

Ans: Inadequate fluid and electrolyte correction would cause intracellular dehydration. This usually happens if the urine output is not adequately monitored and underestimated or if patient has fluid loss because of vomiting, haemorrhage, or inadequate oral intake. On the contrary excess fluid and electrolyte correction would lead to prolonged polyuria.

13. **Would you consider a voiding trial in CUR? What further evaluation would you plan after stabilizing the patient? When?**

Ans: One of the primary CUR outcomes as recommended by the AUA CUR workgroup is successful trial of voiding without catheter (TWOC).[2] Individuals with low residual volume can be offered TWOC.[12] If TWOC is planned, uroflowmetry should be done. It is usually suggested that for uroflowmetry to be representative patient should void minimum 150 ml urine. [13–15]

14. **What about urodynamics? When?**

Ans: As CUR can cause impairment of detrusor function, urodynamic study (UDS) is usually done at least 6 weeks post-catheterization. By 6 weeks most of the patient who initially have impaired detrusor contractility, will have improvement in detrusor contraction.[16] In addition, by this time usually infection and electrolyte imbalance are also taken care of.

15. **How do you decide when to do UDS? Elaborate on the clinical signs of return of detrusor function.**

Ans: Traditionally bladder spasms indicated by pericatheteric urine leak or desire to void urine despite catheter is considered as the sign of recovery of bladder function. But evidence supporting this practice is lacking. The term "bladder spasm" is difficult to define and it is proposed not to use this term in relation to LUTS.[17]

16. **What information will you look for in UDS study? How will UDS triage patients?**

Ans: Urodynamic gives us status of detrusor contractility, detrusor underactivity (DUA), involuntary detrusor contraction (IDC); presence of bladder outlet obstruction, compliance, sensation, bladder capacity and postvoid residue. The important differentiating criteria is P_{det} at Q_{max} (detrusor pressure at peak flow rate). P_{det} at Q_{max} >30 cm H_2O is considered preserved detrusor function and P_{det} at Q_{max} < 30 cm H_2O is considered as impaired detrusor contractility.[18,19]

17. **His UDS was done after four weeks. The tracing is given here. Can you elaborate on the UDS of this patient?**

Ans: During the filling stage, bladder compliance is normal. There are no involuntary detrusor contractions. In the voiding phase, the detrusor pressure is seen rising to 150 cm H_2O. The pressure is fairly sustained. Patient is voiding urine with poor flow. Bladder outlet is urodynamically obstructed and detrusor contractions are good. The UDS tracing is suggestive of bladder outlet obstruction (Fig. 16.2A to C).

18. **What is bladder contractility index and bladder outlet obstruction index?**

Ans: The physiology of bladder contractions and LUTS is complex. Bladder contractility index (BCI)

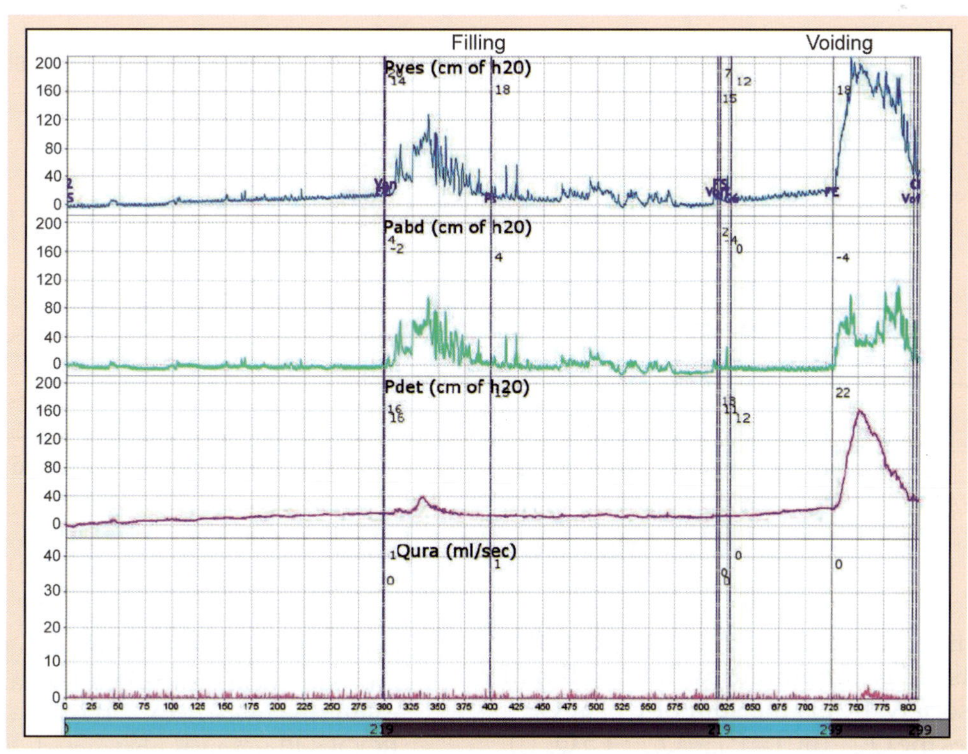

Fig. 16.2A: Urodynamics

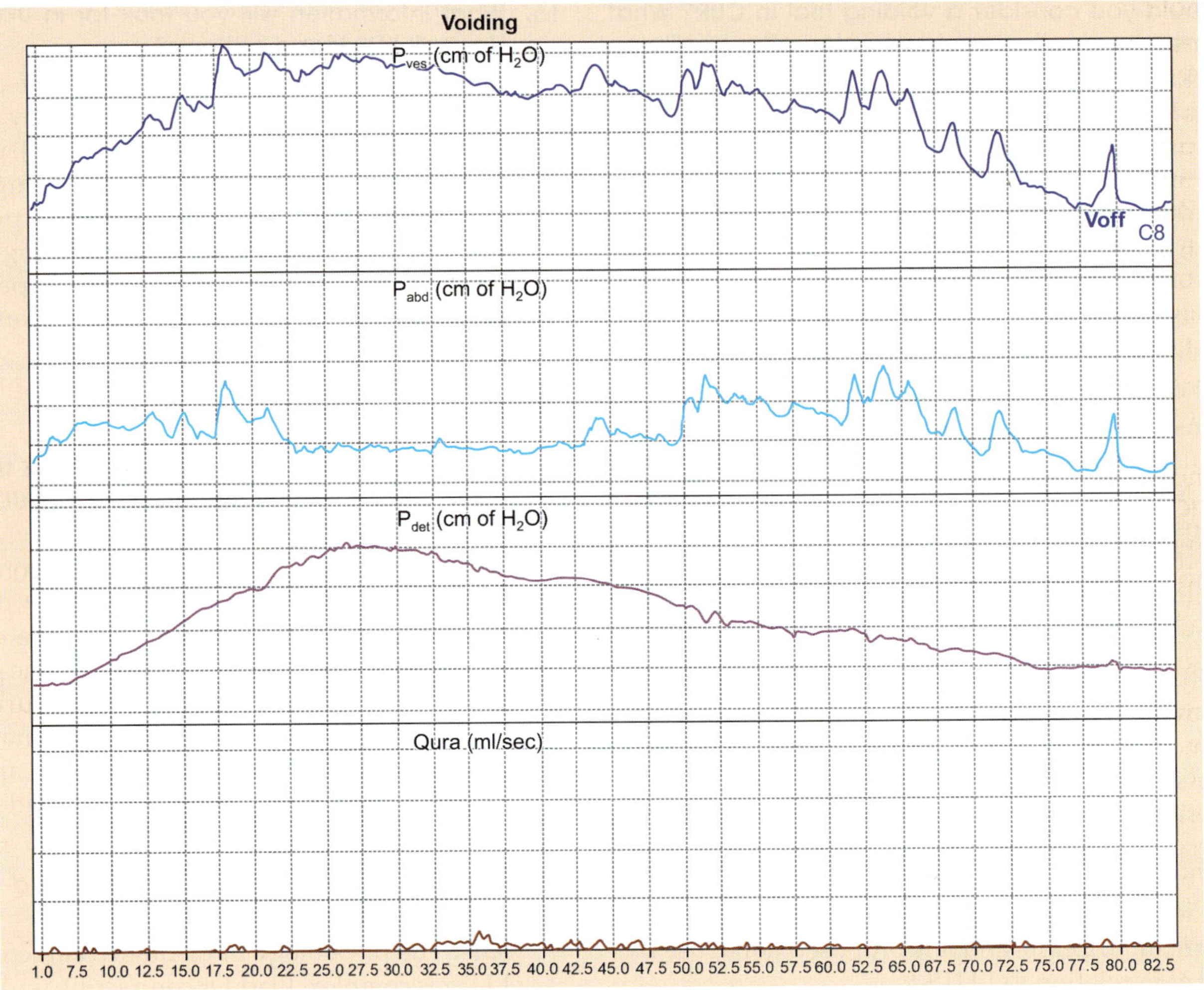

Fig. 16.2B: UDS voiding

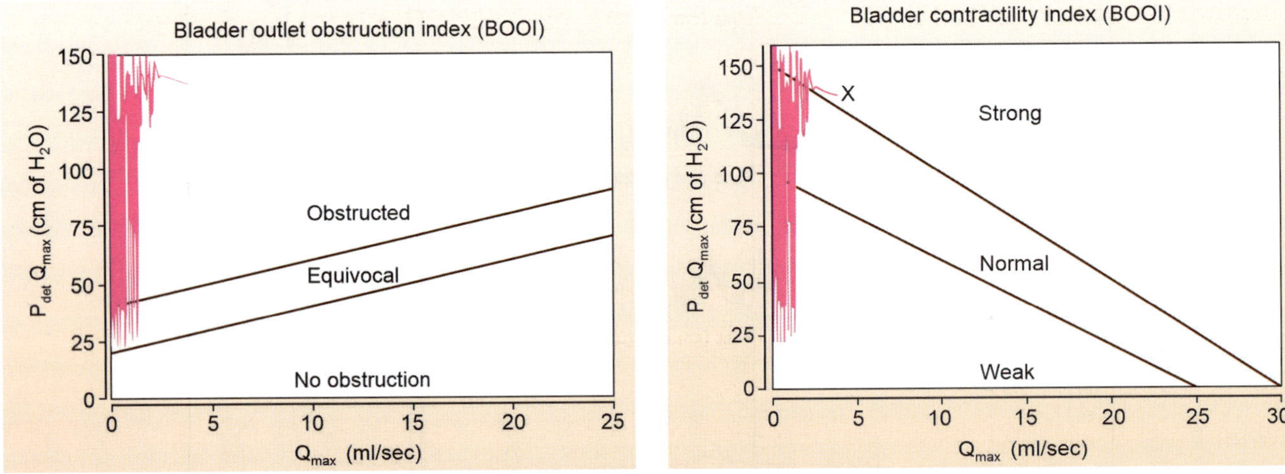

Fig. 16.2C: UDS: BOOI, BCI

is the objective measure of strength of bladder contractions. It is promoted by international continence society. BCI is the sum of P_{det} at Q_{max} and five times the Q_{max} ($BCI = P_{det}@Q_{max} + 5\,Q_{max}$). Bladder outlet obstruction index (BOOI) helps us divide the patients in obstructed, unobstructed and equivocal group. BOOI is calculated $P_{det}@Q_{max}$ minus the twice of Q_{max} ($BOOI = P_{det}@Q_{max} - 2Q_{max}$). BOOI >40 suggests obstructed, 20–40 equivocal and <20 unobstructed.[20]

19. What are the goals of definitive treatment in CUR?

Ans: To improve symptoms and quality of life[21]

- Reduce the risk for complications of impaired bladder emptying (like UTI, bladder stones, ureteric reflux leading to back-pressure on the upper urinary tract, and local skin excoriation due to incontinence)
- Effective treatments to improve detrusor function facilitating bladder emptying are not available.

Management strategies usually aim at bladder drainage techniques (e.g., catheterization/SPC/CIC) or reducing bladder outlet resistance.[21]

20. What is the role of clean-self intermittent catheter (CIC)?

Ans: CIC is useful for dedicated patients with good hand-and-eye coordination with low-risk CUR. The distinct advantages are significantly reduced pain and difficulty of carrying a urethral catheter with a bag, reduced risk of infection, reduced risk of stricture and maintained sexual function. CIC could also be performed for CUR in high-risk patients once the upper tract function is stabilized.[2]

21. What outcome can we expect with bladder outlet surgery?

Ans: A recent meta-analysis assessing a total of 10 comparative studies assessing transurethral bladder outlet surgery found that those with DUA had significantly poorer improvement in I-PSS (International Prostate Symptom Score) and maximal flow rate in comparison with patients who had preserved contractility.[22] Both groups showed similar changes in quality-of-life score, and PVR volumes were equivalent. Although the limited evidence suggests men with DUA and chronic retention do less favourably after bladder outlet surgery,[23] a significant proportion resume spontaneous voiding.[24] In the absence of any other effective treatments, some advocate surgery in the younger, medically fit patient who wishes to become catheter free. Outlet surgery can also help clear the tract and ease CIC after surgery if contemplated.

22. What is the role of Bethanechol in low pressure CUR?

Ans: Bethanechol is a parasympathomimetic agent commonly used to treat postoperative urinary retention and postpartum urinary retention. It is also used in non-obstructive urinary retention. However, as far as its role in detrusor underactivity is concerned, no definite benefit has been observed in an extensive literature search.[25]

23. Had this patient been a female, would you consider urethral dilatation or bladder neck resection?

Ans: The use of urethral dilation for women with DUA and significant residual urine has been advocated but lacks an adequate evidence base to permit clear conclusions to be drawn.[26] Resection or incision of the bladder neck in women with DUA is not recommended, because this may lead to significant problems with either incontinence or bladder neck stenosis.

24. When would you schedule a bladder outlet surgery?

Ans: It is suggested that one should wait till six weeks or beyond for TURP after initial catheterization in these patients because the early operation may not help to improve symptoms.[16]

25. Would you consider resection or enucleation for prostate?

Ans: Since the early experience with HoLEP, it was known, that although clinically not significant, the improvements in urodynamic parameters are better with enucleation than with resection procedures.[27] This led to a lot of studies showing good results of HoLEP in patients with BOO and underactive detrusor irrespective of the technical approach.[28]

26. What about this patient: Resection or enucleation?

Ans: He has a 92 gram prostate as per ultrasound. I would prefer doing his endoscopic enucleation of his prostate with laser (Fig. 16.3).

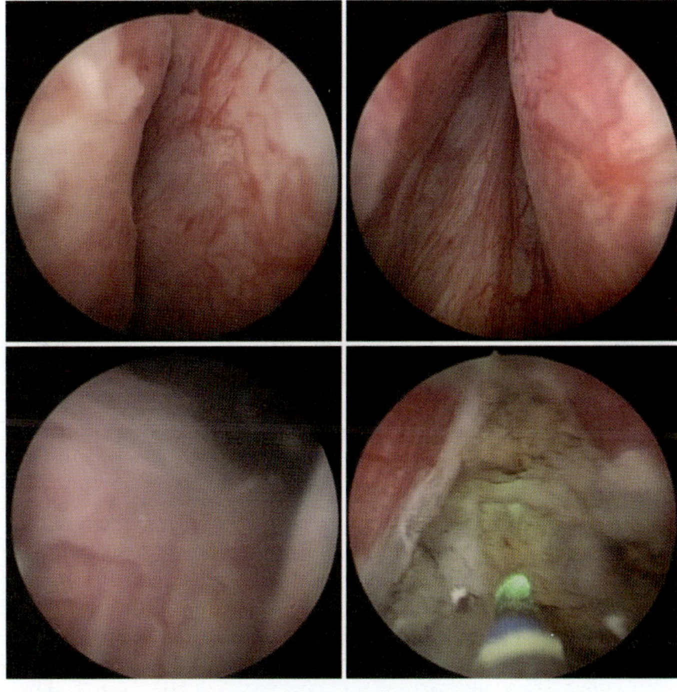

Fig. 16.3: Endoscopic enucleation of prostate

27. What is new in this field?

Ans: It is proposed that the underlying mechanism for detrusor dysfunction in these patients is due to detrusor ischemia and partial denervation. TAC-302 is a novel drug which promotes neurite outgrowth. Phase 2 trial of this molecule showed improvements in bladder contractility index and bladder voiding efficiency.[29] ASP-8302 is a positive allosteric modulator of M3 receptor. In preclinical study it has shown improvement in bladder muscle contractility.[30] Intradetrusor injection of adult muscle-derived cells have shown decreased post-void residual urine volume, increased voiding efficiency, and decreased catheter use in patients with underactive bladder.[31] In addition, sacral neuromodulation[32] and stem cell therapy[33] may hold promising role in future.

Management plan is outlined in Flowchart 16.1.

Flowchart 16.1: Management of chronic retention of urine

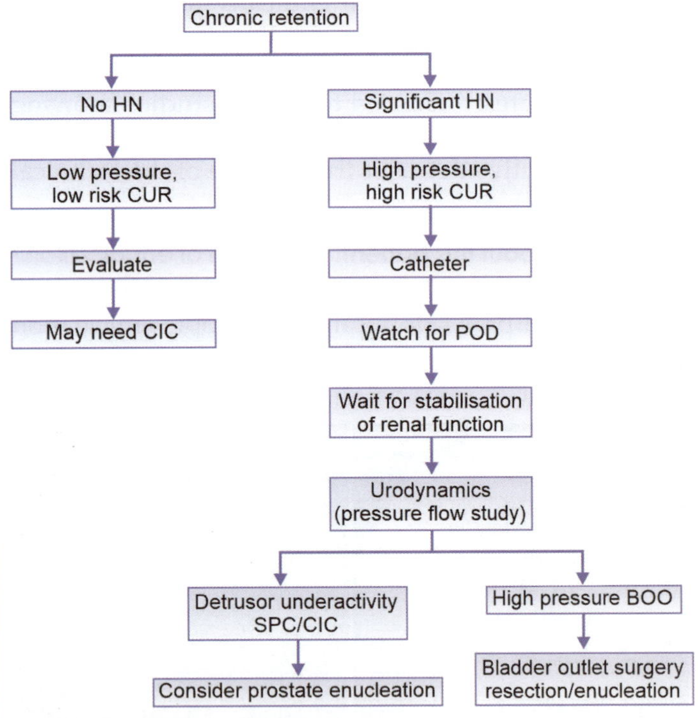

ACKNOWLEDGEMENTS

The authors wish to acknowledge the help received from Dr Sadanand Bhusari, senior nephrologist, Akola in preparation of this manuscript.

SUMMARY

- Chronic urinary retention (CUR) is a non-painful palpable bladder with high residual urine. It is usually classified as low pressure and high pressure. High pressure CRU has risk of upper urinary tract dysfunction. Initial management consists of draining the bladder and effective fluid and electrolyte management. Further evaluation is usually delayed for 2–6 weeks. Urodynamics forms the mainstay in evaluation of CUR. There is no effective medical treatment for management of underactive detrusor. Surgical treatment albeit with sub-optimal outcomes can be offered to some patients with mechanical bladder outlet obstruction. Newer molecules are being evaluated for management of underactive detrusor and may hold promise in future.

REFERENCES

1. Abrams P, Cardozo L, Fall M, Griffiths D, Rosier P, Ulmsten U, *et al*. The standardisation of terminology in lower urinary tract function: report from the standardisation sub-committee of the International Continence Society. Urology. 2003 Jan;61(1):37–49.
2. Stoffel JT, Peterson AC, Sandhu JS, Suskind AM, Wei JT, Lightner DJ. AUA White Paper on Nonneurogenic Chronic Urinary Retention: Consensus Definition, Treatment Algorithm, and Outcome End Points. J Urol. 2017 Jul;198(1):153–60.
3. Abrams PH, Dunn M, George N. Urodynamic findings in chronic retention of urine and their relevance to results of surgery. Br Med J. 1978;2(6147):1258–60.
4. Djavan B, Madersbacher S, Klingler C, Marberger M. Urodynamic assessment of patients with acute urinary retention: is treatment failure after prostatectomy predictable? J Urol. 1997 Nov;158(5):1829–33.
5. George NJ, O'Reilly PH, Barnard RJ, Blacklock NJ. High pressure chronic retention. BMJ. 1983 Jun 4;286(6380):1780–3.
6. Nyman MA, Schwenk NM, Silverstein MD. Management of urinary retention: rapid versus gradual decompression and risk of complications. In: Mayo Clinic Proceedings. Elsevier; 1997. p. 951–6.
7. Naranji I, Bolgeri M. Significant upper urinary tract hematuria as a rare complication of high-pressure chronic retention of urine following decompression: a case report. J Med Case Reports. 2012;6:1–3.
8. Boettcher S, Brandt A, Roth S, Mathers M, Lazica D. Urinary retention: benefit of gradual bladder decompression-myth or truth? A randomized controlled trial. Urol Int. 2013;91(2):140–4.
9. Hunter KF, Bharmal A, Moore KN. Long-term bladder drainage: Suprapubic catheter versus other methods: a scoping review. Neurourol Urodyn. 2013 Sep;32(7):944–51.
10. Harrison S, Lasri A, Jabbour Y, Slaoui A, Djamal J, Karmouni T, *et al*. Post-Obstructive Diuresis: Physiopathology, Diagnosis and Management after Urological Treatment of Obstructive Renal Failure. Open J Urol. 2018;08(09):267–74.
11. Halbgewachs C, Domes T. Postobstructive diuresis: pay close attention to urinary retention. Can Fam Physician. 2015;61(2):137–42.
12. TeachMeSurgery [Internet]. [cited 2023 Aug 7]. Chronic Urinary Retention-Clinical Features-Management. Available from: https://teachmesurgery.com/urology/presentations/chronic-urinary-retention/
13. Garcia-Mora A, Ismail M, Hashim H, Abrams P. 2274 should patients have one or two uroflows, that is the question? J Urol [Internet]. 2013 Apr [cited 2023 Apr 16];189(4S). Available from: http://www.jurology.com/doi/10.1016/j.juro.2013.02.2203.
14. Rosier PFWM, Schaefer W, Lose G, Goldman HB, Guralnick M, Eustice S, *et al*. International Continence Society Good Urodynamic Practices and Terms 2016: Urodynamics, uroflowmetry, cystometry, and pressure-flow study. Neurourol Urodyn. 2017 Jun;36(5):1243–60.

15. Reynard JM, Peters TJ, Lim C, Abrams P. The value of multiple free-flow studies in men with lower urinary tract symptoms. Br J Urol. 1996 Jun;77(6):813–8.
16. Atar KM, Maiti K, Pal DK. Ideal Timing of Prostate Operation in Chronic Urinary Retention due to Benign Prostatic Hyperplasia by Serial Urodynamic Study: A Prospective Longitudinal Study. J Clin Diagn Res [Internet]. 2022 [cited 2023 Apr 16]; Available from: https://www.jcdr.net//article_fulltext.asp?issn=0973–709x&year=2022&month=November&volume=16&issue=11&page=PC11–PC14&id=17172
17. Abrams P. Urodynamics [Internet]. 3rd ed. London: Springer, London; 2006. Available from: DOI https://doi.org/10.1007/1–84628–129–6
18. Osman NI, Chapple CR, Abrams P, Dmochowski R, Haab F, Nitti V, *et al*. Detrusor underactivity and the underactive bladder: a new clinical entity? A review of current terminology, definitions, epidemiology, aetiology, and diagnosis. Eur Urol. 2014;65(2):389–98.
19. Abarbanel J, Marcus EL. Impaired detrusor contractility in community-dwelling elderly presenting with lower urinary tract symptoms. Urology. 2007;69(3):436–40.
20. Abrams P. Bladder outlet obstruction index, bladder contractility index and bladder voiding efficiency: three simple indices to define bladder voiding function. BJU Int. 1999;84:14–5.
21. Brasure M, Fink HA, Risk M, MacDonald R, Shamliyan T, Ouellette J, *et al*. Chronic urinary retention: comparative effectiveness and harms of treatments. 2014.
22. Kim M, Jeong CW, Oh SJ. Effect of Preoperative Urodynamic Detrusor Underactivity on Transurethral Surgery for Benign Prostatic Hyperplasia: A Systematic Review and Meta-Analysis. J Urol. 2018 Jan;199(1):237–44.
23. Ghalayini IF, Al-Ghazo MA, Pickard RS. A prospective randomized trial comparing transurethral prostatic resection and clean intermittent self-catheterization in men with chronic urinary retention. BJU Int. 2005 Jul;96(1):93–7.
24. Monoski MA, Gonzalez RR, Sandhu JS, Reddy B, Te AE. Urodynamic predictors of outcomes with photoselective laser vaporization prostatectomy in patients with benign prostatic hyperplasia and preoperative retention. Urology. 2006 Aug;68(2):312–7.
25. Krishnamoorthy S, Kekre NS. Detrusor underactivity: To tone or not to tone the bladder? Indian J Urol IJU J Urol Soc India. 2009;25(3):407.
26. Basu M, Duckett JRA. Effect of Urethral Dilatation on Women With Voiding Dysfunction. Curr Bladder Dysfunct Rep. 2010 Mar;5(1):23–6.
27. Gilling PJ, Mackey M, Cresswell M, Kennett K, Kabalin JN, Fraundorfer Mr. Holmium laser versus transurethral resection of the prostate: a randomized prospective trial with 1-year followup. J Urol. 1999;162(5):1640–4.
28. Cho MC, Yoo S, Park J, Cho SY, Son H, Oh SJ, *et al*. Effect of preoperative detrusor underactivity on long-term surgical outcomes of photovaporization and holmium laser enucleation in men with benign prostatic hyperplasia: a lesson from 5-year serial follow-up data. BJU Int. 2019;123(5A):E34–42.
29. Yoshida M, Gotoh M, Yokoyama O, Kakizaki H, Yamanishi T, Yamaguchi O. Efficacy of TAC-302 for patients with detrusor underactivity and overactive bladder: a randomized, double-blind, placebo-controlled phase 2 study. World J Urol. 2022;40(11):2799–805.
30. Okimoto R, Ino K, Ishizu K, Takamatsu H, Sakamoto K, Yuyama H, *et al*. Potentiation of muscarinic M3 receptor activation through a new allosteric site with a novel positive allosteric modulator ASP8302. J Pharmacol Exp Ther. 2021;379(1):64–73.
31. Gilleran J, Diokno AC, Ward E, Sirls L, Hasenau D, Giordano J, *et al*. Improved global response outcome after intradetrusor injection of adult muscle-derived cells for the treatment of underactive bladder. Int Urol Nephrol. 2021;53:1331–8.
32. Gupta P, Ehlert MJ, Sirls LT, Peters KM. Percutaneous tibial nerve stimulation and sacral neuromodulation: an update. Curr Urol Rep. 2015;16:1–6.
33. Shin JH, Ryu CM, Yu HY, Shin DM, Choo MS. Current and future directions of stem cell therapy for bladder dysfunction. Stem Cell Rev Rep. 2020;16:82–93.

Chapter
17

Clot Retention

• *Ashish V Rawandale-Patil* • *Lokesh Patni*

LEARNING OBJECTIVES

- Understand the aetiology of clot retention.
- Preliminary evaluation and investigations and plan for further management.
- Armamentarium for management of clot retention.
- Manual clot evacuation.
- Clot evacuation under anaesthesia.
- Preventive measures for recurrent clot formation and precautions to be taken intraoperatively to avoid post-operative haemorrhage.

INTRODUCTION

Clot retention is a common urological emergency. Around 4% of the patients presenting for urologic emergency have gross hematuria.[1] An episode of gross haematuria for a longer duration may lead to formation of clots in the bladder and if the patient is unable to pass the clots, it may give rise to acute urinary retention. Clot retention can present with tachycardia, hypertension, painful bladder spasms. If left unattended, it may further aggravate haemorrhage, cause bladder rupture and perforation.[2] Management of larger clots require intervention. Following are some case scenarios.

Case Scenario

50 years old male known smoker with diabetes mellitus type II on medications presents with history of gross haematuria with large clots off and on for three weeks with frequency, urgency and inability to void. He is vitally stable but has distended bladder palpable up to umbilicus with mild suprapubic tenderness.

Aetiology: Clot retention can occur in the following conditions:

- Carcinoma bladder
- Post-TURP/TURBT/ HoLEP/ PCNL
- UTUC or renal tumours
- Urological trauma
- Antiplatelets/anticoagulants
- Recurrent urinary tract infection (UTI)
- Post-radiotherapy: Actinic cystitis/ haemorrhagic cystitis

1. **What is the plan of management?**

   Ans: The patient appears to be in acute retention of urine. The history of haematuria indicates a possibility of clot retention. It is important to elicit history of trauma, instrumentation, medications including blood thinners, previous history of recurrent urinary tract infection (UTI) or radiotherapy.

Vesical mass: On ultrasound vesical mass appears as an intraluminal nonmobile mass or localized thickened bladder wall. Doppler ultrasound shows flow within the mass which distinguish the tumour from a blood clot.

Initial evaluation would include stabilising the hemodynamics of the patient. Assessment in the form of complete blood count, renal function test, blood grouping (and cross matching if required), bleeding time, clotting time, prothrombin time with international normalised ratio (INR).

An ultrasound helps in diagnosis. The findings of an overdistended bladder with clots in the lumen with no activity on colour Doppler throughout the lesion is diagnostic. Additional information regarding prostatic size, condition of the upper tracts, presence of any mass or hydronephrosis can be obtained. One should also look for presence of any free fluid in the abdominal cavity (in case of trauma, associated hepatic dysfunction) (Figs 17.1 and 17.2).

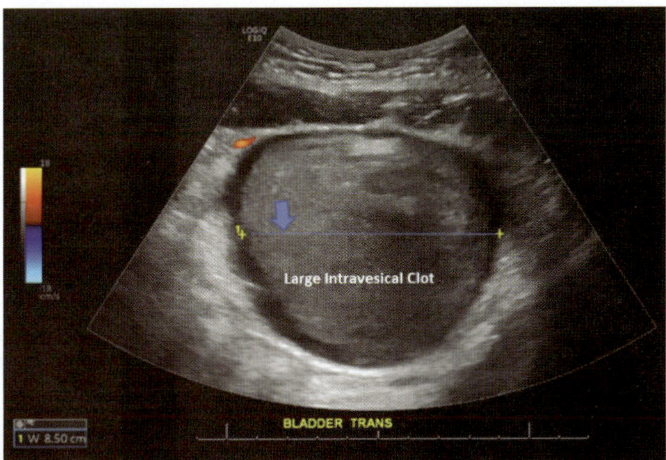

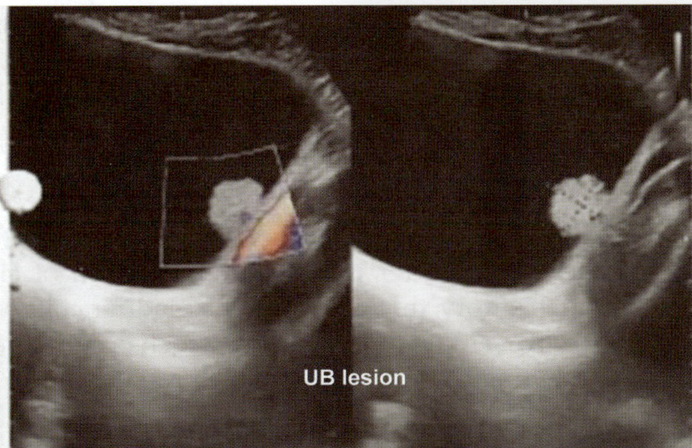

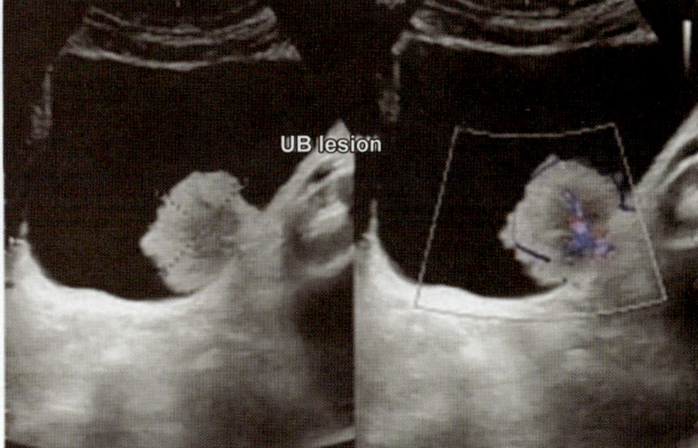

Fig. 17.1: Clots: Blood clots in the urinary bladder are seen as echogenic masses without acoustic shadow. There is no visible blood flow in the Doppler examination. The smaller clots usually move when the patient changes position. Large blood clots are oval and may occupy the entire lumen of the bladder.[3]

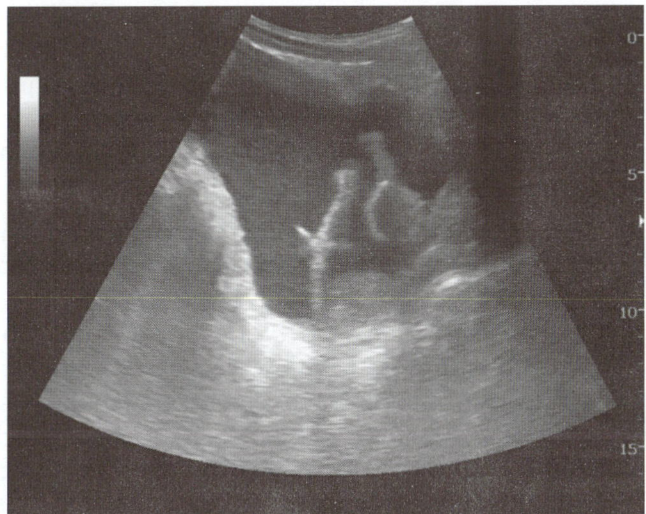

Fig. 17.2: Intra-abdominal fluid with extraperitoneal rupture of bladder

2. **The patient is found to have clot retention with a vesical mass 3 × 3 cm at the posterior wall of the bladder. What would be the next step in management?**

Ans: As the patient is otherwise stable with acute urinary retention, an attempt for catheterisation and evacuation of the clots, i.e. manual bladder wash (MBW) should be attempted. Once the retention is relieved, the patient would be evaluated for further management.

3. **What equipment is required for MBW?**

Manual bladder wash is to be considered in patients with bigger clots that are not amenable for simple manoeuvres like aspiration using a 50 cc/20 cc syringe attached to a Foley's adapter or pinching the catheter and/or the urine bag tubing. Manual bladder wash should be performed in a clean preferably sterile area following universal precautions.

Requirements: Large bore catheter about 20–22 Fr, preferably two way and three way in case as we may require continuous bladder irrigation later or Nelaton's catheter.[4] Sterile normal saline for wash at least 5 litres in case continuous irrigation is contemplated.

Foley's adapter: It is a useful attachment that fits the drainage channel of any catheter and makes the irrigation and aspiration easy and less messy. It has a wide central channel and larger diameter than the commercially available catheter adapters.

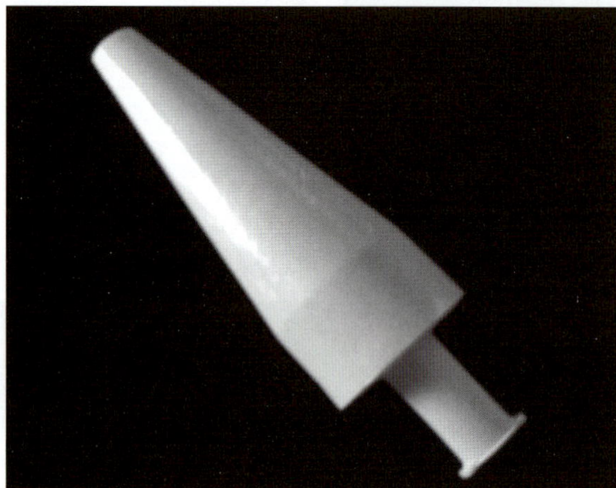

Fig. 17.3: Mega Foley's adapter

4. **What is CATCH-22 protocol?**

Clarebrough et. al. in 2018 proposed a standardized protocol for manual bladder wash which is summarized with the acronym **'CATCH–22'**.[5]

As per the recommendations of the group blood thinners if any should be stopped if possible. Based on the coagulation profile reversal may also be considered. Restarting of antiplatelets can be considered once the haematuria is controlled.

C :	Catheter type and size–A minimum 22 F catheter—upsized, if necessary
A :	Aseptic technique, analgesia, antibiotics
T :	Twisting/catheter manipulation: Catheter manipulation throughout washout Deflation of balloon and retraction of indwelling catheter to clear bladder neck.
C :	**Clot + 1 L rule:** A minimum of 1 L sterile saline washout following the last clot passed.
H :	Help: Have assistance nearby.
22 :	Consider at least a 22 F catheter on initial.

MBW should be done in a clean area using at least a 22 Fr catheter. The procedure should follow the techniques of asepsis. For complete clearance of the clots the catheter could be twisted in all directions to clear the clots from all parts of the bladder. To clear the bladder neck the balloon of the catheter is deflated and the catheter is withdrawn into the bladder neck for better irrigation and aspiration of the region. Around five litres of irrigation fluid should be available. Once the last clot is cleared, i.e. when the urine becomes clear then the bladder wash is continued till at least one litre of saline more is used to ascertain complete clearance of the clots. Assistance should be available in case one need extra equipment or irrigation fluid.

5. **Is there any role of antibiotics?**

Ans: Prophylactic antibiotics should be considered in patients as 80% of nosocomial urinary tract infections are catheter related and repeated instrumentation and the process of a bladder washout also confer an increased risk of introducing microorganisms into the urinary tract.[5]

6. **What about irrigation?**

Ans: Continuous bladder irrigation (CBI) is considered in cases with risk of recurrent haematuria or clot formation. CBI is preferably done using sterile normal saline attached through an intravenous line via a Foley's adapter to the irrigation channel of the three-way catheter. The rate of fluid going in is determined by the colour of fluid coming out, the aim of the irrigation is to keep outflow just clear or light pink in colour (grade I or II)[6] as shown in Fig. 17.4. CBI should be started once the bladder is completely cleared of clots and is empty, this will keep the bladder collapsed and prevent further bleeding which occurs due to stretching of the bladder wall.[5]

7. **In case irrigation is to be given what should be the speed of irrigant?**

Ans: The speed of irrigation should depend upon the color of the returning fluid from the catheter. The irrigation speed should be adjusted so that the irrigant returning from the catheter is light pink in color. At the same time it needs to be observed continuously if the returning fluid is continuously dropping into the urine bag. In case the returning fluid stops, one should check for catheter block and take a decision on the irrigation speed as required.

8. **What is the role of cystoscopy for clot evacuation? What are the other methods described for evacuation of clot during cystoscopy?**

Ans: Large, organized blood clots within the bladder causing urinary retention that are refractory to classic management techniques pose a significant challenge to the surgeon. Clots which are not amenable to aspiration irrigation via a large bore catheter can be managed in the following ways:

- Cystoscopy and aspiration under anaesthesia using a large sheath 25/26 Fr sheath can be attempted. For aspiration Toomey's syringe or Elick's evacuator can be used. Main advantage being complete evacuation of the clots under vision and simultaneous haemostasis of the bleeding point if any found during cystoscopy. Resection of the clots using the TURP loop may

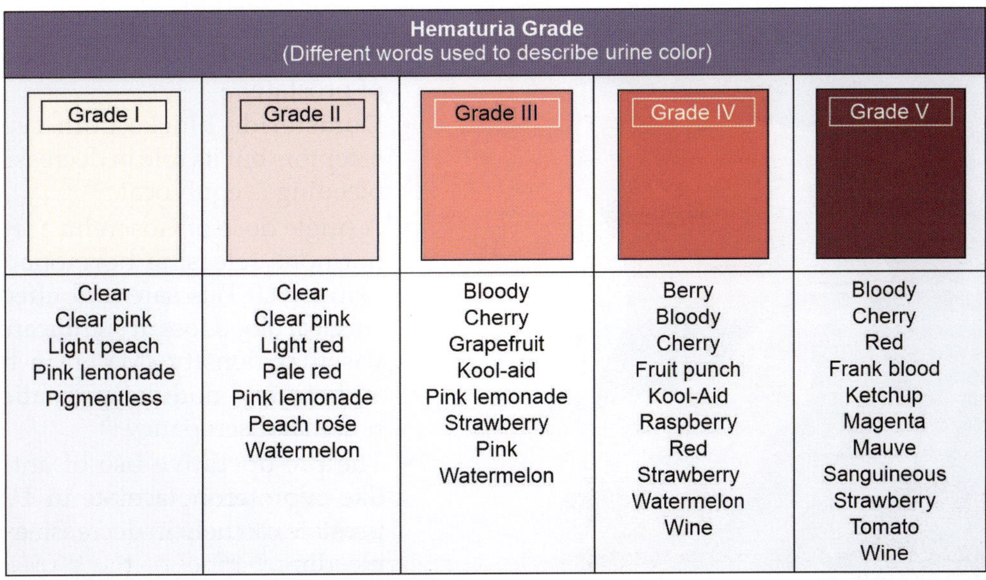

Hematuria Grade
(Different words used to describe urine color)

Grade I	Grade II	Grade III	Grade IV	Grade V
Clear Clear pink Light peach Pink lemonade Pigmentless	Clear Clear pink Light red Pale red Pink lemonade Peach rośe Watermelon	Bloody Cherry Grapefruit Kool-aid Pink lemonade Strawberry Pink Watermelon	Berry Bloody Cherry Fruit punch Kool-Aid Raspberry Red Strawberry Watermelon Wine	Bloody Cherry Red Frank blood Ketchup Magenta Mauve Sanguineous Strawberry Tomato Wine

Fig. 17.4: Hematuria grade

be required in case the clots are organised and not amenable to aspiration (Fig. 17.5).

- Another option is morcellation of the clot using a commercially available HoLEP morcellator.[7]
- Use of hydrogen peroxide,[8] intravesical streptokinase, alteplase—a tissue plasminogen activator[9] have also been described.
- Some authors have described the use of mechanical suction for effective clot evacuation.[10,11]

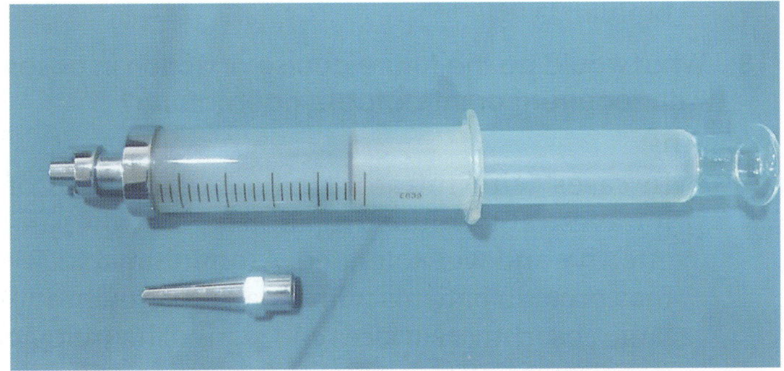

Fig. 17.5: Toomey's syringe with adapter

9. While shifting the patient from the operating room to the ward what are the precautions to be taken?

Ans: It is necessary that the patient is shifted under strict supervision, one should try not to stop the irrigation during the shifting process, for the same the irrigation fluid should be suspended and the urine bag should be placed below the level of the pubic symphysis or attached to the shifting trolley during the whole shifting process. One should continuously observe whether the efflux is coming out into the urine bag.

10. When you apply traction to the Foley's catheter in these cases?

Ans: Traction should be applied only when the bleeding appears to be from the bladder neck and the prostate.[12] Though it is not necessary to apply traction in every such case.

11. You have two options 20 cc and 50 cc. Which syringe would work the best?

Ans: As per authors' personal experience it is easy to apply suction and push irrigation through a 20 cc syringe as it can be easily held in the surgeons' hands and is easily manoeuvrable as compared to a 50 cc syringe.

12. You have all the evacuation devices like Toomey syringe, Elick's evacuator, etc available. Which one would you prefer?

Ans: As per authors' personal experience it is easier to aspirate and push through a Toomey syringe and hence it would be the preferred instrument for clot evacuation through a cystoscope.

13. What is the clue you get from the colour of the irrigation fluid coming out of the catheter?

Ans: One should look at the colour of the returning fluid and categorise it as bright red—arterial, deep red—venous, or dark brown to black—collected liquifying clot.

14. How will you pinch the catheter in case the catheter is blocked?

Ans: Hold the tube of the urine bag so that you have a free 10 cm of segment. Fold this segment at the centre of this segment. Hold both the segments using the first 3 fingers and the thumb of each hand as shown in Fig. 17.6. Pinch the tube using

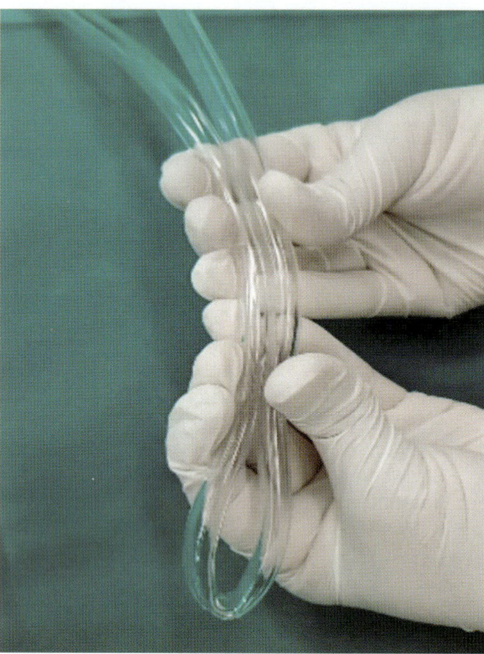

Fig. 17.6: ??

all the six fingers and the thumbs. This manoeuvre would displace a large column of fluid towards the bladder and also the urine bag. This helps displace the clots at both ends of the tube, the eye on the Foley's catheter in the bladder and also the end of the tube in the urine bag (Fig. 17.6).

15. What is the cause of clot retention in a case of chronic retention?

Ans: In a case of chronic retention, the epithelial vessels dilate in order to facilitate blood supply in a bladder which is holding urine at a raised pressure. When this bladder is catheterised, and urine drained instantaneously, there is an acute drop in the intravesical pressure which leads to rupture of the small submucosal vessels.[13,14] This leads to haematuria. The haematuria is generally self-limiting but in authors' experience "slow decompression" can be done if there is bleeding immediately posturine drainage, this keeps the hydrostatic pressure in the bladder maintained and slowly releasing the pressure helps recurrence of further bleeding.

16. What are the preoperative measures you will take to decrease chances of post-operative haemorrhage after TURP?

Ans:

- Finasteride a type II 5α reductase inhibitor, inhibits conversion of testosterone to dihydrotestosterone. It reduces the expression of vascular endothelial growth factor (VEGF) leading to decreased vascularity of the prostate gland. Preoperative finasteride treatment for two to four weeks decreases bleeding during transurethral resection for benign enlargement of prostate.
- Dutasteride blocks both type I and type II receptors but its role in decreasing intraoperative bleeding is equivocal.[15–17]
- A single dose of Goserelin acetate, a luteinizing hormone releasing hormone (LHRH) agonist, before TURP is safe and effective in reducing surgical blood loss. It significantly reduced mean vascular density (MVD) in both suburethral and stromal nodular prostatic tissues without regional discrepancy.[18]
- The pre-operative use of antiandrogen drugs like cyproterone acetate in TURP of large size prostate can help in decreasing the perioperative bleeding.[19,20]

17. Does using different source of energy have any effect on post-operative chances of clot retention?

Ans:

- Bipolar TURP is associated with decreased risk of clot retention compared with monopolar-TURP.[21,22]
- Laser prostatectomy using holmium or potassium-titanyl-phosphate (KTP) have comparable efficacy and overall morbidity to contemporary TURP.[23]
- Photoselective vaporisation PVP with green light laser is said to have less chances of bleeding and clot retention postoperatively as compared to bipolar TURP.[24,25]

18. What would be the future course of action in cases with recurrent or intractable haematuria?

Ans:

- In cases with intractable haematuria use of intravesical 1% alum irrigation is generally safe, effective and well tolerated. Aluminium toxicity may occur in patients with renal impairment and large absorptive surfaces and signs of neurologic impairment such as lethargy, confusion seizures, increased aluminium concentration warrants stoppage of the treatment.[26–28]
- Helmstein first introduced hydrostatic pressure therapy under epidural anaesthesia in 1966 for the treatment of bladder cancer, later he used the therapy or control of haematuria. This therapy is effective for treating severe bleeding from the bladder but seems to have only a temporary effect. However, it has a relatively low morbidity, which makes it ideal for multiple uses and for those patients unable to undergo a general anaesthetic.[28,29]
- Efficacy of intravesical formalin in controlling massive haematuria has been reported in many

studies. However, because of the potential serious complications, it should be used with great caution and only after more conservative measures have failed, use of high concentration of formalin may lead to total loss of bladder function.[28]

- Hyperbaric oxygen therapy, therapeutic embolization and oral sodium pentosanpolysulphate have also been described for cases of intractable or chronic haematuria.[28]
- Intravesical prostaglandins have been used for treating cyclophosphamide-induced haemorrhagic cystitis. It is generally well tolerated but is associated with a high percentage of bladder spasms requires intensive nursing supervision, is costly, and may not be able to control bleeding in all patients.[28]
- Intravesical silver nitrate has also been used for benign as well as haemorrhagic cystitis but with equivocal results.[30,31]
- In some difficult cases suprapubic or open surgery have been described for removal of the clots though extremely rare.

REFERENCES

1. Leon-Mata, J. *et al*. Management of hematuria: all you always wanted to know. Int. Ann. Med. 2018;2(3). https:// doi.org/ 10. 24087/ IAM. 2018.2.3.429.
2. Ritch, C. R. *et al*. Pilot study of Alteplase (tissue plasminogen activator) for treatment of urinary clot retention in an in vitro model. J. Endourol. 23, 1353–1357 (2009).
3. Smereczy ski A, Szopi ski T, Goł bek T, Ostasz O, Bojko S. Sonography of tumors and tumor-like lesions that mimic carcinoma of the urinary bladder. J Ultrason. 2014 Mar;14(56):36–48. doi: 10.15557/JoU.2014.0004. Epub 2014 Mar 30. PMID: 26672732; PMCID: PMC4579734.
4. Kobatake, K., Inoue, S., Takemoto, K. *et al.* Evaluation of urinary catheters for effective manual bladder washout. *Sci Rep* **12**, 14359 (2022). https://doi.org/10.1038/s41598–022–18778–5
5. Clarebrough, E., McGrath, S., Christidis, D. *et al*. CATCH-22: a manual bladder washout protocol to improve care for clot retention. World J Urol 36, 2043–2050 (2018). https://doi.org/10.1007/s00345–018–2346–z.5. Kobatake, K., Inoue, S., Takemoto, K. *et al*. Evaluation of urinary catheters for effective manual bladder washout. Sci Rep 12, 14359 (2022). https://doi.org/10.1038/s41598–022–18778–5.
6. Stout TE, Borofsky M, Soubra A. A Visual Scale for Improving Communication When Describing Gross Hematuria. Urology. 2021 Feb;148:32–36. doi: 10.1016/j.urology.2020.10.054. Epub 2020 Dec 5. PMID: 33285214.
7. Doersch, K. M., Navetta, A. F., Bird, E. T., & El Tayeb, M. M. (2017). Case series: Bladder clot evacuation using a prostate morcellation device. Canadian Urological Association Journal, 11(7), E311–4. https://doi.org/10.5489/cuaj.4219.
8. Warlick CA, Mouli SK, Allaf ME, *et al*. Bladder irrigation using hydrogen peroxide for clot evacuation. Urology, 2006;68:1331–1332.
9. Barry JM. Transurethral clot evacuation from a bladder with a catheter irrigating syringe. J Urol. 1994;151:689. 2. Chad RR, Maria AO, Zhamshid O, *et al*. Pilot study of alteplase (tissue plasminogen activator) for treatment of urinary clot retention in an in vitro model. J Endourol. 2009;23:1353–1357.
10. Goel A, Sengottayan VK, Dwivedi AK. Mechanical suction: an effective and safe method to remove large and tenacious clots from the urinary bladder. Urology. 2011;77:494–496.
11. Song Yu H, Sik Ham W, Soo Hah Y, *et al*. Simple, safe, and successful evacuation of severe organized clot retention using a catheter connected with wall suction: suction and fishing method. Urology. 2011;78:1199–1202.
12. Walker EM, Bera S, Faiz M. Does catheter traction reduce post-transurethral resection of the prostate blood loss? Br J Urol. 1995 May;75(5):614–7. doi: 10.1111/j.1464–410x.1995.tb07419.x. PMID: 7613799.
13. Klamfoth J K, Burtson K M (September 26, 2022) Severe Urinary Retention Resulting in Extreme Post-obstructive Diuresis and Decompressive Hematuria. Cureus 14(9): e29626. doi:10.7759/cureus.29626
14. Muhammed A, Abubakar A: Pathophysiology and management of urinary retention in men. Arch Int Surg. 2012, 2:63–9. 10.4103/2278–9596.110018
15. Zong HT, Peng XX, Yang CC, Zhang Y. A systematic review of the effects and mechanisms of preoperative 5 -reductase inhibitors on intraoperative haemorrhage during surgery for benign prostatic hyperplasia. Asian J Androl. 2011 Nov;13(6):812–8. doi: 10.1038/aja.2011.86. Epub 2011 Sep 5. PMID: 21892196; PMCID: PMC3739552.
16. Zhu YP, Dai B, Zhang HL, Shi GH, Ye DW. Impact of preoperative 5α-reductase inhibitors on perioperative blood loss in patients with benign prostatic hyperplasia: a meta-analysis of randomized controlled trials. BMC Urol. 2015 Jun 2;15:47. doi: 10.1186/s12894–015–0043–4. PMID: 26032962; PMCID: PMC4450838.
17. Kloping YP, Yogiswara N, Azmi Y. The role of preoperative dutasteride in reducing bleeding during transurethral resection of the prostate: A systematic review and meta-analysis of randomized controlled trials. Asian J Urol. 2022 Jan;9(1):18–26. doi: 10.1016/j.ajur.2021.05.011. Epub 2021 Jun 8. PMID: 35198393; PMCID: PMC8841297.
18. Abo El-Enen M, Tawfik A, El-Abd AS, Ragab M, El-Abd S, Elrashidy M, Elmashad N, Rasheed M, El-Abd S. Goserelin acetate before transurethral resection of moderately enlarged benign prostatic hyperplasia: Prospective randomised-controlled clinical trial. Arab J Urol. 2016 Mar;14(1):59–65. doi: 10.1016/j.aju.2015.09.007. Epub 2015 Nov 21. PMID: 26966595; PMCID: PMC4767797.
19. Mohamed, A., Abdelsamad, K., Elgalaly, H., Eliwa, A. Role of Different Types of Anti Androgen in Reduction of Perioperative Bleeding In Transurethral Resection of Prostate for Treatment of Large Size Prostate. Zagazig University Medical Journal, 2023; 29(1.2): 261–267. doi: 10.21608/zumj.2020.21740.1668.
20. Abdelbaki, S.A., Al-Falah, A., Alhefnawy, M. *et al*. The effect of short-term use of finasteride versus cyproterone acetate on perioperative blood loss with monopolar transurethral resection of prostate. Afr J Urol 27, 106 (2021). https://doi.org/10.1186/s12301–021–00211–4.
21. Tang Y, Li J, Pu C, Bai Y, Yuan H, Wei Q, Han P. Bipolar transurethral resection versus monopolar transurethral resection for benign prostatic hypertrophy: a systematic

review and meta-analysis. J Endourol. 2014 Sep;28(9):1107–14. doi: 10.1089/end.2014.0188. Epub 2014 Jun 5. PMID: 24754254; PMCID: PMC4146489.

22. Ahyai SA, Gilling P, Kaplan SA, Kuntz RM, Madersbacher S, Montorsi F, Speakman MJ, Stief CG. Meta-analysis of functional outcomes and complications following transurethral procedures for lower urinary tract symptoms resulting from benign prostatic enlargement. Eur Urol. 2010 Sep;58(3):384–97. doi: 10.1016/j.eururo.2010.06.005. Epub 2010 Jun 11. PMID: 20825758.
23. Gupta NP, Nayyar R. Management of large prostatic adenoma: Lasers versus bipolar transurethral resection of prostate. Indian J Urol 2013;29:225–35.
24. Thangasamy IA, Chalasani V, Bachmann A, Woo HH. Photoselective vaporisation of the prostate using 80-W and 120-W laser versus transurethral resection of the prostate for benign prostatic hyperplasia: a systematic review with meta-analysis from 2002 to 2012. Eur Urol. 2012 Aug;62(2):315–23. doi: 10.1016/j.eururo.2012.04.051. Epub 2012 May 4. PMID: 22575913.
25. Zang YC, Deng XX, Yang DR, Xue BX, Xu LJ, Liu XL, Zhou YB, Shan YX. Photoselective vaporization of the prostate with Green Light 120-W laser versus transurethral resection of the prostate for benign prostatic hyperplasia: a systematic review with meta-analysis of randomized controlled trials. Lasers Med Sci. 2016 Feb;31(2):235–40. doi: 10.1007/s10103–015–1843–1. Epub 2015 Dec 28. PMID: 26712715.
26. Ho CC, Md Zainuddin Z. Alum irrigation for the treatment of intractable haematuria. Malays J Med Sci. 2009 Oct;16(4):66–8. PMID: 22135514; PMCID: PMC3216135.
27. Goel AK, Rao MS, Bhagwat AG, Vaidyanathan S, Goswami AK, Sen TK. Intravesical irrigation with alum for the control of massive bladder haemorrhage. J Urol. 1985 Jun;133(6):956–7. doi: 10.1016/s0022–5347(17)49330–x. PMID: 3999219.
28. Choong SK, Walkden M, Kirby R. The management of intractable haematuria. BJU Int. 2000 Dec;86(9):951–9. doi: 10.1046/j.1464–410x.2000.00900.x. PMID: 11119085.
29. Helmstein K. Treatment of bladder carcinoma by a hydrostatic pressure technique. Br J Urol 1972; 44: 434±50.
30. Diamond DA, Jeffs RD, Marshall FF. Control of prolonged, benign, renal haematuria by silver nitrate instillation. Urology. 1981 Oct;18(4):337–41. doi: 10.1016/0090–4295(81)90384–8. PMID: 7292810.
31. Montgomery BD, Boorjian SA, Ziegelmann MJ, Joyce DD, Linder BJ. Intravesical silver nitrate for refractory haemorrhagic cystitis. Turk J Urol. 2016 Sep;42(3):197–201. doi: 10.5152/tud.2016.38445. PMID: 27635296; PMCID: PMC5012448.

Chapter

18

Voiding LUTS in Young Man

• *Ajay Bhandarkar* • *Nisarg Mehta*

LEARNING OBJECTIVES

- To learn evaluation of a young man with lower urinary tract symptoms (LUTS).
- Specific requirements of young men with BOO.
- Role and indications of urodynamic evaluation in young patient with LUTS.
- Role and type of lifestyle management in LUTS.
- To understand the role and limitations of medical management in benign prostatic obstruction (BPO) in young men.
- To learn when to intervene in young patients with LUTS.
- The clinical value of minimally invasive surgical treatment (MIST) options for BPO.
- To understand the physiology of ejaculation and current role of ejaculation sparing procedures.

INTRODUCTION

In 1994, the phrase "lower urinary tract symptoms" (LUTS) was coined. It describes patients' voiding complaints, which can occur irrespective of underlying cause. They are not sex, age, or disease specific.[1] The incidence and severity of symptoms may increase with age and are divided into those related to storage of urine, voiding symptoms and post-micturition issues. Whereas 64.3% of participants in the EPIC study[2] reported having experienced at least one LUTS, the EpiLUTS study[3] revealed that 72.3% of men and 76.3% of women had experienced at least one LUTS in their lifetime. The International Prostate Symptoms Score (IPSS) is the most popular validated tool for assessing the degree of bother caused by LUTS and the severity of LUTS.

Sense of incomplete emptying, urge incontinence and nocturia are the most bothersome LUTS in men. It is the impact of LUTS on quality-of-life that drives males to seek medical advice and treatment. Unfortunately, perception of severity of symptoms is variable and depends on personal, psychological, societal and economic factors. Urological healthcare providers need to be aware about the complexities of etiopathology of BPE like hormonal alterations, increased sympathetic nervous activity, morphology of prostatic adenoma, relationship of LUTS and sexual function.

According to standard guidelines, including Urological Society of India guidelines,[4] It is advised to treat LUTS/benign prostatic hyperplasia (BPH) in three steps:

1. Conservative methods of management like watchful waiting and changing one's lifestyle.
2. Pharmacological approach (α-blockers, 5α-reductase inhibitors, PDE5 inhibitors, anticholinergics, combinations and herbal therapy)
3. Interventional/surgical options.

As a clinician, it is our duty to understand the needs, concerns and expectations of our patients, especially who are relatively younger and consult us for their LUTS. A variety of different conditions can cause LUTS in young males (age 45 or younger). The focus should be on thorough clinical evaluation to determine the exact etiology and simultaneously understand the expectations from the patient as regards to treatment and its outcomes, since most of the treatment for LUTS have an effect on male sexual functions.

Depending upon the level of bother, men would like relief in their symptoms, but would also accept lower results to avoid deleterious outcomes affecting their sexual life.

In the era of artificial intelligence (AI) and widespread information availability, men are likely to be knowledgeable about the management options. Individualised, patient centric approach for evaluation and management of LUTS is advisable.

Case Scenario

A 40-year-old man comes for consultation. Over last one year he has noticed that he takes longer to pass urine. In his office toilet, his colleagues come after him, finish the act and go back. He is still urinating. This has been quite embarrassing. Since last six months he has difficulty in urination, feels sense of incomplete void, passes urine intermittently. His urine stream is weak and falls between feet. He also strains to pass urine. He has no other illnesses. He is sexually active with a coital frequency of twice per week. He consulted his family physician for urinary trouble. The doctor ordered a urine test and ultrasound. Ultrasound shows prostatic adenoma of 35 grams size with minimal intravesical protrusion and normal upper tracts. His urinalysis shows 8–10 pus cells, but urine culture has not grown any organisms. He has normal renal function.

We have a relatively young male who has severe voiding symptoms, and his ultrasound evaluation shows prostatic adenoma of 35 grams size with minimal intravesical protrusion and normal upper tracts. He has no other illnesses.

He is apprehensive about the diagnostic tests and prefers non-invasive methods for evaluation and treatment, as he is sexually active. We need to counsel him for medical management, minimally invasive therapies/surgical options, their limitations, and costs involved.

1. **What are the various causes of LUTS in young men?**

   Ans:

   There can be one or more than one causes for male LUTS .[5]

   - Benign prostatic obstruction (BPO)
   - Overactive bladder (OAB)
   - Nocturnal polyuria
   - Underactive bladder
   - Chronic pelvic pain syndrome (CPPS)
   - Neurovesical dysfunction
   - Urinary tract infection (UTI)
   - Urethral stricture disease
   - Bladder tumour
   - Distal ureteric calculus

2. **What would you like to ask during history?**

   Ans: Our goal should be to determine the relevant co-morbidities, such as neurological and medical disorders, as well as any probable reasons. An evaluation of existing drugs, lifestyle choices, and psychological and emotional aspects is also necessary. As this is a 40-year-old male patient, one should rule out chronic urinary tract infection. A specific history related to neuro-vesical dysfunction and/or history of spine trauma/surgery also should be sought for.

   One should try to rule out urethral stricture in his particular case with specific points during history like previous recurrent urinary tract infection, history of pelvic trauma, history of genitourinary instrumentation, history of lithuria. Numerous symptom-sensitive questionnaires that can be used to track the effectiveness of treatment have been created. LUTS can be measured and the kind of symptoms that predominate can be identified with the use of symptom scores. Eight questions make up the International Prostate Symptom Score (IPSS),[6] which consists of one question on quality of life (QoL) and seven questions about symptoms. It is also necessary to evaluate sexual function, ideally using validated symptom questionnaires like the International Index of Erectile Function (IIEF).

   One must ask the patient whether his family is complete, since most of the treatments do cause ejaculatory dysfunctions which can affect reproductive potential. Simultaneously it is also important to understand the expectations of the patient as far the outcome of treatment is concerned since this a quality-of-life disorder also.

3. **What are the points that you would like to note during physical examination of this patient?**

   Ans: A physical examination should be conducted, paying special attention to the lower limbs, the perineum, the external genitalia, and the suprapubic area. Rule out penile cancer, balanitis xerotica obliterans (BXO), phimosis, and meatal stenosis. The prostate's volume and texture can be evaluated via digital-rectal examination (DRE), yet there is a little association between the two measurements.

   Specific neurologic assessment is important. Anal tone, peri-anal sensation and bulbocavernosus reflex (BCR) should be assessed.

4. **What other tests are necessary for evaluation of this patient?**

   Ans:

   - **Postvoid residual (PVR)** and uroflowmetry are an optional initial evaluation studies in the management of LUTS. PVR establishes the bladder's initial capacity for emptying. Since there is not a consensus on what constitutes clinically significant PVR, it is advisable to follow the trend.

- **Uroflowmetry is the measurement of how much urine is voided in milliliters (ml) in relation to time (in seconds). The flow curve, the highest flow rate (Q_{max}), and voided volume (greater than 150 ml)—are crucial components of the test. A Q_{max} >15 ml/s is regarded as normal in men. A typical bell-shaped curve may virtually rule out any obstruction. For bladder outlet obstruction, flow rates less than 10 ml/s have demonstrated a 70% specificity, a 70% positive predictive value, and a 47% sensitivity.**[7] Box pattern curve can indicate obstruction due to stricture urethra and straining pattern may suggests detrusor hypoactivity.
- **Prostate specific antigen (PSA):** Patients with LUTS should be informed of the possible advantages and disadvantages of using serum PSA testing to diagnose prostate cancer. If the patient has family history of prostate cancer, PSA testing should be recommended. In younger patients with LUTS, baseline PSA value can guide us to adopt future screening protocols. It can also help to estimate prostate volume; to decide drug of choice in the medical management and predict BPH-related outcomes.
- As ultrasound examination shows normal kidneys without backpressure changes, no further upper tract evaluation is mandatory in this case.
- Ascending urethrogram can be done if we suspect urethral stricture (history of instrumentation or box pattern on uroflowmetry).

5. **Would you like to do a urodynamic study in this patient? If so, why?**

Ans: Urodynamic studies (UDS) are the most definitive tests available to assess the pathophysiology of LUTS. The invasive urodynamic test is the gold standard for the assessment of LUTS pathophysiology and it is used to identify detrusor overactivity (DO), detrusor underactivity (DUA), low bladder compliance, and BOO.

Invasive UDS is not indicated in the above-mentioned patient as a part of initial evaluation. It can be advised, if we suspect any neurovesical or detrusor dysfunction. It is also indicated if we do not observe any improvement on initial medical management or before planning any interventional or surgical treatment.

6. **Are there any non-invasive methods of evaluation for LUTS?**

Ans: The penile cuff test (PCT)[8] involves inflating a pneumatic cuff placed around the penis to disrupt the urine stream. The bladder can be naturally filled prior to the test, therefore, a bladder catheter tube is not required. The test is paired with a urine flow rate measurement utilizing a connected flow meter to produce combined pressure and flow readings during a single void.

Other non-invasive methods like ultrasound techniques[9] include:

- Bladder (BWT) and detrusor wall thickness (DWT)
- Ultrasound estimated bladder weight (UEBW)
- Prostate ultrasound parameters like, prostate volume (PV),
- Intravesical protrusion of prostate (IPP),
- Prostatic artery resistance index (RI)
- Prostatic urethral angle,
- Near infrared spectroscopy

Every one of these methods depends on the operator, requires specialized training, and may involve a learning curve for urologists. DWT and PCT methods of non-invasive evaluation has promising future, however, NIS still remains experimental and yet to prove its clinical usefulness. It can involve additional cost for the centre and patients.

7. **How do we proceed for management in this case?**

Ans: This particular patient is 40 years of age and has severe voiding LUTS with nearly small prostatic adenoma. We need to assess the level of bother and quality-of-life scores too. According to published clinical studies, storage LUTS (like urgency/urge incontinence and sense of incomplete void) are more bothersome symptoms. So, initial treatment advice would be to modify his lifestyle. We need to counsel him about the specific (BPE related) medical management, need for long-term treatment and regular follow-up for assessing the response to drugs. He should be explained about the possible adverse effects of long-term medication.

Following lifestyle modifications should be recommended for the initial management of LUTS[10]:

- Assure the patient that no detectable prostate cancer exists.
- Suggest 1500–2000 ml of fluid each day (smaller amounts may be needed depending on activity and temperature). Can be altered in accordance with the frequency volume chart (FVC).
- Fluid restriction during times when symptoms are most bothersome (long trips, public events). fluid restriction in the evening in the event of troublesome nocturia.
- Avoid caffeine by substituting decaffeinated or caffeine-free beverages for caffeine. If

nocturia troubles you, avoid drinking in the evening and at night.
- With the patient's treating physician, swap out hypertension diuretics for appropriate substitutes that have less of an impact on the urine.
- Avoid constipation.
- To practice distraction techniques for urgency, urethral milking for post-micturition dribbling.

8. Which BPE-specific drug can be used for this patient?

Ans: For a small size prostate (<40 grams) alpha adrenoceptor antagonists[11] are the drug of choice. Alfuzosin (a nonselective alpha blocker) has been shown to be associated with less ejaculatory dysfunction[12] as compared to other selective alpha-1 blockers and should be recommended in this patient.

PDE5 inhibitor (tadalafil) is proved to be a safe and effective drug according to several clinical trials.[13] It significantly improves total IPSS. Tadalafil 5 mg once a day dosage can be a drug of choice in this patient if he has borderline erectile dysfunction. It can be combined with alpha adrenoceptor antagonists for beneficial effect.

9. Would you like to use 5-alpha reductase inhibitors (5-ARIs) in this patient?

Ans: 5-ARIs[14] in young male as a long-term management should be used cautiously, as it is associated with higher sexual adverse events when compared with higher placebo. However, clinically relevant sexual dysfunction following use of 5-ARIs is yet to be established.[15,16] Informed consent, detailed sexual history and patient centric care is advisable for better compliance.

In patients with severe LUTS/with elevated risk of disease progression, prostate volume > 40 ml, high postvoid residual urine (PVR), low Q_{max}, and PSA level 1.5 ng/ml, a combination therapy of 5-ARI and an alpha-1 adrenoceptor antagonist is advised. Combination therapy not only lowers LUTS but has also been shown to be useful in avoiding disease progression and the risk of acute urine retention.

10. What is the role of antimuscarinics in the management of LUTS?

Ans: If storage symptoms are predominant, combination therapy of antimuscarinics with alpha-adrenoceptor antagonists are found to be effective. If baseline PVR is > 150 ml, one has to frequently monitor IPSS and postvoid residual urine to watch for deleterious effect like retention of urine when antimuscarinic drugs are given.[17]

11. Are there any newer drugs available for managing LUTS? How can they be used in this patient?

Ans: Several new drugs (naftopidil, isosorbide dinitrate, botulinum toxin, NX 1207, lonidamine) are already in clinical trials, and a few others (Cetrorelix, peptide receptor agonists/antagonists, S-nitrosothiols, cannabinoid receptor agonists) are in the preclinical stage of development.[18] These medications may be prescribed as a supplement in patients who have persisting symptoms while having an alpha-blocker or a PDE5 inhibitor. Combining various medications to activate several peripheral sites in the prostate and hence maximize intracellular signaling may improve therapy success.

> One should advocate intervention with MIST at an earlier stage in patients who are previously treated with medication that do not show a significant improvement in overall QOL with time.

12. When to Intervene?

Ans: Indications for intervention:

1. Failure of medical therapy to sufficiently ameliorate bothersome LUTS
2. Intolerable pharmaceutical side effects,
3. Progression of the disease despite medical management like, increasing postvoid residual urine/retention of urine, Q_{max} persistently below 10 ml/sec
4. Recurrent urinary tract infections/haematuria due to BPH/BOO.
5. Desire by the patient to avoid taking a daily medications

13. Why should one opt for minimally invasive surgical therapy (MIST) in this patient?

Ans: In an era when patients' quality of life (QoL) is prioritized, we cannot disregard the influence of post-operative retrograde ejaculation (RE) and ejaculatory dysfunction (EjD) on the well-being of patients undergoing elective surgery for BPH.

MIST procedures can bridge the gap for those patients who are not benefiting or who want to discontinue medical management and yet not ready for definitive surgical procedures to remove the prostate adenoma.

14. What are the MIST options available to this patient?

Ans: PUL (prostatic urethral lift) is a minimally invasive operation that uses implants to compress the prostate's lateral lobes. This technology's mode of operation is mechanical rather than ablative or cavitating. At 3–5 years of follow-up, retreatment rates in the PUL studies ranged from 10% to 20%. The Temporary Implantable Nitinol Device (iTIND) is a second-generation mechanical device composed of three struts with double entwined nitinol wires formed as a tulip-shaped stent and is temporarily placed transurethrally.

Water vapor thermal therapy (WVTT) uses radiofrequency-generated convective water vapor thermal energy to trigger instantaneous cell necrosis in the prostate. A retractable needle is introduced into the intended treatment area, and steam at 103 °C is delivered in short 9s bursts via an 18G needle.

When two multi-centre, sham-controlled, double-blind randomized trials[19] for PUL and WVTT were identified and compared, it was observed that, improvements in the bother score by 12–36 months were comparable in both MIST, however, surgical re-treatment rates favoured WVTT over PUL (4.4% vs. 10.7%, respectively).

Robotic waterjet treatment (RWT) can be offered to patients with LUTS. In this technique, robotically controlled waterjet ablates prostate tissue. Resection contour is pre-planned under transrectal ultrasound guidance. As non-thermal energy is used for ablation, post-procedural haemostasis is achieved by catheter traction or cauterization of bleeders with the use of resectoscope. Shorter duration of treatment irrespective of the prostate size, comparable (with TURP) surgical outcome and possible preservation of ejaculation are certain advantages of this procedure.[20]

Prostatic artery embolization (PAE) is superior in ejaculation preservation, but post-procedural improvement in LUTS inferior to other options. It is best indicated in a very high-risk patients. As there is a scarce evidence available in support of PAE, it is not advocated as a standard procedure.[20]

15. What are the limitations of MIST?

Ans: Studies comparing the efficacy of medical therapies versus MISTs, as well as surgical treatments, are scarce and would be extremely beneficial.[21] The cost factor and availability of MIST also needs to be considered before offering these options for eligible patients.

In general, following are the merits and demerits of the MIST procedures:

Pros:

- No sexual side effects
- It can be performed under local anaesthesia. It could be a superior choice for patients who are not ready for invasive surgical therapy or with poor cardiopulmonary function.
- Day care surgery

Cons:

- Not suitable for patients with obstructive large median lobe or with retention of urine.
- Not suitable for large prostates (>80 ml)
- Potential high retreatment rates
- High cost of treatment
- Only mild improvement in Q_{max} and postvoid residual urine.
- Limited long-term data

The cost factor and availability of MIST also needs to be considered before offering these options for eligible patients.

16. How would you advice follow-up in this patient?

Ans: There are no set protocols or guidelines for follow-up of LUTS patients after initial evaluation. If one has advised behavioural modifications or short acting BPE specific drugs like alpha-adrenoceptor antagonists/PDE5 inhibitors, one can assess after 4–6 weeks. IPSS and QoL scores, Q_{max} and PVR should be monitored on every visit to assess the efficacy of management offered. Every three monthly follow-up for the first year is advocated. Frequency of follow-up after one year can be decided based on the response to the management. Detailed or further evaluation like invasive UDS/intervention is advocated only if bothersome LUTS continue or in case of disease progression despite medical management.

Indications of Surgical Treatment:

This patient has a normal sexual function. Surgical or invasive procedures in such young patients should be avoided or delayed due to irreversible sexual adverse effects.

Patients with indications mentioned in "when to intervene" section, who do not want/afford MIST or keen on definitive long-term relief from LUTS and aware about possibility of post-operative irreversible ejaculatory dysfunction should be offered surgical treatment. Uroflowmetry and Pressure flow study[22] (if the age of the patient <50 years or Q_{max} is > 10 ml/sec) should be done before proceeding for the surgical treatment. Bilateral renal hydronephrosis with renal function impairment warrants surgical treatment once initial medical treatment has been given and good detrusor contractility has been ensured. Table 18.1 depicts comparative data on risk of sexual and ejaculatory dysfunction after various BPH treatments.

17. What is the physiological basis of antegrade ejaculation?

Ans: Evidence from ejaculation physiology has shown that the tissues surrounding the

TABLE 18.1: Risk of sexual and ejaculatory dysfunction after various BPH treatments

Procedure	*Risk of postoperative sexual dysfunction*	
Transurethral resection of prostate (TURP)	REj PE DV ED	38.2–89.0% 0–2.0% 18.3–54.0% 13.0–14.0%
Holmium laser enucleation of the prostate (HoLEP)	REj PE DV ED	50.0–76.6% 3.3% 16.7% 5.2–7.9%
Photoselective vaporization of the prostate (PVP)	REj PE ED	21.4–49.9% 5.4% 0–20.9%
Transurethral needle ablation (TUNA)	REj DV ED	0–5.6% 13.0% 5.8%
Transurethral microwave therapy (TUMT)	REj ED	9.2–24.0% 0–18.2%
Prostatic urethral lift (UroLift®)	DV AE	2.9% 2.9%
Aquablation®	REj	10.0%
Prostatic artery embolization (PAE)	REj	24.1%

REj retrograde ejaculation, PE painful ejaculation, DV decreased volume of ejaculate, ED erectile dyfunction, AE anejaculation

verumontanum, rather than the bladder neck, are important for antegrade ejaculation.[23]

Contraction of the musculus ejaculatorious may be responsible for the release of sperm from the ejaculatory ducts into the prostatic urethra as well as the proper movement of the verumontanum during ejaculation.[24] The compromise between adequate BPO alleviation and ejaculation preservation is based on the fact that benign prostatic hyperplasia tissue produces proportionally much less semen than the gland's peripheral area and seminal vesicles.

The idea of the "genital sphincter" is described in Gosling and Thomson's[25] anatomical research. Supramontanal and paracollicular tissue-sparing surgical procedures have been developed in response to these findings.

18. What are the various ejaculation sparing procedures for prostate?

Transurethral incision of prostate (TUIP) and median lobe resection only are some of the established ejaculation preserving procedures. These procedures can be choice of surgical treatment in this patient.

Ejaculation sparing strategies have also been used in TURP and photo-selective prostate vaporization (PVP)[26] with promising results. TURP and PVP, on the other hand, are now only advised for the treatment of small to intermediate-sized prostates.

Given that laser endoscopic enucleation of the prostate (LEEP) techniques have already been shown to be size independent, modified classical ThuLEP surgery[27] by sparing 1.5 cm of tissue above the verumontanum and two hills of tissue at the apex of the lateral lobes can be effective in maintaining ejaculation while improving micturition. On 5-year follow-up, 91% of patients maintained anterograde ejaculation using a modified TURP/HoLEP/ThuLEP technique that spares the paracollicular and supracollicular tissue. Ejaculation-preserving enucleation of the prostate should ideally be performed by a skilled surgeon.[20]

As per the EAU Guidelines, the only recommended ejaculation-sparing (ES) procedure today, is PUL. Recently published clinical data[28] suggests that, both WVTT and PUL in men with middle-size prostates show inferior overall relief in BPO compared to TURP, but sexual function is preserved with better IPSS improvement.

Conclusions

Managing BPE entails far more than a transurethral resection of the prostate. Men with LUTS/BPH should receive a full-sexual examination before being offered any medication or surgical choices, with a clear explanation of the adverse effects impacting sexual QoL that can occur, and should be made aware of the alternatives if applicable. Personalised medicine is quickly becoming a cornerstone of healthcare. Urologists have a quiver full of arrows at their disposal for the total management of LUTS patients, from diagnosis to treatment and follow-up. Innovative drugs/therapies should be utilized in conjunction with a comprehensive approach to patient care. It is the specialist's obligation to be able to provide a treatment that best meets the patient's needs and expectations.

REFERENCES

1. Abrams P. New words for old: lower urinary tract symptoms for "prostatism". Bmj. 1994 Apr 9;308(6934):929–30.
2. Irwin DE, Milsom I, Hunskaar S *et al* (2006) Population-based survey of urinary incontinence, overactive bladder, and other lower urinary tract symptoms in five countries: results of the EPIC study. Eur Urol 50(6):1306–1314. doi:10.1016/j.eururo.2006.09.019.
3. Coyne KS, Sexton CC, Thompson CL *et al* (2009) The prevalence of lower urinary tract symptoms (LUTS) in the USA, the UK and Sweden: results from the Epidemiology of LUTS (EpiLUTS) study. BJU Int 104(3):352–360.doi:10.1111/j.1464-410X.2009.08427.x.

4. Sabnis RB, Mulawkar PM, Joshi RN. The Urological Society of India guidelines on management of benign prostatic hyperplasia/benign prostatic obstruction (Executive summary). Indian J Urol. 2021 Jul-Sep;37(3):210–213. doi: 10.4103/iju.iju_121_21. PMID: 34465948; PMCID: PMC8388351.
5. Gravas, S., Cornu, J. N., Gacci, M., Gratzke, C., Herrmann, T. R. W., Mamoulakis, C., Rieken, M., Speakman, M. J., & Tikkinen, K. A. O. (2019). *Management of non-neurogenic male lower urinary tract symptoms (LUTS), incl. benign prostatic obstruction (BPO)*. (European Association of Urology. Guidelines). European Association of Urology. https://uroweb.org/guideline/treatment-of-non-neurogenic-male-luts.
6. Barry, M.J., *et al*. The American Urological Association symptom index for benign prostatic hyperplasia. The Measurement Committee of the American Urological Association. J Urol, 1992. 148: 1549. https://pubmed.ncbi.nlm.nih.gov/1279218/.
7. Reynard JM, Yang Q, Donovan JL *et al*: The ICS-'BPH' Study: uroflowmetry, lower urinary tract symptoms and bladder outlet obstruction. Br J Urol 1998; 82: 619.
8. Harding C, Robson W, Drinnan M, McIntosh S, Sajeel M, Giffiths C, Pickard R. The penile cuff test: A clinically useful non-invasive urodynamic investigation to diagnose men with lower urinary tract symptoms. Indian J Urol. 2009 Jan;25(1):116–21. doi: 10.4103/0970–1591.45549. PMID: 19468441; PMCID: PMC2684319.
9. Mangat R, Ho HSS, Kuo TLC. Non-invasive evaluation of lower urinary tract symptoms (LUTS) in men. Asian J Urol. 2018 Jan;5(1):42–47. doi:10.1016/j.ajur.2017.12.002. Epub 2017 Dec 8. PMID: 29379736; PMCID:PMC5780291.
10. Yap T, Emberton M: Behaviour modification and benign prostatic hyperplasia: replacement for medications, Curr Opin Urol 20(1):20–27, 2010).
11. Roehrborn CG, Schwinn DA (2004) Alpha1-adrenergic receptor and their inhibitors in lower urinary tract symptoms an benign prostatic hyperplasia. J Urol 171:10291035.
12. HEL Young, SJ Sena *et al*. Alfuzosin and Its Effect on Ejaculatory Dysfunction: A Systematic Review World J Mens Health 2021 Apr 39(2): 186–194).
13. Porst H, Kim ED, CasabE AR *et al* (2011) Efficacy and safety of tadalafil once daily in the treatment of men with lower urinary tract symptoms suggestive of benign prostatic hyperplasia: results of an international randomized, double-blind, placebo-controlled trial. Eur Urol 60:1105–1113.
14. Naslund MJ, Miner M (2007) A review of the clinical efficacy and safety of 5-alpha-reductase inhibitors for the enlarged prostate. Clin Ther 29:17–25.
15. Rosen RC, Roehrborn CG, Manyak MJ *et al*: Evaluation of the impact of dutasteride/tamsulosin combination therapy on libido in sexually active men with lower urinary tract symptoms (LUTS) secondary to benign prostatic hyperplasia (BPH): A post hoc analysis of a prospective randomised placebo-controlled study. Int J Clin Pract. 2019 Sep;73(9):1–9. doi: 10.1111/ijcp.13282. Epub 2018 Nov 5. PMID: 30317693; PMCID: PMC6767409.
16. La Torre A, Giupponi G, Duffy D *et al*: Sexual Dysfunction Related to Drugs: a Critical Review. Part V: -Blocker and 5-ARI Drugs. Pharmacopsychiatry. 2016 Jan;49(1):3–13. doi: 10.1055/s–0035–1565100. Epub 2015 Nov 16. PMID: 26569417.
17. Oelke M, Bachmann A, Descazeaud A, Emberton M, Gravas S, Michel MC, *et al*. EAU guidelines on the treatment and follow-up of non-neurogenic male lower urinary tract symptoms including benign prostatic obstruction. Eur Urol. 2013; 64(1):118–40. doi: 10.1016/j.eururo.2013.03.004 PMID: 23541338.
18. Ückert, S., Kedia, G.T., Tsikas, D. *et al*. Emerging drugs to target lower urinary tract symptomatology (LUTS)/benign prostatic hyperplasia (BPH): focus on the prostate. *World J Urol* **38**, 1423–1435 (2020). https://doi.org/10.1007/s00345–019–02933–1.
19. Elterman D, Shepherd S, Saadat SH, Alshak MN, Bhojani N, Zorn KC, Rijo E, Misrai V, Lajkosz K, Chughtai B. Prostatic urethral lift (UroLift) versus convective water vapor ablation (Rezum) for minimally invasive treatment of BPH: a comparison of improvements and durability in 3-year clinical outcomes. Can J Urol. 2021 Oct;28(5):10824–10833. PMID: 34657655.
20. Ioannis Sokolakis a, Nikolaos Pyrgidis a, Giorgio Ivan Russo b, Petros Sountoulides c, Georgios Hatzichristodoulou. Preserving Ejaculation: A Guide Through the Landscape of Interventional and Surgical Options for Benign Prostatic Obstruction. European Urology Focus, (2022) ISSN: 2405–4569, Vol: 8, Issue: 2, Page: 380–383. DOI:https://doi.org/10.1016/j.euf.2022.03.008.
21. Franco JV, Jung JH, Imamura M, Borofsky M, Omar MI, Escobar Liquitay CM, Young S, Golzarian J, Veroniki AA, Garegnani L, Dahm P. Minimally invasive treatments for lower urinary tract symptoms in men with benign prostatic hyperplasia: a network meta-analysis. Cochrane Database Syst Rev. 2021 Jul 15;7(7):CD013656. doi: 10.1002/14651858.CD013656.pub2. PMID: 34693990; PMCID: PMC8543673.
22. Campbell and Walsh 12th edition, Chapter 145, Evaluation and Nonsurgical Management of Benign Prostatic Hyperplasia.
23. R. Leonardi, The LEST technique: treatment of prostatic obstruction preserving antegrade ejaculation in patients with benign prostatic hyperplasia, Arch. Ital. Urol. Androl. 91 (1) (2019 Mar 29) 35–42,https://doi.org/10.4081/aiua.2019.1.35.
24. Alloussi SH, Lang C, Eichel R, Alloussi S. Ejaculation-preserving transurethral resection of prostate and bladder neck: short-and long-term results of a new innovative resection technique. J Endourol. 2014 Jan;28(1):84–9. doi:10.1089/end.2013.0093. Epub 2013 Oct 10. PMID: 23952037.
25. Gosling J, A, Thompson S, A: A Neurohistochemical and Histological Study of Peripheral Autonomic Neurons of the Human Bladder Neck and Prostate. Urol Int 1977;32:269–276. doi: 10.1159/000280142.
26. Talab SS, Santiago-Lastra YA, Bachmann A, Choi BB, Muir GH, Woo HH, *et al*. V403 the impact of ejaculation-preserving photo-selective vaporization of the prostate (EP-PVP) on lower urinary tract symptoms and ejaculatory function: results of a multi-centre study. J Urol. 2013;189(4S):e164. 10.1016/j.juro.2013.02.1792.
27. Matteo Vittori, Riccardo Bertolo, Francesco Maiorino, Chiara Cipriani, Marco Carilli, Marta Signoretti, Valerio Iacovelli, Michele Antonucci, Pierluigi Bove,: Thulium laser enucleation of prostate: Ejaculation sparing techniques, Urology Video Journal, Volume 13,2022,100129,ISSN 2590–0897,https://doi.org/10.1016/j.urolvj.2022.100129.(https://www.sciencedirect.com/science/article/pii/S2590089722000068).
28. Jean-Nicolas Cornu, Paul Zantek and Glyn Burtt *et al*: Minimally Invasive Treatments for Benign Prostatic Obstruction: A Systematic Review and Network Meta-analysis. European Urology 83 (2023) 534–547. https://doi.org/10.1016/j.eururo.2023.02.028.

Chapter

19

Forgotten DJ

• Abhay Dinkar Mahajan • Poleboyina Vamsi Krishna

LEARNING OBJECTIVES

- Causes of a forgotten DJ stent.
- Pathophysiology of a forgotten DJ stent.
- Complications of forgotten DJ stent.
- Clinical evaluation and grading systems to identify the right approach in a given situation.
- Various treatment options.
- Preventive measures for forgotten stents.
- Advancements in stent devices like drug eluting and biodegradable stents.
- Medicolegal aspects of a forgotten DJ Stent.

INTRODUCTION

Double J stent (DJS) has become an integral part of most of the endourological and open surgical procedures in urology since its first description by Zimskind *et al.* in 1967.[1] The term 'Double J stent' was coined by Finney *et al.* in 1978.[2] In routine practice, the primary use of DJS is to allow adequate drainage of urine from the kidney into the bladder. Stents are commonly deployed after the endourological and percutaneous procedures for kidney and ureteral stone removal. It is also used for non-stone-related diseases like retroperitoneal fibrosis, ureteral stricture, extrinsic compression of the ureter due to tumour or mass, and temporary de-obstruction of the system. In addition, DJS can also be used in ureteric injuries, due to either traumatic or gynaecological surgeries, or for intraoperative identification and protection of the ureter during various pelvic surgeries.[3] Depending upon the indications, DJS can be either placed temporarily or permanently. If there is a need to place the DJS for a longer duration, it needs to be replaced to avoid complications due to prolonged indwelling time. It is recommended to replace the DJS in 3 to 6 months.[4] The material and design of DJS, and the stent being a foreign body, can lead to symptoms like patient discomfort, dysuria, irritative voiding symptoms, infection, and hematuria.[5] The DJ stent is usually removed after a stipulated period once it serves the purpose. As the indwelling time increases, it may lead to an increased incidence of encrustations on the DJ stent and other complications.[6] The long-term complications of DJ stent include encrustation and stone formation, stent fragmentation or migration, sepsis and occasionally deterioration of kidney function.[7]

Case Scenario

A 16-year-old male patient presented to us with symptoms of dysuria, frequency of micturition and mild fever. He had a previous history of ureteroscopy and stone removal with DJ stent placement at some other hospital one year back. The patient was not aware about the DJS placement and did not follow-up with the primary surgeon. Ultrasonography and X-ray KUB showed a retained stent with encrustation on the kidney, ureter and bladder part of the retained DJ stent (Fig. 19.1).

1. **What are the causes of a forgotten DJ stent?**

   Ans: There is a constant improvement in the stent design and material of the stents. The aim is to reduce the discomfort of the stent so that DJS can be kept for a longer time in the body. But the disadvantage of this is it can lead to stent encrustations and further complications. Stent can be forgotten either due to the patient factor

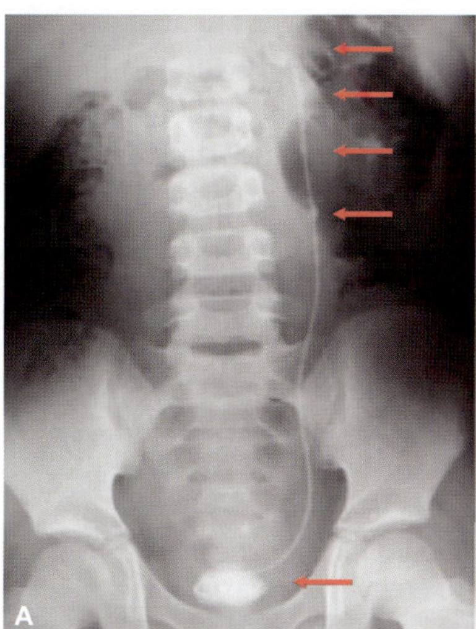
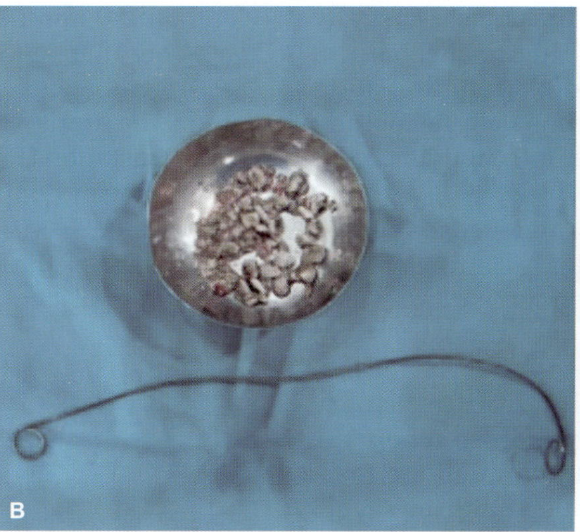
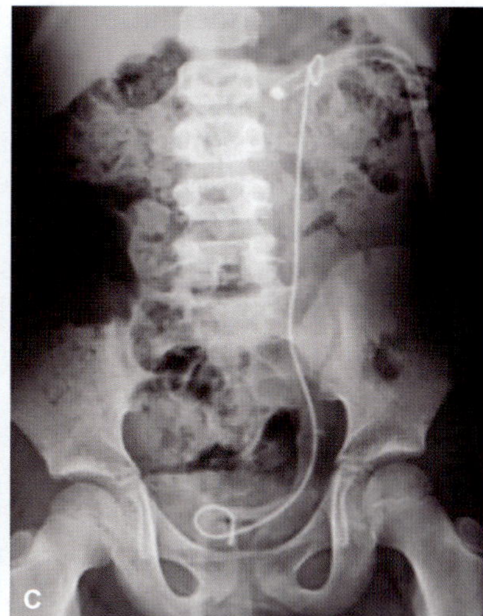

Fig. 19.1A to C: (A) Plain X-ray KUB; (B) Stone fragments and DJ stent; (C) Postoperative X-ray

or the surgeon factor. Patient factors usually consist of lack of information, poor follow-up, low socio-economic status and unawareness of stent placement. Agarwal *et al*. found that poor compliance in follow-up and unawareness of the stent were the commonest reason cited by the patient, followed by the misconception that the stent would last for a lifetime or would dissolve.[8] One study attributes forgotten stent to the socioeconomic background and lack of health insurance.[9] Surgeon or hospital factors are also important which include inadequate information to the patient and relatives regarding the inserted stent and the need for timely stent removal, poor stent registry, and improper follow-up protocols.

2. **What is the pathophysiology of forgotten double J stents?**

Ans: The most common sequelae of forgotten or retained stents is the encrustation that form on the DJS. As the indwelling time increases, the chances of encrustation also increases and it has been observed that the stent encrustation rates are 9.2%, 47.5% and 76.3% if the stent remains indwelling for 6 weeks, 6–12 weeks and more than 12 weeks, respectively.[10] The cause of encrustation is multifactorial. Urinary tract infection is considered the main factor leading to stent encrustation. Urea-splitting organisms in urinary tract infection hydrolyses urea to produce ammonia which in turn makes the urine alkaline to precipitate calcium, magnesium and phosphate over the stone surface. Associated metabolic factors like hypercalcemia, hyperoxaluria, hypocitraturia and hyperuricosuria also contribute to encrustations on the DJS. A biofilm develops due to urease-producing bacteria which further enhances crystal deposition over the stent. The development of the biofilm is a complex procedure which starts with the agglomeration of proteins, polysaccharides and macromolecules with further deposition of bacteria. The biofilm matures and spreads facilitating encrustation over the stent.[11] Malignancy also predisposes to encrustations due to stasis, poor fluid intake, chemotherapy-induced hyperuricosuria and infection.[12] Other causes of stent encrustations are stone disease, congenital abnormalities, pregnancy, sepsis, metabolic factors and chronic renal failure.[13]

Most of the studies show that the encrustations occur on the upper coil of the DJS as the peristalsis sweeps the encrustation from the lower part of the stent.[12] However, Dakkak *et al* reported a higher incidence of stent encrustation in the bladder (68.2%), followed by the ureter (59%) and then the kidney (36.4%), possibly due to prolonged contact time of urine in the bladder.[13]

3. **What are the complications of forgotten DJ stent?**

Ans: The most common complications of forgotten DJ stents are encrustation, migration, breakage, urinary tract infection and renal failure. The complication rates vary in difference series. Nawaz, *et al*. reported stent encrustation in 10.5%, stent migration in 3.5% and stent breakage in 4.5% of cases;[14] and in another study, complications like stent fragmentation (20%), fever (16%), sepsis (8%), and haematuria requiring transfusion (4%) were noted.[15]

The mechanism of stent migration is not clear but probably takes place due to the ureteral peristalsis. It has been observed that the use of proper size of stent and polyurethrane material which has better shape memory, leads to proper coil in the renal pelvis and prevents migration.[16]

Stent fragmentation and breakage is usually seen in long-term stenting due to mechanical stress and decrease in tensile strength due to depolymerisation. Attributing factors include prolonged exposure to urine, infection and poor stent quality.[10]

Urinary tract infections and urosepsis are common complications of urinary stents. Bacterial colonization is very common on chronic indwelling stents almost about 100% and almost 69% in temporary stents leading to bacteria in 45% of patients which can further lead to urinary tract infections in 11% of patients. When the bacteria enter the bloodstream through the renal parenchyma, urosepsis develops and in severe sepsis 30% will further progress septic shock having a high mortality of 30–40%.[17] Recurrent infections can lead to pyonephrosis and deterioration of renal function leading to chronic kidney disease in up to 18.4% of patients and up to 5.2% might require renal replacement therapy.[18]

4. How do you clinically evaluate and investigate patients with forgotten DJS?

Ans: A proper clinical history of stone disease, previous surgery and indwelling time is of utmost importance. Patients with DJS can present with irritative voiding symptoms, dysuria, flank pain, fever and hematuria. Imaging is very crucial in defining the extent of encrustation over the stent (Fig. 19.2). The two most commonly used scoring systems are: Kidney, ureter, bladder (KUB) and forgotten encrusted, calcified (FECal) scoring systems.[19,20] The KUB system identifies stents at risk for requiring multiple surgeries, multimodal surgery, and operative time of more than 180 minutes (Table 19.1). Alex *et al* proposed a forgotten, encrusted, calcified (FECal) Double-J ureteral stents grading system which was based on the stone size, location and degree of stent encrustation (Fig. 19.3). They proposed following grading system:

- Grade I: Minimal linear encrustations along either of the pigtail portions of the indwelling ureteral stent.

TABLE 19.1: KUB grading system for encrusted ureteral stents

K-Kidney
• No evidence of calcification on the renal coil • Visible calcification on the renal coil, maximal width < 5 mm, coil is not filled • Visible calcification on the renal coil, maximal width > 5 mm, coil is not filled • Coil if filled, calcification extends < 5 mm outside of coil • Coil if filled, calcification extends < 5 mm outside of coil (includes staghorn)
U-Ureter
• No evidence of calcification along the ureteral portion of stent • Single calcification along stent, maximal width < 5 mm • Single calcification along stent, maximal width > 5 mm • Multiple calcifications along stent occupying < 50% of length of ureteral portion of stent, maximal width > 5 mm • Multiple calcifications along stent occupying ≥ 50% of length of ureteral portion of stent, maximal width > 5 mm
B-Bladder
• No evidence of calcification on the bladder coil • Visible calcification on the bladder coil, maximal width < 5 mm, coil is not filled • Visible calcification on the bladder coil, maximal width > 5 mm, coil is not filled • Coil is filled, calcification extends < 5 mm outside of coil • Coil is filled, calcification extends > 5 mm outside of coil

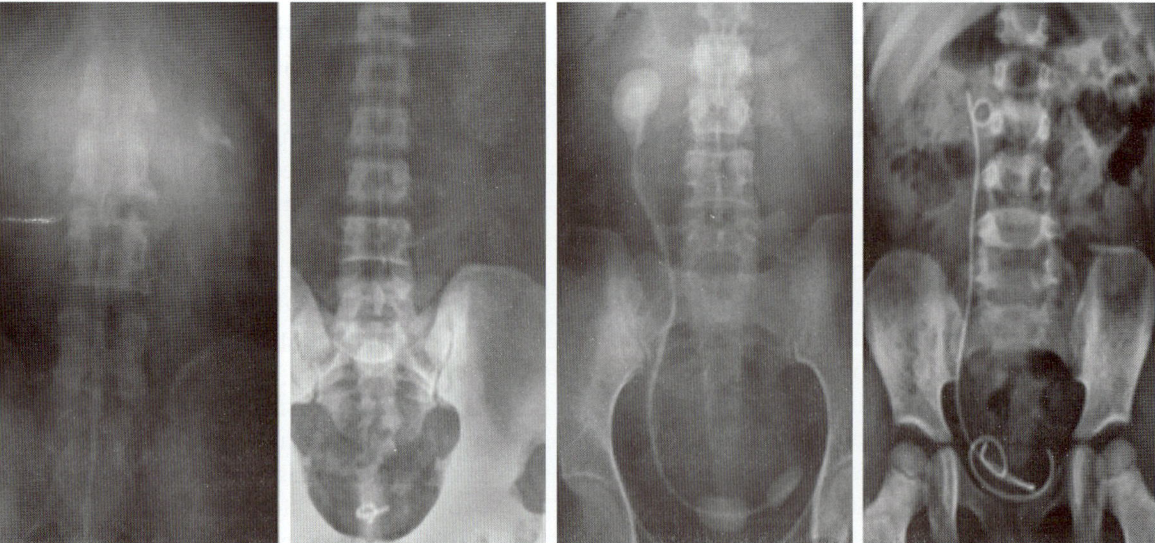

Fig. 19.2: Images of broken, encrusted and stone formations on forgotten stent

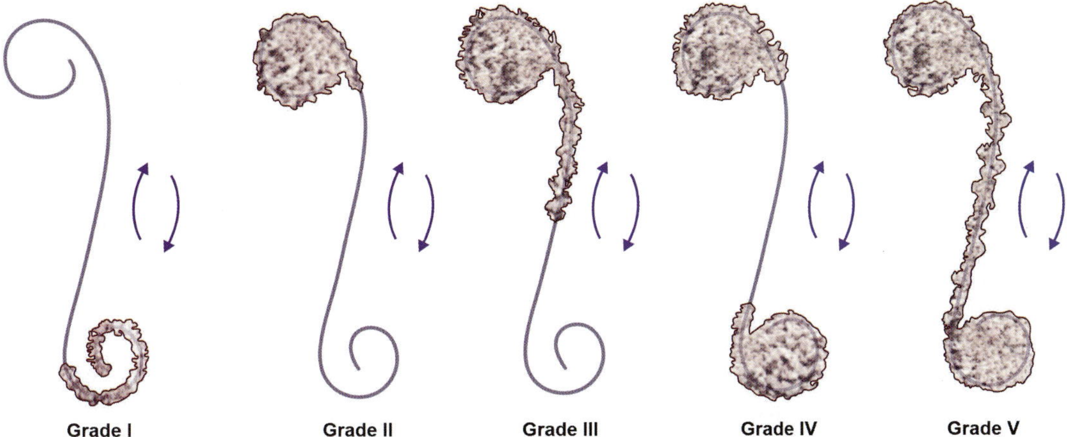

Fig. 19.3: The forgotten, encrusted, calcified (FeCal) grading system

- Grade II: Circular encrustation completely encasing either of the pigtail portions of the indwelling ureteral stent.
- Grade III: Circular encrustation completely encasing either of the pigtail portions as well as linear encrustation of the ureteral aspects of the indwelling ureteral stent.
- Grade IV: Circular encrustations completely encasing both of the pigtail portions of the indwelling ureteral stent.
- Grade V: Diffuse and bulky encrustations completely encasing both of the pigtail and ureteral portions of the indwelling ureteral stent.

Guner *et al* compared these two scoring systems and suggested that the KUB encrusted stent scoring system is better at predicting the number of procedures required to achieve stone and stent-free status.[21] Recently a Visual Grading for Ureteral Encrusted Stent (V-GUES) classification has been proposed which helps to assess the complication rate, treatment success, and the number of sessions required for the patient to be stone and stent-free. It also helps to counsel the patients about the best treatment options and their outcomes[22] (Fig. 19.4).

On CT scan if there is gross hydronephrosis with reduced cortical thickness, evaluation of the function of the kidney is warranted by a radioisotope renal scan. Before any surgical intervention, a sterile urine culture is preferred. If the urine culture shows significant bacterial colony count, it should be treated with appropriate antibiotics prior to surgical intervention. If the urine culture is negative, patient should be operated under proper antibiotic cover.

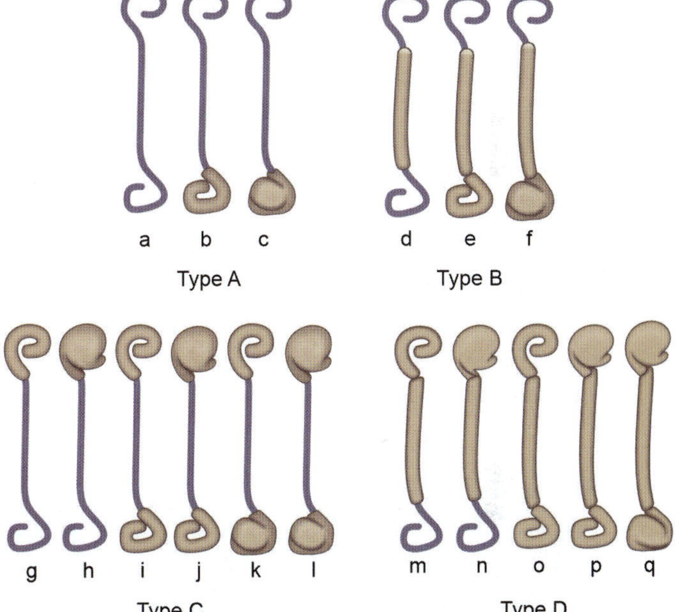

Fig. 19.4: Visual grading for ureteral encrusted stent (V-GUES) classification (Type A: Linear or nonlinear calcification in the distal stent's tail, susceptible to being retrieved with cystolithotripsy; Type B: Linear or nonlinear calcification in the distal stent's tail associated with calcification of the stent's uretheral portion, susceptible to being removed with semirigid ureteroscopy; Type C: Linear or nonlinear calcification of the stent's proximal portion, which could also be associated with distal stent's tail calcification without compromising the uretheral stent's portion, susceptible to being removed with combined access; and Type D: Linear or nonlinear calcification of the proximal stent's portion associated with calcification of the ureteral stent's portion, which could also be calcification of the distal stent's tail, susceptible to removal with combined access. Please check the supplementary video to see a non-enhanced CT scan with a Type C encrusted stent. Color images are available online)

5. What are the treatment options for forgotten DJS?

Ans: Careful assessment of the stent encrustation is essential before any endoscopic intervention. Imaging gives a clue whether the encrustation is present on the kidney coil, bladder coil or on the full length of the ureteric part of the stent. If the encrustation is minimal, simple cystoscopic stent retrieval with forceps is possible. If the encrustation is significant, then additional surgical interventions are required for the removal (Fig 19.5). Sometimes, the stent encrustation is detected intraoperatively during the first attempt of stent removal. In such cases, if the stent is not yielding to removal by forceps, the procedure needs to be abandoned and proper planning for staged endoscopic removal under anaesthesia is contemplated.[23] Bultitude *et al* reported difficulty during cystoscopic removal in 14.3% at 2 months and 42.8% at four months.[7] Sometimes, a single endoscopic procedure is not sufficient and a combination of procedures is required for DJS removal. Forgotten DJS can require multiple procedures and multiple stages for removal. Lam *et al* showed that on average 2.7 procedures are required to clear the encrustations and remove the stent, while Mohan-Pillai *et al* suggested an average of 2.5 endourological procedures for stent-free status.[24,25] Minimally invasive surgery is to be considered the first-line therapy for encrusted stent removal.[13] Fragmented stents usually require combined approach and multiple procedures. Patients with fragmented and bilateral forgotten stents should be counselled for the need for the multiple surgeries.

6. **What would be the role of cystolithotripsy?**

   Ans: This surgery is required when the amount of encrustation is too large over the bladder coil of the stent or when a large stone is present around the lower end of the DJ stent in the bladder. Stone can be fragmented either by pneumatic or by laser energy source. With the use of a holmium laser, there is a distinct advantage of performing dusting for the encrustation or fragmentation of the bladder stone in an attempt to extract the DJ stent in toto. High laser energy of 1–2 J with a frequency of 10–15 Hz is recommended with holmium laser during cystolithotripsy.[22]

7. **When would one need to resort to ureteroscopy?**

   Ans: When the stent encrustation on the ureteric part of the DJ stent hinders removal by cystoscopy, ureteroscopy with either a pneumatic or holmium laser can be used to fragment the encrustation and extract the stent.[26,27] Thomas *et al* have suggested a novel method of using a retrograde approach with a semi-rigid and flexible scope for removing encrusted stent by fragmenting and sequentially cutting the stent with a holmium laser.[28]

8. **Would one need shock wave lithotripsy (SWL)? When?**

   Ans: When the encrustations are located mainly in the upper coil or the upper ureteric segment, shock wave lithotripsy is preferred for stone fragmentation.[29] However, the use of SWL is limited and is indicated only in localized, low-volume encrustations.[30]

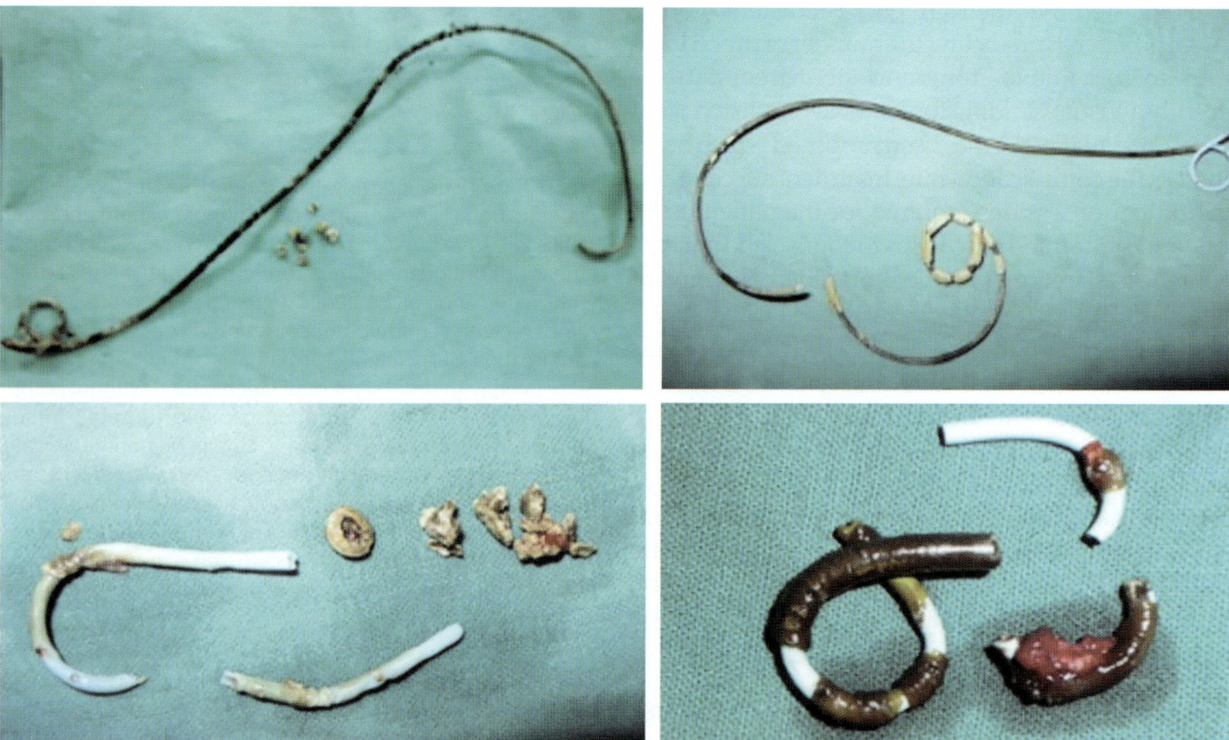

Fig. 19.5: Postoperative images of forgotten stent removed endoscopically

9. **When would you consider percutaneous nephrolithotomy (PCNL)?**
   Ans: A percutaneous approach is usually required for a large stone burden over the stent in the kidney coil or upper ureter wherein the retrograde approach is not feasible. For heavy full-length encrustation, a combined retrograde and antegrade approach is required for complete fragmentation of the encrustations and to make the patient stone and stent-free. The patient should be counselled beforehand regarding the complications and results of this combined approach.[21,29]

10. **Any role of endoscopic combined intrarenal surgery (ECIRS)?**
    Ans: Though there are very few reports of ECIRS in the literature, we feel that ECIRS will become an important procedure for the removal of the forgotten stent. The main advantage will be of a single-stage procedure to make the patient stone and stent-free.

11. **And lastly, would you need to resort to open surgery?**
    Ans: With the availability of newer smaller endoscopes, flexible ureteroscope and lasers, the need for open surgery for encrusted stone removal has significantly gone down. If the endourological approach fails, rarely open surgery is considered. For poorly or non-functioning kidneys due to encrusted stents nephrectomy is performed.[30]

    We suggest an algorithm for management of forgotten stent (Flowchart. 19.1).

Forgotten stents in paediatric patients:

Double J stents are commonly used in paediatric urological surgeries during endoscopic stone removal and after reconstructive surgeries. Special care has to be taken for children as it increases the morbidity, hospital stay and can also affect the renal function. Stent placement should be informed to the parents verbally, should also be mentioned on the discharge card with the tentative time of stent removal and reminder for stent removal on failure to follow-up, to avoid further complications.[31]

Flowchart 19.1: Algorithm for management of forgotten DJ stent

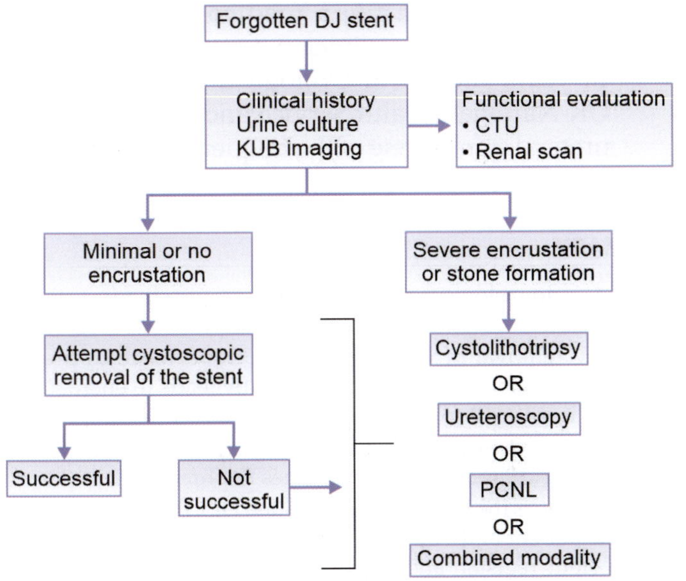

12. **What are the preventive steps for forgotten DJS?**
    Ans: Though there are many reports of successful management of complicated encrusted DJ stents with an aggressive endourological approach, the best primary treatment is prevention. There are various ways for preventive strategies (Table 19.2).

TABLE 19.2: Preventive measures for forgotten stent

Patient-related measures	*Surgeon/hospital measures*
1. Preoperative counselling of the patient and relatives regarding the need for DJS placement	1. Stent register
2. Postoperative XR KUB with DJS shown to the patient	2. Mentioning the DJS placement in the discharge card
3. Importance of follow-up for DJS removal	3. Telephonic call for follow-up and DJS removal
4. Removed DJ stent to be shown to the patients and the relatives	4. Software-based messaging regarding the date of DJS removal
	5. Smartphone-based applications

Patient Education

Before discharge, the patient and relatives should be counselled regarding the DJS removal or change and should be given appointment for the same. The hospital should keep a record of all patients with the DJS, including the date of insertion, follow-up date, and probable time of removal, and in addition, to mention all the details in the discharge summary including the date of stent removal.

Agarwal *et al* suggested a three-steps preventive check method for stent removal in time. The first was to do an X-ray KUB and to show the indwelling stent to the patient and the relatives. The second was to place a stamp on the discharge card mentioning the stent information and thirdly maintain a stent diary. Patients were then called periodically for a visit for stent removal.[9]

Surveillance and record keeping

Record keeping can be done in notebooks, registers or a computer program. The drawback of paper record-keeping is that it remains with the hospital and the patient has to be informed at the time of stent removal. This has a failure rate of 22.4%. To overcome this Ather *et al* has devised a computerised tracking program which reduced the incidence of forgotten DJs from 12.5% to 1.2% in the first year of its application.[32]

Smartphone Applications and Dedicated Applications

Various other methods like sending messages, computer programs, and smartphone apps for stent tracking are used for the timely removal of DJs.[33,34] These applications are dedicated stent trackers. All the patient information like name, date of DJS insertion, expected date of removal and date on which the stent is removed is recorded. Automatic messages and emails are sent to the patients, reminding the date of stent removal or follow-up for DJ stent change. These new applications in future will reduce the incidence of forgotten DJS in a significant way.

13. Ultimately what was done in this case? What was the outcome?

Ans: The patient was treated with appropriate antibiotics as per the urine culture and sensitivity and was planned for endoscopic removal. A combined approach was essential and the patient underwent cystolithotripsy, ureteroscopy and PCNL for stone and stent removal. Stones and encrustations were fragmented with pneumatic lithotripsy and the stent was extracted. Postoperative KUB showed complete clearance (Fig. 19.1). Patient was restented after the procedure and was informed regarding the removal of stent in time. The stent was removed in due course.

14. What are drug eluting and biodegradable stents?

Ans: Drug eluting devices are commonly used in vascular lesions to prevent re-stenosis. The same principle is now applied for urinary stents to prevent re-stenosis as well as stent related complications. Drug eluting stents also has an advantage of preventing drug absorption, distribution and metabolism, thus maintaining the urine drug levels in the optimal therapeutic range.[35] Drug eluting devices can be coated with various materials: Antibiotics like Triclosan, quinolones, silver or Nitrofurazone, RNA-inhibiting peptides and Teicoplanin or heparin, Anti-inflammatory substances like Ketorolac, Indomethacin, Dexamethasone or Simvastatin or anti-proliferative agents like Paclitaxel.[36]

DJ stents used in current practice are biostable in nature. After it has served its purpose it requires removal which incurs additional cost, patient anxiety, anaesthetic risks in pediatric population. Stent encrustation, infection and neglected forgotten DJ stents are some other commonly encountered clinical situations. There has been ever growing need amongst urologists for a biodegradable ureteral stent (BUS). Ideal BUS should glide smoothly over guidewire during insertion, should not migrate or adhere to ureteric wall, should not have local inflammatory response, should not lead to erosion or fistulisation with surrounding organs, should drain urine adequately, should not be carcinogenic, should be radiopaque on radiography and should dissolve completely after weeks without causing hydroureteronephrosis secondary to retained fragment.[37]

Researchers are still in pre-clinical stage to develop ideal BUS with a few promising studies. The main hurdle in developing a biodegradable DJ stent has been unpredictability of degradation rate, challenge of maintaining its mechanical strength, likelihood of obstruction caused by degradation product and difficulty in retrieving partially retained stent products and morbidity associated with it. Synthetic materials like poly-L-lactide-co-glycolide (PLGA), polylactic acid (PLA), polyglycolic acid (PGA), polyglycolic acid/polylactic acid (PGLA), polycaprolactone (PCL), polydioxanone (PDX) has been used in various canine studies with variable success rates. There has been a few studies defining early promising role of magnesium based alloy in developing BUS.[38]

15. What are the medicolegal implications of forgotten DJ stent?

Ans: Apart from the complications of the retained stent, it also has medicolegal implications. If the patient is not informed about the stent placement, follow-up protocol and approximate date of stent removal, he can file a medicolegal suit under negligence by the clinician. Osman *et al* analysed 14 years successful Urological litigations in the UK National Health Service and found forgotten ureteral stent as one of the frequent post-operative-related claims.[39]

SUMMARY

- Most endourological stone surgeries require the insertion of DJS.
- Timely removal of DJS is of utmost importance to prevent complications. Forgotten DJS frequently leads to encrustation which is difficult to manage.
- It usually requires combined endoscopic procedures and rarely open surgical removal or sometimes nephrectomy.
- Prevention is the best cure for forgotten DJS. Proper counselling of the patient and relatives, timely follow-up, record-keeping in a stent register, and regular intimations to the patient by

messaging software or smartphone applications have become important tools to avoid this condition.

REFERENCES

1. Zimskind PD, Fetter TR, Wilkerson JL. Clinical use of long-term indwelling silicone rubber ureteral splints inserted cystoscopically. J Urol. 1967; 97:840–84.
2. Finney RP. Experience with new double J ureteral catheter stent. J Urol 1978;120:678–81.
3. Kuno K, Menzin A, Kauder HH, Sison C, Gal D. Prophylactic ureteral catheterization in gynecologic surgery. Urology. 1998; 52:1004–1008.
4. Dyer RB, Chen MY, Zagoria RJ, Regan JD, Hood CG, Kavanagh PV. Complications of Ureteral Stent Placement. RadioGraphics 2002; 22:1005–1022.
5. Geavlete P, Georgescu D, Multescu R, Stanescu F, Cozma C, Geavlete B. Ureteral stent complications–experience on 50,000 procedures. Journ Med Life. 2021;14(6):769–775.
6. Bultitude MF, Tiptaft RC, Glass JM, Dasgupta P (2003) Management of encrusted ureteral stents impacted in upper tract. Urology 62:622–626.
7. Monga M, Klein E, Castañeda-Zúñiga WR, Thomas R. The forgotten indwelling ureteral stent: A urological dilemma. J Urol 1995; 153:1817–9.
8. Agrawal M, Gite V, Sankapal P, Maheshwari M, Shah A, Dias S *et al*. Retained ureteral stents, an avoidable source of morbidity: 10 years' experience from a single tertiary care centre. Pan African Medical Journal. 2022;42(68). 10.11604/pamj.2022.42.68.29935.
9. Divakaruni N, Palmer CJ, Tek P, Bjurlin MA, Gage MK, Robinson J, *et al*. Forgotten ureteral stents: who's at risk? J Endourol. 2013;27(8):1051–4. https://doi.org/10.1089/end.2012.0754. Epub 2013 Jul 13. PMID: 23590526.
10. El-Faqih SR, Shamsuddin AB, Chakrabarti A, Atassi R, Kardar AH, Osman MK *et al* (1991) Polyurethane internal ureteral stents in the treatment of stone patients: morbidity related to indwelling times. J Urol 146:1487–1491.
11. Castellano C, Nebot A, Romeu J, Soria F, Llopis J. Forgotten ureteral stent syndrome. In: Federico S, Duje R, Graaf. P, editors. Urinary Stents: Current State and Future Perspectives. 1st ed. Switzerland. Springer; 2022. PP. 111–125. ebook. https://doi.org/10.1007/978-3-031-04484-7.
12. Singh I, Gupta NP, Hemal AK, Aron M, Seth A, Dogra PN. Severely encrusted polyurethane ureteral stents: management and analysis of potential risk factors. Urology 2001;58(October (4)):526–31.
13. Dakkak Y, Janane A, Ould-Ismail T, Ghadouane M, Ameur A, Abbar M. Management of encrusted ureteral stents. Afr J Urol 2012;18(3): 131–4.
14. H. Nawaz, M. Hussain, A. Hashmi, Z. Hussain, Experience with indwelling JJ stents, J. Pakistan Med. Assoc. 43 (1993) 147–149.
15. Maher Al-Hajjaj, Oula Abou Alam, Bilal Abu-Hussein, Hasan AL. Muhammad AL Husein. Forgotten Double-J ureteral stent: An analysis of 25 cases in a tertiary hospital. Annals of Med Surg. 80 (2022) 104223. https://doi.org/10.1016/j.amsu.2022.104223.
16. Ramachandra M, Mosayyebi A, Carugo D, Somani BK. Strategies to improve patient outcomes and QOL: current complications of the design and placements of ureteric stents. Res Rep Urol. 2020;12:303–14.
17. Scotland KB, Lo J, Grgic T, Lange D. Ureteral stent-associated infection and sepsis: pathogenesis and prevention: a review. Biofouling. 2019;35:117–27.
18. Murtaza B, Alvi S. Forgotten ureteral stents: an avoidable morbidity. J Coll Physicians Surg Pak. 2016;26(3):208–12.
19. Arenas JL, Shen JK, Keheila M, Abourbih SR, Lee A, Stokes PK, *et al*. Kidney, ureter, and bladder (KUB): a novel grading system for encrusted ureteral stents. Urology. 2016;97:51–5. https://doi.org/10.1016/j.urology.2016.06.050. Epub 2016 Jul 12. PMID: 27421780.
20. Acosta-Miranda AM, Milner J, Turk TM. The FECal double-J: a simplified approach in the management of encrusted and retained ureteral stents. J Endourol. 2009;23:409–15.
21. Guner E, Seker KG. Comparison of Two Different Scoring Systems in Encrusted Ureteral Stent Management: A Single-Center Experience. Urology Journal/Vol 17 No. 3/ May-June 2020/ pp. 248–251. [DOI:10.22037/uj.v0i0.5516].
22. Manzo BO, Alarcon P, Lozada E, Ojeda J, Morales C, Gökce MI, *et al*. A novel visual grading for ureteral encrusted stent classification to help decide the endourologic treatment. J Endourol. 2021;35(9):1314–9. https://doi.org/10.1089/end.2020.1225. Epub 2021 Aug 13. PMID: 33730863.
23. Jones P, Pietropaolo A, Somani B. Endourological Management of Encrusted Ureteral Stents. In: Federico S, Duje R, Graaf. P, editors. Urinary Stents: Current State and Future Perspectives. 1st ed. Switzerland. Springer; 2022. PP. 125–139. ebook. https://doi.org/10.1007/978-3-031-04484-7.
24. Lam JS, Gupta M. Tips and tricks for the management of retained ureteral stents. J Endourol. 2002;16:733–41.
25. Mohan-Pillai K, Keeley FX Jr, Moussa SA, Smith G, Tolley DA. Endourological management of severely encrusted ureteral stents. J Endourol. 1999 Jun;13(5): 377–9.
26. Xu C, Tang H, Gao X, Gao X, Yang B, Sun Y. Management of for-gotten ureteral stents with holmium laser. Lasers in Medical Science 2009;24(March (2)):140–3 [Epub 2008 January 10].
27. Kawahara T, Ito H, Terao H, Ogawa T, Uemura H, Kubota Y, *et al*. Encrusted ureteral stent retrieval using flexible ureteroscopy with a Ho: YAG Laser. Case Reports in Medicine 2012;2012:862539 [Epub 2012 April 3].
28. Thomas A, Cloutier J, Villa L, Letendre J, Ploumidis A, Traxer O. Prospective analysis of a complete retrograde ureteroscopic technique with holmium laser stent cutting for management of encrusted ureteral stents. J Endourol. 2017;31:476–81.
29. Vanderbrink BA, Rastinehad AR, Ost MC, Smith AD. Encrusted urinary stents: evaluation and endourologic management. Journal of Endourology 2008;22(May (5)): 905–12.
30. AravantinosE, GravasS, KaratzasAD, TzortzisV, MelekosM. Forgotten, encrusted ureteral stents: a challenging problem with an endourologic solution. Journal of Endourology 2006;20(December (12)): 1045–9.
31. Nerli RB, Magdum PV, Sharma V, Guntaka AK, Hiremath MB, Ghagane S. Forgotten/retained double J ureteric stents: A source of severe morbidity in children. Afr J Paediatr Surg. 2016 Jan-Mar;13(1):32–5. doi: 10.4103/0189-6725.181704.
32. Ather MH, Talati J, Biyabani R. Physician responsibility for removal of implants: the case for a computerized program for tracking over-due double-J stents. Techniques in Urology 2000;6(September (3)): 189–92.
33. Sancaktutar AA, Tepeler A, Söylemez H, Penbegül N, Atar M, Bozkurt Y, *et al*. A solution for medical and legal problems

arising from forgotten ureteral stents: initial results from a reminder short message service (SMS). Urol Res. 2012;40: 253–8.

34. Ulker V, Atalay HA, Cakmak O, Yucel C, Celik O, Kozacioglu Z. Smartphone-based stent tracking application for prevention of forgotten ureteral double-J stents: a prospective study. Int Braz J Urol. 2019;45:376–83.
35. Barros AA, Browne S, Oliveira C, Lima E, Duarte AR, Healy KE, Reis RL. Drug-eluting bio-degradable ureteral stent: new approach for urothelial tumors of upper urinary tract cancer. Int J Pharm. 2016;513(1–2):227–37. https://doi.org/10.1016/j.ijpharm.2016.08.061.
36. Panagiotis Kallidonis, Athanasios Vagionis, Despoina Liourdi, and Evangelos Liatsikos. Drug Eluting Devices in the Urinary Tract.. In: Federico S, Duje R, Graaf. P, editors. Urinary Stents: Current State and Future Perspectives. 1st ed. Switzerland. Springer; 2022. PP. 387–415. ebook. https://doi.org/10.1007/978-3-031-04484-7.
37. Wang L, Yang G, Xie H, Chen F. Prospects for the research and application of biodegradable ureteral stents: from bench to bedside. J Biomater Sci Polym Ed. 2018 Oct;29(14):1657–1666. doi: 10.1080/09205063.2018.1498184. Epub 2018 Sep 25. PMID: 30141744.
38. Fu WJ, Wang ZX, Li G, Cui FZ, Zhang Y, Zhang X. Comparison of a biodegradable ureteral stent versus the traditional double-J stent for the treatment of ureteral injury: an experimental study. Biomed Mater. 2012 Dec;7(6):065002. doi: 10.1088/1748-6041/7/6/065002. Epub 2012 Oct 9. PMID: 23047290.
39. Osman NI, Collins GN. Urological litigation in the UK National Health Service (NHS): an analysis of 14 years of successful claims. BJU Int. 2011;108:162–5.

Chapter

20

Residual Stones Post-surgery

• *Mallikarjuna Chiruvella* • *Gopal Ramdas Tak*

LEARNING OBJECTIVES

"Post-PCNL small residual fragments" always poses some difficult questions:

- Should it be considered an unsuccessful treatment when small residual fragments are left behind after stone treatment?
- What are the methods available to identify residual fragments, and when is it the best time to assess residual fragments?
- What size of residual fragments that are left behind after stone treatment is acceptable?
- Do all patients and stones have the same risk factors, and are they equally prone to developing complications after stone treatment?
- Is being "stone-free" always the most important outcome after stone treatment, or are there other factors that should also be considered?
- **Imaging:** Imaging plays a vital role in determining the size, location, and number of residual fragments after PCNL. Imaging modalities such as X-ray, ultrasound, and CT scan can be used to assess the residual fragments.
- **Observation:** In some cases, small residual fragments may pass spontaneously without causing any symptoms. Observation can be recommended in these cases, with regular imaging to monitor the size and location of the fragments.
- **Medical management:** Medical management can be considered for small residual fragments that are unlikely to pass spontaneously. Medications such as alpha-blockers, potassium citrate, and thiazide diuretics may be prescribed to facilitate the passage of the fragments.
- **Repeat PCNL:** In cases where the residual fragments are large and cannot pass spontaneously or with medical management, repeat PCNL may be required. Repeat PCNL is a minimally invasive procedure that can be performed to remove the residual fragments.
- **Ureteroscopy:** Ureteroscopy is another minimally invasive procedure that can be used to remove residual fragments.
- **Prevention:** To prevent residual fragments, adequate preoperative evaluation and planning are essential. Appropriate patient selection, proper positioning, and meticulous surgical technique can help reduce the risk of residual fragments. Additionally, postoperative imaging can aid in the detection of residual fragments and postoperative hydration can aid in the management of residual fragments.

INTRODUCTION

Fate of Small Residual Fragments Post-PCNL

Small residual fragments (less than 4 mm) are common after a PCNL procedure, and their fate depends on several factors, such as their size, location, and composition. Here are some possible outcomes for small residual fragments:

Passage: Small fragments may naturally pass out of the body through the urine without causing any symptoms. The urologist may recommend increased fluid intake, diuretics, or alpha-blockers to facilitate the passage of the fragments.

Growth: Some small fragments may grow over time and develop into larger stones. The urologist may prescribe medications to prevent the formation of new stones or to dissolve the existing fragments.

Removal: If the fragments are causing symptoms such as pain, discomfort, or infection, or if they are increasing in size, the urologist may recommend a repeat PCNL, ESWL, or ureteroscopy procedure to remove them.

If the fragments are small, asymptomatic, and not growing, the urologist may recommend observation with regular imaging tests to monitor the size and location of the fragments.

Achieving stone-free status for patients remains challenging, complicated by the inconsistent definition of the term across the urological community. Residual fragments may serve as a source of recurrent stone formation and painful symptoms, leading to significant financial strain for patients. However, conflicting data have also shown that residual fragments may not significantly impact the quality of life of patients and that re-intervention may even worsen their condition.

To make well-informed decisions on how to manage residual fragments, further data is needed to reconcile the discrepant findings and establish clear guidelines.

Case Scenario

A 64-year-old gentleman, a recurrent stone former, presented with right flank pain for six months. On evaluation he was found to have large calculus of 1200 HU in the right renal pelvis measuring 32 × 25 × 11 mm. (Figs 20.1 and 20.2). Multiple calculi, at least 4 in number, were seen in the interpolar and lower pole calyces of the right kidney, the larger one 13.4 × 11.2 mm and 13.1 × 9.3 mm (1200 HU) in the lower pole and 11.6 × 8.5 mm (1100 HU) in the interpolar region. The patient underwent multi-tract PCNL with DJ stent insertion. Post-operative X-ray KUB showed multiple small residual calculi. However, the patient was asymptomatic.

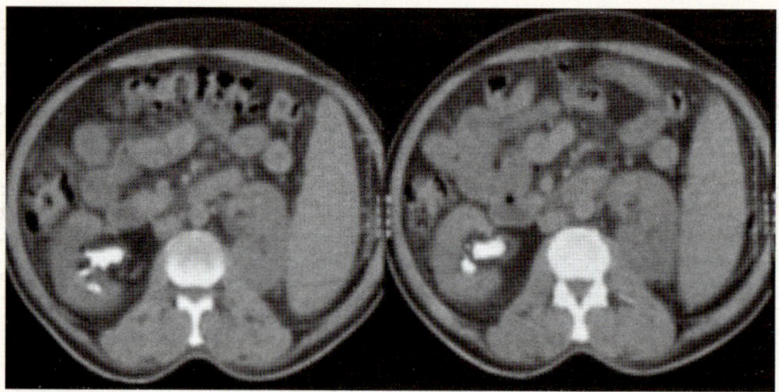

Fig. 20.1: Axial CT image cuts showing right renal staghorn stone

> The management protocol for post-PCNL residual stones can vary depending on several factors such as the size and location of the stone, the composition of the stone, the patient's symptoms, and the surgeon's preference. Urologists will determine the best course of action based on the patient's needs and condition.

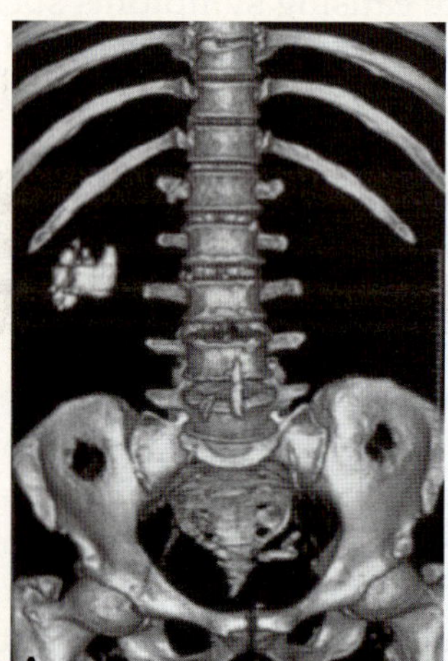

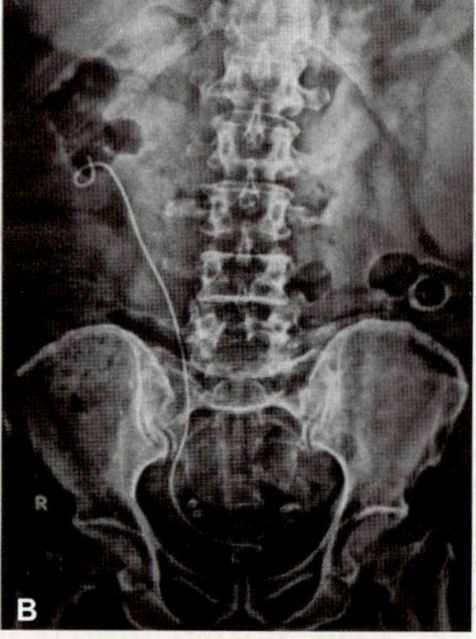

Fig. 20.2A and B: (A) Reconstructed CT image showing right renal staghorn stone; (B) Post Right PCNL residual fragments

1. How important is it to achieve stone-free status during PCNL? What does the literature say?

Ans: According to a study conducted by Krambeck AE *et al*, out of 80 patients who underwent surgery and were followed up for a mean of 19.2 years, 32 patients (36.8%) experienced symptoms related to kidney stones after the surgery. Additionally, among these patients, 8 patients (25%) also developed renal insufficiency.[1]

Altunrende *et al* conducted an interesting study on 430 patients who underwent percutaneous nephrolithotomy (PCNL). A total of 38 patients who had clinically insignificant fragments (CIRFs; 4 mm) were followed for a period of three years. During follow-up, ten (26.3%) patients experienced a symptomatic episode that required medical therapy, while others remained asymptomatic. The radiologic assessment revealed an increase in fragment size in 8 (21.1%) patients, whereas fragment size was steady or decreased in 27 (71.1%) instances. Only three patients (7.9%) experienced spontaneous stone passage.[3] This study proved that fragments 4 mm should not be considered CIRF as the risk of progression in two years is very high.

Raman *et al* went a step further. They followed 42 patients (8%) with residual stones after PCNL. More than 40% (18 out of 42) experienced symptoms related to the stones and 11 of them (61%) required further surgery. The risk of post-operative symptoms that required intervention was higher when the residual stones were larger than 2 mm and located in the renal pelvis or ureter.[2]

It is worth noting that the presence of larger residual fragments is a significant factor in determining the recurrence of stone disease. According to a study conducted by Emmott *et al*, which involved 658 patients, those with residual fragments larger than 4 mm had a higher likelihood of experiencing an earlier recurrence of stone disease compared to those with smaller residuals.[4]

The presence of residual fragments after surgery has been associated with the development of systematic inflammatory response syndrome (SIRS). In a recent study involving 729 patients who underwent percutaneous nephrolithotomy (PCNL), 94 patients (13%) were found to have developed SIRS postoperatively.[5] Residual fragments have also been identified as a risk factor for recurrent urinary tract infections (UTIs). Studies have demonstrated that patients with residual fragments after surgery are more likely to develop UTIs than those without residual fragments. Therefore, residual fragments pose an individual risk factor for recurrent UTIs. ($p < 0.046$).[6]

Treating residual calculi not only reduces the risk of urinary tract infections (UTIs) but also has a positive impact on the overall quality of life (QOL) of patients. By treating residual stones, patients can benefit from the reduced financial burden associated with continued stone treatment and fewer episodes of pain. Therefore, treating residual calculi is crucial for improving patients' physical and financial well-being.

2. Do you mean to say that all residual fragments would be problematic? Does it impact the quality of life? What about cost-effectiveness?

Ans: To fully comprehend the debate surrounding the importance of achieving stone-free status after treatment, it is crucial to acknowledge the inconsistency in defining "stone-free status."

The definition of this term can vary based on factors such as the size of the stone (< 1 mm, < 2 mm, < 4 mm, etc.), the imaging technique used to detect fragments, and the thickness of imaging slices (2 mm slices, 4 mm slices, etc.). Without a consensus on the definition of "stone-free," it is challenging to design strong prospective studies to investigate the potential complications associated with residual fragments.

Despite the significant variation in the definition of stone-free status, a recent study conducted in 2021 revealed that there is no significant difference in disease progression between patients with residual fragments larger than 4 mm and those with smaller fragments.[1] Moreover, from an economic standpoint, pursuing residual fragments is only deemed cost-effective if the fragments after percutaneous nephrolithotomy are larger than 4 mm, as the cost of second-look nephroscopy (approximately $2, 475) is lower than that of long-term management (approximately $4, 674).

Contrary to popular belief, the presence of residual fragments after stone treatment does not significantly impact the quality of life of patients compared to those with no residual fragments. In fact, patients who underwent a re-intervention following initial treatment reported a lower quality of life than those with actively monitored residual fragments.[8]

3. What will you do in this case?

Ans: Since the patient is 64 years old and a recurrent stone former, I will keep this patient on observation.

The observation protocol for post-percutaneous nephrolithotomy (PCNL) residual fragments typically involves the following steps:

1. After PCNL, initial imaging such as ultrasound or CT scan is performed to assess the presence and size of any residual stone fragments.
2. Adequate postoperative hydration is maintained to promote spontaneous passage of small residual fragments.
3. Follow-up imaging is scheduled at specific intervals (e.g., 1–3 months post-PCNL) to monitor the status of residual fragments and any changes in size or location.
4. Patients are monitored for symptoms such as pain, hematuria, or signs of urinary tract infection, which may indicate the presence of residual fragments or complications.
5. Based on the size, location, and clinical significance of residual fragments observed during follow-up imaging, a decision is made regarding the need for additional interventions such as repeat PCNL, ureteroscopy, or extracorporeal shock wave lithotripsy (ESWL).
6. Throughout the observation period, patients are educated about the importance of compliance with follow-up appointments, hydration, and symptom reporting.
7. Any concerns or changes in the patient's condition are promptly communicated to the urologist for further evaluation and management.

This protocol aims to ensure comprehensive monitoring and timely intervention for post-PCNL residual fragments, optimizing patient outcomes and minimizing complications.

4. Which surgery will you do in this case?

Ans: I will keep this patient on observation provided he is asymptomatic, but if the patient insists on complete stone clearance or becomes symptomatic, I will give the option of SWL (which can be done as a daycare procedure under mild sedation or minimal analgesia) or RIRS (which will need general anesthesia, hospital admission, added cost and mild risk of infection).

5. If you choose observation, then how will you follow-up? When to do imaging?

Ans: Since in this case the stone was a radiopaque and small residual stone fragments were clearly seen on post-op X-ray KUB, patient can be followed by a repeat X-ray KUB after 4 weeks and then at 3 months and 6 months provided the patient remains asymptomatic.

If the patient becomes symptomatic then I will intervene and will do either ureterorenoscopy (URS) or RIRS.

6. **Which is your preferred modality for follow-up imaging and why?**

   Ans: Pre-operative X ray KUB is very essential to see whether stone is radiopaque or radiolucent. If stone is radiopaque, then post-surgery I will do X-ray KUB only to check (small) residual stone. If stone is radiolucent I will do USG KUB or NCCT KUB to check stone clearance or (small) residual stone.

7. **What is the indication of PCN in post-PCNL small residual fragments?**

   Ans: In the case of post-PCNL (percutaneous nephrolithotomy) residual fragments, PCN may be indicated if the fragments are causing obstructive pyonephrosis. The fragments may cause obstruction, pain, recurrent urinary tract infection or lead to kidney damage if left untreated. Small PCN tract can be utilized for mini or ultra-mini PCNL to clear residual fragments once infection is controlled.

8. **What is the initial management strategy for small residual stones post-PCNL?**

   Ans: The initial management strategy for small residual stones post-PCNL is observation with serial imaging at 3 months and 6 months and consideration of intervention for stones that are unlikely to pass spontaneously or are causing symptoms.[9]

9. **When is medical therapy recommended for small residual stones post-PCNL?**

   Ans: Medical therapy may be recommended for small residual stones post-PCNL if there is no evidence of stone progression after 3–6 months of observation.[9]

10. **What medications are commonly used to manage small residual stones post-PCNL?**

    Ans: Alpha-blockers and/or thiazide diuretics are commonly used to manage small residual stones post-PCNL.

11. **When is repeat PCNL indicated for small residual stones post-PCNL?**

    Ans: Repeat PCNL may be indicated for small residual stones post-PCNL if there is evidence of stone growth or obstruction on serial imaging, if access to RIRS is not available.

12. **When is shock wave lithotripsy (SWL) indicated for small residual stones post-PCNL?**

    Ans: SWL may be considered for residual fragments greater than 4 mm in size, especially if they are causing symptoms or are not expected to pass spontaneously.

13. **Is there any difference in the management of residual fragments based on stone composition?**

    Ans: Yes, the management of residual fragments after PCNL may vary based on the composition of the stone.[10] For example, if the residual fragments are composed of uric acid, observation may be a reasonable approach as uric acid stones have a higher likelihood of spontaneous passage than other stone types. In contrast, if the residual fragments are composed of calcium oxalate or cystine stones, the risk of spontaneous passage may be lower, and therefore, active intervention may be considered. In addition, certain types of residual fragments, such as those composed of struvite or infection-related stones, may require prompt intervention due to the risk of recurrent urinary tract infections or the formation of new stones.

    The choice of intervention may also depend on the size and location of the residual fragments. For larger or obstructing fragments, interventions such as SWL or ureteroscopy may be more effective in achieving stone clearance, while smaller fragments may be more amenable to observation.

    Therefore, it is important to consider the composition of the residual fragments when determining the appropriate management strategy and to individualize the treatment plan based on the specific case and the patient's preferences and clinical status.[10]

Psychological impact of residual fragments

1. Patients may experience **anxiety and worry** about the presence of residual stones and the potential for recurrence of symptoms such as pain or urinary tract obstruction. The uncertainty about the need for additional treatments or interventions can contribute to heightened anxiety levels.
2. **Concerns about complications** related to residual stones, such as infection, kidney damage, or the need for repeat procedures, can lead to increased stress and fear among patients.
3. Persistent symptoms or the fear of symptom recurrence due to residual stones can **negatively impact a patient's quality of life.** Activities that were once enjoyed may be limited due to discomfort or anxiety.
4. Chronic pain or ongoing urinary symptoms associated with residual stones can contribute to feelings of **sadness, hopelessness, and depression** in some patients. The impact of the condition on daily life and activities can exacerbate these feelings.
5. For patients who undergo multiple procedures or have visible scars from PCNL, there may be

concerns about body image and self-esteem. This can affect social interactions and overall emotional well-being.

6. The stress and emotional burden of dealing with post-PCNL residual stones can also affect **relationships with family members, partners, or caregivers**. Communication and support within these relationships may be impacted.

14. When to assess for post-operative residual fragments (1 month or three months)?

Ans: The timing for assessing postoperative residual fragments after PCNL can vary depending on several factors, including the patient's clinical condition, the size and location of the stones, and the healthcare provider's judgment. However, a common approach is to conduct the initial assessment for post-operative residual fragments within 1 to 3 months after the procedure.

1 Month Post-operative

- Early assessment at 1month post-operative may be suitable for patients who had significant stone burden or complex cases during PCNL.
- It allows for early detection of any large or symptomatic residual fragments that may require prompt intervention or monitoring.

3 Months Post-operative

- Assessment at 3 months post-operative is a more standard timeframe for routine follow-up after PCNL.
- By this time, many small residual fragments may have passed spontaneously or decreased in size, making them easier to manage.
- This timeframe also allows for adequate healing of the urinary tract and reduces the risk of complications associated with early postoperative evaluations.

Significance of profession, metabolic abnormalities, infection stones (struvite calculi), solitary kidney and associated co-morbidities

1. *Profession:* The patient's profession may influence the approach for managing post-PCNL residual fragments. For example, individuals having jobs in army, navy, airforce, pilots will not be allowed to resume their duties or join their duties until they are completely cleared of the stones; which will lead to loss of wages to these individuals. Patients with physically demanding jobs or professions that require heavylifting may experience greater discomfort or limitations if residual fragments cause symptoms or complications.

   Patient occupation can also affect the timing of follow-up assessments and interventions. For instance, individuals with professions that involve frequent travel may require scheduling flexibility for medical appointments.
2. *Metabolic abnormalities:* Patients with underlying metabolic abnormalities such as hypercalciuria, hyperoxaluria, or hypocitraturia may have an increased risk of recurrent stone formation and larger residual fragments post-PCNL.

   Management of metabolic abnormalities through dietary modifications, medication, and lifestyle changes is crucial to reduce the risk of stone recurrence and the formation of new residual fragments.
3. *Infection stones (struvite calculi):* Struvite calculi, commonly associated with urinary tract infections and urease-producing bacteria, can lead to larger and more complex residual fragments after PCNL.

   The presence of infection stones requires comprehensive management, including antibiotic therapy, stone dissolution strategies, and close monitoring for recurrent infections and residual fragments.
4. *Solitary kidney:* Patients with a solitary kidney have unique considerations when dealing with post-PCNL residual fragments. Preservation of renal function and prevention of complications such as ureteral obstruction or recurrent stones are paramount.

   Close monitoring, regular follow-up imaging, and tailored management strategies are essential for patients with a solitary kidney to optimize outcomes and minimize risks.
5. *Associated co-morbidities:* Co-existing medical conditions such as diabetes, hypertension, chronic kidney disease, or autoimmune disorders can impact the management of post-PCNL residual fragments.

   Healthcare providers must consider the patient's overall health status, medication regimen, and potential interactions with stone management strategies when addressing residual fragments in patients with associated co-morbidities.

Significance of prior history of stone disease

Patients with a prior history of stone disease, especially recurrent or multiple episodes, are at a higher risk of developing new stones or residual fragments post-PCNL. This risk is influenced by factors such as stone composition, metabolic abnormalities, dietary habits, and hydration status.

1. *Stone composition:* Patients with a history of calcium oxalate stones may have residual fragments with similar composition, whereas

those with struvite or uric acid stones may have specific considerations in terms of management and prevention.

2. *Underlying metabolic factors:* Patients with a history of stone disease often have underlying metabolic abnormalities such as hypercalciuria, hyperoxaluria, or hypocitraturia. These metabolic factors can contribute to stone formation and affect the size, number, and composition of residual fragments post-PCNL.
3. *Treatment response:* The response to previous stone treatments (e.g., lithotripsy, ureteroscopy, medical therapy) and the outcomes of prior interventions can guide the approach to managing post-PCNL residual fragments. Understanding the patient's treatment history helps in tailoring follow-up plans and preventive measures.
4. *Follow-up monitoring:* Patients with a history of stone disease require regular follow-up and monitoring for stone recurrence, residual fragments, and related complications. Close surveillance allows for early detection of new stones or changes in residual fragments that may necessitate intervention or adjustment of management strategies.
5. *Patient education:* This includes discussing risk factors, lifestyle modifications, dietary recommendations, and adherence to follow-up appointments and preventive measures.

RF in children

Post-percutaneous nephrolithotomy (PCNL) residual fragments in children present unique considerations compared to adults.

1. *Management challenges:* Children may have smaller anatomical structures and different stone compositions compared to adults, which can pose challenges in the management of post-PCNL residual fragments. The size and location of fragments may impact the choice of treatment modalities.
2. *Risk of stone recurrence:* Children with a history of kidney stones are at risk of recurrent stone formation, including the development of new stones or growth of residual fragments post-PCNL. Close monitoring and follow-up are crucial to detect and manage any recurrence early.
3. *Growth and development considerations:* Residual fragments in children may have implications for kidney growth and function, especially in younger patients. Long-term follow-up is necessary to assess the impact of residual fragments on renal health and function as the child grows.
4. *Minimally invasive approaches:* Given the smaller size and unique anatomical considerations in children, minimally invasive approaches such as ureteroscopy or shock wave lithotripsy (SWL) may be preferred for managing post-PCNL residual fragments. These techniques allow for precise targeting of fragments while minimizing potential complications.
5. *Multidisciplinary care:* The management of post-PCNL residual fragments in children often involves a multidisciplinary team approach, including paediatric urologists, nephrologists, radiologists, and paediatricians. Collaboration ensures comprehensive evaluation, treatment, and follow-up care tailored to the child's specific needs.

RF in patients with CKD

Post-percutaneous nephrolithotomy (PCNL) residual fragments in patients with chronic kidney disease (CKD) pose specific challenges and considerations due to the underlying renal impairment.

1. *Risk of complications:* These complications may include urinary tract infections, urinary obstruction, hydronephrosis, and deterioration of renal function.
2. *Impact on renal function:* Residual fragments can contribute to ongoing obstruction, inflammation, and stone-related damage to the kidneys, further impacting renal function in CKD patients. Close monitoring of renal function and imaging studies is essential to assess the impact of residual fragments on kidney health.
3. *Choice of intervention:* The choice of intervention for managing post-PCNL residual fragments in CKD patients depends on various factors, including the size and location of fragments, renal function status, patient symptoms, and comorbidities. Minimally invasive techniques such as ureteroscopy or shock wave lithotripsy (SWL) may be considered to minimize the risk of complications.
4. *Medical management:* CKD patients with residual fragments may benefit from medical management strategies aimed at preventing stone recurrence, promoting fragment clearance, and preserving renal function. This may include dietary modifications, hydration, medications to manage stone composition, and close follow-up with healthcare providers.
5. *Risk of recurrent stones:* CKD patients are prone to recurrent stone formation, necessitating long-term monitoring and preventive measures to reduce the risk of new stones or growth

of residual fragments. Patient education about lifestyle modifications, medication adherence, and regular follow-up is crucial in this population.

Medicolegal implications

1. *Informed consent:* Before undergoing PCNL or any surgical procedure, patients should receive detailed information about the risks, benefits, potential complications, and expected outcomes, including the possibility of residual fragments. Adequate informed consent documentation is essential to ensure that patients understand the potential implications of the procedure, including the risk of residual stones.
2. *Standard of care:* Healthcare providers are expected to adhere to the standard of care when performing PCNL and managing postoperative care, including the detection and management of residual fragments. Deviations from established guidelines or failure to adequately monitor and address residual fragments may raise concerns about the standard of care provided.
3. *Documentation:* Accurate and comprehensive documentation of the PCNL procedure, intraoperative findings, postoperative care, imaging results, patient communication, and follow-up plans is crucial from a medicolegal standpoint. Clear documentation helps establish the rationale for treatment decisions and demonstrates adherence to protocols and guidelines.
4. *Patient communication:* Effective communication with patients regarding the presence of residual fragments, follow-up plans, potential risks, and management options is essential. Poor communication or lack of clarity regarding residual stones can lead to misunderstandings, patient dissatisfaction, and potential medicolegal issues.
5. *Complications and adverse outcomes:* If complications arise due to residual fragments post-PCNL, such as urinary obstruction, recurrent stone formation, infection, or renal impairment, there may be medicolegal implications. Evaluation of the circumstances surrounding the complications, including the management approach and documentation, is crucial in addressing potential medicolegal concerns.

15. Is metabolic evaluation needed?

Ans: Metabolic evaluation is beneficial and often necessary for patients with post-PCNL residual fragments, particularly those with a history of recurrent stone formation or metabolic abnormalities. It plays a crucial role in identifying risk factors, guiding treatment strategies, preventing stone recurrence, optimizing patient outcomes, and guiding follow-up monitoring.

Significance of lifestyle changes and dietary modifications

1. *Prevention of stone recurrence:* Adopting lifestyle changes and dietary modifications can help prevent the recurrence of stones and reduce the risk of new stone formation in patients with post-PCNL residual fragments. These changes target underlying risk factors such as dehydration, high salt intake, and dietary habits that promote stone formation.
2. *Hydration:* Adequate hydration is crucial in preventing stone formation and promoting the clearance of residual fragments. Patients are often advised to increase their fluid intake, particularly water, to maintain dilute urine and reduce the concentration of stone-forming substances.
3. *Dietary modifications:* Low-sodium diet: A low-sodium diet helps reduce urinary calcium excretion, which can contribute to stone formation. Limiting the intake of high-sodium foods and processed foods is recommended.
   Calcium intake: Balancing calcium intake is important. While excessive calcium intake may increase the risk of stones, too little calcium can lead to oxalate absorption and stone formation. A healthcare provider or dietitian can provide guidance on appropriate calcium intake.
   Oxalate-rich foods: Limiting oxalate-rich foods such as spinach, rhubarb, beets, nuts, and chocolate can be beneficial, especially for patients with calcium oxalate stones.
   Purine-rich foods: Patients with uric acid stones may benefit from reducing purine-rich foods like organ meats, shellfish, and certain types of fish.
   Acidic foods: For patients with calcium phosphate stones, reducing the intake of acidic foods and beverages may be recommended.
4. *Weight management:* Maintaining a healthy weight through regular exercise and a balanced diet can help reduce the risk of stone formation and improve overall health. Obesity is a risk factor for stone disease and may exacerbate metabolic abnormalities associated with stone formation.
5. *Regular follow-up:* Patients with post-PCNL residual fragments should have regular follow-up appointments with healthcare providers to monitor stone status, assess metabolic parameters, and adjust lifestyle recommendations as needed.

16. Which are 'high risk' patients for progression of RFs?

Ans:

1. *Large stone burden:* Patients with a large initial stone burden that was only partially treated during PCNL may have a higher risk of residual fragment progression. Large fragments or multiple residual stones are more likely to grow or cause complications over time.
2. *Complex stone composition:* Residual fragments composed of certain materials, such as struvite (infection stones) or cystine stones, are at higher risk of growth and recurrence. These stones may require specific management approaches to prevent progression.
3. *Metabolic abnormalities:* Patients with metabolic abnormalities such as hypercalciuria, hyperoxaluria, hypocitraturia, or hyperuricosuria are at higher risk for stone recurrence and progression of residual fragments. Metabolic evaluation and appropriate management are crucial in these cases.
4. *Underlying renal conditions:* Patients with underlying renal conditions such as chronic kidney disease (CKD), nephrocalcinosis, medullary sponge kidney, or anatomical abnormalities of the urinary tract may be at increased risk for complications related to residual fragments. Close monitoring and specialized care are necessary.
5. *Complicated PCNL procedures:* Patients who experienced complications during the PCNL procedure, such as significant bleeding, perforation, or incomplete stone clearance, are at higher risk for residual fragment progression. These patients may require additional interventions or closer follow-up.

17. How long to keep the patient on follow-up?

Ans: For patients with small residual fragments that are not causing symptoms or complications, short-term follow-up at regular intervals (e.g., every 6 months to 1 year) may be sufficient. During these follow-up visits, imaging studies such as ultrasound or CT scans may be performed to monitor the size and progression of residual fragments.

18. How to prevent residual fragments: planning of tracts, flexible nephroscopy, ECIRS, check nephroscopy?

Ans:

1. **Preoperative Planning:**
   Comprehensive imaging: Utilize high-quality imaging techniques such as CT scans or intravenous urography to accurately assess stone burden, location, complexity, and renal anatomy before PCNL.
   Stone analysis: Perform stone analysis to determine stone composition, which can guide treatment strategies and postoperative management.
   Patient evaluation: Evaluate the patient's medical history, stone history, metabolic profile, and risk factors for stone recurrence to tailor the surgical approach and preventive measures.
2. **Optimized Tract Selection:**
   Tract planning: Plan the PCNL access tract to maximize stone clearance and minimize the risk of residual fragments. Consider factors such as stone location, size, depth, calyceal anatomy, and access angle.
   Access sheath use: Utilize access sheaths during PCNL to facilitate multiple instrument passage, improve irrigation, and enhance stone clearance.
3. **Advanced Techniques and Technologies:**
   Flexible nephroscopy: Use flexible nephroscopy during PCNL to thoroughly inspect all calyces, identify residual fragments, and ensure complete stone clearance.
   Endoscopic combined intrarenal surgery (ECIRS): ECIRS combines flexible nephroscopy with additional techniques such as laser lithotripsy, basket retrieval, or mini-percutaneous approaches to achieve comprehensive stone clearance and minimize residual fragments.
4. **Intraoperative Evaluation:**
   Check nephroscopy: Perform a systematic check nephroscopy at the end of PCNL to visually inspect all calyces, pelvis, and renal parenchyma for any residual fragments. Use angled scopes and flexible instruments as needed for complete visualization.
   Fragment retrieval: Use stone retrieval baskets, graspers, or suction devices to remove any identified residual fragments during check nephroscopy.
5. **Postoperative Management:**
   Imaging follow-up: Schedule postoperative imaging studies (e.g., CT scan, ultrasound) to confirm complete stone clearance and identify any residual fragments early.
   Medical therapy: Consider metabolic evaluation and medical therapy to address underlying metabolic abnormalities, reduce the risk of stone recurrence, and prevent new fragment formation.

By implementing these strategies, urologists can improve the likelihood of achieving complete stone clearance during PCNL and reduce the incidence of post-PCNL residual fragments.

Role of physical therapy (percussion therapy) for RF

It is important to note that physical therapy modalities such as percussion therapy are not established treatments for managing post-PCNL residual fragments. The management approach is primarily focused on urological interventions, medical therapy, lifestyle modifications, and follow-up monitoring under the guidance of healthcare providers specializing in urology and nephrology.

19. Is the incidence of RF dependent on the tract size?

Ans: The incidence of post-PCNL residual fragments may be influenced by factors beyond just the tract size. Stone composition, fragmentation technique, thoroughness of stone clearance, and postoperative management play significant roles in determining the presence of residual fragments.

SUMMARY

Management of post-PCNL small residual fragments seen on imaging

- **Observation:** After a PCNL procedure, imaging tests such as X-ray, CT scan, or ultrasound may be performed to check for any residual stones. If a small residual stone (<4 mm) is seen on imaging, the surgeon may opt for observation with follow-up imaging at regular intervals to monitor the stone's size and location.
- **Medical management:** The patient may be prescribed medications to help dissolve the stone or to prevent the formation of new stones. This may include alpha-blockers, diuretics, or medications to adjust the urine pH levels.
- **SWL (shockwave lithotripsy):** SWL is a non-invasive procedure that uses shock waves to break up kidney stones into smaller pieces that can be passed more easily. This option may be suitable for small residual non-obstructive stones.
- **Ureteroscopy:** Ureteroscopy involves passing rigid or flexible ureteroscope through the urethra and into the bladder and ureter to reach the kidney. The surgeon can then visualize and remove the residual stone using a laser or other specialized tools like baskets or graspers.
- **Percutaneous nephrostomy (PCN) tube placement:** If the residual stone is causing obstruction or infection, a PCN tube may be placed to relieve the obstruction or drain the infected urine before further interventions.
- **Repeat PCNL:** If the residual stone is large or causes symptoms, the patient may need to undergo a repeat PCNL procedure to remove the stone.
- Determining the appropriate management approach for small residual fragments following PCNL requires consideration of factors such as size, location, and composition. Several treatment options are available, including observation, medical management, repeat PCNL, ESWL, and ureteroscopy. It is essential to schedule regular follow-up appointments to monitor the status of the residual fragments and assess the effectiveness of the selected treatment approach.

REFERENCES

1. Krambeck A. AUA 2022: Panel Discussion: Residual Fragments after Stone Surgery: Leave or Chase?
2. Raman JD, Bagrodia A, Gupta A, Bensalah K, Cadeddu JA, Lotan Y, Pearle MS. Natural history of residual fragments following percutaneous nephrolithotomy. The Journal of urology. 2009 Mar;181(3):1163–8.
3. Altunrende F, Tefekli A, Stein RJ, Autorino R, Yuruk E, Laydner H, Binbay M, Muslumanoglu AY. Clinically insignificant residual fragments after percutaneous nephrolithotomy: medium-term follow-up. Journal of endourology. 2011 Jun 1;25(6):941–5.
4. Emmott AS, Brotherhood HL, Paterson RF, Lange D, Chew BH. Complications, re-intervention rates, and natural history of residual stone fragments after percutaneous nephrolithotomy. Journal of endourology. 2018 Jan 1;32(1):28–32.
5. Degirmenci T, Bozkurt IH, Celik S, Yarimoglu S, Basmaci I, Sefik E. Does leaving residual fragments after percutaneous nephrolithotomy in patients with positive stone culture and/or renal pelvic urine culture increase the risk of infectious complications? Urolithiasis. 2019 Aug 1;47:371–5.
6. Agarwal DK, Krambeck AE, Sharma V, Maldonado FJ, Westerman ME, Knoedler JJ, Rivera ME. Treatment of non-obstructive, non-struvite urolithiasis is effective in treatment of recurrent urinary tract infections. World journal of urology. 2020 Aug;38:2029–33.
7. Brain E, Geraghty RM, Lovegrove CE, Yang B, Somani BK. Natural history of post-treatment kidney stone fragments: a systematic review and meta-analysis. The Journal of urology. 2021 Sep;206(3):526–38.
8. Streeper NM, Galida M, Boltz S, Li S, Nakada SY, Raffin EP, Brown DR, Pais VM, Chan JY, Scotland KB, Chew BH. Is stone-free status after surgical intervention for kidney stones associated with better health-related quality of life?-a multicenter study from the north american stone quality of life consortium. Urology. 2021 Feb 1;148:77–82.
9. Ljungberg B, Albiges L, Bedke J, Bex A, Capitanio U, Giles RH, Hora M, Klatte T, Lam T, Marconi L. EAU guidelines, edn. presented at the EAU annual congress Milan 2021. EAU Guidelines Office, Arnhem, The Netherlands. http://uroweb.org/guidelines/compilations-of-all-guidelines. 2021.
10. Özdedeli K, Mete ÇE. Residual fragments after percutaneous nephrolithotomy. Balkan medical journal. 2012 Sep 1;2012(3):230–5.

Chapter 21

BPH in Renal Transplant Patients

• Bipin Chandra Pal • Jyoti Bansal

LEARNING OBJECTIVES

- Pre-transplant evaluation of bladder outflow obstruction.
- Role of pre-transplant TURP.
- Effects of BOO on graft function
- Protocol to avoid renal impairment.
- Role of TURP after transplant

INTRODUCTION

Kidney transplant is the best modality of renal replacement therapy. With increasing pool of older patients (>50 years) awaiting kidney transplant the relevance of lower urinary tract symptoms (LUTS), especially due to benign enlargement of prostate (BEP), holds lot of importance.

Actual incidence and prevalence of BEP in these patients is difficult to assess because of oliguric or anuric state. In pre transplant workup they may be asymptomatic or may not have prior history of LUTS, but they may become symptomatic in post-transplant period after catheter removal. LUTS may exaggerate in the presence of DJ stent. A retrospective study reported an incidence of 9.7% and 7.3% for BEP and TURP 3 years after transplant.[1] Low-pressure storage and low pressure emptying of urinary bladder without residual urine is desirable for the long-term healthy functioning of renal allograft.[2] Thorough evaluation of lower urinary tract is recommended during pre-transplant workup. Regular follow-up in post-transplant period is the key to keeping graft function preserved.

Case Scenario 1

A 60-year-old male with ESRD gets enrolled for the deceased donor kidney transplant. He had LUTS and was taking α-blockers. He has been oliguric for last six months.

1. **What investigations do you suggest?**

   Ans:
   - First and foremost the patient has to be evaluated by transplant surgeon and not only nephrologist before enrolment.
   - Urinalysis (whenever he is passing urine sample can be collected)
   - Serum PSA
   - USG KUB with pre- and post-void
2. **What is the role of urodynamics?**

   Ans: It should be considered if:
   - History of prolonged diabetes (> 10 years)
   - Severe storage symptoms
   - Suspicion or h/o neurological ailment
3. **What is the role of continuing α-blockers in post-transplant?**

   Ans: Continuation of α-blocker in post-transplant period helps in:
   - Increase chances of successful TWOC (trial without catheter)
   - Decrease chances of AUR
   - Decrease chances of UTI
   - Decrease chance of graft dysfunction
4. **Will you do TURP if the waiting period for transplant is prolonged?**

   Ans: No. In an oliguric patient post-TURP complication is high like bladder neck contracture, urethral scarring, bleeding and sepsis.

5. **What precautions will you take during transplant in this patient?**

   Ans:
   - The detrusor may be thick walled, adequate tunnel should be made to have a non-refluxing ureteric reimplant.
   - Neoureterovesical anastomosis should be stented.

6. **What postoperative care has to be taken?**

   Ans: Ensure alpha blocker should be started at least 48 hours before catheter removal besides avoiding constipation and mobilizing the patient.

7. **If required, when will you do TURP?**

   Ans: In post-transplant period.

Case Scenario 2

A 55-year-old male has undergone kidney transplant. After catheter removal he fails to void. How will you proceed?

1. **What investigations do you recommend?**

   Ans: Patient should be assessed with
   1. Review pre-transplant history and workup (USG KUB and uroflowmetry)
   2. Any precipitating factor should be identified like constipation, pain, or DJ stent presence.
   3. USG KUB with pre- and postvoid to access lower tract
   4. Stat output on Foley catheterization.

2. **When will you give a voiding trial?**

   Ans: Start the alpha-blocker and give TWOC after three days.

3. **What will be the choice of α-blocker?**

   Ans: Silodosin should be the drug of choice as it has a short duration of onset of action.

4. **If voiding trial fails what is the next step?**

   Ans: If DJ stent is there, DJ removal to be done as it may also cause stent related LUTS and AUR. Alpha blocker should be started and TWOC should be planned after three days. If this TWOC fails, then proceed surgical management of BPH.

5. **When will you do TURP?**

   Ans: TURP should be done as soon patient's graft function is stable and neoureterovesical anastomosis has been healed. In literature TURP had been done as early as 10th post-operative day of transplant.[15]

6. **What precautions will you take during TURP?**
   - Keep the low-pressure irrigation system.
   - Precise hemostasis.
   - Avoid over cauterization of resection surface.
   - Continue saline irrigation in post-operative period.

7. **Will there be any change in immunosuppression protocols?**

   Ans: Typically, immunosuppression is not altered for elective surgeries. However, there is an important exception for patient receiving mTOR inhibitors (mTORi), as these medications need to be discontinued due to potential complication with wound healing. The alternative regimen is not yet established. Some centers prefer to continue the antimetabolite and slightly increase corticosteroids dose, others prefer a CNI-based regimen until wound healing process is completed.[14]

8. **How long will postoperative antibiotics be given?**

   Ans: Though no standard guideline is there but study suggests continuing antibiotics for three days and catheter removal should be done under antibiotic cover.[12]

9. **What should be the follow-up protocol in post-transplant period?**

   Ans: Though no standard guidelines are available for follow-up specifically in post-transplant patients. Patient with medical management can be followed at three-month interval with specific mention to nephrologist. Similarly, patient who had undergone surgery, follow-up should be done at one month, three months, six months and then yearly.

10. **What are the causes of post-transplant bladder outlet obstruction[3]**

    Ans:
    - Benign enlargement of prostate (BEP): Most common
    - Bladder neck contracture (BNC)
    - Urethral stricture
    - Urinary tract infection
    - Dysfunctional bladder
    - Neurogenic disorder
    - Diabetes mellitus
    - Lymphocele

11. **What would be the important points in history of these patients before transplant?**

    Ans:

    History: Detailed history should be asked for[4–5]

    A. Presence of LUTS (storage and voiding symptoms)

    B. Daily urine output. If anuric, duration of anuria (bladder capacity needs to be assessed if anuria is of more than 1 year)

    C. Presence of constipation (may exaggerate LUTS and may have poor response with medical management)

D. Past or present use of α-blockers
E. History of (h/o) urinary retention
F. H/o UTI
G. H/o urethral instrumentation or catheterisation

12. What about important points in clinical examination?[4–5]

Ans:

A. Local examination of external genitalia (carefully look for presence of phimosis, meatal stenosis).
B. DRE should be done to assess anal tone, prostate size, BCR and presence of fecoliths.

13. How would you evaluate these patients before transplant?[4–5]

Ans:

A. PSA (if age >50 years).
B. Urine routine and urine culture sensitivity
C. USG KUB with prevoid and postvoid residue
D. Uroflowmetry: Voided volume should be at least more than 150 ml for UFM to be representative.
E. MCUG: In patients who are anuric for more than 6 months bladder can be filled with saline and contrast. Filling, voiding and postvoid phase can be done to assess bladder capacity and outflow tract. At the same time uroflowmetry and collection of urine sample for culture and sensitivity can be done.
F. Urodynamic test: Pressure flow study alone or video urodynamic study can be considered if
   - Prior neurological condition suggestive of neurogenic bladder
   - Suspicion of detrusor instability or poor contractility
   - Severe diabetic neuropathy

If patients enrolled for *deceased donor* list, it is prudent to evaluate lower urinary tract yearly. MCUG is desirable if anuria is more than 6 months (will help to assess bladder capacity, outflow tract and PVR).

If required TURP should be avoided in pre-transplant period due to high possibility of developing bladder neck contracture or stricture due to "dry" urethra.[3]

14. How should one plan post-transplant assessment of these patients?

Ans: Patients who had prior diagnosis of BEP in pre-transplant period should continue their alpha-blocker treatment (with or without 5-alpha reductase inhibitor) in post-transplant period. This group of patient has less chance of AUR on Foley catheter removal.[6]

A few patients who neither had LUTS in pre-transplant period nor any finding suggestive of BEP, may become symptomatic in post-transplant period immediately after Foley catheter removal. Symptoms may vary from mild LUTS to repeated failed TWOC to graft dysfunction. Symptoms may exaggerate in presence of DJ stent and/or constipation. Alpha blocker should be started immediately and charting to be done for volume of each void, frequency along with PVR. If symptoms improve and PVR is within acceptable limits, medical management should be continued.

Drug of choice: Silodosin /Tamsulosin / Alfuzosin, any of the medication can be started. In view of short duration of onset of action, silodosin is preferred if started in immediate post-transplant period.

15. Any change in the pharmacokinetics and pharmacodynamics of the transplant medications and prostate medications?[7]

Ans:

1. *Tacrolimus + Silodosin:* Tacrolimus will increase the level or effect of silodosin by P-glycoprotein (MDR1) efflux transporter. Use Caution/ Monitor.
2. *Tacrolimus + Alfuzosin:* Tacrolimus and alfuzosin both increase QTc interval. Use Caution/ Monitor.
3. *Cyclosporine + Silodosin:* Cyclosporine will increase the level or effect of silodosin by affecting hepatic/intestinal enzyme CYP3A4 metabolism. Avoid or use alternate drug.
4. Tacrolimus has no interaction with tamsulosin and or dutasteride.

TABLE 21.1: Initial step to manage LUTS[4–9]

Pre-Tx	*Mild LUTS*	*Mod-Severe LUTS*	*Remark*
Normal urine output	Start AAB and follow with UFM and PVR	Start AAB, if fail then TURP can be considered	TURP should be done 6–8 weeks prior to kidney Tx due to risk of infection
Anuria/oligouria	Start AAB immediately after Tx and at least three days before catheter removal.	Start AAB immediately after Tx. If fail to void, then plan TURP in post-Tx period.	Pre-Tx TURP have high risk of complication like • Bladder neck contracture • Urethral scaring • Bleeding • Sepsis

*AAB: Alpha Adrenergic Blocker, UFM: Uroflowmetry, PVR: Postvoid Residue, Tx: Transplant

If patient fails to void or has persistently high PVR, endoscopic resection should be planned.[8]

16. What would happen if you do not treat BOO?

Ans: After foley catheter removal, high pressure storage and high pressure voiding can severely affect graft function.[3]

In *early post-transplant period* patient can have

- Urinary leak
- Acute urinary retention (AUR)
- Decreased urine output
- Complicated UTI

In *late post-transplant period patient can present with*

- Graft dysfunction
- Recurrent UTI
- Graft pyelonephritis
- Graft VUR

Any unidentified BOO has detrimental impact on graft in short-term and long-term. Apart from routine nephrological evaluation, recipients should be thoroughly assessed for any new onset LUTS. Those who are already on medical management, should be regularly followed with IPSS score, urine analysis and USG PVR.

17. How would you identify a patient who may need BPH surgery after transplant?

Ans: Risk factor for AUR requiring TURP in post-transplant patients:[10]

1. Dialysis duration more than 120 months
2. Age more than 60 years
3. Absence of diabetes mellitus
4. Kidney only transplant

18. When to plan BPH surgery?[3]

Ans: No strict guidelines are present in the literature. Older studies have advised to perform surgery 3–4 weeks after transplant in view of their experience of hazardous complications including death.[2] However, recent studies advise for early intervention (within a month post-transplant) to preserve optimum graft function and at the same time to ensure the ureterovesical anastomosis has had time to fully heal.[11] To strike a balance between preventing unnecessary surgeries for patients with moderate urinary obstruction and identifying those who are most likely to benefit from TURP, it is important to employ an approach that minimizes surgical over-treatment while maximizing the selection of suitable candidates for the procedure. This is appropriate to avoid surgical over treatment of patients with moderate urinary obstruction and at the same time to select patients that are most likely to benefit from TURP.

Surgical modality:[12]

1. TURP: Gold standard procedure either monopoly or bipolar energy.
2. TUIP: Should be considered if[13]
   - Prostate volume <30 gm
   - Patients at risk of detrimental effects of retrograde ejaculation"
3. Laser prostatectomy: No literature available for post-transplant recipient but procedure can be considered if
   - Patient on anti-platelet drugs
   - Large size prostate
4. Other minimally invasive options yet not studied in post-transplant patients.
   - Rezum
   - Urolift

19. What would be the plan for nephrological assessment before TURP?[12]

Ans: Before planning a TURP (transurethral resection of the prostate), it is crucial to exclude other causes of kidney damage. Identifying the optimal timing for TURP is facilitated by this approach. Should there be ongoing issues with kidney function or the presence of proteinuria, the procedure should be postponed. This postponement provides an opportunity for essential interventions like renal biopsy and potential treatments, such as steroid pulse therapy for acute rejection episodes, if needed. TURP is recommended only for those patients who are free from active kidney problems.[10]

20. What should be the immunosuppression (IS) protocol for elective surgery?[14]

Ans: The most frequently used drugs for maintenance IS are

1. Glucocorticoids such as prednisolone.
2. Antimetabolites such as azathioprine, mycophenolate mofetil (MMF), enteric-coated mycophenolate sodium (EC-MPS)
3. Calcineurin inhibitors (CNI) such as cyclosporine A (CsA) or Tacrolimus (Tac)
4. mTOR inhibitors (mTORi) such as Everolimus and Sirolimus

In particular, the first-line recommended triple regimen is Tac, MMF and prednisolone.

Typically, IS is not altered for elective surgeries. However, there is an important exception for patient receiving mTOR inhibitors (mTORi), as these medications need to be discontinued due to potential complication with wound healing. The alternative regimen is not yet established. Some centers prefer to continue the antimetabolite and slightly increase corticosteroids dose, others prefer a CNI-based regimen until wound healing process is completed.[14]

In one of study[12] patients with mTOR-treated, the medication was discontinued at least one week prior to procedure and resumed at leastone week afterwards to prevent interference with surgical healing. To ensure adequate immunosuppression during the perioperative period, dosages of steroid and tacrolimus were increased. Steroid is administered I.V. on the day of surgery (switch from oral prednisone to an equivalent dose of IV methylprednisolone) and then restarted orally as soon as possible.

21. What special precautions would you take during TURP?

Ans:

- Most experienced person in the team should perform the surgery.
- Adequate antibiotic coverage according to urine culture and sensitivity.
- Height of irrigation fluid should be kept at minimum.
- Precise hemostasis.
- Avoid over cauterization of resection surface.
- Continue saline irrigation in post-operative period.
- Antibiotic coverage should be extended in post-operative period.

SUMMARY

- Pre-transplant evaluation of bladder outflow obstruction is of paramount importance.
- Pre-transplant TURP should be avoided.
- Unidentified BOO can result in permanent graft loss.
- Strict adherence to medical management and regular follow-up is needed to avoid renal impairment.
- TURP should be considered if a patient had failed medical management after proper nephrological assessment.

REFERENCES

1. Hurst FP, Neff RT, Falta EM *et al* (2009) Incidence, predictors, and associated outcomes of prostatism after kidney transplantation. Clin J Am Soc Nephrol 4(2):329–336.
2. Tsaur I, Jones J, Melamed RJ, Blaheta RA, Gossmann J, Bentas W. Postoperative voiding dysfunction in older male renal transplant recipients. Transplant Proc. 2009 Jun;41(5):1615–8.
3. de Oliveira Marinho AC, Tavares-da-Silva E, Bastos CA, Roseiro A, Parada B, Retroz E, Marconi L, Moreira P, Nunes P, Simões P, Santos L, Romãozinho C, Figueiredo A. Acute Urinary Retention After Kidney Transplant: Effect on Graft Function, Predictive Factors, and Treatment. Transplant Proc. 2021 Jul–Aug;53(6):1933–1938.
4. EAU Guidelines March 2023. Management of Non-Neurogenis male LUTS. ISBN 978-94-92671-19-6.
5. Power RE, Hickey DP, Little DM. Urological evaluation prior to renal transplantation. Transplant Proc 2004;36:2962–7.
6. Lubetzky M, Ajaimy M, Kamal L, de Boccardo G, Akalin E, Kayler L. Kidney transplant complications from undiagnosed benign prostatic hypertrophy. Clin Transplant. 2015 Jun;29(6):539–42.
7. https://reference.medscape.com/drug-interactionchecker.
8. Sarıer M, Duman, Demir M, Yüksel Y, Emek M, Kukul E. The outcomes of transurethral incision/resection of the prostate (TUIP/TURP) performed early after renal transplantation. Turk J Urol. 2018 Mar;44(2):172–177.
9. Shoskes DA, Hanbury D, Cranston D, Morris PJ. Urological complications in 1,000 consecutive renal transplant recipients. J Urol. 1995 Jan;153(1):18–21.
10. Gratzke C, Pahde A, Dickmann M, Reich O, Seitz M, Jauch K, *et al.* Predictive factors for urinary retention following kidney transplantation in male patients. Scand J Urol Nephrol 2012;46:44–7.
11. Righetto, M., Mancini, M., Modonutti, D. *et al.* Patients with renal transplant and moderate-to-severe LUTS benefit from urodynamic evaluation and early transurethral resection of the prostate. *World J Urol* **39**, 4397–4404 (2021).
12. Volpe A, Billia M, Quaglia M, Vidali M, Marchioro G, Ceratti G, Sogni F, De Lorenzis E, De Angelis P, Airoldi A, Stratta P, Terrone C. Transurethral resection of the prostate in kidney transplant recipients: urological and renal functional outcomes at long-term follow-up. BJU Int. 2013 Aug;112(3):386–93.
13. Gratzke C, Bachmann A, Descazeaud A, Drake MJ, Madersbacher S, Mamoulakis C, *et al.* EAU guidelines on the assessment of non-neurogenic male lower urinary tract symptoms including benign prostatic obstruction. Eur Urol. 2015;67(6):1099–109.
14. Neuwirt, H., Rudnicki, M., Schratzberger, P. *et al.* Immunosuppression after renal transplantation. *memo* **12**, 216–221 (2019).
15. Reinberg Y, Manivel JC *et al.* Transurethral resection of prostate immediately after kidney transplantion. Urology. 1992;39(4):319–321.

Section

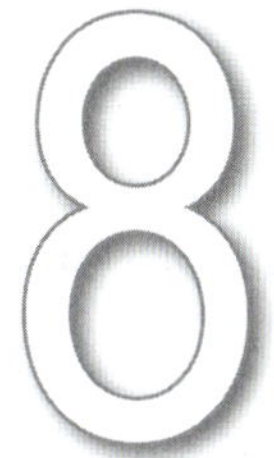

General Urology

Chapter

1

45 Years Man with Milky Urine

• GG Laxman Prabhu

LEARNING OBJECTIVES

- To understand the various presentations of chyluria.
- To understand the pathophysiology of chyluria.
- To detail the various investigations required for diagnosis of chyluria.
- To discuss the various treatment algorithms for chyluria.

INTRODUCTION

Chyle is the result of digestion of fat in the small intestine. While short chain fatty acids are directly absorbed by the intestinal capillaries into the blood stream, medium and long chain fatty acids are first emulsified into fine droplets called chylomicrons, a colloidal suspension of which is called the chyle. In addition, chyle also contains albumin and fibrin. Chyle is collected by specialized lymph vessels in the small bowel called lacteals. It is then carried in the retroperitoneal lymphatics and finally via the thoracic duct transferred to the blood stream. Chyluria results when there is leakage of chyle into the urinary tract. Therefore, chyle is an abnormal constituent of urine. Chyluria can be due to parasitic and non-parasitic causes. Majority of chylurics are seen in areas which are endemic to filariasis. Severe chyluria can cause malnutrition. Evaluation includes confirmation of chyle in urine followed by different types of imaging and cystoscopy with retrograde contrast studies. Most chylurics respond to conservative treatment which comprises diet and anti-parasitic drugs. Sclerotherapy and surgery are reserved for severe forms of chyluria.

Chyluria is an ancient malady. In 300 BC, Charaka, the famous Indian physician called this disease Shuklameha. Hippocrates described this entity in 400 BC.

Case Scenario

A 37-year-old male with milky white urine

A 37-year-old male presents to the urologist's office with history of passing "milky urine", which has been on and off since two years. Of late, he has been finding it difficult to void urine, particularly when urine is not only milky white but thick and viscid. He also reported that whitish discoloration was most prominent in the morning but cleared as the day progressed. There were no other lower urinary tract symptoms. He denied symptoms referable to the upper urinary tract, namely flank pain and colic. He had no history of fever with chills in the last two years but admitted to such episodes about ten years ago during an overseas stint of five years in the African continent. He also reported that during one of these episodes he had pain and swelling on the left side of the scrotum. He had received a course of amoxiclav and diethylcarbamazine citrate (DEC) without any investigations and had been told by the practitioner that treatment for such an illness is only medications. The symptoms had resolved rapidly, but vague discomfort in the scrotum had lingered for a few weeks. He had no loss of weight in the last two years. He denied exposure to the risk of contracting sexually transmitted infections. He was aware of having received BCG vaccine soon after birth but had no contact with individuals diagnosed with tuberculosis at home as well as at work place. He gave no history of major trauma to the flank or abdomen.

He was moderately built and nourished. General examination revealed mild edema of the left foot and the ankle. Abdomen, spine and renal angles were clinically normal. He had a bulky left spermatic cord which neither enhanced nor emptied on standing and lying down. The other organ systems were within normal limits for health. Digital rectal examination was normal.

1. **What are the possible causes of whitish urine in this patient?**

   Ans: A clinician should entertain the following possibilities when a patient gives history of passing whitish or milky urine, viz. A. Chyluria; B. Frank pyuria; C. Phosphaturia; D. Proteinuria; E. Lipiduria and F. Caseouria (Tubercular). Of all these conditions, chyluria can be easily recognized by milky white appearance of the urine (Fig. 1.1). Chyluria is by and large intermittent with intervals of remission. Frank pyuria is characterized by the purulent hue of the urine and constitutional symptoms, namely fever and tenderness in the renal angle as well as suprapubic area. In minor degrees of pyuria, the urine resembles butter milk. Flakes and powdery material is the hallmark of phosphaturia. In proteinurics, the urine is typically foamy or bubbly. Grossly cloudy urine with typical Maltese cross (four "V' or arrowhead-shaped concave quadrilaterals converging at a central point) appearance suggests lipiduria. Presence of cheesy material in the urine should prompt the clinician to consider caseouria.

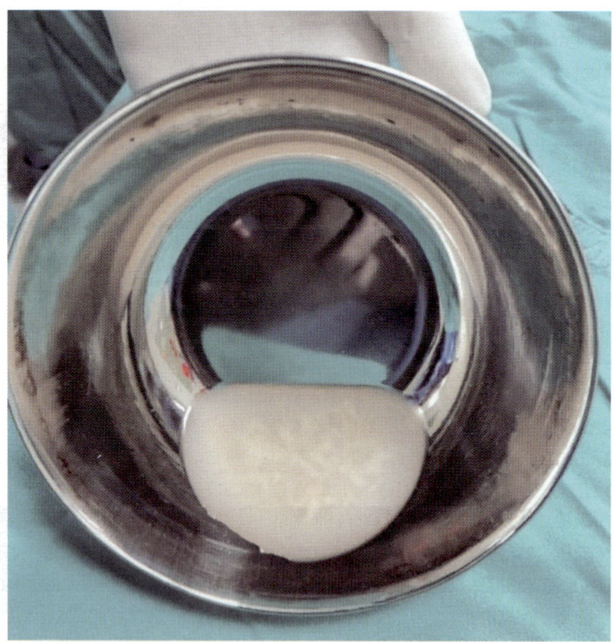

Fig. 1.1: Chylous clots—retrieved from the bladder

2. **How can the clinician ascertain presence of chyle in the urine?**

   Ans: The following tests confirm presence of chyle or fat in the urine:

   1. When made to stand in a receptacle, urine of a chyluric settles into three layers—a top layer of fatty material, the middle layer of pinkish material (clot) and a bottom layer of blood debris.
   2. Ether, chloroform or xylol dissolution test: Addition of ether, chloroform or xylol causes significant reduction in the turbidity of urine.
   3. The conventional heat and acetic acid test done for proteinuria will be negative when there is chyle in the specimen.
   4. A few drops of 1% acetic acid are added to 1 ml of chylous urine. It is then centrifuged at 3000 rpm for 3 minutes. Persistence of turbidity suggests presence of chyle in urine.[1] Urine clears in specimen containing phosphates and pus.
   5. Chylomicrons can be identified under dark ground illumination. Sudan III can be used to stain fat in urine.
   6. Triglycerides are invariably found in the urine of "chylurics". Triglycerides can be measured using a photoelectric colorimeter. This can be done in a patient who gives history of chyluria but when seen in the clinic has clear urine ("intermittent chylurics"). Up to 700 to 900 mg/dl of triglycerides can be found in heavy chylurics. In chylurics with relatively clear urine, 30–90 mg/dl of triglycerides is seen.[1]

3. **What causes chyluria?**

   Ans: The causes of chyluria can be *parasitic* and *non-parasitic*[2]

   Parasitic causes (tropical or endemic): Filariasis (*Wuchereria bancrofti*) causes 95% of parasitic cases.[3]

   Others: Many parasites have been mentioned as causes of chyluria even though a strong cause–effect relationship has not been established in these. Some of them are: *Eustrongylus gigas; Taenia echinococcus; Malarial parasite; Taenia nana; Ascaris; S. haematobium*, and *Ceronomas hominis*. It is also believed that these can coexist with filariasis in the host.[3]

   Non-parasitic causes (non-tropical or European)
   - Congenital: Lymphangiomas (renal and vesical)
   - Neoplastic: Retroperitoneal tumors, lymphomas
   - Traumatic: Injury to retroperitoneal lymphatics
   - Inflammatory: Retroperitoneal lymphangitis causing stenosis of thoracic duct
   - Iatrogenic: Post-radiation, post-partial nephrectomy,[4] post-robotic pyeloplasty[5]
   - Endocrinologic: Diabetes
   - Physiological: Pregnancy

4. **What is the grade of chyluria in the patient under consideration?**

   Ans: Clinical grade is as mentioned in Table 1.1.

TABLE 1.1: Clinical grades of chyluria

Based on the mode of presentation chyluria is graded as Grade 1: Only Milky white urine; Grade 2: White clots with episodes of retention and Grade 3: hematochyluria[6]
In patients with hematochyluria—a large chylous clot admixed with blood adherent to the bladder wall may mimic a urothelial cancer on ultrasound examination[7] (Fig. 1.2).

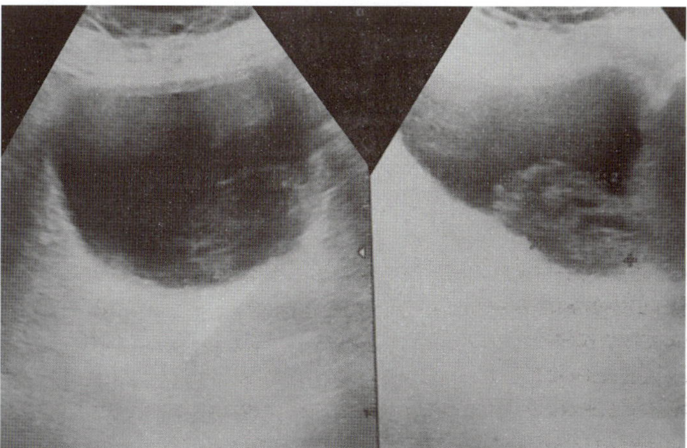

Fig. 1.2: Ultrasound of the bladder showing adherent chylous clot

5. **What could be the most probable cause of chyluria in this patient?**

   Ans: History of living in a country which is endemic for filariasis, the clinical illness alluded to by the patient being highly suggestive of epididymo-orchitis and the medication history point to a parasitic causation, the commonest of which is filariasis.

6. **What is the pathogenesis of chyluria?**

   Ans: Renal lymph is conducted via the retroperitoneal lymphatic channels. These are also responsible for transport of lipids absorbed from the small bowel as chyle. Any obstruction to the flow of lymph in the thoracic duct (of intraluminal, transmural or extraluminal causation) can lead to a pressure build up within the lymphatic vessels draining the organs in the catchment area which include the kidneys. High pressures can cause rupture of these, spilling chyle into the collecting system of the kidneys. Detailed pathophysiology of chyluria enumerated in Table 1.2.

TABLE 1.2: Pathophysiology of chyluria[5]

Two theories have been propounded:
Obstructive Theory
Parasitic infestation (Filarial) causes obliterative lymphangitis. Consequent lymphatic hypertension in the channels proximal to the obstruction (visceral side) will cause dilatation, varicosities and loss of valvular mechanisms leading to backflow into upper lumbar lymph glands which drain the renal lymphatics.
Regurgitative Theory
Toxins released from the dying filarial worms cause transmural inflammation of the lymphatics leading to weakened walls and valves of the larger lymphatic channels with a backlog of lymph in the cisterna chyli from where there will be retrograde flow of lymph into the channels draining the kidneys.
Accumulation of lymph within varicosities whose walls are worn out rupture into the renal collecting system upon attaining a critical intralymphatic pressure is the final common mechanism operational.

7. **What could be the reason for unilateral edema of the foot and ankle in this case?**

   Ans: Laterality of edema is determined by the highly variable anatomical patterns of lymphatic channels draining into the cisterna chyli, which continues as the thoracic duct. The latter conveys most of the body's lymph to the blood stream. The right and left lumbar lymph trunks (kidneys are one of the many structures drained by these) along with intestinal lymph trunks and posterior intercostal lymph vessels drain into the cisterna chyli. In more than 50% of the subjects, the intestinal trunks may drain directly into lumbar trunks or thoracic duct on one side. This may be reason for unilateral edema and more often than not unilateral renal involvement. In practice, this is more commonly seen on the left side.[8]

8. **What are the relevant investigations that are necessary in the initial evaluation of a patient presenting with chyluria?**

   Ans: Majority of the patients presenting with chyluria will not be having active filariasis. In them, a hemogram may only show mild eosinophilia. Serum proteins should always be estimated and hypoproteinemia induced by proteinuria can cause reversal of albumin/ globulin ratio. Filarial antigen in urine and serum can be detected by ELISA method (Fila test). It has a specificity of 85% and sensitivity of 95%.[7] Active filariasis mandates anti-filarial therapy and interventions at the community level for vector control.

   In milder grades of chyluria, especially when interventional procedures are not indicated, abdominal sonography and CECT urogram suffice to rule out compressive retroperitoneal mass lesions.

   In higher grades of chyluria-imaging modalities which can demonstrate *lympho-urinary fistulae* are indicated. The major limitation of imaging modalities is that it is rewarding only in 40% of cases.[3,7]

   Radiological investigations which are done for the diagnosis are mentioned in Table 1.3.

Intravenous urography will be normal in most instances and hence it is not preferred any longer. The dilated lymphatics appear as non-enhancing hypodensities on CECT which are mistaken for lymph nodes. Lymphangiography is an excellent modality of imaging to demonstrate the site, size and number of lympho-urinary fistulae. However, it is an invasive study and calls for the expertise of specialists engaged in its performance routinely. In lieu of conventional lymphangiography, lymphoscintigraphy using Tc-99m diethylenetriamine pentaacetic acid radionucleotides which is a non-invasive study has found preference.[9] Lymphoscintigraphy can show complete or partial obstruction to lymph flow and enhanced flows as well as backflows (reflux). Owing to overlapping reflux, the radio-tracer within the collecting system is oftentimes not discernible.[10]

MR scanning is a useful non-invasive imaging modality in demonstrating pathologic lymphatic channels and scores over CT imaging. On T1 weighted images they are seen as multiple small nodular hypointensities while they appear like a cloak of diffuse homogenous hyperintensities on T2 weighted images.[11]

TABLE 1.3: Imaging studies employed in chyluria evaluation
Ultrasonography—useful in looking for chylous clots in the bladder
Intravenous (excretory) urography (supplanted by CECT urography)
Retrograde uretero-pyelography
Lymphangiography
Magnetic resonance imaging of the retroperitoneum
Lymphoscintigraphy

9. Is cystourethroscopy indicated in every case of chyluria?

Ans: In Grade 1 chyluria, when treatment is essentially conservative, cystourethroscopy is not of much use. In higher grades, it is done for the following reasons: 1. To evacuate chylous clots 2. For lateralization and institution of sclerotherapy, also called renal pelvic instillation of sclerosant (RPIS) and 3. To rule out urothelial disease when imaging studies are equivocal.

When cystourethroscopy is done and the patient is in post-absorptive state, chyluria may be missed. Hence the patient is instructed to have a "fatty meal"six hours prior to the examination to enhance chyluria. Patient may also be asked to ingest 100 mg of butter laden with 100 milligrams of Sudan red III which imparts orange pink color to the urine in chylurics.[12] The coloring agent is expensive and not easily available. Cystourethroscopy should be done meticulously as the source of chylous leak. There can be a "white out" on entry into the bladder which will clear to show chyle in the bladder (Figs 1.3 and 1.4). The chylous leak can also be from the bladder and posterior urethra in addition to be from the upper tract.

Fig. 1.3: White out during cystoscopy

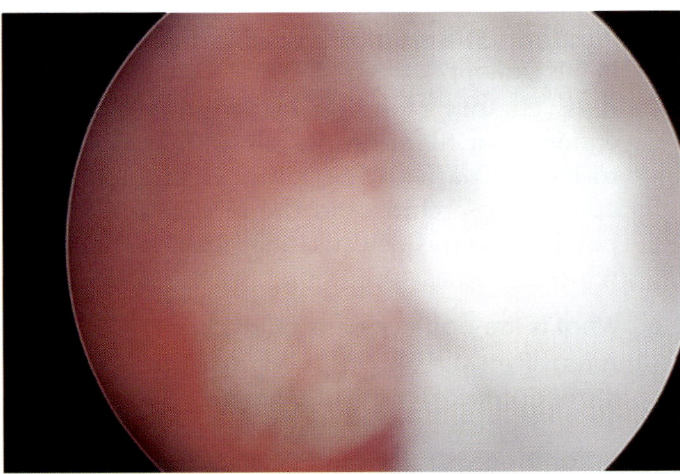

Fig. 1.4: Chyle in the bladder

A chylous efflux is a lateralizing sign (scan QR code to view chylous efflux).

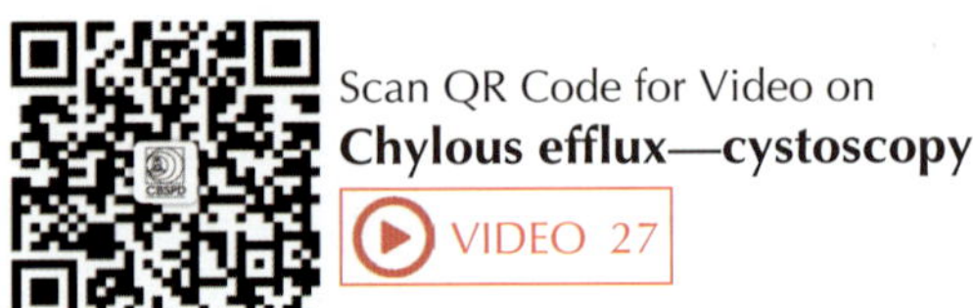

When this is absent, pelvic washings obtained by inserting retrograde catheters on each side can be tested for chyle as well as triglycerides ("split urinalysis").

Cystourethroscopy also provides an opportunity perform retrograde uretero-pyelography which helps in demonstrating pyelo-lymphatic backflow. Retrograde uretero-pyelography should be done with utmost gentleness under fluoroscopic control. Iodinated radio-contrast medium should be trickled into the upper urinary tract (a maximum of 5 to 7 cc which is the average capacity of the renal pelvis) to demonstrate pyelo-lymphatic backflow (Fig. 1.5). Based on the calyceal involvement, three grades of backflows have described. These are mild when a single calyx is involved; moderate when two or more than two calyces are involved and severe when most of the calyces are involved.[13] Forcible instillation may cause intravasation and bacteremic events. Further, distinguishing pyelo-lymphatic backflow from pyelo-venous backflow might be difficult.

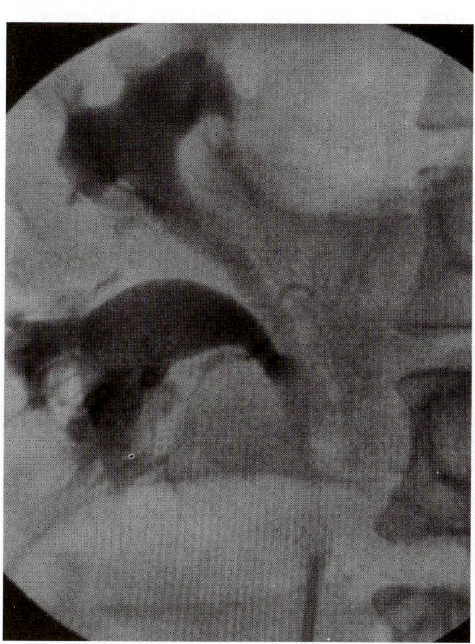

Fig. 1.5: Retrograde pyelography—backflow

Some workers have also tried using gadolinium instead of radio contrast medium for retrograde pyelography claiming that their novel approach obviates ionizing radiation and produces better imaging.[14] In practice, gadolinium MR uretero-pyelography is cumbersome.

10. How is chyluria treated?

Ans: Treatment of chyluria is always done in a stepwise manner (See algorithm of treatment). Majority of the patients are managed conservatively, patients not responding to conservative treatment are offered sclerotherapy (RPIS) and the refractory cases are offered surgery which involves 'chylolymphatic disconnection'.

Conservative Treatment

Majority of patients with mild chyluria are successfully managed by diet and drugs. In the diet, all long chain triglycerides (clarified unsalted butter and mustard seed oil) are replaced with medium chain triglycerides (<12 carbon atoms, e.g. coconut oil). The basis of dietary modification is that small and medium chain triglycerides are directly absorbed into the portal venous system unlike long chain triglycerides which have to be converted into chylomicrons by the enterocytes before being absorbed by the lacteals as chyle. Diet is combined with drugs. Albendazole, diethylcarbamazine citrate (DEC), ivermectin and benzathine penicillin are commonly used in combination and repeated once or twice. Drugs and dosage to manage chyluria are enumerated in Table 1.4.

TABLE 1.4: Antifilarials

Drug	*Action*	*Dose*
Diethylcarbamazine	Larvicidal	6 mg/kg/day × 21 days
Albendazole	Inhibits microtubular proteins of the parasite	400–800 mg/day × 10–14 days
Ivermectin	Blocks neurogenic transmission in the parasites	6–12 mg stat, repeated after 3 weeks
Benzathine penicillin	Inhibits cell wall biosynthesis	1.2 million units weekly for 12 weeks.

More than 70% of patients respond to conservative treatment. Those who do not respond are those with higher grade of chyluria, pretreatment with drugs and those with higher level cholesterol in the urine.[15]

Sclerotherapy

Non-responders to conservative treatment are the candidates for sclerotherapy (RPIS). Sclerosant instilled into the renal pelvis with the aid of retrograde ureteric catheter introduced into the renal pelvis under cystoscopic guidance enters the foci of chylo-lymphatic fistulae, where it causes inflammatory edema (immediate relief) and fibrosis (permanent relief). The procedure is done after a fatty meal under sedation combined with regional or local anesthesia. Chylous efflux guides the clinician to the affected side. 5 to 7 ml (expected renal pelvic capacity in adults) of sclerosant is deposited into the renal pelvis on the affected side in a gentle Trendelenberg position till the patient experiences discomfort.[16] Table 1.5 depicts the common sclerosants used for treating chyluria.

TABLE 1.5: Commonly used sclerosants

Agent	Strength
Silver nitrate[17]	0.1–1%
Povidone iodine	0.2–5%
Potassium bromide	10–25%
Dextrose	50%
Hypertonic saline	3%
Used singly or in combination: 8 hourly instillation for 3 days/ weekly instillation for 6 weeks	

Silver nitrate has been used extensively in the past but has come under the cloud of suspicion in the recent years for three reasons, namely 1. It has to be freshly prepared and medical grade preparation which meets the safety standards is unavailable, 2. Silver nitrate when mixed with normal saline can precipitate as an insoluble silver chloride salt which can be obstructive and 3. A report of mortality following its use.[18] For these reasons, the Urological Society of India issued a directive to all its members to avoid its use.[14]

A mixture of 5% povidone iodine with 50% dextrose, on the other hand, yields a cure rate of around 90% at six months making it a sclerosant of preference.

Surgery

Surgical interventions are reserved for the following patients:

1. Refractory chyluria (those who have not responded to 2 or 3 courses of RPIS)
2. Hypoproteinemia
3. Recurrent clot retention
4. Hematochyluria
5. Recurrent urinary tract infections
6. Altered immune status
7. Psychological disturbances
8. Anasarca
9. Extensive weight loss

Table 1.6 depicts the mnemonic used to remember the definitive indication for surgery.

TABLE 1.6: Indications for surgery

Mnemonic: "***CHYLURIA***"-**C**lot retention, **H**ypoproteinemia/ **H**ematochyluria, **Y**ields easily to stress of illness, **L**oss of weight, **U**rinary tract infections, **R**efractory to sclerotherapy, **I**mmune compromise status, **A**nasarca.

The operations recommended and practiced for chyluria fall broadly under three categories:

A. Disconnection (chylolymphatic)—the various disconnection procedures aim to interrupt most or all of the foci or points of lympho-urinary fistulae. These can be done by open, laparoscopic (transperitoneal/retroperitoneal) and robotic approaches (Fig. 1.6). The various steps are enumerated in Table 1.7. Some or all might be necessary in a given case. Pedal lymphangiography is useful in determining level of disconnection procedures.[22]

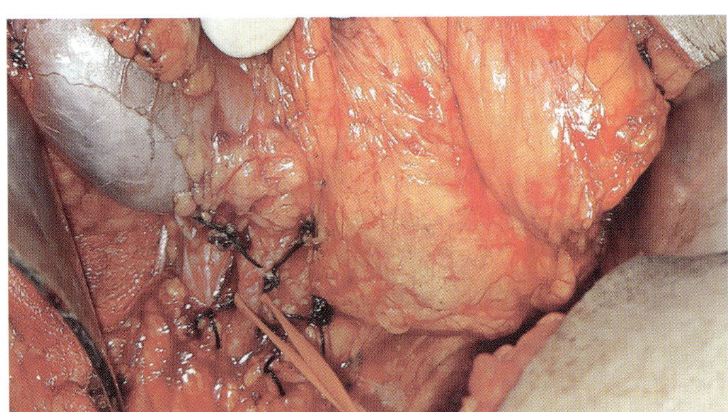

Fig. 1.6: Hilar ligation of lymphatics (Note the skeletonized renal vessels)

B. Diversion (lymphovenous)—the various diversionary procedures aim to divert lymph into anatomically proximate venous channels,

TABLE 1.7: Chylolymphatic disconnection: Steps

Step	What is done	Rationale	What it achieves
Nephrolympholysis	Kidney is dissected free from perirenal fascia	Lymphatic disconnection—perirenal	Tackles Grade III backflow on RGP
Hilar stripping	Skeletonization of hilar vessels after ligation of hilar lymphatics (Fig. 1.6)	Lymphatic disconnection—hilar level	Tackles backflow from hilar site
Ureterolympholysis (Patna Operation)[20]	Stripping of ureteral lymphatics till iliac level	Lymphatic disconnection—ureteral	Clears cloak of lymphatics around the ureter
Fasciectomy	Removal of perirenal tissues	Lymphatic disconnection by excision	Clears most of the abnormal backflow channels
Nephropexy	Fixing the kidney to psaos at 3 points	To prevent hypermobility	Prevents pain due to recurrent ptosis

Additional procedures: A large caliber lymphatic vessel may be anastomosed to the gonadal vein as auxiliary procedure.[21] Omental wrapping after ureterolysis is done with objective providing lymphatic drainage of stripped of its lymphatics

TABLE 1.8: Lymphovenous anastomosis

Cockett and Goodwin's operation[21]	Retroperitoneal lymphovenous anastomosis
Zhao *et al*[23]	Transinguinal spermatic lymphovenous anastomosis
Hou *et al*[24]	Inguinal lymph node—saphenous vein anastomosis

Flowchart 1.1: Algorithm of treatment

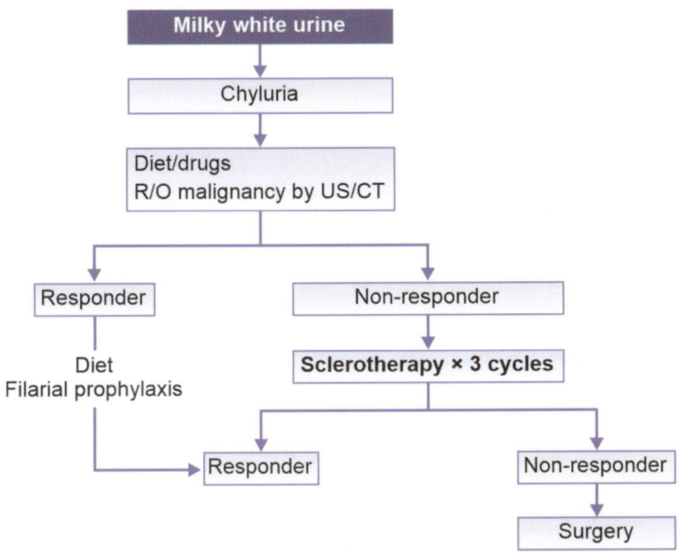

thereby decreasing intralymphatic pressure which helps in minimizing lymphatic leak into the urinary tract. In principle, it seems to be a physiological way of treating chyluria (Table 1.8).

C. Direct procedures on the kidney—autotransplantation[15] is a morbid extension of chylolymphatic disconnection wherein the kidney is disconnected from its vascular connections and transplanted in a suitable bed. It is difficult to justify nephrectomy[12] in chyluria except under very rare situations where the affected kidney turns out to be a source of ineradicable sepsis.

SUMMARY

- Chyle is an abnormal constituent of urine
- Chyluria can be due to parasitic and non-parasitic causes
- Commonest parasitic cause is filariasis
- Chyle leaks into the urinary tract via abnormal lymphatico-urinary fistula which forms the pathologic basis of chyluria
- Clinically, three grades of chyluria are recognized
- MRI and lymphoscintigraphy are the non-invasive methods of demonstrating lympahtico-urinary fistulae
- Most chylurics are managed effectively by diet and anti-parasitic drugs.
- Sclerotherapy and lymphatic disconnection procedures are reserved for severe forms of chyluria
- Severe chyluria can cause anasarca.

REFERENCES

1. Rahman MM. Easy method of detection of chyle in urine. Indian J Nephrol. 2012 Mar; 22(2):147–8.
2. Diamond Eric, Schapira ME, Chyluria. A review of literature, Urology 1985;26:427–31.
3. Sinha RK, Ranjan N, Singh N, Amit K. Chyluria: a scourge of our region. BMJ Case Rep. 2015 Jul 6;2015.
4. Miller Fli, Keppke AL, Yaghmai V, et al. CT dingnosis of chyluria after partial nephrectomy, AlR Am I Roentgenel. 2007:188(1).
5. Rabley A, Pavlinec 1, Kwenda B, Kuo J, Yeung L. Endoscopic Management of Chyluria Caused by Pyelolymphatic Fistula After Robot-Assisted Laparoscopic Pyeloplasty. J Endounl Case Rep. 2020 Det 29; 6(4):409–412.
6. Suri A, Kumar A. Chyluria-SGPGI experience. Indian] Urol 2005; 21:59–62.
7. Dalela D. Issues in etiology and diagnosis making of chyluria. Indian J Urol 2005;21:18–23.
8. Chen KC. Lymphatic abnormalities in patients with chyluria. J Urol 1971;111:106.
9. Singh I, Dargan P, Sharma N. Chyluria—a clinical and diagnostic stepladder algorithm with review of literature. Indian J Urol 2004; 20:79–85.
10. Margaret H. Pui MH., Yueh TC Lymphoscintigraphy in Chyluria, Chyloperitoneum and Chylothorax.] Nucl Med. 1998; 39:1292–1296.
11. Taori, K., Disawal, A., Rathod, J., Puria, R., Waware, P., Bakare, V., Hatgaonkar, A. and Dhakate, S. MRI as Non-Invasive Modality of Choice for Diagnosis of Cause in Case of Chyluria. Open Journal of Nephrology, 2013, 3, 6–10.
12. Yamauchi S. Chyluria: Clinical, laboratory, and statistical study of 45 personal cases observed in Hawaii.] Urol 1945; 54:318.
13. Hemal AK, Kumar M, Wadhwa SN. Retroperitoneoscopic nephrolympholysis and ureterolysis for management of intractable filarial chyluria. J Endourol 1999;13:507.
14. Goel A, Goyal NK, Parihar A, Singh R. Magnetic resonance retrograde pyelography: A novel technique for evaluation of chyluria. Indian] Urology 2014; 30:115–6.
15. Goyal NK, Goel A, Sankhwar Set al. Factors affecting response to medical management in patients of filarial chyluria: a prospective study. Indian] Urol 2014;30:23.
16. Singh KJ, Srivastava A. Nonsurgical management of chyluria (sclerotherapy). Indian] Urol 2005; 21:55–8.
17. Sabnis RB, Punekar SV, Desai RM et al. Instillation of silver nitrate in the treatment of chyluria. Br] Urol 1992.
18. Mandhani A, Kapoor R, Gupta RK et al. Can silver nitrate instillation for the treatment of chyluria be fatal? Br] Urol 1998;82:926.
19. Nandy PR, Dwivedi US, Vyas N et al. Povidone iodine and dextrose solution combination sclerotherapy in chyluria. Urology 2004;64:1107.
20. Prasad PB, Chaudhary DK, Barnwal SM, Jha S, Bharthuar General Urology A. Periureteric lymphovenous stripping in

cases ofchylohematuria-Report of 15 cases (Patna Operation): Indian J Surg 1977:39; 607–12.

21. Cockett AT, Goodwin WE. Chyluria: attempted surgical treatment by lymphatic-venous anastomosis. J Urol 1962;88: 566–8.
22. Karanjavala DK: Technique of clearance of dilated lymphatio in the renal hilum and lower ureter and bladder in cases of intractable chyluria Br] Urol 51:440(1979).
23. Zhao WP, Hou LQ, Shen JL. Summary and prospects of fourteen years' experience with treatment of chyluria by microsurgery. Eur Urol 1988;15:219-22.
24. Hou LQ, Liu QY, Kong QY, Luo CZ, Kong QA, Li LX, et al. Lymphonodovenous anastomosis in the treatment of chyluria. Chin Med J Eng 1991;104:392–4.
25. Brunkwall, Simson O, Berquist D, Jonsson K, Bergentz SE. Chyluria treated with renal autotransplantation: A case report. J Urol 1990;143:793–6.

Chapter

2

25 Years Old Female with Small Capacity Bladder due to GUTB

• *Rahul Gupta*

LEARNING OBJECTIVES

- To understand the presentation of GUTB: Genitourinary tuberculosis also known as GUTB is a complex disorder that may involve any part of the urinary tract and can have varied presentation. It may present from being completely silent resulting in a nonfunctioning kidney to a presentation with severe lower tract symptoms which needs to be differentiated from urinary tract infection or stone disease. Early diagnosis is important as late presentation increases the morbidity.
- To understand the pathophysiology of GUTB: It is imperative to understand and consider the differential diagnosis of GUTB so as to intervene in time. This involves a high degree of suspicion for the disease as it accounts for 10–40% of extra-pulmonary tuberculosis. GUTB invariably has a lag period of 12–24 months from primary infection to clinical presentation and at times can remain dormant for up to 40 years. A higher index of suspicion is needed in immunocompromised patients such as diabetics, patients on immunosuppression (post-renal transplant) and HIV positive patients.
- To understand the evaluation and newer diagnostic methods for GUTB: Diagnosis of GUTB involves isolation of mycobacteria using smear microscopy and GeneXpert MTB/RIF assay. These investigations have a sensitivity of 63–94%. Mycobacterium culture is the gold standard for diagnosing active TB and in addition it gives drug sensitivity to facilitate treatment of GUTB. For a faster diagnosis whole-genome sequencing (WGS) and next-generation sequencing (NGS) can be done. In addition, TB bacilli can be isolated in urine and that gives a clinching evidence regarding the diagnosis. Radiological imaging does play a role in facilitating diagnosis and management of the GUTB but that needs to be tailored according to the patients presentation.
- To understand the treatment protocol: Treatment of GUTB is a mix of medical and surgical intervention to save and optimize the renal function and at the same time alleviate the symptoms of the patient.

Case Scenario

35 years old female laborer presented with anorexia and bilateral flank pain for the last 3 months. Flank pain was dull aching persistent needing oral analgesics off and on. She gave the history of fever on and off with increasing urinary frequency for the last 2 months. Day time frequency was 8–10 times and nighttime 8–9 times. It was associated with urgency, dysuria and occasional urge incontinence. On probing further, she gave history of taking antibiotics off and on (fluoroquinolones and cephalosporins off the counter) with which she felt temporary relief. She had lost about 8 kg weight in the last 3 months. Past medical history was not significant for any prolonged drug intake or any surgical intervention. She has two children which were full term normal deliveries. On evaluation she had anemia, altered renal function (RFT) and raised total counts. Ultrasound revealed bilateral hydronephrosis with hydroureter and small capacity bladder (70 ml). Urine examination revealed sterile pyuria with acidic pH. She was then subjected to radiological investigations; MCUG (micturating cystourethrogram) was suggestive of a small capacity bladder with bilateral vesicoureteral reflux. IVP was done that showed bilateral mild to moderate hydroureteronephrosis with good renal function. On a high suspicion of GUTB she was subjected to urinary PCR for TB which was positive.

1. **What is the etiology of GUTB?**

   Ans: GUTB is a secondary TB caused by infection with *M. tuberculosis*. These days infections with other species of mycobacteria in the MTB complex, including *Mycobacterium bovis*, *Mycobacterium africanum*, *Mycobacterium pinnipedii*, *Mycobacterium microti*, *Mycobacterium caprae*, and the TB vaccine bacillus Calmette-Guérin (BCG) can sometimes cause the disease.

The GU infection is usually hematogenous but can rarely be by lymphatics or by sexual transmission. Reactivation of dormant TB is more common with diabetes, advancing age, low BMI, concurrent cancers, immunosuppression, and kidney failure.

How to Approach a Suspected Case of GUTB

2. **What is differential diagnosis of storage symptoms with low grade fever in a 35-year-old female?**

Ans:
- Urinary tract infection
- Urethritis
- Chronic pyelonephritis
- Chronic cystitis
- Malignancy (CIS or bladder TCC)
- Diabetes mellitus
- GUTB

3. **How would you evaluate such a patient?**

Ans: After taking a detailed history one would request for a voiding diary for 48–72 hours and also start with basic investigation such as complete blood count, urine routine, urine culture sensitivity and renal function tests. This is done to understand the profile of the patient and rule out associated infection as concomitant positive urine culture for aerobic bacteria is present in up to 30% of patients with GUTB.[1]

If the urine culture is positive, the patient should be treated for the same but if it is negative, then one should think of alternative diagnosis such as GUTB/CIS. In that case morning urine sample of the patient can be sent for smear examination with ZN staining to detect mycobacteria and should do urine cytology to rule out malignant or atypical cells.

4. **How to send the urine sample in case of suspected GUTB?**

Ans: Sample should be collected in a glass bottle either sterile or bottle should have been boiled for at least 20 minutes. The sample should be the entire voided first morning urine sample. Collected sample should be transported within four hours of collection. If there is a delay due to any reasons, then this sample needs to be refrigerated. Overall, three such samples need to be sent for evaluation. Samples that are not accepted for evaluation: Less than 40 ml of urine, those collected from catheterized bag and 24 hours pooled sample.[2] One should remember that the diagnostic yield is up to 40% only.[3] This low sensitivity is because for AFB smear microscopy to be positive, it should have at least 5×10^3 bacilli/ml of specimen.[4]

If this sample comes positive for tuberculosis, then it clinches the diagnosis, but since the sensitivity of the test is only 40% so other investigations can be ordered in case of strong suspicion of GUTB.

5. **What are the other investigations for diagnosing GUTB in case of negative urine evaluation?**

Ans: Blood investigations to diagnose TB, GeneXpert MTB/RIF assay, is used for the faster and sensitive diagnosis of TB.[5,6] It is basically a real-time quantitative PCR assay for amplifying Mtb DNA and gives diagnosis as early as 2 hours. *WHO recommends this as investigation of choice* as this can facilitate faster diagnosis and treatment can be started early. Other investigations include mycobacterium culture (considered to be the gold standard for diagnosing TB),[7] whole-genome sequencing (WGS) and next-generation sequencing (NGS) though reliable way of diagnosing TB but are time consuming (2 weeks)[8] are not readily available and not cost effective.

Granulomatous inflammation in biopsy tissue and the presence of acid-fast bacilli are hallmarks of TB.

Once the patient is diagnosed with GUTB on investigations now comes a stage to quantify the damage to the genitourinary system.

6. **What investigations done to quantify the damage to genitourinary system?**

Ans: Initial investigation of choice would be an ultrasonography of the KUB region and that would give information regarding renal architecture in terms of outline, echogenicity and cortico-medullary differentiation. It would delineate degree of hydronephrosis and parenchymal damage such as abscess or perinephric collection. Also, would reflect on the degree of ureteric dilatation and condition of the urinary bladder in terms of the bladder wall thickness and bladder capacity.

After obtaining the information from the ultrasonography, one can proceed with the anatomical and functional studies. If the serum creatinine is within acceptable limits, the investigation of choice in the present era is CT urogram. In cases of compromised renal function or patients allergic to renal contrast an MR urography is recommended.[9–11] Urography can help to quantify the stages of GUTB.

In cases of doubt on contrast study regarding the function of the renal unit a diethylenetriamine pentaacetate renal scan (DTPA) is accrued out to assess the overall GFR.

Degree of renal TB which includes:

1. Stage 1: Nondestructive form wherein renal parenchyma is involved.
2. Stage 2: Small destructive form which refers to TB papillitis.
3. Stage 3: Destructive form which refers to cavernous kidney TB (Figs 2.1A and B).

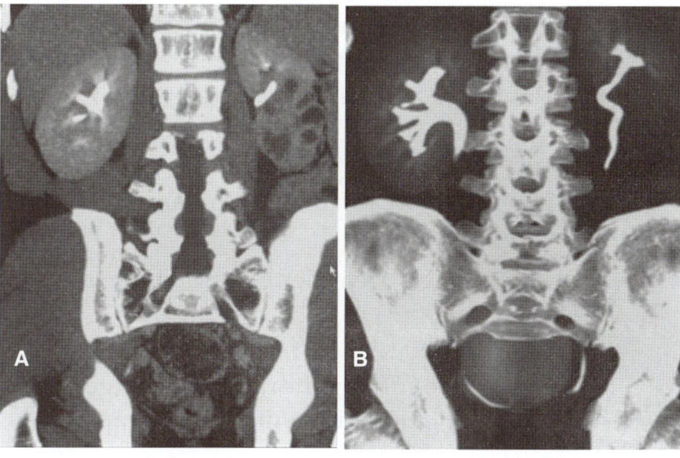

Figs 2.1A and B: (A) Lower polar destruction with non-excretion of contrast; (B) Ghost or phantom lower calyx

4. Stage 4: Widespread destructive form, i.e polycavernous kidney TB.[12] (Figs 2.2A and B).

Degree of ureteric involvement: May present as PUJ obstruction, VUJ obstruction, lower ureteric obstruction or vesicoureteric reflux (Fig. 2.3). Various terminologies have been attributed to such ureters depending on the degree of involvement and outcome.[13]

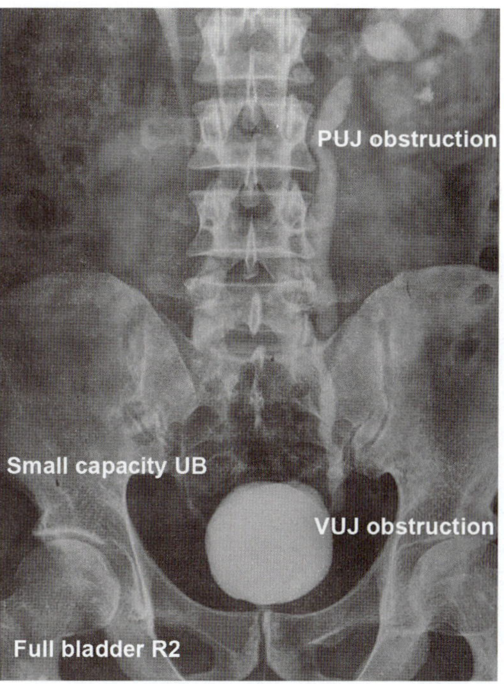

Fig. 2.3: Left PUJ and VUJ obstruction with a small capacity bladder

1. Corkscrew or beaded ureter: Non-confluent areas of dilatations and strictures.
2. Sawtooth ureter: Due to irregularity of the mucosa, dilation and stricture formation.
3. Pipe-stem ureter: Due to ureteral shortening and rigid fibrotic ureter lacking peristaltic movement.

Degree of bladder involvement: Bladder involvement has been classified into four stages[12]:

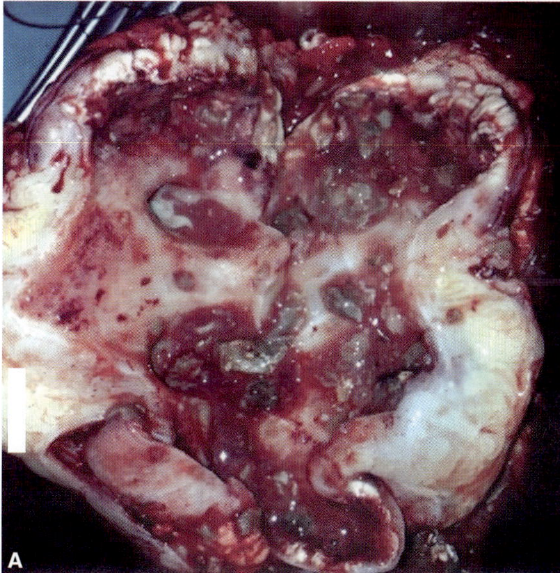

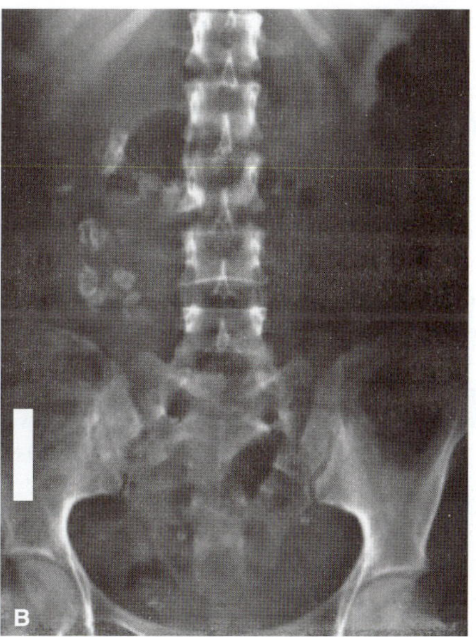

Figs 2.2A and B: (A) Cut open specimen of necrotic kidney; (B) Putty kidney on X-ray KUB

Stage 1: Tubercle-infiltrative bladder TB;
Stage 2: Erosive-ulcerous bladder TB
Stage 3: Interstitial cystitis/painful bladder syndrome
Stage 4: Contracted bladder up to full obliteration: Thimble bladder (Fig. 2.4).

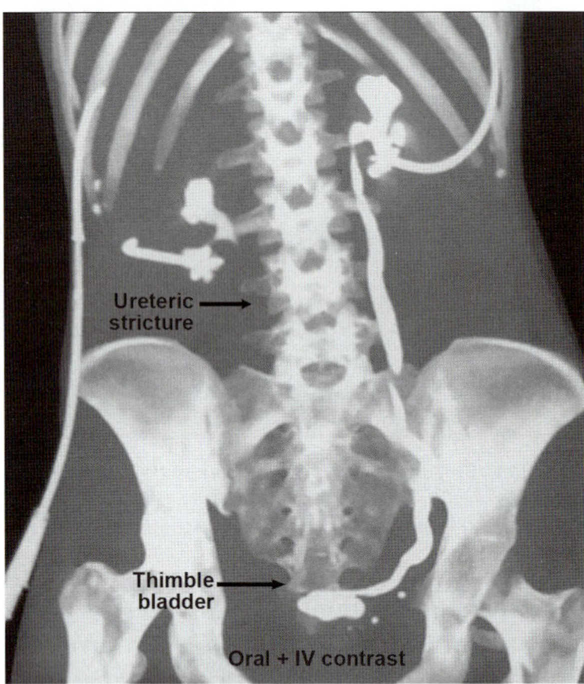

Fig. 2.4: Right ureteric stricture with thimble bladder

Rarely there can be involvement of prostate, scrotum, penis, vulva, vagina, or cervix, uterus, ovary, and fallopian tubes.

7. **What would be the further approach in a patient with GUTB with bilateral hydronephrosis with thimble bladder with compromised renal function?**

Ans: Both medical and surgical intervention must be done in tandem to control the infection and at the same time preserve the renal function. So the medical treatment involves:

i. Definitive anti-tubercular treatment
ii. Symptomatic treatment (anticholinergics/anti-inflammatory/analgesics)
iii. Supportive treatment (multivitamins/appetite enhancers)

And the surgical treatment is stratified into two components:

i. Immediate.
ii. Delayed involving the definitive surgery after the completion of the medical therapy.

8. **What is the recommended anti-tubercular therapy (ATT)?**

Ans: GUTB, in general, is treated with a four-drug regimen for six months: Rifampicin, isoniazid, pyrazinamide and ethambutol for the first two months, then isoniazid and rifampicin for four months (Tables 2.1 to 2.3). Patients with HIV or renal

TABLE 2.1: Recommended regimens for newly diagnosed, relapse or defaulter or multidrug resistant GUTB

Category	*Induction phase*	*Maintenance phase*	
New patient[1]	2 months HRZE	4 months HR	Daily dosing is optimal. Three times per week is acceptable alternative if patient is receiving directly observed medical therapy
Relapse or defaulter[2]	2 months HRZES, 1 month HRZE	5 months HRE	Likelihood of developing drug resistance of low. Advisable to change category after drug sensitivity results available
Rifampicin or multidrug resistant TB[2]	6–9 months Km, Lvx, Eto, Cs, ZE	18 months Lvx, Eto, Cs, E Start empirically.	Start empirically. Perform drug susceptibility for at least HR. Change once results are available

H, Ioniazid; R, rifampicin; Z, pyrazinamide; E, ethambutol; S, streptomycin; Km, kanamycin; Lvx, levoflox; Eto, ethionamide; Cs, cycloserine

Guidelines for treatment of tuberculosis. 4th ed, Geneva: World Health Organization; 2010
Category IV regimen. DOTS-plus guidelines. Revised national tuberculosis program. 2010

TABLE 2.2: Doses of routinely prescribed first line anti-tubercular treatment medication

Drug name	*Daily dose [range (mg/kg)]*	*Three times per week [range (mg/kg)]*
Ioniazid	5 [4–6]	10 [8–12]
Rifampicin	10 [8–12]	10 [8–12]
Pyrazinamide	25 [20–30]	35 [30–40]
Ethambutol	15 [15–20]	30 [25–35]
Streptomycin	15 [12–18]	15 [12–18]

TABLE 2.3: Commonly prescribed second line anti-tubercular drugs and their dosage for adults

Drug name	*Dosage per day (mg)*
Kanamycin	750
Levoflox	750
Ethilonamide	750
Ethambutol	1000
Pyrazinamide	1500
Cycloserine	750
PAS	12000

Dose modification is required in cases of hepatotoxicity and deranged renal function.

abscess would need a longer treatment. Patients who develop multidrug-resistant TB (MDR-TB) require treatment with MDR-TB regimens which include fluoroquinolones, bedaquiline, delaminid, aminoglycosides, etc., The treatment regimen in such cases may extend up to 18 to 24 months [14] (Tables 2.1 to 2.3).

1. Guidelines for treatment of tuberculosis. 4th ed. Geneva: World Health Organization; 2010.
2. Category IV regimen. DOTS-Plus guidelines. Revised national tuberculosis program. 2010.

9. What is the recommended surgical intervention in cases of GUTB?

Ans: Surgical treatment: Can be divided into three categories (Flowchart 2.1 describes summary how to approach GUTB):

i. Initial intervention for functional preservation: Diversion which can either be internal (JJ stent) or external (percutaneous nephrostomy).
ii. Definitive therapy for restoration of the function and anatomy.
iii. Ablative treatment in case of complete loss of function; Nehrectomy/nephroureterectomy.

Ureteric lesions (strictures): Definitive strictures may need appropriate treatment depending on the stricture length and site of the stricture. This may range from pyeloplasty to rarely the replacement of whole ureter using bowel segment (Fig. 2.5).

Urinary bladder: Small capacity thimble bladder may need bowel augmentation or rarely in cases of small scarred urinary bladder, they may need cystectomy and diversion procedure such as ileal conduit.[51]

Ablative procedures are recommended in cases of organ loss which include nephrectomy in cases of nonfunctioning kidney.

10. What was done for the index case?

Ans: This patient was initially initiated on standard ATT (AKT-4) and then simultaneously she was monitored for any deterioration for

Flowchart 2.1: Summary—how to approach GUTB

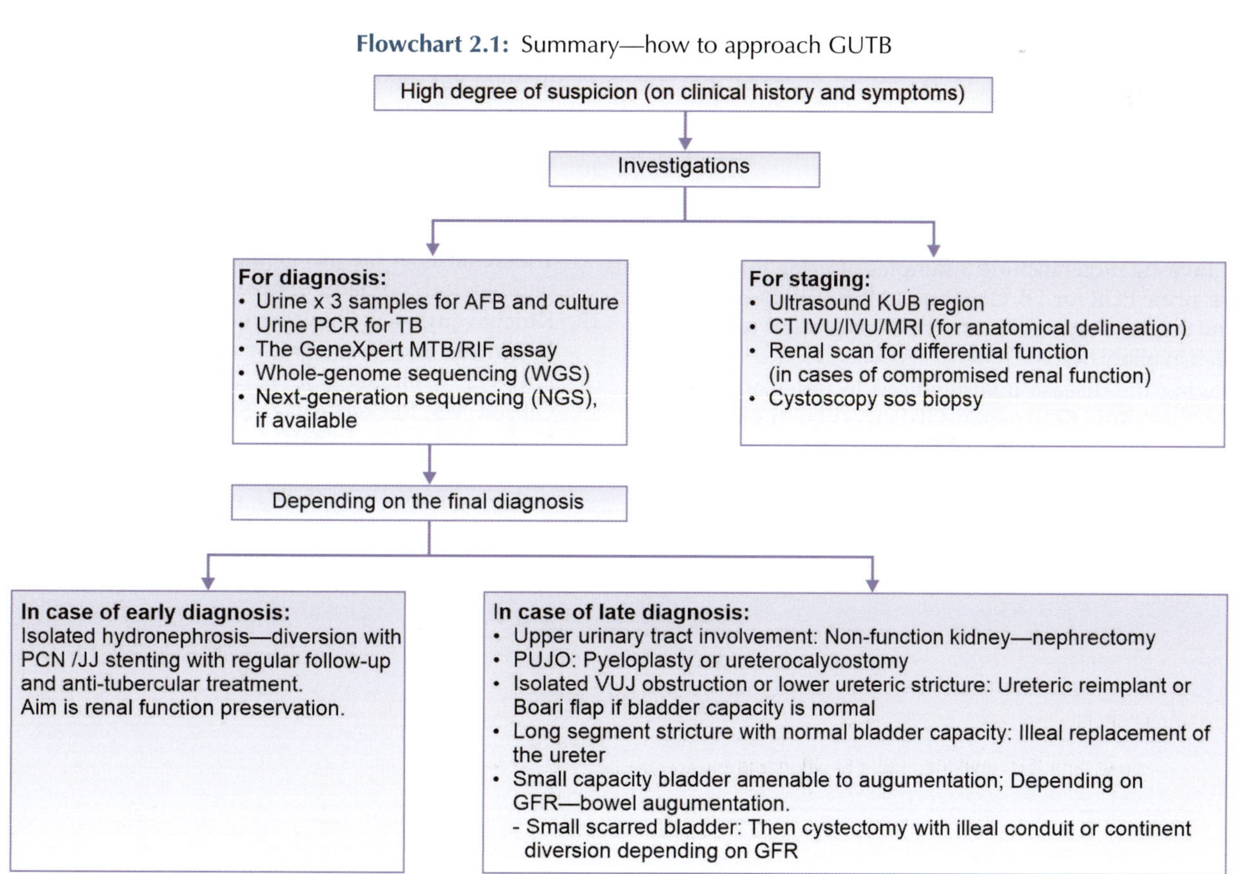

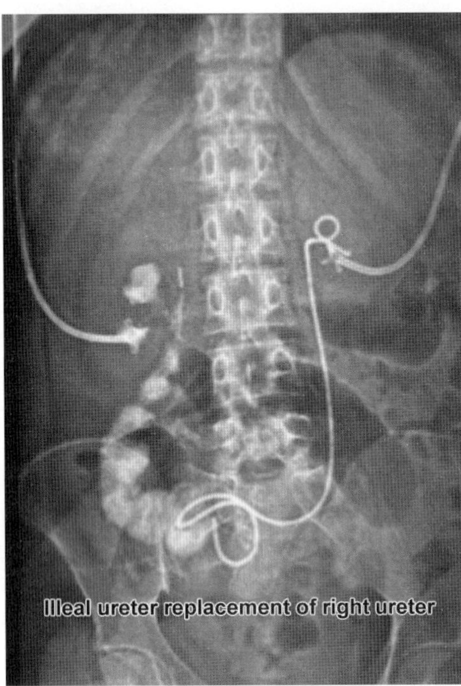

Fig. 2.5: Right nephrostogram showing illeal replacement

hydronephrosis by ultrasonography and serum creatinine. At two months of completion of AKT4 she had improvement in anemia, and she also gained weight. Her renal functions were stable but lower tract symptoms did not improve much. She was subjected to MCUG which showed thimble bladder with bilateral grade II reflux, so she was subjected to augmentation cystoplasty AKT treatment following which her symptoms improved.

SUMMARY

- One should keep a high degree of suspicion for GUTB especially if all other conventional causes have been ruled out.
- Initial investigations include 3 samples of urine for AFB and culture, urine PCR for TB, GeneXpert MTB/RIF assay. Whole-genome sequencing (WGS) and next-generation sequencing (NGS), if available.
- For staging the disease investigations in order of sequence include ultrasound KUB region, CT-IVU/IVU/MR urography (for anatomical delineation), DTPA renal scan for differential function (in cases of compromised renal function), cystoscopy in case of severe symptoms or an adjunct to surgery to rule out active inflammation
- Once diagnosed, then the treatment protocol includes the start of medical management as per guidelines and dose prescribed.
- Surgical intervention can be tailored as per need and should be guided by the finding on the radiological investigations.

REFERENCES

1. Daher *et al.* Review: Renal Tuberculosis in modern era. American Journal of Tropical Medicine 2013.
2. Kulchavenya E, Brizhatyuk E, Khomyakov V. Diagnosis and therapy for prostate tuberculosis. Ther. Adv. Urol. 6, 129–134 (2014).
3. Colabawalla, B. N. Reflections on urogential tuberculosis. Indian J. Urol. 6, 51–59 (1990).
4. Berta, M. *et al.* Bacteriological diagnosis of renal tuberculosis: an experience at the regional tuberculosis laboratory in Córdoba Province. Argentina. Rev. Argentina Microbiología 43, 191–194 (2011).
5. Walzl G, McNerney R, du Plessis N, Bates M, McHugh TD, Chegou NN, Zumla A. Tuberculosis: advances and challenges in development of new diagnostics and biomarkers. Lancet Infect Dis. 2018 Jul;18(7):e199-e210. [PubMed] [Reference list].
6. Pang Y, Shang Y, Lu J, Liang Q, Dong L, Li Y, Zhao L, Jiang G, Huang H. GeneXpert MTB/RIF assay in the diagnosis of urinary tuberculosis from urine specimens. Sci Rep. 2017 Jul 21;7(1):6181. [PMC free article] [PubMed] [Reference list].
7. Walzl, G. *et al.* Tuberculosis: advances and challenges in development of new diagnostics and biomarkers. Lancet Infect. Dis. 18, e199–e210 (2018).
8. Tortoli E, Benedetti M, Fontanelli A and Simonetti MT. Evaluation of automated BACTEC MGIT 960 system for testing susceptibility of Mycobacterium tuberculosis to four major antituberculous drugs: comparison with the radiometric BACTEC 460 TB method and the agar plate method of proportion. J. Clin. Microbiol. 40, 607–610 (2002).
9. Cek, M. *et al.* EAU guidelines for the management of genitourinary tuberculosis. Eur. Urol. 48, 353–362 (2005).
10. Valentini, A. L., Summaria, V. & Marano, P. Diagnostic imaging of uro-genital tuberculosis. Rays 23, 126–143 (1998).
11. Muttarak, M., ChiangMai, W. N. & Lojanapiwat, B. Tuberculosis of the uro-genital tract: imaging features with pathological correlation. Singapore Med. J. 46, 568–574 (2005).
12. Kulchavenya EV, Shevchenko SY & Cherednichenko AG. Diagnosis and treatment of cystitis: more questions than answers? Urologiia 5, 37–42 (2016).
13. Gibson MS, Puckett ML & Shelly ME. Renal tuberculosis. Radiographics 24, 1 (2004).
14. Tiberi, S. *et al.* Tuberculosis: progress and advances in development of new drugs, treatment regimens, and host-directed therapies. Lancet Infect. Dis. 18, e183–e198 (2018).

Chapter

3

Intraoperative Consultation for Gynaecological Injuries

• *Suresh Bhat* • *John Peter*

LEARNING OBJECTIVES

- To navigate unexpected intraoperative complications and difficulties when called in by gynaecology colleagues to avoid patient morbidity/mortality.
- To understand the risk reduction strategies for managing gynaecologic injuries.
- To allude to the algorithm for intra-operative consultation in such injuries.

Intra-operative Bladder Injury

The urinary bladder is spherical when it is full and tetrahedral when it is empty.

The normal capacity of bladder is 400–500 ml. The bladder is covered by the peritoneum only on the dome. As the bladder is close to the uterus and vagina, it is at risk for injury during pelvic surgeries.

High risk factors for bladder injury

- Endometriosis
- Previous pelvic/uterine/transvaginal surgery
- PID
- Large fibroids
- Previous RT
- Malignancies
- Placenta percreta
- Rupture uterus

Prevention

- Anticipate bladder injury in high-risk cases as mentioned above
- Bladder should be kept empty by placing catheter before starting the surgery.
- Sharp dissection is advisable in densely adherent bladders.
- **In bladder base injuries, always suspect associated ureteric injuries and proceed accordingly to detect ureteric injury (discussed elsewhere)**
- When heavy bleeding is encountered, avoid blind clamping/cauterization, instead, try to arrest bleeding with mops and later, do point cauterization.
- In difficult cases, help from a urologist should be obtained

Identification

- High index of suspicion should be there.
- Pooling of clear fluid in the dissection area
- In case of suspicion, distend the bladder with methylene blue mixed with saline solution.

Management

Hutch principles (to prevent VVF) which include the following:

- Immediate detection of bladder injury using vital dyes, if necessary
- Water tight closure of bladder in 2 to 3 layers.
- Satisfactory extravesical drain placement
- Avoidance of vaginal incision, if possible
- Prolonged, uninterrupted post-operative bladder drainage

Case Scenario

A 37-year-old lady undergoes abdominal hysterectomy for endometriosis. During the procedure, the gynecologist suspects bladder/ureteric injury and urologist is called in.

1. **How to proceed?**

Ans: A detailed history of the case is obtained from the gynecologist, the indication for surgery, how difficult was the surgery, how much was the blood loss, suspected site of injury, etc. All the imaging studies available are scrutinized so as to ascertain the characteristics of the primary lesion, distorted anatomy and course of ureter. Once this has been done, the gynecologist and the urologist would go and talk to the relatives of the patient regarding the suspected injury, the procedures that are going to be adopted and the available management options. A detailed consent regarding these would be obtained from the relatives before proceeding with the surgery. If any major reconstructive procedures are required, only temporizing surgeries are done. The major procedures are done later after discussing with the patient.[1]

The urologist should scrub in and do the surgery himself rather than dictating what to do from standing behind the gynecologist.

2. **What should the urologist do to assess bladder injury?**

Ans: First the urologist has to assess the level of hemostasis and the anatomic details of the pelvic organs. If hemostasis is satisfactory, the bladder is inspected for any injury in the form of any obvious cystotomy/loss of detrusor muscle/thermal injuries, etc. The bladder is distended with normal saline to which a few drops of methylene blue is added. If the bladder is intact, there would not be any extravasation. In this context, a ureteric injury is suspected and one has to proceed to find out that. If any bladder injury is detected, bladder is closure in two layers using absorbable sutures. If the detrusor is lost in some areas or lacerated, or thermal injury seen, debridement is done and healthy bladder is closed in 2–3 layers. An SPC is always kept. The integrity of bladder is rechecked before closing. If the hemostasis is not satisfactory, the field is packed with mop for 10 minutes and then slowly removed. Any bleeding is point coagulated or clipped. Then proceed as discussed before.[1]

- **What are the methods to detect viable/healthy bladder wall?**

  Ans: Intravenous injection of fluorescein and inspecting the bladder with Wood's lamp.

- **If bladder is found to be intact, how to proceed?**

  Ans: If the bladder is intact, the urologist should check for ureteral injury. The gynecologist is asked about the side which he/she thinks the ureter is probably injured. If the patient has been positioned in a low lithotomy position in the beginning itself, one has to proceed with cystoscopy provided all instruments are available. Availability of C arm is preferred. **If BP is normal**, the urologist has to ask the anesthesiologist to give 20–40 mg of furosemide IV. This will produce brisk diuresis and a good efflux from the orifice if that ureter is intact. Some use mannitol or 10% dextrose as an irrigant.[2] This improves the visibility of the efflux. Dextrose solution can lead to UTI. IV methylene blue or indigo carmine or sodium fluorescein has been used but are not available in India. This produces blue or red efflux. Methylene blue is a potent reversible inhibitor of monoamine oxidase inhibitor. This inhibition leads to serotonin toxicity when administered to patients on SSRI treatment. It is contraindicated in the patient taking the antidepressant, G6PD deficiency, renal impairment, and full-term pregnancy. Both maternal and fetal deaths have been recorded.

  One can also try bulb ureterogram with cone tipped catheter. Contrast injection will produce extravasation if injury is present. Methylene blue/betadine can be injected through the catheter and this will stain the field if injury is present. If the catheter goes in freely without any hindrance for >17 cm, ureteric injury can be ruled out (this will not rule out ischemic injuries which manifest later).[2]

- **If facilities for cystoscopy are not there how to proceed?**

  Ans: In this scenario, one has to explore the ureter on both the sides. If any laceration or transection has occurred, urine will pool in the field. If ligature or kinking or angulation has occurred, the ureter will distend to the level of injury. If injury is not obvious, the ureter is then carefully dissected from the pelvic brim (where it crosses over the common iliac artery) downwards to the VUJ. Most injuries will be detected by this. Methylene blue or indigo carmine can be given IV. This will stain the field blue. Methylene blue can be injected directly into the abdominal ureter using a very fine needle. Another alternative is to open the bladder and pass infant feeding tube into the ureters to see for any obstruction. If it goes smoothly for > 17 cm, injury is unlikely.[2]

3. **In a case of placenta acreta/percreta if a urologist is called intraoperatively, how to go about?**

- **Ans:** The urologist has to discuss with the anesthesiologist regarding the general condition and vital signs of the patient. If the patient is stable, definitive closure is done after debriding the unhealthy bladder tissues involved by the placental invasion. This may also need a partial segmental cystectomy. As the invasion is usually in the posterior aspect of bladder, one has to take care of the ureters (as discussed previously). Placenta percreta can involve the ureter and rectum as well. If the patient is unstable, bilateral internal iliac artery ligation is done, and proceed as before. In all these patients, a per urethral catheter and an SPC are needed. Post-operatively anticholinergics/beta-3-agonists must be given.[3]

4. **If the condition is diagnosed in the antenatal period, how to proceed?**
   Ans: The obstetrician should get help from interventional radiologist for intraoperative balloon occlusion of the internal iliac artery. Counsel the patient regarding the complications, options available to overcome these.
5. **How long to keep the catheters?**
   Ans: Usually for 2–3 weeks
6. **Which catheter will be removed first?**
   Ans: Depends on the institutional policy.
7. **What is the most important thing one has to take care in post-operative period?**
   Ans: The catheters should not get blocked by any means.
8. **If it is a case of repeat uterine surgery and the gynecologist is finding it difficult to separate bladder from the uterus, what should be done to safeguard the urinary tract?**
   Ans: In such scenarios, sharp dissection is advisable. Sometimes it is prudent to fill the bladder to 200 ml to delineate the bladder and protect it. If still difficult, the bladder is opened and under finger guidance, dissect the bladder carefully away from uterus till cervix.
9. **Is there any role for preoperative DJ stenting?**
   Ans: Studies have shown that there is no difference in incidence of ureteric injury with or without preoperative DJ stenting (1.2%). However, in difficult situations, it is better to stent, as stent helps to identify the ureter.[4] Stent insertion is associated with increased operating time, overall procedure cost, increased length of stay, radiation exposure and potential urinary tract complications including infection, urinary retention, haematuria and perforation.

***Case Scenario** (Contd.)*

Let us go to the post-operative period. Intraoperative everything was fine

10. **What are the red flag signs of urinary tract injury?**
    Ans: Abdominal or loin pain, nausea, vomiting, abdominal distension, fever, leukocytosis, hematuria, anuria, increasing drain from the drain tube.
11. **What is to be done at this point of time?**
    Ans: I will get an ultrasound of the abdomen to look for any fluid collection.
12. **If abdominal US is normal, what next?**
    Ans: Observe her carefully with regular CBC, RFT and US follow-up.
13. **If there is collection, what is to be done?**
    Ans: A urinary tract injury is suspected. The fluid can be aspirated under US guidance and sent for creatinine and potassium estimation. CTU is done for locating any urinary leak. Ureteric fistula manifests later compared to VVF and may take 1 to 4 weeks. Figure 3.1 shows a CTU with urinary leak in the vagina.

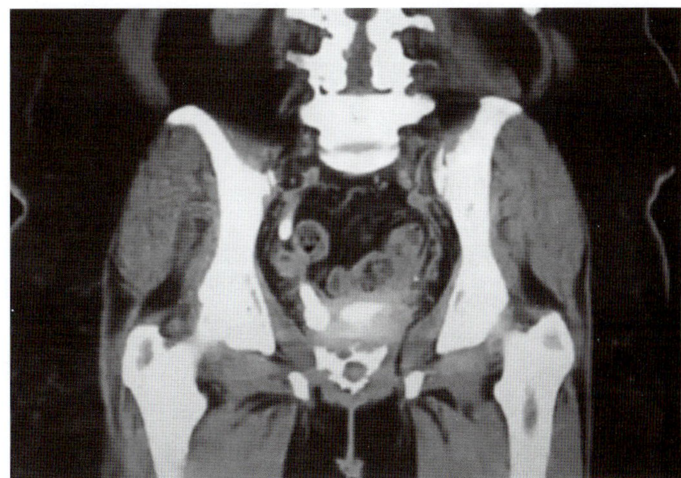

Fig. 3.1: CTU showing urine leak into vagina (If CTU shows ureteric injury, stenting is tried if fails, PCN is done)

SUMMARY

- Hutch principles for management of bladder injury:
  - Immediate detection of bladder injury using vital dyes, if necessary.
  - Water tight closure of bladder.
  - Satisfactory extravesical drain placement.
  - Avoidance of vaginal incision, if possible.
  - Prolonged, uninterrupted post-operative bladder drainage.
- Preoperative DJ stenting may help in easier identification of ureter intraoperatively, but does not decrease the chance of ureteric injury.
- Avoid blunt dissection in separating an adherent bladder.
- Always fill the bladder to check for any leak.
- VVF manifests much earlier than UVF.

REFERENCES

1. Schwarts M.J, Kreshover J.E; Intraoperative consultations in Campbell Walsh Wein Urology ed Partin AW, Dmochowski RR, Kavoussi LR, Peters CA, Wein AJ. 12th ed. Elsevier; 296–304.

2. Gilmour D.; urinary tract injury in gynecologic surgery: Identification and Management; Updates in urology 2023.
3. Kaufman M.R; Urological considereations in pregnancy in Campbell Walsh Wein Urology ed Partin AW, Dmochowski RR, Kavoussi LR, Peters CA, Wein AJ. 12th ed. Elsevier; 282–295.
4. Borghese G, Raimondo D, Esposti E.D *et al*. Preoperative ureteral stenting in women with deep posterior endometriosis and ureteral involvement:is it useful?; international journal of gynecology and obstetrics; 158, 179–186.

Intraoperative Ureteric Injury

Common causes

- Hysterectomy (abdominal/vaginal/laparoscopic/robotic assisted/radical)
- Caesarean section
- Uterine rupture
- Anti-incontinence surgeries
- Other pelvic surgeries

Risk factors

- Difficult pelvis
- Endometriosis
- Pelvic inflammatory disease
- Pelvic mass
- Radiation therapy
- Tuberculosis and
- Previous surgeries.

The lowest 3 cm of the ureter is most commonly injured, and 75% of these injuries occur during gynaecologic surgery, with 3/4 during abdominal surgery and 1/4 during vaginal surgery.

Intraoperative identification: ureteric injuries can be identified by dissecting the ureter outside the adventitia. Cystoscopy with a bulb ureterogram or lighted ureteric catheter is for identification and not for looking at efflux. Cystotomy and cannulating the ureter with infant feeding tube can also be done to identify ureteric injury. In the absence of these tools, an intravenous injection of indigo carmine or methylene blue can be used to assess for urinary flow.

Management: The goals of management for ureteric injuries are the expeditious resolution of urine leak, avoidance of urosepsis, and preservation of renal function. Management depends on the patient's condition, with sick and toxic patients undergoing percutaneous nephrostomy and stable patients undergoing bulb ureterogram, stenting (with a success rate of 60%), or reimplantation.

To manage ureteral injuries, surgeons must anticipate, prevent, recognize, evaluate, repair, test the integrity, and follow-up with patients.

Case Scenario

A 42-year-old lady with a large uterine fibroid was undergoing abdominal hysterectomy. There was heavy bleeding and during dissection, the gynecologist suspected ureteric injury as she was trying to control the bleeding at the vaginal cuff. At this point the gynecologist called for urologists' assistance.

1. **How to proceed?**

   Ans: The initial assessment and discussion with relatives are same as for bladder injury.

   The first step is to attain hemostasis and note the anatomical details. The next step is to try to identify the type and location of ureteric injury. Then proceed with the definitive management. **Always confirm bladder integrity before proceeding.**

2. **Which are the common sites where ureter is injured during abdominal hysterectomy?**

   Ans:
   - Cardinal ligament where the ureter crosses under the uterine artery
   - Dorsal to the infundibulopelvic ligament near or at the pelvic brim
   - Tunnel of Wertheim
   - Intramural portion of the ureter
   - Lateral pelvic sidewall above the uterosacral ligament.

3. **What are the types of ureteric injuries?**

   Ans:
   - Crush
   - Cut
   - Laceration
   - Transection
   - Ligature
   - Kink/angulation
   - Thermal injury.
   - Stripping of adventitia causing ischemic injury

   Figure 3.2 shows right hydroureteronephrosis following iatrogenic injury.

4. **How to identify the ureter in the pelvis?**

   Ans: In females, the pelvic ureter can be identified by its glistening appearance, peristalsis, and longitudinal vessels, as well as a "snapping" feeling while palpating. If there is any difficulty, ureter can be identified at the bifurcation of the common iliac artery (remember the **Luschka's law**: The ureter enters the pelvis 1.5 cm below the common iliac artery bifurcation on the left side and 1.5 cm above the common iliac artery bifurcation on the right[1]). If still ureter is not identified, then one can resort to **Manetta Manoeuvre.**[2] This involves

Fig. 3.2: Right hydroureteronephrosis following surgery, indicating right ureteric injury

incising the lateral peritoneum in a cephalad direction for 10 to 15 cm, and placing index finger on the external iliac artery. As one moves the index finger upwards, the first structure to be felt is the ureter and directly behind the middle phalanx will be the infundibulo pelvic ligament. This way one can safely ligate the infundibulo pelvic ligament safeguarding the ureter.

5. **What will you do to confirm the ureteric injury?**
   - Identify the ureter (given above)
   - Dissect the ureter outside the adventitia from pelvic brim down to identify any
     - Ligature
     - Crush
     - Clean cut
     - Thermal injury
     - Laceration
     - Transection
     - Stripping of adventitia
   - Cystoscopy
     - Bladder injury
     - Ureteric efflux
     - Suture material through bladder
     - Ureteric catheterization and injection of betadine/methylene blue and look for extravasation.
   - RGP (bulb ureterogram)
     - Contrast extravasation
   - Lighted ureteric stent/catheter[3]
   - Cystotomy and pass infant feeding tube into the ureters to confirm patency
   - Intravenous indigo carmine or methylene blue (not available) or indocyanine green

6. **What are the recent additions in the armamentarium to identify ureteric injury?**

   Ans: Fluorescence ureterography where diluted ICG dye is injected directly through the ureteric catheter and visualized with near infrared, using Spies system (Karl Storz)[4]

   Intravenous injection of sodium fluorescein and visualizing with Wood's lamp.[5]

7. **How will you manage ureteric injury?**

   Ans: Management depends on the type and extent of injury:
   - Partial circumferential injury—close the injury and stent the ureter. Keep stent for 6 weeks.
   - Crush injury—check for viability, ureteric reimplantation
   - Thermal injury-ureteric reimplantation
   - Suture passing through the ureter—deligature and stent
   - Complete ligature of the ureter—deligature and stent
   - Complete transection—ureteric reimplantation.

8. **If the injury is higher up, what will you do?**

   Ans: Spatulate the ureter and do uretero-ureterostomy over a DJ stent.

9. **Why do you reimplant instead of uretero-ureterostomy when the injury occurs in lower ureter?**

   Ans: The ureter has two types of blood supply—channel type and plexiform type. Channel type has adjacent vessels anastomosing with each other, whereas in the plexiform type, this does not occur. Lower ureter has mostly plexiform type of blood supply and hence, if uretero-ureterostomy is done, chances of stricture formation is high due to ischemia.[6] If done, later there will be dense fibrosis prohibiting dissection in the area of injury.

10. **How will you follow-up these patients?**

    Ans: Post-operative ultrasound abdomen to look for any hydroureteronephrosis and any collections. The stent is removed after 6 weeks. The urine should be sent for culture and sensitivity after this to rule out infection. Yearly ultrasound for 2–3 years is needed to rule out stricture formation. A functional study is mandatory within 3–6 months.[7]

11. **How will you do ureteric reimplantation?**

    Usually modified Leich-Gregoir procedure is done.

12. **If there is difficulty in bringing the ureter down and you anticipate tension at the anastomotic site, what are the procedures available?**

    This problem can be circumvented by doing a psoas hitch or Boari flap. Other options include transuretero-ureterostomy, ileal ureter, renal descensus and renal auto-transplantation.

13. What precautions will you take while doing these procedures?

Ans: During psoas hitch, the bladder is fixed to the psoas minor tendon taking care not to injure the genitofemoral and the femoral nerves. For Boari flap and Psoas hitch, bladder capacity should be normal.

14. What are the principles of harvesting a Boari flap?[8]

Boari flap should be oriented obliquely downward across the anterior bladder wall such that the base is ipsilateral to the side of ureteral pathology. The base of the flap should measure at least 4 cm in width. The apex of the flap should measure at least 3 cm in width. The length of the flap should approximate the length of the ureteral defect. It is critical that the ratio of length to-base width does not exceed 3: 1 as this risks ischemia to the flap. Flap measurements should be taken with the bladder nondistended. The opposite superior vesical pedicle has to be ligated and divided, whereas the ipsilateral should be preserved.

15. Can you do bilateral psoas hitch/Boari flap?

Ans: Yes, it is possible to do bilateral Psoas hitch[9] and bilateral Boari flap[10]

Rarely females have their distal ureteric supply solely from uterine artery. These blood vessels can get divided during hysterectomy, thereby resulting in ureteral necrosis leading to UVF.[11]

16. Describe the process of development of a UVF from a ureteric injury.

Ans: Ureteric injury causes urinary extravasation resulting in urinoma. It drains through the site of least resistance, i.e. vaginal cuff. Associated necrosis and infection results in formation of fistula. It usually takes 1 week to 1 month for the formation of UVF. The most common symptom is the onset of continuous urinary incontinence one to four weeks after surgery wity normal voiding.

17. What are the clinical features of UVF?

Ans: Fever, lower abdominal pain, flank pain, abdominal distension, nausea/vomiting, diarrhea and continuous urine leak with normal voiding (except in case of bladder injury).

SUMMARY

- Always confirm bladder integrity before proceeding with management of ureteric injuries.
- Identify the ureter properly—in difficult situations, make use of Luscka's law or Manetta manoeuvre.
- Dissect the ureter outside the adventitia.
- Management of ureteric injury depends upon the degree of damage.
- Always reimplant the ureter in case of lower ureteric injuries—plexiform blood vessels in lower ureter result in high incidence of ischemia following injuries.
- Always repair the ureter over a DJ stent.
- Never repair the ureter under tension—use psoas hitch/Boari flap/other techniques to avoid tension.
- Do not delay the repair of a UVF.

REFERENCES

1. Kostov S, Kornovski Y, Slavchev S, Ivanova Y, Dzhenkov D, Dimitrov N, *et al.* Pelvic lymphadenectomy in gynecologic oncology—significance of anatomical variations. Diagnostics. 2021;11(1).
2. Chan JK, Morrow J, Manetta A. Prevention of ureteral injuries in gynecologic surgery. Am J Obstet Gynecol. 2003;188(5):1273–7.
3. Borowiec. The Utility of Lighted Ureteral Stents in Laparoscopic Colorectal Resection: A Survey of Canadian Surgeons. Gastroenterol Res. 2011;4(4):2–6.
4. V. R. Satish V, Acharya A, Ramachandran S, Narasimhan M, Ardhanari R. Fluorescent ureterography with indocyanine green in laparoscopic colorectal surgery: A safe method to prevent intraoperative ureteric injury. J Minim Access Surg. 2022;18(2):320–3.
5. Brown.R.L, Garcia V.F. Genitourinary trauma in Pediatric surgery edited Grosfeld L.J, James.A,O'neil. Jr, Fonkaslsrud.E.W, CoranA.G, 6th Ed; Mosby; 317–37.
6. Shafik A. A study of the arterial pattern of normal ureter. J Urol 1972;107;720–2.
7. Yuvaraja.T. B, Wuntakel.R, Maheshwari. A *et al*; Management and long term follow up of ureteric injuries during Radical hysterectomy; J of Gynec Surgery,2003,19(3), 133–9.
8. Bansal, A., Sinha, R. J., Jhanwar, A., Prakash, G., Purkait, B., & Singh, V; Laparoscopic ureteral reimplantation with Boari flap for the management of long-segment ureteral defect: A case series with review of the literature. Turkish journal of urology, 2017; 43(3): 313–318.
9. Yee DS, Shanberg AM, Ngo AT, Baghdassarian R. Surgical management of bilateral ureteral endometriosis. Int Urol Nephrol. 2006;38(3–4):469–71.
10. Moazin M, Almousa S, Alqasem S, Alhazmi A, Naif aldhaam, Alfakhri A. Management of iatrogenic ureteral injury: Ureteral reimplantation with a bilateral Boari flap. Urol Case Reports. 2020;31–36.
11. Michaels JP. Study of ureteral blood supply and its bearing on necrosis of the ureter following the Wertheim operation. Surg Gynecol Obstet. 1948 Jan;86(1):36–44.

Chapter

4

60 Years Old Man with Fournier Gangrene

• Harprit Singh • Parag Sonawane

LEARNING OBJECTIVES

- To understand the pathophysiology of Fournier's gangrene: Fournier's gangrene (FG) is a devastating infection with prolonged morbidity, in which there is necrotizing infection of the external genitalia, perineal or perianal regions. It is more commonly seen in men with uncontrolled diabetes mellitus, immuno-compromised status, old age, obesity, poor genitourinary or peri-anal hygiene. Identifying the infection early goes a long way in reducing the morbidity and mortality associated with the disease.
  Due to the immunocompromised status of the patients and aggressive bacterial organisms, FG tends to spreads rapidly along the fascial planes. The spread in the subcutaneous plane is more rapid than the overlying skin further complicating the presentation. The synergistic bacterial activity is responsible for tissue necrosis and the putrid smell.
- To understand the microbiology of Fournier's gangrene: The microbial flora responsible for FG is usually polymicrobial and synergistic involving gram-positive, gram-negative and anaerobic organisms. Commonly isolated organisms are: *E. coli*, Enterococci, Klebsiella, *Staph. aureus*, Streptococcal species, and anaerobes like Bacteroides species.
- To understand the evaluation of Fournier's gangrene: Diagnosing FG is usually clinical and involves high degree of suspicion in immunocompromised patients. Role of investigations is very limited. Imaging such as ultrasound, CT scan, and/or MRI of the abdomen-pelvis may be performed to see the spread of the disease, however, surgical intervention should not be delayed.
- To understand the management of Fournier's gangrene: Treatment protocol includes the use of broad spectrum antibiotics with aggressive surgical debridement. These patients also need strict monitoring in HDU till they stabilise.
- To understand the prognostication of Fournier's gangrene: Prognostication of the disease is important both for the treating physician and the patient. There are many scoring systems for FG like LRINEC score, FGSI, and Uludag FGSI scores. These indices help stratify patients into risk categories and indicate the prognosis in such groups of patients.

Case Scenario

A 60-year-old obese man with poorly controlled type 2 diabetes, presents with severe scrotal and perineal pain with swelling on the scrotum. There is blackish discoloration of the overlying skin with a foul-smelling discharge. On presentation, he had tachycardia, was afebrile and was in hypotension.

He has undergone dilatation for stricture urethra a few years back and is currently experiencing bothersome voiding lower urinary tract symptoms (LUTS).

1. **How to approach a case of FG? Give definition of Fournier's gangrene?**

   Ans: FG is a subgroup of necrotising fasciitis (Fig. 4.2) involving the external genitalia, perineum, peri-anal region, and lower abdominal wall.[1] There is a suppurative bacterial infection of the perirectal, perineal, or genital area, which leads to thrombosis of small subcutaneous vessels with infection. This results in the development of gangrene of the overlying skin.[2]

   Fournier's gangrene can be an extension from a genitourinary infection or skin trauma or a peri-anal infectious focus. It spreads rapidly along the superficial dartos and Buck's fascia of the penis, dartos fascia of the scrotum, Colles' fascia of the perineum, and Scarp's fascia of the anterior abdominal wall. The infection spreads more rapidly in the subcutaneous plane than the involvement of the overlying skin. The bacteria produce endotoxin which is responsible for tissue necrosis and the pus produced by anaerobic bacteria (Bacteroides) causes the putrid smell.[2] It is associated with a high mortality rate, in the range of 16–40%.

The disease is named after the famous French venereologist, Jean Alfred Fournier. Dr Jean first reported this condition of the gangrene on a young man's genitals in 1883. He considered genital trauma to be one of the factors predisposing to the disease.

2. **What is your clinical suspicion and what will you look for clinically?**
 Ans: The clinical picture points towards an impending Fournier's gangrene (Fig. 4.1).

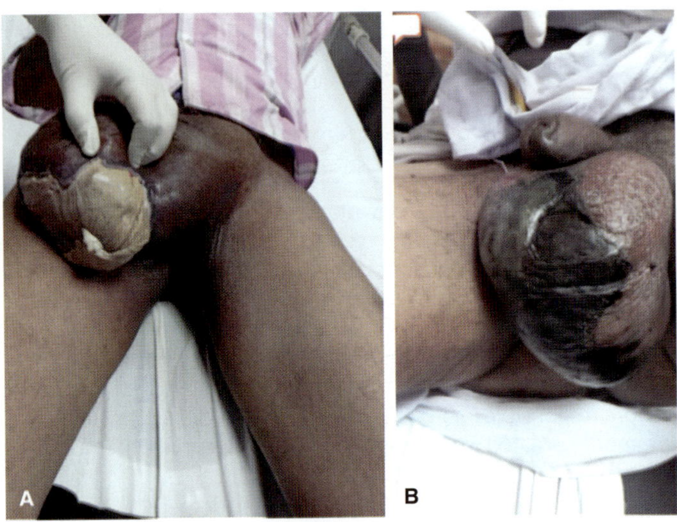

Fig. 4.1A and B: Presentation of FG with a gangrenous patch

A thorough clinical examination of the abdominal-perineal region and genitals should be undertaken especially in obese immunocompromised uncontrolled diabetic patients. Other predisposing factors include

- Chronic alcoholism
- Recent urogenital or colorectal instrumentation,
- Circumcision, paraphimosis
- Peri-anal, peri-rectal infections
- Older age group,
- Peripheral vascular disease
- Higher body mass index (BMI)
- CKD.

The presence of redness (acute inflammation) of the scrotum and adjoining inguinal region along with maceration is a strong pointer towards severe infective process (Fig. 4.2). Appearance of a definitive gangrenous patch and crepitation in the subcutaneous tissue with frank purulent discharge clinches the clinical diagnosis of FG. In these cases, the patient should also be assessed for associated systemic sepsis such as tachycardia and tachypnoea.

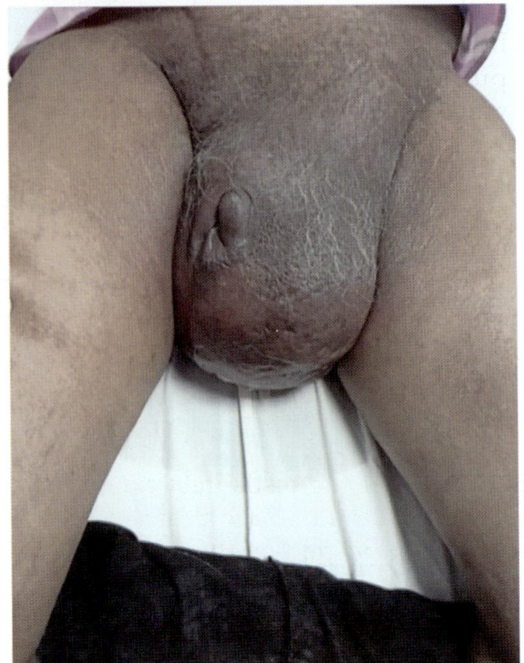

Fig. 4.2: Initial presentation: Redness of the scrotum

3. **Which micro-organisms are commonly involved in FG?**
 Ans: The microbial flora is polymicrobial and synergistic involving gram-positive, gram-negative and anaerobic organisms. Commonly isolated organisms are:
 E. coli, Enterococci, Klebsiella, *Staph aureus*, Streptococcal species, and anaerobes like Bacteroides species. Candida species has also been identified in around 22% of cases in one series.[3]

4. **What would be the differential diagnosis in a patient with FG?**
 Ans: The diagnosis can be confusing only in the early stages of FG. It can be confused with gangrenous balanitis in diabetic men, and among women with gangrenous diabetic vulvitis, ulcerative and gangrenous forms of inguinal lymphogranulomatosis, soft chancre, and acute ulcers of the genitals.

5. **Once a clinical suspicion/diagnosis is made, how to approach the patient?**
 Ans: FG is a surgical emergency.
 - First step is to investigate and stabilise the patient before he can be taken up for definitive intervention. Investigations include complete blood counts, liver function tests, coagulation profile, viral markers and markers for severity of sepsis which include c-reactive proteins, procalcitonin, arterial blood gas analysis and blood cultures. In case of diabetic patients, we should have 4 hourly sugar monitoring.

- Following this patient should be checked for hemodynamic stability (SpO_2, blood pressure, pulse and respiratory rate monitoring) and started on IV fluids in consultation with intensivists.
- Broad-spectrum parenteral antibiotics should be started immediately to cover both gram-positive and gram-negative aerobes and anaerobes, according to local microbiology guidelines.

Patient should be then subjected to aggressive surgical debridement under anaesthesia to ensure that no pocket of purulent or necrotic material is left behind. Debridement should be thorough to the point of reaching viable diffusely bleeding tissue. And if the testis gets exposed, it should be covered by the tough tunica. Orchiectomy is usually not needed as they are rarely involved (Figs 4.3 and 4.4) by infection. Covering the testicles in the medial femoral tissue pocket was previously done but is less effective as it can lead to necrosis of the spermatic cord. A relook debridement is often required in the next 24–48 hours guided by the wound status and degree of clinical improvement.

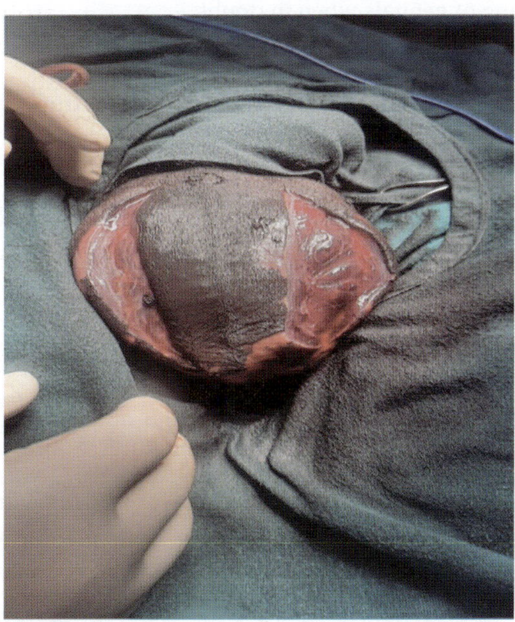

Fig 4.3: Limited and to the point debridement

(*Source:* Figures 4.1 to 4.3: Dr Jo Jo James, Consultant Surgeon, TMH, Jamshedpur)

Literature review of various case series suggests primary or secondary wound closure for scrotal defects < 50%. Flaps or skin grafts would be needed for defects involving > 50% of the scrotum or with extension outside the scrotum.[4] There have been reports suggesting benefits with the use of honey-soaked dressing, vacuum (negative pressure) dressing devices, and hyperbaric oxygen therapy

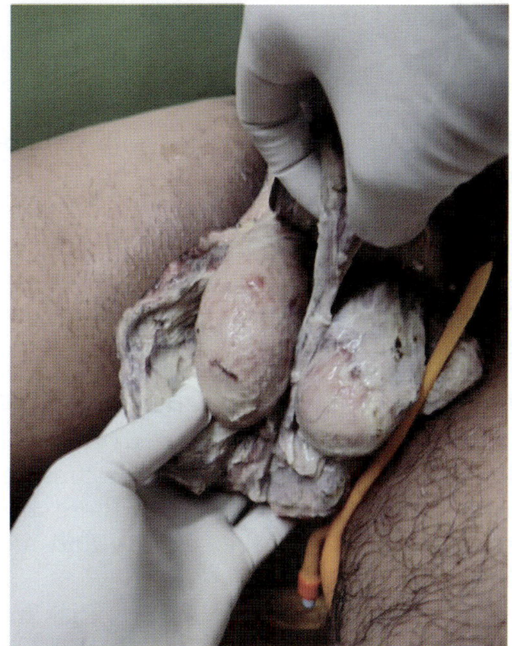

Fig. 4.4: Testis spared during the debridement of FG

but without good quality evidence.[5,6] These options can surely be tried to bring down morbidity.

6. **Is there a need of concurrent orchidectomy in a case of scrotal FG?**

   Ans: Involvement of the testis is rare as the blood supply to the testis if by the gonadal artery which is a branch directly of the aorta, whereas the scrotum receives blood supply from the pudendal artery which is a branch of the femoral artery. The involvement of the testis would suggest a retroperitoneal or intra-abdominal source of infection[7–9] and that is rare.

7. **What are the drugs of choice to manage FG?**

   Ans: The antimicrobial regimen should cover all probable micro-organisms and should penetrate inflammatory tissue. A suggested regime would comprise a broad-spectrum penicillin or third-generation cephalosporin, gentamicin, and metronidazole or clindamycin.[10] Adding an antifungal can be considered based on clinical findings and response to treatment. The antibiotics can subsequently be modified as per culture results.

8. **When would you order imaging in a case of FG?**

   Ans: Imaging can be considered when the diagnosis is in doubt or if the extent of spread is unclear or if a pelvic source of infection is suspected.

   Imaging of the genital region with X-ray and ultrasound may demonstrate air in the subcutaneous tissue. CT scan and MRI of the abdomen-pelvis may be performed to exclude the pararectal spread of infection, which may need bowel diversion.[10] However, surgical treatment should not be delayed for want of imaging confirmation.

9. Discuss the role of diversions with debridement in FG.

Ans: A suprapubic catheter may be required to divert urine and monitor urine output. A temporising colostomy may also be required to divert faeces in case of extensive perineal involvement.

10. What prognostic scores used in case of FG?

Ans: Although elevated urea with low albumin, and hematocrit levels is considered an unfavourable prognostic sign, there are many scores to determine the severity and mortality risk.

1. **LRInEC score:** The Laboratory Risk Indicator for necrotizing Fasciitis (LRInEC) score measures different laboratory parameters (serum CRP, WBC count, Hb, creatinine, sodium, glucose) to give a total score to help stratify patients into risk categories. This may help when the initial clinical assessment is equivocal. An LRInEC score of 6 should raise the suspicion of necrotizing fasciitis, and a score of 8 is strongly predictive; however, this should not be relied on, and clinical assessment should take precedence.[11]
2. **FGSI:** Fournier's gangrene severity index (FGSI) is used to assess the mortality risk. This score is based on nine clinical parameters: Respiratory rate, heart rate, temperature, WBC count, haematocrit, sodium, potassium, creatinine, and sodium bicarbonate levels. Each parameter is valued between 0 and 4, with the higher value given to the greatest deviation from normal. FGSI >9 correlates with high mortality (46–75%); FGSI <9 has a reported 78–96% chance of survival.[12,13]
3. **Simplified FGSI** (SFGSI) to simplify the FGSI score, a simplified score that has only three parameters (potassium, creatinine, and hematocrit) has been used. Sadly it is not yet validated.
4. **Uludag FG Severity Index:** This is a modification to the FGSI index. In addition to FGSI, it includes 2 more parameters relating to the disease severity and patient physiology. These are the dissemination score (depending on the involvement of the anorectal region, pelvic region, or beyond pelvic region) and age index (< or > 60 years).[14]

11. What was done in the index case?

Ans: Patient was hospitalised in HDU and in consultation with endocrinologist, intensivist and an infection disease consultant, he was resuscitated and prepared for an emergency aggressive debridement under antibiotic cover and general anaesthesia. At the end of debridement, a suprapubic urinary diversion catheter was placed. His testis was spared and covered with tunica. Following debridement, he was shifted to HDU and monitored along with daily dressings. He required a skin grafting after 4 weeks once his disease stabilised.

SUMMARY

- Fournier's gangrene (FG) is a life-threatening urosurgical emergency that presents with a necrotizing fasciitis involving external genitalia, perineum, peri-anal region, and abdominal wall.
- The prevalence of the disease is luckily low but the morbidity and mortality still remains high.
- Diabetes, immunocompromised status, genitourinary infections or interventions predisposes to FG.
- The microbial flora is polymicrobial and synergistic.
- Perform routine blood investigations for severity of sepsis and imaging of genitals when in doubt.
- LRInEC, FGSI are some of the prognostic tools to assess severity of FG.
- Aggressive resuscitation along with broad spectrum antibiotics in keeping with local antibiotic policy is vital.
- The cornerstones for the management of FG are timely diagnosis, supportive medical management and complete surgical debridement. They may need to be supported by early and timely re-look debridements and appropriate reconstruction to cover soft tissue defects.

REFERENCES

1. Altarac S, Katušin D, Crnica S, Papeš D, Rajkovi Z, Arslani N. Fournier's gangrene: etiology and outcome analysis of 41 patients. Urologia internationalis. 2012; 88(3):289–93.
2. Eke N. Fournier's gangrene: a review of 1726 cases. British Journal of Surgery. 2000 Jun; 87(6):718–28.
3. Castillejo Becerra CM, Jaeger CD, Rose JR, Beecroft NJ, Shah NC, Posid T, Jenkins LC, Baradaran N. Microorganisms and antibiogram patterns in Fournier's Gangrene: contemporary experience from a single tertiary care center. The Journal of Urology. 2020 Dec;204(6):1249–55.
4. Karian LS, Chung SY, Lee ES. Reconstruction of defects after Fournier gangrene: a systematic review. Eplasty. 2015;15.
5. Subrahmanyam M, Ugane SP. Honey dressing beneficial in treatment of Fournier's gangrene. Indian J Surg. 2004 Mar 1; 66(2):75–7.
6. Jallali N, Withey S, Butler PE. Hyperbaric oxygen as adjuvant therapy in the management of necrotizing fasciitis. The American journal of surgery. 2005 Apr 1;189(4):462–6.
7. Scott SD, Dawes RF, Tate JJ, Royle GT, Karran SJ. The practical management of Fournier's gangrene. Annals of the Royal College of Surgeons of England. 1988 Jan; 70(1):16.

8. Gerber GS, Guss SP, Pielet RW. Fournier's gangrene secondary to intra-abdominal processes. Urology. 1994 Nov 1; 44(5): 779–82.
9. Klutke CG, Miles BJ, Obeid F. Unusual presentation of sigmoid diverticulitis as an acute scrotum. The Journal of urology. 1988 Feb; 139(2):380–1.
10. Chennamsetty A, Khourdaji I, Burks F, Killinger KA. Contemporary diagnosis and management of Fournier's gangrene. Therapeutic Advances in Urology. 2015 Aug; 7(4):203–15.
11. Wong CH, Khin LW, Heng KS, Tan KC, Low CO. The LRINEC (Laboratory Risk Indicator for Necrotizing Fasciitis) score: a tool for distinguishing necrotizing fasciitis from other soft tissue infections. Critical care medicine. 2004 Jul 1; 32(7): 1535–41.
12. Laor E, Palmer LS, Tolia BM, Reid RE, Winter HI. Outcome prediction in patients with Fournier's gangrene. The Journal of urology. 1995 Jul 1; 154(1):89–92.
13. Corcoran AT, Smaldone MC, Gibbons EP, Walsh TJ, Davies BJ. Validation of the Fournier's gangrene severity index in a large contemporary series. The Journal of urology. 2008 Sep 1; 180(3):944–8.
14. Yilmazlar T, Ozturk E, Ozguc H, Ercan I, Vuruskan H, Oktay B. Fournier's gangrene: an analysis of 80 patients and a novel scoring system. Tech Coloproctol. 2010 Sep;14(3):217–23.

Chapter

5

Radiation Cystitis: How to Appraoch

• *Himanshu Pandey*

LEARNING OBJECTIVES

- To understand the etiology and presentation of radiation cystitis: Haemorrhagic radiation cystitis (HRC) usually occurs following radiotherapy (RT) to pelvic for pelvic malignancies. Predominantly gynaecologic neoplasia, urinary bladder cancer and carcinoma prostate.[1]
  Radiation cystitis can be sub-divided into either acute or chronic. Acute radiation cystitis occurs due to acute radiation injury to the rapidly dividing urinary bladder mucosa cells. It can manifest during or soon after radiation treatment. Clinically it presents as predominantly storage symptoms which include dysuria, increased frequency, urgency and rarely as urge incontinence. These symptoms are usually self-limiting and can be managed conservatively with anticholinergic drugs. Late or chronic radiation cystitis, with incidence of 5–10%, and they can manifest anywhere between 6 months and 20 years following pelvic radiation therapy.[2,3]
- To understand the pathophysiology of radiation cystitis: Underlying pathophysiology in HRC involves an obliterative endarteritis that inturn leads to atrophy and fibrosis of the mucosa and submucosa. Following this there is development of dilated and telangiectatic blood vessels that are fragile and prone to bleeding. This irradiated bladder is in variably hypovascular, hypocellular, and hypoxic.[4]
- To understand post-radiation hematuria and its management: The predominant presenting symptom in HRC is haematuria, which may be variable meaning microscopic to mild to severe life-threatening haemorrhage needing hospitalisation. Initial management of such severe cases involves resuscitation with fluid replacement and blood transfusion. Often they also need endoscopic clots evacuation followed by transurethral catheterization and saline irrigation.
- To understand the treatment protocol of radiation cystitis: Treatment of radiation cystitis involves either oral or parenteral agents. The basic aim is to control haematuria and variety of oral drugs such as conjugated oestrogens, pentosan polysulfate or WF10 can be used to achieve the desired result. However, sometimes it warrants intervention which includes cystoscopy and fulguration (laser or electrocoagulation) of bleeding points. Other modalities include injection of botulinum toxin A in the bladder wall may help to relieve irritative bladder symptoms. Other modalities include use of hyperbaric oxygen therapy (HBOT) involves the administration of 100% oxygen at higher than atmospheric pressure. The reported success rate of HBOT for radiation cystitis varies from 60% to 92%. Historically effective use of intravesical instillation of alum and formalin have been reported but good clinical evidence is lacking for its use. Rarely more aggressive treatment options may be required to control intractable haematuria, these include selective embolization or ligation of the internal iliac arteries. Rarely patients may need urinary diversion in the form of percutaneous nephrostomy or bowel conduit, with or without cystectomy.
- To understand the advancement in radiation therapy: Nowadays with advancement in radiation therapy, such as high-energy linear accelerators, conformal radiation therapy (CRT) and intensity-modulated radiation therapy (IMRT), higher doses of radiation to be delivered to the cancer area with simultaneous sparing of the adjoining tissues. Despite these advances, some collateral damage to the adjoining tissue/organs does take place and so, the treating team should be aware of all such modalities available.

Case Scenario

A 53-year-male, a known case of rectal cancer, who received long course chemoradiation (CTRT) three years back: Post-CTRT response scan suggestive of good response in mid-rectal lesion, with no adjacent organ involvement. After completion of CTRT, he underwent anterior resection for his rectal cancer. Patient now complaints of hematuria for 15 days, with passage of clots. There is no history of fever, chills and flank pain. During evaluation, urine culture sterile. USG KUB is suggestive of 50 cc blood clot in bladder, postvoid residual (PVR) 30 ml, prostate 52 g, and no hydronephrosis.

How to approach a case of radiation cystitis with hematuria?

1. **Discuss acute radiation cystitis.**

   Ans: Acute radiation cystitis usually occurs either during or soon after radiation treatment. It is invariably self-limiting and managed conservatively.

2. **What are its symptoms and management?**

Ans: These patients present with storage symptoms predominantly which include include increased urinary frequency, dysuria and urgency. This condition is usually self-limiting, and rarely persists beyond 3 months following radiation therapy. These patients are treated conservatively with the use of anticholinergic drugs (such as oxybutynin chloride) to which they respond adequately. Other drugs which can be used to achieve symptomatic relief include phenazopyridine hydrochloride and flavoxate hydrochloride.[2,3]

3. **What is late radiation cystitis?**

Ans: Late radiation cystitis is one that can develop anytime after about 6 months to 20 years following pelvic radiation therapy with an average latent period of 35 months.[3]

4. **What are its symptoms?**

Ans: The most common presenting symptom is haematuria, which may be variable and range from mild to severe haematuria resulting in clot retention to life-threatening haemorrhage.[7]

5. **What is the incidence of late radiation cystitis[5]?**

Ans: Incidence of late radiation cystitis is usually between 5–10% but may go upto 47%,[3] with bladder cancer patients who had under gone radiation accounting for majority of such cases.

6. **Any differential diagnosis while treating a case of radiation cystitis?**

Ans: Usually the clinical features of late radiation cystitis are not very specific and the presenting symptoms can mimic bladder infection or malignancy. Thus, diagnosis with such symptoms is by the exclusion of other causes of haematuria.

7. **How do you workup a suspected case of radiation cystitis?**

Ans:

1. Urine culture of a mid-stream clean catch is essential to exclude infection.
2. Urine cytology can be done to detect high-grade malignancy.
3. Ultrasonography or intravenous excretory urography is needed to scan upper urinary tract for malignancy in such cases.
4. Lower urinary tract evaluation is mandatory in such cases. Cystoscopy is invariably done under anaesthesia to look for the cause of haematuria. It may reveal erythema, oedema, telangiectasia, bleeding ulcers, fistulas or reduced bladder capacity secondary to fibrosis. At the time of cystoscopy, the suspicious areas need to be biopsied to rule out active malignancy with a special care to not to perforate the bladder wall as these irradiated urinary bladders are very fragile.

8. **Grade the severity of radiation cystitis.**

Ans: Table 5.1 depicts the grades of the radiation cystitis.

9. **Any other grading system you are aware of??**

Ans: The LENT-SOMA scale

10. **What is pathophysiology of radiation cystitis?**

Ans:

Pathophysiology of radiation cystitis involves a progressive end arteritis that results in poor tissue oxygenation and eventual tissue ischemia. This is then followed by tissue necrosis and sloughing resulting in fibroblast deposition on ischemic tissue layers. Later on compensatory neovascularization and telangiectasia occurs and that leads to a friable vascular network resulting in recurrent hematuria (Fig. 5.1).

11. **Enumerate conservative treatment options in a case of radiation cystitis.**

Ans: Refer to Flowchart 5.1.

12. **Discuss the role of alum in radiation cystitis with haematuria?**

Ans:

Aluminium ammonium sulphate or aluminium potassium sulphate (alum) is used for irrigation of HRC cases with active hematuria. It is prepared by dissolving in sterile water (50 g alum in a 5 L bag of sterile water [1% alum solution]) and then

TABLE 5.1: Grades of the radiation cystitis

Hematuria morbidity	*Grade 1*	*Grade II*	*Grade III*	*Grade 1V*	*Grade V*
Acute hemorrhagic radiation cystitis (rTOG scale)	NA	NA	Gross hematuria with or without clot passage	Hematuria requiring transfusion	Death from uncontrolled hematuria
Late hemorrhagic radiation cystitis (rTOG/eOrTC; scale)	Minor telangiectasia (microscopic hematuria)	Generalized telangiectasia (macroscopic hematuria)	Severe generalized telangiectasia (macroscopic hematuria)	Severe hemorrhagic cystitis	Death from uncontrolled hematuria

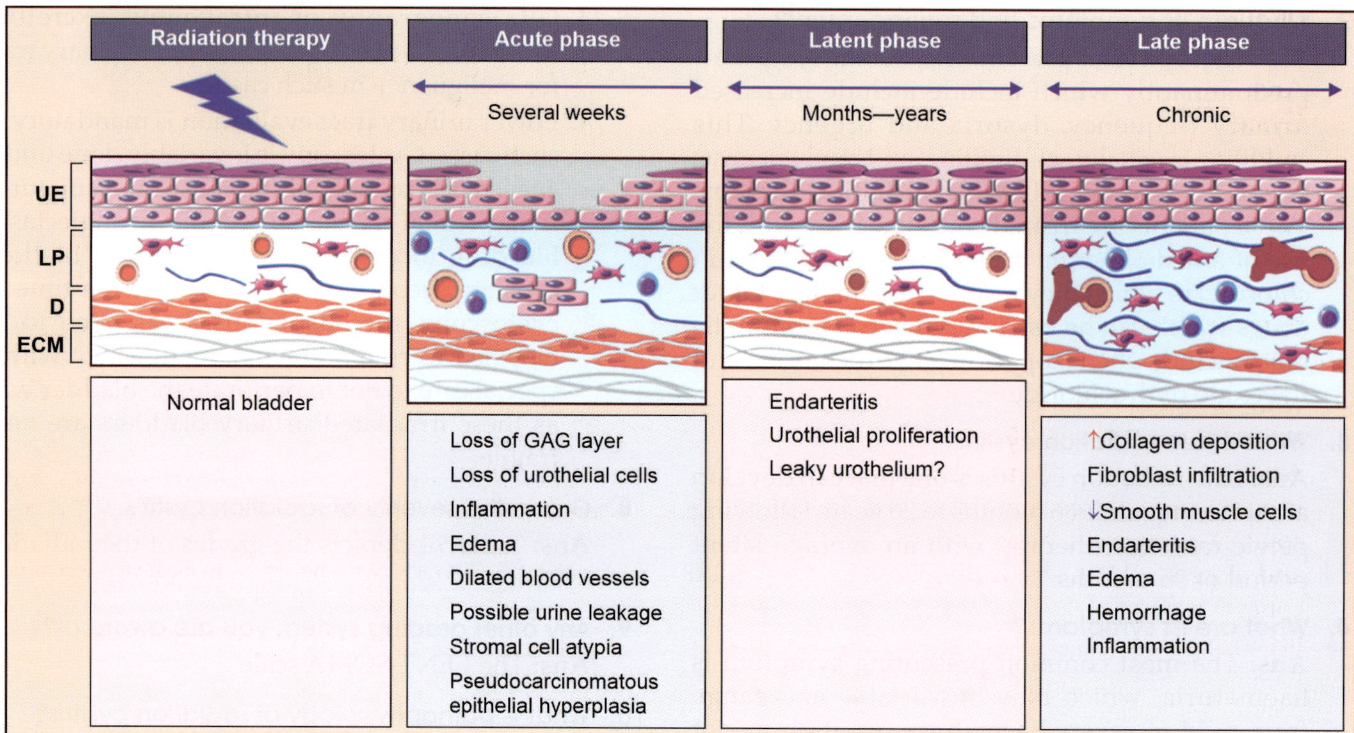

Fig. 5.1: Developmental stages of radiation cystitis (RC). RC progression consists of three phases: A reversible acute inflammatory phase, a latent symptom-free phase, and a late chronic inflammatory phase. Each phase is characterized by specific pathologic changes that contribute to the symptoms associated with RC. UE, uroepithelium; LP, lamina propria; D, detrusor; ECM, extra cellular matrix.

Flowchart 5.1: Radiation cystitis: Treatment algorithm

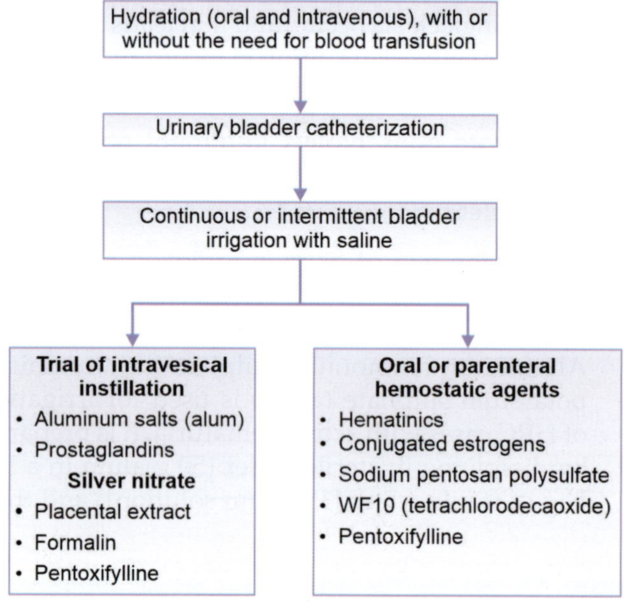

it is used to slowly irrigate the irradiated bladder at a rate of 200 to 300 ml/h. It acts as an astringent at sites of bleeding and may cause protein precipitation on the urothelial lining. This results in stimulating vasoconstriction and decrease in capillary permeability. It has response rates ranging from 50% to 100%.[6]

13. What is the adverse effects associated with the use of alum?

Ans: Adverse effects of use of alum may be localised to bladder in form of suprapubic pain and vesical tenesmus. These can be controlled with antispasmodic and/or analgesic drugs. Systemic side effects include encephalopathy and renal failure have been reported, so one should ensure adequate renal function prior to alum instillation.

14. Enumerate surgical options for management.

Ans:

1. Cystoscopy with fulguration of bleeding points under anaesthesia.
2. Radiological intervention such as selective angio-embolization of iliac arteries.
3. Open ligation of the internal iliac artery
4. Rarely, urinary diversion with or without cystectomy

15. Which kind of urinary diversion will you prefer?

Ans:

Transverse colon conduit is the preferred method of urinary diversion, which has the advantage of using the nonirradiated bowel and ureters for creating the diversion.[7] Percutaneous nephrostomy as a mode of diversion is not preferred at present as it has limited success.

16. Discuss the role of cystectomy at time of urinary diversion.

Ans:

Cystectomy is a preferred option until patient is too morbid not to sustain prolonged surgery as complications related to the defunctionalized bladder which have not been removed can occur in more than 50% of patients.[8–10] These include pyocystis, haemorrhage, pain and neoplastic transformation. So, cystectomy is recommended upfront at the time of urinary diversion.

17. What is HBOT (hyperbaric oxygen therapy) and its rationale of use in HRC?

Ans: It involves the administration of 100% oxygen in a pressurized treatment chamber. This provides condition wherein haemoglobin is fully saturated and oxygen which is now dissolved at a very high concentration in plasma which now circulates in the system to provide therapeutic benefits which includes neo angiogenesis and reduced fibroblastic reaction.[11]

18. What is new in treatment for HRC?

Ans:

1. Amniotic bladder therapy: Herein amniotic membrane which is known to contain proregenerative properties is injected into the detrusor to achieve desired results.[12]
2. Photocoagulation and green light laser for point fulguration of bleeders in case of active hematuria.
3. Phytotherapy: Ich Nieu Khang phytotherapy has been tried with variable success.
4. Use of cranberry in combination with hyaluronic acid and chondroitin sulfate as oral medication has been found to be effective in reducing the severity of HRC.
5. Tacrolimus which is a calcineurin inhibitor and a potent anti-inflammatory agent has also been tried with variable success.[13]

19. What was done in the index case?

Ans: After stabilization of the patient, he was subjected to clot evacuation and a three-way Foley catheter 20 fr was inserted and irrigation started. But since he had recurrent in hospital episodes of hematuria Alum irrigation was started with addition of oral anticholinergic (solifenacin and mirabegron 5/25 mg) once a day and tab pentosan sulphate 100 mg three times a day was added to which the patient responded. Once hematuria settled, he was discharged on catheter which was removed after three days with the warning that the episode may recurrence in which case he should report to emergency room.

SUMMARY

- Radiation cystitis is rare but a morbid complication of pelvic radiation therapy
- Can present any time (> 1–20 years) after radiation therapy
- Hematuria is a common presentation
- Management would depend on severity of hematuria
- A lot of new treatment are being adopted for management and prevention of hematuria

REFERENCES

1. Smit SG, Heyns CF. Management of radiation cystitis. Nat Rev Urol. 2010 Apr;7(4):206–14. doi: 10.1038/nrurol.2010.23. Epub 2010 Mar 9. PMID: 20212517.
2. Levenback C, Eifel PJ, Burke TW, Morris M, Gershenson DM. Hemorrhagic cystitis following radiotherapy for stage Ib cancer of the cervix. Gynecol Oncol. 1994 Nov;55(2):206–10. doi: 10.1006/gyno.1994.1278. PMID: 7959285.
3. Denton AS, Clarke NW, Maher EJ. Non-surgical interventions for late radiation cystitis in patients who have received radical radiotherapy to the pelvis. Cochrane Database Syst Rev. 2002;3:CD001773.
4. Russell NS, Bartelink H. Radiotherapy: the last 25 years. Cancer Treat Rev. 1999 Dec;25(6):365–76. doi: 10.1053/ctrv.1999.0141. PMID: 10644502.
5. Marks LB, Carroll PR, Dugan TC, Anscher MS. The response of the urinary bladder, urethra, and ureter to radiation and chemotherapy. Int J Radiat Oncol Biol Phys. 1995 Mar 30;31(5):1257–80. doi: 10.1016/0360–3016(94)00431–J. PMID: 7713787.
6. Smit SG, Heyns CF. Management of radiation cystitis. Nat Rev Urol. 2010 Apr;7(4):206–14. doi: 10.1038/nrurol.2010.23. Epub 2010 Mar 9. PMID: 20212517.
7. Ravi R, Dewan AK, Pandey KK. Transverse colon conduit urinary diversion in patients treated with very high dose pelvic irradiation. Br J Urol. 1994 Jan;73(1):51–4. doi: 10.1111/j.1464–410x.1994.tb07455.x. PMID: 8298899.
8. Fazili T, Bhat TR, Masood S, Palmer JH, Mufti GR. Fate of the leftover bladder after supravesical urinary diversion for benign disease. J Urol. 2006 Aug;176(2):620–1. doi: 10.1016/j.juro.2006.03.056. PMID: 16813905.
9. Adeyoju AB, Lynch TH, Thornhill JA. The defunctionalized bladder. Int Urogynecol J Pelvic Floor Dysfunct. 1998;9(1):48–51. doi: 10.1007/BF01900542. PMID: 9657178.
10. Adeyoju AB, Thornhill J, Lynch T, Grainger R, McDermott T, Butler MR. The fate of the defunctioned bladder following supravesical urinary diversion. Br J Urol. 1996 Jul;78(1):80–3. doi: 10.1046/j.1464–410x.1996.05615.x. PMID: 8795405.
11. Capelli-Schellpfeffer M, Gerber GS. The use of hyperbaric oxygen in urology. J Urol. 1999 Sep;162(3 Pt 1):647–54. doi: 10.1097/00005392–199909010–00002. PMID: 10458334.
12. Radoiu C, Jeberaeel J, Madan R, Vaishampayan N, Lucas S, Hamada A, Dhar N. A preliminary report assessing the feasibility and effectiveness of amniotic bladder therapy in patients with chronic radiation cystitis. Can J Urol. 2023 Aug;30(4):11607–11612. PMID: 37633288.
13. Dave CN, Chaus F, Chancellor MB, Lajness M, Peters KM. Innovative use of intravesical tacrolimus for hemorrhagic radiation cystitis. Int Urol Nephrol. 2015 Oct;47(10):1679–81. doi: 10.1007/s11255–015–1098–6. Epub 2015 Sep 7. PMID: 26347076.

Chapter

6

Discharging Flank Sinus: Etiology and Approach

• *Milap Shah* • *BM Zeeshan Hameed*

LEARNING OBJECTIVES

- To understand the probable etiology of discharging sinus.
- To understand the pathogenesis of discharging flank sinus.
- To be able to identify the presenting symptoms.
- To understand the investigation and treatment approach in a patient with discharging flank sinus.

Case Scenario

A 46-year-old male presented to the emergency room with a swelling on the right flank. Swelling was present for the last 5 months, and had become painful in the previous 7 days. It was not associated with lower urinary tract symptoms. He denied symptoms referable to the upper urinary tract, namely flank pains and colic. He is a known diabetic on oral hypoglycemic drugs. Patient had history of incision and drainage done previously by a general surgeon for suspected subcutaneous abscess. He was aware of having received BCG vaccine soon after birth but had no contact with individuals diagnosed with tuberculosis in home as well as workplace. He gave no history of major trauma to the flank or abdomen. He was moderately built and nourished. General examination was normal. Abdomen, spine and renal angles were clinically normal. The other organ systems were within normal limits for health. Digital rectal examination was normal.

1. **What are the possible causes for discharging flank sinus?**

   Ans: A clinician should keep the following possibilities in mind while dealing with a patient with discharging flank sinus:[1,2]

   1. Chronic urinary obstructive process with forniceal rupture
   2. Renal (Staghorn stones)/ureteric stones with a possible history of intervention for the same or related symptoms (>85%)
   3. Xanthogranulomatous pyelonephritis (30%)
   4. Tuberculosis (13.3%)
   5. Others such as post-traumatic, iatrogenic (post-PCNL)

2. **In which gender is the incidence higher and why?**

   Ans: The higher incidence of nephron cutaneous fistula (NCF) has been reported in females and that may be related to a smaller muscle mass in women. Moreover, a higher incidence of pyelonephritis has also been reported in females.[3]

3. **What is the pathogenesis of formation of such a discharging sinus/nephron-cutaneous fistula?**

   Ans: The pathogenesis of NCF is attributed to a progressive and chronic inflammatory or degenerative process of the kidney which then extends beyond Gerota's fascia and perinephric fat. Since they are the first barriers and once, they are breached the infection, then directly involves the flank muscle on its posterior rim. Following this the infection then spreads into the lumbar region. Since the lumbar triangle and the lumbar quadrilateral are the site of extremely low anatomical resistance, the infective fistulous tract in this site can easily reach the flank skin. These patients often neglect their signs and symptoms for a long time as it is invariably a painless process. Now this long standing and chronic inflammatory process along with urine stasis supports the continuous infection and the progress of pyelonephritis in such cases. This then results in the destruction of renal parenchyma and the adjoining perinephric fat which finally leads to fistula formation. Thus, by the time diagnosis is made these renal units have become either poorly functioning or even nonfunctioning.[3]

4. What are the presenting symptoms?

Ans: Most common symptoms are:

1. Asymptomatic presentation (63%) with discharging sinus in the flank. Discharge can be pus or clear fluid.
2. Loin pain (30%): Fistulae development after renal pelvicalyceal rupture usually relieves the pain as it diminishes the tensile stress in the collecting system. Invariably these fistulae take the shorter path, generally through the superior or inferior part of lumbar triangle.[4,5]

Characteristic and often diagnostic features of NCF include presence of flank sinus, discharge of fluid, and sometimes a palpable mass or an erythematous area.[2,3]

5. What are the investigations to be done in such a patient?

Ans:

1. Blood analyses: CBC, RFT, CRP—usually are normal unless patient is febrile or has systemic symptoms.
2. Acid-fast bacillus (AFB) test and Mantoux test
3. Pus or the discharge culture and urine culture are usually negative.
4. Imaging:
   a. Initial investigation: Ultrasound abdomen and pelvis and fistulogram. Fistulogram can provide direct evaluation of the fistulous tract and its communication to the deep tissue especially a CT/MRI fistulogram.
   b. Abdominal contrast enhanced computed tomography (CECT) scan. It helps to identify the underlying etiology as well as kidney function which can help to plan further treatment.
   c. Renogram (DTPA/DMSA/EC scan): To determine the differential cortical function and drainage if contrast study is not done or not available.
   d. Role of retrograde pyelography as an initial line of investigation is controversial.[5–7]

6. What are the radiological findings in such a case?

Ans: The following can be the radiological findings in such a case:[1]

1. Diffuse cortical atrophy
2. Hydronephrosis +/- Calculus
3. Renal/peri-renal/parietal abscess
4. Fistulous tract between kidney and skin
5. Functioning/non-functioning kidney

7. Is there any classification of nephron-cutaneous fistulas?

Ans:

1. Direct nephron cutaneous fistula or simple NCF and
2. Indirect NCF, or complex NCF involving other adjoining organs.[9]

8. What is the treatment approach in this patient?

Ans: In complex cases, a planned exploratory laparotomy should be considered. Whereas in case of simple fistula (secondary to stone disease), a trail of antibiotic therapy and with removal of an underlying cause such as stone or foreign body should be carried out.

The first-line antibiotic therapy includes administration of fluoroquinolones, amino-penicillin plus a β-lactamase inhibitor, while second line of therapy involves use of cephalosporins or aminoglycosides.

In cases of documented tuberculosis (typical or atypical mycobacteria) as six months course of anti-tubercular treatment is indicated.[2]

Intervention in the form of placing a percutaneous nephrostomy is sometimes useful and it not only facilitates the passage of urine from the fistula but also helps in reducing the risk of urosepsis. However such cases are difficult to manage conservatively and usually fail. The main treatment is surgical approach in 90% of these patients.[1,3,9]

9. What are the advantages of placing a nephrostomy in such a case?

Ans: After placing a PCN, antegrade pyelography can be done which helps to delineate the renal pelvis and demonstrate the urinary tract in terms of the site of obstruction and the fistulous tract. Moreover, daily urine output and respective creatinine clearance can be measured. This information can also help to decide between an nephron sparing (NS) or non-nephron sparing (NNS) management, especially in case of an initially poorly functioning kidney.[3]

10. What surgical approach is preferred for these cases?

Ans: The crucial point is the choice between renal preservation vs removal in such cases. Invariably these patients end up in nephrectomy (90%) as most of these renal units are either poorly functioning/nonfunctioning at the time of the diagnosis. Other precautions in this case which need to be taken are the complete excision of the perinephric scar and the fistulous tract which needs patience and experience.[2] Due to the extreme complexity of these cases, the preferred modality is open surgery. However, laparoscopic or robot-assisted management should be attempted in experienced hands only.[1,3,8]

Role of partial nephrectomy/NSS is not much reported in such conditions due to overall involvement of renal parenchyma by inflammatory and degenerative processes, the severe reduction of the function of the affected kidney, and technical difficulties.

So, in a nutshell it is very important to define the type of fistula first into either simple or complex. As in the case of a complex fistula multidisciplinary management is necessary, whereas in case of a simple NCF an open nephrectomy for a poorly functioning or nonfunctioning kidney should suffice along with excision of the fistulous tract. Also, completion nephrectomy is recommended in cases of failed NS surgery. Flowchart 6.1 is to be followed.

Flowchart 6.1: Algorithm for approach to spontaneous nephron-cutaneous fistula[2]

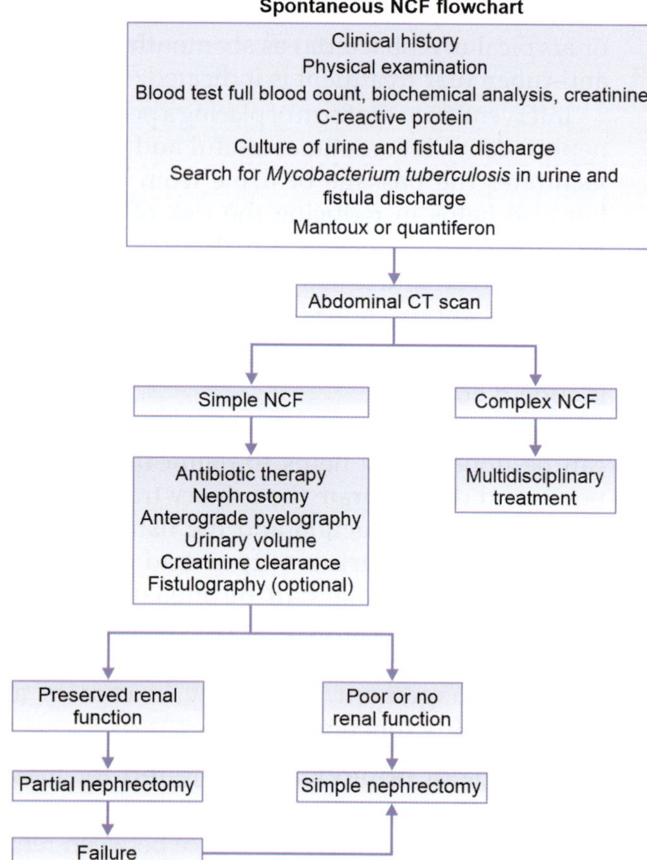

SUMMARY

- Discharging sinus is a rare but a morbid problem.
- Needs thorough evaluation and a proper treatment plan
- Genito-urinary tuberculosis is still a common etiology
- Post-PCNL chronic leak could be due to infection, obstruction or residual calculus.
- Rarely management may need endoscopic deobstruction (infundibulotomy), partial nephrectomy or total simple nephrectomy (if poorly functioning kidney).

REFERENCES

1. Hamard M, Amzalag G, Becker CD, Poletti PA. Asymptomatic Urolithiasis Complicated by Nephrocutaneous Fistula. J Clin Imaging Sci. 2017 Feb 20;7:9. doi: 10.4103/jcis.JCIS_83_16. PMID: 28299237; PMCID: PMC5341303.
2. Gupta R, Mahajan A, Gupta C. Post-percutaneous nephrolithotripsy nephrostomy site tuberculosis: A report of six cases. Urol Ann. 2012 Jan;4(1):41–4. doi: 10.4103/0974-7796.91624. PMID: 22346101; PMCID: PMC3271450.
3. Rubilotta E, Balzarro M, Sarti A, Artibani W. Spontaneous Nephrocutaneous Fistula: A Case Report, Update of the Literature and Management Algorithm. Urol Int. 2016;97(2):241–6. doi: 10.1159/000360403. Epub 2014 Aug 9. PMID: 25115272.
4. Maheshwari PN, Shah HN. Nephrocutaneous fistula through percutaneous nephrolithotomy scar: rare presentation of genitourinary tuberculosis. Urology. 2005 Sep;66(3):655–6. doi: 10.1016/j.urology.2005.04.052. PMID: 16140098.Biyani CS, Torella F, Cornford PA, *et al*: Xanthogranulomatous pyelonephritis with bilateral nephrocutaneous fistulae. Urol Int 1997; 59: 46–47.
5. Das S, Ching V. Nephrocutaneous sinus: a case report. J Urol. 1979 Aug;122(2):232. doi: 10.1016/s0022-5347(17)56341-7. PMID: 459021.Bryniak SR: Primary spontaneous renocutaneous fistula. Urology 1983; 21: 516–517.
6. Karfopoulos AS, Murray W, Stone FJ. Nephrocutaneous fistula. J Med Soc N J. 1981 May;78(5):379–80. PMID: 6945442. Ansari MS, Singh I, Dogra PN: Spontaneous nephrocutaneous fistula: 2 unusual reports with review of literature. Int Urol Nephrol 2004; 36: 239–243.
7. Grabe M, Bjerklund-Johansen TE, Botto H, *et al*: Guidelines on Urological Infections. European Association of Urology, 2013, 4.4.2, p 29.
8. Qureshi MA. Spontaneous nephrocutaneous fistula in tuberculous pyelonephritis. J Coll Physicians Surg Pak. 2007 Jun;17(6):367–8. PMID: 17623591.
9. Ansari MS, Singh I, Dogra PN. Spontaneous nephrocutaneous fistula-2 unusual case reports with review of literature. Int Urol Nephrol. 2004;36(2):239–43. doi: 10.1023/b:urol.0000034685.64057.80. PMID: 15368703.

Chapter 7

Urosepsis Following Endourological Procedures

• Ranjan Kumar Dey • Sumantra Dey

LEARNING OBJECTIVES

- To understand the assessment of the patient in sepsis in the post-operative period for signs and symptoms of systemic inflammatory response.
- To allude to the work up of patients in sepsis and describe the management algorithms for the same.
- To describe the principles of use of empirical broad spectrum followed by culture specific antibiotics, ensuring adequate drainage of urine, aggressive fluid resuscitation with intensive medical monitoring forms the basis of sepsis management.
- To allude to the principles of identification and removal of the source of infection so that they contribute to the management plan.

CLINICAL DEFINITION OF SEPSIS

The previously accepted definition for urosepsis was a systemic inflammatory response syndrome (SIRS) associated with urinary tract infection proven by bacterial cultures. The updated definition states that urosepsis is a life-threatening organ dysfunction caused by body's abnormal response to a urinary tract infection.[1]

Clinically, SIRS is identified by presence of any 3 of the following criteria:

1. Fever, temperature above 38°C, or hypothermia, below 36°C;
2. Tachycardia—over 90/min;
3. Tachypnea—over 20 breaths/min or partial pressure of carbon dioxide in the arterial blood ($PaCO_2$) < 32 mm Hg;
4. Leukocytosis > 12,000/mm^3 or leukopenia < 4000/mm^3, or the presence of immature cells in the periphery < 10%.

SIRS with documented infection is termed sepsis. Biochemical markers have been used for diagnosis and dynamic monitoring of sepsis, e.g. procalcitonin, serum lactate, MR-proADM, C reactive protein, specific cytokines.

Septic shock should be defined as a subset of sepsis in which particularly profound circulatory, cellular and metabolic abnormalities. Patients with septic shock can be clinically identified by a vasopressor requirement to maintain a mean arterial pressure of 65 mmHg or greater and serum lactate level greater than 2 mmol/L (>18 mg/dl) in the absence of hypovolemia.

Urosepsis After Transurethral Prostate Surgery

UTI and other infective complications can be present in 1–26% of patients after TURP. With routine use of antibiotic prophylaxis, the incidence of bacteriuria (26 to 9%) as well as clinical sepsis (4.4 to 0.7%) is reduced. Risk factors like increased operative time, prolonged post-operative catheterisation, preoperative catheterisation, complicated diabetes, age >65 years increases the incidence of infective episodes.

Urosepsis After Ureteric and Renal Stone Surgery

Infection or sepsis is the most common complication affecting patients undergoing surgery for stone disease. With the increasing number of surgeries performed in the current era, burden of infection and associated morbidity is on the rise.[3]

Case Scenario

A 46-year-old female patient underwent left RIRS with DJ stenting for a 1.2 cm upper calyceal stone. Initial post-operative period was uneventful. Foley catheter draining clear urine was removed on morning of POD. Then she had one episode of fever (100.8 °F) in the same

(Contd.)

Case Scenario *(Contd.)*

evening. On examination, pulse rate was 110/min, BP 130/80, respiratory rate 16/min, urine output 550 ml in last 6 hours.

Blood investigations revealed: Total leucocyte count 21,000/cu.mm, raised CRP and procalcitonin.

1. What are the causes of fever in the post-operative period?

Ans: Most early post-operative fever is caused by inflammatory stimulus of tissue damage and exposure to foreign materials (physiologic fever). Differential diagnoses include several non-infectious causes along with infections.

Timing of post-operative fever

1. Immediate post-operative—within hours of surgery
   - Inflammation as a consequence of surgery
   - Trauma or burn-induced inflammation
   - Immune reaction to medications/blood products
   - Malignant hyperthermia
   - Infections predating the operation
2. Early post-operative—0 to 3 days
   - Continued inflammation
   - Infections predating surgery
   - Urinary tract infection
   - Myocardial infarction
   - Early surgical site infection
   - Pneumonia
   - Superficial venous thrombosis
3. Late post-operative fever—4 to 30 days
   - Surgical site infection
   - Surgery specific complications (urine leak, abscess, fistula)
   - Nosocomial infection
4. Delayed post-operative fever—after 4 weeks
   - usually unrelated to surgery

Useful initial screen for post-operative fever: 5W mnemonic—based on day of occurrence[4]

Day 1 WIND—pneumonia, aspiration, pulmonary embolism
Day 2 WATER—urinary tract infection
Day 3 WOUND—surgical site infection
Day 4 WALKING—veinous thrombo-embolism
Day 5 WONDER DRUG—drug related fever

2. How to evaluate such patients?

Ans: Clinical presentation of urosepsis = features of SIRS + documented/clinical evidence of UTI. Signs and symptoms like suprapubic or flank discomfort, dysuria, irritative voiding symptoms must be considered as clinical pointers to urinary tract infection.

The Sepsis Consensus Definition Task Force introduced the sequential (sepsis-related) organ failure assessment (SOFA) score as a mean of operationalizing, this definition of sepsis provided the quick SOFA (qSOFA) scoring system, which facilitates the bedside diagnosis of sepsis.[3]

Assessment of clinical symptoms and strict periodic monitoring of vital signs is mandatory. Routine blood investigations including complete blood counts, renal function test, liver function with coagulation profile should be done. Blood and urine for culture and sensitivity should be sent at the first suspicion of sepsis, prior to starting empirical antibiotics. Specific biochemical markers and cytokines have been used for diagnosis and dynamic assessment (details later). Imaging to assess septic collections is to be considered.

3. What is the role of biomarkers in diagnosing and monitoring urosepsis?

Ans: Commonly used biomarkers in clinical practice are C-reactive protein (CRP) and procalcitonin.

Procalcitonin (PCT) is a peptide precursor of calcitonin. Serum levels of procalcitonin have been shown to increase dramatically in response

TABLE 7.1: Clinical and biochemical assessment for diagnosing sepsis[6]

Appearance	*Inflammatory response*	*Hemodynamic dysfunction*	*Organ dysfunction*	*Tissue malperfusion*
Fever (temp > 38.5 °C)	Leucocytosis (WBC > 11,000/μL)	Hypotension (SBP <90 mmHg, MAP <70 mmHg)	Hypoxemia (PaO_2/FiO_2 <300)	Elevated lactate (>2 m mol/L)
Hypothermia (temp < 36 °C)	Leukopenia (WBC < 4000/μL)	Tachycardia (HR >90/min)	Oliguria (output <0.5 ml/kg/hr for >2 hours despite resuscitation)	Prolonged capillary refill time
Tachypnoea	More than 10% immature forms		Elevated creatinine (increase >0.5 mg/dl from baseline)	Skin mottling
Altered mental status			Disordered coagulation (INR >1.5)	

to bacterial infection. Calcitonin synthesis is normally limited to thyroid C cells. Production is, however, activated in all parenchymal organs in response to bacterial infection, mediated by cytokines. These tissues do not have the ability to cleave PCT to its mature form, calcitonin, leading to the accumulation of procalcitonin. In contrast, PCT production is attenuated by interferon secreted primarily in response to viral infection. This feature makes PCT a specific marker for bacterial infections. PCT becomes detectable within 2–4 hours of the triggering event, reaching peak levels after 12–24 hours. In the absence of a persistent PCT stimulus, it is eliminated, the half-life being 24–35 hours. For this reason, the parameter can be useful for dynamic monitoring of patients.[1]

CRP is an acute phase reactant synthesised in the liver. It is a sensitive marker for sepsis, but not specific as it rises in several non-infectious conditions. Owing to comparatively early rise in blood levels within 2 hours, and short half life of 18 hours, it can be monitored frequently as a marker for resolution/worsening of infection.

Serum lactate is a marker for tissue hypoxia. Rise in serum acetate is associated with increased mortality in sepsis.

Mid-regional proadrenomedulline is another sepsis marker. It has been shown to play a decisive role in the induction of hyperdynamic circulation during the early stages of sepsis and progression to septic shock.

Cytokines are being studied as biomarkers for sepsis. Elevated plasma levels of IL-18 have been correlated with unsatisfactory clinical outcome in patients with sepsis and therefore IL-18 may be an important biomarker in the evaluation of septic patients.

Midline, also known as neuritis growth factor 2, significantly increases in severe sepsis and septic shock, and identifies patients susceptible to cardiovascular failure and shock. Leptin, produced by adipocytes, is involved in expression of several cytokines and is useful for discriminating SIRS from sepsis above a threshold level. Monocyte Chemoattractant Protein 1 (MCP 1) along with IL-18 have been evaluated in studies to diagnose and monitor sepsis in ICU setting, but large scale clinical application not recommended yet.[1]

4. What are the commonly described risk factors for developing sepsis after endourology?

Ans: Commonly described conditions are pre-existing infection/foreign body, anatomical abnormality of urinary tract, diabetes or other immunosuppressed condition.[7] A detailed account is given as follows:

TABLE 7.2: Predisposing factors for urosepsis

Related to patient	*Related to urinary tract disease*	*Related to procedure*
Poor nutritional status	Voiding dysfunction	Stone related surgery
Advanced age	Urinary diversion	Long duration surgery
Immunosuppression: Diabetes, corticosteroid use, autoimmune disease	Obstructed system	Involvement of genital/ gastrointestinal tract
Malignancy	Indwelling catheters/stents	
Liver or renal dysfunction	Anatomic anomalies	
Distant coexistant infection	Chronic bacteriuria	

5. What are the preventive strategies for post-surgical urosepsis?

Ans: General guidelines for prevention of post-surgical sepsis are laid down in detail in EAU[9] guidelines are:

- Isolation of patients with multi-resistant organism infection
- Prudent use of antimicrobial agents for prophylaxis and treatment of established infections.
- Reduction in hospital stay
- Early removal of indwelling urethral catheter
- Use of closed catheter drainage
- Use of least-invasive methods to release urinary tract obstruction until the patient is stabilised.
- Attention to simple everyday techniques to assure asepsis
- Disposable gloves, frequent hand disinfection, and using infection control measures to prevent cross-infections.

Timely administration of prophylactic antibiotics as per centre protocol has a significant impact on reducing post-operative infections.

Midstream urine culture and sensitivity is recommended prior to any endoscopic stone surgery. However, it does not always correlate with obstructed urine or stone cultures, and sepsis may present in one percent of cases with prior negative cultures. Renal pelvic urine culture and stone culture have been considered over voided urine to predict post-operative UTI or sepsis, but their utilisation in guiding clinical practice is limited as it takes several days to obtain culture results.

TABLE 7.3: Recommendation to prevent urosepsis	
Surgery	***Recommendations***[8]
Ureteroscopy/retrograde intra-renal surgery	1. Treat preoperative UTI, do not intervene in presence of active infection. Relieve urinary obstruction, treat infection, perform staged procedure.
	2.If preoperative negative urine culture not possible, administer 3 days of culture sensitive antibiotics before procedure
	3. Antibiotic prophylaxis in all cases
	4. Maintain low intra-renal pressure during procedure—options include periodic drainage through ureteroscope or ureteral access sheath, continuous or intermittent bladder drainage
Percutaneous nephrolithotomy	1. Treat preoperative UTI, do not intervene in presence of active infection.
	2. If preoperative negative urine culture not possible, administer 7 days of culture sensitive antibiotics before procedure
	3. Antibiotic prophylaxis in all cases
	4. Stop procedure if purulent fluid is obtained at puncture, leave a nephrostomy tube, and stage treatment—obtain pelvic urine culture and treat infection completely
	5. Maintain low intrarenal pressure during procedure: Use only enough irrigation to maintain adequate visibility; use a wide renal access sheath, ideally 4 Fr wider than nephroscope.
	6. Limit quantity of irrigation fluid and operative time.
Trans-urethral bladder or prostate surgery	1. Treat preoperative positive urine cultures
	2. If preoperative negative urine cultures not possible, administer culture sensitive antibiotics for 3–7 days
	3. Antibiotic prophylaxis in all cases
	4. Maintain closed urinary drainage system, avoid prolonged catheterisation beyond 3 days

Renal pelvic pressures (RPP) during stone surgery has significant impact on post-operative urosepsis. Pressures greater than 30 mm Hg have shown to result in pyelo-lymphatic back flow. Low RPP during surgery is achieved by using an open low-pressure access system, such as operating through an Amplatz sheath (operating instrument 4 Fr sizes smaller than the access sheath). Inflow of irrigant should be at gravity and never pressurized. Use of forced diuresis with Frusemide 20 mg at the beginning of the procedure and then every 60 minutes of irrigation time may further reduce pyelo-renal reflux that potentially causes fluid overload and bacteremia.

6. What are the principles of antibiotic prophylaxis? What is the recommendation for endourological surgeries?

Ans: Best Practice Statement 2019 (AUA)[10] recommends consideration of antibiotic prophylaxis for all urological procedures in which a tissue breach will occur. It should be initiated 60 minutes before the start of procedure, efficacious levels should be maintained for the duration of the procedure. In special circumstances, it should be extended beyond the limited time of the procedure, maximum up to 24 hours.

Recommendation of antibiotic prophylaxis from European Society of Urology:

TABLE 7.4: Choice of antibiotic regime in urosepsis		
Procedure	***First choice***	***Alternate choice***
Diagnostic cystoscopy or ureteroscopy	Fluroquinolones or 2nd generation cephalosporins or TMP-SMX	Aminoglycoside +/-ampicillin or amoxicillin/clavulanate
TURP or TURBT	Fluroquinolones or TMP-SMX or 2nd/3rd generation cephalosporins or aminopenicillins/beta lactam inhibitors	Aminoglycoside +/-ampicillin or 1st generation cephalosporins or amoxicillin/clavulanate
Ureteroscopy/retrograde renal surgery	2nd/3rd generation cephalosporins or TMP-SMX or aminopenicillins/beta lactam inhibitors or fluroquinolones	Aminoglycoside +/-ampicillin or 1st generation cephalosporins or amoxicillin/clavulanate
Percutaneous renal surgery	2nd/3rd generation cephalosporins or TMP-SMX or aminopenicillins/beta lactam inhibitors	Aminoglycoside +/-ampicillin or 1st generation cephalosporins

7. What are the principles of management of post-surgical urosepsis?[9]

Ans: Management is based on three pillars: Antimicrobial therapy, source control, supportive adjunct measures.

Initial high dose empirical antimicrobial therapy with institute directed protocol of broad spectrum antibiotics is to be started as early as possible, preferably within 1 hour of suspecting sepsis after sending cultures. These should be continued till culture and sensitivity reports are available. Treatment should be continued for 10–14 days, prolonged duration recommended for slow clinical response.

Source control is a key component of management—considered an absolute emergency. Identification of source may be aided by imaging. Once detected, drainage of abscess or obstructed urine; removal of foreign bodies like stones/ catheter/stents should be done without delay.

Adjunctive measures employed are as follows:

- Fluid therapy with crystalloids, vasopressors when needed
- Blood products should be given to target a haemoglobin level of 7–9 g/dl
- Glucose levels should be target at 180 mg/dl
- Deep vein thrombosis prevention
- Stress ulcer prophylaxis

SUMMARY

Measures to prevent urosepsis after endourology:

a. Basic preventive measures:
   - Isolation of patients with multi-drug resistant organism infection
   - Reduction of hospital stay
   - Closed catheter drainage
   - Early removal of indwelling catheters

b. Antibiotic prophylaxis

c. Treatment of prior urinary tract infection

d. Adequate optimisation of the compromised patient

e. Avoiding prolonged surgical time, high intra-pelvic pressures (PCNL, URS, RIRS) , bleeding during surgery

REFERENCES

1. Guliciuc M, Maier AC, Maier IM, Kraft A, Cucuruzac RR, Marinescu M, et al. The Urosepsis—a literature review. Medicina. 2021;57(9):872.
2. Ryan J, O'Neill E, McLornan L. Urosepsis and the urologist! Current Urology. 2021;15(1):39–44.
3. Scotland K, Lange D. Prevention and management of Urosepsis triggered by ureteroscopy. Research and Reports in Urology. 2018;Volume 10:43–9.
4. UpToDate. Available at: https://www.uptodate.com/contents/fever-in-the-surgical-patient#! (Accessed: April 23, 2023).
5. Maiti PK, Chatterjee S, Dey R, Kundu AK, Dey RK. Biofilms on indwelling urologic devices: Microbes and antimicrobial management prospect. Annals of Medical and Health Sciences Research. 2014;4(1):100.
6. Wu P-F. The Association of Sepsis bundles adherence and outcome of sepsis patients with high quick sequential Organ Failure Assessment (qsofa) score. B45 Critical care: Sepsis identification and management. 2020;
7. Smith AD, Preminger GM, Kavoussi LR, Badlani GH, Rastinehad AR. section 1/Preoperative Antibiotics and Prevention of Sepsis. In: Smith's textbook of endourology. Hoboken: Wiley-Blackwell; 2019. p. 58–9.
8. Smith AD, Preminger GM, Kavoussi LR, Badlani GH, Rastinehad AR. section 1/Preoperative Antibiotics and Prevention of Sepsis. In: Smith's textbook of endourology. Hoboken: Wiley-Blackwell; 2019. p. 63–5.
9. EAU Guidelines. Edn. presented at the EAU Annual Congress Milan, Italy 2023. ISBN 978-94-92671-19-6.
10. Lightner DJ, Wymer K, Sanchez J, Kavoussi L. Best practice statement on Urologic Procedures and antimicrobial prophylaxis. Journal of Urology. 2020;203(2):351–6.

Chapter

8

Specimen Handling, Grossing and Processing of Nephrectomy and Prostatectomy Specimen

• *Shruti R Sabnis*

LEARNING OBJECTIVES

- To understand the intricacies of specimen handling for radical nephrectomy and prostatectomy specimens.
- To learn about the sequential journey of tissue processing; From receiving the specimen in the laboratory to the completed slide on the pathologist's desk.
- To understand the importance of macroscopic examination in diagnostic pathology.
- To gain insights into grossing nephrectomy and prostatectomy specimens relevant for the urologists.
- To understand margin assessment and the application of frozen section in radical nephrectomy and prostatectomy.

1. **What is the appropriate workflow for a specimen taken from the patient until it is ready for reporting by the pathologist?**

   Ans:

   - **Labelling and requisition:** A properly labelled specimen should be promptly sent to the laboratory along with the accompanying requisition form, which contains all the relevant clinical details. Any delays in fixation of tissue results in tissue autolysis affecting the proper assessment and reporting of the specimen.
   - **Confirmation of details:** After confirming the patient and specimen identification details, the first step for pathologists is to go through all the clinical and radiological details in the requisition form sent along with the specimen.
   - **Macroscopic examination of the specimen:** The next step is to orient, weigh, measure the specimen and examine and photograph the external surface for relevant gross findings. Afterwards, inking is done wherever indicated. Colored Acrylic ink is used to paint the surface and then fixed with 5% acetic acid.
   - **Dissection:** The next step is to dissect the specimen to expose the tumor. The specimen is photographed and the tumor size, focality and gross appearance is noted. Digital images of the tumors provide a record of the tumor appearance which is helpful in case annotation of tumor sections is required after grossing.
   - **Collection of additional tissue:** If needed, fresh tumor tissue is collected at this stage for molecular studies (e.g. FISH or NGS) or tissue banking for research purposes. Tissue can be placed in special media, snap frozen and stored at –80°C. This results in better RNA and DNA preservation than extraction from FFPE (formalin fixed paraffin embedded) sections.
   - **Fixation:** The specimen is immersed in an adequate amount of 10% neutral buffered formalin for 12–24 hours for "Fixation". 10% neutral buffered formalin is the most widely used fixative. Adequate amount of fixative is 15–20 times the volume of specimen. Formalin vapor is toxic and causes irritation to the eyes, skin and upper respiratory tract on exposure.

     The purpose of tissue fixation is to preserve the tumor tissue by avoiding autolysis by cellular enzymes, prevent bacterial decomposition and make the tissue firm enough to facilitate thin sectioning while grossing.

     Suboptimal fixation affects all downstream procedures and results in suboptimal sections as well as improper results with IHC and molecular studies.

- **Grossing:** Grossing includes noting and documenting gross examination findings and sectioning tissue to be submitted for further microscopic examination. Every laboratory has standardized protocols to be followed for gross sampling of the tumor specimens. Ideal tissue sections are about 3-4 mm in thickness. Tissue sections are subsequently placed into cassettes with appropriate labelling and loaded into the tissue processor for further processing.
- **Tissue Processing:**
  - *Dehydration*: Water content of the tissue is removed and replaced by alcohol/acetone.
  - *Clearing*: Alcohol in tissues is replaced by clearing agent such as xylene which is miscible with both alcohol and paraffin wax, which used for embedding.
  - *Infiltration*: Xylene is replaced by liquid paraffin wax which stiffens tissue enough to enable very thin sectioning.
- **Embedding:** Once processing is complete, the tissues are removed from the cassette and embedded into "blocks" using more liquid paraffin wax. This process is called "embedding". It requires special care to orient and align sections in specific manner as needed for microscopy. Paraffin blocks are then placed over a cooling plate to harden adequately.
- **Microtomy:** Cold blocks are placed in a microtome and 2–3 μ thickness ribbons are cut and floated over water bath containing water at about 70°C, which melts off the excess paraffin wax. These sections are then picked up over glass slides, properly labelled with section number and then sent for staining.
- **Staining:** The most common stain used in histopathology is H and E which contains two dyes: Hematoxylin and eosin. Hematoxylin is a basic dye which has affinity for nucleic acids and thus stains nuclei purple while eosin is an acidic dye which has affinity for cytoplasmic components staining them pink.
- **Mounting:** After staining, the slides are dried and "mounted". Mounting means covering tissue sections with mounting medium like DPX and glass coverslip. This protects tissue sections from damage and provides better optical viewing under microscope. The slides are now ready for microscopic examination.
- **Frozen section:** This technique is used for rapid intraoperative microscopic diagnosis most commonly for evaluating margin status of specimens. It requires an instrument called Cryostat which contains a refrigerated chamber of temperature <–20°C and a microtome inside this chamber. When the tissue sample is placed inside this chamber, the intracellular water hardens to form ice which acts as a matrix enabling thin sectioning of the tissue. These sections are picked up on a slide and stained with a rapid H and E stain. This entire process requires about 20 minutes.
- **Immunohistochemistry (IHC):** This is a technique which can detect presence of specific antigens on FFPE tissue sections using antibodies. With advancement in techniques and automated processors, IHC studies are now commonly used in surgical pathology.[1]
  1. What relevant information should be provided by the urologist within the specimen requisition for radical/partial nephrectomy?
     - Patient identification details: Name, Age, Sex and Identification number.
     - **Specimen details:**
       1. Type of procedure (radical/partial nephrectomy)
       2. Specimen laterality (left/right), type of surgery (open/robotic/laparoscopic)
       3. Tumor site (upper pole/mid pole/ lower pole, etc.)
- **Clinical information:**
  1. Relevant findings suggesting syndromic association or metastatic disease.
  2. Past history/family history of renal cancer
     - Relevant intra-operative findings: Such as breach in capsule/tumor spillage.
     - Pre-operative drug treatment: Such as TKI or immunotherapy/ablative procedure/prior tumor embolization done. These therapies can cause tumor necrosis which will negate the prognostic significance in such cases. Also, necrosis and degeneration may affect histological interpretation of the tumor.

2. How and why to examine external structures of nephrectomy specimen?

Ans:

Radical nephrectomy: Radical nephrectomy specimen encompasses the kidney, perinephric fat along with the surrounding Gerota's fascia and the ureter, with or without the adrenal gland. Adrenal gland, ureter and hilar structures help to properly orient the radical nephrectomy (ureter is present posteriorly at the hilum with respect to renal artery and vein; adrenal is present superiorly).

Measurements of the entire specimen in three dimensions along with length of the ureter and renal vessels are noted for record keeping. Perinephric fat/capsule is not stripped off at any point during examination.

External surface is observed for areas suspicious for involvement by the tumor. The presence of findings such as fissures and rupture on the external surface may indicate involvement of the Gerota's fascia (stage pT4) or presence of residual tumor in the patient (R+ status). Renal vein is observed for the presence of tumor thrombus. Renal vein involvement upstages the tumor to pT3a.[2]

Partial nephrectomy: Partial nephrectomy specimens consist of tumors along with varying amount of renal parenchyma and with or without perinephric fat. Some parts of the pelvicalyceal system and sinus fat may also be included in the specimen.

Specimen should be oriented with respect to surgical resection margin and perinephric fat. The measurements of the entire specimen are noted in the three dimensions. The outer surface and resection margin should be observed for any gross involvement by tumor or area of breach of capsule.[2]

3. **How to ink and dissect the specimen?**

Ans:

Radical nephrectomy: Any suspicious areas of tumor involvement on the external surface are inked (Fig. 8.1). Specimen is bisected along the long axis of the kidney from lateral to medial aspect dividing the kidney into anterior and posterior halves (Figs 8.2 and 8.3).

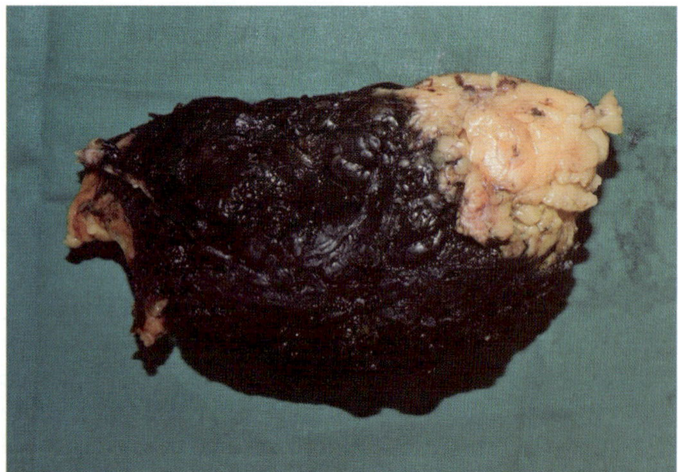

Fig. 8.1: Radical nephrectomy specimen with outer surface showing area suspicious for tumor involvement which is inked

Further incisions may be necessary to adequately expose the tumor along its maximal dimension as well as adequately assess the involvement

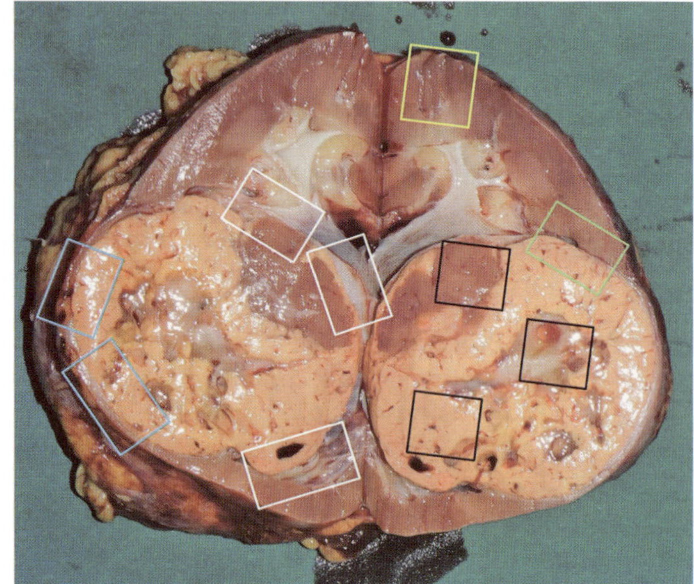

Fig. 8.2: Cut open specimen of radical nephrectomy showing tumor at lower pole. Tumor is solid, well-circumscribed, golden yellow in color, classic for clear cell RCCs. Representative sections to be taken shown with boxes. Representative sections of different appearing areas of tumor (black box), tumor-sinus interface (white box), tumor-perinephric fat interface (blue box), tumor with adjacent kidney (green box), uninvolved renal parenchyma away from tumor (yellow box)

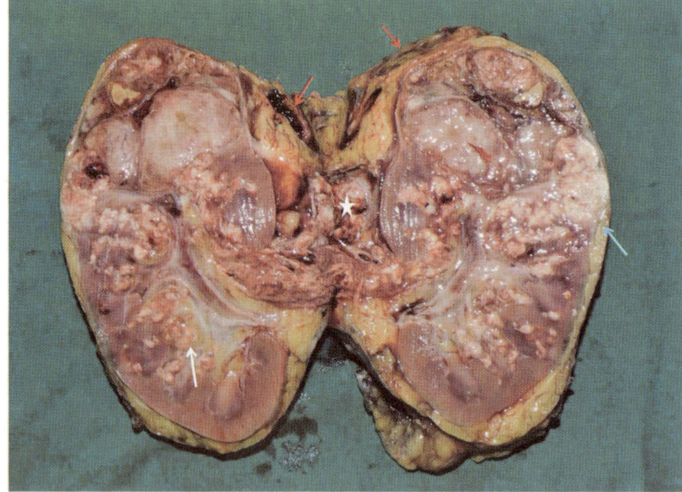

Fig. 8.3: Cut open specimen of radical nephrectomy showing a multifocal whitish tumor with a few hemorrhagic and necrotic areas. Tumor grossly involves perinephric fat (blue arrow), renal vein (white star) and renal sinus fat (white arrow). Adrenal gland visible (red arrow) with areas of haemorrhage

of the renal sinus, renal vein, renal pelvis and perinephric fat. This can be done by making additional cuts in two ways—parallel to the initial incision (*open book method*)[2] or perpendicular to the incision.[3] During this process, perinephric fat or renal capsule is never stripped off from the kidney.[2]

Partial nephrectomy: Surgical margin is inked in all partial nephrectomy specimens. Any other suspicious areas of tumor involvement on the perinephric aspect if present should also be inked.

Specimen is dissected perpendicular to the surgical margin in a *bread-loafing* manner (Figs 8.4A and B). This allows visualization of the maximum tumor size as well as the closest distance of the tumor from the surgical margin. It also helps to assess any visible or suspicious areas of perinephric fat involvement or sinus involvement by the tumor which is important for appropriate staging of the tumor.[2]

4. **What information do we get from macroscopic examination of tumor?**

Ans: Tumor should be measured precisely in millimeters in three dimensions. The cut-off points of 4 cm, 7 cm and 10 cm should be kept in mind which are important for tumor staging (pT1 and pT2). Tumor dimensions should include the part of tumor invading into perinephric fat or renal sinus but not renal vein/IVC thrombus.[4] For multifocal tumors, size of 5 largest nodules to be noted.[4]

The gross appearance of the tumor provides useful insights into the tumor type which is an independent prognostic factor. Tumor type is also important for patient selection for adjuvant therapies, e.g. clear cell RCCs are usually golden yellow in color with variegated appearance and may show some cystic areas as well; papillary RCCs are solid unencapsulated with pale grey to brown color and soft friable cut surface; Multilocular cystic neoplasm of low malignant potential are completely cystic without any solid areas; chromophobe RCC are solid tan brown in colour sometimes with central scar similar to oncocytomas.

Grossly visible areas of hemorrhage, necrosis as well as solid whitish fleshy areas should be noted and sampled during grossing. Solid whitish fleshy areas may show sarcomatoid/rhabdoid differentiation which are independent adverse prognostic indicators regardless of tumor stage and type (Figs 8.2 and 8.3).

5. **How to sample the tumor in radical/partial nephrectomy?**

Ans: Appropriate gross sampling of the tumor is necessary for proper staging and prognostication of any tumor specimen.

The general rule is one section/block per cm of tumor with minimum of 3 sections/blocks.[4]

This includes adequate sampling of the tumor including all solid and cystic areas as well as yellowish or fleshy white areas (for sarcomatoid/rhabdoid differentiation), areas of hemorrhage, necrosis, etc. Necrosis is an important prognostic factor, also perinecrotic areas of tumor usually show higher grade tumor.[3]

For multifocal tumors, sampling of minimum of 5 largest tumors including smaller tumors showing different gross appearance is advised[4] (Fig. 8.2).

6. **What are the other sections taken to assess tumor spread in radical/partial nephrectomy (Fig. 8.2)?**

Ans: The tumor spreads into Gerota's fascia, perinephric fat, renal sinus, pelvicalyceal system, renal vein and adrenal gland is important for staging purposes:

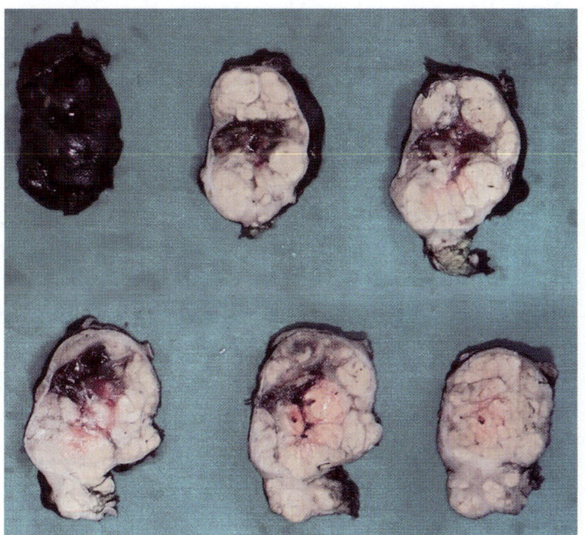

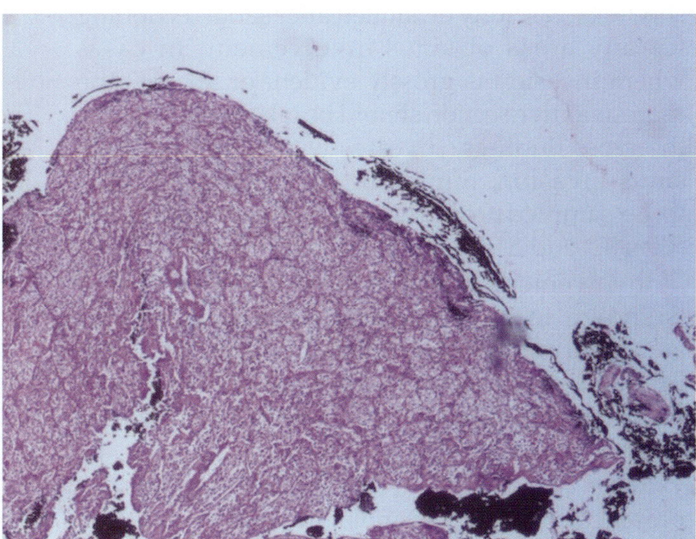

Fig. 8.4A and B: (A) Partial nephrectomy specimen inked and bread-loafed into 3–4 mm serial sections. Tumor is solid, pale yellow in color with areas of hemorrhage. (B) A few areas of surgical resection margin suspicious for involvement by tumor (white arrow), confirmed microscopically showing tumor cells touching the inked margin

Up to stage pT2, tumor is limited to renal parenchyma. Any involvement of adjacent structures upstages the tumor to at least pT3a. Involvement of perinephric fat, renal sinus, renal pelvis or renal vein is staged as pT3a. Involvement of IVC (below the diaphragm) is staged as pT3b and involvement of ipsilateral adrenal gland (contiguous) or Gerota's fascia is staged pT4.

Perinephric fat is present outside the renal capsule but within the Gerota's fascia. After careful sectioning, any areas where the tumor distorts the renal contour by pushing into perinephric fat or nodules of tumor present within the perinephric fat are identified and adequately sampled for perinephric fat invasion.[4] If perinephric fat invasion is grossly absent, one representative section from the area of tumor closest to the perinephric fat is taken for documentation of gross findings. (Figs 8.2 and 8.3).

Gerota's fascia is the plane of surgical dissection. Involvement of Gerota's fascia is considered if the tumor involves the surgical margin of perinephric fat attached to the specimen. It upstages the tumor to pT4.[3]

Renal sinus is the cavity on the medial aspect of the kidney which consists of fat, connective tissue, renal pelvis, branches of renal artery and vein, lymphatics and nerves. There is no capsule separating renal parenchyma and renal pelvis.[3] Involvement of the renal sinus is the principal route for extrarenal spread of tumor.[4] Prognostically, renal sinus involvement predicts a worse outcome compared to perinephric fat involvement.[5] The probability of sinus invasion increases with increase in tumor size. >90% tumors with size 7 cm show sinus invasion.[4] Hence tumor-renal sinus interface should be carefully examined after serial sectioning for any areas of sinus involvement. In cases where invasion is grossly evident or absent, one representative section should be taken to document the gross findings.[2] In cases with uncertain renal sinus invasion, minimum of 3 sections/blocks to be sampled from tumor-renal sinus interface[4] (Figs 8.2 and 8.3).

Involvement of *pelvicalyceal system* by tumor is shown to have negative impact on overall and recurrence free survival. Sections are taken from any areas showing presence of finger like/polypoidal nodule of tumor within the collecting system.[2]

Renal vein invasion (stage pT3a) is defined as presence of tumor thrombus in renal vein or any of its segmental muscle containing branches. Large tumor thrombi in renal vein can be seen grossly. A representative section is taken to confirm gross findings. Frequently, in sections taken from renal sinus, tumor can be seen invading the muscle containing branches which might not be evident on gross examination[4] (Fig. 8.3).

Usually, tumor thrombi if present in the IVC are milked out and separately submitted. In such specimens of caval thrombus, pathologists must look for presence of any adherent vena caval wall which if present upstages the tumor to pT3c. If not grossly visible, minimum of 2 sections/blocks are submitted from thrombi to look for adherent caval wall.[4]

One section of tumor with normal parenchyma interface is submitted. This section aids in assessment of tumor with its surrounding tissue. Also, renal parenchyma acts as an internal control for evaluation by IHC (Fig. 8.2).

Ipsilateral adrenal involvement can be either direct spread from primary tumor or via hematogenous route. Large sized upper pole tumor and presence of vascular involvement are risk factors for adrenal involvement. If there is contiguous invasion of adrenal from the primary tumor, it is staged as pT4. If there is presence of discreet tumor nodules within the gland, it is staged as pM1. Careful examination and serial sectioning of adrenal gland and submitting representative sections is advised.[4] *Contralateral adrenal* involvement is staged pM1.

In nephrectomy specimens, lymph nodes if present are near the hilum. Therefore, hilar tissue fat is examined carefully for any palpable nodes. Palpable lymph nodes have a higher probability of being involved by tumor than small lymph nodes detected microscopically.[2]

7. How to assess margins for radical nephrectomy?

Ans: For radical nephrectomy, the ureter, renal artery, renal vein and soft tissue (Gerota's fascia) margins are assessed and documented. Margin positivity puts the patient at risk for local recurrence and poor overall survival.[3]

For ureter, renal artery and vein, distal most end is cut transversely (shave margin) as to expose the lumen. In case where tumor thrombi are present in the renal vein, renal vein sampling may be done in two ways—either (a) amputating the distal most vein wall in cross section and submitting section with the tumor, or (b) if the wall is freely mobile, trimming and submitting the distal most vein wall separately without tumor.

Renal vein margin is considered positive only if there is tumor attached to the vein wall at the margin. The presence of tumor thrombus within lumen at the margin is not sufficient to be called margin positive[2] (Fig. 8.4).

8. Sections to be submitted (Fig. 8.2):

Ans:

Radical Nephrectomy:

- Margins: Ureter, renal artery, renal vein
- Tumor including all different appearing areas (Min 3 sections)
- Tumor with perinephric fat
- Tumor—renal sinus interface (1–3 sections)
- Tumor with normal renal parenchyma
- Uninvolved parenchyma
- Adrenal gland, if present
- Lymph nodes, if present
- Renal vein thrombus/caval thrombus is submitted (min 2 sections)

Partial Nephrectomy:

- Tumor with surgical margin
- Tumor with perinephric fat
- Tumor: Any other areas not sampled
- Renal parenchyma, if present.

9. How to assess frozen section for margin status of partial nephrectomy?

Ans: Two types of specimens may be received for frozen section evaluation of a partial nephrectomy. Small parenchymal tissue from the tumor bed: It is directly embedded, processed and reported as positive or negative for tumor.

Complete resection specimen—for this, the surgical margin is inked, and the specimen is bisected perpendicular to the surgical margin. Section(s) is taken from the area of tumor closest to the inked margin and submitted for frozen section assessment.

Margin is considered positive only when tumor cells are present touching the inked margin. (Fig. 8.4).

Significance of margin assessment by frozen section for partial nephrectomy remains controversial. Studies have proven that while positive surgical margin does not always co-relate with local recurrence, negative surgical margin does not exclude the risk of local recurrence.[6] There is also some evidence that suggests that even with positive surgical margin on the resection specimen, use of cautery on the resection bed during surgery may destroy the remaining tumor cells.[2]

Due to lack of ability to influence intraoperative management, higher false negative rate and added cost to the patient, frozen sections for margin assessment of partial nephrectomy is not advised.

10. What relevant information should be provided by the urologist within the specimen requisition for a radical prostatectomy?

Ans:

- Patient identification details: Name, age, sex and identification number.
- Type of surgical procedure: Laparoscopic/robotic prostatectomy
- Radiological findings and staging: PSMA PET scan/MRI scan/TRUS.
- Family history: Ca prostate or other BRCA related cancer
- Serum PSA
- TRUS biopsy findings: Gleason scoring, Grade group, number and site of cores involved by tumor, any additional findings present.
- History of any hormonal treatment: ADT/chemotherapy or radiotherapy.

11. How to conduct macroscopic examination of radical prostatectomy specimen?

Ans: Radical prostatectomy consists of prostate with minimal extra-prostatic tissue, both seminal vesicles and segments of both vas deferens.

After properly orienting the specimen (seminal vesicles are superior and posterior, posterior surface is flatter compared to anterior surface) weight and three-dimensional measurements are taken of the prostate as well as seminal vesicles.[7] Specimen is photographed, if indicated.

Fixation of prostatectomy specimen can be done by immersing it in 20 times volume of formalin for 24 hours. Alternatively for larger specimens, to facilitate homogenous fixation, formalin can be injected within the prostate using a syringe and 23G needle and then immersed in formalin for 12–24 hours.[8]

12. How is grossing of radical prostatectomy specimen different (Figs 8.5 and 8.6)?

Ans: After adequate fixation, the prostate specimen is inked entirely with either one color or two colors. Using two different colors for better orientation of right and left side is recommended.[8]

After inking, seminal vesicles are amputated from the prostate gland and submitted entirely. The prostate, without seminal vesicles attached is weighed, measured in the three dimensions and volume is measured by water displacement method. Apical and basal margins are then sectioned.

For apical margin, it is recommended to use modified cone method where 3–4 mm thick "cone" from apical end of the prostate is cut with urethral orifice in the center. This section is further bread-loafed into 2 mm thick sections and submitted into cassettes as right and left apical margins.

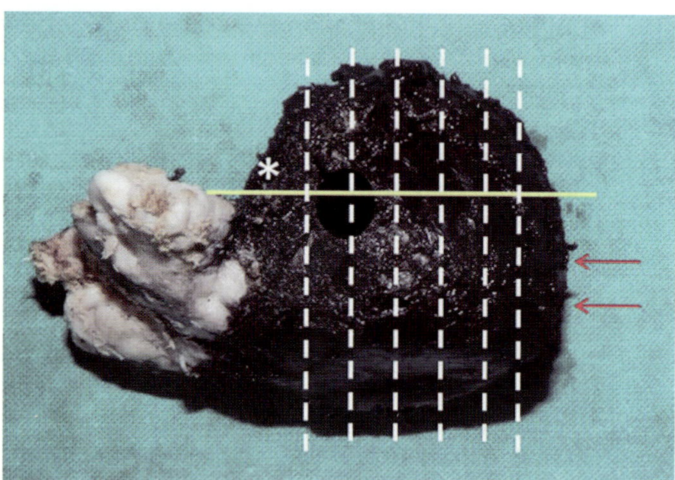

Fig. 8.5: Radical prostatectomy specimen showing inked external surface. For grossing the prostate specimen, serial sectioning is done (white dashed lines) perpendicular to the plane of prostatic urethra (yellow line). Apical margin (red arrow) and bladder base margin (*) sections are further sectioned

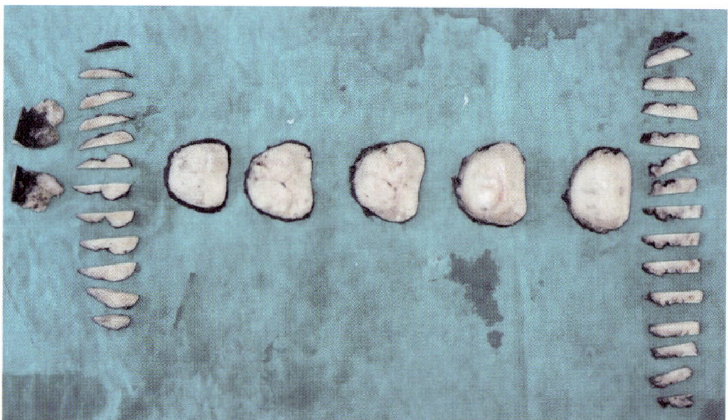

Fig. 8.6: Final sections submitted for microscopic evaluation of radical prostatectomy (in order from left to right)—both seminal vesicles, apical margin sections, whole mount sections and bladder base margin sections

Similarly for bladder base, 3–4 mm thick slice is cut with urethral opening at the center and bread loafed at 2 mm thick sections and submitted int cassettes as right and left bladder base margins. The rest of the prostate is serially sectioned into 3 mm thick slices perpendicular to the prostatic urethra and submitted entirely for microscopic examination.[8,9]

Margin is considered positive only when tumor cells are present touching the inked margin. 3 mm of margin positivity has a higher risk of five-year biochemical recurrence compared to margin negative cases.[7] Apical margin is the most common location for positive margin. Therefore, proper submission of margin sections is vital.[8,9]

Prostate cancer is commonly multifocal and poorly circumscribed. It also varies in colour (from bright yellow to pale to tan to white) and consistency (soft to firm). It is also not easily visible as a mass lesion easily on gross inspection. For these reasons, even with the added cost and labor for technical staff, it is recommended to submit the entire specimen of prostate.[7]

13. What is the role of frozen section in radical prostatectomy?

Ans: Though not routinely practiced, intraoperative frozen sections may be requested to assess margin status (apical or bladder base) or neurovascular bundles (for nerve sparing surgeries) in high-risk cases.[7] Positive margins may prompt a wider excision and final negative margins.

REFERENCES

1. Lester S, Manual of Surgical Pathology, 4th Edition: Elsevier; 2023.
2. Midha D, Menon S, Josephine S, Kumar RM, Kaushal S, Pai SA, Ambekar A, Rao V, Bindhu MR, Patil S, Jagdale R, Soni S, Kulkarni B, Desai S, Sundaram S. Gross reporting of adult kidney tumor specimens: A comprehensive evidence-based review. Indian J Cancer. 2021 Oct-Dec;58(4):493–500. doi: 10.4103/ijc.ijc_354_21. PMID: 34975095.
3. Warren AY, Griffiths D, Fleming S. Standards and datasets for reporting cancers: Dataset for histopathological reporting of adult renal parenchyma neoplasms. 2017.
4. Trpkov K, Grignon DJ, Bonsib SM, Amin MB, Billis A, Lopez-Beltran A, Samaratunga H, Tamboli P, Delahunt B, Egevad L, Montironi R, Srigley JR; members of the ISUP Renal Tumor Panel. Handling and staging of renal cell carcinoma: the International Society of Urological Pathology Consensus (ISUP) conference recommendations. Am J Surg Pathol. 2013 Oct;37(10):1505–17. doi: 10.1097/PAS.0b013e31829a85d0. PMID: 24025521.
5. Srigley J R; Paner G; Zhou M; Harik LR; Allan R; Amin MB; Steven C. Campbell; Chang A; Delahunt B; Grignon D; Humphrey P A; Leibovich B C; Montironi R; Pettus J; Reuter VE Protocol for the Examination of Resection Specimens from Patients with Invasive Carcinoma of Renal Tubular Origin, 2021.
6. Doehn C, Grunwald V, Steiner T, Follmann M, Rexer H, Krege S. The diagnosis, treatment and follow-up of Renal Cell Carcinoma. Dtsch Arztebl Int 2016; 113:590–6.
7. Oxley J, Varma M, Berney D. Standards and datasets for reporting cancers: Dataset for histopathological reporting of Prostatic Carcinomas. 2016.
8. Rao BV, Soni S, Kulkarni B, Bindhu MR, Ambekar A, Midha D *et al*, Grossing and reporting of radical prostatectomy specimens: An evidence-based approach. Indian J Cancer 0;0:0.
9. Samaratunga H, Montironi R, True L, Epstein JI, Griffiths DF, Humphrey PA, van der Kwast T, Wheeler TM, Srigley JR, Delahunt B, Egevad L; ISUP Prostate Cancer Group. International Society of Urological Pathology (ISUP) Consensus Conference on Handling and Staging of Radical Prostatectomy Specimens. Working group 1: specimen handling. Mod Pathol. 2011 Jan;24(1):6–15. doi: 10.1038/modpathol.2010.178. Epub 2010 Sep 10. PMID: 20834234.

Index